Incontinence, functional
Incontinence, reflex
Incontinence, stress
Incontinence, total
Incontinence, urge
Infection, potential for
Injury, potential for (specify): suffocation, poisoning, trauma
Knowledge deficit (specify)
Mobility, impaired physical
Noncompliance (specify)
Nutrition, altered: Less than body requirements
Nutrition, altered: More than body requirements
Nutrition, altered: Potential for more than body requirements
Oral mucous membrane, altered
Parental role conflict
Parenting, altered: Actual
Parenting, altered: Potential
Post trauma response
Powerlessness
Rape trauma syndrome
Role performance, altered
Self-care deficit: Feeding, bathing/hygiene, dressing/grooming, toileting
Self-concept, disturbance in body image, self-esteem, role performance, personal identity
Self-esteem disturbance
   Chronic low self-esteem
   Situational low self-esteem
Sensory/perceptual alteration: Visual, auditory, kinesthetic, gustatory, tactile, olfactory
Sexual dysfunction
Sexuality patterns, altered
Skin integrity, impaired: Actual
Skin integrity, impaired: Potential
Sleep pattern disturbance
Social interaction, impaired
Social isolation
Spiritual distress (distress of the human spirit)
Swallowing, impaired
Thermoregulation, ineffective
Thought processes, altered
Tissue integrity, impaired
Tissue perfusion, altered: Cerebral, cardiopulmonary, renal, gastrointestinal, peripheral
Unilateral neglect
Urinary elimination, altered patterns
Urinary retention
Violence, potential for: Self-directed or directed at others

Textbook of
Pharmacology
and Nursing Care

USING THE NURSING PROCESS

Roger T. Malseed, Ph.D.
Adjunct Associate Professor of Pharmacology
University of Pennsylvania School of Nursing;
Philadelphia College of Pharmacy and Science
Philadelphia, Pennsylvania

Gail S. Harrigan, R.N., M.S.N., C.S.
Formerly, Assistant Director of Nursing for Staff Development
University of Medicine and Dentistry of New Jersey
University Hospital
Newark, New Jersey

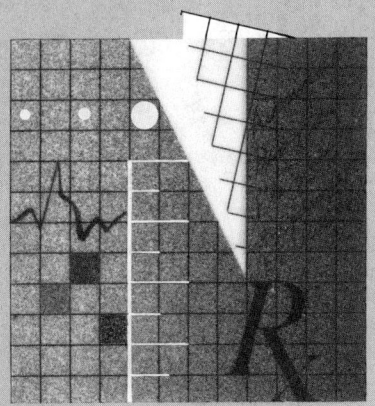

Textbook of
Pharmacology
and Nursing Care

USING THE NURSING PROCESS

J.B. LIPPINCOTT COMPANY

Philadelphia

London   Mexico City
New York   St. Louis
São Paulo   Sydney

Acquisition/Sponsoring Editor:
  Nancy Mullins
Manuscript Editor:
  Virginia Barishek
Indexer: Alexandra Weir
Design Coordinator: Anita Curry
Designer: Tracy Baldwin
Production Coordinator:
  Charlene Squibb
Compositor: TAPSCO, Inc.
Printer/Binder: The Murray
  Printing Company

6 5 4 3 2

Library of Congress Cataloging-in-Publication Data

Malseed, Roger T. (Roger Thomas)
  Textbook of pharmacology and nursing care.

  Includes bibliographies and index.
  1. Pharmacology. 2. Nursing. I. Harrigan, Gail. II. Title. [DNLM: 1.
Drug Therapy—nursing.
2. Pharmacology—nurses' instruction. QV 4 M259t]
RM300.M184 1989   615'.1'.024613   87-35370
ISBN 0-397-54432-4

Any procedure or practice described in this book should be applied by the
health-care practitioner under appropriate supervision in accordance with
professional standards of care used with regard to the unique circumstances
that apply in each practice situation. Care has been taken to confirm the
accuracy of information presented and to describe generally accepted practices.
However, the authors, editors, and publisher cannot accept any responsibility
for errors or omissions or for consequences from application of the information
in this book and make no warranty, express or implied, with respect to the
contents of the book.

Every effort has been made to ensure drug selections and dosages are in
accordance with current recommendations and practice. Because of ongoing
research, changes in government regulations, and the constant flow of
information on drug therapy, reactions, and interactions, the reader is
cautioned to check the package insert for each drug for indications, dosages,
warnings, and precautions, particularly if the drug is new or infrequently used.

To Zoriana,
for her unfailing love and support,
and to Mark and Natalie,
who are a constant source of pride and joy

To Rick and Randy,
who, through their love and laughter,
remind me daily of what is truly important in life

Contributors

Ruth Bindler, R.N., M.S.
Associate Professor
Intercollegiate Center for Nursing Education
Washington State University
Pullman, Washington

Mary E. Cooley, R.N., M.S.N.
Oncology Clinical Nurse Specialist
Hospital of the University of Pennsylvania
Philadelphia, Pennsylvania

Margaret E. Davitt, R.N., M.S.N., C.S.
Head Nurse, Oncology Study Unit
Hospital of the University of Pennsylvania
Philadelphia, Pennsylvania

Frederick J. Goldstein, Ph.D.
Professor of Pharmacology
Philadelphia College of Pharmacy and Science
Philadelphia, Pennsylvania

Freddy Grimm, M.Sc., Pharm. D.
Director, Outpatient Pharmacy
Hospital of the University of Pennsylvania;
Clinical Assistant Professor
Philadelphia College of Pharmacy and Science
Philadelphia, Pennsylvania

Zoriana K. Malseed, Ph.D.
Associate Professor of Anatomy and Physiology
School of Nursing
University of Pennsylvania
Philadelphia, Pennsylvania

Patricia A. Mangan, R.N., B.S.N.
Oncology Nurse Clinician
Hematology–Oncology Outpatient Clinic
Hospital of the University of Pennsylvania
Philadelphia, Pennsylvania

Susan Masoorli, R.N.
President
Perivascular Nurse Consultants
Philadelphia, Pennsylvania

Diane P. Sager
Consultant
Cardiovascular Nursing
Washington, D.C.

Consultants

Michael J. Reichgott, M.D., Ph.D.
Medical Director
Bronx Municipal Hospital Center;
Assistant Dean
Albert Einstein College of Medicine
Bronx, New York

Joan Lynaugh, R.N., Ph.D., F.A.A.N.
Associate Professor
School of Nursing
University of Pennsylvania
Philadelphia, Pennsylvania

Diane P. Sager
Consultant
Cardiovascular Nursing
Washington, D.C.

J. B. Lippincott Company Consultant Board

Preface

Nurses occupy a unique position in the delivery of health care, one that requires broad knowledge encompassing both didactic and practical aspects. A significant responsibility of such a position is the necessity for nurses to be skilled in the clinical pharmacology of the vast array of medicinal agents used in modern pharmacotherapy. Nurses must provide vital monitoring of the safety and efficacy of drug therapy, and responsible and appropriate nursing intervention frequently is a primary determinant of the overall success of drug treatment.

This book was conceived and developed to provide the necessary knowledge for nurses and other health care personnel in both the theoretical aspects of pharmacology as well as the entire nursing process as it relates to drug therapy and patient care.

The nursing process format is strongly emphasized throughout the book in order to encourage readers to utilize all nursing skills in caring for a patient, and not just those required for proper drug administration. Since as many as 20% of patients taking prescribed drugs suffer unexpected drug reactions, nurses need to be provided with the tools necessary to minimize problems and encourage safe drug usage.

The first step in this process is through *Assessment*. The reader is given pertinent historical information including the proper means for obtaining a medical or personal history so that potential problems may be detected at an early stage. This data is culled from the Interactions, Side-Effects/Adverse Reactions, and Contraindications and Precautions sections of the pharmacological profile on each drug or drug class. In addition, suggestions for appropriate physical examinations and laboratory or diagnostic monitoring are included to emphasize the necessity and importance of having a complete data base before administering any drug.

Nursing *Diagnoses* are then listed. They outline the actual and potential reactions a patient may have to a drug and in what areas a nurse may appropriately intervene.

The *Plan* identified in each section outlines goals that assist in ensuring safe drug administration, close monitoring of drug effects, and early detection of side-effects. The goals also provide the framework for patient teaching to optimize drug effectiveness and minimize undesirable reactions.

In the *Intervention* section, common side-effects as well as significant adverse reactions are discussed. Strategies are given for appropriate patient monitoring and those signs and symptoms of potential problems that patients should be taught to report are outlined. In addition, information about specific administration techniques is provided where appropriate.

The *Evaluation* section lists specific outcome criteria that can be used to measure drug effectiveness. Appropriate changes in laboratory values, diagnostic tests, and patient reactions are identified to provide as many objective parameters as possible.

Nursing care plans have been included for 22 major drug categories in order to demonstrate more clearly how drug therapy can affect the *total* patient. These care plans are structured to provide detailed information for the reader about assessment, nursing diagnoses, expected client outcomes, and appropriate interventions, and are designed to complement the narrative in the chapters in which they appear. They are meant to be integrated into the total nursing care plan for a patient, who will obviously have many more needs than simply those related to safe drug administration. Thus, the format intentionally emphasizes the importance of drug therapy in planning total patient care.

Case studies have also been included at the end of many chapters and are largely based on actual experiences with many patients. The case studies are designed to provoke discussion *beyond* the questions asked at the end of each case. Nurses need to discuss the rationale for certain drug regimens, why certain people have difficulty with a particular drug regimen, and how nurses may effectively intervene through demonstration, teaching, and communication with other care givers to minimize a patient's problems with drug therapy.

The book is divided into 12 sections and an appendix. Section I deals with general principles of pharmacology and includes detailed explanations of those concepts needed by the reader to grasp fully the later discussions of the mechanisms, actions, and fate of the individual drugs. A critical aspect of drug therapy is the potential for two or more drugs to interact adversely, and this problem is considered in detail in this section. Given the increasing tendency toward multiple drug therapy, especially in elderly patients, this facet of pharmacology justifiably deserves careful attention. In addition to the general discussion of drug interactions in Section I, extensive listings of documented drug interactions are provided throughout the text for individual drugs or drug groupings.

Section II attempts to define critically the role of the nurse in drug therapy. Techniques of drug administration and patient teaching are reviewed in Chapters 6 and 8. These chapters describe both common and not-so-common drug administration techniques, proper formats for writing drug cards, methods for teaching patients how to take medications properly, and many other aspects of drug administration. Detailed information is given in Chapter 6 about intravenous drug administration, because this route is so often utilized in critical care situations. Through this detailed presentation, readers should be able to obtain the information necessary to ensure safe drug administration from a single resource. Considerable attention is focused on the legal aspects of drug usage, particularly as they relate to the nurse. In addition, considerations of those facets of health care unique to the pediatric and geriatric populations receive careful scrutiny in individual chapters dealing with pediatric pharmacology and geriatric pharmacology. These chapters follow a Nursing Process format, and identify differences in physiological functioning, developmental skills, and learning needs for these populations as well as the many problems inherent in providing safe and effective drug therapy in these patient groups. Finally, a comprehensive review of the mathematics of drug therapy is also presented in this section, where practice problems are provided for many different types of dosage calculations.

Beginning with Section III and continuing through Section XI, the principal classes of drugs the reader is likely to encounter in clinical practice are discussed under their appropriate general headings. Each chapter begins with an overview of the drug class, frequently integrated with a discussion of the physiology of the appropriate organ or body system affected. A detailed account of the pharmacology of the drug class is then presented, followed by specific information relative to the indications, fate, adverse effects, contraindications, precautions, and interactions associated with the class of drugs or, where appropriate, the individual drugs being considered. Tables are used extensively to facilitate comparison of similar drugs. Information provided for every drug includes available preparations, recommended dosages, and other pertinent comments regarding administration. A number of related bibliographic articles are found at the end of each chapter. Finally, a list of review questions based upon the content of the chapter is provided to test the reader's understanding of the material presented.

The problem of drug abuse is addressed at length in a separate chapter in Section XII, where general considerations of the problem are discussed, and guidelines for the recognition and the treatment of abuse of many different drugs are outlined. The Appendix contains many useful tables, such as abbreviations, laboratory values (including international units), and a comprehensive listing of incompatibilities of drugs in solution.

Another unique feature found throughout the text is the presence of many *Disease Briefs*, which provide a concise yet practical review of the etiology and symptoms of a disease that is treatable by a particular drug being discussed.

The scope of this text is an indication of the complexity of modern pharmacotherapeutics. Nurses and other health care providers face an enormous task in keeping informed about the medications that they must administer and monitor. This book is intended to serve as a comprehensive, practical source for that information and to provide the nurse with a single reference from which to obtain sufficient knowledge in both the theoretical and practical aspects of drug therapy and patient care to provide quality health care.

Roger T. Malseed, Ph.D.
Gail S. Harrigan, R.N., M.S.N., C.S.

Acknowledgments

A book of this size and scope is not possible without the assistance and support of many people. The authors would like to express their appreciation to the editors, past and present, at the J.B. Lippincott Company who have overseen various phases of this work and whose advice, direction, and encouragement have helped make the final product a reality. They are Bernice Heller, David Miller, Joyce Mkitarian, Nancy McFarland, and Nancy Mullins.

A variety of nurses, colleagues, and friends gave freely of their time and expertise to ensure that the material in this book is as current and accurate as possible. Thanks are extended to Emily Auermuller, Janet Boury, Margaret Davidson, Dayle Dorsky-Flynn, Anna Ellis, Sally Fedkenheuer, D. Anthony Forrester, Shauna Giggey, Susan Hall-Bruncati, Mary Ellen Hickman, Terri Hollander, Lois Honchurek, Deanna Johnson, Janice Johnston, Margaret Levine, Joan Monahan, Tish Obal, Carole Shea, and Hazel Williams.

A special debt of gratitude is extended to those individuals who spent countless hours typing the manuscript. In particular, Mary Murphy, Lynn Loudy, and the typing service at the J.B. Lippincott Company deserve a sincere thank-you.

It goes without saying that the efforts of the consultants and contributors were of immeasurable importance in sculpturing and refining this book. Their interest, input, and advice are gratefully acknowledged.

The authors would also like to thank the reference librarians at the George Smith Library of the University of Medicine and Dentistry of New Jersey and at the Monmouth County Library, Eastern Branch who provided countless resources and information throughout the development of this book.

A special thank-you is extended to Suzanne Smeltzer for her support, advice, and encouragement throughout this project.

A wife and mother needs additional support when becoming a writer, because many domestic duties begin to fall apart. I would like to thank the Sumski and Harrigan families for helping me hold down the "fort" with support, food, humor, presents, cards, telephone calls, and babysitting services without which I would not have survived. I would especially like to thank my mother, who was always there with a hug, a laugh, and incredible energy just when I needed it most.

Contents

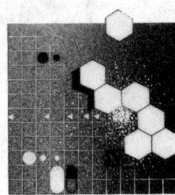
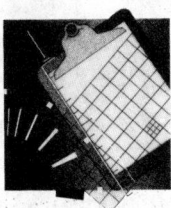

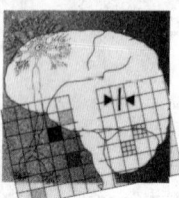

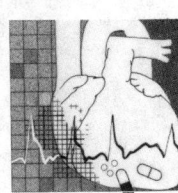

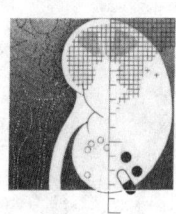
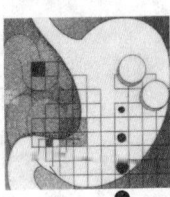

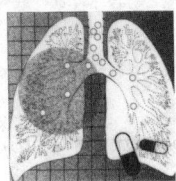
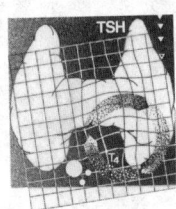

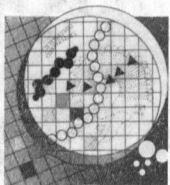

Contents

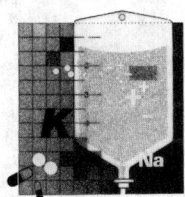
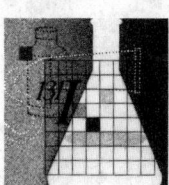

Contents

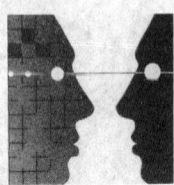

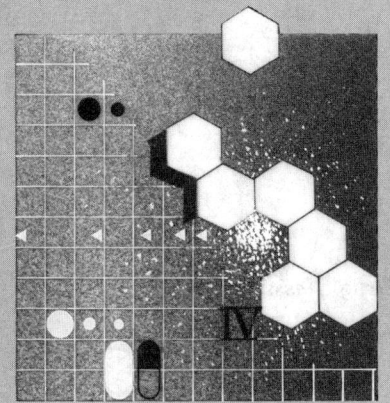

General Principles
of Pharmacology

I

Drug Nomenclature and Classification

Drug Nomenclature
Brand Name vs Generic
Name Prescribing

Drug Classification
Source of the Drug
Organ System Affected
Clinical Use
Chemical Composition

1

Pharmacology may be broadly defined as the study of the *interaction* of drugs with living organisms. As such, it is concerned with the biochemical and physiologic effects of chemical substances on bodily functions, as well as with the various mechanisms by which the body handles the presence of a chemical substance. The scope of pharmacology is immense, encompassing a broad spectrum of subspecialties dealing with the many facets of drug use. The following are several important fields of study falling under the umbrella of pharmacology:

Pharmacokinetics—The study of the principles involved in the absorption, distribution, metabolism, and excretion of drugs

Pharmacodynamics—The study of the biochemical and physiologic mechanisms of action of drugs

Pharmacotherapeutics—The study of drug use for the diagnosis, prevention, and treatment of disease (frequently referred to as *clinical pharmacology*)

Pharmacogenetics—The study of genetic factors as determinants of drug responses

Toxicology—The study of the poisonous effects of drugs and other chemical substances

Pharmacognosy—The study of drugs derived from plant or animal sources

Pharmacy—The study of the art of preparing, compounding, and dispensing medications

Posology—The study of drug dosing

Since the term *drug* has been used in most of the above definitions, it might be well to examine what is meant when this term is used. The official definition of the word *drug*, as proferred by the United States Pure Food and Drug Act, is (1) articles recognized in the *United States Pharmacopeia* or *National Formulary* for internal or external use; (2) articles intended for the diagnosis, cure, mitigation, treatment, or prevention of disease in humans or animals; and (3) articles, other than food, that are intended to affect the structure or function of the body. While certainly impressive, the official definition does not exactly roll from the tongue, and a much simpler, although perhaps oversimplified, definition of *drug* is any substance, other than food, that can affect living processes. It is in this context that the term *drug* will be used throughout this book.

Drug Nomenclature

The introduction of many new drugs in recent years has greatly improved the control of certain disease states (*e.g.*, angina, hypertension, asthma) and provided the clinician with an imposing array of chemicals that can elevate the overall quality of life. These therapeutic advances have not arrived without exacting a toll, however, namely the overwhelming number of new names that now must be committed to the overburdened memories of those health practitioners who must daily prescribe, dispense, and monitor these new drugs. The naming of drug products is at best confusing, but the general concepts relating to drug nomenclature can easily be understood, affording at least a handle with which to grasp this seemingly perplexing area.

As the evolution of a new drug proceeds from the laboratory blackboard to the pharmacy shelf, the substance acquires several different names, some of which remain throughout its clinical life. Initially, the drug is given a chemical name, governed by fairly rigid rules established for the naming of chemical structures. For example, the chemical name of a calcium channel blocker used in angina is 3,5-pyridine-dicarboxylic acid, 1,4-dihydro-2,6-dimethyl-4-(2-nitrophenyl)-, dimethyl ester. This name provides a blueprint for chemists as to the exact structure of the molecule.

In addition to the chemical name, new drugs being investigated in the laboratory are frequently assigned a code name or laboratory designation by the manufacturer. This code name may be an abbreviation, a numerical or alphabetical code, or a coined name. For our calcium channel blocker noted above, the code name used was Bay a 1040. Obviously, this code name has little chemical or pharmacologic significance other than to the laboratory personnel working with the compound, and is seldom used in health-care practice.

Should a laboratory chemical show promise as a potential drug, the manufacturer seeks a *United States Adopted Name* (USAN), which is conferred by the USAN council, composed of representatives from the American Medical Association, American Pharmaceutical Association, and the United States Pharmacopeial Convention. This name is usually synonymous with the *nonproprietary* or *generic name* of the drug assigned by the manufacturer. The generic name is frequently a shortened, simplified term, often derived from the chemical name of the compound, and is the name most often used in the professional literature. The generic name of our calcium channel blocker is nifedipine, which is identical to its USAN.

Should the drug be officially recognized by inclusion into the *United States Pharmacopeia* (USP) or *National Formulary* (NF), the USAN becomes the *official name*, which in many cases is identical with the generic name. While it is possible for a compound to have more than one generic name, although this is rare, it may have only *one* official name.

Finally, each company marketing a new drug selects a *proprietary* or *trade name* for its drug and copyrights it. This name is also referred to as the *brand name*, and is the name most often used in advertising, inasmuch as the company wishes individuals to purchase its brand name product over a similar product by another manufacturer. Thus, in our example, Pfizer Laboratories would advertise their calcium blocker as Procardia, the trade name, rather than as nifedipine, the generic name.

With this multiplicity of drug terminology, it is easy to understand how confusion can arise when discussing a particular drug or group of drugs. Compounding this already perplexing problem are the different generic and trade names given to drugs in other countries. Thus, the same drug marketed by a manufacturer in both the United States and Canada, for example, may have as many as four different names. For this reason, the USAN council and the World Health Organization (WHO), among other agencies, are striving to standardize drug nomenclature worldwide. As a beginning, the USAN for a new drug is now commonly adopted as the nonproprietary or generic name for the drug in most countries of the world. Still much variation in terminology exists with older drugs, and rectifying this confusion in nomenclature will probably never be accomplished completely.

Brand Name vs Generic Name Prescribing

Throughout this text, drugs will be characterized by the generic name followed by the currently available trade names. Readers should acquaint themselves with both names, inasmuch as drugs may be prescribed by either name. Generic vs brand name prescribing has long been a subject of controversy, and valid arguments can be offered for both sides. It is not the intent of this discussion to adopt a position on this delicate issue, since no single answer can be defended completely. Rather, by presenting some of the arguments advanced by proponents of each side, readers should be able to view the controversy from a proper perspective, and make an informed decision *in each individual case* rather than adopt either position totally.

Prescribing a drug by its trade or brand name and indicating "no substitution" on the prescription order form mandates that the order be filled with the exact brand of drug ordered. Use of the nonproprietary or generic name allows the pharmacist to dispense the product of any manufacturer. In some states, a generic drug can also be dispensed if the prescriber writes a trade name, then indicates that "substitution is permissible." Since generic drug laws can differ among states, health practitioners should acquaint themselves with local regulations governing drug prescribing.

Arguments advanced in favor of brand name prescribing include the following:

1. Brand names generally ensure a high-quality product with consistent bioavailability of drug.
2. Brand names usually are subject to high quality control in the manufacturing process, resulting in accurate drug dosing.
3. Brand name tablets and capsules are frequently much easier to identify in the event of a problem, since they are almost always coded or labeled in some manner.
4. Brand names are more widely recognized than generic names, and errors in prescribing and dispensing may therefore be reduced.

Conversely, advocates of generic prescribing point to the following arguments in support of their view:

1. Generic drugs are less costly to the consumer than are brand name drugs.
2. Generic drugs are equivalent therapeutically to brand name drugs, since quality control and manufacturing procedures are comparable.

The decision to prescribe by brand name or generic name must be made based on as much information as obtainable pertaining to the drug as well as to the patient. The factor of cost is certainly important, especially in the older fixed-income population, a major drug-taking group. Yet, cost should not become the sole or even dominant consideration, for one is not purchasing a television set, rather one is buying a medication that has the potential to cause irreparable harm as well as improve health. Thus, safety and efficacy become as important as dollars and cents. In this regard, products of the generic drug industry are probably as safe and effective today as they have ever been, due largely to more stringent control and manufacturing procedures.

While actual drug content is usually remarkably consistent among similar proprietary and nonproprietary products, variability can occur among generically equivalent drugs in bioavailability of the drug once a dose has been taken. Differences in tablet dissolution rates, composition of inert ingredients that make up the tablet or capsule, types of particle coatings used in long-acting formulations, and stability of the drug in various liquid vehicles can all contribute to unequal bioavailability and therapeutic inequivalency among generic drugs. Although these differences are usually slight, they can occasionally result in altered pharmacologic and toxicologic responses when a generic substitution is made.

Only when all factors are weighed can a proper decision be made as to whether to use a brand name or generic name drug. Not to be overlooked in the decision-making process are the wishes of the patients themselves. An informed, satisfied patient is more likely to be a compliant patient, and the importance of apprising the patient of the advantages and disadvantages of the available forms of therapy cannot be overemphasized.

The generic controversy, which is essentially economic in nature, continues unabated, and both sides will continue to attract proponents. Whatever choice is made, however, it is imperative that the patient be monitored to ensure that the desired response is obtained and that the drug chosen is both effective and safe.

Drug Classification

The purpose of classifying drugs is to group compounds possessing similar characteristics (*e.g.*, mechanism of action, effects on body systems, indications for use) so as to facilitate comparisons among them. Understanding the pharmacology of one member of a group imparts a general knowledge of many similar drugs, simply because of the common actions shared by members of a drug group. Moreover, the basic phamacology of new drugs can be quickly understood simply by categorizing them into a group of available drugs. Thus, specific differences among members of a drug group readily become apparent and comparisons between similar drugs, both old and new, can easily be made. This is the unified approach to pharmacology that will be followed throughout this text, a method that greatly facilitates learning and provides the necessary information to assist health-care practitioners in making sensible decisions concerning drug therapy.

There are various ways of classifying drugs, although no single means of classification represents the ideal in terms of completeness and comprehensiveness. Among the common parameters used to classify drug products are (1) source of the drug, (2) organ system affected, (3) clinical usefulness, and (4) chemical composition.

Source of the Drug

Drugs may be obtained from several sources, the principal ones being
1. Plant constituents
2. Animal extracts
3. Inorganic chemicals and minerals
4. Synthetic chemicals
5. Recombinant DNA technology

PLANT CONSTITUENTS
Plants have yielded a wide array of pharmacologically active substances, many of which are widely used in therapy today. *Alkaloids* (*i.e.*, naturally occurring organic chemical compounds) represent the most important group of plant constituents used in medicine and many of these compounds are quite potent and toxic. They may be used as the pure alkaloid but more commonly are administered in the form of the water-soluble salt. Alkaloids such as morphine, codeine, pilocarpine, and atropine have a deservedly important place in drug therapy.

Another clinically important group of plant extracts is made up of the *glycosides*, which contain a sugar as part of the molecule. The most widely used glycosides are the digitalis glycosides, obtained from the seeds and leaves of various species of the foxglove plant. While not necessary for its pharmacologic action, the presence of the sugar in the molecule plays a major role in the absorption of the drug into cardiac muscle cells.

Gums are plant exudates that form thick gelatin-like masses when mixed with water. Some, such as agar and psyllium seed, are used as laxatives, while others, like acacia and tragacanth, are employed primarily as pharmaceutical suspending agents.

Other plant-derived materials useful as therapeutic aids are *tannins*, which serve as astringents and protectives, *resins*, which may have a cathartic action due to a local gastric irritative effect, and *fixed* and *volatile oils*, which have been used as flavoring agents, carminatives, antiseptics, and solubilizing vehicles.

ANIMAL EXTRACTS
Extracts from animal organs are widely used in treating a number of diseases. For example, some insulin products in use today to control the symp-

toms of diabetes mellitus are obtained from the pancreas of cattle and swine, and heparin, a potent anticoagulant, is derived from cow lung or swine intestinal tissue. Some thyroid hormone products used as replacement therapy for hypothyroidism are extracted from the thyroid glands of animals.

INORGANIC CHEMICALS AND MINERALS

Many inorganic elements and minerals are employed in a variety of conditions, both for therapeutic and nutritive value. Iron salts are used for their hematinic action, silver salts are effective antiseptics, and calcium salts are valuable in preventing onset of osteoporosis and rickets. Aluminum and magnesium compounds are very effective antacids, while certain sulfates and citrates can function as saline cathartics. In addition, radioactive isotopes of several elements are vital diagnostic and therapeutic tools.

SYNTHETIC CHEMICALS

The majority of drugs in use today are the result of systematic laboratory synthesis. In addition, several naturally occurring compounds previously used in medicine (e.g., oxytocin, vasopressin) have now been replaced by purer and in many cases less expensive synthetic derivatives. Synthesis of new drugs is usually an expensive and time-consuming process because for every synthetic compound that eventually reaches the market, thousands make it only as far as a numbered bottle in the laboratory storeroom. The cost of nurturing a synthetic chemical from the test tube to the medicine chest is enormous and in some cases the ultimate expenditure is never recouped. Still, the versatility of modern pharmacotherapy is a tribute to the efforts of pharmaceutical chemists.

RECOMBINANT DNA TECHNOLOGY

An innovative procedure for synthesizing certain drugs, recombinant DNA technology, is now being employed in the production of human insulin as well as other drugs. The procedure to produce insulin involves introduction of coded DNA into a well-studied, harmless strain of *Escherichia coli* K12. The A and B chains of the insulin molecule are synthesized by different strains of *E. coli*, then freed and purified individually before being linked by specific disulfide bridges to form an insulin molecule identical in amino acid sequence to endogenous human insulin. Recombinant DNA technology has important implications for the efficient production of many drugs that are now derived solely from animal or human sources and will doubtless become a major technologic advance in drug synthesis. A synthetic human growth hormone is now being prepared through recombinant DNA technology.

Organ System Affected

A general classification of drugs may be based on their effects on a particular body system or function. Thus, there are drugs that act on the nervous system, cardiovascular system, renal function, respiratory function, hormonal function, and so on. A system or functional classification is convenient but provides little information as to the type of drug. For example, although both laxatives and antidiarrheals affect the gastrointestinal system, their pharmacologic actions are opposite. Likewise, both amphetamine and phenobarbital are drugs affecting the central nervous system, but the former is a stimulant whereas the latter is a depressant. Nevertheless, such a classification does permit separation of the vast number of available drugs into broad groups for the purposes of discussion and comparison. This type of classification is used for the section headings in this book and provides a logical grouping format.

Clinical Use

Perhaps the most pertinent means of classifying drugs is based on their clinical application, and this method is used in formulating the individual chapter headings found in this text. Thus, the various drugs that affect gastrointestinal function may be further categorized as antacids, digestants, laxatives, antidiarrheals, emetics, and antiemetics. In addition, drugs used to treat various diseases (e.g., psychoses, anxiety, hypertension, anemia) may be grouped by adding the prefix "anti-." For example, we use antipsychotic agents, antianxiety agents, antihypertensives, and antiemetic drugs. This mode of classification provides the most information as to the actual clinical effects of the compounds and serves to compartmentalize drugs having similar actions. Although applicable to most drugs, this classification method cannot be used for all types of drugs. For example, anti-infective agents act on microorganisms within the body rather than on body systems themselves, and most antibiotics exert similar effects by either slowing the proliferation of the microbe or actually killing the bacterial cells. Therefore, an alternative means for classifying these drugs is necessary. One such means is suggested below.

Chemical Composition

All drugs possess a chemical structure, ranging from simple ions, such as iron and calcium, to complex organic molecules, for example, steroids and polypeptides. In most instances, chemical composition is a quite precise albeit rather unwieldy means of drug classification and is usually of more interest to the research chemist than to the clinician. However, some drug groups do not readily lend themselves to grouping based on source, function, or clinical usefulness. One such group, as noted above, is the anti-infective agents, and these compounds can best be categorized by chemical composition, such as penicillins, tetracyclines, aminoglycosides, and so on.

REVIEW QUESTIONS

1. Distinguish between the terms *pharmacokinetics* and *pharmacodynamics.*
2. What is meant by *toxicology?*
3. List the various means of naming a new drug.
4. Give several arguments both defending and opposing generic and brand name prescribing.
5. Outline various ways for classifying drugs.
6. List some general types of plant constituents that have been used as drugs.
7. What is meant by a "functional classification" of drugs?
8. How might the nurse use a functional classification system to learn about new drugs?

BIBLIOGRAPHY

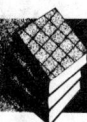

Friend DG: Principles and practices of prescription writing. Clin Pharmacol Ther 6:411, 1965

Jerome JB, Sagan P: The USAN nomenclature system. JAMA 232:294, 1975

Lieberman ML: The Essential Guide to Generic Drugs. New York, Harper & Row, 1986

Trout MF, Lec AM: Generic substitution: A boon or bane to the physician and the consumer? In Melmon KL, et al (eds): Drug Therapeutics: Concepts for Physicians. New York, Elsevier North Holland, 1979

United States Pharmacopeia, 21st ed, and The National Formulary, 16th ed (combined volume). United States Pharmacopeial Convention, 1985

Interaction of Drugs With Body Tissues: Pharmacokinetics

2

Drugs are used to elicit a desired pharmacologic effect. To produce this effect, the molecules of the drug must be present in sufficient concentration at the sites of action of the drug in the body. Many of the processes by which a drug molecule is handled by the body, namely absorption, distribution, biotransformation, and excretion, greatly influence the ultimate concentration of drug that arrives at its active sites in the body. The branch of pharmacology that considers the influence of the above-named processes on drug action is termed *pharmacokinetics*. In this chapter, we will discuss the basic principles underlying the movement of drug molecules throughout the body and review in detail the many factors influencing the absorption, distribution, biotransformation, and excretion of drugs. Their interrelationships are schematically outlined in Figure 2-1.

Passage of Drugs Across Membranes

With the exception of some locally acting compounds, such as gastric antacids, most drugs must cross one or more body membranes to reach their intended site of action. Therefore, to fully under-

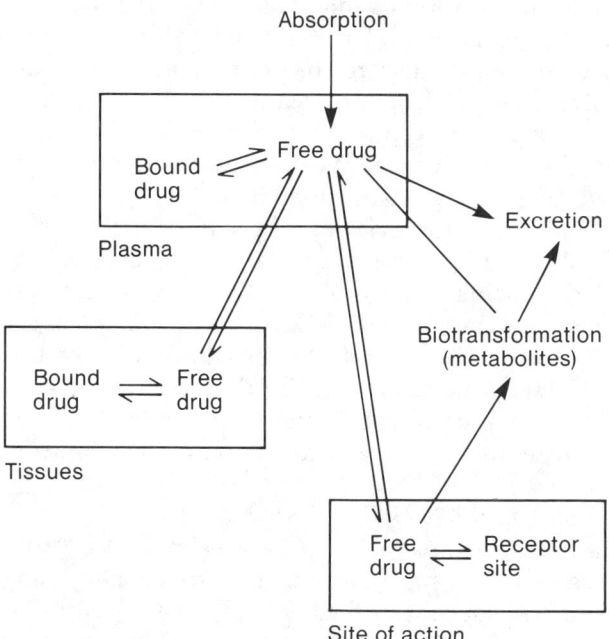

Figure 2-1. Factors influencing concentration of a drug at its site of action. The mechanisms involved in the various processes are discussed in detail throughout Chapter 2.

stand the various factors that can influence the processes of absorption, distribution, biotransformation, and excretion, it is necessary to consider the mechanisms by which drugs can cross membranes and the various properties of drugs that affect this transfer.

Cellular membranes, be they intestinal epithelium, renal tubular cells, vascular epithelium, or membranes enclosing any other type of cell, possess a fairly uniform structure. A typical cellular membrane is illustrated in Figure 2-2, and is composed of phospholipid and protein molecules. The phospholipid molecules are arranged in two parallel rows, termed a *lipid bilayer*. The protein molecules appear to occur randomly, some near the inner or outer surfaces of the membrane and others penetrating the membrane to varying degrees. Recent studies have indicated that this arrangement is dynamic, that is, the phospholipid and protein molecules possess the ability to move in conjunction with each other. This new concept has been termed the *fluid mosaic hypothesis* and may help explain the process whereby certain drugs and neurohormones attach to specific receptor areas on the cellular membrane. At various intervals along the membrane, there also appear to be breaks in the surface, which may represent the so-called pores in the membrane.

Drugs and other substances can cross cellular membranes in several ways. The processes involved are classified as follows:
1. Passive mechanisms
   a. Simple diffusion
   b. Osmosis
   c. Facilitated diffusion
2. Active mechanisms
   a. Active (carrier-mediated) transport
   b. Pinocytosis

Passive Mechanisms

Passive mechanisms refer to the movement of a substance across a membrane from an area of higher concentration to an area of lower concentration, that is, "down a concentration gradient." No energy is required and the movement of substances is either by way of the aqueous pores or by dissolution in the lipid layer of the membrane, depending on the lipid solubility of the substance crossing the membrane.

SIMPLE DIFFUSION
Simple diffusion of a drug from an area of high concentration on one side of a membrane to an area

9

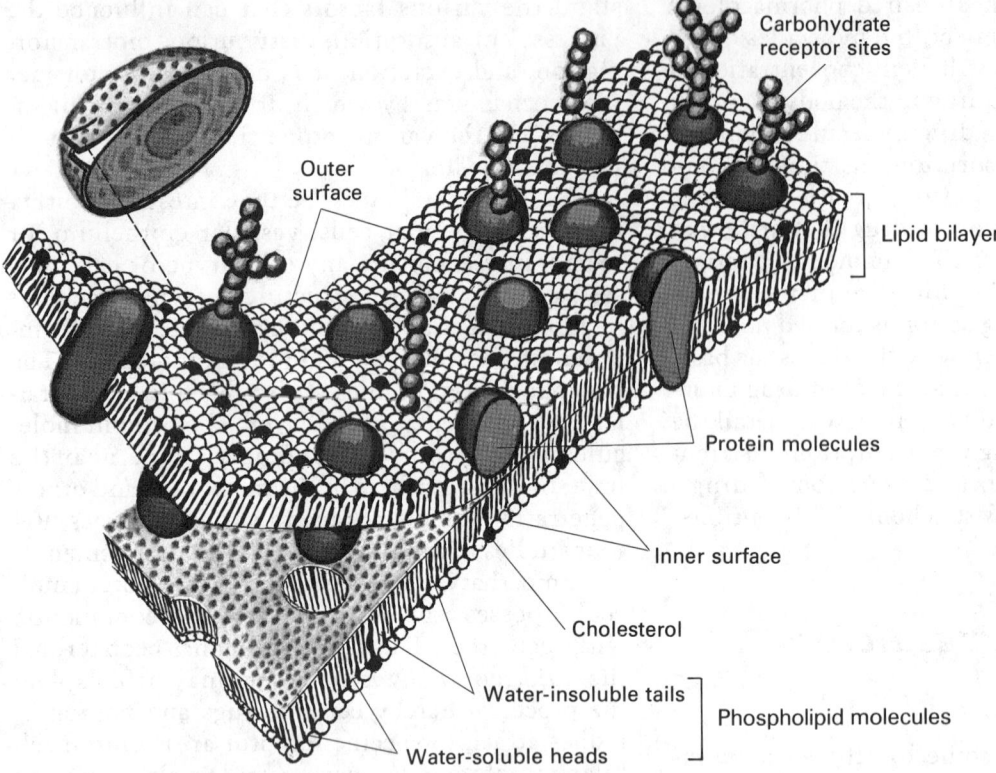

Figure 2-2. *Typical cellular membrane. (Chaffee EE, Lytle IM: Basic Physiology and Anatomy, 4th ed, p 40. Philadelphia, JB Lippincott, 1980)*

of lower concentration on the other side of the membrane is the most common means of membrane transfer of drugs. Movement of drug molecules will continue "down the gradient" as long as a concentration difference exists on either side of the membrane. Once the amount of drug molecules becomes equal on both sides, a *steady-state* concentration is attained, and passive diffusion ceases. Most biologic membranes are relatively permeable to water and allow for bulk flow of water through the membrane pores. This bulk flow may carry with it small water-soluble substances (generally with molecular weights less than 200) and represents an important mechanism for passage of drugs across capillary membranes. This process has also been termed *filtration* when it occurs at the glomerular membranes of the kidney.

OSMOSIS

Osmosis is a form of simple diffusion and describes the movement of a solvent from an area of low solute concentration (*i.e.,* highly diluted area) to an area of high solute concentration (*i.e.,* highly concentrated area). The solvent moves by simple diffusion until the concentration of solvent and hence

the concentration of solute are equal on either side of the membrane. The term *osmotic pressure* is used to define the force or pressure under which a solvent moves from an area of low solute concentration to an area of high solute concentration across a membrane. While osmosis is rarely involved in drug absorption, this concept is being used in developing newer long-acting dosage forms for drugs. For example, a water-soluble drug can be placed inside a capsule surrounded by a semipermeable membrane that allows water molecules in, by osmosis, while not allowing molecules of undissolved drug to escape. The drug is then released slowly as water diffuses into the capsule, dissolves the drug molecules, and then diffuses back out.

FACILITATED DIFFUSION

Facilitated diffusion is similar to simple diffusion, inasmuch as a substance moves across a membrane with the concentration gradient, that is, from an area of higher concentration to an area of lower concentration. In addition, the transfer requires the presence of a *carrier molecule*, which transports the drug substance across the membrane in cases where otherwise the rate of movement by simple diffusion would be too slow. However, since the movement of drugs is "down" the concentration gradient (*i.e.*, from high to low), *no* energy is required unlike the process of active transport described below. For example, glucose is transported across cellular membranes by facilitated diffusion, because glucose itself is insoluble in lipids and in spite of a high concentration gradient could not enter cells without the aid of the carrier molecule. The rate of facilitated diffusion is dependent on the concentration gradient, the number of carrier molecules available, and the affinity of the carrier for the substance to be transported.

Active Mechanisms

Active movement of compounds across a membrane refers to processes requiring the expenditure of energy and the movement of substances *against* the concentration gradient.

ACTIVE (CARRIER-MEDIATED) TRANSPORT

Active transport is a method that uses a carrier molecule to move substances across a membrane from an area of low concentration to an area of high concentration. Because the flow is against the concentration gradient, an energy source is necessary to move the solute molecules "uphill." This energy is usually supplied by the high-energy phosphate compound adenosine triphosphate (ATP). Other features of active transport are the selective nature of the carriers, the saturability of the systems, and the susceptibility to inhibition by drugs that can compete for the available carriers or interfere with the production of energy.

Examples of active transport are the uptake of iodide by thyroid cells, glucose reabsorption by the kidney tubules, and the sodium–potassium pump, which expels sodium ions from cells.

PINOCYTOSIS

Pinocytosis is a mechanism by which large molecules may cross cellular membranes even though they are too large to transit the pores and too insoluble to diffuse through the lipid layer. The surface of the cellular membrane forms an invagination, or "pocket," into which flow extracellular fluid and its constituents. The invaginated membrane then "pinches off" vesicles or round globules, which diffuse across the membrane and deposit their contents on the inside of the cell. The significance of pinocytosis in drug absorption and distribution is probably minimal, although the intrinsic factor, vitamin B_{12} complex, is absorbed from the gastrointestinal tract by the process of pinocytosis. This process is listed under active mechanisms, since it probably requires the expenditure of cellular energy.

The various passive and active mechanisms that control the passage of drugs across cellular membranes are schematically represented in a greatly simplified manner in Figure 2–3.

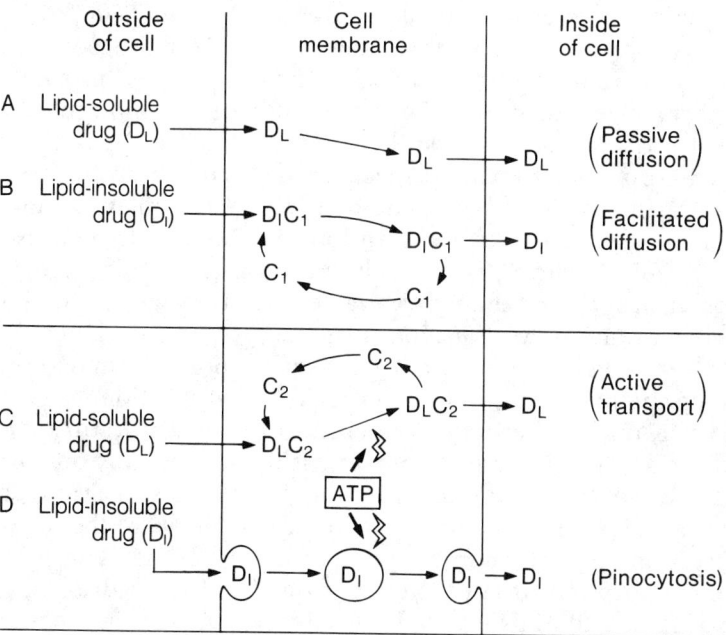

Figure 2-3. Drugs cross cellular membranes by the following mechanisms: (A) a lipid-soluble drug diffuses down the concentration gradient by passive diffusion; (B) a lipid-insoluble drug also moves down the gradient, but requires the assistance of a carrier molecule (C₁) to transport it through the lipid bilayer of the membrane (no energy is necessary); (C) a lipid-soluble drug is transported against the concentration gradient utilizing a different carrier (C₂) and energy supplied by ATP; (D) a lipid-insoluble drug is engulfed by a pinocytotic vesicle and transported in an energy-dependent fashion to the inside of the cell.

Absorption

Absorption refers to the processes by which a drug passes from its location in the body to the circulatory fluids (that is, blood and lymph) immediately following administration. Naturally, the sites and mechanisms involved in absorption will depend to a large extent on the means of administration.

Sites of Absorption from the Gastrointestinal Tract

Drugs may be absorbed from several regions of the gastrointestinal (GI) tract, although most absorption occurs throughout the upper region of the small intestine. The main reasons for this are the presence of many small folds, or *villi*, which greatly increase the absorbing surface area, and the highly permeable nature of the intestinal epithelium. Other factors that make the small intestine the major site for most drug absorption are the presence of special transport systems for absorption of sugars, amino acids, nutrients, and other substances; the fairly rapid gastric emptying of many drugs, which delivers a greater fraction of unabsorbed drug to the upper intestine, and the extensive capillary network of the intestinal villi.

The stomach, on the other hand, functions primarily in the digestion of food and is only involved to a limited extent in drug absorption. The greatest variable in regulating the extent of gastric absorption is the length of time a substance remains in the stomach. However, the extensive blood supply to the gastric mucosa provides a good absorbing medium for drugs that remain in contact with the stomach lining for any length of time. Thus, certain drugs, such as aspirin and alcohol, can be significantly absorbed from the stomach, especially if gastric emptying time is prolonged. The overall contribution of the gastric phase of absorption to total drug absorption, however, is not only quite small with most drugs, but exceedingly variable.

Theoretically, the lining of the mouth or the oral cavity is a very efficient site for drug absorption, since the epithelium is quite thin and highly vascular. However, due to the limited amount of time that orally ingested drugs are in contact with the mucosa of the mouth, absorption is minimal. Conversely, certain dosage forms of a few drugs, such as nitroglycerin and ergotamine, provide for almost complete absorption from the lining of the mouth. These drugs are administered sublingually, that is, under the tongue, in the form of a soluble tablet. The tablet quickly dissolves and the drug is then rapidly absorbed through the thin, highly vascular mucous membrane on the floor of the mouth, yielding a quick onset of action. An added advantage of sublingual absorption is that the drug gains access to the general circulation *without* having to first pass through the liver and being subjected to rapid metabolism. Following absorption from the stomach or intestines, however, drugs initially enter the portal circulation and are immediately transported to the liver, where a portion of the drug may be inactivated before reaching the systemic circulation. This so-called *first-pass inactivation* can reduce the effectiveness of many orally ingested drugs, and is considered further under Biotransformation (Metabolism) later in this chapter.

Mechanisms of Oral Absorption

In general, absorption of most drugs from the GI tract is best explained by simple diffusion of the lipid-soluble form of the drug across the mucosal barrier. Some absorption also occurs by way of aqueous pores in the membrane and by active (energy-requiring) transport mechanisms. These latter two processes can increase the absorption of water-soluble ionized drugs, since they do not involve diffusion of the lipid-soluble form across the fatty membrane.

Absorption of drugs from the GI tract is influenced by several factors.

NATURE OF THE DRUG

Most drugs are either weak acids or weak bases, and exist in solution in both the un-ionized (*i.e.,* intact molecules) and ionized forms. The un-ionized form is the more lipid-soluble form and as such more readily diffuses across the lipid bilayer of cellular membranes. Since most drug molecules are too large to pass through the membrane pores, they must cross the membrane by diffusion through the lipid barrier. Thus, the *lipid solubility* of the un-ionized fraction of drug is of prime importance in determining the rate and extent of oral absorption.

The ratio of un-ionized/ionized fraction of a drug at any one time is dependent on its ionization (or dissociation) constant (known as the pKa) and the pH of the aqueous medium in which the drug is present. The pKa may be defined as the pH at which a drug or other chemical substance exists one half in the un-ionized state and one half in the ionized state. Table 2-1 lists some commonly used drugs and their pKa values. At a *p*H below the pKa, acidic drugs will be predominantly un-ionized whereas basic drugs will be largely ionized. Conversely, if the *p*H of the environment is greater than the pKa of the drug, acidic drugs will exist predominantly in the ionized state, while basic drugs will be largely un-ionized.

For example, acidic drugs such as phenobarbital (pKa = 7.4) and aspirin (pKa = 3.5) are present predominantly in an un-ionized state in areas of low *p*H, such as the stomach (*p*H 1–3). Hence, these drugs would be significantly absorbed at this site. Basic drugs, on the other hand, such as morphine (pKa = 7.9) or amphetamine (pKa = 9.8) would be largely ionized in this *p*H range and not well absorbed. As the drugs move down the intestinal tract, the *p*H increases and acidic drugs become more ionized whereas basic drugs are less ionized. Therefore, the absorption of basic drugs increases as the molecules move through the intestines. The influence of *p*H in the region of the absorbing barrier will be considered more fully later in this chapter.

Another drug-related factor influencing oral absorption is the *stability of the drug* in the fluids of the GI tract. Some drugs, such as insulin, are rapidly destroyed by the enzymes of the digestive tract and thus cannot be given orally.

Finally, the *molecular weight* and *structural configuration* of the molecules can affect the passage of certain drugs through the absorbing membrane of the GI tract. Small-molecular-weight, lipid-insoluble drugs may be significantly absorbed by diffusion through the aqueous pores in the membrane, whereas larger molecules may not be able to "squeeze" through these pores and their absorption is therefore limited.

NATURE OF THE DOSAGE FORM

The dosage form in which a drug is administered (*e.g.*, tablet, capsule, liquid) can be an important determinant of its oral absorption. In order for a drug molecule to cross the absorbing membrane, the molecule must be in solution; therefore, the *dissolution rate* of solid dosage forms such as tablets or capsules may be the limiting factor with regard to rate and extent of drug absorption. Some factors that may influence the dissolution rate of drug formulations are the degree of compression of the tablet or powder within the capsule, the volume and *p*H of gastric fluid, and the presence of specialized coatings around the tablet or capsule that resist breakdown in the stomach. These so-called *enteric-coated* preparations consist of a thin film of material around the tablet or capsule, which is dissolved only in the alkaline environment of the intestines. In this way, drugs that are either irritating to the stomach mucosa or unstable in the presence of gastric digestive enzymes can still be administered orally. The manner in which enteric-coated preparations are formulated is a critical factor in ensuring proper delivery of medication. If the coat is "too resistant" to breakdown even in the intestinal fluids, the drug may pass completely through the GI tract intact.

Table 2-1
Ionization Constants (pKa) of Selected Drugs

Drug	pKa
Acidic	
acetysalicylic acid (aspirin)	3.5
ampicillin	2.5
cephalexin	5.2
dopamine	10.6
furosemide	3.9
ibuprofen	4.4
levodopa	2.3
methotrexate	4.8
phenobarbital	7.4
phenylbutazone	8.3
phenytoin	3.4
probenecid	4.5
thiopental	7.6
tolbutamide	5.3
warfarin	5.0
Basic	
amphetamine	9.8
atropine	9.7
caffeine	0.8
chlorpheniramine	9.2
cocaine	8.5
codeine	8.2
diazepam	3.3
ephedrine	9.6
imipramine	9.5
kanamycin	7.2
methadone	8.4
morphine	7.9
pilocarpine	6.9
propranolol	9.4
scopolamine	8.1

■ NURSING ALERT

Medications are manufactured specifically to maximize their effects by the recommended route of administration. Altering the dosage form may seriously influence the amount of drug that is actually absorbed or the rate at which it is absorbed. In either case, the results may be dangerous to the patient. Therefore, crushing enteric-coated tablets or removing powders or beads from capsules is not appropriate. When a patient has difficulty swallowing pills, seek a liquid form of the medication or an alternative route of administration. Likewise, powders and solutions manufactured for parenteral use should not be given orally or through feeding tubes. Always check with the pharmacist if a question of altering the dosage form arises.

Another important factor in determining the rate of oral absorption is the *concentration* of the drug in solution. Drugs administered in high concentrations in solution or in large amounts as soluble tablets or capsules are more rapidly absorbed than drugs given in low concentrations. This simply reflects the greater movement of drug molecules from a region of high concentration (e.g., stomach) to a region of low concentration (e.g., blood) across the absorbing membrane. Certain drugs, such as digoxin, are sometimes administered in high doses initially, to facilitate rapid attainment of effective plasma levels, and then the dose or rate of administration is reduced to such a point that the desired plasma level is maintained.

Conversely, absorption from the GI tract can be slowed, and thus drug effects prolonged, by use of various *timed-release* or *sustained-action* dosage forms. One type of formulation used to provide a sustained release of medication consists of tablets containing concentric rings of active drug and inert material, providing delayed drug release as each layer disintegrates sequentially. Another type of sustained-release product is capsules containing the active drug in small "beads" that are coated to varying thicknesses with a material that resists rapid disintegration. Thus, the drug is dissolved and released over an extended time as different "beads" disintegrate at different rates. In still another type of slow-release product the active drug is encapsulated in a semipermeable membranous coating. As water seeps into the drug reservoir, it dissolves the particles of drug and then carries the solubilized drug back out into the stomach or intestinal fluid, from which absorption occurs. Finally, some drugs can be combined with resins and

are then released as the drug molecules are exchanged with ions in the gastrointestinal fluids.

NATURE OF THE ABSORBING BARRIER

The characteristics of the barrier, or membrane, across which absorption must take place, can also influence the absorptive process. Two important factors in this regard are the *permeability* of the gastrointestinal epithelium and the *blood flow* in the absorbing region. The thinner and more vascular the mucosal epithelium, the faster the drug is absorbed and carried to its site of action. With GI absorption of orally administered drugs, these factors are difficult to manipulate externally but may be significantly altered in certain disease states, such as gastric ulcer. Absorption of drugs administered subcutaneously or intramuscularly can be markedly improved in many cases, however, by massage or application of heat to the area of injection, thus increasing local blood flow.

The *regional pH of the GI tract* can influence drug solubility as well as the ratio of un-ionized/ionized drug. For example, in the acidic environment of the stomach (pH 1–3), acidic drugs such as barbiturates, salicylates, and penicillins exist largely in the un-ionized state and can readily cross the absorbing membrane. On the other hand, basic drugs such as morphine, ephedrine, and quinidine ionize extensively at low pH, and absorption is thus impaired. As the gastric contents empty into the intestine, the environment becomes progressively more basic (pH 6–8), favoring ionization of acids and hence decreased absorption. Basic drugs, however, ionize less at elevated pH, and their absorption consequently improves.

Perhaps the major factor in determining the rate and extent of GI absorption is the *area of mucosal surface* available for absorption. Since a drug molecule can only cross an absorbing membrane by first coming into contract with the membrane surface, it is obvious that the larger the surface area available, the greater the chance of a drug molecule contacting the surface and subsequently being absorbed. Available absorptive surface area clearly explains why the intestines are the principal site of absorption for most drugs, *irrespective of their chemical make-up*. The absorbing area of the intestinal tract is many times greater than that of the stomach, due both to the length of the intestines and the presence of surface modifications such as microvilli.

MISCELLANEOUS FACTORS

There are a number of other factors that can influence the absorption of orally administered drugs.

Since drugs must come into contact with a membrane in order to be absorbed, the length of time the absorbing surface is exposed to the drug will determine the total absorption. Absorption of drugs from the stomach will be enhanced by delayed gastric emptying, as occurs with a fatty meal, for example. Likewise, drugs absorbed in the intestines will be in contact with the absorbing membrane longer if intestinal peristalsis and motility are slowed, as is seen following administration of anticholinergic drugs or opiates. Conversely, laxatives may impair drug absorption by accelerating drug transit through the intestines. The presence of food in the stomach usually slows absorption of most drugs, although some drugs are better absorbed in the presence of food. Food can also reduce GI irritation resulting from certain drugs and decrease the extent of first-pass hepatic metabolism. The effect of food, where important, on the absorption of individual drugs is considered under the heading Fate in the drug monographs throughout this book.

The presence of other drugs or substances in the GI tract can also retard absorption of some drugs. For example, most tetracycline antibiotics form an insoluble complex with polyvalent metal ions, such as calcium, aluminum, and magnesium. Thus, the absorption of tetracyclines is impaired in the presence of aluminum- and magnesium-containing antacids as well as foods such as dairy products that contain calcium. The various types of drug interactions that may influence gastrointestinal absorption are discussed further in Chapter 5.

Absorption from Parenteral Sites

Absorption following subcutaneous (SC) and intramuscular (IM) injections usually occurs by simple diffusion down a concentration gradient from the injection site to the plasma or lymph. The most important factors controlling absorption from SC or IM sites are the *area of the absorbing capillary membranes* and the *solubility of the drug in the interstitial fluid*. Filtration through channels in the endothelial capillary membrane is very efficient, since these channels are relatively large and can accommodate most lipid-insoluble drugs.

The dosage formulation can also affect absorption from parenteral sites, for example, drugs in aqueous solution are usually absorbed more rapidly than drugs in suspension. Often drugs are suspended in certain vehicles, such as an oil, specifically to retard their rate of absorption and provide a prolonged action. Examples of this are various penicillins (benzathine penicillin and procaine penicillin G) and long-acting hormones and steroidal agents.

Absorption of drugs from IM sites is usually more rapid than from SC areas because of the more extensive vascular supply per unit area of muscle compared with fatty subcutaneous tissue. The decreased peripheral blood flow present during circulatory failure (as in cases of shock) may significantly reduce the rate of absorption of injected drugs and greatly reduce their efficacy. Blood flow to a superficial area can be increased and absorption enhanced by application of heat, local vasodilators, or massage; conversely, decreased blood flow and delayed absorption result from use of cold, a tourniquet, or vasoconstrictors. All these factors can exert a profound influence on the onset as well as the extent of a drug's action.

Intravenous administration, of course, provides the most rapid drug action because the drug enters the bloodstream directly without crossing any membranes.

Absorption from Topical Sites

Absorption of most drugs through the intact skin is very poor, primarily because of the keratinized structure of the epidermis. The extent of absorption through the skin is proportional to the lipid solubility of the drug and the surface area to which the drug is applied. The underlying dermis, however, is quite permeable to many drugs and significant absorption can occur if the overlying skin is abraded or denuded. Enhanced absorption of topically applied drugs can be obtained by dissolving the drug in an oily base, massaging the drug vigorously into the applied area, using an occlusive dressing, or simultaneously applying a keratin-softening agent such as salicyclic acid.

Increasingly, drugs intended for systemic action are being formulated in a way that can utilize topical absorption as the route of administration. For example, the skin of the upper torso is used as the absorbing site for nitroglycerin prepared in the form of a drug-impregnated patch. The drug is sufficiently absorbed in this manner to provide reasonably consistent plasma levels for 12 to 24 hours. This preparation will be reviewed in Chapter 36.

Absorption of most drugs through mucous membranes is usually very rapid, due largely to the thin, highly vascular absorbing surface. However, drugs applied to mucous membranes are usually used for their local action, for example, as nasal decongestants or vaginal anti-infectives. Thus, systemic absorption usually results in unwanted side-effects. A few drugs, however, such as nitroglycerin, ergotamine, and vasopressin, are applied to mucous membranes to facilitate their systemic absorption.

Absorption of inhaled medication depends to a large extent on the particle size of the drug, which determines the extent of penetration into the alveoli of the lungs. This is the primary site of systemic absorption of inhaled medications, because of the close proximity of capillaries to the alveolar membrane. Although most inhaled drugs are intended for their local effects, such as bronchodilators or corticosteroids used in asthma, systemic absorption may be appreciable due to the tremendous surface absorbing area and can result in unwanted adverse effects.

Distribution

After a drug has been absorbed into the circulatory system, its distribution throughout the body is governed by a number of factors. Drug distribution describes the process that transports a drug to its site of action, to other storage sites in the body, and to the organs of metabolism (e.g., liver) and excretion (e.g., kidney). Therefore, the entry of a drug molecule into one of these areas can determine its effectiveness, its duration of action, its mode of metabolism, and its rate of excretion. Since the distribution pattern of a drug is ultimately dependent on its ability to traverse one or more cellular membranes, the principles governing membrane transport of drugs, discussed earlier in this chapter, apply here as well. Thus, lipid-soluble drugs tend to distribute more widely in the body than lipid-insoluble drugs, since they more readily cross cellular membranes and thus can more easily gain access to tissues. Nevertheless, the highly permeable nature of most capillary endothelium (except for brain capillaries) allows ready passage of many drugs, and other than the central nervous system (CNS), most organs can be affected by virtually any drug.

The initial distribution of a drug is primarily dependent on the output of the heart and the local blood flow in the various body organs. Thus, highly perfused organs such as the heart, liver, kidney, and brain tend to receive the largest amount of drug immediately after absorption. Subsequently, other factors come into play that determine the final distribution pattern of a drug. We will consider some of these additional factors in more detail.

Drug Binding

Drugs may bind either to constituents of plasma (e.g., albumin) or of cells (e.g., nucleoproteins). Binding to plasma proteins slows the disappearance of the drug from the plasma, limits its access to cellular sites of action, and prolongs the time the drug remains in the body by slowing its renal filtration. The total amount of drug bound in the plasma is dependent on its plasma concentration, its affinity for the binding sites on albumin, and the total number of available protein-binding sites. The binding is usually reversible and an equilibrium exists between the free and bound forms of a drug, so that

$$\text{Free drug} + \text{plasma protein} \underset{k_1}{\overset{k_2}{\rightleftharpoons}} \text{drug--protein complex}$$

where k_1 reflects the rate at which drug binds to plasma proteins and k_2 is a measure of the rate of dissociation of drug from the plasma proteins.

Since it is only free drug that is capable of crossing cellular membranes, protein binding can interfere with the access of a drug to its sites of action. At the same time, binding slows excretion, and thus a "reservoir" of drug develops in the plasma. As free drug leaves the plasma, either through excretion, metabolism, or diffusion to other tissues, the drug-protein complex dissociates to supply more free drug. Conversely, as the drug concentration increases in the plasma, more free drug becomes bound. However, it is important to keep in mind that the binding capacity of plasma proteins is limited, and saturation can occur, although the amount of drug capable of being bound by plasma proteins is variable and difficult to determine. Once the protein-binding sites are completely occupied, further administration of the drug may result in increased effects or toxic reactions because of the presence of large amounts of non-protein-bound drug. Similarly, many different kinds of drugs are protein bound, and *simultaneous* administration of two or more of these drugs can result in competition for available sites on the binding proteins, displacement of active drug, and subsequently enhanced drug effects. This type of drug interaction is explored more fully in Chapter 5.

For a drug to exert its desired pharmacologic effect, it must either act on abnormal parasites or growths (e.g., microorganisms or neoplasms) or modify existing physiologic processes. The actions of a drug in the body must be viewed as the consequence of a complex series of physical and chemical interactions with certain cellular constituents of the living organism. The net result of a drug's action on a biochemical level is an alteration in the normal physiologic functioning of the organism. If this alteration occurs in an abnormal parasite or growth on the body such as bacteria, virus, or neoplastic tissue, the drug is termed a *chemotherapeutic agent* (e.g., antibiotics, antineoplastics). If a change in the normal physiologic function of the body occurs in response to a drug (e.g., reduction in blood pressure, slowing of the heart rate, increased urine output), the drug is termed a *pharmacodynamic agent*.

Although much remains to be learned concerning the molecular basis of a drug's effects, sufficient information exists to establish a fairly detailed picture of the sites at which drugs act and the biochemical mechanisms involved in their actions.

Virtually all body tissues are exposed to systemically administered drugs, but certain tissues appear to be affected much more than others. Most drugs exert their primary actions at specific sites in the body, although they may affect several tissues or organs, depending on their distribution.

With few exceptions, most drugs exert their effects by first interacting with a functional macromolecular cellular component to initiate a series of biochemical and physiologic changes that ultimately lead to the pharmacologic effect. The cellular component that interacts with the drug molecules is termed a *receptor site* and the chemical bond formed between it and the drug is responsible for the biologic actions of the majority of drugs. Implicit in the "receptor concept" of drug action is the understanding that drugs exert a *quantitative*, not a qualitative, effect at receptor sites. That is, a drug is capable of altering the *rate* of an ongoing physiologic process but cannot create a new function for a cell.

Drug–receptor interactions may or may not result in functional changes in the effector structure (e.g., heart, gastrointestinal smooth muscle, skeletal muscle). Drugs that combine with receptors and elicit a response are termed *agonists*. Drugs that combine with receptors and are devoid of activity, yet prevent an agonist from acting at that particular receptor site, are termed *antagonists*. If the inhibitory action of the antagonist can be overcome by increasing the amount of agonist available to the receptor site, the antagonist is referred to as a *competitive antagonist*. Conversely, if the interaction of the antagonist and the receptor alters the receptor site in such a way that the agonist is ineffective no matter how high the concentration, then the antagonist is termed a *noncompetitive antagonist*. The relationship between agonists and antagonists will be explored more fully later in the chapter.

Principles of Drug–Receptor Interactions

Drug–receptor interactions are governed by several principles, a knowledge of which is important for a better understanding of drug action. Receptors have *specific structural conformations* that correspond spatially to the molecular shape of certain drugs. Thus, the three-dimensional configuration of the reactive area on a cellular constituent greatly determines which drug molecules will be accepted and which are unable to "fit" the receptor. This fit is sometimes significantly altered by a simple chemical modification of the drug molecule, whereas in other cases, extensive molecular substitutions do not appear to impair the ability of the drug to interact with the receptor. This structural specificity has been referred to as the "lock and key" theory of drug–receptor interaction, but the degree of specificity can vary widely at different receptors in the body.

In order for a drug to attach to a reactive area on a cellular component, forces must be present to attract and hold the drug molecule to the receptor site. The *binding forces* in drug–receptor interactions include covalent bonds (usually the strongest, producing essentially irreversible effects), ionic bonds, hydrogen bonds, and van der Waals forces (weakest attractive bonds, yielding a readily reversible effect).

Drugs that "fit" the receptor site can either be agonists or antagonists, as previously discussed. However, an agonist may either stimulate or depress an existing physiologic function, and therefore can be either excitatory or inhibitory. The persistence of occupation of a drug at a receptor site can influence whether the drug functions as a stimulant or a depressant of receptor–mediated activity. For example, succinylcholine initially stimulates cholinergic receptor sites at the neuromuscular junction, resulting in temporary twitching of the muscle. However, by persistently occupying these sites, succinylcholine prevents further receptor activation, resulting in muscle relaxation.

Not all receptors on a particular cell need to be occupied in order for a drug effect to occur; potent drugs may be effective at very low concentrations, occupying only a fraction of the receptors. Thus, *receptor sensitivity* to a particular concentration of drug may determine whether an effect is elicited by a certain level of drug at the receptor site area.

Affinity and Intrinsic Activity

The binding of a drug to a receptor can be represented as follows:

$$\text{Drug (D)} + \text{receptor (R)} \underset{k_2}{\overset{k_1}{\rightleftharpoons}} \underset{\text{complex}}{\text{D–R}} \overset{k_3}{\rightarrow} \text{effect}$$

The rate at which a drug molecule combines with a receptor site is given by the rate constant k_1. Similarly, the rate at which the drug–receptor complex dissociates (*i.e.*, splits apart) is given by the rate constant k_2. The rate at which an effect is generated following a drug–receptor interaction is given by the rate constant k_3. These constants can be utilized to define some basic concepts relating to drug–receptor interactions. The tendency for a drug to form and subsequently maintain a complex with a receptor site is termed *affinity* and may be quantitatively expressed as k_1/k_2, that is, the rate at which the complex forms compared to the rate at which the complex dissociates. Once combined with the receptor, the ability of a drug to evoke a pharmacologic response is termed *intrinsic activity* and can be measured by k_3. Thus, agonists possess both affinity and intrinsic activity, whereas antagonists display only affinity. In other words, the k_3 for antagonists is zero. For example, acetylcholine functions as a cholinergic agonist, but its effects are inhibited by atropine, a cholinergic antagonist capable of occupying the same receptor sites but possessing no intrinsic cholinergic activity of its own. A *partial agonist*, on the other hand, possesses less intrinsic activity than a full agonist, but may have equal affinity. Therefore, the presence of a partial agonist can reduce the effects of a full agonist by competing for the available receptor sites. However, if the partial agonist is present alone, an agonistic action will likely be observed.

Intensity of Drug Effects

The magnitude of the effect elicited by a drug–receptor interaction can vary widely and several

theories have been proposed to explain these variations. The *receptor occupation theory* postulates that the intensity of a drug's effects is directly proportional to the number of receptors occupied. This is probably an oversimplistic view, in that it does not account for differences in absolute milligram potencies among drugs. A second theory is the *rate theory*, which states that the intensity of a drug's effects is proportional to the rate at which drug–receptor interactions occur. A typical curve illustrating the intensity of a drug effect with increasing dosage (conventionally plotted as log dose) is shown in Figure 3-1. The slope of the upward part of the curve is of therapeutic significance in assessing the relative safety of the drug. For example, many central nervous system depressants have a *steep* dose–response curve, indicating that there is a narrow margin between the dose that is effective (e.g., producing mild sedation) and the dose that is potentially toxic (e.g., producing coma). Generally, therefore, the more shallow the slope of a dose–response curve, the greater is the safety margin of that particular drug. Thus, a principal advantage of the benzodiazepine group of antianxiety drugs, such as diazepam (Valium) or oxazepam (Serax) over the barbiturates for the relief of mild anxiety is their much *shallower dose–response curve*, as indicated in Figure 3-2.

Potency vs Efficacy

Potency and *efficacy* are two terms relating to drug action that are often confused. A drug is said to be *potent* when it possesses high intrinsic activity at low unit weight doses. Of the two drugs whose dose–response curves are illustrated in Figure 3-3, drug X is the more potent drug, since it exerts the same intensity of effect as drug Y at much smaller

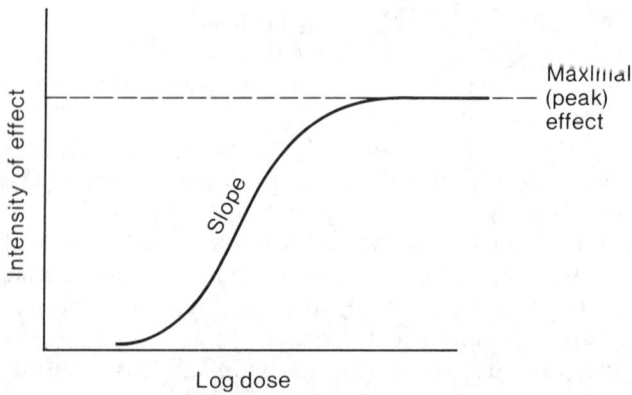

Figure 3-1. Typical dose-response curve for a drug.

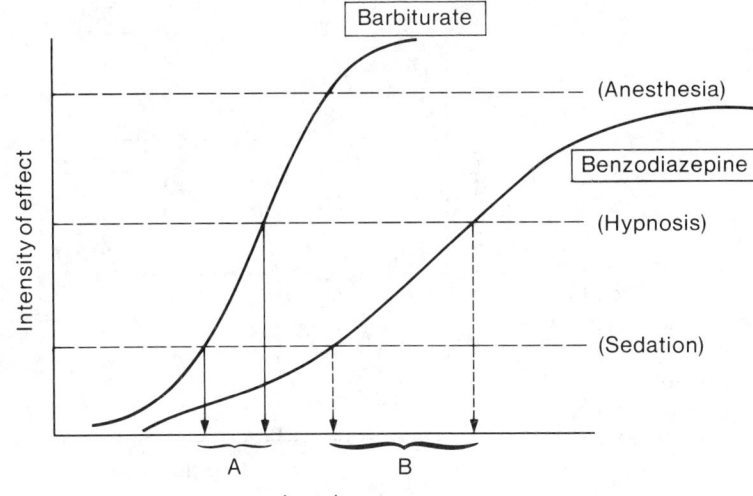

Figure 3-2. *Representative dose-response curves for a benzodiazepine and a barbiturate illustrate the greater margin between the sedative and hypnotic doses of a barbiturate (A) compared to a benzodiazepine (B).*

doses. The maximal effect with each drug, however, is identical. Thus, potencies are compared based on doses that elicit the same intensity of effect. Knowledge of a drug's potency is important for approximating the appropriate dosage level to be administered, but it is relatively unimportant in deciding which of two drugs exhibiting the same maximal effect should be used. It makes little difference if the dose of a drug is 5 mg or 500 mg as long as the dosage is convenient to administer. There is no rationale for believing the more potent drug is the clinically preferred drug, as is sometimes implied in drug advertising.

Efficacy, on the other hand, refers to the maximal (or peak) effect produced by a drug and is an important determinant in the drug selection process. Of the two drugs shown in Figure 3-4, drug X is not only more potent, it also exhibits a greater efficacy, since the maximal effect obtainable with

drug X is greater than that obtainable with drug Y (compare with Fig. 3-3, where the maximal effect of drug X is the same as that of drug Y). For example, oral administration of 4 mg of hydromorphone (Dilaudid) results in much greater pain relief than 65 mg of propoxyphene (Darvon). Therefore, hydromorphone is both more potent and more effective than propoxyphene.

Therapeutic Index

The dose of a drug necessary to produce the desired intensity of effect in one half of all patients is known as the *median effective dose*, or ED_{50}. Similarly, the dose of a drug that elicits an undesirable toxic reaction in one half of all patients is termed the *median toxic dose*, or TD_{50}. In toxicity studies in laboratory animals, the toxic end-point frequently used is death, and the median toxic dose is then referred to as the *median lethal dose*, or LD_{50}. Clinical studies, for obvious reasons, do not attempt to determine the LD_{50} of a drug. Obviously, the larger the difference between the ED_{50} and the TD_{50}, the greater is the safety margin of the drug. One means of expressing a drug's safety is the *therapeutic index*, which is defined as the ratio of the TD_{50} to the ED_{50}. In other words

$$\text{Therapeutic index (TI)} = TD_{50}/ED_{50}$$

The greater the ratio, that is, the lower the ED_{50} or the higher the TD_{50}, the greater is the safety of the drug. Drugs do not have a single TI, since the TD_{50} and ED_{50} values are dependent on the particular end-points measured. Using barbiturates as an ex-

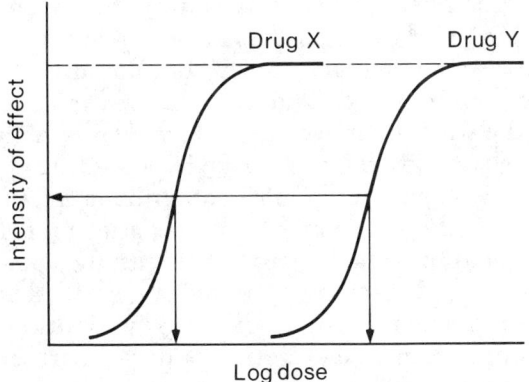

Figure 3-3. *Comparison of potencies of two drugs. Drug X is more potent than drug Y, although both elicit the same maximal effect.*

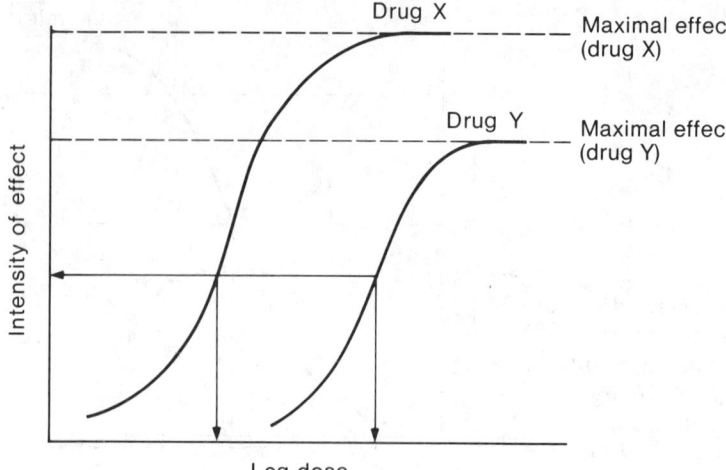

Figure 3-4. *Comparison of efficacies of two drugs. Drug X is more potent than drug Y (produces similar intensity of effect at a lower dose) and exerts a greater maximal effect; thus drug X is more effective.*

ample (see Fig. 3-2), the safety margin between the sedative (ED_{50}) and anesthetic (TD_{50}) doses, is somewhat greater (*i.e.*, a higher TI value) than the safety margin between the hypnotic (a second ED_{50}) and the anesthetic (TD_{50}) doses, since the hypnotic dose is closer to the anesthetic dose than is the sedative dose. It is important to recognize that the TI is simply one measure of a drug's safety and has no bearing on the drug's efficacy. Further, the TI must be viewed in general terms, since certain patients display extreme sensitivity to certain drugs. As an example, aspirin is a very safe drug in normal doses in a majority of individuals; however, severe hypersensitivity reactions to small doses of aspirin have occurred in some patients. Therefore, while the average TI for aspirin is quite high in the general population, some patients are extremely sensitive to very low doses of aspirin.

Non–receptor-Mediated Drug Effects

As indicated earlier, some drugs do not act by combining with receptor sites. For example, *gastric antacids* act largely by neutralizing the hydrochloric acid secreted by gastric parietal cells. *Osmotic diuretics*, such as mannitol, can rid the body of fluid by increasing the osmolarity of plasma, thereby altering the distribution of water in body tissues. Certain *structural analogs of purines and pyrimidines* can be incorporated into cellular constituents such as nucleic acids, thereby disrupting their normal functioning; these drugs are useful in treating many types of cancers. *Metal chelating agents*, such as EDTA, are employed in the treat-

ment of poisoning by several heavy metals. The number of drugs acting by non–receptor-mediated mechanisms is small, however, when compared to the number of drugs that owe their action to a drug–receptor complexation.

Factors Modifying Drug Effects

There are a variety of factors that can influence an individual's response to a drug, and these factors are frequently important for determining the proper drug and dosage to employ in a particular patient.

Age

In general, the pediatric and geriatric populations are more sensitive to the effects of drugs than is the population in between. Infants have immature enzymatic systems and incomplete development of the blood–brain barrier, and these factors, in addition to the small body weight and frequently high percentage of body fat, can markedly alter drug effects in this population. On the other hand, many elderly individuals display reduced hepatic or renal function, and these factors, together with the commonly observed circulatory impairments in this age group, can modify the absorption, distribution, biotransformation, and excretion of drugs. Further consideration of the role that age plays in drug action in the pediatric and geriatric populations is found in Chapters 9 and 10, respectively.

Body Size and Weight

Drug dosages, theoretically, should be adjusted in proportion to the body weight, since the greater the body weight, the more the drug can become diluted in the body. This factor becomes especially critical in infants and small children and will be explored in more detail in Chapter 8. Several formulas for calculating pediatric doses are based on body weight or body surface area. Sample calculations utilizing these formulas are found in Chapter 11. Similarly, the weight loss frequently seen in the elderly makes them more sensitive to the effects of many drugs. Finally, the possibility of altered drug effects in the emaciated or debilitated patient as well as in the very obese patient is obvious.

Sex

Compared to men, some women may exhibit increased sensitivity to certain drugs for a number of reasons, including a relatively smaller body weight, increased ratio of body fat to lean body mass, and possibly hormonal influences.

Route and Time of Administration

Drugs administered orally, subcutaneously, or intramuscularly must be absorbed from the site of administration prior to exerting their effect. Conversely, drugs given intravenously have a very rapid onset of action, since the absorption process is bypassed. A rapid onset of action can be lifesaving in certain instances, such as use of lidocaine to terminate acute arrhythmias associated with a myocardial infarction. However, a rapid action following intravenous injection can be hazardous and possibly fatal if an accidental overdosage or an inappropriate drug is given, as there is very little time to attempt to remove the drug before it can act.

Timing of an oral dose likewise can significantly affect a drug's action. Gastrointestinal absorption of many drugs is slowed in the presence of food, yet some highly irritating drugs must be given with food to reduce the severity of gastrointestinal distress. In such cases, onset of action can be delayed.

Pathologic Conditions

A variety of pathologic states can alter the response to drugs. Rates of metabolism and excretion can be slowed in patients with hepatic and renal dysfunction, respectively, possibly resulting in prolonged drug effects and cumulation toxicity. Therefore, dosage of drugs that depend on renal clearance for their elimination must be reduced in patients with impaired kidney function. Circulatory impairment can also significantly restrict drug distribution, perhaps leading to decreased drug effects or slowed metabolic inactivation or elimination.

Several types of drugs can exhibit altered effects in the presence of certain disease states. For example, many patients with hyperthyroidism are extremely sensitive to the effects of epinephrine. Barbiturates frequently elicit a paradoxic excitatory action in patients experiencing severe pain. Drugs that ordinarily do not cross the blood–brain barrier may attain significant levels in the central nervous system in the presence of meningitis. Fluid and electrolyte imbalances can lead to untoward reactions with the use of cardioactive drugs and diuretics. It is apparent, then, that the existence of an underlying disease process can markedly alter the expected effects of a drug.

Genetic Differences

It is well established that large variations in responsiveness to a particular drug can occur among different individuals. These variations not only require dosage adjustments to obtain the desired therapeutic effect, but are responsible for many instances of adverse reactions in sensitive individuals to doses of drugs that are safe in most other individuals. The term *idiosyncrasy* has frequently been used to describe an abnormal drug response that is not predictable based on a drug's profile of action. Idiosyncrasies can result from a number of factors, but most commonly are related to *genetic abnormalities* that alter the handling of a drug by the body. Some genetic conditions capable of modifying drug responses are aberrant enzymatic activity and altered receptor sensitivity. The study of the genetic factors that can influence drug responsiveness is known as *pharmacogenetics*, and the importance of genetic alterations as determinants of abnormal drug responsiveness is receiving increasing and well-deserved attention.

Psychologic and Emotional State

The attitude and expectations of the person taking the drug can greatly determine its effectiveness. A perfect example of this kind of response is the "placebo effect." This is the appearance of a clinical effect to a dose of a pharmacologically inactive substance (e.g., dextrose) given to a patient who believes he is receiving an active drug. The presence of anxiety accompanying pain frequently necessitates use of larger than normal amounts of an analgesic to quell the pain. Conversely, simultaneous use of an analgesic and a mild sedative may allow a reduction in the analgesic dose, thereby minimizing adverse effects, and in the case of narcotic analgesics, can delay development of tolerance and habituation. The importance of patient reassurance and a positive attitude on the part of the clinician in enhancing the therapeutic efficacy of many drugs cannot be overemphasized.

Repeated Dosage

The frequency and duration of drug dosing can influence the safety as well as the efficacy of therapy. In order to exert a clinical effect, the plasma concentration of a systemically administered drug must attain a certain level so that sufficient drug can be distributed to the site of action. Therefore, plasma level is a frequently employed parameter for measuring drug efficacy, and the dosage of many drugs is adjusted so as to maintain the plasma concentration within a certain range. Should the plasma concentration fall below the bottom of the desired range, effectiveness is reduced or abolished; conversely, an increase in plasma concentration above the upper limit of the desired range frequently is associated with an increased incidence of untoward reactions. A typical plasma concentration curve for a single dose of an orally administered drug is shown in Figure 3-5. The *time to onset of action* reflects the time necessary for the drug to be absorbed to such an extent that the effective plasma level is reached, and the drug is distributed to its site of action in sufficient quantity to elicit a response. As more drug is absorbed, the plasma level rises, more drug reaches the site of action, and the response increases to reflect the attainment of the *peak or maximum plasma level* possible for the particular dose given. As the drug is circulating in the plasma, it begins to be eliminated, either as intact drug molecules or as metabolites. When the rate of elimination exceeds the rate of absorption (due to decreasing amounts of the administered dose remaining to be absorbed), the plasma level begins to decline and the effect of the drug also decreases correspondingly. Once the plasma concentration falls below the minimal level necessary to elicit a pharmacologic effect, drug action ceases, even though some drug still remains in the plasma. Thus, the *duration of action* corresponds to that length of time that the drug is present in the plasma in concentrations sufficient to evoke the desired response.

The use of plasma levels of a drug as an indicator of the intensity of a drug's effects assumes that the concentration of the drug in the blood accurately reflects the concentration of the drug at the site of action. While this correlation does not hold for all drugs, plasma blood levels usually are a fairly reliable indicator of drug concentration at receptor sites. Since blood levels are much more convenient to quantitate than the drug concentration at the

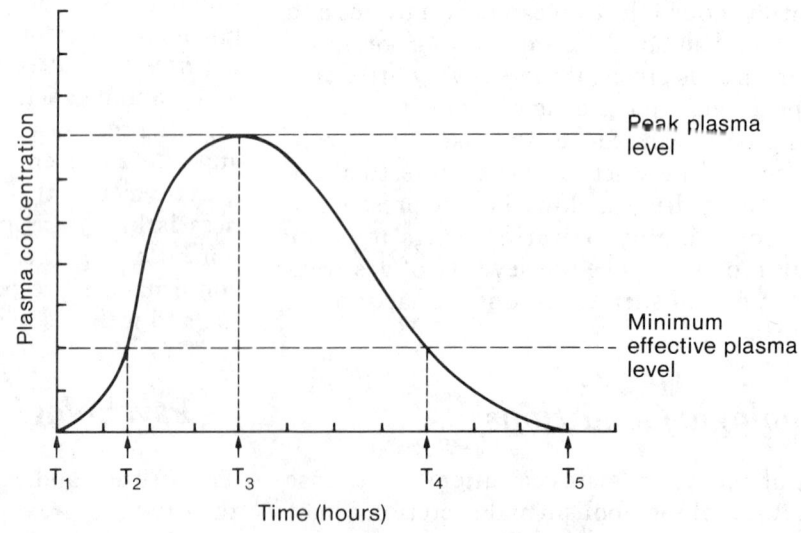

Figure 3-5. Typical plasma-concentration curve for a single dose of an orally administered drug. T_1 = Time of administration; $T_1 \rightarrow T_2$ = Time to onset of action (i.e., 1½ hours); $T_1 \rightarrow T_3$ = Time to attainment of peak plasma concentration (i.e., 4 hours); $T_2 \rightarrow T_4$ = Duration of effective plasma concentration (i.e., 6½ hours); T_5 = Time of complete elimination of drug from the plasma (i.e., 11 hours).

sites of action, blood level data are commonly employed in assessing the effectiveness of a systemically administered drug.

The *elimination half-life* ($T_{1/2}$) is the amount of time required to reduce the plasma level of a drug by one half. Approximately 95% of a dose of a drug is eliminated from the body in four half-lives. Half-life is a value frequently quoted in drug literature, and serves as an indicator of how frequently a drug needs to be administered to ensure maintenance of sufficient plasma concentrations. Hence, a drug with a half-life of 4 to 5 hours may need to be given every 4 hours to maintain its effectiveness, whereas a drug with a half-life of 10 to 12 hours may only require twice-daily administration.

CUMULATION

When a drug is given repeatedly, the absorbed fraction of each dose is added to the amount remaining in the plasma at the time of administration. Thus, the maximum and minimum plasma levels slowly rise until the rate of elimination equals the rate of administration. At that point, assuming the drug is being given in fixed dosage at a constant time interval, a *steady-state* plasma range is attained, and the concentration of the drug in the plasma is said to have reached a *plateau*. The plateau concentration of a drug is dependent on the dose, the frequency of administration, and the elimination half-life. The first two of these factors can be maintained constant; however, the elimina-

tion half-life may decrease as the plasma concentration rises, until, as indicated above, the rate of elimination equals the rate at which the drug is being supplied to the plasma. Once this equilibrium is reached, the plasma levels of a drug can usually be maintained in the desired range by strict adherence to the selected dosage intervals. This concept should be stressed to all patients, and the importance of taking medication on a carefully controlled dosing schedule must be strongly emphasized. Figure 3-6 illustrates the cumulative effect of repeated drug dosage, with the subsequent attainment of a steady-state plasma concentration. All other factors being equal, the plasma level will remain in the effective range as long as the same dose of the drug is administered every 3 hours. Should the dosage be increased or the dosing interval shortened, the plasma level will rise to a new steady-state range, which may be partially above the toxic threshold, and result in the appearance of untoward reactions. Therefore, once the desired steady-state plasma concentration has been attained, changes in dosage or frequency of administration should be avoided.

■ *NURSING ALERT*
To ensure therapeutic plasma levels of drugs
1. Maintain consistent dosage and frequency patterns for drugs that require a

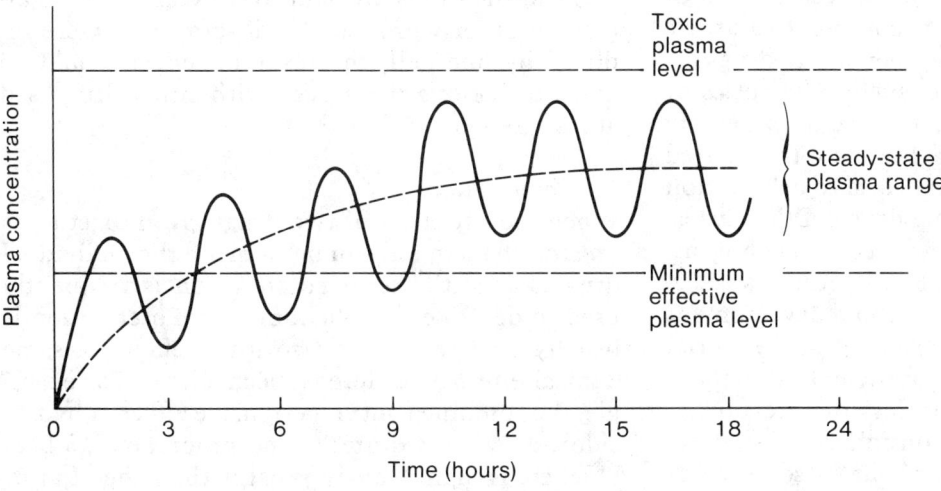

Figure 3-6. Cumulation of drug in the plasma with repeated administration at 3-hour intervals. Maximum and minimum plasma levels initially rise, then reach a plateau when elimination rate equals rate of absorption into the bloodstream. Steady-state plasma concentration (i.e., maintenance of plasma levels within the effective concentration range) persists as long as the drug is administered at the selected dosage intervals.

consistent plasma level to be therapeutic. Antibiotics and cardiotonics fall into this category. Alterations in frequency may affect the therapeutic effect, prolong the treatment, or necessitate a change in drug.

2. Plasma levels of drugs can be tested by blood studies but only if the blood is drawn at a correct time interval after administration of the drug dose. For example, lithium blood levels should be sampled just prior to the subsequent dose, that is, approximately 8 hours to 12 hours following the previous dose. If the patient needs blood samples drawn for plasma level determination, make sure the time is appropriate.

3. Loading doses of drugs may be given to facilitate rapid attainment of therapeutic plasma levels. In this type of dosing, it is just as important to follow a dose and frequency schedule correctly as with other types of drug administration.

TOLERANCE

Repeated administration of some drugs is associated with a progressively decreased response, often leading to the use of increasingly larger doses of the drug to obtain the same clinical effect. Although the mechanism is poorly understood in most cases, it may result from increased rates of drug metabolism or cellular adaptation to a drug's local action. Development of tolerance to drugs capable of causing dependence, such as narcotics or barbiturates, can result with the use of extremely large amounts of these drugs to obtain the desired pain relief or sedation, and may lead to habituation and ultimately physical dependence. Other drugs known to produce tolerance are ethyl alcohol, nitrites, antianxiety agents, and decongestants.

Tachyphylaxis refers to the *rapid* development of tolerance, such that the response to the initial drug administration is the greatest, and subsequent doses produce progressively less of a response. Again, the mechanisms responsible for tachyphylaxis are not well understood, but in some cases may involve a rapid depletion of available neurotransmitter at the nerve ending, as for example with amphetamine injection.

RESISTANCE

The term *resistance* is likewise used to describe a reduced response to a drug dosage that has previously been effective. However, resistance is usually ascribed to anti-infective drugs, where the microorganism becomes resistant to the effects of the drug. The mechanisms by which microorganisms can develop resistance to anti-infective agents are discussed in Chapter 59.

Combined Effects of Drugs

When two or more drugs are used together, they may exert their clinical effects largely independently of one another. For example, a diuretic can be given to a patient to control mild hypertension, while that same patient may also be receiving ampicillin for an infection. Frequently, however, the presence of a second drug alters the response to the first drug, either in a positive or a negative manner. Drug interactions are considered in general terms in Chapter 5 and only a brief review of synergism and antagonism is given here.

SYNERGISM

Two drugs are said to have a *synergistic* action when the therapeutic or toxic effects of the drug combination are considerably greater than those elicited by either drug alone. Two types of synergism are recognized.

Additive Effect

When the net effect of two drugs used together is equal to the *algebraic sum* of the individual drug actions, the drugs are said to have an *additive effect*. In other words, if the dose of each were reduced by one half, the resultant effect would be equal to the effect observed with either drug used at full dosage.

Potentiation

When the net effect of two drugs given together is *greater* than the algebraic sum of the individual drug effects, the term *potentiation* is frequently used to describe this phenomenon. Potentiation is usually seen where the two drugs elicit the same clinical effect by different mechanisms. For example, the combined antihypertensive effect of hydrochlorothiazide, a diuretic, and propranolol, a beta blocker, is significantly greater than the sum of their individual antihypertensive actions.

ANTAGONISM

The effects of one drug can be reduced or abolished by the presence of a second drug, and this effect is termed *antagonism*. Several kinds of drug antagonism have been demonstrated.

Pharmacologic (Competitive)

Two drugs may compete for the same receptor sites; if one drug has equal or greater affinity for the receptor than does the other drug, but lacks intrinsic activity at the receptor site, the effectiveness of the active drug is reduced or abolished. Most instances of pharmacologic antagonism are *competitive* in nature; that is, the antagonism, or receptor blockade, by one drug can be partially or wholly overcome by increasing the amount of active drug at the receptor site. Graphically, competitive antagonism is indicated by a parallel displacement of the dose–response curve to the right, as indicated in Figure 3-7, which illustrates the antagonism of the effects of histamine by an antihistamine.

Chemical

Certain drugs can actually combine chemically with other drugs in the body, thereby resulting in inactivation of the other drug. Several chemical chelating agents (dimercaprol, deferoxamine, edetate calcium disodium) can form stable complexes with certain metals, and are used in the treatment of intoxication or poisoning by substances such as arsenic, lead, mercury, and iron.

Physiologic

If one drug has a biologic effect (*e.g.*, stimulation) that is the opposite of a second drug's effect (*e.g.*, depression), these opposing physiologic actions may cancel one another, and the effects of both drugs are reduced. Examples of such antagonistic actions are the use of a vasoconstrictor (*e.g.*, mephentermine) and a vasodilator (*e.g.*, nitroglycerin) or the use of a mydriatic (*e.g.*, epinephrine) and a miotic (*e.g.*, pilocarpine).

Mechanisms of Drug Action

Although the *clinical* effects of a drug can be described in terms of alterations in physiologic function, the underlying biochemical and biophysical mechanisms of drug action in many instances are not as readily apparent. As discussed earlier in the chapter, the interaction of a drug molecule with a receptor site is the initial event by which the majority of drugs evoke a biologic response. This drug–receptor interaction subsequently initiates a chain of biochemical or physiologic events that determine the ultimate therapeutic response to the drug. Several theories have been advanced to help explain how the chemical complexation between a drug molecule and a reactive site in the body can lead to the enormous range of clinical manifestations that constitute the response to drug therapy.

Enzyme Interaction

Many drugs have been shown to interfere with enzymes necessary for the normal functioning of the organism, by combining with the enzyme molecules in much the same way as the normal enzyme substrates. Since practically all biologic reactions are catalyzed by cellular enzyme systems, alteration of normal enzymatic function can markedly accelerate or retard biologic functions.

Inhibition of tyrosine hydroxylase or aromatic l-amino acid decarboxylase can decrease catecholamine synthesis, and drugs having these actions have been used as antihypertensives and antiparkinsonian agents. Cholinesterase inhibitors increase functional levels of acetylcholine by slowing

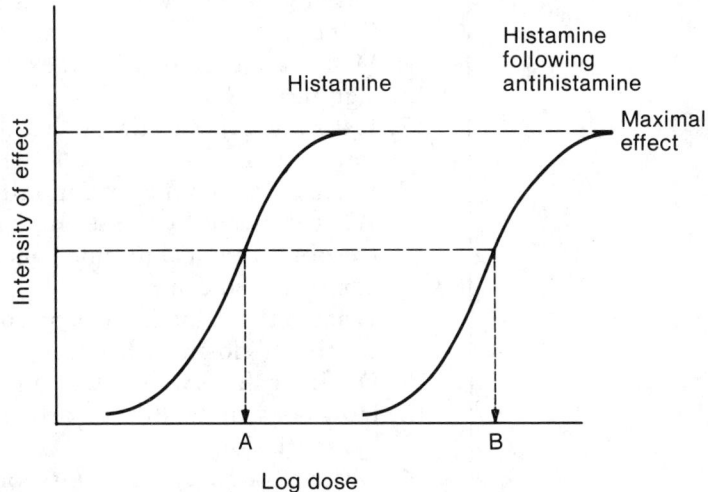

Figure 3-7. Competitive antagonism of histamine by an antihistamine. In the presence of a competitive antagonist (i.e., antihistamine), a much higher dose (Dose B) of histamine is needed to elicit the same intensity of effect as that produced by a small dose (Dose A) of histamine when given alone. The dose-response curve is shifted to the right, but no change is seen in the maximal effect.

its enzymatic inactivation and are effective in treating glaucoma and myasthenia gravis. Inhibitors of hepatic microsomal enzymes can increase the effects of those drugs that depend on microsomal enzymatic function for their metabolic inactivation.

On the other hand, drugs that stimulate the action of adenyl cyclase, the enzyme responsible for the formation of cyclic AMP, have a variety of actions in the body, including bronchodilation, lipolysis, and glycogenolysis. Many drugs can accelerate the activity of the liver microsomal enzymes, thus reducing the effectiveness of other drugs, which are then metabolized at a much faster rate by these catabolic enzymes.

Alterations in Membrane Function

Drugs such as local anesthetics, insulin, or antibiotics may either increase or decrease permeability of cellular membranes, alter active transport processes, or redistribute the concentration of ions on either side of the cellular membrane, thereby changing its resting potential. As discussed previously, passage of drugs across body membranes is essential for most of the interactions between a drug and body tissues. These physicochemical alterations in membrane function can therefore influence a number of biologic activities.

Neurohormonal Interaction

Most physiologic processes are regulated by the activity of neurohormones (e.g., acetylcholine, norepinephrine, serotonin) released from nerve endings. Drugs may modify the actions of these neurohormones in several ways:

1. Altering their rate of synthesis (e.g., carbidopa)
2. Interfering with their binding and storage (e.g., reserpine)
3. Varying their rates of release (e.g., guanethidine, amphetamine)
4. Interfering with their receptor interaction (e.g., propranolol, atropine)
5. Modifying their rate of inactivation (e.g., imipramine, physostigmine)

In addition to the general types of drug mechanisms discussed above, a variety of other mechanisms are responsible for the clinical effects of many drugs. Chemical neutralization of gastric acid, a detergent action on bronchiolar mucus, physical debridement of dead tissue, adsorption of toxins onto the surface of drug particles, and osmotic swelling of mucilloids to provide a laxative action are just a few examples of mechanisms of action for other drugs.

REVIEW QUESTIONS

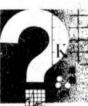

1. Distinguish between an "agonist" and an "antagonist" at a receptor site.
2. What is meant by (1) affinity and (2) intrinsic activity in relation to a drug–receptor interaction?
3. Explain the two theories that attempt to explain the intensity of a drug's effect.
4. What is the significance of a *steep* dose–response curve for a particular drug?
5. Differentiate between what is meant by "potency" and "efficacy."
6. Define the therapeutic index of a drug. What is its significance?
7. List some types of drugs that do *not* act by receptor site interaction.
8. List five factors that can modify drug effects.
9. What is meant by the term *pharmacogenetics*?
10. Describe a typical plasma concentration curve for an orally administered drug.
11. What is the principal reason for taking a drug on a rigidly controlled dosing schedule?
12. Distinguish between "tolerance" and "resistance."
13. How does an "additive" drug effect differ from "potentiation"?
14. Describe three types of antagonism.

BIBLIOGRAPHY

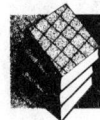

Baxter JD, Fonder JW: Hormone receptors. N Engl J Med 301:1149, 1979

Creese I, Sibley DR: Receptor adaptations to centrally acting drugs. Annu Rev Pharmacol Toxicol 21:357, 1981

Fuller RW: Pharmacology of brain epinephrine neurons. Annu Rev Pharmacol Toxicol 22:31, 1982

Kenakin TP: The classification of drugs and drug receptors in isolated tissues. Pharmacol Rev 36:165, 1984

Smythies JR, Bradley RJ (eds): Receptors in Pharmacology. New York, Marcel Dekker, 1978

Snyder SH: Receptors, neurotransmitters and drug responses. N Engl J Med 300:465, 1979

Starke K: Presynaptic receptors. Annu Rev Pharmacol Toxicol 21:7, 1981

Vessell ES: Why individuals vary in their response to drugs. Trends in Pharmacological Sciences, August:349, 1980

Adverse Drug Effects

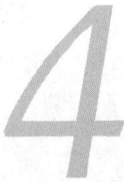

When a drug is administered to a patient, essentially two types of reactions can occur, *desired* drug effects and *undesired* drug effects. The desired drug effects are those clinically beneficial actions for which the drug has been prescribed. Undesired drug effects, on the other hand, represent the pharmacologic actions not sought when the drug is given, and may be further delineated into those that are innocuous and those that are potentially or actually harmful to the patient. The undesired drug effects in this latter group are commonly referred to as *adverse drug effects* or *untoward reactions.*

Much confusion exists regarding the precise terminology applied to undesirable drug reactions. One set of terms frequently but often erroneously interchanged are *side-effects* and *adverse reactions.* Generally, the term *side-effect* should be used to describe mild, often anticipated and usually unavoidable undesirable drug reactions, such as fatigue, drowsiness, nausea, dry mouth, and itching. Although annoying to many individuals, they rarely lead to more serious health problems, and in many instances disappear or ameliorate with continued use of the drug. The term *adverse reactions*, conversely, is used to refer to more serious and sometimes unexpected drug reactions, such as gastric ulceration, blood dyscrasias, respiratory depression, or ocular damage, that may pose a serious threat to the patient's well-being.

Examples of *minor* drug reactions, that is, reactions usually considered to be *side-effects*, include anorexia, cramps, mild diarrhea, dizziness, drowsiness, euphoria, fatigue, low-grade fever, glossitis, headache, hiccups, nausea, mild paresthesias, pruritus ani, mild skin rash, stomatitis, vaginitis, vertigo, weakness, and xerostomia. Some of these reactions can become serious adverse drug effects, however, if they are sufficiently intensified.

Major *adverse drug reactions* can involve many body organs and include addiction, allergic reactions, anaphylactic shock, blood dyscrasias (agranulocytosis, aplastic anemia, bone marrow depression, thrombocytopenia, and so on), cardiac arrhythmias, coma, congestive heart failure, convulsions, diabetes, encephalopathy, hearing impairment, hemorrhage, hypertension/hypotension, kidney or liver dysfunction, mental depression, neoplastic changes, ocular damage, pancreatitis, paralysis, photosensitivity, psychoses, respiratory depression, skin reactions, superinfections, and ulceration.

Throughout this book, the discussion of undesirable drug reactions will be structured in a similar manner; that is, untoward drug reactions will be divided (albeit arbitrarily in many cases) into common side-effects and significant adverse reactions, largely to reflect the more frequent occurrence of many of the common side-effects, as well as the potentially more serious consequences of the significant adverse reactions. It is imperative to recognize, however, that even a trivial side-effect can result in serious pathologic sequelae if it is sufficiently prolonged or intense. Hence, the compartmentalization of untoward drug reactions is tenuous at best.

Changing the dose, dosage form, route of administration, or diet can often reduce or abolish many minor side-effects. Major adverse reactions, however, are frequently dose- and dosage-form independent, and their occurrence is more difficult to control. The propensity for a particular drug to cause reactions, the type of reactions produced, and the frequency of occurrence will determine the utility of the drug for a particular disease state. That is, the possibility of serious toxicity resulting from drug usage is generally acceptable only if the condition being treated is serious enough to warrant the risk. Conversely, drugs causing a high degree of adverse effects should never be used to treat trivial or psychosomatic illnesses. For example, chloramphenicol, a highly toxic antibacterial agent, is acceptable in the treatment of certain salmonella or meningeal infections where other agents have failed or are inappropriate, but the drug should never be used to treat uncomplicated respiratory tract infections. Corticosteroids are invaluable in many types of inflammatory conditions but should not be routinely prescribed for such relatively minor ailments as poison ivy or urticaria.

The incidence of adverse drug reactions (ADRs) is difficult to predict, because it varies widely among different patient populations. It is safe to say, however, that as the drug-taking population increases in number, so does the incidence of untoward reactions. The ever-lengthening life span, the plethora of available drugs, and the increasing abuse of mind-altering drugs can only result in a greater percentage of drug-taking individuals who will experience untoward reactions. Complicating the assessment of ADRs is the fact that in many cases, symptoms of the disease process being treated by drugs closely mimic certain of the drug-induced adverse reactions. For example, nausea, vomiting, and arrhythmias are frequently associated with progressive congestive heart failure. Similarly, these reactions are often noted during therapy with the digitalis glycosides, drugs used in the treatment of congestive heart failure. Differentiation of disease-induced vs drug-induced adverse effects is an obvious necessity in such instances to ensure proper management of the patient. Therefore, knowledge of a drug's possible untoward reaction profile by health-care professionals is of vital importance to ensure the most efficacious, yet safest therapy possible. In addition, the financial consequences of malpractice lawsuits stemming from adverse drug reactions that may have been prevented by greater attention to the toxicologic potential of a prescribed drug can be ruinous. Recognition of the potential for any drug product to elicit equal degrees of good and harm cannot be overemphasized, and anyone prescribing or monitoring drugs has both a professional and a moral responsibility to know the potential consequences of using a particular drug in a patient.

Classification of Adverse Drug Reactions

The multitude of different types of untoward reactions resulting from drug use makes accurate classification of these reactions difficult. While no single means of classification is adequate to categorize the diversity of adverse effects that can occur as a consequence of drug treatment, several general *classes* of adverse drug effects can be delineated. The grouping of the different adverse effects to be followed in this discussion is as follows:
1. Pharmacologic
   a. Extension of therapeutic effect
   b. Nontherapeutic effects
2. Nonpharmacologic
   a. Hypersensitivity
   b. Idiosyncrasy
   c. Photosensitivity
3. Disease-related
4. Multiple-drug reactions
5. Miscellaneous
   a. Carcinogenicity
   b. Teratogenicity
   c. Drug dependence

Pharmacologic Adverse Effects

Many adverse drug effects are the result of a greater than desired intensity of action or elicitation of one or more "secondary" drug effects in addition to the "primary," or intended, drug effect.

EXTENSION OF THERAPEUTIC EFFECT
Overdosage with a therapeutic agent will usually elicit, among other effects, an excessive reaction to the *primary* effect of the drug. For example, tranquilizers used as daytime sedatives in excessive amounts will generally produce drowsiness and possibly hypnosis. In this case, the adverse reaction usually can be overcome by either reducing the dosage or decreasing the frequency of administration. Other common examples of untoward reactions induced by drug overdosage are superficial hemorrhaging with anticoagulants or excessive electrolyte and water depletion secondary to diuretic therapy.

NONTHERAPEUTIC ADVERSE EFFECTS
Since drugs seldom exhibit a single pharmacologic effect, the adverse effects caused by drug administration are frequently the result of manifestation of one or more *secondary* actions produced by a drug molecule. In some cases, these secondary drug effects can be largely eliminated by adjusting the dose carefully in each individual. Many times, however, these adverse reactions are an inescapable consequence of normal therapeutic doses of a drug. For example, using normal doses of many antihistamines is associated with a certain degree of drowsiness, a potentially dangerous occurrence. Even in small, therapeutic doses, anticholinergics used for relief of gastrointestinal (GI) spasm and hypermotility usually produce xerostomia (dry mouth), blurring of vision, and some degree of urinary retention and constipation. Other common examples of drug-induced secondary adverse reactions are constipation with narcotic analgesics, hypokalemia (potassium loss) and hyperuricemia with thiazide diuretics, and orthostatic hypotension with antipsychotic drugs.

Although these secondary effects of a drug usually cannot be controlled by dosage adjustment, since minimal therapeutic doses are already being used, the effects often can be reduced by substituting or adding other drugs to the regimen. For example, the drowsiness seen with many antihistamines can be minimized by using a mild central stimulant such as caffeine, or by switching to an antihistamine possessing minimal central nervous system (CNS) depressant actions, such as terfenadine. Similarly, the hypokalemia associated with thiazide diuretics can be minimized by potassium supplementation.

Secondary adverse reactions may be quite serious, requiring careful patient monitoring and perhaps changes in the drug regimen. Potentially dangerous secondary effects of drugs include the possibility of thrombotic complications with oral contraceptives, arrhythmias with improper digitalis usage, and GI bleeding and ulceration with aspirin and related drugs.

Most pharmacologic adverse reactions have been extensively documented. Thus, in assessing the suitability of a particular therapeutic regimen, the disadvantages of a drug's known predictable toxicity should be weighed against its potential beneficial effects.

Nonpharmacologic Adverse Effects

Another group of adverse drug effects have little relationship to the pharmacologic effects of a drug. Rather, they occur as a result of an abnormal sensitivity or reactivity on the part of the drug recipient to a chemical substance. This aberrant reaction may be termed a *hypersensitivity* (or *allergic*) *reaction* or an *idiosyncratic reaction*. A principal hazard of this type of nonpharmacologic adverse reaction is that it is *not* predictable based on the profile of drug action but occurs only in a fraction of patients receiving the drug. Thus, the onset of an allergic or idiosyncratic drug reaction is often abrupt and unexpected, and can have a serious, and occasionally a fatal, outcome.

HYPERSENSITIVITY

Hypersensitivity or allergic reactions are perhaps the largest single group of untoward drug effects. Allergic reactions are usually *not* dose related and are largely independent of the pharmacologic properties of the drug molecule. These hypersensitivity reactions are associated with an altered reactivity or sensitization of the patient resulting from prior exposure to a drug or chemical that behaves like an allergen. The drug (or metabolite) interacts with a tissue or plasma protein, activating the reticuloendothelial system, resulting in production of antibodies to the drug molecule. A subsequent exposure to the same drug (or in some cases a similar one) elicits an antigen–antibody reaction that produces the symptoms of the allergic response (*e.g.*, itching, edema, congestion, wheezing).

Allergic drug reactions may be classified as either immediate (*e.g.*, anaphylaxis, urticaria) or delayed (*e.g.*, serum sickness).

Immediate

Immediate hypersensitivity or allergic reactions develop within minutes of drug exposure. The drug–antibody reaction probably releases several vasoactive substances, such as histamine and bradykinin, from their tissue stores. These substances can react with the smooth muscle of many body tissues (blood vessels, bronchioles, GI tract) to produce characteristic signs of the allergic reaction, such as bronchoconstriction or vasodilation. The symptoms may be very mild (rash, itching, urticaria) or serious enough (respiratory distress, severe hypotension—frequently termed *anaphylactic shock*) to require immediate attention and swift medical treatment to prevent death. In general, the severity of the reaction is independent of the drug itself but probably depends to a large extent on a patient's sensitivity. It has been documented that even very small doses of common drugs, such as aspirin and penicillin, can produce violent hypersensitivity reactions in susceptible patients. The grave concern about these kinds of reactions is that often they are totally unpredictable, and quick recognition and proper treatment are essential to minimize serious consequences.

Delayed

The delayed type of allergic reaction develops slowly following drug challenge. The clinical picture of delayed hypersensitivity usually includes a diffuse rash, fever, angioedema, swollen lymph nodes, and stiff joints. This syndrome is frequently referred to as *serum sickness*. This name derives from the fact that the allergic response results from damage produced by *circulating* immune complexes that may lodge in small vessels and cause the characteristic symptoms. Sometimes the liver, kidney, and bone marrow may become damaged, although the factors that determine specific organ involvement are largely unknown.

IDIOSYNCRASY

By strict definition, *idiosyncrasy* refers to a peculiarity of bodily function that causes an individual to react in an abnormal manner to a drug. Therefore, idiosyncratic reactions may manifest themselves as either a quantitative (*i.e.*, over- or under-responsiveness) or a qualitative (*e.g.*, paradoxical excitation) change from the norm. These reactions are probably not caused by formation of an antigen–antibody complex but most often result from a genetically determined defect in the patient's ability to handle a particular drug. Idiosyncratic reactions can assume various forms; they may range from the rather mild (erythema, rash, photosensitivity) to the very serious (blood dyscrasias, exfoliative dermatitis, systemic lupus-like reaction, hemolytic anemia, malignant hyperpyrexia). A general description of some of the more important idiosyncratic drug reactions, along with other kinds of adverse drug effects, appears at the end of this chapter.

A specialized field of study termed *pharmacogenetics* deals with those altered drug responses that are under hereditary control; great strides have been made in determining some of the genetic flaws that predispose certain individuals to toxic drug effects. For example, the development of hemolytic anemia on exposure to certain drugs has been linked to a genetic deficiency of the enzyme glucose-6-phosphate dehydrogenase (G-6-PD) in red blood cells. In many other cases, however, the etiology of idiosyncratic drug reactions is less well understood, although a deficiency or excess of drug-metabolizing enzymes is often responsible for the abnormal drug responses seen in certain patients.

PHOTOSENSITIVITY

A unique type of dermatologic hypersensitivity reaction following use of many drugs is observed on exposure to sunlight, and is termed *photosensitization*. Two principal types of reactions can occur in people whose skin has been sensitized by either topical or internal use of photosensitizing drugs. A *photoallergic* reaction presents itself as a papular eruption on sun-exposed areas similar to that resulting from contact dermatitis. It is probably due to the photosensitizing drug forming an antigen by absorption of sunlight and subsequent combination with a skin protein. The resultant antibody formation sensitizes the patient to further synthesis of antigen by continued sun exposure.

A *phototoxic* reaction, on the other hand, is characterized by a severe sunburn, and as such is not always viewed as a hypersensitivity reaction. Nevertheless, it is probably the result of a photosensitizing chemical absorbing ultraviolet radiation energy to such an extent that it becomes toxic to epidermal cells. A representative sampling of drugs and chemicals that are photosensitizing agents is given below:

- aminobenzoic acid
- amitriptyline
- anesthetics (procaine group)
- antimalarials
- barbiturates
- bithionol
- carbamazepine
- chlordiazepoxide
- chlorthalidone
- clindamycin
- coal tar
- contraceptives, oral
- cyproheptadine
- desipramine
- diethylstilbestrol
- digalloyl trioleate (sunscreen)
- diphenhydramine
- doxepin
- estrone
- fluorescein dyes
- 5-fluorouracil
- furosemide
- glyceryl p-aminobenzoate (sunscreen)
- gold salts
- griseofulvin
- haloperidol
- imipramine HCl
- isotretinoin
- lincomycin
- loxapine
- mesoridazine
- mestranol
- methotrimeprazine
- methoxsalen
- 5-methoxypsoralen
- 8-methoxypsoralen
- nalidixic acid
- nortriptyline
- phenolic compounds
- phenothiazines
- phenylbutazone
- phenytoin
- protriptyline
- psoralens
- quinethazone
- quinine
- retinoic acid
- salicylates
- silver salts
- stilbamidine
- sulfonamides
- sulfonylureas
- tetracyclines
- thiazide diuretics
- thiopropazate
- tranylcypromine
- triamterene
- triethylenemelamine
- trimeprazine
- trimethadione
- trimipramine
- triprolidine

Disease-Related Adverse Effects

The pathophysiologic state of a patient is a major determinant of the potential for a drug to cause adverse effects. Underlying disease states, often unrecognized, can greatly increase the possibility of drug toxicity. The more common abnormalities are outlined below.

HEPATIC DISEASE

Since the liver plays a major role in the metabolism and inactivation of many drug molecules, impaired liver function can result in abnormally high plasma levels of a drug for extended periods of time. If normal dosing schedules are followed, accumulation of drug in the body can occur, resulting in symptoms of drug overdosage. Because of the tremendous reserve capacity of the liver, however, near-normal metabolic function usually is present except in the most severe forms of hepatic disease.

RENAL DISEASE

The presence of kidney disease can lead to many adverse reactions with those drugs that are eliminated largely through renal excretory processes. In the presence of renal disease, doses of drugs excreted by the kidney need to be reduced, to avoid accumulation and subsequent toxicity. For example, most aminoglycoside antibiotics are excreted by glomerular filtration as the unchanged drug. Therefore, these drugs are potentially quite toxic even in normal doses in patients with impaired renal function, because their excretion is slowed and their serum half-life is prolonged.

In progressive renal failure, plasma albumin stores may also be decreased, which can reduce the serum protein binding of many drugs, resulting in potentiation of their effects.

EMOTIONAL DISORDERS

Mentally unstable individuals such as those suffering from psychotic disorders should not be allowed to monitor their own drug therapy. Too often, emotionally unsound patients do not comply with proper dosing requirements unless closely monitored, and this can lead to overdosage with many dangerous drugs (e.g., hypnotics, antipsychotics) or use of improper drugs. A major problem exists with misuse of, or overmedication with, the psychotherapeutic group of drugs. Since many individuals taking these drugs exhibit a degree of emotional instability, these drug users represent an extremely high-risk group for potential adverse reactions.

OTHER DISEASE STATES

The existence of many other types of diseases can increase the likelihood for a particular drug to elicit an adverse drug reaction. Patients with bronchial asthma must use nonselective beta-adrenergic blockers (e.g., nadolol, propranolol) with extreme caution, since their bronchospastic action can worsen the already impaired ventilatory flow. Similarly, the beta-adrenergic blockers as well as the calcium channel blocker verapamil should not be given to patients with advanced heart block, because these drugs can reduce myocardial contractility and further slow atrioventricular (AV) conduction. Patients with a healing duodenal ulcer have a high likelihood of experiencing increased gastric bleeding if given one of the nonsteroidal anti-inflammatory drugs, such as indomethacin, naproxen, sulindac, or meclofenamate. Accurate assessment of a patient's overall health status before administration of any medication is perhaps the most important way to ensure the safest and most effective use of a drug.

Multiple-Drug Reactions

The presence of a second drug may greatly modify the actions of a concurrently administered drug. In many instances, drugs are used together to achieve a better clinical response than either drug could achieve alone. This is an example of a positive clinical interaction. On the other hand, indiscriminate multiple drug therapy can be quite hazardous; the chance of untoward reactions increases dramatically as additional drugs are added to a therapeutic regimen. This problem becomes especially acute in the elderly or seriously ill population, where a number of different drugs are frequently being taken simultaneously. Multiple drug regimens should be undertaken cautiously and reevaluated frequently, and the necessity for continuing each drug must be critically weighed against the potential for that drug, not only to elicit untoward reactions itself but also to increase the incidence and severity of adverse reactions to the other drugs comprising the patient's therapeutic regimen.

The mechanisms responsible for multiple drug interactions, both beneficial as well as harmful, will be considered in Chapter 5.

Miscellaneous Adverse Effects

Various other adverse drug effects that do not fall within one of the above groupings have been reported with use of certain drugs and chemicals. Some of the more important of these undesirable effects of drugs and other chemical substances are discussed below.

CARCINOGENICITY

The number of chemical substances, not to mention other factors such as nutritional deficiencies, industrial wastes, microbes, physical trauma, and radiation, that have been classified as potentially carcinogenic is staggering. Many drugs have also been implicated as potential cancer-inducing agents, but the carcinogenic risk ratio for most drug substances is less well established in most instances than, for example, the risk associated with radiation exposure or cigarette smoking. Determination of a drug's cancer-inducing potential is an essential part of preclinical testing, and most drugs have been found to be quite safe in this regard when used in recommended doses. Of course, the long-term risk is impossible to evaluate under acute laboratory conditions, and in some cases the carcinogenic effects of a drug are only realized after years of clinical use. For example, the indications for clofibrate, an antihyperlipidemic drug that has been available for many years, are now greatly restricted, in part due to the findings that on long-term administration of the drug to rodents in doses only five to eight times higher than the human dose, a higher incidence of malignant liver tumors compared to a control population was discovered. It should be realized here that these findings do *not* classify clofibrate as an agent with a high carcinogenic risk in humans; however, they greatly alter the drug's benefit-to-risk ratio, and the drug is now only indicated in treating very selective types of elevated plasma lipids.

On the other hand, several of the currently available antineoplastic drugs used to treat certain carcinomas have been shown to produce other types of cancers. Melphalan has been used successfully in treating multiple myelomas, but acute, nonlymphatic leukemia has developed in some patients during treatment. Thus, the potential benefit to be derived from use of melphalan must be weighed against the possible development of another type of cancer.

Some substances generally recognized as being potentially carcinogenic are
  · androgens
  · antineoplastics
  · asbestos
  · benzene
  · 3.4-benzopyrene

  · busulphan
  · carbon tetrachloride
  · chloroform
  · clofibrate
  · corticosteroids
  · cyclamates
  · dioxane
  · estrogens
  · griseofulvin
  · herbicides
  · metronidazole
  · nitrites
  · nitrofurans
  · nitrosamines
  · oral contraceptives
  · pesticides
  · progestins
  · tobacco smoke
  · TRIS (flame retardant)
  · trypan blue

TERATOGENICITY

Administration of certain drugs to pregnant women, especially during the first trimester of pregnancy, has resulted in fetal deformities. Such drugs are said to be *teratogenic.* In the early 1960s, much publicity was given to the teratogenic effects of thalidomide, a sedative–hypnotic used primarily in Germany. Interestingly, this drug proved extremely safe in adults, with a very low incidence of side-effects. It is obvious, therefore, that a lack of clinically significant adverse drug effects is no assurance that a drug is safe to a developing fetus. Furthermore, animal experimentation is not always able to predict the teratogenic potential of a drug. Since fetal organ development begins quite early in the gestational period, even before many women realize they are pregnant, the use of drugs, especially those known to have a teratogenic potential, should be discouraged in all women attempting to conceive. The Food and Drug Administration (FDA) has established five categories indicating the potential for a drug to cause birth defects. These categories are described in Table 4-1. It should be recognized, however, that regardless of a particular drug's pregnancy category, the benefit-to-risk ratio must be assessed in *each* particular case. However, the potential harm to a developing fetus of not treating a pregnant woman for a serious disease may eclipse the risk of inducing fetal damage. For example, phenytoin is an antiepileptic drug used in the management of grand mal epilepsy, and its use has been associated with fetal abnormalities, especially cleft palate. How-

Table 4-1
FDA Pregnancy Categories

Category	Description
A	No demonstrated fetal risk in humans during any stage of pregnancy
B	No demonstrated fetal risk in animal studies but no adequate studies in pregnant women *or* Animal studies have shown an adverse effect but studies in pregnant women have not demonstrated a risk during any stage of pregnancy.
C	Animal studies have shown an adverse effect on the fetus but there are no adequate studies in humans *or* No animal or human studies are available (use of the drug *may be acceptable* despite the risks).
D	Evidence of human fetal risk *but the* benefits from use of the drug *may be acceptable* despite the risks.
X	Animal or human studies have demonstrated fetal abnormalities or adverse reaction reports give evidence of fetal risk (risk to a pregnant woman clearly outweighs the possible benefit).

ever, the risk to the fetus of a generalized maternal seizure following withdrawal of the medication may be far greater than the risk of developing a congenital abnormality. Similarly, discontinuation of the antineoplastic drug methotrexate may have more serious consequences for the mother in relation to the risk of fetal damage associated with its continued use.

In general, however, no drug (including alcohol and nicotine) should be used during the first trimester of pregnancy unless necessary and only then after a careful assessment of the benefit-to-risk ratio. Thus, there is no justification for using antihistamines to control occasional nausea and vomiting of early pregnancy, in view of the reported cases of fetal damage associated (although *not* definitively linked) with their use. Although fetal damage usually does not occur when drugs are administered late in pregnancy, other complications can occur at this time, such as neonatal bleeding, respiratory depression, and drug addiction. Drugs known to affect the fetus adversely are listed in Table 9-1.

DRUG DEPENDENCE

The ability of many drugs to induce a state of dependence in the patient is well established. Although we generally think of dependence being associated with prolonged abuse of those drugs that have an effect on mood or behavior (*e.g.*, barbiturates, narcotics, amphetamines), dependence can and does result from chronic use of a wide variety of other drugs, including decongestants, antihistamines, and laxatives. Drug dependence varies in intensity and can range from simple habituation (*i.e.*, a pattern of repeated drug use without a physical need for the drug or a strong compulsion to obtain the drug) to psychologic dependence (*i.e.*, *belief* that the drug must be used to function in society) to true physical dependence (*i.e.*, an altered physiologic state that *requires* the presence of the drug to prevent withdrawal symptoms).

The propensity of a drug to elicit dependence is determined not only by the chemical and pharmacologic properties of the drug, but possibly more importantly by the emotional stability of the drug-taking person. The cost to society of drug abuse in terms of reduced productivity, family strife, damaged health, and increased crime is incalculable, and health-care practitioners have a tremendous responsibility not only to educate people to the dangers of improper drug use but also to monitor drug-taking habits carefully whenever possible. An in-depth review of drug abuse, its recognition, and the means for treating drug-dependent individuals is found in Chapter 85.

The "ideal" drug would be one that has a single pharmacologic action, exhibits no adverse drug effects, does not interact with any other drugs, and is inexpensive. It is quite obvious, however, that this type of drug does not exist and probably never will. Therefore, recognition that a drug molecule has deleterious as well as beneficial effects is a perspective that cannot be ignored in the treatment of disease. The task of the clinician, therefore, is an arduous, yet critical one; that is, to design and structure a therapeutic regimen that optimizes the beneficial effects of a drug while minimizing the undesirable actions. This "fine-tuning" of a patient's drug therapy is possible only when a clear understanding exists of both the pharmacologic as well as the toxicologic effects of a drug. The vigilance should not cease, however, once patients have been sent on their way with their medications. Patients are usually the first to notice when something goes wrong while taking a drug, and their attention to detail can often mean the difference between completely avoiding untoward effects or having to treat a serious adverse reaction. Thus, educating patients as to the type and incidence of side-effects that may be expected with the various drugs they are using and informing them of the early signs and symptoms of a more serious developing toxicity are essential to ensure patient compliance and minimize untoward reactions. A thorough knowledge of the types of adverse reactions associated with a particular drug, therefore, is vital to provide both safe and effective drug therapy.

Glossary of Adverse Drug Reactions

Alopecia—A loss of hair, sometimes accompanied by extreme drying of the scalp. A frequent occurrence with many antineoplastic agents, alopecia has also been observed with use of anticoagulants, mephenytoin, methimazole, norethindrone acetate, quinacrine, and trimethadione.

Anaphylactic reaction—A severe systemic allergic reaction that develops suddenly, progresses rapidly, and is frequently fatal if not treated. Symptoms range from itching, hives, nasal congestion, abdominal cramping, and diarrhea to dyspnea, hypotension, fainting, choking sensation, cardiovascular collapse, and possibly death. An anaphylactic reaction can theoretically occur with any drug, but is most commonly observed with those drugs frequently associated with drug allergies, such as penicillins, sulfonamides, and salicylates.

Blood dyscrasias—An abnormal condition of the formed elements or other clotting constituents of the blood. Several types are commonly observed:

1. *Agranulocytosis*—An acute febrile disease, sometimes referred to as *leukopenia*, characterized by an absence of granulocytes (or granular leukocytes) and often a corresponding reduction in monocytes and lymphocytes. Clinical symptoms include chills, fever, and extreme weakness. Because of the lack of white blood cells, the body's defense mechanism is impaired, and severe infection can result. Early warning signs are mucous membrane ulceration, sore throat, skin rash, and fever. Recovery normally occurs within 1 week to 2 weeks after drug is removed. Any existing infection should be vigorously treated. This is the most common drug-induced blood dyscrasia.
2. *Anemia*—A reduction in the number of red blood cells, hemoglobin concentration, and volume of packed red cells. The result is a sharp curtailment in the oxygen-carrying capacity of the blood.

   (a) *Aplastic*—Results from drug-induced damage to the bone marrow and is marked by a deficiency of red cells, hemoglobin, and granular cells, and a predominance of lymphocytes. Clinical signs include fatigue, tachycardia, bleeding, fever, and increased susceptibility to infection. Often fatal due to hemorrhage and overwhelming infection.

   (b) *Hemolytic*—Characterized by a short life span of the red cell. Circulating erythrocytes are destroyed due to increased hemolytic activity induced by certain drugs or poisons. Especially common in individuals with a glucose-6-phosphate dehydrogenase deficiency. Withdrawal of offending agent usually corrects the condition.

3. *Thrombocytopenia*—A decreased blood platelet count, resulting from either platelet destruction or depression of the platelet-forming mechanism in the bone marrow. Onset may be sudden, and symptoms include purpura (petechiae; epistaxis; oral, vaginal, or GI bleeding) and easy bruising. The platelet count returns to normal within a few weeks after cessation of drug therapy, but the count may again rise briefly immediately following stoppage of the drug. Most severe complications can result from excessive cerebral hemorrhage.

Although many currently available drugs can cause one or more of the above blood dyscrasias, it should be recognized that certain drugs are much more likely to elicit a blood dyscrasia than others. Throughout the text, drugs associated with a higher than normal incidence of blood dyscrasias are prominently mentioned.

Erythema multiforme—An acute inflammatory skin disease characterized by lesions consisting of concentric circles of erythema, usually appearing on the neck, face, and legs. Occasionally blisters are observed. It is often accompanied by fever, malaise, arthralgia, and gastric distress. Symptoms may persist for 2 weeks to 6 weeks. The most severe variant, *Stevens-Johnson syndrome*, is characterized by high fever, headache, and inflammatory lesions of the mouth, eyes, and genitalia. Frequently, the bronchial and visceral mucosa are involved. Death can occur because of renal impairment. Drugs that may cause erythema multiforme and the Stevens-Johnson syndrome include

- barbiturates
- carbamazepine
- chloramphenicol
- chlorpropamide
- clindamycin
- ethosuximide
- hydroxyzine
- mephenytoin
- paramethadione
- penicillins
- phensuximide

- phenylbutazone
- phenytoin
- propylthiouracil
- rifampin
- salicylates
- sulfonamides
- tetracycline
- thiazide diuretics
- trimeprazine
- trimethadione

Exfoliative dermatitis—Erythema and scaling of the skin over large parts of the body. Symptoms include itching, weakness, malaise, fever, and weight loss. Exfoliation may include loss of hair and nails as well as skin, and mucosal sloughing can occur. The reaction is generally unpredictable in its duration and recurrence. Relapses are frequent, and secondary infections can be serious. It may occur as a sequela to preexisting dermatoses or contact dermatitis, result from an underlying carcinoma (*e.g.*, leukemia, lymphoma), or be caused by drug use. A listing of some of the drugs that have been linked to development of exfoliative dermatitis is given below:

- aminosalicylic acid (PAS)
- antidiabetics, oral
- barbiturates
- carbamazepine
- chloroquine
- furosemide
- gold salts
- griseofulvin
- hydroflumethiazide
- methotrimeprazine

- methylphenidate
- nitroglycerin
- penicillins
- phenindione
- phenothiazines
- phenylbutazone
- phenytoin
- streptomycin
- sulfonamides
- tetracyclines

Hepatotoxicity—Liver damage frequently resulting from either infections or drug hypersensitivity. The most frequently observed drug-induced manifestation is *jaundice*, characterized by hyperbilirubinemia and deposition of bile pigments in the mucous membranes and skin, which impart the typical yellow appearance. At least three main types of jaundice are recognized.

1. *Cholestatic*—Due to interference with the normal secretion of bile by an obstruction of the biliary passages. It may result from gallstones, tumors, or drug-induced inflammation of the bile channels.
2. *Hepatocellular*—Due to impairment of the function of liver cells. It is also termed *necrotic jaundice,* and it closely resembles severe viral hepatitis.
3. *Hemolytic*—Due to a drug hypersensitivity or a direct toxic effect of the drug on erythrocytes. There may be interference with normal glucose metabolism in the red cells.

In addition to jaundice, a hepatitis-like reaction may be elicited by several kinds of drugs. This effect may either result from a hypersensitivity to the drug or from a direct toxic effect of the drug on liver cells. Since the clinical picture of drug-induced hepatitis closely resembles that of infectious viral hepatitis, a patient history and careful laboratory diagnosis are essential to proper management.

Many drugs have the capacity to alter liver function, thus interfering with a myriad of bodily functions, including drug metabolism, digestion, blood coagulation, gluconeogenesis, glycogenolysis, and cholesterol synthesis. A lengthy but by no means complete listing of potentially hepatotoxic drugs is presented below:

- acetaminophen
- acetanilid
- acetazolamide
- actinomycin
- alcohol
- allopurinol
- amphetamine
- antineoplastics
- capreomycin
- carbamazepine
- carbarsone
- chenodiol
- chloramphenicol
- chlordiazepoxide
- colchicine
- dantrolene
- diazepam
- diethylstilbestrol
- erythromycin estolate
- ethacrynic acid
- ethanol
- ethchlorvynol
- ethionamide
- flurazepam
- fluroxene
- furosemide
- gold salts
- griseofulvin
- haloperidol
- halothane
- indomethacin
- isoniazid
- MAO inhibitors
- mephenytoin

- meprobamate
- methandrostenolone
- methimazole
- methoxyflurane
- methyldopa
- methyltestosterone
- nalidixic acid
- nitrofurantoin
- norethindrone
- novobiocin
- oral contraceptives
- papaverine
- para-aminosalicylic acid (PAS)
- penicillins
- phenacemide
- phenacetin
- phenindione
- phenobarbital
- phenothiazines
- phenylbutazone
- phenytoin
- primaquine
- probenecid
- procainamide
- propoxyphene
- propylthiouracil
- pyrazinamide
- quinacrine
- quinethazone
- quinidine
- quinine
- rifampin
- streptomycin
- sulfonamides

- sulfones
- sulfonylurea anti-diabetics
- tetracyclines
- thiazide diuretics
- thiouracil
- triacetyloleando-mycin

- trichloroethylene
- tricyclic antide-pressants
- trimethadione
- valproic acid

Lupus erythematosus (LE)—An autoimmune inflammatory disorder that can occur in two forms, one affecting only the skin (discoid LE) and the other, more serious, affecting multiple body organs (systemic LE). The etiology of the naturally occurring form is unknown, but both forms occur predominantly in young women. Several drugs, especially hydralazine and procainamide, can also cause a lupus-like reaction. Among the many symptoms are diffuse rash; fever; malaise; alopecia; joint symptoms including stiffness, swelling, and synovitis; conjunctivitis; photophobia; pneumonitis; pleurisy; myocarditis; arrhythmias; lymphadenopathy; splenomegaly; and hemolytic anemia. Renal and neurologic features are absent in drug-induced lupus but are seen in the spontaneously occurring form of the disease. Clinical features generally revert slowly toward normal when the offending drug is withdrawn, but altered laboratory values (*e.g.,* elevated antinuclear antibody titer, leukopenia, thrombocytopenia) indicative of the disease may persist for many months.

Nephrotoxicity—Damage to the functional units of the kidney, such as the glomerular filtration apparatus, blood vessels, or renal tubular cells, or a dysfunction of the components (*e.g.,* enzymes, transport carriers) involved in the tubular secretory and reabsorptive processes. Kidney damage is a serious consequence of therapy with many drugs, as it can result in abnormally high blood levels of drugs and other body constituents normally excreted by the kidney. Drugs that may result in impairment of renal function or worsen existing renal impairment are listed below:

- acetazolamide
- allopurinol
- aminoglycosides
- amitriptyline
- amphotericin B
- bacitracin
- bismuth compounds
- bleomycin
- bumetanide
- carbon tetrachloride
- cephalothin

- chlorinated hydro-carbons (insecticides)
- colchicine
- colistimethate
- colistin
- copper compounds
- corticosteroids
- ethacrynic acid
- ether
- ethylene glycol

- furosemide
- gentamicin
- gold compounds
- griseofulvin
- hydralazine
- isoniazid
- iron salts
- kanamycin
- lithium carbonate
- mannitol
- mefenamic acid
- mercury
- methicillin
- methotrexate
- methoxyflurane
- neomycin
- nitrofurantoin
- para-aminosalicylic acid (PAS)
- paramethadione
- paromomycin
- penicillamine

- phenacetin
- phenazopyridine
- phenindione
- phenylbutazone
- polymyxin B
- probenecid
- propylene glycol
- rifampin
- salicylates
- silver compounds
- spironolactone
- streptomycin
- sulfamethoxazole-trimethoprim
- sulfonamides
- tetracyclines
- thiabendazole
- thiazide diuretics
- thyroid preparations
- triamterene
- trimethadione
- vancomycin

Neurotoxicity—Damage to various nervous system structures, manifested as a wide range of central and peripheral disturbances. Some of the more important neurotoxic effects of drugs are the following:

1. *Extrapyramidal reactions*—Disturbances of the extrapyramidal motor-regulating system in the CNS, resulting in abnormal motor function. Common manifestations include immobility (akinesia), fixed positioning of the limbs (rigidity), sudden violent movement of the arms and head (dystonias), restlessness (akathisia), and rhythmic, clonic muscular activity (tremor). Extrapyramidal reactions are frequently associated with use of antipsychotic drugs.

2. *Myasthenia-like reaction*—Extreme muscle weakness due to an impairment in the transmission of impulses at the neuromuscular junction. This type of a reaction has been seen with use of aminoglycoside antibiotics, colistimethate, and trimethadione.

3. *Ocular toxicity*—Disturbances in the functioning of the eye. Most common manifestation is *blurred vision*, which can occur following use of many drugs, especially those with an anticholinergic action. Drugs possessing an anticholinergic action can also exacerbate *glaucoma*, a condition characterized by increased intraocular pressure secondary to impaired fluid drainage (see Chap. 13). Other drug-in-

duced ocular disorders, along with some representative drugs, causing the particular disorder, are listed below:

Myopia (nearsightedness)—acetazolamide, hydralazine, hydrochlorothiazide, sulfonamides, tetracyclines

Optic neuritis (inflammation of the optic disk)—chloramphenicol, isoniazid, sulfonamides

Pigmentary retinopathy (pigmentation of the retina)—chloroquine, phenothiazines

Toxic amblyopia (chronic optic neuritis)—alcohol, chlorpropamide, nicotinic acid

Cataracts (opacity of the lens)—corticosteroids

Scotomata (an area of impaired vision surrounded by an area of normal or near-normal vision)—hydroxychloroquine, trimethadione

Corneal deposits (deposits of material in the transparent portion of the eyeball)—indomethacin, isotretinoin

4. *Ototoxicity*—Progressive hearing loss and tinnitus caused by damage to the eighth cranial nerve. Often accompanied by vertigo and nystagmus if the vestibular branch of the nerve is affected. Potentially ototoxic drugs that can cause both hearing loss as well as vestibular damage include:

- amikacin
- bumetanide
- chloroquine
- ethacrynic acid
- fenoprofen
- furosemide
- gentamicin
- hydroxychloroquine
- kanamycin
- naproxen
- neomycin
- netilmicin
- phenylbutazone
- quinine
- salicylates
- streptomycin
- tobramycin
- vancomycin

Photosensitivity—An altered responsiveness to light, usually eczematous in nature. Common manifestations are itching, scaling, urticaria, and multiform lesions in severe cases. Drugs that have been associated with photosensitivity reactions are listed earlier in this chapter.

Purpura—Localized hemorrhaging, occurring in the skin, mucous membranes, or serous membranes. The lesions may be petechiae (small blood spots) or ecchymoses (larger areas of bleeding). Commonly seen in patients with thrombocytopenia due to increased platelet destruction. Many drugs can cause purpura, and they are listed below:

- acetazolamide
- ACTH
- allopurinol
- amitriptyline
- anticoagulants
- barbiturates
- chloral hydrate
- chlorpromazine
- chlorpropamide
- corticosteroids
- digitalis glycosides
- fluoxymesterone
- gold salts
- griseofulvin
- iodides
- meprobamate
- para-aminosalicylic acid (PAS)
- penicillins
- phenylbutazone
- quinidine
- rifampin
- sulfonamides
- thiazide diuretics
- trifluoperazine

REVIEW QUESTIONS

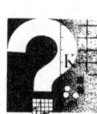

1. How do "side-effects" differ from "adverse reactions"?
2. How can adverse reactions that are an extension of a drug's therapeutic effect be minimized?
3. Distinguish between "immediate" and "delayed" hypersensitivity.
4. What is an idiosyncratic reaction?
5. Give an example of a photoallergic reaction and a phototoxic reaction.
6. Describe what is meant by "teratogenicity."
7. Define the following terms:
   a. Alopecia
   b. Agranulocytosis
   c. Thrombocytopenia
   d. Erythema multiforme
   e. Hepatocellular jaundice
   f. Lupus erythematosus
   g. Extrapyramidal reactions
   h. Purpura

BIBLIOGRAPHY

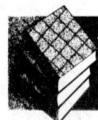

Curtis JR: Drug-induced renal disease. Drugs 18:377, 1979

Jick H, Walker AM, Porter J: Drug-induced liver disease. J Clin Pharmacol 21:359, 1981

Karch FE, Lasagna L: Adverse drug reactions: A critical review. JAMA 234:1236, 1975

Poirier TI: Factors involved in adverse drug reactions. U.S. Pharmacist April:33, 1983

Schiff G: Adverse drug reactions: Recognition of the problem. Facts and Comparisons Drug Newsletter 3:49, 1984

Drug Interactions

5

A drug interaction refers to the process whereby the response to a drug is modified by the presence of another factor, usually a drug or other chemical agent. When two drugs are administered in close sequence to each other, they may interact either to enhance or diminish the intended effect of one or both drugs, or they may produce an unintended and potentially harmful reaction. Depending on the type and intensity of a *beneficial* drug interaction, the clinical effect on the patient may be insignificant or of major consequence. Likewise, *adverse* drug interactions may be inconsequential and readily reversible or serious and permanently disabling. This chapter will offer a detailed look at the reasons why drug interactions occur and the mechanisms that may be involved.

Although the beneficial nature of many drug interactions is firmly established, the clinical significance of adverse drug interactions is greatly understated in many cases. When a patient on multiple drug therapy develops an unusual or disturbing symptom, it is often very difficult to determine if the reaction is caused by an alteration in the disease state being treated, by the presence of a certain drug, by the interaction of two concurrently used drugs, or by some other change in the individual's physiology. What may be a significant drug interaction might simply be viewed as a deterioration in the patient's status or the appearance of a new disease entity. It is apparent, then, that many adverse drug reactions can go completely unheeded or fail to be recognized immediately, especially if the reaction is mild. The clinician must therefore make a careful assessment of *any* change in a patient's condition and possess sufficient knowledge of potential drug interactions to be able to recognize the possibility of a developing drug interaction problem.

The practice of multiple drug therapy is becoming increasingly prevalent as the median age of the population increases, with an attendant increase in the presence of chronic disease conditions requiring drug treatment. It stands to reason that as the number of drugs used concurrently increases, the *potential* for drug interactions increases to an even greater degree. Thus, the benefit-to-risk ratio assumes critical importance in decisions about the number and kinds of drugs to be employed in the therapy of chronic diseases. Occasional episodes of dizziness or tachycardia may be acceptable consequences of drug combinations used to control severe hypertension. On the other hand, use of aspirin is totally unwarranted in coumarin anticoagulant users when other equally effective analgesics are readily available that do not interfere with the action of the anticoagulants. Knowledge of the etiology of drug interactions and the ability to predict possible problems based on drug mechanisms can greatly minimize the toxicity resulting from concurrent drug use.

Attempts to predict drug interactions based on animal experimentation, however, are often unsuccessful, and although laboratory data can occasionally alert the clinician to the possibility that one drug might interact with another drug, animals frequently respond to drugs in a manner quite different from humans. For example, opiates are generally depressants in humans, whereas cats frequently display marked excitation with even small doses of narcotic drugs. Differences in metabolic processes between animals and humans can also result in opposing types of drug interactions. Thus, barbiturates reduce phenytoin metabolism in rats, but accelerate the metabolism in humans. Finally, some animal species lack the ability to display certain human bodily functions. For example, rats are incapable of the vomiting reflex, and therefore would not demonstrate the ability of one drug to potentiate or antagonize the emetic effects of another drug. Thus, the probability of one drug interacting with another drug cannot be accurately predicted by laboratory studies alone or preclinical evaluations. Only after a drug has been available for a number of years does its pattern of drug interactions begin to emerge. Therefore, early detection and prevention of undesirable drug interactions require both an understanding of the pharmacologic profile of a drug as well as careful observation of the patient. Of themselves, most drug interactions are *usually* not serious or life-threatening, especially if detected early and if properly managed, but ignorance of them, through either lack of knowledge or careful observation, can be annoying to the patient and frequently dangerous.

Factors Predisposing to Drug Interactions

There are, of course, numerous reasons why drug interactions occur, and many interactions can be eliminated or at least tempered by recognition of some of the factors that can predispose an individual to the development of an adverse drug interaction.

1. *Insufficient knowledge*—Safe and effective combination drug therapy requires adequate

understanding of the mechanisms of action and potential complications of each type of drug employed. It is the responsibility of the prescriber to select the proper combination of drugs for a particular patient judiciously to maximize the desired therapeutic effects of all the drugs and to minimize the likelihood of the occurrence of adverse drug interactions. In addition, nurses and other health-care professionals who monitor drug responses must possess sufficient knowledge of the pharmacologic profiles of action of drugs used together to assess the efficacy as well as the safety of a drug regimen.

2. *Dietary factors*—Many constituents of an individual's diet can interact with certain drugs. Where such interactions are documented, it is important that the patient be advised to avoid the offending dietary agents. For example, caffeine-containing beverages, if consumed in excess, can increase the central excitatory effects of propoxyphene, possibly leading to convulsions; they may also result in a hypertensive episode with monoamine oxidase (MAO)-inhibitor drugs. Large amounts of licorice, which contains glycyrrhizic acid, can lead to hypokalemia and sodium retention, thus reducing the effectiveness of antihypertensives and diuretics. The toxicity of digitalis glycosides may also be increased by licorice as a consequence of a fall in serum potassium. Other dietary substances that may interact with drugs (and the resultant effects) are tyramine (increased hypertensive response with MAO-inhibitors), dairy products (decreased tetracycline absorption), and green leafy vegetables (decreased anticoagulant response due to increased intake of vitamin K). Some important drug–food interactions are outlined in Table 5-1.

3. *Physiologic state of the individual*—The effect of factors such as age, sex, weight, and genetic abnormalities can greatly influence the occurrence of drug interactions. These various factors have been discussed in detail in Chapter 4 with regard to their influence on the development of adverse drug reactions; refer to that discussion for the general principles that also pertain to the influence of these factors on the development of drug interactions.

4. *Presence of disease states*—The likelihood of a drug interaction is increased in those persons whose pathologic condition (such as liver disease, kidney damage, or altered enzyme systems) may affect the handling of one or more drugs used as part of a therapeutic regimen. Again, the influence of various diseases on the occurrence of adverse drug reactions is considered in Chapter 4, and much of that discussion applies directly to the development of drug interactions as well.

5. *Patient behavior*—The behavioral characteristics of patients are frequently responsible for the occurrence of drug interactions; however, patient behavior is often overlooked as a causative factor in adverse drug interactions. For example, the fairly common practice of seeing more than one physician at a time can increase the risk of a drug interaction if each prescriber is not fully aware of all the drugs being taken by the patient. Self-medication likewise is responsible for a large number of drug interactions that could easily be avoided by proper counseling. The list of over-the-counter (OTC) preparations that can interact with prescription drugs is lengthy and many seemingly innocuous substances such as vitamins and nasal sprays can significantly affect the response to certain drugs. Table 5-2 presents some of the more important potential interactions between OTC and prescription drugs.

Other behavioral problems that can alter a patient's drug responsiveness include poor compliance (*i.e.*, failure to take the prescribed medication as directed), smoking (increases metabolism of many drugs), excessive alcohol consumption (alters drug metabolism and potentiates central nervous system [CNS] depression), and use of street drugs.

6. *Environmental factors*—Often overlooked as a contributory factor in drug interactions is the possibility of exposure to pollutants—industrial, agricultural and other types of chemical agents that are pharmacologically active. Although little direct reliable information exists concerning interactions with these substances, even small amounts of insecticides, fungicides, or industrial wastes can markedly alter the effects of certain therapeutic agents. For example, chlorinated insecticides may stimulate drug metabolism by liver enzymes. Other pesticides are cholinesterase inhibitors, and serious toxicity (*e.g.*, respiratory distress, skeletal muscle weakness, convulsions) can occur in cases of poisoning, especially if another cholinergic drug is being used.

7. *Dosage form factors*—Incompatibility of different dosage forms or improper preparation of a drug may result in drug interactions on either

Table 5-1
Drug–Food Interactions

Drug	Food	Major Effect
acetaminophen	Carbohydrates	Slow drug absorption and onset of therapeutic effect
anticoagulants	Foods rich in vitamin K (*e.g.*, citrus fruits, egg yolks, vegetable oils, green leafy vegetables)	Increase prothrombin time by enhancing hepatic synthesis of clotting factors
antihypertensives; diuretics	Licorice (contains glycyrrhizic acid)	Causes hypokalemia, sodium retention, and elevated blood pressure, antagonizing drug action
digoxin	Dairy products	Slow gastric absorption and decrease therapeutic effect
	Licorice	Hypokalemia; increases digitalis toxicity
griseofulvin	High fat content	Increases rate of absorption
iron salts (*e.g.*, ferrous sulfate)	Citrus fruit juices	Accelerate absorption; may cause nausea, vomiting, anaphylaxis
MAO inhibitors (*e.g.*, pargyline, phenelzine)	Foods rich in tyramine (*e.g.*, aged cheese, red wine, chicken livers)	May result in headache, fever, or hypertensive crisis, as tyramine levels rise
penicillin or erythromycin stearate	Acidic fruit juices	Decompose the drug quickly and may reduce effect
tetracycline	Dairy products containing Ca^{++}	Decrease GI absorption and may inactivate the drug
quinidine	Basic foods (*e.g.*, milk, nuts, most vegetables)	Decrease renal clearance by increasing urine alkalinity; may produce toxic reaction

a physical or a chemical level. Generally, the major concern in this regard is one of *bioavailability*—that is, what fraction of the dose is available through absorption to the fluids of distribution. *In vitro* chemical interactions or *in vivo* alterations in rate or extent of absorption resulting from the presence of a second drug can markedly influence the response to the initially administered agent. Opponents of generic equivalency (*i.e.*, similar efficacy and safety for the same drug manufactured by different companies) often cite the demonstrated differences in absorption rates, dissolution characteristics, and peak blood levels as evidence that not all forms of the same drug are therapeutically or toxicologically equal.

Of particular concern with regard to dosage form considerations are the many "long-acting" or "sustained-release" dosage forms currently available. Many of these products are tablets or capsules

Table 5-2
Over-the-Counter Medications That Can Interact With Prescription Drugs

Drug	Interactants and Major Effects
analgesics	
acetaminophen	Increases hepatotoxic potential of other drugs that also damage the liver
salicylates (*e.g.*, aspirin)	Increase bleeding episodes with anticoagulants and other platelet inhibitors; increase GI ulceration with other gastric irritants (*e.g.*, corticosteroids, anti-inflammatory drugs, alcohol); potentiate effects of oral antidiabetics, barbiturates, phenytoin, and sulfonamides by displacing them from protein-binding sites; decrease effectiveness of vitamin C by increasing its excretion
antacids	Impair absorption of *many* drugs
anticholinergics (*e.g.*, atropine, scopolamine)	Increase side-effects (dry mouth, blurred vision, constipation) of other drugs having an anticholinergic action (*e.g.*, antihistamines, tricyclic antidepressants, carbamazepine, disopyramide)
antidiarrheals	Alter absorption of many drugs by slowing GI motility
antihistamines	Increase sedative effects of CNS depressants; increase anticholinergic side-effects of other drugs (see Anticholinergics, above)
bronchodilators, adrenergic (*e.g.*, epinephrine)	Increase hypertensive effect of pressor agents; decrease effect of oral antidiabetics; increase toxic effects of digitalis glycosides and thyroid drugs; decrease effects of cholinergics in treating glaucoma
cough preparations	See Antihistamines, Decongestants, and Expectorants
decongestants (*i.e.*, phenylephrine, phenylpropanolamine, pseudoephedrine)	Decrease effectiveness of antihypertensive drugs; increase danger of hypertension with MAO inhibitors, other vasopressors, and CNS stimulants (*e.g.*, amphetamines)
expectorants (*e.g.*, guaifenesin)	Increase risk of hemorrhage with heparin
vitamin B_6 (pyridoxine)	Decreases effectiveness of levodopa
vitamin B complex	Increases risk of bleeding with anticoagulants by increasing prothrombin time
vitamin C	Decreases excretion of weak acids (*e.g.*, barbiturates, salicylates, sulfonamides); increases excretion of weak bases (*e.g.*, amphetamine, atropine, quinidine)

that dissolve slowly over many hours, providing a sustained release of medication for a certain period of time and therefore fairly stable plasma levels of drug. The maintenance of steady-state plasma concentrations can be upset, however, by the presence of another drug that might increase gastrointestinal (GI) motility and peristalsis, so that the sustained-release dosage form transits the intestinal tract too quickly to provide for a prolonged drug effect.

Classification and Mechanisms

Interactions between drugs may occur *in vitro* or *in vivo*. An understanding of the basic mechanisms by which drug reactions develop can enable the practitioner either to prevent many interactions from occurring or at least recognize potential interaction problems before they develop into serious complications. Although any classification of drug interactions represents an over-simplification, the following outline will serve as an aid to categorizing many of the important types of drug interactions according to their mechanisms of action.

In Vitro

The term *incompatibility* is often used to designate *in vitro* drug reactions and may refer to either a physical or chemical interaction

1. *Physical*—Occurs if the physical state of either drug is altered when the chemicals are mixed.

For example, amphotericin will precipitate if mixed with normal saline instead of 5% dextrose. Likewise, the anticoagulant effect of heparin, a negatively charged acid, is antagonized by protamine, a positively charged base.

2. *Chemical*—Occurs when the components of a drug mixture interact to form chemically altered products. A few examples of drugs that are chemically incompatible in solution are methicillin and kanamycin, aminophylline and chlorpromazine, dopamine and sodium bicarbonate, and furosemide and ascorbic acid. For a more complete listing of drug incompatibilities, refer to the Appendix.

In most cases, chemical incompatibilities are manifested by a visible sign such as precipitate formation or color change. Occasionally, however, *in vitro* interactions can occur without any observable signs, possibly resulting in undetected loss of potency. Thus, the compatibility of two drugs should always be ascertained by reference to an appropriate source prior to mixing, to ensure that the clinical efficacy of each is not impaired by parenteral admixture.

In Vivo

Most drug interactions occurring in the body can be categorized into one of several classes, depending on the mechanisms responsible for the interaction. It should be repeated that drug interactions can be desirable and expected and often purposely caused, or they may be unwanted and unexpected. The interaction may enhance, retard, or abolish the actions of one or both drugs. Several important mechanisms of *in vivo* drug interactions will be discussed, and pertinent examples will be given. While an understanding of the mechanisms of drug interactions can help the practitioner recognize many potential problems when two or more drugs are combined, it is important that the sections of the book on each individual drug be consulted to obtain a listing of the most likely drug interactions for each agent used. The following classification is intended to serve only as an overview of this tremendously complex field.

ALTERATIONS IN DRUG EFFECTS
Several types of interactions result from alterations in the normal pharmacologic effects of one drug due to the presence of a second drug with similar or different pharmacologic effects.

Similar Pharmacologic Effects
Each of two drugs possessing similar pharmacologic actions will generally enhance the effects of the other. This synergistic interaction can result in either an additive effect or potentiation (see Chap. 3). Thus, combined use of alcohol and a barbiturate would result in an additive CNS-depressant effect. Similarly, the combination of propranolol and clonidine, two antihypertensive drugs, would result in a greater lowering of blood pressure than either drug alone, a clinically desirable interaction. However, when tricyclic antidepressants and carbamazepine, an antiepileptic, are given together, the incidence of anticholinergic side-effects (*e.g.,* dry mouth, blurred vision, urinary hesitancy) is usually greater than when either drug is administered alone, since both drugs have significant cholinergic blocking action. This combination represents an example of an interaction resulting in more pronounced *side-effects.*

Different Pharmacologic Effects
Administration of two drugs with opposing actions usually results in a significant reduction or total abolition of the pharmacologic effects of each. This type of interaction is generally easy to predict if the mechanisms of action of the two drugs are known. Examples might be simultaneous use of a locally acting cholinergic (miotic) and an adrenergic (mydriatic) or the administration of epinephrine (a vasoconstrictor) and histamine (a vasodilator). This type of drug interaction is often purposely induced to reduce or eliminate an undesirable side-effect of one drug by simultaneous use of a second drug. Thus, the reflex tachycardia that frequently accompanies use of peripherally acting vasodilators can be attenuated by concurrent use of a beta-adrenergic blocker, which produces bradycardia as a result of its blocking action on beta receptors in the myocardium.

Competitive Receptor Antagonism
This form of drug interaction is similar to the above because the effects of one drug can be cancelled by the concomitant use of a second drug that blocks access of the first to its receptor site of action. Again, this type of interaction can usually be avoided by an awareness of the mechanisms of action of the two agents. For example, anticholinergic drugs should not be used in patients with glaucoma because they would block the receptor actions of the cholinergic drugs (such as pilocarpine) used to treat this eye disorder. Propranolol, a beta-adrener-

gic blocking drug, would interfere with the bronchodilatory action of isoproterenol in the treatment of chronic obstructive pulmonary disease.

Blockade of Neuronal Uptake or Release
Use of drugs interfering with the uptake or release of other agents by the nerve endings can result in significant interactions that usually decrease the effects of one or both drugs. Phenothiazines and tricyclic antidepressants exert an inhibitory effect on uptake of drugs by the nerve endings. These agents will nullify the antihypertensive effect of guanethidine, which must be taken up by the nerve endings to produce its intended effect. Since many important endogenous pressor amines, such as tyramine and norepinephrine, are partially inactivated by neuronal uptake, these endogenous substances will be potentiated in the presence of neuronal uptake blockers like the phenothiazines and the tricyclics. This potentiation can lead to serious consequences such as severe hypertension or arrhythmias.

Altered Receptor Sensitivity
The sensitivity of a receptor for a particular drug action can be modified by the presence of a second drug. For example, thyroxine may increase the sensitivity of receptors to the anticoagulant effect of the coumarins, so that a dosage adjustment is needed. Likewise, oral antidiabetic drugs such as tolbutamide can increase the sensitivity of insulin receptors on body cells, rendering them more responsive to insulin.

ALTERATIONS IN DRUG HANDLING
Many drug interactions occur as a result of alterations in the handling of one drug caused by the presence of other drugs. These interactions may reflect changes in the absorption, distribution, biotransformation, or excretion of one drug resulting from the actions of a second pharmacologic agent.

Absorption
Any substance capable of altering the normal physiologic processes of the GI tract can markedly impair drug absorption. Alterations in gastric absorption may be caused by the following:

Changes in Gastric pH
Drugs (e.g., sodium bicarbonate or antacids) that can raise the pH of the GI fluid may decrease the absorption of weakly acidic drugs such as salicylates, barbiturates, oral anticoagulants, phenylbutazone, and some sulfonamides, since these drugs become more highly ionized as the pH increases. Conversely, weakly basic drugs such as amphetamines, quinine, and ephedrine tend to remain largely in the un-ionized state at elevated pH levels, and therefore are better absorbed in the presence of an alkalizing drug than at normal gastric pH.

Changes in Intestinal Motility
The faster a drug passes through the stomach and intestines, the less the drug is absorbed. Therefore, drugs that slow GI motility (e.g., anticholinergics, opiates, antidiarrheals) may allow for more complete absorption of some drugs, all other factors being constant. However, if a drug is absorbed more readily from the intestines than from the stomach, slowing GI motility can actually *decrease the rate* of absorption of that drug, as it will remain in the stomach a longer period of time before reaching its site of absorption in the intestines.

On the other hand, drugs that increase the movement of substances through the GI tract, such as laxatives, cholinergic stimulants, or metoclopramide, can reduce absorption of orally administered drugs, since the time the drugs are in contact with the absorbing membrane is diminished. Again, however, if a drug accelerates the emptying of the stomach, it may *increase* the absorption of those drugs that are largely absorbed from the upper intestine. As previously mentioned, the dissolution and subsequent absorption of sustained-release formulations may be significantly impaired by the presence of other drugs that increase GI motility and peristalsis, because the long-acting tablet or capsule would pass through the intestinal tract too rapidly to undergo sufficient disintegration.

Chemical Binding in the Gastrointestinal Tract
Several classes of agents have the capability of forming complexes with many orally administered drugs, thereby impairing their GI absorption. The absorption of tetracyclines is inhibited by the presence of drugs (e.g., antacids) or foods (e.g., milk, cheese) containing calcium, magnesium, or aluminum, substances capable of chemically chelating the tetracycline molecule. Many antacids, as well as cholestyramine (an ionic-exchange resin), may interfere with the absorption of drugs such as warfarin, thyroxine, digitoxin, and phenylbutazone by forming a chemical complex. Charcoal is occasionally used in the treatment of poisoning with various drugs, because it avidly adsorbs many sub-

stances onto the surface of its particles, thereby preventing further drug absorption.

Sequestration
Many fat-soluble drugs, including vitamins A, D, E, and K, will be sequestered in the presence of a fatty vehicle like castor oil or mineral oil, and absorption may be retarded.

Alteration of Intestinal Flora
Alterations in the microbial population of the GI tract can modify the action of certain drugs. For example, broad-spectrum antibiotics can destroy vitamin K-synthesizing organisms in the intestines, thus increasing the action of oral anticoagulants, possibly resulting in bleeding. Drugs metabolized by intestinal microflora, such as methotrexate and levodopa, may exhibit increased effects in the presence of broad-spectrum antibiotics.

Competition for Absorption Mechanisms
Active transport mechanisms function in the absorption of many drugs and can be inhibited by pharmacologic agents that compete for these active absorptive mechanisms. Phenytoin, for example, impedes absorption of folic acid, leading to megaloblastic anemia in many instances. Certain amino acids compete for the same transport mechanisms involved in methyldopa and levodopa absorption, and can therefore retard the absorption of these drugs if present in sufficient amounts.

Miscellaneous Factors
Absorption of many drugs can be influenced by the presence of other drugs or substances that can (1) decrease the rate of mucosal blood flow in the absorbing membranes, (2) influence the volume and content of intestinal secretions, (3) directly damage the absorbing surface, (4) form less lipid-soluble salts with administered drugs, and (5) change the osmotic pressure of the intestinal lumen.

A listing of drugs and other substances that may alter the absorption of other drugs by one or more of the mechanisms outlined above is presented below:
- acetazolamide
- acidifying agents
- alkalizing agents
- aluminum salts
- amino acids
- antacids
- antibiotics
- anticholinergics
- antidiarrheals
- barium salts
- bile salts
- calcium salts
- castor oil
- charcoal
- cholestyramine
- complexing agents (*e.g.*, EDTA)
- dairy products
- food
- iron salts
- laxatives
- magnesium salts
- metoclopramide
- mineral oil
- neomycin
- osmotic diuretics
- p-aminosalicylic acid
- saline cathartics
- sodium bicarbonate

Distribution
The distribution of drugs within the body can be influenced by the presence of other drugs. The following are among the more important mechanisms of drug interactions related to drug distribution.

Competition for Plasma Protein Binding
Drugs bound to plasma proteins are inactive, even though present in the body. On release from the protein-bound stores, the free drug becomes active and is capable of exerting a pharmacologic effect. Many classes of drugs display significant protein-binding capacity, and when any two of these drugs are employed concurrently a drug interaction is likely to occur. This interaction results from the fact that one protein-bound drug generally displays a higher affinity for the binding sites than does the second drug. Thus, one drug is capable of displacing the other from its binding sites, resulting in increased effects of the displaced drug, as well as accelerated elimination, since the displaced drug is now subject to metabolism and excretion. This type of drug interaction becomes especially significant with very highly protein-bound drugs, since a minimal decrease in the fraction of bound drug may be associated with a substantial increase in the plasma level of free drug. For example, oral anticoagulants are approximately 98% protein bound. Concurrent administration of a more avidly bound drug might reduce the fraction of bound anticoagulant to 96%. While this represents only a 2% change in bound drug, the plasma level of free anticoagu-

lant has actually increased *100%* (*i.e.*, 2% unbound to 4% unbound). This large increase in effective plasma concentration can lead to serious bleeding problems in the case of oral anticoagulants, and this type of drug interaction represents a serious consequence of indiscriminate use of other drugs with oral anticoagulants. A list of highly protein-bound drugs that can displace other bound drugs from plasma protein binding sites is given below:

· anticoagulants, oral
· antidiabetics, oral
· barbiturates
· bromocriptine
· calcium channel blockers
· chloral hydrate
· clofibrate
· cyclophosphamide
· diazoxide
· disopyramide
· ethacrynic acid
· furosemide
· indomethacin
· levothyroxine
· methotrexate
· nalidixic acid
· nonsteroidal anti-inflammatory drugs
· phenylbutazone
· prazosin
· probenecid
· propranolol
· quinidine
· salicylates
· sulfinpyrazone
· sulfonamides
· triiodothyronine

However, not all of the drugs listed above have been implicated in *clinically important* drug interactions. Nevertheless, the *potential* for these drugs to interact with other drugs must be recognized.

Displacement from Storage Depots
Many endogenous substances, including neurotransmitters and hormones, are stored by various means in the body. Many drugs exert their effects by either liberating these substances from their storage sites or preventing their release. A drug interaction can occur when two drugs affecting storage mechanisms are given concurrently. The antihypertensive effectiveness of guanethidine, a drug that blocks release of norepinephrine from adrenergic nerve endings, can be reduced by administration of ephedrine or amphetamine, drugs that facilitate norepinephrine release.

Blood Flow Alterations
Pharmacologic agents capable of modifying blood flow to various body organs can greatly influence the distribution and handling of other drugs. For example, epinephrine is often combined with local anesthetics to restrict the spread of the anesthetic by reducing local blood flow. Some cardiovascular drugs can alter blood volume and blood pressure by producing vasoconstriction, thereby restricting the access of other drugs to certain body organs. Decreases in hepatic blood flow by vasoconstrictors likewise can significantly reduce the rate and extent of drug metabolism.

Biotransformation
The process of converting drugs to their respective metabolites is termed *biotransformation*, and it usually occurs in the liver. These reactions are generally mediated by enzymes, so that any drug capable of altering the enzymatic processes involved in the metabolism of other drugs can produce a drug interaction.

Enzyme Inhibition
There are many examples of compounds that interfere with the activity of inactivating enzymes, thereby potentiating other drugs. Monoamine oxidase inhibitors, compounds that inhibit the normal functioning of the endogenous enzyme monoamine oxidase, elevate levels of biogenic amines and may produce severe hypertensive reactions in the presence of pressor amines. Xanthine oxidase inhibitors such as allopurinol increase plasma levels of mercaptopurine by blocking its breakdown. Cholinesterase inhibitors such as physostigmine and neostigmine block degradation of choline esters and can enhance the effects of acetylcholine, succinylcholine and other cholinergic drugs. The anticonvulsant phenytoin is metabolized by hepatic microsomal enzymes, and its effects can be potentiated by microsomal enzyme inhibitors such as p-aminosalicylic acid, disulfiram, isoniazid, and methylphenidate due to accumulation of unmetabolized drug if dosage is not adjusted. These increased levels can result in toxic effects. A therapeutically useful interaction based on enzyme inhibition is the addition of carbidopa to levodopa in the treatment of parkinsonism. Carbidopa competitively inhibits the enzyme dopa decarboxylase in the periphery. This enzyme normally inactivates levodopa before it reaches its site of action in the brain. Thus, peripheral dopa decarboxylase inhibition allows a greater fraction of the levodopa to

enter the CNS intact, resulting in elevated brain levels of levodopa and subsequently increased formation of dopamine to replace the deficient stores of dopamine. Drugs known to inhibit drug-metabolizing enzymes are listed below:

- acetohexamide
- allopurinol
- anabolic steroids
- androgens
- anticoagulants, oral
- antidiabetics, oral
- chloramphenicol
- chlorpromazine
- chlorpropamide
- cholinesterase inhibitors
- clofibrate
- disulfiram
- estrogens
- furazolidone
- isocarboxazid
- isoniazid
- MAO-inhibitors
- methylphenidate
- metronidazole
- nitrofurantoin
- oral contraceptives
- p-aminosalicylic acid
- prednisolone
- prochlorperazine
- quinacrine
- thyroxine

Enzyme Acceleration (Induction)

Liver microsomal enzymes involved in the metabolic breakdown of many classes of drugs can be stimulated by certain pharmacologic agents, including barbiturates, hydantoins, meprobamate, griseofulvin, and chlorinated hydrocarbon insecticides. This is termed *enzyme induction* and results in a decreased therapeutic response to those drugs metabolized by the microsomal enzymes, since the drugs are being metabolized more rapidly. Enzyme induction may occur through increased synthesis of microsomal protein for hepatic metabolic enzymes or possibly through an increase in the size or enzyme content of the endoplasmic reticulum of the liver. There are literally hundreds of drugs and chemicals that can stimulate hepatic enzymatic activity and the range of potential drug interactions along these lines is enormous. For example, coumarin anticoagulants are metabolized at a much faster rate in the presence of a barbiturate, and an appropriate dosage adjustment must be made. Phenytoin reduces the effects of dexamethasone by in-

ducing the microsomal enzymes responsible for its metabolism. Alcohol accelerates the metabolism of barbiturates, isoniazid, tolbutamide, and a variety of other drugs. Some barbiturates can increase the metabolism of androgens, estrogens, and progestins; thus, the efficacy of oral contraceptives may be compromised in barbiturate users.

Enzyme induction can be utilized in an advantageous manner as well. Thus, phenobarbital is used in the treatment of neonatal hyperbilirubinemia, because it accelerates the metabolism of bilirubin to more readily excreted compounds.

Finally, enzyme induction may be responsible for development of tolerance to certain drugs because some drugs may stimulate their own liver metabolism. Examples of such drugs are barbiturates, meprobamate, glutethimide, phenylbutazone, and orphenadrine.

A representative, but by no means complete, listing of metabolic enzyme inducers is presented below:

- alcohol
- anticonvulsants
- antihistamines
- aromatic hydrocarbons, polycyclic
- 3.4 benzpyrene (cigarette smoke, charcoal-broiled foods)
- carbamazepine
- chloral hydrate
- chlordiazepoxide
- chlorinated insecticides (*e.g.*, DDT, Dieldrin, Lindane, Chlordane, Aldrin)
- chlorpromazine
- cortisone
- diphenhydramine
- ethchlorvynol
- glutethimide
- griseofulvin
- haloperidol
- imipramine
- meprobamate
- methoxyflurane
- methyprylon
- nicotine
- nikethamide
- nitrous oxide
- norethynodrel
- orphenadrine
- paramethadione
- phenacetin
- phenobarbital
- phenylbutazone
- phenytoin
- prednisolone

- prednisone
- probenecid
- promazine
- rifampin
- spironolactone
- stilbestrol
- testosterone
- tolbutamide
- triflupromazine

Excretion

Drug interactions occurring with the excretion of drugs may involve any of the renal excretory processes, that is, glomerular filtration, tubular reabsorption, or active tubular secretion. Most clinically important drug interactions occur as a result of either changes in urinary pH, which can alter the fraction of reabsorbed drug, or through competition for active tubular secretory mechanisms.

Changes in Urinary pH

Acidification of the urine with agents such as ammonium chloride can result in reduced effectiveness of basic drugs (*e.g.*, amphetamine and quinidine) because they will be largely ionized at the acidic pH and readily excreted. On the other hand, renal excretion of acidic drugs, such as salicylates, barbiturates, and anticoagulants, will be accelerated by alkalization of the urine with sodium bicarbonate, acetazolamide, or potassium citrate. Manipulation of urinary pH is an effective means of facilitating excretion of drugs in certain cases of overdosage. Thus, ammonium chloride may be given in amphetamine overdosage, whereas sodium bicarbonate might be used in overdosage with phenobarbital or salicylates.

In addition to affecting ionization of drug molecules, urinary pH may influence solubility of drug molecules in the tubular fluid. For example, sulfonamides are poorly soluble in a highly acidic urine. They can precipitate out in the tubules, causing urinary tract obstruction.

Competition for Tubular Mechanisms

Many drugs and metabolites are actively secreted from the renal blood vessels into the tubules of the kidney and subsequently eliminated. Drug interactions may occur when any two actively secreted drugs are used together, due to competition for the active secretory mechanisms. Drugs that may interact by this means, resulting in prolonged therapeutic effects, are salicylates, sulfonamides, penicillins, thiazide diuretics, pyrazolones, dicumarol, indomethacin, probenecid, oral hypoglycemics, ac-

etazolamide, diazoxide, and methotrexate. Small doses of aspirin may impair the uricosuric (uric acid-excreting) action of probenecid by interfering with the active secretion of uric acid into the renal tubules, and can also inhibit the excretion of methotrexate. Competition for active tubular secretion can be used to therapeutic advantage as well. For example, the use of probenecid with penicillin to delay the normally rapid excretion of the penicillin molecule significantly prolongs the effective duration of action of penicillin in the body.

Alterations in Fluid and Electrolyte Balance

Changes in fluid and electrolyte levels induced by certain drugs can markedly affect the therapeutic effectiveness and toxicity of other drugs, particularly those acting on the heart, kidney, and skeletal muscles. Hypokalemia (low serum potassium levels) produced by many diuretic agents and corticosteroids increases the likelihood of digitalis toxicity, and can antagonize the antiarrhythmic effects of quinidine, disopyramide, lidocaine, procainamide, and phenytoin. Potassium loss also may result in prolonged paralysis following use of antidepolarizing skeletal muscle relaxants, such as gallamine or pancuronium.

Another interaction of potential clinical significance is the use of drugs that induce sodium and water retention (*e.g.*, phenylbutazone or corticosteroids) with antihypertensive or diuretic drugs. These fluid-retaining drugs can negate the action of the antihypertensive agents in lowering blood pressure. Conversely, drugs that cause excessive diuresis (*e.g.*, high-ceiling diuretics) may potentiate the hypotensive effects of antihypertensive drugs and of peripheral vasodilators such as papaverine or nitroglycerin.

MISCELLANEOUS DRUG INTERACTIONS

Alterations in the Immune Response

Antibody production can be affected by the presence of certain drugs. Vaccines and toxoids stimulate antibody production, whereas glucocorticoids such as hydrocortisone can inhibit the immune response and should not be used with vaccines.

Although antibiotics are frequently given in combination, drug interactions can occur if both bacteriostatic and bactericidal drugs are given together. For example, penicillins are bactericidal because they interfere with cell wall synthesis in dividing bacteria. They are less effective, however, when used with tetracyclines—drugs which prevent cell division and bacterial growth. This mutual antagonism can cause complications when combination therapy is used to treat severe infections.

Residual Drug Effects

A potential source of drug interactions is the prolonged period of therapeutic effectiveness that is often observed even after a drug is discontinued. Drugs with prolonged actions have the potential to interact with newly introduced drugs even though the first drugs are no longer being administered. For example, a serious delayed interaction occurs when MAO inhibitors are given within two weeks of tricyclic antidepressants. Severe hypertension can occur due to the residual effects of the MAO inhibitors combined with the effects of the tricyclic antidepressants.

It is difficult to simply state the overall clinical importance of drug interactions. Some are beneficial; others represent mild and essentially benign events, requiring merely an adjustment in the dosage of one or more drugs. Most important are potentially life-threatening adverse interactions requiring immediate action. Caution in using multiple drug regimens is especially warranted when the patient is receiving either a drug with a narrow safety margin (*e.g.*, digitalis glycoside, lithium, oral anticoagulant) or a drug for the treatment of a serious disease (*e.g.*, antineoplastic, hypoglycemic, antiarrhythmic), since even slight alterations in the effectiveness of these drugs can have serious consequences. Clinically significant adverse drug interactions can be minimized by an understanding of the various mechanisms involved in their production, awareness of the presence of predisposing factors, and avoidance, where possible, of multiple drug usage (except where expressly designed to capitalize on intended, beneficial interactions).

CASE STUDY

Ms. Johnson, a 70-year-old overweight woman, is being treated for congestive heart failure. She is receiving digoxin and furosemide (Lasix) as part of her treatment. She is also a type II diabetic and has been receiving tolbutamide since she has been unable to remain under control by diet alone. She states that she has difficulty remaining on her diet because she is frequently a dinner guest and does not like to "put the hostess out by not eating what she serves."

While still hospitalized Ms. Johnson develops a high fever and burning sensation on urination. She is diagnosed as having a urinary tract infection and the urology resident on consultation prescribes a sulfonamide-containing drug, Bactrim.

When you make rounds one morning, Ms. Johnson complains of feeling weak and dizzy. She also states that her heart feels like it's pounding in her chest.

Discussion Questions

1. What are the actions of digoxin, furosemide, tolbutamide, and Bactrim? How might they interact to produce untoward effects?
2. What factors might influence Ms. Johnson's response to the drugs she is receiving?
3. What types of communication should you set up to ensure Ms. Johnson's nursing needs are met? Who on the health-care team should become involved?

REVIEW QUESTIONS

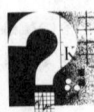

1. List some factors that may predispose an individual to the development of a drug interaction.
2. Give examples of two drugs that may interact based on the following reasons:
   a. Similar pharmacologic effects

    b. Opposing pharmacologic effects

    c. Competitive receptor antagonism

    d. Blockade of neuronal uptake

    e. Altered receptor sensitivity

3. List several reasons why one drug can retard GI absorption of a second drug.

4. Explain why competition for protein-binding sites between two *highly* bound drugs can lead to a more serious drug interaction than competition between two *less avidly* bound drugs.

5. What is meant by "enzyme induction"?

6. How do changes in urinary *p*H alter excretion of highly acidic or highly basic drugs?

BIBLIOGRAPHY

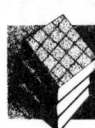

Adverse interactions of drugs. Medical Letter 23(5):17, 1981

Albanese JA, Bond T: Drug Interactions: Basic Principles and Clinical Problems. New York, McGraw-Hill, 1978

Caranasos GJ, Stewart RB, Cluff LE: Clinically desirable drug interactions. Annu Rev Pharmacol Toxicol 25:67, 1985

Carr CJ: Food and drug interactions. Annu Rev Pharmacol Toxicol 22:19, 1982

Cohen SN, Armstrong MF: Drug Interactions: A Handbook for Clinical Use. Baltimore, Williams & Wilkins, 1974

Hansten PD: Drug Interactions, 5th ed. Philadelphia, Lea & Febiger, 1985

Holtzman JL: The role of protein binding in drug therapy. Rational Drug Therapy 18(9):1, 1984

Hussar DA: Drug interactions. American Journal of Pharmacy 145:65, 1973

Koch-Weser J, Greenblatt DJ: Drug interactions in clinical perspective. Eur J Clin Pharmacol 11:405, 1977

Lieber CS: Interaction of ethanol with drugs and vitamin therapy. Ration Drug Ther 19(11):1, 1985

Roe DA: Nutrient and drug interactions. Nutr Rev 42(4): April, 1984

Shinn AF, Shrewsbury RP: Evaluations of Drug Interactions. 3rd ed. St. Louis, CV Mosby, 1985

Sriwatanakul K, Mehta G: Clinically significant drug interactions. Rational Drug Therapy 17(4):1, 1983

Toothaker RD, Welling PG: The effect of food on drug bioavailability. Annu Rev Pharmacol Toxicol 20:173, 1980

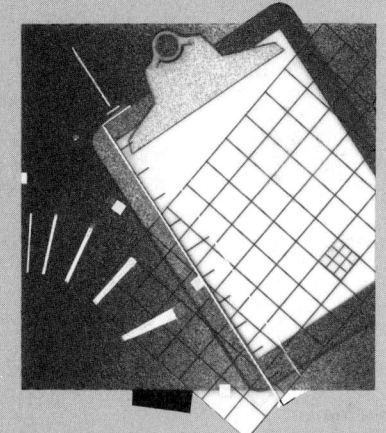

Role of the Nurse in Drug Therapy

II

Use of the Nursing Process in Drug Therapy

6

Drug therapy plays a part in many therapeutic regimens and the nurse's role is crucial in helping the patient manage his care. Sometimes nurses view their roles only in the realm of administration as mere "pill pushers" in a tedious and boring process. Were that the only role, nurses could be replaced by pill-pushing robots, whose margin for error would probably be lower. Such a view demonstrates a lack of understanding about nursing's responsibility and need for accountability in drug therapy. All nurses who administer drugs have the responsibility to

1. Follow the legal guidelines that govern nursing practice and drug therapy
2. Use the nursing process through appropriate
   a. Collection of information about the patient (assessment)
   b. Analysis of data to formulate problem statements and nursing diagnoses
   c. Establishment of goals and objectives for care (plan)
   d. Development and implementation of interventions
   e. Evaluation of the plan's effectiveness

Legal issues surrounding nursing practice as it relates to drug therapy are discussed in detail in Chapter 7. Chapter 8 focuses on safe, correct drug administration. This chapter will discuss the components of the nursing process in relation to the nurse's role in drug therapy.

The nursing process provides a logical framework to assist the nurse in ensuring consistent quality care to all patients. Each component interrelates with the other, as shown in Figure 6-1, so that the process is continuous. Such a framework lends itself well to drug therapy with few exceptions.

Assessment: Data Collection

Assessment of the patient receiving any medication can be divided into two parts to facilitate analysis: subjective and objective data.

Subjective Data

Subjective data collection includes the patient's medical history, medication history, and personal history. The medical history should focus on the organ systems already being treated by drug therapy, the systems or symptoms about to be treated,

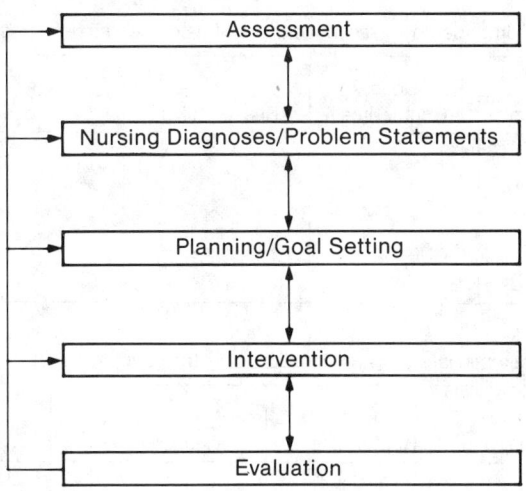

Figure 6-1. *Flow of information through the nursing process is not always stepwise in direction. For example, a change in a patient's physical condition (assessment) may change a drug regimen (plan, intervention) and may change the outcomes sought. Likewise, if on evaluation an intervention is found to have failed (i.e., the patient stopped taking the drug) then the care plan must be reviewed and possibly reorganized.*

and those systems that might be adversely affected by the treatment.

Five questions form the framework for obtaining a medication and personal history of any patient.

1. What other drugs is the patient presently using? Who gives the drugs? What does the patient know about the drugs?
2. What drugs has the patient taken in the past year?
3. What are the patient's symptoms? Which symptoms are being treated by medication?
4. Does the patient have any drug allergies or has he ever had any drug reactions in the past?
5. How does the patient usually follow the directions given for taking prescribed drugs? Does he ever forget?

The first four questions are usually asked specifically on any patient assessment tool (Fig. 6-2). The patient is asked what prescription drugs, over-the-counter medications, and street drugs he takes or has taken within the last year. Many people never think of reporting that they take 4 aspirin a day, a half dozen vitamins, mineral oil for constipation, decongestants for allergy, birth control pills, or that they drink 5 cups of coffee a day unless the interviewer makes a special effort to ask

A. Current drug therapy: Prescription, over-the-counter, street drugs

Medication	Dose Route/Time	Reason taken	Last dose	Prescribing physician	Side-effects	Does patient take medications as prescribed?

B. Drugs taken in last year: Prescription, over-the-counter, street drugs

Medication	Dose Route/Time	Reason taken	Reason stopped	Date stopped	Prescribing physician

C. Drug allergies   Yes _____   No _____   Drugs and reactions _____

_____

Figure 6-2.   Sample medication history (part of a total assessment tool).

appropriate questions. Yet all of these may influence the action and interaction of prescribed drugs.

Most people are also reluctant to share a history of street drug use. Yet many of the street drugs can seriously interfere with drug therapy. The nurse needs to display a nonjudgmental attitude in questioning the patient, allow for privacy during such a discussion, assure confidentiality, and phrase the question tactfully. The nurse should also be prepared for the drugs to be called by their street labels (see Chap. 85) and should ask the patient to clarify the drug name if it sounds unfamiliar. Information about the quantity and frequency of drug use is also important. While listing the drugs the patient takes the nurse also asks what symptoms are being treated by these drugs. From this data the appropriateness of the current therapy can be reviewed, other treatable symptoms may be uncovered, and an outline for physical assessment is established. Such information enables the nurse to decide whether to administer the drugs ordered or to seek clarification before taking legal responsibility for administration. It also provides some indication of the patient's understanding of his drug treatment plan.

Information about drug allergies and drug reactions can alert the nurse to potential problems. If a person is allergic to one drug, he may react to other drugs with similar chemical compositions. For example, the patient who reports a penicillin allergy may also have a reaction to cephalosporins. It is also important to clarify the difference between an allergic reaction and an unpleasant side-effect. A patient may state he is allergic to a drug because it caused vomiting when he actually experienced a side-effect. Allergic responses are detailed in Chapter 4.

Patients who report multiple drug and food allergies or frequent drug reactions need to be monitored carefully when starting a new drug since they are more likely to develop drug allergies. The cause of these multiple allergies is not clear, but the response such patients have may be increased the second or third time an allergy-producing medication is administered. Good history taking can help the nurse avoid giving a medication that could produce disastrous results.

Through the last question, the nurse can discover a patient's previous compliance patterns, an issue that will be discussed in more detail under Patient Teaching and Compliance. This information may be part of the psychosocial assessment on admission or may be uncovered while obtaining a personal history. Through open-ended questions, the nurse can learn about the patient's perception of medicine; what being healthy means to him; how he remembers to take his medicine; and when he is likely to forget. Patients have a tendency to tell what they believe the nurse wants to hear, so use of open-ended questions will avoid "yes/no/go-away" responses.

Objective Data

Objective data collection consists of physical assessment and laboratory or diagnostic tests of the systems most likely to be therapeutically or adversely affected by the drug and is based on the history the patient describes. Physical assessment may focus on the organ or system affected by the disease or producing the symptoms or it may be to establish the pretreatment function of organs most likely to be taxed by the drug, usually the kidney and liver. Tests for mental alertness, memory, and psychomotor skills are also appropriate especially if the patient is expected to learn self-administration or if the prescribed drug will change mental or psychomotor function.

Laboratory tests and diagnostic studies provide a baseline of information valuable throughout drug therapy. These results can be compared with later tests to determine drug effectiveness, development of toxicity, and effect on body systems. Laboratory work typically done for many drugs includes a complete blood count, renal and hepatic function studies, and electrolytes, and may also include blood glucose levels and arterial blood gases.

Assessment of systems and laboratory tests related to the specific drug category will be discussed throughout the text. However, the reader is referred to textbooks on physical assessment and laboratory studies for detailed information. See the Appendix for a list of common laboratory values.

Analysis: Formulation of Nursing Diagnoses

The data collected in the assessment provide multiple clues about the most appropriate nursing actions to take. The data can be categorized into actions the nurse takes independently, called *nursing diagnoses*, or actions the nurse takes in collaboration with other health-care providers, called *collaborative problems.*

A collaborative problem is an actual or potential problem that may result from complications of disease, diagnostic studies, or medical or surgical treatment, and that can be prevented, resolved, or reduced through collaborative nursing interventions (Alfaro, 1986). For example, a patient receiving an intravenous antibiotic may have the problem of *potential complication: phlebitis,* from drug therapy. The nurse will monitor the site for pain, redness, and swelling and initiate changing the IV site on a routine schedule to avoid such problems. In drug therapy most collaborative problems are potential and result from the proposed drug administration or from the side-effects of the drug.

Nursing diagnoses represent those actual or potential problems that the nurse can resolve independently. For example, the patient may be unable to swallow, *impaired swallowing,* which will affect his ability to take pills, or he may have a memory deficit, *an alteration in thought process,* which will prevent him from remembering to take his medication. Most patients will initially have a *knowledge deficit* regarding drug action, rationale for therapy, administration, and side-effects and drug interactions. These are examples of *actual* nursing diagnoses. Potential nursing diagnoses may also be listed. For example, if a medication such as an antihistamine has as a side-effect dizziness or sleepiness, and the patient will be taking such medication for the first time, the patient has the *potential for injury* related to the side-effects of the drug.

The italicized diagnoses are taken from the list of nursing diagnoses developed by the North American Nursing Diagnosis Association (NANDA), and is found on p. 66. These lists, however, are still being refined and debated (see also Lunney, 1982). The beginner should be less concerned with the language in which the problem/diagnosis is stated and more concerned with listing the actual and potential issues in which a nurse can intervene to assist the patient. The most important point to remember is that the diagnoses should assist the nurse to plan for care.

Planning: How to Get the Most Out of Your Time

Setting Goals

Every interaction with a patient is an opportunity to learn and share information. The perfect time to review information with a patient is when he is taking the drug so he can associate what is being

Nursing Diagnoses Approved by the North American Nursing Diagnosis Association, April 1986

Activity intolerance

Activity intolerance, potential

Adjustment, impaired*

Airway clearance, ineffective

Anxiety

Body temperature, potential alteration in*

Bowel elimination, alteration in: constipation

Bowel elimination, alteration in: diarrhea

Bowel elimination, alteration in: incontinence

Breathing pattern, ineffective

Cardiac output, alteration in: decreased

Comfort, alteration in: pain

Comfort, alteration in: chronic pain*

Communication, impaired: verbal

Coping, family: potential for growth

Coping, ineffective family: compromised

Coping, ineffective family: disabling

Coping, ineffective individual

Diversional activity, deficit

Family process, alteration in

Fear

Fluid volume alteration in: excess

Fluid volume deficit, actual

Fluid volume deficit, potential

Gas exchange, impaired

Grieving, anticipatory

Grieving, dysfunctional

Growth and development, altered*

Health maintenance, alteration in

Home maintenance management, impaired

Hopelessness*

Hyperthermia*

Hypothermia*

Incontinence, functional*

Incontinence, reflex*

Incontinence, stress*

Incontinence, total*

Incontinence, urge*

Infection, potential for*

Injury, potential for: (poisoning, potential for; suffocation, potential for; trauma, potential for)

Knowledge deficit (specify)

Mobility, impaired physical

Noncompliance (specify)

Nutrition, alteration in: less than body requirements

Nutrition, alteration in: more than body requirements

Nutrition, alteration in: potential for more than body requirements

Oral mucous membrane, alteration in

Pain, chronic*

Parenting, alteration in: actual

Parenting, alteration in: potential

Post-trauma response*

Powerlessness

Rape trauma syndrome

Self-care deficit: feeding, bathing/hygiene, dressing/grooming, toileting

Self-concept, disturbance in body image, self-esteem, role performance, personal identity

Sensory–perceptual alteration: visual, auditory, kinesthetic, gustatory, tactile, olfactory

Sexual dysfunction

Sexuality patterns, altered*

Skin integrity, impairment of: actual

Skin integrity, impairment of: potential

Sleep pattern disturbance

Social interaction, impaired*

Social isolation

Spiritual distress (distress of the human spirit)

Swallowing, impaired*

Thermoregulation, ineffective*

Thought processes, alteration in

Tissue integrity, impaired*

Tissue perfusion, alteration in: cerebral, cardiopulmonary, renal, gastrointestinal, peripheral

Unilateral neglect

Urinary elimination, alteration in patterns

Urinary retention*

Violence, potential for: self-directed or directed at others

* Diagnoses accepted in 1986

taught with how the drug appears. In order to use time with a patient effectively, a list of patient care goals should be used. Goals are developed from the analysis of data and must relate directly to the nursing diagnoses and collaborative problems that were derived from the data. The goals should meet the following requirements:

1. Goals should be stated as expected outcomes of nursing intervention and emphasize the change desired in physiologic or psychologic behavior.

2. They should be patient-centered, rather than nurse-oriented—what the patient will achieve, not what the nurse will do.

3. They must be realistic, measurable, and mutually acceptable to the patient and the nurse.

4. There should be a built-in time limit for the achievement of the goal where appropriate.

5. All goals set should include other health-care providers as necessary.

Goals may be established by the nurse, by the patient, or through agreement by both parties. If the locus of decision making is the nurse, such as in the care of a comatose patient receiving a lifesaving drug, goals will be stated in terms of what the nurse will do (*e.g.*, titrate lidocaine [an antiarrhythmic drug] drip to maintain premature ventricular contractions [PVCs] at fewer than 3 per minute). If the locus of decision making is the patient, the goals will be stated in terms of what the patient wants (e.g., to incorporate insulin injections into a daily routine at home). Most frequently the goals are mutually agreed on by the nurse and the patient (e.g., by July 10 Mr. R will learn all of the steps of insulin self-injection). Goals must be communicated among all care givers (including family) as appropriate. All nurses caring for the patient should have similar goals. In addition, other care givers must also be aware of certain goals. For example, if a patient is learning to adjust to a new antihypertensive regimen, his physical therapy schedule may need to be revamped to accommodate for periods of dizziness. If the plan is not communicated to the physical therapist, safe care is not guaranteed.

Patient Teaching and Compliance

The success of almost any drug therapy regimen depends on a sound teaching plan. The content of the teaching plan will be similar for patients with the same problems but the goals may differ depending on each patient's needs. Additional goals can be added if needed but, in general, the desired outcomes for any education program provide that the patient and his significant others will be able to

1. State his condition, his therapy, and the rationale and the time frame for the therapy
2. Correctly administer the medication prescribed on an appropriate schedule
3. State expected or common side-effects, how to treat them, and when to seek assistance
4. Obtain whatever drugs and equipment are needed to maintain the therapy
5. Know when to seek follow-up care at an acceptable, accessible facility
6. State the proper storage of drugs for optimal effectiveness and safety
7. State food and drug interactions, if any

A teaching plan designed to meet these goals can easily be developed if the nurse knows what information to teach; therefore, the nurse must be knowledgeable. In fact, many nursing students produce beautiful patient teaching plans for patients early in their training. Unfortunately, many of these plans fail, as do those of their more experienced colleagues, because they do not ask some basic questions when designing the plans. These basic questions give the nurse information about the patient's perception of the events that have occurred and whether or not he is willing to participate in the treatment plan offered, let alone learn anything about it. The nurse who fails to consider the human factors of learning will become frustrated and tend to label some patients as noncompliant. Compliance is a two-way street; much of what a patient decides to do will depend on the teaching he receives, the way it is presented, the trust he develops in the teacher, and how realistic the goals are. The successful nurse teacher will develop a realistic teaching plan that considers the patient's ability to comply. To do this the nurse must consider several questions.

Is the patient ready and willing to learn? Very little teaching can be done if the patient is in pain; if he is preoccupied with all the tubes to which he is connected; or if he is experiencing a family crisis in addition to the personal crisis of being ill. Basic needs must be met first in order to establish a climate for learning.

On the other hand, learning readiness can be expressed by the patient who begins to ask about his condition, his medication, and the procedures being done even before he is able to participate in his care. People vary day to day in learning readiness so the nurse must be ready to assess this on every patient interaction.

What is the patient's perception of health? How does he view his illness? For many patients, to be labeled with a disease for which one must take medicine is to be labeled sick. The pill serves as a reminder that they are not healthy and a logical conclusion is to assume that if they stop taking the pills, they stop being sick. The patient who views illness this way is very apt to stop taking medication once he is unsupervised. The nurse must explore health perceptions with such a patient in order to help the patient achieve successful treatment.

Other patients view medication as an advantage, a badge of illness that gains them sympathy and attention. Many elderly people are not satisfied with their treatment unless they receive medication, yet frequently they abandon the therapy unless others take responsibility for administering it. The nurse needs to explore with such patients their need for companionship and attention in relation to how these needs affect their ability to remain independent. Only when such patients realistically view their resources and the demands placed on them will they begin to learn self-care, including self-medication.

How much can the patient learn? Can he read? Some patients seem to quickly grasp new information and integrate it into their lives. These patients are generally intelligent, motivated to learn, physically well enough to participate, and accepting of whatever they must do to remain independent.

Other patients learn more slowly either because they are not quite ready to learn when the teaching starts or because they have trouble grasping the concepts by the method presented. Patients respond better to visual demonstrations and pictures than to verbal instructions. This is particularly true of the person who cannot read or is a poor reader.

Comprehension of the language used may also be a problem. Patients for whom English is a second language may need to review material more slowly in order to grasp its meaning. If a patient has difficulty understanding concepts or sentences as a result of some neurologic diseases, teaching may have to be completely visual or proceed at a very slow rate. Frequently the technical language a nurse or physician uses to describe a situation will completely confuse the patient. Consider such words as *hypertension, cardiac output, angina pectoris,* and *diuretic.* Do they sound like easily comprehensible English? Imagine the thoughts of a patient who is told he has *hypertension;* taking the word literally, he might believe he is under a lot of stress. The nurse needs to be aware that most patients are not familiar with medical jargon. While it is inappropriate to talk down to any patient, it is important to establish an approach that allows the patient to understand what is being said.

A few patients will retain nothing of what is taught to them no matter how frequently it is repeated or what method is used. This occurs in patients with severe memory deficits or psychiatric conditions that alter the sense of reality. Such patients can be taught to participate in their care but only with close supervision; therefore, the nurse must focus most of her teaching on those who will care for such patients. Such plans should be as simple to follow as possible and teach the care giver how to cope with the patient who refuses to participate.

What does the patient need to know to care for himself safely? While some patients may want to know in anatomic detail what a drug does to their body, others will be overwhelmed with such information. The rule of thumb is to present basic information first. Every patient who is able should achieve the desired outcomes stated at the beginning of this section. However, that information may be more than some people can retain. The nurse needs to develop strategies to help the patient retain the most important information and enlist the help of family or friends with other material.

The patient who cannot remember the name of the drug may still be able to associate its identifying characteristics such as color, markings, or size with its use; for example, the little white scored pill (*i.e.,* digoxin) slows the heart and makes it stronger. Other reminders such as dosage calendars and drug cards have the pills glued to the paper to help the patient remember which drug to take. See Figure 6-3 for a sample drug reminder calendar, and the Guidelines for Developing Patient Drug Cards (p. 70). While the nurse should avoid overloading the patient with too much information, oversimplification about drug action or drug taking can have disastrous results. One elderly lady, admitted with digoxin toxicity, was told digoxin would help her heart. She assumed it was similar to the nitroglycerin she had been taking and proceeded to take it every time she had pain instead of just once a day. To decrease the chance of such problems, the nurse should seek feedback from the patient on what he has learned, preferably several hours or days after the initial teaching. Asking the patient to write or state the information learned in his own words is one method of validating his knowledge. Teaching and the patient's responses should be carefully documented to protect the nurse from liability should the patient forget the information and misrepresent what he has been taught.

Side-effects are also an important part of patient teaching, but restraint should be exercised. The nurse can identify the common side-effects and mention any major adverse reactions the patient needs to monitor. However, too much information can frighten the patient and be as harmful as too little information. If certain side-effects can be avoided, the patient needs to learn appropriate strategies. Information about side-effects should be reinforced over time to ensure the patient remembers signs that could save his life.

The patient will also need to have a plan for what to do if a side-effect or adverse reaction occurs. A family member or close friend can be included so he will know the symptoms and can take action if the patient cannot act independently. If the nurse can help the patient get in tune with his body, he will learn to watch for clues about how he feels. For example, in one case it was helpful to ask

DRUG NAME	DOSE	HOW TO TAKE IT	WHEN TO TAKE IT	IDENTIFYING FEATURES
digoxin	0.125 mg (1 tablet)	By mouth	Once a day (AM)	(e.g., color of tablet or capsule, surface markings, or code number)
propranolol	10 mg (1 tablet)	By mouth	4 times a day	
Septra DS	1 tablet	By mouth	2 times a day × 10 days	

SCHEDULE

HOUR \ DAY	SUNDAY	MONDAY	TUESDAY	WEDNESDAY	THURSDAY	FRIDAY	SATURDAY
9 AM	digoxin 1 pill pulse ____ propranolol 1 pill	same pulse ____ same	same pulse ____ same	same pulse ____ same	same pulse ____ same	same pulse ____ same	same pulse ____ same
10 AM	Day 6 Septra DS 1 pill with 1 full glass water	Day 7 same	Day 8 same	Day 9 same	Day 10 same		
1 PM	propranolol 1 pill	same	same	same	same	same	same
5 PM	propranolol 1 pill	same	same	same	same	same	same
9 PM	propranolol 1 pill	same	same	same	same	same	same
10 PM	Septra DS 1 pill with 1 full glass water	same	same	same	same—last dose if all pills are taken		

Figure 6-3. Sample drug reminder calendar.

Guidelines for Developing Patient Drug Cards

1. List the name of the drug and the dose, route, and frequency of administration in terms the patient can understand.
   Example: Digoxin 0.25 mg (1 pill) by mouth every morning

2. Provide identifying features of the drug. Include color, size, markings, and a picture if available or attach a pill to the drug card. Sources are the pharmacy, the *Physicians' Desk Reference*, and some drug reference books.
   Example: Burroughs Wellcome form of digoxin (Lanoxin) 0.25 mg is a small white pill, plain on one side, scored on the other with the label Burroughs-W x3A

3. Describe the drug's action or use as the patient can understand it.
   Example: Digoxin helps the heart beat slower and stronger.

4. Provide directions for use. Include any foods to be avoided.
   Example: · Try to take digoxin in the morning at the same time every day.
   · If you forget a dose one day don't try to catch up by taking two doses the next day. Take only 1 dose each day.
   · Before taking digoxin, take your pulse, preferably when you first wake up.
   · Weigh yourself every morning and record your weight.
   · Avoid using cough or cold remedies unless you check first with the doctor. Some of these medicines can be harmful to you while you are taking digoxin.

5. List common side-effects and what the patient can do about them.
   Example: Digoxin may cause an upset stomach. If this happens, take the drug with breakfast or other food. If stomach upset persists call the doctor or nurse.

6. List adverse effects and tell the patient what to do about them.
   Example: Call your doctor or nurse immediately if you notice any of the following:
   · Changed pulse rate or irregular pulse
   · Nausea, vomiting, change in appetite, or diarrhea
   · Rapid weight gain or swelling of hands and feet
   · Blurred vision or yellow or green haloes in vision

a new diabetic how she felt just before being admitted to the hospital. Her reports of thirst, hunger, dizziness, and weight loss were signs of elevated blood sugar, and these remembered signals were used to teach her how she would know if her body was getting enough insulin.

How complicated is the drug therapy? The more complex a regimen and the more time it takes in a person's life, the more likely he is to abandon it. If the nurse has difficulty in planning an understandable teaching plan because of the number of drugs the patient must take, then it is likely the plan will fail. The patient will be frustrated and confused and may refuse to do even basic care. When this happens the nurse needs to discuss the difficulty with the physician and attempt to reduce or eliminate some of the medications or treatments ordered. Occasionally less aggressive therapy may be prescribed to ensure the patient will be able to manage it.

What family supports/financial resources does the patient have? If the family unit or other supports are strong, the patient is more likely to comply with the drug therapy. Family members can provide reminders and can relieve the patient of some of the burden that comes from managing alone. Lack of support from loved ones may be a major deterrent to learning and reduce the chance that the patient will follow the drug therapy at home. The nurse should attempt to observe the way a family interacts and plan care accordingly. Whenever possible, the family should be included in any long-term drug treatment plan.

Financial resources need to be evaluated, especially if treatment is long term or costly. Insurance benefits and qualification for special programs must be determined prior to therapy initiation. Lack of resources is a major reason for noncompliance.

Does the patient abuse street drugs or alcohol? The patient who has a history of alcohol abuse or long-term addiction to street drugs is very likely to stop prescribed drug therapy if he returns to his previous pattern of abuse. A history of abuse does not guarantee noncompliance but the nurse needs to explore the importance the patient attaches to prescribed therapy. Family supports can be helpful if they are not part of the patient's circle of drug users. The patient may also agree to begin a treatment program for his addiction. Whatever his reaction, the prescription of drugs that do not mix with alcohol or other drugs such as barbiturate and non-barbiturate sedative–hypnotics, antianxiety agents, and psychotropics should be limited as much as possible. In addition, drug treatment of long duration, such as antituberculosis therapy, is less likely to be carried to completion if the patient lapses back into his abuse habits. Such patients may need extended hospitalization or close outpatient supervision to decrease their chance of spreading the disease to others.

What are the patient's cultural beliefs and personal beliefs about illness and its cure? Patients are guided by their cultural and personal beliefs about what will cure an illness. For example, many Spanish cultures follow a hot/cold theory of illness, and their folk healers prescribe foods and herbs based on the nature of an illness in relation to heat and cold. Therefore, a fever is often considered to be "hot" and would be treated with cool liquids.

Folk remedies are used by many cultures and by people of all socio-economic classes. Vitamins and other products sold in health-food stores represent other forms of folk remedies that may be taken because of a personal belief in their benefit. As long as the folk remedy does not interfere with the prescribed treatment, the nurse should plan to incorporate both regimens into the patient's care rather than to try to get the patient to give it up. When there is a conflict between the treatments, the patient is likely to use the folk cure first or to interchange the two treatments. If his remedy fails to produce results he may follow the established medication regimen, try a new folk cure, or do both. The patient will perceive that he is compliant with the nurse's treatment plan with modifications based on his freedom to make choices.

When evaluating a patient's belief system, the nurse will begin to realize that patients always make choices about their treatment plan. Patients may stop taking medications for many reasons; the side-effects may be worse than the original symptoms; the pill may be associated with being sick. Nurses need to recognize that despite a well-organized teaching plan and much discussion with the patient about his perceptions, the ultimate choice to participate in treatment rests with the patient.

Intervention

Nursing interventions reflect the actual strategies used to implement the plan and meet its goals. Interventions related to drug therapy vary widely. The nurse must learn to interpret, transcribe, and carry out drug orders correctly. This is discussed in detail in Chapter 7. Safe drug administration also involves mastery of a series of techniques and knowledge of when to use them. Chapter 8 provides information on this aspect of nursing intervention.

Implementation of the patient teaching plan is an integral part of the intervention component. Actions may be as complex as setting up an audio-visual demonstration or observing a return demonstration of insulin self-injection or as simple as reminding a patient to drink extra fluids while on antibiotic therapy. Each time a nurse administers a drug there is an opportunity to teach the patient something about that drug.

The nurse must also monitor the patient for the development of side-effects or adverse reactions to a drug. Such monitoring includes observing for symptoms, questioning the patient, and collecting physiologic data. Examples of these may include monitoring the patient's appetite or sleep cycle, taking vital signs, auscultating heart or lung sounds, and collecting laboratory data. A simple flow sheet, usually part of the patient's record, can be used to systematically document the effects of a drug if appropriate parameters are asterisked or noted in some way. If necessary, a separate form may be used, a strategy frequently employed when a specific response is sought such as change in blood pressure or relief from pain.

Psychologic responses to drugs are equally important and monitoring should be diligent. Many drugs seriously alter mental status over time, leading to depression and even suicidal tendencies. The elderly are especially prone to such changes. Drugs can also have paradoxical effects that may manifest as psychologic responses. For example, methylphenidate (Ritalin) used in the treatment of hyperactivity in children can cause an increase in hyperactivity, a sign that the drug is not working. The parents may fail to recognize the change, since hyperactivity is the norm, unless they are given a time frame within which a change should occur and told when to seek help.

Physiologic symptoms may also be misinterpreted as normal psychologic deterioration, especially in the elderly. For example, digoxin toxicity can manifest as a change in vision resulting in the patient seeing green and yellow haloes around objects. Unless the nurse is aware of this symptom such a report might be misconstrued as a hallucination or senility when in fact it demonstrates a life-threatening reaction that must be dealt with immediately.

The manner in which a nurse approaches a patient can enhance the patient's response to any medication. This is a part of the phenomenon called the *placebo response* and refers to any action that produces an effect in a patient because of its implicit or explicit intent (McCaffery, 1982). The placebo response can be used to enhance the effectiveness of any drug because the care giver's approach has been shown to influence drug therapy as well as other regimens. The first step in the process is to establish a climate of trust. Once the nurse has accomplished this, other strategies can also enhance therapy. These are listed in Table 6-1. A thorough discussion of the placebo response and administration of pain medication is found in Chapter 22.

Evaluation

The best way to review the success of a nursing care plan is to determine which nursing interventions succeeded or failed. This can be achieved by looking at the outcome criteria established in the planning phase. The outcomes can be divided into two categories: objective parameters and subjective parameters.

Objective outcomes reflect the physiologic response to a drug and include maintenance of therapeutic drug plasma levels; normal laboratory values (*i.e.*, a return to normal blood glucose); changes in symptoms (*i.e.*, decreased blood pressure, absence of arrhythmias); or absence of adverse reactions. The outcome is easily measured in most cases.

Subjective outcomes reflect the patient's ability to manage the drug regimen. They can measure completion of a prescription within the expected time frame, demonstration of the ability to administer a drug correctly, early reporting of adverse effects, appropriate management of side-effects, and arrival at appointed follow-up visits. While somewhat more difficult to measure, the success of these outcomes can be established by agreement between the nurse and the patient that the outcomes were achieved.

Failure to meet the established outcomes must be explored. New plans and outcomes will be established based on why the first plan failed. Outcome failures can occur because the drug dose was wrong, the side-effects were worse than the symptoms, or the symptoms failed to respond as expected, but the main reason for treatment failure is that the patient stopped taking the drug. Why he

Table 6-1
Nursing Strategies to Enhance Drug Effectiveness

Strategy	Examples
Use a positive approach.	"This antibiotic is usually very effective against bronchitis."
Use convincing stimuli.	The intravenous route of administration is usually more convincing than the oral route.
	"This pain medication is called Demerol and should start giving you relief in about 10 to 15 minutes."
Provide comfort measures.	Backrub, change of position, change of linen, decreasing environmental stimuli such as light or noise can all improve comfort.
Meet basic needs.	Explore the pain or other symptoms with the patient, use active listening techniques, and attempt to show empathy for the patient's condition.

stopped taking the drug may be related to its effects or it may be related to inadequate knowledge, memory deficit, a lack of family support, a loss of faith in the care givers, or a lack of money. He may also have no reason. Nevertheless, the nurse needs to explore these factors with the patient and provide a climate for discussion and for trust if drug therapy is to be successful.

A summary of the nursing process as described in this chapter is provided in Nursing Care Plan 6-1. Throughout the book, sample care plans for selected drug groups are provided that follow these guidelines. Assessment focuses on specific information needed prior to drug therapy. Nursing diagnoses and collaborative problems are listed along with expected outcomes and appropriate nursing interventions. It is hoped these samples will provide the reader with sufficient information to organize care plans for the patient on drug therapy.

The Changing Scope of Practice: Practitioners, Protocols, Prescriptions, and Policies

Most state nurse practice acts contain language that includes the carrying out of physicians' orders as part of the nurse's function, which was previously interpreted to mean that only the physician could prescribe orders. In the 1960s the need for more health-care providers led to the development of programs to prepare nurse practitioners. A nurse practitioner is defined by the American Nurses Association as a licensed, registered nurse who diagnoses and treats potential and actual health problems through such procedures as case finding, health teaching, counseling, and restorative measures in care and prevention. In some states, the nurse practitioner must be master's prepared or earn a certificate from an accredited practitioner program and have passed a certification examination given by the American Nurses Association.

As the role of the practitioner flourished, protocols were developed to guide the nurse's practice. A protocol is a treatment plan developed by nurse practitioners in collaboration with a physician mentor and a pharmacist consultant. The plan describes what actions a nurse practitioner can initiate as a primary care provider in certain disease categories, including the prescription of certain medications, which are approved by the physician mentor. Protocols have been developed for the treatment of such common conditions as colds, sore throats, and flu; stabilized chronic conditions such as hypertension and diabetes; and health-related conditions such as birth control and pregnancy.

Nurse practitioners have been extremely successful in effectively using protocols with prescription of medications. A Michigan study found that nurse practitioners were judicious in their prescription of drugs; tended to emphasize treatment alternatives other than drug therapy; and frequently established therapeutic relationships with clients that were based on improved communication and caring (Munroe et al, 1982). While the report stressed that consumers did not need any more providers to prescribe drugs indiscriminately, it emphasized that the nurse practitioners were careful and appropriate in their prescribing practices.

Recently several states have endorsed the limited prescription of drugs by nurse practitioners and others may follow as nurses seek direct reimbursement for their services from third-party payors. The scope of practice may continue to change as alternatives to the high cost of health care are sought. Nurses have long stated they could economically decrease the cost of health care to consumers. This assertion may be tested in the coming decade.

Scope of practice is also limited by institutional policies regarding the nurse's role in drug therapy. Questions regarding who can administer intravenous push medications, intravenous drips, or certain drugs are decided by various practice, pharmacy, or nursing committees in institutions as well as by the state regulatory board for nursing. Nurses should be aware of who is making decisions on their practice, by what standards the decisions are made, and what input is obtained from the nurses affected. In order to do this, nurses should sit on any institutional committee that develops practice standards for nursing.

Collegial Relationships

Mention has been made throughout this section about the need for adequate communication between physician and nurse to ensure patient safety in medication administration. The volume of drugs

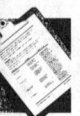

Nursing Care Plan 6-1
Guidelines for Applying the Nursing Process to Medication Administration

Assessment

A. Subjective Data

Perform a nursing assessment specific for medications, which includes the following:

1. Medication History
   a. Current medications being used (prescribed, OTC, borrowed, or street drugs) including the person's knowledge of why the drug is being taken, how it is taken, how often it is taken, and if any side-effects have been noted
   b. Potential for interactions between newly added drug and current regimen
   c. Potential for physical incompatibilities between IV drugs
   d. Past allergies/adverse reactions to drugs
2. Patient's description of symptoms related to drug use
3. Medical history that contraindicates drug use or warrants cautious use (See Contraindications and Precautions section for each drug.) Determine if the patient is pregnant or lactating.
4. Compliance issues/personal history
   a. Compliance with present or past regimens
   b. Cultural, financial, religious, or psychosocial factors that may impede compliance
   c. Ability to read and understand English

B. Objective Data

1. Physical Assessment
   a. Highlight the parameters that must be assessed as a baseline in order to determine drug effectiveness or the onset of side-effects.
   b. Height and weight may be essential in determining accurate drug dose.
   c. Cognitive or psychomotor functioning should be reviewed to determine the patient's ability to manage the regimen.
2. Laboratory data: baseline parameters needed to determine drug effectiveness or onset of side-effects

Nursing Diagnosis	Planning/Evaluation	Intervention
A. Analyze the above data to identify *actual* and *potential* nursing diagnoses and collaborative problems. B. Use NANDA-accepted nursing diagnoses whenever possible. (See the list of approved nursing diagnoses on page 66.) C. Remember that people taking medications will have a high potential for having the nursing diagnosis of "Knowledge Deficit." Only those who have demonstrated a high level of knowledge and familiarity with their medicinal regime can be excluded from having this diagnosis.	A. Write a measurable, client-centered goal (expected outcome) for each nursing diagnosis that you have identified. In the care plans throughout this book, these goals will be found under the heading Expected Client Outcome. Evaluation can only occur in actual practice when a nursing intervention has been tried. B. Be sure that the goals are realistic, have a time frame for achievement, are congruent with other therapies, and are shared with the patient (or caretaker) if appropriate. C. Collaborate with physician/phar-	A. Identify nursing interventions that treat actual nursing diagnoses and prevent potential nursing diagnoses. Most nursing interventions for drug therapy occur in the following areas: 1. Correct, safe drug administration or teaching safe drug taking to the patient 2. Monitoring the person for signs of adverse reactions/side-effects of medications (e.g., follow serum electrolytes levels if the person is taking a diuretic) 3. Patient teaching, which considers previous knowledge,

(continued)

Nursing Diagnosis	Planning/Evaluation	Intervention
	macist to establish the most appropriate medication regime (*e.g.,* consider food and drug interactions, and whether the patient can chew). D. Compare actual observable behaviors with goals/outcome criteria (established in the planning phase) to determine the level of goal achievement. 　1. If goals are not met, determine why, and revise plan. 　2. If goals are met, terminate the plan of care.	learner readiness, and ability to read, write, and communicate. Include the family when appropriate. B. Chart daily what you see, hear, do, and teach the patient regarding medication regime. 　1. Include side-effects/adverse reactions/responses to therapy (*e.g.,* whether pain was relieved). 　2. Remember to chart injection sites, as well as times. 　3. Document site and condition of any IVs (*e.g.,* "right forearm IV infusing well, no redness or pain"). 　4. Document vital signs before and after powerful cardiac drugs, vasodilators, vasopressors, or antipyretics.

available is so large and so frequently changing that knowing everything about all drugs is impossible. Therefore, the pharmacist can also assist by ensuring safe drug-prescribing patterns, acting as a resource for the nurse in the field as well as in the institution, and suggesting alternatives when therapies fail.

Other colleagues will be concerned about a patient's drug therapy, so communication of that information is essential. The physical therapist may need to know if a new antihypertensive drug is causing a patient to have periods of dizziness before getting the patient started on an active physical therapy regimen. The respiratory therapist may want to time certain treatments around a patient's pain medication schedule. The social worker and public health nurse coordinator may want to time interviews with the patient based on medication schedules, particularly if the patient is anxious or in pain. The nurse serves at the center of these interactions since she spends the most time with the patient. Sharing this information with others can positively affect the outcome of their interventions with the patient and should be encouraged.

The Informed Consumer

Much lay literature is now devoted to assisting people to become more knowledgeable about their health care. Articles devoted to cardiac drugs, over-the-counter medications, and the hazards of street drugs have created consumers who will ask more questions about their medications than ever before.

Dealing with informed consumers means that nurses can no longer justify not telling a patient the name of his medication, what the drug does to his body, and what side-effects he might expect. "Your doctor ordered this for you" is no longer the appropriate response to a patient's question about his drug treatment. In this age of knowledge explosion the nurse must give appropriate, correct information to the patient. Nurses are the people most likely to be available when patients have questions about their medicines; therefore, nurses need to be knowledgeable about the drugs they administer. The informed consumer demands it. A pill-pushing robot will not do.

REVIEW QUESTIONS

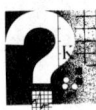

1. What basic information is most important when obtaining a drug history from a patient?
2. Phrase a short dialogue of tactful, open-ended questions to ask a patient about street drug use.
3. What two major categories of problem statements are most frequently used for patients on drug therapy? Give an example of each.
4. What requirements should patient care goals meet? Write two patient care goals that meet all the requirements for a patient who must take an antibiotic medication (Bactrim DS) for a urinary tract infection for two weeks.
5. How can the nurse measure whether a nursing action works? When should a nursing action be measured? State how to evaluate whether the following nursing action worked: "The nurse gave the new diabetic a small booklet that described what insulin does to the body, and what happens when a patient gets too much or too little insulin."
6. What are the five desired outcomes of any medication education program?
7. What variables influence whether the patient will learn about his medication?
8. What part will cultural beliefs play in a medication regimen? How should a nurse plan care with this in mind?
9. What is a treatment protocol? Who may carry out a treatment protocol that includes medication prescriptions?
10. Who determines what medication a nurse can give in the agency where you practice? What role do nurses play in the decision-making process?
11. How can the nurse use other colleagues as resources? What are the nurse's appropriate resources for discussing a patient's drug therapy?

BIBLIOGRAPHY

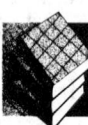

Alfaro R: Application of the Nursing Process. Philadelphia, JB Lippincott, 1986

ASHP and ANA Guidelines for Collaboration of Pharmacists and Nurses in Institutional Care Settings. Am J Hosp Pharm 37:253, 1980

Carnevali DL: Nursing Care Planning: Diagnosis and Management, 3rd ed. Philadelphia, JB Lippincott, 1983

Conway-Rutkowski B: The nurse—also an educator, patient advocate and counselor. Nurs Clin North Am 17(3):41, 1982

Hageman P, Ventura M: Utilizing patient outcome criteria to measure the effects of a medication teaching regimen. West J Nurs Research 3(1):25, 1981

LaBar C: Filling in the blanks on prescription writing. Am J Nurs 86:30, 1986

Lunney M: Nursing diagnoses: Refining the system. Am J Nurs 82:456, 1982

Markowitz JS et al: Nurses, physicians and pharmacists: Their knowledge of hazards of medications. Nurs Res 30:366, 1981

McCaffery M: Would you administer placebos for pain? Nursing '82 12:80, 1982

Moree NA: Nurses speak out: On patients and drug regimens. Am J Nurs 85:51, 1985

Munroe D et al: Prescribing patterns of nurse practitioners. Am J Nurs 82:1538, 1982

Perry SW, Heidrich G: Placebo response: Myth and matter. Am J Nurs 81:720, 1981

Romankiewicz JA: To improve patient adherence to drug regimens: An interdisciplinary approach. Am J Nurs 78:1216, 1978

Trekas J: It takes 2 to achieve compliance. Nursing '84 14:58, 1984

Legal Aspects of Drug Therapy

7

Although many natural products, such as plant extracts, have been used for centuries in treating various disease states, it is only within the last one hundred years that the federal government has become involved in the regulation and standardization of drug products. A number of federal laws have been enacted during the 20th century whose purpose has been to protect the public from fraudulent claims and misbranded medications and to ensure safety as well as efficacy in drug products brought to market. The first part of this chapter will examine the most important federal drug laws in detail.

The safety and efficacy of new drug products is in large measure due to the lengthy and stringent requirements of both preclinical and clinical testing prior to the approval and subsequent marketing of a drug substance. The various phases of the preclinical and clinical trial of a drug will also be described in this chapter. Likewise, the guidelines for rating the efficacy of older drugs already on the market at the time the requirement for clinical testing of new drugs was enacted into law will be outlined.

Finally, the legal implications of drug therapy as they apply to nurses will be given due consideration.

Drug Legislation

While some legislative attempts were made in the late 1800s to regulate adulterated articles used for food or drink, the first important federal law concerning drugs was enacted on June 30, 1906, namely the Wiley-Heyburn Act, more commonly known as the Pure Food and Drug Act, which took effect in 1907. Prompted by public outcry over the lack of purity in food and drugs, the act was passed in an attempt to prohibit adulteration and misbranding of food or drugs in interstate commerce. Sale of preparations containing any of the listed narcotic or habit-forming drugs without a proper label that indicated the name of the drug and the quantity contained in the preparation was prohibited. Under this law, however, accurate labeling was all that the federal government could require. Further provisions were the designation of the *United States Pharmacopeia* (USP) and the *National Formulary* (NF) as the *official* standards for establishing the strength, quality, and purity of medications recognized therein when sold in interstate commerce and the establishment of the Food

and Drug Administration (FDA) as the regulatory agency to enforce the law.

Thus, drugs listed in the USP or NF are designated as *official drugs* and conform to the standards of strength, purity, packaging safety, labeling, and so on, that are set by these compendia. Drugs meeting these standards can be identified by the letters USP or NF following their name. In order to maintain these publications as current as possible, they are revised every 5 years by a committee of scientists from various disciplines, such as pharmacology, pharmaceutical chemistry, medicine, nursing, and microbiology, among others. In the past, the USP and NF were separate entities, but because of their close similarity in style and content, they were combined into a single publication (USP–NF) in 1980. Since this publication is revised only every 5 years, many new drugs do not appear in the USP–NF until several years after they have become available. Thus, it is important to recognize that even though a new drug may not be classified as *official*, having not yet appeared in the official compendium, this should not be viewed as intimating lack of efficacy, safety, or purity; the term *official* merely connotes inclusion in the USP–NF.

The 1906 Pure Food and Drug Act, while certainly a noble attempt to bring some order to drug prescribing, had many shortcomings. For example, under the act, as previously mentioned, accurate *content* labeling was all that was required; thus, fraudulent advertising claims were not controllable. This deficiency was rectified by the passage of the Sherley Amendment in 1912, which prohibited use of fraudulent advertising claims. The 1906 Act, supplemented by the 1912 Amendment, stood as the major piece of federal legislation on drug efficacy for over 30 years, and, while deficient in many aspects, was nevertheless a starting point in the federal government's drive to regulate the sale of drug products more closely.

In 1937, approximately 100 people died following ingestion of a drug labeled "Elixir of Sulfanilamide." It was subsequently determined that the cause of death was not the sulfanilamide, but the solvent diethylene glycol, a poisonous substance, which is now used as an automotive antifreeze. Since at that time the only drug law related to drug labeling, the only charge that could be made against the manufacturer was that the product was mislabeled, since an elixir is by definition an alcoholic solution. This tragedy, however, gave impetus to the passage of the next major piece of drug legislation, the Federal Food, Drug and Cosmetic

Act of 1938. This Act was quite comprehensive in nature and contained a number of provisions intended to ensure both the safety and the efficacy of drug products. Among the important requirements of this act were the following:

1. Required that new drugs be demonstrated to be safe before being marketed, by toxicity testing in the laboratory
2. Required that all drugs (prescription and non-prescription) be properly labeled
3. Designated certain drugs as "habit-forming" and required that these drugs be so labeled
4. Required that "good manufacturing procedures" be followed in the processing of drugs, according to standards set by the FDA

In spite of its comprehensive nature, the 1938 act also had several deficiencies, and a number of amendments were added in later years in an attempt to rectify some of these shortcomings. The first important amendment was enacted in 1952, and termed the *Durham-Humphrey Amendment* after its sponsors. The most important provision of this amendment was the designation of certain drugs as being available by prescription only. These drugs, termed *legend* drugs, must bear the words "Caution: Federal law prohibits dispensing without prescription" on their containers. This amendment also prohibited refilling of such drugs without authorization and presented guidelines about oral and telephone orders for prescription drugs and refills. In addition, the Durham-Humphrey Amendment recognized another class of drugs, namely those that were safe for use without medical prescription, the so-called *over-the-counter* (OTC) drugs. Proper labeling procedures for OTC drugs were also provided in this amendment.

Despite the existing drug laws, federal control over drug advertising and marketing practices was still inadequate, according to many observers, and in 1958, US Senator Estes Kefauver launched a controversial Senate investigation of the drug industry. Although Senator Kefauver received little initial support from the public, another tragic event occurred in the early 1960s, and spurred the investigation. This event, known as the Thalidomide Catastrophe, occurred in Western Europe in 1962. Thalidomide, a seemingly innocuous hypnotic drug, was taken by hundreds of pregnant women; many of the offspring born to these women had severe birth defects. This tragedy helped spur passage of the *Kefauver-Harris Amendment* to the Federal Food, Drug and Cosmetic Act in 1962. Among the important provisions of this amendment was the requirement that

drugs be proven *effective* as well as *safe* before being marketed. The FDA was given authority to oversee and regulate the procedures by which new drugs were tested for safety and efficacy. Prescription drug advertising guidelines were tightened considerably, as were guidelines for investigational use of drugs on humans. Quality control laws for drug manufacturing were upgraded, and the role of the FDA in registering, monitoring and inspecting drug manufacturers was greatly increased. The Kefauver-Harris Amendment was the strongest piece of federal legislation yet enacted to ensure good manufacturing practices, truth in advertising, and safety as well as efficacy of drug products.

Prior to the 1962 Kefauver-Harris Amendment, approval of new drugs was based solely on demonstration of safety, as outlined in the Federal Food, Drug and Cosmetic Act of 1938. One provision of the 1962 amendment granted the FDA the right to regulate the efficacy, as well as the safety, of all drugs marketed since 1938, not just the drugs introduced beginning in 1962. Thus, drug products marketed between 1938 and 1962 had to be reevaluated to determine their efficacy. To facilitate this task, the FDA contracted with the National Academy of Sciences (NAS) and its research division, the National Research Council (NRC), to evaluate the efficacy data and therapeutic claims of the drug products. This study was called the Drug Efficacy Study Implementation (DESI). Based on the results of the evaluation, every drug was classified into one of six categories as follows:

1. *Effective*—Considerable evidence of effectiveness for the designated indications
2. *Probably effective*—More evidence is necessary to conclusively demonstrate effectiveness
3. *Possibly effective*—Little evidence to suggest effectiveness for the recommended indications
4. *Ineffective*—No significant evidence of effectiveness
5. *Ineffective as a fixed combination*—No evidence to suggest all components of the combination are necessary for the claimed effect, although one or more components may be effective if given alone
6. *Effective but*—A restriction or qualification must be added to the labeling

Drugs rated as ineffective were withdrawn from the market. Those rated either probably effective or possibly effective must carry their rating on the label, and their manufacturers are given additional time by the FDA to either substantiate their claims or withdraw the drugs from the market. Throughout this book, drugs rated less than completely effective for a particular indication will be noted in the appropriate section.

Narcotic Drug Laws

Misuse and abuse of mind-altering drugs, such as narcotics, stimulants, and hypnotics, has been a part of human culture for centuries, but it was not until 1914 that the first federal law aimed at controlling traffic in some of these so-called illicit drugs was enacted. The *Harrison Narcotic Act of 1914* established, among other things, the word *narcotic* and legally defined it, and established regulations governing the importation, manufacture, sale, or use of opium, cocaine, and their derivatives. Subsequent revisions of the Harrison Narcotic Act provided similar guidelines relative to marijuana and many newer synthetic opiate drugs. This law, with minor periodic revisions, stood for over 50 years, but, unfortunately, gradually became obsolete and was ineffective in rectifying the burgeoning drug-abuse problem. In an attempt to put more teeth into federal control of habituating drugs, Congress, on May 1, 1971, passed the *Comprehensive Drug Abuse Prevention and Control Act of 1970*, which superseded all previous federal drug laws regulating narcotics and other dangerous drugs. This piece of legislation, commonly referred to as the *Controlled Substances Act*, was designed to control the manufacturing, distribution, administration, and disposition of narcotics, depressants, stimulants, and other drugs having abuse potential as designated by the Drug Enforcement Administration (DEA), a government agency responsible for enforcing the provisions of the Controlled Substances Act.

Among its many provisions, the Controlled Substances Act classified the various drugs subject to abuse into one of five *schedules* according to their medical usefulness and potential for abuse. The drugs comprising the various schedules are given in Table 7-1. Regulations governing each group of drugs are as follows:

Schedule I. Drugs in Schedule I have a *high* abuse potential and *no accepted* medical use in the United States. They are not available for routine prescription use, but may be obtained for investigational studies by proper application to the Drug Enforcement Administration.

Schedule II. Drugs in Schedule II have valid medical indications, but exhibit a *high* abuse potential. Misuse of these substances can lead to profound psychologic and physical dependence.

Schedule III. Drugs in Schedule III have a potential for abuse less than those in Schedule I or II; however, misuse can still lead to moderate to low physical dependence and rather high psychologic dependence.

Schedule IV. Drugs in Schedule IV have a lower abuse potential than Schedule III drugs. Misuse most often results in varying degrees of psychologic dependence, with occasional reports of limited physical dependence.

Schedule V. Schedule V drugs consist mainly of preparations containing moderate amounts of opioid drugs, generally for antitussive or antidiarrheal use. Their abuse potential is less than Schedule IV drugs.

Each commercial container of a controlled substance bears on its label a symbol designating the schedule to which it belongs. Symbols are a large red ''C,'' either enclosing or followed by the Roman numeral I through V referring to the schedule to which the drug belongs.

The following discussion pertains to the various requirements for ordering and dispensing controlled substances. The pharmacology of these substances, together with a review of procedures for recognizing and treating drug abuse will be found in Chapter 85.

Prescribing and Dispensing Controlled Drugs

The requirements for dispensing a controlled drug outlined below are the currently mandated federal regulations. However, it should be stressed that in many instances, individual *state* laws are more stringent than the *federal* law, and must be observed by all practitioners within a particular state. Persons handling controlled substances must therefore acquaint themselves with those specific state regulations, if any, that supersede the federal law.

All prescription orders for Schedule II drugs must be either typewritten or written in ink or indelible pencil and signed by the physician. No prescriptions for Schedule II drugs may be refilled, and all records and inventory information must be maintained separately from the other pharmacy records. A triplicate order form is necessary for ordering Schedule II drugs. Under certain emergency

Table 7-1
Schedules of Controlled Drugs

Schedule I

benzylmorphine
cannabinols (e.g., hashish, marijuana)
dihydromorphine
hallucinogens (e.g., bufotenin, DET,
  DMT, DOB, DOM, ibogaine, LSD,
  MDA, mescaline, peyote, PMA,
  psilocybin, psilocyn)
ketobemidone
levomoramide
nicocodeine
nicomorphine
racemoramide

Schedule II

Depressants
amobarbital
methaqualone
pentobarbital
phencyclidine
secobarbital

Narcotics
alfentanil
alphaprodine
codeine
etorphine
fentanyl
hydromorphone
levorphanol
meperidine
methadone
opium and opium alkaloids (e.g.,
  morphine and codeine)
oxycodone
oxymorphone
phenazocine
sufentanil

Stimulants
amphetamine
coca leaves
cocaine
dextroamphetamine
methamphetamine
methylphenidate
phenmetrazine

Cannabinoids
dronabinol
nabilone

Schedule III

Depressants
aprobarbital
butabarbital
chlorhexadol
glutethimide

Schedule III (continued)

hexobarbital
metharbital
methyprylon
talbutal
thiamylal
thiopental

Narcotics
opiates in combination with other
  non-narcotic drugs (e.g., Empirin
  with Codeine, Tylenol with
  Codeine, Hycodan)
paregoric

Stimulants
benzphetamine
chlorphentermine
mazindol
phendimetrazine

Schedule IV

Depressants
barbital
benzodiazepines (alprazolam,
  chlordiazepoxide, clonazepam,
  clorazepate, diazepam, flurazepam,
  halazepam, lorazepam, midazolam,
  oxazepam, prazepam, temazepam,
  triazolam)
chloral hydrate
ethchlorvynol
ethinamate
mephobarbital
meprobamate
methohexital
paraldehyde
phenobarbital

Narcotics
pentazocine
propoxyphene

Stimulants
diethylpropion
fenfluramine
pemoline
phentermine

Schedule V

buprenorphine
diphenoxylate and atropine (e.g.,
  Lomotil)
loperamide
narcotic drugs in combination with
  other non-narcotic agents,
  generally used as antitussives,
  where the amount of narcotic (e.g.,
  codeine, dihydrocodeine) is limited

situations outlined below, a Schedule II drug may be dispensed on oral authorization.

Orders for Schedule III, IV, and those Schedule V drugs requiring a prescription (see below) may be issued either orally or in writing and may be refilled up to five times within 6 months of the original prescription date if so authorized by the physician. Oral prescription orders must be immediately committed to writing. Prescriptions for drugs in Schedule III, IV, or V must be readily retrievable from the files, and if these controlled substances prescriptions are filed with the remainder of the prescription orders (except Schedule II drugs), each prescription for a Schedule III, IV, or V drug must be marked with the letter "C" in red ink to facilitate retrieval. Records must be maintained for at least 2 years.

Each time a prescription for a Schedule III, IV, or V drug is refilled, the date and amount of drug dispensed must be noted on the back of the order blank and initialed by the dispenser. The label of any controlled drug in Schedule II, III, or IV must contain the following statement "Caution: Federal law prohibits the transfer of this drug to any person other than the patient for whom it was prescribed."

PARTIAL DISTRIBUTION
OF CONTROLLED SUBSTANCES

If the full quantity of a Schedule II drug cannot be supplied with the original prescription order, the remaining portion may be dispensed within 72 hours provided the quantity dispensed with the initial order is noted on the face of the written prescription. Additional partial quantities may not be supplied beyond the 72-hour time limit except on a new prescription order.

Partial dispensing of Schedule III and IV drugs is allowed provided the quantity dispensed is noted on the back of the prescription order. The balance of the partial quantities dispensed may not exceed the total amount authorized (that is, original quantity plus allowable refills), nor extend past the 6-month time limit.

EMERGENCY DISPENSING
OF SCHEDULE II DRUGS

In the event of an emergency situation, a Schedule II controlled substance can be dispensed on oral authorization provided certain conditions are satisfied. An emergency situation is defined as one in which

1. *Immediate* administration of the drug is necessary for proper treatment.

2. No appropriate alternative treatment is available.
3. A written prescription cannot reasonably be provided by the prescribing physician before the drug is required.

The provisions for dispensing a Schedule II drug under an emergency situation are as follows:

1. Quantity dispensed must be limited to the amount necessary to treat the patient during the emergency period.
2. Prescription order must be reduced to writing immediately.
3. All efforts to verify the identity of the prescriber should be made, in the event that he is not known to the dispenser.
4. A written prescription with the notation "Authorization for Emergency Dispensing" must be delivered to the dispenser within 72 hours of the oral authorization, or if mailed, postmarked within 72 hours.

NONPRESCRIPTION DISPENSING
OF SCHEDULE V DRUGS

Certain Schedule V preparations may be dispensed without a prescription providing the following conditions are met:

1. The dispensing is done only by a pharmacist or pharmacist-intern.
2. The purchaser is at least 18 years of age (proof of age is necessary if the purchaser is unknown to the dispenser).
3. Not more than 240 ml or not more than 48 solid dosage units of any substance containing opium, nor more than 120 ml or not more than 24 solid dosage units of any other controlled substance may be distributed to the same purchaser within 48 hours.
4. The name and address of the purchaser, kind and quantity of substance purchased, date of sale, and pharmacist's initials must be recorded for each sale in a Schedule V record book and records maintained for 2 years.

State and local laws often are more stringent with respect to retail distribution of Schedule V substances, and must be observed in lieu of the federal law.

A practitioner (physician, dentist, veterinarian) must apply for permission to dispense controlled drugs by registering with the Drug Enforcement Administration and, on approval, receives a 7-digit registration number (DEA number) that must appear on every order for controlled substances. This registration must be renewed annually. Likewise, every pharmacy that dispenses controlled drugs must register annually with the Drug Enforcement Administration, and their DEA numbers must be available for inspection at the location of business.

The Nurse's Role in Administration of Controlled Drugs

The nurse is guided in the administration of controlled substances by agency policies, which reflect state and federal regulations. In any institution, whether acute or extended care, controlled drugs must be kept in a locked cabinet with access to these medications limited to certain personnel. Agency policy states the frequency with which the stock must be counted (usually every shift); who may give the drugs; how the drugs are to be obtained from the central pharmacy; and who bears ultimate responsibility for loss of any of these drugs. State regulatory agencies generally investigate all losses of controlled substances, so such incidents must be accurately reported.

Institutional policies also reflect the frequency with which controlled drugs are to be reordered. The nurse must comply with these policies and ensure that such drugs are reordered promptly. In acute-care settings, it may be necessary to reorder some Schedule II drugs every 24 hours to 48 hours, whereas orders for drugs in other categories may be valid for 7 days. In extended-care facilities, orders may be written and renewed once every 30 days. Whatever the time limitation, the nurse is responsible for monitoring the response to the drugs administered and for reporting to the physician evidence of change in pain control, development of tolerance, addiction behaviors, or toxic reactions related to the medication. Changes may occur without warning, so the nurse should document the patient's response to the drug each time it is administered.

In the home-care setting, the patient and his family are responsible for obtaining the controlled medication through a local pharmacy. Therefore, the nurse must monitor the patient's response to the drug and report any changes to the physician. If suspicions arise that the patient or another family member has abused the drug, such information should be shared with the physician and the dispensing pharmacist. The frequency of refill requests can then be monitored. Hospice nurses report that this problem occurs occasionally, and is best dealt with by professionals—the physician,

pharmacist, nurse, and regulatory agencies—rather than by a single person making an accusation.

Drug Development

The evolution from laboratory chemical to marketable medication is a slow, tedious, frustrating, and very expensive process. For every 10,000 chemicals tested in the laboratory, approximately ten show sufficient promise to be given a human clinical trial. Of these ten, frequently only one may ultimately receive final approval to be marketed. This extreme attrition rate has a number of important consequences. The main advantage of the process is that the drug that finally emerges is usually the safest and most efficacious for the particular purpose of the many hundreds of compounds tested. However, there are also several disadvantages. The process is so lengthy that some people who might benefit from the drug die before it becomes available. In addition, the process is so costly that companies may opt to develop only drugs that have a reasonable assurance of producing a profit. Consequently, drugs that will be used to treat a small population or a rare disease, those that cannot be patented due to the nature of their chemical composition, or drugs that have a narrow safety margin may never reach the clinical testing stage in spite of their benefit. These are called *orphan drugs*. In 1983, Congress passed the Orphan Drug Act, which provides tax incentives for companies who are willing to manufacture such drugs. In effect, the company can use 73% of the development cost of an orphan drug as a tax credit. New drugs for the treatment of leprosy, severe hirsutism, polycythemia vera, and bleeding esophageal varices are among those recently developed as a result of these incentives.

The following discussion traces the development of a new drug through the various stages of laboratory (*i.e.*, preclinical) and clinical testing. This pathway is represented schematically in Figure 7-1.

Preclinical Testing

SOURCE OF NEW DRUG CANDIDATES
Although new drug candidates can originate in various ways, for example, by empirical screening of chemical compounds, by chemical extraction of naturally occurring substances (*e.g.*, insulin, heparin, thyroid), or simply by serendipity, today most

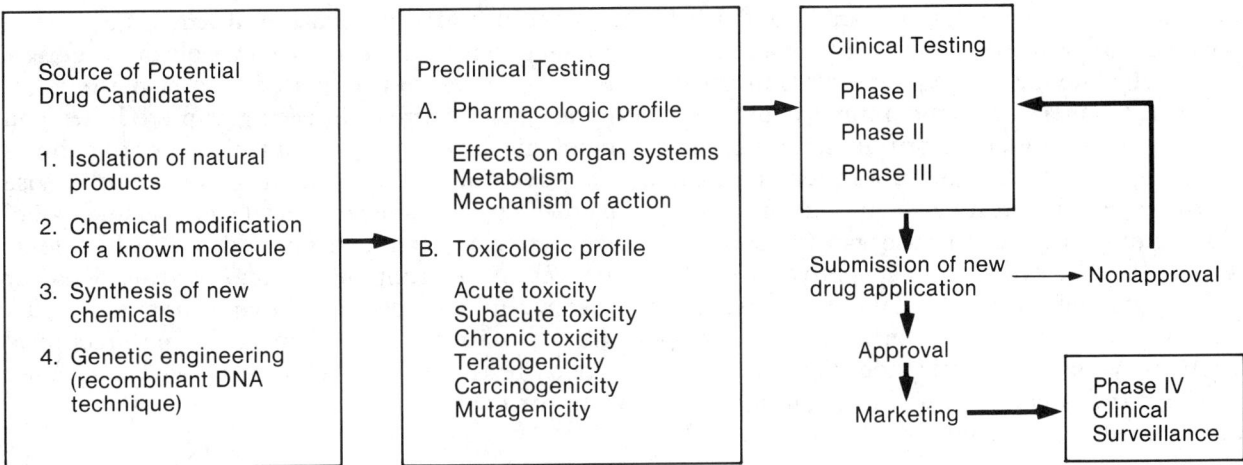

Figure 7-1. Principal stages in drug development.

new drugs result from deliberate modification of an existing drug or from logical chemical synthesis.

Once a compound shows promise as a potentially pharmacologically active agent in a series of preliminary tests, it is subjected to a wide range of *in vitro* and *in vivo* laboratory analyses, representing the *preclinical testing stage* of the candidate. This preclinical evaluation phase is divided into two parts: (1) determination of the pharmacologic profile of the compound; and (2) determination of the toxicologic profile of the compound.

PHARMACOLOGIC PROFILE

The effect of the new compound on a number of organ systems is examined in animal species. The physiologic and biochemical responses that it elicits are evaluated with respect to its potential clinical usefulness in treating certain disease states. Whenever possible, an animal model that closely approximates the human condition for which the drug is being targeted is employed in the preclinical testing phase. For example, certain animals can be made hypertensive experimentally, in order to evaluate the potential effectiveness of a new antihypertensive compound. Likewise, certain strains of mice develop specific tumors, which can be used to assess the efficacy of antitumor drugs. Perhaps the drugs that are most difficult to evaluate in animal models are the psychotherapeutic agents, since there are no reliable means for inducing a psychosis or a psychoneurosis in an animal. As the disease processes afflicting humans become better understood, it may become possible to devise better preclinical animal models.

Finally, it is essential to recognize that drug efficacy or safety as demonstrated in preclinical

animal experiments does not ensure drug efficacy or safety in the treatment of human disease states.

During the preclinical evaluation period the drug's mechanism of action is elucidated. Understanding the mechanism of action is frequently quite helpful in predicting the possible untoward reactions to be expected with use of the drug. Moreover, complications arising as a result of the drug's interactions with other drugs may thus be anticipated and minimized.

Another important element of the preclinical evaluation is the drug's metabolic profile. Various studies are carried out to ascertain its absorption and bioavailability in several animal species, as well as its mode and rate of metabolism and excretion. The extent of protein binding is also determined, and the distribution of the compound throughout the body is mapped. These metabolic studies are helpful in determining the optimal dose and route of administration to be utilized in subsequent clinical studies.

TOXICOLOGIC PROFILE

Once a drug candidate evidences promise of becoming a marketable medication, it is subjected to rigorous toxicity evaluation, according to guidelines established by the FDA. As indicated in Figure 7-1, preclinical toxicity testing encompasses six different areas, each of which is reviewed below.

Acute Toxicity

Acute toxicity testing is done in order to assess the drug's short-term toxic effects and to determine its relative margin of safety in experimental animals. A range of single doses is given to several species by different routes of administration, and the median lethal dose (LD_{50}) in milligrams per kilogram of body weight for each species and route of administration is calculated. The LD_{50} represents the dose that is fatal to one half of the animal population receiving it. This value is helpful in determining a dosage range to be used in subsequent clinical trials. Acute toxicity tests also provide information, at autopsy, of the drug's organ toxicity. By combining the data obtained in acute toxicity tests with those obtained in preclinical efficacy studies, a very important value for each drug can be obtained, namely the therapeutic index (TI). The TI is a measure of the safety margin of a drug in a particular species for a given route of administration. It is defined as follows:

$$TI = LD_{50}/ED_{50}$$

That is, the TI is the ratio of the median lethal dose to the median effective dose (ED_{50}; the dose in milligrams per kilogram of body weight producing the desired effect in 50% of the animal population). The greater the TI, the greater is the relative safety margin of the compound; however, the TI must be viewed as simply an approximation of a drug's safety, since not all animal species mirror the human in the way they handle a particular chemical compound. In addition, the TI does not apply to the occasional hypersensitive patient who may display a toxic reaction to a drug dose considered safe for the general population. Nevertheless, determination of the TI is an important step in the development of a clinical trial.

Subacute Toxicity

Doses of the drug are given to different species of animals for periods ranging from weeks to months, to assess the drug's subacute toxicity. During this period, the animals are closely observed for signs and symptoms of untoward reactions. Laboratory evaluations (e.g., hematology, urinalysis) are performed periodically, and on termination of the study, the animals are killed. Exhaustive histologic studies are then done to determine if any tissue or organ damage has occurred with prolonged use of the drug. These studies are invaluable in deciding whether the drug is sufficiently safe to be given a limited human trial.

Chronic Toxicity

Since many drugs are intended for prolonged use in humans, chronic toxicity studies must be made to assess their potential long-term effects. These studies may continue for a period of years, frequently running concurrently with the clinical trial. They

are conducted in both males and females of several animal species. All the animals are observed closely throughout the testing period, and at periodic intervals, some animals in each group are killed and histologically examined. Control groups of animals that have not received the drug but are otherwise handled in the same manner (e.g., housing, food, light) are also examined for evidence of histologic changes, since spontaneous abnormalities do occur in some animal species. The appearance of drug-induced tissue or organ damage during preclinical toxicity testing will cause the drug to be eliminated from further consideration.

Teratogenicity

Several types of specific toxicity evaluation are made during the preclinical testing. The drug's teratogenic potential, that is, its ability to induce fetal deformities, is an important aspect of the preclinical evaluation. In addition, studies are also performed to measure the drug's effect on fertility, pregnancy, and lactation.

Carcinogenicity

During the chronic toxicity studies, the animals are examined for evidence of carcinogenic changes; any indication that a compound may be capable of inducing a carcinoma in any organ is sufficient to eliminate it from further investigation. These studies are commonly performed in mice and rats, and extend over the average lifetime of the species.

Mutagenicity

Investigational drugs are also screened for mutagenicity, that is, ability to alter the genetic structure of bacteria or cultured mammalian cells. Mutagenicity testing has some value as a prescreening procedure for evidence of carcinogenic potential, but verification of a drug's capability to induce cancer can be done only in the intact animal, and is dependent on the presence of a recognizable tumor or a hematologic change.

Clinical Testing

No matter how exhaustive the preclinical evaluation, it does not afford assurance that the data thereby obtained are applicable to humans. Nevertheless, animal testing is a valuable means of assessing whether a particular compound is sufficiently active and safe to be placed into clinical trial. Very few chemicals that enter preclinical testing emerge as candidates for clinical evaluation; those that do survive preclinical testing have demonstrated a considerable degree of efficacy as well as safety in several animal species.

Once a compound is judged to be ready for evaluation in humans, the manufacturer files with the FDA a "Notice of Claimed Investigational Exemption for a New Drug," also known as an IND. Information contained in the IND includes (1) the chemical structure or composition of the drug; (2) manufacturing information; (3) data on absorption, bioavailability, and metabolism; (4) efficacy and toxicity data in animal species; (5) detailed clinical protocols for testing the drug in humans; and (6) names of the investigators who are to conduct the clinical trials. On reviewing the IND, the FDA advises the manufacturer of its decision; if the decision is favorable, the clinical trials begin.

PHASES OF CLINICAL TESTING

The clinical evaluation of an investigational drug product follows a definite sequence, and is divided into four phases (see Fig. 7-1). Depending on the drug being tested and the results obtained in the initial stages of the clinical trial, the clinical testing period may encompass several years. Throughout the clinical trial, *informed consent* of all participants must be obtained. That is, everyone participating in the clinical trial must be apprised of the purpose of the study, the drugs that are being given, and the potential risks. Not all participants, however, will necessarily receive the active drug. Rather, there is random assignation of volunteers to a treatment group or a control group. This important measure eliminates possible bias and lends credibility to the statistical analysis that will be done at a later time.

The protocols followed in the various phases of clinical testing are described below.

Phase I

Phase I is the exploratory stage of clinical testing in which the potential therapeutic dosage range of the drug is examined in a small number of normal, healthy volunteers. The pharmacokinetics of the drug in humans are compared to the corresponding data from the preclinical animal studies to establish whether humans show significantly different responses to the drug, as well as to establish the clinically useful dosage range to be used in subsequent phases of the trial. Gradually increasing doses are administered to the volunteers, and the appearance of side-effects is noted. Laboratory tests are done to detect adverse effects on the blood and organs. The principal aim of these studies is to evaluate the safety of the anticipated therapeutic dosage range of the drug. Occasionally, an unexpected side-effect occurs, one not noted during preclinical trials, and further testing may be necessary in this phase. Phase I studies are usually *nonblind*, that is, both the investigators (usually clinical pharmacologists) and the subjects know what drug and how much of it is being given.

If the drug's metabolic profile in humans is comparable to that in the experimental animals, if the anticipated dosage range is proven safe and well tolerated, and if no serious or unusual adverse reactions have occurred, Phase II studies are then initiated.

Phase II

The purpose of Phase II studies is to afford initial assessment of the drug's efficacy and safety in a group of subjects having the disease that the drug is intended to treat. The design of the Phase II study is even more important than that of Phase I, and a *double-blind* design is commonly used. That is, neither the investigators nor the subjects know whether drug or placebo is being administered to each participant in the study. This approach is used to eliminate observer bias. Control groups of subjects are employed throughout these studies; they may receive either a pharmacologically inactive substance such as lactose or an available active drug used to treat the same condition as the investigational drug, in forms that appear to be identical. The inactive form, or *placebo*, is very important in clinical drug trials. Subject response to the placebo, termed the *placebo effect*, is observed in approximately one third of all volunteers and may involve both changes in subjective complaints associated with the disease (*e.g.*, pain, anxiety, gastrointestinal distress) as well as actual physiologic changes (*e.g.*, lowered blood pressure, decreased heart rate). This placebo effect must be considered when subject response to the active drug is assessed. Thus, any improvement in the patient's condition following administration of an active drug must be greater than that observed following administration of a placebo in order for the claim to be made that the drug is effective in treating the disease symptoms for which it is intended. On the other hand, use of a currently available active drug in the control group allows the investigator to compare the efficacy of the investigational drug to that of an established drug. In either case, however, whether placebo control or active drug control, both subject and observer bias must be minimized, and double-blind studies are performed wherever possible. Other types of bias in both interpreting and analyzing results of clinical trials can be minimized in the following ways:

1. Random assignation of subjects to the various treatment groups. This results in one of two trial formats:
   a. *Parallel study*—Each subject receives only one treatment (*i.e.*, active drug or control).
   b. *Crossover study*—Each subject receives both the investigational drug and the control drug in random order; the advantage of this format is that each subject serves as his own control.
2. Matching patient population groups with regard to age, sex, and physiologic or pathologic status
3. Development of specific parameters within which drug efficacy and toxicity may be evaluated; reliance on an observer's *subjective* evaluation (*e.g.*, the patient *seems* improved) must be avoided
4. Valid, applicable statistical evaluation of the data when comparing treatment vs control groups

If the safety and efficacy of the investigational drug have been firmly established in the patient population that was tested in Phase II, Phase III studies are then undertaken.

Phase III

Phase III clinical studies represent extensive trials in a large number of patients, with the purpose of firmly establishing the optimal therapeutic regimen for the indicated disease, and obtaining data on the long-term safety and efficacy of the drug. Phase III trials are carried out, where possible, under conditions simulating those anticipated in actual clinical use, and should involve a sufficient number of patients so that any rare or serious toxic effects can be uncovered during this stage. If the investigational drug might be used in specific patient populations (*e.g.*, children, pregnant women), then studies must be performed in these patient subgroups as well. Phase III studies can continue for several years, may involve an extensive patient population, and are quite expensive. Naturally, only those drugs with a strong likelihood of ultimately gaining marketing approval are subjected to the exhaustive Phase III trials.

Once the manufacturer has determined to its satisfaction that the new drug is both safe and effective for the proposed indication, application in the form of a New Drug Application (NDA) is made to the FDA for approval to market the drug.

The NDA is usually a voluminous document containing all the relevant preclinical and clinical data. The FDA then reviews the data, a process that may take several years, although attempts are presently under way to shorten this lag time in cases of important new drugs. If the FDA approves the application, the drug may then be marketed in interstate commerce. If the application is found lacking in certain respects, the manufacturer may choose to perform the necessary additional tests or, in some cases, depending on circumstances, may withdraw the drug, either temporarily or permanently. Once approval to market a drug has been obtained, Phase IV clinical evaluation begins.

Phase IV

The postmarketing monitoring of a drug's efficacy and safety is frequently termed *Phase IV clinical study.* There is no preset duration for Phase IV studies, and the principal rationale for continually monitoring the effects of a drug following its introduction into clinical use is to ensure its safety in situations of more extensive and probably less well-controlled use than prevailed during the clinical trials. Infrequent side-effects may not be manifest during the clinical trial phases, but may become evident once the drug is placed into widespread use. An additional aim of Phase IV evaluation is to detect any drug interactions that could not have occurred during the earlier carefully controlled clinical trials. It is during this extended postmarketing evaluation as well that new indications for a drug frequently suggest themselves. For example, the first beta blocker to be approved was propranolol (Inderal) in the 1960s, and it had a very limited clinical application. Today, however, following almost twenty years of therapeutic use, propranolol has at least six approved indications and several more applications are currently being investigated.

Although it is true that a few drugs have caused serious toxicity following FDA approval and were subsequently withdrawn from the market, the majority of investigational new drugs sanctioned for therapeutic use by the FDA have proven both safe and effective for their intended indications when prescribed in a judicious manner. However, FDA approval of a drug should not be construed as implying that the drug can be employed safely and effectively in whatever manner the clinician deems appropriate. The FDA issues *approved indications* for every drug, and these are the only indications for which the drug may be advertised and dosage recommendations given. Ongoing research frequently uncovers new potential indications for many currently available drugs, but only by submitting to the FDA all the relevant data pertaining to the new indication is a manufacturer able to obtain permission to market the drug for a different condition. Some drugs, however, are commonly used for non-FDA-approved indications, as, for example, the administration of phenytoin, an antiepileptic, for control of digitalis-induced cardiac arrhythmias.

The Nurse's Role in Clinical Testing of Drugs

Nurses will frequently participate in clinical testing of drugs during Phases II, III, and IV. These investigations, classified as clinical research, must receive approval by the institutional committee that oversees human subjects study. A copy of the written approval should be available to the nursing staff before the study begins.

If the nurse is administering medication during Phase II or Phase III double-blind studies, neither she nor the physician will know which medication the patient is given. To reduce the danger arising from this lack of knowledge, all drug trials are conducted according to written protocols that set forth data on the appropriate dose, route of administration, action, and possible side-effects or adverse reactions to the drug. This information should be readily available at all times to the nurse monitoring the patient. Without such data the nurse will be inadequately prepared to make necessary judgments about administrations for which she is liable. Therefore, the nurse has the right to refuse to participate in a drug trial if protocol information has not been made available.

Drug protocols also identify the uses of the drug or drugs being tested, whether for a single drug for pain or a series of drugs for treating a type of cancer. The physician does not have the legal right to change the protocol during a clinical study. If he attempts to do so, the nurse can refuse to participate in the administration of the drug.

As a patient advocate, the nurse should be sure that the patient has given informed consent to participate in a drug trial. According to the code of Federal Regulation no. 45CFR46 (US DHEW, US Government Printing Office, January 11, 1978) there are six elements of informed consent:

1. A fair explanation of the procedures to be followed, their purposes, and the identification of any procedures that are experimental

2. A description of any attendant discomfort and risks reasonably to be expected
3. A description of any benefits reasonably to be expected
4. A disclosure of appropriate alternative procedures that might be advantageous for the subject
5. An offer to answer any inquiries about the procedure
6. An instruction that the subject is free to withdraw consent and to discontinue participation in the project or activity at any time without prejudice to himself

If the nurse believes that the patient has been inadequately informed about a drug trial (or other treatment) or is reluctant to participate, the physician should be asked to give the patient additional information. The nurse can refuse to administer the drug until the patient feels he has been adequately informed and has agreed to participate (Bell, 1981). Drug trials should not begin until the issue of informed consent is clarified.

Some patients, while participating in a drug trial, may feel they are being treated as "guinea pigs." The nurse may be the first to hear such expressions of fear and anger. Such feelings are frequently expressed by patients who have received many types of therapy that have failed. Allowing patients time to verbalize their concerns may be enough to work the problems through. Others may need encouragement to bear the discomfort of drug therapy in order to receive its possible benefit. Occasionally, as a result of multiple factors, a patient may decide to discontinue treatment. The physician should always be included when these decisions are discussed, since he is, by law, responsible for a patient's medical treatment. The nurse has an obligation to make sure that the patient has all the information he wants and needs to come to a decision. Patients and their families also need substantial emotional support, especially when the decision to stop therapy may mean certain death.

Aside from having legal and ethical responsibilities, the nurse provides valuable information about patient response in drug trials. She may be the single professional on the team who can give the highly detailed information that is needed.

Nurses also participate in Phase IV—monitoring of a drug's efficacy and safety—by collecting data about adverse drug reactions. Most institutions require that such data be collated on a special form, which is sent to the pharmacist. Pharmacists report this information to the FDA. Anyone who observes or experiences an adverse drug reaction can report it to the Medical Device and Laboratory Product Problem Reporting Program, US Pharmacopeia, 12601 Townbrook Parkway, Rockville, MD 20852, toll-free number, 800-638-6725. This agency is funded by the FDA.

Medication Orders

Proper ordering of medications is essential for safe and effective drug therapy. Transmission of the physician's wishes as to drug treatment of the patient is usually accomplished by a written order, in either a drug file or a patient chart in the case of hospitalized persons, or in the form of a prescription in the case of an outpatient. Medication orders may be given orally, by telephone, and it is important that such orders be reduced to writing as soon as possible to minimize chance of error.

Generally, persons empowered by state law to write prescriptions include physicians, dentists, and veterinarians. In some states, however, the law has been modified to permit nurse practitioners and physicians' assistants to write prescription orders for certain types of drugs. Since these laws vary from state to state, persons in these situations should acquaint themselves with the regulations in their particular area.

The Prescription

Since the prescription is the most common means for ordering drugs, let us take a closer look at the component parts of a typical prescription, as presented in Figure 7-2.

1. SUPERSCRIPTION
The patient's *full* name and address (not simply Mrs. Jones) should appear at the top of the prescription blank to avoid possible confusion in medication orders. The date of the order should always be displayed prominently, since this is the only indication as to when the order was given. Moreover, in the case of controlled Schedule III and IV drugs, prescriptions cannot be refilled after six months from the date of issuance. The patient's age should be indicated, since this affords the pharmacist a means to assess whether the dose is appropriate.

2. INSCRIPTION
The inscription refers to the name of the drug being ordered, the dosage form, and the strength of the medication. Drugs may be prescribed by either the generic (nonproprietary) name, as in the example of erythromycin in Figure 7-2, or by one of the trade (brand) names, for example, E.E.S. 400, E-Mycin E, Pediamycin 400. The merits and deficiencies of each method of prescribing have been discussed earlier in this text. Legible writing is of utmost importance in drug prescription, since many brand name drugs have similar spellings (*e.g.*, Orinase/Ornade), and medication errors have occurred. It is the responsibility of the pharmacist to clarify the physician's orders whenever a doubt exists. Abbreviations of drug names should be avoided, and when a drug is available in more than one dosage form, the desired form should be clearly specified.

3. SUBSCRIPTION
The subscription contains the dispensing instructions to the pharmacist and usually describes the number of tablets or capsules, the volume of solu-

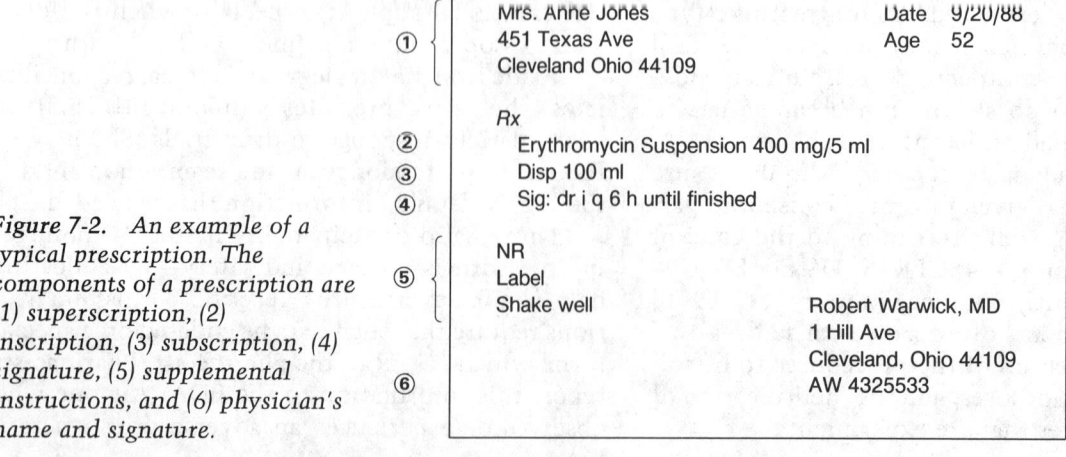

Figure 7-2. An example of a typical prescription. The components of a prescription are (1) superscription, (2) inscription, (3) subscription, (4) signature, (5) supplemental instructions, and (6) physician's name and signature.

tion or suspension, or the weight of ointment or creme. Where more than one drug is prescribed, the subscription may contain orders to mix and make a solution or a powder to be placed into capsules or suspended in a vehicle. This order is frequently abbreviated from the Latin *mistura fiat* as m. ft. (mix and make).

4. SIGNATURE

The directions to the patient make up the signature (Latin *signatura*) of the prescription order, and should contain *explicit* instructions as to how the drug should be used. This section is most often abbreviated; while the use of abbreviations is convenient and time-saving, this may result in dosing errors, inasmuch as many abbreviations are nearly identical. A list of abbreviations is found in the Appendix. For example, *od* can mean either *every day* or *right eye*, and *os* refers to the *left eye* or the *mouth*. Although the type of drug prescribed frequently eliminates such confusion (*e.g., os* in reference to an eye drop obviously means left eye and not by mouth), questions do arise on occasion as to the actual intent of the prescriber. Again, it is imperative that the directions to the patient be clearly stated before any medication is dispensed. Further, dosing instructions should be *orally* conveyed to the patient as well as typed on the prescription label, since many patients may not understand the written directions and may be hesitant to question the doctor, nurse, or pharmacist. Instructions such as "take as directed," "take when needed," and other vague terminology should never be employed; rather, very specific directions should be given. Moreover, the statement "four times a day" can be interpreted to mean anywhere from every 4 hours (*i.e.,* while awake) to every 6 hours (*i.e.,* "round the clock"). Such variation can markedly alter the plasma levels of certain drugs, possibly negating the therapeutic efficacy of very short-acting drugs if taken every 6 hours, and perhaps leading to cumulation toxicity with more slowly excreted drugs if taken every 4 hours. In general, patient directions should be as detailed as necessary to ensure proper compliance, a situation that is seriously deficient in all too many instances.

5. SUPPLEMENTAL INSTRUCTIONS

In addition to the dosing directions, other instructions to the patient as well as to the pharmacist may be included as necessary. The most commonly used supplemental instructions pertain to the number of desired refills, which may range from none (NR—

no refill) to as many as needed (prn—as needed) within the allowance of the law. Refill instructions should *always* be given on the prescription order, for if no instructions are indicated, the pharmacist must check with the physician whenever the patient requests a refill—a time-consuming procedure. Conversely, nonspecific refill instructions such as *when necessary* or *as needed* (prn) are to be discouraged, since control of drug use is then placed in the patient's hands. The federal laws governing allowable refills on controlled drugs were discussed earlier in this chapter.

Other supplemental instructions generally direct the pharmacist to place certain labels on the prescription bottle. Most physicians prefer that the drug name appear on the prescription label; such an instruction is often indicated by the word *label* or *copy* on the medication order. Labeling of prescription drugs affords quick identification in the event of an emergency. Storage and dispensing instructions, such as "Refrigerate after opening," "Shake well," "Take with food," and so on, are also occasionally noted by the physician on the medication order, but most often are supplied by the pharmacist when the prescription is filled. This aspect of patient education can be a vital part of nursing intervention in drug therapy, and nurses should attempt to acquaint themselves with those medications that may require special instructions.

6. PHYSICIAN'S NAME AND SIGNATURE

The physician's name, address, and telephone number are printed at the top of most prescription blanks; therefore, his signature is all that is necessary for most orders. In addition, whenever a controlled substance is prescribed, the physician's Drug Enforcement Administration (DEA) registry number must appear on the order form.

The Nurse's Role in Carrying Out Medication Orders

The components of the medication prescription have been clearly explained above. The rules hold whether the prescriber is writing a prescription for a patient who is at home or prescribing on an order sheet in a health-care institution. The nurse has several legal responsibilities in carrying out medication orders written in the hospital. Nurses must accurately transcribe orders to the medication record sheet, which provides a quick reference for all the medications a patient is receiving. This transcription should be clearly written so that all staff personnel will be able to read the order.

If the order has not been clearly written, the nurse should question the physician to seek clarification. Legally the standard against which nurses are judged is that they will give the *right* medication in the *right* dose, by the *right* route, at the *right* time, to the *right* patient. That standard makes the nurse liable for giving a wrong medication to a patient even if the physician who ordered it committed the error. Therefore, *when in doubt, question the order.*

There are two steps in the process of assessing the physician's order for a medication: first, an initial reading for clarity, and second, a reading for the appropriateness of the order. What has been written must be understandable and free of ambiguities. Any abbreviations, if used, must be correctly interpreted, and the order must contain all parts and information described above. Secondly, before dispensing the medication, the order must be evaluated for appropriateness. The following questions can guide the nurse in making such judgments:

1. Does the medication correspond to the patient's list of problems or diagnoses? For example, has a hypoglycemic agent been ordered for a nondiabetic patient with a normal blood glucose?

2. Does the order call for a drug that the patient may be allergic to? Information on the patient's drug allergies will be in his drug history or profile.

3. Is the dosage appropriate for the patient's body weight, or is it too large for an emaciated patient or too small for a large individual?

4. Does the patient have hepatic or renal dysfunction that may interfere with the drug's metabolism or excretion? Is the drug one that could cause further deterioration of the patient's organ function? An example of this is the order of an aminoglycoside antibiotic for a patient with already existing renal dysfunction.

5. Is the patient concurrently receiving another drug that may interfere with the therapeutic effects of the newly ordered drug? For example, has oral tetracycline been ordered with an antacid?

6. Is the patient physically able to receive the drug? Can he swallow the medication ordered to be given orally? Does he have sufficient muscle mass for a large-volume intramuscular injection? Does he have a patent intravenous line for an infusion?

7. Has there been an abrupt increase or decrease in the dosage from an amount that the patient was previously receiving? Has a drug been abruptly discontinued when it usually requires a gradual reduction of dosage, such as with propranolol or large doses of corticosteroids?

Occasionally, the nurse will be asked to take a telephone order. Institutional policies will identify the context in which this act is permitted. Many institutions require that two nurses listen to telephone orders as they are given, to ensure accuracy and appropriateness, and to protect the nurse. Telephone orders are most appropriate in emergency situations when the physician cannot be present. The accuracy of a telephone order depends on communication between sender and receiver. To ensure that the order is clear, it is always a good idea to write it down and repeat it to the physician before hanging up the telephone. The physician must cosign the order within 24 hours of giving it. Telephone orders can involve risk if the physician later denies having given the order, or if the nurse misinterprets the order. Most institutions discourage the use of telephone orders for these reasons, and nurses should be cautious about accepting them.

Lastly, nurses are responsible for administering most of the medications ordered. In order to meet the legal standard, they must be knowledgeable about the medications given, careful in administration, and alert to potential problems that may result in errors. In one study of 3000 medication errors, the most frequently committed ones were (1) failing to give a dose, (2) giving a wrong dose, and (3) giving the wrong medication. About 6% of the errors gave rise to complications (Long, 1982).

Most errors occur because nurses fail to adhere to institutional policies. Policies are designed to protect both the nurse and the patient, so familiarity with them is important. Safe medication administration depends on responsible action by a team of colleagues, all of whom are legally accountable. The interaction of all of these people will determine whether or not the patient receives safe care. Nurses should take an active role in ensuring patient safety by using caution in medication administration, and by participating in discussions of committees that formulate guidelines for patient care.

A general outline of hospital policies to guide drug administration by nurses and guidelines for avoiding medication errors are given in Chapter 8.

REVIEW QUESTIONS

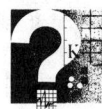

1. Describe the provisions of the Pure Food and Drug Act of 1906.
2. What was the main purpose of the Sherley Amendment of 1912?
3. Outline the major parts of the Federal Food, Drug and Cosmetic Act of 1938.
4. What statement must appear on the containers of prescription drugs as a result of the Durham-Humphrey Amendment?
5. What are the provisions of the Kefauver-Harris Amendment of 1962?
6. What does the abbreviation DESI mean?
7. List the six categories into which drugs marketed between 1938 and 1962 must be categorized according to the DESI.
8. Describe the five schedules of controlled drugs designated by the Comprehensive Drug Abuse Prevention and Control Act of 1970.
9. What procedures must be followed in order to dispense a Schedule II controlled substance via an oral order in an emergency situation?
10. Give some sources for potential drug candidates.
11. What areas does preclinical toxicity testing of a new drug candidate encompass?
12. What is an IND and what information does it contain?
13. Briefly describe the four phases of clinical drug evaluation.
14. What is the placebo effect?
15. Distinguish between a "parallel" and a "crossover" study in clinical drug testing.
16. How can a nurse ensure that a patient has given informed consent to participate in a clinical drug trial?
17. Under what circumstances can a patient end his participation in a clinical drug study?
18. What are the three most common medication errors committed by nurses? How can they be avoided?
19. What is the standard of care on which nurses are held liable for safe administration of medications?
20. What two elements are most important in the accurate transcription of medication orders?

BIBLIOGRAPHY

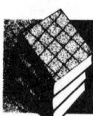

Bell NK: Whose autonomy is at stake? Am J Nurs June:1170, 1981

Bowers JZ, Velo GP (eds): Drug Assessment: Criteria and Methods. New York, Elsevier North Holland, 1979

Cushing M: Drug errors can be bitter pills. Am J Nurs 86:895, 1986

Davis N, Cohen M: Learning from mistakes: 20 tips for avoiding medication errors. Nursing '82 12:65, 1982

Department of Justice: Regulations implementing the Comprehensive Drug Abuse Prevention and Control Act of 1970. Federal Register 36(80):1, 1971

Fink JL (ed): Pharmacy Law Digest. Media, PA, Harwal Publishing, 1981

Kennedy D: A calm look at "drug lag." JAMA 239:423, 1978

Lasagna L: Historical viewpoint of clinical trials. Drug Information J 16:7, 1982

Long G: The effect of medication distribution systems on medication errors. Nurs Res 31(3):182, 1982

Nealon E et al: What do patients know about clinical trials. Am J Nurs 85:807, 1985

A Primer on New Drug Development. Rockville, MD, HEW publication No. (FDA) 74-3021, Department of Health, Education and Welfare, 1974

Schafer A: The ethics of the randomized clinical trial. N Engl J Med 307:719, 1982

Sheiner LB: Clinical trials and the illusion of objectivity. In Melmon KL et al (eds): Drug Therapeutics: Concepts for Physicians, p. 167. New York, Elsevier North Holland, 1979

Slone D, Shapiro S, Miettinen OS, Finkle WD, Stolley PD: Drug evaluation after marketing. Ann Intern Med 90:257, 1979

Stites L: Protecting research subjects. Am J Nurs June:1139, 1979

Wertheimer AI: The placebo effect. Pharmacy International 1:12, 1980

Drug Administration: Nursing Intervention Strategies

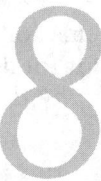

The administration of medications is one of the most exacting of all nursing responsibilities because it demands complete accuracy. The nurse must be familiar with the institution policies on storage and distribution of drugs. For each drug the nurse administers, she must thoroughly understand the indications for its use, the drug's actions within the body, the dosage, side-effects, and the expected therapeutic response. She also needs to understand the patient's condition and past drug history. This chapter emphasizes principles of nursing actions that enable the nurse to apply her knowledge to any patient situation.

Drug Preparation and Storage

An orderly, quiet, clean, well-equipped, and well-lighted area is essential for the proper preparation of medications. Each nursing unit or clinic should make available an isolated area designated solely for the preparation and storage of drugs. Federal, state, and local regulations, as well as those imposed by accrediting bodies such as the Joint Commission for Accreditation of Hospitals, must be met in the design and construction of the medication area.

Because most medications are perishable, labels on all drug containers must carry an *expiration date*, the date after which the drug will no longer retain full potency. The potency period varies among drugs. Some drugs are stable for a period of years, others for only hours after preparation. Though a drug may not become useless immediately on the expiration date, the decomposition of some drugs may result in the formation of new compounds. Therefore, for legal reasons, an expired drug should not be administered after that date. The pharmacy is required to maintain an adequate stock of fresh medications; however, the nurse should know the drug's expiration date and verify this before giving the drug to a patient. When storing drugs at the nursing station, the nurse should make sure that the date on the label is visible, use older stock first, and return outdated drugs to the pharmacy.

Temperature, light, humidity, and exposure to air can affect the deterioration of stored drugs. The manufacturer's label usually indicates storage temperature requirements or limits for the drug. Drugs that are to be kept frozen are stored in the pharmacy and thawed just before they are to be given on the patient unit. Products requiring refrigeration are kept in a refrigerator in the patient care area, and this refrigerator is used *only* for drug storage.

It is advisable to keep a thermometer in the medication storage and preparation area. A rule of thumb is that an environment that is comfortable for personnel is safe for any agent that can be stored at *room temperature*. Some drugs, however, such as magnesium sulfate, require a *warm* ambient temperature to prevent their cystallization.

Exposure to *light* can cause some drugs to degenerate quickly; these drugs are supplied in amber-colored containers, where they must be kept until they are administered. Some drugs for parenteral use must be protected from light while being administered.

Atmospheric moisture can also hasten the deterioration of some medications, especially those prepared in tablet, capsule, or powder form; these medications are supplied in air-tight containers. Tablets and capsules that are particularly susceptible to damage from humidity are supplied with a *desiccant capsule*, which absorbs moisture. Care must be taken to keep the desiccant in the container until the last of the medication has been administered, and then to discard it.

Some drugs in liquid form, such as aqueous solutions, must be protected from *exposure to air*, and these drugs are supplied in air-tight, single-dose ampules. Once the ampule has been opened, the medication must be used or discarded.

Drug storage must also be planned to prevent drug misuse. Controlled drugs, such as narcotics and barbiturates, are stored in a separate, locked, permanently affixed, wall compartment in the medication preparation area. (This requirement is mandated by the Controlled Substances Act of 1970.) Other potentially dangerous drugs, such as curare-like substances, should also be kept in a locked cabinet. Drugs classified as *investigational* must be stored separately, to prevent inadvertent use. The medication room itself should be enclosed and locked and used for the sole purpose of storing and preparing medications. If the drug storage system consists of a mobile cart, the cart must contain a locked compartment for storage of controlled drugs and other potentially dangerous substances.

Drug Supply Systems

There are three systems for supplying drugs to or within the nursing unit for distribution to patients: *floor stock system; individual patient supply sys-*

tem; and *unit-dose system.* A combination of these systems may sometimes be followed to meet individual patient or nursing needs. Regardless of the system used, the objective of all systems is the safe delivery of medications to the patient and the prevention of errors.

All drug supply systems require that the physician's order for all drugs be transcribed to a medication administration record (MAR), one page for scheduled medications and one for as-needed and single doses. All drug orders on the MAR are checked following transcription and then daily against the original orders by the nurse. With the floor stock and individual patient supply methods, the nurse must also transcribe the order to a drug card or ticket used to label each individual dose of medication; with the unit-dose method, the MAR is taken to the patient's bedside.

Floor Stock System

In the floor stock system, all routine medications for the type of patient usually assigned to the nursing unit are kept on the shelves. This arrangement was widely used before the 1960s but now is used rarely, primarily in extended-care facilities. Since all drugs are kept in large, similar-appearing containers, the potential for selecting the wrong drug is greater than with other systems. In addition, the likelihood of theft is greater since it is difficult to know how much is in each container, and the nurse must spend an inordinate amount of time checking expiration dates on all of the stock.

Individual Patient Supply System

The individual patient supply system is an improvement over the floor stock system in that there are fewer drugs to be stored, and the pharmacist plays an active role. With the physician's order, drugs are prepared by the pharmacist in individual packages, usually a 3-day or 4-day supply. The packages are labeled with the drug name and the patient's name and room number, and are delivered to the nursing unit to be stored in an individual drawer or in the refrigerator. At the time of administration, the nurse checks the MAR against the physician's order; checks medication cards against the MAR to be sure there is a card for every drug listed; takes the medication card to the medication

room; and prepares the drug for administration. The medication card serves as the drug label until the drug is brought to the patient. After the drug has been given, the nurse indicates the drug was given on the MAR using the card as a reference, and the card is then returned to a storage area to be available for use with the next dose. This system is the one most often used in extended-care facilities.

Unit-Dose System

The unit-dose system is currently the method of choice because it is economical, saves the nurse's time, and helps to prevent errors. The physician writes his order on carbonized paper. The nurse reviews the order and then sends the carbon copy of the drug order to the pharmacy where the pharmacist evaluates the order. If the pharmacist finds the order to be appropriate, he dispenses the drug in a single-dose package, usually providing enough packages for a 24-hour period. The pharmacist labels each package, or the manufacturer's prefilled and labeled packages are used.

On the nursing unit, all drugs except those requiring refrigeration are stored in a locked medication cart with individual compartments for each patient's drugs. All drug orders on the MAR are checked daily against the original written orders in the patient's chart. The MAR is taken with the drug cart to the patient. Before giving the drug, the nurse reads the order on the MAR and compares it with the drug supplied; after giving the drug, the nurse makes the appropriate notation in the MAR, and proceeds to the next patient.

There are both advantages and disadvantages to the unit-dose system. One disadvantage is that the nurse must administer medications prepared by another person—a fact that highlights the necessity for the nurse to have reliable knowledge of the appearance of all drugs she administers. Another disadvantage is that if a dose of medication is dropped or destroyed, the nurse must replace it before she can give a dose.

The advantages of the unit-dose system are many: (1) two persons who are knowledgeable about drugs check the written order; (2) medication cards are eliminated, thereby reducing transcription time and possible error; (3) medications remain labeled until the moment they are administered; (4) dose calculations are kept to a minimum; (5) liquid oral medications will not be erroneously combined; (6) with the nurse's help, patients can learn to check their labeled medications in preparation for self-administration at home; (7) drugs can be returned for credit if not used, because they have not been opened and contaminated; (8) the sterility of parenteral drugs is easier to maintain in prefilled syringes; and (9) the nurse is freed from the responsibility of diluting and preparing drugs for parenteral administration, and of compounding large-volume parenteral fluid–drug combinations —legally, the duty of the pharmacist.

Developing a Schedule of Drug Administration

The nurse is responsible for designing a schedule that ensures the patient will receive each prescribed drug or drugs at the ordered frequency so as to produce the optimal therapeutic effect. This schedule takes into account the institution's prearranged schedule, the patient's meal schedule, the patient's sleeping pattern, and a knowledge of the drug's action within the body.

Prearranged hospital dosing schedules are designed to simplify drug administration for large groups of patients and usually fit the needs of those patients (see Table 8-1 for examples). Prearranged

schedules must not be used blindly; occasionally a deviation may be called for that is related to the drug itself or to the patient's condition. When a schedule has been determined, it is advisable to administer drugs within at least one-half hour of the designated time.

When writing an order for a medication, the physician should indicate how many individual doses he wants the patient to receive in 24 hours and at what time intervals. If, for example, he writes "tetracycline 250 mg PO qid," the nurse, using her knowledge of the drug's action within the body, should clarify the order since the drug should be given at 6-hour intervals, such as 6 AM, 12 PM, 6 PM, and 12 AM, and not four times a day as qid indicates. The physician should rewrite the order unless he had other reasons for writing the original order, such as not wanting the patient awakened for the late and early doses.

Drugs prescribed to control, prevent, or suppress a pathologic condition are best given continuously or at evenly spaced intervals. This type of administration helps to maintain a desired drug level in the blood. The drug form as well as the route of administration will determine if the drug concentration is to be maintained at a constant level in the plasma (see Chap. 2).

Table 8-1
Commonly Used Dosing Schedules*

Frequency of Administration	Abbreviation	Times to Be Administered
Once daily	qd	10 AM
Twice daily	bid	10 AM, 6 PM
Every 12 hours	q12h	10 AM, 10 PM
Three times daily (during waking hours)	tid	10 AM, 2 PM, 6 PM
Every 8 hours	q8h	6 AM, 2 PM, 10 PM
Four times daily (during waking hours)	qid	10 AM, 2 PM, 6 PM, 10 PM
Every 6 hours	q6h	6 AM, 12 PM, 6 PM, 12 AM
Every 4 hours	q4h	6 AM, 10 AM, 2 PM, 6 PM, 10 PM, 2 AM
Bedtime (hour of sleep)	hs	10 PM (should be flexible to meet patient needs)
Before meals	ac	1 hour before meals
After meals	pc	2 hours after meals or with meals

* Time schedules are arbitrarily set by institution and may vary. An alternate time schedule might be one that uses 9 AM as its base. A drug given bid might then be given 9 AM, 5 PM; one given qid might be given 9 AM, 1 PM, 5 PM, and 9 PM.

Nursing Intervention in the Administration of Drugs

With the nursing process in mind, administration of drugs can begin. At the start of the shift, the nurse collects data on each patient's current status and any recent change in condition or therapy. A brief visit to each patient will confirm information found in the nursing report at the beginning of the shift. It is helpful to make notes of specific needs or problems that may affect drug administration. For example, "Patient has been vomiting since 2 AM, unable to take oral medications"; "Patient's IV is infiltrated"; "Nasogastric tube accidentally removed by patient at 6 AM"; "Patient to have upper GI x-ray this AM and is now NPO."

After completing an initial assessment of the patients under her care, the nurse can identify and prioritize any problems and plan the administration of appropriate medications.

Each institution has its own policies governing drug administration aimed at promoting safety and preventing medication errors. The nurse should be familiar with all of the following policy categories.

1. A definite policy regarding who administers medications to various patients. Where the team nursing concept is practiced, each nurse in charge of a particular group of patients may be assigned to administer drugs to the entire group. Or, each person on the team who is licensed to give medications may administer only to those patients to whom she is assigned. The same routine may apply where primary nursing is practiced. Some institutions find it best to designate one person to be responsible for giving medications to the whole group of patients, while the nurse responsible for the physical care of the patients also monitors for drug effects once the drugs have been given.
2. The checking of all medication orders every 24 hours (in some institutions this must be done on every shift). The order on the MAR (and medication card if that system is used) should be carefully compared with the originating physician's orders for errors in transcription or interpretation of dosage, route, time of administration, and so on.
3. The questioning of unusual or unfamiliar drug names carried in an order. If the drug name doesn't appear in the *Physician's Desk Reference* or other resource, the pharmacy should be called before the drug is given. This is especially true when there is more than one form

of the drug. For example, Darvon is different in dose and chemical composition from Darvon N.
4. A specific policy on what medications a nurse is allowed to give, the acceptable dosage ranges permitted, and routes of administration

In addition, to minimize medication errors, the nurse should develop certain habits of administration:

1. When preparing medications to be given, the label should be carefully checked before removing the drug from its container, whether it is a stock container or single-unit dose. Make sure that the order and medication correspond *exactly*. *Never* use a medication from an unlabeled or an illegibly labeled container.
2. If a calculation is required for dosage preparation, the mathematics should be checked carefully. If you are uncertain about your figures, consult an experienced colleague or the pharmacist. Keep in mind that the drug manufacturer usually supplies drugs in containers or dosage forms in the size of the most frequently prescribed dosage. Question any order or calculation that requires the use of a large number of tablets or ampules.
3. When measuring liquid oral medications from a stock supply, use appropriate equipment. In most cases, liquid drugs should be ordered and measured in milliliters, rather than teaspoons or tablespoons. Regardless of the unit of measurement, either convert to milliliters or use a graduated container to measure the unit ordered. Convert 1 teaspoon to 5 ml and use a milliliter measuring device. If drops are ordered, use only the dropper provided by the manufacturer. Do not use the same dropper for more than one medication. The viscosity of a liquid and the design of the dropper govern the size of the drop formed. Do not use a noncalibrated dropper to "guess measure" a drug ordered in milliliters. A noncalibrated dropper can be used only to measure a drug ordered in drops.
4. Never administer medications prepared by someone else, except when using the unit-dose system in which the pharmacist has prepared and labeled the doses. If you administer a drug prepared in error by another person, you will be liable for any harm that the patient experiences.
5. Become familiar with the appearance of tablets and capsules. When in doubt about the identification of a drug, use the manufacturer's code

number on the tablet or capsule, and consult the *Physician's Desk Reference.* Do not use a drug or unit dose that looks as if it has been tampered with or damaged. A unit dose should reach the patient *sealed* in its single-dose container.

6. When administering any potentially dangerous drug, have another nurse, who is certified to administer drugs and whose judgment you trust, check the dose you have drawn into the syringe. Show the other nurse the order, the drug bottle, and the syringe with the dose. Drugs that fall into this category include insulin, heparin, experimental chemotherapeutic agents, and any toxic drug used in titrated intravenous solutions such as dobutamine, ritodrine, lidocaine, nitroprusside, and many others.

7. Question unexpected alterations in dosage, especially fractional ones. For example, assume that a patient had been receiving clonidine 0.2 mg bid for about two weeks, and a new order is written for clonidine 2 mg bid. The latter is ten times the former dose. The nurse should immediately call the physician's attention to this discrepancy. If such an error were uncorrected, the patient receiving the medication could be harmed.

8. Be aware that some drug doses must be decreased stepwise before being discontinued, and transcribe orders accordingly. Most steroids and propranolol fall into this category. Abruptly discontinuing administration of such drugs can cause serious adverse effects.

9. Avoid the use of ambiguous abbreviations in transcribing orders, and clarify all unusual physician drug orders. Common abbreviations that can cause confusion include:

    DC, D/C—This can be used to mean discharge *or* discontinue.

    o.d.—Appropriately used means daily (with periods present) but can be misinterpreted to mean *right eye* (written without periods). The order "daily" should be written out.

    qd—Means every day. However, if large periods are used after the letters, the period between the "q" and the "d" may appear as the letter "i" and the order may thus be misinterpreted as "qid" or four times a day.

    μg—Is sometimes used for abbreviating *microgram*, but can be misinterpreted as "mg" or milligram, causing a large error in the amount of drug given. The preferred abbreviation for microgram is mcg.

10. Always question illegible handwriting. Never attempt to interpret questionable orders. It is the legal responsibility of nurses and physicians to write legibly.

When all drugs have been checked and prepared for administration, they can be taken to the patients. A professional approach to medication administration is essential. Most persons are aware that medication errors do occur in hospitals and will feel more secure about receiving drugs from a nurse who shows professional concern toward both patient well-being and medication responsibilities.

Identify the patient by examining his *identification band.* Never rely on the patient answering to his name, the presence of a name card at the foot of the bed, or the word of a roommate. These are notoriously unreliable means of patient identification. Once the person has been correctly identified, tell him what medication he is to receive and what it is for. Not only do these measures prepare the patient to receive information about his medications, they also help to prevent medication errors. Listen to the patient who says he has already received the medication you are about to give him, or who states that he should not receive the drug. Regardless of his mental state, always double check the medication record and verify it with another staff member caring for the patient before you give the medication. Double check for known drug allergies at this time.

Immediately after the patient has received the medication, document this fact according to hospital procedure, so that another person will not mistakenly repeat the dose. Chart any adverse reactions and notify the physician if any serious problems have developed. If fluid intake is to be recorded, any fluids given with the drug must be charted. Follow policy regarding unused drugs. Never return unused drugs to stock containers.

When the Patient Refuses a Medication

The patient has the right to refuse any treatment offered to him. If this happens, take time to find out why he refuses to take the medication, since refusal is usually the result of anxiety or of a misunderstanding, or it may signal a change in the patient's mental status. Allow the patient to discuss his concerns in a nonthreatening atmosphere. If the problem cannot be resolved quickly, notify the physician and document the refusal and your opinion as to why it has occurred. Communicate the problem to appropriate members of the nursing staff.

Bedside Medications

Never be tempted to leave oral medications or topical agents such as antiseptic solutions at the bedside. If the patient wishes to take a medication later, and if this is permissible, replace the dose in the medication cart with an appropriate label. Instruct the patient to ask for the drug when he is ready.

If a patient is learning to self-medicate, certain medications may be kept at the bedside according to institution policy and with a physician's order. Examples of such medications include nitroglycerin, antacids, and topical agents. Before a patient is entrusted with independent drug taking, an assessment of his knowledge base about the drug and his ability to take it correctly should be completed. Self-medication should be carefully monitored and documented by the nurse. Efforts should be made to keep these medications only for the patient for whom they were prescribed. In some institutions a locked bedside drawer is available to which the patient has a key.

Techniques of Drug Administration

Additional information relative to pediatric drug administration is presented in Chapter 9.

There are three routes by which a drug enters the body; oral–gastrointestinal, topical, and parenteral. The factors that help determine which route is appropriate for a particular drug and the patient are described in detail in other chapters, and are only summarized here:

1. The *chemical and physical properties* of the drug
2. The *intended site of drug action.* Some drugs exert different effects at various body sites, depending on the route of administration.
3. The desired *rapidity and duration of drug action.* Drugs administered intramuscularly may exert their effects over a longer period of time

than when given intravenously. The anticipated blood level of the drug also enters into the decision about the route of administration.
4. The *patient's tolerance* for the drug. For example, an emaciated person or very small child may not have sufficient muscle mass for a drug to be given repeatedly by the intramuscular route.

The physician decides, in most instances, which route is preferable, but the nurse should understand the reason why a particular route was chosen. It is within the nurse's role to inform the physician if difficulties arise related to a route of administration and to suggest alternatives based on knowledge of the drug and the patient. Unless the physician has indicated that either of two routes may be used, the nurse should never make a change without consulting the physician.

Administration of Drugs by the Oral–Gastrointestinal Route

An oral drug is one that is swallowed or is mechanically introduced into the stomach or upper gastrointestinal tract through a tube. Either solid dosage forms (tablets, capsules) or liquids can be administered by the oral–gastrointestinal route. Drugs administered in this manner can exert local or systemic effects. The onset of drug action may be rapid or relatively slow, depending on its physical form (capsule or tablet), which affects its dissolution rate and the time necessary for absorption through the gastric or intestinal mucosa into the circulation.

Instruct patients to take their medications only with water unless specifically instructed otherwise, and to avoid the use of carbonated drinks and fruit juices. Remember that some medications must be taken with a large quantity of water to aid dissolution.

With oral preparations, be cognizant of the patient's ability or inability to swallow before you administer them. If you have reason to believe that the patient may have dysphagia, test for its presence by offering him a few sips of water. Patients who may have dysphagia include those identified as having difficulty chewing and swallowing; those with muscular weakness secondary to a cerebral vascular accident, multiple sclerosis, Parkinson's disease, and other disease states; those whose speech is slurred; those who have had an endotracheal or a nasogastric tube inserted; and those who are confused, agitated, or semiconscious. Anticipate problems of swallowing in persons whose oropharynx or esophagus has been traumatized or subjected to surgery, and those who have obstructive lesions of the oropharynx or esophagus. If a patient is unable to swallow solids safely, a drug may be supplied in liquid form or an alternative route may be chosen.

SOLID PREPARATIONS
When administering tablets or capsules, the nurse should never break an unscored tablet or open a capsule to divide it for a specified dose, because the resulting dose may be incorrect. Likewise, tablets should never be crushed or dissolved, nor should capsules be opened and their contents dropped into a liquid or food without the specific approval and guidance from the pharmacist.

If the pharmacist has given approval for you to crush a tablet, always use clean techniques for this procedure and dilute the drug in a liquid approved by the pharmacist. If the drug is not supplied in liquid form or cannot be crushed, and the patient is unable to swallow the preparation safely, a different means of administration may be required, for example, by nasogastric tube or parenteral administration.

Drugs in powder or granular form may be dissolved in water or another liquid to facilitate their being swallowed. Sometimes, with medications that have a disagreeable taste, it may be permissible to add fruit juice, but always ask the pharmacist first.

Some tablets and capsules are manufactured in forms that cannot be altered without compromising drug action.

An enteric-coated drug dissolves and is released only when it enters the alkaline environment of the small intestine. The purpose of the coating is to prevent drug inactivation in the acidic gastric fluid and to prevent irritation to the gastric mucosa, and these benefits are lost if an enteric-coated medication is crushed.

Capsules containing time-release beads should not be emptied and mixed with food or fluids; to do so could cause them to break up and dissolve, with subsequent altered absorption. Instruct the patient to swallow all tablets and capsules without first chewing them, unless a preparation is designed to be chewed. The foregoing information applies also to patients who will be self-medicating at home.

Trade names often give information as to whether the medications can be crushed or dissolved. Drugs with names that include "bid," "Dur," "SA" (sustained-action), "SR" (sustained release), or "Span," "Repetabs," "Sequels," "Spansules," "Film-seal," or "Extentabs" should never be altered prior to being administered.

LIQUID PREPARATIONS
Some liquid drug forms for oral administration separate on standing. The solution must be thoroughly mixed to ensure even dispersion. This applies to aqueous suspensions, magmas, gels, and suspensions. If the suspension has a disagreeable taste, dilute with water or juice with the approval of the pharmacist.

Tinctures and spirits, being highly concentrated, are prescribed in small quantities, usually drops, to be added to a specified quantity of water. Never dilute elixirs or extracts, as to do so may cause the drug to precipitate out of the solution.

NASOGASTRIC OR GASTROSTOMY TUBE
Patients who are unable to swallow are sometimes given a nasogastric or, in some cases, a gastrostomy tube. Before giving medications via these tubes, ask yourself the following questions:
1. Should the medication be given with food or on an empty stomach?
2. If the drug is to be given with food, are there any foods that should be avoided (such as milk products)?
3. What volume of liquid feeding has the patient tolerated during the preceding few hours? Has he vomited?
4. Is the tube in place? Check placement of a nasogastric tube by aspirating for gastric contents or by inserting a small amount of air in the tube and listening at the gastric hiatus for a characteristic bubble sound. Check the placement of a gastrostomy tube by aspiration or, if dislodging is suspected, by x-ray film.

Do not administer a drug by tube with a feeding if there is a possibility that the patient will vomit. Do not put the medication in the liquid food itself because the patient may not tolerate the entire volume. Administer the drug first, either on an empty stomach or an hour before feeding or immediately prior to a feeding, depending on the drug. The medication must be in liquid form. Remember that a heavy suspension passed through a tube could occlude the tube if the tube has not been carefully rinsed. All medications, feedings, and water must be warmed to room temperature before being instilled to prevent gas formation, cramping, and nausea.

Drug administration via nasogastric or gastrostomy tube is not an innocuous procedure. The instillation of a large volume of fluid or an irritating medication can cause gastric distention or nausea and vomiting. The gastric contents may then be aspirated into the respiratory tract, resulting in lung tissue damage and respiratory distress. If a drug is administered through a nasogastric tube inadvertently placed in the trachea or bronchus, respiratory distress and lung damage, and possibly death, may follow.

Procedure

Place the patient in semi-Fowler's position to help prevent regurgitation. Determine the position of the tip of the tube if using a nasogastric tube. Keep the tube clamped while attaching the administration device, usually a 50-ml syringe. Add medication. Unclamp the tube and allow medication to flow by gravity. As with any tube infusion, do not force the medication fluid into the tube. Carefully observe the patient for signs of respiratory distress or gagging that may be secondary to nausea. Stop the instillation immediately on noting any sign of distress. Flush the tube carefully with warm water to ensure that the entire dose has been given and to prevent the tube from becoming clogged, and reclamp the tube. Keep the patient in semi-Fowler's position for at least 30 minutes following administration, and continue to observe his reactions.

Administration of Drugs by the Topical Route

Topical administration means that the drug is applied to the surface of the skin or the mucous membranes. Ointments, aqueous liquids, lotions or creams, and aerosols or sprays are applied topically.

The types of drugs generally applied to the skin are antiseptics and anti-infectives, anti-inflammatory agents, astringents, antipruritics, emollients, keratolytics, enzymes, counterirritants, and vasodilators.

Topical agents may exert their effects only on the surface of the skin and on the tissues immediately below the surface, or systemically by absorption through the skin, and through the surface of the mucous membranes of the mouth and rectum. Absorption directly into the blood can also occur if the keratin surface layer of the skin has been broken as in the case of wounds or burns.

Conditions commonly treated with topical agents include acne; some localized skin cancers; psoriasis; rashes; infections of the skin and wounds; infestations of the skin and hair by lice or other insects; ulcers of the skin; decubitus ulcers; burns; and angina pectoris.

Procedure

When administering a topical agent, provide privacy and give the patient a thorough explanation of the procedure. This step will help to prepare the patient to self-administer the agent at home, and is especially important in the case of chronic conditions.

Follow the physician's or manufacturer's recommendations for cleansing the skin and using sterile or clean technique, according to the situation. Sterile or aseptic technique is indicated whenever the skin is broken, as with wounds or burns. Do not assume that because a wound or burn is infected, sterile technique is unnecessary. The objective is to prevent further contamination of the area. Sterile technique will also protect the nurse from exposure to the infection.

Never remove the drug from its container with your fingers, unless you are wearing sterile gloves. When applying an ointment or a cream from a tube, squeeze out a small portion and remove it from the tube opening onto a sterile surface, such as a gauze pad. Then squeeze out the desired amount of drug for use. This measure avoids using material that may have been contaminated when it touched the tube lid. When administering a topical vasodilator ointment, always use a dosage-guide paper when applying the drug to the skin, to ensure correct dosage.

Apply only a thin layer of drug to the skin, unless the nature of the drug dictates otherwise, as with topical burn preparations that are applied to a specified depth over the affected area.

Cover the medicated area with a sterile dressing if this has been ordered; if a cover is necessary to keep the drug on the lesion; and to prevent the medication from staining clothing or unaffected skin. Take care when using adhesive tape near a wound or rash—it may cause skin breakdown. Even if the surrounding skin appears normal, it may be fragile and vulnerable to damage.

Wet dressings, soaks, and compresses are sometimes used in the treatment of skin ulcers. Infected or contaminated wounds may also be treated with dressings or soaks containing antiseptics or antibiotic solutions. These applications are usually sterile and are applied for a specified length of time, followed by a dry sterile dressing.

Applying drugs to the skin is not without hazards. Patients are just as susceptible to drug reactions and allergies by this route as with other routes. Observe the area for any signs that suggest drug intolerance; if systemic effects are expected, observe for changes in blood pressure, or for the development of nausea or vomiting. If an adverse reaction occurs, notify the physician, remove the drug, and withhold the next dose until the physician gives further instructions.

The nurse should wash her hands after application to prevent potential absorption from administration of topical agents.

MUCOUS MEMBRANES

Drugs applied to the mucous membranes can also exert local or systemic effects. Tablets, lozenges, powders, and suppositories are all applied to mucous membranes. Eyes, ears, nose, oropharynx, lower respiratory tract, vagina, and rectum are sites of such application and afford effective absorption into the circulation.

Oral Mucous Membranes

As with application of drugs to mucous membranes elsewhere in the body, both local and systemic effects are possible with drugs applied to the mucous membranes of the oral cavity. Local effects are exerted by mouth washes, gargles, and lozenges; systemic effects, by buccal or sublingual tablets and sprays (nitroglycerin).

Procedure

The procedure to be followed with these drugs is self-explanatory; however, a few precautions are in order.

With washes and gargles, instruct the patient not to swallow any of the solution, and to gargle all of the specified dose. A topical solution such as gentian violet is probably best applied initially by the nurse, with care taken to apply the medication to all of the lesions. The patient can then be instructed in self-medication, including the reminder not to swallow any of the drug. Sublingual tablets are rapidly absorbed through the highly vascular floor of the mouth as are buccal tablets placed inside the space between the cheek and teeth. The patient must be instructed not to chew or swallow these kinds of tablets, for swallowing would cause the drug to be inactivated by the gastric fluids.

Ophthalmic Medications

Topical ophthalmic preparations and the conditions for which they are generally prescribed include the following: corticosteroids and vasoconstrictors for inflammation secondary to allergy or irritation; antibiotics and antifungals for infections; miotics and decongestants for glaucoma. In addition, mydriatics and cycloplegics are used in eye examinations; methylcellulose and saline are used to lubricate the eyes; and proparacaine and similar drugs are used as local anesthetics.

Drugs for use in the eye may be applied in the form of drops, ointments, or sustained-release disks.

The patient will probably be apprehensive about eye treatments. Take time to tell the patient the name of the drug and its purpose, as well as how it is to be applied. Offer to instruct him in the proper technique, and correct his technique if necessary. Explain what sensation he might expect when the drug touches the eye.

Wash your hands, use aseptic technique, and *avoid touching the eye.*

Procedure

Ask the patient to lie down or sit in a chair and lean back. To instill drops, have the patient look up; then drop the prescribed number of drops into the conjunctival sac, not onto the cornea. Have the patient blink to spread the medication over the surface of the eye. He can then close his eyes if he wishes to. Note any immediate untoward reactions, undue pain, or redness or swelling of the eye or conjunctival tissues. Keep the patient at rest for a few minutes, and instruct him not to blot the eye for at least 4 to 5 minutes. If a local anesthetic has been administered for a diagnostic procedure, remind the patient to close his eyes before blotting them to avoid scratching the now insensitive cornea.

To apply an ophthalmic ointment, have the patient look up. Apply gentle traction to the skin below the eye to hold the eye open. Place a quantity of ointment onto a sterile surface, then squeeze a short ribbon of it onto the inside rim of the lower lid. Instruct the patient to then blink to spread the ointment over the surface of the eye. Warn him that the ointment may make his vision blurred. Apply ointments at bedtime if possible.

Otic Medications

Conditions limited to the external canal and the outer tympanic membrane may be treated by instillation of drops and solutions. Infection, inflammation and its associated pain, and ceruminal obstruction are commonly treated by instillations.

Local effects are the rule, but systemic effects may occur rarely.

Ear Drops
The physician will order the number of drops to be instilled. Follow sterile technique if the tympanic membrane is not intact. Inform the patient that he may experience a rush of sound as the fluid enters the canal.

Warm the solution by holding the bottle in your hands or keeping it in your pocket for a few minutes. The canal must be straightened manually, so that the drug can reach the end of the canal and the tympanic membrane. In an adult, gently pull the external ear *back and up*; in a child, pull the lower part of the external ear *back and down*. It is sometimes necessary to place a small ball of cotton loosely at the opening of the ear to protect the canal and the membrane.

Ear Irrigations
Irrigations are ordered for the purpose of removing cerumen or foreign objects from the canal. Many of the procedures and precautions described above under Ear Drops apply also to irrigations, and may be referred to as needed. It is especially important to warm the irrigation solution to 100°F (37.8°C) to prevent stimulation of the inner ear, which could cause the patient to experience vertigo.

Place an emesis basin under the ear; then with an ear syringe gently direct the stream of irrigation fluid toward the wall of the canal (never directly toward the tympanic membrane). Stop the irrigation if the patient has pain or becomes dizzy. Allow the solution to flow out freely into the basin, observing for the passage of the foreign object, cerumen, or blood. Have the patient lie on the affected side for 5 to 10 minutes after the irrigation, to promote drainage.

Nasal Medications
Aqueous solutions of decongestants, antihistamines, and topical corticosteroids are used in the treatment of nasal congestion and itching due to allergy or viral infection, and in the treatment of idiopathic rhinitis. Bacterial infections of the nasal passages or the sinuses are usually treated with systemic antibiotics administered orally.

In the correct dose, these medications exert their effects on the nasal passages, whereas overdoses can exert systemic effects, including rebound congestion and hypertension. Desirable systemic effects are produced by the application of oxytocin powder to the nasal membranes.

Procedure
Be sure the solution is at room temperature and that it is clear rather than cloudy. Use one bottle of solution for one patient only, to prevent cross-contamination.

Have the patient blow his nose to remove secretions, and then have him lie down or sit in a chair, and tilt his head back to facilitate the passage of drops into the nasal canal. Place the dropper near the nasal opening and instill the dose. *Do not touch the dropper to the skin* to prevent the patient from sneezing and to avoid contaminating the dropper.

If a spray is ordered, insert the nozzle into the nasal opening until a seal is created between the nozzle and the skin. Have the patient sniff to disperse the medication into the passages. Instruct the patient to report any undue discomfort and to remain at rest with his head tilted back, or to lean forward and then back, for several minutes.

When teaching patients how to self-medicate with nasal preparations, remind them about the importance of taking the prescribed dose and avoiding contamination of the solution.

Inhaled Respiratory Medications
The membranes lining the respiratory passages permit absorption of certain drugs into the general circulation, while the effects of other agents are confined to the surface tissues. Locally, obstructive pulmonary diseases such as asthma and chronic bronchitis are treated with bronchodilators, corticosteroids, mucolytics, and moisturizing agents; systemically, nitrous oxide, halothane, and similar drugs are used to achieve general anesthesia, and oxygen is used to treat hypoxia.

Bronchodilators, corticosteroids, mucolytics, halothane, and nitrous oxide are all delivered to the respiratory membrane by inhalation of the liquid or gas, which has been nebulized into a fine spray under pressure. Nebulization is achieved by use of an intermittent positive-pressure breathing (IPPB) apparatus, a small portable nebulizer, or by a similar device. Some drugs are supplied in metered-dose nebulizers that release a premeasured dose by push button. Volatile liquid and gas anesthetics are vaporized with oxygen in a special apparatus housing a nebulizer. Nebulization delivers a fine mist onto the surface endothelium of the respiratory passages. The drug exerts its effects either on the surface tissues only, or is absorbed into the circulating blood and exerts systemic effects.

Medications in powder form are delivered by *insufflation*, in which the powder is blown into the respiratory passages. Insufflation is accomplished through the use of pressurized containers that release measured doses by push button. See Chapters 15 and 48 for use of specific nebulizers.

Procedure

Administration of drugs by inhalation or insufflation requires a knowledge of the drug that is to be used and the diluent, if any, to be used and its required volume. The patient will need to be instructed in the technique required to use the nebulizing apparatus; how to inhale, when to inhale, whether or not to hold the breath after the drug has been delivered; and how to exhale. Instruction must be individualized because each of the several types of apparatus available is distinctive in features and operation. Treatments for respiratory disorders may cause the patient to cough; this is desirable because it aids in removing secretions and clearing the respiratory passages.

Help the patient to cough and reassure him that coughing is expected and beneficial. Observe for adverse reactions as indicated by an excessive rise in heart rate; nausea and abdominal distention (secondary to air being forced into the stomach by the apparatus); and dizziness or rapid shallow respirations that may presage respiratory alkalosis due to rapid inhalations. If any of these occur, stop the treatment and notify the physician. Stay with the patient, and continue to observe him. Patients who will be self-medicating at home will require careful instruction about both the drug and the method of administration.

In emergency situations, some drugs in an aqueous liquid form can be placed into the trachea through an endotracheal tube, to be rapidly absorbed into the circulation. Atropine, lidocaine, and epinephrine can be administered *intratracheally* to obtain rapid results without causing damage to the endotracheal tissues. On the other hand, sodium bicarbonate, which is used in cardiopulmonary resuscitation, must *never* be administered by tube because it deactivates the alveolar surfactant in the lungs and leads to atelectasis.

Rectal Medications

Medications applied to the mucous membranes of the rectum can exert local or systemic effects. The forms commonly used are suppositories, creams or ointments, and aqueous or oily liquids.

Locally, peristalsis is stimulated by suppositories to treat constipation or to prepare the lower gastrointestinal tract for surgery, examination, or the administration of other drugs. Saline or soap-solution enemas may be given for the same pur-

pose. Corticosteroids, astringents, and local anesthetics are applied in suppository, cream, or ointment form to relieve the discomfort of hemorrhoids. Antibiotics and corticosteroids may be used in enemas to treat inflammatory diseases of the colon.

Rectally administered sedatives, analgesics, antiemetics, antipyretics, and bronchodilators, in the form of suppositories or solutions, can exert systemic effects. There are some advantages to this route: (1) in the case of the patient who is unable to take an oral medication because of the nature of the drug, the condition of the upper gastrointestinal tract, or his mental state; (2) medication readily enters the general circulation because of the vascular nature of the colon; and (3) it offers an alternative to invasive routes of administration.

The rectal route also has some disadvantages: (1) absorption may be unpredictable because the patient may not be able to retain the suppository or solution; and (2) as the solution leaves the colon and enters the circulating blood, it may reach the portal circulation and be inactivated by the liver.

Procedure

Many patients find rectal drug administration embarrassing. It is helpful for the nurse to maintain a professional, straightforward approach throughout the procedure, to give the patient a complete explanation about the procedure, and to ensure patient privacy to the extent possible. It is best to administer the drug before the patient eats, since peristaltic stimulation can cause nausea if the patient's stomach is full. A cleansing enema may be given before a drug is instilled, to remove fecal material that might otherwise prevent the medication from contacting the mucosa, where absorption into the blood occurs. Suppositories melt slowly at body temperature, so they should be kept cold until just before they are inserted into the rectum. The nurse, or the patient if he is able, should insert the suppository beyond the internal rectal sphincter to prevent it from slipping out. The suppository must be retained as long as possible to ensure complete absorption, so the patient should be instructed to lie on his left side, and to take deep breaths when he feels cramping. In the case of suppositories administered to induce peristalsis, expulsion of lower bowel contents should occur within 20 minutes. Stay with the patient if he needs assistance.

When administering an enema, whether given to cleanse the lower gastrointestinal tract or to instill drugs, remember that the solution must be retained until it can exert its effect or until absorption is complete. Warm the solution to body temperature, keep the volume of drug-containing solution to 120 ml or less, and unless a prepackaged enema is being used, use a small rectal tube or urinary catheter (rather than a conventional rectal tube) to promote patient comfort. Inform the patient about any discomfort he might be expected to feel. Instruct him to lie on his left side with his knees comfortably flexed. Insert the tube 10 cm to 15 cm, then *slowly* infuse the solution. When the entire dose has been given, slowly remove the catheter. Stay with the patient and help him to deep breathe if he has cramps. If the patient finds it difficult to retain the solution, a Foley catheter may be inserted into the rectum beyond the internal sphincter and the retention balloon inflated. Consult institutional policy to learn if this procedure is permissible and what size catheter and balloon is permitted. To prevent damage to the rectum, the inflated balloon should be left in place only long enough for drug absorption to take place.

Vaginal Medications
Antiseptics and anti-infectives are instilled into the vaginal canal in the form of aqueous solutions, suppositories, creams, or foams.

Procedure
Most women have had the experience of self-administering a douche or a cream, so they should be permitted to perform this procedure if they feel comfortable about it. The nurse should lend assistance as needed. If the patient is young and feels apprehensive about the procedure, take the time to allay her fears as much as possible. A few points should be kept in mind when a vaginal irrigation is being administered: (1) the warm solution must enter the vagina under very low pressure to prevent tissue damage and to prevent the drug from entering the cervical canal; (2) the tip of the nozzle must be rotated to ensure that the medication reaches all parts of the vaginal canal.

Administration of Drugs by the Parenteral Route

Parenteral drugs are those that are injected into body tissues. All medications and equipment used for this route of administration must be sterile. Either local or systemic effects are exerted depending on the mode of administration and the drug. Parenteral administration encompasses intradermal

(intracutaneous), subcutaneous, intramuscular, intravenous, intra-arterial, intraperitoneal, intrathoracic (intrapleural), intrathecal (intraspinal), intracardiac, and intrasynovial (intra-articular) modes. Only those procedures that are performed by the nurse will be discussed in detail here; those that are usually performed by the physician will be described briefly in relation to their nursing implications.

PREPARATION FOR ADMINISTRATION
The size of the syringe to be used is dictated by the amount of solution to be administered. All syringes are calibrated in milliliters or fractions thereof. The amount of solution contained in the needle shaft and needle hub, the so-called dead space of the syringe–needle system, has been calculated into the calibrations on the syringe barrel. Hence, it is not necessary to draw any air into the filled syringe to push behind the drug solution, emptying the dead space.

DRUG INCOMPATIBILITY
Drug solutions can be incompatible with one another, resulting in drug inactivation, chemical breakdown, or the development of a toxic compound. Even drugs that can be safely combined may have limited compatibility based on duration of contact, temperature, light, and humidity. To minimize the risk of dangerous drug incompatibilities, the nurse should use the following guidelines:

1. Become familiar with compatibility charts issued by the institution where you work. When in doubt about any drug combination, refer to the pharmacist or drug manufacturer for clarification. Do not rely on the word of other professionals, or combine drugs because "it has always been done that way." Chapter 5 has several lists of drug incompatibilities. See also the Appendix.
2. Never assume that since one drug can be combined with another that related drugs can also be combined.
3. To limit vial contamination, withdraw doses from a multidose vial into an empty syringe; then withdraw the second medication from a single-dose vial. If both doses are to be withdrawn from multidose vials, withdraw each separately and then combine them.

SKIN PREPARATION
To prepare the skin for injection, it must be thoroughly cleansed. A brief gentle scrubbing with iso-

propyl alcohol or a germicide such as iodophor is recommended if the needle is to be inserted and then removed; if the needle or a catheter is to remain in the tissues, the skin should be scrubbed for several minutes with iodophor. Follow institutional policy. Regardless of which technique is indicated, the scrub is done by application of the antiseptic or germicide to the center of the site where the needle is to be inserted, followed by application of the solution in a circular pattern outward from that site. The solution should then be allowed to dry before the needle is inserted.

PATIENT PREPARATION

The nurse must assess the patient's level of anxiety and design an approach that can help to alleviate discomfort. Thorough explanation, coupled with an efficient and professional approach, and good technique are the best tools. Inform the patient of the steps you plan to take to reduce his discomfort and explain the anticipated benefits of the drug and the procedure. The psychologic and emotional preparation of the patient is detailed in Chapter 6.

INTRADERMAL INJECTION

Intradermal or intracutaneous injection is the injection of a drug into the outer layers of the skin, between the outermost or epidermis layer above the subcutaneous layer, into the dermis (Fig. 8-1). It is primarily used to anesthetize the skin for other invasive procedures; to test for tuberculosis, histoplasmosis, and similar diseases; and to test for allergy. The volume of drug is usually less than 0.5 ml. The 1-ml syringe, calibrated in 0.01-ml increments, is usually used where accurate calibrations

are needed for drug measurement. A 26-gauge or 27-gauge needle that is ½ inch to ⅝ inch long is used (Table 8-2).

Procedure

Following skin preparation, the skin is stretched taut with one hand and the needle is quickly inserted at a 10-degree to 15-degree angle to a depth of about 0.5 cm. The drug is then injected, creating a small wheal under the skin.

In skin testing, the tissue must be observed for signs of sensitivity reaction. Local reactions are characterized by the formation of a wheal or hive, redness, swelling, and possibly itching. Systemic allergic reactions are rare but can occur.

SUBCUTANEOUS INJECTION

In subcutaneous injection, the drug is placed into the tissues below the dermis but above the muscle layer (see Fig. 8-1). Absorption is more rapid from this layer than from the intradermal layer because of the increased capillary supply, though it is slower than absorption by the intramuscular route. This characteristic is desirable when a sustained drug effect is needed. Such factors as peripheral edema, vasoconstriction, and the presence of burns can slow absorption; therefore, subcutaneous injections should not be administered to patients with hypotension, edema in the injection areas, severe skin lesions such as burns and psoriasis, or severe arterial occlusive disease in the affected extremity.

Procedure

In most clinical circumstances, drugs administered subcutaneously include insulin, aqueous epinephrine, tetanus toxoid, heparin, small volumes of narcotics, vaccines, vitamin B_{12}, and allergen serums. Only small volumes, 0.5 ml to 1.5 ml, of soluble, well-diluted, nonirritating drugs should be given. The recommended needle sizes are 25 gauge to 27 gauge, ½ inch to ⅝ inch long (see Table 8-2). The lateral aspect of the upper arms and thighs, the abdomen below, above, and lateral to the umbilicus, and the upper back are the sites of injection.

After the skin has been prepared, the injection can be done in one of two ways. If the patient is lean, pinch up an area of skin between the index finger and thumb of one hand and insert the needle at a 45-degree angle with the other; if the patient is obese, or if a fatty site such as the abdomen is used, simply insert the needle at a 90-degree angle. The purpose of these steps is to ensure that the drug has

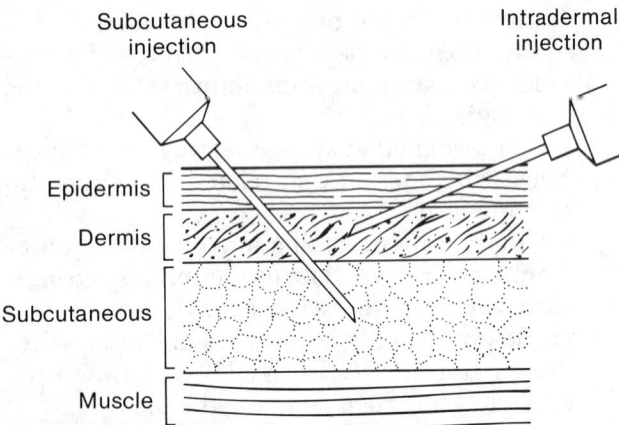

Figure 8-1. Diagrammatic representation of the tissue layers below the epidermis and the sites for intradermal and subcutaneous injections.

Table 8-2
Parameters for Parenteral Injections

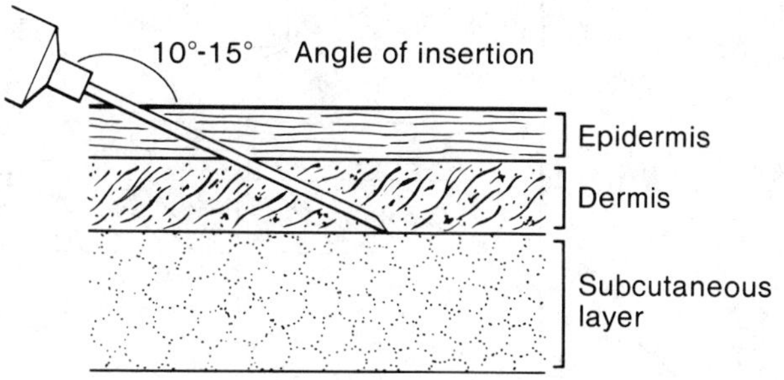

Needle Size	Needle Length	Syringe Type	Volume of Solution
Intradermal Injection			
26 gauge–27 gauge	½ inch–⅝ inch	1 ml with 0.01-ml increments (*i.e.*, tuberculin type)	<0.5 ml

10°–15° Angle of insertion

Epidermis

Dermis

Subcutaneous layer

Subcutaneous Injection			
25 gauge–27 gauge	½ inch–⅝ inch	1-ml–3-ml syringe (insulin syringe; tuberculin syringe)	0.5 ml–1.5 ml

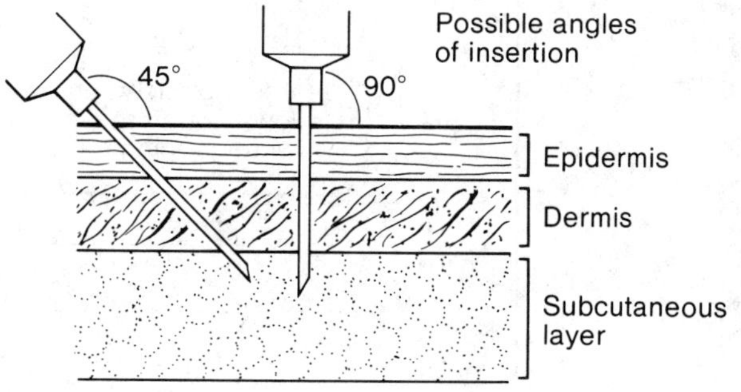

Possible angles of insertion

45°   90°

Epidermis

Dermis

Subcutaneous layer

(continued)

reached the subcutaneous tissues. Once the needle is in place, pull back on the plunger to aspirate for blood; if none is present, slowly inject the drug. Remove the needle quickly and apply pressure to the site. Massage the area to enhance absorption. The procedure differs for injection of heparin and is explained in Chapter 39. Variations on this technique are also used in injection of insulin and are explained in Chapter 54.

INTRAMUSCULAR INJECTION

In intramuscular injections, the medication is injected into the body of a muscle. This route may be used to administer irritating drugs, aqueous suspensions, and solutions in oils in volumes of 1.5 ml to 5 ml. Absorption is faster than with the subcutaneous route because muscle is richly supplied with blood. Systemic effects occur within 15 to 30 minutes of injection, depending on the drug and the

Table 8-2 (continued)
Parameters for Parenteral Injections

Needle Size	Needle Length	Syringe Type	Volume of Solution

Intramuscular Injection

| See Table 8-3. Varies according to muscle used. See Figure 8-2. | See Table 8-3; varies according to muscle used | 3-ml–5-ml syringe | 1.5 ml–5 ml |

Intravenous Injection or Infusion

| 14 gauge–27 gauge; depends on drug viscosity, size of patient | ½ inch–3½ inches; depends on type; intracatheters may be longer. | Varies: See text. | Varies: See text. |

efficiency of the systemic circulation. Several factors affect drug absorption and therapeutic effect, as follows:

1. *Composition and solubility of the drug and the carrying vehicle.* In some instances, the rate of drug absorption can be controlled by how the drug is dissolved and what fluid vehicle is used.
2. *Site of injection.* The rapidity with which the drug is absorbed into the circulation depends on the blood flow to the muscle. The *deltoid* muscle has the richest blood flow of any muscle used for injection.
3. *Injection technique and depth of needle insertion.* Care must be taken to select an appropriate needle length for the size of the muscle and the depth of the fatty tissue above the muscle body (Table 8-3). Care must be taken to insert the needle into the center of the muscle, where blood flow is best and there is no subcutaneous fat. The intramuscular route should not be used when the patient is in shock or has severe tissue edema.

Procedure

Using the information in Table 8-3, determine the appropriate muscle group to be used for the injection. Then determine the specific injection site by locating the anatomic landmarks shown in Figure 8-2. Assess the muscle mass and fatty tissue at the selected site. In the obese patient, the area over the muscle may need to be stretched before the needle is injected to reduce the thickness of overlying tissues. In an infant, child, or thin adult, the muscle mass can be pinched to raise it from the bone. These preliminary steps are important to ensure correct anatomic placement of the needle, thus avoiding blood vessels and nerves.

Once the location of the injection site is determined, administer the drug in a syringe with a clean, dry needle to minimize irritation. Cleanse the injection site according to institution policy and insert the needle with a quick dart-like action, usually at a 75-degree to a 90-degree angle, depending on the size of the muscle. Pull back on the plunger before injecting to test accidental injection into a blood vessel. If blood is seen in the syringe, withdraw the needle, apply pressure to the site, and prepare a new dose of the drug. Do not reinject the contaminated drug in a different site. If a nerve is punctured on needle insertion, the patient will complain of immediate severe pain or a tingling numbness along the nerve tract. If this occurs, withdraw the needle and notify the physician.

If needle insertion is correct, inject the solution by firmly pushing the plunger and keeping the syringe steady. Sources vary on how quickly to inject the solution, but most patients will report they prefer the procedure to be over as quickly as possible. After all the solution is injected, withdraw the needle straight out of the site and apply mild pressure.

A variation on this technique, called the *Z-track method*, can be used to prevent a large-volume injection from oozing out of the muscle and

Table 8-3
A Guide to Intramuscular Injection

Muscle	Injection Volume	Needle Size	Comments
Gluteus medius, gluteus minimus	1.0 ml–5.0 ml	20 gauge–23 gauge, 1½ inches–3 inches	Deep IM; Z-track (Fig. 8-3); large volume; any drug that can be given IM
Vastus lateralis	1.0 ml–5.0 ml	22 gauge–25 gauge, 1½ inches–2 inches (adults)	Any drug that can be given IM; not for Z-track
Rectus femoris	1.0 ml–2.0 ml	22 gauge–25 gauge, ½ inch–1 inch	Small-volume injections; used for infants
Deltoid (not used in children under 3 years of age)	0.5 ml–1.5 ml	23 gauge–25 gauge, ⅝ inch–1 inch	Small volume; often used for narcotics, sedatives, or vaccines

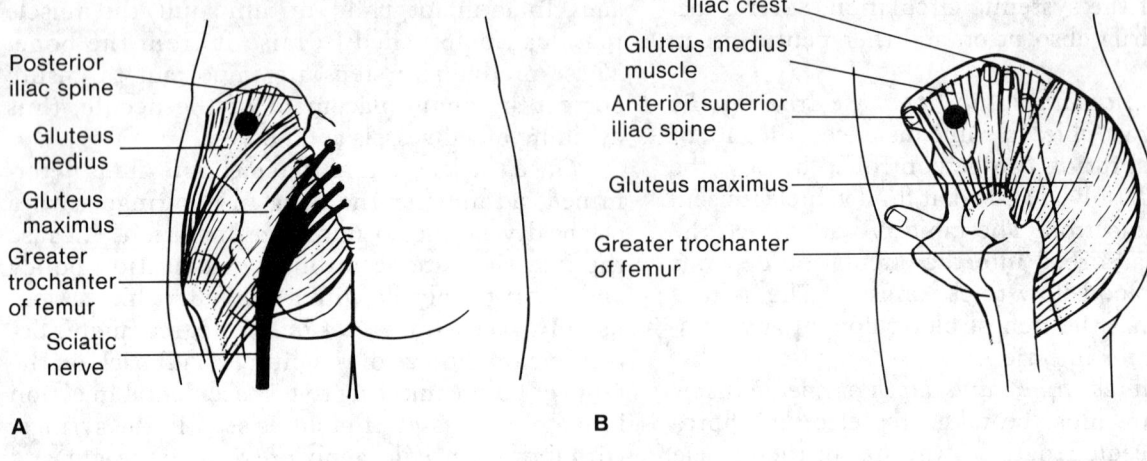

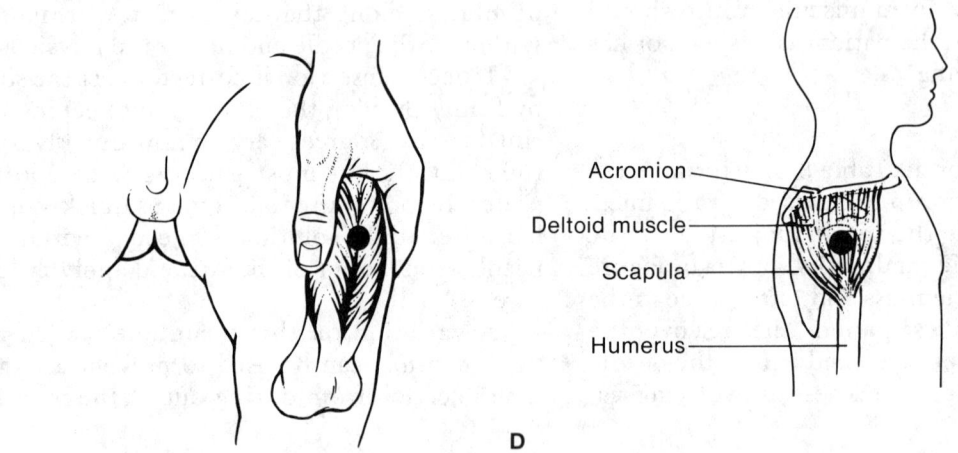

Figure 8-2.   *Anatomical landmarks used for determining sites for IM injections. (A) Dorsogluteal site. Injection is made above and lateral to a line drawn from the greater trochanter of the femur to the posterior superior iliac spine to avoid the sciatic nerve. (B) Ventrogluteal site. Injection is made into the center of a triangle formed between the second and third fingers when the palm is placed on the greater trochanter, the index finger on the anterior superior iliac spine, and the middle finger on the iliac crest. (C) Midlateral thigh site (especially in children). Injection is made equidistant between the greater trochanter and the patella and halfway between the front and side of the thigh. (D) Mid-deltoid site. Injection is made into the mid-deltoid area, below the acromion and lateral to the axilla.*

out through the needle track. With this method, the injection area is pulled to one side with gentle traction and the needle is inserted into the muscle. After the solution is injected, traction on the skin is released. The solution is thus deposited in the muscle but not directly under the needle track (see Fig. 8-3).

If multiple injections must be given, rotation of injection sites should be systematic to avoid unnec-

essary tissue trauma. The illustration on p. 114 provides directions for using a body map to rotate intramuscular injections.

INTRAVENOUS ADMINISTRATION

Intravenous (IV) injection—the injection of a drug solution directly into a vein—is not always performed by the nurse. Nurse practice acts, policy statements formulated by nurses' associations and

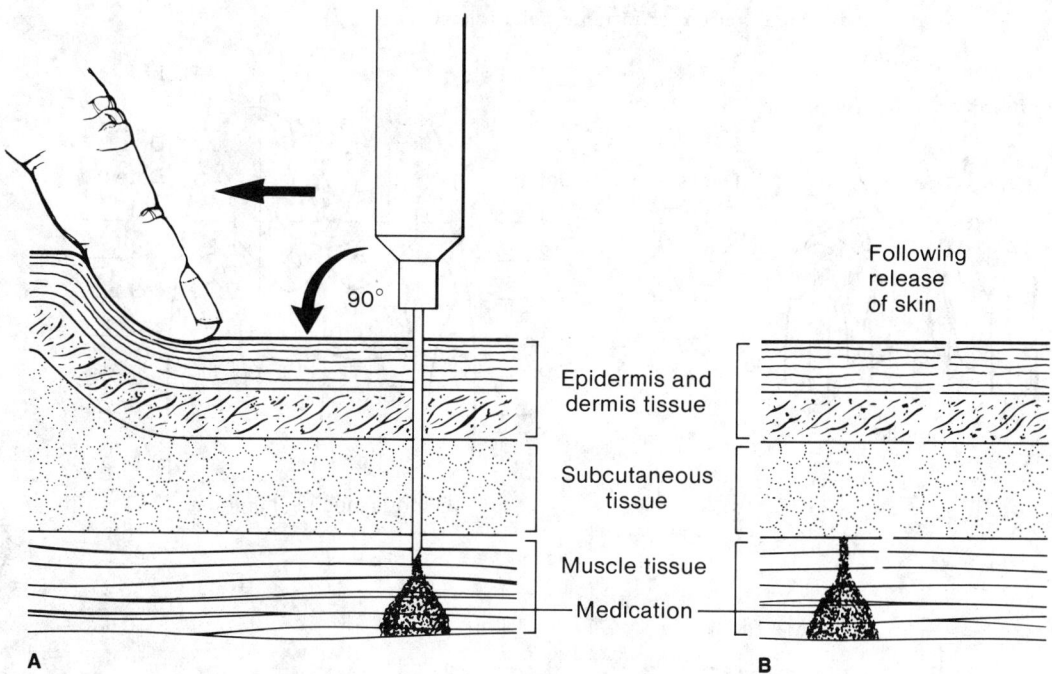

Figure 8-3. Procedure for Z-track intramuscular injection used for
administration of medication known to cause staining of superficial tissues.
(A) Skin is stretched to one side, and medication is injected. (B) When needle
is removed, skin is allowed to return to normal position, sealing off the
deposited drug from the track of the needle.

medical societies, and specific institutional policies govern this method of drug administration, and the practitioner must be aware of these policies.

Hospitals manage IV drug administration in several ways. Designated persons practice only in specialized areas of the hospital or clinic, for example, in critical care units or the emergency room, or as members of an IV team, and they are usually required to attend classes and undergo supervised practice to ensure competence. IV therapy teams may be authorized to insert and maintain IV lines. When possible, these teams are on duty 24 hours a day, 7 days a week.

Hospitals formulate written policies to guide personnel performing these functions. The procedure for safe and competent IV drug administration includes (1) preparing the IV line, which includes selecting the appropriate apparatus; (2) selecting an appropriate venous site and inserting the IV line; (3) preparing IV drugs and admixtures (in many institutions this is done by the pharmacist); (4) administering the drugs and admixtures and monitoring their effects; and (5) managing any complications.

Whether or not the nurse is a member of the IV team, it is highly likely that at some time in her career she will be called on to administer drugs intravenously. She should thoroughly familiarize herself with IV therapy so that she will feel confident of her ability to perform it.

Procedure

Preparing the Line
The IV line consists of the fluid container, the administration set (tubing, drip chamber, and flow-control device), in some instances an in-line filter, and the needle or cannula. When preparing an IV line, select a fluid that is compatible with the drugs to be administered, or verify that the fluid ordered by the physician is compatible with the drugs. Consult an up-to-date reference or call the pharmacist. Select the correct size container according to the physician's order, the volume needed for correct drug dilution, or predicted patient need. Inspect the container for defects such as foreign bodies or discoloration of the fluid, cracks in the glass, or leaks (if a bag), and check the expiration date.

The type of set to be used depends on the type of infusion to be administered. All sets have a drip chamber that is calibrated to deliver a specific number of drops per milliliter of fluid. Most standard sets provide 10 drops, 15 drops, or 20 drops per

Body Map Rotation for Intramuscular Injections

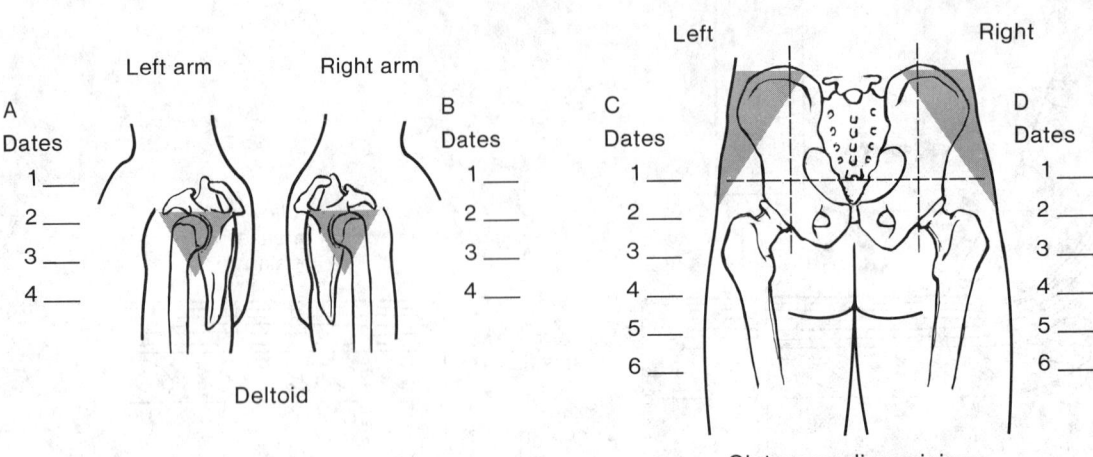

Deltoid

Gluteus medius; minimus

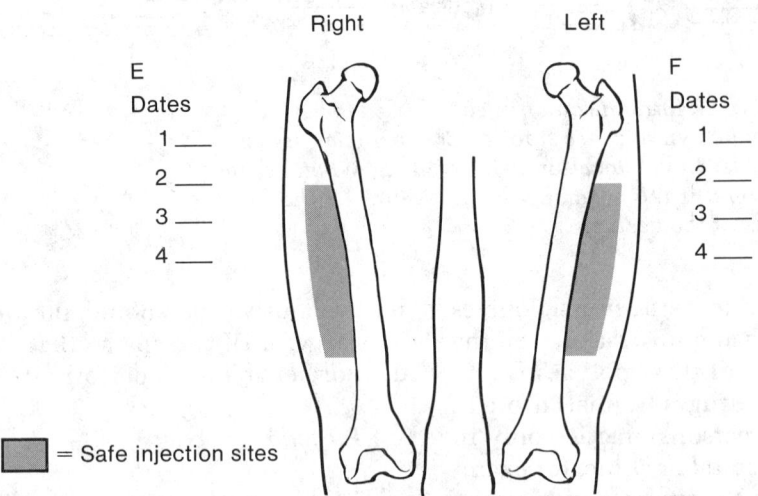

= Safe injection sites

Vastus lateralis/rectus femoris

1. Refer to Table 8-3 for site selection based on drug volume and to Figure 8-2 to determine anatomic landmarks.
2. Start with the preferred site, depending on the age of the patient, or with site *A* if no preference is given. After giving the injection, mark the date after the number 1 at site *A*. Rotate to site *B* for the next injection, then to *C*, and so on using all appropriate sites. Return to site *A* only after all other appropriate sites have been used.
3. The second injection at any site should be approximately 1½ inches or one knuckle width from the first needle mark; the third should be 1½ inches from the second, and so on. The number of injections possible at a specific site depends on the patient's size and muscle mass.
4. Anatomic landmarks should be determined before each injection. The site should be thoroughly examined, and pain, redness, swelling, induration, or sponginess should be noted. Any of these changes should be reported to the physician, because they indicate damaged tissue. The site should not be used for further injections.

milliliter, depending on the manufacturer; these are identified as *regular drip chambers. Microdrop* sets, which produce smaller drops, 60 drops per milliliter, allow for precise control of the dose. It is essential that the nurse know the drop calibration, also called the *drop factor,* so that the flow rate can be accurately calculated and monitored. Every set has rubber-stopped injection ports designed for the addition of IV secondary lines and for drug injection.

Some sets include volume-control chambers. In this type of set, the chamber is filled with a measured amount of fluid, up to 150 ml, from the main container. With this arrangement, the patient receives fluid from this chamber only, thus limiting the volume. Volume-control arrangements are especially useful in pediatric IV administration, in which inadvertent fluid overload could be hazardous. Some drugs may be injected into the volume-control chambers and infused after being diluted in a measured amount of fluid (Fig. 8-4A).

Another type of set is used in conjunction with a volume-control infusion pump. In this set-up, a special pumping chamber is incorporated into the tubing. When the administration set is connected to the pump and filled with fluid, the pump draws a measured amount of fluid into the chamber, then injects it into the patient. This is the most accurate type of infusion pump available.

Certain basic features are found in all IV tubing: a piercing pin whose function is to insert the tubing into the fluid container; the drip chamber; a flow-control clamp; and a needle adapter at the patient end of the tubing, which is inserted into the IV needle or cannula.

An in-line filtration device may also be used as a means of removing contaminates and particulate matter from drug-containing admixtures. In-line filters are incorporated into some IV administration sets, while others are added to the tubing when necessary. The pharmacist should determine the need for and the type and size of the filter used.

To prepare the fluid container and administration set for use, close the flow-control clamp and insert the piercing pin into the container opening. If a glass bottle is used, listen for a hissing sound, which occurs with insertion; it indicates that the bottle vacuum is intact. No sound will be heard when piercing an IV bag. Then invert the bottle or bag and suspend it on the pole. Fill the drip chamber by squeezing it, filling it only halfway. Open the flow-control clamp and allow fluid to fill the tubing up to the end. When it is full, close the clamp.

Inserting the Line

Factors that must be considered in vein selection (Table 8-4) include
1. The type of *medication* to be administered. Most drugs can be given by peripheral veins where blood flow is sufficient to dilute the solution and prevent venous wall irritation. Hypertonic or caustic drug solutions should, in most cases, be given through a large central vein. When possible, these drugs as well as vasopressors should not be given through the small veins of the hand because tissue damage

leading to necrosis could occur if the drug were to leak from the vein.
2. The *availability of veins.* Some veins that would routinely be used may be unavailable because of trauma, surgery, or burns, or because circulation has been compromised. Avoid the use of the lower extremities because IV therapy may promote venous thrombosis; if the lower extremity must be used, use the veins of the foot rather than those of the leg.
3. The *patient's ability to cooperate.* If the patient is confused or combative, use a vein that is less likely to be disrupted such as a central line in the subclavian or an extremity vein that can be restrained.

The lumen of the vein must be large enough to accommodate the IV line, and the blood flow must be adequate to transport drug and fluid into the circulation. Parts of the body involved in movement, such as joints, should be avoided, but if a vein in a joint must be used, a splint will be required to prevent displacement of the line.

After the site has been selected, a suitable needle or IV catheter is chosen. Most catheters are radiopaque and are made of polyethylene, polyvinylchloride (PVC), or Teflon. They are equipped with an inserting needle, which is removed once the tube is inside the vein. Catheter size ranges from 14 gauge to 22 gauge with a length of 1¼ inches to 2 inches; a larger or smaller device is used when the size of the vein requires this. Stainless-steel, wing-grip, "butterfly" needle units are popular; they range in size from 14 gauge to 27 gauge, ¾ inch to 1 inch in length. Insertion technique varies with the vein used and the device.

Preparing the Drugs

As a rule, drug reconstitution and admixture preparation are done in the pharmacy where strict adherence to aseptic technique can be maintained. This is a highly technical function that requires complete accuracy; it is also occasionally dangerous. Certain drug compounds prepared for IV administration, especially some drugs used in cancer chemotherapy, can produce particles that are irritating to the eyes and the nose; certain others can cause skin irritation or contact burns. These drugs constitute an environmental hazard and unnecessarily jeopardize the nurse's safety. A laminar flow hood, which provides nonrecirculated air flow, decreases the number of circulating particles. If the nurse must prepare such drugs, she should insist that flow hoods or specially ventilated areas be

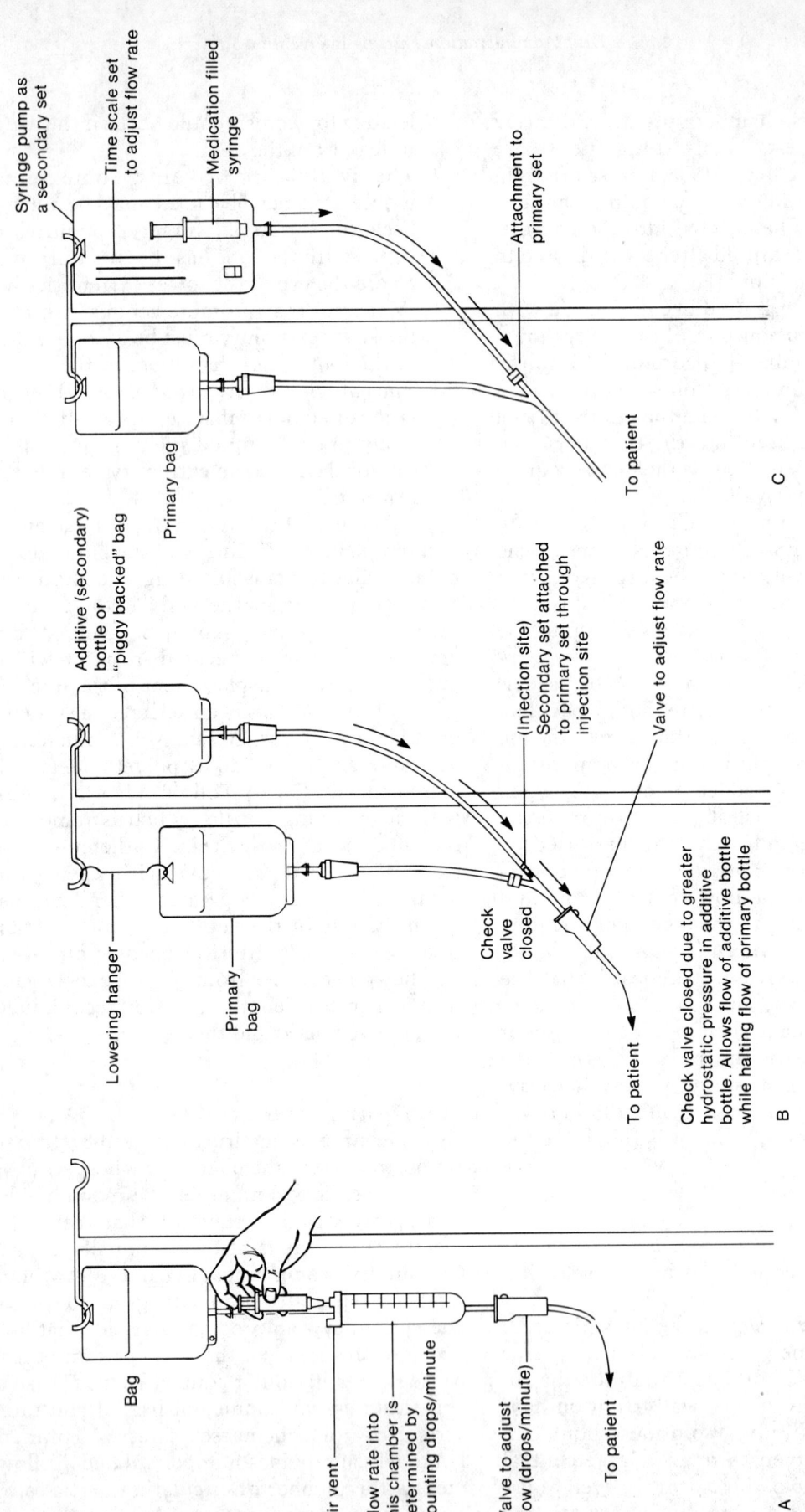

Figure 8-4. *Methods of intermittent intravenous infusion. (A) The drug is injected into a secondary chamber located between the bag of solution and the patient. (B) The drug is administered from a secondary or "piggybacked" bag into an established IV line. (C) The drug is placed in a syringe, which is then attached to an infusion pump, and is administered either directly into a heparin lock or "piggybacked" into an established IV line.*

Syringe pump as a secondary set

Time scale set to adjust flow rate

Medication filled syringe

Attachment to primary set

Primary bag

To patient

C

Additive (secondary) bottle or "piggy backed" bag

Lowering hanger

Primary bag

Check valve closed

(Injection site) Secondary set attached to primary set through injection site

Valve to adjust flow rate

To patient

Check valve closed due to greater hydrostatic pressure in additive bottle. Allows flow of additive bottle while halting flow of primary bottle

B

Bag

Air vent

Flow rate into this chamber is determined by counting drops/minute

Valve to adjust flow (drops/minute)

To patient

A

Table 8-4
Factors in the Selection of Peripheral or Central Sites for Intravenous Insertion

Factor	Peripheral Veins		Central Veins	
	Suitable	Unsuitable	Suitable	Unsuitable
Type of drug or solution	Most drugs, isotonic fluids	Irritating drugs or hypertonic fluids that require maximal dilution	Irritating drugs or hypertonic fluids	Drugs that if injected centrally could cause arrhythmias, shock, or other complications
Duration of therapy	Short-term or intermittent therapy	Long-term therapy, in which all available veins would be used up	Moderate to long-term continuous therapy	Short-term therapy; the patient is subjected to greater risks
Accessibility of veins	Patients with adequate peripheral veins	Very obese patients; intravenous drug abusers; conditions that impair peripheral circulation	When peripheral veins inaccessible, especially if intravenous line is needed in an emergency	At times not accessible after repeated use (e.g., pacemaker). May be accessible, but increased risks due to location near lungs
Cooperation of patient	Extremity can usually be restrained sufficiently to allow insertion and maintenance of line	Disoriented or agitated adult or child may be more likely to attempt removal of intravenous line located in upper extremity	Central lines, especially subclavian, are less likely to be disrupted, once inserted	Patient must lie absolutely still during the insertion to prevent pneumothorax and other complications

provided for reconstitution. In addition, all nurses should wear protective clothing, such as a mask, gown, or gloves, when mixing dangerous drug compounds.

If the nurse is required to prepare drugs or admixtures, she should keep the following guidelines in mind:

1. Wash hands and work in a quiet, clean area.
2. Calculate the dose carefully (*i.e.*, the amount of drug dilution and final solution needed). See Chapter 11 on dosage calculation.
3. Inspect the drug vial for the presence of cracks, foreign bodies or contamination, precipitates, or color changes.
4. Check the drug's expiration date and be certain that the drug is intended for IV use.
5. When reconstituting a drug from powder, carefully follow the *manufacturer's* recommendations about the diluent. Use *only* that diluent since any other could render the drug less active or could produce an unwanted compound. Read the package insert or consult the pharmacist. Use *sterile water for injection* and normal

saline for injection with or without a preservative, as dictated by the drug literature. Most manufacturers suggest volumes of diluent that will create a drug solution of a particular concentration to facilitate the measurement of an accurate dose.

6. Maintain sterility of the rubber stopper on the drug bottle or vial, the needle and plunger of the syringe used to transfer fluids and the drug, and the top of the IV fluid bottle or its medication port at all times.
7. Clean the rubber stopper before inserting the needle. To prevent particulate matter, such as minute bits of rubber, glass, metal, or plastic, from entering the patient's body during an injection or infusion, place a syringe filter on the syringe used to transfer the drug from the drug container to the patient. There are several types of filters available with varying filtering capacities; the pharmacist is the best source of information on which to use. An admixture prepared in the pharmacy will be accompanied by the appropriate filter for the specific pur-

pose and drug used. Using the wrong filter could reduce the amount of drug delivered to the patient.

8. When adding a drug to a bottle or bag of IV fluid or when injecting a drug into an IV line, be certain that the drug is compatible with the fluid and any other drug present in the system. Consult a compatibility chart or the pharmacist. If two incompatible drugs are to be given by infusion or injection, flush the IV line with a compatible fluid after the first drug has been infused, and flush following the second.

9. When adding a drug to a container of IV fluids for infusion, protect the bottle from light if the manufacturer so advises. A foil bag is supplied by the manufacturer to cover the bottle or bag. It is not necessary to cover the infusion tubing because the drug is in the tubing for only a brief time.

10. Prepared drugs and solutions should be used shortly after being prepared. Date and store vials of reconstituted drugs as indicated by the manufacturer, and discard them as indicated. Date all prepared multidose vials.

11. Some antibiotics intended for use in intermittent infusions are supplied in powder form for reconstitution in a container that accommodates a large volume of diluent. Read the label to be certain that the amount of drug and diluent added is correct.

12. When adding drugs to infusion fluid, agitate the container to mix the solution thoroughly. When adding a drug to fluids that are being infused, inject the drug into the injection port at the top of the IV tubing, then *quickly* invert the container to mix the drug throughout the solution, and agitate the container. Failure to agitate a solution properly could allow a large amount of the drug to be infused all at once in a concentrated form.

Specific Methods for Administration of Intravenous Drugs

IV drugs are administered by direct injection, intermittent infusion, or continuous infusion, according to the nature of the drug and the effects anticipated.

Injection Method

Injection, or IV "push," is the administration of a relatively small volume of a concentrated solution directly into the venous system by syringe, through the IV tubing or directly into the IV cannula or needle. The medications are given over a period of several minutes or as a *bolus* within a short period of time. The injection method is used to administer drugs that are not diluted in large volumes of fluid because dilution would inactivate them. Examples are diazepam, digoxin, and furosemide. This method is also used when an immediate effect is necessary; an example is lidocaine (also used in long-term infusion to control cardiac dysrhythmias).

In the first of these methods, the drug is given slowly within 1 to 5 minutes, the actual speed of the injection being measured in milligrams of drug per minute. The period of injection is timed by a watch. Adverse reactions are possible nevertheless; thorough knowledge of the drug and of the patient's physiologic state are required for safe administration.

In the second, or *bolus*, method, the drug is administered rapidly by instantaneous injection to deliver the drug in high concentration to vital organs, such as the heart, brain, or kidney. Most drugs are not administered as a bolus, however, because the rapid rise in drug concentration in the blood can cause adverse reactions, including *speed shock*. Speed shock is the body's reaction to the sudden presence of a high concentration of a foreign substance; it can lead to seizures, respiratory arrest, and cardiac arrest. The possibility of speed shock occurring has traditionally made the administration of IV injections the responsibility of the physician.

Before injection proceeds, the placement of the IV cannula or needle in the vein must be verified. The reason for this is that some drugs can cause serious tissue damage if inadvertently injected into the tissues surrounding the vein. To check on placement when injecting directly into the vein, retract the syringe plunger to pull blood into the chamber, then inject. If blood does not enter the syringe, use another vein. This should be done whether the needle has been inserted directly into the vein or has been inserted into the tubing of a running IV system. When the needle position is checked in a functioning infusion system, the needle containing the drug is inserted into an injection port in the tubing; then the tubing above the port is pinched before the syringe plunger is retracted.

Once the placement of the needle or cannula has been confirmed, the drug is injected at the *manufacturer's suggested rate* in milliliters per minute. If an incompatibility exists between the drug and the primary fluid in a line, flush the lower tubing (nearer the patient) with a compatible solution before injecting the drug. An alternative to this procedure is to inject the drug directly into the needle or cannula after the infusion line has been removed. Care must be taken not to contaminate the cannula or tubing.

A heparin lock or intermittent infusion set with a resealable rubber injection port is used in patients who require direct IV injections but do not need an IV infusion line. This method allows the patient who requires medication for extended periods of time to have more mobility and eliminates the need for a KVO (keep vein open) IV drip. Drugs given by this method include heparin and antibiotics as well as some cancer chemotherapy agents. Patency of the line is maintained by injection of a heparin and saline solution at regular intervals. The drug injected must be compatible with heparin. If it is not, flush the system with a compatible fluid before injecting, then replace the heparin solution. (See also Chap. 39 for further discussion.)

Infusion Method

IV infusion differs from injection in that a relatively large volume of fluid or drug-containing fluid is instilled through the line over a period of time. Maintenance of the correct rate of infusion is one of the main nursing responsibilities in IV administration. Medications and the fluid vehicle must be infused at an appropriate rate and in an accurate manner to achieve the desired therapeutic response and to prevent adverse reactions and complications. See Chapter 11 for a complete discussion on how to calculate flow rates of IV solutions. Flow rate of a solution should be checked hourly while an IV is being administered and more frequently when a new or dangerous drug is being infused.

Several factors affect the rate of flow of an IV infusion: (1) viscosity of the fluid; (2) amount of fluid in the container (since a full container produces a more rapid infusion rate than a nearly empty one); (3) height of the container (the higher the container is placed, the more rapidly it will infuse); (4) the presence or absence of an in-line filter; and (5) the size of the IV cannula or needle (the larger the size, the more rapid the flow).

When *precise* control of the infusion is needed, one of several devices may be used. A *controller* is an electronic device that regulates the passage of fluid through the tubing by means of a magnetically activated metal ball valve that is synchronized with a drop detector. It is not a true pump, and it is therefore potentially inaccurate. A *pump* operates by exerting pressure on the tubing or on the fluid inside a special tubing. The pump may be *nonvo-*

lumetric (measures rate in drops per minute) or *volumetric* (measures milliliters per minute).

Under most circumstances, the volumetric pump is the most accurate flow rate control device. Most such pumps are designed to prevent air from being pumped into the patient and to sound an alarm when resistance to pumping is met because of a clotted cannula, pinched tubing, or other cause. It takes time and practice to learn how to operate these pumps. The nurse will find it helpful to read and study the manual that is provided with the device. Other special pumps are available for specific situations.

There are two methods of IV infusion: *intermittent* and *continuous*.

1. Intermittent infusion. An intermittent infusion consists of a specific dose of a drug added to a small volume of fluid that is infused over a period of time, ranging from 20 minutes to 2 hours. Its purpose is to produce drug level peaks in the blood. Piggyback, volume-control infusion sets, and syringe infusion pumps may be used (see Fig. 8-4). Usually, when this method of administration is required, it is because the drug must be diluted before it enters the patient's body; it is most effective when given over a definite period of time at fixed intervals around the clock. The volume of diluent usually ranges from 20 ml to 250 ml, depending on the amount of drug and its properties. Many antibiotics and antineoplastic drugs are given in this manner.

   The drug is placed in a secondary infusion set, which may be a small (piggyback) bottle or bag of fluid with administration tubing; diluted in a volume-control set in the calibrated chamber; or mixed in a syringe and infused via a pump mechanism. With any type of secondary infusion apparatus, the tubing is inserted into the existing IV line or into a heparin lock through a needle. The solution is then infused at the prescribed rate. Care must be taken to maintain an open line once the infusion has been completed. A heparin lock or a system without a primary IV line will clot if the intermittent infusion has been completed and there is no fluid remaining to run into the needle and vein. Most administration tubing used for a primary infusion has an automatic valve that opens and allows fluid from the primary fluid container to run when the secondary, intermittent infusion has been completed.

2. Continuous infusion. In continuous infusion, the drug is added to a relatively large volume of

fluid (250 ml to 1000 ml) and infused continuously over a period of several hours or days. Continuous infusion is preferred when the drug must be highly diluted before entering the body (e.g., potassium chloride, dobutamine, amphotericin B). This method maintains a steady blood level of the drug. Replacement therapy with fluids and electrolytes is provided in this manner, as is total parenteral nutrition.

Drugs needed to control certain pathologies are often infused continuously, but at varying rates, the rate being determined by need to control a vital sign or to effect a desired outcome. Examples include the use of lidocaine infusion to control ventricular dysrhythmias; oxytocin to initiate and maintain uterine contractions during labor or to maintain uterine contractions to control postpartum bleeding; and dopamine to regulate systemic arterial blood pressure. In all such cases, physiologic parameters are established by which the infusion rate can be adjusted or *titrated*. In the examples cited, these parameters are the frequency of abnormal heartbeats, the strength and frequency of uterine contractions or amount of bleeding, and the arterial blood pressure, respectively.

In titrating drugs, the physician prescribes the starting dose or infusion rate (in milliliters or milligrams per minute), and the values of the desired physiologic parameters. For example, the order could be written: "dobutamine hydrochloride by continuous infusion, using a 500 mcg/ml solution; begin with a rate of 3 mcg/min, and maintain an arterial blood pressure of 110 mm Hg." The titrated drug should always be connected as a *secondary infusion* in case it must be discontinued. It is recommended that an accurate rate-control device be used, because most drugs administered in this manner can cause serious toxicity if administered too rapidly.

PREVENTING AND MANAGING ADVERSE REACTIONS IN INTRAVENOUS ADMINISTRATION

Untoward reactions can occur more rapidly following IV drug administration than with other modes of administration. In general, it is advisable to remain with the patient for the first 5 to 15 minutes following initial administration to observe for changes in vital signs or early signs and symptoms of an allergic reaction. Instruct the alert patient to report any unusual symptoms, and keep the call

bell within his reach. Continue to check the patient at 10- to 15-minute intervals for the next hour or so, except when more frequent observations of vital signs are dictated by the drug being given. Once the patient has safely received the drug several times, or his condition has stabilized, the patient can be checked hourly. Keep emergency drugs and equipment always ready for use. Be knowledgeable about adverse drug reactions that might develop, and at the first indication of an allergic reaction or other adverse effect, discontinue the drug and notify the physician immediately. If the drug is being used to control a serious condition such as shock, reduce or stop the infusion and carefully monitor vital signs. In some instances, another drug may be needed, while in other instances it may be necessary only to allow sufficient time for the offending drug to be eliminated from the body.

Controlling Infection

Strict adherence to aseptic insertion techniques is essential in IV therapy. IV solutions are ideal media for the growth of bacteria; this is especially true of parenteral nutrition solutions. Septicemia, an extremely serious condition characterized by fever, chills, and hypotension, is a possible dire complication caused by the introduction of pathogenic microorganisms into the patient's bloodstream.

The National Centers for Disease Control recommends that IV fluids and containers be changed every 24 hours to 48 hours and tubings be changed every 48 hours to help prevent bacterial growth. The IV cannula or needle must be changed every 48 hours to 72 hours, unless signs of inflammation or infiltration occur. To aid in the process of changing tubing and cannulas, many institutions label these devices as to date and time of insertion. Long-term indwelling catheters, such as the double-lumen Hickman or Broviac catheter, can be left in place indefinitely so long as daily aseptic technique is followed. Tubing changes should be performed aseptically, and all new devices dated and labeled.

Preventing and Managing Phlebitis and Venous Thrombosis

Venous inflammation and the subsequent development of a venous clot or thrombosis can occur whenever a cannula or a needle is inserted into a vein. These complications are usually the result of bacterial invasion of the area or irritation of the interior wall of the vein. The signs and symptoms of this development include pain at the insertion site and along the venous tract, swelling, redness, purulent drainage, and fever (late). Monitor every patient carefully. Should signs and symptoms develop, however, remove the IV equipment, and provide proper nursing care to the area, including application of moist heat and elevation of the extremity.

Preventing and Managing Air Embolism
A large volume of air introduced into the venous system can cause an air embolism, a potentially fatal complication that is entirely preventable. Air can be introduced during IV line insertion, especially when central veins (subclavian and jugular) are used. This occurs when a cannula has been inserted that is not equipped with a plug at the external end or is not attached to a fluid-filled tubing system or the tubing is not properly primed. Thus, with the cannula in the vein, air enters through the open-ended tubing as the patient inhales; the negative pressure within the chest is sufficient to create suction. Air from a fluid container can also be sucked into the vein if the infusion system has run dry and the venous pressure is lower than that in the tubing. The amount of air estimated to cause a significant air embolism is between 70 ml and 150 ml.

When a bubble of air of this size enters the venous system, it moves to the heart; in the right ventricle, it impedes the heart's pumping ability. Flow of blood to the lungs and subsequently to the arterial system is reduced. Small air bubbles are pumped into the lungs, occluding the pulmonary arterioles and causing cyanosis. The resulting reduced cardiac output can cause syncope. The immediate signs of a significant air embolism are rapid, labored breathing; pallor; a fall in blood pressure; and a churning murmur audible over the entire chest. The patient will then become unresponsive, eventually cyanotic, and possibly experience cardiac arrest if prompt treatment is not initiated.

If an air embolism is suspected, *immediately* remove the entry way for the air by closing whatever opening exists in the IV line, turn the patient onto his left side, and lower the head of the bed. This maneuver moves the air to the apex of the right ventricle and allows blood to bypass the obstruction bubble and flow into the pulmonary outflow tract. Try to maintain patency of the IV line during these maneuvers; it will be needed for the administration of emergency drugs. Administer oxygen by mask, monitor vital signs, and call for medical assistance. This dire complication can be prevented: never leave the hub of the catheter open during insertion into the vein; have the patient perform the Valsalva maneuver during IV tubing changes and when central venous lines are being cared for; avoid removing the tubing from a cannula whenever the patient is short of breath; and carefully tape the tubing to avoid disconnecting it.

INTRAVENOUS THERAPY AT HOME
When IV drugs, fluid, or nutritional therapy is ordered for the patient in his home, several nursing considerations arise. These patients and their families will require comprehensive instruction prior to discharge and at home during the course of therapy. Ongoing professional care by a visiting nurse is also advisable. Information on the drug, its preparation, storage, administration, and after-care should be covered. Procedures for infection control must be included as well as information on the signs and symptoms of complications. All guidelines should be given to the patient in writing, along with the name and telephone number of the person to contact for questions or problems. (See Chap. 79 for guidelines for the patient to receive home TPN.)

Home IV therapy may be administered either through a central venous line or through a heparin lock inserted into a peripheral vein. (See Chapter 79, Table 79-4, for a discussion of the advantages and disadvantages of various infusion sites.) Administration is usually by intermittent infusion using one of the three methods shown in Figure 8-4.

OTHER METHODS OF PARENTERAL DRUG ADMINISTRATION
Less frequently used methods of parenteral drug administration include intra-arterial, intraperitoneal, intrapleural, intrathecal, intracardiac, and intrasynovial. All of these routes are the responsibility of the physician, with the exception of the intrathecal route when it is used for regional anesthesia. In this case, the certified nurse anesthetist may perform the procedure in some institutions.

Intra-arterial Infusion (Regional Arterial Perfusion)
Intra-arterial infusion is usually used for the delivery of antineoplastic agents directly into the arterial blood supply of an inoperable malignant tumor or into an organ containing such a tumor. Localized lesions of the liver, head, neck, or bone may be treated in this manner. The drug is administered in high concentrations directly into the lesion or re-

gion, without dilution, and thence into the general circulatory system; it does not pass into the liver, where it could be metabolized and inactivated, or into the kidneys, from which it would be excreted. With a higher drug concentration in the affected area and a lower systemic level of the drug, fewer adverse effects are seen.

The catheters are placed into an appropriate artery, either surgically or angiographically. If placed surgically, the catheter is left permanently throughout the treatment period, with patency maintained by infusion of a heparinized fluid under pressure. A volumetric infusion pump infuses the drug under pressure.

Patients with a surgically placed arterial catheter may be ambulatory, and may receive chemotherapy on an outpatient basis. Some patients wear a small, portable infusion pump, which allows greater mobility. Totally implantable arterial pumps are also in use.

Nurses do not implant arterial lines but are usually responsible for maintaining catheter patency, adding medication to the infusion, preventing infection, and teaching the patient self-care, including drug administration. Meticulous care is required to prevent infection and skin erosion, as well as to provide daily cleansing of the catheter exit wound; application of an antimicrobial ointment; use of sterile dressings; and patient and family teaching, including daily temperature readings and wound observation.

Both nurse and patient must observe for signs and symptoms of catheter dislodgement, artery wall damage and tearing, occlusion of the catheter by thrombus, and emboli. The patient must keep clamps at hand to control arterial bleeding if the catheter breaks or the tubing is disconnected.

Intraperitoneal Instillation

Intraperitoneal instillation is most widely used in renal dysfunction. This procedure, commonly called *dialysis*, involves the instillation of large volumes (1500 ml–2000 ml) of isotonic (usually) electrolyte solution into the peritoneal cavity through a surgically placed Tenckhoff catheter in the abdominal wall. When the fluid comes in contact with the peritoneal membranes, substances to which the membrane is permeable, such as electrolytes, nitrogenous compounds, and water, diffuse passively through the membrane and into the dialysis fluid. Although the substances can diffuse in both directions (from the blood or back into the blood from the fluid), the net transfer is in the direction of the instilled fluid where the concentra-

tion of most substances is lower. The fluid is drained out of the peritoneal cavity and discarded. Thus, some substances that would be removed by normal kidney function are removed with the fluid. Patients can receive these treatments in the hospital, in an outpatient dialysis center, or at home.

Other disorders in which intraperitoneal instillation may be administered include severe peritonitis in which antibiotics are instilled directly into the cavity, certain types of abdominal cancer in which antineoplastic agents are injected directly into the cavity and thence to the tumor mass, and ovarian and colorectal cancer.

Care of the patient and of the abdominal catheter is the same in all types of dialysis. Sterile technique is maintained at all times. Surgical face masks and sterile gloves should be worn whenever the catheter is handled. The insertion site is cleaned daily with an iodophor solution and hydrogen peroxide. A germicidal ointment is applied after the cleansing, along with a sterile occlusive dressing. The area is examined for signs of infection. Patient and family should receive instruction in these procedures.

Premixed dialysis solutions with preconnected drainage bags are commercially available. Fluids to be instilled into the peritoneal cavity must be warmed to body temperature (98.6°F, 37°C) to prevent abdominal cramping and discomfort. After the medications are added to the fluid, the fluid is instilled by gravity flow. The fluid remains in the cavity for the prescribed period of time. The drainage bag is placed below the level of the patient's abdomen, and the fluid drains out. The patient may need to change his position to promote fluid drainage. The catheter insertion site must be checked to ensure that there is no leakage of fluid.

Dialysis may cause some discomfort, and there may be irritation and discomfort due to the catheter until the insertion site is well healed. If discomfort is accompanied by fever, malaise, rigidity of the abdominal wall, or rebound tenderness, an infection is the probable cause.

Intrapleural (Intrathoracic) Administration

Antibiotics and antineoplastic drugs are sometimes injected into the chest cavity to treat pleural conditions unresponsive to drugs given by other routes. Antibiotics may be administered to treat resistant infections within the pleural space, and antineoplastic drugs may be instilled to inhibit a cancer that has invaded the pleura. Instillation of these drugs can cause considerable pain, and the patient will need adequate psychologic preparation and support, as well as pain relief measures.

Intraspinal and Epidural Administration

A *spinal* injection instills a drug into the subarachnoid space of the spinal canal. The purpose of this type of administration is to place a drug directly into the cerebrospinal fluid and obtain anesthesia of the nerve tracts above and below the site of injection, or to administer antibiotics or antineoplastic agents. X-ray contrast media can also be injected into the subarachnoid space to detect lesions of the spinal cord, canal, and supporting structures.

Usually a 2-inch to 3-inch needle is used and the injection made through the second, third, or fourth interspace of the lumbar vertebrae. A plastic intravenous catheter is sometimes left in place to provide access for a prolonged period of time such as for anesthesia during labor and delivery. In addition, a device called the *Ommaya reservoir* has been developed to provide a reusable direct access to the cerebrospinal fluid for the administration of antibiotics, analgesics, and antineoplastic drugs into the brain. This reservoir also offers a way of measuring cerebrospinal fluid pressure, draining excess fluid to reduce intracranial pressure, or for sampling the fluid for analysis.

The Ommaya reservoir is a round, dome-shaped chamber, made of silicone, with a tube attached to the bottom. This device is implanted surgically beneath the scalp over a burr hole into the skull, usually on the top of the head. The tube of the reservoir is inserted into the lateral ventricle of the brain through a so-called silent area of the nondominant frontal lobe, to reduce the likelihood of a neurologic deficit. Following healing of the incision, this reservoir may then be punctured by a needle through the scalp and injected with the drug. It may function for many months, an average of 200 punctures, without leakage. The student is encouraged to refer to articles on this device in the Bibliography.

Epidural drug administration is the placement of medications immediately *above* the dural covering of the spinal canal, outside the subarachnoid space. It is the most frequently used technique or route of administration for anesthesia of the lower one half of the body because there are fewer complications and reactions than seen with the spinal injection of anesthetic agents.

While nurses (except certified nurse anesthetists) usually do not administer drugs by these routes, nursing support of the patient is essential, since many persons fear they will experience complications of spinal and epidural injections such as paralysis or chronic back pain. These myths should be dispelled beforehand to help relieve the patient's anxiety. Inform the patient that the needle is placed in or above the spinal canal, but *below* the level of the spinal cord; a diagram will help the patient understand the procedure. These injections are painful and uncomfortable, and the patient will need supportive care.

Nursing responsibilities will also include care following anesthesia and drug administration. Such injections can affect vital signs; hypotension and bradycardia can occur, necessitating careful monitoring of blood pressure and heart rate. Spinal anesthesia can affect respiratory function in that the anesthetic agent, if it reaches high enough, can paralyze the diaphragm. In addition, patients who have received spinal injections of anesthetic drugs or x-ray contrast media may experience postinjection headache that can be relieved with analgesics and fluids. See Chapter 20 for further discussion.

Intracardiac Administration

In cardiac *standstill* or *ventricular fibrillation*, epinephrine and calcium chloride may be injected directly into the right or left ventricular cavity. The resultant high concentration of these drugs may stimulate cardiac activity sufficiently that the heart will respond to electrical cardioversion, cardiac massage, or other components of cardiopulmonary resuscitation. This procedure is performed by the physician.

Intrasynovial (Intra-articular) Administration

Drugs, usually corticosteroids, can be injected into joint spaces to treat inflammatory conditions such as arthritis. Most joints can be treated in this manner. While the physician administers the injection, the nurse assists by positioning the patient, offering explanations about the procedure, and providing supportive care.

Nursing Evaluation of Drug Administration

Evaluation of drug effectiveness begins as soon as the drug has been given. The nurse evaluates for positive effects and observes for adverse reactions. This can be done competently only if the nurse understands the patient's pathology, the drug's actions within the body, and the drug–disease relationship. She learns to anticipate signs, symptoms, and behaviors that point to progress or its absence. She needs to understand the drug's usual duration of action, as well as the possible adverse reactions to which it can give rise. Finally, she should be alert to any indications that a patient is unable to tolerate a specified route of drug administration and should notify the physician of the problem.

REVIEW QUESTIONS

1. Create a flow sheet that would help a nurse ensure proper drug storage in an institution or in a patient's home.
2. Compare the advantages and disadvantages of the three major drug supply systems: floor stock, individual patient supply, and unit dose.
3. What institution policies must a nurse become familiar with in order to ensure safe administration of drugs?
4. What habits of drug administration does the nurse need to learn to administer drugs safely?
5. Outline a procedure for administering a drug
   a. Orally
   b. Through a nasogastric tube
   c. Topically
   d. In the eye
   e. In the ear
   f. Through the nose
6. Define parenteral administration of drugs.
7. Outline a procedure for administration of drugs by the following routes, including patient preparation:
   a. Intradermal route
   b. Subcutaneous route
   c. Intramuscular route
8. Outline the five steps necessary to provide safe intravenous drug administration.
9. What are the dangers of administering a drug by the IV push method?
10. Describe nursing actions to prevent and manage adverse reactions to IV drug therapy.

BIBLIOGRAPHY

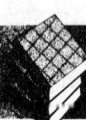

Anderson MA, Aker SN, Hickman RO: The double-lumen Hickman catheter. Am J Nurs 82:272, 1982

Burke E: Insulin injection: Site and technique. Am J Nurs 72:2194, 1972

Cantwell R, Hollis R, Rogers MP: What do you know about cardiac drugs for a code? Nursing '82 12(10):34, 1982

Coblio NA: Don't combine those drugs. Nursing '81 11(8):48, 1981

Cockshott W et al: Intramuscular or intralipomatous injections? N Engl J Med 307:356, 1982

Cohen MR: Medication errors. Nursing '80 10(3):28, 1980

Cohen MR: Medication errors. Nursing '81 11(5):17, 1981

Cohen MR: Play it safe: Don't use these abbreviations. Nursing '82 12(10):66, 1982

Davis NM, Cohen MR: Learning from mistakes: Twenty tips for avoiding medication errors. Nursing '82 12(3):65, 1982

Dedrick R et al: Pharmacokinetic rationale for peritoneal drug administration in the treatment of ovarian cancer. Cancer Treat Rep 62:1, 1978

DeMoss CJ: Giving intravenous chemotherapy at home. Am J Nurs 80:2188, 1980

Esparza DM, Weyland JB: Nursing care for the patient with an Ommaya reservoir. Oncology Nursing Forum 9:17, 1982

Flanagan JP et al: Air embolus—A lethal complication of subclavian venipuncture. N Engl J Med 281:488, 1969

Fredholm NZ: The insulin pump: A new method of insulin delivery. Am J Nurs 81:2024, 1981

Geolot P, McKinney H: Administering parenteral drugs. Am J Nurs 75:788, 1975

Greenblatt D, Kock-Weser J: Intramuscular injection of drugs. N Engl J Med 295:542, 1976

Hamby WB, Terry RN: Air embolism in operations done in the sitting position: A report of five fatal cases and one rescue by a simple maneuver. Surgery 31:212, 1952

Hanson D: Intramuscular injection injuries and complications. Am J Nurs 73:99, 1973

Hobbs B, Ness S: Rationale for and longterm care of indwelling arterial infusion systems. Oncology Nursing Forum 4:6, 1977

Jenkins JF, Hubbard SM, Howser DM: Managing intraperitoneal chemotherapy—A new assault in ovarian cancer. Nursing '82 12(5):76, 1982

Johnston S, Patt YZ: Caring for the patient on intraarterial chemotherapy. Nursing '81 11(11):108, 1981

Johnston-Early A, Cohen MH, White KS: Venipuncture and problem veins. Am J Nurs 81:1636, 1981

Kirilloff LH, Tibbals SC: Drugs for asthma—A complete guide. Am J Nurs 83:55, 1983

Lawson M, Bottino JC, McCredie KB: Long-term I.V. therapy: A new approach. Am J Nurs 79:1100, 1979

Lenz CL: Make your needle selection right to the point. Nursing '83 13(2):50, 1983

Leutzinger R, Judson A: Drawing blood from a Hickman catheter. Nursing '81 11(12):65, 1981

Nawrocki HR: The ins and outs of administering I.V. bolus injections. Nursing '81 11(11):124, 1981

Newton DW, Newton M: Route, site and technique—Three key decisions in giving parenteral medication. Nursing '79 9(7):18, 1979

Norheim C: Spinal anesthesia. Nursing '86 16(4):42, 1986

Ommaya AK: Subcutaneous reservoir and pump for sterile access to ventricular cerebrospinal fluid. Lancet 2:983, 1963

Ostrow LS: Air embolism and central venous lines. Am J Nurs 81(11):2036, 1981

Pitel M: The subcutaneous injection. Am J Nurs 71:76, 1971

Richard C: Nursing implications in the prevention of complications in peritoneal dialysis. Heart Lung 4:890, 1975

Saunders WH et al: Nursing Care in Eye, Ear, Nose and Throat Disorders, 4th ed. St Louis, CV Mosby, 1979

Tenckhoff H, Schechter H: A bacteriologically safe peritoneal access device. American Society of Internal Artificial Organs 14:181, 1968

Travel J: Factors affecting pain of injection. JAMA 158:368, 1955

Trissel LA: Handbook on Injectable Drugs, 4th ed. Washington, DC, American Society of Hospital Pharmacists, 1986

Vogel TC, McSkimming SA: Teaching parents to give indwelling C.V. catheter care. Nursing '83 13(1):55, 1983

Wong DL: Significance of dead space in syringes. Am J Nurs 82:1237, 1982

Wordell DC: Should you crush that tablet? Nursing '82 12(9):76, 1982

Wordell DC: Report on intravenous therapy national survey. Nursing '81 11(1):80, 1981

Wordell DC: Giving medication through a nasogastric tube. Nursing '80 10(5):71, 1980

Pediatric Pharmacology

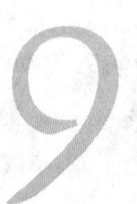

Many of the general principles of pharmacology and pharmacokinetics apply to the child as they do to the adult. However, the progressive physiologic and psychologic stages of childhood often present varying responses and needs regarding medications. These unique aspects of pediatric pharmacology will be discussed in this chapter, using a nursing process approach. Indeed, even before birth, the developing fetus can be exposed to the effects of drugs ingested by the mother during the very vulnerable gestational period. Most drugs readily cross the placental barrier, and there are a number of drugs known to have a damaging effect on the fetus. These so-called teratogenic drugs are listed in Table 9-1.

Assessment of Growth and Development by System

A child's body systems grow at varying rates; thus, the reaction to drugs at various ages is often not predictable from age or weight alone. For example, the infant's kidney function improves throughout the first few months of life so that by 1 year of age, renal function is fairly mature. Conversely, myelinization of the central nervous system, which creates the blood–brain barrier to passage of drugs, is not mature until 2 years of age. A review of body systems development follows, with emphasis on common needs for certain medications at various ages and the impact of development on pharmacokinetics.

Integumentary System

The skin of the infant, in particular the premature infant, is very permeable to passage of substances. The thinness of the infant's skin is apparent in the color changes from pallor to redness to cyanosis that are evident in response to changes in blood dynamics. For this reason, use of potentially toxic substances such as hexachlorophene to bathe infants should be discouraged, and milder and less toxic substances should be substituted. Early in infancy, the skin begins to increase in thickness, and its permeability decreases as the child advances in age. Eccrine sweat glands are not fully functional until 2 years of age, and apocrine sweat glands are nonfunctional until puberty. This results in a scanty lipoid or oily skin surface during childhood,

sometimes causing dryness, and absorption of substances through the skin may be enhanced.

The skin of infants and children is more sensitive than that of adults, leading to a greater likelihood of eczema and allergic responses to medications. For example, a maculopapular erythematous rash in response to administered ampicillin is more common in children under 10 years of age than in older persons, and skin surfaces altered by the presence of a rash are more permeable to substances in general. Another change noted in the skin of the developing adolescent is increased sebaceous gland activity, which often leads to development of acne vulgaris.

Head and Neck

MOUTH

The infant under 3 to 4 months of age pushes solid foods out of the mouth because of tongue movements. Thus, liquid medications should be given through a nipple or oral syringe. Since the young infant's taste buds are poorly developed, bitter medications are rarely refused until over 4 months of age.

Tooth development begins at about the sixth week of fetal life and continues through age 16 to 20 years. The periods of calcification are critical for formation of strong, healthy teeth. Although nutrition plays a crucial role in this development, there are periods when ingestion of certain medications can permanently influence dentition. For example, tetracycline antibiotics can be deposited in the dentin and enamel of teeth, causing stains, caries, and hypoplasia. Since the calcification of all permanent teeth except the third molars is completed by age 8 years, the use of tetracycline should be avoided in children under this age.

One of the most effective methods of strengthening tooth enamel has been the addition of fluoride to water supplies. Some cities and towns have naturally occurring fluoride or add this mineral to water supplies, whereas others do not have natural or added fluoride. Thus, the nurse should be aware of the dosages of fluoride recommended by the American Academy of Pediatrics and the American Dental Association (Table 9-2). She can then determine if the local water supply contains sufficient fluoride and advise parents as to the quantity of supplemental fluoride needed. Nurses in schools and day-care centers are often instrumental in in-

Table 9-1
Drugs Known to Affect the Fetus and Newborn Infant Adversely

Drug	Effect on Fetus
alcohol	Intrauterine growth retardation, physical abnormalities, mental retardation, neonatal alcohol withdrawal, fetal alcohol syndrome
aminoglycosides	Ototoxicity
aminopterin	Abortion, malformations
amphetamines	Congenital heart disease, transposition of the great vessels
androgens	Masculinization of female fetus
corticosteroids	Multiple malformations
dicumarol	Fetal bleeding and death, hypoplastic nasal structures
diethylstilbestrol	Genital abnormalities, adenocarcinoma of vagina and cervix
haloperidol	Limb abnormalities
insulin	Skeletal malformations can occur with insulin shock.
iodine, radioactive (^{131}I)	Destruction of fetal thyroid
lithium	Multiple malformations
mepivacaine	Bradycardia
methimazole	Goiter
methotrexate	Multiple malformations
nicotine	Decreased growth rate
norethindrone (Norlutin)	Masculinization of female fetus
paramethadione	Fetal death, multiple malformations, mental retardation
phenmetrazine	Skeletal and visceral abnormalities
phenytoin	Multiple malformations, anemia
potassium iodide	Goiter
propylthiouracil	Goiter
quinine	Abortion, thrombocytopenia
rifampin	Cleft palate, skeletal abnormalities
sulfonamide	Anemia, skeletal defects
tetracycline	Pigmentation of teeth, hypoplasia of enamel
thalidomide	Phocomelia, other limb malformations
thiazide diuretics	Thrombocytopenia
tricyclic antidepressants	Limb abnormalities
trimethadione	Abortion, multiple malformations, mental retardation

Table 9-2
Recommended Fluoride Dosages

Fluoride in Water Supply (parts per million)	Age in Years	Fluoride Dosage (mg/day)
Under 0.3	Birth–2	0.25
	2–3	0.5
	3–14	1.0
0.3–0.7	Birth–2	0
	2–3	0.25
	3–14	0.5
Over 0.7	Birth–2	0
	2–3	0
	3–14	0

stituting school fluoride administration to children whose parents desire and sign permission for such a program. Oral liquid and tablets as well as topical fluoride applications are available. The nurse must also teach parents to avoid use of fluoride above the recommended levels, since this may result in white or brown discoloration of the teeth.

Older preschoolers and school-age children may have loose deciduous teeth. The nurse should assess for loose teeth, especially before allowing a child to chew a tablet.

EYES

The eyes of newborns are routinely treated with an application of silver nitrate or other agent to prevent ophthalmia neonatorum. Many infants develop a conjunctivitis and watery discharge for approximately 24 hours following application, but there are no permanent side-effects to this medication. The nurse involved in newborn care should carefully observe the eyes of infants, since a conjunctivitis that lasts 3 days beyond application of silver nitrate is likely due to other causes.

Retinal vascularization is complete at about 8 months of gestation, so the premature infant is at high risk for retinal damage. The premature infant who is administered high levels of oxygen may react with vasoconstriction and later vasodilation of retinal vessels, resulting in varying degrees of vision loss. The risk of this problem, retrolental fibroplasia, is believed to be lessened if plasma oxygen (PO_2) levels are maintained between 50 mm Hg to 100 mm Hg. All infants who are less than 36 weeks' gestation or weigh less than 2000 g and re-

ceive oxygen therapy after birth should have an eye examination immediately following therapy and again approximately 6 months later.

Another side-effect of ophthalmic drugs may be observed in children when eye medications such as atropine or phenylephrine are absorbed systemically through the lacrimal duct. A dose that may not create observable systemic effects in adults may be sufficient to do so in children, and for this reason, ointments rather than liquid solutions are often used when ophthalmic medication is required since ointments are not as easily absorbed through the nasolacrimal duct.

EARS

The ear canal of the young child is anatomically different from that of the adult. Whereas the adult's ear canal curves downward and the tympanic membrane lies vertically, the young child's ear canal curves upward and the tympanic membrane lies more horizontally. Thus, when examining the ear with an otoscope or when instilling ear medication, the nurse pulls the pinna up and back for adults and older children but down and back for children under 6 years of age (Fig. 9-1).

In addition, the eustachian tube is wider and more horizontal in children; thus, microorganisms can ascend into the middle ear more readily. Therefore, many young children suffer repeated cases of otitis media, or middle ear infection. This illness may be treated by a variety of antibiotics. Although decongestants and antihistamines have often been used to decrease middle ear fluid, the efficacy of this practice is questionable. The incidence of otitis media can be decreased if parents are advised to avoid giving a child a bottle immediately before sleep since the liquid pools at the back of the mouth during sleep where it can ascend through the eustachian tube.

Brain and Nervous System

Brain growth occurs in spurts during the first 3 months of fetal life, the last trimester, and then again after birth until about age 4 years. Since the myelinization that prevents many substances in the circulation from entering the brain is not mature in the first 2 to 4 years of life, the young child is more susceptible to adverse effects of drugs that can influence the central nervous system. For example, antipsychotic agents such as the phenothiazines

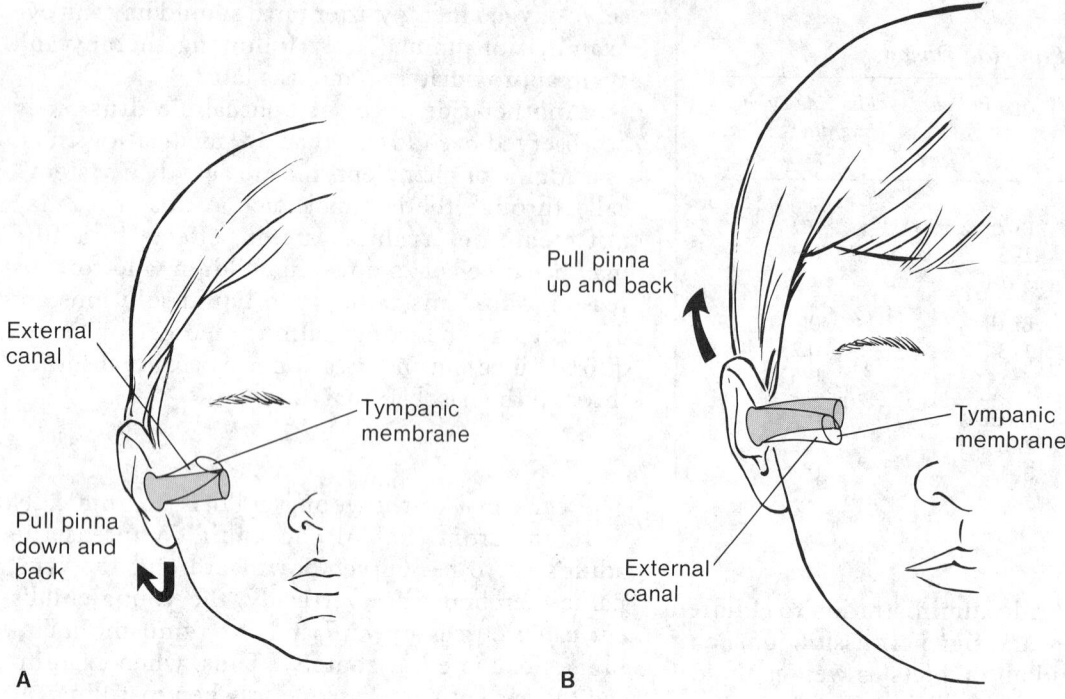

Figure 9-1. Method of otic administration to (A) infant and toddler and (B) older child.

often cause extrapyramidal reactions in children (involuntary muscle contractions, lack of muscle tone, impairment of voluntary movement) more frequently than in adults. The nurse who administers drugs with potential nervous system effects must carefully observe the child for such adverse reactions.

Aspirin used to treat symptoms of certain viral infections has been associated with an increased incidence of a neurologic disease termed *Reye's syndrome* in children. For this reason, acetaminophen is preferred to relieve pain and reduce fever in children with influenza or suspected chickenpox.

Respiratory System

The nurse should determine if the respiratory rate of young children is within the range expected for the child's age (*i.e.*, newborn, 30–80/min; 1 year, 20–40/min; 2–5 years, 20–30/min). The nurse in a newborn nursery should observe infants (especially if premature) for signs of respiratory distress syndrome such as a resting respiratory rate over 60/minute, an expiratory grunt, intercostal retrac-

tions, nasal flaring, xiphoid retraction, lag of chest movement on inspiration, and cyanosis. The newborn may breathe normally until several hours after birth when the disease may first manifest itself.

Since the upper respiratory passages of young children are shorter than in adults; and since protective mechanisms such as the presence of cilia and the ability to cough are not as well developed, the child experiences more upper and lower respiratory infections. Most children have one or two upper respiratory infections (colds) per year. Children also have a higher incidence of respiratory allergic conditions than do adults. Nurses should note the child's respiratory rate and rhythm; presence of adventitious sounds such as rales, rhonchi, and wheezing; production of mucus; cough; retractions; and nasal flaring. Unusual findings should be referred for diagnosis and treatment to a physician or nurse practitioner. Drugs such as antihistamines, decongestants, antitussives, expectorants, and bronchodilators may be useful in these conditions.

Children with congenital diseases such as cystic fibrosis will require frequent monitoring and teaching regarding other medications, such as mucolytic agents, that they may routinely take by respiratory inhalation.

Cardiovascular System

The premature newborn and the young infant have poor peripheral circulation, leading to slower absorption of intramuscularly or subcutaneously administered drugs. The intravenous route, on the other hand, is more direct and therefore more predictable.

The body fluid of the infant is proportionally much greater than that of the adult (80% to 85% of body weight for infants vs 60% for children over 2 years of age and for adults). Thus, a comparatively larger dose of water-soluble drugs per body weight is often required to achieve desired therapeutic effects in the infant due to the greater proportion of extracellular fluid.

The heart grows steadily throughout childhood, reaching adult size and capacity sometime during adolescence.

The nurse must be familiar with normal pulse and blood pressure values for children of different ages. For example, while the nurse will not give digoxin to an adult whose apical pulse is below 60, she will not give the drug to a young child whose apical pulse is lower than 100. Alteration in vital signs may be one of the first indications of side-effects to such medications, especially in young children who cannot verbalize other subjective symptoms. See Table 9-3 for normal pulse rate and blood pressure values for children of different ages.

Anesthetic agents administered to the mother during delivery may adversely affect fetal cardiovascular functioning. Delivery room nurses should observe newborns closely for signs of cardiovascular distress.

Gastrointestinal Tract and Liver

Premature and newborn infants have a relatively long gastric emptying time. Thus, active forms of drugs such as acetaminophen that are destroyed by gastric acid will be absorbed in smaller amounts since they are exposed for longer periods of time. Other drugs that are not destroyed by gastric acid will be absorbed more slowly but the total amount will eventually become available to the systemic

Table 9-3
Average Pulse Rates and Blood Pressure
Values for Children of Different Ages

Age	Resting Pulse Rate	Average Blood Pressure
Newborn	120–160	80/45
1–6 mo	115–150	85/55
7–12 mo	110–140	90/60
1–2 yr	100–130	95/65
2–4 yr	90–120	100/65
4–6 yr	80–115	100/65
6–10 yr	75–110	110/65
10–14 yr	70–100	115/65
14–18 yr	65–90	120/70

circulation. The more adult-like, shorter gastric emptying time is reached by infants at 6 to 8 months of age.

The more acidic gastric pH of young infants permits better absorption of acidic drugs such as penicillin, since these drugs are largely un-ionized at low pH (see Chap. 2). Other factors affecting absorption of orally administered drugs include presence of food (generally slows absorption), bacterial flora, mucus, bile salts, and enzymes. Infants lack some enzymes and transport systems that may cause altered absorption of many drugs. The presence of diarrhea or vomiting can also decrease drug absorption; thus, the nurse who administers oral medication must observe the child for presence of gastrointestinal illness.

The most common symptoms of gastrointestinal illness in childhood are regurgitation, vomiting, diarrhea, and constipation. Regurgitation is fairly common in infants up to 9 to 12 months of age and is usually treated by positioning (keeping upper body elevated following feedings) rather than with medications. Mild vomiting and diarrhea are usually self-limiting disorders that also seldom require medication. More severe forms of these disorders, however, require medical attention; diarrhea continues to be a major cause of debilitation and death in children. Treatment frequently centers on identifying the cause and restoring fluid and electrolyte balance. In treating constipation, on the other hand, parents should be encouraged to increase fluids, juices, and fiber in the child's diet rather than administer laxatives.

Infants may ingest drugs during breast-feeding. Although occasional medications taken by a lactating mother are usually not harmful, some drugs may be highly concentrated in breast milk and cause undesired symptoms in the infant. Examples of some potentially harmful drugs excreted in breast milk are atropine, anticoagulants, thyroid medications, and narcotics. Lactating mothers should be instructed to check with their physician before taking any medication and to read product insert information before taking any drug.

The liver, in addition to serving as the major organ of drug metabolism, also plays a key role in drug distribution, since the plasma proteins it produces become bound to many drugs. The liver of the infant, particularly of the premature or newborn infant, produces substantially smaller proportions of these proteins. Therefore, proportionately larger amounts of drugs are unbound in the circulation, increasing the incidence of side-effects. In addition, many of the liver enzymes that metabolize drugs are present in smaller amounts during infancy. This leads to an increased half-life of drugs and therefore a need for longer dosing intervals to avoid cumulation and development of toxic effects. The infant who is taking multiple drugs is at a higher risk since this further stresses the inadequate mechanisms for drug metabolism. The nurse's role in observing for medication side-effects in infants is extremely important.

Musculoskeletal System

Several drugs have the potential for altering the skeletal growth rate of children. The effect is usually magnified with large doses and prolonged periods of drug administration. For example, adrenocorticosteroids can slow growth by impairing epiphyseal maturation, an effect not prevented by growth hormone. Further, evidence suggests that prolonged use of methylphenidate (Ritalin) can suppress height and weight gain. These effects appear to be reversible when the drugs are discontinued after short-term administration. Height and weight measurements should be taken frequently, recorded on growth grids, and reviewed by a pediatrician or nurse.

Muscle development increases steadily throughout childhood, and the amount of subcutaneous fat increases during the first year of life and then remains fairly stable. The nurse should carefully assess muscle development and the amount of subcutaneous fat prior to selecting sites for administration of intramuscular and subcutaneous injec-

tions. The small amount of fat in the young infant means that the child will not store large amounts of highly lipid-soluble drugs in fatty tissue depots in the body and thus will need smaller doses of these lipid-soluble medications, such as diazepam (Valium) and barbiturates, to achieve therapeutic blood levels.

Infants under 4 months of age are unable to support their heads and thus should be held in an upright position with the head elevated to about 45 degrees when oral medications are administered. This position is preferred to a supine position, which may result in aspiration or choking. The toddler usually sits well without support and may feel more in control if allowed to sit upright when oral medications are administered.

Genitourinary System

The urinary system plays a primary role in eliminating many drugs from the body, and the functioning of an infant's urinary system is substantially different from that of older children and adults. The glomerular filtration rate of newborn and young infants may be nearly 50% less than that of the adult, not reaching adult values until about 5 months of age. Tubular secreting ability is reduced about 30% compared to adults in infants under 7 months of age. Therefore, the young infant's inability to excrete many drugs quickly contributes to a longer half-life of the drugs. The infant who is ill becomes dehydrated quickly because of the large amount of circulating extracellular fluid. The dehydration and resultant oliguria may further impair drug elimination. Nurses should carefully assess children for signs of dehydration such as intake and output ratio and specific gravity or concentration of urine. Total water requirements per 24 hours are approximately 400 ml to 500 ml at 10 days, 750 ml to 900 ml at 3 months, 1000 ml to 1100 ml at 6 months, 1200 ml to 1300 ml at 1 year, 1400 ml to 1500 ml at 2 years, and 1600 ml to 2000 ml at 4 to 6 years. The specific gravity of urine is between 1.001 and 1.020 in the newborn and may range up to 1.030 as the child grows.

Urinary tract infections are fairly common in children. Since many of these infections are asymptomatic or induce nonspecific symptoms such as lethargy and vomiting, routine urine screenings should be performed periodically. Infections are treated with an antibiotic specific for the disease-causing organism. Predisposing factors to development of urinary infections include contamination from feces due to incorrect wiping and use of chemical irritants such as bubble bath.

Assessment of Psychologic Development

Just as the child's rate of physiologic growth influences the ability to absorb, distribute, biotransform, and eliminate drugs, psychologic development often determines the methods of drug administration that must be used by the nurse. Normal social, motor, and language development can be assessed by a number of developmental screening tests. The reader is referred to the section Approaching the Child, later in this chapter, for further application of the knowledge regarding psychologic development to the administration of medications to the child.

Infant

Although the infant does not understand the purpose of receiving medications, bodily contact and speech are important methods of communicating security and love. Parents and nurses can provide for these relationship needs during and following medication administration, particularly when it is painful. Having a parent present during medication administration often increases the infant's trust in the nurse. This is particularly true in the infant over 6 to 7 months of age who clearly identifies the parents and becomes anxious when strangers approach him.

Toddler

The toddler is able to use verbal communication and understand short, appropriate explanations as to why medicine is needed. Negative behavior can be minimized by providing positive statements such as, "It's time for you to drink your medicine now." Since rituals and routines are important at this age, administering a pill at the same time daily (*e.g.*, just before a favorite television show) or putting a star on a chart each time a medicine is taken will facilitate compliance. Toddlers begin to imitate adults, and this can provide a method for teaching safe and effective means of drug administration. For example, parents should not take a

medicine in front of a toddler, then place the container where the child can easily reach it, since the child may imitate the parent and ingest the medicine, as well. Likewise, children should never be told a medicine is candy since they may then want more of it, possibly resulting in poisoning.

Preschooler

Preschool children can understand the purpose of medications, and can be questioned regarding their knowledge of drugs such as immunizations or antibiotics prior to their administration. Pictures or other audiovisual–tactile aids can assist in this instruction. Body line drawings and the Gellert Index of Body Knowledge (Gellert, 1978) are helpful tools to assess a preschooler's knowledge about the body and to teach by pictures where and how a medicine will work in the body. Books such as *No Measles, No Mumps for Me, Curious George Goes to the Hospital, Nicky Goes to the Doctor,* and *Color Me Diabetic,* as well as books and tapes by Mr. Rogers on health-care experiences, are helpful teaching tools (see Bibliography, Sample Books for Children, at the end of this chapter). The importance of careful assessment of the preschooler's understanding of why medications are needed cannot be overestimated. For example, a child may believe an injection received at the doctor's office is punishment for fighting that day with a sibling or may not understand why drinking a medicine can help an ear infection and worry that something else may be wrong. Since a child often views the body as a balloon-like object filled with blood and bones, a bandage applied after an injection may be used to "hold the blood inside the body." Since preschoolers exercise increasing control over their bodies, they can be instructed to count, recite the alphabet, or tell about their pets to provide distraction during an injection. Verbal praise after drug administration and use of rewards can help make the experience a positive one. For example, the nurse might say, "It does hurt to get that shot but you helped so much by holding still and counting during it." Likewise, prior to the injection, the nurse can promote control by telling the child "This shot may hurt, but it will be over quickly. Your Mom will hold your arm so you'll remember to hold real still. Can you count to ten while I give the shot? I'll tell you when to start counting." The nurse should not lie to the child, such as by saying an injection will not hurt, for to do so would risk loss of the child's trust in all future encounters.

School-Age Child and Adolescent

The school-age child and adolescent have increasing cognitive ability and can thus appreciate explanations concerning use of medications. With appropriate teaching, they are usually able to carry out self-administration, even with drugs such as insulin given daily. Self-management of drug administration can contribute to increased bodily control and independence.

The peer group becomes more important as the child becomes less dependent on the family; thus, the influence of friends on a child taking medications should be carefully assessed. Identification with a peer group can be used beneficially by introducing the school-age child to another child taking similar medications. For example, support and information groups for teenage diabetics or hemophiliacs may assist in providing information and coping skills and help adolescents feel less isolated from peers. Increased compliance with the prescribed treatment may result.

Some examples of helpful statements that may facilitate discussion with health-care providers are, "Some teenage diabetics find it hard to stay on their diets when their friends are going out after school or to parties at night. Is that a problem for you?" Or "Tell me the two times when it's hardest for you to stay on your diet." Or "Some people feel uncomfortable when they have to take medicine at school and their friends might see them. Tell me about whether that happens to you." It is important to provide a forum where the child can express feelings without fear of scolding. As importantly, the nurse must provide appropriate information about any risks the child may create by incorrect self-medication. Written information that the child can read at home is often a useful approach with school-age children and adolescents.

The adolescent and possibly the school-age child may use street drugs, alcohol, over-the-counter medications, or oral contraceptives. When obtaining a drug history, it is important that the nurse inquire about such use, assuring confidentiality and asking open-ended questions.

Nursing Diagnosis

Nursing diagnoses for children receiving medications are similar to those for adults. See Chapter 6.

Plan

The nursing care goals for all pediatric patients receiving medication include the following:

1. To calculate the prescribed medication correctly
2. To administer the drug safely so the patient gets the maximum benefit from the drug
3. To use an approach when administering medication that considers the child's developmental level and helps the child to build trust toward the care givers
4. To provide the patient and family with appropriate information on the effects of the medication, storage of the drug, and administration techniques
5. To work with parents to provide a safe environment for their children in order to minimize the danger of accidental poisoning

Intervention

Dosage Forms, Measuring Devices, and Computation

A general overview of drug administration can be found in Chapter 8. Several dosage forms are more frequently used in children due to their relative ease of administration and are considered in greater detail below. Since most infants, toddlers, and preschoolers have difficulty swallowing tablets, liquid oral preparations such as suspensions, syrups, and elixirs are commonly used. Such liquids can be measured by using either a calibrated dropper, which may be provided with the medication; a syringe without a needle; a medication spoon that is accurately calibrated; or a medicine cup. Use of household teaspoons and tablespoons should be discouraged, since their actual volume can vary significantly. The dropper supplied with a particular medicine should be used only with that medicine and not transferred to others, since its calibration for measuring drug products of differing viscosity or temperature can lead to dose variation.

When liquid oral medications are not available, tablets or capsules can be crushed or opened and the contents placed in a small amount of a food such as applesauce or ice cream to disguise taste. Although variation in blood levels can occur using this method with some medications, the pharmacist can be consulted about the specific medicine and the vehicle to be used. Enteric-coated or sustained-release tablets, on the other hand, should *not* be crushed since their delayed action depends on a slow dissolution of the outer coating.

Although general principles of dosage computation apply to pediatric dosing as well as to adult dosing, the small amounts of medication usually given and the difficulty in ascertaining safe pediatric doses offer particular challenges. The reader should review the section in Chapter 11 on pediatric dosage. Although rules exist for calculating pediatric dosages based on those given to adults, these rules do not always take into account the varying rates of growth of body systems during childhood. Thus, it is preferable to calculate pediatric dosages on the basis of specific pediatric doses (mg/kg or mg/m^2). The mg/m^2 dosage calculation method uses the body surface area (m^2), a measure of the relationship between height and weight (see Fig. 11-1, Chap. 11). This is the most accurate method of pediatric dosage calculation since it most clearly reflects the growth of body systems that are responsible for metabolizing and excreting drugs.

Pediatric Drug Administration

Administration of medications by all routes is discussed in Chapter 8. Therefore, only the variations unique to pediatric administration are discussed in this section. Before administering any drug, proper identification of the child should be made (e.g., name band), since young children are often unable to identify themselves. The potential for adverse effects resulting from a wrong medication and possible long-term consequences are obvious, particularly with very young children.

ORAL ADMINISTRATION
Most oral medications administered to children under school age are in liquid form; thus, proper volume measurement is of great importance. The infant is generally held at a 45-degree angle in an adult's lap or in an infant seat with both hands restrained and given the medicine through an oral syringe, dropper, or nipple. Older infants may occasionally spit out a medication that is distasteful; in this case, an oral syringe can be placed across the tongue diagonally and the medicine directed to the side and back of the mouth. Directing medication directly at the throat and placing the child completely supine should be avoided because of the danger of aspiration.

The toddler and preschooler will usually cooperate in receiving oral medications by tipping the head back so that the proper volume can be administered or they will drink from a medicine cup. Occasionally, the child may refuse to take the medication and will have to be restrained and given the dose using the technique described above for the infant.

Many liquid preparations have a high sugar content and the child should therefore receive oral care following administration. Preparations with no sugar are commonly available or, if not, can be prepared on request by pharmacies for children who are diabetic or who should otherwise limit sugar intake. The same medication may be available with different flavoring from a different company, so that if a medication is refused due to objectionable taste, a preparation with a more acceptable taste may be available.

Another method of administering oral medications is by crushing tablets or opening capsules and mixing the contents with a small amount of food. This procedure is acceptable for many drugs, but some drug preparations do not readily lend themselves to administration in this manner. Usually a teaspoon or two of applesauce or jello will suffice as a medium for combining with a drug. A medicine should not be added to a bottle or glass of milk or juice, since if the child does not drink the total amount, the actual amount of medicine cannot be determined accurately. In addition, the rate of ingestion in such a case may be prolonged, resulting in very slow absorption. Foods that are nonessential are usually chosen for delivery of medicines because the child may develop an aversion to the food owing to the taste of the medicine it includes. Thus, foods such as applesauce, jello, ice cream, or jelly are frequently used, whereas essential foods such as milk, formula, or orange juice are avoided as medication delivery vehicles.

OTIC ADMINISTRATION
The tympanic membrane should be checked initially for intactness by viewing with an otoscope before administration of medication into the ear canal. Administration proceeds as for adults, with one important variation: the pinna should be pulled *down* and *back* for children under 6 years of age, whereas it is pulled up and back for children above that age and for adults (see Figure 9-1). The head of the infant and toddler should be adequately

restrained to avoid movement during administration.

RECTAL ADMINISTRATION
Although rectal suppository instillation procedures are the same for children as for adults, the smaller anal opening and rectum necessitate use of smaller fingers. The fifth digit is used to insert suppositories for infants. The buttocks are held together for a few minutes following insertion to discourage expelling the suppository.

Occasionally, therapeutic enemas are used. Once again, the procedure is similar to that for adults except that smaller tubing is used and the catheter is inserted only 1½ to 3 inches, depending on the child's size. Only very small amounts of fluid can be accommodated by the young child's rectum, so a 50-ml syringe barrel attached to enema tubing is often used for very small children. Volumes of enema solutions in older children should not exceed 250 ml in toddlers, 500 ml in children 5 to 10 years of age, and 750 ml in children 10 to 15 years of age. Only isotonic saline solutions should be used.

PARENTERAL ADMINISTRATION
Principles of parenteral administration in children are virtually the same as those discussed in Chapter 8 for adults. However, a child's size and metabolic function may necessitate changes in site selection and needle size, as well as provision for adequate restraint. In addition, microdrip infusion sets and infusion pumps are more frequently used for children than for adults since control of fluid volume is essential.

Subcutaneous and Intramuscular
Subcutaneous injection sites in children are generally the same as those used in adults. Intramuscular injection sites are also the same with two variations. First, a dorsal injection into the gluteus maximus muscle should not be used until the child has been walking for at least a year. Prior to that time (about age 2 years), the gluteus maximus is not sufficiently developed and the sciatic nerve is relatively close to the site of injection. Therefore, the vastus lateralis is the preferred site of injection in young children. Secondly, the deltoid is rarely used in very young children because of its small size, although it may occasionally be used for a small dose (0.5 ml) of an immunizing drug after 1½ years of age. Table 9-4 presents guidelines for the maximal volume of injectable solutions that may be given to different age populations.

A small-gauge needle (usually 22–26 gauge) should be used to administer pediatric medications whenever possible. The length of the needle used for injection may vary from as short as ½ to ⅝ inch for infants, up to 1 inch for school-age children, and 1½ inches for adolescents, if necessary.

Restraint may be necessary when administering parenteral medications to children. Usually only in infancy can one nurse adequately restrain a

Table 9-4
Guidelines for Maximal Amounts of Solutions to Be Injected into Muscle Tissues

Muscle Group	Birth to 1½ Years (ml)	1½ to 3 Years (ml)	3 to 6 Years (ml)	6 to 15 Years (ml)	15 Years to Adulthood (ml)
Deltoid	Not recommended	Not recommended unless other sites are not available 0.5	0.5	0.5	1
Gluteus maximus	Not recommended	Not recommended unless other sites are not available 1	1.5	1.5–2	2–2.5
Ventrogluteal	Not recommended	Not recommended unless other sites are not available 1	1.5	1.5–2	2–2.5
Vastus lateralis	0.5–1	1	1.5	1.5–2	2–2.5

(Howry LB, Bindler RM, Tso Y: Pediatric Medications, p 62. Philadelphia, JB Lippincott, 1981)

child in order to give a medication, since the child's arms and legs must both be immobilized (Fig. 9-2). A parent or another nurse can assist in restraining the older infant or child to minimize movement (Fig. 9-3). The child is usually kept lying for administration, although sitting on the side of a bed or in an adult's lap for injections into the deltoid may be allowed (Fig. 9-4). During injection, the nurse should rest her dorsal hand surface on the skin near the injection site and grasp the bottom of the syringe between the thumb and forefinger of the same hand so that the syringe does not inadvertently become dislodged if the child moves during administration.

Intravenous

Intravenous injection sites are the same for children as for adults except in very young infants. Due to reduced peripheral circulation in the very young infant, veins in extremities are often difficult to locate; thus, the frontal or superficial scalp veins are frequently sites of choice (Fig. 9-5). A small area of scalp is shaved and prepared; following insertion

of a 23-gauge or 25-gauge butterfly needle, the area may be covered with a medicine cup or other protective device. If a vein on an extremity is to be used for intravenous infusion, a small Penrose drain or rubber band is used as a tourniquet and the extremity is temporarily restrained by taping it to a sandbag. This will free both of the nurse's hands for intravenous insertion. The infant's vein rarely "pops" on entry as does an adult's; therefore, special caution and patience are needed during intravenous insertion.

A means of restraint that can be used to immobilize an older child during intravenous administration is termed a *mummy restraint.* This involves wrapping the child in material such that the extremity to be used may be left free and, if necessary, held by another nurse. This procedure is usually done in a separate treatment room to avoid performing painful procedures in a room with other children as much as possible and to help the child feel safe and secure in his hospital room because painful procedures are not performed there. Usually one physician or nurse should make no

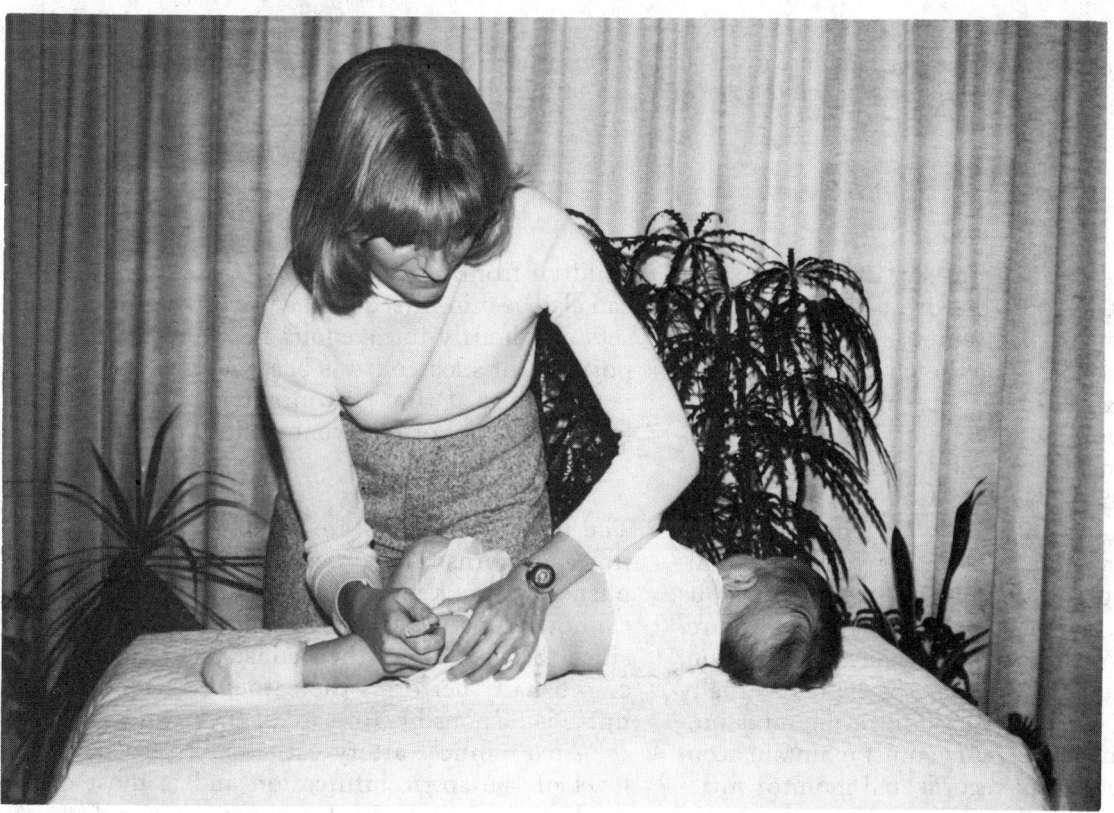

Figure 9-2.   One nurse restrains an infant for IM administration into vastus lateralis muscle. Both arms and legs are immobilized by the nurse's arms.

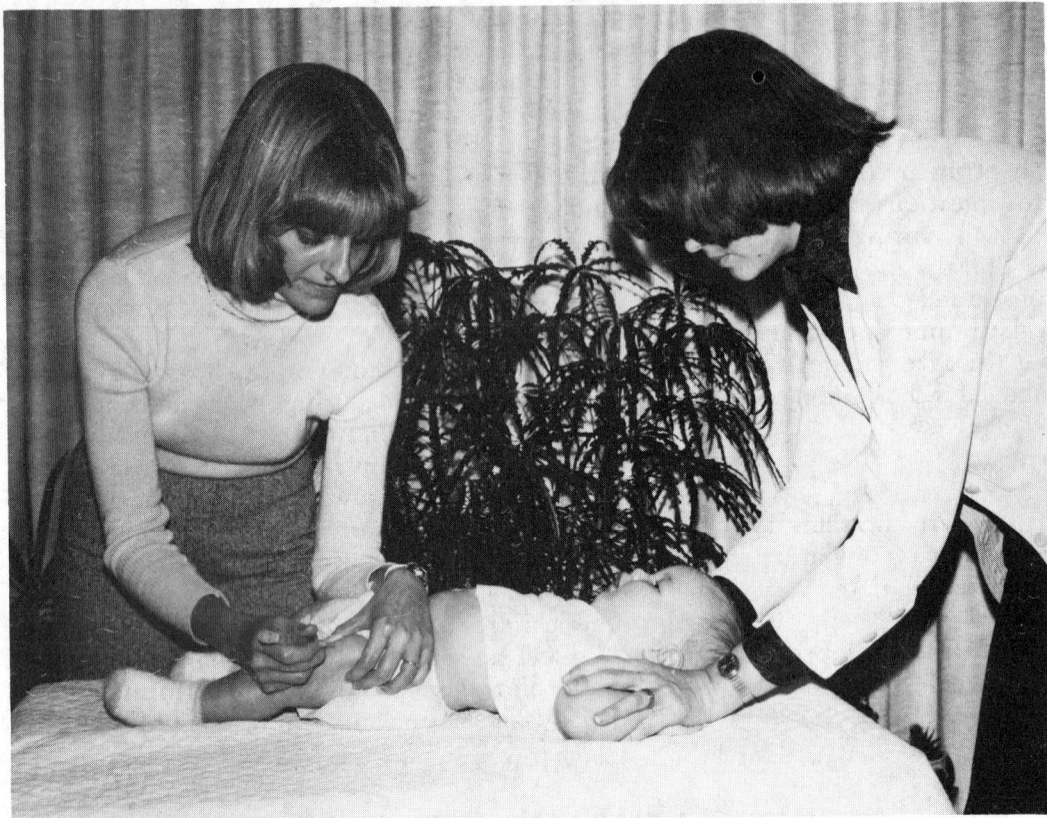

Figure 9-3. *Infant restrained for injection into vastus lateralis muscle by two individuals. One restrains the upper torso while other gives the injection.*

more than two or three unsuccessful attempts at starting an intravenous before calling for assistance. All unsuccessful attempts as well as the successful one are charted on the child's record, with time, needle size and type, site, and infusion solution type, amount, and rate recorded as well.

The extremities of a child receiving intravenous therapy must be adequately restrained. Restraints are removed at least every 2 hours, color is checked, and range of motion is given to extremities so that circulation is not impaired. Intravenous patency is checked at least hourly and even more often during infusion of intravenous medication. The young child will not be able to express verbally the discomfort created by an infiltrating infusion.

During infusion the nurse must maintain accurate intake and output records and monitor intravenous bottles carefully so that fluid overload does not inadvertently occur. Generally, bottles larger than 250 ml are not used in children under 2 years of age and those larger than 500 ml are not used in

children from 2 to 10 years of age. Fluid overload can also be minimized by the use of volume control sets and hourly intravenous flow sheets. The importance of such controls becomes clear when one realizes that at times an infant may require even less than 10 ml of intravenous fluid per hour!

Umbilical Catheters

The umbilical vessels are sometimes catheterized in ill newborns. This process is most easily accomplished within a few moments of birth and usually cannot be instituted later than 4 days after birth since the vessels are then constricted. The physician usually performs the catheterization and the nurse is responsible for care of the catheter.

An umbilical artery catheter is placed at the level of the aortic bifurcation and is most often used to obtain samples for blood gases and *p*H. A heparinized flush solution is used to maintain patency between blood draws. On occasion, percutaneous catheterization of other arteries, such as the

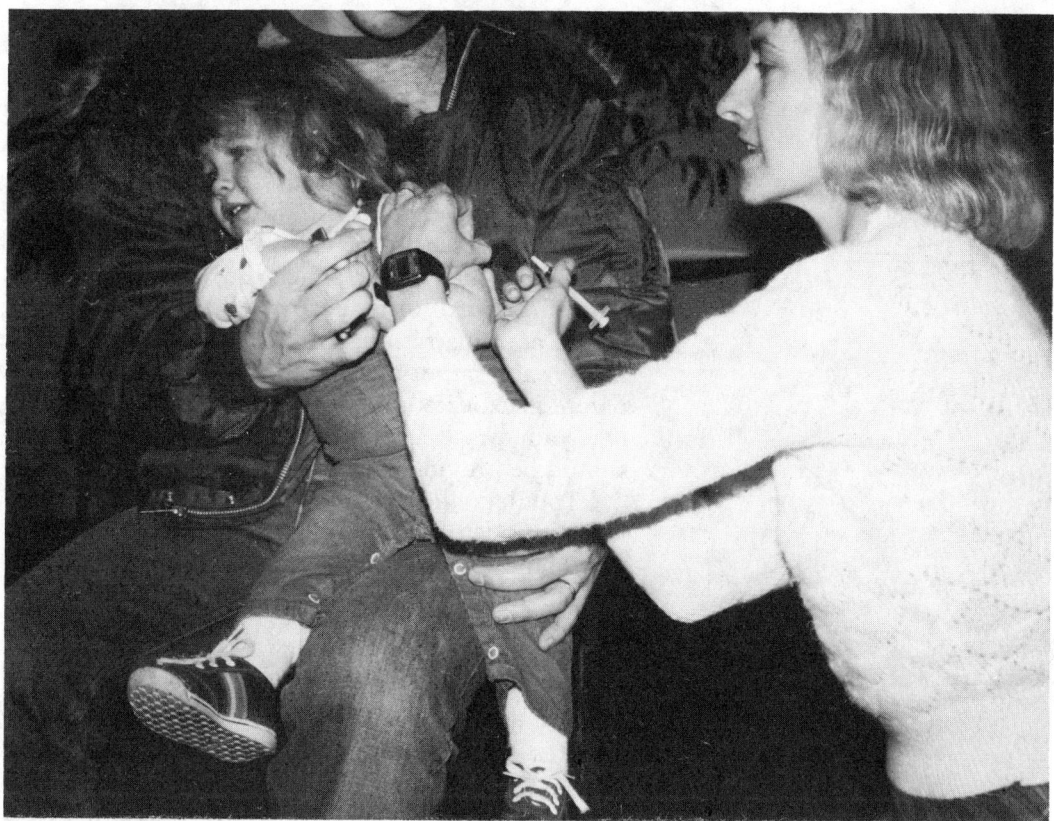

Figure 9-4. The child may be seated in the parent's lap for injections.

radial artery or a scalp artery, is used instead of a catheterization of an umbilical artery for blood draws.

The umbilical venous catheter is placed in the inferior vena cava near the right atrium and is used to obtain central venous pressure measurements. Catheters may also be used for exchange transfusions and infusion of fluids. The use of umbilical arterial catheters for infusion of medications such as antibiotics and calcium gluconate increases the incidence of complications so these catheters are not generally used for this purpose.

Harmful effects of umbilical catheters include thrombus and embolus formation, vascular damage from perforation or hypertonic solutions, hemorrhage, infection, and spasm of iliac arteries. Table 9-5 outlines appropriate nursing care to prevent these dangerous side-effects.

OTHER ADMINISTRATION ROUTES

There are no significant variations in techniques for administration of topical, ophthalmic, nasal, re-

spiratory, or vaginal medications from those described for adults. However, the nurse must provide adequate restraint when necessary to avoid injury and ensure proper administration. The physiologic characteristics of young children, discussed earlier in this chapter, should be taken into account before administering medications by any route.

SPECIAL ADMINISTRATION PROBLEMS

Occasionally a child will refuse to take a medication. If the dose is oral, he will need to be adequately restrained with his head elevated to a 45-degree angle. Pressure over the cheeks will usually open the mouth so that the medicine can be slowly instilled toward the back and side of the mouth with an oral syringe. The mouth is then held closed until the medicine is swallowed. The older child who refuses a medicine needs time to express fears, for example, in play sessions with administration equipment. Clear, short explanations and a firm approach usually work best. For other routes of administration, an agitated child should be re-

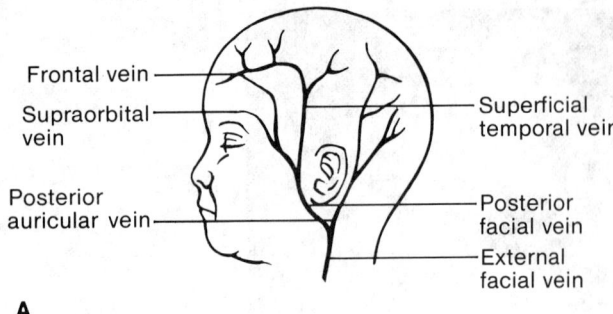

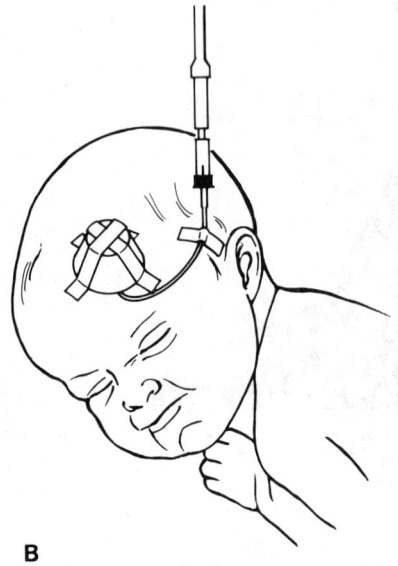

Figure 9-5.   Placement of infant scalp intravenous. (A) Venous system of infant scalp. (B) Paper cup used to protect IV site.

strained so that the procedure can be carried out quickly and with the least amount of trauma.

If a child immediately spits out or vomits an entire dose of medication, it should be administered again. If more than approximately one half but not the whole dose is expelled, one half of the dose is usually administered again. If the nurse cannot accurately estimate the amount that is spit out or vomited, or if there is a narrow therapeutic index (e.g., digoxin) for the drug, the prescriber should be contacted for instructions.

Approaching the Child

Variations in methods of restraint, sites of drug administration, and dosage forms have been dis-

cussed but one of the most important factors in administering medications to children is the approach a nurse uses with a child, and this approach may determine the degree of trauma a child experiences.

During infancy, administration is best done quickly, and the child should be comforted if the procedure was painful. Parents can be encouraged to provide this comfort when they are present. The older infant can often easily be held on a parent's lap for administration of polio vaccine or other oral medication rather than on the examining table. If a parent is expected to restrain the infant's arms and legs, adequate explanation and demonstration should be provided so it is securely done.

Toddlers and preschoolers require short, clear explanations of what will happen, why it is being done, and what is expected of them. The nurse should not lie, for example, ''This shot won't hurt,'' but rather should give truthful information and suggest coping methods, such as ''I'm going to give you this shot to help your sore throat get better. It will hurt for a minute. We'll hold your legs still while we give it and you can squeeze Mommy's hand.'' Parents should be instructed never to use a visit to the doctor or possibility of a shot as a threat of punishment for the child's behavior, such as ''If you don't stop fighting I'll take you to the doctor and he'll give you a shot.'' This serves only to destroy trust in health professionals and causes the child to believe that visits to a health-care giver for an injection are punishment for bad behavior.

The child should be given an opportunity to play act with a syringe (without the needle unless closely supervised) and other equipment on dolls to help him become familiar with the equipment. This play is best provided before the time of administration, but if this is not feasible, parents can be sent home with an empty, needleless syringe and cotton ball, or a medicine cup and encouraged to provide play sessions for the child. The child can also be encouraged to draw pictures of ''getting your shots (immunizations) so you can go to school'' or read stories about trips to the hospital or doctor's office (see Bibliography, Sample Books for Children, at the end of this chapter). Such play sessions help the child to replay important events of life, thereby gaining a better understanding of them and feeling more in control. Children may often want to give repeated shots to a doll and may be heard giving the same directions they received; the control and mastery gained by such experiences

Table 9-5
Nursing Measures to Prevent Complications
of Umbilical Catheters

Complications	Preventive Measures
Thrombus, embolus, vascular damage	Use heparinized solutions for infusion. Use heparinized flush hourly and after each blood draw. Assess circulation of extremities hourly up to 24 hours after removal of catheter. Maintain intake and output record. Observe stools for blood. Assess bowel sounds and abdominal girth.
Hemorrhage	Leave cord exposed for observation. Monitor vital signs.
Infection	Use sterile technique in inserting and caring for catheter. Use antibiotic pad at site. Replace antibiotic pad daily.

decrease the child's fears and fantasies on subsequent visits for health care.

School-age children and adolescents also require explanations of medications; they usually need to know the drug's actions, some common side-effects to watch for, and how the drug will make them feel. Discussions with illustrations of pertinent body parts and material for them to read are appropriate methods of teaching.

Family Teaching Needs

KNOWLEDGE OF MEDICATIONS
One of the primary reasons persons fail to comply with a prescribed course of medication is lack of knowledge regarding the purpose or technique of therapy. It is important for the nurse to evaluate the knowledge of parents and children who are old enough to be responsible for self-medication. Patients should be taught the name, basic purpose, desired effects, common side-effects, dosage, and administration times for all medications they are receiving. The name and telephone number of the clinic, office, or hospital to call if questions arise concerning the medication or if unexpected side-effects occur should be provided. Specific instructions for a particular type of drug should be emphasized. For example, parents should be told that the entire course of an antibiotic must be administered even though symptoms disappear in the first few days and that the doses should be given at the stated intervals (even if this means waking the child at night) in order to maintain therapeutic blood levels. On the other hand, the nurse can assist the parents in planning the administration of a one-time-daily medication so that it need not be given during school hours and fits best into the family's schedule. Information such as expected action and time of peak level should be included in such teaching.

Whenever a medication is administered in a clinic, parents should be apprised of possible side-effects that may occur later at home and taught what to do for them. For example, parents should be advised of the common side-effects of diphtheria–pertussis–tetanus (DPT) vaccine (slight fever and erythema or induration at the injection site) and told to call the clinic immediately if other symptoms such as uncontrolled crying or screaming should occur. Another example of parent education is advising parents to wash hands thoroughly after changing diapers following administration of oral polio vaccine since the live virus multiplies in the gastrointestinal tract and is excreted in the feces. Some clinics and hospital pediatric units have handouts for parents describing important information about drugs frequently administered in the area such as immunizations, antibiotics, or chemotherapeutic agents. Such materials are valuable for reference at home but a verbal discussion should also take place and the parent's ability to read English should be assessed as well.

Nurses in the hospital have a unique opportunity to teach parents as they visit and assist with care of their hospitalized children. The names of medications the child is receiving can be stated, with explanations of effects and other information. If the child will continue to need a particular medicine after discharge, the parent can be included in the administration process while the child is still hospitalized. Parents who will be giving medications at home should receive information on any special storage requirements, such as whether the drug should be protected from light, heat, or cold, or, conversely, if the bottle should be kept refrigerated.

ADMINISTRATION OF MEDICATIONS AT HOME

Health personnel often wrongly assume that a patient will automatically know how to administer medications. If two or three nurses have difficulty restraining a child for drug administration, one can hardly expect a parent to do the job at home. The parent should be instructed as to proper methods of holding the child and administering oral liquids or tablets and be able to demonstrate these methods to the satisfaction of the instructor. Parents should be discouraged from using household spoons for administering liquid medications and told to use the dropper that comes with a particular medication. If the medicine has no dropper, parents should be given a medication spoon or syringe without the needle to measure and administer the drug accurately. Many liquid medications need vigorous shaking before administration, and this information should be provided when necessary. Parents are encouraged to destroy leftover prescription medicines and to avoid using one child's prescription for someone else unless recommended by the prescriber.

When parents return for a later health-care visit, the nurse should inquire about the administration of the previously prescribed medication. Statements such as "It's often hard to get two-year-olds to take medicine. How did it go when you gave the ampicillin to Sherry?" or "What position and procedure worked best to give the medicine to Josh?" are nonthreatening and encourage parents to share their experiences.

If drugs must be administered in school or a day-care center, it is essential that the medicine be clearly labeled with name, dosage, prescriber's name, and pharmacy name and telephone number. Medicines should be left in their original containers. Parents and prescribers may have to sign a permission form for the drug to be administered by the teacher or school nurse. All leftover medicine should be sent home with the parent. Schools should establish a safe place to keep such medicines and clearly state who is responsible for administration.

SELECTION OF MEDICINES AND DRUG HISTORY

Parents are encouraged to keep accurate medication records for their children from the time of birth. These records should include information on all drugs received. When any medicine is administered in a clinic or doctor's office, the name, dosage, and expected effect should be written down and given to the parent. The parent should be encouraged to keep a notebook listing these medications with dates and responses. Any allergic reactions are especially important to note and should be reported to future health-care providers. If a child has a severe allergy, whether to a medication or to other substances (such as a bee sting), or has a chronic disease (such as diabetes), the child should wear an identifying Medic-Alert bracelet.

The consumer is faced with a wide array of nonprescription medicines. Parents usually need assistance in selecting an appropriate analgesic/antipyretic and mild decongestant for common childhood illnesses. Such teaching should be a part of regular health maintenance. When need for other over-the-counter medicines is felt, parents should be encouraged to contact their pediatrician, nurse practitioner, family physician, or pharmacist. Such medicines should only be taken as directed and further medical help should be sought if symptoms do not improve within a few days. When taking drug histories, the nurse should ask specific questions regarding use of over-the-counter medicines and vitamins.

POISONING

Poisoning remains a leading cause of death in childhood. There are over two million accidental poisonings annually in this country, more than 60% of which occur in children under 5 years of age, with a peak occurring at 2 years. Approximately 25% of children who ingest a poison will be involved in a second poison ingestion within 1 year. Common poisonings include ingestion of medications and household substances; thus, the nurse needs to emphasize proper storage of all medicines and other potential poisons. Child-resistant caps can be requested from pharmacies but they may provide a false sense of security since many toddlers and preschoolers can open these

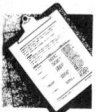

Nursing Care Plan 9-1
Guidelines for Applying the Nursing Process to Medication Administration for Children*

Assessment

A. Subjective Data

1. Medication History:
   a. Include a history of immunizations.
   b. Exposure to teratogenic agents *in utero*
   c. If child is breast-fed, ask the mother is she is taking any medications.
2. Child's perception of events/drug therapy based on age-related psychologic growth and development.
3. Compliance issues: Parent's past success in helping child to complete drug therapy.
4. Safety issues: Parent's knowledge of safe storage of medications and "child proofing" of home.

B. Objective Data

1. Focus the physical assessment on the differences in growth and development of body system.
2. An *accurate* height and weight must be recorded in order to determine safe drug dosage.
3. Laboratory values may be different for children in different age categories.

Nursing Diagnosis	*Planning/Evaluation*	*Intervention*
A. Include nursing diagnoses that reflect parental/family problems, as well as those of the child (*e.g.*, "Knowledge deficit: Mother does not know how to give injections," and "Fear related to bad past experience with injections"). B. Identify problems with safety for children, including storing medications and changes in administration technique.	Writing goals (expected outcomes) for children is the same as for adults, although parents are more likely to be included. (See the guidelines listed in Chapter 6 for goals for adults.) The evaluation phase is the same for children as for adults. However, it may be more complex because it is more likely to include not only an evaluation of the child, but also of the parents and family.	A. Administration techniques may vary. Be aware of those routes and techniques specific to children which are designed to ensure safe, correct drug administration (*e.g.*, use of volume control chamber for administering an IV drug). B. Observe carefully for side-effects/adverse reactions because children vary in ability to give verbal cues, depending on age. (Observing for subtle physical changes and slight changes in mood, appetite, and activity becomes more important.) C. Use creative approaches to implement nursing interventions, remembering to take the time to establish trust: 1. Use play as a method of teaching and to elicit feedback. 2. Encourage and observe parent/child interactions. 3. Include the family unit when teaching about medications.

* These are in addition to the general guidelines listed in Chapter 6.

containers. While proper storage of harmful items should be emphasized with parents, teaching can also be done with children in schools and day-care centers so they begin to identify substances harmful for ingestion. For example, they can be given "Mr. Yuk" stickers to bring home and place on harmful items.

When potential poisoning has occurred, parents should first call the nearest poison control center. The telephone number of the poison control center should be listed near each telephone for emergency access. Based on the recommendations of the center, it may be necessary to induce vomiting. All homes should contain a bottle of syrup of ipecac for this purpose. Syrup of ipecac is available in 1 fluid ounce (30 ml) containers without a prescription. The dosage to be administered is 1 to 2 teaspoons (5 ml–10 ml) for children under 1 year of age; 2 to 3 teaspoons (10 ml–15 ml) for children 1 to 5 years of age; and 3 teaspoons or 1 tablespoon (15 ml) for persons over 5 years of age and weighing more than 25 pounds. The dosage may be repeated once in 20 to 30 minutes if vomiting has not occurred. If vomiting still does not occur, the child should be taken to a physician or to the hospital, since the stomach contents may have to be removed by lavage. At least 4 to 8 ounces (120 ml–240 ml) of fluid, preferably water, should be administered with syrup of ipecac. This drug should only be given when directed, since vomiting can be harmful if a corrosive poison was ingested. If parents take the child to an emergency room, they should bring any vomitus and the container of the ingested substance with them. Once opened, syrup of ipecac should not be used for future episodes since evaporation may have occurred. Parents should be told to obtain a new bottle to replace the used one. Expiration dates should be checked periodically.

Evaluation

Pediatric patients are clearly unique in their response to medications. Each child requires careful assessment of physiologic and psychologic developmental functioning to ensure safe and effective drug therapy. Although infants, especially the premature, are at highest risk for complications due to medications largely because of the low level of liver and urinary drug clearance, unexpected reactions can occur at any age. The outcomes sought for all children receiving medication are safe administration and careful monitoring of responses.

In addition, the approach of the care provider can markedly influence the response of children to the medication experience. Thus, the role of the nurse in using restraint when necessary, using age-related explanations, and providing play experiences is vital in fostering compliance and assisting the child in developing a positive attitude about the experience.

The pediatric client has often been called a "therapeutic orphan" in regard to medications. The unique developmental needs make it difficult to predict and recommend pediatric dosages. Since drugs without specific childhood dosages must often be prescribed to treat children, the nurse's role in observation is of obvious importance.

Indeed, the field of pediatric pharmacology offers particular challenges and rewards, providing an opportunity for long-term impact on clients. See Nursing Care Plan 9-1, Guidelines for Applying the Nursing Process to Medication Administration for Children.

REVIEW QUESTIONS

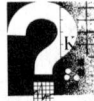

1. A 6-month-old child was treated for otitis media 3 days ago with an oral antibiotic that is being administered four times daily. The child returns to the clinic today with a rash over the entire body. What questions will you ask? What further assessments will you make?
2. A newborn is receiving four medications. Discuss the effect her organ development and the number of medications will have on her ability to metabolize and excrete the medications.
3. You must administer a 0.5-ml intramuscular injection of DTP vaccine to 6-month-old Sara. Describe the history you will obtain, the injection site you will use, how you will hold and comfort Sara, and the instructions you will give the parent.

4. Seven-year-old Tim has an intravenous infusion flowing. Describe the observations you will make of the infusion flow, the infusion site, and Tim. How will you record your observations?

5. Fourteen-year-old Sue is a recently diagnosed diabetic. What teaching techniques are likely to work best at her age?

6. You have been asked to present a class to a group of second graders about the experience of being hospitalized. What information about hospitalization and medications will you want to relay? Prepare the lesson plan listing your objectives for student learning, class content, and learning experiences.

7. Two-year-old Billy has had two episodes of accidental poisoning at home. How is the likelihood of poisoning influenced by his musculoskeletal maturation at this time? How should Billy's parents plan to "poison-proof" their home? What instructions will you give the parents related to emergency administration of syrup of ipecac?

BIBLIOGRAPHY

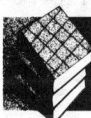

Barnett H, Vesterdal J: The physiologic and clinical significance of immaturity of kidney function in young infants. J Pediatr 42:99, 1953

Blake S: The bright side of phototherapy. MCN 8(1):23, 1983

Cantekin E et al: Lack of efficacy of a decongestant-antihistamine combination for otitis media with effusion ("secretory otitis media") in children. N Engl J Med 308(6):297, 1983

Chudzik G, Yaffee S: Introduction to the special problems of pediatric drug therapy. Drug Therapy, July:17, 1973

Committee on Infectious Diseases Report: Aspirin and Reye syndrome. Pediatrics 69(6):810, 1982

Done A: Developmental pharmacology. Clin Pharmacol Ther 5(4):432, 1964

Dunne R, Perez R: Reye's syndrome: A challenge not limited to critical care nurses. Issues in Comprehensive Pediatric Nursing 5(4):253, 1981

Foster S: Administering medications to children. Issues in Comp Ped Nsg 3(5):1, 1978

Fujita MT: The impact of illness or surgery on the body image of the child. Nurs Clin North Am 7(4):41, 1972

Gellert E: Psychosocial aspects of pediatric care. New York, Grune & Stratton, 1978

Giacoia G, Gorodisher R: Pharmacologic principles in neonatal drug therapy. Clin Perinatol 2(1):125, 1975

Golden N et al: Maternal alcohol use and infant development. Pediatrics 70(6):931, 1982

Hingson R et al: Effects of maternal drinking and marijuana use on fetal growth and development. Pediatrics 70(4):539, 1982

Howry L, Bindler R, Tso Y: Pediatric Medications. Philadelphia, JB Lippincott, 1981

Hurwitz E, Goodman R: A cluster of cases of Reye syndrome associated with chickenpox. Pediatrics 70(6):901, 1982

Jusko W: Pharmacokinetic principles in pediatric pharmacology. Pediatr Clin North Am 19(1):81, 1972

Kitterman J, Phibbs R, Tooley W: Catheterization of umbilical vessels in newborn infants. Pediatr Clin North Am 17(4):895, 1970

Kunzman L: Some factors influencing a young child's mastery of hospitalization. Nurs Clin North Am 7(1):13, 1972

Masaki B: Physiologic basis for pediatric drug therapy. US Pharmacist Nov/Dec:36, 1978

Mirkin B: Developmental pharmacology. Annu Rev Pharmacol 10:255, 1970

Mokrohsky S et al: Low positioning of umbilical-artery catheters increases associated complications in newborn infants. N Engl J Med 299(11):561, 1978

Ormond E, Caulfield C: A practical guide to giving oral medications to young children. MCN 1(5):320, 1976

Rajani K et al: Effect of heparinization of fluids infused through an umbilical artery catheter on catheter patency and frequency of complications. Pediatrics 63(4):552, 1979

Rane A, Sjoqvist F: Drug metabolism in the human fetus and newborn infant. Pediatr Clin North Am 19(1):37, 1972

Rane A, Wilson J: Clinical pharmacokinetics in infants and children. Clinical Pharmacokinetics 1:2, 1976

Shepard T: Teratogenicity of therapeutic agents. Curr Probl Pediatr 10(2):5, 1979

Trauner D: Reye's syndrome. Curr Probl Pediatr 12(7):5, 1982

Tyrala E et al: Clinical pharmacology of hexachlorophene in newborn infants. J Pediatr 81(3):481, 1977

Wei S (ed): Pediatric Dental Care, New York, Medcom, 1978

Winters R, Lewis A: Neonatal I.V. Therapy. Chicago, Abbott Laboratories, 1970

Sample Books for Children

Cooper A et al: Color Me Diabetic. San Marcos, Calif: Palomar College, 1976

Rey M, Rey H: Curious George Goes to the Hospital. Boston, Houghton-Mifflin, 1966

Scary R: Nicky Goes to the Doctor. New York, Golden Press, 1978

Shay A: What Happens When You Go to the Hospital. Chicago, Reilly & Lee, 1969

Showers P: No Measles, No Mumps for Me. New York, Thomas Y Crowell, 1980

Sobol H: Jeff's Hospital Book. New York, HZ Walck, 1975

Tamburine J: I Think I Will Go to the Hospital. Nashville, Abingdon Press, 1965

Wever A: Elizabeth Gets Well. New York, Thomas Y Crowell, 1970

Wenger D: Mr. Hypo Is My Friend. Elkhart, IN, Ames, 1973

Geriatric Pharmacology

10

The aging process is associated with certain recognizable physical changes, among them decreased body weight, loss of hair, and alterations in posture and in contour of external features. More important in terms of drug therapy, however, are the less obvious changes occurring in the internal body organs and in physiologic functions. With advancing age, there are decreases in the number of cells in most body tissues; changes in the activity of the remaining cells (e.g., metabolic function, permeability, respiration); increased proliferation of connective tissue and fat; impaired adaptation to stress; and decreases in muscle strength, circulation, oxygen utilization, and sensory perception. Age-related changes in the functioning of various organ systems are summarized in Table 10-1. These deteriorations in organ and tissue functioning can result in altered responsiveness to many drugs; therefore, effects of drug therapy in the aged are often unpredictable, and untoward reactions are quite common and frequently serious.

Complicating the picture is the multiplicity of drugs that may comprise an elderly individual's therapeutic regimen. A progressively increasing life span has resulted in a greater proportion of the population reaching advanced age, with a corresponding increase in the use of drugs for treating chronic disease conditions such as congestive heart failure, hypertension, cerebrovascular disease, and carcinomas. Average life expectancy in Western countries now stands at nearly 70 years for men and almost 80 years for women. Since the frequency of drug therapy and the average number of drugs taken per person usually increase progressively with age, it is not surprising that the incidence of adverse drug reactions and drug interactions in the geriatric population has undergone a tremendous proliferation.

It has been estimated that in the United States the elderly account for almost one third of all drug taking. They often take several drugs at one time; many nursing home patients routinely receive up to six drugs on a daily basis. With such widespread multiple drug use, it is easy to understand why close to 90% of elderly patients experience one or more episodes of adverse reactions to their drug therapy. Therefore, the necessity for a careful, conservative approach to geriatric drug therapy is obvious, and constant attention to the response of the elderly patient to drugs is essential if maximum benefit is to be derived with minimal adverse effects.

Table 10-1
Age-Related Changes in Organ Function*

Heart

Increased size
Decreased heart rate
Decreased cardiac output
Impaired adaptation to stress

Cardiovascular System

Decreased peripheral blood flow
Increased systemic resistance
Loss of vessel elasticity

Nervous system

Loss of neuronal function
Decreased brain weight
Impaired neuronal conduction
Reduced sensory perception (vision, hearing)

Musculoskeletal System

Osteoporosis
Loss of muscle mass

Lungs

Loss of elasticity

Kidneys

Decreased renal blood flow
Decreased glomerular filtration rate
Loss of functioning nephrons

Liver

Reduced enzymatic activity
Impaired hepatic perfusion

Hormonal

Loss of gonadal steroidal function
Decreased anabolic activity

Gastrointestinal

Decreased digestive secretions
Decreased motility and peristalsis
Decreased gastric acidity

* Frequency and severity of changes vary widely among individuals.

Determinants of Altered Drug Responses in the Elderly

The frequent presence of multiple disease states in the elderly and the attendant use of several different drugs concurrently, as well as the wide variability in the development of organ and tissue pathology, make determination of proper drug dosage a difficult matter. The safe and effective use of drugs in the aged depends on individualized therapy and requires constant reevaluation. There are a number of variables that influence the response to drugs in the geriatric population. In general, drugs tend to be absorbed, distributed, metabolized and excreted much less efficiently in elderly patients, compared with younger adults. Thus, the danger of untoward reactions as well as drug interactions is magnified. In addition, elderly patients are sometimes physically incapacitated or mentally confused, and compliance with the prescribed drug regimen can be poor, especially if the patient lives alone. This latter aspect of geriatric drug usage will be considered later in this chapter.

Changes in the pharmacokinetic fate of drugs in the geriatric population are often responsible for undesirable drug effects. Some of the more important alterations that occur are discussed below.

Absorption

Many changes in the gastrointestinal (GI) tract that occur with age may impair absorptive capacity. Gastric secretory cell function is reduced, leading to impaired acid release and an elevation in gastric pH. Although secretions are rarely reduced to the extent that digestion is seriously compromised, the elevated pH can slow absorption of weak acids such as salicylates, since they are more highly ionized in a less acidic environment and less readily pass the absorptive barrier (see Chap. 2). Impaired active transport mechanisms in the small intestine can also reduce absorption of those substances dependent on such mechanisms for transfer across absorbing membranes. The number of epithelial absorbing cells may be reduced with advancing age, and mucosal blood flow is frequently decreased, thus slowing the rate at which drugs may pass from the intestinal lumen to the bloodstream. Gastric emptying time is often prolonged, due to reduced GI motility, thus slowing absorption of drugs from the small intestine. Although the *rate* of drug absorption may be somewhat less consistent in the elderly, the *extent* to which a drug is absorbed is probably not markedly different from that in younger patients, provided there is no serious underlying disease. This has important implications regarding onset of action and time to peak effect,

which may be significantly slowed in the older patient.

Distribution

Unlike absorption, the distribution of drugs in the elderly is often significantly different from that observed in younger adults. A major factor that can restrict drug distribution in the geriatric patient is reduced cardiac output, which results in decreased perfusion of many bodily organs. Impaired peripheral blood flow, possibly due to atherosclerotic deposits within vessel walls, also influences the final distribution of a drug. Lowered serum albumin levels reduce the availability of drug binding sites in the plasma and may not only alter the transport of highly protein-bound drugs such as barbiturates, phenytoin, phenylbutazone, quinidine, tolbutamide, and warfarin, but also increase their likelihood to elicit adverse effects. Geriatric patients usually exhibit a diminished lean body mass and lowered proportion of body water compared to younger patients. Conversely, the percentage of body fat usually increases with advancing age, from approximately 20% to 35% in men and from 35% to 50% in women. These increases in adipose tissue fractions can result in more extensive distribution of highly lipid-soluble drugs (*e.g.*, barbiturates, diazepam, lidocaine) and more extensive storage of these drugs in the adipose tissue reservoirs. This latter phenomenon is frequently responsible for the prolonged residual effects of many drugs in elderly patients, and can be a serious hazard in the case of central nervous system (CNS) depressants.

Metabolism

Significant changes in liver function generally do not occur until rather late in life (after age 70), due in part to the tremendous reserve capacity of the organ. However, decreases in hepatic function at an earlier age can often develop secondary to the presence of chronic disease states, and the decreases are frequently responsible for the toxic effects of drugs used to treat these states. Reduced metabolism of many drugs in the elderly may be a consequence of progressive loss of liver cells as well as impaired enzyme function but more commonly is a result of decreased perfusion of the liver secondary to diminished cardiac output and compromised circulatory function. Hepatic blood flow may be reduced as much as 50% in the elderly compared to young adults; thus, the hepatic clearance of drugs may be significantly slowed in the geriatric patient. The important implication here is that doses of many drugs need to be reduced in the elderly, since the retarded rate of metabolism can result in a prolonged duration of action and danger of accumulation. Of course, patients with liver disease (cirrhosis, hepatitis, fatty infiltration) or decreased hepatic blood flow (congestive heart failure, pulmonary hypertension, arteriosclerosis) are extremely sensitive to those drugs that are primarily detoxified by the hepatic enzyme systems.

Excretion

Glomerular filtration rate declines by approximately one third by age 65, largely due to reduced renal blood flow and loss of functioning nephrons. Likewise, tubular reabsorption and active tubular secretion, the other important renal mechanisms, are somewhat reduced in the geriatric patient. The reduced clearance of those drugs eliminated largely by the kidney correlates with the decline in glomerular filtration. Examples of such drugs are the aminoglycoside antibiotics, cimetidine, chlorpropamide, digoxin, lithium, and procainamide. It is essential that the dosage of these and other drugs undergoing extensive renal clearance be reduced in the presence of diminished kidney function. Similarly, drugs eliminated by active tubular secretory processes (e.g., penicillin, probenecid) may exhibit decreased rates of elimination in the elderly.

Serum creatinine levels are useful as an indicator of glomerular function, especially in young patients. However, the serum creatinine concentration depends on the level of creatinine production by the body as well as on its clearance by the kidney. With advancing age, the decline in total body mass, particularly muscle, is reflected in a reduction in creatinine synthesis and turnover. Thus, despite the decrease in creatinine clearance resulting from reduced kidney function in the geriatric patient, the fact that creatinine production is lowered as well frequently results in no significant change in serum creatinine levels. It is apparent, then, that *serum* creatinine levels do not always accurately reflect kidney function (i.e., glomerular filtration) in the elderly patient, and reliance on serum creatinine as a sole indicator of kidney functioning can be misleading. Creatinine clearance based on calculations using 24-hour urinary excretion in addition to serum levels is a much

more reliable indicator of glomerular filtration in the geriatric patient.

Miscellaneous Factors

In addition to changes in the absorption, distribution, metabolism, and excretion of drugs, many other factors contribute to altered drug responsiveness in the geriatric population. Some of the more important of these are discussed here.

ALTERED RECEPTOR SENSITIVITY

Altered susceptibility to the effects of certain drugs is noted in many geriatric patients. While the pharmacokinetic alterations described above are frequently responsible for this hypersusceptibility, the altered drug responsiveness often observed following a single dose of a drug suggests that there is in some cases an actual alteration in the receptor sensitivity to the drug. For example, some elderly patients may be particularly resistant to certain drugs, such as barbiturates. These changes may be due in part to a reduced number or sensitivity of barbiturate receptors in the elderly patient. Conversely, increased responsiveness to many drugs also occurs in some elderly patients and is probably the result of both altered pharmacokinetic responses (e.g., reduced metabolism or excretion, decreased serum protein binding) as well as impaired homeostatic mechanisms, which normally serve to limit the response to a particular drug to a clinically relevant extent.

PRESENCE OF CHRONIC DISEASE STATES

As mentioned earlier, many elderly patients exhibit one or more chronic pathologic conditions, such as hypertension, diabetes, angina, congestive heart failure, or peripheral vascular disease. These diseases can often markedly affect the responsiveness to a particular drug. Altered drug responses in elderly patients presenting one or more of these disease states may result from an impairment in the handling of a drug by the body (i.e., reduced absorption, restricted distribution, decreased metabolism, slowed excretion) or can be due to impaired compensatory mechanisms secondary to a decrease in the function of a particular organ, such as the heart or adrenal glands. For example, postural (or orthostatic) hypotension is a common occurrence in the elderly, due to blunted homeostatic mechanisms normally operative in the maintenance of blood pressure. This condition is frequently exacerbated by a number of drugs taken by the elderly, such as antihypertensives, antipsychotics, and vasodilators.

HORMONAL CHANGES
Many drugs act through hormonal mechanisms and thus may elicit altered responses because of reduced endocrine secretion as the aging process continues. Decreases are often observed in thyroid function, glucose tolerance, adrenal cortical activity, and gonadal hormone release in the geriatric population. Replacement drug therapy is frequently indicated in these instances but can result in greatly enhanced effects early in the course of therapy due to an initial supersensitivity of the hormonal receptor sites following prolonged lack of sufficient stimulation. Thus, hormonal replacement must be undertaken cautiously, and initial dosage levels should be kept to a minimum to avoid excessive receptor activation and possible development of adverse reactions.

Atrophic changes in certain structures (bones and genital organs) due to lack of hormonal action may likewise modify a drug's effect or increase its toxicity. For example, use of steroids in the aged can result in enhanced breakdown of bone and increased susceptibility to infection, compared to that observed in younger patients.

BEHAVORIAL CHANGES
Often overlooked, but critically important as a major determinant of drug responses in the aged, is the mental condition of the patient. Cerebral arteriosclerosis can result in confusion, loss of memory, and even dementia. These behavioral abnormalities may adversely affect normal physiologic functioning. Also, impaired memory and disorientation frequently are responsible for poor dosage compliance, accidental overdosage, and ingestion of the wrong drug.

Drug Therapy in the Elderly: The Nursing Process

Assessment

Drug therapy in the geriatric population is at best difficult and in many instances quite hazardous. A thorough understanding of the altered physiology of this age group, as described earlier in the chapter, is essential for proper drug prescribing.

Likewise, an awareness not only of the expected effects of a drug, but also of the usual unto-

ward effects and possible paradoxical reactions, is vital for assessing both the efficacy and the safety of geriatric drug therapy. Baseline data collection can be divided into four areas: necessity of therapy, duration of therapy, adequacy of therapy, and the patient's level of competence. Each of these will be discussed separately.

NECESSITY OF THERAPY
Many afflictions besetting the elderly do not require drug intervention. Therefore, the clinician needs to explore why the geriatric patient is seeking treatment. Changes in life status, loss of income, death of spouse or friends, and generalized feelings of growing old are all reasons why some elderly seek medical intervention. Our culture has always searched for the "Fountain of Youth," so it may be with this in mind that the older person enters the health-care system looking for the youthful cure. Careful attention to the elderly patient's complaints may avert unnecessary treatment with drugs.

The decision to treat a geriatric patient who complains of bothersome symptoms with either drug therapy or some other form of therapy is often a difficult one, and requires patience, compassion, and, above all, an understanding of the pharmacology and toxicology of the drugs considered for use. The patient's symptoms may be due to an underlying disease state, but they may also result from other medications, both prescription and over-the-counter, that the patient may be taking. The necessity of obtaining a drug history is obvious, therefore, in assessing the need for additional drug treatment. A general, yet very useful rule of thumb in deciding whether a drug is necessary is that, with few exceptions, drugs that have a profile of potential untoward reactions that are worse than the current symptoms described by the patient should be avoided. The benefit-to-risk ratio of drug use in the elderly assumes critical dimensions in view of the greater likelihood of older patients to experience untoward reactions to drug therapy. All care givers should advocate a conservative approach to therapy for the elderly patient.

DURATION OF THERAPY
Equally important as deciding which drug or drugs to prescribe is determining how long therapy with a particular drug should be continued. Too often, drugs are prescribed on a prn (*i.e.*, as needed) refill basis, and the decision as to the length of time the drug is to be taken is left to the patient. The danger

inherent in such a practice is enormous, and no patient (geriatric or otherwise) should be allowed to regulate his drug therapy without professional monitoring and assessment. The problem of non-compliance with the optimal duration of therapy for a particular drug is twofold: insufficient ther-apy or overly prolonged therapy. The first problem is commonly encountered with anti-infective drugs, where with minimal exceptions, treatment must be continued for at least seven, and preferably ten days. Premature termination of anti-infective drug therapy frequently leads to recurrence of the infection, often of a more serious and resistant na-ture, and this can have serious consequences in el-derly or debilitated patients. This is particularly true of urinary tract infections, which represent a very common affliction of the elderly.

The other noncompliance problem relating to duration of drug therapy is continuation of treat-ment past the point of need. This is especially criti-cal in the case of centrally acting drugs such as hypnotics, tranquilizers, and narcotic analgesics, due to the danger of dependence with prolonged use of these agents. Strict monitoring of these kinds of medications in the geriatric patient is of utmost importance, since the CNS-depressant ac-tion of the drugs can further impair the possibly compromised judgment and psychomotor coordi-nation of the elderly patient. Although no drug should be withheld from a patient simply because of the possibility of habituation or deleterious CNS effects if truly needed, treatment with such drugs must be closely monitored and therapy terminated once the desired effect is attained or it becomes obvious that the drug is either ineffective or poorly tolerated. Confounding the problem of accurately assessing the effect of psychoactive drugs in the elderly is the pattern of drug-induced side-effects, which frequently closely mimic signs of advancing age, such as confusion, weakness, tremor, malaise, and so on.

The nurse must collect data on each encounter with the patient to determine whether drug ther-apy should continue and whether the elderly pa-tient is complying with the prescribed regimen. The nurse can sometimes serve as an advocate for the patient when multiple care givers have been involved and a regimen has become too compli-cated.

ADEQUACY OF THERAPY
Overprescribing of medications is as deleterious as inadequate therapy. The presence of multiple dis-eases in many geriatric patients occasionally leads

to a "shotgun" approach to prescribing that greatly increases the danger of drug toxicity and especially drug interactions. In addition, the reduced mental capacity of many older people makes it very diffi-cult for them to manage multiple drug therapy. Thus, the smallest number of drugs that are ade-quate to serve the patient's needs should be pre-scribed. Dosing of geriatric patients should be con-servative as well. As previously mentioned, elderly patients are frequently more sensitive to the effects of a drug than are younger patients; thus, they will require lower doses and longer dosage intervals for many drugs. Drug therapy should be initiated with small doses, and the dose gradually increased until an optimal effect is observed. Complex dosage schedules should be avoided if at all possible, be-cause many geriatric patients find it difficult to adhere to such schedules; single daily dosage is usually preferred. Abrupt alterations in dosage should be avoided. Whenever additional drugs are added to the regimen, the current dosage schedule should be reviewed and appropriate modifications made. The nurse can facilitate this process by col-lecting a drug history at each encounter with the patient. This should include information about the use of other drugs, both over-the-counter and pre-scription, and whether the patient has been treated by another physician or dentist since he was last seen.

LEVEL OF COMPETENCE
Lastly, the patient's ability to manage any drug reg-imen must be assessed. This is critical before any teaching can begin or the decision made that the patient is capable of medicating himself. The pa-tient's level of alertness, independence in care, memory for recent events, and retention of infor-mation are all parameters that will help the nurse plan medication administration and home care. Sometimes, the elderly person's memory will be the cause of later compliance problems. If such problems can be uncovered early, many methods can be employed to help the person continue the regimen.

Nursing Diagnosis

Nursing diagnoses for elderly patients receiving medications are similar to those for other adults. Refer to Chapter 6 as well as the accompanying Nursing Care Plan 10-1, Guidelines for Applying the Nursing Process to Medication Administration for Gerontologic Clients, for more information.

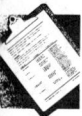

Assessment

A. Subjective Data

1. Medication History
   a. Include questions concerning use of folk remedies.
   b. Determine the number of health-care providers seen by the patient, and who has written which prescriptions to be sure of appropriate therapies.
2. Medical history: Be systematic because elderly people often have multisystem problems that may require long and detailed assessment (e.g., decreased liver, renal, and cardiac function may affect drug action and duration).
3. Personal history: Explore financial resources, availability of support systems, and client's view of illness. All are critical with the elderly.

B. Objective Data

1. Physical Assessment
   a. Examine mental alertness, memory, and motor skills to determine how independent the person can be in managing his own drug administration.
   b. Establish baseline vital signs: norms may vary from the adult ranges.
2. Laboratory data: Values may vary from the normal adult (e.g., older people may have a higher urine creatinine clearance level).

Nursing Diagnosis	Planning/Evaluation	Intervention
Gerontologic clients are at risk for many nursing diagnoses that can influence drug therapy. Below are some common examples: · Alteration in bowel elimination: constipation · Alteration in comfort: chronic pain · Alteration in nutrition: less than body requirements · Alteration in oral mucous membrane · Alteration in thought processes · Fluid volume excess · Impairment of skin integrity · Self-care deficit · Sensory–perceptual alterations · Impaired physical mobility · Ineffective individual coping related to loneliness	The planning phase for the elderly client is the same as for the adult (see Chapter 6), although goals are more likely to include family members/caretakers. The evaluation phase is the same as for the adult (see Chapter 6), although family members/caretakers are more likely to be evaluated as well.	A. Develop a trust relationship and encourage the person to seek help when he needs it. B. Provide a system to monitor for side-effects/adverse reactions carefully, because these are more likely in the elderly. C. Be aware that small doses of sedatives, analgesics, and narcotics can have *significant effects* on the elderly. Some drugs may also cause *opposite* effects from those intended (e.g., a sedative may cause an elderly person to become agitated and confused). D. Provide teaching sessions that keep the regimen as simple as possible, consider the patient's limitations in motor skills, and provide for memory cues that are tied to daily routines.

* These are in addition to the general guidelines listed in Chapter 6.

Plan

The nursing care goals for the elderly patient taking medications should include
  · Reducing anxiety surrounding medication administration
  · Establishing a regimen with which the patient can comply
  · Developing strategies that will help the patient take prescribed medication safely and consistently

Intervention

REDUCING ANXIETY SURROUNDING MEDICATION ADMINISTRATION

To reduce anxiety, the nurse should establish an open-ended dialogue with the patient, allowing the patient time to express his fears. Questions about specific problems such as memory may be useful, but the nurse also needs to explore how the patient feels about taking medicine. Some patients expect drugs will cure them or make them feel better (or more valuable), and become anxious when medications are decreased or discontinued. Others may see medicine as a sign of weakness or aging and may be resistant to the prescribed therapy. The nurse can improve the chances the elderly patient will comply by establishing perceptions early and planning care to incorporate the patient's beliefs into the drug regimen.

ESTABLISHING A VIABLE REGIMEN AND DEVELOPING SAFETY STRATEGIES

Success in compliance depends on the patient's ability to follow the regimen. Compliance decreases as complexity increases. One way to establish whether the patient will be able to follow the regimen is to establish a supervised routine similar to the one the patient will follow at home. The routine should tie drug taking to memory joggers. Memory joggers may be daily routines such as mealtimes or sleep times, calendars on which the drugs are listed, or pill boxes in which the correct number of pills are placed in appropriate time slots (see Chap. 6 for some examples). Pill boxes can be made of muffin tins, egg cartons, or commercially available boxes. Establishment of a routine that the patient finds easy to use and remember is critical to success.

The viable regimen is also one the patient can understand. Before the patient can be allowed independence in drug taking, he should know, at least on a basic level, which symptoms are being treated by the prescribed medicine and what side-effects he should watch for. This information may be better used if it is written down or described in pictures (for the nonreader) or on a tape (for the blind). Memory fails even the younger person on a complex drug regimen, so the elderly person will benefit from such assistance.

The regimen should also be initially supervised in order to ensure the patient's safety. The bottles the patient will use must be clearly labeled in lettering large enough to be easily read. If drugs have a similar appearance, they should be placed in different types of containers in order to avoid confusion. Sometimes an elderly patient will have diffi-

culty swallowing a drug. The formulation may be easier to manage if smaller pills or liquids can be given. Again, by reviewing these parameters before the patient goes home, the regimen may be more easily managed.

Vials and bottles containing the drugs may need to have easily opened caps for use by elderly patients with arthritic changes. "Child-proof" closures are best avoided. Medicine droppers, measuring cups, and syringes need to have lettering clear enough for the patient to read. Magnifiers can be used if necessary, but the patient will need practice in order to master their use.

The patient should have a written list of all the medicines he is currently taking that can be carried with him at all times. The date the list was made and the prescribing physician should also be recorded. This information can be valuable if the patient is treated by another health-care giver or in an emergency.

As a final precaution to ensure regimen safety, the nurse should check multiple drug regimens for potential drug interactions before sending a patient home, to avoid unnecessary toxic reactions. Patients should be counseled not to add new drugs, even over-the-counter preparations, alcohol, or street drugs, without seeking advice from a health professional.

Evaluation

For the elderly, there are several outcome criteria for measuring the success of a medication regimen. Most of these are best checked on a home visit and include the use of the memory joggers such as calendars and boxes, the number of pills left in a prescription bottle, the development of toxicity or other side-effects from the drugs taken, and the patient's perception of his success or happiness with his ability to manage the regimen.

A summary of the use of the nursing process in the care of the elderly patient on drug therapy can be found in Nursing Care Plan 10-1.

REVIEW QUESTIONS

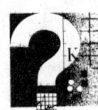

1. Describe some age-related changes in organ functions frequently seen in the elderly.
2. What factors can reduce total drug distribution in the geriatric patient?
3. Why don't reduced serum creatinine levels always accurately reflect impaired kidney function in many elderly patients?
4. What assessment factors should be considered in deciding (1) the necessity, (2) the adequacy, and (3) the duration of drug therapy in elderly patients? How can the nurse establish the patient's level of competence?
5. How can the nurse reduce a patient's anxiety surrounding a drug regimen?
6. Why are memory joggers important for elderly patients on a complex drug regimen? What useful strategies can help them remember to take drugs at the prescribed time?
7. What are some outcome criteria the nurse can use to determine if the elderly patient is successful in following a prescribed drug regimen?
8. What precautions should be taken in labeling and dispensing medications to geriatric patients?

BIBLIOGRAPHY

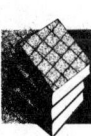

Abrams WB: Drugs and the elderly. Ration Drug Ther 19(6):1, 1985
Alford DM, Moll JA: Helping elderly patients in ambulatory settings cope with drug therapy. Nurs Clin North Am 17:275, 1982
Dall CE, Gresham L: Promoting effective drug-taking behavior in the elderly. Nurs Clin North Am 17:283, 1982
Gotz BE, Gotz VP: Drugs and the elderly. Am J Nurs 78:1347, 1978
Greenblatt DJ, Sellers EM, Shader RI: Drug disposition in old age. N Engl J Med 306:1081, 1982
Holloway DA: Drug problems in the geriatric patient. Drug Intell Clin Pharm 8:632, 1974
Hudson MF: Drugs and the older adult: Take special care. Nursing '84 14(8):47, 1984
Jarvik L (ed): Clinical Pharmacology and the Aged Patient. New York, Raven Press, 1981
Kenny AD: Designing therapy for the elderly. Drug Ther 9(7):49, 1978
Pagliaro LA, Pagliaro AM (eds): Pharmacologic Aspects of Aging. St Louis, CV Mosby, 1983
Poe WD, Holloway DA: Drugs and the Aged. New York, McGraw-Hill, 1980
Richey DP, Bender DA: Pharmacokinetic consequences of aging. Annu Rev Pharmacol Toxicol 17:49, 1977
Riley GA: How aging influences drug therapy. U.S. Pharmacist 2(10):28, 1977
Rowe JW: Health care of the elderly. N Engl J Med 312:827, 1985
Salzman C: Geriatric psychoparmacology. Annu Rev Med 36:217, 1981
Sivertson L, Fletcher J: Assisting the elderly with drug therapy in the home. Nurs Clin North Am 17:293, 1982
Vestal RE (ed): Drug Treatment in the Elderly. Sydney, Australia, ADIS Health Science Press, 1984
Ward M, Baltman M: Drug therapy in the elderly. Am Fam Physician 19:143, 1979

Mathematics of Drug Therapy

Weights and Measures
  Metric System
  Apothecaries' System
  Household Measurement
    Systems
  Conversions

Solutions
  Concentration of Solutions
  Preparation of Solutions

Dosage Calculations
  Oral Dosage
  Parenteral Dosage
  Pediatric Dosage

11

Administration of medications in the proper amount is an important aspect of patient care, and the nurse's responsibility in this task is evident. Nurses are a vital link between physician and patient and, in the hospital setting, are directly responsible for administering drugs. Since safe and effective drug therapy depends on the use of the right drug in the proper amount, it is imperative that nurses have a firm grasp of the principles of drug dosage. Thus, in addition to a basic working knowledge of arithmetic, the nurse must have an understanding of the systems used for weight and measurement and the principles behind preparation of drug solutions for both oral and parenteral use, as well as the ability to calculate and verify drug dosages. To say that it is no longer necessary for nurses to be skilled in the mathematics of drug preparation and dosing because most drugs are now administered in a prepackaged, ready-to-use form is to shun a responsibility that may someday save a life or prevent serious toxicity. All health-care professionals handling drugs must possess a fundamental understanding of dosage measurement and have the ability to calculate the proper drug dose. Although the following discussion does not purport to be an in-depth exercise in dosage calculations, sufficient basic information and sample calculations will be provided so that the reader should emerge with a fundamental working knowledge of the mathematics of drug therapy. To further the reader's skills in this area, several books devoted entirely to dosage calculations and preparation of solutions are listed in the bibliography at the end of the chapter. Should the reader feel it necessary to review some of the basic mechanics of arithmetic, such as fractions, decimals, percentages, ratios, and so on, it is recommended one of these specialized books be consulted. The focus in this chapter will be on the application of basic arithmetic principles in the calculation of drug doses and the preparation of drug solutions.

Weights and Measures

There are several means by which drugs and chemicals can be weighed and measured, and this diversity of methods can lead to confusion and dosage errors. Thus, it is important for the nurse as well as other health-care professionals to understand the differences among the various measurement systems, and to be able to convert from one system to another.

The systems of weighing and measuring in use today in the United States are (1) the metric system, (2) the apothecaries' (or apothecary) system, and (3) the household measurement system. Of these, the metric system is the most widely used and the easiest to master. It is the system almost exclusively used throughout the rest of the world, and the United States is gradually converting to the metric system as well. The apothecaries' system was employed in England at one time, and its use was carried over into some other English-speaking countries, such as the United States, where its vestige remains. Medications are still being ordered occasionally in apothecaries' units (*e.g.*, grains, fluid drams) although this practice should be discouraged. Finally, household measures such as the teaspoon and tablespoon are frequently used to designate drug doses, although this practice should be discouraged because of the lack of uniformity in such household items as the teaspoon and tablespoon. A closer look at each of these systems will serve to point out the major similarities as well as the differences among them. Tables of conversion values will also be given.

Metric System

As indicated, the metric system is gradually becoming the standard system of measurement worldwide and for good reason. It is the most logical system, since it is based entirely on multiples of 10. The basic units of metric measurement are the *meter*, *liter*, and *gram*, representing length, volume, and weight, respectively. Being a decimal system, these basic units can be multiplied or divided by multiples of 10 to yield all the units of measurement. These secondary units are then named by adding Greek or Latin prefixes to the name of the basic unit. The following diagram illustrates the terminology:

1000.0 kilo- one thousand	100.0 hecto- one hundred	10.0 deca- ten	1.0 meter liter gram	0.1 deci- one tenth	0.01 centi- one hundredth	0.001 mill- one thousandth	0.000001 micro- one millionth

Thus, a centimeter is one hundredth of a meter, and a kilogram is one thousand grams. The metric system is a very simple form of measurement, for one need only know three basic units and several prefixes in order to name all the units of weight, volume, and length. The most commonly used measures of weight and volume in the metric system are given below:

Metric Weights

1000 micrograms (mcg or μg) = 1 milligram (mg)
1000 milligrams (mg) = 1 gram (g or gm)
1000 grams (g or gm) = 1 kilogram (kg)

Metric Volumes

1000 milliliters (ml) = 1 liter (l)
1000 liters (l) = 1 kiloliter (kl)

Since the liter represents the volume of a cube whose sides measure 10 centimeters, it is frequently said to contain 1000 cubic centimeters (cc or cm³). Thus, for practical purposes, 1 ml = 1 cc, and these units are used interchangeably. To illustrate the size of the basic metric units in relation to more commonly used units of measurement, the following relationship may be given:

1 quart *approximately equals* 1 liter
1 yard *approximately equals* 1 meter
1 ounce *approximately equals* 30 grams

Practice Problems

Fill in the blanks. (See Appendix for answers.)

a. 0.5 kg = _____ mg   f. 3.0 g = _____ mg
b. 100 ml = _____ L   g. 0.1 L = _____ cc
c. 3.0 mg = _____ mcg   h. 4000 mcg = _____ g
d. 2.5 L = _____ ml   i. 0.05 mg = _____ mcg
e. 500 cc = _____ ml   j. 500 L = _____ kl

Apothecaries' System

The apothecaries' system is much older than the metric system, is quite a bit more confusing, and requires memorization of a number of terms used to designate various units. For these reasons, the apothecaries' system is virtually obsolete in this country, although it is still occasionally used for older drugs, in which case the metric equivalent must be given.

The basic unit of weight in this system is the *grain*, originally defined as the weight of a plump grain of wheat, a rather imprecise standard at best. Other larger units of weight include the scruple,

dram, ounce, and pound. These units are commonly abbreviated as follows:

grain = gr
scruple = Э
dram = Ʒ or dr
ounce = Ʒ or oz
pound = lb

The smallest unit of fluid measure in the apothecaries' system in the *minim*, which is the approximate volume of water weighing 1 grain. Larger units of apothecary volume include the fluid dram, fluid ounce, and pint. These units are abbreviated as follows:

minim = ♏
fluid dram = fƷ
fluid ounce = fƷ
pint = O or pt

When the various symbols are used for apothecary units, the quantity of each unit is frequently expressed in Roman numerals and written *following* the unit. Thus, 10 grains may be written as "gr x," 6 fluid ounces as "fƷ vi," and 8 drams as "Ʒ viii." Fractional numbers are usually given in Arabic numerals (e.g., $\frac{1}{6}$, $\frac{1}{10}$) except for one half, which is often designated as $\overline{ss}$. For example, 7$\frac{1}{2}$ minims might be written "♏ viiss," obviously a rather archaic, unwieldly, and possibly confusing method.

The apothecaries' measurements of weight and volume used in medicine are illustrated below:

Apothecaries' Weights

20 grains (gr) = 1 scruple (Э)
60 grains (gr) = 3 scruples (Э) = 1 dram (Ʒ)
8 drams (Ʒ) = 1 ounce (Ʒ)
12 ounces (Ʒ) = 1 pound (lb)

Note: The apothecaries' pound contains 12 ounces, whereas in the *avoirdupois* system of weights commonly used for most items in the United States, there are 16 ounces in 1 pound.

Apothecaries' Volumes

60 minims (♏) = 1 fluid dram (fƷ)
8 fluid drams (fƷ) = 1 fluid ounce (fƷ)
16 fluid ounces (fƷ) = 1 pint (O or pt)
2 pints (O or pt) = 1 quart (qt)
4 quarts (qt) = 1 gallon (C or gal)

In the apothecaries' system, a minim (♏) is approximately equivalent to a drop (gtt—Latin, gutta) of water, but may not necessarily be equal to a drop of another substance (e.g., alcohol, ether, oil) due to differences in density. Further, due to the variability in the *size* of droplets (and hence the total volume) of different liquids, minims should be measured using a calibrated pipet or flask and *not* estimated based on drops.

Practice Problems

See Appendix for answers.

1. Interpret the following:
    a. ℥ xii
    b. ♏ xxxii
    c. f℥ vi
    d. gr xxx
    e. f℥ iiss̄
    f. 0 iv
2. Fill in the blanks.
    a. ℥ s̄s = _____ gr
    b. _____ f℥ = 0.5 f℥
    c. 0 ÷ = _____ ♏
    d. 6 ℈ = _____ ℥
    e. _____ C = 32 f℥

    f. 4 ℥ = _____ gr
    g. 480 ♏ = _____ f℥
    h. _____ qt = 16 f℥
    i. 2 lb = _____ ℥
    j. 240 gr = _____ ℈

household measuring devices, some equivalents are only approximate.

$$1 \text{ drop (gtt)} = 1 \text{ minim } (♏)$$
$$1 \text{ teaspoon (tsp)} = 60 \text{ drops}$$
$$= 60 \text{ minims } (♏)$$
$$= 1 \text{ fluid dram (f℥)}$$
$$= 4\text{--}5 \text{ milliliters (ml) or}$$
$$\text{cubic centimeters (cm}^3 \text{ or cc)}$$
$$1 \text{ tablespoon (tbsp)} = 4 \text{ fluid drams (f℥)}$$
$$= 4 \text{ teaspoons (tsp)}$$
$$= 16\text{--}20 \text{ milliliters (ml) or}$$
$$\text{cubic centimeters (cm}^3 \text{ or cc)}$$

Practice Problems

See Appendix for answers.

a. 240 ♏ = _____ tsp
b. 2 tsp = _____ gtt
c. _____ f℥ = 4 tbsp
d. 20 cc = _____ tsp
e. _____ f℥ = 2 tsp

Household Measurement Systems

Since many medications are administered in the home, household measures such as the teaspoon are frequently used, and prescription drugs are often dispensed with instructions to take a teaspoon or a tablespoon of a liquid at certain time intervals. Household measures are certainly convenient and there is no doubt that they are widely used for administering drugs in the home. However, their use should be discouraged whenever possible, since significant variability in actual volume can occur among household teaspoons (*e.g.,* 4 ml–6 ml) and tablespoons (*e.g.,* 12 ml–18 ml).

It is preferable to provide patients with a *standardized* teaspoon or other type of measuring device for oral liquids rather than to rely on use of a household utensil. Such devices are frequently available commercially or are provided with the medication bottle. Although certainly not critical for most drugs, a slight variation in dosage of some of the more potent medications can result in development of toxic reactions. For this reason, oral dosages should be given in milliliters or cubic centimeters, not in teaspoons or tablespoons, and the medication should be measured with the aid of calibrated containers to ensure accurate dosage. Approximate equivalent volumes of common household utensils in comparison with units of volume in the metric and apothecaries' systems are given below. Note that because of the variability in

Conversions

Since all three systems of measurement may still be used today under some circumstances, knowledge of the approximate equivalent weights and volumes between any two of the systems is imperative. In performing dosage calculations, it is often necessary to convert from the metric to the apothecary system or *vice versa*. For example, a drug dosage strength may be given in milligrams but the prescriber may order the drug dosage in grains. Thus, an understanding of the relationship between milligram (metric weight) and grain (apothecary weight) is required to make the proper conversion. All necessary conversions can easily be made by using a few basic equivalents, which are listed in Table 11-1.

While the equivalents given in Table 11-1 are frequently used in converting from one system to another, they are only *approximate* relationships in most cases. *Exact* equivalents, such as

1 grain = 64.8 milligrams
1 gram = 15.432 grains
1 milliliter = 16.23 minims

are cumbersome to use in everyday calculations, and the differences between the exact and approximate values are too slight to be of significance except perhaps in the case of precise laboratory determinations or preparation of pharmaceutical formulations and prescription compounding. Therefore, use of approximate equivalents is the

Table 11-1
Commonly Used Equivalents

Weight

1 grain (gr) = 60 milligrams (mg)
1 gram (g) = 15 or 16 grains (gr)
1 dram (ℨ) = 4 grams (g)
1 ounce (℥) = 30 grams (g)
1 kilogram (kg) = 2.2 pounds (lb)

Volume

1 milliliter (ml) = 15 or 16 minims (♏)
1 fluid dram (fℨ) = 4 milliliters (ml) = 1 teaspoon (tsp)
1 fluid ounce (fℨ) = 30 milliliters (ml) = 2 tablespoons (tbsp)
1 quart (qt) = 1000 milliliters (ml)

established procedure for converting among systems of measurement.

A comprehensive listing of approximate equivalent weights and volumes among the three systems of measurement is presented in Table 11-2.

Practice Problems
See Appendix for answers.

1. Convert the following to apothecary equivalents.
   a. 30 mg = _____ gr   g. 600 mcg = _____ gr
   b. 6 ml = _____ fℨ   h. 120 ml = _____ fℨ
   c. 5 mg = _____ gr   i. 0.6 ml = _____ ♏
   d. 0.5 L = _____ fℨ   j. 3 g = _____ ℨ
   e. 8 ml = _____ ♏   k. 20 ml = _____ fℨ
   f. 0.1 g = _____ gr   l. 1 mg = _____ gr

2. Convert the following to metric equivalents.
   a. 120 ♏ = _____ ml   g. 0.5 fℨ = _____ ml
   b. 4 fℨ = _____ ml   h. 75 gr = _____ mg
   c. 8 ℨ = _____ g   i. $^1/_{150}$ gr = _____ mcg
   d. $^1/_{500}$ gr = _____ mg   j. 3 gr = _____ g
   e. 5 gr = _____ g   k. 1 gr = _____ mg
   f. 4 pints = _____ L   l. 30 fℨ = _____ ml

3. Fill in the blanks.
   a. 4 ml = _____ tsp
   b. 2 tbsp = _____ fℨ
   c. _____ gtt = 2 ml
   d. 8 fℨ = _____ tsp
   e. _____ L = 1 pint
   f. _____ tsp = 60 ♏

4. Fill in the blanks.
   a. 1 fℨ = _____ ml = _____ quart
   b. 2 fℨ = _____ ♏ = _____ ml
   c. gr s̄s̄ = _____ mcg = _____ mg
   d. 15 g = _____ ℨ = _____ ℥
   e. 4 tsp = _____ fℨ = _____ ml

f. 120 g = _____ ℥ = _____ ℨ
g. 4 mg = _____ gr = _____ g
h. 3 L = _____ fℨ = _____ pints
i. 0.6 ml = _____ gtt = _____ ♏

Solutions

Solutions are clear mixtures prepared by dissolving either a solid, liquid, or gas in a liquid. The substance dissolved is termed the *solute* and the liquid in which the substance is dissolved is the *solvent*. Since most solutions in clinical use today are premixed by the manufacturer or compounded by the pharmacist, the nurse seldom is required to prepare a solution. Nevertheless, it is important to understand the basic principles underlying solution preparation and be able to calculate the concentration of active drug per unit volume of solution. In addition, stock solutions of highly concentrated substances often need to be diluted before use; thus, it is necessary to understand this type of calculation as well.

Before reviewing the mathematics of solution preparation, we will describe some terms commonly used in association with solutions.

Dilute—Solution containing small amount of solute compared to solvent

Concentrated—Solution with large quantity of solute in the solution

Saturated—Solution containing maximum amount of solute capable of dissolving in the solvent at a given pressure and temperature

Stock solution—A highly concentrated

Table 11-2
Metric Doses With Approximate Apothecary and Household Equivalents

Metric	Approximate Apothecary Equivalent	Approximate Household Equivalent
Volume		
1000 ml (1 liter)	1 quart	
500 ml	1 pint	
250 ml	8 fluid ounces	1 glassful
120 ml	4 fluid ounces	
30 ml	1 fluid ounce	2 tablespoons
15 ml	4 fluid drams	1 tablespoon
8 ml	2 fluid drams	2 teaspoons
4 ml	1 fluid dram	1 teaspoon
1 ml	15 minims	
0.5 ml	8 minims	
0.06 ml	1 minim	1 drop
Weight		
30 g	1 ounce	
15 g	4 drams	
4 g	1 dram (60 grains)	
1 g	15 grains	
0.1 g (100 mg)	$1\frac{1}{2}$ grains	
60 mg	1 grain	
30 mg	$\frac{1}{2}$ grain	
15 mg	$\frac{1}{4}$ grain	
10 mg	$\frac{1}{6}$ grain	
5 mg	$\frac{1}{12}$ grain	
1 mg (1000 mcg)	$\frac{1}{60}$ grain	
600 mcg	$\frac{1}{100}$ grain	
300 mcg	$\frac{1}{200}$ grain	
100 mcg	$\frac{1}{600}$ grain	

solution, often commercially prepared, which must be diluted prior to use

There are three methods of preparing solutions, based on the units used to describe the component parts:

1. *Weight in weight (W/W)*—A certain weight of solute is dissolved in a certain weight of solvent. This is probably the most accurate method for preparing solutions, but is infrequently used outside the laboratory.
2. *Weight in volume (W/V)*—A certain weight of solute is dissolved in a certain volume of solvent to make the necessary amount of solution. This is the most commonly used procedure for preparing solutions in medicine and pharmacy.
3. *Volume in volume (V/V)*—A given volume of solute is added to a given volume of solvent to make the desired final solution volume.

Concentration of Solutions

The concentration, or strength, of a solution may be expressed in several ways. Thus, a solution of boric acid, for example, can be described as all of the following:

1. 1:25
2. 4%
3. 0.6 gr/ml

All three of these solutions are *identical*. A 1:25 solution means that there is 1 g of drug in every 25 ml of solution. Likewise, a 4% solution contains 4 g of drug in 100 ml of solution, or 1 g in 25 ml. Finally, 0.6 gr/ml means that there are 0.6 gr in 1 ml, or 15 gr (equal to 1 g) in 25 ml. Keep in mind that these concentrations can refer to any of the above three means of describing solutions. For example, a 4% boric acid solution refers to 4 g of boric acid powder in 100 ml of solution (W/V), and a 5% alcohol solution means that there are 5 ml of alcohol in 100 ml of solution (V/V). Further, a 2% boric acid ointment is prepared by adding 2 g of boric acid powder to a sufficient weight of ointment base to make a total of 100 g of ointment (W/W).

Practice Problems
See Appendix for answers.
  a. 2% = 1:_____
  b. 5 mg/ml = _____%
  c. 1:4000 = _____ mg/ml
  d. 4% = _____ gr/ml
  e. 0.1 mg/ml = 1:_____

Strength of solutions can also be spoken of in terms of *molarity* and *normality*. A *molar solution* contains 1 gram molecular weight of solute in a liter (*i.e.*, 1000 ml) of solution. The molecular weight of a solute is obtained by adding together the atomic weights of the constituents. Thus, a 1 molar (1M) solution of sodium chloride (NaCl) contains 58 g of sodium chloride (atomic weights: Na = 23, Cl = 35) in 1 liter, and a 1M sulfuric acid (H_2SO_4) solution contains 98 g of hydrogen sulfate per liter (atomic weights: H = 1, S = 32, O = 16).

A *normal solution*, on the other hand, contains 1 gram equivalent weight/liter of solution. An *equivalent weight* represents the weight of an element in grams that is equal in reacting power to 1 g of hydrogen or 8 g of oxygen, and is obtained by dividing the atomic weight of the element by its valence. Thus, the equivalent weight of sodium and chloride is the same as their molecular weight, since the valence of both Na^+ and Cl^- is 1; therefore, a 1 normal solution of NaCl is exactly the same as a 1 molar solution, since the valence of each element is 1. However, the equivalent weight of sulfuric acid (H_2SO_4) is *one-half* that of the molecular weight, since there are two hydrogen ions, representing a total valence of +2. Thus, the molecular weight must be divided by 2 in order to obtain the equivalent weight. Therefore, a 1N sulfuric acid is only one-half the strength of a 1M sulfuric acid, since it contains only 49 g of H_2SO_4, the equivalent weight.

Another term frequently used in medicine to describe the strength or concentration of certain drugs is *milliequivalents* (mEq). For example, a solution of potassium chloride (KCl) may be given as 20 mEq/15 ml, to indicate the dose of potassium and chloride in each tablespoonful. A milliequivalent is simply *one thousandth of an equivalent weight*; thus, 20 mEq of potassium chloride equals 1480 mg, as shown below:
  Molecular weight KCl = 74
  Equivalent weight KCl = 74 g (valence is 1)
  Milliequivalent weight KCl = 74 mg *(1/1000 × 74 g)*
Thus, 20 mEq = 20 × 74 mg = $\boxed{1480 \text{ mg KCl}}$

Preparation of Solutions

Although the calculations necessary to prepare drug solutions can be carried out using either the metric or apothecary system, it is usually easier to convert all units to the metric system before beginning the calculations. Thus, whenever possible, that is the method that will be followed in this chapter for all sample problems. When reviewing the sample problems or doing the practice problems, refer to the tables of conversions earlier in the chapter as necessary.

CALCULATION OF SOLUTION STRENGTH
The strength of a solution can be determined in percent, as a ratio strength, or as a W/V concentration. A few examples will serve to illustrate the neccessary arithmetic.

Example
What is the percent concentration of a 1:2000 solution of mercuric chloride?

1:2000 = 1 g/2000 ml

$$\frac{1 \text{ g}}{2000 \text{ ml}} = \frac{x \text{ g}}{100 \text{ ml}}$$

x = 0.05g

Thus, 0.05 g/100 ml = $\boxed{0.05\% \text{ solution}}$

Example
If 300 gr of sodium chloride is dissolved in 500 ml of water, express the concentration as (1) percent and (2) ratio.

Convert gr to g:

15 gr = 1 g

Therefore, 300 gr = 20 g

The solution strength can now be given as 20 g/500 ml

$$\frac{20 \text{ g}}{500 \text{ ml}} = \frac{x \text{ g}}{100 \text{ ml}}$$

x = 4 g

Thus, 4 g/100 ml = ┃ 4% solution ┃

To find the ratio

$$\frac{4 \text{ g}}{100 \text{ ml}} = \frac{1 \text{ g}}{x \text{ ml}}$$

x = 25 ml

Thus, 4% = $\frac{1 \text{ g}}{25 \text{ ml}}$ = ┃ 1:25 solution ┃

Example
120 ml of a 6% iodine solution contains how many grains of iodine?

6% = 6 g/100 ml

We have 120 ml of solution, therefore

$$\frac{6 \text{ g}}{100 \text{ ml}} = \frac{x \text{ g}}{120 \text{ ml}}$$

x = 7.2 g of iodine in 120 ml

Convert g to gr:

1 g = 15 gr

Therefore, 7.2 g = 108 gr

Thus, 120 ml of a 6% solution contains ┃ 108 gr ┃ of iodine

Example
Calculate the percent concentrations of a solution resulting from the addition of f3 viii of pure alcohol to 200 ml of water.

Convert f3 to ml:

1 f3 = 4 ml

Therefore, 8 f3 = 32 ml

Addition of 32 ml to 200 ml gives a total volume of solution = 232 ml

To calculate the percent concentration

$$\frac{32 \text{ ml alcohol}}{232 \text{ ml solution}} = \frac{x \text{ ml}}{100 \text{ ml}}$$

x = 13.8 ml pure alcohol in 100 ml

Thus, 13.8 ml/100 ml = ┃ 13.8% solution ┃

Practice Problems (See Appendix for answers)
1. Give the percent strength of the following solutions:
   a. 1:400 _____   e. 40 mg/ml _____
   b. 1:10,000 _____ f. 0.6 g/ml _____
   c. 1:3 _____   g. 8 g/L _____
   d. 1:25 _____   h. 20 mg/5 ml _____

2. Give the ratio strength of the following solutions:
   a. 20% _____   e. 10 mg/ml _____
   b. 0.4% _____   f. 0.2 g/100 ml _____
   c. 80% _____   g. 4 g/L _____
   d. 0.05% _____   h. 2 mg/ml _____
3. If 0.5 g of thimerosal is dissolved in 120 ml, what is the percent concentration?
4. What is the ratio strength of a glucose in water solution containing 8 drams in 500 ml?
5. Give the concentration of the following solutions in (1) percent and (2) ratio.
   a. 30 mg in f3 vi _____ ; _____
   b. $\frac{1}{30}$ gr in 2 ml _____ ; _____
   c. 1 ounce in 1 L _____ ; _____
   d. f3 ⁓⁓ in 600 ml _____ ; _____
   e. 0.2 g in f3 xvi _____ ; _____

CALCULATION OF SOLUTE CONCENTRATION
The amount of solute (*e.g.*, drug) contained in a solution can easily be ascertained from the volume of solution and the solution strength. Likewise, the amount of drug needed to prepare a solution of desired strength can also be calculated. A few examples will illustrate.

Example
How many grams of potassium iodide are needed to prepare 200 ml of a 2% solution?

Need 2% = 2 g/100 ml

$$\frac{2 \text{ g}}{100 \text{ ml}} = \frac{x \text{ g}}{200 \text{ ml}}$$

x = ┃ 4 g ┃ needed

Example
In order to make 30 ml of a 1:500 solution, how many grains are necessary?

1:500 = 1 g/500 ml

Need 30 ml

$$\frac{1 \text{ g}}{500 \text{ ml}} = \frac{x \text{ g}}{30 \text{ ml}}$$

x = 0.06 g = 60 mg

Convert mg to gr:

60 mg = 1 gr

Thus, need ┃ 1 gr ┃

Example

A 12% solution of Zephiran Chloride is available in 8 fluid ounce bottles. How many milligrams of Zephiran Chloride are contained in the bottle?

12% = 12 g/100 ml

Have 8 f℥

Convert f℥ to ml:

1 f℥ = 30 ml

Therefore, 8 f℥ = 240 ml

$$\frac{12\ g}{100\ ml} = \frac{x\ g}{240\ ml}$$

x = 28.8 g in 8 f℥ of a 12% solution

Thus, 28.8 g = $\boxed{28,800\ mg}$

Example

How many fluid drams of propylene glycol are required to prepare 500 ml of a 20% solution? (Since propylene glycol is a liquid, we use a volume-to-volume ratio.)

20% = 20 ml/100 ml (V/V)

$$\frac{20\ ml}{100\ ml} = \frac{x\ ml}{500\ ml}$$

x = 100 ml of propylene glycol needed for solution.

Convert milliliters to fluid drams:

4 ml = 1 fℨ

Therefore, 100 ml = 25 fℨ

Thus, need $\boxed{25\ fℨ}$

Practice Problems

See Appendix for answers.
1. How many grams of solute are contained in the following solutions?
   a. 400 ml of a 2% solution
   b. 30 ml of a 50% solution
   c. 200 ml of a 1:2000 solution
   d. 0.6 L of a 1:10,000 solution
   e. 8 f℥ of a 40% solution
   f. 1 pint of a 1:250 solution
2. To prepare 100 ml of a 1:1000 silver nitrate solution, how many grains are required?
3. How many milliliters of absolute alcohol are found in f℥ vi of a 1:20 solution?

CALCULATION OF SOLUTION VOLUME

Knowing the quantity of solute available, we can determine the total volume of a solution of a specified concentration that can be prepared. Again, several examples will demonstrate the calculations involved.

Example

What volume of 5% dextrose in water can be prepared from 40 g of dextrose powder?

5% = 5 g/100 ml

Have 40 g

$$\frac{5\ g}{100\ ml} = \frac{40\ g}{x\ ml}$$

$\boxed{x = 800\ ml}$

Example

How many fluid drams of a 4% solution of cocaine hydrochloride can be made with 2 g of powder?

4% = 4 g/100 ml

Have 2 g

$$\frac{4\ g}{100\ ml} = \frac{2\ g}{x\ ml}$$

x = 50 ml

Convert milliliters to fluid drams:

4 ml = 1 fℨ

Therefore, 50 ml = $\boxed{12.5\ fℨ}$

Example

How much 1:500 solution can be prepared from two 15-gr codeine phosphate tablets?

1:500 = 1 g/500 ml

Have 30 gr (2 × 15 gr)

Convert grains to grams:

15 gr = 1 g

Therefore, 30 gr = 2 g

$$\frac{1\ g}{500\ ml} = \frac{2\ g}{x\ ml}$$

x = $\boxed{1000\ ml}$ can be prepared

Practice Problems

See Appendix for answers.
1. How many milliliters of a 20% solution can be prepared from 6 g of drug?
2. What volume of 1:600 solution can be made from gr v of pure drug?
3. How many fluid ounces of a 0.5% drug solution can be prepared from 300 mg of drug powder?

4. Using three $\frac{1}{2}$-gr codeine tablets, how many milliliters of a 1:10,000 solution can be made?

DILUTING STOCK SOLUTIONS

If a drug is already in solution in fairly high concentration, weaker solutions can be prepared by diluting the more concentrated, or *stock solution.* A simple formula may be used in making the necessary calculations:

Quantity of stock solution

$$= \frac{\text{strength of} \atop \text{solution} \times {\text{quantity of} \atop \text{desired solution}}}{\text{strength of stock solution}}$$

Example

How many milliliters of 40% potassium permanganate solution are needed to prepare 1 L of a 2% solution?

Need 1 L of 2%

Have 40% on hand

1 L = 1000 ml

Using the above formula

$$\text{x ml} = \frac{2\% \times 1000 \text{ ml}}{40\%}$$

x = $\boxed{50 \text{ ml}}$ of stock solution needed

Therefore, the diluted solution is prepared by taking 50 ml of the 40% solution and adding sufficient vehicle (*e.g.,* water or saline) to make 1000 ml.

Example

What quantity of a 1:5000 solution can be made by diluting 100 ml of a 1:100 solution? Again, using the formula

$$100 \text{ ml} = \frac{1/5000 \times \text{x ml}}{1/100}$$

$$100 \text{ ml} = 1/50 \times \text{x ml}$$

$$\frac{100 \text{ ml}}{1/50} = \text{x ml}$$

$\boxed{5000 \text{ ml}}$ = x

Therefore, 5000 ml or 5 L of a 1:5000 solution can be prepared from 100 ml of a 1:100 solution.

Example

You have a bottle of Zephiran Chloride solution, 12%, on hand, and wish to prepare a pint of a 1:1000 dilution. How many milliliters of stock solution must you use?

Have 12% solution

Want 1:1000 solution = $\dfrac{1 \text{ g}}{1000 \text{ ml}} = \dfrac{0.1 \text{ g}}{100 \text{ ml}} = 0.1\%$

Convert pints to milliliters (approximate):

1 pint = 500 ml (actual = 473 ml)

Use the formula

$$\text{x ml} = \frac{0.1\% \times 500 \text{ ml}}{12\%}$$

$$\text{x ml} = \frac{50}{12}$$

x = $\boxed{4.2 \text{ ml}}$

Therefore, diluting 4.2 ml of a 12% solution up to 500 ml yields a 1:1000 solution.

Example

In order to prepare 4 L of an 0.1% solution of epinephrine, what volume of 1:20 stock solution must be used?

Have 1:20 solution = $\dfrac{1 \text{ g}}{20 \text{ ml}} = \dfrac{5 \text{ g}}{100 \text{ ml}} = 5\%$

Need 0.1%

Using the formula

$$\text{x ml} = \frac{0.1\% \times 4000 \text{ ml}}{5\%}$$

$$\text{x ml} = 400/5$$

x = $\boxed{80 \text{ ml}}$

Therefore, 80 ml of a 1:20 solution diluted to 4 L (4000 ml) yields a 0.1% solution.

Practice Problems

See Appendix for answers.

1. How much 1% neomycin sulfate solution can be prepared from 30 ml of a 20% stock solution?
2. What quantity of diluent must be added to f℥ viii of 20% stock solution to yield a final concentration of 1:200?
3. How many milliliters of a 0.5% gentian violet solution are required to make f℥ iv of a 1:100,000 solution?
4. Using 15 ml of a 1% stock solution of atropine sulfate, how many fluid ounces of a 0.2% solution can be prepared?
5. How many minims of a 2% solution of pilocarpine hydrochloride are required to formulate f℥ i of a 0.1% solution.

Dosage Calculations

The most common method for administering drugs is by mouth, usually in the form of either tablets, capsules, or liquids. Although most drugs are prescribed in doses that simply require the patient to take a specified number of tablets or capsules or a certain volume of liquid, there are some instances where a calculation must be made in order to arrive at the proper dosage. For example, if the drug strength is labeled in units different from those prescribed, a conversion is needed to determine the correct amount of drug to be given. Likewise, if the dose of the drug ordered is not an even multiple of the dosage strengths available, the number of fractional tablets, capsules, teaspoons, and so on must be calculated. A dosage calculation must also be done to determine the volume of an injectable drug that must be administered to provide the desired dose of drug. It is evident, therefore, that in order to ensure accurate drug dosing the nurse should understand the basic principles involved in dosage calculations.

This section will review a variety of dosing situations in which a dosage calculation is required by presenting a number of different examples, followed by similar practice problems to test the reader's understanding. Remember, most dosage calculations are common sense arithmetic manipulations, and should not be viewed with trepidation or frustration. Many require a simple conversion between systems of measurement, and again the reader should refer to the conversion tables earlier in the chapter.

Oral Dosage

As previously mentioned, most oral drugs are prescribed in doses that represent exact multiples of the available dosage forms. Thus, it is simply a matter of giving a certain number of tablets or capsules. For example, if a physician orders 500 mg of ampicillin and the capsules available are 250 mg each, two capsules would be given. Similarly, if 1 gr of phenobarbital is prescribed, and only $\frac{1}{4}$-gr and $\frac{1}{2}$-gr tablets are available, you would administer preferably two $\frac{1}{2}$-gr tablets or perhaps four $\frac{1}{4}$-gr tablets. On occasion, a fractional amount of drug is required. For example, if 2.5 mg of diazepam is ordered, one would give one-half of a 5-mg tablet. Similarly, if a patient requires 300 mg of quinidine, this dose could be given as one and one-half 200-mg tablets. Recognize, however, that only tablets

that are scored, that is, "creased" along the diameter, should be broken. Even with scored tablets, however, the break is not always "clean," resulting in a slightly larger or smaller amount of drug administered. Thus, whenever possible, it is best to administer whole tablets, even if more than one strength preparation must be taken concurrently.

Occasionally, the physician will order a tablet or capsule in units other than the units in which the drug is marketed. In this case, a conversion is required.

Example
Codeine sulfate is prescribed in a dose of gr $\frac{1}{4}$ four times a day. How many 30-mg codeine tablets should be taken?
Need $\frac{1}{4}$ gr
Have 30 mg
Convert grains to milligrams:

1 gr = 60 mg

Therefore, $\frac{1}{4}$ gr = 15 mg
Since 15 mg is needed and we have 30-mg tablets, $\boxed{\frac{1}{2} \text{ tablet}}$ is given four times a day.

Example
The prescription calls for $\frac{1}{300}$ gr of atropine. The atropine tablets on hand are 0.2 mg. How many tablets are needed?

Need $\dfrac{1}{300}$ gr = 200 mcg = 0.2 mg

Have 0.2-mg tablets

Therefore, $\boxed{1 \text{ tablet}}$ is required.

When oral *liquids* are prescribed, it is necessary to know the concentration of drug per unit volume as stated on the label. Oral liquids will usually have the drug concentration given as weight/volume, such as mg/ml, mg/5 ml, and so forth. Again, most drugs are prescribed so that a convenient volume of liquid is given, such as a teaspoonful or a tablespoonful. However, calculations are frequently necessary to determine the correct volume of liquid to be administered for each dose as well as to convert between units of measurement when required.

Example
Elixir of potassium chloride is prescribed in a dose of 15 mEq four times a day. The preparation available contains 5 mEq/5 cc. How many teaspoons are needed for each dose?

Recall 5 cc = 5 ml

Need 15 mEq

Have 5 mEq/5 ml

Therefore, 15 ml are required

Convert milliliters to teaspoons (tsp):

4 ml–5 ml = 1 tsp

Therefore, 15 ml = 3 tsp–4 tsp

Note: Since 3 to 4 teaspoons equals a tablespoon, 15 ml is usually given as 1 tablespoon.

Example

A patient is to receive 5 gr of acetaminophen every 4 hours. Acetaminophen elixir contains 120 mg/5 ml. How many teaspoons must be given?

Need 5 gr

Have 120 mg/5 ml

Convert milligrams to grains:

60 mg = 1 gr

Therefore, 120 mg = 2 gr

Since there are 2 gr/5 ml and the patient requires 5 gr

$$\frac{2 \text{ gr}}{5 \text{ ml}} = \frac{5 \text{ gr}}{x \text{ ml}}$$

x = 12.5 ml needed

Convert milliliters to teaspoons:

4 ml–5 ml = 1 tsp

Therefore, 12.5 ml = 3 tsp (approximately). Again, 3 teaspoons is most often administered as 1 tablespoon.

Note: The above two problems clearly demonstrate the imprecision of household measures. In the first example, the required volume was *15 ml*, which would be given as a tablespoon. In the second example, a tablespoon would also commonly be used, although the actual volume of elixir calculated was only *12.5 ml*, a 20% difference. These examples underscore the necessity for using accurately calibrated measuring devices rather than household utensils whenever possible in administering drugs.

Example

How many fluid drams of penicillin VK suspension, 250 mg/5 ml, are needed to provide a dose of 1 g?

Need 1 g = 1000 mg

Have 250 mg/5 ml

$$\frac{250 \text{ mg}}{5 \text{ ml}} = \frac{1000 \text{ mg}}{x \text{ ml}}$$

x = 20 ml needed

Convert milliliters to fluid drams:

4 ml = 1 f℥

Therefore, 20 ml = 5 f℥

Practice Problems

See Appendix for answers.

1. How many 0.125-mg digoxin tablets are needed for one week if the daily dose is 0.25 mg?
2. If the dose of sulfamethoxazole is gr xv three times a day, how many 0.5-g tablets are needed in one day?
3. In order to administer 1/150 gr of atropine, how many 1/600-gr tablets are needed?
4. How many 1½-gr secobarbital capsules are required for 14 days if the dose is 200 mg at bedtime daily?
5. Ampicillin, 250 mg/5 ml, is prescribed for 10 days at a dose of 1 teaspoon four times a day. How many grams of ampicillin are consumed in that time?
6. A cough syrup contains 240 mg codeine/4 f℥. How many grains of codeine are in each teaspoon?
7. If the dose of erythromycin is 200 mg three times a day, how many milliliters of a 400 mg/5 ml suspension are needed for a 10-day supply?
8. Ammonium chloride is available as a 10% solution. If the dose is 1 teaspoon in water three times a day as an expectorant, how many milligrams does the patient receive in one day?
9. A 4-f℥ bottle of cough syrup contains 25 mg diphenhydramine/5 ml. How much drug would be consumed if the patient used one half of the bottle?
10. Elixir of phenobarbital is labeled 4 mg/ml. A patient attempts to overdose by swallowing the contents of two 6-f℥ bottles at once. How many grains of phenobarbital does the patient consume?

Parenteral Dosage

Calculations involving drugs to be given parenterally are based on the same principles as those used above for determining oral dosages. Thus, an understanding of the methods used for diluting concentrated solutions is necessary, as is a knowledge of the various conversion factors. Of the various methods for administering drugs parenterally, as discussed in Chapter 8, the most hazardous of the commonly used routes is intravenous (IV).

Therefore, the calculations involving IV dosage forms of drugs take on added significance when viewed in this perspective. A calculation error involving an IV dosage can be potentially more hazardous to the patient than, for example, an error in an oral dosage calculation, since the drug has an immediate onset of action and overdoses are generally more difficult to manage because retrieval of the drug is virtually impossible. In addition, the rate at which an intravenous medication is given is equally important to safe administration. Thus, it is imperative that calculations involving use of IV drugs be correct, although errors in any type of drug calculations are serious matters and should be avoided. Whenever doubt exists as to the correctness of a calculation, the drug should never be administered without having the calculation figures checked.

Drugs for injection are usually supplied in single-dose or multiple-dose vials, either already in solution or as a dry (i.e., desiccated) powder to which the specified diluent (e.g., sterile water for injection, sterile saline) is added. Occasionally, a drug is available in an ampule, a sealed glass container usually holding a single dose. Examples of calculations involving use of both drugs in solution as well as powdered drugs will be given. Calculation of intravenous solution rates will also be demonstrated. In addition, a brief discussion of insulin dosage, which is based on measurement in USP *units* rather than by conventional methods, such as milligrams or grains, is included. Dosages of various other drugs, such as some penicillins, vasopressin, oxytocin, and corticotropin, are also given in *units*, and calculations are performed as if the dosage was given by any other means.

DRUGS IN SOLUTION

Drugs contained in solution in multiple dose vials are labeled according to the amount of drug per unit volume of injectable solution. Thus, chlorpromazine injection might be labeled 25 mg/ml, and the vial may contain 10 ml or 20 ml. Likewise, vitamin B_{12} injection is available as 100 mcg/ml and 1000 mcg/ml, in 10-ml and 30-ml sizes. Seldom are the entire contents of the vial used at one time; thus, a calculation of the required volume is often necessary.

Example
How many milliliters of chlorpromazine injection, 25 mg/ml, must be given to provide a dose of 75 mg?

Need 75 mg

Have 25 mg/ml

$$\frac{25 \text{ mg}}{1 \text{ ml}} = \frac{75 \text{ mg}}{x \text{ ml}}$$

x = $\boxed{3 \text{ ml}}$

Example
What volume of vitamin B_{12} injection, 1000 mcg/ml, is needed to administer a dose of 0.6 mg?

Need 0.6 mg = 600 mcg

Have 1000 mcg/ml

$$\frac{1000 \text{ mcg}}{1 \text{ ml}} = \frac{600 \text{ mcg}}{x \text{ ml}}$$

x = $\boxed{0.6 \text{ ml}}$

Example
Digoxin is available in ampules containing 0.5 mg/2 ml. The prescribed dose is 0.125 mg daily. How many milliliters are needed?

Need 0.125 mg

Have 0.5 mg/2 ml

$$\frac{0.5 \text{ mg}}{2 \text{ ml}} = \frac{0.125 \text{ mg}}{x \text{ ml}}$$

x = $\boxed{0.5 \text{ ml}}$

Example
How many milliliters of a solution of atropine sulfate, 0.6 mg/ml, must be used to provide a dose of 1/200 gr?

Need 1/200 gr

Have 0.6 mg/ml

Convert grains to milligrams:

1 gr = 60 mg

Therefore, 1/200 gr = 0.3 mg = 300 mcg

$$\frac{0.6 \text{ mg}}{1 \text{ ml}} = \frac{0.3 \text{ mg}}{x \text{ ml}}$$

x = $\boxed{0.5 \text{ ml}}$

Practice Problems
See Appendix for answers.
 1. Vials of morphine sulfate are labeled 5 mg/ml. How many milliliters are required to yield a dose of 1/10 gr?
 2. Secobarbital sodium is available in vials con-

taining 50 mg/ml. In order to administer 80 mg, what volume must be given?

3. A drug is prescribed in a dose of gr 1/150. The solution is labeled 4 mg/10 ml. How much of the solution must be used?

4. In order to inject 1 g of streptomycin IM, it is necessary to give how many milliliters of a solution containing 400 mg/ml?

DRUGS AS POWDERS

Many drugs are unstable for any length of time in solution and hence are packaged as a dry powder in a multiple-dose vial. In order to inject these drugs, a diluent is added to the vial in a specified volume so that each unit of solution (*e.g.*, 1 ml) contains the desired dose of the drug. The recommended diluents are always given in the package literature, since some drugs are incompatible with or insoluble in certain diluents. Always refer to the instructions enclosed with the drug when preparing an injectable solution. If the amount of diluent to be added is not given, an appropriate source should be consulted before the solution is prepared. Usually, the volume of the dry powder does not significantly contribute to the final solution volume unless otherwise indicated in the instructions.

Another package format used with some powdered drugs for injection is the so-called piggyback vial. This consists of a two-chambered glass vial with a separation in between. The powdered drug is contained in one chamber and the diluent in the other. At the time of use, the separation between the chambers is removed, usually by exerting force at the top and bottom of the vial, and the drug mixes with the diluent. This method ensures that the precise quantities of drug and diluent are combined and eliminates the possibility of contamination during mixing by introduction of nonsterile diluent or needles.

Calculations with powdered drugs for injection most often involve the amount of diluent to be added in order to achieve the desired concentration.

Example

A vial of powder for injection is labeled 50 mg. How much diluent should be added so that a 20-mg dose is contained in 0.5 ml?

Need 20 mg/0.5 ml

Have 50 mg powder

$$\frac{20 \text{ mg}}{0.5 \text{ ml}} = \frac{50 \text{ mg}}{x \text{ ml}}$$

$x = \boxed{1.25 \text{ ml}}$

Note: It is assumed that the volume of the powder is not significant.

Example

Cephradine for injection is packaged in vials containing 250 mg of powder. The recommended volume of diluent for intramuscular injection is 1.2 ml. What volume of injection should be used to administer 125 mg to a child?

Need 125 mg

Have 250 mg/1.2 ml

$$\frac{250 \text{ mg}}{1.2 \text{ ml}} = \frac{125 \text{ mg}}{x \text{ ml}}$$

$x = \boxed{0.6 \text{ ml}}$

Example

A multiple-dose vial of penicillin G contains 1 million units (U) of powdered drug. How much diluent must be added so that 200,000 U will be administered with each 0.5 ml of injection volume?

Need 200,000 U/0.5 ml

Have 1,000,000 U powder

$$\frac{200,000 \text{ U}}{0.5 \text{ ml}} = \frac{1,000,000 \text{ U}}{x \text{ ml}}$$

$x = \boxed{2.5 \text{ ml}}$

Again, the volume of the penicillin powder is assumed to be negligible.

Practice Problems

See Appendix for answers.

1. How much diluent must be added to a vial of carbenicillin disodium, 5 g, so that a dose of 1.5 g is contained in 1 ml?

2. A vial of powder for injection is labeled 500 mg. If 4 ml is the recommended diluent volume, how much drug is contained in an injection volume of 0.5 ml?

3. Benzathine penicillin G powder for injection is available in 10-ml vials containing 300,000 units/ml. How many units of powder are in each vial?

RATES OF ADMINISTRATION OF INTRAVENOUS SOLUTIONS

Intravenous medication may be given in solution through an already established intravenous line. The rate at which the solution is administered is critical since medication given too quickly can cause toxic reactions and medication given too slowly may crystallize or decompose before it is absorbed. The rate of flow of a volume of medication is usually given for a time period when a prescription is written, such as, for example, 50 ml in 30 minutes or 500 ml in 4 hours. Since IV medications are given through an IV tubing set that contains a drop chamber, the "drop factor" or number of drops per milliliter must be known in order to calculate rate. Most intravenous tubing sets contain drop chambers that deliver either 10 drops or 15 drops per milliliter. Microdrop tubing is also available that delivers 60 drops per milliliter. To calculate solution rates, the easiest formula to remember is

$$\frac{\text{Volume of solution in milliliters} \times \text{drop factor}}{\text{time (in minutes)}}$$

Example
The physician orders 250 mg of ampicillin in 50 ml of 5% dextrose in water to be given IV over 30 minutes. The drop factor for the intravenous set is 15 drops = 1 ml. At how many drops per minute should the medication be given?

Convert milliliters to drops:

50 ml × 15 drops/ml = 750 gtt

Divide by time:

$$\frac{750 \text{ gtt}}{30 \text{ min}} = \boxed{25 \text{ gtt/min}} \text{ for 30 minutes}$$

Example
The physician orders intravenous fluid, 5% dextrose in water, 500 ml every 12 hours. The fluid is to be run through a microdrip tubing. The drop factor is 60 gtt = 1 ml. At what rate (drops per minute) should the IV be set?

Convert milliliters to drops:

500 ml × 60 gtt/ml = 30,000 gtt

Convert hours to minutes:

12 h × 60 min/h = 720 minutes

Use formula

$$\frac{30,000 \text{ gtt}}{720 \text{ min}} = 42 \text{ gtt/min}$$

Practice Problems
See Appendix for answers.
1. The physician orders Solu-Cortef, 100 mg in 50 ml of 5% dextrose in water, to be given by IV secondary set over 1 hour. The drop factor for the IV set is 10 drops (gtt) = 1 ml. At what rate of infusion (drops/minute) should the IV be set?
2. IV orders on Mr. Jones are for 1000 ml of 5% dextrose and normal saline to be infused every 8 hours. The drop factor on the IV set is 15 drops = 1 ml. At what rate of infusion (drops/minute) should the IV be set?
3. Baby Michael, age 1 year, has an IV infusion of 250 ml 5% dextrose and 0.25% normal saline with 2.5 mEq KCl. It is to infuse through a measured-volume cylinder at 25 ml per hour. The IV cylinder has a drop factor of 60 gtt = 1 ml. At what rate of infusion (drops/minute) should the IV be set?

INSULIN

Insulin dosage has been greatly simplified with the nearly universal adoption of the U100 (*i.e.*, 100 units/ml) strength as the standard insulin preparation. Previously, several different strengths (U40, U80, U100) were available and dosage errors occasionally arose when the wrong syringe size was employed (*e.g.*, giving U80 insulin with a syringe calibrated in U40 units). Today, with the almost exclusive use of U100 insulins and the corresponding U100 calibrated syringes, dosage errors have been largely eliminated. Thus, no calculations are necessary as long as the proper insulin syringe is used. The units are indicated on the barrel of the syringe and the insulin solution is simply drawn into the syringe to the proper mark corresponding to the prescribed dose. An insulin syringe (*not* a tuberculin syringe) must *always* be used in dispensing insulin.

Another syringe that is available for use with U100 insulin contains a volume of only 0.35 ml, and is termed a *micro-dose* or *lo-dose* insulin syringe. This particular syringe is intended for patients who require less than 35 units of U100 insulin, and is claimed to be more accurate for measuring small volumes of insulin, thereby reducing the chance of dosage errors. This lo-dose insulin syringe has a 35-unit scale graduated in 1-unit increments, thus allowing for exact dosage measurement.

Pediatric Dosage

Drug doses for infants and young children are usually smaller than those given to adults; however, there is no universally accepted method for calculating a pediatric dose as a fraction of an adult dose. Pediatric doses therefore are commonly given on a weight basis (that is, mg/kg or mg/lb) and the amount of drug needed can then be determined by knowing the weight of the child. A useful conversion in calculating pediatric doses is the relationship between kilograms and pounds, that is, 1 kg = 2.2 lb.

Example

The recommended dose of doxycycline in children is 2 mg/lb. How many milligrams should a 42-lb child receive?

2 mg per 1 lb

x mg per 42 lb

$$\frac{2 \text{ mg}}{1 \text{ lb}} = \frac{x \text{ mg}}{42 \text{ lb}}$$

x = $\boxed{84 \text{ mg}}$

Example

How many milligrams of diphenhydramine per day should a 55-lb child receive if the recommended pediatric dose is 5 mg/kg/day?

1 kg = 2.2 lb

x kg = 55 lb

$$\frac{1 \text{ kg}}{2.2 \text{ lb}} = \frac{x \text{ kg}}{55 \text{ lb}}$$

x = 25 kg

Daily dose = 5 mg/kg

$$\frac{5 \text{ mg}}{1 \text{ kg}} = \frac{x \text{ mg}}{25 \text{ kg}}$$

x = $\boxed{125 \text{ mg}}$

Example

The recommended pediatric dose of amoxicillin for an ear infection is 20 mg/kg/day in three divided doses. How many milligrams would a 33-lb child receive in each dose?

1 kg = 2.2 lb

x kg = 33 lb

$$\frac{1 \text{ kg}}{2.2 \text{ lb}} = \frac{x \text{ kg}}{33 \text{ lb}}$$

x = 15 kg

Daily dose = 20 mg/kg

$$\frac{20 \text{ mg}}{1 \text{ kg}} = \frac{x \text{ mg}}{15 \text{ kg}}$$

x = 300 mg per day

If total amount is taken in 3 doses, each dose = $\boxed{100 \text{ mg}}$

Example

How many mg/kg/day of phenobarbital would a 44-lb child receive if the dose is gr$\overline{\overline{ss}}$ four times a day?

1 kg = 2.2 lb

x kg = 44 lb

$$\frac{1 \text{ kg}}{2.2 \text{ lb}} = \frac{x \text{ kg}}{44 \text{ lb}}$$

x = 20 kg

Drug dose = 2 gr/day ($\frac{1}{2}$ gr × 4)

Convert grains to milligrams:

1 gr = 60 mg

Therefore 2 gr = 120 mg = daily dose in milligrams

The 20-kg child is taking 120 mg/day.

To find mg/kg/day

$$\frac{120 \text{ mg}}{20 \text{ kg}} = \frac{x \text{ mg}}{1 \text{ kg}}$$

x = $\boxed{6 \text{ mg/kg}}$

There have been several attempts in the past to devise formulas for calculating pediatric doses from the standard adult dose. In each case, the adult dose is multiplied by a fraction that is calculated based on a child's weight, age, or body surface area. The four pediatric dosage rules are given below, with an example of how each is used. The first three are only of theoretical interest. Most children's dosages are determined based on the child's weight (*i.e.*, on a mg of drug/kg of body weight basis) or occasionally on the basis of body surface area.

YOUNG'S RULE

Young's rule applies to children over 2 years of age and is only an approximation, due to considerable variation in body weight among children of the same age.

$$\text{Child dose} = \frac{\text{age (yr)}}{\text{age (yr)} + 12} \times \text{adult dose}$$

Example

Calculate the dose of phenytoin for a 5-year-old child if the average adult dose is 300 mg daily.

$$\text{Child dose} = \frac{5}{5 + 12} \times 300 \text{ mg}$$

$$= \frac{5}{17} \times 300 \text{ mg}$$

$$= \boxed{88 \text{ mg}}$$

FRIED'S RULE

Fried's rule is mainly applicable to children under 1 year of age.

$$\text{Child dose} = \frac{\text{age (months)}}{150} \times \text{adult dose}$$

Example

The usual adult dose of paregoric is 75 minims. What is the dose for a 9-month-old child?

$$\text{Child dose} = \frac{9}{150} \times 75 \text{ m}$$

$$= \boxed{4.5 \text{ m}}$$

This dose could be dispensed as 5 drops.

CLARK'S RULE

Clark's rule applies to young children and uses weight of the child in pounds, rather than the child's age.

$$\text{Child dose} = \frac{\text{weight (pounds)}}{150} \times \text{adult dose}$$

Example

If the adult dose of acetaminophen is 650 mg, how many milligrams should be given to a 25-lb child?

$$\text{Child dose} = \frac{25}{150} \times 650 \text{ mg}$$

$$= \boxed{108 \text{ mg}}$$

BODY SURFACE AREA RULE

This method depends on first determining the child's body surface area in square meters. This is usually done by referring to special charts, called *body surface nomograms*, from which the surface area of the body is estimated using the child's height and weight. Such a nomogram is illustrated in Figure 11-1. This is a somewhat unwieldy method, but is probably more exact than the other methods outlined above.

$$\text{Child dose} = \frac{\text{surface area of child (square meters)}}{1.7 \text{ square meters}} \times \text{adult dose}$$

Note: 1.7 square meters is the average adult body surface area.

Example

How many units of penicillin VK should a child with a body surface area of 0.48 square meters be given if the adult dose is 400,000 units?

$$\text{Child dose} = \frac{0.48}{1.7} \times 400,000 \text{ U}$$

$$= \boxed{113,000 \text{ U}} \text{ (approximately)}$$

Practice Problems

See Appendix for answers.

1. The pediatric dose of dyphylline is 3 mg/lb IM. How many milligrams will a 42-lb child receive?
2. The oral dose range of erythromycin in children is 30 mg to 50 mg/kg/day. How many milligrams will a 66-lb child receive if given the highest recommended dose?
3. The maximum recommended pediatric dose of thioridazine is 3 mg/kg/day in three divided doses. How many grains of thioridazine would a 66-lb child receive at each dose?
4. How many mg/kg/day would a 50-kg child receive if the recommended children's dose is 500 mg three times a day?
5. Determine the dose of gentamicin for a 3-year-old child if the adult dose is 80 mg.
6. Calculate the dosage of pentobarbital for a 15-month-old child if the adult dose is 30 mg.
7. If the adult dose of sulfisoxazole is 4 g to 8 g/day, what is the dosage range for an infant weighing 30 lb?
8. The adult dose of cefadroxil is 2 g/day. How many milligrams would be required for a 7½-month-old infant?
9. How many grains of meperidine should a 4-year-old child receive if the average adult dose is 240 mg?
10. The recommended average adult dose of guaifenesin is 200 mg every 4 hours. Calculate the dose for a 3-year-old child weighing 42 lb who is 40 inches in height. Use as many formulas as possible and compare the results. What are your conclusions?

After having read this chapter, studied the examples given, and worked the practice problems, you should possess a basic understanding of the mathematics of drug therapy. While every possible dosage situation has not been explored, a sufficient sampling of various types of problems has been presented to enable the reader to grasp the essential elements of dosage calculations. Remember that computing doses requires common sense as well as the mathematical tools. If a dose looks strange, question it! It could be wrong, but even if it is an unusual correct dose, the physician should appreciate your concern in questioning something unusual. Many potential law suits have been avoided by careful calculation before giving a dose of a drug that "didn't seem quite right." Speak up whenever you are not comfortable about a dose you are giving—it is part of your obligation to your patients.

West nomogram for estimation of body surface area

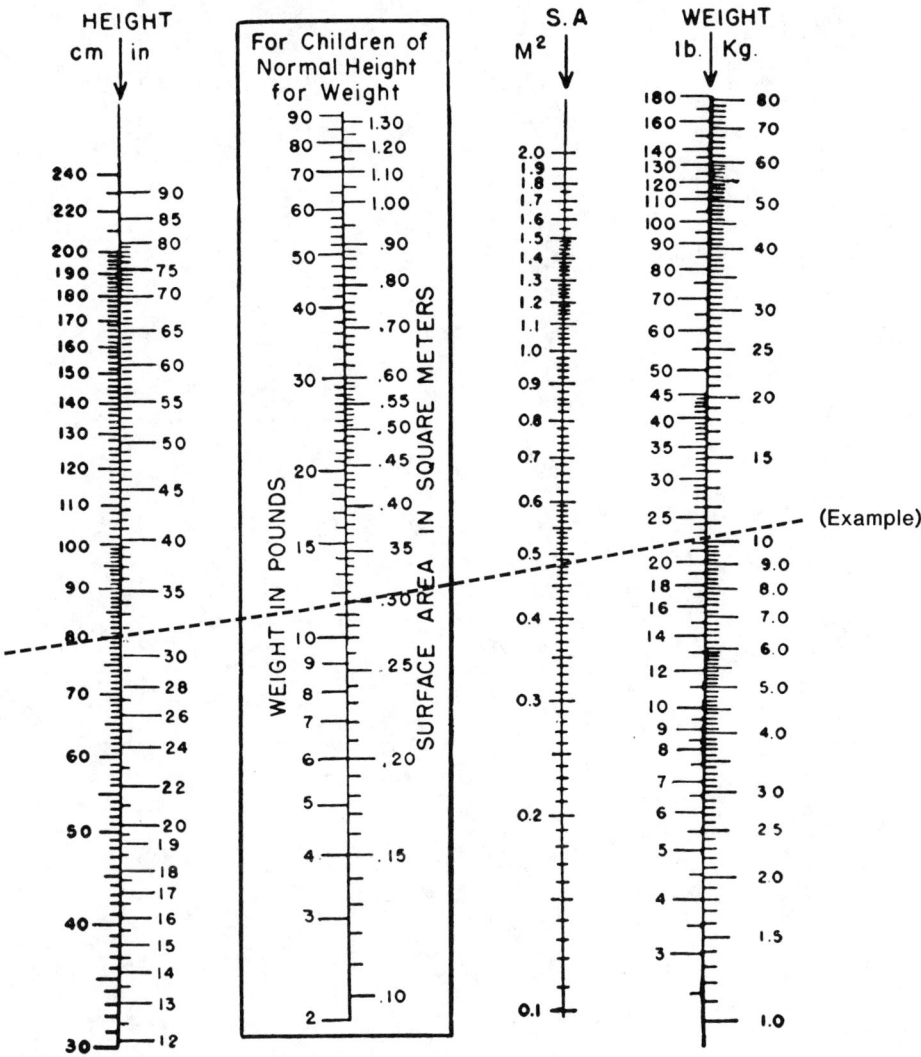

Figure 11-1. Body surface area nomogram. The surface area is indicated at the intersection of a straight line connecting the height and weight column with the surface area column. If the patient is of roughly average size, it is determined by the weight alone (enclosed area). (From Shirkey HC: Drug therapy. In Vaughan VC. McKay RJ. Behrman RE (eds): Nelson Textbook of Pediatrics, 11th ed. Philadelphia. WB Saunders, 1979)

BIBLIOGRAPHY

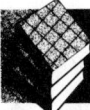

Anderson EM, Vervoren TM: Workbook of Solutions and Dosage of Drugs. St Louis, CV Mosby, 1976

Blume DM: Dosages and Solutions. Philadelphia, FA Davis, 1980

Keane C, Fletcher S: Drugs and Solutions. Philadelphia, WB Saunders, 1980

Medici GA: Drug Dosage Calculations: A Guide for Current Clinical Practice. Englewood Cliffs, NJ, Prentice Hall, 1980

Richardson LI, Richardson JK: The Mathematics of Drugs and Solutions with Clinical Applications. New York, McGraw-Hill, 1980

Verner L: Mathematics for Health Practitioners: Basic Concepts and Clinical Applications. Philadelphia, JB Lippincott, 1978

Whisler BL: Mathematics for Health Professionsals. North Scituate, MA, Duxbury Press, 1979

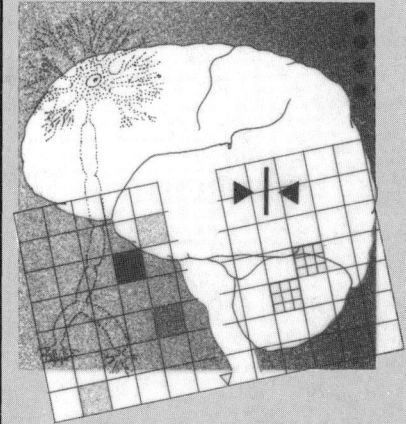

Drugs Acting on the Nervous System

III

The Nervous System

Peripheral Nervous System
  Neurohormonal Function
  Receptor Concept

Central Nervous System

12

The human nervous system is an immensely complex structure, encompassing more than 12 billion nerve cells or neurons. Along with the endocrine system, it regulates and coordinates the functioning of the various organs of the body. Transmission of information in the endocrine system is by way of circulating hormones, and this system provides for slowly developing but long-lasting control. The nervous system, on the other hand, can evoke rapid changes in body function since transmission of information is through electrical conduction of impulses along nerve fibers and chemical transmission of these impulses between nerve fibers. This system, therefore, provides "moment-to-moment" control.

The human nervous system can be divided in the following manner:

1. Peripheral nervous system
   a. Somatic system
   b. Autonomic system
      (1) Sympathetic division
      (2) Parasympathetic division
2. Central nervous system
   a. Brain
   b. Spinal cord

Peripheral Nervous System

The peripheral nervous system is divided into the somatic and autonomic branches, and several important differences exist between these two systems, as outlined in Table 12-1. The somatic system is mainly concerned with conveying to the central nervous system sensory information relative to the external environment, such as light, heat, and pressure, and mediating those skeletal muscle responses that represent one's reaction to the environment. Thus, the somatic system is viewed as a voluntary system—one over which a person exerts conscious control.

In contrast, the autonomic system includes those sensory and motor nerves that primarily innervate organs (smooth muscle, heart, glands) that usually function independently of our volition. This system is classified as an involuntary system. While responses of the somatic system such as contraction of skeletal muscle are almost always excitatory, those of the autonomic system can be either excitatory (e.g., vasoconstriction) or inhibitory (e.g., bradycardia and bronchodilation), depending on the organ and neurohormone involved.

The autonomic system may be further subclassified anatomically and functionally into the sympathetic and parasympathetic divisions. The characteristics of each division are listed in Table 12-2.

The parasympathetic division is sometimes referred to as a *cholinergic system* because the neurotransmitter at its postganglionic nerve endings is the cholinergic neurohormone acetylcholine, whereas the sympathetic system may be termed an *adrenergic system* because its postganglionic neu-

Table 12-1
Comparison of the Somatic and Autonomic Nervous Systems

Parameter	*Somatic Nervous System*	*Autonomic Nervous System*
Nature of the response	Voluntary	Involuntary
Centers of neuronal origin in the CNS	Cerebrum, cerebellum, midbrain, basal ganglia, spinal cord	Midbrain, hypothalamus, pons, medulla, spinal cord
Structures innervated by efferent nerve fibers	Skeletal muscles, sensory organs	Smooth muscle, cardiac muscle, exocrine and endocrine glands
Efferent nerve pathways	Single neuron with cell body in CNS and axon terminal at effector structure (e.g., skeletal muscle fiber)	Two-neuron chain, with body of preganglionic neuron in CNS and axon terminal in a peripheral ganglia. Postganglionic neuron has cell body in ganglia (synapses with preganglionic nerve ending) and axon terminal at effector structure (e.g., heart, GI tract, bronchioles, glands)
Effect of nerve impulse on innervated structures	Excitation (e.g., skeletal muscle contraction)	Excitation (e.g., vasoconstriction, salivation) or inhibition (e.g., bradycardia, bronchodilation)

Table 12-2

Comparison of the Parasympathetic and Sympathetic Divisions of the Autonomic Nervous System

Parameter	Parasympathetic Division	Sympathetic Division
Outflow from CNS	Craniosacral	Thoracolumbar
	Cranial nerves (3, 7, 9, 10; i.e., oculomotor, facial, glossopharyngeal, and vagus) and sacral (S2–S4) segments of the spinal cord	Thoracic (T1–T12) and lumbar (L1–L3) segments of the spinal cord
Ganglia	Near or within structure innervated	Close to spinal cord
Preganglionic fiber	Long and myelinated	Short and myelinated
Postganglionic fiber	Short and nonmyelinated	Long and nonmyelinated
Response to stimulation	Localized to a restricted area	Generalized and widespread
Neurotransmitter at all ganglia	Acetylcholine	Acetylcholine
Neurotransmitter at postganglionic nerve ending	Acetylcholine	Norepinephrine

rotransmitter *in most cases* is the adrenergic neurohormone norepinephrine.

A schematic representation of somatic and autonomic nerve fibers and their neurotransmitters is presented in Figure 12-1. As indicated, some effector structures (i.e., heart, smooth muscle, some glands) are innervated by both divisions of the autonomic system, and in dually innervated structures the pharmacologic effects of the two divisions are opposite. That is, if sympathetic activation causes excitation, parasympathetic activation causes inhibition. However, it is important to recognize that the two divisions do not exert equal control over all dually innervated structures. For example, the sympathetic division controls blood vessel tone, and hence blood pressure, to a much greater degree than the parasympathetic system, whereas the reverse is true in the functioning of the gastrointestinal tract.

Other structures are singly innervated, including the adrenal medulla, sweat glands, certain blood vessels, intrinsic eye muscles, and pilomotor muscles of the skin. The response of these structures is always excitatory, irrespective of their innervation. The effects of sympathetic versus parasympathetic stimulation on various structures of the body and the receptor types involved, which are

discussed later in this chapter, are outlined in Table 12-3, in which the opposing nature of most responses and the excitatory nature of singly innervated structures are clearly indicated. As indicated in Figure 12-1, although the sweat glands and skeletal muscle blood vessels are innervated by sympathetic fibers, the neurotransmitter released at the nerve ending is acetylcholine, not norepinephrine. In the adrenal medulla, where the innervation is parasympathetic, the neurohormone acetylcholine triggers secretion of epinephrine and in smaller amounts norepinephrine from the chromaffin cells. Thus, peripheral nerves are probably best classified chemically; that is, on the basis of the principal neurohormone released from their nerve endings. Nerves releasing acetylcholine are thus termed *cholinergic*, and those releasing norepinephrine are called *adrenergic*. The terms *sympathetic* and *parasympathetic* are primarily used in an anatomic sense. The various mechanisms by which these neurohormones function at nerve endings are reviewed below.

Neurohormonal Function

The functional unit of the nervous system is the neuron, a specialized cell capable of generating and transmitting electrical impulses. The passage of an impulse along a neuron, termed *conduction*, is an electrical process involving changes in the potential difference across the neuronal membrane caused by alterations in the flow of ions through the membrane. Drugs such as local anesthetics are capable of interrupting conduction of nerve impulses along a neuron by interfering with ionic flow across the membrane.

On the other hand, the transmission of an impulse between adjacent neurons is a chemical process mediated by substances termed *neurohormones* or *neurotransmitters* (e.g., acetylcholine, norepinephrine) that are stored within the nerve ending and diffuse from one neuron to another across the interneuronal space or synaptic junction. It should be remembered that the postsynaptic structure can be either a second neuron or some other type of organ or tissue, such as a muscle fiber or gland. The transmission of nerve impulses is an essential step in the functioning of the nervous system, and because it is a chemically (neurohormonally) mediated process, it is readily affected by many different classes of drugs.

In order to understand how drugs can affect nerve impulse transmission, it is necessary to first review the sequence of events that occur during the transmission of impulses between neurons.

1. *Biosynthesis of neurotransmitter.* Chemical substances that mediate transmission are formed from precursor substances within the nerve ending. Acetylcholine is synthesized from choline and acetyl coenzyme A by the action of the enzyme choline acetyltransferase (see Chap. 13). Norepinephrine is formed from the amino acid phenylalanine through a series of enzymatic conversions (see Chap. 15). In the adrenal medulla, as well as in certain brain areas, norepinephrine is further converted to epinephrine.

2. *Storage of neurotransmitter.* On formation, the neurotransmitter is taken up into specialized sites (such as vesicles) within the nerve endings and stored. This allows the neuron to "build up" a surplus of the transmitter in anticipation of its need. Thousands of molecules of acetylcholine are stored in each vesicle. These vesicles are thought to be membranous sacs derived from the neuronal membrane. Some norepinephrine is stored in granules bound to ATP, the so-called *reserve pool*, whereas other norepinephrine exists in the cytoplasm and is not contained within vesicles. This latter fraction is known as the *mobile pool*, and is not

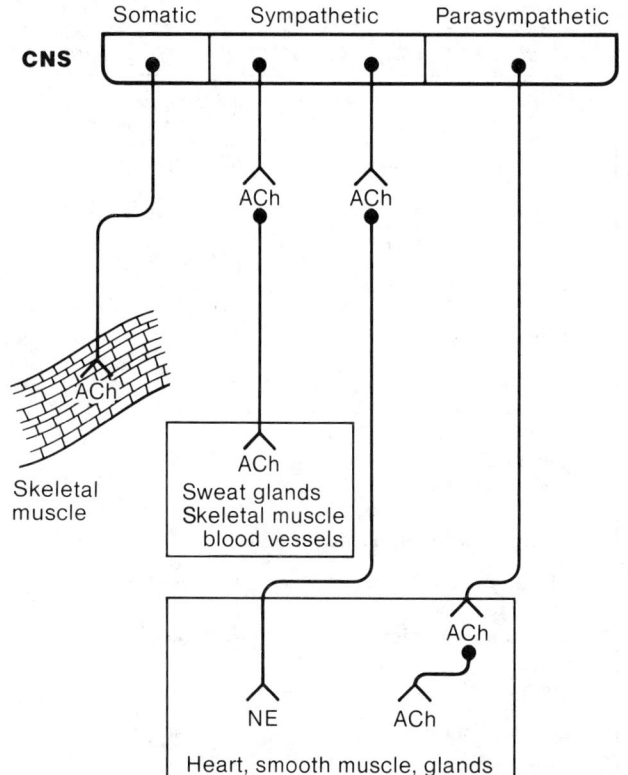

Figure 12-1. *A comparison of the somatic and autonomic nervous systems. The somatic system innervates skeletal muscles and the single neuron from the CNS releases the cholinergic neurohormone acetylcholine (ACh) at the neuromuscular junction. In the sympathetic system, short preganglionic neurons synapse with longer postganglionic neurons at ganglia where ACh is the neurotransmitter. The postganglionic neurons then innervate various effector organs, where the postganglionic neurohormone is usually norepinephrine (NE), although ACh is released from sympathetic nerves innervating sweat glands and skeletal muscle blood vessels. The parasympathetic system is composed of long preganglionic fibers that synapse with very short postganglionic fibers at ganglia in effector structures. ACh is the neurohormone released from both preganglionic and postganglionic parasympathetic fibers. (See text and Tables 12-1 and 12-2 for additional information.)*

released by a nerve action potential (see below), but can be expelled by various drugs, such as tyramine.

3. *Release of neurotransmitter.* With the arrival of a nerve action potential at the nerve ending, depolarization of the presynaptic membrane occurs, resulting in release of the neurotransmitter from its storage site into the synaptic junction. Release of the neurohormones proba-

Table 12-3
Responses of Effector Structures to Autonomic Nervous System Activation

Effector	Parasympathetic Activation		Sympathetic Activation	
	Action	Receptor	Action	Receptor
Heart				
Rate	Decreased	M	Increased	β_1
Contractility			Increased	β_1
Blood Vessels				
Coronary			Dilated	
Skeletal muscle			Dilated	β_2, M
Skin and mucosa			Constricted	α
Cerebral, pulmonary, abdominal viscera	Dilated		Constricted	α
Stomach and Intestine				
Motility and tone	Increased	M	Decreased	β_2
Sphincters	Relaxed	M	Contracted	α
Glandular secretion	Increased	M	Decreased	
Urinary Bladder				
Detrusor muscle	Contracted	M	Relaxed	β_2
Trigone and sphincter	Relaxed	M	Contracted	α
Other Smooth Muscle				
Bronchial muscle, ureters, gallbladder, and ducts	Contracted	M	Relaxed	β_2
Salivary Glands				
	Stimulated (profuse, watery secretion)	M	Stimulated (sparse, thick, mucinous secretion)	α
Eye				
Radial muscle of iris			Contracted (mydriasis)	α
Sphincter muscle of iris	Contracted (miosis)	M		
Ciliary muscle	Contracted (accommodated for near vision)	M	Relaxed (for far vision)	β
Spleen Capsule				
			Contracted	α
Liver				
			Glycogenolysis; gluconeogenesis	α, β_2
Uterus (Pregnant)				
			Relaxed	β_2
Kidney				
			Renin secretion	β_1

(continued)

Table 12-3 (continued)
Responses of Effector Structures to Autonomic Nervous System Activation

Effector	Parasympathetic Activation		Sympathetic Activation	
	Action	Receptor	Action	Receptor
Skin				
Sweat glands			Stimulated	M, α
Pilomotor muscles			Contracted	α
Pancreas				
Islet cells			Decreased insulin secretion	α_2
Acinar cells	Increased enzyme secretion	M		
Adrenal Medulla				
	Secretion of E and NE	N		
Fat Cells				
			Lipolysis	α, β_1

Key: M, muscarinic; N, nicotinic; α, alpha; β, beta.

bly is due to influx of calcium ions into the nerve ending, resulting in destabilization of the storage vesicles, subsequent fusion with the terminal plasma membrane, and extrusion of the neurotransmitter into the synaptic cleft.

The release of presynaptic stores of norepinephrine can be regulated by a negative feedback mechanism that is mediated by alpha-2 receptor sites (see Table 12-4) on the presynaptic nerve ending. When the level of norepinephrine released from the nerve ending becomes excessive, increased activation of prejunctional alpha-2 receptor sites occurs on the terminal nerve ending, thereby attenuating further release of norepinephrine. In this way, the neurotransmitter can regulate its own rate of release through a negative feedback mechanism. A number of other clinically useful drugs also influence the release of norepinephrine by either activating (*e.g.*, clonidine) or blocking (*e.g.*, imipramine) presynaptic alpha-2 receptor sites. Conversely, activation of presynaptic beta receptor sites has been postulated to facilitate neurohormonal release.

Prejunctional regulation of neurotransmitter release is not limited to norepinephrine. Evidence suggests that most substances that function as neurotransmitters (*e.g.*, serotonin, histamine, polypeptides) can regulate their own release through a negative feedback mechanism.

4. *Interaction with postsynaptic membrane.* The released neurohormone diffuses across the synaptic junction and interacts (complexes) with specific reactive areas (receptor sites) on the postsynaptic membrane. This interaction can result in either depolarization (activation) or hyperpolarization (inhibition) of the neuron or effector structure and subsequent facilitation or blockade of nerve impulse transmission.

5. *Inactivation of neurotransmitter.* Neurohormonal action can be terminated in several ways:

   a. Diffusion of the released neurotransmitter away from the synaptic area; probably important in removing excess or "overflow" but of little consequence for terminating the effects of physiologically released amounts of neurohormones

   b. Enzymatic breakdown of neurohormone; plays a greater role for acetylcholine than for norepinephrine. Acetylcholinesterase cleaves the neurotransmitter into choline and acetate, thus terminating its action. Two enzymes, monoamide oxidase (MAO), which is found in the prejunctional nerve ending, and catechol-O-methyl transferase

(COMT), which is localized postjunctionally, function to inactivate norepinephrine, but these are of little significance in *initially* terminating the action of the endogenously released hormone.

   c. Uptake of released neurotransmitter, either into the presynaptic nerve terminal from where it was released (uptake I) or into surrounding non-neural glial or smooth muscle cells (uptake II). Uptake I represents the principal means by which norepinephrine is inactivated following its extrusion from the prejunctional nerve ending.

6. *Repolarization of postsynaptic membrane.* Following termination of neurotransmitter action, the postsynaptic receptor area membrane is repolarized, that is, returned to its original ionic polarity and responsiveness.

Drugs acting on the nervous system may affect the transmission of impulses in one or more of the preceding steps. Types of drug action at each step are listed below, along with examples of drugs described in the text that have the particular type of action specified:

1. Inhibition of biosynthesis (*e.g.,* carbidopa, metyrosine)
2. Interference with intraneuronal binding or storage (*e.g.,* reserpine)
3. Interference with transmitter release (*e.g.,* guanethidine, clonidine)
4. Enhancement of transmitter release (*e.g.,* amphetamine, amantadine, guanidine)
5. Activation of postsynaptic receptor sites (*e.g.,* pilocarpine, isoproterenol, bromocriptine)
6. Blockade of postsynaptic receptor sites (*e.g.,* atropine, propranolol, tubocurarine)
7. Interference with neurotransmitter inactivation (*e.g.,* physostigmine, imipramine, tranylcypromine)
8. Prevention of postsynaptic membrane repolarization (*e.g.,* succinylcholine)

Receptor Concept

A receptor site may be viewed as a chemically reactive area on the surface of a cell membrane that is capable of complexing with specific neurohormones. This interaction initiates a sequence of events that alters the ionic permeability of the membrane, eliciting biochemical changes in the postsynaptic structure that result in either stimulation or inhibition of the functional activity of the effector structure, such as a muscle fiber, gland, or neuron. A more extensive discussion of drug–receptor interactions can be found in Chapter 3.

Receptors may be classified on the basis of their location, their selective responsiveness to various activators or blockers, and their differences in effector structure responses.

Table 12-4 lists several criteria that can be used to distinguish the various kinds of cholinergic and adrenergic receptor sites found in the peripheral nervous system. Cholinergic receptors are differentiated primarily on the basis of their anatomic location and the relative selectivity of cholinergic antagonists. The cholinergic receptor subtypes are named after the alkaloids that were originally used in their identification, and are referred to as muscarinic (M) sites, which respond to the alkaloid muscarine, and nicotinic (N) sites, which are activated by nicotine. M sites are located on effector structures innervated by *post*ganglionic parasympathetic and a *few* sympathetic fibers and may be found typically in the heart, smooth muscle cells, some glands, and skeletal muscle blood vessels. In addition, M receptors have also been characterized in the brain and in autonomic ganglia (see below). N sites are situated on postjunctional membranes of *all* autonomic ganglia (these receptors were previously termed NI sites) and in the neuromuscular end-plate of skeletal muscle (these receptors were previously named NII sites). The nicotinic receptors in autonomic ganglia are *not* identical to those in skeletal muscle, inasmuch as they respond differently to certain agonists and antagonists. Further complicating the picture is the existence of evidence suggesting that muscarinic receptors may be subdivided further into M_1 and M_2 sites based on the selectivity of various cholinergic agonists and antagonists.

Adrenergic receptors have traditionally been grouped into *alpha* and *beta* receptor sites according to their location, their differential activation or blockade by various drugs, and the types of responses they mediate. Each receptor type is further subdivided to reflect differences in location and function (see Table 12-4). Alpha-1 receptors are found postsynaptically in vascular smooth muscle, GI and urinary sphincter muscles, and in the eye, skin, pancreas, and salivary glands. Alpha-2 receptors occur on presynaptic nerve endings (where they control the release of norepinephrine), as well as in platelets, fat cells, and possibly also in vascular smooth muscle. Beta-1 receptors occur primarily in the heart and adipose tissue, and may also be found in the central nervous system and on presynaptic noradrenergic nerve endings. Beta-2 sites are present in the bronchioles, skeletal muscle vas-

Table 12-4
Characteristics of Autonomic Receptor Sites

Type	Location	Activators	Blockers
Cholinergic			
Muscarinic (M)	Sites innervated by postganglionic parasympathetic fibers (heart, smooth muscle cells, exocrine gland); brain; autonomic ganglia (?)	acetylcholine; pilocarpine	atropine
Nicotinic (N)	Autonomic ganglia; neuromuscular end-plate of skeletal muscle	acetylcholine; nicotine	trimethaphan (ganglia); d-tubocurare (neuromuscular junction)
Adrenergic			
Alpha-1	Most blood vessels, gastrointestinal tract, pancreas, eye, skin	norepinephrine; epinephrine; phenylephrine	phentolamine; tolazoline
Alpha-2	Presynaptic terminal ending of adrenergic nerve fibers; platelets; fat cells; vascular smooth muscle	norepinephrine; epinephrine; clonidine	imipramine
Beta-1	Heart; gastrointestinal tract; urinary bladder; eye; adipose tissue; presynaptic sympathetic nerve endings	epinephrine; isoproterenol	propranolol; metoprolol
Beta-2	Bronchioles, uterus, skeletal muscle, blood vessels, liver	epinephrine; isoproterenol; metaproterenol	propranolol
Dopamine	Renal, visceral and coronary blood vessels; brain; presynaptic nerve terminals	dopamine	haloperidol

culature, liver, kidney, and urinary bladder. A fifth type of adrenergic receptor responds selectively to the neurohormone dopamine, and is found on visceral and splanchnic blood vessels, in various brain areas, and also possibly on presynaptic sympathetic nerve terminals. A review of the responses elicited by activation of the various adrenergic receptors is presented in Table 15-1.

In addition to the receptor sites for the cholinergic and adrenergic neurohormones outlined above, other specialized types of receptors exist in peripheral and central structures. For example, two types of histamine receptors (H_1 and H_2 sites) are present in various body tissues, and these receptors selectively mediate the diverse actions of endogenous histamine on different body organs. A further discussion of histamine receptor sites is found in Chapter 18, which deals with antihistamine drugs. Serotonin, another endogenous neurohormone, interacts with at least two kinds of specific reactive sites to elicit its pharmacologic effects, and these effects can be abolished by agents that are capable of selectively blocking the different serotonin receptor sites. Antiserotonin drugs are also discussed

in Chapter 18. Many other putative neurotransmitters, including glycine, glutamic acid, gamma-aminobutyric acid (GABA), and bradykinin, are also believed to exert their effects by chemically combining with a corresponding receptor site.

Receptor sensitivity can be altered depending on the degree of activity at a particular receptor site. Persistent activation of a receptor results in a gradual loss of sensitivity; thus, when the agonist is removed, the receptor is less reactive to additional agonists for some time. The term *down-regulation* has been coined to describe this phenomenon and helps explain the action of several drugs, such as the tricyclic antidepressants (for a further description of the mechanisms involved in down-regulation of receptor sites, see Chap. 29). Similarly, persistent receptor antagonism can result in a state of receptor supersensitivity, leading to exaggerated responses once the antagonist is removed. For example, prolonged dopamine blockade by antipsychotic drugs results in hypersensitivity of central dopamine receptors. This dopamine supersensitivity or *up-regulation* of dopamine receptor sites is believed to be responsible for the appearance of the characteristic orofacial movements seen with long-term antipsychotic drug therapy.

Central Nervous System

The central nervous system (CNS) is composed of the brain and the spinal cord and together they serve to integrate and regulate a tremendous range of sensory, motor, and emotional activities. Thus, drugs that affect central neuronal function have the potential to alter the behavior of an individual markedly. The mechanisms of action of centrally acting drugs are similar to those of peripherally acting drugs, and, in fact, many drugs exert simultaneous effects on both the central and peripheral nervous systems. Moreover, because of the complex neuronal interconnections among various CNS areas, drugs acting at a specific central locus may exert widespread pharmacologic effects throughout the body and simultaneously alter the functioning of several physiologic systems.

The diversity of functions regulated by the CNS can best be illustrated by outlining the major subdivisions of the brain and the principal physiologic functions controlled by each area. Many of these functions are considered in more detail in the various chapters of the book dealing with drugs that can influence the various central nervous system areas controlling many bodily functions.

A. Forebrain
  1. Telencephalon
    a. Cerebral cortex
      (1) Analysis of sensory input—reception, integration, organization, facilitation of appropriate action (primary sensory areas)
      (2) Memory development (temporal lobe)
      (3) Storage of short-term information and elaboration of thought (temporal and frontal lobe)
      (4) Analysis and control of muscular coordination (superior temporal gyrus and frontal lobe)
      (5) Speech (temporal lobe)
      (6) Hearing (superior temporal lobe)
      (7) Vision (occipital lobe)
    b. Corpus striatum (caudate, putamen)
      (1) Planning, programming, and modulation of motor movement
      (2) Control of muscle tone
    c. Corpus callosum
      (1) Connects two hemispheres of the cerebral cortex, permitting functional integration
  2. Diencephalon
    a. Thalamus
      (1) Relay center for discrimination of incoming sensory signals (e.g., pain, temperature, touch)
      (2) Modulation of motor impulses from cerebral cortex
      (3) Integration of emotional behavior
    b. Hypothalamus
      (1) Regulation of cardiovascular function
      (2) Regulation of body water and electrolytes
      (3) Regulation of temperature
      (4) Regulation of food intake and satiety
      (5) Control of endocrine functioning
      (6) Control of sleep–wake mechanisms
      (7) Modification of behavior
B. Midbrain
  1. Mesencephalon
    a. Corpora quadrigemina (superior and inferior colliculus)
      (1) Relay centers for visual and hearing reflexes
    b. Cerebral peduncles
      (1) Control of motor coordination and postural reflexes
    c. Red nucleus
      (1) Regulation of motor functioning
    d. Substantia nigra
      (1) Regulation of motor functioning
C. Hindbrain
  1. Metencephalon
    a. Cerebellum
      (1) Coordination of muscle activity (synergia)
      (2) Maintenance of equilibrium and posture
    b. Pons
      (1) Relay center for impulses from the medulla to higher cortical centers
      (2) Regulation of respiration
  2. Myelencephalon
    a. Medulla oblongata
      (1) Control of respiration and cardiovascular function (heart and blood vessels)
      (2) Regulation of certain reflex activity (swallowing, salivation, vomiting)
      (3) Modulation of gastrointestinal function

In addition to the specific areas outlined above, mention should be made of several groups of CNS structures that function as integrated systems to control certain aspects of behavior. The *reticular formation* is a diffuse network of cells and nuclei scattered throughout the brain stem and extending upward into the midbrain. Impulses from spinal cord ascending pathways (by way of collateral neurons) and the cerebellum impinge on the reticular formation, which in turn makes diffuse connections with the cerebral cortex by way of relay nuclei in many subcortical areas. The reticular formation functions as part of the so-called extrapyramidal system and is capable of modifying motor activity, but the principal role of the reticular formation is the maintenance of a state of alertness or arousal in the organism. The functioning of the reticular formation and, in fact, of the entire reticular-activating system (RAS) can be markedly impaired by many classes of drugs, including barbiturates, anesthetics, and antipsychotics, resulting in varying degrees of CNS depression.

The principal group of structures controlling emotional behavior is collectively termed the *limbic system*, which is composed of several subcortical areas (thalamus, hypothalamus, hippocampus, amygdala, septum, preoptic area, and portions of the basal ganglia) and a surrounding ring of cortical tissue on the medial and ventral surfaces of each cerebral hemisphere. The limbic system functions to regulate many aspects of behavior, such as feelings of pleasure, anger, rage, and fear. It also functions in regulating biologic rhythms, sexual activity, feeding, and learning. Many portions of the limbic circuit transmit their impulses through the hypothalamus, so their output is frequently expressed in the form of autonomic manifestations, such as changes in blood pressure or respiration, hormonal changes, and expressions of pain, anger, and pleasure. Drugs used in the treatment of emotional disorders, such as antipsychotics, antidepressants, and lithium, exert at least a part of their action on the structures of the limbic system.

The *basal ganglia* are composed of three areas in the forebrain—the caudate nucleus, putamen, and globus pallidus—as well as several areas in the midbrain, such as the substantia nigra, red nucleus, and subthalamic nucleus. These structures are important for the integration and regulation of locomotor activity and postural reflexes. Pathologic changes in these ganglia result in the appearance of many types of movement disorders, the most common of which is parkinsonism.

REVIEW QUESTIONS

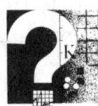

1. What are the major divisions and subdivisions of the human nervous system?
2. Why is the parasympathetic system often referred to as a *cholinergic system*?
3. Briefly distinguish between the somatic and autonomic nervous systems with respect to (1) nature of the response, (2) structures innervated, and (3) type of efferent nerve pathway.
4. What are the major differences between the sympathetic and parasympathetic branches of the autonomic nervous system?
5. Contrast the functions of *conduction vs transmission* in a neuronal pathway.
6. Give the principal steps in the sequence of events occurring during transmission of a nerve impulse.
7. Briefly describe presynaptic feedback as a modulator of neurohormone release from nerve endings.
8. List the various means by which the action of released neurohormones can be terminated.
9. Define what is meant by a *receptor site*.
10. How are cholinergic receptors classified? Where is each type located?
11. Distinguish between the various alpha and beta receptors with regard to the principal locations in the body.
12. Give the major functions of the following central nervous system structures: (1) corpus striatum, (2) hypothalamus, (3) substantia nigra, (4) cerebellum, (5) medulla oblongata, and (6) limbic system.

BIBLIOGRAPHY

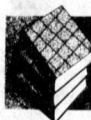

Appenzeller O: The Autonomic Nervous System. 3rd ed, Amsterdam, Elsevier, 1982

Cooper JR, Bloom FE, Roth RH: The Biochemical Basis of Neuropharmacology, 4th ed. New York, Oxford University Press, 1982

Cooper JR, Meyer FM: Possible mechanisms involved in the release and modulation of release of neuroactive agents. Neurochem Int 6:419, 1984

Gootman PM: Development of the autonomic nervous system. Fed Proc 42:1619, 1983

Hakanson R, Sundler F: The design of the neuroendocrine system: A unifying concept and its consequences. Trends Pharmacol Sci 4:41, 1983

Hirschowitz BI, Hammer R, Giachetti A, Keirns JJ, Levine RR (eds): Subtypes of muscarnic receptors. Trends Pharmacol Sci Suppl 1, 1984

Kilbinger H: Presynaptic muscarinic receptors modulating acetylcholine release. Trends Pharmacol Sci 5:103, 1984

Iversen LL, Iversen SD, Synder SH (eds): Handbook of Psychopharmacology. New York, Plenum Press, 1983

Langer SZ: Presynaptic receptors and modulation of neurotransmission: Pharmacological implications and therapeutic relevance. Trends in Neuroscience, 3:110, 1980

Lefkowitz RJ, Caron MG, Stiles GL: Mechanisms of membrane-receptor regulation. Biochemical, physiological and clinical insights derived from studies of the adrenergic receptors. N Engl J Med 310:1570, 1984

Motulsky HJ, Insel PA: Adrenergic receptors in man: Direct identification, physiologic regulation and clinical alteration. N Engl J Med 307:18, 1982

Salama AI: Presynaptic modulation of postsynaptic receptors in mental disease. Ann NY Acad Sci 430:1, 1984

Starke K: Pre-synaptic receptors. Annu Rev Pharmacol Toxicol 21:7, 1981

Su C: Purinergic neurotransmission and neuromodulation. Annu Rev Pharmacol Toxicol 23:397, 1983

Cholinergic Drugs

Direct-Acting Cholinergic Drugs

Choline Esters
    Acetylcholine Chloride
        Intraocular
    Carbachol Intraocular
    Carbachol Topical
    Bethanechol Chloride

Cholinomimetic Alkaloids
    Pilocarpine Hydrochloride
    Pilocarpine Nitrate
    Pilocarpine Ocular
        Therapeutic System

Indirect-Acting Cholinergic Drugs

Reversible Cholinesterase Inhibitors
    Physostigmine, Ophthalmic
    Physostigmine, Systemic
    Demecarium Bromide
    Ambenonium
    Edrophonium
    Neostigmine
    Pyridostigmine

Irreversible Cholinesterase Inhibitors
    Echothiophate Iodide
    Isoflurophate

Cholinesterase Inhibitor Antidote
    Pralidoxime Chloride

13

Cholinergic drugs are substances capable of evoking biologic responses similar to those elicited by the endogenous cholinergic neurotransmitter acetylcholine (ACh). The biologic effects produced by these drugs in many ways mimic those evoked by stimulation of cholinergic nerves and for this reason the cholinergic drugs are frequently referred to as *cholinomimetic* agents.

On the basis of their principal mechanism of action, the cholinergic drugs may be classified as either *direct-acting* or *indirect-acting*. The direct-acting cholinergics produce their cholinomimetic effects by directly binding to and activating the various muscarinic and nicotinic cholinergic receptor sites on postjunctional membranes (see Chap. 12). The indirect-acting drugs, on the other hand, do not combine with cholinergic receptor sites; rather, they inhibit the functioning of the cholinesterase enzymes responsible for the inactivation of endogenously released ACh. By retarding the enzymatic breakdown of ACh, these indirect-acting cholinergic drugs cause accumulation of ACh in the vicinity of cholinergic receptors, thus enhancing and prolonging the action of the cholinergic neurohormone. A schematic outline of the function of ACh in nerve transmission and the actions of the two classes of cholinergic drugs is presented in Figure 13-1.

Direct-Acting Cholinergic Drugs

The direct-acting cholinergic drugs can be categorized based on their chemical structures into *choline esters* (*e.g.*, acetylcholine, bethanechol) and *cholinomimetic alkaloids* (*e.g.*, pilocarpine, nicotine).

Acetylcholine is a neurohormone that mediates nerve impulse transmission at the various cholinergic sites. It is synthesized in cholinergic neurons in the following manner:

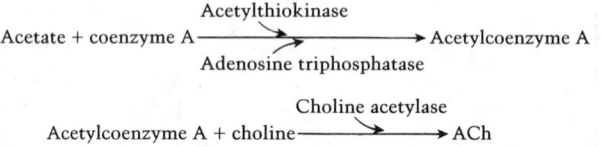

Once formed, ACh is stored in packets or vesicles within the nerve ending, presumably in combination with adenosine triphosphatase (ATP) and a

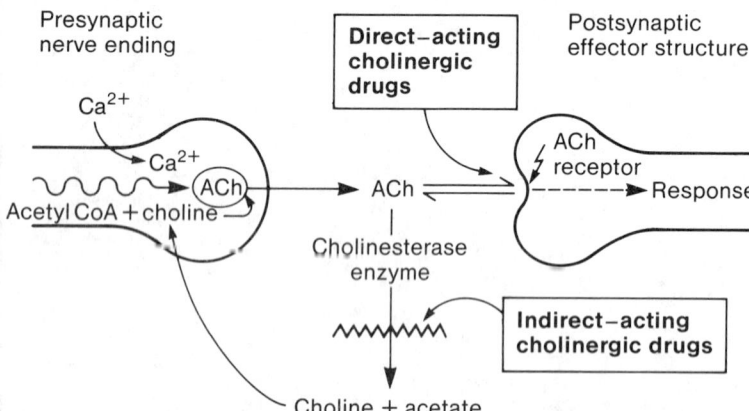

Figure 13-1. *Effects of direct-acting and indirect-acting cholinergic drugs on cholinergic function. Upon arrival of a nerve impulse at the presynaptic nerve ending, there is influx of Ca^{2+} ions and ACh is released. It then diffuses across the synaptic cleft and interacts with the cholinergic receptor site on the postsynaptic effector structure. Following its receptor complexation, the ACh molecule leaves the site and is enzymatically broken down by acetylcholinesterase to choline and acetate. Direct-acting cholinergic drugs complex with the cholinergic receptor site themselves, whereas indirect-acting cholinergic drugs inhibit the enzymatic degradation of ACh.*

proteoglycan. On arrival of an action potential at the cholinergic nerve ending, there is an influx of calcium ions (see Fig. 13-1), which facilitates the expulsion of ACh from the storage vesicle into the synaptic cleft. Following release, the molecules of ACh diffuse to the receptor sites on the effector structure and bind to these reactive membrane areas, eliciting an appropriate response in the postsynaptic structure. The action of ACh is then rapidly terminated in the synaptic area by the acetylcholinesterase enzyme. Body fluids contain two major enzymes capable of hydrolyzing ACh, *acetylcholinesterase* (AChE) and *butyrocholinesterase* (BuChE). Acetylcholinesterase is present in very high concentrations in cholinergic neurons, exhibits a high degree of specificity for ACh, and represents the principal biochemical mechanism for inactivating ACh at cholinergic nerve endings. Conversely, butyrocholinesterase is found in largest amounts in the plasma and liver, is relatively nonspecific in its actions, and, while it may play a minor role in the catabolism of ACh, probably is mainly involved in the degradation of other cholinergic-like compounds in the systemic circulation.

Paralleling the extensive distribution of cholinergic nerve fibers in the body, the pharmacologic actions of ACh are many and varied. Table 13-1 lists the principal pharmacologic effects of ACh, along with some expected clinical consequences. However, despite the obvious physiologic importance of endogenous ACh, the clinical usefulness of this substance as a drug is greatly restricted, largely because of its rapid inactivation by cholinesterase enzymes and its nonselective effects on all three types of cholinergic receptor sites. The rapid enzymatic hydrolysis of ACh results in a very transient action when given systemically, whereas the receptor nonspecificity leads to the development of a diverse range of undesirable side-effects. The clinically effective direct-acting cholinergic drugs comprise a group of both natural and synthetic drugs that possess most, if not all, of the pharmacologic actions of endogenous ACh, but exhibit greater resistance to enzymatic inactivation and, in some cases, greater selectivity of action at particular cholinergic receptor sites.

Choline Esters

The three clinically available choline esters (acetylcholine, bethanechol, carbamylcholine) differ with respect to their susceptibility to inactivation by cholinesterase enzymes and in their specificity for the various cholinergic receptor sites. These differences are outlined in Table 13-2. Acetylcholine, as

Table 13-1
Pharmacologic Effects of Acetylcholine and Clinical Consequences

Effect	Clinical Consequence
Gastrointestinal tract	
Increased peristalsis	Diarrhea
Relaxation of sphincter muscles	
Increased glandular secretions	
Cardiovascular system	
Decreased heart rate	
Vasodilation	Hypotension
Urinary tract	
Contraction of detrusor muscle	Urination
Relaxation of trigone and sphincter	
Other smooth muscle	
Contraction of bronchiolar smooth muscle	Bronchoconstriction
Contraction of gallbladder and ducts	
Contraction of ureter	
Contraction of sphincter muscle of iris	Miosis
Contraction of ciliary muscle	Accommodation for near vision
Glands	
Stimulation of exocrine gland secretion (lacrimal, sweat, salivary, bronchial)	Sweating Salivation

Table 13-2
Pharmacologic Properties of Choline Esters

	Muscarinic Receptor Activation			Nicotinic Receptor Activation	Inactivation by Cholinesterase
	GI/Urinary	Cardiovascular	Ocular		
Acetylcholine	Moderate	Moderate	Weak	Moderate	Yes
Bethanechol	Strong	Weak	Moderate	None	No
Carbamylcholine	Strong	Weak	Moderate	Strong	No

previously noted, is rapidly hydrolyzed by cholinesterase enzymes, and its effects are very short-lived. In addition, it is relatively nonselective in its effects, and can activate all cholinergic receptor sites. The clinical use of acetylcholine is confined to a few specific applications in the eye. Carbamylcholine, or carbachol, like acetylcholine, is largely nonselective in its receptor effects and possesses a very strong nicotinic receptor-activating effect. Its use is likewise limited to ophthalmic application. However, carbamylcholine is almost totally resistant to the action of cholinesterase and exhibits a much longer duration of action than acetylcholine following instillation into the eye. Bethanechol is largely unaffected by cholinesterase as well, but exhibits little nicotinic receptor activity. Rather, its receptor action appears to be somewhat selective for the muscarinic sites on gastrointestinal and urinary smooth muscle, and bethanechol is principally used in treating postoperative urinary retention and abdominal distention.

Acetylcholine Chloride Intraocular

(Miochol)

MECHANISM AND ACTIONS
Acetylcholine elicits contraction of the smooth muscle of the iris sphincter, resulting in constriction of the pupil and contraction of the ciliary muscle, leading to accommodation for near vision.

USES
1. To promote rapid miosis during cataract surgery, iridectomy, penetrating keratoplasty, and other anterior chamber procedures

ADMINISTRATION AND DOSAGE
The solution is aseptically prepared by dissolving the contents of the lower half of a dual-chamber vial (20 mg lyophilized ACh and 60 mg mannitol) with the diluent in the upper half (2 ml sterile water for injection) by breaking the seal between the chambers. The resultant 1:100 ACh solution is very unstable and should be used immediately. Any solution remaining must be discarded.

The solution is gently instilled into the anterior chamber parallel to the face of the iris, generally by the surgeon. In most cases, 0.5 ml to 2 ml of solution produces satisfactory miosis. Following instillation, the peripheral iris is drawn away from the angle of the anterior chamber. The solution need not be flushed from the eye, since the miotic action of acetylcholine persists for only about 10 minutes. Miosis can be maintained following surgery by topical application of a longer-acting miotic such as pilocarpine.

NURSING CONSIDERATIONS
Acetylcholine is used exclusively during surgical procedures. Therefore, the amount of intervention by the nurse in the operating room is somewhat limited. The primary concern will be appropriate sterilization of the vial, so the solution may be mixed during the surgical procedure. To sterilize, immerse the whole vial (both chambers) in a sterilizing solution such as 70% ethanol for a half hour prior to use. Do not gas sterilize the vial.

Carbachol Intraocular

(Miostat)

Carbamylcholine, or carbachol, can also be employed to produce pupillary miosis during surgery. For this application, 0.5 ml of a 0.01% sterile solution is instilled by the surgeon into the anterior chamber. Miosis usually is complete within 2 minutes to 5 minutes.

Carbachol Topical

(Isopto Carbachol)

Carbachol topical is a potent, long-acting cholinergic used in the form of eye drops for the treatment of resistant cases of glaucoma (see Disease Brief: Glaucoma.).

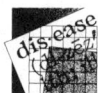

DISEASE BRIEF

■ *Glaucoma*

Glaucoma is characterized by elevated pressure within the chambers of the eye due to excessive production of aqueous humor or reduced outflow or both. If unchecked, this increased intraocular pressure eventually can result in blindness. There are two *major* types of primary glaucoma, open or wide angle (chronic, simple) and narrow angle (acute, congestive), as well as secondary (*e.g.*, surgically induced) and congenital glaucoma. The "angle" in question is that formed by the iris and the cornea, and it is within this angle that the channels for drainage of fluid from the anterior chamber are located, the so-called trabecular network. In chronic, wide-angle glaucoma, the impaired drainage is often the consequence of a degeneration of the channels by which the aqueous humor drains from the chamber. This form of glaucoma can be controlled in most cases by proper drug treatment. Narrow-angle glaucoma results from a closure of the angle between the iris and cornea, thus reducing access of the aqueous humor to the drainage channels. This condition may be amenable to drug treatment, but frequently requires surgery.

MECHANISM AND ACTIONS

Activation of muscarinic receptors in the eye contracts the ciliary muscle, which facilitates drainage of the aqueous humor from the chamber through the trabecular network and accommodates the eye for near vision. In addition, the sphincter muscle contracts, producing miosis. The enhanced drainage of aqueous humor lowers elevated intraocular pressure.

USES

1. To reduce intraocular pressure in cases of open-angle or narrow-angle glaucoma resistant to other cholinergic drugs such as pilocarpine

ADMINISTRATION AND DOSAGE

One or two drops of a 0.75% to 3% solution are instilled into the lower conjunctival sac two or four times a day. The frequency of application and the strength of solution employed are determined by the patient's condition and response.

FATE

The miotic effect is noted within several minutes and persists for 4 hours to 8 hours following application.

SIDE-EFFECTS/ADVERSE REACTIONS

With topical application, the most commonly reported side-effects are headache, pain over the eyebrow, reddening of the conjuctiva, and a temporary reduction in visual acuity due to ciliary spasm. With large doses or prolonged usage, significant systemic absorption can occur, resulting in a wide range of cholinergic effects such as sweating, flushing, abdominal cramping, diarrhea, urinary urgency, and hypotension.

CONTRAINDICATIONS AND PRECAUTIONS

Carbachol is contraindicated in the presence of corneal abrasions and acute iritis (*i.e.*, inflammation of the iris).

Due to the possibility of systemic absorption, carbachol should be used *cautiously* in patients with asthma, ulcers, gastrointestinal (GI) or urinary distress, hyperthyroidism, parkinsonism, and acute cardiac failure.

■ *Nursing Process*

□ *ASSESSMENT*

□ *Subjective Data*

With any long-acting cholinergic, nursing assessment must focus on all body systems, not just on the muscle group for which the drug is prescribed. The systemic effects listed in Table 13-1 can apply to any long-term user of carbachol, so when interviewing such a patient initially, the nurse should inquire about changes in the function of the GI and genitourinary (GU) systems, cardiovascular system, and other smooth muscles besides the eye.

□ *Objective Data*

Over time, nursing assessment should focus on changes in side-effects. Encourage the patient to report recurring symptoms so dose adjustments can be made. Doses can be altered to minimize side-effects while still maintaining therapeutic levels. Nursing intervention here may improve patient compliance.

☐ *NURSING DIAGNOSES*

Actual nursing diagnoses for this drug may include
Knowledge deficit: action, administration, and side-effects of the drug.

Potential nursing diagnoses are related to the side-effects of the drug and may include
Alteration in bowel elimination: diarrhea
Alteration in cardiac output: decreased
Ineffective breathing patterns related to bronchoconstriction
Sensory–perceptual alterations: vision changes related to inappropriate dosing or miotic effect
Alteration in patterns of urinary elimination: urgency

☐ *PLAN*

The nursing goal for the patient receiving carbachol should be to plan administration with the patient in order to minimize side-effects and maximize the patient's safety.

☐ *INTERVENTION*

The miotic effect of carbachol results in its most common side-effect, blurred vision. Patients need to know this will diminish over time, generally within 2 hours. However, during the period of blurred vision, the patient should be encouraged to avoid activities requiring clear vision, such as driving, using sharp instruments, or doing detail work. Helping the patient plan his dosage administration at times when there is a minimal need for such activity will reduce frustration and also foster compliance.

Carbachol is used primarily in cases where the patient is not responding to the use of pilocarpine. Although carbachol is more potent than pilocarpine, both drugs act by the same mechanism and are rarely used together. Any time concurrent therapy with both drugs is ordered, clarify the prescription. In most cases, the pilocarpine order should be discontinued.

☐ *EVALUATION*

Outcome criteria against which to measure the success of therapy may be the patient's ability to use the drug correctly, reports that the time of administration works well to minimize the side-effect of blurred vision, and the patient's report of symptoms that would require dosage adjustments.

Bethanechol Chloride

(Duvoid, Myotonachol, Urabeth, Urecholine)

MECHANISM AND ACTIONS

Bethanechol is a synthetic choline ester with predominantly muscarinic actions on the GI and urinary systems. The drug selectively activates cholinergic receptor sites in the GI and urinary tract musculature, increases tone and peristalsis of the stomach and intestines, and contracts the detrusor muscle of the urinary bladder sufficiently to initiate micturition and to empty the bladder. Bethanechol possesses minimal nicotinic action; thus, it does not stimulate autonomic ganglia or voluntary muscles at recommended doses. Bethanechol has little effect on heart rate, blood pressure, or peripheral circulation.

USES

1. Treatment of acute postoperative or postpartum nonobstructive urinary retention and neurogenic atony of the bladder
2. Relief of postoperative abdominal distention and adynamic ileus
3. Management of reflux esophagitis (investigational use)

ADMINISTRATION AND DOSAGE

Bethanechol may be administered orally as tablets (5 mg, 10 mg, 25 mg, 50 mg) or subcutaneously as an injection solution containing 5 mg/ml. The dose should be individualized based on severity of the condition. Orally, the usual adult dose is 10 mg to 50 mg two to four times a day to a maximum of 200 mg daily. *Children* should receive 0.2 mg/kg three times a day.

The usual subcutaneous dose is 2.5 mg to 5 mg three to four times a day, as required. Rarely, single doses up to 10 mg may be needed, but the possibility of serious adverse reactions should be recognized.

The pediatric subcutaneous dose ranges from 0.15 mg to 0.2 mg/kg three times a day. The injectable form should never be given intramuscularly (IM) or intravenously (IV), only subcutaneously (SC) because severe cholinergic overstimulation (hypotension, diarrhea, abdominal cramps, shock, cardiac arrest) can occur.

FATE

The onset of action occurs within 30 minutes to 60 minutes following oral administration and within 5 minutes to 15 minutes with SC injection. Effects persist for approximately 2 hours to 4 hours with both oral and SC administration, but may last for up to 6 hours.

SIDE-EFFECTS/ADVERSE REACTIONS
Adverse reactions are usually the result of excessive dosage. Early indications of excessive dosage include salivation, sweating, flushing, abdominal cramping, and nausea and vomiting. Urinary urgency, involuntary defecation, headache, hypotension, and asthmatic-like attacks have also been reported with large doses. Other untoward reactions have included transient syncope, transient heart block, bronchospasm, and dyspnea.

CONTRAINDICATIONS AND PRECAUTIONS
Bethanechol is contraindicated in patients with bronchial asthma, peptic ulcer, coronary artery disease, epilepsy, parkinsonism, pronounced bradycardia, hyperthyroidism, atrioventricular (A–V) conduction defects, or coronary occlusion, and in pregnancy. The drug must be used with extreme *caution,* and only where possible benefit clearly outweighs risk, in the presence of urinary bladder neck or intestinal obstruction, acute inflammatory lesions of the GI tract, or peritonitis, and following recent urinary bladder surgery or GI resection.

INTERACTIONS
1. Concurrent use with other cholinergics may increase the potential for toxic reactions.
2. A severe drop in blood pressure may occur if ganglionic blocking agents are given with bethanechol.
3. Quinidine, procainamide, and disopyramide can antagonize the action of bethanechol.

NURSING CONSIDERATIONS
Watch patients closely for the adverse reactions listed since the margin of safety for the therapeutic dose of this drug is narrow. At the first sign of toxicity (nausea, dyspnea, substernal pain, irregular pulse), notify the physician. The treatment of overdose is with atropine; a syringe containing 0.6 mg of atropine should be readily available, and the drug given subcutaneously if required.

The dosage range for oral and subcutaneous administration of bethanechol is very different. Clarify ambiguous orders since the doses for the two routes cannot be interchanged. Administering an oral dose subcutaneously would result in a dangerous overdose to the patient.

Administer oral bethanechol on an empty stomach since it can cause nausea and vomiting if given after meals. Also, remember this is a rapid-acting cholinergic; absorption is enhanced by administration orally to an empty GI tract. Keep a bedpan close to the patient or be certain he will have rapid access to a bathroom when he needs it. Helping the patient plan for the response to the drug will reduce the chance of accidents and the embarrassment that can result.

Cholinomimetic Alkaloids

Several naturally occurring alkaloidal substances possess acetylcholine-like activity at muscarinic receptor sites. Muscarine is found in certain mushrooms and exerts a strong agonistic action at the muscarinic receptor sites (see Chap. 12). In fact, these receptors derive their name from the fact that they are selectively activated by the alkaloid muscarine. This substance is primarily of toxicologic importance and is responsible for the symptoms of poisoning with many species of mushrooms. Atropine is a specific antidote to the effects of muscarine.

The only cholinomimetic alkaloid of therapeutic importance is pilocarpine.

Pilocarpine Hydrochloride
(Adsorbocarpine, Akarpine, Almocarpine, Isopto-Carpine, Pilocar, Pilopine HS)

Pilocarpine Nitrate
(P.V. Carpine)

Pilocarpine is the most commonly used direct-acting cholinergic miotic. It is employed exclusively in the eye for its potent miotic and antiglaucoma effects. Systemic absorption of pilocarpine can result in profuse salivation and sweating.

MECHANISM AND ACTIONS
The effects of pilocarpine are due to a muscarinic action in the eye, resulting in contraction of the iris sphincter (miosis) and constriction of the ciliary muscle (accommodation for near vision). Ciliary muscle contraction is also thought to facilitate aqueous humor outflow in chronic open-angle glaucoma by increasing drainage through the trabecular network. In angle-closure glaucoma, pupillary constriction pulls the iris away from the trabecular network, thus reducing the mechanical obstruction to drainage.

USES

1. Treatment of chronic simple glaucoma, especially open-angle
2. Treatment of acute congestive glaucoma (prior to surgery), usually combined with other miotics, beta-blockers, hyperosmotic agents, or carbonic anhydrase inhibitors
3. To reverse effects of mydriatics and cycloplegics following surgery or ophthalmic examinations

ADMINISTRATION AND DOSAGE

Various solutions of pilocarpine ranging from 0.25% to 10% are available for ophthalmic use. In addition, a 4% gel is also available. Pilocarpine is also used in a fixed combination with epinephrine (P.E., E-Pilo) or physostigmine (Isopto P-ES). In treating chronic simple glaucoma, the initial pilocarpine dose is usually 1 drop of a 1% or 2% solution up to six times a day depending on the condition. Concentrations of between 0.5% and 4% are most frequently employed. Solutions of 5% or stronger are less commonly used, since the incidence of adverse reactions is much higher. Acute narrow-angle glaucoma is managed with 1 drop of a 1% or 2% solution every 5 minutes to 10 minutes for 3 to 6 doses, then every 1 hour to 3 hours thereafter. To prevent a bilateral attack of angle-closure glaucoma, 1 drop is instilled in the unaffected eye every 6 hours to 8 hours. To counteract the mydriatic and cycloplegic effects of other drugs, 1 drop of a 1% solution is commonly prescribed.

Pilocarpine appears to bind to iris melanin, a pigment, which affects the rate of movement of the drug to an active receptor site. Blue-eyed patients may absorb more of the drug than their brown-eyed counterparts, and black patients with very dark pigmentation may absorb little or none of the drug. This fact is especially important when determining the concentration of the drug to be used during initial therapy and may influence the success of the treatment.

FATE

Miosis begins within 10 minutes to 30 minutes and lasts 4 hours to 8 hours. The maximal reduction in intraocular pressure usually occurs in 60 minutes to 90 minutes, and persists for 4 hours to 12 hours.

SIDE-EFFECTS/ADVERSE REACTIONS

The most frequently observed side-effects are eye pain and difficulty in focusing. Headache and local irritation have also been reported, as well as decreased night vision and altered distance vision.

Systemic absorption of significant quantities of drug can lead to a cholinergic syndrome characterized by flushing, sweating, abdominal cramping, diarrhea, and urinary urgency.

CONTRAINDICATIONS AND PRECAUTIONS

Pilocarpine should not be used where miosis is undesirable, such as in acute iritis or other acute inflammatory disease of the anterior chamber. *Cautious use* is warranted in patients with severe bronchial asthma, peptic ulcer, hyperthyroidism, urinary tract obstruction, or Parkinson's disease.

Pilocarpine Ocular Therapeutic System
(Ocusert Pilo)

Ocusert Pilo is a continuous-release form of pilocarpine (20 mcg/hour or 40 mcg/hour) placed into the lower conjunctival cul-de-sac. The pilocarpine ocular therapeutic system provides for the maintenance of therapeutically effective concentrations of pilocarpine over extended periods of time. It is used primarily for continuous therapy of open-angle glaucoma. A system unit is inserted into the conjunctival sac once a week. Release rate of pilocarpine is not affected by presence of other locally acting drugs (*e.g.,* epinephrine, carbonic anhydrase inhibitors). Myopia can occur for several hours following insertion of the system but is usually mild. The system can be moved to the upper conjunctival sac before sleep, to aid in retention during the night.

The drug should be used cautiously in the presence of infectious conjunctivitis or keratitis. Safety of use in the presence of retinal detachments has not been established. Signs of conjunctival irritation, erythema, and increased secretions may occur when first used but tend to lessen after the first 1 week to 2 weeks. The system is frequently poorly tolerated by patients, and its usefulness is somewhat limited. The user's ability to manage the placement and removal of the system must be monitored to ensure proper drug delivery.

■ Nursing Process

□ ASSESSMENT

As with other ocular cholinergics, the nurse must assess the patient for systemic smooth muscle effects of the drug, as well as for the local effects to the eye. This will be an ongoing process while the drug therapy is supervised.

Medical history taking should include questions about asthma, ulcer disease, thyroid problems, and Parkinson's disease, since a positive history may preclude use of the drug.

A drug history is also helpful in establishing a baseline. Any patient receiving pilocarpine should *not* be given mydriatics, which increase intraocular pressure.

Glaucoma therapy, the main indication for pilocarpine, is a life-long problem and requires consistent participation by the patient. Therefore, early in the therapy, the nurse needs to assess whether the patient will be able to administer the drug independently, what family resources or community supports will be able to assist, and how well the patient will be able to absorb necessary information and maintain a routine in order to ensure successful treatment.

☐ *NURSING DIAGNOSES*
Actual nursing diagnosis for this drug is
　Knowledge deficit: about action, administration, and side-effects of pilocarpine
Potential nursing diagnoses include
　Noncompliance: failure to maintain the drug regimen, which must continue for life
　Alteration in bowel elimination: diarrhea related to systemic absorption
　Alteration in comfort: eye pain or headache from the drug effects
　Sensory–perceptual changes in vision related to changes in night and distance vision
　Alteration in patterns of urinary elimination: urgency related to systemic absorption of the drug

☐ *PLAN*
Nursing care goals should focus on establishing a teaching plan that enables the patient to learn appropriate administration and storage techniques and how to handle side-effects if they should occur.

☐ *INTERVENTION*
The following are basic teaching guidelines for the patient taking pilocarpine:
1. Careful administration. Give the patient plenty of time to practice. See also Table 13-3, Teaching Self-Administration of Eye Drops and Ointments, and Chapter 8, section on eye drops.

Table 13-3
Teaching Self-Administration of Eye Drops and Ointments

Inserting eye medication requires some practice. These are some major points to follow when inserting eye drops or ointments:
1. Wash your hands.
2. Sit in a comfortable chair.
3. Lean your head back so you are comfortable.
4. Open your eye; pull down your lower lid.
5. Apply the prescribed ribbon of ointment along the lower conjunctival surface (inside the lid) or apply the number of drops prescribed into the conjunctival sac (the space created by pulling the lower lid down). Avoid touching the eyelid with the medication applicator to prevent contamination.
6. Close eyes and immediately compress the inner canthus (the space where the lacrimal duct is visible). Doing so will decrease the amount of medication lost through drainage into the nasal chamber and will minimize systemic absorption.
7. Rest for at least 1 minute to give the medication time to absorb.

2. Even spacing of doses. Pilocarpine levels in the eye should be maintained as consistent as possible to ensure reduction of intraocular pressure and avoid fluctuations that could result in irreversible nerve damage. Therefore, optimal dosing schedules are every 6 hours to every 8 hours. Question any order that is written qid and reinforce with patients the importance of even-spaced dosing at home.
3. The symptoms of systemic toxicity. Basic symptoms patients should watch for are sweating, salivation, cramping, and nausea. Help the patient to develop a plan for reaching help immediately if such symptoms occur. Include family or other supports so everyone knows what symptoms to watch for.
4. Establishing a place where the drug can be stored. Pilocarpine should be protected from light since it is very unstable.
5. Incorporating the drug into the patient's lifestyle. The glaucoma patient needs to get into the habit of taking eye drops with him wherever he goes so that doses are never delayed. He also needs to plan for an emergency should a bottle be lost or accidentally destroyed. Patients can plan for this by keeping an extra bottle in a handbag or in the home and establishing an account with a pharmacy that will provide 24-hour emergency service.

□ *EVALUATION*

Once the patient teaching on pilocarpine has been completed, encourage the patient and support people to give return demonstrations on the instillation of the drug and to explain how they will handle emergencies and how and when they will seek help. The patient and family who show evidence of this type of planning before discharge are more likely to follow the prescribed regimen successfully at home.

Indirect-Acting Cholinergic Drugs

The indirect-acting cholinergic drugs are termed *cholinesterase inhibitors*, inasmuch as they inhibit the enzymatic hydrolysis of acetylcholine by the cholinesterase enzymes, thereby elevating the levels and prolonging the action of the cholinergic neurohormone at its receptor sites (see Fig. 13-1). Based on the length of time that these substances interfere with the functioning of the cholinesterase enzyme, they are categorized as *reversible* or *irreversible* cholinesterase inhibitors. The duration of action of the reversible cholinesterase inhibitors is measured in terms of hours, whereas the action of the irreversible cholinesterase inhibitors is usually given in terms of weeks or months.

Reversible Cholinesterase Inhibitors

The reversible cholinesterase inhibitors are generally short-acting compounds that are capable of increasing the levels of functional acetylcholine at the cholinergic receptor sites. By facilitating cholinergic neurotransmission, these agents have a range of clinical applications. They may be employed in the treatment of glaucoma following local instillation into the eye, but their principal uses are for the diagnosis and treatment of myasthenia gravis and as antidotes for overdoses with anticholinergic or curariform drugs (*e.g.*, gallamine, pancuronium).

Physostigmine is used both topically and systemically, and its indications are outlined below. Demecarium is only applied topically as a miotic. The remaining four drugs (ambenonium, edrophonium, neostigmine, pyridostigmine) are given systemically for the diagnosis and treatment of myasthenia gravis.

Physostigmine, Ophthalmic
(Eserine, Isopto-Eserine)

Physostigmine, Systemic
(Antilirium)

MECHANISM AND ACTIONS

Physostigmine competes with ACh for active sites on the surface of the cholinesterase enzyme; as a result, the hydrolytic cleavage of the ACh molecule is retarded. Thus, functional levels of ACh are increased and its action is prolonged at muscarinic and nicotinic receptor sites throughout the body. Systemic administration of physostigmine elicits the typical range of "cholinergic" side-effects. The drug is highly lipid soluble, unlike other cholinesterase inhibitors; hence, it penetrates easily into the central nervous system (CNS) and is therefore of value in the symptomatic treatment of overdosage with centrally acting anticholinergic drugs.

USES

Topical
1. Reduction of elevated intraocular pressure in open-angle glaucoma
2. To reverse mydriasis caused by anticholinergic drugs
3. Treatment of lice infestations of eyelid and accessory structures

Systemic
1. To reverse the toxic peripheral and central effects resulting from overdosage or poisoning with drugs having an anticholinergic action (*e.g.*, tricyclic antidepressants, scopolamine)
2. To antagonize the CNS-depressant effects of diazepam and overcome the respiratory-de-

pressant effects of morphine (investigational uses)

3. Treatment of delirium tremens and Alzheimer's disease (investigational uses)

ADMINISTRATION AND DOSAGE
Physostigmine is available as an ophthalmic ointment (0.25%), ophthalmic solution (0.25%, 0.5%), and as an injectable solution containing 1 mg/ml.

Topically, 2 drops of the 0.25% or 0.5% solution is applied two to four times a day as needed. Alternately, a 1-cm strip of the 0.25% ophthalmic ointment may be used one to three times a day.

For antidoting toxic effects of anticholinergic drugs, 2 mg is given IM or IV and repeated as necessary as life-threatening signs (arrhythmias, convulsions) recur. IV injection should be given slowly, over 1 minute to 2 minutes, to prevent adverse reactions.

Pediatric
In life-threatening situations only, a dose of 0.5 mg may be given by slow IV injection and repeated at 5-minute to 10-minute intervals as needed, to a maximum dose of 2 mg.

FATE
Following topical application, the peak miotic effect occurs in 1 hour to 2 hours, lasting 12 hours to 24 hours. Absorption is rapid following IM administration. Systemic doses are rapidly metabolized by cholinesterases. Effects following IV administration are seen within 5 minutes and persist up to 1 hour. The drug readily enters the CNS. The plasma half-life is approximately 1 hour to 2 hours.

SIDE-EFFECTS/ADVERSE REACTIONS
Common side-effects following ophthalmic use are decreased visual acuity, eyelid twitching, increased tearing, and mild headache. More serious untoward reactions resulting from ophthalmic administration are altered pigmentation of the iris, conjunctival irritation, and follicular cysts.

Systemic application frequently results in sweating, nausea, cramping, salivation, and urinary urgency. Excessive systemic doses or too rapid IV injection can lead to a "cholinergic crisis," characterized by a wide range of cholinergic effects including dyspnea, bradycardia, palpitations, muscle cramping, excessive weakness, vomiting, hypotension, bronchospasm, convulsions, and ultimately respiratory paralysis. (Refer to the discussion of

antimyasthenic drugs, which follows, for further information on diagnosing a cholinergic crisis.)

CONTRAINDICATIONS AND PRECAUTIONS
Ophthalmic use of physostigmine is contraindicated in the presence of iris or ciliary body inflammation or narrow-angle glaucoma prior to iridectomy. Contraindications to the systemic use of physostigmine include bronchial asthma, gangrene, severe cardiovascular (CV) disease, diabetes, and intestinal or urinary bladder obstruction, and patients receiving choline esters or depolarizing neuromuscular blocking agents. Cautious use is warranted in patients with epilepsy, parkinsonism, or bradycardia.

INTERACTIONS
1. The systemic effects of physostigmine can be potentiated by choline esters, other systemically acting cholinesterase inhibitors, and depolarizing neuro-muscular blocking agents, such as succinylcholine or decamethonium.

Demecarium Bromide
(Humorsol)

MECHANISM AND ACTIONS
Demecarium inhibits enzymatic breakdown of ACh, thus prolonging its effects at cholinergic receptor sites. Local application in the eye elicits an intense miosis and contracts the ciliary muscle, facilitating outflow of aqueous humor. It is usually classified as a reversible cholinesterase inhibitor, but its action is significantly longer than that of other reversible inhibitors.

USES
1. Treatment of open-angle glaucoma
2. Diagnosis and treatment of accommodative esotropia (convergent strabismus)

ADMINISTRATION AND DOSAGE
Demecarium is used as an ophthalmic solution (0.125% or 0.25%).

Recommended doses are:

Glaucoma—initially, 1 to 2 drops of a 0.125% solution. Increase from 1 to 2 drops twice a week to 1 to 2 drops twice a day as condition warrants. Usual dosage for open-angle glaucoma is 1 drop twice a day.

Accommodative esotropia—1 drop of 0.125%

solution daily for 2 weeks, then 1 drop every other day for 2 weeks to 3 weeks. Reduce dosage frequency as condition improves to twice a week, then once a week. Discontinue and evaluate patient status regularly (*i.e.*, every 4 weeks–12 weeks). If after 4 months patient still requires 1 drop every 2 days to control condition, discontinue therapy.

FATE
Following topical application, miosis develops within 30 minutes and is maximal within 2 hours to 3 hours. Residual miosis may persist up to 1 week following a single instillation. Intraocular pressure is lowered within 12 hours.

SIDE-EFFECTS/ADVERSE REACTIONS
The most frequently observed side-effects are blurred vision, eyelid twitching, brow pain, and lacrimation. Photophobia has also been commonly reported. More serious local effects include cysts on the iris, conjunctival hyperemia and thickening, lens opacities, activation of latent iritis, and, rarely, retinal detachment.

Significant systemic absorption can result in cholinergic stimulation, characterized by nausea, vomiting, abdominal pain, urinary frequency, sweating, muscular weakness, hypotension, and bradycardia.

CONTRAINDICATIONS AND PRECAUTIONS
Demercarium is contraindicated in narrow-angle glaucoma, ocular hypertension, and inflammatory conditions of the eye. *Cautious use* is indicated in patients with bronchial asthma, peptic ulcer, pronounced bradycardia, recent myocardial infarction, parkinsonism, and epilepsy. Safe use in pregnancy has not been established.

INTERACTIONS
See under Physostigmine for possible interactions following systemic absorption of demecarium.

NURSING CONSIDERATIONS
Optimal doses of physostigmine and demecarium require frequent initial tonometer readings. The nurse should let the patient know the reasons for these frequent tests and observe him carefully for side-effects. The advantage of these drugs is that they are longer lasting and need to be taken less frequently.

Since both drugs are long acting, patients need to know that headache and dimness of vision may persist for some time after initiation of treatment. Another bothersome side-effect, localized twitching, may occur following instillation of the medication. Preparing the patient for these events will help him cope with the therapy.

The patient taking physostigmine or demecarium must also be taught careful self-administration of medication (see Table 13-3 and also Chap. 8). In addition, patients must be careful in storing these drugs. Help them to identify a storage place at home where the medication will not be exposed to high or excessive heat. See also the nursing considerations for cholinesterase inhibitors later in this chapter.

Table 13-4
Comparison of Onset and Duration of Action Among Antimyasthenic Cholinesterase Inhibitors

Drug	Route of Administration	Onset	Duration
Ambenonium	PO	30 min	4 h–6 h
Edrophonium	IM	2 min–10 min	10 min–40 min
	IV	1 min	5 min–20 min
Neostigmine	PO	30 min–60 min	2 h–4 h
	IM	15 min–30 min	2 h–4 h
	IV	5 min–10 min	2 h–4 h
Pyridostigmine	PO	20 min–40 min	3 h–6 h
	IM	10 min–15 min	2 h–4 h
	IV	2 min–5 min	2 h–4 h

Ambenonium
(Mytelase)

Edrophonium
(Tensilon)

Neostigmine
(Prostigmin)

Pyridostigmine
(Mestinon, Regonol)

These four reversible cholinesterase inhibitors are primarily used for the diagnosis and treatment of

myasthenia gravis (see Disease Brief: Myasthenia Gravis). While they all function in a similar manner (*i.e.*, facilitation of cholinergic neurotransmission at the neuromuscular junction), thus improving the muscle weakness characteristic of myasthenia, significant differences exist among the four drugs with regard to onset and duration of action and incidence and severity of side-effects. Table 13-4 lists the onset and duration of each of these drugs when administered by various routes. However, since many similarities also exist among these four drugs, they will be discussed here as a group. Individual characteristics and dosage ranges are presented in Table 13-5.

 DISEASE BRIEF

■ *Myasthenia Gravis*

Myasthenia gravis is a disease affecting skeletal muscles, and is characterized by muscular weakness and rapid fatigability that lessen with rest and worsen with exercise. Any skeletal muscle may be affected (and severe cases involve most skeletal muscles) but those most commonly involved initially are the smaller muscles of the head, neck, and extremities. Early indications, therefore, include ptosis, diplopia, and difficulty in speaking or swallowing. Involvement of the respiratory muscles is usually the ultimate cause of death. The basic defect in myasthenia is a significant reduction (70%–90%) in the number of functional cholinergic receptors on the postjunctional muscle end-plate, which greatly impairs normal cholinergic activation of the muscle fibers. This receptor deficit is believed to occur as a result of an autoimmune process that produces antibodies against the body's own cholinergic receptors. Treatment is directed toward elevating the levels of functional ACh at the neuromuscular junction in an attempt to improve cholinergic stimulation of the available receptors.

    The nursing care goals for which medication may be used are aimed at decreasing the symptoms and limitations caused by the muscle weakness. Provision for respiratory support and creative responses to difficulties in swallowing and the resulting problems in meeting nutritional needs, as well as dealing with the depression that results from coping with this chronic, progressive illness are the focus of the nurse's attention.

MECHANISM AND ACTIONS
The reversible cholinesterase inhibitors transiently inhibit cholinesterase enzymes, allowing an intensification and prolongation of the actions of ACh at cholinergic receptors throughout the body, including the neuromuscular junction. In addition, neostigmine exhibits a direct ACh-like stimulating effect at cholinergic receptors on skeletal muscle and may also increase the release of presynaptic stores of ACh. These drugs all improve muscle strength and delay fatigue. Generalized cholinergic responses are frequently noted at the outset of ther-

apy, and may require use of a muscarinic antagonist (see Chap. 14) to minimize disturbing side-effects. Tolerance to the muscarinic effects frequently develops, however.

USES
1. Diagnosis of myasthenia gravis (edrophonium)
2. Treatment of myasthenia gravis (ambenonium, neostigmine, pyridostigmine)
3. Symptomatic management of the symptoms of poisoning with nondepolarizing skeletal mus-

Table 13-5
Antimyasthenic Cholinesterase Inhibitors

Drug	Preparations	Usual Dosage Range	Clinical Considerations
Ambenonium chloride (Mytelase)	Tablets—10 mg	Adults: 5 mg–25 mg 3 to 4 times/day (up to 75 mg/dose has been used in certain instances but is highly dangerous) Children: 0.5 mg–1.5 mg/kg day in 3 or 4 divided doses	Longest acting of the orally effective antimyasthenic drugs; lower incidence of GI, respiratory, and CV side-effects than neostigmine. Cumulative effects have occurred due to prolonged action; thus, be alert for early signs of overdosage (*e.g.*, salivation, difficulty in chewing or swallowing, muscle weakness). Warning of overdosage may be minimal, moving quickly from the first appearance of side-effects to serious toxic manifestations. Teach the patient and family to contact the physician at the first sign of side-effects. This is a major concern for patients taking over 150 mg daily. To maximize the advantage of this drug's prolonged duration of action, teach the patient to take the drug at bedtime so he can sleep through the night without recurrence of symptoms.
Edrophonium chloride (Tensilon)	Injection—10 mg/ml	*Diagnosis* Adults: 2 mg IV over 15 sec–30 sec. If no reaction in 45 sec, inject additional 8 mg; alternately, give 10 mg IM if veins are inaccessible. Children IV-1 mg if weight is less than 75 lb; 2 mg if more than 75 lb; administer within 45 sec; titrate up to 5 mg in small children and up to 10 mg in larger children. IM—2 mg if weight is less than 75 lb; 5 mg if more than 75 lb *Curariform Antagonists* 10 mg IV over 30–45 sec; repeat as necessary to a maximum of 40 mg.	Short-acting drug primarily used for differential diagnosis of myasthenia and for reversing neuromuscular block produced by curariform drugs (*e.g.*, tubocurarine, gallamine). *Not* indicated for chronic therapy of myasthenia. Positive response to diagnostic test is a brief improvement in muscle strength without muscle fasciculations. Nonmyasthenic patients evidence transient fasciculations and temporary muscle weakness. Patients in cholinergic crisis show further muscle weakness and marked increase in oropharyngeal secretions; anticholinesterase drugs should be discontinued. Atropine sulfate and facilities for respiratory assistance should be immediately available. Transient bradycardia can occur, and cardiac arrest has been reported. Check pulse frequently during therapy
Neostigmine bromide (Prostigmin)	Tablets—15 mg	*Oral* Adults: 15 mg–30 mg 3–4 times/day. Increase gradually until maximum benefit, up	Reversible cholinesterase inhibitor that also has a direct agonistic action on cholinergic receptor sites. Parenteral form can be used to diagnose myasthenia, but edrophonium is

(continued)

Table 13-5 (continued)
Antimyasthenic Cholinesterase Inhibitors

Drug	Preparations	Usual Dosage Range	Clinical Considerations
Neostigmine bromide (Prostigmin) (continued)		to 375 mg/day. Dosage interval must be individualized. Children: 2 mg/kg/day every 3 h–4 h	preferred due to more rapid onset and shorter duration. Also indicated for symptomatic treatment of curariform drug overdosage. Poorly absorbed orally. Higher incidence of muscarinic side-effects than other orally effective antimyasthenics. Monitor changes in muscle strength and side-effects in relation to each dose and document accordingly. Keep atropine on hand at all times and be prepared to support respiration.
Neostigmine methylsulfate (Prostigmin)	Injection—1:1000, 1:2000, 1:4000	*SC, IM* *Myasthenia* Adults: 0.5 mg; repeat as necessary based on response. Children: 10 mcg–40 mcg/kg every 2 to 3 h *Diagnosis of Myasthenia* Adults: 0.022 mg/kg IM Children: 0.04 mg/kg IM *IV* *Curariform antidote* Adults: 0.5 mg–2 mg by slow IV injection. Repeat to a total dose of 5 mg. Children: 0.07 mg–0.08 mg/kg/dose	See above.
Pyridostigmine bromide (Mestinon, Regonol)	Tablets—60 mg Sustained release tablets—180 mg Syrup—60 mg/5 ml Injection—5 mg/ml	*Oral* Adults: 60 mg–120 mg every 3 h–4 h initially. Maintenance dose can range from 60 mg to 1.5 g a day. Average is 600 mg daily. Children: 7 mg/kg/day in 5 or 6 divided doses. *IM, IV* *Curare antidote* 10 mg–20 mg *Myasthenia* 2 mg every 2 h–3 h IM or IV	Most commonly used medication in treatment of myasthenia. Shorter acting than ambenonium, and has a slower onset but longer duration of action than neostigmine. Lower incidence of GI side-effects, salivation, and bradycardia than neostigmine and ambenonium. Long-acting tablets are used every 6 h for maintenance therapy but increase the risk of cholinergic crisis. When using sustained-release tablets, reinforce with the patient the need for accurate scheduling of administration at least every 6 h, at the same time every day. The first signs of overdose may be twitching of muscles around the eyes, mouth, or upper arms. Teach the patient to report these symptoms as soon as they occur.

cle relaxants (IV pyridostigmine, neostigmine, or edrophonium)
4. Relief of postoperative abdominal distention and urinary retention (neostigmine; infrequent use)

ADMINISTRATION AND DOSAGE
See Table 13-5.

FATE
Oral absorption of all drugs is generally poor and erratic. Edrophonium is given by injection only and has a rapid onset and short duration of action. Ambenonium exhibits the longest duration of action with oral administration (see Table 13-4), followed by pyridostigmine and neostigmine. Penetration of all drugs into the CNS is minimal. Metabolism is by way of hepatic enzymes, and metabolites are eliminated by the kidneys.

SIDE-EFFECTS/ADVERSE REACTIONS
The most frequently encountered side-effects represent generalized activation of muscarinic and ganglionic nicotinic receptor sites by the elevated levels of ACh and include nausea, diarrhea, abdominal discomfort, salivation, sweating, urinary urgency, and muscle twitching. The incidence of muscarinic side-effects is greatest with neostigmine, less with ambenonium, and least with pyridostigmine among the chronically used oral medications.

A range of other adverse reactions has been reported with use of these drugs, although not every drug has been associated with each adverse effect.

CNS—dysphonia, irritability, restlessness, convulsions
Respiratory—increased bronchial secretions, laryngospasm, bronchoconstriction, respiratory paralysis
Ocular—miosis, cycloplegia, diplopia, lacrimation
Cardiovascular—bradycardia, arrhythmias, hypotension
GI—increased salivary, gastric, and intestinal secretions, dysphagia, cramping
Other—muscle weakness, urinary frequency or incontinence, skin rash (neostigmine, pyridostigmine); thrombophlebitis with IV use

Overdosage may lead to a cholinergic crisis, characterized by intensified muscarinic and nicotinic effects such as diarrhea, profuse sweating, bradycardia, increased secretions, and profound muscle weakness, perhaps leading to respiratory paralysis and death. In patients with myasthenia, it may be difficult to distinguish a *myasthenic* crisis from a *cholinergic* crisis, inasmuch as the major symptom is extreme muscle weakness. Differentiation is extremely critical, however, since the treatment of the two conditions differs radically. Generally, if the weakness develops within 1 hour after drug administration, cholinergic drug overdosage is probable, and a cholinergic crisis should be suspected. More slowly developing weakness (*e.g.*, 3 hours–4 hours) usually indicates underdosage or patient resistance to the drug, and a myasthenic crisis is likely. If symptomatic determination cannot be made, edrophonium IV may be used to distinguish a cholinergic crisis from a myasthenic crisis. In the former, the symptoms are temporarily worsened, whereas in the latter, muscle weakness improves following drug injection. Obviously, this is a hazardous procedure and should be undertaken only by personnel skilled in the administration of the drug and assessment of the patient.

Treatment of a myasthenic crisis requires increased amounts of cholinesterase inhibitor drugs, whereas a cholinergic crisis necessitates immediate withdrawal of all cholinergic drugs and administration of atropine.

CONTRAINDICATIONS AND PRECAUTIONS
Mechanical intestinal or urinary obstruction is a contraindication for all four drugs in this group. In addition, neostigmine and pyridostigmine are contraindicated in patients with bromide sensitivity (because they are bromide salts) or with urinary tract infections. *Cautious use* is indicated in patients with bronchial asthma, peptic ulcer, cardiac arrhythmias, hypotension, epilepsy, and following a recent coronary occlusion. Safety for use in pregnancy has not been determined. When given IV to women near term, the drugs may induce premature labor.

INTERACTIONS
1. The actions of the antimyasthenic cholinesterase inhibitors can be antagonized by drugs having a neuromuscular blocking action, such as aminoglycoside antibiotics, general and local anesthetics, and certain antiarrhythmic agents (quinidine, procainamide).
2. Neostigmine may prolong the action of depolarizing muscle relaxants such as succinylcholine (see Chap. 19).

3. Neostigmine can antagonize the effects of nondepolarizing neuromuscular blocking agents, such as as gallamine, pancuronium, and metocurine.
4. Magnesium can antagonize the effects of anticholinesterase drugs on skeletal muscle, since it exerts a direct muscle-relaxing effect.

■ *Nursing Process*

□ *ASSESSMENT*

□ *Subjective Data*
A careful drug history should be obtained in order to avoid potentially dangerous drug interactions.

The most important baseline data for the nurse will be the patient's motivation to use the drug therapy to remain independent. In addition, family support and interaction will be critical when teaching the patient and other family members about the complex and potentially frightening management of the disease process.

□ *Objective Data*
Motor skills testing and muscle strength assessments will also be done to determine the type and dosage of drug to be prescribed.

□ *NURSING DIAGNOSES*
Actual nursing diagnoses include
   Knowledge deficit: about the action, administration schedule, and side-effects of the drug
Potential nursing diagnoses related to the drug therapy for the patient with myasthenia include
   Alteration in bowel elimination: diarrhea or incontinence depending on drug reaction
   Ineffective breathing patterns related to inadequate dose or development of drug tolerance
   Alteration in cardiac output: decreased related to drug side-effect or inadequacy of dose
   Impaired verbal communication related to drug failure or development of tolerance
   Ineffective family or individual coping (may range from compromised to disabling depending on how members view role changes related to the illness and how they respond to the complex regimen)
   Noncompliance with the prescribed regimen (could be related to hopelessness, depression, death wish, or other factors)
   Alteration in nutrition: less than body requirements related to drug's inability to reduce symptoms of dysphagia
   Powerlessness related to the inability to control symptoms completely with drug therapy
   Self-care deficit (will vary depending on the degree to which the drug restores muscle function)
   Alteration in patterns of urinary elimination (ranging from increased urgency to incontinence related to drug side-effects)

□ *PLAN*
The nursing care goals should focus on teaching the patient how to manage his drug regimen within the prescribed range, how to recognize the symptoms of overdose or toxicity, and how to deal with emergencies.

□ *INTERVENTION*
Drug therapy with reversible cholinesterase inhibitors is potentially dangerous. The patient must know what drug he is taking and what other drugs he must avoid (see Interactions, above). The myasthenic patient should be encouraged to wear a Medic-Alert bracelet or some other form of identification so any care giver would readily know what drug he is taking.

To some extent, the myasthenic patient will exercise control over his drug regimen. Doses of the drug will be altered in order to reduce disease effects without inducing side-effects, and the patient should have a say in determining the dose to meet his needs. Doses are also adjusted to correspond to times of the day when stress is increased or activity is increased, such as at mealtimes and before shopping. However, the timing of doses should remain consistent so blood levels are not allowed to fall. The patient should be placed on a schedule that suits his life-style and then encouraged to adhere to it faithfully. The patient or his family, or both, must become "clock-watchers," and reminders such as the alarms on a digital watch may become very useful.

The margin of safety on all of these drugs is narrow. Therefore, combinations of cholinesterase inhibitors should never be used nor should the patient be exposed to insecticides that are chemically similar to the cholinesterase inhibitors (Malathion, Diazinon). More importantly, the patient and his family need to learn to recognize the symptoms of overdose: salivation, sweating, diarrhea, muscle weakness, bradycardia, nausea, vomiting, vivid dreams, and hallucinations. The antidote is atropine, and respiratory assistance should always be available. Family members must be willing to participate, since rapid action must be taken if overdose occurs. The family or support person must know how to rapidly access emergency medical assistance, how and when to give atropine, and how to do cardiopulmonary resuscitation should the patient go into respiratory arrest.

Just the idea that such an event could occur will be frightening to most families. The nurse needs to give the family and patient emotional support and allow them time to verbalize their concerns. Role-playing an emergency scene with the family may help them anticipate what to expect and how they will need to help.

☐ **EVALUATION**
Evaluate such outcomes as the patient's and family's ability to monitor the drug, to know and watch for side-effects, and to incorporate the regimen into daily life. Learning how to act in an emergency will take time but many families will learn in order to help the patient to survive and to decrease their own sense of helplessness. As with any chronic disease, acceptance of the disease and its regimen for control will be an ongoing process.

Irreversible Cholinesterase Inhibitors

The "irreversible" cholinesterase inhibitors are organophosphorus compounds that cause phosphorylation of the cholinesterase enzyme. This permanently inactivates the enzyme, and enzymatic activity remains impaired until new enzyme can be synthesized, often requiring weeks or even months for full restoration of function. These compounds were developed as potential chemical warfare agents (e.g., Soman, a nerve gas) and are now extensively used as pesticides and insecticides (e.g., Malathion, Parathion). Carelessness in their application annually results in many cases of intoxication and even death. Most of these compounds are quite lipid soluble and are therefore well absorbed from the skin, lungs, and GI tract. Acute intoxication with one of the organophosphorus insecticides following accidental environmental exposure results in symptoms of cholinergic (i.e., muscarinic) excess, such as miosis, sweating, salivation, bronchoconstriction, bradycardia, urinary incontinence, vomiting, and diarrhea. CNS excitation (e.g., insomnia, tremors, confusion, convulsions) is promi-

nent initially because these compounds readily traverse the blood–brain barrier; however, in severe poisoning, the major danger lies in a secondary CNS depression, leading to respiratory paralysis and cardiovascular collapse. While the organophosphorus inhibitors preferentially attack plasma cholinesterase (i.e., butyrocholinesterase), their pharmacologic and toxicologic effects are due almost entirely to increasing inhibition of neuronal acetylcholinesterase when the inhibitors attain sufficient levels. Plasma cholinesterase is synthesized by the liver within a few days, whereas regeneration of acetylcholinesterase at cholinergic receptors requires several weeks to months. Thus, the long duration of action of these compounds makes poisoning a serious matter, and prompt antidotal measures are necessary to prevent fatalities.

Supportive measures in cases of organophosphate poisoning include (1) maintenance of vital signs and respiratory assistance by artificial means if necessary; (2) prevention of further absorption by removal of contaminated clothing and by thorough washing of the skin; (3) control of convulsions (e.g., IV diazepam or sodium thiopental) and maintenance of blood pressure (e.g., adrenergic pressor amines); (4) treatment of symptoms of muscarinic excess with atropine, 1 mg to 2 mg IV every 5 minutes to 15 minutes as needed; and (5) specific antidoting of cholinesterase inhibitors with pralidoxime, as described later in this chapter.

The commercial importance of the toxicology of the irreversible cholinesterase inhibitors used in agriculture is well established. Conversely, due to their extreme potency, lack of receptor specificity, and persistent action, the clinical usefulness of this type of chemical compound is quite limited. Currently, only two irreversible cholinesterase inhibitors are available for therapeutic application, echothiophate iodide and isofluorophate, and their use is confined to local instillation in the eye for the production of prolonged miosis and for the reduction of elevated intraocular pressure in glaucoma.

Echothiophate Iodide
(Phospholine Iodide)

MECHANISM AND ACTIONS
Echothiophate produces a long-lasting inhibition of cholinesterase enzymatic function, thereby potentiating the action of endogenous ACh at the cholinergic receptor sites. Enzymatic activity returns only upon synthesis of new enzyme. Local

instillation into the eye results in miosis, increased accommodation because of ciliary muscle contraction, and reduced intraocular pressure resulting from enhanced outflow of aqueous humor.

USES
1. Treatment of chronic, open-angle glaucoma in patients not adequately controlled by shorter-acting miotics
2. Treatment of angle-closure glaucoma following iridectomy
3. Diagnosis and treatment of accommodative esotropia (convergent strabismus), a condition in which one eye is fixed on an object while the other eye deviates inward

ADMINISTRATION AND DOSAGE
Echothiophate is available as a powder with an aqueous diluent for reconstitution into 0.03%, 0.06%, 0.125%, or 0.25% solution. Once prepared, solutions are stable for several weeks at room temperature and much longer if refrigerated. Dosage is as follows:

Glaucoma—1 drop of a 0.03% to 0.25% solution once or twice a day, depending on response

Accommodative esotropia

Diagnosis—1 drop of a 0.125% solution once a day in both eyes for 2 weeks to 3 weeks. A favorable response may begin within a few hours.

Treatment—1 drop of a 0.06% solution daily or a 0.125% solution every other day. Reduce dose as treatment progresses.

FATE
Miosis develops within 10 minutes to 20 minutes, becomes maximal within 30 minutes, and may persist for up to 1 month. Intraocular pressure is reduced within 6 hours, peak effect occurs within 24 hours, and effects persist for up to 1 month.

SIDE-EFFECTS/ADVERSE REACTIONS
Commonly encountered side-effects include stinging and burning in the eye, lacrimation, blurred vision, brow ache, hyperemia, and eyelid twitching. Other local effects noted are headache, photosensitivity, iris cysts, conjunctival thickening, lenticular opacities, iritis, and, rarely, retinal detachment. Systemic absorption, if significant, can result in a wide range of cholinergic symptoms, as outlined previously.

CONTRAINDICATIONS AND PRECAUTIONS
Echothiophate is contraindicated in acute angle-closure glaucoma and uveitis. *Cautious use* is indicated in patients with corneal abrasions, retinal detachment, bronchial asthma, GI spasticity, epilepsy, parkinsonism, and severe bradycardia.

INTERACTIONS
1. Use of echothiophate may result in increased toxic effects with organophosphate insecticide exposure.
2. Other cholinesterase inhibitors may potentiate the effects of echothiophate.
3. Effects of succinylcholine, a skeletal muscle relaxant which is also hydrolyzed by cholinesterase, may be increased in patients receiving echothiophate, possibly resulting in respiratory and cardiovascular depression.

NURSING CONSIDERATIONS
Echothiophate iodide can produce cholinergic crisis if overdosage occurs. As with all cholinesterase inhibitors, the patient must learn to watch for the development of side-effects and signs of toxicity. The patient must also learn that increasing the dosage increases the chance of toxicity so the prescribed treatment and timing must be strictly adhered to. Most patients will take just one dose per day; advise administration at bedtime to minimize the inconvenience of blurred vision during the day.

The patient may develop tolerance to this drug with prolonged use. For this reason, the physician may alternate therapy with another miotic or discontinue the drug for a period of time. The patient needs to understand that this does not mean he is "cured" and must start the drug again when prescribed.

Isoflurophate
(Floropryl)

Isoflurophate is similar to echothiophate in actions, indications, and toxicity. However, since it is insoluble in water, it is only available as an ophthalmic ointment (0.25%), which many patients find inconvenient to use. Following application to the lower conjunctival sac, miosis occurs within 15 minutes to 30 minutes, and becomes maximal within 4 hours. Effects may persist for several weeks because of the permanent inactivation of cholinesterase enzyme. Isoflurophate is unstable in water. Potency is lost if the ointment comes in contact with moisture; thus, the tip of the tube should not be allowed to come into contact with any moist surface. The drug is readily absorbed from the skin, and systemic effects have occurred following topical contact. Refer to the discussion of echothiophate, above, for applicable adverse effects, cautions, and drug interactions.

ADMINISTRATION AND DOSAGE
Isoflurophate should be applied at bedtime, if possible, since blurred vision is common. The cornea should not be touched with the tube, and hands should be washed immediately after use. Avoid excessive application, since systemic side-effects are more likely with frequent usage.

Glaucoma—¼-inch strip of 0.025% ointment every 8 hours to 12 hours. Frequency of application is then adjusted based on tonometric readings of intraocular pressure. For maintenance therapy, the drug may be applied once every 8 hours to 72 hours.

Accommodative esotropia—not more than a ¼-inch strip of ointment every night for 2 weeks. Dosage is then reduced gradually to once-a-week application, as the patient's condition warrants. Therapy may need to be continued indefinitely.

NURSING CONSIDERATIONS
Since isoflurophate is rapidly absorbed through the skin and can cause systemic effects, the nurse may want to wear gloves when administering the ointment to a patient. After learning self-administering, the patient may also wish to do this to decrease the risk of toxicity. The drug is also somewhat unstable; keep the tube tightly closed and refrigerated to prevent moisture absorption and loss of potency.

Instruct the patient to report the use of this drug to any surgeon contemplating surgery. The drug should be discontinued preoperatively because it causes vasodilation, a surgical risk.

Cholinesterase Inhibitor Antidote

A specific antidote, pralidoxime (PAM), is available primarily for treating overdosage with organophosphorus cholinesterase inhibitors, which usually occurs as a result of insecticide poisoning. It is also capable of antagonizing the effects of the reversible cholinesterase inhibitors (e.g., neostigmine) used in the treatment of myasthenia gravis, although its effectiveness is much less with these

compounds. Treatment with PAM should be initiated as soon as possible following poisoning because the enzyme–inhibitor complex that has formed undergoes a fairly rapid process of "aging." Thus, within hours, the complex becomes extremely stable and largely resistant to the action of the reactivator PAM.

Pralidoxime Chloride
(PAM, Protopam)

MECHANISM AND ACTIONS
Pralidoxime disrupts the bond between the phosphorus group of the cholinesterase enzyme inhibitor and the esteratic site of the cholinesterase, thus displacing the molecules of the cholinesterase inhibitor from the enzymatic binding sites. Enzymatic activity is restored, and ACh is then inactivated normally. The drug may detoxify certain organophosphate compounds by a direct chemical reaction. Reactivation of the cholinesterase enzyme markedly diminishes the respiratory paralysis resulting from organophosphate intoxication.

USES
1. Antidote to poisoning with pesticides and insecticides of the organophosphate class, such as diazinon, malathion, parathion, dichlorvos, and TEPP, among others
2. Treatment of overdosage with anticholinesterase drugs used in myasthenia gravis

ADMINISTRATION AND DOSAGE
The drug is available as a powder with diluent (1 g/20 ml), injection solution (300 mg/ml), and also as 500-mg tablets. Dosing recommendations are

Insecticide poisoning
Adults—1 g to 2 g as IV infusion in 100 ml saline over 15 minutes to 30 minutes, often with atropine (2 mg–4 mg IV). Repeat dosage in 1 hour if muscle weakness persists. If IV administration is not feasible, drug may be given IM or SC. In the absence of severe GI symptoms, 1 g to 3 g may be given orally every 5 hours.

Treatment is most effective if begun within a few hours after poisoning. Effectiveness is greatly diminished if begun later than 36 hours after exposure.
Children—20 mg to 40 mg/kg by IV infusion with 0.5 mg to 1 mg atropine IV

Anticholinesterase overdosage—initially, 1 g to 2 g by IV injection followed by increments of 250 mg every 5 minutes until symptoms subside

FATE
Oral absorption is slow and highly erratic. Peak plasma levels occur in 5 minutes to 10 minutes IV and 10 minutes to 20 minutes IM. The drug is distributed throughout the extracellular fluid spaces and is not bound to plasma proteins. Pralidoxime is relatively short acting (plasma half-life is approximately 2 hours) and rapidly excreted in the urine as both metabolites and unchanged drug.

SIDE-EFFECTS/ADVERSE REACTIONS
The most common side-effects following parenteral use are dizziness, blurred vision, headache, drowsiness, and nausea. Other adverse reactions include tachycardia, laryngospasm, muscle weakness, and hyperventilation, especially with too rapid IV administration. Excitement and mania have been reported following recovery of consciousness. It is frequently difficult, however, to differentiate the toxic effects resulting from organophosphate poisoning from those due to administration of pralidoxime.

CONTRAINDICATIONS AND PRECAUTIONS
There are really no absolute contraindications, depending on the severity of the poisoning. Pralidoxime is not effective, however, in antidoting poisoning by phosphate compounds having no anticholinesterase activity.

Cautious use is indicated in patients with myasthenia gravis, impaired renal function, severe cardiac disease, bronchial asthma, or peptic ulcers.

INTERACTIONS
1. Barbiturates may be potentiated by cholinesterase inhibitors, and should be used cautiously in treating convulsions.

■ Nursing Process

□ ASSESSMENT
Determine what insecticide is involved in the poisoning. PAM is ineffective in cases of carbamate (Sevin) poisoning and should not be used against an insecticide that does not have anticholinesterase activity because the treatment could be deadly.

Initial laboratory work may include red blood cell count and plasma cholinesterase levels.

□ NURSING DIAGNOSES
All are *potential* diagnoses based on the response to drug therapy and include
   Anxiety related to symptoms of poisoning
   Ineffective breathing patterns related to laryngospasm or hyperventilation from too rapid IV administration
   Alteration in cardiac output: decreased related to tachycardia resulting from drug toxicity
   Impaired gas exchange related to laryngospasm or hyperventilation
   Sensory—perceptual alteration in vision: dizziness from rapid IV administration
   Alteration in thought processes related to drug response or effect of poison

□ PLAN
The nursing care goals should be aimed at facilitating rapid treatment before the poisonous insecticide becomes a stable compound in the body and at protecting the patient. An equally important goal is to provide protection for the nurse from systemic absorption of the insecticide.

□ INTERVENTION
In caring for the patient with poisoning, thoroughly wash the skin with alcohol if the skin is the route of contamination; dispose of clothing and wear gloves when initially undressing and bathing the patient. Discard linens used in bathing. If the poison was ingested, gastric lavage must be performed.

When administering the prescribed dose of PAM, infuse slowly, via IV pump if possible, at the prescribed rate, because tachycardia, muscle rigidity, and laryngospasm can occur if the infusion is too rapid. Symptoms of poisoning and of drug toxicity are similar, so monitor carefully.

Protect the patient during treatment since hyperactivity and excitement may occur during recovery from the poisoning. The physician will probably also want blood drawn for red blood cell and plasma cholinesterase level determinations at intervals to monitor the patient's progress.

If used in the presence of myasthenia, be aware that PAM can cause a myasthenic crisis. Have edrophonium on hand and be prepared to support respiration.

PAM can also potentiate atropine toxicity when used with that drug. Watch for signs of xerostomia, blurred vision, flushing, and excitement, and discontinue atropine immediately if symptoms occur.

□ *EVALUATION*

The outcomes against which to judge the success of the therapy would be a return to normal of the cholinesterase plasma levels, adequate respiratory function and blood gas values, and adequate recovery with minimal side-effects from the drug.

CASE STUDY

Glaucoma

Mr. Johnson, aged 50, has been wearing glasses for 3 years. He complains to his doctor that his vision seems worse with the glasses and that he has pain in his eyes, particularly in the right eye, especially in the morning. On tonometric examination, the ophthalmologist discovers that Mr. Johnson has glaucoma in both eyes, but it is more pronounced in the right. He prescribes pilocarpine 1% solution, 1 drop in the left eye and 2 drops in the right eye four times a day. You are asked to teach Mr. Johnson, who lives alone and works as an accountant, how to take his medication.

Discussion Questions

1. What information about Mr. Johnson's life-style and support systems do you need to know to plan appropriate teaching?
2. Mr. Johnson was seen in his doctor's office on an outpatient basis. What information will you give him at this initial meeting? How will you plan for follow-up?
3. What changes must Mr. Johnson make in his life-style to incorporate administration of this drug? Are these changes realistic?
4. How will you know if Mr. Johnson complies with the prescribed regimen?

REVIEW QUESTIONS

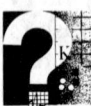

1. How are cholinergic drugs classified?
2. List the principal pharmacologic effects of acetylcholine.
3. What are the principal indications for the acetylcholine preparation used clinically?
4. Briefly describe the pathology of glaucoma.
5. What is the mechanism of action of cholinergic drugs used in treating glaucoma?
6. What are the common side-effects of pilocarpine when used in treating glaucoma? How may the patient be taught to manage these side-effects?
7. List several uses for the reversible cholinesterase inhibitors.
8. How may a cholinergic crisis be distinguished from a worsening of myasthenia gravis during therapy with a cholinesterase inhibitor?
9. Describe the symptoms of myasthenia gravis. Briefly discuss the etiology of this disease.
10. What is the principal application today for irreversible cholinesterase inhibitors?
11. Give the clinical indications for use of echothiophate iodide.

12. Name the cholinesterase inhibitor antidote. Briefly describe its mechanism of action.
13. What outcomes should be sought by the nurse when planning a teaching guide for the patient who will be taking cholinergic eye drops at home?
14. What action of the drugs listed in this chapter precipitates a cholinergic crisis?
15. What nursing intervention can effectively reduce the systemic absorption of most cholinergic eye drops after instillation?
16. Outline an initial plan for teaching the myasthenic patient and his family how to manage his illness with drug therapy.

BIBLIOGRAPHY

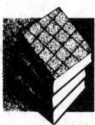

Drachman DB: Myasthenia gravis. N Engl J Med 298:136; 186, 1978
Drachman DB: The biology of myasthenia gravis. Annu Rev Neurosci 4:227, 1981
Fields WS: Myasthenia gravis. Ann NY Acad Sci 183:1, 1971
Gershon MD: The enteric nervous system. Annu Rev Neurosci 4:227, 1981
Hrovath M: Myasthenia gravis: A nursing approach. J Neurosurg February: 7, 1982
Jeglum E: Ocular therapeutics. Nurs Clin North Am September: 453, 1982
Kaufman PL, Weidman T, Robinson JR: Cholinergics. In Sears ML (ed): Pharmacology of the Eye. Handbook of Experimental Pharmacology, vol 69, p 149. Berlin, Springer-Verlag, 1984
Lindstrom J, Dau P: The biology of myasthenia gravis. Annu Rev Pharmacol 20:337, 1980
Nilsson E: Physostigmine treatment in various drug-induced intoxications. Ann Clin Res 14:165, 1982
Phelps CD: The treatment of open-angle glaucoma. Drug Ther 7:68, 1977
Quail C, Waddleton C: Treating the glaucomas. Nurses' Drug Alert 4:93, 1980
Schwartz B: Current concepts in ophthalmology: The glaucomas. N Engl J Med 299:182, 1978
Todd B: Using eye drops and ointments safely. Geriatric Nursing Jan/Feb:53, 1983
Watanabe AM: Cholinergic agonists and antagonists. In Rosen MR, Hoffman BF (eds): Cardiac Therapy, p 95. Hingham, MA, Nijhoff, 1983
Webster GD: Advances in treating lower urinary tract dysfunction. Drug Ther 12:113, 1982

Cholinergic Blocking (Parasympatholytic) Drugs

Classification and Actions

Characteristics of Anticholinergic Drugs

14

Cholinergic blocking drugs inhibit the actions of acetylcholine (ACh) and other cholinergic drugs at receptor sites on effector structures innervated by cholinergic nerve fibers and are frequently referred to as *anticholinergics.* In addition, the term *parasympatholytic* has also been used to describe these drugs, reflecting their ability to interfere with the functioning of the parasympathetic nervous system.

Classification and Actions

The diverse group of drugs classified as anticholinergics may be arbitrarily divided into three subgroups based on their *relative* specificity for the different types of cholinergic receptor sites (see Chap. 12).

1. *Muscarinic blockers* (e.g., atropine, propantheline). These compose the "classical" group of anticholinergic drugs that inhibit cholinergic transmission at post-ganglionic parasympathetic receptor sites (muscarinic; M), such as those found on smooth muscle, cardiac muscle, and exocrine glands.
2. *Ganglionic blockers* (e.g., mecamylamine, trimethaphan). These drugs inhibit cholinergic transmission at autonomic ganglia (nicotinic; N) sites in both parasympathetic and sympathetic nerve fibers.
3. *Neuromuscular blockers* (e.g., tubocurare, pancuronium). These drugs inhibit cholinergic transmission at the neuromuscular end-plate of skeletal muscle (nicotinic; N) receptor sites.

As indicated, the term *anticholinergic* has come to be associated primarily with the muscarinic blockers, since most of the commonly used anticholinergic drugs exert a relatively selective blocking action at M sites when used at normal dose levels. Considerable overlap in receptor blocking effects is observed, however, when large doses of any one of the three types of cholinergic blockers are administered. This extension of cholinergic blockage to all cholinergic receptors is frequently responsible for a disturbing range of side-effects when any of the cholinergic blocking agents is used in large amounts.

The distribution of cholinergic nerves in the body is vast; hence, cholinergic blockers can exert a wide range of pharmacologic effects depending on the extent of receptor antagonism at the various cholinergic receptor sites.

Major organs affected by the anticholinergic group of drugs include the eye, respiratory tract, gastrointestinal (GI) tract, urinary bladder, most nonvascular smooth muscle, exocrine glands, and, to varying degrees, the central nervous system (CNS). The principal pharmacologic actions of the anticholinergic group of drugs are listed in Table 14-1.

The effectiveness of cholinergic blockers as receptor antagonists varies considerably with the tissue under study. Thus, some cholinergically mediated effects (e.g., salivary and bronchial secretions) are blocked by very small doses of anticholinergics, whereas other effects (e.g., gastric acid secretion) are relatively resistant to antagonism by even large amounts of these drugs. The *decreasing order of sensitivity* (i.e., most sensitive listed first) of cholinergically innervated structures to blockade by atropine, the prototype anticholinergic drug, is listed below, with the corresponding result of blockade by atropine on each structure shown in parentheses:

1. Salivary, bronchial, and sweat glands (decreased secretions)
2. Iris sphincter (mydriasis), ciliary muscle (cycloplegia), and cardiac vagal nerve endings (tachycardia)
3. Urinary bladder detrusor (relaxation) and sphincter (contraction) muscles and GI smooth muscle (relaxation)
4. Gastric secretory cells (decreased secretion of hydrochloric acid, mucin, and digestive enzymes)

The efficacy of the various anticholinergic drugs in blocking activation of the cholinergic receptor sites is significantly *greater* when the agonist is an exogenous, or externally administered, cholinergic drug rather than endogenous ACh released from the cholinergic nerve ending. Thus, a higher concentration (i.e., larger dose) of cholinergic antagonist is needed to block effector structure responses to endogenous cholinergic nerve stimulation (i.e., effects due to release of ACh from presynaptic cholinergic nerve endings) than the actions of an exogenous cholinergic agonist. A similar situation exists with most other types of pharmacologic antagonists, for example, adrenergic blockers or antihistamines.

Atropine and scopolamine represent the principal naturally occurring anticholinergic drugs; along with hyoscyamine, they are known as the *belladonna alkaloids* (see Table 14-2). These compounds are rapidly absorbed orally, exert a relatively selective blocking action at muscarinic re-

Table 14-1
Pharmacologic Actions of Anticholinergics

Effects	Clinical Consequences
Cardiovascular	
Decreased heart rate in small doses (central vagal stimulation)	
Increased heart rate in large doses (peripheral vagal blockade)	Prevention of reflex bradycardia
Gastrointestinal Tract	
Decreased motility	Delayed gastric emptying, constipation
Decreased smooth muscle tone	
Decreased secretions	
Urinary Tract	
Relaxation of detrusor muscle	Urinary retention
Contraction of sphincter muscle	
Eye	
Mydriasis (decreased response of sphincter muscle)	Blurred vision
Cycloplegia (decreased response of ciliary muscle)	
Smooth Muscle	
Slight relaxation of nonvascular smooth muscle (e.g., biliary, bronchiolar, intestinal, uterine)	Relief of biliary or intestinal colic
Exocrine Glands	
Decreased sweat gland secretion	Anhidrosis, xerostomia, hyperthermia
Decreased salivation	
Decreased mucous gland secretion (nasopharynx and bronchioles)	
Central Nervous System	
Drowsiness, disorientation, hallucinations (large doses)	
Decreased tremor and rigidity of parkinsonism	Treatment of Parkinson's disease
Decreased vestibular activation	Prevention of motion sickness

ceptor sites, and readily enter the CNS, where atropine is primarily a stimulant and scopolamine functions as a depressant. The major disadvantage of the belladonna alkaloids is elicitation of a wide range of undesirable peripheral and central effects when the drugs are given in doses sufficient to reduce GI motility and secretions.

Therefore, a number of tertiary and quaternary ammonium compounds have been synthesized in an attempt to reduce the incidence of side-effects, while at the same time to provide a degree of cholinergic receptor site specificity. These goals, however, have only been partially realized.

The synthetic *tertiary amines* may be further subdivided into antispasmodics, mydriatics, and antiparkinsonian drugs (see Table 14-2). The antispasmodics demonstrate very little cholinergic blocking action; rather, their effects appear to re-

Table 14-2
Classification of Antimuscarinic Drugs

Belladonna Alkaloids

atropine
hyoscyamine
scopolamine

Tertiary Amine Antispasmodics

dicyclomine
oxybutynin
oxyphencyclimine

Tertiary Amine Mydriatics

cyclopentolate
tropicamide

Tertiary Amine Antiparkinsonian Agents

benztropine
biperiden
ethopropazine
orphenadrine hydrochloride
procyclidine
trihexyphenidyl

Quarternary Amine Anticholinergics

anisotropine
clidinium
glycopyrrolate
hexocyclium
homatropine
isopropamide
mepenzolate
methantheline
methscopolamine
oxyphenonium
propantheline
tridihexethyl

sult from a direct relaxant effect on GI smooth muscle. Thus, gastric acid secretion is relatively unimpaired, and these drugs are more properly termed *smooth muscle relaxants* rather than anticholinergics. The antiparkinsonian tertiary amines, on the other hand, are affective cholinergic antagonists with a higher ratio of central to peripheral action than other systemically administered cholinergic blocking drugs. Their use is therefore associated with a smaller incidence of peripheral anticholinergic side-effects.

The *quaternary amine* anticholinergics (see Table 14-2), unlike the belladonna alkaloids and tertiary amines, are poorly and erratically absorbed orally, and have a low lipid/water partition coeffi-

cient (*i.e.*, are less lipid soluble). Therefore, they do not readily cross lipid membranes, and their distribution to the GI mucosa, eye, and CNS is limited. They are of little value as mydriatics in the eye, and their central effects are minimal. Quaternization of the compounds increases their ganglionic blocking and neuromuscular blocking effects, however, and large doses may affect ganglionic and neuromuscular transmission.

Nevertheless, since the overall pharmacology of the various anticholinergic drugs is quite similar, the discussion of these drugs focuses on them as a group. Likewise, general nursing considerations are given for all cholinergic blocking drugs. The many individual drugs are listed in Table 14-3 later in the chapter, where specific characteristics and appropriate nursing applications for each drug are presented.

Characteristics of Anticholinergic Drugs

MECHANISM AND ACTIONS

In normal doses, there is inhibition of the muscarinic actions of ACh and related cholinergic agents at postganglionic parasympathetic receptor sites, including smooth muscle, cardiac muscle, and secretory glands. Larger doses, especially of quaternary amines, result in inhibition of transmission at ganglionic and neuromuscular cholinergic receptors as well. Effects (see Table 14-1) include decreased salivary and bronchial secretions and sweating, mydriasis, tachycardia, reduced GI and urinary motility, and decreased gastric acid secretion. Clinical responses include dry mouth, blurred vision, palpitations, constipation, and urinary hesitancy. Naturally occurring alkaloids and tertiary amines have an effect on the CNS as well, which may range from excitation to depression, depending on drug and dosage.

USES

Refer to Table 14-3 for specific uses for each drug.
1. Production of mydriasis and cycloplegia as an aid to ophthalmic examinations
2. Preoperative medication to reduce excess salivation and prevent bradycardia (scopolamine additionally produces a tranquilizing effect.)
3. Decrease GI motility and secretions in cases of peptic ulcer, GI spasms, irritable bowel syn-

drome, or other GI disorders (Large doses are necessary.)

4. Minimize muscarinic side-effects associated with cholinesterase inhibitor treatment of myasthenia
5. Relief of nasopharyngeal and bronchial secretions accompanying upper respiratory and allergic disorders
6. Relief of bronchoconstriction due to excessive parasympathetic function in bronchial asthma, chronic bronchitis, and other chronic obstructive pulmonary diseases
7. Prevention and relief of motion sickness
8. Treatment of enuresis in children, and relief of urinary frequency or urgency
9. Treatment of sinus bradycardia and conduction block due to excessive vagal tone
10. Production of obstetric amnesia in conjunction with analgesics (scopolamine—infrequent use)
11. Relief of dysmenorrhea—infrequent use
12. Antidote to overdosage with cholinergic agents (anticholinesterases, organophosphate insecticides and pesticides)
13. Relief of symptoms of parkinsonism (especially tremor and rigidity), and control of extrapyramidal disorders resulting from antipsychotic drug usage (see Chap. 31)

ADMINISTRATION AND DOSAGE
See Table 14-3.

FATE
Natural alkaloids and most tertiary amines are well absorbed in the GI tract and in the eye. Scopolamine is also absorbed significantly through the postauricular skin when applied in the form of a transdermal patch (see Table 14-3). Quaternary amines are poorly and erratically absorbed orally. The extent of distribution largely depends on lipid solubility; the more lipid-soluble alkaloids and tertiary amines are widely distributed peripherally and centrally, while quaternary amines have a more limited peripheral distribution. The duration of action of quaternary amines is somewhat longer than that of tertiary amines.

SIDE-EFFECTS/ADVERSE REACTIONS
The most frequently encountered side-effects with anticholinergic drugs are the result of nonselective receptor antagonism, and include xerostomia, blurred vision, urinary hesitancy, constipation, palpitations, and flushing. The occurrence of other adverse reactions depends in large measure on the dosage of the drug and the individual sensitivity of the patient. Adverse reactions associated with use of anticholinergics include:

GI—Vomiting, dysphagia, bloating, paralytic ileus, and possibly gastroesophageal reflux

Cardiovascular—Tachycardia, hypertension

CNS—Headache, nervousness, drowsiness, confusion, restlessness, insomnia, delirium, hallucinations, elevated body temperature

Ocular—Photophobia, cycloplegia, increased intraocular tension

Dermatologic—Rash, urticaria, systemic allergic reactions

Other—Urinary retention, dysuria, impotence, suppression of lactation, respiratory difficulties, muscular incoordination

Overdosage is characterized by many of the above symptoms; however, CNS effects are not generally observed with overdosage with quaternary amines. Treatment consists of removal of unabsorbed drug by emesis or gastric lavage, together with symptomatic therapy if necessary. Physostigmine (0.5 mg–2 mg IV repeated up to 5 mg), neostigmine (0.5 mg–1 mg IM every 2 hours–3 hours or 0.5 mg–2 mg IV), or pilocarpine (5 mg SC) can be used to relieve peripheral symptoms, while CNS excitation can also be controlled with physostigmine (see Chap. 13) as well as with a short-acting benzodiazepine (*e.g.*, diazepam) or barbiturate IV. Hypotension can be reversed with pressor amines such as levarterenol or metaraminol.

CONTRAINDICATIONS AND PRECAUTIONS
Contraindications to the use of systemic anticholinergics include narrow-angle glaucoma, adhesions between the iris and lens, tachycardia, severe coronary artery disease, obstructive GI disorders, paralytic ileus, severe ulcerative colitis, toxic megacolon, hiatal hernia with reflux esophagitis, urinary obstruction, myasthenia gravis, and serious renal or hepatic disease. *Cautious use* is warranted in patients with peptic ulcer, chronic obstructive pulmonary disease, hypertension, hyperthyroidism, congestive heart failure, spastic paralysis, ulcerative colitis, or biliary tract disease, and in infants, small children, and elderly or debilitated patients.

INTERACTIONS
1. The following drugs may increase the effects of anticholinergics: antihistamines, tricyclic anti-

depressants, antipsychotics, antiarrhythmics (quinidine, procainamide, disopyramide), benzodiazepine antianxiety drugs, meperidine, nitrates, methylphenidate, orphenadrine, primidone, monoamine oxidase inhibitors, and amantadine.

2. Guanethidine, histamine, and reserpine can antagonize the inhibitory effects of anticholinergics on gastric acid secretion.

3. Anticholinergics may enhance the bronchodilation produced by adrenergic drugs.

4. Antacids may impair the GI absorption of anticholinergics.

5. Anticholinergics may decrease the effects of cholinergics (*e.g.*, pilocarpine or physostigmine) used locally in the eye. Concurrent use of anticholinergics with haloperidol or corticosteroids may elevate intraocular pressure.

6. The effect of levodopa may be decreased by anticholinergics due to accelerated gastric breakdown.

7. The effect of metoclopramide on GI motility is antagonized by anticholinergics.

8. IV administration of anticholinergics can result in ventricular arrhythmias in patients receiving cyclopropane.

■ *Nursing Process*

□ *ASSESSMENT*
Careful history taking and physical assessment are important for any patient receiving anticholinergics. The patient with a history of hypertension, cardiovascular disease, recurrent or migraine headaches, glaucoma, or prostatic hypertrophy may not be an appropriate candidate for these drugs. Certainly the risks must be weighed against the benefits before therapy is started.

□ *NURSING DIAGNOSES*
Actual nursing diagnoses for these drugs include
Knowledge deficit regarding the action, administration, and side-effects of these drugs
Potential nursing diagnoses are all related to the side-effects of these drugs and may include
Alteration in bowel elimination: constipation
Alteration in cardiac output: decreased
Alteration in comfort related to xerostomia, flushing, palpitations

Sensory–perceptual alterations in vision and taste
Alteration in sexual function: impotence
Sleep pattern disturbance: insomnia
Urinary retention

□ *PLAN*
Nursing care goals should be aimed at assisting the patient to manage or report the many side-effects associated with these drugs.

□ *INTERVENTION*
Side-effects can frequently be decreased but not eliminated by altering the drug's dose. For dry mouth and thirst the nurse can recommend sucking on sourball candy or hard candy, or chewing gum. Encourage fluid intake, particularly in hot weather, since the patient will be more susceptible to dehydration.

The patient may need to learn when dizziness, drowsiness, or blurred vision is most likely to occur so he can space activities accordingly and he should be cautioned against driving or operating machinery at such times. The elderly patient is even more susceptible to such symptoms and should be cautioned to be even more careful when they occur. Climbing stairs and taking hot baths may actually enhance the symptoms, creating grave safety dangers, and should be avoided when symptoms occur.

The hospitalized patient should have vital signs taken regularly. Bradycardia and hypertension are possible side-effects, which should be reported. Teach the patient to recognize how his body feels if these symptoms occur. Once he is home he will be more likely to report them if such symptoms occur again.

Urinary output should also be monitored since urinary retention can occur. Remind the patient to be aware of the frequency of urination and the quantity. Teach him to report any changes.

Remember that the safety margin for anticholinergics is very narrow. Check the dosage ordered carefully to avoid toxicity. Most parenteral doses are less than 1 ml. If appropriate, use a tuberculin syringe to ensure an accurate amount is drawn from the vial.

□ *EVALUATION*
The best criterion for judging the success of therapy is the patient's ability to manage the symptoms for which the drug is prescribed and to handle the side-effects.

(*Text continues on p. 224.*)

Table 14-3
Anticholinergics

Drug	Preparations	Usual Dosage Range	Major Uses	Clinical Considerations
Belladonna Alkaloids				
atropine	Tablets—0.4 mg Hypodermic tablets —0.3 mg, 0.4 mg, 0.6 mg Ophthalmic drop—0.5%, 1%, 2%, 3% Ophthalmic oint- ment—0.5%, 1% Injection—0.05 mg/ml, 0.1 mg/ml, 0.3 mg/ml, 0.4 mg/ml, 0.5 mg/ml, 0.8 mg/ml, 1.2 mg/ml Solution for inhala- tion—0.2%, 0.5%	*Systemic* Adults: 0.4 mg–0.6 mg every 4 h–6 h Children: 0.1 mg–0.6 mg depending on weight *Ophthalmic* Adults: 1–2 drops 4 times/day Children: 1 drop 0.5%–1% 1–3 times/day *Refraction* 1–2 drops 1 h before examination *Inhalation (oral)* Adults: 0.025 mg/kg diluted with 3 ml–5 ml saline by nebulizer 3–4 times/day Children: 0.05 mg/ml diluted in saline by nebulizer 3–4 times/day	See general discus- sion of anticholin- ergics in text.	Atropine flush due to peripheral vaso- dilation is a nor- mal effect of the drug. When used in the eye, prevent systemic absorp- tion by compress- ing lacrimal sac following instilla- tion. Do not use in children under 6 years of age. Re- duce systemic dose in elderly patients, to minimize danger of tachycar- dia and elevated intraocular pres- sure. Inhaled atro- pine produces a se- lective bronchodi- latory effect with minimal tachycar- dia and drying of secretions. Oph- thalmic drops available with prednisolone (My- drapred). IV doses of greater than 2 mg may initially result in bradycar- dia, which will subside within minutes. Give oral doses no less than half hour before mealtimes for best response and give the nighttime dose at least 2 hours after the last meal.
belladonna alkaloids, levorotatory (Bella- foline)	Tablets—0.25 mg Injection—0.5 mg/ml	Adults Tablets—0.25 mg–0.5 mg 3 times/day Injection—0.25 mg–0.5 mg SC 1–2 times/day Children Tablets—0.125 mg–0.25 mg 3 times/day	Preoperative medica- tion, GI hypermo- tility, dysmenor- rhea, respiratory hypersecretion and bronchial asthma, motion sickness, enuresis, nocturia	Infrequently used preparation. Bella- dona tincture is also available for GI disturbances (spasms, hypermo- tility), 0.6 ml–1 ml 3–4 times/day.

(continued)

Table 14-3 (continued)
Anticholinergics

Drug	Preparations	Usual Dosage Range	Major Uses	Clinical Considerations
Belladonna Alkaloids (continued)				
belladonna extract	Tablets—15 mg Liquid—30 mg belladonna alkaloids/100 ml	Tablets—15 mg 3–4 times/day Liquid—0.6–1.0 ml 3–4 times/day	GI hypermotility, dysmenorrhea, parkinsonism, enuresis, motion sickness	Crude botanical preparation containing hyoscyamine, atropine, and scopolamine. Available in combination with phenobarbital (Chardonna-2, Belap) or butabarbital (Butibel). Used for GI disorders.
hyoscyamine sulfate (Anaspaz, Bellaspaz, Cystospaz, Cystospaz-M, Levsinex, Neoquess)	Tablets—0.125 mg, 0.13 mg, 0.15 mg Time-release capsules—0.375 mg Elixir—0.125 mg/5 ml Oral drops—0.125 mg/ml Injection—0.5 mg/ml	*Oral/Sublingual* Adults: 0.125 mg–0.25 mg 3–4 times/day Children: 2 yr–10 yr: ½ adult dose *Parenteral* SC, IM, or IV: 0.25 mg–0.5 mg 3–4 times/day	GI spasm and hypersecretion, cholinergic poisoning, dysmenorrhea, urinary spasm, acute rhinitis	Well absorbed orally. May be useful in controlling diarrhea. Tablets, elixir, and drops are also available with phenobarbital (Levsin PB).
scopolamine hydrobromide (Isopto Hyoscine, and various manufacturers)	Capsules—0.25 mg Injection—0.3 mg/ml, 0.4 mg/ml, 0.86 mg/ml, 1.0 mg/ml Ophthalmic drops—0.25%	*Systemic* Adults: (SC, IM) 0.3 mg–0.6 mg Children: (SC, IM) 0.1 mg–0.3 mg *Ophthalmic* 1–2 drops; adjust dosage to requirements *Motion Sickness* 0.25-mg capsule 1 h before travel; repeat in 4 h if necessary	Preanesthetic medication, motion sickness, spastic states, obstetric analgesia (with narcotics), ophthalmic mydriatic and cycloplegic, hyperhidrosis, excess salivation and secretion	CNS depression can occur with systemic use. Overdosage results in excitement, confusion, and delirium. Produces amnesia when given with narcotics. May produce delirium if used alone in severe pain. Effects generally persist 4 h to 6 h. Neostigmine and physostigmine are effective antidotes. Initial response to the drug may be a paradoxical excitation that will subside as the patient becomes more sedated. Do not be misled by such activity; guard the patient's safety by using side rails and other protective measures as needed.

(continued)

Table 14-3 (continued)
Anticholinergics

Drug	Preparations	Usual Dosage Range	Major Uses	Clinical Considerations
Belladonna Alkaloids (continued)				
scopolamine transdermal therapeutic system (Transderm-Scop)	Adhesive patch containing 1.5 mg scopolamine and delivering 0.5 mg over 3 days at a constant rate	Apply 1 system to the postauricular skin once every 3 days, several hours before exposure	Prevention of motion sickness	Circular adhesive patch that delivers steady-state blood levels of scopolamine over 3 days. An initial priming dose is released from the adhesive layer and quickly brings the plasma level to the desired steady state, which is maintained by continuous release of drug from the reservoir through the rate-controlling membrane. Most frequent side-effects are dry mouth, blurred vision, and drowsiness. Use with caution in the presence of glaucoma, urinary or GI obstruction, impaired liver or kidney function, and in the elderly. Safe use in children has not been established. Response to this drug will vary from person to person so the patient should be advised to put the disk on at least 3 hours before experiencing the aggravating motion. This way he will know if drowsiness is going to occur before operating a vehicle. Best results are obtained when the disk is applied the night before motion is experienced. Disk can be cut if a smaller dose is desired but may not

(continued)

Table 14-3 (continued)
Anticholinergics

Drug	Preparations	Usual Dosage Range	Major Uses	Clinical Considerations
Belladonna Alkaloids *(continued)*				
scopolamine transdermal therapeutic system (Transderm-Scop) *(continued)*				be effective for 3 days. Wash hands after application and after removal to decrease chance of drug contact with eyes. Wash site before application to improve adhesion and after removal to stop systemic absorption. Use a new site for a second application. Ask potential users about allergies to adhesives before applying patch.
Tertiary Amine Antispasmodics				
dicyclomine hydrochloride (Bentyl, and various other manufacturers)	Tablets—20 mg Capsules—10 mg, 20 mg Liquid—10 mg/5 ml Injection—10 mg/ml	Adults Oral—10 mg–20 mg 3–4 times/day IM—20 mg every 4–6 h Children: 5 mg–10 mg 3–4 times/day orally	GI spasm and hyper-irritability, ulcerative colitis, infant colic	Usually administered with antacids in GI disorders, since it does not reduce gastric secretions. Common side-effects are dizziness, abdominal fullness, and slight euphoria. Has fewer side-effects than atropine but is still contraindicated for any patient with the potential for an adverse response to anticholinergics.
oxybutynin chloride (Ditropan)	Tablets—5 mg Syrup—5 mg/5 ml	Adults: 5 mg 2–3 times/day Children: 5 mg twice a day	Urinary incontinence (reflex neurogenic bladder)	Exhibits both a direct smooth muscle relaxing action and a weak antimuscarinic action on smooth muscle. Has only one-fifth the anticholinergic activity of atropine but is 5–10 times more potent as an antispasmodic. Delays desire to void. Do not use in children under 5 years or in patients

(continued)

Table 14-3 (continued)
Anticholinergics

Drug	Preparations	Usual Dosage Range	Major Uses	Clinical Considerations
Tertiary Amine Antispasmodics (continued)				
oxybutynin chloride (Ditropan) (continued)				with paralytic ileus, colitis, intestinal atony, megacolon, myasthenia, or obstructive uropathy.
oxyphencyclimine hydrochloride (Daricon)	Tablets—10 mg	5 mg–10 mg 2–3 times/day	Adjunctive treatment of peptic ulcer	May induce CNS stimulation. Do not use in children under 12 years. Available with pentobarbital (Daricon-PB) and hydroxyzine (Vistrax).

Tertiary Amine Mydriatics

General Considerations

Both drugs often cause stinging on instillation. Prepare patient for this occurrence, which is transient. The cycloplegia and mydriasis that are induced by these drugs can result in transient photophobia. Instruct patients to wear dark glasses to reduce discomfort. Tell the patient to make arrangements for transportation when having one of these drugs instilled on an outpatient basis. It is unsafe for this person to drive for 2–3 hours after drug administration. Systemic effects can occur but are minimized if lacrimal sac is compressed for 2–3 min. Watch for flushing, tachycardia, confusion, fever, and ataxia after instillation, especially in children.

Drug	Preparations	Usual Dosage Range	Major Uses	Clinical Considerations
cyclopentolate hydrochloride (AK-Pentolate, Cyclogyl)	Ophthalmic drops—0.5%, 1%, 2%	*Refraction* Adults—1 drop 1%–2% solution, followed by a second drop in 5 min	Ophthalmic refraction for diagnostic purposes	Effects can persist for up to 24 h. Pilocarpine (1–2 drops 1%–2% solution) reduces recovery time to 3–6 h. Can produce behavioral disturbances in children (ataxia, disorientation, restlessness, incoherent speech) if absorbed systemically. Ophthalmic drops available with phenylephrine (Cyclomydril) for increased mydriatic effect
tropicamide (Mydriacyl)	Ophthalmic drops—0.5%, 1%	*Refraction* 1–2 drops of 1%; repeat in 5 min and every 20 min–30 min as needed to maintain mydriasis *Examination of Fundus* 1–2 drops 0.5% 20 min–30 min prior to examination	Ophthalmic refraction for diagnostic purposes	Effects occur in 20 min–30 min. Recovery takes 4 h–6 h. Larger doses may be necessary if iris is heavily pigmented.

(continued)

Table 14-3 (continued)
Anticholinergics

Drug	Preparations	Usual Dosage Range	Major Uses	Clinical Considerations

Tertiary Amine Antiparkinson Drugs

General Considerations

These drugs are generally used as adjuncts to other medications and are most effective in decreasing rigidity and excessive salivation associated with parkinsonism. The drugs should always be gradually withdrawn if prescription is discontinued; abrupt withdrawal may increase rigidity and tremors. Patients develop tolerance to these drugs with continued use. Inform patients that optimal effects may take several days to develop. Drugs should be taken with food or milk to reduce GI upset. Caution patients to avoid exertion in hot weather, since these drugs can cause hyperthermia.

Drug	Preparations	Usual Dosage Range	Major Uses	Clinical Considerations
benztropine mesylate (Cogentin)	Tablets—0.5 mg, 1 mg, 2 mg Injection—1 mg/ml	*Parkinsonism* 1 mg–2 mg daily to a maximum of 6 mg *Extrapyramidal Reactions* 1 mg–4 mg 1–2 times/day *Acute Dystonic Reactions* 1 mg–2 mg IM or IV followed by 1 mg–2 mg orally twice/day	Parkinsonism, extrapyramidal reactions	If used with L-dopa, adjust dose of each medication accordingly. Start with low dose and gradually increase. No significant difference in onset of action IM or IV. Sedative effect can occur. Withdraw gradually. See Chapter 31.
biperiden (Akineton)	Tablets—2 mg Injection—5 mg/ml	*Parkinsonism* 2 mg 3–4 times/day with meals *Extrapyramidal Reactions* 2 mg 1–3 times/day orally or 2 mg IM or IV, repeated every half hour to a maximum of 4 doses	Parkinsonism, extrapyramidal reactions	Most effective on akinesia and rigidity. May elevate mood. Can produce incoordination following IV or IM use. See Chapter 31.
ethopropazine hydrochloride (Parsidol)	Tablets—10 mg, 50 mg	Initially 50 mg 1–2 times/day to a maximum of 600 mg/day in severe cases	Parkinsonism, extrapyramidal reactions	Does not potentiate CNS depressants. Drug causes high incidence of dose-related side-effects, including drowsiness, hypotension, confusion, and GI distress. See Chapter 31.
orphenadrine hydrochloride (Disipal)	Tablets—50 mg	*Parkinsonism* 50 mg 3 times/day up to 250 mg daily	Parkinsonism, extrapyramidal reactions	Major effect is on rigidity of parkinsonism. See Chapter 31. Also available as *citrate* salt for muscle spasms (see below).
orphenadrine citrate (Banflex, Flexoject, Flexon, K-Flex, Marflex, Myolin, Norflex, O'Flex)	Tablets—100 mg Sustained-release tablets—100 mg Injection—30 mg/ml	*Muscle Spasms* 100 mg orally twice a day or 60 mg IV or IM every 12 h as necessary	Skeletal muscle spasms	Muscle relaxant (probably centrally acting) used to relieve acute musculoskeletal dis-

(continued)

Table 14-3 (continued)
Anticholinergics

Drug	Preparations	Usual Dosage Range	Major Uses	Clinical Considerations
Tertiary Amine Antiparkinson Drugs (continued)				
orphenadrine citrate (Banflex, Flexoject, Flexon, K-Flex, Marflex, Myolin, Norflex, O'Flex) (continued)				orders. See Chapter 19. May produce dizziness in addition to normal anticholinergic side-effects in large doses.
procyclidine (Kemadrin)	Tablets—5 mg	*Parkinsonism* 2.5 mg–5 mg 3 times/day *Extrapyramidal Reactions* 2.5 mg–5 mg 3–4 times/day	Parkinsonism, extrapyramidal reactions	Most effective against rigidity. May temporarily worsen tremor. In elderly, may induce confusion and psychotic reactions. Note decreased urinary output and reduce dose if necessary. See Chapter 31.
trihexyphenidyl hydrochloride (Aphen, Artane, Trihexane, Trihexidyl, Trihexy)	Tablets—2 mg, 5 mg Elixir—2 mg/5 ml Capsules (sustained release)—5 mg	*Parkinsonism* 1 mg initially, increased by 2-mg increments every 3–5 days to a total dose of 6 mg–10 mg/day; usual maintenance dose is 6 mg–12 mg daily in divided doses *Extrapyramidal Reactions* 5 mg–15 mg in divided doses	Parkinsonism, extrapyramidal reactions	When used with L-dopa, reduce dose of each drug proportionately. Major effect is on rigidity, with minimal effects on tremor. Sustained-release capsules are *not* intended for initial therapy but may be used once patient is stabilized. May produce CNS stimulation and excessive drying of the mouth. Often given before meals. See Chapter 31.
Quaternary Amine Anticholinergics				
anisotropine methylbromide (Valpin 50)	Tablets—50 mg	Adults: 50 mg 3 times/day	GI spasms, adjunctive therapy in peptic ulcer	Oral absorption is erratic.
clidinium bromide (Quarzan)	Capsules—2.5 mg, 5 mg	2.5 mg–5 mg 3–4 times/day	GI hypermotility and hypersecretion	Erratically absorbed orally. Reduce dosage in geriatric or debilitated patients. Also available in combination with chlordiazepoxide as Librax.

(continued)

Table 14-3 (continued)
Anticholinergics

Drug	Preparations	Usual Dosage Range	Major Uses	Clinical Considerations
Quarternary Amine Anticholinergics (continued)				
glycopyrrolate (Robinul)	Tablets—1 mg, 2 mg Injection—0.2 mg/ml	*Oral* 1 mg–2 mg 2–3 times/day *Parenteral* (IM, IV)—0.1 mg–0.2 mg 3–4 times/day *Reversal of Neuromuscular Blockade* 0.2 mg IV for every 1 mg neostigmine or equivalent received	GI disorders, preoperative medication, cholinergic overdosage	Not indicated in children. May cause burning at site of injection. Do not mix with solutions of sodium chloride or bicarbonate. Oral absorption is irregular.
hexocyclium methylsulfate (Tral)	Tablets—25 mg Timed-release tablets—50 mg	25 mg 4 times/day; alternately, 50 mg twice a day	GI hypermotility, hypersecretion	Oral absorption is unpredictable. Do not chew tablets. Do not use in children. Watch for hypersensitivity.
homatropine hydrobromide (Ak-Homatropine, Isopto Homatropine)	Ophthalmic drops—2%, 5%	*Refraction* 1–2 drops 2% every 10 min–15 min if necessary *Uveitis* 1–2 drops 2%–5% every 3 h–4 h	Refraction, uveitis, relief of ciliary spasm, preoperative cycloplegic, and mydriatic	Cycloplegia may be prolonged and caution in driving is recommended.
isopropamide iodide (Darbid)	Tablets—5 mg	5 mg–10 mg twice a day (every 12 h)	GI spasm and hypersecretion, diarrhea, urinary spasm	Not for use in children under 12 years. Erratically absorbed orally. Iodine skin rash may occur. May alter protein-bound iodine and ^{131}I tests, since drug is an iodide salt.
mepenzolate bromide (Cantil)	Tablets—25 mg	25 mg–50 mg 4 times/day	GI hypermotility, diarrhea, ulcerative colitis	Urinary hesitancy and constipation can occur, especially at larger doses. Oral absorption is very erratic.
methantheline bromide (Banthine)	Tablets—50 mg	Adults: 50 mg–100 mg 4 times/day Children, less than 1 year: 12 mg–25 mg 4 times/day over 1 year: 25 mg–50 mg 4 times/day	Preoperative medication, uretral spasm, urinary frequency	Less effective than many other similar agents. Tablets are very bitter. Poorly absorbed orally.

(continued)

Table 14-3 (continued)
Anticholinergics

Drug	Preparations	Usual Dosage Range	Major Uses	Clinical Considerations
Quarternary Amine Anticholinergics (continued)				
methscopolamine bromide (Pamine)	Tablets—2.5 mg	2.5 mg 3 times/day and 5 mg at bedtime	GI hypermotility, adjunctive therapy in peptic ulcer	Take drug one-half hour before meals. May exert curare-like relaxant effect on smooth muscle.
oxyphenonium bromide (Antrenyl)	Tablets—5 mg	10 mg 4 times/day	GI hyperacidity and hypermotility	Erratically absorbed; high incidence of common anticholinergic side-effects. Not for use in children.
propantheline bromide (Pro-Banthine, Norpanth)	Tablets—7.5 mg, 15 mg	*Oral* 7.5 mg–15 mg 3 times/day and 30 mg at bedtime Children: 1.5 mg–3 mg/kg/day in 3–4 divided doses	GI spasm and hypersecretion, adjunctive therapy in peptic ulcer	Increased fluid intake may minimize fecal impaction and urinary hesitancy. Blurring of vision and dizziness can occur.
tridihexethyl chloride (Pathilon)	Tablets—25 mg	Adults: 25 mg–50 mg 3–4 times/day	Adjunctive therapy of peptic ulcer	Also available with meprobamate (Pathibamate)

CASE STUDY

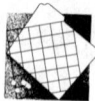

Helen Carroll was planning a sailing trip in the Caribbean but was nervous about suffering motion sickness during the 5 days she expected to be on board. At the suggestion of a friend she contacted her physician to ask him about possible medications to avoid this discomfort. He prescribed scopolamine transdermal therapeutic system, 1 patch every 3 days to be applied before boarding the boat.

During the second day of the trip, after applying the patch Mrs. Carroll began to feel drowsy and complained of dry mouth. After taking a nap she awoke feeling dizzy and nauseous. She removed the patch but symptoms continued to persist for several hours. The following day she felt fine.

When she returned from her vacation, she reported this reaction to her physician.

Discussion Questions

1. What side-effects of scopolamine did Mrs. Carroll experience?
2. What should she have done at the first sign of symptoms?
3. What strategies could the physician suggest to Mrs. Carroll to avoid these symptoms in the future?

REVIEW QUESTIONS

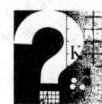

1. How are cholinergic blocking drugs classified?
2. List the major effects of anticholinergic drugs on (1) the GI tract, (2) the eye, (3) the exocrine glands, and (4) the urinary tract.
3. Are all cholinergic receptors equally sensitive to blockade by anticholinergic drugs? Explain.
4. What are the principal differences between tertiary and quaternary amine anticholinergics?
5. Give at least seven (7) uses for anticholinergic drugs.
6. In what situations is use of systemic anticholinergic drugs contraindicated?
7. What must patients receiving an anticholinergic drug for urinary incontinence be told?
8. In what form is scopolamine most often used for prevention of motion sickness? What are the common side-effects of this treatment?
9. What cautions must persons receiving an anticholinergic drug locally in the eye be aware of?
10. What treatment options are available for managing anticholinergic drug overdose?

BIBLIOGRAPHY

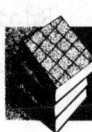

Greenblatt DJ, Shader RI: Anticholinergics. N Engl J Med 288:1215, 1973

Ingelfinger FJ: Anticholinergic therapy of gastrointestinal disorders. N Engl J Med 268:1454, 1963

Price NM, Schmitt LG, McGuire J, Shaw JE, Trobough G: Transdermal scopolamine in the prevention of motion sickness at sea. Clin Pharmacol Ther 29:414, 1981

Rumack BH: Anticholinergic poisoning: Treatment with physostigmine. Pediatrics 52:449, 1973

Shader RI, Greenblatt DJ: Belladonna alkaloids and synthetic anticholinergics: Uses and toxicity. In Shader RI (ed): Psychiatric Complications of Medical Drugs, p 103. New York, Raven Press, 1972

Stockbruegger RW, Jaup BH, Abrahamsson H, Dotevall G: Clinical pharmacology of muscarinic antagonists. Trends Pharmacol Sci, Suppl:74, 1984

Adrenergic Drugs

Endogenous Catecholamines
  Epinephrine
  Dipivefrin
  Norepinephrine (NE)
  Dopamine

Synthetic Catecholamines
  Isoproterenol
  Dobutamine

Vasopressor Amines
  Mephentermine
  Metaraminol
  Methoxamine
  Phenylephrine Parenteral

Nasal Decongestants

Ophthalmic Decongestants

Bronchodilators
  Ephedrine
  Ethylnorepinephrine
  Selective Beta$_2$ Agonists:
    Albuterol, Bitolterol,
    Isoetharine,
    Metaproterenol,
    Terbutaline

Smooth Muscle Relaxants
  Isoxsuprine
  Nylidrin
  Ritodrine

CNS Stimulants and Anorexiants

15

Adrenergic drugs are compounds, either natural or synthetic, which are capable of eliciting biologic responses similar to those produced by activation of the sympathetic nervous system or resulting from adrenal medullary discharge. For this reason, these agents may also be termed *sympathomimetic* drugs—that is, drugs that mimic sympathetic nerve stimulation.

The principal adrenergic compounds naturally occurring in the body are the endogenous catecholamines epinephrine (E), norepinephrine (NE), and dopamine (DA). *Epinephrine* is the major secretory product of the adrenal medulla and is released during periods of physical or emotional stress. It plays an important role in the body's adaptation to the stressful situation. It is also found in other organs of the body, but its role is less clear. *Norepineph-rine* is found in adrenergic nerve endings and is the principal mediator of transmission at adrenergic neuroeffector junctions. In addition, norepineph-rine is found in certain central brain regions and in peripheral sympathetic ganglia, where it probably serves a modulatory function. *Dopamine's* primary role in the body is as a central neurotransmitter involved in regulation of motor function and pituitary hormone secretion. It also acts peripherally in certain vascular beds to cause vasodilation of mesenteric and renal blood vessels.

The synthesis of the three endogenous catecholamines proceeds as outlined in Fig. 15-1. Conversion of norepinephrine to epinephrine only occurs to a significant extent in chromaffin tissue of the adrenal medulla and possibly in certain brain areas. In other adrenergic nerve endings, the pri-

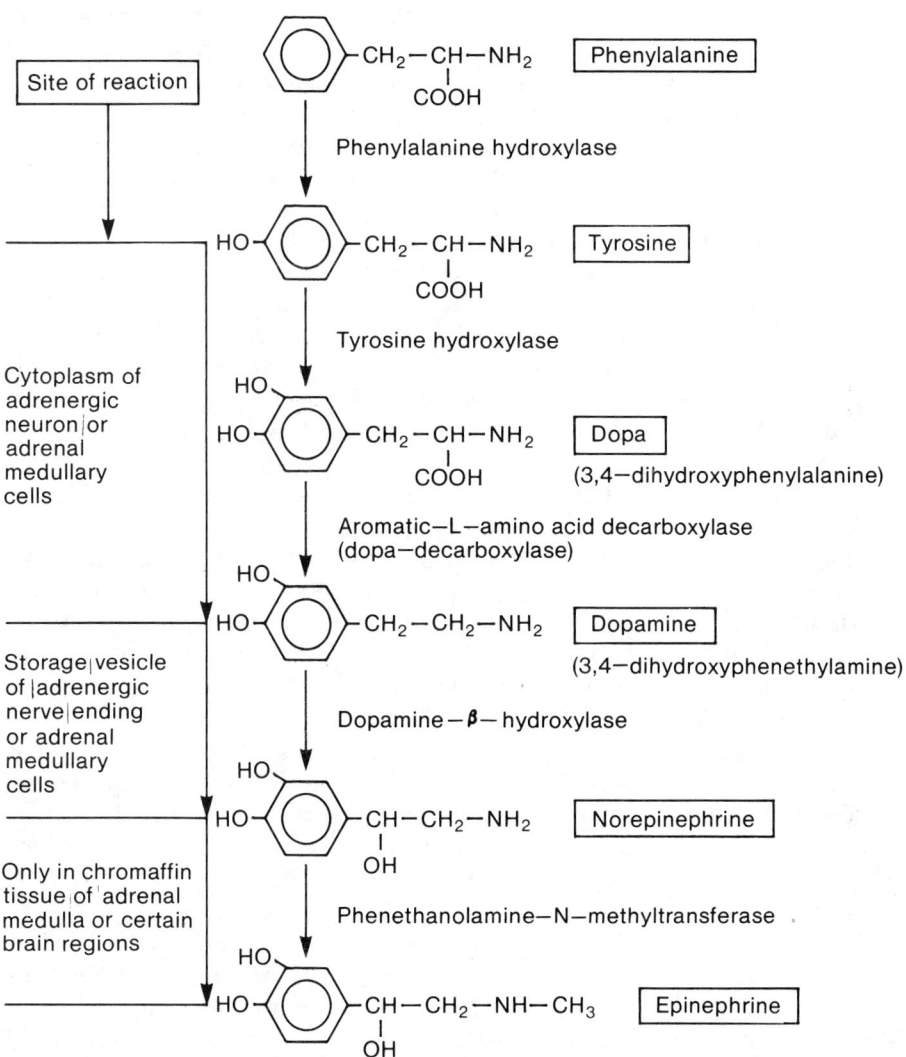

Figure 15-1.   Sites and mechanisms in the biosynthesis of catecholamines.

mary synthetic product is norepinephrine. The synthesis of norepinephrine can be controlled by a negative feedback inhibitory mechanism which depends on the level of available neurohormone in the adrenergic nerve endings. Elevated levels of norepinephrine apparently inhibit a cofactor necessary for the function of tyrosine hydroxylase, the enzyme which converts tyrosine to DOPA (see Figs. 15-1 and 15-2).

Once formed, a portion of the norepinephrine is stored in granules (vesicles) bound to ATP; this constitutes the "reserve pool" of neurohormone, and it is in dynamic equilibrium with one (or probably many more) "mobile" or functional pools. These functional pools exist in a "protected" form in the cytoplasm of the nerve ending and the norepinephrine contained therein is *not* released by a nerve action potential (see below) but may be extruded by the action of certain sympathomimetic amines such as tyramine.

Arrival of a nerve action potential at the nerve ending causes an influx of calcium into the nerve terminal, resulting in fusion of the norepinephrine-containing vesicles with the plasma membrane and subsequent extrusion of the neurohormone into the synaptic cleft.

The norepinephrine then diffuses across the synaptic cleft and interacts with adrenergic receptor sites on the surface of the effector cell, eliciting the response. The action of released norepinephrine can be terminated by (1) enzymatic breakdown, (2) uptake into either adrenergic neurons or non-neural surrounding cells, and (3) diffusion into the extracellular fluid. Enzymatic inactivation of norepinephrine is probably of little significance in initially terminating the action of the endogenously released neurohormone. The two principal enzymes involved in catecholamine metabolism are monoamine oxidase (MAO), located in the mitochondria of the nerve endings and catechol-o-methyltransferase (COMT), found in the cytoplasm of postjunctional effector structures. MAO functions mainly in the regulation of the levels of norepinephrine in the presynaptic nerve ending, whereas COMT may play a minor role in the inactivation of norepinephrine once it has interacted with postjunctional receptor sites.

Diffusion away from the synaptic area becomes important in removing the "overflow" of neurotransmitter resulting from excessive release, but its role in terminating the effects of normally released amounts of norepinephrine is probably minor.

The major mechanism for inactivating neuronally released norepinephrine is active uptake of the neurotransmitter molecules, either back into the adrenergic nerve endings from where release occurred or into surrounding non-neural cells (e.g., glial or smooth muscle). Reuptake into the nerve terminal is termed *uptake-1* and is of prime importance in maintaining an adequate store of neurohormone within the nerve ending. Uptake-1 can be blocked by tricyclic antidepressants and cocaine among other drugs. Non-neural cell uptake of norepinephrine is termed *uptake-2*, and is blocked by corticosteroids. A neurohormonal concentrating system exists within the adrenergic nerve ending which transports the free neurotransmitter molecules that have re-entered the nerve ending back into the storage vesicles. This transport system is blocked by the reserpine alkaloids.

These neuronal uptake mechanisms are not necessarily restricted to norepinephrine, because other adrenergic compounds (e.g., metaraminol methylnorepinephrine and octopamine) are also taken up and stored in much the same manner as norepinephrine. A diagrammatic representation of the events occurring at an adrenergic neuroeffector junction is presented in Fig. 15-2.

Differences in the responses of effector structures to the various adrenergic agents led to the concept of the existence of two distinct types of adrenergic receptor sites, first designated by Ahlquist in 1948 as alpha (α) and beta (β). Distinction is made between these two receptor types based on (1) differential activation by various catecholamines and (2) selective inhibition by various adrenergic blocking agents. Thus, among the endogenous catecholamines, epinephrine and norepinephrine generally show similar potencies at the alpha receptor sites (although epinephrine may be more potent in some instances). Both substances, however, are considerably more potent at alpha sites than isoproterenol, a frequently used synthetic catecholamine. Conversely, at beta sites, isoproterenol is generally the most potent agonist, followed by epinephrine. Norepinephrine is only weakly active at beta receptors.

The above relationships, in reality, represent somewhat of an oversimplification, because the two basic types of adrenergic receptors can be further subdivided. That is, there are two distinct types of alpha receptors (alpha$_1$, alpha$_2$) as well as two types of beta receptors (beta$_1$, beta$_2$) (see Chap. 12) and the distinction is based primarily on their location. Thus, *alpha$_1$* receptors are found postsynaptically on vascular smooth muscle and gastrointestinal (GI) and urinary sphincters, as well as in the eye, pancreas, spleen, and on certain glands. *Alpha$_2$* receptors are located on presynaptic adrenergic nerve endings, where they control the release

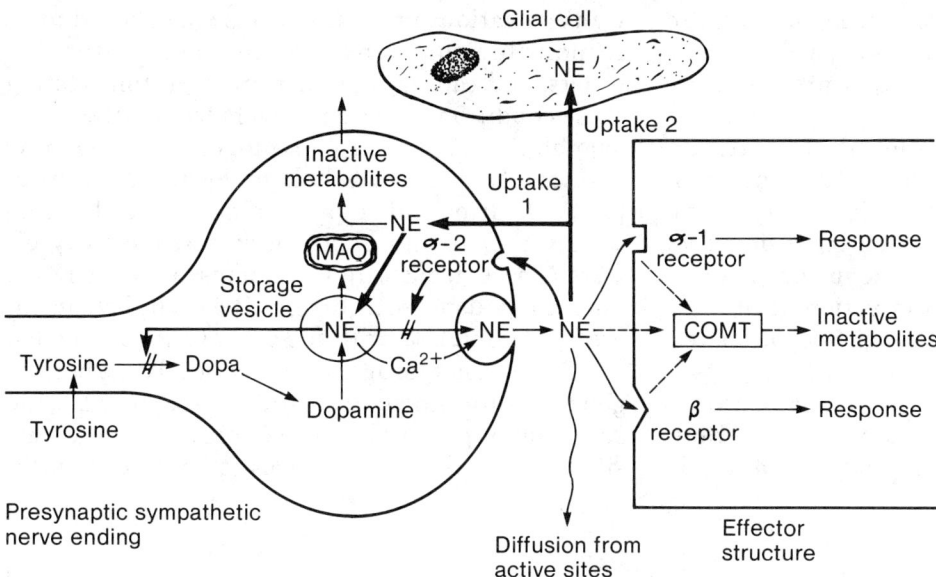

Figure 15-2. *Diagrammatic representation of events occurring at a sympathetic neuroeffector junction (see text for complete description). Following its synthesis from tyrosine, norepinephrine (NE) is stored in vesicles in the nerve ending. Arrival of a nerve impulse at the nerve ending results in an influx of Ca^{2+} which facilitates fusion of vesicles to the plasma membrane and subsequent extrusion of NE into the synaptic cleft. The neurotransmitter then interacts with adrenergic receptor sites on the effector structure membrane. The action of NE is terminated in several ways. The neurohormone may (1) diffuse away from the junctional area, (2) interact with COMT enzymes in the cytoplasm of the effector cells, resulting in formation of inactive metabolites, or (3) be actively taken up by either the presynaptic nerve terminal (uptake 1) or surrounding cells (uptake 2). Within the nerve terminal, free NE can be enzymatically inactivated by MAO found in mitochondria. The synthesis of NE is regulated by a negative feedback, which blocks the conversion of tyrosine to dopa, and the release of NE is also regulated by a negative feedback activated by interaction with presynaptic α-2 receptor sites.*

of norepinephrine by a negative feedback mechanism. Other sites where alpha$_2$ receptors have been demonstrated include platelets, fat cells, and certain vascular smooth muscle cells. *Beta$_1$* receptors exist primarily in the heart and adipose tissue, while *beta$_2$* receptors are located on GI, uterine, urinary, and bronchiolar smooth muscle, skeletal muscle, blood vessels, and in the liver and kidney.

When the order of sensitivity of the adrenergic receptor *subtypes* to the catecholamines is examined, the following rank order of potencies is obtained:

Alpha$_1$
epinephrine $\geqq$ norepinephrine $\gg$ isoproterenol
Alpha$_2$
epinephrine = norepinephrine (isoproterenol is ineffective)
Beta$_1$
isoproterenol > epinephrine = norepinephrine

Beta$_2$
isoproterenol $\geqq$ epinephrine $\gg$ norepinephrine

In addition to the adrenergic alpha and beta receptors described above, there are also specific *dopaminergic* receptors located on renal and visceral blood vessels. Activation of these receptor sites by the catecholamine dopamine results in vasodilation and reduced vascular resistance in the renal and mesenteric circulation. This selective dopaminergic effect is present only with small doses of exogenously administered dopamine; as the dose is increased and the serum drug level rises, dopamine is also capable of activating cardiac beta$_1$ sites and systemic alpha$_1$ sites, producing typical catecholamine effects. Dopamine receptors are also found in various areas of the central nervous system (CNS), where they function in the regulation of motor activity, and in autonomic ganglia as well, where their role is less well understood.

A summary of the various adrenergic receptor sites, their locations, and the principal responses mediated by each receptor type is presented in Table 15-1.

The pharmacologic actions of the various adrenergic agents depend to a large extent on their affinity and specificity for the different types of adrenergic receptors, as well as their intrinsic activity at each site. An overview of the major pharmacologic effects resulting from activation of the different kinds of peripheral adrenergic receptor sites is presented in Table 15-2.

In addition to their many peripheral actions, many adrenergic compounds exert profound effects on the CNS. Alterations in catecholamine activity in various brain structures are believed to be responsible for many affective and motor disorders, and those drugs that are useful in treating these conditions function largely by modifying the availability or action of endogenous adrenergic amines. Many noncatecholamine adrenergic drugs (e.g., ephedrine and amphetamine) can easily penetrate the CNS and elicit marked stimulatory effects. These agents are often abused and they are potentially dangerous drugs. They will be considered in Chapter 32 with the other CNS stimulants.

The adrenergic agents comprise a large, heterogeneous group of compounds possessing a wide spectrum of pharmacologic actions. Adequate classification of these substances, therefore, is diffi-

Table 15-1
Adrenergic Receptor Sites

	ALPHA$_1$	ALPHA$_2$	BETA$_1$	BETA$_2$	DOPAMINERGIC
Activated by:	Epinephrine Norepinephrine	Epinephrine Norepinephrine	Epinephrine Isoproterenol	Epinephrine Isoproterenol	Dopamine*

Major Peripheral Locations

	ALPHA$_1$	ALPHA$_2$	BETA$_1$	BETA$_2$	DOPAMINERGIC
	Vascular smooth muscle; GI and urinary sphincters; Eye (radial muscles); Pancreas; Spleen; Salivary glands; Skin (sweat glands, pilomotor muscles)	Presynaptic adrenergic and cholinergic nerve terminals; Platelets; Fat cells; Vascular smooth muscle	Heart; Adipose tissue; Intestinal smooth muscle	Smooth muscle (bronchiolar, GI, uterine, urinary); Skeletal muscle vasculature; Liver; Kidney	Renal, coronary, and visceral blood vessels

Responses

	ALPHA$_1$	ALPHA$_2$	BETA$_1$	BETA$_2$	DOPAMINERGIC
Excitatory	Vasoconstriction (rapid onset—short lived); Contraction of GI and urinary sphincters; Mydriasis (contraction of radial muscle); Salivary and sweat gland secretion	Platelet aggregation; Vasoconstriction (slow onset—long lived)	Cardiac stimulation; Lipolysis	Glycogenolysis, gluconeogenesis; Increased renin secretion	
Inhibitory	Decreased pancreatic secretions	Decreased neurotransmitter release; Inhibition of lipolysis; Decreased GI motility	Decreased GI motility	Bronchodilation; Uterine relaxation; Decreased GI motility; Relaxation of urinary bladder; Vasodilation of skeletal muscle vessels	Dilation of renal, coronary, and visceral blood vessels

* Note: Dopamine can also activate cardiac beta$_1$ receptors and vascular alpha$_1$ receptors in higher doses.

Table 15-2
Adrenergic Drug Effects

Structure	Response	Receptor Type
Cardiovascular system		
Heart	Increased rate	Beta$_1$
	Increased force	Beta$_1$
	Increased A-V conduction velocity	
Blood vessels		
Skeletal muscle	Vasoconstriction	Alpha$_1$, alpha$_2$
	Vasodilation	Beta$_2$
Mucosal	Vasoconstriction	Alpha$_1$
Mesenteric	Vasoconstriction	Alpha$_1$
	Vasodilation	Dopaminergic
Coronary and Renal	Vasodilation	Dopaminergic
Bronchioles	Smooth muscle relaxation	Beta$_2$
GI tract		
Smooth muscle	Relaxation	Beta$_2$
Sphincters	Contraction	Alpha$_1$
Uterus		
Smooth muscle	Relaxation	Beta$_2$
Eye		
Radial muscle	Contraction	Alpha$_1$
Ciliary muscle	Relaxation (weak)	Beta$_1$
Skin		
Pilomotor muscles	Contraction	Alpha$_1$
Sweat glands	Secretion (weak)	Alpha$_1$
Liver	Glycogenolysis	Beta$_2$
	Gluconeogenesis	Beta$_2$
Adipose tissue	Lipolysis	Beta$_1$
	Inhibition of lipolysis	Alpha$_2$
Pancreas	Decreased insulin secretion	Alpha$_2$
Kidney	Secretion of renin	Beta$_1$
Platelets	Aggregation	Alpha$_2$

cult. Based on their predominant mechanism of action, adrenergic drugs can be divided into three groups.

1. Direct-acting—Compounds acting directly at the postsynaptic adrenergic receptor sites (e.g., norepinephrine, dopamine)
2. Indirect-acting—Compounds acting on the presynaptic adrenergic nerve terminals to promote the release of stored adrenergic neurohormones (e.g., tyramine)
3. Dual-acting—Compounds possessing a mixture of both direct and indirect actions (e.g., ephedrine, amphetamine)

This mechanistic grouping of adrenergic agents, however, does not differentiate among the many different types of drugs to a sufficient extent. Thus, in order to discuss the adrenergic drugs in a more reasonable order, the following arbitrary classification will be used with the realization that many drugs fall into more than one of the proposed categories.

  I. Endogenous catecholamines (e.g., epinephrine, norepinephrine, dopamine)
 II. Synthetic catecholamines (e.g., isoproterenol, dobutamine)
III. Vasopressor amines (e.g., metaraminol)

IV. Nasal decongestants (*e.g.,* phenylephrine)
V. Ophthalmic decongestants (*e.g.,* naphazoline)
VI. Bronchodilators (*e.g.,* ephedrine, metaproterenol)
VII. Smooth muscle relaxants (*e.g.,* isoxsuprine, ritodrine)
VIII. CNS stimulants and anorexiants (*e.g.,* amphetamine)

Endogenous Catecholamines

The three major endogenous catecholamines, epinephrine, norepinephrine, and dopamine, serve to mediate the functioning of the sympathetic nervous system and are found widely throughout the body. Moreover, many other classes of pharmacologic agents exert their effects by modifying the action of one or more of these endogenous substances, so that the catecholamines participate in the action of a wide range of drugs. Catecholamines can also be prepared synthetically and are widely used in the treatment of many disease states. The therapeutic indications for the catecholamines are primarily based on their vasoconstrictive, bronchodilatory, and cardiac stimulatory actions.

Epinephrine

Parenteral solution (Adrenalin)

Parenteral suspension (Asmolin, Sus-Phrine)

Inhalation (Asthmahaler, Asthmanefrin, Bronitin, Bronkaid Mist, Medihaler-Epi, Micronefrin, Primatene, Vaponefrin)

Nasal (Adrenalin)

Ophthalmic (Adrenalin, Epifrin, E1, E2, Epinal, Epitrate, Eppy/N, Glaucon, Mytrate)

MECHANISM AND ACTIONS
Epinephrine acts on both alpha- and beta-adrenergic receptors to varying degrees. In physiologic amounts, its predominant actions are on the heart and on vascular and nonvascular smooth muscle. Heart rate, force of contraction, and cardiac output are increased and atrioventricular (A–V) conduction is accelerated, while the A–V refractory period is shortened. The latter two actions are responsible for epinephrine-induced cardiac arrhythmias. Epinephrine constricts arterioles, primarily in the skin, mucous membranes, and viscera due to an alpha-activating action, but dilates skeletal muscle and hepatic blood vessels as a result of a beta$_2$ receptor action. Effects on blood pressure are largely dependent on the dose. Rapid intravenous (IV) injection usually evokes a prompt elevation of blood pressure, mainly systolic, which is rather transient and does not exhibit tolerance. Slow IV infusion of epinephrine usually elicits a moderate rise in systolic pressure (increased force of contraction) and a decrease in diastolic pressure (vasodilation of skeletal muscle vasculature). Pulse pressure may increase significantly, but mean blood pressure is minimally affected. Epinephrine stimulates adenyl cyclase enzyme by an action on beta$_2$ receptors, resulting in formation of cyclic AMP, which relaxes bronchiolar smooth muscle. Bronchiolar arterioles are constricted, and the effects of histamine are physiologically antagonized. Uterine smooth muscle is generally contracted, except in the latter stages of pregnancy, when myometrial tone is decreased (beta$_2$ activation). Blood glucose is elevated, due to glycogenolysis and gluconeogenesis. In the eye, epinephrine induces mydriasis and also lowers intraocular pressure by decreasing formation and increasing outflow of aqueous humor. Effects on the CNS are minimal at normal doses, as the drug does not pass the blood–brain barrier in significant amounts.

USES
1. Symptomatic relief of anaphylactic, allergic, and other hypersensitivity reactions
2. Pressor agent for acute hypotensive states
3. Nasal decongestion
4. Bronchodilation and pulmonary decongestion (relaxes bronchial smooth muscle and constricts mucosal blood vessels). May be used in emergency management of acute epiglottiditis and croup
5. Aid to restoration of normal cardiac rhythm in cases of cardiac arrest
6. Management of simple, open-angle glaucoma (decreases production and increases outflow of aqueous humor)
7. Ocular decongestion (vasoconstriction and production of mydriasis
8. Topical hemostasis (controls superficial bleeding)
9. Potentiation and prolongation of the action of local anesthetics

ADMINISTRATION AND DOSAGE

Parenteral

For parenteral administration, epinephrine is available as a 1:1000, 1:10,000, and 1:100,000 (pediatric) solution, as well as a 1:200 suspension, which provides a more prolonged action (up to 8 hours) than the solution, for use as a bronchodilator.

Cardiac arrest—5 ml to 10 ml 1:10,000 by IV injection; may repeat at 5 ml every 5 minutes, until normal rhythm is restored

Intracardiac—3 ml to 5 ml 1:10,000

Intraspinal—0.2 ml to 0.4 ml 1:1000 added to anesthetic solution

With local anesthetic—1:20,000 to 1:100,000 dilution

Bronchospasm—0.3 ml to 0.5 ml 1:1000 SC or IM; repeat every 20 minutes up to 4 hours *or*

0.1 ml to 0.3 ml 1:200 suspension SC (children—0.01 mg/kg 1:1000 SC; repeat every 20 minutes up to 4 hours)

Inhalation

Eight to 15 drops of a 1% to 2% solution in a nebulizer or metered aerosol as directed. Allow 1 minute to 5 minutes between inhalations, and use least number of inhalations that are effective. May be used in a mist nebulizer for young children who cannot cooperate in using a nebulizer with a mouthpiece.

Topical

Nasal—1 to 2 drops 0.1% solution every 4 hours to 6 hours

Hemostatic—1:1000 to 1:10,000 applied locally

Ophthalmic

Epinephrine is used ophthalmically in solutions of various strengths (0.1%, 0.25%, 0.5%, 1%, 2%).

Glaucoma—1 to 2 drops 0.25% to 2% solution one to two times/day individualized to patient needs

Ocular mydriasis and hemostasis—1 to 2 drops of a 0.1% solution; repeat as necessary

FATE

Epinephrine is readily absorbed by mucous membranes but is rapidly destroyed by digestive enzymes, thus it is useless orally. Aqueous solutions are very unstable and oxidize readily, forming an amber or yellow color in solution. They should be used immediately. Effects occur quickly when given SC, IM, intraocularly, or by inhalation. For example, bronchodilation is seen 5 minutes to 10 minutes after SC administration, and maximal effects are noted within 20 minutes. The duration of action following injection of the solution is short; suspension forms provide more prolonged actions (6 hours to 12 hours). The drug is usually rapidly inactivated by uptake into adrenergic nerve endings or through enzymatic (MAO, COMT) hydrolysis. Circulating drug is hydrolyzed in the liver, and the metabolites, chiefly vanillylmandelic acid (VMA), are excreted in the urine. Penetration of drug into the CNS is minimal.

SIDE-EFFECTS/ADVERSE REACTIONS

The most frequently observed side-effects following systemic administration of epinephrine are nervousness, anxiety, headache, palpitations, sweating, and nausea. Local ophthalmic application frequently results in headache, lacrimation, and stinging. Nasal instillation often leads to burning, mucosal dryness, and sneezing. More serious adverse reactions are listed below:

Systemic—Weakness, dizziness, hypertension, anginal pain, tachycardia and arrhythmias, pulmonary edema, dyspnea, urinary retention, cerebral or subarachnoid hemorrhage, delusions, tremor, psychoses, lactic acidosis

Ophthalmic—Conjunctival irritation; pigmentation of eyelids, cornea, or conjunctiva; iritis; shedding of eyelashes; scotomas

Overdosage can result in a marked elevation in the blood pressure, and treatment consists of a rapid-acting vasodilator or alpha-adrenergic blocker.

CONTRAINDICATIONS AND PRECAUTIONS

Systemic epinephrine is contraindicated in the presence of severe hypertension, arrhythmias, coronary artery disease, shock, porphyria, narrow-angle glaucoma, organic brain damage, during labor (delays second stage), and in combination with general anesthetics, especially halogenated hydrocarbons.

Administer very cautiously to elderly patients or those with hypertension, hyperthyroidism, diabetes, parkinsonism, cardiovascular disease, long-term bronchial asthma or emphysema, psychoneuroses, prostatic hypertrophy, or tuberculosis.

Safe use in pregnancy or during lactation has not been established.

INTERACTIONS

1. Epinephrine may be potentiated by other sympathomimetic agents (e.g., phenylephrine, mephentermine), tricyclic antidepressants, MAO inhibitors, antihistamines, thyroxine, guanethidine.
2. Epinephrine may produce arrhythmias when used in combination with digitalis, general anesthetics, or isoproterenol, and may produce bradycardia when used with propranolol.
3. Epinephrine may produce hyperglycemia, altering the requirements for insulin or oral hypoglycemic agents.
4. The cardiac and bronchodilatory effects of epinephrine are antagonized by propranolol and other nonselective beta-blockers. Pressor effects are blocked by alpha-adrenergic blockers (e.g., phentolamine), but may be intensified in the presence of beta-blockers (e.g., propranolol).
5. Diuretics may increase the vascular pressor response to epinephrine.

■ Nursing Process

□ ASSESSMENT

Epinephrine is an emergency drug. It may be used to prevent a situation from escalating into a life-threatening event, such as inhalation during an asthmatic attack or injection after a bee sting, or it may be used in the treatment of respiratory or cardiac arrest.

In a respiratory or cardiac emergency, the patient must receive basic life support including cardiopulmonary resuscitation (CPR) as necessary. Assessment of this patient must be done rapidly and continuously with emphasis on the systems malfunctioning. Epinephrine may be given during cardiac arrest if ventricular fibrillation or cardiac standstill has occurred, so continuous cardiac monitoring is essential.

If the patient has not reached the stage of respiratory or cardiac arrest, vital signs will be even more closely monitored. Heart rate, blood pressure, respiratory rate, and peripheral tissue perfusion as evidenced by color and temperature of face and extremities must be frequently evaluated. Continuous ECG monitoring is also essential because arrhythmias may develop which will contraindi-

cate further use of epinephrine. The cycle of assessment, intervention, evaluation, and reassessment is continuous with epinephrine therapy, and parameters change much more quickly than with many other drugs.

Epinephrine may be used by a patient at home either as an inhalant or subcutaneous injection during an asthma attack or as a subcutaneous injection to prevent anaphylaxis and subsequent cardiac or respiratory arrest in a person who is highly allergic to an animal or insect toxin. The person and his family must learn how to administer the drug in a situation in which quick action is crucial. The nurse must carefully assess this family for their ability to respond and act calmly in emergency situations before deciding whether they will be able to manage drug administration.

For any patient who may take epinephrine at home, a careful drug history and medical history should be obtained. Epinephrine adversely interacts with other prescription drugs used for cardiac and respiratory problems as well as many over-the-counter cold and allergy remedies. Once an outline of drugs is developed the patient must learn which drugs are compatible with epinephrine and which ones to avoid if he must take epinephrine in an emergency. Any patient with a history of cardiac disease or hypertension, long-term bronchial asthma, or other respiratory diseases may need epinephrine in an emergency but is also at high risk for adverse reactions to the drug.

□ NURSING DIAGNOSES

Actual and potential nursing diagnoses for the patient receiving epinephrine will vary widely depending on the reason the drug is used. For example, the *actual* nursing diagnoses for a patient who will keep epinephrine in an anaphylaxis kit at home for use in case of bee sting might include:

  Knowledge deficit regarding the action, dose, administration, and response to the drug as well as what to do after the drug is administered

  Anxiety about the ability to respond to such an emergency

Potential diagnoses once the event occurs and the drug is given may include:

  Anxiety about drug effectiveness and the ability to reach emergency help in time

  Alteration in cardiac output: decreased output related to palpitations which frequently occur after drug administration

  Alteration in comfort related to headache and nausea which are also common side-effects

□ *PLAN*

The nursing goals also vary with the different uses of epinephrine.

In cardiac arrest: To prepare the drug correctly for physician administration in order to reverse cardiac arrest.

For home administration regardless of route: To establish a teaching plan which enables the patient and/or family member to correctly and safely administer the drug while minimizing the side-effects.

□ *INTERVENTION*

Parenteral epinephrine should be kept as an emergency drug in any facility where patients are seen. Prefilled syringes may be preferred because they take less time to prepare in an emergency.

Epinephrine is an unstable drug, and regardless of the route by which it is given it must be stored away from heat, light, and air. When checking the emergency cart the nurse must regularly examine epinephrine vials for color changes to yellow or amber, formation of precipitates, and the manufacturer's expiration date. Patients taking the drug at home should also be taught to routinely check for these changes.

□ *Intravenous/Intracardiac Administration*

Once the need for epinephrine has been determined the administration guidelines given above should be closely followed. The drug alone will not eliminate cardiac standstill or ventricular fibrillation but can coarsen the heart pattern so cardiac muscle will be more responsive to electrical defibrillation. This drug is easily destroyed by alkalis, oxidizing agents, and salts of zinc, copper, and iron. Epinephrine should be given through an IV line containing 5% dextrose and water, normal saline, or 5% dextrose and saline. The IV line should be flushed completely before administering epinephrine if any drug has been given before it. This is especially important if sodium bicarbonate, frequently used during arrests, has been given.

Epinephrine should be given in small strengths ranging from 1:1000 to 1:100,000, which indicate dose as follows: 1:1000 contains 1 mg/ml, 1:10,000 contains 0.1 mg/ml, 1:100,000 contains 0.01 mg/ml. Watch the zeros closely when selecting a vial. Giving the wrong dose can quickly result in an overdose. Repeat injections will only be given until a viable cardiac rhythm or adequate air exchange has been established. Antidotal drugs such as phentolamine, propranolol, and nitrates should be kept on hand when giving epinephrine by either the intravenous or intracardiac route to treat arrhythmias secondary to epinephrine administration.

□ *Systemic Use for Hypersensitivity Reaction*

The patient with a history of hypersensitivity or anaphylactic reaction, for example to bee stings, may need to self-administer epinephrine subcutaneously to avert respiratory arrest. The drug is also used to treat acute cases of bronchospasm resulting from bronchial asthma. The nurse must determine whether the patient or another family member must take responsibility for learning this potential life-saving technique.

Even for the patient willing to learn self-administration of epinephrine, backup support from family and friends must be strong and readily available. In some instances the patient will lose strength too rapidly to act for himself, and the main objective is to act quickly. When teaching administration of epinephrine emphasize the following points:

1. Measure exactly the prescribed dose. Epinephrine is given in small amounts, and overdosage can easily occur. Usually administration will be through a tuberculin syringe.
2. Always aspirate the syringe prior to injection to ensure the needle is not in a vein.
3. Massage the injection site to hasten absorption. Carefully rotate sites. This action will prevent tissue necrosis from local vasoconstriction.
4. Epinephrine SC is short-acting (20 minutes to 30 minutes) and one dose may not abort an attack. Seek medical attention if immediate relief is not noted.
5. Tolerance to this drug will develop over time if used repeatedly. Notify physician if response to drug diminishes.
6. The drug's side-effects, nervousness, tremulousness, nausea, and palpitations, are frightening symptoms which will pass quickly.
7. Encourage the patient's family to put together an anaphylaxis kit (some are available ready-made) so everything needed is in one spot. Encourage the family to go through a dry run of the emergency so they have a sense of what to expect should the event actually occur.

□ *Use by Inhalation*

Other types of inhalants are used more frequently than epinephrine; nevertheless, for the patient using an epinephrine inhalant (see p. 259 for details on using oral inhalers) in an acute asthmatic attack the following are the most important considerations:

1. If symptoms are not relieved in 15 minutes to 30 minutes, consult the physician immediately. Allow 1 to 2 minutes between inhalations to reduce the chance of overdose. Use only the minimal number of inhalations to relieve symptoms. Overdosage can produce severe systemic effects.
2. Many patients are prescribed routine isoproterenol as regular therapy. This medication should not be used for at least 4 hours after administration of epinephrine to avoid cardiac arrhythmias.
3. Bronchial irritation, nervousness, or insomnia are signs that the patient should reduce the dosage.
4. Encourage good mouth care, such as rinsing the mouth with water after inhalation to prevent excessive drying effects.

□ *Ophthalmic Use*
In addition to information about instillation of eye drops, the patient taking epinephrine eye drops should know the following:
1. Taking the drops at night will minimize the discomfort of the mydriasis and photophobia which are uncomfortable side-effects. Because of these effects the patient should not drive or engage in any activity requiring clear vision immediately after taking the drug.
2. Although initial tearing, stinging, burning of eyes and headaches are not uncommon, the patient should report the persistence of such symptoms to the physician.
3. If hypersensitivity to the drug occurs, manifested by itching, edema, and watery discharge, the patient should discontinue the drug and contact the physician immediately.
4. The drug should be discontinued prior to surgery in which general anesthetics such as halothane or other halogenated hydrocarbons will be used because of the danger of arrhythmias from systemic absorption of epinephrine. Encourage the patient to report all drug use to any physician or dentist, but particularly when surgery is involved.
5. Epinephrine eye drops may stain soft contact lenses.

□ *Nasal Use*
The patient taking an epinephrine nasal inhalant should know the following:
1. Avoid contaminating dropper tip. Rinse dropper in hot water after each application.

2. Avoid prolonged use of nasal decongestants, because rebound congestion frequently occurs.
3. Give nose drops with head low or tilted back to prevent passage into throat or systemic absorption.
4. Instillation of nasal solution will sting, but the discomfort will be temporary.

□ *EVALUATION*
The main outcome criteria for evaluating the success of epinephrine in a cardiac arrest is the restoration of a viable cardiac rhythm. Epinephrine is only one of a series of emergency drugs used to achieve this end so it will be difficult to judge its effectiveness apart from the others.

The outcome criteria for subcutaneous administration of epinephrine is the ability of the patient or family member to give the drug correctly and whether the drug effectively averts or improves symptoms of a hypersensitivity reaction or asthmatic attack.

For the other methods of administration the nurse can judge success by the patient's ability to self-administer the drug with minimal side-effects.

Dipivefrin
(Propine)

Dipivefrin is a lipid-soluble prodrug of epinephrine—that is, it is converted to epinephrine by enzymatic hydrolysis following instillation into the eye. Due to its highly lipophilic nature, it penetrates into the anterior chamber more readily than epinephrine, thus allowing use of a much smaller amount of drug. Onset of action is within 30 minutes. Dipivefrin is indicated for the control of intraocular pressure in chronic, open-angle glaucoma, and its use is associated with fewer side-effects than conventional epinephrine therapy, because less drug is required due to improved absorption. Therapeutic response to twice daily administration of dipivefrin is approximately equivalent to that of 2% pilocarpine given four times a day, without the miosis and cycloplegia characteristic of cholinergic therapy. However, the response is somewhat inferior to that observed with 2% epinephrine. Due to its mydriatic action, dipivefrin, like epinephrine, is contraindicated in narrow-angle glaucoma.

The side-effects associated with dipivefrin therapy are similar to those noted previously for ophthalmic epinephrine administration but occur with lower frequency. Burning and stinging following instillation are the most common side-effects. In addition, systemic effects (tachycardia, increased blood pressure, arrhythmias) have been reported following ocular administration of epinephrine and can occur with use of dipivefrin as well. Dipivefrin is available as a 0.1% solution, and the usual dosage is 1 drop every 12 hours.

Norepinephrine (NE)
(Levarterenol, Levophed)

MECHANISM AND ACTIONS
Norepinephrine exerts both an alpha-adrenergic action, resulting in powerful vasoconstriction of peripheral vessels, and a somewhat less intense beta$_1$ agonistic effect, which enhances the force of contraction. Blood pressure is elevated, coronary blood flow is improved, and cardiac output is usually increased as the blood pressure is raised. A reflex bradycardia can occur in response to peripheral vasoconstriction. CNS and metabolic effects are minimal.

USES
1. Restoration of blood pressure in acute hypotensive states, such as sympathectomy, poliomyelitis, myocardial infarction, spinal anesthesia, septicemia, and drug or transfusion reactions
2. Adjunctive treatment of cardiac arrest and extreme hypotension

ADMINISTRATION AND DOSAGE
Norepinephrine is available as an injection solution (1 mg/ml). The drug is inactive orally and is given by IV infusion. The initial dose is 8 to 12 mcg/min (*i.e.*, 2–3 ml/min) of a 4 mcg/ml dilution (4 mg NE in 1000 ml 5% dextrose). The average maintenance dose is 2 to 4 mcg/min, and the infusion is continued until adequate blood pressure and tissue perfusion are maintained without therapy.

FATE
Norepinephrine is ineffective when given orally. Pressor effects occur rapidly with IV infusion and disappear within 2 minutes after termination of the infusion. The drug is taken up by adrenergic nerve endings and is also rapidly inactivated in the liver and other tissues by catechol-o-methyl transferase. Excretion is by way of the kidney, largely as metabolites and some (5%–15%) unchanged drug.

SIDE-EFFECTS/ADVERSE REACTIONS
Side-effects are less common with norepinephrine than with epinephrine, but may include reflex bradycardia, headache, palpitations, and nervousness. More serious adverse reactions usually result from excessive doses and encompass hypertension, respiratory distress, tremors, arrhythmias in the presence of certain anesthetics, and tissue necrosis following extravasation. Large doses can also cause chest pain, photophobia, hyperglycemia, vomiting, severe hypertension, cerebral hemorrhage, and convulsions.

CONTRAINDICATIONS AND PRECAUTIONS
Contraindications to the use of norepinephrine include hypovolemic shock, vascular thrombosis, use during general anesthesia when halogenated hydrocarbons (*e.g.*, halothane) are employed, extreme hypoxia or hypercapnia, and pregnancy. *Cautious use* is indicated in the presence of hypertension, hyperthyroidism, progressive heart disease, and in elderly patients.

INTERACTIONS
1. The pressor effects of norepinephrine may be potentiated in the presence of tricyclic antidepressants, MAO inhibitors, other sympathomimetic drugs, beta-blockers, antihistamines, guanethidine, and methyldopa.
2. Norepinephrine together with oxytocic drugs may result in severe hypertension.
3. Norepinephrine may precipitate cardiac arrhythmias in the presence of cyclopropane and the halogenated hydrocarbon general anesthetics.
4. Diuretics may reduce arterial responsiveness to norepinephrine.

■ Nursing Process

(See Dopamine)

Dopamine
(Dopastat, Intropin)

MECHANISM AND ACTIONS
Dopamine acts both directly on adrenergic receptor sites and indirectly on presynaptic nerve terminals to release norepinephrine. These effects are dose-

dependent. In low doses (up to 2 mcg/kg/min), the drug predominately activates selective dopaminergic receptors on renal and mesenteric blood vessels to cause vasodilation. This action is accompanied by increases in renal blood flow, glomerular filtration rate, and sodium excretion. In slightly larger amounts (2–10 mcg/kg/min), dopamine also exerts a beta$_1$ agonistic effect on the myocardium, resulting in increased force of contraction, stroke volume, and cardiac output. Heart rate is usually unchanged. Oxygen consumption is somewhat less than with isoproterenol. Large doses (greater than 10 mcg/kg/min) further stimulate alpha-adrenergic receptors, producing generalized vasoconstriction and elevated blood pressure.

USES

1. Correction of the hemodynamic imbalances associated with various forms of shock (e.g., trauma, heart surgery, myocardial infarction, renal failure, septicemia)

ADMINISTRATION AND DOSAGE

Dopamine is available as several strengths of injection solution (0.8 mg/ml, 1.6 mg/ml, 40 mg/ml, 80 mg/ml, 160 mg/ml).

Initially, 2 to 5 mcg/kg/min of diluted solution is administered by IV infusion. Dosage may be increased by 5 to 10 mcg/kg/min increments up to 20 to 50 mcg/kg/min in severely ill patients. Most patients can be maintained on a dose of 20 mcg/kg/min or less.

As indicated, the drug is available as injectable solutions. These are prepared by dilution in an appropriate IV solution, usually 5% dextrose or sodium chloride injection, according to the package instructions. Dopamine is also available as previously prepared infusion solutions containing 80 mg/100 ml or 160 mg/100 ml in 5% dextrose. The 160 mg/100 ml solution may be preferable when a slower rate of infusion is desired or in patients with significant fluid retention.

FATE

The onset of action is within 2 minutes to 4 minutes, and effects persist for less than 10 minutes. Distribution is extensive, but the drug does not cross the blood–brain barrier. Approximately 75% of a dose is metabolized in the liver, kidney, and plasma, while the remainder is converted to norepinephrine in adrenergic nerve terminals. The drug is excreted in the urine, mainly as metabolites.

SIDE-EFFECTS/ADVERSE REACTIONS

Common side-effects during infusion are headache, nausea, palpitations, tachycardia, dyspnea, hypotension, and ectopic beats. Other adverse reactions, principally observed at high doses, include hypertension, conduction irregularities, azotemia, decreased urinary outflow, nervousness, vomiting, and numbness or pain in the hands or feet. Necrosis and tissue sloughing can occur following extravasation.

CONTRAINDICATIONS AND PRECAUTIONS

Dopamine is contraindicated in the presence of tachyarrhythmias and pheochromocytoma. *Cautious use* is indicated in patients with occlusive vascular diseases such as arterial embolism, cold injury, diabetic endarteritis, and atherosclerosis, as well as in pregnant women, children, and patients who have recently received an MAO inhibitor.

INTERACTIONS

1. The pressor effects of dopamine may be potentiated by MAO inhibitors, tricyclic antidepressants, other sympathomimetics, ergot alkaloids, oxytocics, furazolidone, and guanethidine.
2. The actions of dopamine and diuretics may be mutually additive.
3. Dopamine may produce arrhythmias in the presence of cyclopropane and halogenated hydrocarbon anesthetics.
4. Use of phenytoin with dopamine may lead to hypotension, bradycardia, and seizures.
5. Dopamine may reverse the effects of beta-blockers.

■ Nursing Process for Norepinephrine and Dopamine

Many of dopamine's actions, especially in larger amounts, resemble those of norepinephrine in the body, so the nursing considerations are similar for both drugs. In the following discussion, norepinephrine will be used as the prototype.

□ ASSESSMENT

Both drugs are used in acute hypotensive situations and are therefore considered emergency drugs. Initial assessment and nursing intervention may occur simultaneously. Data may not be collected in the interest of time or may be followed more closely after the patient is stabilized.

□ *Subjective Data*

If possible, a medication history should be obtained because many drugs that lower blood pressure will be affected by norepinephrine. For example, if a patient with hypertension treated with a beta-blocker develops a toxic, hypotensive reaction to the drug this may be successfully treated with dopamine. Conversely, if a patient is hypotensive from an adverse reaction to diuretics, hypovolemia may actually be the problem and dopamine is not the drug of choice. Such differentiation, even in the midst of an emergency, will facilitate safe drug therapy.

Medical history is also important because hypertension, coronary or peripheral artery diseases, and cardiac arrhythmias may contraindicate use of either drug.

□ *Objective Data*

In an emergency, the essential baseline assessment is cardiovascular status. Heart rate and blood pressure must be known. If possible, a direct arterial line should be inserted for accurate monitoring. Pulmonary wedge pressure or central venous pressure may also be used.

Laboratory data may not be collected until the patient is stabilized, but electrolytes are essential to determine fluid volume and electrolyte status. A blood urea nitrogen or creatinine study may be ordered to determine renal function and to give an idea of the patient's fluid volume and the drug's effect on renal perfusion.

□ *NURSING DIAGNOSES*

Actual nursing diagnoses may include:

 Knowledge deficit related to the action and effects of the drug and the reason for extensive monitoring

 Anxiety related to the life-threatening event

Potential nursing diagnoses include:

 Impaired tissue integrity due to extravasation of the drug

 Alteration in tissue perfusion related to drug effects on peripheral and renal circulation

□ *PLAN*

Nursing care goals for the patient receiving norepinephrine should include accurate:

 Provision of life support as necessary

 Safe administration paying particular attention to patency of infusion site

 Monitoring for side-effects such as rapid blood pressure changes, decreased urine output, toxic interactions, and arrhythmias

□ *INTERVENTION*

During initial infusion of the drug, blood pressure readings should be monitored continuously. In the event only indirect sphygmomanometer readings can be obtained they should be done every 2 minutes to 5 minutes. As vital signs stabilize, readings can be taken every 15 minutes to 20 minutes. The drug must be slowly tapered to avoid hypotensive crisis. During this process, blood pressure readings should again be taken every 2 minutes to 5 minutes. Other parameters to watch closely include pulse, color, and skin temperature.

The drug should be infused as a secondary IV which can be disconnected from the main IV line without interrupting the intravenous site. Infusion should be monitored on an infusion pump with an infiltration alarm to ensure accurate dosing. Blood pressure goals should be set by the physician, and the infusion will be titrated to maintain those goals.

One of the adverse effects of norepinephrine is peripheral vasoconstriction, which can rapidly lead to gangrene. Tissue perfusion should be checked hourly by examining the fingers and toes and pressing the nailbeds to test for capillary refill. Peripheral pulses and skin temperature and sensation should also be monitored.

Another of the adverse effects of norepinephrine is renal necrosis because the drug decreases renal perfusion. Output should be monitored at least every hour; if output decreases, the physician should be notified immediately.

Both drugs are extremely irritating to tissue, and extravasation can lead to tissue necrosis and possibly limb loss. To decrease the chance of extravasation, the nurse should make sure the infusion is given in a large vein and that alternate infusion sites are used as necessary. Leg veins should be avoided, especially in the elderly, because occlusion of the vasculature can occur. Signs of extravasation include skin blanching, swelling, and hardness around the site. If these occur, the infusion must be stopped and the physician notified at once. Each institution has its own protocol for treatment of extravasation but most include instillation of 10 ml to 15 ml of normal saline mixed with 5 mg to 10 mg of phentolamine into the *infiltrated* area, not the IV line.

Another danger with the use of IV norepinephrine is physical incompatabilities with other emergency drugs such as sodium bicarbonate, phenytoin, and barbiturates. In order to minimize such interactions IV lines should be thoroughly flushed before infusing this drug. If possible a second line should be inserted exclusively for norepinephrine administration.

Norepinephrine also interacts with normal saline resulting in oxidation and loss of potency. Therefore, the drug should be infused through a line containing a dextrose and water or dextrose and saline solution.

The margin of safety for norepinephrine is extremely narrow. Bradycardia and other arrhythmias are not uncommon as a result of large doses. To combat these, atropine, lidocaine, and propranolol should be on hand at all times so prompt action can be taken if necessary.

□ *EVALUATION*

The outcome sought with these drugs is restoration of viable blood pressure, maintenance of a patent IV site, and minimal side-effects. Nursing Care Plan 15-1 is a summary of the nursing process for patients receiving norepinephrine or dopamine. Many of its points can be applied in the use of isoproterenol as well.

Synthetic Catecholamines

In addition to the three catecholamines found endogenously, two synthetic derivatives, isoproterenol and dobutamine, are also available clinically. They are almost exclusively activators of beta-adrenergic receptor sites. Isoproterenol nonselectively activates all beta receptors, and dobutamine exerts a relatively specific activation of cardiac beta₁ receptors.

Isoproterenol

Oral/parenteral (Isuprel)

Inhalation (Aerolone, Medihaler-Iso, Norisodrine, Vapo-Iso)

MECHANISM AND ACTIONS

Isoproterenol is a direct-acting sympathomimetic with a preferential effect on beta-adrenergic receptors. Activation of beta₁ sites in the heart increases heart rate, force of contraction, and A–V conduction velocity, with a corresponding increase in cardiac output and systolic blood pressure. Beta₂ activation of peripheral blood vessels causes vasodilation, which lowers peripheral vascular resistance and diastolic blood pressure. Isoproterenol relaxes most smooth muscle (beta₂ effect), the most pronounced effects being on the bronchioles and GI tract. Antigen-induced histamine release may also be blocked. Uterine smooth muscle is also relaxed. CNS effects are usually slight, but central excitation can occur.

USES
1. Relief of bronchospasm associated with respiratory disorders and general anesthesia
2. Adjunct in management of shock, cardiac arrest, Adams-Stokes syndrome, ventricular arrhythmias due to A–V block, and carotid sinus hypersensitivity

ADMINISTRATION AND DOSAGE
Isoproterenol is available as an injection solution (0.2 mg/ml), sublingual tablets (10 mg, 15 mg), aerosol (0.2%, 0.25%), and a solution for nebulization (0.03%, 0.06%, 0.25%, 0.5%, 1%).

Isoproterenol may be administered by IV infusion, direct IV, intramuscular (IM) or subcutaneous (SC) injection, sublingually, and by inhalation. Recommended doses are as follows:

Parenteral
Shock—0.25 ml to 2.5 ml/min of 1:500,000 dilution in dextrose 5% by IV infusion (0.5–5 mcg/min)
Cardiac arrest—
  IV injection—1 ml to 3 ml of a 1:50,000 dilution (0.02 mg–0.06 mg)
  IV infusion—1.25 ml/min of a 1:250,000 dilution (5 mcg/min)
  IM, SC—1 ml of a 1:5,000 solution (0.2 mg)
  Intracardiac—0.1 ml of a 1:5,000 solution (0.02 mg)
Bronchospasm (during anesthesia)—0.01 mg to 0.02 mg IV of a 1:50,000 solution in saline or dextrose 5%

Sublingual
Bronchospasm—10 mg to 20 mg three to four times/day (children—5 mg three to four times/day)
Heart block—10 mg initially (range 5 mg–50 mg) as maintenance therapy (*not* used in emergency treatment)

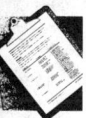

Nursing Care Plan 15-1
The Patient Receiving Adrenergic Vasopressors (e.g., dopamine, norepinephrine)

Assessment

Subjective Data

1. Medication history: refer to Interactions section to formulate pertinent questions.
   a. Current drugs being taken that may be physically incompatible with a vasopressor; that when combined with a vasopressor may cause an undesired effect; or that require an alteration in dosage of either drug
   b. Drug allergies/hypersensitivity to vasopressors
2. Medical history: refer to Contraindications sections for specific drug.
   a. Check for pre-existing conditions that may precipitate adverse reactions, such as renal disease, arterial insufficiency problems (*e.g.*, embolic disease, Raynaud's disease, cold injury, diabetes), and cardiac dysrhythmias.
   b. Current pregnancy
   c. History of obstructive urinary disease or prostatic enlargement

Objective Data

1. Physical Assessment focusing on:
   a. Cardiovascular status: arterial blood pressure, cardiac output, CVP or PWP, heart rate, EKG monitoring
   b. Peripheral vascular status: color, temperature, and pulses in the extremities
   c. Renal vascular status: urinary output, input/output ratio
   d. Neurovascular status: mental alertness, ability to communicate
   e. Body weight in kilograms
   f. IV access established
2. Laboratory Data
   a. BUN, creatinine, electrolytes
   b. Arterial blood gases, mixed venous oxygen saturation

Nursing Diagnosis	Expected Client Outcome	Intervention
Potential alteration in cardiac output: decreased, related to drug effect	Blood pressure will be maintained within desired range (usual prescribed goal for the adult is a mean pressure of between 80–90 mm Hg) and desired CVP/PWP and cardiac output will be achieved.	Initiate drug administration in mcg/kg/min as prescribed, starting with lowest dose and gradually increasing IV rate until desired blood pressure is achieved, or adverse reaction is noted. Monitor the signs of drug effectiveness, including BP within set goals, ↑ urinary output, improved mental status, ↓ pallor, improved peripheral vascular status. As optimal response is noted, titrate dose downward as prescribed and note any deterioration in vital signs.
	Normal sinus rhythm will be maintained.	Monitor heart rate on continuous EKG. Be prepared to treat dysrhythmias with lidocaine; bradycardia with atropine; angina with nitroglycerine. Notify physician of any changes. Rule out other causes of dysrhythmias (fear, pain, hypoxia, electrolyte imbalance).

(continued)

Nursing Care Plan 15-1 (continued)
The Patient Receiving Adrenergic Vasopressors (e.g., dopamine, norepinephrine)

Nursing Diagnosis	Expected Client Outcome	Intervention
Potential alteration in tissue perfusion: renal, related to drug effect	Urinary output will be at least 30 ml/h.	Monitor input and output hourly through drug infusion. Notify physician if output falls below 30 ml/h. Reduce infusion rate as prescribed. Output may improve.
Potential alteration in tissue perfusion: peripheral, related to drug effect	Temperature, nail bed capillary filling, color, sensation, and pulses will remain within normal limits.	Monitor temperature of extremities, nail bed capillary refill in fingers and toes, skin color and peripheral pulses and presence of pain or sensation every 15 min–60 min, depending on patient's response to drug. Notify physician of any changes. Reduce infusion rate as prescribed. Peripheral tissue perfusion may improve.
Potential alteration in tissue perfusion: cerebral, related to drug effect.	The patient will remain alert and oriented.	Monitor BP, changes in mental alertness, headache, and blurring of vision, which are signs of increased intracranial pressure. Notify physician of any changes. Reduce infusion rate as prescribed. Mental status may improve.
Potential alteration in tissue perfusion: cardiovascular, related to drug effect	Symptoms of angina will be prevented if detected early.	Monitor signs of angina (*i.e.*, substernal pain). Notify physician. Obtain arterial blood gases to rule out hypoxemia, as ordered. Reduce infusion rate as ordered. Pain may disappear. Be prepared to administer nitroglycerin or analgesic as prescribed.
Knowledge deficit related to how the drug is working, why intensive monitoring is essential	Patient will verbalize understanding of how the drug works and why monitoring is essential.	Teach the person that drug helps to promote heart function. Monitoring is necessary to "fine tune" drug administration.
Anxiety related to life-threatening illness	Patient will express concerns and verbalize desired comfort measures.	Provide basic explanations of actions on each intervention. Encourage verbalization about condition, feeling other stressors. Provide diversions through family visits, radio, something patient enjoys. Provide bodily comfort measures.
Potential impaired tissue integrity related to drug extravasation	Good skin integrity will be maintained.	Control infusion rate by an infusion device that has an infiltration alarm. Use a central line if possible; if a peripheral line is used, avoid hands or feet. Monitor IV site every hour for pain, skin blanching, reduced temperature, swelling.

(continued)

Nursing Diagnosis	Expected Client Outcome	Intervention
Potential impaired tissue integrity related to drug extravasation (continued)		If infiltration is suspected notify physicians, discontinue line, start new line immediately; drug cannot be abruptly discontinued.
Potential alteration in comfort: nausea/vomiting related to drug effect	Vomiting will be prevented or promptly managed.	Be prepared to administer anti-emetics as prescribed if patient complains of nausea. Be prepared to suction to prevent aspiration if patient is semiconscious or immobilized.
Sleep pattern disturbance related to frequent assessments and treatments	Patient will be allowed rest periods whenever possible.	Arrange uninterrupted rest periods once drug has produced stabilization of symptoms.

Inhalation

Solution—3 to 7 inhalations of 1:100 solution or 5 to 15 inhalations of 1:200 solution in a hand-held nebulizer; repeat in 5 minutes to 10 minutes, if needed; may be given up to five times/day.

Aerosol—1 to 2 inhalations of metered dose aerosol four to six times/day.

FATE

Isoproterenol is readily absorbed when given parenterally or by inhalation; however, sublingual absorption and rectal absorption are unreliable. Onset of action is immediate with IV injection, and within 30 minutes sublingually. Duration of action is less than 1 hour IV and 1 hour to 2 hours sublingually. The drug is metabolized in the GI tract, liver, lungs, and other tissues, and metabolites are excreted in the urine within 24 hours to 48 hours. Approximately 50% of an IV dose is excreted unchanged by the kidney.

SIDE-EFFECTS/ADVERSE REACTIONS

The most frequently encountered side-effects are nervousness, headache, palpitations, flushing, nausea, dizziness, and, following inhalation, dryness of the oropharynx. Other less common adverse reactions include buccal ulcerations (sublingual), bronchial irritation and edema (especially with inhalation of the powder), cardiac distress (tachycardia, dysrhythmias, anginal pain), and, rarely, parotid gland enlargement. Overdosage may result in severe bronchoconstriction, cardiac excitability, and possibly cardiac arrest.

CONTRAINDICATIONS AND PRECAUTIONS

Isoproterenol is contraindicated in patients with arrhythmias associated with tachycardia, other than those that require increased inotropic activity. *Cautious administration* is recommended in the presence of hypertension, coronary insufficiency, diabetes, hyperthyroidism, renal dysfunction, or prostatic hypertrophy and in elderly or debilitated patients or patients unusually sensitive to sympathomimetic amines.

INTERACTIONS

1. Combined use of isoproterenol with epinephrine may lead to serious arrhythmias.
2. Arrhythmias may develop if isoproterenol is used with cyclopropane or halogenated hydrocarbon anesthetics.
3. The effects of isoproterenol are specifically antagonized by propranolol and other beta-adrenergic blockers.

■ Nursing Process

(See also Nursing Care Plan 15-1 and Nursing Process for Norepinephrine and Dopamine; much of the care is similar.)

□ ASSESSMENT

Isoproterenol, when used parenterally, requires the same close monitoring as the other catecholamines (see Nursing Process for Norepinephrine and Dopamine). In addition, the nurse must be careful in selecting formulations of the drug because solutions for injection and inhalation are different, as are tablets for oral and sublingual use. Check the bottle label carefully before administration.

□ *NURSING DIAGNOSES*
(See Nursing Care Plan 15-1.)

□ *PLAN*
The nursing care goals should focus on teaching patients the correct administration methods and how to manage tolerance and side-effects. These are discussed below.

In emergencies, the goal is to maintain heart rate until a cardiac pacemaker can be installed. Intervention is then the same as for norepinephrine.

□ *INTERVENTION*

□ *Inhalation*
The major problem that occurs with the use of the inhalation product is tolerance. As tolerance develops, the patient becomes more dependent on frequent doses of isoproterenol and may repeat treatments three to five times in a 12-hour period. At this point, the patient may develop rebound bronchospasm and suffer a cardiac arrest. The nurse should warn the patient to contact the physician if the relief time between doses decreases before the dangerous level is reached.

Patients should also be taught to properly use the inhaler (see Chap. 8). When inhaling isoproterenol, the patient should not breathe deeply but with normal force and depth. The solution is not to be used if it is cloudy or discolored.

□ *Oral/Sublingual*
Oral and sublingual tablets are not interchangable so the nurse using both should learn to recognize the difference between them. Some of the isoproterenol products are sustained-release tablets; these should never be crushed because doing so will adversely affect absorption.

The patient using sublingual tablets should allow the tablet to dissolve under the tongue without sucking or swallowing, until the drug has been absorbed. Prolonged use of sublingual tablets can damage teeth so the patient should also be told to rinse his mouth after each administration, after the drug has been completely absorbed.

□ *EVALUATION*
The outcome sought is symptom relief of bronchospasm. For the patient using an inhaler, the out-

come should be management of tolerance, if it occurs, and correct use of the inhaler. For the patient taking oral or sublingual tablets the outcome should be that the patient takes the medicine correctly and protects his teeth from damage.

Dobutamine
(Dobutrex)

MECHANISM AND ACTIONS
Dobutamine directly activates beta$_1$ receptor sites on the myocardium with little or no interaction at beta$_2$ or alpha receptors. It does not cause release of norepinephrine. Contractile force is increased, as is stroke volume and cardiac output. These actions are usually accomplished *without* a marked increase in heart rate. Systemic vascular resistance is frequently decreased, however systolic blood pressure may remain unchanged or be slightly increased.

USES
1. Short-term treatment of acute cardiac decompensation due to depressed contractility resulting from organic heart disease or cardiac surgery

ADMINISTRATION AND DOSAGE
Dobutamine is supplied as a powder for injection (250 mg/vial). The drug is administered by IV infusion following dilution in sterile water for injection or 5% dextrose injection. The usual dosage range is 2.5 to 10 mcg/kg/min of either a 250, 500 or 1,000 mcg/ml solution. Doses up to 40 mcg/kg/min have been used on occasion. The rate of administration and duration of infusion are determined by the patient's response as measured by heart rate, blood pressure, urine flow, ectopic activity, and, whenever possible, cardiac output and central venous or pulmonary wedge pressure.

FATE
Effects are noted within 1 minute to 2 minutes, but maximal effect may require 10 minutes to develop. Dobutamine has a very short duration of action (plasma half-life is 2 minutes) and is rapidly metabolized and excreted.

SIDE-EFFECTS/ADVERSE REACTIONS
Most patients experience a slight increase in systolic blood pressure (10 mm Hg to 20 mm Hg) and heart rate (5 to 15 beats/min), and these effects are dose-dependent. Premature ventricular beats occur

in approximately 5% of patients. Less frequent adverse reactions are headache, palpitations, nausea, anginal pain, and dyspnea. Very large doses can significantly increase blood pressure and heart rate, and the infusion should be slowed or terminated temporarily if excessive pressure elevation is seen.

CONTRAINDICATIONS AND PRECAUTIONS
Idiopathic hypertrophic subaortic stenosis is a contraindication to use of dobutamine. The drug should be given *cautiously* to patients with preexisting hypertension, cardiac valvular obstruction, and cardiac arrhythmias.

INTERACTIONS
1. Cyclopropane and halogenated hydrocarbons may increase the incidence of arrhythmias with dobutamine.
2. Pressor effects of dobutamine can be enhanced by MAO inhibitors, tricyclic antidepressants, oxytocic drugs, and sympathomimetic amines.
3. Dobutamine may be ineffective in a patient receiving a beta-blocker.
4. The combination of dobutamine and nitroprusside results in a higher cardiac output and lower pulmonary wedge pressure than use of either drug alone.

NURSING CONSIDERATIONS
The parenteral use of dobutamine requires careful monitoring of ECG, blood pressure, cardiac rate and rhythm, urinary output, and, where possible, cardiac output and pulmonary wedge pressure. Because the drug's major action is to improve cardiac output, the nurse should more closely monitor any patient with a recent MI, atrial fibrillation, or preexisting hypertension. In fact, in patients with atrial fibrillation and rapid ventricular responses, digitalis may be ordered prior to initiation of dobutamine.

The infusion of dobutamine should be monitored by use of an infusion pump. The patient should be closely monitored for signs of infiltration at the IV site, and the drug should be discontinued if infiltration occurs.

Once diluted, dobutamine is an unstable drug and will lose its potency after 24 hours, although a slight color change during this period is not uncommon and does not indicate loss of potency. However, watch the solution closely.

The duration of the drug is very brief; effects are terminated shortly after discontinuation of therapy. This is an advantage if the patient suffers an overdose. Should the nurse observe tachycardia or an excessive increase in blood pressure, the infusion rate should be decreased or stopped. Usually the side-effects will disappear.

Vasopressor Amines

Sympathomimetic vasopressor agents comprise a group of synthetic substances possessing both direct and indirect adrenergic activity. Their predominant pharmacologic effect is the production of generalized vasoconstriction, and they are primarily indicated for the management of acute hypotensive situations, such as those associated with cardiac arrest, circulatory shock, drug reactions, and complications of general anesthesia. However, hypotension alone is not always a sufficient reason to use a vasopressor amine. Many hypotensive states are associated with shock, accompanied by reflex vasoconstriction, which reduces perfusion of vital organs. In such situations, administration of a vasoconstrictor may exacerbate, rather than relieve, the tissue hypoxia in the vital organs. Thus, in most acute hypotensive conditions, primary efforts are directed toward restoration of circulating blood volume, improvement in cardiac output, and maintenance of adequate tissue perfusion. For many forms of shock, dopamine is the preferred drug, inasmuch as it dilates the renal and visceral blood vessels and improves cardiac output. Use of vasopressor amines must be decided on an individual basis, and administered only in the presence of adequate circulating blood volume. Further, vasopressor amines must be given with extreme caution in patients under general anesthesia with a halogenated hydrocarbon, because these anesthetics sensitize the myocardium to the arrhythmic actions of adrenergic amines.

The adrenergic amines used for their acute pressor effects include the previously discussed endogenous and synthetic catecholamines, as well as the four vasopressor drugs reviewed below.

Mephentermine
(Wyamine)

MECHANISM AND ACTIONS
Mephentermine acts both directly on adrenergic receptors and also indirectly by releasing norepinephrine. Cardiac output is elevated and both systolic and diastolic pressures are increased. Its pressor action is due primarily to the increased cardiac

output (beta-adrenergic effect) and also to peripheral vasoconstriction.

USES
1. Hypotension secondary to ganglionic blockade or spinal anesthesia
2. Maintenance of blood pressure in shock following hemorrhage while fluid replacement is accomplished

ADMINISTRATION AND DOSAGE
Mephentermine is used as an injection solution (15 mg/ml, 30 mg/ml) that may be given IM or IV as an undiluted solution or by IV infusion of a 5% dextrose in water dilution.

IM, IV—30 mg to 45 mg in a single injection (30-mg supplements as needed to maintain blood pressure)

IV infusion—0.1% (1 mg/ml) in 5% dextrose in water by continuous infusion at a rate of 1 mg/min; two 10-ml vials (30 mg/ml) added to 500 ml of 5% dextrose in water.

FATE
Following IM injection, effects occur in 5 minutes to 15 minutes and persist for 2 hours to 4 hours. Onset with IV injection is immediate, and duration is 30 minutes to 60 minutes. The drug is rapidly metabolized and is excreted in the urine. CNS effects are minimal at normal doses.

SIDE-EFFECTS/ADVERSE REACTIONS
Side-effects occur infrequently, although occasional anxiety has been reported. With large doses, adverse reactions can include tremors, drowsiness, confusion, incoherence, hypertension, arrhythmias, and, rarely, convulsions.

CONTRAINDICATIONS AND PRECAUTIONS
The drug should not be given to patients receiving MAO inhibitors, or chlorpromazine (See under Interactions). *Cautious use* is recommended in the presence of hypertension, hyperthyroidism, cardiovascular disease, arteriosclerosis, and in chronically debilitated persons.

INTERACTIONS
1. Pressor effects may be potentiated by MAO inhibitors, tricyclic antidepressants, sympathomimetic amines, and oxytocic drugs.
2. Arrhythmias may result if used in combination with cyclopropane, halothane, or digitalis.

3. Pressor effects can be antagonized by guanethidine and reserpine.
4. The hypotension secondary to chlorpromazine may be potentiated by mephentermine.

NURSING CONSIDERATIONS
Blood pressure, pulse, and EKG should be monitored constantly during IV administration beginning with every 2 minutes on initiation of therapy and until vital signs are stabilized, then every 5 minutes to 15 minutes for the duration of therapy. Regulation of the rate of infusion and duration of therapy depends on patient response. Use of an infusion pump is recommended to maintain an accurate rate. The IV site should be checked regularly for infiltration because extravasation can occur causing tissue necrosis.

Because side-effects can result, causing anxiety, confusion, and seizures, the nurse should monitor the patient closely and provide a protective environment during infusion. Patients can develop tolerance to mephentermine with repeated injections; increases in doses should not be used to compensate.

Metaraminol
(Aramine)

MECHANISM AND ACTIONS
The pressor effect of metaraminol is largely due to peripheral vasoconstriction resulting from a direct alpha-adrenergic receptor agonistic action. Cardiac beta stimulation probably only plays a minor role in the pressor response. Reflex bradycardia is common. The drug can also deplete norepinephrine stores in adrenergic nerve endings. Systolic and diastolic blood pressure rises, but perfusion of vital organs may decrease.

USES
1. Prevention and treatment of acute hypotensive states associated with spinal anesthesia
2. Adjunctive management of hypotension caused by brain damage, hemorrhage, surgery, drug reactions, septicemia, or cardiogenic shock

ADMINISTRATION AND DOSAGE
Metaraminol is administered SC, IM, or IV, either by direct injection of a 1% solution or by IV infusion of a dilution in 5% dextrose injection or so-

dium chloride injection. Dosage ranges are as follows:

IM, SC—2 mg to 10 mg (prevention of hypotension)

IV injection—0.5 mg to 5 mg followed by infusion of 15 mg to 100 mg in 500 ml 5% dextrose

IV infusion (preferred in shock)—15 to 100 mg/500 ml 5% dextrose; rate is adjusted to maintain desired blood pressure; range is usually 0.2 to 0.6 mg/min.

Pediatric—0.01 mg/kg as a single dose

FATE

The onset of action is within 1 minute to 2 minutes with IV infusion, 10 minutes with IM injection, and 10 minutes to 20 minutes following SC injection. The effects may persist from 15 minutes to 60 minutes, depending on the route of administration. Metabolism occurs chiefly in the liver and excretion in the urine. Some drug may be taken up by adrenergic nerve endings.

SIDE-EFFECTS/ADVERSE REACTIONS

Most commonly observed side-effects are restlessness, sweating, and palpitations. In large doses, tachycardia, anginal pain, arrhythmias, severe hypertension, convulsions, cardiac arrest, and cerebral hemorrhage can occur. Tissue necrosis and sloughing at the injection site have been reported.

Prolonged use may perpetuate the shock state by preventing volume expansion. Hypotension may occur following termination of the drug.

CONTRAINDICATIONS AND PRECAUTIONS

Contraindications to the use of metaraminol include pulmonary edema, metabolic acidosis, and combined use with halogenated hydrocarbon anesthetics or MAO inhibitors. In addition, metaraminol should not be used as the sole therapy in hypovolemic shock.

Cautious use is indicated in patients with hypertension, hyperthyroidism, diabetes, or cirrhosis, and in patients taking digitalis drugs.

INTERACTIONS

1. The pressor effects of metaraminol may be enhanced by sympathomimetics, MAO inhibitors, tricyclic antidepressants, guanethidine, reserpine, oxytocics, and ergot alkaloids.
2. Arrhythmias may develop in combination with halogenated hydrocarbon anesthetics, digitalis, or mercurial diuretics.
3. Metaraminol can reverse the effect of beta-adrenergic blocking agents.

NURSING CONSIDERATIONS

Metaraminol has a prolonged effect so careful monitoring is essential to avoid excess blood pressure response and the other adverse effects. Blood pressure should be taken every 2 to 5 minutes during the infusion; a continuous ECG is necessary to monitor arrhythmias secondary to drug use and the flow rate should be as exact as possible. An infusion pump should be used and infusion carefully adjusted as the blood pressure responds to the drug. Metaraminol causes many of the same problems as norepinephrine so all previously mentioned nursing considerations with regard to vital signs, urinary output, infiltration, and withdrawal of the drug should be observed.

In addition, response to metaraminol may be erratic in patients with coexistent shock and acidosis. The physician should try to correct blood volume, if possible, before initiating the drug. During administration the nurse should closely watch urinary output and obtain sodium and potassium levels to monitor renal function.

Arrhythmias are common in patients receiving metaraminol who are also digitalized, but bradycardia can occur in any patient being treated. Atropine should be readily available to counteract this side-effect should it occur.

Methoxamine

(Vasoxyl)

MECHANISM AND ACTIONS

Methoxamine is a direct alpha-adrenergic receptor stimulant, producing extensive vasoconstriction with little or no stimulant effects on the heart or the CNS. Reflex bradycardia is a common occurrence and may be attenuated by atropine. Cardiac output may be decreased slightly or remain unchanged. Renal blood flow is reduced. Methoxamine is not useful when cardiac failure is the principal cause of hypotension.

USES

1. Restoration or maintenance of blood pressure during anesthesia
2. Termination of paroxysmal supraventricular tachycardia

ADMINISTRATION AND DOSAGE

Methoxamine is used as an injection solution (20 mg/ml) and may be given by IM or slow IV injection, depending on the situation, as outlined below:

Hypotension
IV—3 mg to 5 mg by slow injection
IM (usual route)—10 mg to 15 mg just prior to anesthesia or to correct a fall in blood pressure; repeat if necessary in 15 minutes
Children—0.25 mg/kg IM

Paroxysmal Supraventricular Tachycardia
IV—10 mg by slow injection
Children—0.8 mg/kg

FATE
Effects are noted within 15 minutes after IM injection and may persist for 1 hour to 2 hours. Onset is almost immediate following IV injection, and the duration is 60 minutes. The drug does not enter the CNS, and excretion is by way of the kidneys.

SIDE-EFFECTS/ADVERSE REACTIONS
The most frequently reported side-effects are paresthesias, coldness in the extremities, and pilomotor stimulation. Other adverse reactions, most commonly seen with large doses, are urinary urgency, sustained hypertension, bradycardia, severe headache, and vomiting.

CONTRAINDICATIONS AND PRECAUTIONS
Methoxamine should not be given in combination with local anesthetics to prolong their action at local sites. *Cautious use* is necessary in patients with advanced cardiovascular disease, hyperthyroidism, myocardial damage, and following use of the ergot alkaloids (e.g., ergotamine, ergonovine).

INTERACTIONS
(See under Metaraminol.)

NURSING CONSIDERATIONS
(See under Metaraminol.)

Phenylephrine Parenteral
(Neo-Synephrine)

MECHANISM AND ACTIONS
Phenylephrine exerts a direct, powerful activation of alpha-adrenergic receptors, resulting in marked vasoconstriction and reflex bradycardia. The drug has only a minimal effect on cardiac beta receptors, therefore, cardiac irregularities are rare. Most vascular beds are constricted, thus, blood flow is restricted to vital organs as well as cutaneous and limb sites. Tachyphylaxis is uncommon, hence repeated injections elicit comparable responses. CNS effects are minimal.

USES
1. Maintenance of blood pressure during spinal and inhalation anesthesia
2. Treatment of shock or drug-induced hypotension
3. Management of paroxysmal supraventricular tachycardia
4. Production of vasoconstriction for regional analgesia (added to local anesthetic solution)

ADMINISTRATION AND DOSAGE
Phenylephrine parenteral (1% injection solution) may be administered by SC, IM, or slow IV injection, or as a continuous IV infusion in a dilute solution. Doses for the various indications are as follows:

Hypotension
SC, IM—2 mg to 5 mg of a 1% solution
IV—0.1 mg to 0.5 mg of a 0.1% solution (may repeat in 15 minutes)
IV infusion—100 to 200 drops/min of a 1:50,000 solution until pressure is stabilized, then 40 to 60 drops/min for maintenance
Pediatric—0.1 mg/kg SC or IM

Prolong Spinal Anesthesia
2 mg to 5 mg added to anesthetic solution

Paroxysmal Supraventricular Tachycardia
0.5 mg IV injection over 20 seconds to 30 seconds; may increase by 0.1-mg increments as needed

FATE
Onset of action is immediate with IV injection, and within 10 minutes to 15 minutes with SC or IM injection. Effects last 15 minutes to 20 minutes following IV administration, 30 minutes to 2 hours with IM injection and 45 minutes to 60 minutes following SC injection.

SIDE-EFFECTS/ADVERSE REACTIONS
Palpitations, paresthesias, and reflex bradycardia are the most commonly noted side-effects; large

doses may result in the appearance of headache, excitability, dizziness, restlessness, vomiting, and an unusually rapid or irregular heart beat, especially following IV injection. Markedly elevated blood pressure can occur in cases of overdosage.

CONTRAINDICATIONS AND PRECAUTIONS

Phenylephrine is contraindicated in severe hypertension, cardiac arrhythmias, and coronary artery disease. The drug should be given *cautiously* in the presence of hypertension, hyperthyroidism, myocardial disease, partial heart block, severe arteriosclerosis, and bradycardia.

INTERACTIONS

(See under Metaraminol.)

NURSING CONSIDERATIONS

While most of the nursing considerations are the same as those for metaraminol, there is one exception. The early signs of overdose for phenylephrine are fullness in the head, tachycardia, and numbness or tingling of extremities. Blood pressure can also rise rapidly so an alpha-adrenergic blocker such as phentolamine should be on hand during drug administration.

Nasal Decongestants

Adrenergic drugs used for the relief of nasal congestion provide a prompt decongestant effect when applied topically to the nasal mucosa. They exert a direct vasoconstrictive action on the arterioles in the mucosa, thus reducing local blood flow, fluid exudation, and mucosal edema. Nasal decongestants are most often used in the form of drops or sprays, and this method of administration is usually effective in the *acute* management of rhinorrhea associated with allergies or the common cold. Oral dosage forms of several adrenergic decongestants are also available, but the incidence of systemic side-effects (*e.g.*, increased blood pressure, tachycardia, CNS excitation) is considerably higher with these drugs compared to the locally applied drugs.

With all decongestants, and especially those used as nasal sprays or nose drops, tolerance to the decongestant effect develops rapidly. Continued use of these drugs frequently results in the appearance of "rebound congestion," characterized by hyperemia and edema of the mucosal membrane. This condition can occur in as short a period of time as 1 week, especially if drug use is frequent or excessive. For this reason use of nasal decongestants for longer than 5 days to 7 days should be strongly discouraged. Should rebound congestion develop, drug usage should be discontinued, and the patient should be instructed to use saline nose drops and a humidifier to help relieve the discomfort. In cases of severe hyperemia and edema, locally applied corticosteroids may be necessary.

Most of the intranasal decongestants have a long duration of action and are only used twice a day. Too frequent application, as noted above, is a major cause of rebound congestion. A general discussion of adrenergic nasal decongestants will follow. For more specific prescribing information concerning each individual drug see Table 15-3.

MECHANISM AND ACTIONS

Most adrenergic decongestants, except for epinephrine and ephedrine, possess relatively selective alpha-adrenergic receptor activity, which produces vasoconstriction of mucosal blood vessels. Thus, shrinkage of swollen tissue occurs, and mucus secretion is decreased.

The orally effective decongestants (phenylpropanolamine, pseudoephedrine, ephedrine, phenylephrine) exert a more generalized vasoconstrictive effect and a less intense mucosal decongestion compared to the locally applied drug. Blood pressure changes are usually minimal, however CNS stimulation can occur.

USES

1. Relief of nasal congestion associated with allergic reactions, colds, acute and chronic inflammatory states, and hay fever (oral or topical application)
2. Adjunctive therapy in middle ear infections (decreases congestion around eustachian tubes) (oral or topical application)
3. Relief of pressure and pain due to ear block during air travel (nasal sprays)

ADMINISTRATION AND DOSAGE

See Table 15-3.

FATE

Topically applied drugs exert a rapid effect which may persist from several hours up to 12 hours. Most drugs are readily absorbed through mucous membranes, and large doses may exert systemic effects, such as increased blood pressure and CNS stimulation.

Table 15-3
Nasal Decongestants

Drug	Preparations	Usual Dosage Range	Clinical Considerations
desoxyephedrine (Vicks Inhaler)	Inhaler—50 mg	1 to 2 inhalations as needed	Avoid excessive use. Headache can occur.
ephedrine (Efed-II, Efedron, Vatronol)	Drops—0.5% Jelly—0.6% Capsules—25 mg, 50 mg Syrup—11, 20 mg/ml	*Topical*—2 to 3 drops or small amount of jelly in nostril every 3 h to 4 h *Oral*—25 mg to 50 mg every 3 h to 4 h (children —3 mg/kg/day in four to six divided doses)	Avoid swallowing nose drops because systemic effects can occur. Do not use drops or jelly longer than 4 days. Do not give to children under age 6. Other uses are discussed in text under Ephedrine.
epinephrine (Adrenalin)	Drops—0.1%	1 to 2 drops every 4 h to 6 h	Do not give to children under age 6. Avoid prolonged or excessive use. See also text under Endogenous Catecholamines and in Table 15-4.
naphazoline (Privine)	Drops—0.5% Spray—0.5%	2 drops or sprays each nostril every 3 h to 6 h	Insomnia is not a problem, so drug may be given at bedtime. Naphazoline is incompatible with aluminum. May produce CNS depression. Ophthalmic drops also available; see Table 15-4 also.
oxymetazoline (Afrin, Dristan Long-Lasting Nasal Mist, Neo-Synephrine 12 H, Sinex Long Acting, and various other manufacturers)	Drops—0.025%, 0.05% Spray—0.05%	*Adults*—2 to 3 drops or sprays of 0.05% twice a day *Children under 6*—2 to 3 drops of 0.025% twice a day	Long-acting preparation; do not exceed twice-a-day dosage and limit use to 7 days to 14 days. Do not use in children under age 2. Package insert suggests patient should bend head forward, sniff the spray, then bend head back.
phenylephrine (various manufacturers)	Drops—0.125%, 0.16%, 0.2%, 0.25%, 0.5%, 1% Spray—0.2%, 0.25%, 0.5% Jelly—0.5%	*Adults*—0.25% to 0.5% solution or spray every 3 h to 4 h *Children (6–12)*—0.25% solution or spray every 3 h to 4 h *Infants*—0.125% to 0.2% solution or spray every 2 h to 4 h	Jelly is placed into nasal cavity and gently inhaled. Do not use for prolonged periods, especially in children. Avoid swallowing solution because systemic effects can occur.
phenylpropanolamine (Propagest, Rhindecon, Sucrets Cold Decongestant Lozenge)	Tablets—25 mg, 50 mg Lozenges—25 mg Timed-release capsules— 75 mg Syrup—12.5 mg/5 ml	*Adults*—25 mg every 4 h or 50 mg every 8 h or 75 mg (long acting) every 12 h *Children (6–12)*—12.5 mg every 4 h; (2–6 years) 6.25 mg every 4 h	Do not exceed recommended dosage, especially in children, because side-effects are likely to occur. Reserpine can antagonize effects of phenylpropanolamine. Also available over the counter as an anorexiant of questionable efficacy. See discussion in text.
propylhexedrine (Benzedrex)	Inhaler—250 mg	1 to 2 inhalations as needed	Do not overuse because CNS stimulation can occur. May produce headache and temporary elevation of blood pressure.
pseudoephedrine (Afrinol, Novafed,	Tablets—30 mg, 60 mg	*Adults*—60 mg every 4 h to 6 h or 120 mg sustained-	Fewer side-effects, less pressor action and longer duration than

(continued)

Table 15-3 (continued)
Nasal Decongestants

Drug	Preparations	Usual Dosage Range	Clinical Considerations
Sudafed, and various other manufacturers)	Repeat action tablets—120 mg Capsules—120 mg (timed-release) Liquid—15 mg/5 ml, 30 mg/5 ml	release every 12 h Children—15 mg to 30 mg every 4 h to 6 h depending on age	ephedrine. Rebound congestion is minimal. Avoid taking drug near bedtime because stimulation can occur. Do not use if restlessness, dizziness, tremors, or other signs of CNS excitation occur.
tetrahydrozoline (Tyzine)	Drops—0.05%, 0.1%	*Adults*—2 to 4 drops 0.1% every 3 h to 4 h *Children (2–6 yrs)*—2 to 3 drops 0.05% every 3 h to 4 h	Large doses may produce CNS depression. Not recommended in children under age 2. Ophthalmic drops also available. See Table 15-4.
xylometazoline (Chlorohist Long Acting, Neo-Spray Long Acting, NeoSynephrine II, Otrivin)	Drops—0.05%, 0.1% Spray—0.1%	*Adults*—2 to 3 drops or sprays every 8 h to 10 h *Children*—2 to 3 drops 0.05% every 8 h to 10 h	Effects persist 4 h to 8 h. Do not use in aluminum containers. Do not exceed recommended dosage because systemic effects are likely.

SIDE-EFFECTS/ADVERSE REACTIONS

The commonly encountered side-effects following local instillation of the drugs into the nasal cavity are stinging and burning of the mucosa, sneezing, and dryness of the nasal membranes.

Rebound congestion is common with prolonged use of nasal decongestants. With use of the oral drugs, especially at high doses or with significant systemic absorption of intranasally applied drugs, adverse reactions include palpitations, tachycardia, hypertension, arrhythmias, nervousness, insomnia, dizziness, blurred vision, dysuria, sweating, respiratory difficulty, tremor, and convulsions. Severe overdosage may result in marked somnolence, sedation, severe hypotension, bradycardia, respiratory depression, and coma.

CONTRAINDICATIONS AND PRECAUTIONS

Adrenergic nasal decongestants should not be used in patients with narrow-angle glaucoma, or in patients concurrently receiving MAO inhibitors or tricyclic antidepressants. Due to the possibility of generalized vasoconstriction and tachycardia, oral decongestants are contraindicated in persons with severe hypertension or coronary artery disease. *Cautious use* of decongestants is warranted in the presence of arrhythmias, hyperthyroidism, diabetes, severe arteriosclerosis, glaucoma, prostatic hypertrophy, and chronic cough accompanied by productive secretions. Safe usage in pregnancy or in nursing mothers has not been established, and elderly or debilitated patients may be more prone to develop CNS excitation.

INTERACTIONS

1. The systemic effects of nasal decongestants may be potentiated by other sympathomimetics, MAO inhibitors, tricyclic antidepressants, antihistamines, and thyroxine.

NURSING CONSIDERATIONS

See Chapter 8 for correct administration of nasal medications.

Patients should be aware that many of these drugs can result in rebound congestion if treatment is prolonged or exceeds the recommended dose. While this condition is not life-threatening, it is uncomfortable and can be avoided. The nurse can instruct the patient not to use the medication for more than 5 days without consulting the physician and to gradually attempt to go longer periods of time between doses. Treatment consists of gradually withdrawing the drug by initially discontinuing the medication on one nostril, then both. Substitution of an *oral* decongestant for the nasal spray is occasionally helpful in withdrawing from the medication completely.

Patients also need to know these drugs can cause systemic toxicity. Drowsiness, decreased respiration, and dizziness resulting from a drop in pulse and blood pressure should be immediately reported.

Ophthalmic Decongestants

The sympathomimetics used in ophthalmology are employed primarily to produce arteriolar vasoconstriction and pupillary dilation due to their strong alpha-adrenergic effects. The various adrenergic drugs used locally in the eye are listed in Table 15-4. Depending on the strength of the various preparations, these drugs have a number of indications. The stronger solutions of phenylephrine (2.5%, 10%) as well as 1% hydroxyamphetamine are primarily used in diagnostic eye examinations, during ocular surgery, and to prevent synechiae formation in uveitis. Medium strength solutions (0.5%, 1%, and 2% epinephrine) are indicated in open-angle glaucoma, while the weaker solutions (0.1% epinephrine, 0.012% and 0.02% naphazoline, 0.08%, 0.12%, and 0.15% phenylephrine, and 0.05% tetrahydrozoline) are principally employed for symptomatic relief of minor eye irritations due to allergies, colds, wind, pollens, and so forth. These weaker solutions are available over the counter, whereas the stronger solutions require a prescription.

The major advantages of adrenergic ophthalmics over anticholinergics having many of the same actions in the eye are that ophthalmic decongestants do not produce cycloplegia (i.e., paralysis of accommodation), nor do they increase intraocular pressure. Due to their mydriatic effect, however, they are contraindicated in narrow-angle glaucoma because retraction of the iris would further impair the already reduced drainage of aqueous humor resulting from occlusion of the channels by the abnormally positioned iris. A general review of this class of drugs will be followed by the listing of individual drugs in Table 15-4.

MECHANISM AND ACTIONS
The major effect of ophthalmic decongestants is a direct activation of alpha receptor sites in the eye, resulting in vasoconstriction of small blood vessels and contraction of the radial muscle, which leads to mydriasis. Some locally applied adrenergics (e.g., epinephrine, hydroxyamphetamine) also possess a beta-adrenergic action, which relaxes the ciliary muscle and decreases the formation of aqueous humor.

USES
(Not all drugs are used for every indication—see Table 15-4.)
1. Facilitate examination of the fundus of the eye
2. Reduce the incidence of synechiae formation in uveitis
3. Dilation of the pupil prior to intraocular surgery
4. Treatment of open-angle glaucoma (increases outflow and decreases production of aqueous humor)
5. Symptomatic relief of minor eye irritations due to colds, hay fever, dust, wind, and so forth

ADMINISTRATION AND DOSAGE
See Table 15-4.

FATE
Following local instillation into the eye, the onset of mydriasis is rapid, and maximal dilation is attained within 30 minutes to 60 minutes. Effects usually persist for several hours.

SIDE-EFFECTS/ADVERSE REACTIONS
Common side-effects with use of adrenergic ophthalmics are stinging or burning in the eyes, headache or browache, and temporary blurred vision. More serious local adverse reactions include conjunctival irritation, pigmentary deposits in the lids, conjunctiva, or cornea, and, rarely, maculopathy with a central scotoma. Systemic absorption of significant amounts may lead to palpitations, tachycardia, hypertension, anxiety, sweating, insomnia, dizziness, and pallor.

CONTRAINDICATIONS AND PRECAUTIONS
Ocular decongestants are contraindicated in patients with narrow-angle glaucoma, and prior to iridectomy in eyes capable of angle closure. Phenylephrine 10% is contraindicated in infants. Due to the possibility of significant systemic absorption, these drugs should be used cautiously in patients with hypertension, hyperthyroidism, diabetes, arteriosclerosis, heart disease, and bronchial asthma.

NURSING CONSIDERATIONS
See Clinical Considerations in Table 15-4.

Bronchodilators

Sympathomimetic bronchodilators are employed in the treatment of bronchial asthma and other

Table 15-4
Ophthalmic Decongestants

Drug	Preparations	Usual Dosage Range	Clinical Considerations
epinephrine (various manufacturers)	Drops—0.1%, 0.25%, 0.5%, 1.0%, 2%	1 to 2 drops 0.1% to 0.25% individualized to condition	Used in conjunctivitis, to control bleeding in surgery and to elicit mydriasis. Effects last 1 h to 3 h. Solutions of 0.5% and stronger are also used for open-angle glaucoma. Weaker solutions are used as decongestants. Solutions are unstable; keep closed and protect from light and heat; discard if solution is brown. See general discussion of epinephrine in text.
hydroxyamphetamine (Paredrine)	Drops—1%	1 to 2 drops as needed	Primarily used to dilate pupil for eye exams, surgery, and uveitis. Effects last up to 4 h to 6 h.
naphazoline (AK-Con, Albalon, Allerest, Clear Eyes, Comfort, Degest-2, Muro's Opcon, Naphcon, Vasoclear, Vasocon)	Drops—0.012%, 0.02%, 0.03%, 0.05%, 0.1%	1 to 2 drops every 3 h to 4 h	Primarily used as an ocular decongestant. 0.012% to 0.05% solutions available over the counter, 0.1% by prescription only. Available in combination with pheniramine (Naphcon A) and antazoline (Albalon-A, Vasocon-A). Can cause rebound congestion if use exceeds recommended dose. May sting on initial instillation, but discomfort will pass within minutes.
phenylephrine (AK-Dilate, AK-Nefrin, Isopto Frin, Mydfrin, Neo-Synephrine)	Drops—0.12%, 2.5%, 10%	10%—uveitis, open-angle glaucoma, prior to intraocular surgery 2.5%—refraction, ophthalmic exams, prior to surgery, uveitis 0.2%—ocular decongestion, relief of minor eye irritations (available over the counter)	Do not use 10% solution in children. Prior instillation of a local anesthetic in the eye may alleviate much of the stinging and burning caused by phenylephrine. The 2.5% solution may be used as a diagnostic test for narrow-angle glaucoma. The 0.12% solution is also available over the counter combined with zinc sulfate (*e.g.,* Zincfrin), or as prescription only combined with pyrilamine (Prefrin-A) or pheniramine (AK-Vernacon). May cause rebound hypertension in patients with orthostatic hypertension. Safety margin is narrow; watch for overdosage. Can cause rebound miosis in the elderly; readministration will be less effective.
tetrahydrozoline (Murine Plus, Optigene-3, Soothe, Visine)	Drops—0.05%	1 to 2 drops two to three times/day	Primarily used to relieve minor symptoms of eye irritation. Available over the counter. Can cause rebound congestion if use exceeds recommended dose.

chronic obstructive pulmonary diseases (COPDs) (see Chap. 48 for Disease Briefs). Parenteral (i.e., SC, IM) injections of epinephrine are usually very effective in relieving respiratory distress (dyspnea, wheezing, chest tightness) during an acute asthmatic attack. However, some patients respond poorly to epinephrine during an acute attack; such patients are often successfully treated by IV infusion of aminophylline, a xanthine bronchodilator discussed in Chapter 48. Continual symptomatic management of chronic asthma may be accomplished with oral or inhaled use of one of the adrenergic bronchodilators, although several other types of drugs (e.g., theophylline, corticosteroids, cromolyn) are employed as well. These other drugs will also be considered in Chapter 48.

Sympathomimetic agents used as bronchodilators possess prominent beta-adrenergic activity that elicits relaxation of the smooth muscle of the bronchioles. Several drugs in this category (epinephrine, isoproterenol, ephedrine) activate *all* beta-adrenergic receptor sites, and their use is associated with a disturbing range of side-effects, particularly involving activation of $beta_1$ receptor sites in the cardiovascular system. Newer adrenergic bronchodilators (e.g., albuterol, metaproterenol, terbutaline) exhibit a greater degree of selectivity with regard to the $beta_2$ receptors located on bronchiolar smooth muscle, and thus produce a lower incidence of cardiac side-effects, although *complete* separation of $beta_1$ and $beta_2$ activity has still not been realized, especially at elevated doses. In addition to direct relaxation of bronchiolar smooth muscle, the adrenergic bronchodilators may inhibit the release of endogenous bronchoconstricting allergens from the mast cells and increase bronchiolar ciliary activity, thus facilitating expulsion of mucus. These actions of the bronchodilating sympathomimetics are due in part to an elevation in the levels of cyclic AMP resulting from stimulation of adenyl cyclase, the enzyme that catalyzes formation of cyclic AMP. Finally, those agents (epinephrine, ephedrine), possessing alpha-adrenergic action as well as beta activity, exert a secondary vasoconstrictive effect on bronchiolar blood vessels, and the resultant mucosal decongestant action also contributes to their effectiveness in treating chronic lung diseases.

The relative popularity of the various adrenergic bronchodilators is determined by many factors, including the type and severity of the condition being treated, physician preference, patient acceptance, and cost. Epinephrine and isoproterenol are potent bronchodilators whose use is somewhat restricted by the fact that they cause a considerable amount of cardiac excitation in many patients. They have been discussed earlier in the chapter. Ephedrine is a less potent bronchodilator which exhibits more pronounced central excitatory effects than other adrenergic drugs. It is discussed below, along with the remaining sympathomimetic bronchodilators that exert a more selective action on $beta_2$ receptor sites in the bronchioles. Other types of drugs used as bronchodilators (e.g., theophylline) are discussed in Chapter 48.

Ephedrine

MECHANISM AND ACTIONS

Ephedrine is a dual-acting adrenergic amine which is less potent and has a slower onset and longer duration than epinephrine. Its effects result from a direct activation of both alpha- and beta-adrenergic receptor sites as well as presynaptic release of norepinephrine. Ephedrine produces tachycardia, increased blood pressure and cardiac output, causes mydriasis, and relaxes bronchiolar and GI smooth muscle. The bronchodilation is less intense than that produced by epinephrine but is more prolonged. Central stimulatory effects are also more pronounced than with epinephrine. Local application to the nasal mucosa constricts small arterioles, thus reducing engorgement and facilitating drainage (see Table 15-3). The urinary bladder sphincter is contracted, promoting urinary retention; this effect, coupled with the central stimulatory action which decreases the depth of sleep, forms the basis for its use in enuresis. Ephedrine may potentiate the action of acetylcholine at the neuromuscular junction, an action possibly of benefit in myasthenia gravis (see Chap. 13).

USES

1. Bronchodilation in milder forms of chronic pulmonary diseases (e.g., bronchial asthma, bronchitis).
   Note: Ephedrine is available in many fixed combinations with theophylline and phenobarbital (e.g., Tedral), and theophylline and hydroxyzine (e.g., Marax), often including other expectorants and sedatives. Use of these fixed combination products in asthma should be discouraged, as titration of *individual* doses is frequently necessary, yet is not possible in fixed combinations.
2. Relief of nasal mucosal congestion (see Table 15-3)

3. Maintenance of blood pressure during spinal anesthesia and control of postural hypotension (injection only)
4. Treatment of enuresis (with atropine)
5. Treatment of narcolepsy
6. Support of ventricular rate in Adams-Stokes syndrome
7. Treatment of overdosage with CNS depressants
8. Adjunctive treatment of myasthenia gravis (with cholinesterase inhibitor)

ADMINISTRATION AND DOSAGE

Ephedrine for systemic use is available as 25-mg and 50-mg capsules, syrup containing 11 mg or 20 mg per 5 ml, and injection solution containing 25 mg/ml and 50 mg/ml. Oral administration is preferred when possible for most nonemergency indications, although ephedrine can also be given IM, SC, or by slow IV injection.

Adults
25 mg to 50 mg PO, SC, IM, or slow IV every 3 hours to 4 hours as necessary (not to exceed 150 mg/24 h)
Intranasal—see Table 15-3

Children
2 to 3 mg/kg/day in four to six divided doses, PO, SC, or IV

FATE

Ephedrine is readily absorbed orally and parenterally. Bronchodilation is maximal within 30 minutes to 60 minutes of oral administration and within 10 minutes to 20 minutes of IM injection. Effects persist for 3 hours to 5 hours orally and 1 hour to 2 hours IM and SC. The drug is distributed widely in the body, and readily crosses the blood–brain barrier, exerting a rather marked stimulating effect. The drug is largely (60%–70%) excreted unchanged in the urine.

SIDE-EFFECTS/ADVERSE REACTIONS

The most frequently encountered side-effects result from the central stimulatory effects of ephedrine, and include nervousness, insomnia, and occasional anxiety. Other adverse reactions most often occur with large doses, such as headache, tremor, confusion, vertigo, sweating, nausea, palpitations, tachycardia, arrhythmias, transient hypertension, dysuria, and urinary retention. Overdosage is characterized by euphoria, delirium, CNS depression, respiratory depression, and occasionally hallucinations.

CONTRAINDICATIONS AND PRECAUTIONS

Ephedrine is contraindicated in severe hypertension, narrow-angle glaucoma, arrhythmias in patients receiving MAO inhibitors, and during anesthesia with a halogenated hydrocarbon such as halothane. The drug should be used with *caution* in patients with coronary artery disease, hyperthyroidism, diabetes, prostatic hypertrophy, arteriosclerosis, and chronic heart disease.

INTERACTIONS

1. The pressor effects of ephedrine may be increased by ergot alkaloids, oxytocics, MAO inhibitors, other sympathomimetics, and furazolidone.
2. Ephedrine may reduce the effectiveness of guanethidine.
3. Ephedrine may be less effective in the presence of methyldopa or reserpine.
4. Arrhythmias can occur if used in combination with halothane and related anesthetics or digitalis drugs.

NURSING CONSIDERATIONS

See also Chapter 48.

The primary concern with this drug is dosage control. Patients should be taught to follow the recommended dosage carefully because the central stimulatory effect of this drug can lead to tolerance and abuse. To maintain effectiveness, patients may need several drug-free days interspersed with the therapy.

Elderly persons are very susceptible to the effects of this drug. They are more prone to developing hallucinations, convulsions, and CNS depression as well as insomnia and urinary retention. Timing of administration and monitoring output can be important strategies in guiding use of ephedrine.

When ephedrine is used IV it will affect blood pressure. This vital sign must be monitored closely until the patient is stabilized. In addition, the effectiveness of ephedrine will diminish in the presence of respiratory acidosis. Consequently, arterial blood gases should be regularly monitored while the patient is receiving this drug.

Ethylnorepinephrine

(Bronkephrine)

Ethylnorepinephrine is an adrenergic bronchodilator similar in most respects to isoproterenol. It primarily activates beta-adrenergic receptor sites; its

Table 15-5
Selective Beta$_2$ Adrenergic Bronchodilators

Drug	Preparations	Usual Dosage Range	Clinical Considerations
			General: Observe for development of paradoxical bronchospasm with any of the drugs; the physician should be notified immediately.
albuterol (Proventil, Ventolin)	Inhaler—90 mcg/metered dose Tablets—2 mg, 4 mg Syrup—2 mg/5 ml Sustained-release tablets—4 mg Solution for inhalation—0.83 mg/ml, 5 mg/ml	Inhalation—1 to 2 inhalations every 4 h to 6 h Prevention of exercise-induced bronchospasm—2 inhalations 15 min prior to exercise Oral—2 mg to 4 mg three to four times/day (maximum 32 mg/day) *Children (6–14)*—2 mg three to four times/day *Children (2–6)*—0.1 mg/kg three times/day	Gradually absorbed from the bronchioles. Onset occurs within 15 min following inhalation and persists for 3 h to 4 h. With oral use, onset is 30 min and effects persist for 4 to 6 h. Most common side-effects are nervousness and tremor (20%), headache (7%), and tachycardia (5%). May delay preterm labor. Drug has displayed a tumorogenic potential in animals at high doses. Do not use with other sympathomimetic drugs (danger of increased CV side-effects).
bitolterol (Tornalate)	Aerosol—0.8% (delivers 0.37 mg per inhalation)	2 inhalations at an interval of 1 min to 3 min; a third inhalation may be given if necessary Prevention of bronchospasm—2 inhalations every 8 h	Used for prophylaxis or treatment of bronchospasm. Effects occur within 5 min and persist up to 8 h. Longest acting inhaled beta$_2$ agonist; may be used with theophylline or corticosteroids.
isoetharine (Arm-a-Med Isoetharine, Beta-2, Bronkometer, Bronkosol, Dey-Dose Isoetharine, Dey-lute, Disorine, Dispos-a Med Isoetharine)	Solution for nebulization—0.062%, 0.08%, 0.1%, 0.125%, 0.14%, 0.167%, 0.17%, 0.2%, 0.25%, 0.5%, 1% Aerosol—340 mcg delivered per metered dose	*Solution*—3 to 7 inhalations of undiluted solution by a hand nebulizer or 0.25 ml to 0.5 ml of a 0.5% or 1% solution diluted 1:3 with saline or other diluent (lower strength solutions are given undiluted) by oxygen aerosolization or IPPB apparatus *Aerosol nebulizer*—1 to 2 inhalations as needed	Relaxes bronchial smooth muscle by an action on beta$_2$ receptors. May also inhibit histamine release. Can be administered by IPPB apparatus—see package instructions. Do not use if solution is brown or contains a precipitate. Avoid contact with the eyes. Oxygen flow rate is adjusted to 4 to 6 liter/min over 15 min to 20 min for oxygen aerosolization. Pediatric dosage has not been established.
metaproterenol (Alupent, Metaprel)	Tablets—10 mg, 20 mg Syrup—10 mg/5 ml Aerosol inhaler—225 mg (0.65 mg/dose) Solution for nebulization—0.6%, 5%	*Oral* Adults—20 mg three to four times/day Children (6–9)—10 mg three to four times/day Children (under 6)—1.3 to 2.6 mg/kg/day *Inhalation* 10 inhalations of 5% solution by hand nebulizer or 2 to 3	Effects appear almost immediately with inhalation and within 15 min to 30 min orally. Duration is 2 h to 4 h with inhaler and 4 h to 5 h orally. Nervousness, tremor, and weakness are common with oral administration of 20 mg. Bad taste can occur with oral inhalation but will gradually disappear with repeated use.

(continued)

Table 15-5 (continued)
Selective Beta₂ Adrenergic Bronchodilators

Drug	Preparations	Usual Dosage Range	Clinical Considerations
metaproterenol (Alupent, Metaprel) (*continued*)		inhalations of metered dose aerosol inhaler every 3 h to 4 h to a maximum of 12 inhalations/day	Overdose can lead to cardiac arrest; encourage adherence to prescribed dose.
terbutaline (Brethaire, Brethine, Bricanyl)	Tablets—2.5 mg, 5 mg Injection—1 mg/ml Aerosol—0.2 mg delivered per dose	*Oral* Adults—2.5 mg to 5 mg three times/day (maximum 15 mg/day) Children (over 12)—2.5 mg three times/day *SC*—0.25 mg; repeat in 15 min to 30 min if needed. If no response after two doses, seek alternate measures *Aerosol*—2 inhalations, 1 min apart, every 4 h to 6 h *Delay premature labor* (investigational) 10 mcg/min IV infusion titrated upward to a maximum of 80 mcg/ min. Oral doses of 2.5 mg every 4 h to 6 h have been used until term.	Slowly absorbed orally and parenterally. Effects appear within 15 min to 30 min and persist 2 h to 4 h with SC injection, up to 6 h with inhalation, and 4 to 8 h with oral administration. Muscle tremor is common with 5-mg oral dose. Used by IV infusion to delay premature labor (investigational use); see Nursing Process for ritodrine. Cardiovascular side-effects are more common with SC injection.

alpha effect is considerably less than that of epinephrine, hence the effect on blood pressure is less marked.

The principal application of ethylnorepinephrine is relief of bronchospasm; however, it is usually reserved for acute attacks, inasmuch as it must be administered IM or SC. Onset of action is 5 minutes to 10 minutes, and effects last 1 hour to 2 hours. The adult dose is 1 mg to 2 mg (0.5 ml–1 ml), while children receive 0.1 ml to 0.5 ml depending on weight. Refer to the discussion of isoproterenol earlier in the chapter for additional information.

Selective Beta₂ Agonists: Albuterol, Bitolterol, Isoetharine, Metaproterenol, Terbutaline

The selective beta₂ bronchodilators preferentially activate beta₂ receptor sites on bronchiolar and other smooth muscle at normal dose levels, leading to relaxation. The absence of significant beta₁-receptor activity at recommended doses reduces the degree of cardiac excitability frequently observed with nonselective beta agonists such as isoproterenol or epinephrine. When administered by inhalation, bronchodilation observed with beta₂ agonists is comparable to that seen with isoproterenol. Certain beta₂ agonists are also available for oral or parenteral use (see Table 15-5) for either chronic (oral) or acute (SC) symptomatic management of bronchial asthma. The beta₂ agonists will be reviewed as a group, then detailed individually in Table 15-5.

MECHANISM AND ACTIONS
In recommended doses, beta₂-adrenergic receptor sites are preferentially activated, resulting in relaxation of bronchiolar, vascular, and uterine smooth muscle to varying degrees. Action at cardiac beta₁ receptors is generally minimal, thus tachycardia and increased cardiac output are rarely significant.

USES

1. Relief of reversible bronchospasm associated with asthma and other bronchospastic disorders
2. Delay premature labor (investigational use only)

ADMINISTRATION AND DOSAGE

See Table 15-5.

FATE

Inhaled drugs have a rapid onset of action, generally within 5 minutes. Following oral or SC administration, effects are noted within 15 minutes to 30 minutes. Duration of action ranges from 2 hours to 4 hours with inhalation (up to 8 hours with bitolterol); effects persist 4 hours to 8 hours following oral administration. Excretion is largely by the kidney, both as unchanged drug and metabolites.

SIDE-EFFECTS/ADVERSE REACTIONS

Side-effects following inhalation are minimal. Oral doses can elicit mild muscle tremor, nervousness, weakness, headache, flushing, sweating, insomnia, vertigo, and irritability. *Excessive* oral dosage or significant systemic absorption following inhalation can lead to cardiovascular reactions such as palpitations, tachycardia, arrhythmias, chest discomfort, and increased blood pressure, although these reactions are much less common than with use of the nonspecific beta agonists, such as epinephrine and ephedrine. Nausea, vomiting, muscle cramping, coughing, and difficulty in urination have also occurred. Drying of the oropharynx may accompany inhalation.

CONTRAINDICATIONS AND PRECAUTIONS

Principal contraindications to use of beta$_2$ agonists are tachyarrhythmias, severe coronary artery disease, and administration in combination with halogenated hydrocarbon anesthetics. These drugs must be given *with caution* to patients with hypertension, hyperthyroidism, diabetes, prostatic hypertrophy, narrow-angle glaucoma, and a history of seizures.

INTERACTIONS

1. The cardiovascular effects of beta$_2$ agonists may be enhanced by other sympathomimetics, MAO inhibitors, and tricyclic antidepressants.
2. The bronchodilating effect of beta$_2$ agonists is antagonized by nonselective beta-blockers (*e.g.*, propranolol, nadolol, timolol, pindolol).

NURSING CONSIDERATIONS

See Chapter 48 for more complete nursing process information about bronchodilators.

The beta$_2$ agonists are generally used as adjunctive therapy with theophylline products. Such combinations exert additive effects, but individual responses are extremely variable. Consequently the nurse's most important role is to teach the patient the action of the drug and to help him learn to adjust the therapy to his own symptoms. He can be encouraged to use the lowest dose possible to obtain relief, to monitor his symptoms closely, to monitor how long the medication provides relief, and report changes in symptoms promptly to the physician. The asthmatic patient who takes such an active role will generally use drug therapy more effectively and manage his illness better.

See Chapter 8 for directions on administering bronchodilators by inhaler. See the box "Teaching Self-Administration of Bronchodilators by Metered-Dose Inhaler" for points on teaching patients self-administration with metered dose nebulizers.

For the most part beta$_2$ agonist bronchodilators are not used in combination. Any orders that call for treatments with more than one drug from this category should be clarified with the prescriber.

Smooth Muscle Relaxants

Several adrenergic drugs have the ability to relax smooth muscle, and this action has led to their use in the treatment of peripheral vascular insufficiency and premature labor.

Nylidrin and isoxsuprine are two orally effective sympathomimetics that exhibit a beta-adrenergic receptor agonistic action. Activation of beta$_2$ receptor sites in skeletal muscle vasculature can lead to vasodilation of normal vessels. However, the vasodilator effects of nylidrin and isoxsuprine on muscle blood flow are *not* prevented by beta-blockers. Thus, these drugs probably also exert a direct relaxant effect on vascular smooth muscle in addition to their beta-agonistic action. Despite the fact that blood flow in normal resting skeletal muscle can be increased by these drugs, there is no conclusive evidence that they have a beneficial effect in chronic occlusive vascular conditions such as arteriosclerosis or thromboangiitis obliterans. Because skeletal muscle and cerebral vascular beds are probably already reflexly dilated by the ischemia resulting from a vascular occlusion, peripheral vasodilator drugs primarily increase blood supply to *nondilated, nonischemic* areas not in

Teaching Self-Administration of Bronchodilators by Metered-Dose Inhaler (Canister Nebulizer)

It is extremely important for the patient to learn the correct use of these administration tools. If used incorrectly serious overdose can occur. When teaching this technique, allow the patient plenty of time for supervised practice (refer to the product insert) and emphasize the following points:

1. Place the drug container in the short end of the plastic mouthpiece. The container nozzle must fit in the small hole provided. For albuterol and metaproterenol, shake the container before beginning the treatment. Refer to product information to learn number of doses in each canister. Also, teach the patient how to detach the mouthpiece from the metal canister and to rinse the mouthpiece daily with hot water.
2. Hold the inhaler so the drug container is upside down.
3. Insert the mouthpiece into mouth and close lips tightly around it.
4. Exhale deeply through the nose.
5. Inhale deeply through the mouth. At the same time, press down on the container to release the medication. (Check package instructions before teaching this item. For some medications a regular breath is indicated instead of a deep one.)
6. Hold breath a few seconds then exhale slowly.
7. Allow 2 minutes before repeating the medication inhalation. Remember that the patient may be short of breath at the time he is taking this medication. He may need to learn to use a relaxation–focusing technique, a slow mental-counting technique, or a watch with a second-hand or digital second-counter in order to follow the required timing.

critical need of improved perfusion. Further compromising the efficacy of these drugs is the fall in blood pressure which frequently accompanies their administration. Thus, their hypotensive effect may actually *reduce* cerebral blood flow and perfusion of vital organs. Therefore, use of nylidrin and isoxsuprine for treating peripheral and cerebral vascular insufficiency should be discouraged.

Isoxsuprine has also been used to delay premature labor, as it also exerts a uterine smooth muscle relaxant effect. Its effects are nonselective, however, and side-effects due to beta-receptor activation elsewhere in the body are frequent. Use of isoxsuprine as a uterine relaxant has been largely supplanted by ritodrine, another beta agonist which exerts a somewhat more selective effect on beta$_2$ receptors in the uterus. These three sympathomimetic smooth muscle relaxants are discussed below.

Isoxsuprine
(Vasodilan, Voxsuprine)

MECHANISM AND ACTIONS
Isoxsuprine exerts a beta-adrenergic receptor activating effect, however, its vasodilating action is not blocked by beta-blockers, suggesting that the drug also has a direct relaxant effect on vascular smooth muscle. Isoxsuprine may also possess some alpha-adrenergic blocking action. Resting blood flow in skeletal muscle is increased, whereas cutaneous blood flow is unaltered. Cardiac stimulation is common, resulting in increased heart rate, force of contraction, and cardiac output. Uterine smooth muscle is relaxed. High doses may inhibit platelet aggregation and decrease blood viscosity.

USES
(*Note:* Clinical effectiveness has *not* been established for any of the indications below.)
1. Symptomatic treatment of peripheral vascular insufficiency (*e.g.*, Raynaud's disease, thromboangiitis obliterans, arteriosclerotic obliterans)
2. Treatment of premature labor and threatened abortion (experimental use only)

ADMINISTRATION AND DOSAGE
Isoxsuprine is available for oral administration as 10-mg and 20-mg tablets. The recommended dosage is 10 mg to 20 mg three to four times a day.

FATE
The drug is well absorbed orally. Peak blood levels are attained in approximately 1 hour and persist for 2 hours to 3 hours. Excretion is primarily in the urine.

SIDE-EFFECTS/ADVERSE REACTIONS

The most frequently encountered side-effect with isoxsuprine administration is facial flushing. Other adverse reactions are primarily dose-related and include tachycardia, chest pain, hypotension, irregular heartbeat, nervousness, weakness, dizziness, nausea, vomiting, and abdominal distress. There have been rare reports of a skin rash.

CONTRAINDICATIONS AND PRECAUTIONS

Isoxsuprine should not be given in the presence of arterial bleeding or immediately postpartum. *Cautious use* is warranted in patients with bleeding disorders, coronary artery disease, glaucoma, severe cerebrovascular disease, and following a recent myocardial infarction.

INTERACTIONS

1. The effects of isoxsuprine can be antagonized by sympathomimetic drugs having a significant alpha-adrenergic activity.

NURSING CONSIDERATIONS

The use of isoxsuprine in arterial vascular disease is an adjunct to appropriate physical care. The patient must also be taught to control his or her weight, to exercise, to stop smoking, to wear proper footwear, to keep extremities warm, and to provide prompt attention to any skin lesion. The drug may not help the patient with extensive circulatory impairment. If over several weeks of therapy the patient notices no change or a worsening of symptoms, these should be reported to the doctor. Cessation of numbness, coldness, or tingling in the affected extremities is evidence the drug is working.

Blood pressure should be closely monitored throughout therapy to observe the hypotensive effects of the drug and prevent the occurrence of systemic damage.

Vasodilan is being used experimentally for relief of premature labor. See Nursing Considerations discussion under Ritodrine.

Nylidrin

(Arlidin, Adrin)

MECHANISM AND ACTIONS

Nylidrin increases blood flow in skeletal muscles by stimulating beta-adrenergic receptors and by exerting a direct relaxant effect on vascular smooth muscle. Cerebral blood flow is usually not increased, because the vasodilation of cerebral blood vessels is offset by the fall in blood pressure. Cutaneous blood flow is unaffected. Cardiac output is slightly increased, and heart rate may also increase. Systolic pressure may rise slightly, but diastolic pressure is reduced.

USES

(*Note:* Clinical effectiveness has *not* been established for any of the indications below.)

1. Symptomatic relief of peripheral vasospastic disorders (*e.g.,* diabetic vascular disease, acrocyanosis, Raynaud's disease, night leg cramps, ischemic ulcer, frostbite, thrombophlebitis)
2. Relief of circulatory disturbances of the inner ear (*e.g.,* cochlear cell, macular, or ampullar ischemia; labyrinthine artery spasm)

ADMINISTRATION AND DOSAGE

Nylidrin as 6-mg and 12-mg tablets is used orally in a dosage range of 3 mg to 12 mg given three or four times a day.

FATE

Oral absorption is good. Effects are noted within 10 minutes, attain a maximum at 30 minutes to 40 minutes, and last approximately 2 hours. The drug is slowly excreted in the urine.

SIDE-EFFECTS/ADVERSE REACTIONS

Adverse reactions associated with nylidrin are nervousness, trembling, nausea, vomiting, weakness, dizziness, palpitations, tachycardia, and hypotension.

CONTRAINDICATIONS AND PRECAUTIONS

Nylidrin is contraindicated during an acute myocardial infarction and in patients with severe angina, tachyarrhythmias, uncompensated heart failure, and thyrotoxicosis. The drug must be given *cautiously* in the presence of hypertension, peptic ulcer, and cardiac disorders.

INTERACTIONS

(See under Isoxsuprine.)

NURSING CONSIDERATIONS

(See under Isoxsuprine.) In addition, nylidrin may cause palpitations in some patients. Patients should report this symptom to their physician. The condition may subside by itself; if not the treatment will be discontinued.

Ritodrine

(Yutopar)

Ritodrine is a fairly selective beta$_2$-adrenergic receptor agonist which can inhibit uterine contractions, and therefore is used in the management of premature labor. It is administered initially by IV infusion to arrest contractions, then orally for as long as necessary to prolong pregnancy the desired extent. Its overall toxicity is somewhat lower than other agents employed in premature labor (alcohol, magnesium sulfate, isoxsuprine).

MECHANISM AND ACTIONS

Ritodrine activates beta$_2$ receptor sites on uterine smooth muscle, thus increasing levels of cyclic AMP which reduces the contractile response. It also affects cardiac beta$_1$ receptors, especially following IV administration, resulting in tachycardia and widening of the pulse pressure. With oral administration, the increase in heart rate is mild and slow to develop. Transient elevations of serum glucose, insulin, and free fatty acids have been observed, especially with IV use. Serum potassium may also be reduced.

USES

1. Management of preterm labor in suitable patients, when the gestation is greater than 20 weeks. IV administration arrests the acute response, and oral administration is then used to prevent recurrence.

ADMINISTRATION AND DOSAGE

Ritodrine is available as tablets (10 mg) and injection solution (10 mg/ml). A controlled infusion device is recommended so the rate of flow can be adjusted in drops/minute. To prepare the infusion solution, 150 mg (3 ampules) are diluted in 500 ml of diluent to yield a final solution of 0.3 mg/ml.

Drug administration is begun as a slow IV infusion. The initial dose is 0.1 mg/min of a 0.3 mg/ml dilution at a rate of 0.33 ml/min or 20 drops/min using a microdrip chamber. Depending on the response, the dose may be increased gradually in increments of 0.05 mg/min every 10 minutes until the desired result is attained. The usual effective dosage range is 0.15 mg/min to 0.35 mg/min. The infusion should be carried on for 12 hours after labor has ceased.

Approximately 30 minutes prior to ending the infusion, an oral dose of 10 mg should be given. For the next 24 hours, 10 mg should be given every 2 hours. Thereafter, 10 mg to 20 mg are administered every 4 hours to 6 hours for as long as is necessary to prolong pregnancy. The maximum oral dose is 120 mg/day.

FATE

Peak serum levels following oral administration occur in 30 minutes to 60 minutes. Oral bioavailability is approximately 30% of the administered dose. Food may inhibit the effectiveness of oral ritodrine. Ritodrine is metabolized in the liver and excreted in the urine, 70% to 90% of a dose within 24 hours. Protein binding is approximately 30%.

SIDE-EFFECTS/ADVERSE REACTIONS

The most common side-effects encountered with use of ritodrine, especially following IV infusion, are increases in maternal and fetal heart rates, alterations in maternal blood pressure (i.e., increased systolic and decreased diastolic), transient elevation in blood glucose and insulin, hypokalemia, palpitations, tremor, nausea, headache, and erythema. Less frequently observed adverse reactions are vomiting, nervousness, restlessness, anxiety, emotional changes, chest pain or tightness, arrhythmias, and rash. Infrequently noted effects include epigastric distress, constipation or diarrhea, sweating, chills, dyspnea, hyperventilation, glycosuria, lactic acidosis, heart murmur, and anaphylactic reaction.

CONTRAINDICATIONS AND PRECAUTIONS

Contraindications to use of ritodrine include conditions in which continuation of pregnancy would be hazardous for the health of mother or fetus, such as antepartum hemorrhage, eclampsia, fetal death, maternal cardiac disease, pulmonary hypertension, hyperthyroidism, or uncontrolled diabetes. In addition, ritodrine is contraindicated in the presence of cardiac tachyarrhythmias, uncontrolled hypertension, bronchial asthma, and hypovolemia, and prior to the twentieth week of pregnancy. Cautious use is indicated in patients with controlled diabetes, hypertension, or cardiac impairment.

INTERACTIONS

1. Combined administration of ritodrine and corticosteroids may lead to pulmonary edema.
2. Effects of other adrenergic amines may be potentiated by ritodrine.
3. Beta-blockers will reduce the effectiveness of ritodrine.

4. Ritodrine may increase the hypokalemia observed with various diuretics.

■ Nursing Process

Note: Terbutaline is also being used to delay premature labor (see Table 15-5). The following discussion applies to use of that drug as well.

□ Assessment

Baseline maternal pulse and blood pressure should be obtained, and a vaginal examination should be performed to determine the degree of cervical dilation. A fetal heart rate should also be obtained and if the medication is to be administered intravenously, fetal monitoring will be started. All of these parameters will provide a baseline. If the physician questions the viability of the fetus, ultrasound may also be ordered. Laboratory studies should be done to determine adequacy of renal and liver function. Clotting studies also should be done to rule out abruptio placentae.

The woman who is in premature labor may be extremely frightened of losing her child. She will need to have a clear understanding of what the drug can and cannot do and what the risks are. If she is going home on the medication she needs to know how limited her mobility will be, because drug therapy is only part of a total regimen which usually includes bedrest until the thirty-sixth week. In addition, she also needs to plan how she will pay for the medication, which is extremely expensive. The mother who agrees to ritodrine therapy must be aware of the commitment necessary to facilitate success.

□ Nursing Diagnoses

Actual nursing diagnoses for the patient receiving ritodrine include:

Knowledge deficit regarding action, administration, and side-effects of the drug

Fear of losing the unborn child

Alteration in family process resulting from physical limitations placed on the mother on home drug therapy

Impaired home maintenance management due to activity restrictions

Potential nursing diagnoses usually related to the side-effects of the drug include:

Alteration in cardiac output (decreased)

□ Plan

The nursing care goals vary depending on whether the drug is given intravenously or on an outpatient basis. If parenteral therapy is in order, the main goal is to ensure adequate dosing with minimal side-effects. This is also the goal for the woman taking ritodrine at home. In addition, the woman needs an opportunity to express and deal with her anxiety and if going home, needs to establish an administration routine that will ensure stable blood levels at all times.

□ Intervention

Intravenous infusion of ritodrine can be best monitored through an infusion pump. Because the dose given usually requires fluid administration over at least a 24-hour period, the nurse must also watch this patient for signs of fluid overload which can manifest as edema, rales, and decreased output. In addition, pulse and blood pressure should be closely monitored and the patient may need to be on a cardiac monitor to watch for signs of tachycardia or other arrhythmias.

Emotional support will be essential. The woman will be attached to a fetal monitor, a cardiac monitor, and an IV line, and will be constantly worried that the drug will not work and she will continue in labor. It is important to keep her informed about her progress and what the monitors are showing. Time should be taken to talk realistically about her fears because it is possible the ritodrine will not work or that side-effects will become severe and the drug will have to be discontinued.

The woman who will take ritodrine at home needs to plan how to limit her activities, which may be very difficult if she has other children. She needs to know what side-effects to watch for, especially signs of fluid retention and edema. This patient will be closely monitored at home, may be taught to use a portable fetal monitor to check contractions, and will probably need the assistance of a visiting nurse.

□ Evaluation

The outcome criteria against which the patient will judge successful treatment is the elimination of premature labor. Most patients will tolerate the side-effects if this outcome is achieved and they are able to deliver close to normal term. However, ethical concerns may also be at issue. Many clinicians and parents feel premature labor is a natural method of aborting an abnormal fetus and have concerns about the use of ritodrine. The mother may worry about fetal deformity until a normal baby is actually delivered.

CNS Stimulants and Anorexiants

The principal adrenergic drugs used for their central stimulatory effects are the amphetamine derivatives and ephedrine. The major indications for these compounds are control of obesity, relief of depression, and treatment of attention deficit disorder in children. Due to their profound central excitatory action, they are an often abused class of drugs. These compounds will be discussed in Chapter 32, and aspects of their abuse potential will be reviewed in Chapter 85.

A number of products containing phenylpropanolamine, a sympathomimetic decongestant, in amounts ranging from 25 mg to 75 mg are promoted as over-the-counter nonprescription diet aids (*e.g.*, Acutrim, Control, Dexatrim, Prolamine) as an adjunct to caloric restriction. Many of these preparations contain various other substances as well, such as vitamins, minerals, and grapefruit ex-

tract. Phenylpropanolamine is claimed to exert an anorexiant effect by a central action at the level of the appetite control center in the hypothalamus. However, its efficacy as an appetite suppressant is subject to considerable doubt by many health professionals, and use of the drug, especially at high dose levels, should be strictly controlled. Due to its cardiac-stimulating and blood pressure–elevating effects, phenylpropanolamine should not be used by patients with cardiovascular disease, hypertension, diabetes, hyperthyroidism, glaucoma, or renal impairment. Combined use with other sympathomimetics, MAO inhibitors, and tricyclic antidepressants should also be avoided. Phenylpropanolamine administration must be discontinued at once should palpitations, dizziness, or rapid pulse occur. Recommended doses are 25 mg phenylpropanolamine three times a day or 50 mg to 75 mg of the long-acting preparations once daily. Continuous use for longer than 3 months is not recommended. The drug must be used in conjunction with a restricted caloric intake.

CASE STUDY

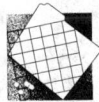

Jackie Kilmer, a 28-year-old woman, is 24 weeks pregnant. She calls her obstetrician when she begins having labor pains 3 minutes to 4 minutes apart. Jackie has a history of premature labor, had a miscarriage with her first pregnancy, and was treated with ritodrine in her second pregnancy from week 26 to week 36. She delivered a normal baby girl, Elise, at 38 weeks. Elise is now 2 years old.

The doctor advises Jackie to go to the emergency room immediately. She is admitted to the labor room and examined. Her cervix is 2 cm dilated and contractions are now 1 minute to 2 minutes apart. Blood work is drawn and abruptio placentae is ruled out. The doctor orders a ritodrine drip at a rate of 0.1 mg/min to be increased 50 mcg/min every 10 minutes until the labor ceases.

Jackie remains on ritodrine IV for 5 hours before labor pains cease. The decision is made to titrate the dose and begin oral ritodrine. She is told she will be discharged on the drug.

Discussion Questions

1. What data were needed before ritodrine was started on this patient? Why must abruptio placentae be ruled out?
2. What are the major side-effects of the drug on the mother and fetus? What should the nursing care goals be during this acute phase of treatment?
3. What would be an appropriate home care plan for Jackie? What complications must be dealt with in planning her discharge?

REVIEW QUESTIONS

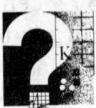

1. What are the principal physiologic roles for the three endogenous catecholamines?
2. Describe the biosynthesis of epinephrine.
3. Norepinephrine released from an adrenergic nerve ending can be inactivated in what three ways?
4. Distinguish between *uptake-1* and *uptake-2* with regard to inactivation of epinephrine.
5. List a brief plan for teaching a family home administration of epinephrine.
6. Contrast alpha$_1$ and alpha$_2$ receptor sites with respect to (a) location and (b) responses following activation.
7. Distinguish between the two types of beta-adrenergic receptor sites using the same parameters as in Question 6.
8. Where are dopaminergic receptors located and what responses do they mediate?
9. How does dipivefrin (Propine) differ from epinephrine? What are its advantages over epinephrine?
10. Describe the major cardiovascular effects of dopamine infusion as the dosage is increased.
11. List the major assessment parameters for the patient who receives norepinephrine or dopamine.
12. What are the effects of isoproterenol on (a) the heart, (b) the bronchioles, and (c) the uterus?
13. Why are vasopressor amines not always indicated in the treatment of shock? What precautions must be taken when they are used?
14. What is the principal danger associated with prolonged use of nasal decongestants?
15. What problems result from the development of tolerence to adrenergic drugs? How can the nurse reduce the rate at which tolerance develops?
16. List the major indications for adrenergic ophthalmic decongestants.
17. What is the advantage of selective beta$_2$ agonists over epinephrine and isoproterenol as bronchodilators?
18. Describe the two major types of asthma.
19. What are the principal disadvantages of nylidrin and isoxsuprine in the treatment of peripheral vascular disorders?
20. Review the following administration methods. Outline a patient-teaching guide for the patient taking:
    a. an inhalant—isoproterenol
    b. nose drops—oxymetazoline
    c. eye drops—naphazoline
21. What are the main nursing goals for the patient in premature labor receiving ritodrine or terbutaline?

BIBLIOGRAPHY

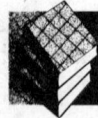

Abundis J: Hazards of metered-dose bronchodilator inhalers. J Emerg Nsg 11:252, 1985

Adrenergics. Nursing 83, January 1983 (Suppl.)

Axelrod J: Noradrenaline: Fate and control of its biosynthesis. Science 173:598, 1971

Balkam JA: Allergic rhinitis therapy and the nursing mother. Pediatr Nursing March/April: 47, 1981

Berthelsen S, Pettinger WA: A functional basis for classification of alpha-adrenergic receptors. Life Sci 21:595, 1977

Caritis SN: Treatment of preterm labor: A review of therapeutic options. Drugs 26:243, 1983

Dixon WR, Mosimann WF, Weiner N: The role of presynaptic feedback mechanisms in regulation of norepinephrine release by nerve stimulation. J Pharmacol Exp Ther 209:196, 1979

Eckstein JW, Abboud FM: Circulatory effects of sympathomimetic amines. Am Heart J 63:119, 1962

Feely J, DeVane PJ, MacLean D: Beta-blockers and sympathomimetics. Br Med J 286:1043, 1983

Goldberg LI: Dopamine—Clinical uses of an endogenous catecholamine. N Engl J Med 291:707, 1974

Goldberg LT: Cardiovascular and renal actions of dopamine: Potential clinical applications. Pharmacol Rev 24:1, 1972

Henney HR: Knowledge of nurses and respiratory therapists about using cannister nebulizers. Am J Hosp Pharm 41:2403, 1984

Hoffman BB, Lefkowitz RJ: Alpha-adrenergic receptor subtypes. N Engl J Med 302:1390, 1980

Huss P, et al: The new inotropic drug, dobutamine. Heart Lung January/February:121, 1981

Kelly RB, Deutsch JW, Carlson SS, Wagner JA: Biochemistry of neurotransmitter release. Annu Rev Neuroscience 2:399, 1979

Langer SZ: Presynaptic receptors and their role in the regulation of transmitter release. Br J Pharmacol 60:481, 1977

McGrath JC: Evidence for more than one type of post-junctional alpha-adrenoceptor. Biochem Pharmacol 31:467, 1982

Minneman KP, Pittman RN, Molinoff PB: Beta-adrenergic receptor subtypes: Properties, distribution, and regulations. Annu Rev Neuroscience 4:419, 1981

Motulsky HJ, Insel PA: Adrenergic receptors in man. N Engl J Med 307:18, 1982

Nelson HS: Beta-adrenergic agonists. Chest 82:335, 1982

Rogers T: Clinical problems in the adult with asthma. Nurs Clin North Am June:293, 1981

Sonnenblick EH, Frishman WH, LeJemtel TH: Dobutamine: A new synthetic cardioactive sympathetic amine. N Engl J Med 300:17, 1978

Webb-Johnson DC, Andrews JL: Bronchodilator therapy. N Engl J Med 297:476, 1977

Zaimis E: Vasopressor drugs and catecholamines. Anesthesiology 29:732, 1968

Adrenergic Blocking Agents (Sympatholytic Drugs)

16

Several types of pharmacologic agents are capable of interfering with the functioning of the sympathetic nervous system as well as the actions of exogenous adrenergic drugs. Certain compounds can either deplete the catecholamine stores in adrenergic nerve endings or retard release of the catecholamine neurotransmitters (e.g., norepinephrine) from the nerve ending in response to a nerve impulse. Drugs of this type which act presynaptically to inhibit synthesis, storage, or release of adrenergic neurohormones are frequently referred to as *adrenergic neuronal blockers* and are frequently employed as antihypertensives. These drugs, such as guanethidine, reserpine, and methyldopa, are principally used as antihypertensives and will be considered in Chapter 35.

Other antiadrenergic agents inhibit the interaction of endogenously released adrenergic neurohormones (i.e., norepinephrine, epinephrine) or exogenously administered sympathomimetic amines with the various types of adrenergic receptor sites. These drugs are termed *adrenergic receptor blockers.* As is the case with most other receptor antagonists, such as anticholinergics and antihistamines, adrenergic receptor blockers more effectively antagonize the actions of circulating adrenergic neurohormones or exogenously administered adrenergic drugs than the responses of the various body organs to sympathetic nerve stimulation.

Reflecting the generally accepted classification of adrenergic receptor sites into alpha and beta types (see Table 15-1), the adrenergic receptor blockers are likewise separated into alpha-adrenergic and beta-adrenergic blocking agents, and the delineation is essentially complete for the majority of currently available drugs. That is, alpha blockers do not generally block beta sites and *vice versa.* Some alpha blockers, such as phenoxybenzamine and prazosin, are relatively selective postsynaptic $alpha_1$ antagonists, whereas others, like phentolamine and tolazoline, are largely nonspecific in their blocking actions and interfere with the activation of both $alpha_1$ and presynaptic $alpha_2$ sites. Similarly, beta-adrenergic blocking agents can be grouped into selective $beta_1$ blockers (e.g., atenolol and metoprolol) and nonselective (i.e., $beta_1$ and $beta_2$) blockers such as nadolol, propranolol, pindolol, and timolol. With both alpha and beta blockers, the greater specificity of action of the selective blockers reduces many of the undesirable side-effects that can result from nonselective adrenergic blockade.

Alpha-Adrenergic Blocking Agents

Compounds capable of blocking the actions of either endogenous or exogenous agonists at the alpha-adrenergic receptor sites are termed alpha-blockers. Alpha-adrenergic receptor antagonists may be classified into one of two groups based on their duration of action.
1. Irreversible, noncompetitive antagonist (e.g., phenoxybenzamine)
2. Reversible, competitive antagonists (e.g., phentolamine, prazosin, tolazoline)

Phenoxybenzamine forms a stable, covalent bond with the $alpha_1$ receptor sites, resulting in a prolonged (i.e., 3 days to 4 days) blockade of the receptor site. Daily administration of the drug leads to permanent inhibition of receptor activity. Phenoxybenzamine exerts little effect on presynaptic $alpha_2$ sites.

The remaining alpha-blockers are reversible competitive antagonists whose effects persist at most for only several hours. The antagonistic action of these reversible inhibitors can easily be overcome by larger concentrations of agonist (i.e., norepinephrine) at the receptor site.

Prazosin is an $alpha_1$ selective antagonist used in the management of mild to moderate hypertension. Its principal advantage over nonselective alpha antagonists is the relative absence of reflex tachycardia commonly associated with other alpha-blockers (see below). Prazosin will be considered in detail in Chapter 35 with the other antihypertensive agents. Phentolamine and tolazoline, on the other hand, are largely nonspecific in their blocking action, and interfere with activation of both $alpha_1$ and $alpha_2$ sites. In addition, these latter two drugs exert a direct relaxant effect on vascular smooth muscle and possess muscarinic cholinergic and histaminergic agonistic activity.

Another group of compounds, the ergot alkaloids, exhibit alpha-adrenergic blocking activity. However, these drugs, such as ergotamine and dihydroergotoxine mesylates, a mixture of three alkaloidal substances, also possess a direct smooth-muscle spasmogenic effect as well as a serotonin-blocking action and a central dopamine agonistic effect. This complex pattern of pharmacologic actions greatly limits the clinical usefulness of these drugs as vasodilators. In fact, the major danger associated with most ergot alkaloids is severe *vasospasm* in cases of overdosage, due to their marked spasmogenic action at high doses. Ergotamine is primarily used in the relief of vascular headaches and is reviewed in Chapter 18. Dihydroergotoxine mesylates, commonly referred to as ergoloid mesylates, is indicated for treatment of reduced mental capacity in the elderly, often reflected as forgetfulness, lack of self-care, disorganization, and mood changes. Its action is presumably due to reduced cerebral blood flow and blunted metabolism. The drug purportedly has a more favorable ratio of alpha-blocking activity to direct vasospastic activity and hence is claimed to improve blood flow to the CNS and increase central metabolic activity. The clinical effectiveness of dihydroergotoxine mesylates is subject to considerable doubt, however, although improvements in some subjective CNS disturbances have been reported. Nausea and vomiting are frequent occurrences with use of the drug, especially in large amounts. Moreover, tolerance to the vasodilator effects develops rapidly. The drug is considered in more detail in Chapter 36.

Other ergot alkaloids, such as ergonovine and bromocriptine, have additional clinical applications and will be considered in the appropriate chapters throughout the book.

Pharmacologic Effects of Alpha-Blockers

The principal effects of alpha-blockers are on the cardiovascular system, where they decrease peripheral vascular resistance and thus lower blood pressure due to an antagonistic action at vascular alpha$_1$ receptor sites. However, by interfering with sympathetic control of vasomotor function, alpha-blockers frequently result in a marked degree of orthostatic or postural hypotension, often leading to dizziness, lightheadedness, and vertigo upon assumption of a standing position. Heart rate and cardiac output are usually increased as a consequence of an uninhibited reflex response to blood pressure reduction. The reflex tachycardia is fur-

ther magnified when the nonspecific alpha-blockers, which also block presynaptic alpha$_2$ sites, are used, inasmuch as the release of norepinephrine from prejunctional adrenergic nerve endings is augmented due to removal of the inhibitory alpha$_2$-mediated negative feedback mechanism (see Fig. 15-2). This controlled release of neurohormone can even further stimulate chronotropic beta receptors in the heart leading to excessive tachycardia. Excessive reflex tachycardia also commonly occurs with phenoxybenzamine, because this drug not only causes vasodilation but also inhibits neuronal and extraneuronal uptake of norepinephrine, thus retarding its inactivation. However, prazosin does not usually exhibit significant reflex tachycardia, as it does not block presynaptic alpha$_2$ receptors as does phentolamine and tolazoline, nor does it reduce norepinephrine uptake as does phenoxybenzamine.

It is difficult to generalize concerning other pharmacologic effects of alpha-blockers, because some drugs possess various other actions (*e.g.*, cholinomimetic, histaminic, direct spasmolytic) in addition to alpha-receptor antagonism. Generally, however, alpha-blockers cause miosis by blocking catecholamine-mediated contraction of the radial muscle of the iris. In the GI tract, the alpha-blockers possessing cholinomimetic and histaminergic activity frequently cause hypersecretion and increased peristalsis. The effect of alpha-blockers on the CNS is highly variable, and both stimulant and depressant effects have been noted. Certain nonvascular smooth muscle may be relaxed, and salivary and sweat gland secretions can be reduced.

Phenoxybenzamine
(Dibenzyline)

MECHANISM AND ACTIONS
Phenoxybenzamine forms a stable bond with alpha-adrenergic receptor sites, resulting in a long-lasting, noncompetitive blockade. Receptor blockage persists for several days. The drug appears to be somewhat more selective in blocking alpha$_1$ than alpha$_2$ receptors, although it can inhibit the effects of both alpha$_1$ and alpha$_2$ agonists. Phenoxybenzamine reduces neuronal uptake of catecholamines, increases release of norepinephrine from presynaptic adrenergic nerve terminals (by presynaptic alpha$_2$ blockade), and also possesses anticholinergic, antihistamine, and antiserotonin actions, primarily at high doses. Clinical effects of the drug include increased blood flow to the skin, mucosa,

and abdominal viscera and decreased blood pressure, both in the supine and erect positions, but primarily of the orthostatic type. Reflex increases in cardiac output and heart rate can occur.

USES

1. Control hypertension and sweating associated with pheochromocytoma (see Disease Brief: Pheochromocytoma), frequently in combination with a beta-blocker if tachycardia is prominent.
2. Improve circulation in vasospastic (*not* occlusive) peripheral vascular diseases (*e.g.*, Raynaud's, acrocyanosis, frostbite).
3. Treatment of micturition dysfunction due to neurogenic bladder, outlet obstruction, or prostatic obstruction). (Effectiveness has not yet been conclusively determined.)

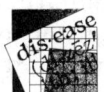

DISEASE BRIEF

■ Pheochromocytoma

Pheochromocytoma is a chromaffin cell tumor, usually of the adrenal medulla, which actively secretes excessive amounts of catecholamines. Clinical signs include hypertension (frequently of a severe and sustained nature) tachycardia, and arrhythmias. Diagnosis is usually made based on a chemical analysis of urinary concentrations of catecholamines and their metabolites, primarily vanillylmandelic acid (VMA), metanephrine, and normetanephrine. Surgical removal of the tumor is the preferred treatment, but alpha-adrenergic blockers are frequently used, both preoperatively to control the elevated pressure and tachycardia and during surgery, together with beta-blockers, to prevent excessive blood pressure elevation, tachycardia, and arrhythmias which may result from release of excess catecholamines as a consequence of surgical manipulation of the tumor.

ADMINISTRATION AND DOSAGE

Phenoxybenzamine is available as 10-mg capsules. Dosage should be individualized and adjusted to meet the needs of each patient. Initially, 10 mg is administered once a day. The dosage may then be increased by 10 mg at 4-day intervals until an optimum response is attained, which usually takes about 2 weeks. The usual maintenance dosage range is 20 mg to 60 mg/day.

FATE

Oral absorption is incomplete; only 20% to 30% of the dose is absorbed in an active form. Peak effects occur within 4 hours to 6 hours, and the blocking action persists for 3 days to 4 days with a single dose. Excretion is primarily by the kidney and bile, approximately 80% of the dose within 24 hours.

SIDE-EFFECTS/ADVERSE REACTIONS

Lightheadedness and dizziness commonly occur when the patient rises from a lying or sitting position. Other frequently observed side-effects are rapid heart beat, nasal congestion, and miosis, with possible blurring of vision. Additional adverse effects include dry mouth, drowsiness, weakness, confusion, headache, inability to ejaculate and, rarely, diarrhea, vomiting, and skin rash.

CONTRAINDICATIONS AND PRECAUTIONS

Phenoxybenzamine is contraindicated in conditions in which a sudden fall in blood pressure would prove dangerous. *Cautious use* is indicated in patients with cerebral or coronary arteriosclerosis, renal insufficiency, compensated congestive heart failure, and respiratory infections, the symptoms of which may be aggravated by phenoxybenzamine. The elderly patient may be more sensitive to the hypotensive action of phenoxybenzamine because of the progressive decrease in cardiovascular reflex responsiveness with aging.

INTERACTIONS

1. Adrenergic compounds that stimulate both alpha and beta receptors, such as epinephrine, may produce an exaggerated drop in blood pressure and tachycardia in the presence of an alpha-blocker, the so-called epinephrine reversal.

2. Phenoxybenzamine can have an additive hypotensive effect with other types of antihypertensive drugs.

■ Nursing Process

□ ASSESSMENT
Diagnosis of pheochromocytoma will have been made before this drug is started, so all of the laboratory studies mentioned in the pheochromocytoma disease brief will be part of the pretreatment assessment. Baseline blood pressure in sitting, lying, and standing positions must be done to measure the effectiveness of the drug.

In addition, for the patient with peripheral vascular disease, peripheral pulses should be measured and skin color and temperature assessed.

□ NURSING DIAGNOSIS
The *actual* nursing diagnoses for the patient taking phenoxybenzamine include:
   Knowledge deficit related to action, administration, and side-effects of the drug
   Potential for injury related to orthostatic hypotension which occurs early in therapy
Potential nursing diagnoses related to side-effects of the drug include:
   Alteration in cardiac output: decreased
   Impaired gas exchange
   Sensory–perceptual alteration in vision and smell
   Sexual dysfunction related to inability to ejaculate
   Alteration in tissue perfusion

□ PLAN
Nursing care goals for the patient receiving phenoxybenzamine include careful monitoring of blood pressure during dosage adjustment and assisting the patient to manage the drug's side-effects.

□ INTERVENTION
Dosage of phenoxybenzamine will be carefully titrated to achieve lowered blood pressure; each change will be monitored for approximately 4 days to determine the effect on the patient. A flow sheet for blood pressure, pulse rate and rhythm, and other responses to the drug may be a useful tool for keeping all vital information in one place.

Phenoxybenzamine has a dramatic effect on blood pressure and can cause significant orthostatic hypotension especially in the elderly. Nursing responsibilities include teaching the patient to sit up very slowly and remain sitting for a few minutes before standing. If weakness or faintness occur the patient needs to lie down. Occasionally severe hypotension will occur. To deal with this the patient will be put flat in bed for 24 hours, have leg bandages applied to facilitate peripheral vascular return, and if necessary a norepinephrine drip will be started.

The patient also needs to be aware of what symptoms to expect and how to deal with them. Palpitations, tachycardia, orthostatic hypotension, nasal congestion, and impaired ejaculation are bothersome effects which may disappear as the body adjusts to the drug. If these symptoms do not disappear over several weeks, the patient should be advised to call the physician. The patient also needs to watch for symptoms of respiratory infections because the drug will aggravate such conditions. If the patient takes the drug with meals he can minimize gastrointestinal irritation.

□ EVALUATION
For the patient with vascular disease, a decrease in cyanosis or pallor in the extremities, return of normal skin color, increase in skin temperature, improved capillary filling in the nail beds, and lessened sensitivity to cold are all indicators that the drug is working. In the patient with pheochromocytoma, decrease in blood pressure and pulse rate are indicators of effectiveness.

Phentolamine
(Regitine)

MECHANISM AND ACTIONS
Phentolamine exerts a reversible, competitive, short-acting block of both alpha₂ and alpha₁ receptor sites. In addition, it has a direct relaxant effect on the vascular smooth muscle and may also exert a muscarinic and histamine-like agonistic effect and an antiserotonin action. Peripheral vascular resistance is decreased, and venous return to the heart is reduced. Reflex tachycardia commonly occurs, and the cardiac output may be increased. GI motility can be stimulated, and an increase in gastric secretion of hydrochloric acid and pepsin has been observed.

USES
1. Control of hypertension in patients with pheochromocytoma during stress periods, and prior to or during surgical excision of tumor, frequently in combination with a beta-blocker
2. Prevent tissue necrosis and sloughing resulting

from extravasation of norepinephrine or other vasopressors such as dopamine or metaraminol

3. Diagnosis of pheochromocytoma (measurement of urinary catecholamines is the preferred technique for diagnosis and phentolamine is seldom used)

4. Experimental uses include treatment of hypertensive crises resulting from an interaction between sympathomimetic amines and MAO inhibitors, or rebound hypertension following withdrawal of clonidine or other antihypertensive agents.

ADMINISTRATION AND DOSAGE

Phentolamine is available as an injection containing 5 mg/ml. Recommended doses for the various indications are as follows:

Pheochromocytoma

Preoperative reduction of blood pressure in pheochromocytoma

Adults—5 mg IM or IV 1 hour or 2 hours before surgery

Children—1 mg IM or IV 1 hour to 2 hours before surgery

Repeat if necessary. During surgery, 5 mg (adults) or 1 mg (children) may be given IV to control episodes of hypertension, tachycardia, and other signs of epinephrine toxicity.

Prevention of dermal necrosis due to extravasation of norepinephrine or other potent vasopressors

10 mg added to each liter of norepinephrine solution or 5 mg to 10 mg in 10 ml saline injected into the area of extravasation within 12 hours

FATE

Onset of action following IM injection is rapid. Peak effects occur within 2 minutes with IV injection and within 10 minutes to 15 minutes with IM administration. Action persists for 15 minutes with IV use and up to 4 hours following IM injection. Phentolamine is excreted largely as metabolites in the urine.

SIDE-EFFECTS/ADVERSE REACTIONS

Most commonly occurring side-effects are flushing, nasal congestion, and GI distress. In addition, tachycardia is usually present. Other adverse reactions are hypotension (usually orthostatic), anginal pain, arrhythmias, weakness, dizziness, vomiting, and diarrhea. If evidence of shock occurs, the patient should be treated vigorously, as myocardial infarction and cerebrovascular occlusion have resulted from the severe hypotension occasionally seen with IV injection.

CONTRAINDICATIONS AND PRECAUTIONS

Phentolamine is contraindicated following a recent myocardial infarction, and in the presence of angina or other types of coronary insufficiency. The drug must be administered *cautiously* in patients using digitalis drugs because tachycardia and arrhythmias can occur. The safety of the drug in pregnant or nursing women has not been established, and elderly persons may demonstrate an exaggerated hypotensive effect.

INTERACTIONS

See under Phenoxybenzamine.

NURSING CONSIDERATIONS

Phentolamine is given parenterally; during such a procedure nursing care will center on monitoring blood pressure and pulse because they will be the indicators of severe hypotension. Keep the patient supine during the infusion and be ready to treat overdosage rigorously and promptly. Norepinephrine is the drug of choice in treating overdosage, *not* epinephrine. Epinephrine will unmask the beta effect of the drug and cause a further drop in blood pressure. If the patient has a history of cardiac arrhythmias, ECG monitoring may also be appropriate.

The use of phentolamine as a diagnostic aid in pheochromocytoma is appropriate only to confirm the results of other tests, not as a procedure of choice. If the physician decides to do such a test, emergency resuscitation equipment and norepinephrine should be close at hand.

Patient teaching for this patient includes instruction on how to reduce the effects of orthostatic hypotension and how to minimize gastrointestinal irritation by taking the drug with milk or meals. (See under Nursing Process for phenoxybenzamine.)

The parenteral form of this drug should be mixed immediately before using it because it is an unstable solution.

Tolazoline

(Priscoline)

MECHANISM AND ACTIONS

Tolazoline exhibits a variety of actions, including a weak, nonselective (*i.e.*, alpha₁ and alpha₂) alpha-adrenergic blocking effect, a direct relaxant effect on vascular smooth muscle, cholinergic-like and histamine-like activity and beta-adrenergic activity. Peripheral vasodilation results primarily from the musculotropic spasmolytic and histamine-like actions; the alpha-blocking effect is weak and transient. GI motility is increased due to the cholinergic action, and gastric secretions are stimulated due to the histaminergic action. Improvement in blood flow is primarily in the cutaneous vessels.

USES
1. Adjunctive management of persistent pulmonary hypertension in the newborn when sufficient oxygenation cannot be maintained by usual supportive care
2. Improved blood flow in spastic peripheral vascular disorders associated with acrocyanosis, arteriosclerosis obliterans, thromboangiitis obliterans, gangrene, and various other conditions. (Efficacy has not been established, and the drug is rated only "possibly effective.")

ADMINISTRATION AND DOSAGE
The drug is used parenterally as a 25-mg/ml injection solution. The recommended dosage for pulmonary hypertension is 1 to 2 mg/kg by scalp vein initially, followed by an infusion of 1 to 2 mg/kg/hr to increase arterial oxygen. Response generally occurs within 30 minutes. There has been only limited experience with infusions lasting longer than 36 to 48 hours. IV administration is often accompanied by flushing and tachycardia.

FATE
The drug is slowly but well absorbed by all routes of administration. Maximal effects following IV occur in 30 minutes to 60 minutes. In neonates, the half-life ranges from 3 hours to 10 hours. Tolazoline is excreted largely unchanged by the kidney.

SIDE-EFFECTS/ADVERSE REACTIONS
Common side-effects include flushing, tingling, or numbness in extremities, nausea, and reflex tachycardia. Additional adverse reactions are:

CV—Anginal pain, arrhythmias, orthostatic hypotension
GI—Nausea, vomiting, diarrhea, gastric discomfort, ulcer-like pain
CNS—Apprehension, mydriasis, headache
Other—Pulmonary hemorrhage, rash, edema, oliguria, hematuria, leukopenia, thrombocytopenia

CONTRAINDICATIONS AND PRECAUTIONS
Tolazoline is contraindicated in patients with coronary artery disease and cerebrovascular insufficiency. The drug should be used with *caution* in the presence of peptic ulcer and other GI disorders, and mitral stenosis.

INTERACTIONS
See under Phenoxybenzamine.

NURSING CONSIDERATIONS
Although not frequently done, a patient may be discharged on IM injections of this drug. If so, he will need to know the following:
- Ingestion of alcohol with tolazoline can result in a disulfiram-like reaction (tachycardia, sweating, dyspnea, vomiting) (see Chap. 26).
- Overexposure to cold environments should be avoided; drug effectiveness is enhanced by warm surroundings.
- Side-effects such as orthostatic hypotension, nausea, headache, and reflex tachycardia will disappear with continued therapy.
- Flushing, increased skin temperature, and piloerection indicate the drug is working and that the dose is optimal.

If the patient is receiving tolazoline in the hospital, the side-effect requiring nursing intervention most frequently will be hypotension. This patient should be placed supine, given IV fluids, and treated for overdose with ephedrine. Epinephrine should not be given because the beta effect of the drug will be unmasked resulting in a further drop in blood pressure.

Intra-arterial injection of tolazoline should be discouraged. This procedure is performed only by physicians who are familiar with the drug's action, and then only for carefully selected patients whose conditions warrant such measures. The route is to be used only when IV administration has failed to produce desired results and then only when emergency equipment, including ephedrine is immediately available.

Beta-Adrenergic Blocking Agents

Acebutolol, Atenolol, Betaxolol, Esmolol, Labetalol,* Levobunolol, Metoprolol, Nadolol, Pindolol, Propranolol, Timolol

Drugs capable of exerting a reversible competitive blocking action at beta-adrenergic receptor sites, thereby antagonizing the action of catecholamines and other beta-agonists, are termed beta-adrenergic blocking agents. The beta-blockers can be divided into nonselective and selective antagonists. Nonselective beta antagonists (levobunolol, nadolol, pindolol, propranolol, timolol) block both beta$_1$ and beta$_2$ receptor sites, whereas selective beta-blockers (acebutolol, atenolol, betaxolol, esmolol, metoprolol) exert their blocking effects predominantly at beta$_1$ receptors in the usually administered doses. The selectivity of certain drugs for cardiac beta$_1$ sites is relative and dose dependent. That is, in high concentrations, the beta-blocking ac-

tions of the "selective" beta$_1$ blockers can extend to the beta$_2$ receptors as well, such as those in the bronchioles.

While all the available beta-receptor blockers are effective competitive antagonists at the various beta-receptors, a number of differences exist in the properties of the individual drugs. A brief comparison of some of the pharmacologic and pharmacokinetic properties of the various beta-blockers is presented in Table 16-1. Labetalol, a combined beta- and alpha-blocker, is also included in Table 16-1, and is discussed at length in Chapter 35 because it is used as an antihypertensive drug. Finally, esmolol, a rapid acting beta-blocker used to control excessive heart rate is discussed following the general monograph on beta blockers.

Pharmacologic Effects of Beta-Blockers

Most of the pharmacologic effects of beta-blockers are the direct result of beta-receptor antagonism.

* Also an alpha$_1$ blocker.

Table 16-1
Pharmacologic and Pharmacokinetic Properties of Beta-Blockers

Drug	Receptor Activity	Oral Absorption	Protein Binding	Elimination Half-Life	Membrane-Stabilizing Activity*	Intrinsic Sympathomimetic Activity*	Interpatient Variations in Plasma Levels*
acebutolol (Sectral)	β_1	90%	25%	3 h to 4 h	0	+	
atenolol (Tenormin)	β_1	50%	5%–15%	6 h to 9 h	0	0	4-fold
betaxolol (Betoptic)	β_1	(ophthalmic use only)			0	0	
levobunolol (Betagan)	β_1, β_2	(ophthalmic use only)			0	0	
metoprolol (Lopressor)	β_1	95%–100%	10%–15%	3 h to 6 h	+	0	10-fold
nadolol (Corgard)	β_1, β_2	30%	30%	18 h to 24 h	0	0	7-fold
pindolol (Visken)	β_1, β_2	95%–100%	40%–50%	3 h to 4 h	+	+++	4-fold
propranolol (Inderal)	$\beta_1\ \beta_2$	90%–100%	90%–95%	3 h to 6 h	++	0	20-fold
timolol (Blocadren, Timoptic)	β_1, β_2	90%–95%	10%	3 h to 4 h	0	0	7-fold
labetalol† (Normodyne, Trandate)	$\beta_1\ \beta_2$	100%	50%	6 h to 8 h	+	0	

* Refer to the discussion of beta-blockers in the text for an explanation of these characteristics.
† Also possesses alpha$_1$ blocking activity and beta$_2$ agonistic activity.

The principal effects of blockade of beta$_1$ receptors in the heart are a slowing of heart rate and a decrease in force on contraction, that is, a negative chronotropic and inotropic action, respectively. Other cardiac effects of the beta-blockers include slowed A-V conduction velocity and prolonged A-V refractory period. Pindolol, and to a lesser extent acebutolol, possess a partial agonistic action at beta$_1$ cardiac receptors (termed an intrinsic sympathomimetic action or ISA) which results in *less* reduction in heart rate and cardiac output than other beta-blockers. This ISA action can be blocked by other beta-blocking drugs because it is a direct receptor action. The clinical significance of this slightly reduced heart rate and cardiac output remains to be definitely established, however.

Beta-blockers effectively lower blood pressure, although the various mechanisms involved in this antihypertensive effect are not completely known. Among the actions of beta blockers that may contribute to the blood pressure lowering effect are (1) decreased cardiac output, (2) interference with the release of renin and subsequent activation of angiotensin and release of aldosterone, (3) reduced sympathetic outflow from central vasomotor regulatory sites, and (4) impaired presynaptic release of NE from adrenergic nerve endings. The antihypertensive actions of the beta-blocking agents will be explored more fully in Chapter 35. Interestingly, blockade of peripheral vascular beta$_2$ receptors subserving vasodilation can result in *increased* peripheral vascular resistance. Yet, despite the initial rise in peripheral resistance, blood pressure is consistently lowered by beta antagonists.

Blockage of beta$_2$ receptor sites in the bronchioles can increase airway resistance due to elevated tone of bronchial smooth muscle. While this effect of the nonselective beta-blockers is usually not clinically significant in persons with normal ventilatory function, increased airway resistance may prove dangerous in patients with asthma or other chronic obstructive pulmonary diseases. The potential advantage of using one of the beta$_1$ selective blockers in these patients is obvious, as they have less tendency to interact with bronchiolar beta$_2$ sites in normal doses than do the nonselective blockers.

Beta-receptor blockade in the eye has been shown to decrease formation of aqueous humor and thus lower elevated intraocular pressure in the anterior chamber. Several beta-blockers (betaxolol, levobunolol, timolol) are applied locally as eye drops and are effective in the management of chronic, open-angle glaucoma.

Beta-adrenergic antagonists, especially the nonselective agents, can inhibit sympathetic stimulation of lipolysis and also glycogenolysis in the liver. Thus, the compensatory mobilization of glucose and free fatty acids in response to hypoglycemia may be blocked. This action is of little consequence in the nondiabetic, but may result in severe hypoglycemia in insulin-dependent diabetics.

Propranolol and, to a certain extent, metoprolol and pindolol possess a degree of quinidine-like local anesthetic activity, also known as a *membrane-stabilizing* action on several types of tissues, including skeletal muscle, neurons, and the myocardium. This effect may contribute to the antiarrhythmic action of these agents in certain types of cardiac arrhythmias although in normal doses the concentration of drug attained in the myocardium is probably insufficient to provide a significant local anesthetic effect.

Beta-blockers have been demonstrated to reduce platelet aggregation, perhaps by inhibiting the synthesis of thromboxane A$_2$, a powerful vasoconstrictor and platelet aggregatory agent.

The major adverse reactions associated with administration of beta-blockers are, in many cases, an extension of the predictable pharmacologic actions. Thus, decreased cardiac functioning (*i.e.*, depressed contractility, reduced cardiac output, bradycardia) may prove hazardous in patients with compensated congestive heart failure or sinus node disease, while the bronchoconstrictive effects of the nonselective blockers are undesirable in asthmatics. In the diabetic, not only might beta-blockade increase the degree of hypoglycemia in response to insulin but can also mask the early symptoms of hypoglycemia, such as tremor, sweating, and increased heart rate. Thus, use of a beta-blocker for any indication should only be undertaken after obtaining a complete patient medical history and carefully assessing the benefit-to-risk ratio in patients with conditions such as impaired cardiac or respiratory function or diabetes.

Although most beta-blockers exhibit a reasonably comparable profile of action, the recognized indications for the different compounds vary. Approved and investigational uses for the individual beta-blockers are listed in Table 16-2.

The beta-blockers will be discussed as a group, although characteristics of individual drugs will be noted where the differences from the other drugs in the group are important. Each individual beta-blocker will then be listed in Table 16-3, where dosage ranges and pertinent information will be

Table 16-2
Approved and Investigational Uses for Beta-Blockers

Indication	Drugs
Approved Uses	
Hypertension	acebutolol, atenolol, metoprolol, labetalol, nadolol, pindolol, propranolol, timolol (oral)
Angina	atenolol, nadolol, propranolol
Arrhythmias	acebutolol, esmolol, propranolol
Migraine prophylaxis	propranolol
Hypertrophic Subaortic stenosis	propranolol
Reduce risk of reinfection after acute infarct	propranolol, timolol (oral)
Glaucoma	betaxolol, levobunolol, timolol (ophthalmic)
Pheochromocytoma (adjunctive therapy)	propranolol
Hyperthyroidism (to control cardiac stimulation)	propranolol

Investigational Uses

One or more of the beta-blockers has been reported to be of benefit in the following conditions:

Acute pain symptoms	Hypothermia	Spastic colon
Alcohol withdrawal	Insulinoma	Tardive dyskinesia
Anxiety	Lithium-induced tremor	Tetanus
Cardiogenic shock	Mitral stenosis	Tetralogy of Fallot
Digitalis intoxication	Narcolepsy	Ureteral colic
Disseminated intravascular coagulation	Narcotic withdrawal	Urinary incontinence
	Parkinsonism	
Dissecting aorta	Phantom limb pain	
Essential tremor	Pulmonary stenosis	
GI bleeding in cirrhosis	Schizophrenia	
Hemorrhagic shock		

provided. Additional information relating to the respective uses (*e.g.*, antianginal, antihypertensive, antiarrhythmic) of specific blockers can be found in the appropriate chapters dealing with these particular classes of drugs.

MECHANISM AND ACTIONS
(See general discussion above.)

USES
(See Tables 16-2 and 16-3.)

ADMINISTRATION AND DOSAGE
(See Table 16-3.)

FATE
(See also Table 16-1 and 16-3.)

Oral absorption is virtually complete except for atenolol and nadolol, however, systemic bioavailability of acebutolol, metoprolol, propranolol, and timolol is low because of extensive first-pass hepatic metabolism (see Chap. 2).

Thus, plasma levels can vary widely from patient to patient depending on the extent of metabolism (see Table 16-1). Food enhances the bioavailability of propranolol and metoprolol. Protein binding is minimal with the exception of propranolol. Acebutolol, atenolol, and nadolol do not readily pass the blood–brain barrier due to low

(*Text continues on p. 279.*)

Table 16-3
Beta-Adrenergic Blocking Agents

Drug	Preparations	Usual Dosage Range	Clinical Considerations
acebutolol (Sectral)	Capsules—200 mg, 400 mg	*Hypertension* Initially 400 mg daily in one single or two divided doses. Usual maintenance dose range is 400 mg–800 mg daily. *Ventricular Arrhythmias* 200 mg twice a day initially. Increase gradually until optimal response; usual dosage range is 600 mg–1200 mg daily.	Selective beta$_1$-blocker used for hypertension and controlling ventricular premature beats. May be taken without regard to meals. Reduce dosage in elderly persons because plasma levels are higher. Use cautiously in impaired renal or hepatic function. Low lipid solubility; does not significantly pass blood–brain barrier.
atenolol (Tenormin)	Tablets—50 mg, 100 mg	*Hypertension* Initially, 50 mg once a day. Increase to 100 mg once a day if necessary after 1–2 weeks. *Angina* 50 mg once a day. May increase to 100 mg once a day if necessary.	Long-acting, selective beta$_1$ antagonist. Minimal protein binding. Dosage may have to be reduced in patients with significant renal failure because drug is excreted unchanged in the urine. Does not pass blood–brain barrier. Long half-life allows once daily dosing—drug should be taken same time every day. Available with chlorthalidone as Tenoretic.
betaxolol (Betoptic)	Ophthalmic solution —0.5%	1 drop twice a day	Used for treating ocular hypertension and chronic open-angle glaucoma. May be given alone or in combination with other antiglaucoma drugs. Onset of action is 30 min and effects persist up to 12 hr. Little effect on pupil size or accommodation. Discomfort and tearing may occur upon instillation. Virtually devoid of systemic side-effects.
labetalol (Normodyne, Trandate)	Tablets—100 mg, 200 mg, 300 mg Injection—5 mg/ml	*Hypertension* Oral—Initially, 100 mg twice a day; increase in 100-mg twice daily increments until desired response; usual maintenance dose is 200 mg–400 mg, twice daily. IV—20 mg by slow IV injection initially; repeat at 10-min intervals with 40 mg or 80 mg to a maximum of 300 mg or 2 mg/min of a 1-mg/ml dilution by IV infusion to a maximum of 300 mg (usual dosage range is 50 mg–200 mg).	Combined nonselective beta-blocker and alpha$_1$-blocker; may also exhibit beta$_2$ agonistic activity; used as an anti-hypertensive in both acute (IV) and chronic situations. Does not elicit marked changes in heart rate, renal function, or cardiac output. Postural hypotension can occur. Complete discussion of the drug is found in Chapter 35.
levobunolol (Betagan)	Ophthalmic solution —0.5%	1 drop once or twice a day	(See betaxolol.) Onset of action is 30 min–60 min, and effects persist up to 24 h. Greater likelihood of systemic side-effects than with betaxolol (*e.g.,*

(continued)

Table 16-3 (continued)
Beta-Adrenergic Blocking Agents

Drug	Preparations	Usual Dosage Range	Clinical Considerations
levobunolol (Betagan) (continued)			bradycardia, hypotension). Frequently causes burning or stinging upon instillation in the eyes; headache and dizziness have also been reported.
metoprolol (Lopressor)	Tablets—50 mg, 100 mg Injection—1 mg/ml	*Hypertension* Initially, 50 mg orally, twice a day. Increase at weekly intervals until optimum effect is attained. Usual maintenance dose is 100 mg twice a day (range 100 mg–450 mg/day). *Myocardial infarction* Three IV bolus injections of 5 mg each at 2-min intervals; then 50 mg orally every 6 h thereafter for 48 h, then 100 mg twice a day.	Selective beta$_1$-blocker. Well absorbed orally but undergoes significant first-pass hepatic metabolism. Weakly protein bound. Readily enters the CNS. If twice daily administration does not provide sufficient blood pressure control due to short half-life of drug, give three times/day in divided doses. Ingestion of food enhances oral absorption. During early phase of myocardial infarction, treatment should be initiated as soon as possible. If immediate IV administration is not possible or not tolerated, begin oral therapy (100 mg twice/day) as soon as clinical condition allows. Treatment may be continued for months if deemed beneficial. Prevention of reinfarction is most dramatic in patients suffering first infarction and presenting with left ventricular failure, cardiomegaly, or atrial fibrillation.
nadolol (Corgard)	Tablets—20 mg, 40 mg, 80 mg, 120 mg, 160 mg	*Hypertension* Initially, 40 mg once daily. Increase gradually in 40-mg–80-mg increments. Usual dosage range 40 mg–80 mg once daily. Maximum dose is 320 mg/day. *Angina* Initially, 40 mg once daily. Increase at 3–7-day intervals until desired effect. Usual dosage range is 40 mg–80 mg once daily. Maximum dose is 240 mg/day.	Long-acting, nonselective beta-blocker. Does not enter the CNS. Excreted essentially unchanged by the kidney, therefore dosage may need to be reduced in renal failure. Presence of food does not affect rate or extent (approximately 30%) of absorption. If drug is to be discontinued, taper dosage gradually over 1 wk–2 wk. Do not administer more often than once a day.
pindolol (Visken)	Tablets—5 mg, 10 mg	*Hypertension* Initially 5 mg two to three times/day. Adjust dosage at 2–3-week intervals in increments of 10 mg to obtain the desired reduction in pressure. Maximum dose is 60 mg/day.	Nonselective beta antagonist with intrinsic sympathomimetic activity, thus exhibits slightly less slowing of heart rate than other beta-blockers. Rapidly absorbed orally. Peak plasma levels in 1 hr. Short acting. Excreted both as unchanged drug and metabolites. No significant first-pass hepatic metabolism. Use is frequently associated with slight weight gain.
propranolol (Inderal)	Tablets—10 mg, 20 mg, 40 mg, 60 mg, 80 mg, 90 mg	*Hypertension* Initially, 40 mg twice a day or 80 mg SR once daily.	Widely used, nonselective beta-blocker. Also possesses a quinidine-like cardiac membrane depressant action.

(continued)

Table 16-3 (continued)
Beta-Adrenergic Blocking Agents

Drug	Preparations	Usual Dosage Range	Clinical Considerations
propranolol (Inderal) *(continued)*	Capsules (sustained release-SR) 60 mg, 80 mg, 120 mg, 160 mg Oral solution—20 mg/5 ml, 40 mg/5 ml Concentrated oral solution (Intensol)—80 mg/ml Injection—1 mg/ml	Increase gradually until desired response; usual dosage range is 120 mg–240 mg/day in two to three divided doses or 120 mg–160 mg SR once daily *Angina* Initially, 10 mg–20 mg three to four times/day or 80 mg SR once daily. Increase at 3–7-day intervals. Usual dose is 160 mg/day in single or divided doses. *Arrhythmias* 10 mg to 30 mg three to four times/day *Hypertrophic subaortic stenosis* 20 mg to 40 mg three to four times/day or 80 mg to 160 mg once daily *Migraine* Initially, 80 mg once daily or in divided doses. Usual dosage range is 160–240 mg/day.	Well absorbed orally (food enhances absorption), but undergoes extensive first-pass hepatic metabolism, and variations in plasma levels among patients are wide. Highly protein bound. Excreted largely as metabolites in the urine. If treatment of angina is to be discontinued, decrease dose gradually over several weeks as severe angina or myocardial infarction can be precipitated by abrupt termination. If a satisfactory response in the treatment of migraine is not achieved within 4–6 wk after reaching the maximum dose, (*i.e.*, 240 mg/day), drug should be discontinued. IV injection should be undertaken with extreme caution, and central venous pressure and ECG closely monitored. Transfer to oral therapy as soon as possible.
timolol *Oral* (Blocadren) *Ophthalmic* (Timoptic)	Tablets—5 mg, 10 mg, 20 mg Ophthalmic drops—0.25%, 0.5%	*Oral:* *Hypertension* Initially, 10 mg twice a day. Usual maintenance range is 20 mg–40 mg/day in two divided doses. *Myocardial infarction* 10 mg twice a day for long-term prophylaxis following the acute phase. *Ophthalmic:* Glaucoma—1 drop of 0.25%–0.5% solution twice a day.	Nonselective beta antagonist used orally for hypertension and as prophylaxis following an acute myocardial infarction and as eye drops for the management of chronic open-angle glaucoma. Oral absorption is good, and protein binding is minimal. Oral drug is short acting and may have to be given three times/day if response is inadequate. Effects in eye begin in 30 min, peak in 1 h–2 h, and persist up to 24 h. Do not give more than 1 drop 0.5% twice a day. Add other antiglaucoma drugs if necessary (see Chap. 13). When used intraocularly, systemic effects can occur frequently, especially with prolonged use. Systemic absorption can be minimized by instructing patients to press gently on the lacrimal duct after drug administration. Ocular use is contraindicated in patients with bradycardia, second or third degree heart block, congestive heart failure, pulmonary edema, or bronchial asthma.

lipid solubility. Atenolol and nadolol are excreted unchanged by the kidney; the remaining beta-blockers are partially to almost completely metabolized in the liver and excreted as both metabolites and unchanged drug by the kidney. Elimination half-lives are rather short (3–6 hours), except for atenolol (6–9 hours), labetalol (6–8 hours), and nadolol (16–24 hours).

SIDE-EFFECTS/ADVERSE REACTIONS

The most frequently observed side-effects with the majority of beta-blocking agents are drowsiness, lightheadedness, dizziness, numbness or tingling of the fingers and/or toes, nausea, and bradycardia. A wide range of other adverse reactions have been reported in patients taking beta-blockers, and these are listed below organized by organ system. Not all of the following adverse effects have been related to all of the beta-blockers but it should be recognized that the *potential* for the occurrence of any of these adverse reactions exists for all members of the group.

CV—Tachyarrhythmias, chest pain, AV block, sinoatrial block, peripheral arterial insufficiency, pulmonary edema, syncope, cerebrovascular accident, cardiac failure

CNS—(Incidence is significantly lower with acebutolol, atenolol, and nadolol because they do not readily pass the blood–brain barrier) dizziness, vertigo, depression, weakness, behavioral disturbances, agitation, disorientation, memory loss, emotional instability, sleep disturbances, bizarre dreams, catatonia, hallucinations

GI—Diarrhea, vomiting, gastric pain, anorexia, bloating, dry mouth, ischemic colitis, hepatomegaly

Respiratory—Bronchospasm, dyspnea, cough, rales, nasal congestion

Musculoskeletal—Joint pain, muscle cramping

Dermatologic—Rash, pruritus, skin irritation, sweating, dry skin, increased pigmentation

Other—Hypoglycemia, alopecia, acute pancreatitis, agranulocytosis, thrombocytopenia, eosinophilia, urinary difficulty, fever, sore throat, psoriasis-like rash and blurred vision. Elevated BUN, serum transaminases, alkaline phosphatase, and lactate dehydrogenase have been noted with propranolol and timolol and may occur with other beta-blockers as well. These elevations are usually not progressive or associated with clinical manifestations.

CONTRAINDICATIONS AND PRECAUTIONS

Beta-adrenergic blocking agents are contraindicated in the presence of cardiogenic shock, greater than first-degree heart block, overt cardiac failure, sinus bradycardia, and severe congestive heart failure. In addition, beta-blockers should not be given to patients receiving other drugs that augment alpha-adrenergic activity, such as MAO inhibitors or adrenergic pressor amines. *Nonselective* beta-blockers are also contraindicated in bronchial asthma. All beta-blocking agents should be used *cautiously* in the presence of nonallergic bronchospasm, peripheral vascular insufficiency, allergic rhinitis, or a history of allergies, impaired renal or hepatic function, diabetes, and myasthenia gravis. Abrupt withdrawal of a beta-blocker has resulted in hypersensitivity to catecholamines, resulting in worsening of angina, intensification of symptoms of hyperthyroidism, myocardial infarction, and arrhythmias. Thus, *gradual* withdrawal with close monitoring of the patient is recommended whenever therapy with a beta-blocker is terminated.

INTERACTIONS

1. Beta-blockers can have additive cardiac depressant effect with digitalis, phenytoin, verapamil, or quinidine.
2. The effects of beta-blockers can be reversed by norepinephrine, isoproterenol, dopamine, dobutamine, and other sympathomimetic drugs.
3. Plasma levels of propranolol and possibly other beta-blockers can be elevated by chlorpromazine, cimetidine, furosemide, and hydralazine.
4. Beta-blockers can antagonize the bronchodilating action of theophylline and may decrease theophylline clearance.
5. The hypotensive action of beta-blockers can be increased by diuretics and other antihypertensives, and decreased by indomethacin, salicylates, and nonsteroidal anti-inflammatory agents, possibly due to inhibition of prostaglandin synthesis.
6. Phenobarbital and phenytoin can reduce plasma levels of beta-blockers by the process of enzyme induction.
7. Beta-blockers may prolong insulin-induced hypoglycemia and mask the symptoms of lowered blood glucose.
8. Beta-adrenergic blockage may increase the incidence of the "first-dose" orthostatic hypotensive response to prazosin (see Chap. 35), and the severity of "rebound hypertension" on clonidine withdrawal.

9. Propranolol or metoprolol may impair the clearance by lidocaine.
10. Beta-blockers may enhance muscle-relaxing actions of succinylcholine and tubocurarine.
11. IV phenytoin may potentiate the cardiac depressant action of beta-blockers.

Esmolol

(Brevibloc)

MECHANISM AND ACTIONS
Esmolol is a beta₁ adrenergic blocker possessing a rapid onset and very short duration of action. It decreases blood pressure and heart rate in a dose-related fashion when given by IV infusion.

USES
1. Rapid control of ventricular rate in patients with atrial fibrillation or flutter
2. Control of noncompensatory tachycardia

ADMINISTRATION AND DOSAGE
Esmolol is available as a concentrated solution for injection (250 mg/ml) that must be diluted prior to infusion to a concentration of 10 mg/ml or less to avoid venous irritation.

Treatment is initiated with a loading dose infusion of 500 mcg/kg/min for 1 minute, followed by a 4-minute infusion of 50 mcg/kg/min. If an adequate therapeutic response is not attained, repeat the loading dose and follow with an infusion of 100 mcg/kg/min for 4 minutes. Continue the loading dose/maintenance dose procedure by increasing the maintenance dose in 50 mcg/kg/min increments until the desired heart rate is attained. The average dose is 100 mcg/kg/min.

After adequate control of the heart rate has been attained, transition to alternate antiarrhythmic drugs should be undertaken, with gradual reduction in the esmolol dosage. Esmolol is well tolerated for at least 24 hours to 48 hours.

SIDE-EFFECTS/ADVERSE REACTIONS
Induration and irritation at the infusion site are the most frequently encountered side-effects with esmolol. Other untoward effects include edema, erythema, skin discoloration and burning, urinary retention, fever, flushing, pallor, speech disorders, somnolence, confusion, paresthesias, lightheadedness, taste alteration, midscapular pain, and asthenia.

CONTRAINDICATIONS AND PRECAUTIONS
Hypotension occurs in up to 50% of patients and is generally dose related. Patients must be closely monitored during infusion. Because of the short action of esmolol, hypotension is reversed within 20 minutes to 30 minutes after stopping the infusion. If a reaction develops at the infusion site, an alternative site should be used.

INTERACTIONS
1. Concomitant IV administration of esmolol and digoxin may reduce digoxin blood levels 10% to 20%.
2. IV morphine administration can increase esmolol steady-state plasma levels up to 50%.

■ Nursing Process

(See also Chap. 35.)

□ ASSESSMENT

□ Subjective Data
A drug history should be obtained because beta-blockers adversely interact with many other drugs. A system review should also be done, and any history of renal or liver problems should be reported.

Treatment with beta-blockers requires the patient to be consistent and responsible in following the regimen. The nurse needs to assess the patient's memory, motivation, and support systems to determine whether compliance will be a problem.

□ Objective Data
Baseline vital signs should be obtained on any patient starting a beta-blocker. Blood pressure should be taken with the patient sitting and lying down. Pretreatment weight should also be charted. Laboratory assessment may include baseline renal and hepatic function studies.

□ NURSING DIAGNOSES
The *actual* nursing diagnoses for any patient receiving beta-blocker drugs include:
   Knowledge deficit related to action administration and side-effects of the drug
   Potential for injury related to transient dizziness from orthostatic hypotension
Potential nursing diagnoses are related to side-effects for the most part and include:
   Alteration in bowel elimination: diarrhea
   Ineffective breathing pattern

Alteration in cardiac output: decreased
Alteration in fluid volume: excess
Noncompliance with drug regimen—may
  occur for a variety of reasons (e.g.,
  side-effects, cost, disappearance of
  symptoms) (see also Chap. 35)
Sleep pattern disturbance
Alteration in thought processes

□ PLAN

Nursing care goals should focus on teaching the patient administration techniques that will enhance the drug's effects and how to monitor and respond to the side-effects of the drug.

□ INTERVENTION

To ensure achievement of adequate plasma levels, the patient needs to learn to take a beta-blocker drug at the same time every day and before meals to enhance absorption. Memory joggers or pill calendars or boxes may be helpful in facilitating this process early in therapy. Abrupt cessation of the drug can have serious consequences even with as few as two missed doses. Rapid falls in plasma levels can lead to a rapid hypertension, angina, arrhythmias, and myocardial infarction. The patient needs to notify the physician if he becomes ill or unable to take the drug for any reason. If side-effects become unmanageable, the drug will still have to be withdrawn gradually.

Early in therapy the dose may have to be adjusted to minimize side-effects. An apical pulse is an accurate indicator of dose because a fall in pulse below 60 beats per minute may mean the dosage is too high. If the patient has been very sensitive to changes in dose, he may learn to take his own pulse at home to monitor the drug's effect.

Patients on beta-blockers must also be aware of the drug's effects on glucose metabolism. Prolonged fasting may greatly potentiate the hypoglycemic effects of the beta-blocker drugs. Therefore, patients should be taught the importance of eating regular balanced meals when on this drug. Smoking may reduce a beta-blocker's effectiveness, and alcohol may enhance its hypotensive and CNS depres-

sant effect. The patient should be aware this will occur and encouraged to reduce or eliminate his use of both.

Fluid retention may be a side-effect of the drug. The patient should be encouraged to monitor his weight and urine output and to watch for signs of swelling of hands and feet. If a beta-blocker is started in the hospital, the patient should be placed on intake and output because a shift in fluid balance can easily be measured and will be an early sign of heart failure.

Orthostatic hypotension is also a problem for many patients on beta-blockers. The nurse should aim intervention at teaching the patient to rise slowly from a lying position or sitting position and to avoid prolonged standing. Patients need to be aware of lightheadedness and dizziness and to sit down as soon as these sensations occur. Some patients are more lightheaded about an hour after a dose of the medicine. If the patient can become aware of these body signals he will be able to plan his activities accordingly. For example, if dizziness occurs soon after a dose, the patient ought not to plan driving or operating other machinery during that time.

The patient on prolonged therapy should have regular hematologic, hepatic, and renal function studies drawn. (See under Side-Effects/Adverse Reactions.) Beta-blockers can result in toxicity over time, and their effects should be closely monitored.

The patient who is having surgery should always be asked what other drugs he is taking. Some clinicians recommend patients be taken off beta-blockers 48 hours before any surgery, although this procedure has become controversial. If this decision is made the dose may need to be gradually withdrawn beginning about 1 week before surgery. The nurse finding such a patient should contact the physician.

□ EVALUATION

The outcome criteria for measuring successful drug therapy with beta-blockers is that the patient's symptoms (blood pressure, headaches) are controlled with minimal side-effects and that the patient is consistent in taking the drug.

CASE STUDY

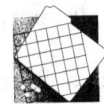

Sally Brooker, age 72, was recovering from her second myocardial infarction in 5 years. Mrs. Brooker was a patient on a cardiac step-down unit and was being managed on a drug regimen which included digoxin, hydrodiuril, nitroglycerin, and propranolol, 20 mg PO qid (10^A-2^P-6^P-10^P) for angina.

During transcription of a drug order a nurse on the evening

shift neglected to recopy the propranolol order to the medication administration record (MAR). Subsequently, Mrs. Brooker missed two doses of propranolol.

The error was uncovered when the record was reviewed after Mrs. Brooker awakened at 2 AM complaining of chest pain. The physician was notified, and the patient was given morphine. She was placed on a cardiac monitor, and the propranolol was restarted. Mrs. Brooker suffered no further effects from the error and was discharged 3 days later.

Discussion Questions

1. What vital signs must be monitored while Mrs. Brooker recovers from this abrupt withdrawal?
2. How should the patient be told about the incident?
3. How could the nurse have avoided committing the transcription error?
4. In preparing Mrs. Brooker for discharge what information about propranolol should be reviewed? Outline a basic teaching plan and drug card.

REVIEW QUESTIONS

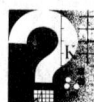

1. Distinguish between the terms "adrenergic neuronal blocker" and "adrenergic receptor blocker."
2. How are alpha-adrenergic blockers classified? Give an example of a drug in each class.
3. How does prazosin differ from phentolamine in its alpha-blocking action?
4. Why are the ergot alkaloids not always suitable for use as vasodilators in spite of their alpha-adrenergic blocking activity?
5. List the principal effects of alpha-blockers on the cardiovascular system.
6. What other actions of phentolamine and tolazoline, in addition to alpha-blockade, may contribute to the hypotensive effect of the drugs?
7. What is meant by a selective vs nonselective beta-blocker?
8. List the major approved indications for beta-blockers.
9. Which beta-adrenergic blocker is:
   a. poorest absorbed orally?
   b. most extensively protein bound?
   c. longest acting orally?
   d. a partial agonist as well as an antagonist?
   e. used both orally and locally in the eye?
   f. useful to control rapid ventricular rate
10. What are the effects of nonselective beta-blockers on (a) the heart, (b) the bronchioles, and (c) blood levels of glucose and free fatty acids?
11. Why must beta-blockers be used with caution in patients with (a) congestive heart failure, (b) peripheral vascular insufficiency, and (c) diabetes?
12. What actions can the nurse teach a patient to take when suffering from orthostatic hypertension as a result of taking an alpha- or a beta-blocker?

13. How should a patient be withdrawn from a beta-blocker drug?

BIBLIOGRAPHY

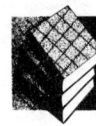

Cruickshank JM: The clinical importance of cardioselectivity and lipophilicity in beta blockers. Am Heart J 100:160, 1980

Doxey JC, Smith CFC, Walker JM: Selectivity of blocking agents for pre- and postsynaptic alpha-adrenoceptors. Br J Pharmacol 60:91, 1977

Drug data: Timoptic. Am J Nurs February:329, 1979

Fischer RG, Byrd HJ: Beta-adrenergic blocking agents. US Pharmacist 46:Aug. 1982

Frishman WH: Beta-adrenoceptor antagonists: New drugs and new indications. N Engl J Med 305:500, 1981

Frishman WH, Furberg CD, Friedenwald WT: Beta-adrenergic blockade for survivors of acute myocardial infarction. N Engl J Med 310:830, 1984

Graham RM: The physiology and pharmacology of alpha and beta blockade. J Cardiovasc Med (suppl), April 1981

Johnson GP, Johanson BC: Beta blockers: An expert's guide to what's on the market. Am J Nurs 83:1034, 1983

McDevitt DG: Beta-adrenergic blocking drugs and partial agonist activity: Is it clinically relevant. Drugs 25:331, 1983

Ople LH: Drugs and the heart. I. Beta blocking agents: Lancet 1:693, 1980

Singh BN, Laddu AR: Esmolol: A novel ultra-short acting beta-adrenoceptor blocking agent. Ration Drug Ther 20(8):1, 1986

Snyder DW: A clinical approach to beta blocker use following myocardial infarction. Modern Medicine 55(6):44, 1987

Vedin JA, Wilhelmsson CE: Beta receptor blocking agents in the secondary prevention of coronary heart disease. Am Rev Pharmacol Toxicol 23:29, 1983

Wood AJJ: How the beta-blockers differ: A pharmacologic comparison. Drug Therapy 13:59, 1983

Ganglionic Blocking Agents

Depolarizing Blockers
    Nicotine
    Nicotine Resin Complex

Antidepolarizing Blockers
    Mecamylamine
    Trimethaphan

17

Synaptic transmission at the ganglia of the autonomic nervous system is mediated by acetylcholine (ACh), and thus can be impeded by drugs capable of blocking the actions of the cholinergic neurotransmitter. Those specific anticholinergic compounds acting primarily at autonomic ganglia are termed *ganglionic blocking agents*. Although many experimental substances are employed to alter ganglionic function in the laboratory, there are presently only two therapeutically useful agents, and their clinical applicability is restricted to the production of hypotensive states for specialized circumstances. Because the agents are nonselective in their blocking action, transmission is reduced in both sympathetic and parasympathetic ganglia. Thus, in addition to interfering with those sympathetic impulses that constrict vascular smooth muscle, the agents likewise block impulses to many other body organs, resulting in a wide range of side-effects. Typical effects caused by parasympathetic blockade include tachycardia, decreased gastrointestinal (GI) motility and secretions, dryness of the mouth, urinary retention, constipation, paralysis of ocular accommodation, mydriasis, and impotence. It is evident that the scope of possible adverse reactions greatly limits the clinical utility of these drugs.

Neurotransmission of the ganglia can be blocked in one of two ways. Ganglionic blockers may either occupy the excitatory cholinergic (*i.e.,* nicotinic) receptor sites and elicit a persistent depolarization of the postsynaptic membrane or competitively antagonize the action of acetylcholine at the receptor site, thus preventing depolarization. The former group of drugs are termed *depolarizing blockers;* the latter drugs are referred to as *antidepolarizing blockers.*

Depolarizing Blockers

Depolarizing blockers, of which the alkaloid nicotine is an example, exert an initial stimulation of the postganglionic receptors, then block further receptor activation by persistently occupying the site and preventing repolarization of the postsynaptic membrane.

Nicotine

Nicotine is the principal alkaloid of the leaves of the tobacco plant, *Nicotiana tabacum.* Although of no therapeutic value, nicotine is of considerable toxicologic importance because it is systemically absorbed from tobacco smoke and may be accidentally inhaled from nicotine-containing insecticides. The pharmacologic effects of nicotine are quite variable and depend largely on the amount absorbed, extent and level of exposure, and physiologic state of the individual—that is, the presence of underlying disease states such as peripheral vascular disorders, hypertension, coronary artery disease, or congestive heart failure. Nicotine is potentially one of the most toxic of all alkaloids, although the amount found in cigarettes is quite small. The drug is readily absorbed from the mucosal surfaces of the GI and respiratory tracts; the liquid form of the alkaloid, occasionally used as insecticide, is also well absorbed through the intact skin. Nicotine is excreted in the urine, primarily as inactive metabolites. Urinary excretion is facilitated if the urine is acidic. Some excretion also occurs in the milk of lactating women who are cigarette smokers.

CNS EFFECTS

Small doses of nicotine stimulate the CNS, whereas large doses produce an initial central excitation followed by a depression. Respiration is increased by moderate amounts of nicotine due to stimulation of carotid body and aortic chemoreceptors. Increasing doses initially stimulate the medullary respiratory center directly; however, respiration is eventually paralyzed by toxic doses due to overall CNS depression and a peripheral neuromuscular blocking action.

Nausea and vomiting can result from activation of the chemoreceptor trigger zone in the medulla and possibly by vagal stimulation of the medullary vomiting center itself.

Increased release of the antidiuretic hormone (ADH) can occur as a result of stimulation of the hypothalamic nuclei controlling posterior pituitary function. As a consequence, increased water reabsorption occurs in the renal tubules.

Large doses of nicotine can result in muscle tremor, and in sufficiently high concentrations, the drug can produce convulsions.

CARDIOVASCULAR EFFECTS

The principal cardiovascular effects of nicotine, in usual amounts, result from the initial stimulation of sympathetic ganglionic function. Thus, heart rate is moderately increased due to a predominant sympathetic ganglionic stimulation. Likewise, peripheral blood vessels are constricted, and blood pressure tends to be slightly elevated. The potential consequences of chronic tobacco smoking in persons with peripheral vascular disease, angina, hypertension, or congestive heart failure, therefore, are quite obvious. In fact, patients who smoke and who take vasodilators for any of these conditions may have a variable response to the medications as a result of the vasoconstrictive effect of nicotine.

GASTROINTESTINAL EFFECTS

Unlike the cardiovascular system, the predominant autonomic regulation of the GI tract is parasympathetic and thus the effects of nicotine on GI function are the result of increased parasympathetic stimulation. Intestinal motility is slightly increased by small amounts of nicotine; however, the concentration of the alkaloid in cigarette smoke has little effect on volume or acidity of gastric secretions. Salivation, nausea, and, occasionally, vomiting can occur with occasional ingestion of nicotine, primarily due to stimulation of emetic centers in the brain stem.

RESPIRATORY EFFECTS

Other than a slight stimulation of the medullary respiratory center, the effects of nicotine on respiration are minimal. Of far greater significance in this respect is the potential danger of prolonged exposure to the combustion products found in cigarette smoke, and the relationship of smoking to chronic irritative pulmonary disease, lung carcinoma, and coronary heart disease.

NICOTINE POISONING

Nicotine is an extremely potent and rapid-acting toxic substance. Acute nicotine poisoning most often results from accidental ingestion of insecticides containing liquid nicotine, although severe toxic effects have resulted from topical absorption of the alkaloid as well. An initial period of CNS excitation is usually quickly followed by profound central depression of vital functions. Symptoms of poisoning may include salivation, diarrhea, abdominal cramping, vomiting, hypotension, fainting, and rapid pulse. Death usually results from respiratory paralysis, a consequence of both depression of the respiratory center and peripheral blockade of motor impulses to the diaphragm and respiratory muscles.

There is no specific antidote to nicotine, and treatment of overdosage is symptomatic. Necessary measures can include (1) gastric lavage with a 1:10,000 solution of potassium permanganate, an alkaloidal oxidant, (2) artificial respiration, with oxygen if needed, (3) control of convulsions with IV diazepam or barbiturates, and (4) support of blood pressure and cardiovascular function with vasopressors and IV fluids.

NURSING CONSIDERATIONS AND SMOKING

The effects of nicotine on body systems should be incentive enough for any person to quit. The statistics on the development of lung cancer, chronic pulmonary disease, and heart disease as well as the Surgeon General's report and the specific warnings now required on all cigarette packages should be other incentives. But while the smoker is cognitively aware of all this evidence, the smoking habit is not an intellectual pursuit and cannot be stopped by simply giving the smoker information.

Smoking is a physical and emotional addiction. Withdrawal symptoms include irritability, insomnia, fidgetiness, decreased libido, and increased appetite. Most frequently, the irritability, especially when accompanied by life stresses, is what makes a smoker go back after quitting. Quitting smoking also means giving up an attachment to a habit and has been equated with the grief experienced during the loss of a close friend (Richard and Shepard, 1981). Quitting smoking is not an easy thing to do.

Nursing intervention may include discussions with the patient about possible actions to take and helping him develop methods of behavior modification. Many people report success through support groups such as Smoke Enders or others sponsored by local hospitals and organizations, by hypnosis, and, infrequently, by just quitting "cold turkey."

Success at quitting may depend on motivation, current life stresses, a supportive network at home and work, and being able to substitute other behaviors during times that used to be spent smoking such as with a cup of coffee or with a drink. The smoker also needs time to work through the loss. The nurse who is quitting or trying to help another to quit must recognize that the smoker will need time and help to find a sequence of supports which will help him quit. Punitive remarks will not serve any purpose except to produce anger and information is not always useful. Supportive assistance seems to be the key to success.

Nicotine Resin Complex
(Nicorette)

Recently, a prescription chewing gum, nicotine resin complex, has been used to help smokers quit. The gum contains 2 mg of nicotine which is bound to an ion-exchange resin. As the person chews the gum, nicotine is slowly released and absorbed through the buccal mucosa. Blood levels of nicotine produced by this method are thought to help the smoker cope with the physical side-effects of withdrawal.

Most patients require about 10 pieces of gum per day but should not exceed 30 pieces. The patient is told to take one piece of gum when he feels the urge to smoke, and chew it approximately 10 to 15 times until a tingling sensation develops and the urge passes. He leaves the gum in the buccal pouch and chews only when the urge returns. The gum can be chewed up to 30 minutes before losing its effect. Treatment generally lasts several weeks.

Side-effects are rare but may occur if the patient chews too many pieces or chews the gum too rapidly. Common side-effects include dizziness, hiccups, nausea, and mouth irritation.

Antidepolarizing Blockers

The antidepolarizing group of ganglionic blocking agents, to which all the clinically useful drugs belong, function as competitive antagonists of ACh at the postganglionic receptor sites. Their predominant effect is to reduce sympathetic vascular tone, producing marked vasodilation and hypotension (primarily orthostatic), and decreasing venous return to the heart and consequently cardiac output. They are potent blood pressure–lowering drugs, but their extensive range of side-effects due to nonselective receptor blockade limits their clinical usefulness to a few specific indications.

The two antidepolarizing blockers in clinical use differ in chemical structure and properties. Mecamylamine is a secondary amine which is reliably absorbed from the GI tract and can be administered orally. Trimethaphan, on the other hand, is a quaternary ammonium derivative with a low lipid/water partition coefficient and therefore poor oral absorption; it must be administered parenterally. These drugs are reviewed below.

Mecamylamine
(Inversine)

MECHANISM AND ACTIONS
Mecamylamine is a competitive antagonist of acetylcholine at autonomic ganglia. The drug produces prolonged blood pressure lowering in both normotensive and hypertensive patients. The antihypertensive action is primarily orthostatic, although supine blood pressure is also significantly reduced.

USES
1. Management of moderately severe to severe essential hypertension and uncomplicated malignant hypertension
   Note: Mecamylamine is virtually obsolete and should only be used in rare instances when all other agents have failed.

ADMINISTRATION AND DOSAGE
Mecamylamine is given orally, as 2.5-mg tablets. The initial dose is 2.5 mg, twice a day. Dosage increments of 2.5 mg may be added every two days until the desired blood pressure reduction has been attained. The usual daily maintenance dose is 25 mg/day in three divided doses. Administration following meals may result in more gradual absorption and better control of the blood pressure. When control is particularly difficult, dividing the total daily dosage into four or even more doses may be beneficial. Occasionally, a larger fraction of the daily dosage may need to be given in the afternoon or evening because the response to the morning dose is sometimes greater than to the other doses.

FATE
Oral absorption is complete. The onset of action occurs 30 to 90 minutes after administration, and the effects persist for up to 12 hours, and occasionally longer. The drug is widely distributed throughout the body, and it readily crosses the blood–brain barrier. Excretion is slow by way of the kidneys, but is increased by an acidic urine.

SIDE-EFFECTS/ADVERSE REACTIONS
The most frequently reported side-effects are dryness of the mouth, constipation, drowsiness, blurred vision, dizziness, and lightheadedness. Other dose-related adverse reactions are urinary hesitancy, impotence, weakness, anorexia, nausea, vomiting, paralytic ileus, and rarely, confusion, depression, tremor, dyspnea, and convulsions.

CONTRAINDICATIONS AND PRECAUTIONS
Mecamylamine should not be used in patients with coronary or renal insufficiency, uremia, glaucoma, pyloric stenosis, and following a recent myocardial infarction. *Cautious use* is warranted in the presence of elevated BUN, bladder neck obstruction, prostatic hypertrophy, and urethral stricture. A

number of conditions have been shown to enhance the hypotensive effects of mecamylamine, including fever, infection, high ambient temperature, hemorrhage, pregnancy, surgery, vigorous exercise, and salt depletion (as may result from diarrhea, vomiting, sweating, or diuretics). The drug crosses the placental barrier, and safety for use in pregnancy is not established.

INTERACTIONS

1. The hypotensive effect of mecamylamine can be enhanced by alcohol, other antihypertensive agents, diuretics, anesthetics, MAO inhibitors, and bethanechol.
2. Mecamylamine may potentiate sympathomimetic drugs, resulting in a diminished hypotensive response.
3. The effects of mecamylamine may be prolonged by sodium bicarbonate and other urinary alkalinizers.
4. Enhanced neuromuscular blockade and muscle weakness may result from combined use of mecamylamine and neuromuscular blocking agents.

NURSING CONSIDERATIONS
(See also Chapter 35.)

Sudden discontinuation of mecamylamine can result in rebound hypertension and possible cerebrovascular accident. Therefore, the nurse should never withhold the drug if side-effects occur. Instead the physician should be contacted and the drug should be discontinued gradually while other antihypertensives are substituted. For the same reason, the patient should also be taught never to abruptly stop taking the drug but to immediately contact the physician should side-effects become difficult to manage.

Nursing intervention in early administration of this drug should be aimed at assisting the physician to titrate the doses to obtain optimal responses. Blood pressure should be monitored while the patient is both sitting and lying, and the patient should be asked to report signs of orthostatic hypotension (faintness or dizziness, especially on rising). The physician will use these observations to establish an effective maintenance dose. The goal is to use a dose of the drug just below that which produces orthostatic hypotension.

The drug should be taken after meals, which assists in achieving smoother control of the blood levels of mecamylamine. In addition, because response to the drug is greater in the morning, smaller doses should be given in the morning and larger ones in the afternoon.

Another early nursing intervention is to monitor fluid intake and output, watching for urinary retention and edema. Observations of changes in these parameters should be reported promptly because dosage adjustment may be required.

In addition, the patient taking this drug should not use over-the-counter drugs containing sodium bicarbonate (e.g., remedies to relieve stomach upset) because these drugs will increase urinary pH which can cause drug toxicity.

The patient must also watch for constipation. If this occurs use of a laxative such as milk of magnesia or the like is advised; bulk laxatives will be ineffective. If constipation becomes a problem or is accompanied by abdominal distention or nausea, the patient needs to contact the physician. These are signs of paralytic ileus and must be treated promptly. Generally the physician will discontinue the drug slowly and use another antihypertensive agent.

Trimethaphan
(Arfonad)

MECHANISM AND ACTIONS
The blocking action of trimethaphan is exerted at postsynaptic cholinergic receptor sites in sympathetic and parasympathetic ganglia, and results in stabilization of the postganglionic membranes. The competitive antagonism at the ganglia is short-lived. A direct relaxant effect on vascular smooth muscle is also seen. Peripheral venous pooling of blood occurs, and cardiac output is reduced. Blood pressure is markedly lowered, especially in the upright position. Trimethaphan can cause release of histamine, which can also dilate peripheral vessels.

USES
1. Production of controlled hypotension during surgery
2. Acute regulation of blood pressure in hypertensive emergencies
3. Emergency treatment of pulmonary edema resulting from pulmonary hypertension
4. Management of dissecting aortic aneurysm or ischemic heart disease when other drugs cannot be used (investigational use only)

ADMINISTRATION AND DOSAGE
Trimethaphan is available as an injection solution containing 50 mg/ml and is administered by IV infusion. A 1-mg/ml infusion solution is prepared by diluting 10 ml (500 mg) of injection solution to 500 ml in 5% dextrose injection. The IV drip is

started at a rate of 3 to 4 ml/min, then adjusted to maintain the desired degree of hypotension. If a patient's blood pressure does not begin to decrease with the initial infusion rate within 10 minutes, the rate should be increased by 0.5 mg every 10 minutes until a response is seen. Frequent blood pressure determinations are necessary. Infusion rates ranging from 0.3 to 6 ml/min have been used. Children may be administered 50 to 150 mcg/kg/min.

FATE

The onset of action is almost immediate following initiation of the infusion. Effects persist for approximately 10 minutes to 20 minutes after infusion is terminated. Tachyphylaxis can occur, requiring increased doses to maintain the desired effect. Trimethaphan is excreted by the kidneys, largely as intact drug.

SIDE-EFFECTS/ADVERSE REACTIONS

The incidence and severity of adverse reactions following administration of trimethaphan are related to the extent of ganglionic blockade, which in turn depends on the dose. Among the adverse effects reported with the drug are changes in heart rate, orthostatic hypotension, angina-like pain, urinary retention, nausea, vomiting, constipation, mydriasis, cycloplegia, dry mouth, anhidrosis, itching, urticaria, restlessness, and weakness. Respiratory depression has occurred with large doses, although a causal effect has not been established.

CONTRAINDICATIONS AND PRECAUTIONS

Contraindications to trimethaphan include conditions in which hypotension may be hazardous to the patient, such as shock, hypovolemia, anemia, asphyxia, and respiratory insufficiency. *Cautious use* is warranted in patients with arteriosclerosis; renal, hepatic, or cardiac disease; degenerative CNS disease, Addison's disease, diabetes, glaucoma, or a history of allergies (drug releases histamine). Caution must also be used in the very young and in elderly or debilitated persons.

INTERACTIONS

1. The hypotensive effects of trimethaphan can be potentiated by antihypertensive agents, anesthetics, vasodilators, and diuretics.
2. Trimethaphan can prolong the muscle-relaxing action of neuromuscular blocking agents.

NURSING CONSIDERATIONS

The response to trimethaphan is usually rapid so monitoring is critically important. Frequent measurements of blood pressure, pulse, and respiratory rate will identify the stability of the patient's response to the drug. Urinary output in relation to intake and abdominal distention can indicate urinary retention. Changes should be reported immediately.

Titration of this drug to achieve desired effects and avoid untoward effects is important. Patients on trimethaphan should receive the drug IV through an infusion pump to be certain the infusion rate is accurately monitored. Use of the pump will also assist the nurse to terminate the infusion gradually while watching the blood pressure closely. Tolerance can develop within 48 hours and may affect the ability of the drug to continue to lower blood pressure.

As with any antihypertensive agent administered by titrated infusion, the dose must be titrated carefully; avoiding rapid falls in blood pressure, especially in patients with cardiovascular or cerebrovascular disease. A rapid fall in blood pressure can produce cardiac or cerebral anoxia. The physician should set a blood pressure goal and a time limit for reaching it. When infusion is used to lower blood pressure during a surgical procedure, the drug should be terminated prior to wound closure to allow the pressure to return to normal, usually within 10 minutes.

Therapeutic doses of trimethaphan can quickly become toxic. The nurse should have on hand adequate amounts of oxygen, replacement fluids, respiratory aids, and vasopressor agents to treat adverse reactions. Phenylephrine, mephentermine, and dopamine are the vasopressor drugs of choice.

REVIEW QUESTIONS

1. How may ganglionic blocking agents can be classified?
2. Briefly describe the cardiovascular and CNS effects of nicotine.
3. What measures may be necessary in the management of nicotine poisoning?
4. How can nicotine resin complex gum be used to help a patient to quit smoking?
5. How does mecamylamine differ from trimethaphan?

6. Describe appropriate nursing interventions to assist a patient to respond to the orthostatic hypotension caused by mecamylamine.
7. What equipment and medications should the circulating nurse have on hand in the operating room when a patient is receiving trimethaphan intraoperatively?

BIBLIOGRAPHY

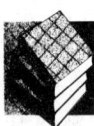

Fisher ML: Helping acutely ill patients put out the fire. Am J Nurs 79:1104, June 1979

Halpern JS: Effects of cigarette smoking on drugs. J Educ Nursing 11:211, 1985

Miletick DJ, Ivankovich AD: Cardiovascular effects of ganglionic blocking drugs. Int Anesthesiol Clin 16:151, 1978

Moree NA: New drugs: Hands on experience. Am J Nurs 85:252, 1985

Richard E, Shepard AC: Giving up smoking: A lesson in loss therapy. Am J Nurs 81:755, 1981

Salem MR: Therapeutic uses of ganglionic blocking drugs. Int Anesthesiol Clin 16:171, 1978

Volle RL: Ganglionic transmission. Ann Rev Pharmacol 9:135, 1969

Antihistamine–Antiserotonin Agents

18

Histamine and serotonin are two endogenous, biologically active amines which are widely distributed throughout the body and possess a myriad of physiologic and pharmacologic actions. The clinical usefulness of these amines, however, is greatly limited, due in part to their instability in gastric secretions, their lack of specificity, and, perhaps most importantly, the lack of precisely defined roles for the compounds in normal physiologic processes. Conversely, drugs that antagonize the actions of histamine and serotonin have a number of important therapeutic applications, including management of allergic reactions, gastric hypersecretion, and vascular headaches. This chapter will examine the basic pharmacology of these endogenous amines and review the clinical pharmacology and therapeutic applications of the antihistamine and antiserotonin drugs, as well as the ergot alkaloids, compounds possessing activity at serotonin receptor sites.

Histamine and Antihistamines

Histamine

Histamine is present in virtually all mammalian tissues, with highest amounts found in the skin, gastrointestinal (GI) mucosa, and lungs. Histamine is formed from the decarboxylation of the amino acid histidine. Sites of histamine localization in the body include (1) mast cells and basophils, the fixed tissue and circulating histaminocytes, respectively, where histamine is probably bound in a complex with heparin and an acidic protein; (2) gastric mucosal cells, where histamine is not extensively bound; and (3) CNS histamine-containing cells, located primarily in the hypothalamus. The bound form of histamine in the mast cells and basophils can be released by a variety of stimuli, both mechanical and chemical, including antigen–antibody reactions and exposure to a wide range of drugs. Upon release from binding sites or tissue stores, histamine is capable of eliciting a tremendous range of pharmacologic effects, from mild itching to circulatory shock.

The major pharmacologic actions of histamine are centered on the cardiovascular system, nonvascular smooth muscle, exocrine glands, and the adrenal medulla. The effects of histamine are mediated by an action on two distinct types of histaminergic receptors, termed H_1- and H_2-receptor sites. H_1 receptors are those associated with the smooth muscle of the blood vessels, bronchioles, and the GI tract, while H_2 receptors are found on gastric parietal cells (which secrete hydrochloric acid), the myocardium, and certain blood vessels. It appears that the contraction of nonvascular smooth muscle is an H_1-receptor effect, the secretion of gastric acid and acceleration of the heart rate are caused by H_2-receptor activation, and vascular dilation and increased permeability result from a combined action of histamine on both H_1 and H_2 sites.

PHARMACOLOGIC EFFECTS OF HISTAMINE

Histamine is capable of exerting powerful effects on certain organ systems of the body. However, considerable species difference exists with regard to histamine responsiveness. Thus, humans, along with dogs, cats, and guinea pigs, display significant sensitivity to the actions of histamine, whereas certain lower species, such as mice and rats, are much less responsive to the compound.

Cardiovascular System

Histamine relaxes smooth muscle of the arterioles and precapillary sphincter, thus increasing blood flow and capillary permeability. These effects can be demonstrated quite nicely by an intradermal injection of 10 mcg to 20 mcg of histamine, which results in a characteristic response termed the *triple reaction of Lewis*. The initial event is an area of *erythema* due to dilation of small microcirculatory vessels in the area of injection. This is followed by a *flare*, an irregular widening area of redness due to surrounding arteriolar dilation, and also by the appearance of a *wheal* or edematous swelling at the injection site, the result of capillary leakage of fluid due to increased permeability.

While small amounts of histamine have little effect on blood pressure or heart rate, large doses can elicit a hypotensive reaction, primarily due to generalized vasodilation. This effect is inhibited only by a combination of H_1- and H_2-blockers, suggesting that both types of histamine receptors are operative in vascular smooth muscle. Heart rate may be increased by histamine, a result of both a direct effect on myocardial H_2 receptors and a reflex response to the generalized vasodilation. Force of contraction may be slightly augmented as well by an H_2-receptor interaction.

Smooth Muscle

Most nonvascular smooth muscle is contracted by histamine due to a direct spasmogenic effect resulting largely from H_1-receptor activation. While organ sensitivity to the smooth muscle spasmogenic action of histamine varies considerably among species, human bronchiolar smooth muscle is highly reactive to histamine, especially in the asthmatic patient. Conversely, most other smooth muscle (e.g., GI, uterine, gallbladder, urinary bladder) is much less sensitive. In fact, some asthmatics are several hundred times more sensitive to the bronchoconstrictive effects of histamine than nonasthmatics.

Secretory Glands

Histamine is a potent stimulus for the secretion of hydrochloric acid by parietal cells of the gastric mucosa. This effect is mediated by H_2-receptor sites. The fact that H_2-receptor antagonists can inhibit the gastric secretory response to gastrin and to cholinergic stimulation as well suggests an interdependence of several secretory mechanisms involving gastric parietal cells, with histamine possibly serving as a common neurohormonal mediator.

In contrast to its marked secretory action on gastric acid-producing cells, histamine has much less of an effect on other types of exocrine glands, such as salivary, lacrimal, pancreatic, and respiratory.

Likewise, endocrine glands are largely unresponsive to histamine, with the exception of the adrenal medulla, where the release of the catecholamines epinephrine and norepinephrine is enhanced by histamine.

PHYSIOLOGIC FUNCTIONS OF HISTAMINE

In spite of the profound effects elicited by endogenous histamine, the physiologic functions of this amine remain largely speculative. Perhaps the best established function for histamine is its role in *gastric secretion*. However, it remains to be determined whether histamine itself is the final common mediator of hydrochloric acid secretion or whether it simply functions as one of several mediators.

Histamine may have an important function in regulating regional blood flow due to its *local vasodilatory action* on the microcirculation. During periods of stress, increased histamine release may serve to channel blood flow to needed areas by its circulatory actions.

Evidence indicates that histamine serves as a *neurotransmitter subserving the sensory phenomena of pain and especially of itching*. This action is probably an important component of the response to insect stings and bites; namely, pruritus, burning, and localized pain and irritation.

Finally, histamine is produced in large amounts by tissues undergoing a rapid rate of growth or repair, suggesting a possible role in cellular growth or regeneration. This *tissue-anabolic* action remains to be definitely established.

PATHOLOGIC SIGNIFICANCE OF HISTAMINE

While the physiologic functions of endogenous histamine remain largely speculative (e.g., neurotransmission, gastric acid secretion, tissue growth and repair), its role in several pathologic processes associated with acute and chronic allergic and hypersensitivity reactions and adverse drug reactions is much more clearly established.

Histamine can be released from cells by physical and chemical agents, a variety of drugs and toxins, and antigen–antibody reactions; therefore it plays a critical role in the symptomatology of many allergic, anaphylactic, and hypersensitivity reactions. Likewise, a number of drugs that can either block histamine release, competitively antagonize its receptor activation, or elicit actions opposite those of histamine (such as bronchodilation and vasoconstriction) are useful in the prophylaxis and treatment of many allergic reactions.

A variety of drugs can evoke histamine release from intracellular binding sites, and this releasing effect may contribute to the dermatologic, respiratory, cardiovascular, and gastrointestinal side-effects associated with many drugs. Representative histamine-releasing drugs include the following:

atropine
codeine
hydralazine
meperidine
morphine
papaverine
polymyxin

quinidine
sympathomimetic amines
trimethaphan
tubocurarine

CLINICAL USES OF HISTAMINE

The use of histamine in clinical medicine is essentially obsolete. Its therapeutic application is limited by its nonspecific range of pharmacologic actions and its rapid inactivation when given orally.

Histamine itself and its structural analogue betazole (Histalog) were once commonly used to test for functional achlorhydria (lack of gastric hydrochloric acid), but they have now largely been replaced by a more effective and less toxic diagnostic agent, pentagastrin (Peptavlon), which is discussed in Chapter 80. Histamine phosphate injection (0.275 mg) has occasionally been used for presumptive diagnosis of pheochromocytoma (see Chap. 80), but this is a dangerous procedure which is rarely employed today, due to the availability of more reliable chemical assays for detecting elevated catecholamine levels in the urine (see Disease Brief in Chap. 16). The principal importance of histamine, therefore, lies in its role as mediator of certain pathologic conditions and in the therapeutic value of its antagonism by antihistamine drugs.

Antihistamines

Drugs that competitively block the effects of histamine at various receptor sites in the body are termed *antihistamines*. Antihistamines are classified as either H_1- or H_2-receptor antagonists, although the H_1-blockers comprise the overwhelming majority of drugs, and the term antihistamine has come to be associated synonymously with H_1-antagonists. The H_2-blockers were first developed in the early 1970s and represent a major advance in the treatment of peptic ulcers, inasmuch as they exert a specific blocking effect on gastric parietal cell H_2-receptor sites, markedly reducing their output of hydrochloric acid.

H_1-Receptor Antagonists

The H_1-receptor blockers can be categorized chemically into one of several groups, each of which demonstrates slightly different pharmacologic properties, although most antihistamine drugs are comparably effective histamine antagonists when used at their recommended dosage levels. How-

ever, the *clinical* efficacy of the different antihistamines may vary widely among individuals: thus, drugs from one group may be significantly more effective in a certain patient than drugs from another group. Likewise, therapeutic effectiveness of one drug may diminish with time, and switching to another drug may restore clinical efficacy.

The chemical classification of H_1-receptor antagonists, the relative incidence of some common side-effects, and comparative potency ratios are shown in Table 18-1.

It is important to recognize that although H_1-receptor antagonists can theoretically prevent effector cell responses to both exogenous and endogenous histamine, the antagonists are significantly more effective against the former. However, endogenous histamine is responsible for most allergic reactions. Moreover, antihistamines are much more useful when given before a histamine challenge rather than after an allergic attack has begun. Finally, antihistamines are effective only to the extent that histamine is the primary causative factor in the allergic response. Therefore, H_1 antagonists are most effective in prevention of seasonal pollinosis and urticaria, somewhat less effective in allergic dermatoses, contact dermatitis, vasomotor rhinitis, serum sickness, and allergic transfusion reactions, and seldom useful alone in bronchial asthma, GI allergies, and systemic anaphylactic reactions.

PHARMACOLOGIC EFFECTS OF H_1 ANTAGONISTS

The term antihistamine is perhaps an oversimplification in that most H_1-receptor antagonists display a range of other pharmacologic actions unrelated to histamine antagonism.

Anticholinergic

Virtually all antihistamines possess some antimuscarinic (i.e., atropine-like) activity, which is probably of minimal therapeutic importance but may account for many of the side-effects, such as dryness of the mouth, blurred vision, tachycardia, and urinary hesitancy.

Local Anesthetic

Most H_1-receptor antagonists exhibit a degree of local anesthesia; some drugs, such as diphenhydramine and promethazine are more potent in this regard than procaine. Use of topical antihistamines as local anesthetics is restricted, however, by a high degree of local irritation and sensitization.

Table 18-1
Classification of Antihistamines

Chemical Category	Drugs	Usual Adult Dose (mg)*	Remarks
Alkylamines	brompheniramine	8	Low incidence of drowsiness and moderate GI upset. Most widely used antihistamine group.
	chlorpheniramine	4	
	dexchlorpheniramine	2	
	triprolidine	2.5	
Ethanolamines	carbinoxamine	4	Moderate to high incidence of drowsiness. Minimal GI upset. Dimenhydrinate is used for prophylaxis of motion sickness; diphenhydramine and doxylamine used in OTC sleep aids
	clemastine	1.34	
	dimenhydrinate	50	
	diphenhydramine	50	
	doxylamine	25	
Ethylenediamines	pyrilamine	50	Moderately sedating. High incidence of GI upset. Pyrilamine used in some OTC sleep aids.
	tripelennamine	50	
Phenothiazines	methdilazine	8	High degree of drowsiness. Trimeprazine also blocks serotonin. Many side-effects and contraindications. Can be used for motion sickness.
	promethazine	25	
	trimeprazine	2.5	
Piperazines	cyclizine	50	Primarily used for prophylaxis of motion sickness.
	meclizine	50	
Miscellaneous	azatadine	2	Sedation is moderate with cyproheptadine and azatadine which also block serotonin. Terfenadine is largely nonsedating.
	cyproheptadine	4	
	diphenylpyraline	2	
	phenindamine	25	
	terfenadine	60	

* Usual *single* oral adult dose in milligrams.

Cardiac Depressant
Due to their local anesthetic or membrane-stabilizing action, antihistamines possess a quinidine-like action on the myocardium, although in most instances it is too weak to be of clinical significance.

CNS Depressant
The most commonly encountered side-effects with most antihistamines are sedation and drowsiness (see Table 18-1 for the incidence among the various groups of drugs). This sedative action is the basis for the use of antihistamines as sleep aids, and is also responsible for the often undesirable daytime drowsiness experienced by many patients taking these drugs. With recommended doses, occasional episodes of paradoxical restlessness, nervousness, and central excitation are noted, especially in children. These central stimulatory effects become significantly more prevalent at very high doses and can lead to convulsions and extreme agitation.

In addition to the above actions of antihistamines, other properties of some of the compounds include an antiserotonin effect, an alpha-adrener-

gic blocking action and an antinauseant effect in preventing motion sickness.

The clinical pharmacology of the H_1-receptor antagonists will be discussed as a group, as they are remarkably similar in most of their actions, with a listing of individual drugs given in Table 18-2. The H_2-receptor blockers will be considered individually later in the chapter.

MECHANISM AND ACTIONS
Antihistamines classified as H_1-receptor antagonists exert a competitive blocking action on histamine at H_1-receptor sites on effector structures such as vascular and nonvascular smooth muscle. Other actions exhibited by most antihistamines include antimuscarinic, antiserotonin, antiadrenergic, local anesthetic, and CNS depressant. Among the clinical effects of H_1-receptor blockers are amelioration of symptoms of allergic reactions such as increased secretions, bronchiolar smooth muscle contraction, increased capillary leakage, and edema formation. The central actions of antihistamines include sedation, drowsiness, decreased extrapyra-

(Text continues on p. 300.)

Table 18-2
Antihistamines

Drug	Preparations	Usual Dosage Range	Major Use	Clinical Considerations
azatadine (Opti-mine)	Tablets—1 mg	1 mg–2 mg twice a day	Allergic disorders	Do not use in children under age 12. Has antiserotonin effects as well.
brompheniramine (Bromphen, Dimetane, and various other manufacturers)	Tablets—4 mg Tablets (timed-release)—8 mg, 12 mg Elixir—2 mg/5 ml Injection—10 mg/ml, 100 mg/ml	*Oral:* Adults—4 mg–8 mg three to four times/day or 8 mg–12 mg timed-release twice a day Children over 6—2 mg–4 mg three to four times/day Children under 6—0.5 mg/kg daily in divided doses *Parenteral:* Adults—5 mg–20 mg IV, IM, or SC twice a day (maximum 40 mg/day) Children–0.5 mg/kg/day	Allergic disorders Cough	Keep patient lying down during IV administration. Sweating, hypotension, and faintness may occur with IV use. Do not use solutions with preservatives for IV use. Monitor blood levels; can produce agranulocytosis. (See chlorpheniramine.)
buclizine (Bucladin-S)	Tablets—50 mg	Nausea—50 mg to 150 mg/day Motion sickness—50 mg one-half hour before travel, and 50 mg every 4–6 hr as needed	Nausea, vomiting, and vertigo; Prevention of motion sickness	Tablets may be chewed or swallowed whole; can also be dissolved under tongue. Do not use during pregnancy or in small cildren. May produce headache, nervousness, drowsiness, and dryness of the mouth.
carbinoxamine (Clistin)	Tablets—4 mg	Adults—4 mg–8 mg three to four times/day Children—2 mg–6 mg three to four times/day depending on age	Allergic disorders	Mildly sedating, strong anticholinergic action; good antiemetic.
chlorpheniramine (Chlor-Trimeton, Teldrin, and various other manufacturers)	Chewable tablets—2 mg Tablets—4 mg Timed-release tablets—8 mg, 12 mg Timed-release capsules—8 mg, 12 mg Syrup—2 mg/5 ml Injection—10, 100 mg/ml	*Oral:* Adults—4 mg three to six times day or 8 mg–12 mg twice a day (timed-release) Children 6–12—2 mg three to six times/day Children 2–6—1 mg three to four times/day *Parenteral:* Allergy—5 mg–20 mg IM, SC (maximum 40 mg/day) Anaphylaxis—10 mg–20 mg IV	Allergic disorders Transfusion and drug reactions Anaphylactic reactions	May be used prophylactically for blood transfusion. *Only* injection solution used IV is 10 mg/ml; when given IV or added directly to stored blood, do not use solution with preservatives. Low incidence of drowsiness and other side-effects. Has antiemetic, antitussive, and some local anesthetic action. Timed-release preparations are not recommended in children under age 12. May produce increased drowsiness, particularly in elderly persons.
clemastine (Tavist)	Tablets—1.34 mg, 2.68 mg Syrup—0.67 mg/5 ml	Adults–1.34 mg–2.68 mg two to three times/day (maximum three tablets daily)	Allergic disorders	Not recommended in children under age 12. Monitor blood levels; can produce hemolytic anemia. Use cautiously in the elderly.

(continued)

Table 18-2 (continued)
Antihistamines

Drug	Preparations	Usual Dosage Range	Major Use	Clinical Considerations
cyclizine (Marezine)	Tablets—50 mg Injection—50 mg/ml	*Oral:* 50 mg one-half hour before travel; repeat every 4–6 hr to a maximum of 300 mg/day (children 6–10 yr—½ adult dose) *IM:* 50 mg every 4–6 hr	Prevention and treatment of motion sickness and postoperative nausea and vomiting	Do not use in pregnancy or in children under age 6. Produces frequent drowsiness. For postoperative nausea and vomiting give 20 min to 30 min before end of surgery. Overdosage may produce hyperexcitability and convulsions. Claimed to reduce the sensitivity of the labyrinthine apparatus to motion. Store in a cool place; may discolor to light yellow; does not affect potency.
dexchlorpheniramine (Dexchlor, Poladex, T.D. Polaramine, Polargen)	Tablets—2 mg Repeat-action tablets—4 mg, 6 mg Syrup—2 mg/5 ml	Adults—2 mg three to four times a day or 4 mg–6 mg repeat-action tablets twice a day Child—½ adult dose Infant—¼ adult dose	Allergic disorders	Low incidence of many common side-effects. Do not use repeat-action tablets in children. Available as an expectorant with pseudoephedrine and guaifenesin.
dimenhydrinate (Dramamine and various other manufacturers)	Tablets—50 mg Liquid—12.5 mg/ml Injection—50 mg/ml	*Oral:* Adults—50 mg–100 mg every 4 hr Children (6 yr–12 yr)—25 mg to 50 mg three times/day Children (2 yr–6 yr)—up to 25 mg every 6–8 hr *IM:* Adults—50 mg as needed Children—1.25 mg/kg four times a day up to 300 mg/day *IV (adults only)*—50 mg in 10 ml sodium chloride given over 2 min	Prevention and treatment of nausea, vomiting and vertigo of motion sickness, radiation sickness, or anesthesia	Drowsiness is common, especially at higher doses. Caution when used in combination with aminoglycoside antibiotics, because it may mask signs of ototoxicity, leading to permanent damage. Tolerance develops with continued use. Do not mix parenteral solutions with other drugs because many are incompatible. Dilute IV solutions with maximum allowable fluid. This drug is very irritating to veins.
diphenhydramine (Benadryl and various other manufacturers)	Tablets—25 mg, 50 mg Capsules—25 mg, 50 mg Elixir—12.5 mg/5 ml Syrup—12.5, 13.3 mg/5 ml Injection—10, 50 mg/ml Cream—1%, 2%	*Oral:* Adults—25 mg–50 mg three to four times/day Children (over 20 lb)—5 mg/kg/day in divided doses *Parenteral—IV or deep IM* Adults—10 mg–50 mg as needed (maximum 400 mg/day) Children—5 mg/kg/day in four divided doses	Allergic disorders Motion sickness Adjunctive therapy in anaphylactic reactions Prevention of reactions to blood or plasma Sedative in pediatric patients Cough due to colds or allergies	Topical preparations may cause hypersensitivity reactions. High incidence of drowsiness initially, which decreases with use. Monitor blood pressure carefully with parenteral use. Very low incidence of GI disturbances. Found in several OTC sleep aids—Sleep EZE, Sominex 2, Twilite). Solution is very irritating to tissue. Give deep IM and rotate injection sites with every dose.

(continued)

Table 18-2 (continued)
Antihistamines

Drug	Preparations	Usual Dosage Range	Major Use	Clinical Considerations
diphenhydramine (Benadryl and various other manufacturers) (*continued*)			Oral anesthesia in dental practice Parkinsonism Acute dystonias Insomnia	
diphenylpyraline (Hispril)	Timed-release capsules—5 mg	Adults—5 mg twice a day Children (over 6)—5 mg daily	Alergic disorders	Do not use in children under age 6.
doxylamine (Unisom)	Tablets—25 mg	Adults—25 mg 20–30 min before bedtime	Insomnia	Drowsiness is very common; indicated as a nonprescription sleep aid.
meclizine (Antivert, Antrizine, Bonine, Dizmiss, Motion Cure, Ru-Vert M, Wehvert)	Tablets—12.5 mg, 50 mg Chewable tablets—25 mg	*Motion Sickness*—25 mg–50 mg 1 hr prior to travel. Repeat every 24 h. *Vertigo*—25 mg–100 mg daily in divided doses as needed	Motion sickness Vertigo due to disease of the vestibular system	Do not use in pregnancy or young children. Commonly causes dry mouth and drowsiness. Weak anticholinergic action. Tablets are oral or chewable. This drug has a slower onset and longer duration than many others. Watch for delayed development of side-effects.
methdilazine (Tacaryl)	Chewable tablets—4 mg Tablets—8 mg Syrup—4 mg/5 ml	Adults—8 mg two to four times/day Children—4 mg two to four times/day	Pruritus Urticaria	Tablets may be chewed (4 mg) or swallowed whole (8 mg). Structurally a phenothiazine (see Chap. 27 for possible adverse reactions). Strong anticholinergic and antiemetic. Do not use in children under age 3.
promethazine (Phenergan and various other manufacturers)	Tablets—12.5 mg, 25 mg, 50 mg Syrup—6.25, 25 mg/5 ml Suppositories—12.5 mg, 25 mg, 50 mg Injection—25, 50 mg/ml	*Oral:* Adults—12.5 mg–50 mg every 4 h–6 h as necessary Children—6.25 mg–12.5 mg three times/day as needed *Rectal*—12.5 mg–25 mg every 4 h–6 h as necessary *Parenteral (usually IM)*—12.5 mg–25 mg individualized to condition (children—0.6–1.2 mg/kg) When used IV, maximum concentration is 25 mg/ml/min	Allergic disorders and reactions to blood plasma Motion sickness Nausea and vomiting due to anesthesia, drugs, or surgery Preoperative and obstetrical sedation Adjunct to analgesics in postoperative or	Phenothiazine derivative (see Chap. 27). Potent antihistamine and sedative with prolonged effects. May cause false-positive on urine pregnancy tests (immunologic type). Avoid intra-arterial injection because severe arteriospasm can result. Irritating to tissue if given SC. Give deep IM and rotate sites with every dose. Photosensitivity is a problem. Caution patient to use dark glasses and avoid bright light. Reduce dose of analgesics and other sedative-hypnotics if used in combination with promethazine. Injection is

Table 18-2 (continued)
Antihistamines

Drug	Preparations	Usual Dosage Range	Major Use	Clinical Considerations
promethazine (Phenergan and various other manufacturers) (*continued*)			chronic pain Sedation and light sleep Cough	incompatible with alkaline drugs; should be diluted with saline prior to injection. Flush heparin lock with saline prior to and after injecting drug because it is incompatible with heparin. Avoid contact with skin or eyes. Good antiemetic, but may mask vomiting caused by other drugs. Protect injectible form from light and do not use if cloudy or darkened. Available with expectorant, either plain or with codeine and/or decongestants.
pyrilamine (Dormarex)	Tablets—25 mg Capsules—25 mg	Adults—25 mg–50 mg three times/day Insomnia—50 mg at bedtime	Allergic disorders Insomnia	Not recommended in children under age 6; found in several OTC cough formulations, drug is only mildly sedating and weakly anticholinergic.
terfenadine (Seldane)	Tablets—60 mg	Adults and children over 12—60 mg twice a day	Allergic disorders (especially rhinitis)	Long-acting oral antihistamine used for control of chronic allergic disorders; very minimally sedating.
tripelennamine (Pyribenzamine, Pelamine, PBZ)	Tablets—25 mg, 50 mg Long-acting tablets —100 mg Elixir—37.5 mg/5 ml	Adults—25 mg–50 mg every 4 h–6 h (maximum 600 mg/day or 100 mg two to three times/day) Children—5 mg/kg/day in four to six doses (maximum 300 mg/day)	Allergic disorders and reactions to blood or plasma Pruritus and other topical skin disorders Mucuous membrane analgesia and anesthesia in the mouth cough	Do not use 100-mg sustained-acting form in children. Used as mouthwash for herpetic gingivostomatitis in children. Caution in elderly because dizziness, sedation, and hypotension are more likely to occur. Possesses some antitussive and local anesthetic activity.
triprolidine (Actidil, Bayidyl)	Tablets—2.5 mg Syrup—1.25 mg/5 ml	Adults—2.5 mg three to four times/day Children (6–12)—1.25 mg three to five times/day Children (2–6)—0.6 mg three to four times/day Children (under 2)—0.3 mg three to four times/day	Allergic disorders	Low degree of drowsiness and most other side-effects. Rapid onset of action. May cause paradoxical excitation and irritability. Combined with pseudoephedrine as Actifed; this combination is also available with codeine and guaifenesin as Actifed-C. Children under age 6 should be given syrup only.

midal motor activity, and reduced nausea and vomiting associated with motion sickness, anesthesia, or surgery. A central antitussive action has also been proposed. H_1-blockers do *not* reduce gastric acid secretion.

USES

Note: Not all of the available antihistamines have all the following indications—see Table 18-2 for respective uses of each drug.

1. Relief of symptoms of various allergic disorders (*e.g.*, allergic rhinitis, vasomotor rhinitis, uncomplicated urticaria and angioedema, allergic reactions to blood or plasma)
2. Adjunctive treatment in anaphylactic reactions (with epinephrine and other measures)
3. Prevention and treatment of motion sickness
4. Relief of insomnia (short-term basis only)
5. Adjunctive therapy for parkinsonism and extrapyramidal reactions due to antipsychotic drug therapy
6. Relief of coughs caused by colds, allergies, or minor throat irritations
7. Prevention and control of nausea and vomiting due to anesthesia or surgery
8. Adjunct to analgesics for obstetrics and postoperative pain, and for preoperative sedation and relief of apprehension
9. Production of local oral anesthesia in dentistry

ADMINISTRATION AND DOSAGE
See Table 18-2.

FATE

Most antihistamines are well-absorbed from the GI tract and are administered orally. Peak blood levels are usually attained within 1 hour to 2 hours. Most drugs have an effective duration of 3 hours to 5 hours following a single dose; the duration of action with sustained-release forms of the drugs is 8 hours to 12 hours. Distribution is extensive throughout the body, including the CNS. Antihistamines are primarily metabolized in the liver or kidney and excreted in the urine, principally as metabolites. The efficacy of the H_1-blockers is *not* appreciably enhanced by parenteral administration. Topical application provides effective local anesthesia, but the risk of sensitization is high.

SIDE-EFFECTS/ADVERSE REACTIONS

The side-effects occurring with greatest frequency following use of a systemic antihistamine are drowsiness, dizziness, epigastric distress, and thickening of bronchial secretions. A wide range of other adverse reactions have been reported with antihistamine usage, although the frequency and severity of the adverse reactions listed below vary greatly among the available preparations, and most are relatively rare at recommended doses.

CV—Hypotension, palpitations, tachycardia, arrhythmias

GI—Anorexia, nausea, vomiting, diarrhea, or constipation

CNS—Confusion, restlessness, impaired coordination, blurred vision, vertigo, tinnitus, heaviness and weakness of the hands, nervousness, tremors, paresthesias, irritability, excitation, insomnia, hysteria

Hematologic—Hemolytic anemia, thrombocytopenia, leukopenia, pancytopenia, agranulocytosis

Urinary—Urinary frequency or retention, dysuria

Respiratory—Wheezing, chest tightness, nasal congestion

Hypersensitivity—Urticaria, drug rash, photosensitivity, anaphylactic shock

Other—Headache, diplopia, sweating, pallor, stinging or burning at site of injection

With overdosage—Fever, ataxia, hallucinations, convulsions, coma, cardiovascular and respiratory collapse (children are especially susceptible)

CONTRAINDICATIONS AND PRECAUTIONS

Antihistamines should not be used in nursing mothers because they are readily excreted in breast milk and can lead to adverse affects, such as excessive drowsiness in newborn infants. Although not absolutely contraindicated, the drugs should be avoided in early pregnancy unless absolutely necessary because a possible link to fetal malformations has been suggested. Other contraindications to use of antihistamines are premature or newborn infants and patients on MAO-inhibitor therapy (see under Interactions). In addition, phenothiazine antihistamines (methdilazine, promethazine, trimeprazine) are contraindicated in comatose patients, states of CNS depression due to drug overdosage, jaundice, bone marrow depression, and acutely ill or dehydrated children. All antihistamines should be used with *caution* in the following conditions: asthma, narrow-angle glaucoma, peptic ulcer, prostatic hypertrophy, bladder neck obstruction, convulsive disorders, hyperthyroidism, cardiovascular or renal disease, hypertension, and diabetes.

INTERACTIONS

1. The sedative effects of antihistamines may be enhanced by concurrent use of other CNS depressants (e.g., alcohol, barbiturates, narcotics, antianxiety drugs).
2. Atropine-like side-effects (e.g., dryness of mouth, blurred vision, urinary retention, constipation) are potentiated by other anticholinergics, tricyclic antidepressants, and MAO inhibitors.
3. The effects of epinephrine may be increased by certain commonly used antihistamines, such as diphenhydramine, chlorpheniramine, and tripelennamine.

(In addition, several antihistamines are phenothiazines and have the potential to interact in other ways with many drugs—refer to chapter 27 for a complete discussion of phenothiazines.)

■ *Nursing Process*

□ *ASSESSMENT*

Sometimes the nurse may have difficulty determining if the patient is using antihistamines because most are over-the-counter medications which patients frequently forget to report. When obtaining a drug history the nurse should remember to specifically ask about such drugs so care can be more appropriately planned. Antihistamines interact with several other drugs, including alcohol, and may be dangerous with some combinations.

□ *NURSING DIAGNOSES*

Actual nursing diagnosis for patients taking antihistamines is:

Knowledge deficit related to safe
    administration, side-effects, and
    contraindications for this drug.

Potential nursing diagnoses for this drug, based on common side-effects, include:

Ineffective airway clearance related to
    thickened bronchial secretions
Alteration in nutrition related to epigastric
    distress
Potential for injury related to dizziness
Sensory–perceptual alteration in vision related
    to dizziness
Impairment of skin integrity (especially in
    children who are more susceptible to rashes)
Sleep pattern disturbance
Urinary retention

□ *PLAN*

The nursing care goal is to teach the patient how to manage administration of these drugs to minimize side-effects and maximize their therapeutic effect.

□ *INTERVENTION*

The main nursing intervention is teaching users to watch for side-effects. Users should not drive or operate machinery when the drug has taken effect because of the CNS side-effect of drowsiness. Drowsiness may subside as the body adjusts to the drug. Coffee or tea may also help. For elderly persons, the CNS effects can result in sedation, confusion, and hypertension so all antihistamines should be used cautiously in this age group. Children are also susceptible to varying CNS effects of these drugs. A child may become mentally dulled or paradoxically excited when the drug is given. Overdosage is more dangerous in children and can result in hallucinations, convulsions, and, rarely, death. These drugs should be used with caution.

Another problem with antihistamines is development of tolerance, thus reducing the effectiveness of the drug. The user may be tempted to take more of the drug when the effectiveness diminishes, but a better strategy is to change to a different type or attempt to go drug-free for several days.

Bronchial secretions may become thickened and difficult to expectorate during antihistamine therapy. As a precaution, patients should be encouraged to drink extra fluids and to use a cool mist vaporizer, humidifier, or open pan of water in the bedroom. A mother who is breast-feeding should be encouraged to continue when her infant is receiving antihistamines because breast milk will provide an excellent source of fluids and will not thicken secretions.

For the patient who complains of GI upset the drug can be taken with milk or food to decrease side-effects.

Antihistamines should be discontinued several days before allergy skin testing because the drug may mask positive results.

Topical antihistamine preparations can produce serious hypersensitivity reactions due to their chemical composition. The drug should be discontinued at the first sign of rash, redness, or itching. Topical preparations are not to be applied to broken, exposed, or weeping skin areas.

□ *EVALUATION*

The outcome most patients seek is control of symptoms with minimal side-affects. Drowsiness is the most uncomfortable side-effect, and many

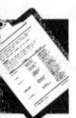

Assessment

Subjective Data

1. Medication history
   a. Refer to Interactions sections to formulate pertinent questions.
   b. Many are OTC drugs, which can be overlooked on history taking. Determine if other antihistamines are currently being used and length of time used, because tolerance can develop when drugs are taken for extended periods.
   c. Drug allergies/hypersensitivity to antihistamines
2. Symptoms the parent/patient desires to be treated with the drug
3. Medical history
   a. Check for preexisting conditions that may precipitate adverse reactions, such as multiple allergies, CNS disease, heart disease/defect, gastrointestinal disorders, narrow angle glaucoma, hyperthyroidism, hypertension, diabetes.
   b. Current pregnancy/lactation. Such patients should avoid antihistamine use.
4. Compliance issues
   a. Parent's/child's knowledge of what the drug should do and how to take the drug
   b. Parent's past experiences in getting the child to take the drug; methods used to give the child the drug

Objective Data

1. Physical assessment
   a. Vital signs
   b. Height and weight
   c. Urinary output
   d. Nasopharyngeal examination
   e. Neurologic status: mental alertness, psychomotor skills
2. Laboratory/diagnostic data: glaucoma tonometry if appropriate

Nursing Diagnosis	Expected Client Outcome	Intervention
Knowledge deficit related to correct drug taking, side-effects, and time frame for safe use	Will obtain relief from symptoms of allergy, motion sickness, or insomnia by following the recommended administration schedule for the specific drug	Teach the patient to start by taking the drug as recommended, usually no more than every 6 h.
		Recommend a change in dosage or drug if tolerance develops as a more effective strategy than taking the same dose more frequently.
		Recommend drug taking for no more than 5–7 days. If symptoms persist, the physician should be contacted.
		Teach the patient to monitor for common side effects as described below and follow preventive or reactive strategies given.
Potential for injury related to drowsiness, dizziness	Will use safety precautions to avoid injury	Caution users to avoid driving, climbing heights, operating machinery until drug effects are known.
		Caffeine beverages or continued use may reduce drowsiness.
		Teach parents to be prepared for extreme drowsiness or paradoxical excitation in young children and to protect from injury and reduce dose or stop drug if symptom is severe.

(continued)

Nursing Diagnosis	Expected Client Outcome	Intervention
Potential ineffective airway clearance related to thickened secretions	Will liquify and expel secretions.	Encourage use of a cool-mist vaporizer or an ultrasonic humidifier if secretions are thick, dry, and difficult to expel.
		Encourage increased clear fluid intake.
Potential alteration in comfort: nausea, dry mouth	Will prevent or obtain relief from nausea, dry mouth	Encourage patient to take drug with meals or milk to decrease GI upset.
		Encourage fluid intake and frequent mouth care.
Potential for injury: related to poisoning	Access to drug by child will be prevented	Encourage breast-feeding mother to avoid use of drug.
		Teach proper storage to keep drug out of child's reach.

patients will change drugs until they find one they can take without becoming drowsy. Because most people will try to continue their daily activities while taking the drug, this outcome may be critical. Nursing Care Plan 18-1 contains guidelines for developing nursing care plans for patients receiving antihistamines. While the plan is geared toward children, most parameters apply to adults as well.

H_2-Receptor Antagonists

Certain actions of histamine, namely its gastric secretory, myocardial stimulant, and certain vascular dilatory effects are mediated by receptors designated as histamine-2 sites that are *not* blocked by the classic antihistamine drugs. These observations led to the development of selective H_2-receptor antagonists. Clinical studies with H_2-blockers have demonstrated marked, and in some instances almost complete reduction in gastric secretory volume, total acidity, and pepsin activity following administration of an H_2-receptor antagonist. Therefore, these substances (cimetidine, famotidine, ranitidine) have an important role in the therapeutic management of peptic ulcers and various gastric hypersecretory states.

PHARMACOLOGIC EFFECTS OF H_2 ANTAGONISTS

H_2-receptor blockers markedly reduce the secretion of gastric hydrochloric acid evoked by histamine, pentagastrin, vagal nerve stimulation, caffeine, food, and insulin-induced hypoglycemia. Thus, it appears that H_2-receptor blockade on gas-

tric parietal cells not only prevents the secretory response to histamine itself, but also impairs the ability of other stimuli, both chemical and neuronal, to evoke a full secretory response. An interdependence of several mechanisms that operate to control hydrochloric acid release from the gastric mucosa is therefore probable, with histamine possibly serving as a final common neurohormonal mediator.

H_2-receptor blockers have little effect on other gastrointestinal secretions and do not significantly alter GI motility or lower esophageal sphincter tone. Likewise, at doses that effectively suppress gastric acid secretion, H_2-blockers have no significant effect on the heart or blood pressure, probably reflecting the minimal role played by endogenous histamine in the normal regulation of cardiovascular functioning. An antiandrogenic action has been demonstrated for cimetidine, one of the H_2-blockers, and several cases of gynecomastia and reduced sperm count in men and galactorrhea in women have been noted. The clinical significance of this antiandrogenic action remains to be completely established.

In the treatment of active peptic ulcer, several types of drugs have been employed, including antacids, anticholinergics, H_2-blockers, and sucralfate. Of these various drugs, H_2-blockers probably represent the agents that are most effective in and best tolerated by most patients. Systemic anticholinergics can decrease acid secretion, but large doses are generally necessary, and side-effects are common; thus, patient compliance is usually poor. High-potency liquid antacids promote ulcer healing rates similar to those obtained with H_2-blockers, but frequent dosing (*i.e.*, every 2 hours to 3 hours) is necessary, and again compliance is poor, except perhaps during the acute, painful phase of the condition. Sucralfate is a sulfated sucrose–aluminum hydroxide compound which forms an ulcer-adherent complex with exudative material at the ulcer site, thus producing a protective barrier over the ulcerated area, protecting it from further acid and pepsin attack. Its efficacy is reportedly similar to that of cimetidine, and the drug represents an alternative in the management of duodenal ulcers. A complete discussion of sucralfate is found in Chapter 42.

Cimetidine

(Tagamet)

MECHANISM AND ACTIONS

Cimetidine exerts a selective competitive antagonistic action at histamine$_2$-receptor sites. Blockade of H$_2$-receptors in the gastric mucosa reduces daytime and nocturnal gastric acid secretion by 90% to 100% as well as acid secretion in response to food, caffeine, pentagastrin, and insulin. Secretory volume is also markedly decreased, and total pepsin output is reduced. Gastric *p*H is elevated to 5.0 or greater for 3 hours to 4 hours.

USES

1. Treatment of gastric and duodenal ulcers
2. Reduction of acid levels in acute or recurrent gastric hypersecretory conditions (*e.g.*, stress ulcers in hospitalized patients)
3. Prevention of recurrence of ulcers in high-risk patients
4. Treatment of pathologic hypersecretory conditions (*e.g.*, Zollinger-Ellison syndrome, systemic mastocytosis, multiple endocrine adenomas)
5. Investigational uses include prevention of aspiration pneumonitis during general anesthesia, control of hyperparathyroidism in chronic hemodialysis patients, and as adjunctive therapy in treating gastroesophageal reflux, herpes virus infection, and tinea capitis, and in hirsute women (due to its antiandrogenic action).

ADMINISTRATION AND DOSAGE

Cimetidine is available for oral usage as tablets (200 mg, 300 mg, 400 mg, 800 mg), as liquid (300 mg/5 ml), and as an injectable solution for IM (300 mg/2 ml) or IV (300 mg/50 ml) use. In the treatment of active peptic ulcer, 800 mg is given orally at bedtime or 400 mg is given twice a day for 4 weeks to 6 weeks. Once healing has occurred, a maintenance dose of 400 mg at bedtime is usually sufficient to prevent recurrence, and is frequently given on a chronic basis in high-risk patients. In other hypersecretory conditions (see under Uses), the recommended dosage is 300 mg four to six times a day to a maximum of 2400 mg per day, continued for as long as is clinically necessary.

Parenteral administration is indicated in hospitalized patients with intractable ulcers or pathologic hypersecretory conditions and in patients unable to take oral medications. The parenteral dose is 300 mg diluted in 20 ml Sodium Chloride Injection and administered over 1 minute to 2 minutes or 300 mg in 100 ml 5% Dextrose Injection by infusion over 15 minutes to 20 minutes. Cimetidine injection is stable for 48 hours at room temperature if mixed with 9% normal saline or a 5% or 10% dextrose solution. It should not be mixed with sterile water for injection. In patients with impaired renal function, 300 mg is given every 8 hours to 12 hours. The drug has not been widely used in children, but a dosage of 20 to 40 mg/kg/day in divided doses has been recommended.

FATE

Oral absorption is rapid, and the drug is not subject to first-pass inactivation. Food delays but does not reduce the extent of oral absorption. Oral bioavailability is approximately 70% to 80%. Peak serum levels are attained within 45 minutes to 90 minutes. Half-life is about 2 hours in persons with normal renal function. Duration of effective inhibition of basal gastric secretion is 4 to 5 hours. Plasma protein binding is minimal (15%–20%). Excretion is mainly in the urine, largely as unchanged drug (75%), especially following parenteral administration. Following IM or IV administration, approximately 75% of the drug is excreted within 24 hours.

SIDE-EFFECTS/ADVERSE REACTIONS

Side-effects are rather infrequent with normal doses of cimetidine, and only 1% to 2% of patients experience adverse reactions, the most common of which are mild and transient diarrhea, nausea, dizziness, rash, and muscular ache. Transient pain is often noted at the site of IM injection. Other reported adverse effects include headache, confusion, gynecomastia, alopecia, galactorrhea, decreased sperm count, impotence, altered heartbeat, delirium, ataxia, dysarthria, hallucinations, increased plasma creatinine and serum transaminases, and rarely blood dyscrasias, such as neutropenia, agranulocytosis, thrombocytopenia, and aplastic or hemolytic anemia. IV bolus injection has resulted in cardiac arrhythmias and hypotension.

CONTRAINDICATIONS AND PREVENTIONS
There are no known absolute contraindications to use of cimetidine. *Cautious use,* however, is warranted in pregnant or nursing women, in elderly or severely ill patients, in patients with impaired renal or hepatic function, and in children under age 16.

INTERACTIONS
1. Antacids and metoclopramide may impair oral absorption of cimetidine if administered simultaneously.
2. Cimetidine may increase the half-life of certain benzodiazepine drugs (alprazolam, chlordiazepoxide, diazepam, flurazepam, triazolam), beta-blockers, caffeine, theophylline, lidocaine, salicylates, phenytoin, quinidine, and other drugs metabolized in the liver due to slowed hepatic metabolic functioning.
3. Cimetidine may increase the pharmacologic effects of procainamide by reducing its renal clearance.
4. Concurrent use of cimetidine and morphine may result in muscle twitching, confusion, and apnea.
5. The effectiveness of sucralfate may be reduced by cimetidine, because sucralfate requires an acid medium to be most effective.
6. Decreased oral absorption of ketoconazole may occur in the presence of cimetidine due to increased *p*H.
7. Increased effects of carbamazepine have been reported when it was given in conjunction with cimetidine.
8. Concurrent administration of cimetidine and digoxin have resulted in decreased serum levels of digoxin.

■ Nursing Process

□ ASSESSMENT

□ Subjective Data
A drug history is essential because cimetidine interacts with many compounds. See Interactions above for help in formulating appropriate questions. A medical history should also be obtained with emphasis on past episodes of gastrointestinal problems and renal or hepatic disease. Frequently the patient on cimetidine has had a variety of treatments for ulcer and may have taken the drug before.

Patients frequently see cimetidine as a "wonder drug" and have high expectations about its effectiveness. The patient needs to discuss his perception of what this drug is and what it will do. Cimetidine is more effective in treating duodenal ulcers than gastric ulcers, and relapse is common after discontinuation of therapy. If the patient has realistic expectations about this drug he is more likely to use it effectively.

□ Objective Data
Physical assessment should include review of the liver, abdomen, kidney, and cardiovascular system to check for the presence of arrhythmias. Laboratory tests may include renal and hepatic function studies as well as a complete blood count. The patient may also have an ECG (if cardiovascular status is questionable) and an upper GI series.

□ NURSING DIAGNOSES
Actual nursing diagnoses for the patient starting on cimetidine may include:
> Knowledge deficit related to correct dose and administration of the drug as well as to side-effects
> Alteration in comfort related to epigastric distress

Potential nursing diagnoses are related to the drug's side-effects and may include:
> Alteration in bowel elimination: diarrhea
> Potential for injury related to dizziness

□ PLAN
Nursing care goals should focus on assisting the patient to learn safe drug-taking practices with cimetidine and how to monitor for common and dangerous reactions to the drug.

□ INTERVENTION
To safely administer cimetidine intravenously the nurse must remember that cimetidine may be incompatible when mixed in the same IV line with other drugs such as aminophylline or barbiturates. To minimize the risk of precipitation, the IV line should be completely flushed before cimetidine is administered, and the dosing schedule should be adjusted so the drug is not given immediately before or after other intravenous drugs.

Given the range of side-effects and lack of information about the long-term safety of this drug, long-term and indiscriminate use of cimetidine should be discouraged. Patients should understand that they should not take cimetidine as they would antacids (*i.e.*, for relief of symptoms) but on a scheduled basis. Self-dosing should be discouraged and prescriptions limited. Antacids can be used to treat episodic pain but should be taken at least 1 hour before or after cimetidine administration.

Elderly and renal-impaired patients are particularly prone to confusion associated with cimetidine administration. Patients and families should be taught to monitor such effects closely and report changes to the physician.

Hematologic, renal, and hepatic studies should be done periodically if the patient has been on cimetidine for more than 4 weeks because the incidence of serious reactions increases over time.

Common side-effects such as dizziness, nausea, and diarrhea are frequently transient and will resolve as the body adjusts to the drug. If these symptoms do not abate after a week or if they continue to worsen the patient should notify the prescriber.

□ EVALUATION

The outcomes sought are reduction or elimination of epigastric pain, radiographic validation that the ulcer heals, evidence that the patient complies with the drug regimen as prescribed, and absence of significant side-effects.

Famotidine

(Pepcid)

MECHANISM AND ACTIONS

Famotidine is a competitive inhibitor of histamine$_2$ receptors. It reduces basal and nocturnal gastric acid secretion as well as acid secretion stimulated by food and pentagastrin. Intragastric *p*H is elevated to between 5 and 6. Pepsin secretion is also reduced and its action is depressed. Famotidine is long acting and is suitable for once daily dosing. The drug does not appear to have antiandrogenic activity, nor does it affect the CNS or interfere with hepatic metabolism of other drugs.

USES

1. Short-term treatment of active duodenal ulcer
2. Maintenance therapy of duodenal ulcer after healing has occurred
3. Treatment of pathological hypersecretory conditions (*e.g.*, Zollinger-Ellison syndrome)

ADMINISTRATION AND DOSAGE

Famotidine is available as 20-mg or 40-mg tablets, as an oral suspension containing 40 mg/5 ml, and as an IV solution (10 mg/ml) that may be diluted for IV infusion.

For active duodenal ulcer, 40 mg is given once daily at bedtime for 4 weeks to 6 weeks. Alternately, 20 mg may be given twice a day. For maintenance therapy, 20 mg once daily is usually prescribed.

In treating pathological hypersecretory conditions, the usual starting dose is 20 mg every 6 hours for as long as necessary. Some patients with severe hypersecretory states may require up to 160 mg every 6 hours. In hospitalized patients who cannot tolerate oral medications, 20 mg may be given by slow IV injection or infusion every 12 hours. IV injections should be performed over at least 2 minutes in a volume of 5 ml to 10 ml. For infusion, 2 ml (10 mg) is diluted with 100 ml of 5% dextrose and given over 15 minutes to 30 minutes.

FATE

Oral absorption is incomplete and bioavailability is less than 50%. First pass metabolism is minimal. Peak plasma levels occur in 1 hour to 3 hours. Plasma protein binding averages 15% to 20%. The elimination half-life is 2 hours to 4 hours. Famotidine is eliminated by both renal (60%–70%) and metabolic (30%–35%) routes. Up to 70% of a dose may appear unchanged in the urine. In severe renal insufficiency, the half-life may exceed 20 hours.

SIDE-EFFECTS/ADVERSE REACTIONS

Side-effects occurring during famotidine therapy are headache, diarrhea, dizziness, and constipation. Although many other untoward reactions have occurred in patients receiving famotidine, a direct cause-and-effect relationship cannot be established.

CONTRAINDICATIONS AND PRECAUTIONS

There are no absolute contraindications to use of famotidine. The drug should be used *cautiously* in patients with renal dysfunction and in pregnant or nursing women.

Ranitidine

(Zantac)

Ranitidine is a long-acting H$_2$ antagonist used for treatment of duodenal and gastric ulcers. Unlike cimetidine, its oral absorption is not impaired by antacids, it possesses no antiandrogenic activity, there is no observable potentiation of warfarin-type anticoagulants, and drug-metabolizing activity of liver enzymes is not impaired.

MECHANISM AND ACTIONS
Ranitidine exerts a competitive inhibition of the action of histamine at H_2-receptor sites, including those on the gastric parietal cells. This action markedly reduces daytime and nocturnal gastric acid secretion. Pepsin secretion is largely unaffected, and fasting or postprandial gastrin serum levels are not changed. Hepatic blood flow is slightly reduced.

USES
1. Short-term (*i.e.*, 4–8 weeks) treatment of active gastric or duodenal ulcers
2. Maintenance therapy for duodenal ulcer (up to 1 year)
3. Treatment of pathologic hypersecretory condition (*e.g.*, Zollinger-Ellison syndrome, systemic mastocytosis)
4. Management of gastroesophageal reflux disease
5. Prevention of pulmonary aspiration of acid during anesthesia (investigational use)

ADMINISTRATION AND DOSAGE
Ranitidine is available as 150-mg and 300-mg tablets and as an injectable solution containing 25 mg/ml. Oral doses are usually 150 mg, twice a day, although up to 6 g/day have been used in severe pathologic hypersecretory conditions. Alternately, 300 mg at bedtime has been effective as a single daily dose. For maintenance therapy, 150 mg may be given at bedtime. IM doses are 50 mg every 6 hours to 8 hours, given undiluted, whereas the same dose may be administered IV diluted to 20 ml in sodium chloride injection and given over at least 5 minutes. The diluted solution is stable for up to 48 hours at room temperature.

FATE
Oral absorption is good and is not significantly affected by the presence of food or antacids. Peak serum levels occur in 1 hour to 3 hours, and effects persist 8 hours to 12 hours. The drug is metabolized in the liver, and the major route of excretion is the kidney, with approximately 30% of an oral dose being eliminated unchanged.

SIDE-EFFECTS/ADVERSE REACTIONS
Side-effects are relatively infrequent with ranitidine: headache, nausea, and constipation are the most frequently reported. Other adverse reactions seen on occasion with ranitidine are dizziness, insomnia, tachycardia, premature ventricular beats, arthralgia, gynecomastia, impotence, rash, alopecia, hepatitis, and, rarely, blood dyscrasias. Transient pain at IM injection sites and local burning or itching with IV administration have also been noted.

CONTRAINDICATIONS AND PRECAUTIONS
There are no absolute contraindications to the use of ranitidine. The drug should be used with *caution*, however, in patients with impaired liver or kidney function and in pregnant or nursing mothers.

INTERACTIONS
1. Ranitidine may decrease the renal clearance of procainamide.
2. The oral absorption of ranitidine may be impaired by antacids, although this effect is minimal.
3. Ranitidine may enhance the hypoglycemic action of glipizide.

NURSING CONSIDERATIONS
(See also Nursing Process for cimetidine.)

Ranitidine may be used after therapy with cimetidine has been unsuccessful. Therefore it is extremely important to obtain a brief drug history and disease course to review how the patient has managed his illness. The patient must be encouraged to view the drug as part of a total therapeutic regimen. The patient must learn how his eating habits and life-style affect the disease and what outcomes should be sought through therapy.

To reduce nausea and constipation the patient should be instructed to take ranitidine with meals and to include adequate roughage in his diet. If the patient also takes antacids he should avoid taking them at the same time as ranitidine.

As with cimetidine, the long-term effects of ranitidine have yet to be established. Consequently, therapy should be of short duration with minimum prescription refills. The patient should be encouraged to take the drug as prescribed—not only when he has symptoms. The elderly patient or one on a limited income may be tempted to use ranitidine as a PRN drug because it is relatively expensive.

Serotonin and Antiserotonin Drugs

Serotonin

Serotonin, or 5-hydroxytryptamine (5-HT), is a naturally occurring amine which is found in various sites in the body and participates in a number of important biologic functions, such as vascular tone, emotional stability and mood, and gastrointestinal function. In addition, it probably serves as a neurohormone or neuromodulator in the sensory phenomena of pain and itching.

In humans, over 90% of the serotonin in the body is located in enterochromaffin cells of the gastrointestinal tract, approximately 7% to 8% is found in platelets, and the remainder in the CNS. Serotonin is synthesized from the amino acid l-tryptophan; normally, however, only a small fraction of dietary tryptophan is utilized for serotonin synthesis. Upon formation, serotonin is either stored or rapidly inactivated, principally by monoamine oxidase. The turnover rate of serotonin in the CNS is quite rapid but somewhat slower in the intestines. Platelets lack the enzymes necessary for serotonin synthesis but have the ability to concentrate the amine by means of an active carrier mechanism.

PHARMACOLOGIC EFFECTS OF SEROTONIN

The pharmacologic effects of serotonin are complex and variable, and depend on many factors, such as species, dose, frequency of administration, and presence of reflex compensatory mechanisms in certain organ systems. The following discussion must therefore be viewed as a general overview of the pharmacology of serotonin.

Cardiovascular System

A direct spasmogenic effect on vascular smooth muscle, resulting in vasoconstriction, is the classic response to serotonin, yet it is seldom observed in its "pure" form. Depending on the vascular bed studied, the activity of reflex mechanisms, the resting tone of the blood vessels, and the modification of autonomic ganglionic function, serotonin can elicit either vasoconstriction or vasodilation. For example, pulmonary and renal vessels seem especially sensitive to the constrictor action of the amine, whereas vessels in skeletal muscle and the heart usually respond by dilating. Veins are commonly constricted, but capillary permeability is not significantly altered. An intravenous injection of serotonin often results in a *triphasic* effect on blood pressure, (1) an initial brief decrease due to a coronary chemoreceptor reflex, (2) a succeeding pressor response due mainly to peripheral vasoconstriction and possibly a positive inotropic action, and (3) a prolonged depressor response, probably the result of slowly developing vasodilation of skeletal muscle vasculature.

Serotonin has both positive inotropic (increased force of contraction) and chronotropic (increased heart rate) effects on the heart, but these are seldom of significance because activation of baro- and chemoreceptor reflexes quickly blunt any direct effects of serotonin. Platelet aggregation is enhanced by serotonin, but the platelet stores of serotonin are not released; again, the significance of this effect is not known.

Smooth Muscle

Gastrointestinal smooth muscle is contracted by serotonin, and peristalsis is increased. These effects are due to a direct action of serotonin on smooth muscle cells and an activation of ganglion cells innervating intestinal smooth muscle. Secretions are usually unaffected.

Bronchiolar smooth muscle is also somewhat weakly contracted by serotonin, but this effect is of little significance except in the asthmatic patient. Other smooth muscles, such as biliary and uterine, are not significantly affected by serotonin in normal amounts.

Nervous System

In the peripheral nervous system, serotonin participates in the phenomena of pain and itching, probably by stimulating sensory nerve endings. In addition, it is an activator of certain cardiovascular and respiratory reflexes by stimulation of chemoreceptor nerve endings. Large amounts of serotonin elicit ganglion cell firing, whereas lesser amounts have variable ganglionic effects.

In the CNS, serotonin is found in many regions, although most cell bodies of serotonergic neurons are located in the midline brain stem areas known as the raphe nuclei, from which nerve fibers project to the spinal cord, other brain stem regions, and many forebrain structures. Serotonin plays an important role in such diverse CNS-mediated functions as mood, sleep, appetite, temperature regulation, pain-perception, vision, and neuroendocrine control. Moreover, serotonin is found in large amounts in the pineal gland, where it serves as a precursor for the synthesis of melatonin.

The principal interest in serotonin lies in its role as a mediator of a number of physiologic and pathologic processes, some of which have been described above. Other pathologic conditions in which there is evidence of a contributory role for serotonin include allergic reactions, inflammatory processes, complications associated with myocardial infarction, and the carcinoid syndrome. To date, however, serotonin itself has no *therapeutic* value, as it is rapidly degraded orally, does not pass the blood–brain barrier, and is largely nonspecific in its effects. Several serotonin antagonists have demonstrated a clinical usefulness in preventing or treating certain disorders, and these drugs will be reviewed individually below.

Antiserotonin Drugs

Several drugs have the capability of competitively antagonizing the action of serotonin at its receptor sites, although most of these antiserotonin drugs have other pharmacologic actions as well and therefore their clinical effects are not always entirely due to serotonin receptor blockade. Serotonin antagonists have a number of indications, although in most cases there are other more effective or less toxic drugs available to treat the condition in question; thus, the clinical application of the serotonin receptor blockers is somewhat limited. Their principal use is in the symptomatic management of certain allergic conditions (they are especially effective in relieving itching), in the prophylaxis of migraine headache (see Disease Brief: Migraine) in which their mechanism is not entirely understood, and for treatment of the carcinoid syndrome (see Disease Brief: Carcinoid Syndrome) in which they reduce the diarrhea and abdominal cramping characteristic of this condition.

Cyproheptadine
(Periactin)

MECHANISM AND ACTIONS
The pharmacologic actions exhibited by cyproheptadine include antiserotonergic, antihistaminic, anticholinergic, local anesthetic, and an appetite-

stimulating effect; this latter effect is probably due to an action on hypothalamic appetite-regulating centers. A mild CNS depressive effect is also noted, and platelet aggregation may be impaired. Most of the recognized uses for cyproheptadine are based on its fairly strong histamine-blocking activity. The contribution of its antiserotonin action is probably of importance in relieving pruritus and in the prophylaxis of migraine, but remains to be established for the other indications.

USES
1. Relief of various allergic disorders, especially rhinitis, allergic conjunctivitis, and allergic skin manifestations such as urticaria, pruritus, and angioedema (including cold urticaria)
2. Prevention or reduction of allergic reactions to blood and plasma
3. Adjunctive therapy for anaphylactic reactions
4. Relief of pruritus resulting from drug or serum reactions, physical allergies, or insect bites
5. Prophylaxis of migraine (somewhat less effective than methysergide)
6. Symptomatic treatment of the carcinoid syndrome
7. Stimulate appetite in underweight and anorexia nervosa patients (investigational use only and usually discouraged)

ADMINISTRATION AND DOSAGE
Cyproheptadine is administered orally as tablets (4 mg) or syrup (2 mg/5 ml). The usual adult dose is 12 mg to 16 mg/day in three or four divided doses, with a range of 4 mg to 32 mg/day. Children's dosage is recommended at 0.25 mg/kg/day. Thus, children 2 to 6 years old are given 2 mg, two to three times/day, and those 7 to 14 years old receive 4 mg, two to three times/day. Maximum dosage in children is 16 mg/day.

FATE
Oral absorption is adequate. Onset of action is within 60 minutes, and effects persist for 4 hours to 6 hours.

SIDE-EFFECTS/ADVERSE REACTIONS
The most commonly occurring side-effects resemble those seen with use of antihistamines: sedation, dryness of the mouth, nose, and throat, thickening of bronchial secretions, dizziness, and epigastric distress. Other reactions associated with cyproheptadine include impaired coordination, urinary difficulty, nausea, skin rash, CNS excitation (especially in children), irritability, confusion, ataxia, hypotension, and bradycardia. (Refer also to the

discussion of adverse reactions under Histamine₁-Blockers for other possible adverse reactions resulting from the histamine-blocking action of cyproheptadine.)

CONTRAINDICATIONS AND PRECAUTIONS

Cyproheptadine is contraindicated in patients with lower respiratory disease, urinary retention, bladder obstruction, narrow-angle glaucoma, peptic ulcer, prostatic hypertrophy, and in elderly or debilitated patients, newborn or premature infants, and nursing mothers. Cyproheptadine should also not be used in combination with MAO inhibitors. *Cautious use* is indicated in the presence of asthma, open-angle glaucoma, hyperthyroidism, hypertension, and cardiovascular disease. This drug should be used in pregnant women only when apparent benefit clearly outweighs potential risks (*i.e.*, fetal damage).

INTERACTIONS

1. MAO inhibitors or anticholinergics may intensify many of the side-effects of cyproheptadine.
2. The drug has additive CNS depressant effects with other depressants (*e.g.*, alcohols, narcotics, barbiturates).

NURSING CONSIDERATIONS

Nursing intervention centers on monitoring dosage and managing symptoms. Drowsiness is a common side-effect which will usually subside in several days. Patients can use caffeinated beverages to decrease drowsiness in the interim but need to be cautious about driving and operating machinery.

Dosing needs to be carefully adjusted depending on the patient's needs and responses. This may be more easily accomplished with the liquid form of the drug, especially in small children. Children

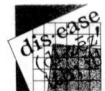

DISEASE BRIEF

■ Migraine

Migraine is a severe, throbbing, frequently unilateral headache which may last from several hours to several days, and may be accompanied by anorexia, nausea, and vomiting. In some instances (*i.e.*, 10%–20%), the attack is preceded by prodromal symptoms (the so-called aura) which may involve visual, sensory, auditory, or motor disturbances, and this type of attack is termed "classic" migraine. However, the majority of cases (*i.e.*, up to 80%) are of sudden onset but may not be associated with nausea or vomiting. This latter type has been referred to as "common" or "atypical" migraine. Migraine is more common in women, is familial in about two thirds of patients, and most often has its onset in adolescence. The pathophysiology is not completely understood, but the symptoms may be ascribed to changes in vascular function in cerebral arteries, often described as an initial constriction, which produces the prodromal symptoms, followed by dilation, increased pulsation, and possible eventual rigidity of the cerebral vessels, all of which are responsible for the excruciating pain. The neurotransmitter most implicated in these vascular alterations is serotonin, a vasoconstrictor, although its precise role in regulating cerebral arterial function remains to be completely established. Plasma serotonin levels are elevated during the prodromal phase but are decreased during the subsequent pain phase.

In addition to the drugs listed in this chapter, the reader may want to refer to other sections of the book as listed below for discussion of other drugs used both experimentally and as adjunctive therapy in the prevention and treatment of migraine:

    Prevention:
            Propranolol (Chap. 16)
            Clonidine (Chap. 35)
            Calcium Channel Blockers (Chap. 36)
    Treatment:
            Analgesics (Chaps. 22, 23)

are more susceptible to developing a paradoxical excitatory state from the drug and should be watched for agitation, confusion, and hallucinations. Elderly patients, conversely, may be more drowsy, dizzy, or hypotensive. Both groups should be closely monitored.

(See also Nursing Process for ergotamine.)

Ergot Alkaloids

The ergot alkaloids are a group of natural and semisynthetic drugs derived from a fungus, *Claviceps purpurea*, which infests the rye plant. These drugs possess a variety of pharmacologic action, such as a smooth muscle spasmogenic effect, an adrenergic-blocking effect, and both agonistic and antagonistic actions at serotonin receptor sites. Moreover, certain ergot alkaloids, especially the hallucinogen lysergic acid diethylamide (LSD) and bromocriptine, exert a significant action in the CNS. In addition to bromocriptine (discussed in Chap. 31), which is used in parkinsonism and to suppress postpartum lactation, the most commonly used ergot alkaloids are ergonovine and ergotamine. Ergonovine is primarily employed in obstetrics to facilitate uterine involution and suppress postpartum hemorrhage. It is reviewed in Chapter 51 together with oxytocin, a similarly acting drug. Ergotamine is mainly indicated for the relief of vascular headache and, together with its structural analogue, dihydroergotamine, is discussed here.

Ergotamine

(Ergomar, Ergostat, Medihaler-Ergotamine, Wigrettes)

MECHANISM AND ACTIONS
Ergotamine exerts a direct spasmogenic effect on smooth muscle of peripheral and cranial blood vessels. In addition, it is an alpha-adrenergic blocking agent and also exhibits a serotonin-blocking action. Ergotamine is a potent uterine stimulant. The drug is not an analgesic, and the relief of pain associated with a migraine attack is due to cerebral vasoconstriction, with a resultant decrease in the amplitude of pulsations of cranial vessels. Ergotamine is considered a specific agent for relief of vascular headaches and is frequently administered in combination with caffeine (*e.g.,* Cafergot, Cafetrate, ErgoCaf, Wigraine) which contributes to the effectiveness of the treatment. This combination is also available with pentobarbital and belladonna alkaloids as Cafergot P-B.

USES
1. Relief of pain associated with vascular headaches, such as migraine and histamine cephalgia (most effective if given early in an attack)

ADMINISTRATION AND DOSAGE
Ergotamine itself is available as sublingual tablets (2 mg) or for inhalation (9 mg/ml aerosol which delivers 0.36 mg/dose). In addition, ergotamine and caffeine are also available as suppositories containing 2 mg ergotamine and 100 mg caffeine, and as oral tablets containing 1 mg ergotamine and 100 mg caffeine. For *sublingual* use, one tablet (2 mg) is placed under the tongue at the onset of the migraine attack. Subsequent tablets may be taken at 30-minute intervals. Maximum dosage is three tablets/24 h and five tablets/week. With ergotamine *aerosol*, one inhalation (0.36 mg) is given at the onset of the attack, and may be repeated at 5-minute intervals to a maximum of six inhalations/24 h.

Two *oral* tablets of ergotamine and caffeine, with or without belladonna and sodium pentobarbital, may be taken at the first sign of an attack,

---

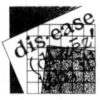

DISEASE BRIEF

■ *Carcinoid Syndrome*

The carcinoid syndrome is the result of a tumor of serotonin-containing enterochromaffin cells, usually found in the ileum, stomach, or bronchi. As a result of release of large quantities of serotonin, along with other vasoactive compounds such as histamine, catecholamines, and peptides, there is development of intense flushing, abdominal cramping, and diarrhea, along with asthmatic symptoms, edema, and possibly cardiac lesions. Treatment may be undertaken with oral corticosteroids, as well as serotonin antagonists, the latter drugs being most effective in abolishing the GI manifestations but largely ineffective in treating the flushing and other cardiovascular-related symptoms.

followed by one tablet every half hour as needed, to a maximum of six tablets per attack or ten tablets per week.

Alternately, one suppository may be given initially, followed by a second dose in 1 hour. No more than five suppositories should be used within 7 days.

FATE

GI absorption is slow and incomplete, and the response is unpredictable. Following oral administration, 2 hours are required to attain peak blood levels. Concurrent administration of caffeine may increase absorption rate and peak plasma levels. Absorption following sublingual and aerosol administration is generally good, and effects appear quickly. Rectal absorption is slow but fairly constant. The duration of action may persist for up to 24 hours. The drug is metabolized in the liver, and 90% of the metabolites are excreted in the bile.

SIDE-EFFECTS/ADVERSE REACTIONS

The incidence and severity of adverse effects are largely dose-dependent, although individual sensitivity varies greatly, and a reduction in dosage will usually eliminate most undesirable reactions. The most commonly observed side-effects of larger than recommended doses of ergotamine are numbness or tingling in the extremities, GI discomfort, diarrhea, muscle pain, weakness in the legs, cold hands or feet, and dizziness. Other reported adverse reactions have been localized edema, bradycardia (especially with large doses), angina-like pain, intermittent claudication, itching, anxiety, confusion, and changes in vision. Overdosage can result in ergotism and may be characterized by vomiting, weak pulse, worsening headache, hypertension, chest pain, extreme thirst, cyanotic skin, and gangrene. Severe peripheral vaso-constriction can be treated with a peripherally acting vasodilator such as nitroprusside.

CONTRAINDICATIONS AND PRECAUTIONS

Ergotamine has a number of contraindications, such as peripheral vascular disease, hypertension, hepatic or renal disease, severe pruritus, sepsis, coronary artery disease, infectious states, malnutrition, pregnancy, and in young children. The drug should be used with *caution* in elderly patients and in nursing mothers because the drug is excreted into breast milk and may cause vomiting and diarrhea in the infant. Prolonged administration should be avoided due to the danger of ergotism and development of gangrene.

INTERACTIONS

1. The vasoconstrictor action of ergotamine may be enhanced by beta-blockers, vasopressor amines, alpha$_1$-adrenergic agonists, and other peripheral vasoconstrictors.
2. The effects of ergotamine may be potentiated by nitroglycerin (increased bioavailability) and troleandomycin (decreased metabolism).

■ Nursing Process

□ ASSESSMENT

□ Subjective Data

The patient who suffers migraine headaches must learn to become aware of the symptoms or events that lead to headache, even the patient who does not have prodromal symptoms. The earlier the patient takes the drug the more likely it is to be effective. To help him become more aware the patient can keep a headache diary which should include surrounding events which occurred on the day of the headache; the date of the onset, how long the headache lasted; what and how much medication was taken; what the symptoms were; what actions, other than medication, the patient took to relieve the symptoms. This information is helpful in identifying precipitating events for the headaches and the effectiveness of treatment. The effectiveness of drug therapy is very variable among migraine sufferers and should be reevaluated regularly.

A complete medical history focusing on cardiovascular and peripheral vascular problems should be obtained as well as a medication and food history. Some foods, such as wine, cheese, and caffeine-containing beverages, have been associated with migraines.

□ NURSING DIAGNOSES

Actual nursing diagnoses for the patient taking drug therapy for migraine include:

Knowledge deficit related to the dose and side-effects of the drug as well as how best to plan a strategy to use the drug for effective pain relief

Alteration in comfort: pain

Alteration in individual coping related to debilitation caused by migraines and to the degree it interferes in one's life

Potential nursing diagnoses for the drug are based on side-effects and vary from drug to drug. As an example, the following is a partial list of diagnoses resulting from the many side-effects of ergotamine:

Alteration in bowel elimination: diarrhea
Alteration in comfort: epigastric pain
Alteration in fluid volume: excess
Alteration in tissue perfusion

□ PLAN
The nursing care goal is to find a series of actions, including drug therapy, which will help the patient manage the pain. The long-term goal is to find a regimen which will prevent the headaches from occurring.

□ INTERVENTION
This patient needs to learn relaxation techniques to reduce stress levels. If he can identify areas of stress in his life and develop coping skills more useful than the physical symptoms of a migraine, the symptoms may occur less frequently, although they rarely disappear completely. Regardless of the cause, migraine headaches are not "psychosomatic" or "faked." Headache sufferers need positive strategies to help them cope with their life situations and medication to reduce symptoms once they occur. Most are fearful that they "cause" their own symptoms.

Once symptoms begin, the person should lie down in a darkened, quiet room following drug administration because relief of pain may be expedited under such conditions. Stimuli must be reduced as much as possible.

Symptoms are generally self-limiting, but continuous vomiting during an attack may lead to severe dehydration and electrolyte imbalance. If symptoms, especially vomiting, do not abate the patient should seek immediate medical attention.

□ EVALUATION
The outcome sought is control of headache pain and normalization of daily activities. The patient may need to vary doses and timing of the drug in the sequence of pain development to achieve success.

Dihydroergotamine
(D.H.E. 45)
Dihydroergotamine is an ergot alkaloid possessing pharmacologic and toxicologic properties similar to those of ergotamine; however, its adrenergic-blocking action is more pronounced, whereas its vasoconstrictive emetic and oxytocic actions are less intense. Dihydroergotamine may be given IM (1 mg at 1-hour intervals to a total dose of 3 mg) or IV (1 mg–2 mg) to abort or control vascular headaches when a rapid action is desired and other routes of administration (*e.g.*, sublingual) are not generally effective or feasible. Effects are noted within 15 to 30 minutes with IM injection (more rapidly with IV) and persist for 3 to 4 hours. (Refer to the previous discussion of ergotamine for additional information on adverse reactions, contraindications, precautions, interactions, and nursing considerations.)

Methysergide
(Sansert)

MECHANISM AND ACTIONS
Methysergide is a semisynthetic ergot alkaloid which primarily functions as a serotonin receptor antagonist, although it also possesses moderate agonistic action at serotonin receptors and may exert some direct smooth muscle stimulation as well. Although methysergide has little direct vasoconstrictive action itself, it appears to interact with serotonin in such a way as to facilitate its vasoconstrictive activity on cranial arteries, thus reducing excessive pulsations (see Disease Brief: Migraine). However, the exact mechanism(s) involved in the antimigraine effect of methysergide have not been conclusively determined. The drug is strictly a prophylactic agent and has no effect during an acute attack.

USES
1. Prevention or reduction in frequency of vascular (migraine-type) headaches, especially if frequency exceeds one per week or if severity is intense. (*Not* used in treating acute attacks)

ADMINISTRATION AND DOSAGE
Methysergide is available as 2-mg tablets for oral use. The usual adult dose is 4 mg to 8 mg (two to four tablets) daily in divided doses, given with meals. Doses for children have not been established. The drug must be discontinued for 3- to 4-week intervals every 6 months to minimize the danger of toxicity (see under Side-Effects/Adverse Reactions). If effects are not apparent within 3 weeks after beginning therapy, further benefit is

unlikely and the drug should be discontinued. Dosage should be reduced gradually over the last 2 to 3 weeks of each treatment course to avoid "rebound headaches."

FATE
Little is known of the actual metabolic fate of methysergide. Oral absorption is probably adequate. One to two days are required to produce an optimal protective effect, and the action requires several days to subside following termination of drug therapy.

SIDE-EFFECTS/ADVERSE REACTIONS

■ **Warning**
Long-term administration of methysergide has resulted in retroperitoneal and pleuro-pulmonary fibrosis and fibrotic thickening of cardiac valves (see below). Thus, therapy must be suspended for 3- to 4-week intervals every 6 months, and chronic prophylactic administration of methysergide should only be undertaken in patients with frequent or severe migraine attacks.

The most frequently occurring side-effects during methysergide treatment are GI distress, heartburn, nausea, abdominal pain, diarrhea, drowsiness, lightheadedness, flushing, and occasionally muscle and joint pains. An extensive range of other adverse effects have been associated with methysergide therapy, especially prolonged usage, and these are listed below by organ system:

Fibrotic complications—Retroperitoneal fibrosis (associated with fatigue, weight loss, fever, backache, urinary obstruction, lower limb vascular insufficiency), pleural fibrosis (dyspnea, chest tightness, pleural effusion), and cardiac fibrosis (thickening of aortic root, aortic and mitral valves)

CV—Chest or abdominal pain, numbness in extremities, paresthesias, peripheral edema, postural hypotension, tachycardia, thrombophlebitis, claudication

GI—Vomiting, constipation, increased gastric acid

CNS—Insomnia, euphoria, feelings of dissociation, hallucinations, nightmares (may be related to vascular headache and not the drug)

Dermatologic/Hematologic—Nonspecific rash, telangiectasia, alopecia, neutropenia, eosinophilia

Other—Weight gain, peripheral edema, weakness, scotomas

CONTRAINDICATIONS AND PRECAUTIONS
Methysergide should not be given to persons with peripheral vascular disease, arteriosclerosis, severe hypertension, coronary artery disease, phlebitis, cellulitis, pulmonary disease, impaired liver or renal function, collagen diseases, or valvular heart disorders. Pregnancy, debilitated states, and serious infections also constitute contraindications to methysergide. *Cautious use* of methysergide is necessary in nursing mothers, because the drug can cause vomiting, diarrhea, and seizures in infants.

NURSING CONSIDERATIONS
(Refer also to Nursing Process for ergotamine.)

The important nursing responsibility with this drug is to teach the patient to manage minor side-effects and to be aware of ones that should be reported.

A patient can learn how to check for edema, and how to maintain a low salt intake and adjust calorie intake if weight gain or edema is noticed. If these measures do not bring weight loss and resolution of swelling the physician should be notified.

Orthostatic hypotension is a potential problem which can be dealt with by lying down with legs elevated. The patient should be reminded to rise slowly from a supine position and rest momentarily before standing.

Fibrotic and cardiovascular changes are the symptoms of drug toxicity. To monitor these closely the patient should have periodic cardiac, renal, and kidney blood studies. He must immediately report any coldness or numbness in the extremities; leg cramps; edema; girdle, flank, or chest pain; or dysuria because these are early signs of toxicity.

Trimeprazine
(Temaril)

MECHANISM AND ACTIONS
A phenothiazine derivative, trimeprazine possesses antiserotonergic, antihistaminic, and anticholinergic actions. A moderate CNS depressant effect is also present, and drowsiness is quite common.

USES

1. Symptomatic relief of pruritus in urticaria and possibly in other dermatologic disorders
2. Preoperative sedation in children (investigational use)

ADMINISTRATION AND DOSAGE

Trimeprazine is used orally as tablets (2.5 mg), sustained-release capsules (5 mg), or syrup (2.5 mg/5 ml). The usual adult dose is 2.5 mg four times a day or 5 mg (long-acting capsules) twice a day. Children over age 3 should receive 2.5 mg one to three times a day, and younger children are given 1.25 mg one to three times a day as required.

FATE

Oral absorption is good. Effects of tablets or syrup begin in 15 minutes to 60 minutes, peak in 1 hour to 2 hours, and persist for 3 hours to 6 hours. Sustained-release capsules evidence a slower onset, but a prolonged duration of action (up to 12 hours). The drug is metabolized in the liver and excreted in the urine.

SIDE-EFFECTS/ADVERSE REACTIONS

Drowsiness, lightheadedness, and weakness represent the most commonly occurring side-effects. Among the other reported adverse reactions are orthostatic hypotension, tachycardia, dizziness, dryness of bronchial and other secretions, urinary and respiratory difficulty, allergic skin reactions, GI upset, and cholestatic jaundice. In addition, because trimeprazine is a phenothiazine derivative, the adverse reactions for phenothiazines, detailed in Chapter 27, are *theoretically* possible, although the incidence is minimal at recommended doses.

CONTRAINDICATIONS AND PRECAUTIONS

Trimeprazine should not be used in newborns, pregnant women, in acutely ill or dehydrated children, or in patients with bone marrow depression. A *cautious* approach to therapy should be undertaken in persons with hepatic or renal disease, a history of convulsive disorders, CNS depression, asthma, cardiovascular disease, narrow-angle glaucoma, prostatic hypertrophy, hypertension, duodenal or bladder neck obstruction, or respiratory disease. (See Chap. 27 for additional precautions.)

INTERACTIONS

(See also Chap. 27 and under Antihistamines earlier in this chapter.)

1. The anticholingeric effects may be intensified by MAO inhibitors, tricyclic antidepressants, and thiazide diuretics.
2. The incidence of phenothiazine-related adverse effects (see Chap. 27) may be increased by reserpine, nylidrin, oral contraceptives, and progesterone.
3. The sedative effects of trimeprazine may be intensified by other CNS depressants, such as alcohol, barbiturates, hypnotics, narcotics, or anesthetics.

NURSING CONSIDERATIONS

Side-effects may be dose-related, so the patient may need to experiment to find a balance. The most common side-effects, drowsiness, dizziness, and lightheadedness, are usually transient and will subside after a few days. In the interim, patients need to avoid hazardous activities such as driving or operating dangerous equipment until the effects of the drug are known. Some side-effects can be reduced or eliminated by taking the drug with meals or milk. This will slow absorption but will not decrease drug effectiveness.

Elderly persons and young children are much more susceptible to the adverse effects of this drug. In elderly persons, trimeprazine may produce hypertension, syncope, confusion, and excess sedation. To minimize adverse effects in children under 6 years old, long-acting capsules should be avoided.

CASE STUDY **Migraine Headaches**

Ms. Ann Dorlas is a 30-year-old woman who comes to the headache clinic of a large university center for evaluation of migraine. She states she has a 15-year history of headaches and reports her mother had headaches all her life. Ms. Dorlas came to the clinic because her headaches seem to be getting worse, lasting longer than 24 hours and occurring more frequently than ever before. Ms. Dorlas, the mother of two toddlers, a boy 3 years old and a girl 1½ years old recently returned to work full time as a secretary in a busy law firm. The migraine headaches have caused her to miss work 4 days in the last 2 months. During the time she has the headaches, she is unable to adequately care for her children, and her husband and mother-in-law must assist her.

After evaluation of her symptoms and assessment of the ways she has previously treated her headaches, the physician decides to start Ms. Dorlas on ergotamine (Ergomar), 2 mg sublingual for migraine attacks.

Discussion Questions

1. What new life stress has Ms. Dorlas recently added? How can the nurse discuss them with this patient? List some coping strategies to suggest.
2. Plan a headache diary. Describe how such a tool should be explained to this patient and how to encourage its successful use after migraine attacks.
3. What information should Ms. Dorlas be given about ergotamine?
   a. What is the maximum dose of drug she should take?
   b. What are the signs of ergotism (*e.g.*, toxicity) she should watch for?
   c. When should the drug be taken?

REVIEW QUESTIONS

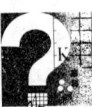

1. In what sites in the body is most endogenous histamine found?
2. Briefly list the major pharmacologic effects of histamine.
3. Distinguish between the two types of histamine receptors.
4. Describe some possible physiologic functions for histamine.
5. What pharmacologic actions are displayed by most H_1 antagonists in addition to blocking histamine?
6. Give some uses for H_1-receptor blockers.
7. List five major nursing considerations for patients using H_1 antagonists.
8. Discuss the pharmacologic effects of cimetidine.
9. What are the principal indications for cimetidine?
10. How does (a) ranitidine and (b) famotidine differ from cimetidine?
11. Detail the major effects of serotonin in the body.
12. What are the important uses for serotonin antagonists?
13. List several ergot alkaloids and the principal indications for each.
14. What is the major caution to be observed with use of methysergide?

BIBLIOGRAPHY

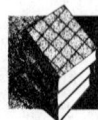

Aghajanian GK, Wang RY: Physiology and pharmacology of central serotonergic neurons. In Lipton MA, DiMascio A, Killam KF (eds) Psychopharmacology: A Generation of Progress, p 171. New York, Raven Press, 1978

Ambielli MP: Drug stop. J Neurosurg Nursing 15:370, 1983

Beaven M: Histamine. N Engl J Med 294:320, 1976
Berde B: Ergot compounds: A synopsis. Adv Biochem Psychopharmacol 23:3, 1980
Brogden RN, Hed RC, Speight TM, Avery GS: Cimetidine: A review of its pharmacological properties and therapeutic efficacy in peptic ulcer disease. Drugs 15:93, 1978
Forssman B, et al.: Propranolol for migraine prophylaxis. Headache 238:45, Nov 1976
Green JP, Johnson CL, Weinstein H: Histamine as a neurotransmitter. In Lipton MA, Dimascio A, Killam KF (eds): Psychopharmacology: A Generation of Progress, p 319. New York, Raven Press, 1978
Hirschowitz BI: H-2 histamine receptors. Ann Rev Pharmacol Toxicol 19:203, 1979
Lagunoff D, Martin TW: Agents that release histamine from mast cells. Ann Rev Pharmacol Toxicol, 23:331, 1983
Moree NA, et al.: How do the new drugs measure up? Am J Nurs 84:902, 1984
Pearlman DS: Antihistamines: Pharmacology and clinical use. Drugs 12:258, 1976
Raskin NH: Pharmacology of migraine. Ann Rev Pharmacol Toxicol 21:463, 1981
Todd B: Drugs and the elderly: Antiulcer preparations. Geriatric Nursing 122:March/April, 1983
Zakusov VV (ed): Pharmacology of Central Synapses: 5-hydroxytryptamine Antagonists. New York, Pergamon Press, 1980, p 143.

Skeletal Muscle Relaxants

Peripherally Acting Muscle Relaxants

Neuromuscular Blocking Agents
  Antidepolarizing Blockers
    d-Tubocurarine
    Metocurine
    Gallamine
    Pancuronium
    Atracurium
    Vecuronium
  Depolarizing Blockers
    Succinylcholine
  Hexafluorenium

Direct Myotropic-Acting Agent
  Dantrolene

Centrally Acting Muscle Relaxants
  Baclofen, Carisoprodol,
    Chlorphenesin,
    Chlorzoxazone,
    Cyclobenzaprine,
    Metaxalone,
    Methocarbamol,
    Orphenadrine

19

Skeletal muscle activity can be affected by a diverse group of pharmacologic agents capable of acting either at the neuromuscular junction or at various levels within the spinal cord and brain stem. Those agents that interfere with transmission of cholinergic impulses at the neuromuscular junction generally produce paralysis of the skeletal muscles involved. Those drugs that act either directly on the contractile mechanism of the skeletal musculature or on transmission within spinal cord motor reflex pathways primarily elicit varying degrees of skeletal muscle relaxation. The former group are employed principally as adjuncts to general anesthetics and in minor surgical procedures or shock therapy, whereas the latter group are used to afford a degree of relief from muscle spasms and hyperreflexia resulting from conditions such as inflammation, anxiety, stress, and neurologic disorders.

Based on their site of action, skeletal muscle relaxants may be classified in the following manner:

I. Peripherally acting muscle relaxants
  A. Neuromuscular blocking agents
    1. Antidepolarizing blockers (*e.g.,* tubocurarine gallamine, vecuronium)
    2. Depolarizing blockers (succinylcholine)
  B. Direct myotropic-acting agents (*e.g.,* dantrolene)
II. Centrally acting muscle relaxants (*e.g.,* carisoprodol, methocarbamol)

Peripherally Acting Muscle Relaxants

Neuromuscular Blocking Agents

Drugs in this category interfere with the transmission of cholinergic impulses between somatic motor neurons and skeletal muscle fibers—that is, at the neuromuscular junction.

Figure 19-1 depicts the general anatomic arrangement of the neuromuscular junction and details the innervation of the motor end-plate by a terminal branch of the motor neuron. In order to better understand the mechanisms involved in the action of the neuromuscular blockers, a brief overview of the sequence of events occurring during excitation of skeletal muscle by a nerve impulse is presented below.

NEUROMUSCULAR TRANSMISSION— SEQUENCE OF EVENTS

1. Arrival of a nerve action potential at the motor nerve terminal, resulting in depolarization of the terminal axonal membrane
2. Influx of Ca^{++} and resultant release of acetylcholine (ACh) from its storage vesicles in the presynaptic nerve ending into the synaptic junction
3. Diffusion of ACh across the synaptic junction to the postsynaptic membrane (*i.e.,* motor end-plate of skeletal muscle) and interaction of ACh with postjunctional cholinergic receptor sites
4. Increased permeability of the postjunctional membrane to sodium and potassium, and resulting depolarization of the motor end-plate region, giving rise to a local end-plate potential (EPP)
5. If the EPP is of sufficient strength (magnitude of the EPP is directly related to amount of ACh released), generation of a muscle action potential (MAP) occurs, which is propagated throughout the conduction system of the muscle fibers
6. Release of Ca^{++} from binding sites in the sarcoplasmic reticulum of the muscle fibers into the sarcoplasm surrounding the myofilaments actin and myosin
7. Sliding of myosin and actin filaments together, eliciting contraction of the muscle fiber, the so-called excitation–contraction coupling
8. Inactivation of ACh by acetylcholinesterase enzyme, relaxation of the muscle fiber, and depolarization of the terminal axonal membrane and motor end-plate region

ACTION OF NEUROMUSCULAR BLOCKING AGENTS

Two mechanisms may be involved in the inhibition of transmission at the neuromuscular junction, both involving the postsynaptic receptor site. One

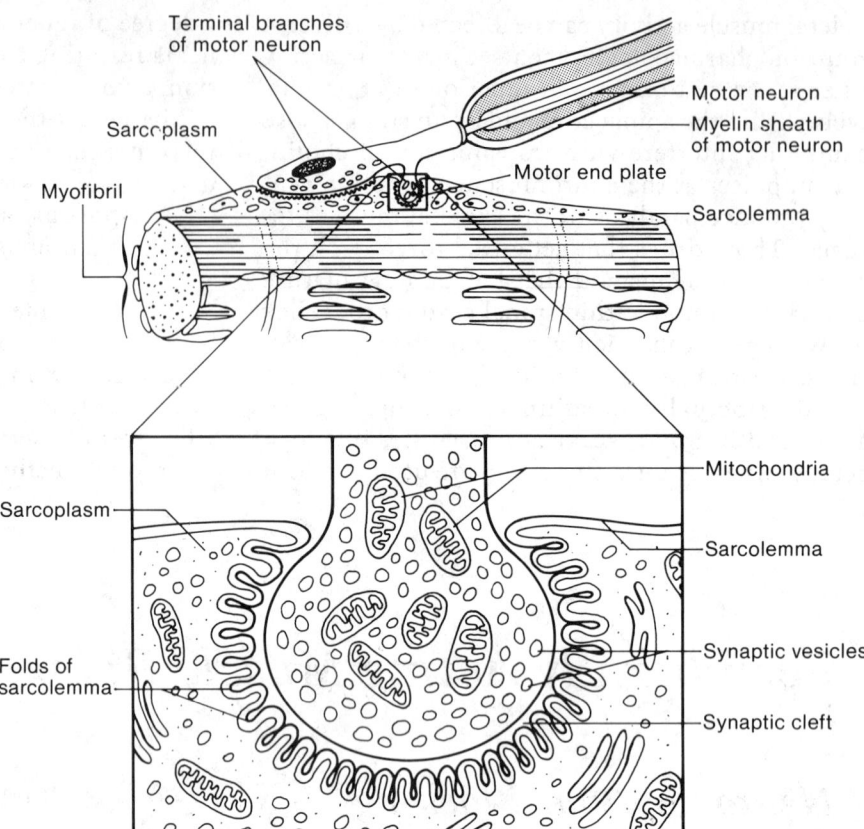

Figure 19-1. A neuromuscular junction, showing the detailed innervation of the motor end-plate region by a terminal branch of the motor neuron. (After Tortora GJ, Anagnostakos NP: Principles of Anatomy and Physiology, 5th ed. New York, Harper & Row, 1987)

group of drugs, typified by d-tubocurarine, functions as antidepolarizing (or nondepolarizing) agents, competitively antagonizing the action of acetylcholine at the receptor site and preventing depolarization of the postsynaptic membrane. The second group of drugs, exemplified by succinylcholine, acts as depolarizing agents, producing an initial activation (depolarization) of the receptor followed by a persistent occupation that markedly delays repolarization, thus blocking further receptor stimulation. These mechanisms are essentially similar to those displayed by the various ganglionic blocking agents (see Chap. 17), where both antidepolarizing (e.g., trimethaphan) and depolarizing (e.g., nicotine) blocking actions are evident as well.

The competitive blockade effected by the antidepolarizing drugs may be surmounted by increasing the local concentration of ACh at the neuromuscular junction. Use of cholinesterase inhibitors, such as neostigmine or edrophonium, is frequently effective in managing overdosage with the antidepolarizing blocking agents. Due to the nonselective action of the cholinesterase inhibitors, however, atropine sulfate is frequently administered in combination with the cholinesterase inhibitor drugs when they are used to treat over-

dosage with skeletal muscle relaxants. Atropine blocks the undesired muscarinic (M) effects such as bradycardia and salivation that can occur with drugs like neostigmine or edrophonium. Conversely, use of cholinesterase inhibitors is contraindicated in cases of overdosage with depolarizing neuromuscular blockers, inasmuch as the resultant elevated levels of ACh may intensify, rather than ameliorate, the muscle paralysis.

Neuromuscular blocking agents are essentially anticholinergic agents; however their specificity for the neuromuscular junction is realized only at normal therapeutic doses. If present in excessive amounts, their cholinergic antagonism may extend to other sites as well, namely autonomic ganglia and postganglionic parasympathetic (atropine-sensitive) endings. This overlapping of effects is responsible for certain adverse reactions exhibited by these drugs at high dose levels (e.g., cardioacceleration, arrhythmias, hypotension). On the other hand, these drugs do not effectively penetrate the blood–brain barrier at therapeutic concentrations, so their CNS effects are minimal. Consciousness and perception remain unimpaired, and pain is not affected. Certain neuromuscular blockers, most notably d-tubocurarine and, to a lesser extent, metocurine and succinylcholine, can release histamine from intracellular stores, and the increased levels of circulating histamine may cause varying degrees of bronchospasm, salivary and mucosal secretions, hypotension, and other unwanted effects.

The skeletal muscles are not all equally susceptible to the paralytic effects of neuromuscular blocking agents. The smaller muscles of the eye and eyelids, along with the muscles involved in talking and swallowing, are the first to be affected, followed by progressive weakening of the muscles of the neck and extremities. Fortunately, the muscles of respiration (intercostals, diaphragm) are the most resistant. However, differences in sensitivity among many of the muscles are very slight, and the margin between the effective dose and the toxic dose of most of the neuromuscular blocking drugs is quite small. Therefore, these drugs should only be used by persons trained and experienced in their use, and close patient monitoring is essential.

A slight overdose can result in serious impairment of respiration and marked hypotension. Overdosage with neuromuscular blocking agents is treated by artificial respiration with oxygen and use of vasopressors (*e.g.*, levarterenol). Cholinesterase inhibitors (*e.g.*, edrophonium) as noted above, can also be employed in cases of poisoning with antidepolarizing blockers (tubocurarine, atracurium, gallamine, metocurine, pancuronium, vecuronium) to overcome the competitive blockade, but these inhibitors are contraindicated in cases of overdosage with depolarizing blockers (succinylcholine) for the reasons stated earlier.

Antidepolarizing Blockers

Drugs belonging to the group classified as antidepolarizing blocking agents are also known as nondepolarizing, stabilizing, or curariform drugs. This latter designation derives from the fact that the first antidepolarizing muscle relaxant was the alkaloid d-tubocurarine, the active principle of a group of South American arrow poisons collectively called curare. Several synthetic and semisynthetic products (atracurium, metocurine, gallamine, pancuronium, vecuronium) have since been developed which all possess a similar action at the neuromuscular junction, although their potencies vary somewhat, and the range of adverse effects differs among these curare-like compounds. However, all of the antidepolarizing muscle relaxants function as reversible competitive antagonists of ACh at the postjunctional neuromuscular cholin-

geric receptor sites. When the ACh-induced EPP (excitatory postsynaptic potential) is reduced to less than 70% of its normal amplitude by the presence of a cholinergic antagonist, skeletal muscle contraction in response to somatic nerve stimulation is blocked, and a temporary state of muscle paralysis develops. Inasmuch as differences exist among the antidepolarizing neuromuscular blockers with regard to duration of action, range of side-effects, and potency, the drugs will be considered individually.

d-Tubocurarine

Metocurine
(Metubine)

The curare preparations include d-tubocurarine, an alkaloid extracted from the plant *Chondodendron tomentosum*, and metocurine, a semisynthetic derivative of d-tubocurarine.

MECHANISM AND ACTIONS
The curare drugs produce temporary skeletal muscle paralysis by blocking cholinergic nerve impulses to skeletal muscle. They function as competitive antagonists of acetylcholine at nicotinic receptor sites on the postsynaptic membrane of the neuromuscular junction. Metocurine does not possess the degree of autonomic ganglionic-blocking action of d-tubocurarine and is associated with much less histamine release, thus, the incidence of hypotension and bronchospasm is lower, compared to d-tubocurarine. In addition, following its administration, metocurine reaches the neuromuscular junction more quickly than d-tubocurarine, and is approximately twice as potent. Repeated doses of both drugs may lead to a cumulative effect because some drug is retained by the body for long periods of time. These curare drugs do not alter the perception of pain and have no effect on higher intellectual function or consciousness.

USES
1. Adjunct to general anesthetics to provide adequate muscle relaxation
2. Reduce intensity of muscle contractions during shock therapy
3. Facilitate management of patients undergoing mechanical ventilation
4. Diagnosis of myasthenia gravis when results of other tests are inconclusive (tubocurarine only —rarely used)

ADMINISTRATION AND DOSAGE

Tubocurarine is available as a 3-mg/ml (20 units/ml) injection solution, and metocurine is used as a 2-mg/ml injection. Both curare drugs are usually administered by slow IV injection; in addition, tubocurarine may be given IM, but this route is not recommended for metocurine. Dosage is highly individualized and depends on patient sensitivity, presence of other drugs, and type of general anesthetic used. The margin for error is small, and dosage should be carefully controlled. Recommended doses are:

Tubocurarine

· Adjunct to anesthesia—40 units to 60 units (6 mg–9 mg) IV at the time incision is made. Supplements of 20 units to 30 units (3 mg–4.5 mg) may be given as needed. Dosage may be calculated based on weight, (i.e., 1.1 units/kg).
· Shock therapy—1.1 units/kg IV prior to shock over 60 seconds to 90 seconds.
· Diagnosis of myasthenia—$\frac{1}{15}$ to $\frac{1}{5}$ of the average adult electroshock dose

Metocurine

· Adjunct to anesthesia—The dosage depends on the type of general anesthesia used. The usual range is 0.2 to 0.4 mg/kg IV over 30 seconds to 60 seconds based on the degree of potentiation of the muscle-relaxing action of metocurine expected from the anesthetic. Supplemental doses average 0.5 mg to 1 mg and are given as needed.
· Shock therapy—2 mg to 4 mg by slow IV injection, until a head-drop response occurs

FATE

Onset of paralysis occurs within 3 minutes to 5 minutes following IV injection. Maximal effects persist approximately 30 minutes to 60 minutes, and effective muscle paralysis may last for up to 90 minutes. Complete recovery of muscle function may require several hours. Both drugs are approximately 30% to 40% protein bound. Half-lives range from 1 hour to 3 hours for d-tubocurarine and 3 hours to 4 hours for metocurine. Approximately 45% to 50% of each dose is excreted unchanged in the urine. IM absorption is variable and unpredictable. Metocurine readily crosses the placental barrier.

SIDE-EFFECTS/ADVERSE REACTIONS

Dizziness is frequently noted upon injection of the curare drugs. Other adverse reactions associated with these agents are profound muscle weakness, feelings of warmth, hypotension, bronchospasm, respiratory depression, hypoxia, apnea (rare), increased bronchial and salivary secretions, hypersensitivity reactions, and malignant hyperthermia. Overdosage may be characterized by prolonged and profound apnea and sudden release of histamine, resulting in marked hypotension and cardiovascular collapse.

CONTRAINDICATIONS AND PRECAUTIONS

Curare drugs are contraindicated in patients in whom histamine release would prove hazardous (for example, asthmatics) and in patients with severe myasthenia gravis, hyperthermia, electrolyte imbalance, or acidosis. In addition, metocurine is contraindicated in persons with iodide hypersensitivity because it is an iodide salt. *Cautious use* is necessary in persons with impaired cardiovascular, pulmonary, endocrine, renal, or hepatic function, hypotension, thyroid or collagen disorders, a history of allergies in elderly or debilitated patients, and pregnant or nursing mothers.

INTERACTIONS

1. The intensity and duration of action of the curare drugs may be increased by administration of inhalation anesthetics (halothane, ether, enflurane, methoxyflurane) but *not* by thiobarbiturates, nitrous oxide, droperidol, or narcotics.
2. The effects of the curare compounds may also be intensified by aminoglycosides, amphotericin B, clindamycin, lincomycin, lithium, potassium-depleting diuretics, antiarrythmics (quinidine, procainamide, propranolol), phenothiazines, diazepam, calcium and magnesium salts, and trimethaphan.
3. The effects of the curare drugs can be antagonized by cholinesterase inhibitors and other cholinergic drugs.
4. The tachycardia frequently noted with anticholinergic drugs, tricyclic antidepressants, antihistamines, and phenothiazines may be augmented by curare compounds.

■ Nursing Process

□ ASSESSMENT

□ Subjective Data

Baseline information collected is related to the body systems that influence clearance of the drugs, body systems affected by the drugs, and concomitant drug therapy. The nurse needs to ascertain the presence of chronic illnesses such as hypertension, respiratory diseases such as COPD or asthma and myasthenia gravis because symptoms can be exacerbated by the antidepolarizing agents. A history of allergy to bromides will also complicate therapy.

Medications taken, such as diuretics or antiarrhythmics can further complicate therapy because they can intensify the relaxant action of antidepolarizing agents. Other areas of concern in obtaining a drug history are treatment with aminoglycosides, phenothiazines, or tricyclic antidepressants, all of which interact with antidepolarizing agents.

□ *Objective Data*
Baseline assessment of liver and kidney function can be done, and laboratory studies indicate any impairments in these areas. Careful attention should be given to elderly and very young patients because liver and kidney function in these age groups is not optimum. Electrolyte levels should also be drawn with special attention given to magnesium and potassium levels because these can also affect the action.

Baseline vital signs will also be important because significant changes in respiration, pulse, and blood pressure may occur.

□ *NURSING DIAGNOSES*
Actual nursing diagnoses for the patient receiving an antidepolarizing agent are related to the drug-induced voluntary muscle paralysis and include:
   Airway clearance, ineffective (which is also related to a drug-induced increase in bronchial secretions)
   Breathing pattern, ineffective
   Impaired physical mobility
   Knowledge deficit regarding how the drug will affect his body
   Functional incontinence
Potential nursing diagnoses are related to drug-induced paralysis or the side-effects of the drug and include:
   Anxiety related to the drug's lack of effect on the sensorium
   Injury, potential for trauma or suffocation
   Hyperthermia

□ *PLAN*
In most institutions general nursing staff will not administer these drugs. Administration is limited to anesthesiologists, nurse anesthetists, and, occasionally, nursing staff involved in the care of patients on ventilators. For most, the nursing care goals will be centered on accurate preoperative assessment, preoperative availability of equipment

and medication, and postoperative monitoring of the recovery patient. The principles mentioned here for operative care also apply to the patient being prepared for electroshock therapy. For the intubated, ventilated patient the nursing care goals center on relief of anxiety and close monitoring of the patient to ensure that he remains intubated and adequately ventilated.

□ *INTERVENTION*
The patient entering the recovery room after administration of one of the curare agents will be intubated. As the drug wears off and the patient awakens skeletal muscle paralysis and weakness will completely reverse and the patient will want to be extubated as soon as possible. The nurse must observe for the possibility of apnea or recurrence of the paralytic effects during the early recovery phase and should monitor respirations closely. The patient should be extubated only when the respiratory function and other signs (eyelid droop and eye movement loss) seem to be disappearing. Ways to assess return of strength are to ask the patient to lift his head, open his eyes, swallow, cough, and perform a finger grip with both hands.

Another problem in the recovery room or during the perioperative anesthesia period is the evidence of overdose which will be manifested by severe hypotension, prolonged apnea, and cardiovascular collapse. Response should be immediate and includes neostigmine or edrophonium to reverse the drug effects; atropine, fluids, and vasopressors to respond to the cardiovascular changes and antihistamines to counteract the histamine released.

If the curare-type drugs are used on a ventilator-dependent patient the nurse will have other responsibilities. These drugs paralyze the skeletal muscles but do not induce unconsciousness nor relieve anxiety or pain. Imagine, therefore, what it must feel like to be unable to breathe and be completely awake. While the drug helps the patient get optimum benefit from respiration by a ventilator he will feel very anxious and out of control. The patient needs one-on-one nursing care for reassurance that he will not be abandoned. In some facilities sedation is given to reduce anxiety. In others, the curare drugs are withheld long enough for the patient to recover some function to enable him to let his needs for pain relief or other comfort measures be known. The form of communication is usually by nodding or blinking in response to questions.

Artificial tears should be instilled in the eyes of this patient on a regular basis, usually every 2 hours

(Text continues on p. 326.)

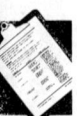

Nursing Care Plan 19-1
The Patient Receiving a Neuromuscular Blocking Agent for Controlled Ventilation

Assessment

Subjective Data	1. Medication history
	  a. Refer to Interactions section to formulate pertinent questions
	  b. Determine the potential for physical incompatibilities with other IV drugs.
	  c. Allergy to bromides
	2. Medical history
	  a. Presence of conditions that may increase respiratory deficit, such as acute or chronic respiratory disease, myasthenia gravis, cardiac disease, extremes in age
	  b. History of malignant hyperthermia

Objective Data	1. Physical assessment focusing on
	  a. Respiratory function: air exchange, breath sounds
	  b. Vital signs
	  c. Skin integrity
	  d. Presence of musculoskeletal injuries
	  e. Renal function: urinary output, I/O ratio
	2. Laboratory/diagnostic data
	  a. Renal, hepatic function studies: baseline and periodic to detect problems
	  b. Arterial blood gases
	  c. Electrolytes, especially K^+ and Mg^{2+}

Nursing Diagnosis	*Expected Client Outcome*	*Intervention*
Ineffective airway clearance related to drug effect (paralysis) and drug-induced increase in respiratory tract secretions	Airway will remain clear	Suction patient frequently. Administer anticholinergic drugs as prescribed to reduce secretions.
Ineffective breathing pattern related to drug-induced paralysis	Arterial blood gas (ABG) levels will remain within normal limits while the patient is on mechanical ventilation	Monitor for drug effectiveness in preventing the patient from resisting the action of the ventilator. Measure ABGs as prescribed. Secure endotracheal tube/tracheostomy to prevent accidental extubation. Keep ventilator alarms on at all times.
Functional incontinence related to drug-induced paralysis	Urine-induced skin breakdown will be prevented Urinary tract infection will be avoided	Insert urinary catheter as ordered to avoid incontinence Monitor for leakage around catheter site Maintain fluid intake (IV) of 2000 ml/day Avoid opening catheter system Obtain periodic urine C and S samples to detect early any infections
Impaired physical mobility related to drug-induced paralysis	Range of motion of extremities will be maintained	Perform passive range-of-motion exercises to all joint areas several times a day unless contraindicated due to injury. Initiate physical therapy consultation as prescribed. Use caution when turning to avoid injury to muscles and joints if limitations in mobility exist.

(continued)

Nursing Care Plan 19-1 (continued)
The Patient Receiving a Neuromuscular Blocking Agent for Controlled Ventilation

Nursing Diagnosis	Expected Client Outcome	Intervention
Knowledge deficit related to drug effect and required constant monitoring	Will communicate (during drug-free periods) understanding of need for drug and for monitoring	Explain the drug's effect of inducing total paralysis so that ventilation can be controlled.
		Provide constant nursing attendance to meet needs.
		Provide short drug-free periods, so needs can be communicated.
		Explain that the effects of the drug are temporary.
Anxiety related to drug's lack of effect on sensorium while inducing total paralysis	Will verbalize effectiveness of interventions (either during drug-free periods or after therapy is completed)	Provide basic explanations of all actions.
		Assume the patient is awake and able to hear.
		Provide touch to comfort the patient and make him aware of your presence.
		Orient the patient to time.
		Provide distractions such as a radio or visitors.
Potential alteration in skin integrity related to drug-induced paralysis	Skin surfaces will remain intact	Establish a q 1–2 h turning schedule.
		Use padding, special bedding to decrease pressure on bony prominences.
		Provide frequent skin care to decrease contact of moisture and feces with skin.
		Promote venous return in lower extremities by passive range-of-motion exercises, occasional leg elevation, use of support stockings.
Potential hyperthermia	Temperature will remain within normal limits	Monitor temperature every 2–4 h as prescribed.
		Report any elevations to physician immediately.
		Be prepared to treat malignant hyperthermia with hypothermia blanket, dantrolene, emergency equipment as prescribed.
Potential for injury to eyes related to drug-induced paralysis	Corneal damage will be prevented	Apply moisture-providing agents (e.g., artificial tears) to eyes every 1–2 h as prescribed.
		Apply eye covers to protect eyes from environmental irritants (patient unable to blink).
Potential sleep pattern disturbance related to frequent nursing care	Will be allowed rest periods whenever possible	Decrease environmental stimuli as much as possible during sleep periods.
		Minimize interventions during rest periods.

to 4 hours. Eyes should be taped closed to prevent corneal damage and to allow the patient to sleep. The patient should also be afforded time to have his eyes open.

For the patient receiving the curare drugs, extubation would be fatal. Therefore, the nurse needs to ensure the tracheostomy or endotracheal tube is securely placed. In addition, the alarm system on the ventilator is the only method by which the nurse will know anything is wrong because the patient will no longer be able to fight the machine. Therefore, the ventilator alarms should *never* be turned off for any reason.

Atropine may be used to decrease respiratory secretions from the drug. However, frequent suctioning and mouthcare are also essential to prevent complications.

Supportive care should include skin care, frequent turning, and positioning to prevent sores. The patient may also benefit by having a radio as a source of stimulation. All nursing staff and visitors should be encouraged to talk and touch the patient as another method of stimulation. Personnel and visitors must always assume the patient is awake and avoid conversations that might increase the patient's anxiety.

These drugs are extremely hazardous. In most institutions, especially in areas where suicidal patients are present, these drugs should be kept locked and counted like narcotics.

Normally, the effects of the antidepolarizing agents disappear within 60 minutes to 90 minutes. However, after a patient has received repeated doses high enough to paralyze the diaphragm, complete recovery may take up to 4 days. Respiratory function usually returns quickly, but extremity weakness may continue.

□ *EVALUATION*
The outcome sought with this drug is muscle relaxation, but the nursing outcomes sought are adequate protection of the patient, safe management of respiration while the patient is unable to breathe, and the return of adequate ventilation once the effects of the drug have worn off. Nursing Care Plan 19-1 contains a care plan for the patient receiving a neuromuscular blocking agent for controlled ventilation.

Gallamine
(Flaxedil)

MECHANISM AND ACTIONS
Gallamine is a synthetic neuromuscular blocking agent which competes with ACh at the nicotinic cholinergic receptor sites on the motor end-plate of skeletal muscles. It is somewhat less potent than d-tubocurarine, but does not cause bronchospasm nor release histamine. Also, gallamine does not appear to affect transmission in autonomic ganglia, alter GI tone or motility, or change the pain threshold. However, it does exert a strong vagal blocking action, which may be responsible for the development of tachycardia and increased blood pressure.

USES
1. Production of skeletal muscle relaxation as an adjunct to general anesthesia
2. Facilitate management of patients undergoing mechanical ventilation
3. Reduce intensity of muscle contractions during electro- or chemoshock therapy

ADMINISTRATION AND DOSAGE
Gallamine is used as a 20-mg/ml injection solution and is given by slow IV injection. Dosage is highly individualized and based on weight, age, presence of other drugs, and pathologic conditions. The recommended initial dose is 1 mg/kg, a dose that produces approximately a 50% reduction in respiratory minute volume. The maximum single dose is 100 mg. For prolonged procedures, 0.5 to 1 mg/kg can be given at 30- to 40-minute intervals.

FATE
The onset of effect is almost immediate following IV injection, and the duration of action is usually 15 minutes to 30 minutes although the range is dose-dependent. Cumulation can occur with repeated injections. Gallamine is excreted unchanged by the kidney.

SIDE-EFFECTS/ADVERSE REACTIONS
Tachycardia regularly occurs with doses of 0.5 mg/kg and higher, reaches a maximum about 3 minutes after injection, and then gradually subsides. Dizziness may also develop. Other less common adverse effects are primarily an extension of the drug's action and include extreme muscle weakness, respiratory depression, and apnea. Hypersensitivity reactions, including severe anaphylaxis, have also been reported infrequently.

CONTRAINDICATIONS AND PRECAUTIONS
Contraindications to gallamine include myasthenia gravis, conditions in which tachycardia might be hazardous (*e.g.*, hyperthyroidism, cardiac disease), renal impairment, shock, decreased pulmonary function, and patients who are sensitive to iodides

(drug is a triethiodide salt). Gallamine should not be used in infants under 11 pounds. Gallamine must be used *cautiously* in patients with impaired pulmonary function, coronary artery disease, electrolyte imbalance, dehydration, elevated body temperature, and in elderly or debilitated patients.

INTERACTIONS
(See under d-Tubocurarine and Metocurine.)

Pancuronium
(Pavulon)

MECHANISM AND ACTIONS
Pancuronium is a synthetic nondepolarizing neuromuscular blocker which competitively antagonizes the action of ACh at the cholinergic receptor sites on the motor end-plate of skeletal muscle. The drug is approximately five times more potent than d-tubocurarine, but has minimal effects on the circulatory system in normal doses and produces little or no histamine release or ganglionic blockade. High doses exert a vagal blocking action, resulting in tachycardia and increased blood pressure, although to a lesser extent than that seen with gallamine.

USES
1. Adjunct to anesthetics during surgery
2. Assist patients receiving mechanical ventilation

ADMINISTRATION AND DOSAGE
The initial IV dose of pancuronium ranges between 0.04 and 0.1 mg/kg depending on other drugs being used and condition of the patient. The drug is available as 1-mg/ml and 2-mg/ml solutions. For prolonged procedures, incremental doses of 0.01 mg/kg may be given every 30 minutes to 60 minutes, if necessary. Children, other than neonates, should receive the same mg/kg dosage as adults. However, a test dose of 0.02 mg/kg may be given initially in the pediatric population.

FATE
Onset of action with pancuronium is within 1 minute, and peak effects occur within 3 minutes to 5 minutes. Recovery occurs within 45 minutes to 60 minutes. The drug is excreted primarily unchanged by the kidney.

SIDE-EFFECTS/ADVERSE REACTIONS
Tachycardia is the most frequently encountered side-effect, along with salivation and prolonged muscle weakness. Other adverse effects that have been reported are respiratory difficulty, apnea, rash, increased blood pressure, and, rarely, cardiac arrhythmias.

CONTRAINDICATIONS AND PRECAUTIONS
Pancuronium is contraindicated in myasthenia gravis, conditions in which tachycardia might be hazardous (such as coronary artery disease), and bromide hypersensitivity. The drug must be administered with *caution* to persons with impaired renal, pulmonary, or cardiovascular functioning, electrolyte imbalance, and to debilitated or dehydrated patients. When used during a cesarean section, recovery may be delayed if the patient has received magnesium for preeclampsia because magnesium salts enhance neuromuscular blockade.

INTERACTIONS
(See under d-Tubocurarine and Metocurine.)

Atracurium
(Tracrium)

MECHANISM AND ACTIONS
Atracurium is a nondepolarizing skeletal muscle relaxant which functions as a competitive antagonist of cholinergic receptor sites on the motor and plate. Histamine release is minimal at recommended doses, and significant hemodynamic changes seldom occur within the usual dosage range.

USES
1. Adjunct to general anesthesia to relax skeletal muscle during surgery or mechanical intubation

ADMINISTRATION AND DOSAGE
Atracurium is used as an IV injection solution containing 10 mg/ml. The recommended initial dose is 0.4 to 0.5 mg/kg as an IV bolus. Maintenance doses of 0.08 to 0.2 mg/kg may then be given at regular intervals depending on the length of the surgical procedure. Children over 2 years of age are given the adult dosage. Younger children may receive 0.3 to 0.4 mg/kg as an initial dose.

FATE
An initial dose of 0.4 mg/kg produces neuromuscular blockade within 2 minutes to 5 minutes, with recovery beginning approximately 20 minutes to 30 minutes after injection. Complete recovery

occurs in about 60 minutes to 75 minutes. The first maintenance dose is usually required within 20 minutes to 45 minutes after the initial injection, and then at 15- to 25-minute intervals. The elimination half-life is approximately 20 minutes, and the drug is inactivated in the plasma.

SIDE-EFFECTS/ADVERSE REACTIONS
Most adverse reactions reported with atracurium are the consequence of histamine release. Most often encountered side-effects are skin flushing and tachycardia. Other adverse reactions include skin rash, urticaria, erythema, dyspnea, bronchospasm, laryngospasm, hypotension, and prolonged muscle relaxation. IM injection is not recommended because it is likely to result in tissue irritation.

CONTRAINDICATIONS AND PRECAUTIONS
Atracurium should be used with *caution* in patients with myasthenia gravis or other neuromuscular diseases, severe electrolyte disorders, and in pregnant or nursing mothers. The drug solution is acid and should not be mixed with alkaline solutions (*e.g.*, barbiturates) because atracurium can be precipitated and inactivated.

INTERACTIONS
1. The neuromuscular blocking action of atracurium may be enhanced by halothane, isoflurane, enflurane, aminoglycoside antibiotics, clindamycin, procainamide, quinidine, and trimethaphan.
2. Phenytoin and theophylline may antagonize or reverse the neuromuscular blocking action of atracurium.
3. Concurrent use of succinylcholine may increase the depth of atracurium-induced neuromuscular blockage.

Vecuronium
(Norcuron)

MECHANISM AND ACTIONS
Vecuronium is a nondepolarizing neuromuscular blocking agent which competitively blocks cholinergic receptors at the motor end-plate in skeletal muscle. The onset of action is shorter and the duration of paralysis longer with increasing doses. Hemodynamic function is largely unchanged with use of recommended doses.

USES
1. Adjunct to general anesthesia to provide skeletal muscle relaxation during surgery or mechanical intubation

ADMINISTRATION AND DOSAGE
Vecuronium is available as powder for IV injection containing 10 mg/5-ml vial. The initial adult dosage is 0.08 to 0.1 mg/kg given as an IV bolus. During prolonged procedures, additional doses of 0.01 to 0.015 mg/kg may be given at 15-minute to 25-minute intervals as necessary. Children over 10 years of age receive the adult dosage; children under 10 may require a slightly higher initial dosage and more frequent supplementation. Usage in neonates is not recommended.

FATE
Following IV administration, maximal neuromuscular blockade occurs within 3 minutes to 5 minutes. Recovery is nearly complete within 45 minutes to 60 minutes. The drug is approximately 75% protein bound. The elimination half-life is 60 minutes to 75 minutes, and vecuronium is eliminated both in the urine and bile.

SIDE-EFFECTS/ADVERSE REACTIONS
Side-effects are infrequent with recommended doses of vecuronium. Excessive skeletal muscle weakness can occur if the effects of the drug are prolonged. Very large doses can produce decreased respiratory reserve, reduced tidal volume, and apnea, although these reactions are rare with normal usage.

CONTRAINDICATIONS AND PRECAUTIONS
Cautious use of vecuronium should be exercised in patients with myasthenia gravis or other neuromuscular disorders, hepatic disease (prolongs recovery time), electrolyte imbalances, obesity (may impair normal ventilation), and in pregnant or nursing mothers. The drug should not be used in neonates. Delayed onset can occur if circulation is reduced, as in patients with cardiovascular disease, edema, and in elderly persons.

INTERACTIONS
1. An intensified neuromuscular blockade can occur if vecuronium is administered in combination with succinylcholine, inhalation anesthetics (*e.g.*, halothane, enflurane, isoflurane), aminoglycoside antibiotics, tetracyclines, polymyxin, colistin, bacitracin, quinidine, and magnesium.

Depolarizing Blockers

Currently, succinylcholine is the only depolarizing neuromuscular blocker in clinical use. Its action is essentially a biphasic one. Initially, the drug acts like ACh at the neuromuscular nicotinic receptors, producing depolarization of the motor end-plate. However, succinylcholine is not metabolized as rapidly as ACh, thus the state of depolarization is prolonged and the muscle remains unresponsive to further stimulation as long as the drug occupies the receptor sites. The immediate transient excitatory phase when the drug first interacts with receptors results in the appearance of muscle fasciculations or twitching for a brief period of time following injection. This phase is quickly followed by muscle relaxation and a *flaccid* paralysis.

Succinylcholine is rapidly inactivated by plasma pseudocholinesterase, resulting in a rather brief duration of action, approximately 5 minutes to 10 minutes. However, some patients exhibit an abnormal plasma pseudocholinesterase pattern, and a prolonged muscular paralysis can occur in these patients following even a single dose of succinylcholine. In addition, there is some evidence that neuromuscular blockade following succinylcholine may persist beyond the actual presence of the drug at the receptor; this suggests the possibility of desensitization of the receptor caused by conformational changes of the reactive area.

One means of delaying enzymatic hydrolysis of succinylcholine and prolonging its effects is the prior administration of hexafluorenium, a potent, relatively selective inhibitor of plasma cholinesterase. Hexafluorenium will be discussed following succinylcholine.

Succinylcholine

(Anectine, Quelicin, Sucostrin)

MECHANISM AND ACTIONS

Following an initial stimulation of the cholinergic receptors on the motor end-plate, succinylcholine exerts a persistent depolarization of the skeletal muscle membrane as long as the drug remains in contact with the receptor. Thus, transient muscle fasciculations are seen initially, but quickly give way to flaccid paralysis. Succinylcholine is rapidly hydrolyzed by plasma cholinesterase enzymes, thus the normal duration of action of the drug is quite short (see under Fate). When given repeatedly over extended periods of time, the depolarizing character of the block (*i.e.*, Phase I block) may change to a nondepolarizing (curare-like) block (*i.e.*, Phase II block) which may be associated with profound respiratory depression or apnea. Other effects of succinylcholine include a slight initial increase in vagal tone, especially in children, resulting in hypotension and possibly arrhythmias, and a slight elevation in intraocular pressure. The drug may stimulate autonomic ganglia, producing tachycardia and elevated blood pressure following the initial vagal effect. Histamine release can occur, although the effect is usually not clinically significant. The drug does not affect consciousness or the pain threshold, and does not cross the blood–brain barrier or placental barrier to a significant extent. Succinylcholine has no direct effect on the uterus or other smooth muscle. Tachyphylaxis (*i.e.*, loss of efficacy) occurs with repeated dosing.

USES

1. Production of skeletal muscle relaxation as an adjunct to general anesthesia or mechanical ventilation
2. Reduction of the intensity of muscle contractions during shock therapy
3. Facilitation of intubation procedures

ADMINISTRATION AND DOSAGE

Succinylcholine is available in several concentrations as an injection solution (20 mg/ml, 50 mg/ml, 100 mg/ml) or as a powder for reconstitution (100 mg/vial, 500 mg/vial, 1000 mg/vial). Succinylcholine is usually given IV, although the IM route may be used in infants and others in whom a suitable vein is inaccessible. The effective dosage range is 0.3 mg/kg to 1.1 mg/kg IV given over 10 seconds to 30 seconds which produces muscle paralysis lasting approximately 5 minutes to 10 minutes. Prolonged muscle relaxation is achieved by subsequent IV injections of 0.04 mg/kg to 0.07 mg/kg at appropriate intervals. Children's dosage ranges from 1 to 2 mg/kg by IV injection or 2.5 to 4 mg/kg IM. IM injections should be given deep into the deltoid muscle. An initial test dose of 0.1 mg/kg can be given to assess the sensitivity of the patient. To avoid patient distress, the drug is administered only after consciousness has been lost. Solutions are highly unstable, and should be prepared fresh, and any unused portion should be discarded within 24 hours. For electroshock therapy, the drug is given 1 minute prior to administration of the shock.

FATE

Onset of muscle relaxation is within 1 minute IV and within 3 minutes IM. Effects generally last 4 minutes to 8 minutes following IV injection and up to 20 minutes with IM administration. The drug is rapidly hydrolyzed by plasma pseudocholinesterase, initially to succinylmonocholine, a weak nondepolarizing muscle relaxant, which is more slowly inactivated and can accumulate with frequent dosing, resulting in prolonged paralysis. Excretion is by way of the kidney, mostly as metabolites and approximately 10% as unchanged drug.

SIDE-EFFECTS/ADVERSE REACTIONS
Adverse reactions usually represent an extension of the pharmacologic effects of the drug. Most frequently noted side-effects are transient muscle twitching and bradycardia (especially in children). Other adverse effects seen with succinylcholine injection are prolonged muscle weakness, muscle pain, tachycardia, hypertension, arrhythmias, respiratory depression, apnea, excessive salivation, increased intraocular pressure, hyperkalemia, rash, myoglobinemia, decreased GI motility, anaphylactoid reactions, and cardiac arrest. Abrupt onset of malignant hyperthermia, a hypermetabolic disease of skeletal muscle, can occur with succinylcholine. Early signs include muscle rigidity, tachycardia, rising body temperature, and metabolic acidosis (see Disease Brief: Malignant Hyperthermia).

DISEASE BRIEF

■ Malignant Hyperthermia

Malignant hyperthermia is a relatively rare disorder, and may be due to a defect in the patient's ability to sequester calcium ions in the sarcoplasmic reticulum. The condition is triggered by various stimuli, most notably exposure to general anesthetics or neuromuscular blocking agents (especially succinylcholine) which cause a sudden increase in free myoplasmic calcium. This elevated calcium level evokes massive muscle contraction, and accelerated catabolic processes, which greatly increase lactic acid production and sharply elevate body temperature. Other clinical signs of malignant hyperthermia are tachycardia, tachypnea, metabolic acidosis, cyanosis, and extreme skeletal muscle rigidity. Prompt treatment is essential to prevent death and involves supportive measures such as administration of oxygen and sodium bicarbonate, restoration of fluid and electrolyte balance, and maintenance of an adequate urinary output. Currently, dantrolene IV is the only approved drug treatment, but verapamil and other calcium-channel blockers (see Chap. 36) have been used experimentally.

CONTRAINDICATIONS AND PRECAUTIONS
Contraindications to the use of succinylcholine include familial history of malignant hyperthermia, acute narrow-angle glaucoma, penetrating eye injuries, and genetically determined disorders of plasma pseudocholinesterase. The drug should be used with *caution* in patients with renal, cardiovascular, hepatic, pulmonary, or metabolic disorders, severe burns, electrolyte imbalance, glaucoma, spinal cord injury, degenerative neuromuscular diseases, fractures, and respiratory depression. In addition, *caution* is warranted in patients undergoing eye surgery, patients receiving quinidine or digitalis drugs, and patients with low levels of plasma cholinesterase such as dehydrated or anemic patients, patients exposed to neurotoxic insecticides, patients with liver disease, cancer, collagen disorders, or myxedema, and patients receiving MAO inhibitors, oral contraceptives, antimalarial drugs, or chlorpromazine.

INTERACTIONS
1. The neuromuscular blocking action of succinylcholine may be enhanced by aminoglycosides, beta-blockers, chloroquine, furosemide, lidocaine, lithium, isoflurane, magnesium salts, oxytocin, phenothiazines, polymyxin antibiotics, procainamide, quinidine, and trimethaphan.
2. The effects of succinylcholine may be prolonged and intensified by drugs that interfere with the action of plasma cholinesterase enzyme (*e.g.*, cholinesterase inhibitors, cyclo-

phosphamide, thio-TEPA, MAO inhibitors, procaine, antimalarial drugs).
3. Diazepam may reduce the duration of the neuromuscular blockade elicited by succinylcholine.
4. Succinylcholine can cause arrhythmias in the digitalized patient by causing a sudden release of potassium from muscle cells.

NURSING CONSIDERATIONS
Although the composition of the drug is different, most of its uses and actions are the same as those of the curare drugs; therefore, the nursing considerations are the same. A few factors need emphasis. Succinylcholine is extremely rapid in action, consequently, all equipment for intubation and respiratory support should be ready for use as soon as the drug is given. While its rapid onset and short duration are its main advantages, repeated doses can result in the prolongation of respiratory depression seen with curare drugs, so nursing concerns are similar.

Unlike the curare drugs, succinylcholine has been associated with malignant hyperthermia. Monitor body temperature closely during drug administration. (See Disease Brief for further information.)

Hexafluorenium

(Mylaxen)

Hexafluorenium prolongs the neuromuscular blocking action of succinylcholine and reduces the muscle fasciculations commonly associated with its injection. Hexafluorenium exerts a relatively selective inhibitory effect on plasma cholinesterases, unlike other cholinesterase inhibitors (see Chap. 13). The drug is administered in a ratio of 2 mg hexafluorenium for each 1 mg succinylcholine. Initially, 0.4 mg/kg are given IV 3 minutes before a 0.2-mg/kg dose of succinylcholine. Muscle relaxation following this combination usually persists 20 minutes to 30 minutes. Repeat doses of hexafluorenium (0.1–0.2 mg/kg) may be given during long procedures when it becomes apparent that the effects of succinylcholine injections are becoming progressively shorter. The intensity and duration of action of the hexafluorenium–succinylcholine drug combination is largely unaffected by the general anesthetic used.

Adverse reactions are generally due to increased succinylcholine activity. (See the previous discussion of succinylcholine for untoward effects, precautions, and interactions.)

Direct Myotropic-Acting Agent

Dantrolene
(Dantrium)

A different type of peripherally acting skeletal muscle relaxant is typified by the drug dantrolene; unlike the classic neuromuscular blocking agents, dantrolene does not interfere with transmission of impulses between somatic motor nerves and skeletal muscle. Its action appears to be the consequence of a direct effect on the skeletal muscle fibers to interfere with their contractile mechanisms. Specifically, the drug retards the release of a contraction-activating substance, probably calcium, from its binding sites in the sarcoplasmic reticulum. Dantrolene is available in oral form for treatment of muscle spasticity resulting from chronic neurologic disorders such as cerebral palsy, multiple sclerosis, or stroke, and as an IV injection for the emergency management of malignant hyperthermia such as that resulting from general anesthesia. (see Disease Brief.)

The principal danger with dantrolene therapy is hepatotoxicity, especially with high doses (i.e., above 400 mg/day) or long-term treatment. The risk of hepatic injury appears to be greater in females, in patients over 35 years of age, and in patients taking other medications as well. Appropriate monitoring of hepatic function, including frequent SGOT and SGPT determinations, are necessary during therapy. Should abnormal values occur or should symptoms of hepatitis develop, the drug should be discontinued. The lowest effective dose should always be used, and if no observable benefit occurs within 45 days, the drug must be discontinued.

MECHANISM AND ACTIONS
Dantrolene produces direct relaxation of skeletal muscle fibers, probably by interference with the release of calcium ions from the sarcoplasmic reticulum. The effects on smooth and cardiac muscles are inconsistent. The drug also impairs catabolism within muscle cells by blocking increases in myoplasmic calcium, and therefore prevents the abnormal rise in body temperature. Dantrolene may pos-

sess some central nervous system action as well, resulting in drowsiness, dizziness, and weakness.

USES

1. Relief of muscle spasticity associated with chronic neurologic disorders (*e.g.*, cerebral palsy, stroke, spinal cord injury, or multiple sclerosis). (Most effective where spasticity is painful and limits muscle performance.) Not indicated in the treatment of skeletal muscle spasm associated with rheumatic disorders
2. Emergency treatment of malignant hyperthermia (IV injection)
3. Preoperative prophylaxis of malignant hyperthermia in known or suspected high-risk patients (oral use)
4. Treatment of exercise-induced muscle pain (investigational use)

ADMINISTRATION AND DOSAGE

Dantrolene is available as capsules (25 mg, 50 mg, 100 mg) for oral use and as a powder for IV injection (20 mg/vial). Oral dosage must be titrated to obtain the optimal effect at the lowest dose possible, in view of the increased potential for hepatotoxicity at high doses. To reduce gastric upset from the drug, administer with meals or give with milk. Doses are as follows:

Muscle Spasticity

Adults—Initially 25 mg orally, once daily. Increase gradually in 25-mg increments to a maximum of 100 mg two to four times/day. Maintain each dose for 4 days to 7 days before increasing.

Children—Initially 0.5 mg/kg orally, twice a day; increase by 0.5-mg/kg increments to a maximum of 3 mg/kg two to four times/day.

Malignant Hyperthermia

Treatment—Initially, 1 mg/kg IV. If abnormalities persist or reappear, repeat up to a cumulative dose of 10 mg/kg. Usual required dose is 2 to 5 mg/kg. Child's dosage is the same as adults. Administration should be continuous until symptoms subside.

Preoperative: Prophylaxis—4 to 8 mg/kg/day orally in three to four divided doses for 1 day to 2 days prior to surgery. Last dose is given 3 hours to 4 hours before start of surgery.

Postcrisis follow-up—4 to 8 mg/kg/day orally in four divided doses for 1 day to 3

days following a malignant hyperthermia crisis to prevent recurrence of symptoms.

FATE

Oral absorption is slow and incomplete but consistent. The drug is significantly bound to plasma proteins. Optimal effects following oral use may take several days to become manifest. Elimination half-life is 8 hours to 9 hours with oral administration and 5 hours following IV injection. Dantrolene is metabolized primarily in the liver, and both metabolites and unaltered drug are excreted in the urine.

SIDE-EFFECTS/ADVERSE REACTIONS

Untoward reactions to dantrolene are seldom noted with IV injection to treat malignant hyperthermia, but primarily occur with oral use. The most common side-effects are drowsiness, dizziness, weakness, malaise, fatigue, and diarrhea. These are usually transient effects, and can usually be minimized or avoided completely by initiating therapy at low doses. A wide range of other adverse reactions have been reported with dantrolene and they are listed below by organ system:

GI—Constipation, bleeding, cramping, anorexia, difficulty in swallowing, gastric irritation, severe diarrhea

CNS—Headache, lightheadedness, insomnia, visual and speech disturbances, taste alterations, seizures, depression, confusion, nervousness

CV—Tachycardia, phlebitis, erratic blood pressure

Urinary—Urinary frequency, crystalluria, incontinence, nocturia, urinary retention, impotence

Dermatologic—Abnormal hair growth, rash, pruritus, urticaria, eczema-like reaction, photosensitization

Other—Hepatitis, backache, myalgia, tearing, chills, fever, respiratory distress. The drug is highly alkaline and may be irritating upon extravasation during IV administration.

CONTRAINDICATIONS AND PRECAUTIONS

Oral dantrolene is contraindicated in active hepatic disease, and in conditions where muscle spasticity is necessary to maintain an upright posture or balance. *Cautious use* is necessary in the presence of impaired pulmonary function, cardiac impairment caused by myocardial disease, a history of hepatic dysfunction, and in pregnant or lactating women or children under age 5. Caution is also indicated in females and in patients over 35 years of age in whom there exists a greater likelihood of developing hepatotoxicity.

INTERACTIONS

1. Estrogens may increase the danger of hepatotoxicity, especially in women over 35 years of age.
2. CNS depression may be potentiated by other tranquilizing agents. For this reason discourage patients from using alcohol while taking this drug.
3. Warfarin and clofibrate reduce the protein binding of dantrolene and may potentiate its effects.

■ Nursing Process

□ ASSESSMENT

□ Subjective Data
A thorough drug history should be obtained as well as a medical history of hepatic dysfunction and gastrointestinal problems or cardiovascular disease. Patients must understand the limits of the drug in relieving muscle spasticity because it is most effective when symptoms are pain and severe mobility limitation.

□ Objective Data
Pregnancy and lactation should be ruled out. Laboratory studies should also include hepatic function studies. These parameters may not be tested when the drug is used in an emergency for treating malignant hyperthemia but are appropriate for other indications.

Physical assessment should focus on musculoskeletal functioning to provide a baseline against which to judge drug effectiveness.

□ NURSING DIAGNOSES
Actual nursing diagnoses for the patient receiving dantrolene may include:

Knowledge deficit related to the action, administration, and side-effects of the drug
In an emergency, diagnoses may include:
Hyperthermia
Potential for injury

Alteration in cardiac output: decreased
Impaired gas exchange
Potential nursing diagnoses are related, primarily, to the common side-effects of the drug and may include:

Alteration in bowel elimination: diarrhea
Potential for injury: trauma; related to CNS effects of dizziness and weakness
Noncompliance related to slow achievement of drug effects

□ PLAN
Nursing care goals for the patient receiving dantrolene for muscle spasms include assisting the patient to achieve an optimum dosage level and to manage the side-effects. For the patient suffering malignant hyperthermia the goals are to provide supportive care to reduce temperature as rapidly as possible.

□ INTERVENTION
Early in the treatment the physician may order titrated doses to determine the lowest effective dose and reduce the chance of toxicity. The nurse will assist the patient to manage these dosage changes and monitor changes in spasticity. Patients also need encouragement to continue the drug for at least 1 week to 2 weeks before beneficial effects will be noted. During the transition period they may be discouraged by the development of dizziness and drowsiness. These symptoms subside with time but patients should be cautioned to limit driving or other hazardous activities until their comfort level increases. Other activities that will enhance the drug are exercise programs and use of braces to reduce the spasms. Patients need to be aware that dantrolene is only part of a total therapeutic program designed to alleviate symptoms.

Nursing care for the patient with malignant hyperthermia receiving dantrolene would include careful monitoring of the IV infusion, use of cooling blankets, alcohol baths, and other body cooling techniques, continuous temperature monitoring, and evaluation of output because renal failure is a danger with this disorder.

Any person with a family history of malignant hyperthermia should be encouraged to wear a Medic-Alert bracelet.

□ EVALUATION
Relief of muscle spasticity or reduction of dangerous hyperthermia are the main outcomes sought when dantrolene is administered.

Centrally Acting Muscle Relaxants

Baclofen, Carisoprodol, Chlorphenesin, Chlorzoxazone, Cyclobenzaprine, Metaxalone, Methocarbamol, Orphenadrine

The aim of the centrally acting muscle relaxants is to decrease skeletel muscle tone, thereby relieving pain associated with acute musculoskeletal disorders without causing a loss of voluntary motor function or consciousness. Many central nervous system depressants (e.g., alcohol, antianxiety drugs, barbiturates) can elicit varying degrees of muscle relaxation but are of little use clinically because they also produce marked sedation and other undesirable effects. Attempts to dissociate this CNS depressant action from the muscle-relaxing effect by synthesis of various centrally acting muscle relaxants thus far, with the occasional exception to be noted below, have met with very limited success, and most currently useful central muscle relaxants evoke a degree of sedation that makes long-term use of these drugs undesirable.

Agents in this class have been termed *interneuronal* or *polysynaptic* blocking drugs, such designations offering an explanation of their mechanism of action. These compounds act in part at various levels within the CNS (i.e., brain stem or spinal cord interneurons) to depress synaptic transmission in motor reflex pathways. They appear to exert a weak synaptic blocking action between neurons of these motor circuits, the degree of impairment being proportional to the number of synapses involved in the pathway. In addition to their neuronal blocking action, most of these drugs directly depress higher centers, such as the basal ganglia, that function in the regulation of motor activity. This CNS depressant action probably contributes a significant amount to the muscle relaxant effects of most of the centrally acting drugs.

With the exception of baclofen and diazepam (a widely used antianxiety agent to be discussed in Chap. 28), the drugs comprising the centrally acting muscle relaxants are remarkably similar in their pharmacology and toxicology. No one agent possesses a significant therapeutic advantage over any other agent, and for the most part, choice of a drug is a personal preference.

Because these drugs share many common properties, they will be discussed as a group. Individual drugs will then be listed in Table 19-1, where the characteristics of each drug will be presented in greater detail.

MECHANISM AND ACTIONS

The principal mechanism of action of centrally acting skeletal muscle relaxants is interference with transmission of impulses in motor reflex pathways involving the spinal cord, brain stem, and basal ganglia. These drugs appear to prolong synaptic recovery time and decrease repetitive spinal interneuronal discharges. Centrally acting muscle relaxants do not directly affect the skeletal muscle fibers nor block the cholinergic receptors on the motor end-plate. A general CNS depressant effect probably contributes to the degree of muscle relaxation observed with these drugs. Diazepam (see Chap. 28) and baclofen are particularly effective in the control of skeletal muscle spasticity associated with neurologic disorders such as multiple sclerosis, cerebral palsy, or spinal cord damage. This probably reflects an additional action of these drugs to facilitate the effects of GABA, an inhibitory neurotransmitter, which results in reduced efferent spinal cord motor neuron activity and depressed brain stem reticular function.

USES
1. Relief of pain and discomfort of muscle spasms associated with acute musculoskeletal disorders (e.g., inflammatory states, peripheral injury (sprain, strains), connective tissue disorders)
2. Alleviation of spasticity resulting from multiple sclerosis, spinal cord disease, and other neurologic conditions (diazepam and baclofen *only*)

ADMINISTRATION AND DOSAGE
Most of the centrally acting muscle relaxants are administered orally, for periods of one to several weeks. Diazepam (see Chap. 28), methocarbamol,

Table 19-1
Centrally Acting Skeletal Muscle Relaxants

Drug	Preparations	Usual Dosage Range	Clinical Considerations
baclofen (Lioresal)	Tablets—10 mg, 20 mg	5 mg three times/day. Increase by 5 mg every 3 days to optimal effect (maximum 80 mg/day)	Primarily used for relief of spasticity due to multiple sclerosis or spinal cord diseases. Drug has been used investigationally to treat trigeminal neuralgia. Sedation is usually transient. Absorption is reduced at higher doses. Half-life is 3 h–4 h. May increase urinary frequency. Do not use in patients with stroke or rheumatic disorders, in children under age 12, pregnant women, nursing mothers. Cautious use in epileptics and in presence of renal impairment. Reduce dose slowly to avoid possibility of hallucinations on abrupt withdrawal. May alter laboratory tests for SGOT, alkaline phosphatase, and blood sugar. Give with milk to decrease GI distress.
carisoprodol (Rela, Soma, Soprodol)	Tablets—350 mg	350 mg four times/day	Contraindicated in acute intermittent porphyria and in persons with meprobamate sensitivity. Allergic reactions can develop to early doses (rash, erythema, pruritus, eosinophilia). Stop drug and treat symptomatically. Carefully monitor urine output and avoid overhydration. Use cautiously in addiction-prone individuals. Reduce dose slowly as withdrawal symptoms can include headache, nausea, malaise, and insomnia. Also available with aspirin as Soma Compound and with codeine as Soma Compound with Codeine.
chlorphenesin (Maolate)	Tablets—400 mg	Initially 800 mg three times/day. Reduce to 400 mg three to four times/day for maintenance.	Cautious use in pregnancy, children, liver disease, or for periods exceeding 8 weeks. Discontinue at first sign of allergic reaction. Paradoxical excitation may occur but is usually controlled by dosage reduction. Administer with milk or with meals to reduce gastric distress. Blood dyscrasias are a possible hazard. Patient should have routine blood studies.
chlorzoxazone (Paraflex)	Tablets—250 mg	Adults—250 mg–500 mg three to four times/day. Reduce gradually as improvement is noted. Children—125 mg–500 mg three to four times/day. May be crushed and mixed with food or other vehicle.	Use cautiously in pregnancy, history of drug allergy, hepatic dysfunction. May discolor urine, but is not nephrotoxic. Give with meals to minimize GI irritation. Also available with acetaminophen as Parafon Forte and others.

(continued)

Table 19-1 (continued)
Centrally Acting Skeletal Muscle Relaxants

Drug	Preparations	Usual Dosage Range	Clinical Considerations
cyclobenzaprine (Flexeril)	Tablets—10 mg	10 mg three times/day to a maximum of 60 mg/day (not in children under age 15)	Do not use for longer than 2 wk–3 wk. *Not* effective in spasticity due to cerebral or spinal cord disease or cerebral palsy. Contraindicated in hyperthyroidism, arrhythmias, congestive heart failure, acute recovery phase of myocardial infarction, or with MAO inhibitors. Similar to tricyclic antidepressants in action (see Chap. 29) and may have similar central effects. High incidence of drowsiness, dry mouth, and dizziness. Possesses anticholinergic activity, responsible for atropine-like side-effects and interactions (see Chap. 14). Caution in glaucoma and urinary retention. Reduce dose slowly; do not stop abruptly. Withdrawal symptoms include headache, nausea, malaise. Antidote for overdose is physostigmine.
metaxolone (Skelaxin)	Tablets—400 mg	800 mg three to four times/day (not in children under age 12)	Contraindicated in anemia, renal or hepatic impairment, nursing mothers. Liver function studies should be done regularly. Observe for yellowish coloration of skin or eyes. Cautious use in epilepsy, pregnancy, allergic states. GI upset is common, as is headache, nervousness, and irritability. May interfere with Benedict's test (false positive).
methocarbamol (Delaxin, Marbaxin, Robaxin)	Tablets—500 mg, 750 mg Injection—100 mg/ml	*Oral:* Adults—1.5 g four times/day initially; reduce to 750 mg–1000 mg four times/day Children—60 to 75 mg/kg/day *IM:* 0.5 g–1 g every 8 h *IV:* 300 mg/min to a total daily dose of 1 g–3 g for maximum 3 days *IV infusion:* 1 g (10 ml) diluted to 250 ml saline or 5% dextrose given by IV drip *Tetanus:* 1 g–3 g directly into IV tubing every 6 h (Children 15 mg/kg every 6 h)	May control the neuromuscular manifestations of tetanus when given IV. Substitute oral administration for injection as soon as possible. Avoid extravasation, because irritability and thrombophlebitis can result. Do not give SC. Contraindicated in renal dysfunction (vehicle may cause acidosis and urea retention), children under age 12 (except for tetanus), epilepsy (especially IV). Keep patient recumbent during and at least 15 min after IV usage to minimize orthostatic hypotension and other side-effects. May interfere with laboratory tests for 5-HIAA and VMA. Too rapid IV injection may cause CNS side-effects (*e.g.*, dizziness, vertigo, syncope, headache, blurred vision) as well as bradycardia, hypotension, flushing, and anaphylactic reaction. Cautious use in myasthenia gravis. Check IV infusion for proper flow to minimize danger of thrombophlebitis and sloughing. Urine may darken upon standing. Also available orally with aspirin as Robaxisal.

(continued)

Table 19-1 (continued)
Centrally Acting Skeletal Muscle Relaxants

Drug	Preparations	Usual Dosage Range	Clinical Considerations
orphenadrine citrate (Banflex, Flexoject, Flexon, K-Flex, Marflex, Myolin, Neocyten, Norflex, O-Flex, Orphanate)	Tablets—100 mg Sustained-release tablets—100 mg Injection—30 mg/ml	*Oral:* 100 mg twice a day *IV, IM:* 60 mg every 12 h as needed (inject IV over 5 min with patient supine)	Strong anticholinergic with high incidence of atropine-like side-effects (see Chap. 14). Contraindicated in narrow-angle glaucoma, myasthenia, duodenal obstruction, ulcers, prostatic hypertrophy, bladder obstruction. Cautious use in pregnant women and children. Periodic monitoring of blood, urine, and liver function is recommended with prolonged use. Caution in urinary retention, tachycardia, coronary insufficiency, arrhythmias. Also available as the HCl salt (Disipal) for control of parkinsonism. (See Chap. 31) Narrow margin of safety. Watch for signs of toxicity which include flushing, fever, dry mouth, blurred vision. Stop drug and notify physician if this occurs. Available with aspirin and caffeine as Norgesic.

and orphenadrine can also be given parenterally (usually IM or IV) for acute muscle spasm. Refer to Table 19-1 for the dosage recommendations for all of the drugs.

FATE
In general, oral absorption is rapid. Peak plasma levels are usually attained in 1 hour to 3 hours, and effects persist for 3 hours to 6 hours. The drugs are largely metabolized in the liver, and metabolites are primarily excreted in the urine.

SIDE-EFFECTS/ADVERSE REACTIONS
(See Table 19-1 for specific information about each drug.) The most frequently occurring side-effects of the centrally acting skeletal muscle relaxants are drowsiness, fatigue, dizziness, lightheadedness, and GI upset. Anticholinergic side-effects, such as dry mouth and blurred vision, are frequently encountered with orphenadrine and cyclobenzaprine. A wide variety of other adverse reactions have been noted on occasion with use of the central skeletal muscle relaxants and are listed below. It is important to recognize, however, that not all of the adverse reactions given below have been associated with every drug.
GI—Anorexia, nausea, diarrhea, hiccups, bleeding, abdominal pain
CNS—Ataxia, headache, blurred vision, insomnia, confusion, irritability, paresthesias
CV—Tachycardia, hypotension, flushing, petechiae, thrombophlebitis, chest pain, palpitations, syncope
Urinary—Urinary retention, dysuria, enuresis
Hematologic—Leukopenia, pancytopenia, thrombocytopenia, agranulocytosis, hemolytic anemia
Hypersensitivity—Rash, erythema, pruritus, fever, asthma-like reaction, dermatoses, angioedema, anaphylactic reactions
Hepatic—Abnormal liver function tests, jaundice
Respiratory—Nasal congestion, dyspnea
Other—Dysarthria, dyspepsia, tremors, euphoria, metallic taste, pain or sloughing at site of injection, increased intraocular tension, conjunctivitis, tinnitus, slurred speech

CONTRAINDICATIONS AND PRECAUTIONS
The contraindications for the various central skeletal muscle relaxants differ among the individual drugs and therefore will be given for each drug in Table 19-1. Use of these drugs should be undertaken with *caution* in persons with impaired renal or hepatic function or respiratory depression, in

persons who must drive or operate machinery, in patients taking other CNS depressants, in young children, in elderly or debilitated patients, and in pregnant or lactating women. In addition, orphenadrine and cyclobenzaprine should be used cautiously in the presence of glaucoma, urinary retention, arrhythmias, and tachycardia, because they possess significant anticholinergic activity.

INTERACTIONS
1. The CNS depressive effects of centrally acting muscle relaxants and other CNS depressants (e.g., alcohol, barbiturates, narcotics, antianxiety agents) are additive.
2. MAO inhibitors may increase the toxicity of cyclobenzaprine.
3. Atropine-like side-effects can be intensified by use of anticholinergic drugs with cyclobenzaprine and orphenadrine.
4. Cyclobenzaprine may interfere with the antihypertensive action of guanethidine and similarly acting compounds.

■ Nursing Process

□ ASSESSMENT

□ Subjective Data
A history of the illness must be obtained so the degree of pain, spasm, and limitation of movement and muscle strength is known. These parameters will be used throughout drug therapy to determine drug effectiveness and adjust dosage.

History taking will vary with different drugs (see Table 19-1) but all patients should be asked about renal, hepatic, or respiratory disease. A drug history should also be obtained because significant adverse reactions can occur.

□ Objective Data
Physical assessment of musculoskeletal function is essential. Laboratory data on renal or hepatic function should be obtained if problems are suspected or if the patient is elderly. Pregnancy should also be ruled out.

□ NURSING DIAGNOSES
Actual nursing diagnoses for the patient receiving skeletal muscle relaxants may include:

Knowledge deficit related to the action, administration, and side-effects of the drug
Sensory-perceptual alterations in vision related to the central depressant action of the drug

Potential nursing diagnoses, based on common side-effects, may include:

Alteration in comfort: gastrointestinal upset or dry mouth
Potential for injury: trauma related to dizziness and slowed reaction time

□ PLAN
Nursing goals are focused on helping the patient achieve a drug regimen that reduces muscle spasticity without eliminating the ability to perform daily functions. Other goals may be geared toward teaching the patient to monitor for side-effects and to safely withdraw from the drug.

□ INTERVENTION
Early in the administration of these muscle relaxants, the nurse needs to observe the drug's effect on motor function. Does the drug reduce or eliminate the patient's ability to move independently? If the relaxant reduces spasticity to such a degree that the patient cannot perform functions, such as walking or lifting, that he was able to do prior to the drug's administration, then the dose may be too high or the drug may be too strong. Baseline data on the patient's motor function and careful observation by the nurse while the patient is in early stages of drug therapy will assist the physician and patient to reach a compromise on dosage, the goal of which is to reduce spasticity without eliminating function.

Is the dizziness or drowsiness produced by the drug incapacitating? These are common side-effects which should subside as the patient builds tolerance to the drug. Until such time as the symptoms disappear, the patient should be cautioned against driving or engaging in other activities that require mental alertness. If the symptoms do not subside, the dosage or time of day the drug is taken may need to be adjusted so the patient can resume normal activities. Some patients may limit their doses to after the evening meal and at bedtime to minimize the time when they will be awake and dizzy or will take the drug prior to physical therapy or exercise when the effect is lessened.

As noted in Table 19-1, many of these drugs cause moderate to severe withdrawal symptoms if stopped abruptly. Patients need to know this early in the treatment so if debilitating side-effects occur they will contact the physician to begin a withdrawal regimen.

□ EVALUATION
Outcomes which can be used to measure drug effectiveness include a decrease in pain or spasm, improved motor function, early reporting of side-effects, and requests for supervised alterations in drug dose to accommodate changes in motor function or to initiate drug withdrawal.

CASE STUDY

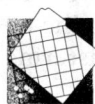

Bennett Stevens, age 19, is rushed to the emergency room after a motor vehicle accident in which his motorcycle was hit from behind by a car. He was thrown about 75 feet into an embankment. Bennett was not wearing a helmet. At the scene he was placed on a spinal-stabilizing stretcher.

When seen in the emergency room he was found to have a crushing chest injury and multiple fractures of both legs. During emergency care he developed respiratory arrest and was intubated and placed on a mechanical ventilator. He was transferred to the trauma unit.

Due to the nature of his chest injuries the trauma team decided to keep Bennett on the ventilator for several days. However, whenever Bennett arouses he begins to fight the machine. In addition, he is difficult to suction because of his resistance; consequently his secretions are building rapidly. The decision is made to put him on pancuronium to temporarily suppress his ventilation in order to stabilize him.

Discussion Questions

1. What explanations must be given to this patient before administering this drug?
2. Outline a nursing care plan for this patient to manage his care while the drug is working. Remember all skeletal muscle function will be lost. What needs must be met?
3. What are the major side-effects to watch for? What monitoring must be done to ensure any changes will be observed?

REVIEW QUESTIONS

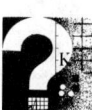

1. What are the principal uses for (a) neuromuscular blocking agents and (b) centrally acting skeletal muscle relaxants?
2. Briefly outline the sequence of events occurring during neuromuscular transmission.
3. Distinguish between *antidepolarizing* and *depolarizing* neuromuscular blocking agents.
4. What other pharmacologic actions of the neuromuscular blockers are responsible for many of the side-effects observed with these drugs?
5. What is the approximate sequence of paralysis of skeletal muscles following administration of a neuromuscular blocker?
6. In what ways does the synthetic curare derivative metocurine possess an advantage over d-tubocurarine?
7. List some other drugs that can potentiate the muscle-relaxing action of neuromuscular blocking agents.
8. What is the mechanism of action of succinylcholine?
9. How does the action of dantrolene differ from other muscle relaxants?
10. What are the principal indications for dantrolene?
11. Briefly discuss the site and mechanism of action of the centrally acting relaxants.
12. By what criteria can the nurse help a patient determine the effectiveness of a centrally acting muscle relaxant?

13. What criteria should the nurse use to determine when a patient can safely leave the recovery room after anesthesia that included use of succinylcholine or tubocurare?
14. What are the reasons for administering curare drugs to a patient on a ventilator?
15. What critical nursing interventions must be taken when a ventilator patient is given a neuromuscular blocking agent?

BIBLIOGRAPHY

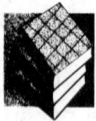

Bowman WC: Non-relaxant properties of neuromuscular blocking drugs. Br J Anesthesia 54:147, 1982

Davidoff RA: Pharmacology of spasticity. Neurology 28:46, 1980

Dennis MJ: Development of the neuromuscular junction: Inductive interactions between cells. Ann Rev Neuroscience 4:43, 1981

Drug Data: Lioresal. Am J Nurs 78:1945, November 1978

Feldman S: Neuromuscular blocking drugs. In Churchill-Davidson HC and Wylie WD (eds): A Practice of Anesthesia, 5th ed, p 727. Chicago, Year Book Medical Publishers, 1984

Fraulini KE, Gorski DW: Don't let preoperative medications put you in a spin. Nursing 83 13:26–30, December 1983

Herrold RK: The drug connection. Am J Nurs 84:1389, November 1984

Miller RD, Savarese JJ: Pharmacology of muscle relaxants, their antagonists, and monitoring of neuromuscular function. In Miller RD (ed): Anesthesia, p 487. New York, Churchill Livingstone, 1981

Young RR, Delwaide PJ: Spasticity (2 parts). N Engl J Med 304:28,96, 1981

Zaimis E (ed): Neuromuscular Junction. Berlin, Springer-Verlag, 1976

Local Anesthetics

20

Local anesthetics reversibly block conduction of nerve impulses along the axons of all sensory, motor, and autonomic nerve fibers. They are employed to elicit a transient loss of sensation, usually in a delimited area, most often for the purpose of eliminating pain. The first local anesthetic to be introduced was cocaine, and it was widely used in ophthalmology from the late 1800s to the early 1900s, when a second local anesthetic, procaine, was synthesized. Procaine, although commonly employed since that time, has several disadvantages, such as slow onset of action, short duration, and frequent allergic reactions. A number of other drugs having local anesthetic properties have been synthesized in the intervening years in an attempt to minimize some of the undesirable effects of these early agents, and although many newer agents show some significant advantages over the older drugs, no single local anesthetic currently available represents the ideal drug in terms of potency, efficacy, and safety.

Classification of Local Anesthetics

Classification of local anesthetics can be based either on chemical structure or principal clinical usage. Structurally, most local anesthetic drugs belong to one of three categories:
1. Esters of benzoic or aminobenzoic acid
2. Amides
3. Ethers
The individual drugs belonging to each of these classes of local anesthetics are listed in Table 20-1. Structurally, most local anesthetics consist of a lipophilic group (usually an aromatic ring); an intermediate chain, which contains either an ester, amide, or other linkage; and an amine group, which is hydrophilic. The balance between the lipophilic and hydrophilic strengths of the respective groups is a major determinant of the activity of the compound, and this aspect will be discussed further below. The type of linkage in the intermediate chain, on the other hand, is important in determining the duration of action of the drug. For example, esters are hydrolyzed rapidly by plasma cholinesterase and thus are short-acting. Amides are largely metabolized in the liver, although the rate of inactivation varies widely among the different amides. Ethers are generally long-acting compounds and are only used topically.

Table 20-1
Chemical Classification of Local Anesthetics

Esters of Benzoic or Aminobenzoic Acid

benoxinate
benzocaine
butamben
chloroprocaine
cocaine
cyclomethycaine
dyclonine
procaine
proparacaine
tetracaine

Amides

bupivacaine
dibucaine
etidocaine
lidocaine
mepivacaine
prilocaine

Ether

pramoxine

Local anesthetics have several clinical applications, both topically and parenterally, and thus can also be classified as follows:
1. Surface anesthetics (skin, mucous membrane, eye, ear—e.g., benzocaine, cocaine, diperodon, pramoxine)
2. Infiltration anesthetics (local intradermal or subcutaneous injection—e.g., etidocaine, lidocaine, prilocaine, procaine)
3. Spinal anesthetics (subarachnoid injection—e.g., procaine, tetracaine)
4. Epidural anesthetics (injection into area surrounding the dura mater of spinal cord—e.g., bupivacaine, etidocaine, lidocaine, mepivacaine, prilocaine)

While some local anesthetics are only employed by one route of administration (e.g., butamben, proparacaine), it should be noted that several of these drugs can be given by more than one route. These include lidocaine (topical, infiltration, epidural, caudal, spinal) and tetracaine (topical, ophthalmic, spinal, caudal). An overview of the different routes by which local anesthetics can be administered is presented in Table 20-2. An illustration of sites used for injection of local anesthetics is found in Figure 20-1.

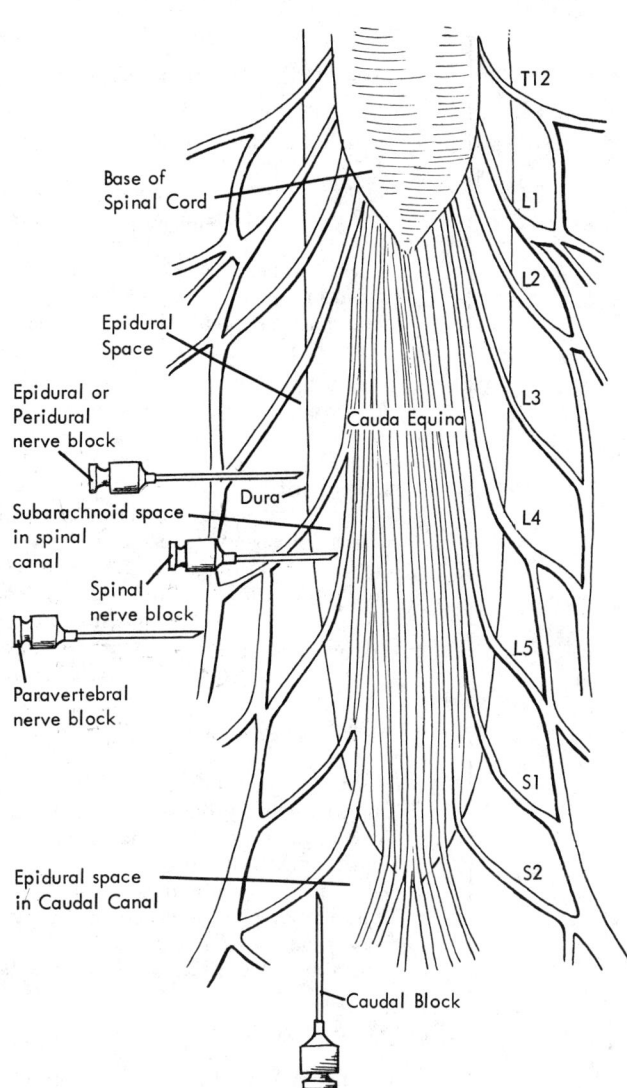

Figure 20-1. *Injection sites for paravertebral, spinal, epidural, and caudal administration of local anesthetics. (Rodman MJ, Smith DW: Pharmacology and Drug Therapy in Nursing, 2nd ed. Philadelphia, JB Lippincott, 1979)*

Mechanism of Local Anesthetic Action

Local anesthetics are weak bases (*i.e.*, secondary or tertiary amines) which are injected in the form of their water-soluble, cationic salts. However, in order to penetrate the nerve membrane and reach their site of action within the nerve fiber, the drugs need to be in the nonionic, lipid-soluble state. The ratio of the cationic to the nonionic form of the drug is dependent on several factors, such as the ionization constant of the molecules and the regional *p*H. The uncharged, nonionic fraction of drug diffuses across the nerve membrane, then re-equilibrates between the nonionic and cationic forms within the nerve fiber. This reequilibration is believed essential for the pharmacologic activity

of local anesthetics because the cationic form of the drug is the active form within the nerve fiber. Thus, penetration to the site of action is dependent on the presence of sufficient amount of lipid-soluble, nonionic drug; once inside the nerve membrane, however, activity depends on conversion to the cationic state. This relationship explains why local anesthetics are frequently much less effective when injected into regions of inflammation. Such sites have a low extracellular *p*H due to the presence of acidic cellular breakdown products. The low *p*H favors ionization of the basic drug to the cationic form in the extracellular fluid, thereby decreasing penetration into the nerve fiber.

The cationic form of the local anesthetic functions to stabilize the nerve membrane, increasing the threshold for excitation and slowing the rate of rise and the amplitude of the nerve action poten-

Table 20-2
Routes of Administration of Local Anesthetics

Topical or Surface

· Applied as lotion, cream, spray, gel, solution, or powder
· Used to anesthetize mucous membranes for minor surgery, or to relieve pain and itching on topical areas
· Poorly absorbed through intact skin, but may attain significant systemic concentrations following applicaton to highly vascular mucous membranes, especially the tracheobronchial tree or nasal mucosa
· Major adverse effect is a local allergic reaction.

Infiltration

· Injection of a local anesthetic solution *directly* into a tissue area to be manipulated
· Sensory nerve endings are numbed temporarily, allowing minor surgery such as drainage or excision of a cyst, suturing, and dental work.
· Epinephrine (1:200,000) is frequently added to the local anesthetic solution to be infiltrated in order to prolong the duration of anesthesia and restrict spread of the anesthetic drug.
· Systemic toxicity is usually minimal, except when large doses of the drug are necessary for extensive surgical purposes.

Nerve Block (Paravertebral)

· Injection of a local anesthetic into the vicinity of a nerve trunk that supplies the operative site (*e.g.,* pudendal block for obstetrical delivery)
· Single or multiple nerves may be blocked depending on the site of injection.
· Higher concentrations of solution are generally necessary in order to penetrate the larger diameter nerve trunk fibers.
· Thorough knowledge of neuroanatomy is necessary to obtain the desired area and degree of anesthesia.
· Pain from injection can be reduced if the injection is administered slowly.

Spinal (Subarachnoid)

· Injection of local anesthetic solution into the subarachnoid space surrounding the spinal column, usually at the level of the second lumbar vertebrae
· Spread of the drug upward or downward is dependent on the specific gravity (*i.e.,* density) of solution and positioning of the patient (*e.g.,* use of low specific gravity solution [*i.e.,* solution that would "float" in spinal fluid] necessitates patient in head-downward position to facilitate caudal diffusion of drug in the spinal column; similarly high density solution with patient in head-upward position also moves "downward" in spinal column, anesthetizing only lower part of the body).
· Patient is awake, muscle relaxation in lower extremities is usually good and cardiovascular function is normal; however, hypotension occurs frequently, especially if sympathetic nerves are affected.
· Primarily used for lower abdominal surgical procedures and obstetrics
· Headache is a frequent complication, due to puncture of the dura and loss of cerebrospinal fluid pressure.
· A low spinal (*i.e.,* 3rd or 4th lumbar space puncture) administered while the patient is seated is termed a "saddle block." The patient must remain seated upright for 30 to 60 seconds after injection to allow movement of drug to lower areas of the spinal column; procedure affects only those parts of the lower body that would contact a saddle; primarily used in obstetrics to reduce the pain from episiotomy, delivery, and repair.

(continued)

Table 20-2 (continued)
Routes of Administration of Local Anesthetics

Epidural (Peridural)

· Injection of local anesthetic into the region *outside* of the subarachnoid space; usually in the 2nd lumbar space; thus, the drug (a) diffuses across the dura, acting on nerve roots and the spinal cord, and (b) blocks the nerve fibers as they emerge from the subarachnoid space.
· Because the dura is not punctured, no spinal fluid escapes; therefore, the likelihood of headache is minimized.
· Extent and duration of anesthesia are dependent on the volume and concentration of local anesthetic used and will determine effect on fetus.
· Hypertension is common.

Caudal

· A form of epidural anesthesia in which the local anesthetic is injected into the caudal canal at the base of the spinal column, the area containing the efferent spinal nerves innervating the pelvic viscera
· Side-effects are minimal, and respiration and blood pressure are largely unaffected.
· Primarily used in obstetrics and for lower pelvic and rectal surgery

tial. These effects are accomplished by competing with calcium for a phospholipid binding site on the nerve membrane that controls the inward flow of sodium ions. Thus, sodium influx is decreased, depolarization is prevented, and propagation of the impulse along the axon is blocked. The normal resting potential of the neuron is largely unaltered. Increased extracellular calcium can partially antagonize the action of local anesthetics, whereas elevated levels of extracellular potassium can enhance local anesthetic activity.

Effects on Nerve Fibers of Different Size

Nerve fibers may be classified into three major types depending on diameter, conduction velocity, myelination, and function. Table 20-3 outlines the characteristics of the principal types of nerve fibers. When a local anesthetic is injected into the region of mixed nerve fibers, differential effects with respect to onset and recovery as well as clinical efficacy are observed, depending on the size and state of myelination of the nerve fibers. In general, small nonmyelinated C fibers (*e.g.*, dorsal root and sympathetic postganglionic) mediating pain and vasoconstriction are affected first by local anesthetics, followed by the small, myelinated A-delta fibers mediating pain and temperature. Larger

fibers carrying sensory impulses (*e.g.*, A-alpha, A-beta) are blocked next, and finally motor nerves (*e.g.*, A-gamma) are anesthetized, resulting in decreased skeletal muscle tone. Recovery proceeds in the opposite direction (*i.e.*, motor function is restored before sensory function).

Pharmacokinetics

Although the predominant effects of local anesthetics are confined to the circumscribed area adjacent to the injection or application site, systemic absorption does occur to varying degrees and may produce undesirable reactions. Large doses or inadvertent intravascular injection of local anesthetics may result in cardiovascular effects, such as hypotension or cardiac depression, or central nervous system effects, such as stimulation and convulsions followed by depression. Systemic absorption of most local anesthetics can be minimized by addition of a local vasoconstrictor (*e.g.*, 1:200,000 epinephrine) to the injection solution; this constricts the vessels in the immediate area, and prevents spread of the administered anesthetic. Vasoconstrictors also prolong the duration of action of local anesthetics, reduce the amount of drug needed, and may help slow local hemorrhaging if surgery is performed. Use of vasoconstrictors, however, is less effective in prolonging the action

Table 20-3
Classification and Characteristics of Nerve Fibers

Type	Diameter (μm)	Conduction Velocity (m/sec)	Myelination	Major Function
A-alpha	12–22	70–120	Yes	Somatic motor, proprioception
A-beta	5–12	30–70	Yes	Touch, pressure
A-gamma	3–7	15–40	Yes	Motor, touch
A-delta	1–4	12–30	Yes	Pain, temperature
B	1–3	3–15	Minimal	Autonomic preganglionic
C				
Dorsal root	0.2–1.2	0.3–2.3		Pain, spinal reflexes
Sympathetic	0.2–1.2	0.7–2.5		Postganglionic sympathetic

of highly lipid-soluble, longer acting local anesthetics, such as bupivacaine and etidocaine.

As previously mentioned, the ester-type local anesthetics are usually very short acting because they are rapidly hydrolyzed by plasma cholinesterase. Amide drugs, however, are primarily inactivated in the liver, although there is considerable variation in the rates of hepatic degradation. Thus, lidocaine and prilocaine exhibit the shortest duration of action, whereas etidocaine and bupivacaine have a significantly longer duration. The presence of impaired hepatic function can markedly prolong the half-lives of the amide local anesthetics dependent on the liver for metabolism, and can result in a higher incidence of adverse effects.

Adverse Effects

The majority of adverse effects seen with use of local anesthetics are the result of excessive doses and hence increased systemic absorption. CNS excitation can occur with large doses of local anesthetics, leading to a variety of symptoms, including restlessness, anxiety, tremor, and occasionally convulsions. The central excitatory effect is usually followed by CNS depression with very large amounts of drug, frequently resulting in cardiovascular and respiratory depression, extreme drowsiness, and sometimes unconsciousness and coma; if untreated, death can ensue.

Vascular smooth muscle may be relaxed (except by cocaine, a potent vasoconstrictor), and many aspects of cardiac functioning are depressed by local anesthetics. In this regard, lidocaine is extensively employed as an antiarrhythmic agent by IV administration. (This aspect of its pharmacology is reviewed in Chap. 34.)

Ester-type local anesthetics (e.g., procaine, tetracaine) can produce allergic reactions, most often a contact dermatitis upon topical application, although bronchospasm and anaphylaxis have been reported following injection. Allergic reactions with amide or ether-type drugs are not as common.

Local anesthetics readily cross the placental barrier and, when used during labor and delivery, can cause varying degrees of maternal, fetal, and neonatal toxicity. Fetal bradycardia may occur in approximately 25% of patients receiving amide-type anesthetics for paracervical block, and the risk is increased in premature or postmature delivery, preeclampsia fetal distress, and when large doses are required. Other fetal untoward reactions following local anesthetic use can include depressed respiration, seizures, weakness, and convulsions. A complete review of local anesthetic-induced adverse reactions is presented in the monograph which follows.

The general pharmacology and clinical implications of local anesthetics will be discussed as a group. Specific characteristics of individual drugs will then be detailed in Table 20-4 along with prescribing information and available preparations.

Local Anesthetics

MECHANISM AND ACTIONS
(See general discussion above.)

Local anesthetics cross the membrane of nerve fibers and appear to compete with calcium for a site on the nerve membrane controlling the passage of sodium. By reducing sodium permeability, the drugs slow the rate of depolarization and decrease the amplitude of the nerve impulse below the threshold level for firing. Thus, propagation of the impulse along the nerve fiber is blocked. Loss of nerve function proceeds in an orderly fashion: pain is lost first, followed by the sensations of temperature, touch, proprioception, and finally skeletal muscle tone. Systemic effects of local anesthetics include CNS stimulation followed by depression, cardiac depression, and relaxation of vascular smooth muscle.

USES

1. Relief of pain, soreness, irritation, and itching associated with various skin and mucous membrane disorders (e.g., minor burns, rashes, wounds, allergic conditions, fungus infections, skin ulcers, hemorrhoids, fissures) (topical administration)
2. Production of corneal and conjunctival anesthesia to facilitate ophthalmic procedures, such as tonometry, gonioscopy, removal of foreign bodies, and minor ocular surgery
3. Production of infiltration, nerve block, spinal, epidural, or caudal anesthesia in surgery, obstetrics, or dental work
4. Treatment of cardiac arrhythmias (see Chap. 34)

ADMINISTRATION AND DOSAGE
(See Table 20-4.)

FATE
Absorption is largely dependent on site of administration, dose, degree of vasoconstriction, and blood flow to the area. Onset of action is variable but is usually within 5 minutes to 10 minutes for most injections. Surface anesthesia develops rapidly upon topical application. Duration of action varies widely and following injection may range from 0.5 hour to 1 hour (procaine) up to 4 hours (bupivacaine, dibucaine, etidocaine, tetracaine). Table 20-5 lists the average onset and duration of action for the various local anesthetic drugs. Some agents are rapidly hydrolyzed by plasma cholinesterases (e.g., procaine) or liver enzymes (e.g., lidocaine, etidocaine), while others are more resistant to inactivation. Excretion is primarily in the urine, mainly as metabolites, but some unchanged drug as well. Bupivacaine, tetracaine, and etidocaine are highly protein-bound, whereas binding is minimal with procaine.

SIDE-EFFECTS/ADVERSE REACTIONS
The most frequently noted side-effects with topical application of local anesthetics are localized allergic reactions, such as contact dermatitis, whereas ophthalmic application is commonly associated with a stinging or burning sensation. Parenteral administration is usually very well tolerated by most patients, and most adverse reactions to injection of local anesthetics are the result of hypersensitivity, decreased tolerance, or excessive dosage. Significant systemic absorption of a local anesthetic drug can lead to CNS stimulation (dizziness, blurred vision, confusion, irritability, tinnitus, convulsions, tremors) followed by CNS depression (drowsiness, unconsciousness, respiratory arrest), difficulty in speaking, hearing, swallowing, or breathing, muscle twitching, hypotension, myocardial depression, bradycardia, and cardiac arrest.

Epidural or caudal injection may provoke spinal block, urinary retention, incontinence, loss of sexual function, paresthesias, weakness, headache, backache, and loss of sphincter control, whereas spinal anesthesia may cause hypotension, severe headache or backache, neck stiffness, respiratory depression, or nerve root damage.

Other adverse reactions that have occurred following topical drug application are keratitis, fissuring of fingertips, urticaria, cutaneous lesions, edema, urethritis, skin sloughing and necrosis, and anaphylactic reaction. Remember, a nurse who is hypersensitive to these drugs may suffer an adverse reaction after applying the drug to the patient. Anyone with known hypersensitivity or recurrent dermatitis should wear gloves when administering these drugs topically. Corneal opacities have resulted from instillation of local anesthetics into the eye.

Adverse reactions specific to an individual local anesthetic drug are listed under clinical considerations in Table 20-4.

CONTRAINDICATIONS AND PRECAUTIONS
Local anesthetics should not be given in dentistry where inflammation or sepsis exists at the site of injection. Spinal anesthesia is contraindicated in the presence of arthritis, meningitis, poliomyelitis, septicemia, spondylitis, or other spinal column conditions such as lumbar tuberculosis, metastatic lesions, or pyogenic infections. Epidural anesthesia should not be induced where abruptio placentae or placenta previa are present. Prilocaine is contraindicated in patients with methemoglobinemia, and

(Text continues on p. 351.)

Table 20-4
Local Anesthesics

Drug	Preparations	Usual Dosage Range	Clinical Considerations
benoxinate and sodium fluorescein (Fluress)	Drops—0.4% benoxinate and 0.25% sodium fluorescein	Tonometry and removal of sutures and foreign bodies—1 to 2 drops before operation. Ophthalmic anesthesia—2 drops 90 sec apart for three installations.	Short-acting anesthetic, with possible bacteriostatic action; no effect on pupil size or accommodation; minimal stinging or burning; fluorescein sodium stains abraded or ulcerated areas, facilitating visualization of foreign bodies; fluorescein is also available *alone* as ophthalmic drops or strips which are moistened and touched against the cornea as an aid in diagnosing corneal abrasions or presence of foreign bodies or for fitting hard contact lenses.
benzocaine (various manufacturers)	Ointment—1%, 2%, 5%, 20% Cream—1%, 5%, 6% Lotion—0.5% Aerosol solution—3%, 5%, 9.4%, 20% Oral Liquid—2%, 20% Otic solution—1.5%, 5%, 20% Gel—7.5%, 10%, 20% Candy—5 mg Gum—6 mg Lozenges—3 mg, 5 mg, 6.25 mg, 10 mg, 15 mg, 32 mg (with additives)	Apply to area several times a day as required. Suppositories and rectal ointment given morning and night, and after each bowel movement. Gel used as a lubricant on catheters, specula, etc. Liquid, gel, or aerosol for oral mucous membrane anesthesia in dentistry or topical anesthesia. Oral candy/gum as an aid in weight loss—6 mg–15 mg just prior to food consumption (maximum 45 mg/day) Lozenges for sore throat and mouth irritation	Slowly absorbed from mucous membranes and exerts a fairly prolonged action. Drug is a component of many combination products (*e.g.*, oral, anorectal, otic, topical). Produces hypersensitivity reactions in some individuals. Stop drug at first sign of allergic response. Avoid contact with eyes. May be used for temporary relief of toothache and other dental procedures. Employed to lubricate catheters, endoscopic tubes, sigmoidoscopes, proctoscopes, and vaginal specula. Not intended for use on infants under 1 year. Caution parent not to use such products on a teething child. Also used as gum or candy (Ayds, Slim-Line) to decrease taste sensation as an adjunct in weight reduction programs.
bupivacaine (Marcaine, Sensorcaine)	Injection—0.25%, 0.5%, 0.75% alone or with 1:200,000 epinephrine	Infiltration—0.25% Epidural/caudal—0.25% to 0.5% Peripheral Nerve Block—0.25% to 0.5% Retrobular block—0.75% Sympathetic block—0.25%; Dental block—0.5%	Onset slower than lidocaine, but more prolonged duration. Widely used for nerve block, epidural or caudal for long surgical or obstetrical procedures, and relief of pain during labor. (*Caution:* 0.75% concentration should not be used for obstetrical anesthesia; cardiac arrest and death have occurred.) Maximum dose 400 mg (with epinephrine) in 24 h. Do not use for spinal block. Not for use in children under 12 years old. Also use cautiously in elderly or patients with hepatic disease.

(continued)

Table 20-4 (continued)
Local Anesthesics

Drug	Preparations	Usual Dosage Range	Clinical Considerations
butamben (Butesin)	Ointment—1%	Apply two to three times/ day as needed	Used primarily in minor burns and skin irritations
chloroprocaine (Nesa-caine)	Injection—1%, 2%, 3%	Infiltration/nerve block— 1% to 2% Caudal/epidural—2% to 3%	Onset is within 10 min and effects persist 30 min–90 min. Available without preservatives for caudal or epidural block. More rapid acting and less toxic than pro-caine. IV use may produce thrombophlebitis. Prior use of chloroprocaine may interfere with subsequent use of bupiva-caine.
cocaine (various man-ufacturers)	Soluble tablets—135 mg Topical solution—40 mg/ml, 100 mg/ml	Surface anesthesia—1% to 4%	Class II Controlled Substance (see Chap. 7). Central stimulant that can lead to overwhelming psy-chological dependence when re-peatedly inhaled or injected. Pro-duces vasoconstriction when ap-plied to mucous membrane. Not used by injection or in the eyes. Onset of action is rapid when ap-plied locally, and duration is about 1 h–2 h. A 4% solution is prepared by dissolving 135 mg in 3.4 ml of distilled water. Widely abused drug (See Chap. 85.)
dibucaine (Nuper-cainal, Nupercaine)	Ointment—1% Cream—5%	Apply locally two to three times/day	Approximately 8 to 10 times more potent than procaine. Onset about 15 min and duration 3 h to 4 h. Primarily used for topical anesthesia in local skin disorders.
dyclonine (Dyclone)	Solution—0.5%, 1%	Apply topically to skin or mucous membranes	Used prior to endoscopic proce-dures, to block the gag reflex and to relieve pain of oral or anogeni-tal lesions. Onset is about 10 min, and duration approximately 60 min. May be used in patients hypersensitive to other local an-esthetics.
etidocaine (Duranest)	Injection—1% alone or 1% and 1.5% with 1:200,000 epinephrine	Infiltration, lumbar, central nerve block—1% Caudal—1% Caesarean, intra-abdominal surgery—1% to 1.5% Maxillary—1.5%	Onset of action within 3 min to 5 min. Duration may last up to 8 h with epinephrine (caution in am-bulatory patients). Induces pro-found motor blockade when given peridurally. Not for use in children under 14 years old. Use caution in elderly persons.
lidocaine (Xylocaine, and various other manufacturers)	Ointment—2.5%, 5% Jelly—2% Solution—2%, 4%, 10%	Apply topically as needed. Solution for pain and in-flammation of mouth,	Slightly more potent than procaine. Rapid onset of action (1 min–2 min), lasting up to 2 h. Widely

(continued)

Table 20-4 (continued)
Local Anesthesics

Drug	Preparations	Usual Dosage Range	Clinical Considerations
lidocaine (Xylocaine, and various other manufacturers) (continued)	Injection—0.5%, 1%, 1.5%, 2%, 4%, 10%, 20% alone Injection—0.5%, 1%, 1.5%, 2% with epinephrine Injection—1.5% with 7.5% dextrose Injection—5% with 7.5% glucose	throat, pharynx, and urethra, as needed. *Injection:* Infiltration—0.5% to 1% *Nerve block:* Dental—2% Intercostal—1% Brachial—1.5% Paracervical—1% *Epidural:* Thoracic—1% Lumbar—1% to 2% *Caudal:* Obstetric—1% Surgical—1.5% Spinal—5% with glucose Saddle block—1.5% with dextrose	used as antiarrhythmic agent (see Chap. 34). Do *not* use solution with epinephrine for arrhythmias, or solutions with preservatives for spinal or epidural block. Oral solutions can interfere with swallowing reflex; caution in pediatric and geriatric patients. Can enhance muscle-relaxing action of neuromuscular blocking agents. Contraindicated in persons with blood dyscrasias.
mepivacaine (Carbocaine, Isocaine, Polocaine)	Injection—1%, 1.5%, 2%, 3% Injection—2% with 1:20,000 levonordefrin	Nerve block—1% to 2% Paracervical block—1% Caudal/epidural—1% to 2% Infiltration—1% Analgesia—1% to 2% Dental block—3% or 2% with levonordefrin	Twice as potent as procaine, with comparable onset, but more prolonged duration of action. Possesses some vasoconstrictive action. Therefore, does not usually require a vasoconstrictor. Injection containing levonordefrin is used in dental procedures *only*. Not used topically. Less drowsiness and depression than observed with lidocaine. Use with caution in renal dysfunction and elderly patients.
pramoxine (Tronothane, Prax, Proctofoam)	Cream—1% Lotion—1% Suppositories—1% Aerosal foam—(rectal use)—1% Rectal ointment—1%	Apply topically or rectally two to three times/day as needed.	Not used by injection, or applied to the eye or nasal mucosa. Component of many anorectal preparations (*e.g.*, ointments, foams, suppositories). Used mainly to relieve pain and itching, especially of hemorrhoids, and to facilitate endotracheal, intragastric, and rectal intubation procedures.
prilocaine (Citanest)	Injection—4% Injection—4% with 1:200,000 epinephrine	Nerve block/infiltration in dental procedures—4%	Similar to lidocaine in its actions, but has a slower onset of action. May induce drowsiness and sleepiness. Associated with some cases of methemoglobinemia and not widely used for this reason. Use is largely restricted to dental procedures.
procaine (Novocain)	Injection—1%, 2%, 10% (plain)	Infiltration—0.25% to 0.5% Nerve block—0.5% to 2% Spinal—10%	Not employed topically. Rapidly eliminated, short-acting (30 min–60 min), no central stimula-

(continued)

Table 20-4 (continued)
Local Anesthesics

Drug	Preparations	Usual Dosage Range	Clinical Considerations
procaine (Novocain) (continued)			tion, and relatively nontoxic, although fairly high incidence of allergic reactions. Metabolic product may interfere with actions of sulfonamides, and other local anesthetics should be used in presence of sulfonamide antibiotics. The amide of procaine is an effective antiarrhythmic agent (see Chap. 34).
proparacaine (Ak-taine, Alcaine, I-Paracaine, Kainair, Ophthaine, Ophthetic)	Ophthalmic drops—0.5%	Cataract surgery—1 drop every 5 min to 10 min Removal of sutures—1 to 2 drops 2 min to 3 min prior to surgery Foreign bodies—1 to 2 drops prior to extraction Tonometry—1 to 2 drops before measurement	Used in the eye exclusively. Produces minimal irritation. May produce allergic contact dermatitis with drying and fissuring of the fingertips. Also available in combination with fluorescein (0.25%) as fluorocaine or I-Parescein (see Benoxinate and sodium fluorescein).
tetracaine (Ponto-caine)	Cream—1% Ointment—0.5% Oral solution—2% Ophthalmic ointment—0.5% Ophthalmic solution—0.5% Injection—1% Injection—0.2%, 0.3%, with 6% dextrose Powder—20 mg in Niphanoid (snowlike crystals) ampules	Apply locally (0.5% to 2%) as needed for pain, burning, itching. Cataract surgery—1 drop (0.5%) every 5 min to 10 min Suture removal—1 to 2 drops (0.5%) 2 min to 3 min prior to procedure Foreign bodies—1 to 2 drops prior to operating Tonometry—1 to 2 drops before measurement Ophthalmic inflammation—Apply ointment two to three times/day Spinal anesthesia—0.2% to 1% Caudal anesthesia—0.2% to 0.3% with dextrose Nasal or pharyngeal anesthesia—2% solution	More potent (8–10 times) and longer acting than procaine, but more toxic as well. Onset of action is relatively slow with a duration between 2 h and 3 h. Employed in rather low concentrations for surface anesthesia of eye, nose, and throat, as well as spinal and caudal anesthesia. Produces prolonged spinal anesthesia for operations requiring 2 h to 3 h; doses exceeding 15 mg are rarely required. Do not reuse leftover autoclaved ampules because crystals may form.

bupivacaine should not be used for obstetrical paracervical block, because fetal bradycardia and death have occurred.

Conditions that demand *cautious use* of local anesthetics include heart block, liver or kidney disease, hyperthyroidism, shock, malignant hyperthermia, and inflammation at the intended site of injection. Vasoconstrictor-containing preparations should be used cautiously in patients with hypertension or peripheral vascular disease. Caution is also warranted when performing spinal anesthesia in patients with chronic backache, frequent headache, or a history of migraine and hypotension.

INTERACTIONS
1. Certain local anesthetic drugs (*e.g.*, lidocaine) may enhance muscle-relaxing effects of neuromuscular blocking agents.

Table 20-5
Onset and Duration of Action of Local Anesthetics Following
Topical and Parenteral Administration

	Onset (Min)	Duration (H)
Topical Only		
benoxinate (eye)	0.5	0.25–0.5
benzocaine	0.5–1	0.5–1
butamben	2–5	0.5–1
cocaine	2–5	0.5–2
dibucaine	5–15	2–4
dyclonine	5–10	0.5–1
pramoxine	2–5	0.5–1
proparacaine (eye)	0.5–1	0.25–0.5
Parenteral Only		
bupivacaine	2–5	2–4
chloroprocaine	5–10	0.25–0.5
etidocaine	3–5	2–3
mepivacaine	2–5	1–2
prilocaine	1–3	0.5–1.5
procaine	2–4	0.25–0.5
Topical and Parenteral		
lidocaine		
Topical	1–2	0.5–1
Parenteral	0.5–1	0.5–1
tetracaine		
Topical	2–5	0.5–1
Parenteral	5–10	2–3

2. Additive cardiac depressant effects may occur when local anesthetics and other cardiac depressant drugs (e.g., quinidine, propranolol, phenytoin) are given together.

3. Solutions of local anesthetics containing a vasoconstrictor (e.g., epinephrine) can produce blood pressure alterations in combination with MAO inhibitors, tricyclic antidepressants, phenothiazines, and pressor agents.

4. Vasoconstrictors in local anesthetic solutions may precipitate arrhythmias in combination with chloroform, cyclopropane, halothane, and related general anesthetics.

5. Procaine, chloroprocaine, and proparacaine may retard the action of sulfonamide antibiotics, because they are derivatives of PABA.

6. Local anesthetics may have additive effects with sedatives or other CNS depressants.

7. The metabolism of the ester-type local anesthetics (see Table 20-1) may be slowed by cholinesterase inhibitors.

■ Nursing Process

□ ASSESSMENT

□ Subjective Data

For any patient receiving a local anesthetic a thorough drug history must be obtained with attention to use of street drugs, cardiac depressants, or antidepressants which can adversely affect the action of the anesthetics. In addition, questions should be asked about drug allergies, particularly to any "-caine" medications or to PABA-containing products (sun screens). There is a high incidence of cross-hypersensitivity to these products. If a patient has been allergic to procaine (Novocain) for example, there is an increased chance he will be allergic to others in the group. A history of renal or liver disease is also noteworthy because alteration in function may decrease the person's ability to get rid of the anesthetic once administered. Elderly persons and children are particularly susceptible to such problems in using local anesthetics. A history of migraine, chronic headache or backache, or hypotension is also noteworthy.

If the patient is facing an operative procedure with a local anesthetic the nurse should inquire about the patient's perception of what the drug will do and what will happen to him while in surgery. The patient needs to know that he will be awake, that another drug will probably be given to relax him, and that he will be aware of what is going on during the procedure. Many patients are nervous about being awake and will need reassurance. The patient facing surgery under local anesthesia is more in need of a preoperative visit by OR nurses than any other patient and will benefit greatly from having a nurse as his resource during the procedure.

□ *Objective Data*
Physical assessment should note the presence of any arthritic or structural deformities in the site to be injected as well as any evidence of inflammation or edema. A cardiovascular and respiratory assessment should also be completed. A baseline blood pressure should be recorded in a prominent location.

Laboratory studies may be based on history but will probably assess renal and hepatic function. An ECG may also be performed if surgery is to be done.

□ *NURSING DIAGNOSES*
Actual nursing diagnoses for the patient receiving a local anesthetic may include:
    Knowledge deficit about the effect of the drug on the body
    Sensory–perceptual alterations in tactile and kinesthetic receptors
    Impaired physical mobility in affected body part
Potential nursing diagnoses may be related to side-effects based on route of administration or on drug effects and can include:
    Potential for injury: trauma related to loss of sensation
    Impaired tissue integrity related to allergic response (most frequent with topical applications)
    Alteration in comfort related to burning or stinging (most frequent with ophthalmic applications)
Potential nursing diagnoses related to side-effects of parenteral administration are very serious and include:

Alteration in thought processes related to alternating CNS excitation and depression
Alteration in cardiac output: decreased
Ineffective breathing pattern
Impaired gas exchange
} may develop if significant systemic absorption occurs

□ *PLAN*
The nursing goals for this patient should include:
1. Having all necessary equipment available for resuscitation when systemic absorption is a possibility; cardiac or respiratory arrest is more likely to occur when a local anesthetic is administered in large doses to elderly or debilitated patients or in patients receiving the drug in traumatized or debrided areas, because increased systemic absorption can occur.
2. Attempting to administer the medications safely to minimize the danger of systemic effects.
3. Monitoring closely for allergic responses; with topical application itching and rash may be the only symptoms; with injection, an anaphylactic reaction may occur necessitating resuscitation.
4. Providing the patient with adequate comfort for delivery, operative, or diagnostic procedure.

□ *INTERVENTION*

□ *Topical Applications*
In most cases the patient may participate in application of the anesthetic and should be taught the amount to apply and what systemic side-effects are indicators that too much of the drug is being absorbed. These include changes in motor function in the area since that is the last level of local anesthesia. If an allergic reaction occurs, the drug should be immediately discontinued, the physician notified, and symptomatic treatment of itching or rash begun.

Patients should be warned to avoid contact with large areas of their skin when applying topical anesthetics because they are easily absorbed. Gloves may be worn, hands should be washed thoroughly, and patients should be encouraged not to rub their eyes after anesthetic drops have been instilled. This applies to nurses as well as to patients.

If the patient has been given an oral anesthetic spray, the gag reflex and ability to swallow must be tested before the patient is allowed to eat or drink. Without a gag reflex a patient will aspirate anything ingested. Nurses should be careful not to inhale the spray while administering it because absorption through the nasal mucosa is rapid and an anesthetic effect can occur.

□ Injections

After administration of a local anesthetic to a patient having an operative or diagnostic procedure, the OR nurse should assure that environmental stimuli including light, noise, and conversation be kept to a minimum. Many anesthetized patients are hypersensitive to such stimuli and can become anxious and excited. The patient can hear everything so conversation about the procedure should be limited and information should be directly shared with him. Patients under local anesthesia frequently complain they were treated as though they were not present at their own operation. OR staff, accustomed to completely anesthetized patients, must be cognizant of their behavior when the patient receives a local anesthetic.

The sequence of anesthesia with local injection is, in order of occurrence, loss or pain, temperature, sensation of touch, and motor function. Those functions will return in reverse order and provide a method by which the nurse can monitor the effect of anesthesia and, consequently, when the anesthesia is wearing off. For the patient receiving an epidural block this is particularly important because his perception of pain indicates that more of the drug is needed immediately because the block will be more effective if the drug is administered again before the pain returns.

Development of systemic effects must be closely monitored during local anesthesia especially for the drugs used in obstetrical delivery. Symptoms such as hypotension, bradycardia, light-headedness, and excitation can lead to convulsions and are serious. In addition, hypotension in a laboring mother can lead to fetal hypoxia within 4 minutes to 5 minutes. Therefore, maternal and fetal vital signs should be closely monitored. Fluids are usually administered *prior* to epidural or spinal anesthesia to prevent the development of hypotension. If hypotension occurs, the mother will be placed on her left side to displace the uterus and assist vasodilation of abdominal vessels. Fluids will be forced intravenously to rapidly increase fluid volume, legs will be elevated, and oxygen may be administered to maintain adequate levels to the fetus. If the blood pressure does not return to normal, vasoconstrictors such as ephedrine or mephentermine may be administered. Similar actions should be taken in any patient who suffers hypotension as a result of local anesthesia during a procedure.

In any block in which the dura mater has been punctured, the patient may suffer a "spinal headache" as a result of spinal fluid leakage. These headaches are generally not responsive to analgesics, thus the best nursing intervention is to prevent them. Fluids should be forced, up to 3000 ml pre- and postoperatively, and the patient should remain in bed for several hours after anesthesia. Analgesics may provide some relief, at least psychologically. The headache will disappear when the spinal fluid volume returns to normal.

Most local anesthetics for spinal or nerve injection do not contain preservatives. As a result they are unstable, and vials should be discarded after each patient administration, avoiding re-use.

□ EVALUATION

The outcome sought is adequate local anesthesia with minimal systemic absorption and few or no side-effects.

CASE STUDY

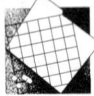

Gwen Harris, age 35, is admitted to the labor room in active labor. Over the next 6 hours her cervix dilates from 3 cm to 8 cm, and the labor pains begin to get very intense coming every 1 minute to 2 minutes and lasting about 1 minute. When the pain seems constant to her and she begins having the urge to push, she and her obstetrician agree to use epidural anesthesia for the delivery.

The anesthesiologist inserts an epidural catheter and an intravenous drip is started and 2% lidocaine is administered. Mrs. Harris is placed on a cardiac monitor and a fetal monitor.

Discussion Questions

1. What information should be collected before Mrs. Harris receives lidocaine?

2. How will epidural anesthesia affect this patient's ability to push during delivery? What strategies must the nurse use to help her?
3. What nursing interventions are necessary during the IV infusion into the epidural space?
4. Postanesthesia, what steps should be taken to protect Mrs. Harris from injury?

REVIEW QUESTIONS

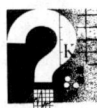

1. How may local anesthetics be classified?
2. Why do local anesthetics need to be converted to the nonionic state following administration?
3. What factors can influence the ratio of cationic/nonionic form of the drug present at any one time in the body?
4. Why are local anesthetics usually less effective when injected into an inflamed area?
5. *Briefly* describe the following routes of injection for local anesthetics: (a) spinal, (b) paravertebral, (c) epidural, (d) caudal, and (e) "saddle block."
6. What is the general sequence by which the various types of nerve fibers are depressed following injection of a local anesthetic?
7. Give several reasons why a vasoconstrictor (*e.g.*, epinephrine) may be added to a local anesthetic solution.
8. What are the major adverse effects associated with local anesthetic usage?
9. Under what conditions should caution be exercised when injecting local anesthetics?
10. What dangers exist for the nurse administering a local anesthetic? How can the nurse protect him- or herself?
11. How can patient anxiety over being awake during an operative procedure be reduced?
12. What nursing interventions should be taken if an obstetrical patient with an epidural block develops hypotension?

BIBLIOGRAPHY

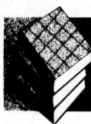

Catteral WA: The molecular basis of neuronal excitability. Science 223:653, 1984
Covino BG: Pharmacology of local anesthetic agents. Ration Drug Ther 21(8):1, 1987
Dahle JS: Caring for the patient with local anesthesia. AORN Journal 27:985, April 1978
deJong RH: Toxic effects of local anesthetics. JAMA 239:1166, 1978
Fink BR (ed): Progress in Anesthesiology: Molecular Mechanisms of Anesthesia, Vol. 2. New York, Raven Press, 1980
Floyd CC: Drugs for childbirth: Your guide to their benefits and risks. RN 41:May 1977
Grad RK, Woodside J: Obstetrical analgesics and anesthesia: Methods of relief for the patient in labor. Am J Nurs 77:242, February 1977
Jensen D: The Human Nervous System. New York, Appleton-Century-Crofts, 1980
Mather LE, Cousins MJ: Local anesthetics and their current clinical use. Drugs 18:185, 1979
Nicolls ET, Corke BC, Osthermer GW: Epidural anesthesia for the woman in labor. Am J Nurs 81:1826, October 1981
Strichartz GR (ed): Local Anesthetics. Handbook of Experimental Pharmacology. Berlin, Springer-Verlag, 1985

General Anesthetics

21

Although alcohols and opiates have been used for centuries in attempts to suppress the pain of surgical procedures, it was not until the mid-1800s that the first demonstrations of drug-induced general anesthesia utilizing the volatile liquids chloroform and diethyl ether were reported. Somewhat later, the anesthetic properties of nitrous oxide gas, originally suggested by Priestley as early as 1776, were revealed. However, the modern age of anesthesia did not begin until the introduction of the intravenous barbiturate, thiopental, in the 1930s, and the skeletal muscle relaxant d-tubocurarine about a decade later. Since that time, a number of general anesthetic agents, both intravenous and inhalational, have been developed, and while certain newer drugs possess distinct advantages over older drugs, no single general anesthetic represents the "ideal" drug in terms of potency, efficacy, stability, and safety. Thus, the practice of general anesthesia commonly involves use of two or more drugs in combination to take advantage of their desirable attributes (e.g., speed of induction, skeletal muscle relaxation), while at the same time minimizing their undesirable characteristics (e.g., respiratory depression, hepatotoxicity). In addition, other types of drugs, such as muscle relaxants, sedatives, and anticholinergics are frequently given either prior to or in conjunction with general anesthetics to provide an adequate degree of skeletal muscle relaxation, calm the anxious patient, and minimize excessive salivary and bronchial secretions, respectively. Selection of a total general anesthetic regimen depends on a number of factors, such as the nature and length of the anticipated surgical procedure, and the pathophysiologic status of the patient. The term "balanced anesthesia" is sometimes applied to the practice of administering two or more anesthetics together with other ancillary medications (e.g., anticholinergics, muscle relaxants, and so forth) to provide smooth induction, sufficient depth and duration of anesthesia, adequate muscle relaxation, decreased tracheobronchial secretions, and minimal hazards to the vital systems. This concept will be reviewed again later in the chapter.

Stages of Anesthesia

As the degree of general anesthesia deepens, a series of physiologic changes ensues which provide an indication of the depth of depression of the CNS. Traditionally, these changes have been categorized into four stages, each of which displays a characteristic physiologic pattern. These stages were originally described for diethyl ether, a drug having a very slow onset of action, and thus exhibiting a distinct separation between the various stages. In modern anesthesiology, however, the distinctive signs of each stage of anesthesia are frequently obscured because many currently used general anesthetics have a very rapid onset of action and quickly bypass the early stages of anesthesia. In addition, mechanical respiratory assistance eliminates the variability in respiratory rate and depth seen with progressive deepening of anesthesia. Finally, certain characteristic signs of the various stages, such as pupillary diameter, tear secretion, and muscle relaxation, can be influenced by the use of preanesthetic medications like anticholinergics and succinylcholine. Therefore, the delineation of anesthesia into distinct stages is imprecise at best with most modern-day general anesthetics, and the appearance and duration of the effects noted in each stage vary widely, depending on the choice of anesthetic, speed of induction, and technique of the anesthesiologist. Table 21-1 presents an overview of the more important physiologic changes that occur as general anesthesia deepens.

Stage I, lasting until consciousness is lost, is characterized by absence of pain (analgesia), increasingly difficult speech, and, frequently, euphoria, vivid dreaming, and some motor excitability. Amnesia is usually present.

Stage II begins with loss of consciousness and is often referred to as the stage of delirium. Respiration is irregular, heart rate and blood pressure increase, and the patient is frequently tense and may struggle, retch, vomit, or urinate. Behavior is very variable in this stage, depending on the speed of induction, type of preanesthetic medication, and the amount of external sensory stimuli. This stage is often quickly bypassed with use of intravenous anesthetics displaying a rapid onset of action.

Stage III is the stage of surgical anesthesia and begins with the return of regular respiration and the appearance of some muscle relaxation. The stage is further subdivided into four *planes*, reflecting an increasing depth of CNS depression and degree of muscle relaxation. The particular plane of anesthesia in stage III is usually determined by several parameters, including pupil size, presence or absence of reflexes, eye movements, and tear secretion. Most surgery is performed in plane 2 or 3 of stage III, because muscle relaxation is optimal at this depth. As the patient passes from plane 1 to plane 4, respiration becomes shallower and more

Table 21-1
Stages and Characteristics of Anesthesia

Stage/plane	Respiration	Cardiovascular	Muscle Tone	Reflexes	Other
Stage 1	Regular	Normal	Normal	Normal	Analgesia, euphoria, amnesia
Stage II	Rapid, irregular	Heart rate and blood pressure increased	Tense Struggling	Swallowing, retching, gagging, vomiting	Mydriasis, roving eyeballs, loss of consciousness, decreased eyelid reflex
Stage III					
Plane 1	Regular	Heart rate and blood pressure normal	Smaller muscles relaxed	Lid and pharyngeal (gag) reflex absent	Increase tear secretion, miosis, some eye movement, increased respiration and blood pressure with incision
Plane 2	Regular but shallower	Heart rate and blood pressure normal	Large muscles relaxed	Corneal and laryngeal reflex absent	Eyes stilled, miosis, decreased tear secretion, no response to incision
Plane 3	Shallow and mainly abdominal	Blood pressure falls slightly; some tachycardia	Complete relaxation	Pupillary (light) and cough reflex disappear	Mydriasis, decreased tear secretion
Plane 4	Abdominal and very shallow	Hypotension and some tachycardia	Complete relaxation	No reflexes	Mydriasis, no lacrimation
Stage IV	Respiratory paralysis	Marked hypotension and failing circulation	Complete relaxation	No reflexes	Extreme mydriasis, medullary paralysis, and eventual death

abdominal, the eyeballs cease roving, reflexes disappear, and skeletal muscles become increasingly relaxed.

When spontaneous respiration ceases, the patient enters stage IV. This stage represents an undesired depth of anesthesia, in which the respiratory and vasomotor centers become depressed to the extent that respiration and circulation fail. Circulatory and respiratory support must be provided at this depth to prevent death.

Mechanisms of General Anesthesia

Although it is well established that general anesthetics act on the CNS to reduce the perception on painful stimuli, the mechanisms by which this action is accomplished have not been precisely determined. In all probability, due to the great diversity in chemical structure among the many general anesthetics, no single mechanism will be able to ade-

quately explain the effects of these drugs. General anesthetics do not interact with specific receptor sites as do many other types of drugs. Rather, they appear to alter the structure or functioning of nerve cell components, thereby reducing neuronal excitability and increasing the firing threshold. One theory as to how this effect is accomplished is the *conformational distortion theory*, which postulates that the physical presence of the anesthetic molecules within the nerve membrane distorts the conformation of the membrane and impedes ionic flow through the channels. The decrease in sodium influx therefore reduces neuronal excitability and slows the rate of rise of the nerve-action potential. While attractive from a mechanistic point of view, this theory probably cannot be applied to all general anesthetics, because the poor lipid solubility of some drugs restricts their access to the nerve membrane. The *Meyer–Overton theory* correlates the potency of a general anesthetic with its lipid solubility; that is, the more lipid soluble a drug is, the greater its anesthetic potency. While this theory can explain differences in uptake of general anesthetics by fatty nerve cell membranes, it does not offer an explanation of how the drugs act once at their site of action. Further, not all highly lipid-soluble substances are anesthetic, and some potent anesthetics are not fat-soluble.

The *hydrate* or *water crystal* theory was proposed in the early 1960s, and states that an anesthetic drug reacts with water in brain tissue to form hydrates or microcrystals of ice which can inhibit nerve cell functioning, perhaps by coating the neuronal membrane, thus impeding ion passage. Although the general correlation between the ability of an anesthetic drug to form hydrates and its potency is rather weak, this theory may offer at least partial explanation for the observation that cold or hypothermia can decrease feeling and sensation, and may allow a smaller dose of general anesthetic to be given with comparable results.

A number of *biochemical theories* have been advanced to explain the generation of anesthesia. Anesthetics have been postulated to inhibit glucose metabolism in brain cells, to block production of high-energy phosphate compounds (ATP), and to impair oxygen utilization and thus cellular respiration. While these effects have been demonstrated *in vitro*, there is no conclusive evidence that such mechanisms occur in the brain when general anesthetics are administered. Therefore, the precise mechanism whereby general anesthetic drugs abolish pain and produce unconsciousness is still largely unknown, in spite of the many interesting theories that have evolved over the years. One can only state with certainty that these drugs decrease the normal level of activity of CNS.

Adjunctive Anesthetic Medications

Production of safe and efficient general anesthesia depends to a great extent on the proper preparation of the patient. As previously mentioned, several other classes of drugs are routinely administered either before, during, or after surgical procedures to facilitate the induction and maintenance of anesthesia and to minimize the occurrence of undesirable reactions. Among the classes of drugs utilized as adjuncts to general anesthesia are the following:

· *Sedatives*—Generally a benzodiazepine (*e.g.*, diazepam, lorazepam, midazolam) is administered prior to surgery to calm the anxious patient. Short-acting barbiturates (*e.g.*, pentobarbital, secobarbital) have also been used for this purpose, but the danger of increased respiratory depression is greater with barbiturates than with benzodiazepines. Hydroxyzine is also employed for preoperative sedation, and produces minimal circulatory and respiratory depression but does not prolong anesthesia.

· *Anticholinergics*—Atropine or one of the synthetic anticholinergics is usually given prior to a general anesthetic to reduce salivary and bronchial secretions, which can be excessive with certain inhaled anesthetics. In addition, atropine decreases cardiac vagal tone and thus limits the reflex bradycardia frequently associated with general anesthetics.

· *Narcotics*—Various narcotic drugs (*e.g.*, morphine, meperidine, sufentanil, fentanyl) have been employed prior to surgery to reduce anxiety, provide an additional degree of analgesia, decrease the cough reflex, and reduce the amount of anesthetic needed. The use of narcotics for preoperative sedation and analgesia is subject to some controversy, however, inasmuch as they may depress respiration and cough, prolong the anesthetic state, and induce postoperative nausea and vomiting. Their use is largely a matter of physician preference.

· *Skeletal Muscle Relaxants*—Neuromuscular blocking agents, such as succinylcholine, pancuronium, and gallamine, are frequently included in the anesthetic regimen to provide an additional degree of skeletal muscle relaxation and therefore allow a lower dose of general anesthetic to be used, reducing the incidence of adverse reactions. Because they are all relatively short-acting drugs, good control of skeletal muscle activity can be maintained by an experienced anesthetist. (For a more complete description of the peripherally acting skeletal muscle relaxants, see Chap. 19.)

· *Antiemetics*—Postoperative nausea and vomiting can be controlled by use of an antiemetic during the recovery period. A commonly used drug for this purpose is the phenothiazine, prochlorperazine; other useful antiemetics include scopolamine, cyclizine, and trimethobenzamide.

Other types of drugs that are occasionally administered postoperatively are cholinergics such as bethanechol for the relief of abdominal distention and urinary retention, analgesics to provide necessary pain relief, and laxatives to relieve constipation.

Classification of General Anesthetics

The clinically useful general anesthetics may be classified in the following manner:
 I. Inhalation anesthetics
   A. Gases (e.g., nitrous oxide, cyclopropane)
   B. Volatile liquids (e.g., halothane, isoflurane)
 II. Intravenous anesthetics
   A. Ultra short-acting barbiturates (e.g., thiopental, methohexital)
   B. Nonbarbiturate hypnotics (e.g., etomidate)
   C. Dissociative agents (e.g., ketamine, Innovar—may also be given IM)

Although the basic clinical pharmacology of each general anesthetic drug will be reviewed here, anyone handling these drugs on a routine basis should become thoroughly familiar with the advantages and disadvantages of each preparation and the procedures for their proper administration (i.e., open–drop, semiclosed, or complete rebreathing methods) by consulting specific literature sources pertaining to each agent. The following monographs will attempt to provide the essential information concerning the more widely used drugs but should not be viewed as a complete description of the pharmacologic properties and clinical implications of the compounds.

■ Nursing Process

Note: Specific comment will be offered on individual drugs where appropriate, but most nursing intervention is similar for all general anesthetics.

□ PREOPERATIVE ASSESSMENT

□ Subjective Data
A detailed family history, including questions about malignant hyperthermia, porphyria, cardiovascular disease, diabetes, and kidney disease should be obtained preoperatively. Because the effect of anesthesia is widespread among all body systems, identification of any problems will help the operating room staff better plan care.

A history of alcohol or drug abuse is also significant in assessing the patient about to be anesthetized. A person suffering from alcohol or drug withdrawal is a poor risk for anesthesia because these street drugs will affect the predictability of the anesthesia's effect. Once such a variable is discovered, alternate plans for local methods of anesthesia may be preferred.

If the patient has been under anesthesia before, the nurse should ask about past reactions or perceptions of the event. Some people will report difficulty in "going under" or emerging from anesthesia. Because response to doses of anesthetic by people even of similar size is widely variable this factor may help the anesthesiologist facilitate easier induction and emergence.

Each patient undergoing surgery has a variety of perceptions of what will happen and harbors many fears about bodily mutilation. These mind–body fears are frequently coupled with unvoiced anxiety about loss of self-control, never again waking up, brain damage, and death. Fears and anxieties are better discussed preoperatively; doing so may actually make induction of anesthesia easier. If this information is obtained early in assessment, the nurse will be better able to plan the kind of information to share so as not to overwhelm the patient and increase his anxiety.

□ Objective Data
A complete physical assessment should be completed for anyone undergoing general anesthesia so an adequate functional baseline can be established. Usually the site of surgery will be subject to the most detailed review but cardiovascular, respiratory, renal, and hepatic function must be known.

□ NURSING DIAGNOSES
Actual preoperative nursing diagnoses for the patient receiving general anesthesia include:
   Knowledge deficit related to the effects of anesthesia on the body and what postoperative care will be like
   Anxiety or fear related to unknown events surrounding surgery
Potential nursing diagnoses for the patient during and after anesthesia may include:
   Potential alteration in body temperature related to effects of emergence
   Ineffective breathing pattern related to depth of anesthesia and effect on respiratory muscles
   Alteration in cardiac output: decreased, related to an adverse response to anesthesia
   Impaired gas exchange related to inadequate respiratory drive if a toxic reaction to anesthesia occurs

Functional incontinence
Potential for injury: trauma
Sensory–perceptual alteration of all senses
Impaired swallowing related to intubation

□ *PLAN*

The goals for preoperative discussion about anesthesia may include the following:
1. The patient will meet the anesthesiologist and operating room nurse who will care for him so he sees some familiar faces in a frightening environment.
2. The type of anesthesia and its effects will be discussed.
3. The patient will be allowed to verbalize what he thinks will happen as he is anesthetized.
4. The patient will be taught preoperatively some early postoperative activities so he will know what care will be rendered as he emerges from anesthesia.

The goals for intraoperative care of the patient should include:
1. The patient will be protected from injury and disturbing environmental stimuli to ensure safety throughout the procedure.
2. Measures will be taken to have all necessary drugs and equipment on hand in case of cardiac or respiratory arrest, development of malignant hyperthermia, or other emergencies.

The goals for recovery room care of the patient emerging from anesthesia include:
1. Systematic, frequent assessment of vital signs, level of consciousness, side-effects of anesthesia to ensure safe emergence
2. Protection from injury
3. Maintenance of emergency equipment for use if needed

□ *INTERVENTION*

□ *Patient Education about Anesthesia*

The patient needs an opportunity to meet the anesthesiologist to know who will be responsible for "putting him to sleep" and what anesthetic will be given. The anesthesiologist can obtain a medical history, particularly of respiratory disorders and medication taken, including use of alcohol or street drugs which may influence anesthesia induction. He will usually give an explanation of the anesthesia process. However, the patient may be left with unanswered questions especially if the interview was short, or if the patient was anxious or did not know what questions to ask.

Preoperative teaching by the nurse after the anesthesiology visit can allay patient anxiety. Frequent questions patients ask include: Will I talk during anesthesia? Will I be paralyzed? How will I be protected? How do you keep me from falling off the table? Will they take my gown off? Will I fight when I'm going under? Will I suffocate with the mask over my face? These should provide the nurse with clues about the patient's multiple fears. By discussing these fears, past experiences, and a little about how anesthesia feels, many of a patient's concerns can be alleviated. If the same nurse doing the preoperative teaching is available to be at the patient's side during anesthesia induction, anxiety and panic in the patient tend to be greatly reduced.

Preoperative teaching should also discuss what will happen as the patient emerges from anesthesia. An explanation of the various equipment to be attached, particularly the use of an endotracheal tube or other airway may help decrease the panic the patient feels when he wakes up. A patient is more likely to be cooperative in the early postoperative period if he is given information about the tubes, blood pressure readings, IVs, and his role in a preoperative teaching discussion. Many patients have some short-term memory loss following anesthesia but will usually remember preoperative explanations before any drugs have been administered.

□ *Intraoperative Care*

The circulating nurse in the operating room is responsible for ensuring that all emergency equipment is available should anything untoward occur during surgery. Cardiac arrest is a possibility when general anesthesia is administered, and, while the patient will already be mechanically ventilated, emergency cardiac drugs, EKG machine, and defibrillator should be easily accessible.

Another emergency the circulating nurse may need to plan for is the onset of malignant hyperthermia which can occur after the initial induction of anesthesia. Treatment must be rapid and will include sponge baths, use of a hypothermia blanket, and rapid administration of dantrolene. (See Chap. 19.)

□ *Postoperative Care*

In the recovery room, postoperative care should focus on careful monitoring of the patient's vital signs. As anesthesia wears off, any of these parameters can change quickly so vital signs taken every 5 minutes to 15 minutes may be the standard procedure until the patient is discharged to his room.

Assessment of airway and breathing is most critical in the recovery phase because respiration is the source of many postoperative complications. The nurse should monitor rate, depth of breathing, and presence of wheezing, snoring, coughing, or stridor. Tracheal irritation from the endotracheal tube or the anesthetic gases can result in laryngospasm; poor excretion of the gases may reduce the respiratory rate. Any of these can result in respiratory distress and arrest. Emergency resuscitative equipment should be in the recovery room including a ventilator to provide mechanical assistance, if necessary.

Temperature should also be monitored. Malignant hyperthermia can occur up through the early recovery phase from anesthesia. More frequently, the patient will develop slight hypothermia resulting in a severe shivering response. This symptom will disappear as the anesthesia wears off, but providing extra blankets will increase patient comfort. In severe cases, the patient may need oxygen to compensate for that lost due to the metabolic exertion of shivering.

Pulse and blood pressure will slowly return to pre-anesthesia levels. Vital signs in the initial recovery stage will indicate bradycardia and hypotension. If hypotension persists, the legs should be elevated to promote venous return, and the physician should be notified. Oxygen may be administered to improve cellular oxygen saturation during the period of reduced cardiac output and respiratory drive.

Patients also experience changes in level of consciousness as they emerge from anesthesia. These may range from sleepy but arousable to highly combative. Although the latter behavior is not frequent, patients have been known to thrash and throw punches. Occasionally, such a patient may need some sedation and restraints to protect himself and others from injury. Usually the patient will have no recollection of such behavior once fully aroused. More frequently, the patient will be lethargic although arousable. The nurse can facilitate awakening by calling the patient's name and reorienting him to time, place, and the sequence of events that have occurred.

Patients also occasionally experience nausea and vomiting on emergence from anesthesia. Placing the patient in a sidelying position, if not contraindicated by surgery, will reduce the chance of aspiration if vomiting does occur. An antiemetic may be ordered by the anesthesiologist if vomiting persists.

When vital signs are stable, the anesthesiologist will discharge the patient, and the recovery room nurse will be responsible for passing information on to the nurse receiving the patient in his room. Information about vital signs, level of consciousness, fluids, type of anesthesia, and urinary output will help the floor nurse continue the careful monitoring of the patient emerging from anesthesia.

□ EVALUATION

The outcomes by which to judge success of general anesthesia are safe emergence from anesthesia with minimal side-effects and return of normal vital signs.

Occupational Hazards for Nursing Staff

During anesthesia, anesthetic waste gas (i.e., that lost from the anesthesia machine and equipment and the vapors that expire from the patient) enters the operating room environment. All operating room personnel are then exposed to the waste gas, and such exposure constitutes an occupational hazard.

The side-effects reported are more frequently related to exposure to halothane and nitrous oxide, the most commonly used anesthetic gases. Evidence exists that the prolonged exposure to gases may lead to symptoms that range from headaches, fatigue, and irritability to spontaneous abortion, congenital anomalies, hepatic disease, renal disease, and cancer of lymph glands and other parts of the immunologic system. Congenital anomalies have appeared in children born to parents when only the father is exposed to the gases (Seuffert, 1976).

Nurses who work in operating room settings need to be aware of the risks and to advocate a safe environment for all. Methods to reduce exposure to anesthetic waste gases include scavenging techniques to detect and eliminate gases, nonrecirculating ventilating systems in surgical suites so the gases are eliminated soon after they escape, periodic maintenance of anesthesia equipment, use of low-leak equipment, and a safe work technique by the anesthetist to keep concentrations of the gases at safe levels. State departments of health generally set guidelines for safe practice, but nurses should know how the operating room administration enacts those guidelines to monitor employee safety.

Inhalation Anesthetics

The inhalation anesthetics include gases and volatile liquids. Both types enter the circulation rapidly following absorption from the alveoli of the lungs. However, in order for anesthesia to occur, the drug must be transferred from the alveoli to the blood, then to the brain. Many factors determine the rapidity and efficiency of this transfer. Among the more important are the lipid-solubility of the drug, its concentration in inspired air, the pulmonary ventilation rate and blood flow, and the blood gas partition coefficient. Because it is not practical to measure the anesthetic concentration in brain tissue directly, a frequently used measure of anesthetic potency is the minimum alveolar concentration (MAC), which is defined as the concentration of anesthetic in the alveoli of the lungs which prevents response to painful stimuli (e.g., incision) in 50% of patients. The lower the MAC, the more potent is the anesthetic drug. Table 21-2 lists some representative MACs for commonly used general anesthetics, along with other characteristics of these drugs. It should be remembered that MAC values are based on the presence of the general anesthetic alone, without adjunctive medication. The use of sedatives, narcotics, or other preanesthetic medications will lower the effective MAC, and thus the inspired concentration of drug should be lowered accordingly. In general, most surgery is performed between 0.8 and 1.2 times the MAC, although as low as one half the MAC may be used, depending on the presence of adjunctive medications that may enhance the response to the general anesthetic drug.

Gases

Three gases (cyclopropane, ethylene, nitrous oxide) are currently available for use as general anesthetics, and of these, only nitrous oxide is used to any extent. In fact, it is one of the most widely used of all general anesthetics, most often as part of a total anesthetic regimen which may include sedatives, other anesthetics, narcotics, barbiturates, and muscle relaxants. Such a regimen, termed *balanced anesthesia*, usually produces rapid induction

---

Table 21-2
Characteristics of Inhalation Anesthetics

Drug	Minimum Alveolar Concentration (MAC)* %	Onset of Anesthesia	Muscle-Relaxing Action
Gases			
cyclopropane	10	Rapid	Fair
ethylene	80	Rapid	Poor
nitrous oxide	>100†	Rapid	Fair
Volatile Liquids			
enflurane	1.68	Rapid	Good
ether	2.0	Slow	Excellent
halothane	0.75	Rapid	Fair
isoflurane	1.2	Rapid	Good
methoxyflurane	0.16	Slow	Fair/Good

* MAC = minimum concentration of inhalational anesthetic drug (in percent) in the alveoli that prevents a response to surgical incision in 50% of patients; serves as a standard for comparison of the potency among general anesthetics; the lower the MAC, the more potent the drug.
† A MAC of greater than 100% indicates that not even one MAC can be attained at normal barometric pressure; nitrous oxide is the least potent general anesthetic.

with minimal adverse effects, and it allows a significant reduction in the amount of each drug required.

The other two gases, cyclopropane and ethylene, are seldom used today because of their highly flammable and explosive nature.

Cyclopropane

Cyclopropane is an anesthetic gas which has a rapid onset of action and a good safety margin and produces satisfactory analgesia and skeletal muscle relaxation in full anesthetic doses. Due to its explosive nature, it must be administered in a closed, rebreathing system with oxygen. Respiratory irritation is minimal, although occasional laryngospasm has occurred, and blood pressure is well maintained during anesthesia. However, the drug does sensitize the myocardium to the arrhythmogenic effects of catecholamines, and this can result in sudden death. Maintenance of adequate ventilation will minimize the possibility of arrhythmias. Postoperative nausea, vomiting, and headaches occur frequently following use of cyclopropane. Malignant hyperthermia has been associated with cyclopropane administration.

Previously, cyclopropane has been used for a variety of operative procedures, especially in patients with cardiovascular complications, respiratory difficulty, or impending shock. It has also been used in obstetrics because the drug does not affect uterine contractions.

For induction, concentrations up to 50% have been employed, whereas maintenance levels are usually 10% to 50%. Emergence excitement can occur, which can be reduced by administering a sedative or narcotic prior to discontinuing the drug. Extreme caution such as use of antistatic equipment must be exercised during administration of cyclopropane to prevent an explosion. The drug is essentially obsolete today.

Ethylene

Ethylene is a highly volatile gas which produces rapid induction and recovery, exhibits low toxicity, and possesses a wide safety margin. It is similar to, but slightly more potent than nitrous oxide; however, unlike nitrous oxide, it is highly explosive and has an unpleasant odor. Muscle relaxation is poor. Ethylene must be given in high concentrations (80%) with oxygen in a closed system, and the

major danger is hypoxia. Due to the availability of more potent and less hazardous general anesthetics, the use of ethylene today is almost nonexistent.

Nitrous Oxide (N_2O)

MECHANISM AND ACTIONS
Nitrous oxide, also known as laughing gas, is an inorganic general anesthetic gas commonly used as a component of "balanced anesthesia" and as a supplement to more potent inhalational anesthetics. It is nonexplosive and displays a very rapid onset of action (due to its low solubility in blood and hence faster penetration into the CNS) and a correspondingly short duration. Nitrous oxide is a poor skeletal muscle relaxant and due to its lack of potency, can only induce a very light plane of surgical anesthesia. Thus, anesthesia of sufficient depth to perform most surgical procedures cannot be attained with nitrous oxide alone without seriously depriving the patient of oxygen. Hypoxia will result if concentrations of nitrous oxide greater than 80% are used for any length of time, so at least 20% oxygen is provided whenever nitrous oxide is administered. Moderate analgesia can be obtained with 20% to 30% nitrous oxide, and concentrations of 60% to 70% are sufficient to prolong surgical anesthesia in the presence of another general anesthetic in the properly premedicated patient.

USES
1. Induction of anesthesia
2. Supplemental maintenance of general anesthesia
3. Production of analgesia for minor surgical or dental procedures

ADMINISTRATION AND DOSAGE
Nitrous oxide is given by inhalation, in oxygen mixture. For analgesia, 20% to 50% of N_2O may be used in brief surgical or dental procedures in which muscle relaxation is not required, or in obstetrics. As a component of balanced anesthesia, it is used in concentrations of 50% to 70% to prolong the anesthetic state and reduce the amount of other general anesthetics required. For rapid induction of anesthesia, concentrations of 80% and occasionally higher may be given for brief periods of time.

FATE
Onset of anesthesia is rapid, and the duration of action is short. Excretion is almost entirely by exhalation.

SIDE-EFFECTS/ADVERSE REACTIONS

Untoward reactions to nitrous oxide are infrequent, but some patients may experience dizziness, vivid dreaming, and possibly hallucinations while the drug is being administered. Serious consequences may occur if a state of hypoxia develops for any length of time, and cyanosis, convulsions, leukopenia, and bone marrow depression can occur. Very high concentrations of nitrous oxide may result in vomiting, myocardial and respiratory depression, and ultimately death.

Because nitrous oxide is normally used at high concentrations and is considerably more soluble in blood than nitrogen, it will enter pockets of trapped gas, replacing nitrogen and expanding the volume of gas. This situation can occur in the bowel, lung, or middle ear, resulting in possible damage to the organs as a consequence of rapid expansion. Likewise, a significant elevation in cerebrospinal fluid pressure has occurred with nitrous oxide following injection of air into the cerebral ventricles during a pneumoencephalogram.

NURSING CONSIDERATIONS

Nitrous oxide is favored because of its short duration and is frequently used in outpatient surgery and dental work. However, the nurse should exercise caution in releasing such a patient by asking the patient orienting questions and monitoring alertness and attention span. These patients should not drive until the effect of the medication has worn off; such responses are extremely individual.

Volatile Liquids

Other than nitrous oxide, the most commonly used inhalational general anesthetics are the volatile liquids. They are administered by inhalation of the vapors given off by the liquid along with adequate amounts of oxygen. The depth of anesthesia can be fairly well controlled by varying the concentration, because these agents are generally short acting. Recovery begins as soon as the drug is removed, because most drugs are excreted largely through the lungs.

The first volatile liquid to be used was diethyl ether, and for many years, it represented the preferred inhalational anesthetic. Today, however, ether is essentially obsolete, owing to the availability of more potent, more rapid acting, and safer general anesthetics. Therefore, ether will be discussed briefly below, primarily because of its historical importance. The four other currently available volatile liquid general anesthetics possess distinct advantages and disadvantages relative to one another and will be reviewed individually.

Ether (Diethyl Ether)

Diethyl ether was the first clinically useful volatile liquid anesthetic. Among its advantages are a good safety margin, excellent skeletal muscle-relaxing ability, minimal effects on the cardiovascular system, and substantial analgesic effect. These advantages, however, are considerably outweighed by the drug's disadvantages, which include a noxious odor, slow and often unpleasant induction, prolonged emergence, respiratory irritation, increased salivary and bronchial secretions, high incidence of postoperative nausea and vomiting, and its extreme flammability.

Ether is occasionally used where sophisticated patient-monitoring equipment is not available, primarily due to its good safety margin. The various stages of anesthesia (see Table 21-1) are well delineated with ether due to its slow induction and recovery, and this level of anesthesia can be fairly well controlled by patient observation.

Concentrations of 5% to 10% have previously been used to induce anesthesia, although the induction process is slow and uncomfortable, and the drug is rarely used in this manner. Good surgical anesthesia can be maintained with concentrations of 3% to 5% in combination with other general anesthetics.

The clinical use of diethyl ether has declined markedly in recent years, and the drug is becoming obsolete.

NURSING CONSIDERATIONS

Nursing intervention aims to deal with the slow emergence from ether anesthesia and the nausea associated with the anesthetic.

To control nausea, preoperative administration of anticholinergics will reduce the secretions and the chance of aspiration. Postoperatively, the patient should be positioned on his side, especially if he is nauseous, to reduce the chance of aspiration should he begin to vomit. Turning only the head to the side will do little to avoid aspiration.

During the emergence phase the patient should be adequately protected because his sensations will be altered for a prolonged period of time. Careful positioning to avoid undue pressure on any body part and padding to prevent injury will help because the patient will have little sense of his position in space or of pain or pressure until the anesthesia wears off.

Enflurane
(Ethrane)

MECHANISM AND ACTIONS

Enflurane is a potent, volatile liquid anesthetic widely used today for many surgical procedures. Induction and recovery are rapid, skeletal muscle relaxation is good (only minimal amounts of muscle relaxants are needed for more extensive surgery), and the drug is nonflammable. Salivary and bronchial secretions are increased, myocardial contractility is somewhat depressed while the heart rate is unchanged, and blood pressure is usually reduced. High concentrations of enflurane have a CNS stimulant effect and can result in increased muscle contractions and possibly seizures. For this reason, enflurane is frequently given in combination with nitrous oxide, which allows use of a smaller amount of enflurane and hence less danger of CNS excitation.

USES
1. Induction and maintenance of general anesthesia, frequently in combination with nitrous oxide and/or minimal amounts of skeletal muscle relaxants
2. Provide analgesia for vaginal delivery or supplement other anesthetics for cesarean section

ADMINISTRATION AND DOSAGE

Enflurane may be administered at concentrations of 2% to 4.5% for 7 minutes to 10 minutes to induce anesthesia. Surgical levels of anesthesia can usually be maintained with concentrations between 0.5% and 3%.

FATE

Onset of anesthesia and recovery are very rapid. Due to its fairly low solubility, it is excreted largely unchanged through the lungs, with only minimal amounts (2%–3%) of a dose absorbed and metabolized in the liver, partially to fluoride ion, and excreted in the kidney.

SIDE-EFFECTS/ADVERSE REACTIONS

A slight fall in blood pressure is frequently observed following enflurane administration, and shivering can occur during emergence. With increasing depth of anesthesia, decreases in force of cardiac muscle contraction have been observed, and CNS stimulation can occur with prolonged use, possibly resulting in muscle spasm, tremors, and convulsions. Kidney function may be impaired if the concentration of fluoride ion resulting from drug metabolism becomes excessive.

CONTRAINDICATIONS AND PRECAUTIONS

Enflurane should be administered with *caution* to persons with impaired kidney function, a history of epilepsy or other convulsive states, cardiac disease, or arrhythmias.

INTERACTIONS
1. An increased potential for arrhythmias resulting from the effects of catecholamines on the myocardium may occur in the presence of enflurane.
2. Additive myocardial depression can occur when enflurane is used in combination with beta-blockers, quinidine, procainamide, disopyramide, digitalis drugs, and verapamil.
3. Enflurane may potentiate the muscle-relaxing effects of antidepolarizing neuromuscular blockers.

Halothane
(Fluothane)

MECHANISM AND ACTIONS

Halothane is a potent, nonflammable, pleasant-smelling volatile liquid anesthetic, and is one of the most widely used anesthetic drugs. It is nonirritating to the respiratory tract, dilates the bronchioles, and does not increase salivary or bronchial secretions. Muscle relaxation is only fair with halothane, and a skeletal muscle relaxant is almost always used. Halothane is a myocardial depressant and cardiac output, contractile force, and blood pressure all decrease following administration. In addition, the drug sensitizes the myocardium to the arrhythmogenic effects of catecholamines, and serious arrhythmias can result if a catecholamine is used in the presence of halothane. Respiratory depression is marked, and apnea, hypoxia, and acidosis may develop during deep anesthesia; controlled ventilation is commonly employed with halothane. Postanesthetic nausea and vomiting are rare.

USES
1. Induction and maintenance of general anesthesia

ADMINISTRATION AND DOSAGE

Halothane is commonly administered by closed inhalation, frequently with either oxygen or a mixture of nitrous oxide and oxygen. The concentration of drug necessary for induction varies among different patients, usually within a range of 1% to 4%. Concentrations of 0.5% to 1.5% are adequate to maintain the desired level of surgical anesthesia.

FATE

Induction and recovery are rapid. Elimination is primarily by way of the lungs, although some drug is metabolized in the liver (some metabolites may be responsible for toxic effects—see below). The metabolites are excreted in the urine.

SIDE-EFFECTS/ADVERSE REACTIONS

Halothane frequently produces rapid, shallow respiration, slight fall in blood pressure, and transient bradycardia. These effects may become more intense as the level of anesthesia deepens. Severe hypotension and respiratory depression have occurred with elevated levels of halothane. Arrhythmias can be precipitated in the presence of catecholamines. A potential complication of halothane administration is liver damage, and this is thought to be due to a hypersensitivity reaction, perhaps to one of the metabolic products. The incidence of hepatic damage is higher in persons with prior hepatic disease, and increases with repetitive doses, although the hepatotoxic effects do not appear to occur in children. The drug should not be used a second time in persons who show evidence of liver dysfunction following initial use of halothane, or who show such reactions as fever, anorexia, vomiting, or abdominal pain (see under Contraindications and Precautions). Malignant hyperthermia is possible with halothane, although the occurrence is rare.

CONTRAINDICATIONS AND PRECAUTIONS

Halothane should not be used for obstetrical anesthesia because the drug is a potent uterine relaxant. Other contraindications include active hepatic or biliary disease and in combination with catecholamines. *Cautious use* of halothane is indicated in persons with cardiac disease or preexisting liver dysfunction and during pregnancy.

INTERACTIONS

1. Halothane may potentiate the effects of antidepolarizing skeletal muscle relaxants such as gallamine or pancuronium and also ganglionic blockers.
2. The combination of halothane and catecholamines may result in development of arrhythmias.
3. Halothane may prevent uterine response to ergot drugs or oxytocin.

NURSING CONSIDERATIONS

If marked hypotension occurs postoperatively from halothane anesthesia, the physician should be contacted immediately. Vasopressors such as ephedrine and phenylephrine may be used to treat the hypotension; atropine should be available to treat associated bradycardia.

Shivering is frequently a side-effect of halothane anesthesia. The patient may need to be warmed by controlling environmental temperature and providing extra blankets to completely cover him. Oxygen may be administered if shivering is sufficient to increase metabolism. Symptoms of oxygen deprivation may include change in sensorium and rapid breathing.

Isoflurane
(Forane)

MECHANISM AND ACTIONS

Isoflurane is a volatile liquid general anesthetic structurally similar to enflurane, but with several advantages. It exhibits a rapid onset and quick recovery, possesses good muscle-relaxing ability, but has minimal CNS excitatory effects. Isoflurane does not sensitize the heart to the arrhythmogenic effects of catecholamines. Blood pressure progressively decreases with increasing dosage, and respiratory depression may be significant with larger than recommended doses.

USES

1. Induction and maintenance of general anesthesia

DOSAGE

For induction of anesthesia, concentrations between 1.5% and 3% are administered over 5 minutes to 10 minutes. To maintain the desired depth of anesthesia, 1% to 2.5% concentrations are given together with nitrous oxide.

FATE

Both induction and recovery from anesthesia are quite rapid. Excretion is primarily through the lungs. Less than 1% of the total amount absorbed is metabolized.

SIDE-EFFECTS/ADVERSE REACTIONS
A mild decrease in blood pressure is occasionally noted during administration. Other untoward reactions attributable to isoflurane are respiratory depression, tachycardia, and, rarely, malignant hyperthermia.

CONTRAINDICATIONS AND PRECAUTIONS
There are no absolute contraindications to isoflurane. The agent must be used *cautiously*, however, in persons with respiratory disease or cardiac failure.

INTERACTIONS
1. The muscle relaxant effect of isoflurane may be augmented by concomitant use of other skeletal muscle relaxants.
2. Increased respiratory depression can occur if isoflurane is used in combination with barbiturates, narcotics, and other respiratory depressants.

Methoxyflurane
(Penthrane)

MECHANISM AND ACTIONS
A potent volatile liquid anesthetic, methoxyflurane is highly soluble in blood, thus exhibiting a rather slow onset and prolonged recovery. Analgesia is quite marked, even before consciousness is lost and persists for some time following the regaining of consciousness, reducing the need for postsurgical analgesics. Muscle relaxation is only fair when the drug is used at safe anesthetic concentrations, but becomes quite good at higher concentration levels. Cardiovascular function is depressed similar to halothane; however, methoxyflurane does not sensitize the myocardium to catecholamines.

USES
1. Maintenance of surgical anesthesia of less than 4 hours' duration (usually with nitrous oxide and oxygen)
2. Analgesia in obstetrics and minor surgical procedures

ADMINISTRATION AND DOSAGE
To provide adequate analgesia for minor surgical procedures, concentrations of 0.3% to 0.8% are administered by inhalation. To induce general anesthesia, the drug has been given at concentrations of up to 2% for short periods of time (2 minutes–5 minutes). Lower levels (0.1%–2%) are then used to maintain an adequate level of anesthesia, together with oxygen and at least 50% nitrous oxide.

FATE
Onset of surgical anesthesia is slow, but analgesia develops more rapidly. Emergence is prolonged, and drowsiness often persists after consciousness is regained. Excretion is primarily through the lungs, but some metabolism occurs in the liver, yielding free fluoride ion, which may be nephrotoxic (see below).

SIDE-EFFECTS/ADVERSE REACTIONS
The most common side-effects with methoxyflurane are slight hypotension, nausea, and postanesthetic drowsiness. Other adverse reactions include respiratory depression, delirium, hepatic dysfunction (*e.g.*, jaundice, necrosis), malignant hyperthermia (rare), and renal dysfunction, possibly resulting in renal failure. This latter complication is due to the fact that the drug is stored in body fat and slowly metabolized to the free fluoride ion over several days. If the fluoride ion concentration becomes large enough, a high output (polyuric) renal failure can develop, as the kidney loses its concentrating ability. The potential nephrotoxicity of methoxyflurane is the major reason for its rather limited usage today.

CONTRAINDICATIONS AND PRECAUTIONS
Methoxyflurane is contraindicated in renal disease, cirrhosis, and viral hepatitis. It should not be given to patients with a history of hepatotoxicity to other inhalational anesthetics, to patients who have recently received methoxyflurane or to patients undergoing vascular surgery near the renal vessels. The drug must be administered with *caution* to persons with diabetes or altered liver function values, during pregnancy, and for surgical procedures lasting beyond four hours, because the danger of fluoride ion accumulation increases progressively with the length of time the drug is given.

INTERACTIONS
1. Use of methoxyflurane with certain nephrotoxic antibiotics (*e.g.*, vancomycin, aminoglycosides, amphotericin) may result in fatal renal toxicity.
2. The muscle-relaxing action of antidepolarizing neuromuscular blocking agents may be aug-

mented by methoxyflurane; reduce dose of each accordingly.

NURSING CONSIDERATIONS
Postoperative evaluation of renal function including urine output, creatinine levels, and electrolytes should be ordered to monitor the development of nephrotoxicity. Narcotic administration for pain will be given conservatively in the first 6 postoperative hours because the effects of narcotics and methoxyflurane may result in respiratory depression.

Intravenous Anesthetics

The general anesthetics administered IV include three ultra-short-acting barbiturates, which are used mainly for induction of anesthesia but may also be employed as the sole general anesthetic in short surgical procedures associated with minimal pain. The barbiturates can also serve as supplements to other anesthetic agents during longer procedures.

They are rapidly taken up by the brain following IV injection and almost as rapidly redistributed to other parts of the body. Therefore, within 5 minutes after injection, the brain level of the barbiturate has declined to about one half of its peak attained shortly (30 sec–45 sec) after injection, and only about one tenth of the initial concentration remains in the brain at 30 minutes following injection because the drug has been redistributed to other fatty stores in the body. Emergence occurs during this period of declining brain levels, even though the rate of metabolism and excretion of the drug from the body is quite constant and rather slow (10%–15%/hour).

A rapid-acting, nonbarbiturate hypnotic, etomidate, is also available for IV use as an induction anesthetic and may also be useful for supplementing other anesthetics such as nitrous oxide.

Two other drugs that can be administered either IV or IM are categorized as dissociative anesthetics because they induce a neuroleptic-like effect characterized by analgesia, quietude, and detachment from the environment without loss of consciousness. These two drugs, ketamine and Innovar, differ slightly in some of their pharmacologic properties, and will be discussed separately below.

Ultra-Short-Acting Barbiturates

The barbiturates employed in general anesthesia are those having an extremely rapid onset and rela-

tively short duration (15 min–30 min) of action. The response of the CNS to these drugs is essentially the same as that following an inhalation anesthetic—in succeeding order, loss of consciousness, diminished reflexes, loss of motor tone, and ultimately failure of the vital medullary centers. Recovery proceeds in the reverse direction.

The major advantages of the IV barbiturates compared to many inhalation anesthetics are the rapidity and smoothness of onset, absence of salivation, greater patient acceptance (no occlusive face mask), short duration (allowing better control), speedy recovery, nonflammability, absence of bronchial irritation, and little danger of arrhythmias.

Disadvantages of the IV anesthetics include higher incidences of respiratory and circulatory depression, laryngospasm, bronchospasm, and the danger of tissue necrosis if leakage occurs. Prolonged or repeated administration may result in cumulative toxicity because the drugs are removed slowly from the body.

As there are many similarities among the three anesthetic barbiturates, they will be discussed as a group. Dosages, as well as specific information pertaining to each drug, will then be given in Table 21-3.

Methohexital
(Brevital)

Thiamylal
(Surital)

Thiopental
(Pentothal)

MECHANISM AND ACTIONS
The intravenous barbiturates exert a CNS-depressant effect to produce hypnosis and anesthesia without analgesia. Muscle relaxation is generally

Table 21-3
Intravenous Barbiturate Anesthetics

Drug	Preparations	Usual Dosage Range	Clinical Considerations
methohexital (Brevital)	Powder for injection— 500 mg, 2.5 g, 5 g	*Induction*—5 ml–12 ml of a 1% solution by infusion at a rate of 1 ml/5 sec *Maintenance*—2 ml–4 ml of a 1% solution every 4 min–7 min	Shortest-acting IV barbiturate, poor muscle-relaxing ability; proper preanesthetic medication should be given. Sterile water for injection is the preferred diluent. Do not use dilutions that are not clear and colorless. Dilutions in sterile water are stable at room temperature for 6 weeks. Do not mix with acid solutions or allow contact with silicone. Incompatible with lactated Ringer's solution.
thiamylal (Surital)	Powder for injection— 1 g, 5 g, 10 g	*Induction*—3 ml–6 ml of a 2.5% solution at a rate of 1 ml/5 sec *Maintenance*—2.5% solution by intermittent IV injection as needed or 0.3% solution by continuous drip	Similar to methohexital with a longer duration of action (10–30 min). Do not mix with atropine, tubocurarine, or succinylcholine; do not reconstitute with Ringer's solution or solutions containing bacteriostatic agents or buffers. Sterile water for injection is the preferred diluent for IV injection solutions. Continuous drip solutions are prepared with 5% dextrose or isotonic sodium chloride to avoid hypotonicity. Use only clear solutions. Stable at room temperature for 24 h and refrigerated for 6 days.
thiopental (Pentothal)	Injection—250 mg, 400 mg, 500 mg syringes Powder for injection— 500 mg, 1 g, 2.5 g, 5 g Rectal suspension— 400 mg/g of suspension	Anesthesia *Induction*—2 ml–3 ml of 2.5% solution IV at 20-sec– 40-sec intervals *Maintenance*—1 ml–2 ml 2.5% solution as needed (IV drip 0.2%–0.4%) *Convulsions*—3 ml–5 ml of 2.5% solution *Psychiatry*—4 ml–5 ml of 2.5% solution (IV drip—0.2% at a rate of 50 ml/min) *Rectal*—1 g/75 lb (30 mg/kg) to a maximum of 1.5 g for children and 4 g for adults	Most widely used IV barbiturate anesthetic. Rectal administration can result in irritation, diarrhea, cramping, and bleeding. Do not give rectally in the presence of inflammatory, ulcerative, or bleeding lesions of the lower bowel. Do not use concentrations less than 2% in sterile water for injection for IV administration, because hemolysis can occur. Use freshly prepared solutions; discard unused portions after 24 h. Avoid mixing with other solutions having an acid pH (e.g., tubocurarine or succinylcholine solutions).

inadequate, even with deep anesthesia. These drugs are potent respiratory depressants, and the degree of respiratory depression is dose-dependent. Large doses can also decrease cardiac output and lower arterial blood pressure, due to a direct myocardial depressant action. Hepatic blood flow and glomerular filtration rates may be temporarily decreased.

USES
1. Induction of anesthesia
2. Supplementation of other general anesthetics
3. Production of anesthesia for short surgical procedures with minimal painful stimuli
4. Induction of hypnosis
5. Control of convulsive states during and following general or local anesthesia or other causes (thiopental)
6. Aid to narcoanalysis and narcosynthesis in psychiatric disorders (thiopental)

ADMINISTRATION AND DOSAGE
(See Table 21-3.)

FATE

Induction is smooth and rapid. Onset of anesthesia occurs within 30 seconds to 60 seconds following IV injection. The drugs quickly cross the blood–brain barrier but are then rapidly redistributed to other parts of the body, first to highly vascular organs, then subsequently to fatty tissue, where they are stored. The duration of anesthesia with methohexital is 5 minutes to 8 minutes, whereas anesthesia lasts 15 minutes to 30 minutes with thiamylal and thiopental. Rectal absorption of thiopental is good, and onset of effect occurs within 10 minutes. The plasma half-life of the drug ranges between 4 hours and 8 hours. Repeated dosing or continuous infusion results in accumulation of the drug in lipid storage sites, which can lead to prolonged drowsiness and respiratory or circulatory depression.

SIDE-EFFECTS/ADVERSE REACTIONS

A dose-dependent respiratory depression occurs with use of IV barbiturates. Other common side-effects are laryngospasm, coughing, and yawning. The remaining adverse reactions listed below vary in their frequency of occurrence, and most are noted with prolonged administration.

CV—Myocardial and circulatory depression, arrhythmias, thrombophlebitis, pain on injection, necrosis or sloughing of tissue upon extravasation, arteriospasm upon inadvertent intra-arterial injection

Respiratory—Hiccups, sneezing, bronchospasm, apnea, dyspnea

CNS—Prolonged somnolence, headache, emergence delirium, anxiety

Other—Nausea, vomiting, allergic reactions (pruritus, urticaria, rhinitis), abdominal pain, salivation, shivering, muscle twitching

CONTRAINDICATIONS AND PRECAUTIONS

Absolute contraindications include latent or manifest porphyria and the absence of suitable veins for IV administration. Additionally, thiopental is contraindicated in status asthmaticus. *Extreme caution* is necessary when IV barbiturates are given in the presence of severe cardiovascular disease, bronchial asthma, hypotension, shock, Addison's disease, hepatic or renal dysfunction, myxedema, increased blood urea, severe anemia, increased intracranial pressure, and myasthenia gravis.

INTERACTIONS

1. Additive CNS depressive effects can occur when IV barbiturates are given in combination with narcotics, hypnotics, alcohol, or other CNS depressant drugs.
2. Orthostatic hypotension may be elicited or aggravated by concomitant administration of IV barbiturates and furosemide, bumetanide, or ethacrynic acid.

NURSING CONSIDERATIONS

Careful monitoring of the IV insertion site is essential because extravasation of the barbiturates can cause tissue necrosis. An anesthetized patient is unlikely to complain of site pain until after anesthesia wears off. Procaine 1% can be injected locally to reduce pain should extravasation occur.

Because these drugs are slowly metabolized, any patient receiving them, including outpatients, should be closely monitored and protected during the recovery period until sensory and motor function returns. Sensory function will be somewhat altered for several hours so a patient should not be allowed to drive himself home after an outpatient procedure. In addition, respiratory depression is a possibility during and after anesthesia administration. Resuscitative equipment needs to be available in case of an emergency.

Nonbarbiturate Hypnotics

In addition to the three IV barbiturates reviewed above, a rapid-acting nonbarbiturate hypnotic, etomidate, is available for induction or supplementation of general anesthesia.

Etomidate

(Amidate)

MECHANISM AND ACTIONS

Etomidate produces rapid hypnosis following IV injection, but it is not analgesic. The hemodynamic effects are similar to those of thiopental, but the drug has little or no effect on cardiac output, heart rate, and peripheral circulation. Cerebral blood flow is slightly reduced, as are intracranial and intraocular pressure. Respiratory depression is minimal at normal dosage ranges. Injection of etomidate is frequently associated with pain, and there is a high incidence of transient skeletal muscle hyperactivity, mainly myoclonic in nature.

USES

1. Induction of general anesthesia
2. Supplementation of subpotent anesthetic

agents (*e.g.,* nitrous oxide/O$_2$) agents during short operative procedures
3. Prolonged sedation of critically ill patients (investigational use only)

ADMINISTRATION AND DOSAGE
Etomidate is used by IV injection only (2 mg/ml). Doses between 0.2 and 0.6 mg/kg given over 30 seconds to 60 seconds are used to induce an anesthetic state. To supplement other anesthetics (*e.g.,* nitrous oxide), smaller increments may be administered as needed.

FATE
Following IV injection, anesthesia occurs within 1 minute and persists for approximately 3 minutes to 5 minutes. The drug is approximately 75% protein bound. Etomidate is rapidly metabolized in the liver, and about 75% of the administered dose is excreted in the urine within 24 hours. Plasma half-life is approximately 60 to 90 minutes. The drug is lipid-soluble and has a large volume of distribution in the body.

SIDE-EFFECTS/ADVERSE REACTIONS
The common untoward reactions associated with etomidate are transient venous pain upon injection (20%–25%), myoclonic and tonic muscle movements (30%–35%), and eye movements (8%–10%). Less frequently noted adverse effects are hypotension, tachycardia or bradycardia, arrhythmias, hyperventilation, laryngospasm, hiccups, transient apnea, and postoperative nausea and vomiting.

CONTRAINDICATIONS AND PRECAUTIONS
Use of etomidate in children under age 10 is not recommended. *Cautious use* is warranted in pregnant and nursing mothers (drug has embryocidal effects in rats), in skeletal muscle hyperactivity states, and in the presence of respiratory disease.

INTERACTIONS
1. Etomidate can have an additive depressant effect on the CNS when used in combination with narcotics, other hypnotics, alcohol, and other CNS depressants.

Dissociative Agents

Two drugs, ketamine and Innovar, can be used in certain situations where an anesthetic-like state is desired, but unconsciousness might prove disadvantageous. These agents are employed alone for certain indications or combined with other anesthetics or analgesics. They differ sufficiently in their actions and pharmacologic properties that they will be discussed separately.

Ketamine
(Ketalar)

MECHANISM AND ACTIONS
Ketamine is a rapid-acting anesthetic producing a state of dissociation, characterized by profound analgesia, normal skeletal muscle tone and laryngeal reflexes, and variable cardiovascular and respiratory stimulation. The patient appears to be awake, but does not respond to pain and does not recall the experience following recovery. The actions of ketamine are presumed to result from an interruption of association pathways in the brain prior to an effect on specific sensory pathways. Blood pressure is usually elevated within a few minutes after injection (10%–50% above preanesthetic levels) but returns to normal within 15 minutes. Ketamine possesses a rather wide margin of safety and is compatible with commonly used general and local anesthetics. Emergence from ketamine anesthesia is prolonged, and in 10% to 15% of patients is marked by psychological manifestations ranging from pleasant (dream-like states, vivid imagery) to quite disagreeable (nightmare-like effects, hallucinations). These may be accompanied by confusion, excitement, and irrational behavior. Duration is usually no more than several hours, although recurrences have taken place up to 24 hours postoperatively. The incidence of emergence reactions may be reduced by lowering the dosage, giving IV diazepam (see dosage) and minimizing sensory stimulation during the recovery phase.

USES
1. Diagnostic and short surgical procedures not requiring skeletal muscle relaxation (*e.g.,* treatment of burns) especially in children
2. Induction of anesthesia before administration of other general anesthetics
3. Supplementation of low-potency agents such as nitrous oxide

ADMINISTRATION AND DOSAGE
Ketamine is available in three strengths (10 mg/ml, 50 mg/ml, 100 mg/ml) for IV or IM injection. Recommended dosage ranges are fairly wide, and the

needs of each patient must be titrated individually. For anesthesia induction, doses are 1 to 4.5 mg/kg IV given over 60 seconds or 6.5 to 13 mg/kg IM. Induction may also be accomplished by slow IV injection (0.5 mg/kg/min) of 1 to 2 mg/kg in combination with diazepam (2 to 5 mg IV over 60 seconds) in a separate syringe. To maintain anesthesia or supplement other low-potency agents, one half to the full induction dose may be repeated as needed, titrated to the patient's needs.

Adult patients induced with ketamine and supplemental diazepam can be maintained with a slow microdrip infusion of ketamine in a dose of 0.1 to 0.5 mg/min, augmented by 2 mg to 5 mg of diazepam IV as needed.

FATE

The onset of surgical anesthesia is 30 seconds with IV injection and 3 minutes to 4 minutes with IM administration. Effects persist for 5 minutes to 10 minutes IV and 15 minutes to 25 minutes IM. Blood pressure elevation begins shortly after IV injection, peaks within several minutes, and generally returns to normal within 15 minutes. Ketamine is metabolized in the liver and excreted in the urine.

SIDE-EFFECTS/ADVERSE REACTIONS

Ketamine can cause numerous untoward reactions, and close patient monitoring is essential. The most commonly elicited side-effects are elevated blood pressure and heart rate, mild respiratory stimulation, and intensified muscle tone. Anorexia, nausea, vomiting, diplopia, nystagmus, transient erythema, and rash and pain at the injection site have also been reported. Large doses may produce respiratory depression, hypotension, and arrhythmias. Emergence reactions, more common in adults than in children, can include dreaming, vivid imagery, hallucinations, confusion, excitement, nightmares, irrational behavior, and delirium. A short-acting barbiturate may be needed to terminate a severe emergence reaction.

CONTRAINDICATIONS AND PRECAUTIONS

The use of ketamine is contraindicated in those patients in whom an elevation in blood pressure would constitute a health hazard. The drug should not be given alone in surgical or diagnostic procedures involving the pharynx, larynx, or bronchial tree, because pharyngeal and laryngeal reflexes remain active. *Caution* must be observed in using ketamine in patients with hypertension, convulsive disorders, cardiac disease, and elevated cerebrospinal fluid pressure. The drug is also used with caution in pregnant women, chronic or acutely intoxicated persons, and psychotic or neurotic patients.

INTERACTIONS

1. Barbiturates or narcotics may prolong ketamine recovery time.
2. Severe hypertension and tachycardia can occur in the presence of thyroid replacement drugs.
3. Ketamine may increase the neuromuscular blocking effects of nondepolarizing muscle relaxants (*e.g.*, tubocurarine, atracurium, vecuronium).

NURSING CONSIDERATIONS

The patient who has received ketamine needs to be placed in a recovery area where sensory stimulation is minimal because the patient's perception of speech, touch, and visual stimuli may be grossly exaggerated and irrational behavior may develop. The nurse should approach him calmly, speak quietly, and touch him as little as possible until he is aroused. If the patient is a child, warn the parents about possible behavior and encourage them to use a similar approach. A rapid-acting barbiturate may be ordered if the emergence reaction becomes severe. Safety measures such as padded side rails may be used to increase protection.

Blood pressure must be monitored because severe hypertension can occur. Ketamine and barbiturates should not be mixed in the same syringe because they are incompatible.

Fentanyl/Droperidol

(Innovar)

MECHANISM AND ACTIONS

Innovar is a drug combination which contains 0.05 mg of fentanyl, a narcotic analgesic (see Chap. 22) and 2.5 mg of droperidol, a neuroleptic or major tranquilizer (see Chap. 27). This combination produces an effect termed *neuroleptanalgesia*, which is characterized by general quiescence, reduced motor activity, and profound analgesia. Innovar is employed in a number of ways to produce tranquilization and analgesia. Consciousness is not lost, and the use of Innovar can greatly facilitate intubation procedures, where a conscious, cooperative patient is an asset. Hypotension and bradycardia can occur, as well as respiratory depression and extrapyramidal symptoms, most often muscle rigidity. Anesthesia can be induced during Innovar use by concurrent administration of 65% nitrous oxide in oxygen.

USES

1. Production of tranquilization and analgesia for diagnostic and minor surgical procedures
2. Induction of anesthesia or anesthetic premedication
3. Adjunct for the maintenance of general and regional anesthesia, in combination with nitrous oxide and oxygen

ADMINISTRATION AND DOSAGE

Innovar may be administered either IM or IV. The following doses are generally recommended ranges, but individual dosage titration is necessary, depending on the application and the status of the patient. Vital signs must be monitored during administration. Reduce the initial dose in elderly, debilitated, or poor risk patients.

Premedication—0.5 ml to 2.0 ml IM 45 minutes to 60 minutes prior to surgery (children—0.25 ml/20 lb IM)

Induction—1 ml/20 to 25 lb by slow IV injection (3 min–5 min), or 10 ml/250 ml 5% dextrose by IV drip. (Children—0.5 ml/20 lb IM)

Diagnostic procedures—0.5 ml to 2.0 ml IM 45 minutes to 60 minutes before procedure. Increments of 0.5 ml to 1.0 ml IV may be used for prolonged procedures as needed. Topical anesthesia will also be needed as an adjunct to produce numbing in such procedures as bronchoscopies and to reduce the gag reflex.

FATE

The drug combination exhibits a rather slow onset and prolonged duration of analgesia, although each component has different characteristics. Fentanyl possesses a rapid action (onset 5 min–10 min) and short duration (up to 1 h), whereas droperidol exhibits a slower onset (30 min) and a more sustained effect (up to 6 h).

SIDE-EFFECTS/ADVERSE REACTIONS

The most frequently noted side-effects of Innovar are muscle rigidity, hypotension, slight respiratory depression, and post-drug drowsiness. Other adverse reactions reported with use of Innovar are dizziness, shivering, tachycardia, delirium, hallucinations, vomiting, laryngospasm, and bronchospasm. In addition, droperidol can elicit extrapyramidal reactions (see Chap. 27) because it is a neuroleptic drug.

CONTRAINDICATIONS AND PRECAUTIONS

Contraindications to use of Innovar are parkinsonism, presence of MAO-inhibitor drugs, and children under 2 years of age. *Cautious use* is necessary in patients with arrhythmias, chronic obstructive pulmonary disease, liver or kidney dysfunction, and in trauma patients, because muscle rigidity may occur.

INTERACTIONS

1. CNS depressants (*e.g.*, barbiturates, narcotics, alcohol) may have additive depressant effects with Innovar.

NURSING CONSIDERATIONS

Because the postoperative complications include respiratory depression and hypotension, narcotic antagonists (such as naloxone), fluids, and pressor agents should be readily available if such effects occur.

REVIEW QUESTIONS

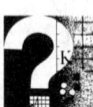

1. Briefly define the concept of "balanced anesthesia."
2. Trace the changes in (a) respiration, (b) cardiovascular function, and (c) muscle tone as general anesthesia passes through the four major stages.
3. What effects are noted as the patient passes from plane 1 through plane 4 of stage III anesthesia?
4. Explain briefly the following theories of action of general anesthetics:
   (a) Meyer–Overton theory
   (b) Water-crystal theory
   (c) Conformational distortion theory
5. Briefly give the reasons for the use of the following preanesthetic medications:

(a) anticholinergics
(b) narcotics
(c) skeletal muscle relaxants

6. What is the significance of the MAC in conjunction with inhalational anesthetics?
7. What are the principal *disadvantages* of the following inhalational anesthetics:
    (a) cyclopropane
    (b) nitrous oxide
    (c) enflurane
    (d) methoxyflurane
8. How are the intravenous general anesthetics classified?
9. Briefly list the advantages and disadvantages of the intravenous barbiturate anesthetics.
10. What is "neuroleptanalgesia"?
11. List the major effects of ketamine. Briefly describe the emergence reaction frequently observed in adults who have received ketamine.
12. What are the principal indications for Innovar?
13. Explain how preoperative teaching can reduce anesthesia induction panic for many patients.
14. Explain the rationale for frequent postanesthesia recovery room measurement of temperature, pulse, respiration, and blood pressure.
15. How can nurses working in operating room environments protect themselves from the hazards of waste gases?

BIBLIOGRAPHY

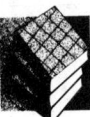

Andrews DR, Taylor C: Documenting post-anesthesia recovery. Am J Nurs 85:290, 1985

Cohen EN: Toxicity of inhalation anesthetic agents. Br J Anesth 50:665, 1978

Dripps RD, Eckenhoff JE, Vandam LD: Introduction to Anesthesia: The Principles of Safe Practice. Philadelphia, WB Saunders, 1982

Fink BR (ed): Molecular Mechanisms of Anesthesia. New York, Raven Press, 1980

Ngai SH: Effects of anesthesia on various organs. N Engl J Med 302:564, 1980

Roth SH: Physical mechanisms of anesthesia. Annu Rev Pharmacol Toxicol 19:159, 1979

Seufert HJ: A review of occupational health hazards associated with anesthetic waste gases. AORN Journal 24:744, October 1976

Smith RM: Anesthesia for Infants and Children. St. Louis, CV Mosby, 1980

White MJ, Wolf-Wilets VC: Memory loss following halothane anesthesia. AORN Journal 26:1053, December 1977

White PF, Way WL, Trevor AJ: Ketamine: Its pharmacology and therapeutic uses. Anesthesiology 56:119, 1982

Narcotic Analgesics and Antagonists

22

The narcotic analgesics encompass a group of both naturally occurring and synthetic agents capable of interacting with specific receptor sites in the CNS to relieve pain in conscious persons. Narcotic antagonists, on the other hand, are those compounds that can occupy these same receptor sites, but act to interfere with many of the actions of the narcotic analgesics.

Narcotic Analgesics

Drugs used in the management of severe pain have traditionally been referred to as "narcotic" analgesics to distinguish them from less potent analgesic drugs such as aspirin or acetaminophen. However, use of the term "narcotic" is not entirely appropriate because it is derived from a Greek word meaning "stuporous" or "unconscious," although narcotic analgesics relieve pain without inducing sleep or loss of consciousness. Since the prototype of these drugs is morphine, a substance obtained from the opium poppy, these compounds are also referred to as "opiates," and this has become the preferred term.

The naturally occurring alkaloids of opium (morphine and codeine) are themselves commonly used, or they may be modified chemically to form semisynthetic derivatives which are significantly more potent in some cases than the two natural alkaloids. In addition, a group of purely synthetic opiate compounds have also been prepared. These produce many pharmacologic effects similar to those of morphine but differ slightly in some of their actions and are, in certain instances, significantly more potent on a milligram basis.

Classification of Narcotic Drugs

Drugs possessing an opiate-like action fall into one of two broad categories, the narcotic agonist analgesics and the narcotic agonist–antagonist analgesics. The former group comprises most of the opiates, both natural and synthetic, commonly used for the relief of pain. These drugs exert an agonistic action at the various opiate receptor sites in the CNS (see discussion of opiate receptors below) and differ among themselves primarily in potency, addiction liability, and duration of action.

The narcotic agonist–antagonist analgesics are also effective pain relievers, but by virtue of their partial antagonistic action at certain opiate receptor sites, they are claimed to have a lower abuse potential than the potent narcotic agonist analgesics and to produce somewhat less respiratory depression in large doses than the other opiate drugs. These differences will be explored more fully later in the chapter.

Within the grouping of narcotic agonist analgesics, the individual drugs can be further categorized on the basis of their chemical structures. While chemical classification provides a convenient means of separating the agonist analgesics into distinct categories for discussion purposes, further differences exist even within each class with regard to potency and toxicity. For example, although morphine and codeine belong to the same chemical classification, the former is quite potent and highly addicting, while the latter is much less potent and addicting. The various narcotic analgesic drugs can be classified in the following manner:

I. Narcotic Agonist Analgesics
  A. Phenanthrenes
    1. Naturally occurring opium alkaloids (morphine, codeine)
    2. Semisynthetic derivatives of morphine (hydromorphone, oxymorphone)
    3. Semisynthetic derivatives of codeine (hydrocodone, oxycodone)
  B. Methadones (methadone, propoxyphene)
  C. Morphinans (levorphanol)
  D. Phenylpiperidine (meperidine, fentanyl, alfentanil, sufentanil)
II. Narcotic Agonist–Antagonist Analgesics
  A. Phenanthrenes (nalbuphine, buprenorphine)
  B. Morphinans (butorphanol)
  C. Benzomorphans (pentazocine)

Pharmacokinetics of Opiate Drugs

The various opiates differ markedly in their relative potencies, their duration of action, their oral/parenteral potency ratio, and their addiction liability. Table 22-1 lists several properties of the clinically available opiates. Although gastrointestinal absorption of most narcotic drugs is good, their potency following oral administration is considerably less in most cases than following parenteral use, the result primarily of significant first-pass hepatic inactivation immediately following absorption. Opiates having high oral/parenteral potency ratios (*i.e.*, nearly as potent orally as parenterally) include levorphanol, methadone, oxycodone and codeine, whereas low oral/parenteral potency ratios are characteristic of morphine, hydromorphone, and meperidine. In general, addiction liabil-

Table 22-1
Comparative Pharmacologic Properties of Opiates

	Equianalgesic Doses (mg)*		Onset of Action (min)†	Duration of Action (h)†	Analgesic Efficacy	Addictive Liability
	PO	SC, IM				
Agonists						
morphine (MS Contin, Roxanol)	60	10	10–20	4–6	High	High
fentanyl (Sublimaze)	—	0.1–0.2	5–15	1–2	High	High
sufentanil (Sufenta)	—	—	2–4 (IV)	0.5–1	High	High
alfentanil (Alfenta)	—	—	2–4 (IV)	0.5–1	High	High
hydromorphone (Dilaudid)	8	1–2	15–30	4–5	High	High
oxymorphone (Numorphan)	6	1–1.5	5–10	3–5	High	High
levorphanol (Levo-Dromoran)	4	2–3	15–30	4–6	High	High
methadone (Dolophine)	20	7–10	10–15	4–6	High	High
oxycodone	30	15	15–30	3–5	Medium	Medium–High
meperidine (Demerol, Pethadol)	300	75–100	10–20	2–4	Medium	High
codeine	200	120	15–30	3–5	Low	Medium
propoxyphene (Darvon)	‡	—	15–30 (PO)	4–6	Low	Low
Agonist-Antagonists						
buprenorphine (Buprenex)	—	0.3	10–15	4–6	High	Low
butorphanol (Stadol)	—	2–4	5–10	3–4	High	Low
nalbuphine (Nubain)	—	10	10–15	3–6	High	Low
pentazocine (Talwin)	150	30–60	15–30	3–4	Medium	Medium–Low

* All doses as stated are approximately equivalent to 10 mg morphine IM or SC. Note that chronic administration of narcotics alters pharmacokinetics and decreases the parenteral/oral dose ratio. For example, chronic administration of morphine decreases the ratio from 6:1 to 2:1.
† Onset and duration of action based on IM or SC administration, unless otherwise noted.
‡ Propoxyphene is a very weak analgesic that cannot be compared to other opiates in equianalgesic doses.

ity, a major problem inherent in the repeated use of narcotics, closely parallels potency, and habituation is an almost inescapable consequence of prolonged use of the potent opiates. The topic of drug addiction will be discussed more fully in Chapter 85.

Pharmacologic Actions of Opiate Drugs

The pharmacologic effects of therapeutic doses of opiates extend to many different systems of the body. An outline of the major pharmacologic actions of narcotic analgesics is presented in Table

Table 22-2
Pharmacologic Effects of Narcotic Analgesics

CNS

Analgesia
Sedation
Euphoria
Emesis (*anti*emetic at very high doses)
Depressed cough reflex
Respiratory depression (depression of medullary respiratory center)

Cardiovascular

Orthostatic hypotension (depression of medullary vasomotor center; peripheral vascular dilation)

GI Tract

Decreased peristalsis and stomach motility
Delayed gastric emptying time
Constipation

Smooth Muscle

Increased tone of most nonvascular smooth muscle (*e.g.*, GI, urinary, biliary)

Urinary System

Urinary tract spasm
Contraction of urinary sphincter
Decreased renal blood flow
Release of antidiuretic hormone

Eye

Miosis

Neuroendocrine

Release of prolactin and somatotropin
Decreased release of luteinizing hormone and thyrotropin

Table 22-3
Opiate Receptors

Receptor Type	Pharmacologic Effects
Mu (μ)	Supraspinal analgesia Euphoria Respiratory depression Addiction
Kappa (κ)	Spinal analgesia Sedation Miosis
Sigma (σ)	Dysphoria Hallucinations Respiratory/vasomotor stimulation
Delta (δ)	Affective behavior

22-2. It should be noted that considerable variation exists among the different opiate drugs with regard to the frequency and intensity of many of the effects shown in Table 22-2. Not only are most of the actions of narcotics dose-dependent and thus more intense at high doses, but some effects are seen to a much greater degree with certain drugs; for example, sedation is much stronger with the combined agonists–antagonists than with the pure agonists.

The opiate drugs exert their effects by combining with specific narcotic receptor sites, and several types of receptors have been identified in the central and peripheral nervous systems. Sites of high opiate receptor concentration include the dorsal horn of the spinal cord and several subcortical brain areas, such as the periaqueductal gray, hypothalamus, thalamus, locus ceruleus, and raphe nuclei. Characterization of opiate receptors is based on the type of responses mediated by interaction of a narcotic drug at each receptor site, as outlined in Table 22-3.

The narcotic drugs bind to the different receptors to varying degrees, and the relative preference of an opiate for certain receptor types over others will determine the overall pharmacologic profile of the drug. For example, most narcotic agonists will interact at both the *mu* and *kappa* receptors, and therefore elicit the characteristic narcotic actions. The mixed agonist–antagonist drugs, however, appear to more avidly bind to the *kappa* and *sigma* than to the *mu* receptors; in fact, they may act as partial antagonists at the *mu* sites. This differential receptor action of the mixed agonist–antagonist drugs may help explain their lower abuse potential, reduced euphoric effects, and greater sedative action compared to the narcotic agonists. In addition, antagonism of the *mu* receptors can at least partially reverse the effects of other narcotic agonists acting at these sites, and lead to the appearance of withdrawal symptoms should a mixed agonist–antagonist be given in the presence of an agonist.

Central nervous system sites that contain opiate receptors also contain endogenous morphine-like peptides which interact with the opiate receptor sites to elicit physiologic effects similar to those of the exogenous narcotic agonists. Three distinct groups of endogenous opioid-like peptides have been isolated thus far and have been termed *endorphins, enkephalins,* and *dynorphins.* Each group is derived from a distinct precursor polypeptide and exhibits a characteristic distribution pattern in the CNS.

Beta-endorphin is a 31-amino-acid peptide derived from pro-opiomelanocortin. Beta-endorphin is primarily found in the pituitary, with much smaller amounts in many other brain sites. It is a very potent endogenous opioid which is involved in a variety of behavioral and physiologic actions beyond the analgesic effects of the opiates.

The smallest peptides exhibiting endogenous opiate activity are the enkephalins, pentapeptides named methionine-enkephalin (or met-enkephalin) and leucine-enkephalin (or leu-enkephalin). Although beta-endorphin contains the amino-acid sequence for met-enkephalin, it is *not* converted to this peptide; rather, the enkephalins are derived from a larger polypeptide termed proenkephalin.

The enkephalins are located in nerve endings throughout the central nervous system and are particularly abundant in the brain stem and dorsal horn of the spinal cord, as well as the basal ganglia and portions of the limbic system. These enkephalin-containing regions have virtually no beta-endorphin; thus, neurons that contain enkephalins seem to be quite distinct from those that contain beta-endorphin. Enkephalins are believed to act by modifying impulse transmission in pain pathways by combining with opiate receptor sites in a manner similar to that of the narcotic analgesics. Enkephalins may be released by a variety of stimuli, such as sensory stimulation or emotional upset; therefore, the body appears to possess a natural mechanism for pain control and other behavioral modifications. Activity of enkephalins may also be enhanced by the presence of narcotic drugs, and these pentapeptides may play a major role in the development of analgesia resulting from use of exogenous opiate drugs.

The dynorphins are formed from prodynorphin and the most potent appears to be a 17-amino-acid peptide termed dynorphin A; other dynorphins are alpha and beta neoendorphins and dynorphin B. Dynorphins are present in many brain regions as well.

The endogenous opioid peptides display various affinities for the opioid receptor sites. Enkephalins appear to bind to both *delta* and to *mu* sites with approximately equal affinity. Beta-endorphin likewise binds predominantly to *mu* and *delta* sites although it can interact with more specialized sites as well. Dynorphins appear to interact primarily at *kappa* sites, although some may bind to *mu* and *delta* receptors as well. The clinical significance of this differential receptor interaction among the various endogenous opiates remains to be established.

Although both beta-endorphin and the enkephalins can mimic the action of narcotic drugs in various pharmacologic test systems, they are of little clinical value because they are not absorbed orally and are rapidly degraded by metabolizing enzymes in the brain, blood, and other tissues. The development of synthetic analogues of these endogenous substances that would retain their analgesic action while conferring oral effectiveness and resistance to rapid inactivation would be a major advance in the area of pain management. An alternative avenue of drug development already underway is the synthesis of inhibitors of the enzymes responsible for the rapid inactivation of the enkephalins. Such drugs might serve to potentiate the analgesic efficacy of the endogenously released enkephalins.

Modification of neurotransmitter function may also play a role in the action of narcotic analgesics. The release of several neurohormones, including norepinephrine, dopamine, acetylcholine, serotonin, and substance P can be inhibited by opiate drugs, possibly due to interference with the influx of calcium ions into neuronal cells, an essential step for neurotransmitter release. While the neurohormonal modifying action of narcotics probably contributes to the pharmacologic effects of these drugs, the varied clinical actions of opiates cannot be ascribed solely to an interaction with a single neurotransmitter.

Several of the more important pharmacologic effects of narcotic drugs outlined in Table 22-2 will now be reviewed in greater detail.

Central Effects

ANALGESIA
Multiple sites and mechanisms of action are involved in narcotic-induced analgesia. Opiate drugs

may impair the transmission of incoming noxious impulses in the substantia gelatinosa of the spinal column, probably by blocking release of an excitatory neurotransmitter such as substance P. Pain-transmitting sensory afferent neurons appear to release a peptide, substance P, from their terminals within the spinal cord, and this release can be attenuated by opiate drugs and by enkephalins acting at opioid receptor sites within the spinal cord.

In certain midbrain areas, most notably the periaqueductal gray region, narcotics also appear to enhance the activity of neurons that project to the spinal cord by way of several descending fiber tracts involved in the modulation of painful impulses. Impaired synthesis of cyclic AMP due to decreased activity of the enzyme adenylate cyclase in certain brain areas has also been postulated to play a role in opiate-induced analgesia.

It is generally accepted that a painful experience of any origin includes both the actual sensation of pain *and* the individual perception of and reaction to the presence of the painful stimulus.

Narcotic analgesics have the ability not only to modify the actual *sensation* of the painful input by blocking conduction in pain pathways in the spinal cord, brain stem, and midbrain, as described above, but also to alter the *perception* of the noxious sensation by decreasing sensory responsiveness at higher cortical centers. Following an effective dose of an opiate, the threshold for pain is elevated, but even if the painful stimulus is still sufficient to be perceived, it becomes less threatening and the patient is considerably less affected, because the usual reaction to pain (*i.e.*, anxiety, fear, panic) is obtunded. However, this resulting tranquility and release from tension frequently is associated with an exaggerated sense of well-being, which is often responsible for the desire to repeat the drug, which may ultimately lead to habituation. Euphoria is commonly experienced by someone in pain who is given a narcotic analgesic, but occasionally some patients may develop the opposite reaction, namely dysphoria, a distinctly unpleasant state characterized by restlessness, agitation, malaise, and depression. Dysphoria is also seen quite often when opiates are given to pain-free persons.

SEDATION
Therapeutic doses of opiate analgesics commonly induce a state of quietude and drowsiness. The extremities become heavy, a sensation of warmth is felt, the mouth becomes dry, and sleep sometimes ensues, from which the patient is easily aroused. Sedation is considerably more prominent with the

mixed narcotic agonist–antagonists than with the other narcotic drugs.

RESPIRATORY DEPRESSION
All narcotic agonist drugs induce dose-dependent respiratory depression, and respiratory paralysis is the principal cause of death in cases of narcotic overdosage. The major mechanism by which opiates decrease respiration is a reduced sensitivity of the neurons of the brain stem respiratory centers to carbon dioxide. All phases of respiratory activity are depressed (rate, minute volume, tidal exchange), and the retention of carbon dioxide can result in cerebral vasodilation and increased intracranial pressure. Although the mixed narcotic agonist–antagonists are claimed to elicit less respiratory depression than other narcotic drugs, their advantage in this respect is little more than therapeutic window dressing. In reality, the mixed agonist–antagonists display a "ceiling effect" with regard to the degree of respiratory depression associated with increasing dosage. Thus, at high doses, the extent of respiratory depression is no longer dose-dependent as with lower doses, but "flattens out." This is shown graphically in Figure 22-1. In contrast, the narcotic agonists exhibit a true dose-dependent depression of respiration *even with very large doses* (see Fig. 22-1). While the degree of respiratory depression resulting from large doses of the mixed agonist–antagonists is less than

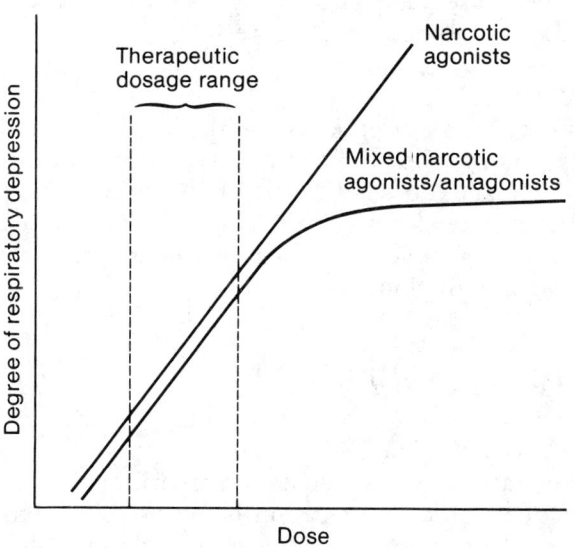

Figure 22-1. Comparison of respiratory depressant effects of narcotic agonists and mixed narcotic agonists/antagonists (see text for explanation).

that seen with *large* doses of the pure narcotic agonists, there is essentially *no* difference in the degree of depression *within the commonly employed therapeutic dosage ranges* of the drugs.

EMESIS

Narcotic analgesics can elicit nausea and vomiting in therapeutic doses, primarily due to their ability to directly stimulate the chemoreceptor trigger zone (CTZ) in the medulla. Although the incidence of nausea and vomiting is relatively small in recumbent patients, a significantly greater degree of nausea and vomiting is observed in ambulatory patients. This suggests the involvement of the vestibular apparatus as well, perhaps reflected as increased vestibular sensitivity following a narcotic drug. Phenothiazines (*e.g.*, prochlorperazine) are frequently effective in overcoming narcotic-induced nausea and vomiting.

COUGH SUPPRESSION

Inhibition of the cough reflex is an action shared by all narcotic analgesics; however, only a few opiate drugs are routinely used as antitussives. Codeine and hydrocodone, in particular, are frequently used to relieve persistent coughing and are quite effective in most cases. The mechanism appears to be a direct depression of the medullary cough center. Routine use of narcotic antitussives results in a high degree of tolerance, and these drugs should only be employed on a short-term basis under close supervision. Habituation to codeine or hydrocodone can occur with routine use, and dependence has been observed. (The narcotic antitussives will be reviewed in detail in Chapter 47.)

MIOSIS

Pupillary constriction is seen with all narcotic agonists, and may be marked in the event of overdosage. Tolerance does not develop to the miotic effect of the opiates, and the presence of constricted pupils is a valuable aid in diagnosing narcotic overdosage or addiction.

Peripheral Effects

CARDIOVASCULAR

In general, therapeutic doses of narcotic analgesics have no significant effects on blood pressure, cardiac rate or rhythm, or cardiac output in the supine patient. Resistance (*i.e.*, arteriolar) and capacitance (*i.e.*, venular) vessels are dilated slightly by opiates, probably due to a release of histamine and a depression of adrenergic tone at the level of the brain stem vasomotor center. This peripheral arteriolar and venular dilation can result in orthostatic hypotension, especially when a supine patient arises, and proper assistance must be provided to these patients. Similarly, persons with decreased blood volume are more prone to develop hypotension with use of narcotic drugs.

Cerebral circulation is not directly affected by opiates, but as noted above, retention of carbon dioxide subsequent to narcotic-induced respiratory depression can lead to cerebral vasodilation, and possibly increased cerebrospinal and intracranial fluid pressure.

Morphine and other opiates can reduce the left ventricular end-diastolic pressure (LVEDP), thus decreasing oxygen consumption and cardiac workload. These effects are beneficial in patients experiencing a myocardial infarction and therefore contribute to the usefulness of morphine during the acute stages of infarction.

GASTROINTESTINAL

The effects of narcotic drugs on gastrointestinal function are variable depending on the level of the GI tract affected. In the stomach, motility is usually reduced while the tone of the antral and upper duodenum is increased. Passage of gastric contents through the duodenum can therefore be markedly slowed, and absorption of many drugs is delayed. Hydrochloric acid secretion may be slightly decreased.

Resting tone of the small intestine is increased, and periodic spasms are noted. The amplitude of propulsive contractions is greatly reduced both in the small and large intestines. Tone in the large intestine is greatly increased, which delays fecal passage, facilitates absorption of water from the fecal mass, and results in constipation. Anal sphincter tone is enhanced. Little tolerance develops to the constipating action of narcotic drugs. While all opiates elicit qualitatively similar effects on the GI tract, there is considerable variability in potency among the different opiate derivatives with regard to their constipating action.

SMOOTH MUSCLE

Most other nonvascular smooth muscle is contracted by opiates. Therapeutic doses of most narcotics greatly increase pressure in the biliary tract by contracting biliary smooth muscle, and can result in biliary colic. While narcotics can relieve the pain associated with biliary spasm, their smooth muscle spasmogenic action may actually exacerbate an underlying cause of the pain. Some evidence indicates that low doses of meperidine and pentazocine are slightly less spasmogenic than most other narcotic drugs; however, these doses are probably only marginally analgesic as well.

Ureteral and urinary bladder tone are increased by opiates as is tone of the vesicle sphincter, and urinary retention has occurred, especially in the postoperative patient. The central effects of narcotics to decrease perception of stimuli for urination also contribute to opiate-induced urinary retention, as can decreased renal blood flow. Narcotics can also increase the release of antidiuretic hormone from the neurohypophysis.

Uterine tone may be decreased somewhat, especially by large doses of narcotic drugs and the intensity of uterine contractions may be diminished. In addition, decreased central perceptive ability secondary to narcotic usage may interfere with normal patient cooperation during labor; the combination of these effects can significantly prolong labor and delivery.

HORMONAL

Release by prolactin (LTH) and possibly also somatotropin (growth hormone) are enhanced by narcotics, whereas secretion of luteinizing hormone (LH) and thyrotropin (TSH) are inhibited. While the hormonal effects resulting from acute administration of opiate drugs are probably of little clinical consequence, the potential role played by endogenous opioids (e.g., endorphins) in the control of pituitary hormonal secretion is of considerable interest.

Tolerance and Habituation

Repeated administration of a narcotic drug invariably results in a gradual loss of analgesic effectiveness as well as increasing degrees of tolerance (i.e., need for increasingly larger doses to obtain a comparable effect) to several other effects of the opiates. The development of tolerance to the actions of narcotic drugs is dependent on several factors, including the drug itself, as well as the dosage, dosing intervals, and duration of therapy. The mechanisms that may be responsible for tolerance to opiate drugs include increased rates of metabolic degradation or clearance with continued use and a reduced receptor sensitivity over time with chronic drug administration. Tolerance most readily develops to the analgesic, euphoric, and respiratory

depressant effects of narcotics, but tolerance has also been observed in connection with the sedative, antidiuretic, hypotensive, antitussive, and emetic actions of these drugs. Conversely, little or no tolerance has been reported to the miotic or constipating effects of narcotics. Clinically recognizable tolerance can occur after 1 week to 2 weeks of regular narcotic usage, and leads to the necessity of administering larger doses to obtain the same degree of pain relief. As doses are continually increased, the degree of tolerance increases dramatically, and the patient may require many times the initial dose of narcotic to obtain a comparable effect. A person dependent on narcotics may in fact require doses that would prove fatal in a nontolerant individual. Continued use of increasing amounts of a narcotic drug almost invariably leads to a physical dependence, in which a constant supply of drug is necessary to avoid precipitation of withdrawal symptoms. (A more complete discussion of the abuse potential of narcotic drugs is presented in Chap. 85.)

Although dependence is a very real problem with chronic use of opiate drugs, the fear of making a person dependent too often results in the administration of insufficient amounts of drug to adequately control severe pain. For example, there is virtually no danger of addicting a postoperative patient by administering large doses of an opiate drug for several days during a surgical recovery stage. Undertreatment in such circumstances may subject the patient to unnecessary suffering, with the mistaken idea of preventing the development of habituation, which is rarely of concern with short-term treatment.

Similarly, patients suffering from intractable cancer pain should never be denied adequate analgesic drug treatment because of a fear of addiction or respiratory depression. The newer, long-acting oral forms of morphine, as well as other potent, orally effective narcotic drugs, should be given on a *regularly scheduled basis* in the terminal phases of cancer, in order to keep the patient comfortable and pain free. Under no circumstances should subtherapeutic amounts of analgesic drugs be given because of a fear of addiction in such patients.

The tendency to undertreat rather than overtreat with narcotic drugs derives from the concern of making patients dependent on these drugs. The likelihood of creating dependency with therapeutic use of the narcotic drugs is minimal and patients in severe pain should be given adequate amounts of these drugs to quell the pain for as long as is necessary.

In a person physically dependent on narcotics, discontinuation of the drug results in the appearance of withdrawal or abstinence symptoms. The type and severity of the symptoms are dependent on the length of time the drug has been used, the dosage, and the means of discontinuing the drug (*i.e.*, sudden cessation vs gradual tapering). The more rapidly the drug level in the body is decreased, the more intense is the withdrawal reaction. Acute cessation of a narcotic drug following prolonged use leads to a fairly predictable pattern of reactions; lacrimation, rhinorrhea, sweating, yawning, chills, and goose pimples usually occur within 8 hours to 16 hours after the last dose. Peak withdrawal effects are generally observed within 36 hours to 48 hours, and include abdominal cramping, muscle aching, nausea, vomiting, diarrhea, hyperthermia, and hyperventilation. Most symptoms subside within 3 days to 5 days, but some may persist for much longer periods of time. Variations in the onset and duration of symptoms are noted among the different opiates. For example, withdrawal symptoms associated with chronic meperidine usage frequently subside within 18 hours to 24 hours, whereas those seen with methadone are much slower in developing, requiring several days to attain a peak effect, and often persist for several weeks. However, the abstinence syndrome with methadone is somewhat less intense than that associated with morphine or heroin, and this is one reason that methadone is substituted for heroin in some detoxification programs.

A sudden, severe abstinence reaction can be precipitated in chronic opiate users by the administration of a narcotic antagonist such as naloxone. Within several minutes after injection of the antagonist, the withdrawal symptoms described above are observed, and persist for up to one-half hour, that is, until the antagonistic effects of naloxone have dissipated. A similar, but frequently less severe withdrawal reaction has occurred when one of the mixed narcotic agonist–antagonists has been administered to a patient already receiving one of the pure narcotic agonists. The partial blocking action of the agonist–antagonist drug on opiate *mu* receptors can elicit a withdrawal syndrome characterized by cramping, nausea, lacrimation, rhinorrhea, anxiety, and restlessness.

Although the abuse potential of the mixed agonist–antagonists is less than that of the potent narcotic agonists, prolonged use, especially in emotionally unstable individuals or persons with a history of drug abuse, can lead to psychological and in some cases physical dependence. Abrupt discontinuation of these drugs in such instances will result in withdrawal reactions similar to those seen with the other narcotic agonists, although the intensity and duration of the symptoms are usually less than with the more potent narcotic drugs. The intensity of narcotic withdrawal symptoms can be ameliorated by use of clonidine, an orally effective antihypertensive drug discussed in Chapter 35.

The various narcotic drugs will be reviewed as a group because much of their pharmacology is similar. Characteristics of each drug will then be detailed in Table 22-4 (agonists) and Table 22-5 (agonist–antagonists).

Agonists

Alfentanil, Codeine, Fentanyl, Hydromorphone, Levorphanol, Meperidine, Methadone, Morphine, Opium, Oxycodone, Oxymorphone, Propoxyphene, Sufentanil

Agonist–Antagonists

Buprenorphine, Butorphanol, Nalbuphine, Pentazocine

MECHANISM AND ACTIONS

The actions of narcotic drugs are complex and involve multiple sites and mechanisms of action. Opiates can elevate the pain threshold, alter the perception of pain, obtund the anxiety or apprehension associated with the presence of pain, and induce somnolence and clouding of mentation. Several mechanisms are operative in the above actions, and include (1) direct activation of opiate receptor sites in the spinal cord, brain stem, and subcortical brain nuclei; (2) potentiation of the effects of endogenous opiates; and (3) activation of descending spinal cord pathways, which reduces the level of incoming sensory pain impulses at various segmental levels of the cord. Narcotics can reduce calcium influx into neuronal cells, thereby impairing release of neurohormones such as norepinephrine, dopamine, serotonin, and substance P. The latter compound is found in many primary sensory afferent neurons, especially in the spinal

(Text continues on p. 394.)

Table 22-4
Narcotic Agonist Analgesics

Drug	Preparations	Usual Dosage Range	Clinical Considerations
Phenanthrenes			
morphine (Astramorph-PF, Duramorph, MS Contin, MSIR, Roxanol, Roxanol SR, RMS)	Soluble tablets—10 mg, 15 mg, 30 mg Oral tablets—15 mg, 30 mg Substained-release tablets —30 mg Oral solution—10 mg/5 ml, 20 mg/5 ml, 20 mg/ml Injection—0.5 mg/ml, 1 mg/ml, 2 mg/ml, 4 mg/ml, 5 mg/ml, 8 mg/ml, 10 mg/ml, 15 mg/ml Drops—20 mg/ml Suppositories—5 mg, 10 mg, 20 mg, 30 mg	Oral—10 mg to 30 mg every 4 h–6 h Sustained-release—30 mg every 8 h–12 h SC, IM—(Adults) 5 mg to 20 mg every 4 h (usual 10 mg); (Children) 0.1 mg/kg to 0.2 mg/kg every 4 h IV—4 mg to 10 mg injected slowly Rectal—10 mg to 20 mg every 4 h Epidural—5 mg in lumbar region once daily *or* 2 mg to 4 mg by continuous infusion over 24 h Intrathecal—usually $1/10$ of epidural dose	Principal opium alkaloid, and standard to which other opiates are compared. Most effective parenterally because oral availability may be somewhat limited. Commonly produces drowsiness and relief from anxiety; large doses induce deep sleep and profound respiratory depression. Oral form (especially sustained-release tablets) is very effective in controlling chronic pain when given *on a regular schedule*. Oral solution may be combined with other medications (sedatives, alcohol, amphetamine, phenothiazines) as a "cocktail" for relief of severe pain; such mixtures have been termed Brompton's mixtures (*i.e.*, any alcoholic mixture containing morphine and other additives). Although use of Brompton's mixture has been effective in controlling chronic severe pain, current recommendations are for use of a single narcotic analgesic (*e.g.*, morphine), with sufficient dosage on a regular basis being as effective as a mixture with fewer side-effects. Adjunctive medications (*e.g.*, sedatives, tricyclic antidepressants, stimulants) may be given individually as desired, but fixed combinations should be avoided. Schedule II.
codeine (Codeine Phosphate, Codeine Sulfate)	Soluble tablets—15 mg, 30 mg, 60 mg Tablets—15 mg, 30 mg, 60 mg Injection—30 mg/ml, 60 mg/ml	*Analgesia* Adults—15 mg to 60 mg 4 times/day orally; SC, IM, or IV Children—0.5 mg/kg every 4 h–6 h orally, SC, or IM	Less potent and less abuse potential than morphine. Widely used in cough medications. Suppresses cough by direct depressant effect on medullary

(continued)

Table 22-4 (continued)
Narcotic Agonist Analgesics

Drug	Preparations	Usual Dosage Range	Clinical Considerations
Phenanthrenes (continued)			
codeine (Codeine Phosphate, Codeine Sulfate) (continued)		*Antitussive* Adults—10 mg to 20 mg every 4 h–6 h to a maximum of 120 mg/24 h Children—(6 yr to 12 yr) 5 mg to 10 mg every 4 h–6 h (maximum 60 mg/day) (2 yr to 6 yr) 2.5 mg to 5 mg every 4 h–6 h (maximum 30 mg/day)	cough center. As an analgesic, most frequently used in combination with aspirin, acetaminophen, or other analgesics. High doses (e.g., 60 mg) may cause restlessness and excitement. Rapid onset of action following oral administration (10 min to 15 min) and effects persist for up to 6 h. Used in combination with centrally acting muscle relaxants for pain of muscle spasm and rigidity. Schedule II.
hydromorphone (Dilaudid)	Tablets—1 mg, 2 mg, 3 mg, 4 mg Injection—1 mg/ml, 2 mg/ml, 3 mg/ml, 4 mg/ml, 10 mg/ml Suppositories—3 mg	SC, IM—2 mg to 4 mg every 4 h–6 h (may also be given by *slow* IV injection) Oral—2 mg to 4 mg every 4 h–6 h Rectal—1 suppository every 6 h–8 h	Very potent (8× to 10× morphine) analgesic, producing less sedation, vomiting, and nausea than morphine. Elicits marked respiratory depression; therefore, use smallest dose possible. Suppositories may give prolonged effect. High abuse potential and popular "street drug" due to extreme potency and lack of strong hypnotic effect. Oral form is very useful in treating severe chronic pain but drug is relatively short-acting. Schedule II.
oxymorphone (Numorphan)	Injection—1 mg/ml, 1.5 mg/ml Suppositories—5 mg	SC, IM—1 mg to 1.5 mg every 4 h–6 h IV—0.5 mg as needed Rectal—5 mg every 4 h–6 h Analgesic during labor—0.5 mg to 1 mg IM every 4 h–6 h	Rapid-acting (5 min to 10 min), potent (5× to 10× morphine) analgesic. Used for preoperative sedation, obstetrical analgesia and relief of anxiety in patients with dyspnea due to pulmonary edema or left ventricular failure. High incidence of nausea, vomiting, and euphoria. Little constipation or antitussive action. Not recommended in children less than 12 years old. Schedule II.
oxycodone (Roxicodone)	Tablets—5 mg Oral solution—5 mg/5 ml	Adults—5 mg every 6 h	Orally effective analgesic used for relief of moderate to severe pain; good

(continued)

Table 22-4 (continued)
Narcotic Agonist Analgesics

Drug	Preparations	Usual Dosage Range	Clinical Considerations
Phenanthrenes (continued)			
oxycodone (Roxicodone) (continued)			antitussive action. Not recommended for use in children. Frequently given in combination with aspirin (Percodan) or acetaminophen (Percocet, Tylox).
opium (Paregoric, Pantopon)	Injection (Pantopon)—20 mg opium alkaloids hydrochlorides/ml (equivalent to 15 mg morphine/ml) Tincture—10% opium in 19% alcohol Camphorated Tincture (Paregoric)—2 mg morphine equivalent/5 ml with 45% alcohol	*Injection* IM, SC—5 mg to 20 mg every 4 h–5 h *Tincture* 0.6 ml (6 mg morphine) 4 times/day *Camphorated Tincture* Adults—5 ml to 10 ml (2 mg–4 mg morphine) one to four times/day Children—0.25 to 0.5 ml/kg one to four times/day	Activity is primarily due to morphine content. Use has been largely replaced by morphine or other narcotics, except for paregoric, which is widely used for cramps, diarrhea, and teething pain in infants (topical application). Discontinue drug once diarrhea has been controlled to prevent excessive dosage. Do not confuse paregoric (camphorated opium tincture containing 2 mg morphine/5 ml) with opium tincture itself (50 mg morphine/5 ml). Absorption of drug from GI tract is improved if diluted in a little water. Injection and tincture are Schedule II and camphorated tincture is Schedule III.
Methadones			
methadone (Dolophine)	Injection—10 mg/ml Tablets—5 mg, 10 mg Oral solution—5 mg/5 ml, 10 mg/5 ml Dispersible tablets—40 mg (for detoxification *only*)	*Analgesia* IM, SC, orally—2.5 mg–10 mg every 3 h–4 h (Children 0.7 mg/kg/day) *Chronic pain regimen* 5 mg every 12 h to 20 mg every 5 h. Start with 5 mg every 5 h–6 h and titrate according to patient's needs. *Narcotic detoxification* (Highly individualized depending on severity of withdrawal symptoms) 15 mg to 20 mg orally (up to 40 mg) to suppress symptoms. Treatment not to exceed 21 days,	May be used to relieve severe pain, usually orally or IM; SC administration may be painful. Longer-acting and less sedating than morphine, especially when given on a chronic basis. Exerts a similar degree of respiratory depression and addiction liability as morphine. Not recommended for obstetrics or as an analgesic in young children except in cancer-related pain, where it is very effective. Also used for detoxification and maintenance of

(continued)

Table 22-4 (continued)
Narcotic Agonist Analgesics

Drug	Preparations	Usual Dosage Range	Clinical Considerations
Methadones (continued)			
methadone (Dolophine) (*continued*)		during which time the dose is gradually reduced *Maintenance therapy* 20 mg to 120 mg daily, individualized to control abstinence symptoms but not produce sedation or respiratory depression	narcotic addiction in approved programs. Administered orally on a daily basis; abstinence syndrome is qualitatively similar to morphine, but onset is slower, course is more prolonged, and symptoms are less severe. With prolonged oral use, most side-effects disappear, but constipation and sweating often persist. Euphoria is much less prominent with methadone, and addict may eventually overcome compulsive need for the narcotic "high." Should be used in combination with other psychiatric and social counseling (see Chapter 85). Schedule II.
propoxyphene (Darvon, Dolene, Doxaphene, Prophene 65)	Capsules—32 mg, 65 mg (HCl salt) Tablets—100 mg (napsylate salt) Suspension—10 mg/ml (napsylate salt)	Adults—65 mg to 100 mg every 4 h *Note:* 65 mg of the HCl salt is equivalent to 100 mg of the napsylate salt.	Very weak analgesic, structurally related to methadone. Little antitussive activity. Has many of the side-effects of narcotics and can produce habituation and physical dependence to approximately the same degree as codeine. Restlessness, tremor, and mild euphoria commonly occur. Usually administered in fixed combination with aspirin and caffeine (*e.g.,* Darvon Compound), acetaminophen (*e.g.,* Darvocet, Dolene AP, Wygesic) or aspirin (*e.g.,* Darvon w/ASA). Will potentiate CNS depressant effects of alcohol and tranquilizers; such combinations are a major cause of drug-related fatalities. Symptoms of overdosage resemble those of narcotics, with the addition of convulsions. Treatment consists of respiratory assistance, narcotic antagonists, anti-

(continued)

Table 22-4 (continued)
Narcotic Agonist Analgesics

Drug	Preparations	Usual Dosage Range	Clinical Considerations
Methadones (continued)			
propoxyphene (Darvon, Dolene, Doxaphene, Prophene 65) (continued)			convulsants, and circulatory support (fluids, vasopressors). Use with caution, and avoid prolonged or excessive dosage and concurrent use of tranquilizers or alcohol. Maximum recommended doses are 390 mg/day of the HCl salt and 600 mg/day of the napsylate salt. Schedule IV.
Morphinans			
levorphanol (Levo-Dromoran)	Injection—2 mg/ml Tablets—2 mg	2 mg to 3 mg orally or SC every 4 h–6 h	Very potent analgesic (4× to 5× morphine); almost as effective orally as parenterally. Used preoperatively to potentiate and prolong general anesthesia, and to shorten recovery time. Also is a useful supplement to nitrous oxide–oxygen anesthesia. Low incidence of nausea, vomiting, and constipation, but strong sedative and respiratory depressant. Slow onset of peak effect (60 min–90 min) but prolonged duration (6 h–8 h). Reduce dose in pediatric and geriatric population and in poor-risk patients. Has a bitter taste. Protect from light. Schedule II.
Phenylpiperidines			
meperidine (Demerol, Pethadol)	Injection—10, 25, 50, 75, 100 mg/ml Tablets—50 mg, 100 mg Syrup—50 mg/5 ml	*Analgesia* IM, SC, Orally—50 mg to 150 mg every 3 h–4 h (Children—1 to 2 mg/kg IM, SC or orally every 3 h–4 h) *Preoperative medication* Adults—50 mg to 100 mg IM or SC 30 min–90 min before anesthesia Children—1 to 2 mg/kg IM or SC *Obstetrical analgesia* 50 mg to 100 mg IM or SC; repeat at 1-h to 3-h intervals	Moderately potent analgesic ($^1/_{10}$ morphine) with weak antitussive activity. Less spasmogenic and constipating than most other narcotics; more rapid onset and shorter duration of action (2 h–4 h) compared to morphine. Significantly less effective orally than parenterally. Frequent dizziness and occasional tremors, uncoordinated muscle movements, and other signs of CNS exci-

(continued)

Table 22-4 (continued)
Narcotic Agonist Analgesics

Drug	Preparations	Usual Dosage Range	Clinical Considerations
Phenylpiperidines (continued)			
meperidine (Demerol, Pethadol) (continued)			tation can occur. Attains high levels in breast milk. Used for moderate pain, often associated with diagnostic procedures, minor surgical procedures, or obstetrics. Also for preanesthetic medication and by slow IV infusion (1 mg/ml) for support of anesthesia. Solutions of meperidine and barbiturates are incompatible. Prolonged therapy may result in elevated normeperidine levels (detectable by plasma sample) which can result in CNS symptoms ranging from shakiness to seizures. If such toxicity occurs, withdraw the drug. Do not use naloxone because it may precipitate seizures. Schedule II.
fentanyl (Sublimaze)	Injection—0.05 mg/ml	*Preoperative* 0.05 mg to 0.1 mg IM *General anesthesia* Induction—0.05 mg to 0.1 mg IV (repeat at 2-min to 3-min intervals) Maintenance—0.025 mg to 0.1 mg IV or IM as needed *Adjunct to general anesthesia* 0.002 to 0.05 mg/kg as needed *Postoperative* 0.05 mg to 0.1 mg IM every 1 h to 2 h for pain, tachypnea, and delirium Children (2 yr to 12 yr)—0.02 to 0.03 mg/20 to 25 lb	Very potent (100× morphine) analgesic used for short durations (e.g., preoperative, during surgery, or postoperative to relieve pain and anxiety and as an anesthetic agent with oxygen in selected high-risk patients such as open-heart surgery, complicated neurologic procedures). Rapid onset (10 min–15 min IM) and short duration (1 h–2 h). Respiratory depression often outlasts analgesia. Have antidotal measures (e.g., oxygen, endotracheal tube, narcotic antagonist, muscle relaxant) on hand. Rapid IV administration may cause muscle spasm or rigidity. Also available in combination with the neuroleptic droperidol as Innovar, which is used to produce analgesia and tranquilization (neuro-

(continued)

Table 22-4 (continued)
Narcotic Agonist Analgesics

Drug	Preparations	Usual Dosage Range	Clinical Considerations
Phenylpiperidines (continued)			
fentanyl (Sublimaze) (continued)			leptanalgesia) for short surgical and diagnostic procedures (see Chapter 21). Combination may result in restlessness, hallucinations, extrapyramidal symptoms, and postoperative drowsiness. Vital signs should be monitored continuously during use. Schedule II.
alfentanil (Alfenta)	Injection—0.5 mg/ml	*Analgesia adjunct* 8 to 50 mcg/kg IV, followed by increments of 3 to 15 mcg/kg as required (maximum 75 mcg/kg) *Induction anesthetic* 130 to 245 mcg/kg IV followed by 0.5 to 1.5 mcg/kg/min IV infusion	Rapid-acting narcotic used IV as an analgesic adjunct during N_2O/O_2/barbiturate anesthesia. Also used as a primary induction anesthetic in general surgery where intubation and mechanical ventilation are required. Determine dose based on *lean* body weight in obese individuals; reduce dose in elderly or debilitated persons. Not recommended in children under 12. Vital signs must be closely monitored.
sufentanil (Sufenta)	Injection—50 mcg/ml	*Adults* For general surgery in which intubation and mechanical ventilation are required 1–2 mcg/kg with N_2O/O_2; maintenance dose of 10 mcg–25 mcg as analgesia lightens For more complicated surgery 2–8 mcg/kg with N_2O/O_2; maintenance doses of 25 mcg–50 mcg as needed For complete anesthesia 8–30 mcg/kg with 100% O_2 and a muscle relaxant; maintenance doses of 25 mcg–50 mcg as anesthesia lightens *Children* (under 12)—10–25 mcg/kg with 100% O_2 for general anesthesia in children undergoing cardiovascular surgery	An anesthetic agent that can induce and maintain anesthesia with 100% O_2 in patients undergoing major surgical procedures, such as cardiovascular surgery or neurosurgery in the sitting position. Also used as an analgesic adjunct at doses less than 8 mcg/kg to maintain balanced general anesthesia. Dosage should be based on lean body weight and reduced in the elderly or debilitated. Doses above 8 mcg/kg produce sleep. Catecholamine release is suppressed at doses up to 25 mcg/kg, and sympathetic responses are attenuated at doses between 25 mcg/kg and 35 mcg/kg. Postoperative mechanical ventilation is necessary due to extended respiratory depression. Schedule II.

Table 22-5
Narcotic Agonist-Antagonist Analgesics

Drug	Preparations	Usual Dosage Range	Clinical Considerations
Phenanthrenes			
nalbuphine (Nubain)	Injection—10 mg/ml, 20 mg/ml	SC, IM, IV—10 mg/70 kg individual; repeat every 3 h–6 h as necessary. Maximum 160 mg/day	Chemically related to oxycodone and naloxone, and possesses both agonistic activity at *kappa* and *delta* receptors and weak antagonistic activity at *mu* receptors. Analgesia is approximately equivalent to morphine on a milligram basis, with somewhat lower abuse potential (less than that of codeine or propoxyphene). May precipitate withdrawal symptoms in patients on chronic narcotic therapy; use one fourth normal dose initially in these patients. High incidence of sedation. Does not increase systemic vascular resistance or cardiac workload like other narcotic agonist–antagonists. At usual adult dose, respiratory depression is equal to that seen with morphine; larger doses (*i.e.*, above 30 mg), however, do not result in appreciable increases in degree of respiratory depression, unlike morphine. Duration of analgesia ranges from 3 h–6 h. Do not use in pregnant women or children under 18 years of age. *Not* a controlled drug.
buprenorphine (Buprenex)	Injection—0.3 mg/ml	Adults and children over 12 yr—0.3 mg–0.6 mg IM or slow IV every 6 h as needed	Semisynthetic derivative of thebaine that has a high affinity for *mu* receptors and dissociates from them slowly. Exhibits a long duration of action (up to 6 h), low degree of dependence, and is approximately 20×–30× more potent than morphine. Possesses antagonist activity equal to that of naloxone. May reduce blood pressure and heart rate and produces respiratory depression equal to that of morphine at normal dosage ranges. Sedation is very common. Use cautiously in elderly or debilitated patients, or patients with impaired hepatic, renal, or pulmonary function. May precipitate withdrawal symptoms in narcotic-dependent patients. Schedule V.
Morphinan			
butorphanol (Stadol)	Injection—1 mg/ml, 2 mg/ml	IM—2 mg every 3 h–4 h (maximum 4 mg/dose) IV—1 mg every 3 h–4 h	Potent analgesic (4×–7× morphine on a weight basis). Respiratory depression with 2-mg dose is equivalent to that achieved with 10 mg of morphine, but does not increase appreciably at 4 mg. Possesses weak narcotic antagonistic

(continued)

Table 22-5 (continued)
Narcotic Agonist-Antagonist Analgesics

Drug	Preparations	Usual Dosage Range	Clinical Considerations
Morphinan (continued)			
butorphanol (Stadol) (continued)			activity (considerably less than that of naloxone); use with caution in patients dependent on narcotics because withdrawal symptoms can occur. Most frequent side-effect is sedation. Peak analgesia occurs in 1 h with IM use and persists for 3 h–4 h. Not recommended in children less than 18 years of age or in nursing mothers. Use cautiously in the presence of liver or kidney disease, coronary artery insufficiency (increases cardiac workload), respiratory impairment, and in persons physically dependent on narcotic drugs.
Benzomorphan			
pentazocine (Talwin)	Tablets—50 mg Injection—30 mg/ml	Oral—50 mg every 3 h–4 h (maximum dose—600 mg/day) IM, SC, IV—30 mg every 3 h–4 h (maximum dose—360 mg/day) Obstetrics—30 mg IM or 20 mg IV every 2 h–3 h	One third as potent as morphine parenterally. Possesses some narcotic antagonist activity as well, therefore, can antagonize the effects of other opiates and may elicit withdrawal symptoms in patients who have been taking other narcotics regularly. Onset is 15 min–30 min after IM, SC, or oral use and 2 min–3 min IV. Duration from 2 h–3 h parenterally and up to 5 h with oral use. Has sedative activity and widely used preoperatively in obstetrics as well as for moderate and severe pain. Addiction liability about equal to codeine. Tablets are marketed as Talwin-Nx and contain 0.5 mg of naloxone, a potent narcotic antagonist. Although inactive orally, naloxone has profound antagonistic actions against narcotics when injected, and its inclusion in the tablet is intended to curb a form of pentazocine abuse in which the tablets are dissolved and injected. Can induce tachycardia, hypertension, confusion, hallucinations, bizarre thought processes, and other CNS effects in large doses. Abrupt discontinuation of drug may result in muscle cramping, chills, restlessness, anxiety, and other symptoms of narcotic withdrawal. Do not mix with soluble barbiturates because a precipitate will form. Rotate injection sites if used chronically to minimize sclerosis of skin and subcutaneous tissues. Severe respiratory depression is treated with naloxone and other supportive measures. Schedule IV.

cord, and may function as an excitatory neurotransmitter at postsynaptic nerve endings transmitting painful sensations.

Narcotics reduce the sensitivity of medullary respiratory center neurons to carbon dioxide, leading to a dose-dependent respiratory depression, although there appears to be a "ceiling" effect to the respiratory depression with the combined agonist–antagonist drugs (see Fig. 22-1). The chemoreceptor trigger zone (CTZ) in the medulla is activated by opiate drugs which may result in nausea and vomiting.

The responsiveness of peripheral alpha-adrenergic receptors is decreased, leading to visceral pooling of blood and possible orthostatic hypotension. The hypotensive effect may also be due to depression of the medullary vasomotor center and to release of histamine, a peripheral vasodilator. The reduced venous tone and decreased peripheral resistance may contribute to the effectiveness of opiates in relieving dyspnea secondary to left ventricular failure, because both would reduce left ventricular work.

Other actions of narcotic drugs are a direct inhibitory effect on propulsive activity in the GI tract, biliary constriction, increased tone of the urinary sphincter, and reduced uterine tone. Neuroendocrine effects are usually not clinically significant, but may include decreased release of luteinizing hormone (LH) and thyrotropin (TSH), and increased secretion of prolactin (LTH), somatotropin (growth hormone), and antidiuretic hormone (ADH).

USES
Note: Not all drugs are indicated for all of the following uses. Refer to Tables 22-4 and 22-5 for specific applications of individual drugs.
1. Relief of moderate to severe pain, such as that associated with carcinomas, myocardial infarction, burns, fractures, and postsurgical trauma (Narcotics are usually more effective against the constant, "visceral" type of pain than against sharp, intermittent pain.)
2. Reduce anxiety and enhance effectiveness of anesthetics in patients undergoing surgery
3. Relief of acute dyspnea resulting from pulmonary edema in persons with left ventricular failure (see under Mechanism and Actions)
4. Suppression of coughing (especially codeine and hydrocodone)
5. Treatment of diarrhea and abdominal cramping

6. Detoxification and maintenance therapy of narcotic addiction (methadone only)

ADMINISTRATION AND DOSAGE
See Tables 22-4 and 22-5.

FATE
Absorption from SC and IM injection sites as well as GI mucosa is generally good. Some drugs undergo significant first-pass hepatic metabolism immediately upon absorption and therefore the effective oral dose is considerably higher than the parenteral dose (see Table 22-1). The compounds are widely distributed in the body and localize in highest amounts in the liver, kidneys, lungs, and spleen. Brain concentrations are usually low compared to other body organs; highly lipophilic drugs (e.g., fentanyl) cross the blood–brain barrier more readily than weakly lipophilic agents such as morphine. Analgesic effects are noted within 30 minutes after oral administration and 5 minutes to 15 minutes following parenteral injection. (See Table 22-1 for duration of analgesia with each narcotic drug.) Narcotic drugs are converted primarily to polar metabolites which are readily excreted by the kidneys. Small quantities of unchanged drug may also be eliminated in the urine and feces.

SIDE-EFFECTS/ADVERSE REACTIONS
Dizziness, lightheadedness, nausea, sedation, and sweating are the most frequently noted side-effects with narcotic analgesics. Many other adverse reactions have occurred with narcotic drugs, and are listed by organ system below:
CNS—Euphoria or dysphoria, headache, agitation, tremor, disorientation, delirium, uncoordinated movements, transient hallucinations
CV—Bradycardia, palpitation, hypotension, syncope, phlebitis with IV injection
GI—Dry mouth, anorexia, constipation, vomiting, biliary tract spasm
Respiratory—Respiratory depression (observed in fetus and newborn as well), laryngospasm
Genitourinary—Urinary hesitancy or retention, dysuria, antidiuretic effect, loss of potency or libido
Hypersensitivity—Urticaria, pruritus, sneezing, edema, hemorrhagic urticaria, wheal and flare at IV injection site
Other—Pain at injection site, local tissue irritation, porphyria, muscular rigidity

Acute overdosage is characterized by extreme miosis, hypothermia, oliguria, bradycardia, hypotension, deep sleep, marked respiratory depression, pulmonary edema, coma, and cardiac arrest.

CONTRAINDICATIONS AND PRECAUTIONS

In all but extreme cases of need, the narcotic analgesics are contraindicated in patients with increased intracranial pressure because the retention of CO_2 resulting from depressed respiration can lead to cerebral vasodilation. Other contraindications include severe respiratory disease, hepatic cirrhosis, severe ulcerative colitis, and kyphoscoliosis. Opiates are also usually contraindicated in undiagnosed acute abdominal conditions, severe diarrhea due to ingestion of a toxic substance (until the toxin has been removed), in premature infants, and during labor when a premature infant is anticipated. Meperidine is also contraindicated in patients who are taking or have recently received an MAO-inhibitor (see under Interactions).

Narcotic drugs must be used with *caution* in patients with adrenal insufficiency, hypothyroidism, impaired hepatic or renal function, cerebral arteriosclerosis, prostatic hypertrophy, acute alcoholism, supraventricular tachycardia, diabetic acidosis, and in elderly or debilitated persons and pregnant or lactating women.

INTERACTIONS

1. The CNS-depressant effects of narcotics may be potentiated or prolonged by concurrent use of other CNS depressants (*e.g.*, barbiturates, alcohol, anesthetics, phenothiazines, sedatives, tricyclic antidepressants).
2. Muscle relaxation and respiratory depression may be intensified by concurrent use of narcotics and neuromuscular blocking agents (*e.g.*, succinylcholine).
3. Symptoms of acute narcotic overdose, possibly causing death, may occur with use of meperidine within 14 days of an MAO inhibitor.
4. Withdrawal symptoms may occur in patients addicted to narcotics if the narcotic agonist–antagonist drugs (see Table 22-5) are added, because they may antagonize the actions of the pure agonists.
5. Meperidine has anticholinergic effects that may be additive with those of other drugs (*e.g.*, atropine-like agents, tricyclic antidepressants, disopyramide).

6. The analgesic efficacy of narcotic drugs can be potentiated by tricyclic antidepressants, phenothiazines, amphetamines, and methocarbamol.
7. Phenytoin or rifampin may reduce blood concentrations of methadone to such an extent as to precipitate withdrawal symptoms.
8. Orthostatic hypotension may be intensified by concurrent use of narcotic analgesics and high-ceiling diuretics, such as furosemide, bumetanide, and ethacrynic acid.

■ Nursing Process

The nursing care for the patient receiving narcotic analgesics is inseparably linked to the treatment of pain and will influence how the medication is used, what effect it will have, and how the patient will perceive the experience.

□ ASSESSMENT

□ Subjective Data

Because pain is a subjective phenomenon, discovering a patient's need for pain medication will not always be easy. The expression of pain is colored by a person's cultural background as well as what he thinks others expect him to do or say. Facial grimaces, crying, holding the site of pain, writhing in bed are all visual cues of pain. However, some patients refuse to engage in these activities because they believe in stoicism. This approach is frequently found in elderly persons and others who suffer chronic pain; hence, visual cues will not be helpful. Cues also color the health-care staff's perception of pain as well as their response to it. In addition, health-care personnel establish "norms" of what should and should not be painful. These are also subjective responses and have nothing to do with actual pain. The nurse needs to surmount the obstacles created by preconceived notions of what a person in pain should look like or what constitutes a painful experience, in order to adequately assess a patient's pain and design appropriate interventions. Statistically, patients usually rate their pain higher than the staff perceives it to be.

Given that subjective cues may be misleading, the nurse needs to establish some guidelines for assessing pain which may include determining where the pain is located and asking the patient to describe it. Some patients will deny having pain but will admit to cramping, discomfort, or itching. By determining the source of the pain, the nurse can work with the patient to determine what will relieve it. Hence, a backrub may be more effective than meperidine once muscular aching from bedrest is identified as the source. Drugs do not necessarily ease all pain. This assessment might also determine what medication will relieve the pain. For example, the patient with a headache does not need morphine even though it may be the only pain medication currently ordered.

Once the location of the pain is determined, the patient should be asked to rate it on a scale of 0 to 10; 0 being no pain and 10 being unbearable pain. This data will help the nurse determine how the patient is coping with the perceived discomfort and may actually help the patient put it into perspective.

A health history and assessment of psychosocial functioning should be obtained when the patient is comfortable or pain free. Such information is useful in later interactions when a patient is in pain. A patient who has been suffering multiple illnesses of long duration is very likely to have little ability to cope with pain. Life stresses, such as suffering a loss of family or of bodily function and general anxiety, will also make it difficult for a patient to manage pain.

When assessing the need for medication for children in pain, the above parameters may be used, but more frequently a different assessment technique is appropriate. Many health-care personnel feel it is unnecessary to assess or medicate children in pain because of children's limited perception. The fallacy of this thinking can be quickly documented by observing any child in pain. In the child under 2 years old, signs will include irritability, crying, or loss of appetite. Although the child may not verbalize pain, a nurse should consider medicating any child suffering from the same condition for which pain medication would be offered to an adult. In the child over age 2, the level of communication will vary. Using play, the nurse can ask the child to paint on a doll, or to draw on a simple figure where he hurts. Parents can also aid as resources in determining pain. Although the child may not tell a nurse about pain, he may describe it to his parents whom he trusts to take care of him. The child's activity, attention span, and appetite are all indicators of the level of discomfort.

A medication history is also important before narcotic analgesics are administered. Many patients in chronic pain will use a variety of over-the-counter remedies, some of which may continue to be useful when narcotics are started. *All* drug use should be identified, including use of alcohol and street drugs, so that appropriate strategies for relief can be mapped out. In addition, narcotics interact with a variety of other drugs and can result in toxic interactions. Therefore, knowledge of the total drug regimen is essential for safe care and is especially important with elderly patients on multiple drug therapy.

□ *Objective Data*
Physical assessment of cardiovascular, respiratory, and psychomotor function is essential. Assessment of musculoskeletal mass is important if intramuscular or subcutaneous administration of narcotics is being considered. Ability to swallow should also be tested. Other systems may be examined if affected by the pain or if the history reveals significant problems. Laboratory data may include assessment of renal and hepatic function especially in children and elderly persons, but response to medication will be very individualized regardless of function and will have to be evaluated throughout therapy.

□ *NURSING DIAGNOSES*
Actual nursing diagnoses for patients receiving narcotic analgesics may include:

Knowledge deficit related to the action, administration, and side-effects of the drug
Alteration in comfort: pain or chronic pain

Potential nursing diagnoses may be based on the way pain is affecting the patient's life, the way the drug influences the patient's activity, or the side-effects of the drug and may include:

Potential activity intolerance
Impaired adjustment
Anxiety
Alteration in bowel elimination: constipation
Alteration in cardiac output: decreased
Ineffective individual (or family) coping
Impaired gas exchange
Hopelessness
Impaired physical mobility
Noncompliance with the regimen as prescribed, especially if it fails to provide relief
Alteration in nutrition: less than body requirements related to pain or drug side-effects
Self-care deficit related to all activities of daily living depending on degree of mobility pain relief provides

Sensory–perceptual alteration of any of the senses as a drug side-effect
Sexual dysfunction from pain or drug side-effects
Sleep pattern disturbance
Alteration in thought processes
Urinary retention

In fact, almost all of the listed NANDA Nursing Diagnoses may apply to one or more patients seeking pain relief.

□ *PLAN*

The main goal of pain medication is to provide a patient with adequate relief from discomfort while maintaining his ability to be in control of his environment and participate in his care. In terminal cancer pain, achievement of relief and comfort may outweigh the desire to keep a patient functionally independent.

□ *INTERVENTION*

The nurse needs to develop intervention strategies which will meet the stated goal of adequate pain relief without side-effects, if possible. First it is important to choose an appropriate route. A variety of routes are used to administer pain medication; several factors should be considered before a route is chosen.

1. Expected duration of therapy. If the patient has terminal cancer, oral medication may be tried first, then IM or SC, then intravenous injections, continuous intravenous infusions, and, occasionally, intraspinal or epidural infusion of narcotics. In the immediate postoperative period, the intramuscular route may be most appropriate, but injections should not be given for more than 2 weeks, even when sites are carefully rotated, because tissue damage occurs rapidly.

2. Size, muscle mass, and condition of the skin or veins. If the patient is extremely thin, intramuscular injections may be inappropriate regardless of other parameters. If edema is present, as frequently occurs in the patient with congestive heart failure or who is burned, the drug will be inadequately absorbed unless administered by the oral or intravenous route. If veins are fragile, intravenous routes may be precluded unless a central vein can be used.

3. Ability to swallow. A young child, a debilitated adult, or a terminally ill patient may be unable to swallow pills but may be able to swallow liquids. If the patient is unable to swallow con-

sistently, then an alternate route should be sought.

All of these factors will influence absorption of the narcotic and subsequent pain relief. The nurse needs to review pain medication orders early for appropriateness of route of administration so that time is not wasted clarifying or changing orders when the patient is in pain.

The nurse must also be clear on the techniques of administration, particularly if the intravenous or intraspinal route is used. Institutions usually provide specific policies regarding administration by these routes. Rate of infusion, use of infusion pumps, and responsibilities of the physician and nurse should be clearly stated. Procedures for administration of drug therapy, calculation of dosages, and care of catheters and IV lines should be identified. These routes are generally used for patients whose pain has been unrelieved by other methods. While the potential for toxicity is high, most patients receiving drugs by these routes, including young children, will have developed a high tolerance for narcotics and will probably experience few adverse effects. Likewise, the desire for pain relief may preclude concern about sedation.

Perception of pain colors the nurse's administration of pain medication as well as how the physician orders it. The most frequent reason health professionals give for undermedication of pain is fear of addicting the patient and the subsequent development of tolerance requiring more medication. Less than 1% of addictions are the result of receiving narcotic pain medications, so statistically this concern is invalid. Because tolerance and addiction usually occur with repeated administration over at least a 10-day period, the chance is low that the patient in acute pain will suffer any consequences.

Positive nursing strategies for treating pain with narcotics can greatly increase patient comfort. Administration of an adequate dose to relieve pain is important. Except in the immediate postanesthesia period where interaction with anesthetic drugs precludes it, the dose should be high enough to provide relief without producing side-effects. In fact, the dose may be started at a slightly higher level and titrated down based on the symptoms which occur. This is a particularly good practice with cancer patients who have a high tolerance for pain medication and with addicts in acute pain, but may be helpful for any patient in acute pain.

Early in an acute pain episode, or in treating chronic pain of terminal patients, medication should be given on a regular schedule rather than on a p.r.n. basis. The patient may think when the physician tells him he can have something for pain every 4 hours that it will automatically be brought to him. He will be confused if he later finds out he must ask for it, so establishing a regimen can build trust. In acute pain episodes of short or long duration, adequate analgesia before the pain becomes severe is more effective in reducing pain than attempting to alleviate the pain after it has peaked. (This is especially important in the acute postoperative period.) If the dose becomes ineffective or the patient complains of pain before the time interval has passed, then tolerance is beginning, and the physician should be notified. Strategies to deal with tolerance include changing the type of medication to another of equal analgesic value (see Tables 22-1 and 22-6), increasing the dosage of the same medication, or decreasing the time interval between doses.

As the pain diminishes the medication may be changed again and the patient eased off the drug. Refer to Tables 22-1 and 22-6 for equianalgesic rates. Reducing the strength of medication too quickly can cause acute withdrawal and should be avoided. If problems persist in removing the patient from a drug, methadone can be used in reducing doses until it can be eliminated.

To enhance the effectiveness of pain medication, the nurse can use positive reinforcement. This may include explaining how long it will take before the medication begins to work, eliciting how the patient feels after the medication takes effect, and consciously planning with the patient to give medication before he gets out of bed or does

coughing and deep breathing exercises. These activities help the patient perceive the drug's benefit and may positively affect the drug's placebo effect (i.e., a psychological effect beyond that expected of the drug).

Administration of pain medication to elderly persons will vary somewhat from administration to the younger adult because function of the body systems diminishes with age. Pain is dangerous to the elderly; it can cause shallow breathing which will lead to fluid accumulation in the lungs, cause fatigue leading to decreased cardiac output and the possibility of heart failure, and produce anxiety which will decrease coping ability. Although respiratory depression from analgesics is a particular concern with elderly persons, giving smaller, more frequent doses will reduce the risk. Narcotic duration of action may be longer in elderly persons, giving some patients a longer period of relief with a drug. Observation of this effect early in therapy can help determine dosage frequency.

For the elderly person suffering chronic pain, timing administration of medications around activities requiring exertion such as dressing or walking may help him cope.

In children, administration by any route other than injection is always preferable. However, the nurse should not avoid giving the medication simply because it is painful. If it will hurt, the best strategy is to be honest about the pain, give the injection as quickly as possible, and return when the child has gotten relief to remind him how much better he felt after the shot.

For all patients, side-effects may be a problem, but most common side-effects do not preclude continued drug use. Many patients will complain of dizziness and lightheadedness. This central nervous system effect will usually pass as the patient adjusts to the dose. In the interim, outpatients should be cautioned to avoid driving or operating any potentially dangerous machinery until such effects pass. The hospitalized patient should be protected from injury if such effects occur. The patient should be told to remain in bed or should be assisted out of bed. Side rails should be kept up and a call bell placed within easy reach because equilibrium can be greatly affected.

Gastrointestinal side-effects most common with narcotics include nausea and constipation. The patient should take the drug with food or after meals if gastrointestinal upset occurs. Constipation is a problem with prolonged therapy because peristalsis is slowed by this drug group. The patient should be encouraged to increase fluid intake and

---

Table 22-6

Approximate Equivalent Doses of Analgesics Employed Orally for Less Severe Pain*

Name	PO dose (mg)
Non-Narcotics	
aspirin	650
acetaminophen	650
Controlled Substances	
codeine	32
meperidine	50
oxycodone	5
pentazocine	30
propoxyphene	65

* All doses are approximately equivalent to aspirin 650 mg. (Adapted with permission from Rogers AG: Pharmacology of analgesics. J Neurosurg Nurs 10(4):182, 1978)

add bulk foods and roughage to his diet. A bulk laxative may also be prescribed.

□ *EVALUATION*

The outcome criteria for pain management may be different for the nurse and the patient unless they reach some agreement. For the patient the outcome sought may range from total relief to some relief enabling him to manage his daily activities. This latter outcome may be sought by patients in chronic pain. The nurse may seek to minimize side-effects and prevent addiction or tolerance in addition to providing relief. The importance of achieving these outcomes varies with the individual, the disease state, the cause of pain, and other variables connected with pain previously mentioned. Nursing Care Plan 22-1 summarizes the nursing process described above and provides guidelines for establishing a nursing care plan for the patient receiving narcotic analgesics.

The Use of Placebos in Pain Management

A placebo is any form of treatment that produces an effect in a patient because of its implicit or explicit intent, not because of its specific physical or chemical properties (McCaffery, 1982). The placebo response is used to enhance any drug therapy by the positive attributes the care givers relate (e.g., "This medicine should help relieve your pain"). Placebos (e.g., sugar pills or saline solutions) are sometimes given as part of double-blind clinical trials of new drugs (see Chap. 7).

Unfortunately, many health-care professionals use the placebo effect in a negative sense, particularly in pain medication administration. When a patient complains of pain beyond that which staff expect him to have, placebo injections or pills may be given. Reasons health-care professionals use for administering placebos include determining real vs imaginary pain, preventing addiction, proving the patient is wrong or exaggerating his symptoms. More than likely the real reason may be that the staff is frustrated by the patient's demands for pain medication and they are unable or unwilling to use any other strategy to cope with the patient's needs.

In fact, placebos do not determine real pain, prevent addiction, or prove that patients are wrong, exaggerating, or psychologically maladapted. Often, patients can perceive a difference between a potent analgesic drug, with its sedative side-effects, and a placebo medication, which of

course is devoid of drug-induced side-effects. However, about 85% of all patients in pain might receive relief from a placebo at one time or another, and placebos are capable of relieving severe pain in some persons.

Placebo therapy only indicates whether a person is a placebo reactor or a nonreactor. Characteristics of reactors are cooperation, positive attitude about care, fewer complaints of pain, and increased responsiveness to morphine. Characteristics of nonreactors include rigid, suspicious personality and nonresponsiveness to many active drugs. Most drug addicts fall into this category, so placebo therapy for them is usually futile.

Placebos may be used to help in the treatment of long-term pain but the nurse must consider the ethics of this deceptive therapy before agreeing to participate. The patient could be asked to give his consent to participate in the treatment. Although the physician may argue that this defeats the purpose of the treatment, studies have shown that a placebo reactor will get positive benefits from the placebo even when he knows what it is. This strategy could be coupled with double-blind administration in which the patient gets an active drug occasionally, but neither he nor the nurse knows when. Such activity takes more effort on the part of the whole health team but reduces the chance that placebos will be used as punitive therapy. If the patient refuses to participate, as is his right, then titration and gradual withdrawal of drugs or exploration of alternate pain-relieving strategies such as transcutaneous nerve stimulation can be used.

The nurse must ethically feel placebo therapy is justified, agree to participate, and find some way to justify its use, especially if the physician refuses to seek the patient's consent. One theory of placebo therapy is that it helps stimulate the body's own endorphins, particularly in placebo-reactive patients. A placebo might then be called an endorphin-reactor. The label is more positive among professionals than the use of the term placebo, but the practice of placebo treatment for pain without consent is a deception to the patient regardless of what it is called.

A patient who has difficulty withdrawing from pain medication needs extensive counseling and support from staff. Consultations with a psychiatric clinical nurse specialist, psychiatrist, or physician specializing in pain management may be needed. A placebo is never a permanent solution in pain management. At best it is an occasional tool, sometimes overused and abused in the process of patient care.

(*Text continues on p. 402.*)

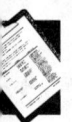

Nursing Care Plan 22-1
The Patient Receiving Narcotic Analgesics

Assessment

Subjective Data

1. Medication history: refer to Interactions section to formulate pertinent questions
   a. Ask about OTC analgesic use, use of alcohol, use of street drugs, especially patients with chronic pain and elderly clients
   b. Differentiate reports of drug allergy/hypersensitivity versus drug reaction (*e.g.*, vomiting from codeine)
2. Ask patient to describe the pain in specific terms: expression, description of sensation, location, rating on a scale of 1–10, history, and progress; observe irritability, play, and appetite in children
3. Medical history
   a. Check for preexisting conditions, such as severe respiratory disease, cardiac dysrhythmias, impaired renal or hepatic function, hypothyroidism, that may precipitate adverse reactions
   b. Determine cause of pain; use is contraindicated in undiagnosed acute abdomen, increased intracranial pressure
4. Personal history: coping patterns used for pain management, family supports, recent life stressors, ability to understand and manage prescribed regimen, as appropriate

Objective Data

1. Physical assessment
   a. Neurologic status: level of consciousness, memory, mental alertness, psychomotor skills, vision
   b. Cardiovascular status: heart rate, heart rhythm, blood pressure
   c. Respiratory function: lung sounds, respiratory rate and effort
   d. Musculoskeletal: muscle mass if multiple injections are anticipated
2. Laboratory data: varies; perform renal and hepatic function studies in elderly patients and young children

Nursing Diagnosis*	Expected Client Outcome	Intervention
Alteration in comfort: acute or chronic pain	Will obtain relief from acute pain	Administer medication as prescribed, preferably on a round-the-clock schedule rather than prn when pain is intolerable or unremitting. Ensure dose ordered is adequate for the size and age of the patient. Provide comfort measures such as back rub, change in positioning, decrease in environmental stimuli, and fewer interruptions during peak drug periods.
	Will tolerate chronic pain through adequate medication	Arrange a prn schedule so the patient has maximum pain relief during stressful situations (*e.g.*, early post-operative ambulation, dressing). Chart changes in drug response time due to tolerance. Encourage physician to change to another drug of equal analgesic value if necessary. Encourage activity; permit distractors as tolerated.
Knowledge deficit related to drug effect, frequency of administration, potential side-effects, withdrawal	Will verbalize knowledge of drug's action, correct administration schedule, and common side-effects	Teach patient what drug can do (*i.e.*, relieve pain perception) versus what it cannot do (*i.e.*, remove source of pain).

(continued)

* Most NANDA diagnoses can be applied. A sample of common problems has been chosen.

Nursing Diagnosis*	Expected Client Outcome	Intervention
		Establish with patient and physician the time frame for administration (*e.g.*, prn or every 3–4 hours).
		Teach the patient to monitor common side-effects as described below and follow preventive/reactive strategies given.
	Will withdraw from long-term therapy with minimal adverse effects	Initiate gradual reduction in dose; move from parenteral to oral drugs as prescribed.
		Observe for hyperventilation, hyperthermia, lacrimation, rhinorrhea. Notify physician of changes; dose reduction may need to be more gradual.
		Assure patient that symptoms are transient.
Potential for injury related to dizziness, drowsiness	Will avoid injury	Keep side rails up so that bedridden patients can avoid falls from bed due to changes in spatial perceptions caused by dizziness.
		Assist patient in getting out of bed or ambulating until effect of drug is known.
		Caution outpatients to avoid driving, climbing, or operating machinery until drug effects are known.
		Be prepared for paradoxical or exaggerated reactions in elderly patients or young children.
Potential alteration in bowel elimination: constipation related to drug-induced slowed peristalsis	Will maintain regular bowel schedule	Encourage the patient to increase fluids, fiber, and roughage food intake throughout drug therapy.
		Administer laxatives as prescribed.
Potential alteration in cardiac output related to drug effect or pain	Heart rate, rhythm will remain within normal limits	Determine effectiveness of medication in providing relief. Pain can cause fatigue leading to decreased cardiac output, especially in the elderly. Dose or drug may need to be changed.
		Monitor heart rate, rhythm every 4 hours during medication therapy.
		Report changes in heart rate, persistent dizziness, and chest pain to physician immediately.
Potential ineffective breathing pattern related to drug effect or pain	Respiratory rate, effort will remain within normal limits	Determine medication effectiveness in providing relief. Pain can cause shallow breathing, which will cause CO_2 trapping and acid–base imbalance.
		Monitor respiratory rate, effort at least every 4 hours during drug therapy.
		Notify physician immediately if dyspnea, shallow breathing, rales, or change of consciousness is noted.
		(continued)

Nursing Care Plan 22-1 (continued)
The Patient Receiving Narcotic Analgesics

Nursing Diagnosis*	Expected Client Outcome	Intervention
Potential alteration in tissue integrity related to multiple injections	Will maintain intact tissue at all injection sites	If long-term pain management is anticipated, work with physician to start patient on effective oral medication, moving to parenteral administration as needed.
		Rotate sites using a body map (see Chapter 8).
		Palpate sites for redness, pain, swelling, and induration before each injection and avoid site if these symptoms develop.
		Seek change in route to intravenous or intrathecal for seriously ill or debilitated patients before tissue breakdown occurs.

Narcotic Antagonists

Drugs capable of reversing the effects of the narcotic agonists are termed *narcotic antagonists.* Both of the drugs in this category, naloxone and naltrexone, are viewed as "pure" antagonists because they possess no intrinsic agonistic activity, unlike the mixed agonist–antagonist drugs discussed previously.

Naloxone is a rapid-acting drug given parenterally to reverse (or prevent, in some cases) the effects of opioid drugs, especially in the event of overdosage. It is capable of reversing the respiratory depressant, sedative, hypotensive, analgesic, and psychotomimetic effects of opiate drugs. In the absence of narcotics, naloxone exhibits essentially no pharmacologic activity.

Naltrexone is an orally administered narcotic antagonist which can attenuate or block the subjective effects of opioid drugs and reduce the physical dependence on these agents. It is used as an adjunct in maintaining an opioid-free state in detoxified former addicts.

Naloxone

(Narcan)

MECHANISM AND ACTIONS
Naloxone exhibits a very high affinity for the *mu* receptor sites and is capable of displacing narcotic drugs from these receptors, thus reversing their effects. Naloxone can also reverse the dysphoric and psychotomimetic effects of the mixed agonist–antagonists such as pentazocine. In the absence of narcotics, naloxone exhibits essentially no pharmacologic activity except for a mild sedative effect at very high doses. No tolerance or dependence has been reported with use of naloxone. Naloxone is specific for treating poisoning with opioid drugs and will not reverse the respiratory depression induced by other CNS depressants (*e.g.,* barbiturates, anesthetics).

USES
1. Reversal of respiratory depression and other adverse reactions induced by excessive doses of opioid drugs
2. Diagnosis of suspected acute opiate overdosage
3. *Investigational* uses include reversal of alcoholic coma and improvement of circulation in refractory shock.

ADMINISTRATION AND DOSAGE
Naloxone is used as an injection for adults (0.4 mg/ml) or neonates (0.02 mg/ml). It may be administered IV, IM, or SC, although it is usually given IV in emergency situations. It is a relatively short-acting drug (serum half-life = 1 hour) and may need to be given repeatedly in cases of poisoning with longer-acting opioid drugs. To treat known or suspected narcotic overdosage, adults are given an initial dose of 0.4 mg to 2 mg, IV, with

additional doses repeated at 2-minute to 3-minute intervals as needed for up to three doses. If no response occurs after a total dosage of 10 mg, the involvement of a narcotic drug must be questioned. Subsequent doses may then be given, IV, at 1-hour to 2-hour intervals as necessary until the patient has stabilized.

In children and neonates, the initial dose is 0.01 mg/kg, IV, SC, or IM. A subsequent dose of 0.1 mg/kg may be administered if needed.

The management of postoperative narcotic depression in adults can be accomplished with doses of 0.1 mg to 0.2 mg IV every 2 minutes to 3 minutes until the desired degree of reversal is attained (*i.e.,* sufficient ventilation and alertness). Repeat doses may be needed at 1-hour to 2-hour intervals. To reverse postoperative narcotic depression in children, 0.005 mg to 0.01 mg is given IV at 2-minute to 5-minute intervals.

FATE

Naloxone is virtually inactive orally. Following injection, naloxone is rapidly distributed in the body, and the antagonistic effects are evident within 1 minute to 2 minutes of IV administration and only slightly longer following SC or IM injection. The action persists for 1 hour to 4 hours depending on the dose and route of administration (IM and SC doses are longer-acting than IV). The drug is metabolized in the liver and excreted in the urine. The serum half-life ranges from 30 minutes to 90 minutes.

SIDE-EFFECTS/ADVERSE REACTIONS

The principal adverse reactions observed with naloxone treatment result from a too-rapid reversal of narcotic depression and can include nausea, sweating, vomiting, tachycardia, increased blood pressure, and tremors. In postoperative patients, occasional reports of hypertension, ventricular tachycardia, and pulmonary edema have appeared. Excessive naloxone dosage can reverse analgesia and result in excitement.

CONTRAINDICATIONS AND PRECAUTIONS

Naloxone should be given *cautiously* to known or suspected narcotic addicts, because a withdrawal syndrome will be precipitated. Safe use has not been established in pregnant women or nursing mothers.

NURSING CONSIDERATIONS

A narcotic antagonist is usually administered during a critical situation when respiratory failure or cardiac arrest is either imminent or occurring.

Therefore, all resuscitative equipment should be available.

If the drug is effective in reversing the overdose, withdrawal symptoms will occur depending on the amount or type of narcotic used. Symptoms are severe in methadone users but virtually nonexistent in meperidine users unless the dose is 1.6 g or more per day. The action of the antagonists is short in comparison to narcotics, and repeated injections and respiratory support may be necessary. If the patient fails to respond to three doses of naloxone, overdose by drugs other than narcotics (*i.e.,* barbiturates) should be suspected.

Naltrexone

(Trexan)

MECHANISM AND ACTIONS

Naltrexone blocks the effects of opiate drugs by a competitive binding at opioid receptors. It is a pure antagonist and is devoid of agonistic action at the receptor. When given concurrently with opiate drugs, it markedly attenuates their euphoria and other subjective effects and in the properly motivated individual, provides an adjunctive means for maintaining an opioid-free state. The receptor-blocking action persists for at least 24 hours, and may be extended up to 72 hours with increasing dosage. Because it is a competitive blocking action, the blockade can be surmounted by large doses of opiate drugs; thus the need for additional measures, such as counseling and other supportive endeavors, to ensure that the patient's opioid-free state is maintained. The drug should *not* be administered until a person has remained opioid-free for at least 7 days to prevent the elicitation of withdrawal symptoms by the antagonist.

USES

1. Adjunctive therapy, as an aid in the maintenance of an opioid-free state in detoxified former addicts

ADMINISTRATION AND DOSAGE

Naltrexone is available as 50-mg tablets. Treatment should not be initiated until a test dose of naloxone does *not* result in signs of opioid withdrawal. The initial dose of naltrexone is 25 mg and the patient is observed closely for 1 hour. If no withdrawal signs occur, an additional 25 mg is given. Thereafter, 50 mg once a day will provide a clinically effective blocking action of orally or parenterally administered opiates. The dosage schedule is flexible, and improved patient compliance sometimes can be obtained by giving 100 mg every other day or perhaps 150 mg every third day.

FATE

Following oral administration, peak blood levels occur within 1 hour. Naltrexone undergoes extensive first-pass hepatic metabolism, and some of the metabolites are active antagonists as well. Effects persist from 24 hours to 72 hours and are apparently independent of dosage. Naltrexone and its metabolites are excreted primarily by the kidneys.

SIDE-EFFECTS/ADVERSE REACTIONS

Because naltrexone is a pure antagonist, the majority of side-effects are due to its ability to precipitate a withdrawal syndrome. Effects most often observed include nervousness, headache, difficulty sleeping, abdominal pain, cramping, nausea, vomiting, joint and muscle pain, and nasal congestion.

Many other adverse effects have been noted with naltrexone, largely the result of withdrawal from the opioid state. Naltrexone has been reported to cause dose-related hepatocellular damage and should be used with extreme caution in persons with preexisting liver disease.

CONTRAINDICATIONS AND PRECAUTIONS

Use of naltrexone is contraindicated in patients receiving opioid drugs or in acute opioid withdrawal, and in patients with acute hepatitis or liver failure. A *cautious* approach to therapy should be undertaken in pregnant women or nursing mothers and in children under 18 years of age.

CASE STUDY

Mrs. Martin suffered a low back injury when she fell off a horse about 7 years ago. She is 35 and the mother of two teenage sons aged 15 and 13 years. She has been in and out of the hospital over the past 7 years for pain and immobility, but has refused surgery because, with each hospitalization, the pain is relieved after 1 week in traction.

On this admission, however, Mrs. Martin is still on bedrest and in pain after 14 days of traction. Dr. Johnson, her attending physician, suggests a lumbar laminectomy once again.

The nurses on 4 South know Mrs. Martin from her previous admissions. In the past she has always been stoic and taken pain medication only when "she really needed it." Now they find her to be demanding and abrupt. She requests the ordered pain medication, Demerol 75 mg IM, every 4 hours to the minute and has done so for the past 5 days. She complains about the care given and has gotten into several fights with the nurses and her sons. Although Dr. Johnson has ordered the addition of Valium 5 mg qid, Mrs. Martin is still uncooperative and demanding.

Discussion Questions

1. What assessments need to be made regarding Mrs. Martin's pain and her need for medication?
2. What factors are influencing Mrs. Martin's reaction to pain medications?
3. What strategies can the nurses use to attempt to reduce Mrs. Martin's pain?
4. Should this patient receive placebos? Under what circumstances?

REVIEW QUESTIONS

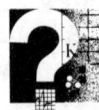

1. Distinguish between narcotic agonists and mixed narcotic agonist–antagonists in terms of their pharmacologic effects.
2. Describe the major pharmacologic effects of narcotic drugs mediated by interaction with *each* of the three major opiate receptor sites.

3. List the principal groups of endogenous opioid-like peptides and briefly compare their functions.

4. Why are the endogenous opiates found in the CNS unsuitable for clinical use?

5. Briefly explain the mechanisms involved in the analgesic action of narcotic drugs. What is the role of substance P?

6. How do narcotic drugs depress respiratory function? Do the mixed narcotic agonist–antagonists exhibit the same degree of respiratory depression as the narcotic agonists at all doses? Explain your answer.

7. *Briefly* state the mechanisms responsible for the (a) emetic, (b) hypotensive, (c) constipating, and (d) urinary retentive actions of narcotic drugs.

8. List the primary withdrawal symptoms observed when opiate drugs are suddenly discontinued.

9. Discuss the rationale for administering opiates on a regularly scheduled basis rather than "as needed" for controlling chronic pain.

10. What is Brompton's mixture? What other types of drugs have been given concurrently with opiates to enhance their effectiveness?

11. In what ways may sufentanil be used?

12. What are the two available "pure" narcotic antagonists? How do they differ in their usage?

13. Give the major contraindications to use of naloxone.

14. What four basic questions can the nurse ask to make a reasonable assessment of a patient's pain?

15. What are your perceptions of pain cues? How might they bias you against providing pain relief to a patient?

16. How can the nurse adequately assess pain in a child under 2 years? Over 2 years?

17. When should pain medication be given PRN (as needed)? When should such practice be avoided?

18. How can the use of an equianalgesic table help the patient in pain?

19. How can the nurse use positive reinforcement to enhance the placebo effect of narcotic analgesics?

20. What are the characteristics of placebo reactors and nonreactors?

21. What are the nurse's ethical responsibilities in administration of placebos for pain?

BIBLIOGRAPHY

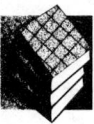

Akil H, Watson SJ, Young E et al: Endogenous opioids: Biology and function. Annu Rev Neurosci 7:223, 1984

Bloom FE: The endorphins: A growing family of pharmacologically pertinent peptides. Annu Rev Pharmacol 23:151, 1983

Brena SF: Chronic pain: A structured approach to drug therapy. Mod Medicine 52:124, 1984

Chang KJ, Cuatrecasas P: Heterogenicity and properties of opiate receptors. Fed Proc 40:2729, 1981

Chapman CR, Bonica JJ: Acute Pain, Current Concepts. Upjohn, 1983

Collier HOJ, Hughes J, Rance MJ et al (eds): Opioids: Past, Present and Future. London, Taylor and Frances, 1984

Fraser DG: Intravenous morphine infusion for chronic pain. Ann Intern Med 93:781, 1980

Iwamoto ET, Martin W: Multiple opiate receptors. Med Res Rev 1:411, 1981

Jacox A: Assessing pain. Am J Nurs 79:895, 1979

Kosterlitz HW, Collier HOJ, Villarreal JE (eds): Agonist and Antagonist Reactions of Narcotic Analgesic Drugs. Baltimore, University Park Press, 1973

Martin WR: Pharmacology of opioids. Pharmacol Rev 35:283, 1983

Martinson IM et al: Nursing care in childhood cancer: Methadone. Am J Nurs 82:432, 1982

Maxwell M: How to use methadone for the cancer patient's pain. Am J Nurs 80:1606, 1980

McCaffery M: Narcotic analgesia for the elderly. Am J Nurs 85:296, 1985

McCaffery M: Problems with meperidine. PRN Forum 3:1, 1984

McCaffery M: Placebos for Pain? Nursing 12:80, 1982

McCaffery M, Hart L: Undertreatment of acute pain with narcotics. Am J Nurs 76:1586, 1976

McGuire L, Dizard S: Managing pain in the young patient. Nursing 12:521, 1982

Muller RA, Pelczynski L: You can control cancer pain with drugs. Nursing 12:50, 1982

Panayotoff K: Managing pain in the elderly patient. Nursing 12:531, 1982

Pernow B: Substance P. Pharmacol Rev 35:85, 1983

Perry S, Heidrich WG: Placebo response: Myth and matter. Am J Nurs 81:720, 1981

Pert CB, Snyder SH: Opiate receptor: Demonstration in nervous tissue. Science 179:1011, 1973

Portenoy RK: Continuous infusion of opioids. Am J Nurs 86:318, 1986

Rogers A: Analgesic consultation. Am J Nurs 85:296, 1985

Rogers A: Pharmacology of analgesics. J Neurosurg Nurs 10:180, 1978

Schechter NL: Pain and pain control in children. Curr Probl Pediatr 15:1, 1985

Verebey K (ed): Opioids in mental illness. Ann NY Acad Sci 398:1, 1982

Wall PD, Melzack R (eds): Textbook of Pain. New York, Churchill-Livingstone, 1984

Woolverton WL, Schuster CR: Behavioral and pharmacological aspects of opioid dependence: Mixed agonists-antagonists. Pharmacol Rev 35:33, 1983

Yaksh TL, Noveihed R: The physiology and pharmacology of spinal opiates. Annu Rev Pharmacol Toxicol 25:433, 1985

Yaksh TL, Rudy TA: Narcotic analgesics: CNS sites and mechanisms of action as revealed by intracerebral injection techniques. Pain 4:299, 1978

Non-Narcotic Analgesic and Anti-Inflammatory Drugs

Salicylates

Para-Aminophenol Derivatives
  Acetaminophen

Pyrazolones
  Phenylbutazone

Nonsteroidal Anti-Inflammatory Drugs
  Indomethacin
  Fenoprofen
  Flurbiprofen
  Ibuprofen
  Ketoprofen
  Meclofenamate
  Mefenamic Acid
  Naproxen
  Naproxen Sodium
  Piroxicam
  Sulindac
  Suprofen
  Tolmetin

Gold Compounds
  Auranofin
  Aurothioglucose
  Gold Sodium Thiomalate

Miscellaneous Anti-Inflammatory Agents
  Penicillamine

Antigout Drugs
  Colchicine
  Probenecid
  Sulfinpyrazone
  Allopurinol

23

Drugs that exhibit an analgesic, antipyretic, or anti-inflammatory action but are devoid of the undesirable properties of narcotic analgesics, such as respiratory depression, dependence, and sedation are referred to as the non-narcotic analgesic/anti-inflammatory agents. This chemically and pharmacologically diverse group of drugs has a variety of indications. These include relief of mild to moderate pain; reduction of elevated body temperature (antipyresis); symptomatic relief of the manifestations of inflammation; inhibition of platelet aggregation, which may provide protection against transient ischemic attacks and other thromboembolic complications; and prevention or relief of the symptoms of gout.

Classification of the heterogeneous group of non-narcotic analgesic and anti-inflammatory drugs is difficult, owing to the considerable variation in chemical structure and pharmacologic action among the drugs. Hence, any categorization of these agents is arbitrary at best. The following listing represents one such classification to enable the reader to consider these drugs in somewhat logical sequence:

Non-Narcotic Analgesic and Anti-Inflammatory Drugs
A. Salicylates (e.g., aspirin, choline salicylate)
B. Para-aminophenol derivatives (e.g., acetaminophen)
C. Pyrazolones (e.g., phenylbutazone)
D. Nonsteroidal anti-inflammatory agents (e.g., ibuprofen, naproxen, piroxicam)
E. Gold compounds (e.g., aurothioglucose, auranofin)
F. Miscellaneous anti-inflammatory agents (e.g., penicillamine)
G. Antigout drugs (e.g., allopurinol, probenecid)

In addition to the drugs outlined above, several other pharmacologic agents have been employed in certain types of inflammatory states, but are discussed elsewhere in the book because they primarily are used for treating other conditions. For example, the antimalarial drugs chloroquine and hydroxychloroquine are sometimes used to treat severe, refractory cases of rheumatoid arthritis but are principally indicated for the suppression and treatment of acute attacks of malaria. They are considered only briefly here and discussed in detail in Chapter 70. Similarly, immunosuppressive agents have long been used in severe inflammatory conditions, although their major indications currently are to prevent organ rejection and as adjuncts in the chemotherapy of cancer. Drugs such as cyclophos-

phamide and methotrexate are reviewed in Chapter 75 with other antineoplastic drugs, while azathioprine is discussed in Chapter 84.

Salicylates

Drugs in this category are derivatives of salicylic acid and possess analgesic, antipyretic, and anti-inflammatory actions. In addition, many of these drugs are capable of inhibiting platelet aggregation; the decreased platelet aggregatory effects suggest a potential clinical value for these compounds in protecting against certain thrombotic events thought to be associated with cerebrovascular and ischemic heart diseases. This aspect of salicylate pharmacology is currently receiving much attention. Finally, in large doses, salicylates can decrease prothrombin production and impair renal tubular reabsorption of uric acid.

Aspirin, the most widely used of the salicylates, was first synthesized in the mid-1800s but was not introduced into clinical medicine until the beginning of the twentieth century. Since its introduction, aspirin has been employed in a number of disease states with remarkable success and a minimal degree of serious toxicity. Despite the relative absence of major untoward reactions, however, aspirin is responsible for more instances of poisoning than is generally recognized. In fact, aspirin is the leading cause of drug poisoning in young children, and only barbiturates, alcohol, and carbon monoxide are responsible for more accidental fatalities among the general population. Due to its ready availability and therefore its proclivity toward unsupervised self-medication, aspirin has apparently never received the respect that such an important therapeutic agent deserves, and the drug is frequently misused. It is imperative, therefore, that health-care professionals place aspirin in proper perspective relative to its multiplicity of pharmacologic effects and its potential to cause a substantial number of undesirable reactions.

Because differences among the currently available salicylate preparations are primarily quantitative, they will be discussed as a group. Characteristics of individual drugs are listed in Table 23-1.

MECHANISM AND ACTIONS

Analgesia
Mild to moderate pain of diverse origin (e.g., musculoskeletal, dental, postoperative) generally responds well to salicylates. The mechanism of their

(Text continues on p. 412.)

Table 23-1
Salicylates

Drug	Preparations	Usual Dosage Range	Clinical Considerations
Aspirin (various manufacturers)	Tablets—65 mg, 81 mg, 325 mg, 500 mg Gum tablets—227.5 mg Enteric-coated tablets—325 mg, 500 mg, 650 mg, 975 mg Timed-release tablets—650 mg, 800 mg Enteric-coated capsules—325 mg, 500 mg Suppositories—60 mg, 120 mg, 130 mg, 195 mg, 200 mg, 300 mg, 325 mg, 600 mg, 650 mg, 1200 mg	*Adults:* Pain, fever— 325 mg to 650 mg Inflammation—2.6 to 7.8 g/day Transient ischemic attacks —40 to 1300 mg/day (highly variable—see text) Prevention of myocardial infarction—325 mg/day *Children:* Pain, fever—65 mg/kg/day in divided doses Inflammation—90 to 130 mg/kg/day in divided doses at 4-h to 6-h intervals	See general discussion of salicylates. In addition: Keep aspirin in a cool, dry place. Do not use if vinegar-like odor is detectable because potency is likely to be reduced. Use of suppositories may be best route for a vomiting patient, but absorption will be more variable. Do not use controlled-release preparations for short-term analgesia or antipyresis, because the onset of action is slow.
choline salicylate (Arthropan)	Liquid—870 mg/5 ml (870 mg equivalent to 650 mg aspirin)	1 teaspoonful (870 mg) every 3 h to 4 h to a maximum of six times/day For rheumatoid arthritis—1 tsp to 2 tsp up to four times/day	Liquid preparation giving more rapid absorption and less gastric irritation than aspirin. Useful in patients with difficulty in swallowing tablets or capsules, in patients who experience gastric distress with regular aspirin, and in patients who should avoid sodium-containing salicylates. Taste may be objectionable; drug can be mixed with fruit juice or other vehicle if desired; do not give with antacids.
diflunisal (Dolobid)	Tablets—250 mg, 500 mg	Pain—500 mg to 1 mg initially, followed by 250 mg to 500 mg every 8 h to 12 h Rheumatoid arthritis/osteoarthritis—500 mg to 1000 mg daily in two divided doses (maximum 1500 mg/day)	A salicylic acid derivative *not* metabolized to salicylic acid. Used for mild to moderate pain and osteoarthritis. Long-acting (used twice a day) analgesic comparable in potency to aspirin or acetaminophen at a dose of 500 mg and equivalent to acetaminophen plus codeine at a dose of 1000 mg. Platelet-inhibitory effect is dose-related and usually transient and reversible. At 1 g/day, bleeding time is only slightly increased. Anti-inflammatory efficacy is equal to 2 to 3 g/day of aspirin, with less GI distress in some patients.

(continued)

Table 23-1 (continued)
Salicylates

Drug	Preparations	Usual Dosage Range	Clinical Considerations
diflunisal (Dolobid) (*continued*)			Do not use in children under age 12. Use cautiously in patients with impaired cardiac function or hypertension, because fluid retention can occur. Do not take aspirin, acetaminophen, or a nonsteroidal anti-inflammatory drug with diflunisal.
magnesium salicylate (Doan's Pills, Magan, Mobidin)	Tablets—325 mg, 545 mg, 600 mg	650 mg four times/day or 1090 mg three times/day. Increase to 3.6 to 4.8 g/day at 3-h to 6-h intervals as needed. Up to 9.6 g/day have been used in rheumatic fever.	Not recommended in children under age 12. A sodium-free salicylate having a somewhat lower incidence of GI upset than regular aspirin. Use with caution in patients with impaired renal function. Contraindicated in advanced renal insufficiency.
methyl salicylate (oil of wintergreen)	10% to 50% in ointment and liniments	Applied topically as a counterirritant to relieve pain associated with muscular and rheumatic conditions	Significant absorption can occur through the skin and may produce untoward effects. Very toxic if orally ingested, especially by children. Liquids containing more than 5% methylsalicylate must be in child-resistant containers. Use cautiously on irritated skin.
salicylamide (Uromide)	Tablets—325 mg, 667 mg	*Adults*—325 mg to 667 mg three to four times/day *Children:*—65 mg/kg/day in six divided doses on advice of physician	An amide of salicylic acid that is less effective than aspirin, but also slightly less toxic. Shorter-acting than other salicylates because it is largely metabolized before entering systemic circulation. May be useful in aspirin-allergic individuals. Drowsiness and dizziness can occur. No significant anti-inflammatory action.
salicylic acid (Calicylic, Compound W, Derma-Soft, Freezone, Gordofilm, Hydrisalic, Keralyt, Mediplast, Occlusal, Off-Ezy, Oxyclean, Salacid, Salonil, Wart-off)	Cream—2.5%, 10% Ointment—25%, 40%, 60% Gel—6%, 17% Soap—3.5% Liquid—13.6%, 17% Plaster—40%	Apply to affected area, usually at night, and wash off in the morning. Following remission, use occasionally to maintain clearing effect.	Primarily used topically as a keratolytic agent for conditions such as psoriasis, keratosis, acne, fungal infections, or any other condition requiring removal of excessive dead skin. Skin should be hydrated at least 5 min prior to use with wet packs or soaks. May

(continued)

Table 23-1 (continued)
Salicylates

Drug	Preparations	Usual Dosage Range	Clinical Considerations
salicylic acid (Calicylic, Compound W, Derma-soft, Freezone, Gordo-film, Hydrisalic, Keralyt, Mediplast, Occlusal, Off-Ezy, Oxyclean, Salacid, Salonil, Wart-off) (continued)			cause irritation and burning of skin. Systemic absorption can occur to a significant extent. Also may be applied as an ether-alcohol or a colloidian solution (Freezone, Compound W, Occlusal, Off-Ezy, Wart-off) for removal of corns, warts, and calluses. Use cautiously in children under age 12. Avoid contact with eyes or mucous membranes.
salsalate (Artha-G, Disal-cid, Mono-Gesic, Salflex)	Tablets—500 mg, 750 mg Capsules—500 mg	3 g/day in divided doses	Primarily used for relief of signs and symptoms of rheumatoid arthritis and other rheumatic conditions. Minimal effect on platelet aggregation. Following absorption, drug is hydrolyzed to two molecules of salicylic acid. Drug is insoluble in gastric juice and not absorbed until it reaches small intestine. Low incidence of GI upset. Not for use in children under age 12. Do not combine with other salicylates.
sodium salicylate (Uracel)	Tablets—325 mg, 650 mg Enteric-coated tablets— 325 mg, 650 mg Injection—1 g/10 ml	325 mg to 650 mg every 4 h to 8 h as needed	Less effective than an equal dose of aspirin. Irritating to GI mucosa because free salicylic acid is liberated. Use cautiously in renal dysfunction or in individuals on a low-sodium diet. Sodium bicarbonate given concurrently may reduce gastric irritation, but increases rate of excretion as well. When giving injection, avoid extravasation because drug will cause sloughing and necrosis of tissues.
sodium thiosalicylate (Thiocyl, Tusal)	Injection—50 mg/ml	Analgesia—50 mg to 100 mg daily or alternate days Rheumatic fever—100 mg to 150 mg every 4 h to 6 h for 3 days, then 100 mg twice/day Acute gout—100 mg every 3 h to 4 h for 2 days, then 100 mg/day	Readily absorbed following IM administration. Occasionally used in inflammatory conditions and acute stages of rheumatic fever

analgesic effect is not entirely clear, but probably is the result of their interaction with prostaglandins. Salicylates inhibit prostaglandin synthesis by impairing the activity of the enzyme cyclo-oxygenase, which catalyzes the conversion of arachidonic acid to a series of intermediate compounds known as prostaglandin endoperoxides in cell membranes. These unstable endoperoxide intermediates are then further transformed, depending on regional enzymatic activity, to a variety of prostaglandins or related substances known as thromboxanes or leukotrienes which exert a range of pharmacologic effects (see Chap. 82). Prostaglandin E_2 (PGE_2) increases the sensitivity of peripheral pain receptors to endogenous pain-producing substances, such as bradykinin; therefore, inhibition of PGE_2 production by salicylates lowers the sensitivity of peripheral pain receptors and reduces the intensity of the noxious stimulus. Other mechanisms that may be involved in the analgesic action of salicylates include enhanced absorption of fluid from edematous, inflamed areas, which may be a focus of pain, and perhaps an action in the CNS as well.

Aspirin irreversibly acetylates cyclo-oxygenase, whereas the effects of the other salicylates are more transient. However, there is little difference in the inhibitory action of aspirin vs the other salicylates on prostaglandin synthesis on an acute basis.

Antipyresis

Salicylates lower elevated temperatures but do not affect normal body temperature. The mechanisms involved in this antipyretic action are (1) vasodilation of superficial blood vessels, resulting in increased dissipation of body heat by sweating and (2) decreased production of prostaglandin E, which can be produced in response to the presence of bacterial pyrogens during a course of infection; increased production of prostaglandin E in the hypothalamus may impair the normal temperature-regulating mechanism in this CNS site.

Anti-inflammatory

The anti-inflammatory effects of salicylates also are the result of several mechanisms. The principal action of these drugs in relieving swelling and joint stiffness resides in their ability to decrease prostaglandin synthesis. The level of prostaglandin E is elevated in synovial fluid of inflamed joints, where it probably contributes to the swelling (by increased capillary permeability), pain (by sensitization of pain receptors), and gradual erosion of bone. Other mechanisms that may contribute to the anti-inflammatory action of salicylates are (1)

interference with release of tissue-destructive lysosomal enzymes, (2) inhibition of granulocyte adherence to damaged vessels in the inflammatory focus, and (3) reduction of leukocyte and macrophage migration into the site of inflammation.

Whereas the analgesic and antipyretic actions of aspirin are realized at doses of 0.6 g, considerably larger amounts (i.e., 2.5 to 7.5 g/day) are necessary to adequately control the symptoms of inflammation. The principal disadvantage of these large doses is the frequent development of gastric irritation, and this aspect of aspirin usage will be considered below.

Platelet Antiaggregatory Action

Platelet aggregation appears to be inhibited by aspirin but not to a significant extent by other salicylates. This difference is probably due to the acetyl group of aspirin, which is capable of *irreversibly* inhibiting platelet cyclo-oxygenase and the subsequent synthesis of thromboxane A_2 for the life of the platelet (i.e., 8–11 days). Because thromboxane A_2 is a vasoconstrictor and facilitates platelet aggregation, inhibition of its synthesis in platelets reduces their tendency to aggregate. Other salicylates have only a weak and transient inhibitory effect on platelet cyclo-oxygenase, and thromboxane synthesis is only briefly interrupted.

Low doses of aspirin appear to be more effective in reducing platelet aggregation than higher doses, presumably due to the fact that synthesis of platelet thromboxane is more sensitive to inhibition by aspirin than synthesis of vessel wall prostacyclin (PGI_2), a substance that inhibits platelet aggregation. Doses of aspirin in the range of 40 to 80 mg/day have been shown to reduce thromboxane levels up to 95%, while prostacyclin levels are decreased by only 35%. Therefore, the prostacyclin-to-thromboxane ratio is markedly increased, and platelet aggregation is prevented. Higher doses of aspirin (e.g., 325 mg/day) almost completely block *both* vessel wall prostacyclin and platelet thromboxane synthesis, and the acute antiaggregatory effects of prostacyclin are lost. However, because prostacyclin activity is only temporarily interrupted, while thromboxane A_2 activity is impaired for the life of the platelet, even larger doses of aspirin can result in a favorable prostacyclin-to-thromboxane A_2 ratio with continued use, especially if given every 2 to 3 days rather than once or twice daily.

Several other nonsalicylate drugs, such as dipyridamole and sulfinpyrazone, also display the ability to impair platelet aggregation, but their actions differ in certain respects from those of aspirin. A complete discussion of sulfinpyrazone is found later in this chapter, whereas dipyridamole is considered in Chapter 36.

Aspirin is being used increasingly as a prophylactic agent against thromboembolic complications associated with cardiovascular diseases. Low doses have demonstrated effectiveness in reducing the risk of recurrent transient cerebral ischemic attacks resulting from embolic episodes and such an application will represent a major use for aspirin in the future. Dosage levels appear to be critical, however, in order to obtain the most favorable prostacyclin-to-thromboxane ratio (see above), and considerable work remains to be done to establish the optimal dose of aspirin for preventing thromboembolic occurrences.

Gastrointestinal

Salicylates can cause gastric irritation and the most common side-effect experienced by persons taking aspirin is GI upset, usually manifested as nausea and heartburn. Gastric irritation resulting from aspirin use may be due to a direct irritative effect of the undissolved tablet on the gastric mucosa, to absorption of the salicylate moiety by the mucosal cells, or to a reduced level of prostaglandins, which serve a protective function in preventing erosion of the gastric wall.

The incidence of GI irritation with aspirin is considerably greater when large doses are used regularly to control symptoms of inflammation than when the drug is taken occasionally for pain or fever. Nearly 50% of persons taking several grams of aspirin a day find the drug intolerable because of gastric upset, and this is most often the limiting factor in the use of aspirin as an anti-inflammatory agent. Even persons without symptomatic GI irritation may have aspirin-induced trace GI bleeding.

The use of commercially buffered aspirin tablets is seldom effective in significantly reducing the incidence of GI upset, because the quantity of buffer in the tablet is minimal. Liquid antacids can ameliorate the irritative effects of aspirin if taken concurrently, however, the increased alkalinity resulting from the antacid may retard the rate of absorption of aspirin and absorbable antacids may accelerate the renal excretion of aspirin in the form of salicylic acid, thereby reducing its effectiveness. Gastric distress can also be reduced by use of enteric-coated aspirin tablets, which resist dissolution in gastric fluids, but are slowly dissolved during intestinal transit. Problems with tablets not dissolving have occurred, and patients taking these enteric-coated dosage forms should be instructed to periodically examine their stools for the presence of intact tablets.

Minor GI bleeding is frequently associated with routine use of aspirin, and may become significant at high doses. Fecal blood loss should be monitored during chronic high-dose aspirin therapy and use of alcohol should be restricted, because it can significantly enhance the gastric erosive effects of aspirin. Prolonged blood loss associated with aspirin usage can result in anemia.

While many of the other salicylate preparations (see Table 23-1) are claimed to be less irritating to the GI tract than aspirin, the differences in most people are too small to be clinically significant. Patients intolerant of aspirin will rarely be able to take one or the other salicylates.

Other Actions

Large doses of salicylates can increase the rate and depth of respiration by stimulating the medullary respiratory center. The loss of CO_2, if excessive, can lead to respiratory alkalosis.

Decreased production of prothrombin has been reported with very high doses of aspirin and may alter oral anticoagulant requirements if the drugs are used together. Normal doses do not affect synthesis of prothrombin.

Daily doses of 2 g or less of aspirin increase serum uric acid levels by competing for the tubular secretory mechanism responsible for uric acid elimination from the plasma. Conversely, doses of aspirin exceeding 4 to 5 g/day can reduce serum urate levels by blocking renal tubular reabsorption of uric acid. These actions can interfere with the maintenance of stable serum uric acid levels in patients being treated for gout.

Salicylates can decrease blood glucose levels and impair glucose tolerance in the diabetic. Slight dosage adjustments of insulin or oral antidiabetic drugs may be necessary.

USES

1. Relief of mild to moderate pain, especially of musculoskeletal origin (e.g., headache, myalgia, neuralgia)
2. Reduction of elevated body temperature
3. Symptomatic treatment of various inflammatory conditions (e.g., rheumatoid arthritis and osteoarthritis, bursitis, rheumatic fever). Large doses (3 g–7 g/day) are usually necessary, and therapy is palliative, not curative.
4. *Prophylaxis* of thromboembolic complications (*e.g.*, venous emboli, cerebral ischemia) asso-

ciated with cardiovascular disorders (no benefit in completed stroke) and reduction of the risk of transient ischemic attacks in men (effectiveness in women has not been conclusively demonstrated)

5. Prevention of acute myocardial infarction in men with previous infarction or unstable angina (investigational use)

ADMINISTRATION AND DOSAGE
See Table 23-1.

FATE
Salicylates are rapidly absorbed from the stomach and proximal sections of the small intestine. Peak serum levels are attained within 1 hour to 2 hours. The acidic environment of the stomach favors absorption of salicylates by keeping the largest fraction of the drug in the un-ionized, lipid-diffusible form. Increasing gastric pH with alkaline buffers used to reduce GI irritation accelerates dissolution rates of the tablet, favoring absorption, but also increases the ionized/un-ionized fraction of drug, which retards absorption. The net effect on salicylate absorption of commercial buffers and other weak alkalies is minimal, however. Most salicylates are hydrolyzed following absorption, forming salicylic acid, which is found in the blood as the salicylate ion bound to serum albumin in varying amounts. Salicylate is largely converted to watersoluble, conjugated metabolites and excreted by the kidney. Alkalinization of the urine, for example with antacids or sodium bicarbonate, increases the rate of excretion of salicylates by favoring ionization in the tubular fluid. Large doses are excreted more slowly than small doses, probably due to slower metabolism as a result of saturation of hepatic enzymes.

SIDE-EFFECTS/ADVERSE REACTIONS
The most frequently encountered side-effects with salicylates are heartburn, nausea, and other minor symptoms of gastric distress. This problem can often be overcome by taking the drug with food, a *full* glass of water, a small amount of antacid, or in one of the enteric-coated dosage forms (see Table 23-1). More serious GI reactions are seen at high doses, and can include bleeding and mucosal ulceration. Large doses of salicylates often result in a syndrome known as *salicylism*, characterized by headache, dizziness, tinnitus, confusion, sweating, hearing loss, palpitations, and hyperventilation. These symptoms are reversible by reducing the dosage and can be used as an indicator of the upper limit of tolerable dosage levels.

Although salicylate-induced hyperventilation may lead to respiratory alkalosis by loss of CO_2, acute intoxication in children frequently presents as *acidosis*, because of the high levels of acidic salicylate ion that have accumulated.

Hypersensitivity reactions have occurred with salicylate usage, and range from mild symptoms such as rash and pruritus to serious manifestations like bronchoconstriction, edema, and shock. The occurrence of salicylate hypersensitivity is more common in persons with a history of allergic conditions from childhood, and the drugs should be used with caution in such individuals.

Use of salicylates, especially aspirin, in children with influenza or chickenpox has been associated with development of Reye's syndrome, an acute life-threatening condition marked by initial severe vomiting and lethargy and progressing to delirium, coma, and death. Mortality rate is approximately 25%, and permanent brain damage is common in survivors. Although a *definite* causal relationship to salicylates has not been confirmed, aspirin and other salicylates are not recommended in children with influenza or chickenpox.

Other adverse reactions noted with use of salicylates include renal dysfunction, asymptomatic hepatitis, elevations in serum amylase, SGOT and SGPT levels, and anorexia.

Severe intoxication may lead to CNS stimulation (delirium, hallucinations), respiratory alkalosis followed by acidosis, acid–base disturbances, petechial hemorrhaging, hyperthermia, hypokalemia, oliguria, convulsions, respiratory failure, and coma.

CONTRAINDICATIONS AND PRECAUTIONS
Salicylates are contraindicated in patients with hemophilia, bleeding ulcers, and other hemorrhagic states. Salicylates are not recommended in children with influenza or chickenpox (see under Side-Effects/Adverse Reactions). *Cautious use* is warranted in the presence of gastric ulcers, anemia, impaired hepatic function, chronic renal insufficiency, asthma, and nasal polyps (higher incidence of allergic reactions in these conditions), in patients taking oral anticoagulants, and in pregnant or nursing women.

INTERACTIONS
1. The effects of aspirin may be enhanced or prolonged by drugs that acidify the urine (*e.g.*, am-

monium chloride, ascorbic acid), and decreased by urinary alkalinizers (e.g., absorbable antacids, sodium bicarbonate).

2. By competing for protein-binding sites, the salicylate metabolite of aspirin may enhance the actions and toxicity of oral anticoagulants, heparin, naproxen, oral antidiabetics, phenytoin, thiopental, indomethacin, methotrexate, thyroid hormones, sulfonamide antibiotics, valproic acid, and penicillins.

3. Aspirin in small doses can inhibit the uricosuric effects of probenecid and sulfinpyrazone.

4. Aspirin may increase the risk of bleeding with oral anticoagulants and drugs that interfere with platelet aggregation.

5. Phenobarbital may decrease aspirin's efficacy by enzyme induction.

6. The antihypertensive action of beta-blockers may be blunted by concurrent use of salicylates, possibly due to prostaglandin inhibition.

7. The incidence of GI distress and bleeding may be increased by steroids, alcohol, indomethacin, pyrazolones, and other anti-inflammatory drugs.

8. Furosemide may decrease salicylate excretion, resulting in toxicity at lower doses.

9. Salicylates in high doses have a hypoglycemic action and may potentiate the effects of insulin and sulfonylurea antidiabetic drugs.

10. Antacids and activated charcoal can reduce the oral absorption of aspirin.

11. Aspirin may lower the clinical effectiveness of nonsteroidal anti-inflammatory agents.

■ Nursing Process

(Most information will deal with aspirin; differences are noted when indicated.)

□ ASSESSMENT

□ Subjective Data
Aspirin is a frequently used medication, and its toxicity is somewhat underestimated. Many people use aspirin so frequently they forget it is a drug and may be unaware of how much they take. For these reasons, a drug history should include questions about over-the-counter medications and specifically about aspirin. It may be helpful to ask the patient when he takes aspirin and how often symptoms occur in a week or a month. Estimates of aspirin use may then be more accurately determined. Such information will be important to the

physician ordering anticoagulant or anti-inflammatory drug therapy because aspirin intake may need to be reduced or eliminated. This information is also important in preoperative assessments because long-term aspirin use may increase the chance of postoperative hemorrhage. A patient should be asked to avoid all aspirin and aspirin-containing products for 2 to 7 days before any type of surgery, including dental work.

Lastly, a patient about to receive salicylates should always be asked about allergy to aspirin because cross-hypersensitivity is common. History taking should also include questions about GI upset from aspirin ingestion, ulcers, bleeding pathology, and renal disease because the presence of any of these problems makes the patient a poor candidate for salicylate therapy.

□ Objective Data
Physical assessment of the gastrointestinal and cardiovascular systems is appropriate to establish a baseline. Laboratory evaluation to establish bleeding time may be ordered if therapy will be long term.

□ NURSING DIAGNOSES
Actual nursing diagnoses for the patient taking a salicylate may include:

Knowledge deficit related to the action, dose, and side-effects of the drug

Potential nursing diagnoses are based on side-effects which vary according to the dose and duration of therapy. Common diagnoses may include:

Alteration in comfort; heartburn or nausea
Alteration in oral mucous membrane related to irritation

□ PLAN
1. Patients will take salicylates with a minimum of GI upset and toxic side-effects.
2. Families will learn safe use of salicylates to avoid aspirin overdose.
3. Patients with hypersensitivity to the drug will learn the hidden dangers to watch for to avoid accidental ingestion.

□ INTERVENTION
Although most patients experience few side-effects with aspirin, several warnings are important. When high doses of aspirin are used, patients need to learn the signs of overdose such as tinnitus, dizziness, and impaired vision or hearing. If these symptoms occur, the drug should be immediately discontinued. These symptoms may rapidly de-

velop if the patient takes the "extra-strength" aspirin compounds.

Continual self-medication with aspirin for fever or pain may mask signs of infection. Encourage any patient to seek physician consultation if the need for aspirin continues for more than 3 or 4 days.

The use of aspirin in children has decreased considerably with the fear of Reye's syndrome; however, there may be occasions when a parent may treat a child with aspirin. Children with fever and dehydration are more prone to the development of toxicity from aspirin, even at low doses, and parents should be warned of the danger. Acetaminophen use should be encouraged whenever possible.

If aspirin intoxication occurs, the patient must be brought to the hospital. Emergency treatment will include prompt emesis, gastric lavage, use of fluids and electrolytes, and, in severe cases, oxygen with mechanical ventilation and dialysis for renal failure. Because of easy availability, aspirin overdose is frequently seen in children and in suicide attempts. Families need to learn to keep all medications out of reach of children and others who might misuse them.

Patients with acute aspirin hypersensitivity should be encouraged to have it recorded on all health-care records or to wear a Medic-Alert bracelet. These patients should also be taught to read over-the-counter medication labels carefully. Many cold preparations and pain relievers contain salicylates which may or may not be listed as aspirin.

Aspirin is an effective remedy in the treatment of mild to moderate pain and can provide considerable relief if used correctly. For the patient suffering from acute or chronic inflammation, aspirin will work best if taken on a constant dosage schedule to minimize fluctuations in plasma levels and maximize relief. This method is also applicable to the patient suffering mild to moderate pain from other conditions such as musculoskeletal injuries. If pain is not relieved by aspirin, narcotics may be ordered. However, aspirin administration should probably continue because the combination may reduce the quantity or frequency of oral narcotic needed to achieve adequate pain relief.

Many people underestimate the effectiveness of non-narcotics such as aspirin and acetaminophen. Aspirin or acetaminophen have been found to be equally effective when compared to several oral narcotic drugs in double-blind studies. (Approximate dosage equivalencies are shown in Table 22-6.)

Many non-narcotic/narcotic combinations exist (e.g., Tylenol with Codeine, Empirin with Codeine, Fiorinal with Codeine, Vicodin, Percodan, Percocet-5, Tylox) usually containing a narcotic drug (codeine or oxycodone) and aspirin or acetaminophen, occasionally in combination with caffeine and/or a barbiturate. These combination products are usually prescribed for moderate to severe pain associated with fractures, dental extractions, postoperative pain, and so forth. While these combinations may be somewhat more effective than aspirin or acetaminophen alone, their continued use may result in development of dependence, because they all contain a narcotic drug. Control of most pain should be attempted with a non-narcotic analgesic prior to use of a narcotic drug, simply because of the reduced incidence of adverse effects and the lessened likelihood of habituation.

□ EVALUATION

The outcome sought is adequate pain relief or improved mobility or changed blood values with minimal side-effects. The patient should be able to demonstrate safe dosing techniques and be aware of toxic reactions. Nursing Care Plan 23-1 summarizes the nursing process for patients receiving salicylates.

Para-Aminophenol Derivatives

There are two important compounds in this category, phenacetin and N-acetyl-p-aminophenol (acetaminophen). Phenacetin may still be found in an occasional analgesic drug combination, but its use should be strictly avoided. Phenacetin has been associated with anemia, acidosis, methemoglobinemia, and kidney damage, and the use of any combination containing phenacetin should be strongly discouraged because other equally effective and less toxic analgesics and antipyretics exist. All phenacetin-containing preparations must carry a warning against the dangers of kidney damage with chronic use of the drug.

The other clinically useful para-aminophenol derivative is acetaminophen, the principal metabolite of phenacetin. Widely employed as an aspirin substitute, acetaminophen is considerably less toxic than phenacetin. Moreover, compared to aspirin, acetaminophen has the following advantages:

1. Lower incidence of GI upset and bleeding
2. Lower incidence of hypersensitivity reactions

3. No significant interaction with oral anticoagulants or uricosuric drugs
4. Availability in a palatable liquid form for pediatric use

The principal disadvantage of acetaminophen relative to aspirin is that it possesses no significant anti-inflammatory action, presumably due to its lack of significant inhibitory effect on prostaglandin synthesis in the periphery. When used on an occasional basis as directed, acetaminophen is essentially free of serious toxicity. However, large doses have resulted in hepatotoxicity, and liver damage can also occur with chronic ingestion of normal doses in alcoholics and persons with impaired hepatic function (see Side-Effects/Adverse Reactions below).

Acetaminophen

(Datril, Tempra, Tylenol, and various other manufacturers)

MECHANISM AND ACTIONS
The mechanism of acetaminophen in relieving pain and reducing fever is not completely established although its efficacy is comparable to that of aspirin. Elevated body temperatures are reduced, possibly by a direct action on hypothalamic heat regulatory centers, leading to vasodilation and sweating, as well as by an inhibitory effect on endogenous pyrogens. Acetaminophen possesses *no* significant anti-inflammatory activity, presumably due to a lack of significant inhibition of *peripheral* prostaglandin synthesis, although it appears to be very effective in blocking prostaglandin synthetase enzymatic activity in the CNS. Acetaminophen does not exhibit uricosuric, platelet antiaggregatory, ulcerative, or prothrombin-inhibitory actions as aspirin does.

USES
1. Relief of mild to moderate pain of various origins, (*e.g.*, musculoskeletal, headache, toothache, teething, tonsillectomy, dysmenorrhea, "flu", and so forth). Also indicated in patients with aspirin hypersensitivity, upper GI disorders, and bleeding disorders
2. Reduction of elevated temperature associated with colds and other bacterial and viral infections

ADMINISTRATION AND DOSAGE
Acetaminophen is usually given orally, as tablets (80 mg, 160 mg, 325 mg, 500 mg, 650 mg), capsules (325 mg, 500 mg), elixir (120 mg/5 ml, 160 mg/5 ml, 325 mg/5 ml) or alcohol-free solution (100 mg/ml, 120 mg/2.5 ml, 160 mg/5 ml, 167 mg/5 ml). Rectal suppositories containing 120 mg, 125 mg, 325 mg or 650 mg are also available, although bioavailability is more variable with rectal administration. Adult dosage is 325 mg to 650 mg every 4 hours to 6 hours to a maximum of 4 g/day.

For long-term therapy, doses should not exceed 2.6 g/day due to the danger of hepatotoxicity. Children's doses are based on age and body weight and the following are recommended dosages:
  0 to 1 year: 40 to 80 mg four to five times/day
  1 to 3 years: 120 to 160 mg four to five times/day
  4 to 8 years: 240 to 320 mg four to five times/day
  9 to 12 years: 400 to 480 mg four to five times/day

FATE
Acetaminophen is well absorbed orally; peak plasma concentrations occur within 30 minutes to 90 minutes. Effects last for 3 hours to 5 hours. Protein binding is variable but usually not clinically significant. The drug is metabolized in the liver, and 80% to 90% is excreted in the urine as conjugated metabolites. A minor intermediate metabolite is converted to a hepatotoxic substance, but is normally rapidly detoxified by conjugation with glutathione via sulfhydryl groups, and excreted as the conjugated product. Large acute doses or chronic dosing with acetaminophen can deplete hepatic stores of glutathione, the substance which quickly detoxifies the potentially hepatotoxic intermediate. In these situations, hepatic necrosis can occur (see below).

SIDE-EFFECTS/ADVERSE REACTIONS
Occasional acetaminophen usage is remarkably free of untoward reactions. Chronic administration of acetaminophen, particularly in high doses, may rarely lead to CNS stimulation, hypoglycemia, drowsiness, skin eruptions, urticaria, erythematous rash, and blood dyscrasias (leukopenia, thrombocytopenia, hemolytic anemia, neutropenia).

Acute overdosage with acetaminophen can result in hepatotoxicity. Initial signs of hepatotoxicity include nausea, vomiting, malaise, sweating, diarrhea, and abdominal pain. Other symptoms of acute poisoning include chills, fever, skin eruptions, palpitations, weakness, cyanosis, and CNS stimulation (excitement, delirium, toxic psychosis) followed by CNS depression, vascular collapse, convulsions, and coma.

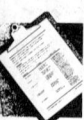

Nursing Care Plan 23-1
The Patient Receiving Salicylates

Assessment

Subjective Data

1. Medication history: Refer to *Interactions* section to formulate pertinent questions
   a. Ask about extent, frequency, and type of OTC analgesic use, especially in elderly patients
   b. Allergies/hypersensitivity to aspirin
2. Determine symptoms for which patient takes aspirin; such a determination may facilitate accurate estimate of use
3. Medical history:
   a. Check for preexisting conditions which may precipitate adverse reactions such as: gastrointestinal disorders, bleeding problems, renal or hepatic disease
   b. Current pregnancy or lactation

Objective Data

1. Physical assessment
   a. Gastrointestinal function: appearance of stools, GI motility
   b. Cardiovascular status: heart rate, blood pressure
   c. Neurologic status: memory, mental acuity, psychomotor skills
2. Laboratory data: coagulation studies should be performed if extended therapy is anticipated

Nursing Diagnosis	Expected Client Outcome	Intervention
Knowledge deficit related to drug effect, frequency of administration, potential side-effects	Will verbalize knowledge of drug's action, correct method of administration to relieve symptoms, and common side-effects	Explain how salicylates work to reduce pain, inflammation, or elevated temperature or how they may be used to prevent thromboembolic episodes. Administer or teach patient to take dose as prescribed preferably on a round-the-clock schedule rather than prn during acute pain or inflammation or if the drug is used to prevent thromboembolism. Administer dose or teach patient to take dose for febrile episodes on a prn schedule based on a predetermined elevation limit, usually 101°F. Teach patient to monitor common side-effects as described below and follow preventive/reactive strategies given.
Potential impairment of skin integrity related to a drug hypersensitivity reaction	Will report immediately any symptoms of hypersensitivity	Administer minimum dosage to person receiving salicylates for the first time. Monitor patients receiving high doses very closely. Report immediately any rash or pruritus to physician. Drug must be discontinued to avoid more serious side-effects. Have antihistamines, corticosteroids, epinephrine on hand for use as required.
	Will wear a Medicalert device if hypersensitivity is known	Teach patient to alert all caregivers of allergy. Identify resources where Medicalert device can be obtained.

(continued)

Nursing Diagnosis	Expected Client Outcome	Intervention
Potential alteration in comfort: heartburn or nausea related to gastric irritation	Will prevent or obtain relief from common GI symptoms	Encourage patient to take drug with food, with a full glass of water, or with antacid if necessary. Enteric-coated dosage form may be used. Teach patient to contact physician if heartburn persists or if stools appear dark, because GI mucosal bleeding can occur.
Potential sensory-perceptual alteration related to salicylate intoxication	Salicylate intoxication will be avoided	Teach patients to take prescribed dose or dose recommended on package instructions. Intoxication is more likely with "extra strength" compounds Encourage patient to force fluids. Toxicity is more likely when the patient is dehydrated. Teach the symptoms of toxicity: dizziness, tinnitus, confusion, hyperventilation. Dose must be reduced or drug must be discontinued. Be prepared for emergency treatment, especially if toxicity is induced by accidental poisoning. Vomiting must be induced. Other measures may include gastric lavage, fluids and electrolyte administration, oxygen or mechanical ventilation, and possibly dialysis. Encourage keeping medication out of reach of children to prevent accidental poisoning.

The degree of liver damage following acute overdosage can be estimated by determining the serum half-life of acetaminophen or acetaminophen plasma levels. Hepatic damage is likely if the half-life is greater than 4 hours or if plasma levels exceed 250 to 300 μg/ml 4 hours after ingestion or 50 μg/ml 12 hours after ingestion. In addition, chronic use of 5 to 8 g/day over several weeks has resulted in liver damage, although hepatotoxicity is more likely following a *single* ingestion of as low as 6 g of drug.

Treatment of acute overdosage includes emesis, gastric lavage, and activated charcoal. Hepatic damage can be minimized or prevented by administration (*within the first 10 hours to 12 hours* after ingestion of acetaminophen) of acetylcysteine (see Chap. 49), either IV or orally. A loading dose of 140 mg/kg is given initially, followed by 70 mg/kg every 4 hours for 17 doses. Acetylcysteine supplies sulfhydryl groups to facilitate detoxification of the hepatotoxic intermediate of acetaminophen (see under Fate). Because activated charcoal can absorb acetylcysteine and block its absorption, any activated charcoal in the stomach should be lavaged prior to giving acetylcysteine.

CONTRAINDICATIONS AND PRECAUTIONS

Acetaminophen should not be given to persons with a glucose-6-phosphate dehydrogenase deficiency or severe anemia. *Cautious use* is indicated in patients with impaired liver or kidney function and in very young children.

INTERACTIONS

1. The rate of absorption of acetaminophen may be slowed by anticholinergics, narcotics, activated charcoal, and antacids.
2. Oral contraceptives may increase the hepatic metabolism of acetaminophen.
3. Concurrent use of diflunisal has resulted in increased plasma levels of acetaminophen.

4. Chronic alcohol ingestion increases the likelihood of toxicity with large doses of acetaminophen.
5. Caffeine increases the analgesic effectiveness of acetaminophen.

NURSING CONSIDERATIONS
(Refer to the Nursing Process for salicylates.)

The use of acetaminophen has increased in recent years so that it is frequently part of the household pharmacy. Its ready availability makes it a source of overdose in children and suicidal patients. The sooner an overdose victim is seen and treated the less the chance that he will suffer hepatic damage, the most dangerous sequela to overdose.

The nurse's responsibility in acetaminophen overdose is to attempt to gain as accurate a picture of ingestion of the drug as possible from the victim or family. This will be difficult to do because the patient may be uncooperative. It will be helpful to know if the patient also ingested other drugs which may increase the chance of hepatotoxicity. Drugs in this category include barbiturates, alcohol, nicotine, chloral hydrate, glutethimide, and meprobamate.

The patient will usually be hospitalized to monitor potential hepatic toxicity. Liver studies need to be completed regularly, because changes in SGOT, SGPT, bilirubin, and PT will be the first signs of hepatic dysfunction. The presence of dark urine and clay-colored stools will also signal problems.

If acetylcysteine (Mucomyst) is ordered, the main nursing concern will be to convince the patient to swallow the unpleasant-tasting and -smelling drug. Chilling acetylcysteine may help as will mixing it in beverages such as soft drinks, orange juice, or grapefruit juice.

Pyrazolones

The pyrazolones are currently represented by two drugs (phenylbutazone and sulfinpyrazone) that have pharmacologic effects similar to those of the salicylates, but are more potent anti-inflammatory agents. Sulfinpyrazone, however, is much more effective as a uricosuric drug than as an anti-inflammatory agent and is used in maintenance therapy for gout. It is discussed at the end of this chapter with other antigout medications.

Phenylbutazone is a very effective anti-inflammatory agent, but it is highly toxic. Therefore, its use should be restricted to severe acute inflammatory conditions not benefited by other less toxic agents such as the salicylates. Generally, use of phenylbutazone should be limited to 1 week. In the absence of a favorable response, the drug should be discontinued. If clinical benefit is noted, however, longer term use may be employed, although the lowest effective dose must be given and the dosage gradually reduced. The drug should be withdrawn as soon as possible. Although phenylbutazone possesses analgesic and antipyretic actions as well, it should *never* be used in place of aspirin or acetaminophen as a general-purpose pain reliever or fever reducer.

Phenylbutazone
(Azolid, Butazolidin)

MECHANISM AND ACTIONS
Phenylbutazone possesses significant analgesic, antipyretic, and anti-inflammatory activity and weak uricosuric activity. Its anti-inflammatory effects result from several mechanisms, which may include interference with prostaglandin synthesis, decreased leukocyte migration, and impaired release and activity of lysosomal enzymes. Phenylbutazone increases sodium and water retention and may interfere with platelet aggregation. Iodine uptake by thyroid cells is reduced, and hepatic microsomal enzyme activity is accelerated (see under Interactions).

USES
1. Relief of acute symptoms of active rheumatoid arthritis, ankylosing spondylitis, osteoarthritis, psoriatic arthritis, and painful shoulder conditions (*e.g.*, peritendinitis, bursitis, capsulitis), where other less toxic agents are ineffective
2. Short-term treatment of acute attacks of degenerative joint disease of the hips and knees
3. Symptomatic treatment of acute gout (*short-term* use only; not for maintenance therapy)
4. Symptomatic treatment of acute superficial thrombophlebitis (unapproved use)

Caution: Do not use pyrazolones to treat minor painful conditions or fever.

ADMINISTRATION AND DOSAGE
Phenylbutazone is available as tablets or capsules containing 100 mg, which are administered with food, milk, or antacids to minimize the gastric

upset that frequently accompanies their use. The recommended doses are as follows:

Arthritis, degenerative joint disease, spondylitis, painful shoulder—Initially, 300 mg to 600 mg daily in three to four divided doses (maximum 600 mg/day). When improvement is realized, decrease dosage promptly to minimum effective level. Usual maintenance dose is 100 to 200 mg/day to a maximum of 400 mg/day.

Acute Gout—Initially, 400 mg, followed by 100 mg every 4 hours. Treatment is usually terminated within 4 days, but should never be continued longer than 1 week.

FATE
Phenylbutazone is rapidly and completely absorbed orally. Effects appear within 30 minutes to 60 minutes. Peak plasma levels occur within 2 hours to 4 hours. The drug exhibits a long half-life (70 hours–80 hours), and cumulation toxicity can occur with repeated administration. It is highly bound to plasma proteins (95%–98%). The principal site of biotransformation is the liver and the major metabolite of phenylbutazone is oxyphenbutazone, which is also active. Excretion is by way of the kidney, largely as conjugated metabolites.

SIDE-EFFECTS/ADVERSE REACTIONS
The most frequently encountered side-effects of phenylbutazone are abdominal discomfort, edema, weight gain, nausea, indigestion, heartburn, rash, and diarrhea. A wide variety of other adverse effects have been reported with use of phenylbutazone, and they are listed below by system. The incidence of most adverse reactions increases dramatically with prolonged use or use of high doses.

GI—Ulceration of esophagus, stomach, small intestine, bowel; occult GI bleeding, gastritis, abdominal distention, hematemesis, vomiting, salivary gland enlargement, hepatitis

Hematologic—Aplastic anemia, agranulcytosis, leukopenia, thrombocytopenia, bone marrow depression

Allergic/dermatologic (Require prompt withdrawal of drug)—petechiae, toxic pruritus, erythema nodosum, erythema multiforme, asthmatic attacks, exfoliative dermatitis, Stevens–Johnson syndrome, serum sickness, polyarteritis, urticaria, arthralgia, fever, anaphylactic shock

Renal/metabolic—Proteinuria, hematuria, oliguria, anuria, glomerulonephritis, renal stones, tubular necrosis, ureteral obstruction, sodium and chloride retention, edema, metabolic acidosis, hyperglycemia, thyroid hyperplasia, toxic goiter

CV—Hypertension, pericarditis, myocarditis with muscle necrosis, cardiac decompensation

Ocular/otic—Diplopia, optic neuritis, retinal hemorrhage, retinal detachment, hearing loss

CNS (seen primarily with overdose)—Agitation, confusion, lethargy, depression, hallucinations, convulsions, psychosis, hyperventilation

CONTRAINDICATIONS AND PRECAUTIONS
Phenylbutazone is contraindicated in the presence of GI inflammation, ulceration or bleeding, blood dyscrasias, hypertension, thyroid disease, renal, hepatic, or cardiac dysfunction, pancreatitis, temporal arteritis, or systemic edema, in patients receiving anticoagulants, in children under age 14, and in senile persons. The drug must be *used cautiously* in alcoholics, patients with chronic obstructive respiratory disease, visual disturbances, edema, unexplained bleeding, glaucoma, during pregnancy or nursing, and in older persons.

In general, phenylbutazone should not be given to patients in whom other less toxic therapeutic measures can be successfully undertaken. The drug should be discontinued at the first sign of developing hematologic toxicity, such as fever, bruising or bleeding, sore throat, oral mucosal lesions, or symptoms of anemia. Likewise, therapy must be terminated if the patient reports severe epigastric pain, black/tarry stools, skin rash, edema, or significant weight gain. Complete laboratory examinations (*e.g.*, blood count, urinalysis, liver function) should be performed at the initiation of therapy and at regular, frequent intervals during treatment. Phenylbutazone is a very effective anti-inflammatory drug but is potentially extremely toxic. Strict supervision is necessary to ensure safe and effective therapy.

INTERACTIONS
1. Phenylbutazone may potentiate the effects of other protein-bound drugs (oral anticoagulants, sulfonamides, phenytoin, oral hypoglycemics, other anti-inflammatory drugs such as salicylates and indomethacin).
2. Phenylbutazone may decrease the effects of di-

gitoxin, dicumarol, and cortisone by accelerating their enzymatic degradation.

3. The effects of phenylbutazone may be decreased by tricyclic antidepressants and by cholestyramine, which inhibits its gastric absorption.

4. The effects of insulin and oral antidiabetics can be enhanced by phenylbutazone.

5. Metabolic enzyme inducers such as phenobarbital, rifampin, or corticosteroids may decrease the half-life of phenylbutazone.

6. Methylphenidate may prolong the half-life of phenylbutazone.

NURSING CONSIDERATIONS

These are not drugs of choice in the treatment of gout or arthritis but are used only when less toxic drugs are ineffective or poorly tolerated. Therefore, patients starting on them need much encouragement and a lot of teaching to ensure that they gain benefits with minimal toxicity. Patients need to adhere to the prescribed dosage schedule because the chance of toxicity increases as the dose increases, and to have follow-up blood and liver studies done as ordered. If the patient perceives no therapeutic relief from the drug in 1 week of therapy, he should contact the physician and discontinue the drug. Patients may need support if this was considered a "last effort" and fails.

Pyrazolones induce sodium retention. The patient should be taught to restrict sodium intake, to watch for signs of edema in legs, feet, or hands, and to weigh himself daily. Any changes should be reported to the physician immediately.

Nonsteroidal Anti-Inflammatory Drugs

In a search for effective anti-inflammatory drugs that might prove less toxic than many of the older, established agents, several organic acids were shown to have a somewhat lower incidence of side-effects (*e.g.,* tinnitus, GI distress) than comparably effective doses of the salicylates or pyrazolones. These compounds have been termed the *nonsteroidal anti-inflammatory drugs* (NSAIDs), and they are approximately equal to large doses of aspirin in relieving symptoms of common inflammatory conditions. Of these substances, indomethacin is considerably more toxic than the others and will be discussed separately. The remaining drugs belong to various chemical classes, and display significant differences with respect to their pharmacokinetic properties, such as onset of action and duration of effects. Their principal advantage relative to other anti-inflammatory agents (*e.g.,* aspirin, salicylates, pyrazolones) is that they are slightly better tolerated by some patients.

These compounds possess analgesic and antipyretic activity but should *not* be used for the relief of minor headache pain or reduction of elevated body temperature in place of more commonly prescribed drugs (aspirin, acetaminophen). However, with the exception of indomethacin and meclofenamate, they may be employed for relieving other types of mild to moderate pain such as dysmenorrhea, postextraction dental pain, postsurgical episiotomy, and soft-tissue athletic injuries, in addition to their use as anti-inflammatory drugs. Their action in inflammatory states is to reduce joint swelling, pain, and stiffness, and to increase the functional capacity of the joint; however, they do not alter the progressive course of the underlying disease state.

While the NSAIDs may be somewhat more effective than high doses of aspirin or other salicylates in the symptomatic management of acute gouty arthritis, psoriatic arthropathy, and ankylosing spondylitis, their efficacy in treating the commonly encountered forms of rheumatoid and osteoarthritis is essentially equivalent to that of aspirin. Because several of the NSAIDs (*e.g.,* naproxen, piroxicam, sulindac) exhibit a longer duration of action than aspirin, they are prescribed in single or twice-daily doses (Table 23-2) which may facilitate better patient compliance compared to the multiple daily dosing necessary with aspirin.

On the other hand, these compounds are expensive, so there is little justification for their use in treating inflammatory states in persons who can tolerate the large daily doses of salicylates needed to control inflammation. Rather, the compounds are logical alternatives to the salicylates in patients unable to take large doses of aspirin-like drugs on a continual basis, and certainly should be employed as aspirin substitutes instead of the more toxic pyrazolones and corticosteroids.

These drugs (other than indomethacin and meclofenamate) exhibit a somewhat lower incidence of the milder forms of GI distress that commonly occur with high-dose salicylate use. It must be noted, however, that most of the other untoward reactions and drug interactions associated with large doses of aspirin and related compounds are also evident to a similar degree with the nonsteroidal, anti-inflammatory agents. In addition, aspirin

Table 23-2
Pharmacokinetic Properties of Nonsteroidal Anti-Inflammatory Agents

Drug	Peak Blood Levels (h)	Plasma Half-Life (h)	Single Dosage Range (mg)	Dosage Interval (h)
Proprionic Acids				
fenoprofen (Nalfon)	1.5–2	2–3	300–600	6–8
flurbiprofen (Ocufen)*	—	—	—	—
ibuprofen (Motrin)	1–2	1.5–2.5	400–800	6–8
ketoprofen (Orudis)	0.5–1.5	2–4	150–300	6–8
naproxen (Naprosyn)	2–4	12–15	250–375	8–12
naproxen sodium (Anaprox)	1–2	12–15	275–550	8–12
suprofen (Suprol)	0.5–2	2–4	200	4–6
Indoles				
indomethacin (Indocin)	1–2	4–6	25–50	6–8
sulindac (Clinoril)	1–2	8–16	150–200	12
tolmetin (Tolectin)	0.5–1	1–2	200–400	4–6
Fenamates				
meclofenamate (Meclomen)	0.5–1.5	2–3	200–400	4–6
mefenamic acid (Ponstel)	2–4	2–4	250–500	4–6
Oxicams				
piroxicam (Feldene)	3–5	30–75	10–20	24

* Only used as an ophthalmic solution. See Table 23-3.

itself should not be given with these nonsteroidal drugs because it can decrease the blood level and activity of the nonaspirin drugs. Likewise, combinations of the nonsteroidal drugs with low doses of corticosteroids are probably not significantly more effective than either drug alone.

Indomethacin

(Indameth, Indocin, Indo-Lemmon, Indomed)

Indomethacin is a potent anti-inflammatory agent which is somewhat more effective than salicylates or NSAIDs in treating moderate to severe inflammatory conditions. Due to its fairly high incidence of untoward reactions, however, its use should be restricted to those inflammatory states that do not respond to other less toxic drugs. Indomethacin can relieve the symptoms of acute gout within a short period of time, and the drug has become widely used in treating this condition.

MECHANISM AND ACTIONS
Inhibition of prostaglandin synthesis probably accounts for much of the anti-inflammatory effec-

tiveness of indomethacin, although the drug has also been claimed to decrease capillary permeability, block release of lysosomal enzymes, and retard the migration of polymorphonuclear leukocytes.

USES
1. Symptomatic management of
   a. Moderate to severe rheumatoid arthritis
   b. Ankylosing (rheumatoid) spondylitis
   c. Osteoarthritis of large joints (e.g., hip, shoulder)
   d. Acute gouty arthritis (short-term use only —maximum 5 days)
2. Assist closure of persistent patent ductus arteriosus in premature infants (investigational use only)

ADMINISTRATION AND DOSAGE
Indomethacin is used orally or rectally as 25-mg and 50-mg capsules, 75-mg sustained-release capsules (Indocin-SR), oral suspension (25 mg/5 ml), and suppositories (50 mg). Indomethacin is not approved for use in children under age 14. Due to its gastric-irritating effect, the drug should be given with food. Initial dosage in chronic inflammatory

conditions is 25 mg two to three times a day. Dosage may be increased by 25 mg to 50 mg/week to a maximum daily dosage of 200 mg. Depending on dosage requirements, the 75-mg sustained-release capsules may be administered one to two times a day for maintenance therapy, but this formulation is not indicated for acute gouty arthritis.

For the symptomatic management of acute gout, 50 mg is given three times a day until the pain is tolerable, then the dose is rapidly reduced over the next 3 to 5 days until therapy is terminated.

In treating patent ductus arteriosus in premature infants, indomethacin is given IV as three doses at 12-hour to 24-hour intervals. Dosage is based on the age of the infant. The *initial* IV dose in all children is 0.2 mg/kg. Children under 48 hours of age are then given two succeeding doses of 0.1 mg/kg each. Children from 2 to 7 days old receive succeeding doses of 0.2 mg/kg, while children over 7 days of age may be given 0.25 mg/kg in two succeeding doses.

FATE

Indomethacin is readily absorbed orally and widely distributed in the body. The onset of action is 1 hour to 2 hours, and the half-life is 4 hours to 6 hours. The drug is highly protein-bound (90%) in the plasma. Indomethacin is metabolized in the liver and kidney and excreted in the urine (60%) as conjugates and unchanged drug. The remainder is eliminated through the bile in the feces.

SIDE-EFFECTS/ADVERSE REACTIONS

The most commonly encountered side-effects with indomethacin usage are headache (20%–30%), dizziness, heartburn, nausea, stomach pain, diarrhea, and tinnitus. A myriad of other adverse effects have been associated with indomethacin, especially with chronic use of high doses, and these are listed below by organ system.

GI—Anorexia, vomiting, bloating, ulceration, perforation and hemorrhage of the esophagus, stomach, and small intestine; gastroenteritis, proctitis, rectal bleeding

CNS—Fatigue, depression, anxiety, confusion, muscle weakness syncope, involuntary movements, psychic disturbances, convulsions, peripheral neuropathy, depersonalization

Hematologic—Leukopenia, bone marrow depression, anemia secondary to bleeding, aplastic anemia, agranulocytosis, thrombocytopenic purpura

CV—Hypertension, tachycardia, chest pain, palpitations

Eye/ear—Retinal changes including macula, corneal deposits, blurred vision, hearing disturbances, tinnitus

Dermatologic—Pruritus, rash, urticaria, petechiae, alopecia, exfoliative dermatitis

Allergic—Hypotension, angioedema, respiratory distress, asthma-like attack

Other—Epistaxis, vaginal bleeding, dysuria, urinary urgency, hematuria, and increased BUN, SGOT, SGPT, alkaline phosphatase, and serum amylase

CONTRAINDICATIONS AND PRECAUTIONS

Use of indomethacin is contraindicated in patients with salicylate allergy, nasal polyps associated with angioedema, GI lesions or ulceration, and in pregnant women, nursing mothers, and young children. The drug must be used *with caution* in persons with epilepsy or parkinsonism, because these conditions can be aggravated by indomethacin. *Cautious use* is also warranted in patients with renal or hepatic dysfunction, coagulation defects, severe infections, and psychotic disturbances, as well as in elderly or debilitated persons.

INTERACTIONS

1. GI bleeding due to indomethacin can be intensified by use of corticosteroids, salicylates, and pyrazolones.
2. Indomethacin may interfere with the action of furosemide (Lasix) and thiazide diuretics and may reduce the anti-hypertensive efficacy of beta-blockers, presumably as a result of increased fluid retention.
3. Concurrent use of diflunisal and indomethacin may result in significantly elevated plasma levels of indomethacin and increased toxicity.
4. Large doses of aspirin may decrease indomethacin blood levels.
5. Probenecid may increase plasma levels of indomethacin.
6. Indomethacin may alter oral anticoagulant requirements, either by decreasing plasma protein binding, thereby elevating anticoagulant blood levels, or by causing excessive bleeding due to GI ulceration.
7. Lithium excretion may be impaired by indomethacin, possibly leading to lithium toxicity.
8. Indomethacin together with triamterene can result in acute, reversible renal failure.

■ *Nursing Process*

Indomethacin is frequently used in the treatment of arthritis that has become unresponsive to aspirin. Because its potential for toxicity is high, given the range of side-effects listed, care must be taken to reduce the chance of problems.

□ *ASSESSMENT*

The patient's history of arthritis and how it affects him will be important. The patient must be able to hold and take the medication unless assistance is available and must have sufficient memory or memory joggers to prevent possible overdose. In addition, preliminary blood count, renal and hepatic function tests, and hearing and ophthalmologic examinations should be done before the medication is begun to establish a baseline for monitoring potential serious side-effects during therapy.

□ *NURSING DIAGNOSES AND PLAN*
(See Nursing Process for salicylates.)

□ *INTERVENTION*

The dose of indomethacin may be titrated by the physician until an effective therapeutic level is maintained. Within the therapy plan the patient may wish to vary the dose to respond to periods of pain or stiffness. For example, if symptoms are worse at night or in the morning then the largest dose may be taken at bedtime, but this dose should never exceed 100 mg. If symptoms do not respond to indomethacin in 2 weeks to 3 weeks, the physician should be notified and the drug discontinued.

Patients should be encouraged to take the drug with food, milk, or antacids to decrease gastric irritability. They should also learn the major side-effects to watch for: rectal bleeding, confusion, tachycardia, pruritus and dysuria; and to report these to the physician immediately. He will probably discontinue the drug.

□ *EVALUATION*

Outcomes sought are pain relief, increased mobility, and minimal side-effects.

Fenoprofen
(Nalfon)

Flurbiprofen
(Ocufen)

Ibuprofen
(Motrin and others)

Ketoprofen
(Orudis)

Meclofenamate
(Meclomen)

Mefenamic Acid
(Ponstel)

Naproxen
(Naprosyn)

Naproxen Sodium
(Anaprox)

Piroxicam
(Feldene)

Sulindac
(Clinoril)

Suprofen
(Suprol)

Tolmetin
(Tolectin)

The above group of nonsteroidal anti-inflammatory drugs (NSAIDs) is composed of chemically dissimilar agents possessing a pharmacologic spectrum of action similar to that of aspirin. With one notable exception (meclofenamate), they exhibit a slightly lower incidence of minor gastric disturbances than the salicylates and do not appear to interfere with platelet aggregation to the extent that aspirin does. Most of the above NSAIDs are primarily used both for rheumatoid arthritis and osteoarthritis and for relief of mild to moderate pain of various origins. In addition, flurbiprofen is employed as an ophthalmic solution during cataract surgery.

MECHANISM AND ACTIONS

The principal mechanism of action of the NSAIDs is inhibition of prostaglandin synthesis, which decreases the sensitivity of peripheral pain receptors and reduces capillary leakage. Other actions attributed to the NSAIDs are decreased release of cellular, tissue-destructive enzymes, and impaired migration of polymorphonuclear leukocytes. These agents also lower the sensitivity of the temperature-regulating center in the hypothalamus, transiently interfere with platelet aggregation, and decrease uterine tone (by blockade of prostaglandin synthesis and release in the myometrium).

USES

1. Symptomatic relief of rheumatoid and osteoarthritis, ankylosing spondylitis, and psoriatic arthropathy
2. Treatment of acute gout and gouty arthritis (especially naproxen and sulindac)
3. Treatment of juvenile rheumatoid arthritis (tolmetin *only* agent approved; ibuprofen and naproxen have been used investigationally)
4. Relief of mild to moderate pain associated with dysmenorrhea, dental extractions, episiotomy, and athletic injuries such as sprains and strains (*except* meclofenamate)
5. Inhibition of intraoperative miosis during ocular surgery (flurbiprofen only)

ADMINISTRATION AND DOSAGE
(See Table 23-4.)

FATE

The NSAIDs are rapidly and nearly completely absorbed orally. Food generally delays absorption but does not affect the total amount absorbed (except suprofen, whose oral absorption is reduced 10%–20%). Table 23-2 contains a pharmacokinetic profile (*i.e.*, time to peak blood levels, plasma half-life, and dosage intervals) of each drug. All drugs are highly bound to plasma proteins (90%–98%). Excretion is generally by way of the kidney, largely as conjugated metabolites. Some biliary excretion occurs.

SIDE-EFFECTS/ADVERSE REACTIONS

GI distress (indigestion, burning, diarrhea, nausea, abdominal discomfort) is frequently noted with use of the NSAIDs (highest incidence with meclofenamate), as well as dizziness, headache (highest incidence with fenoprofen), tinnitus, and sometimes constipation. A variety of other untoward reactions have also been associated with NSAIDs and are listed below, although the incidence and severity differ among the drugs (see Table 23-3).

GI—Vomiting, cramping, bloating, epigastric pain, gastric or duodenal ulceration, bleeding, gastroenteritis, proctitis, ulcerative stomatitis
Allergic—Pruritus, skin rash, urticaria, erythema multiforme (rare), purpura (rare)

CNS—Drowsiness, nervousness, insomnia, confusion, depression, tremor, muscle weakness, peripheral neuropathy
Eye/ear—Blurred vision, diplopia, decreased hearing
CV—Palpitation, tachycardia, edema, prolonged bleeding time, arrhythmias, chest pain
Hepatic—Abnormal liver function tests, cholestatic hepatitis, jaundice
Renal—Hematuria, proteinuria, cystitis, urinary tract infection, azotemia, dysuria, polyuria, oliguria, fluid retention, nephrosis, glomerular and interstitial nephritis, renal papillary necrosis anuria

Note: Relative nephrotoxicity among NSAIDs is indomethacin > fenoprofen > ibuprofen = mefenamic acid = naproxen > piroxicam = sulindac = tolmetin.

CONTRAINDICATIONS AND PRECAUTIONS

NSAIDs are contraindicated in patients hypersensitive to aspirin and in the presence of active peptic ulcer. In addition, fenoprofen and mefenamic acid should not be used in the presence of impaired renal function. *Caution* should be exercised when administering one of the drugs to patients with epilepsy or parkinsonism, because these conditions may be exacerbated. NSAIDs are also to be used cautiously in persons with GI pain, rectal bleeding, hemostatic or coagulation defects, compromised cardiac functioning or hypertension (drugs may increase fluid retention), infections, and in elderly or debilitated patients.

INTERACTIONS

1. Effects of other protein-bound drugs (*e.g.*, hydantoins, sulfonamides, oral anticoagulants, pyrazolones) may be increased by nonsteroidal anti-inflammatory drugs.
2. GI adverse reactions may be intensified by concurrent administration of indomethacin, pyrazolones, salicylates, or corticosteroids.
3. Aspirin and other salicylates may decrease the blood level of nonsteroidal drugs.
4. Barbiturates may decrease the effects of fenoprofen by promoting its metabolism by the liver.
5. Plasma levels of NSAIDs can be increased by probenecid.
6. Piroxicam can increase steady-state plasma lithium levels. However, sulindac has been shown to decrease lithium levels.

7. NSAIDs may impair the antihypertensive effect of beta-blockers and of converting enzyme inhibitors (*e.g., captopril*).

NURSING CONSIDERATIONS

Individuals with arthritis may respond to one or more of the NSAIDs but may obtain no relief from others. Such patients will need support and encouragement as various drugs and dosage levels are used to attempt to achieve relief. For each of the drugs, the patient needs to know what toxic effects to watch for, but for most of the NSAIDs, GI symptoms and central nervous system changes represent the greatest hazard to treatment.

During such treatment experiments the patient may be tempted to resume using aspirin to obtain relief. However, salicylates will decrease the therapeutic blood level of most NSAIDs and should be avoided. Acetaminophen can be used without antagonism of the nonsteroidal drugs.

Gold Compounds

Injectable preparations containing approximately 50% elemental gold have been used for many years as part of the regimen for treating severe rheumatoid arthritis. Aurothioglucose and gold sodium thiomalate are two such preparations used intramuscularly in active arthritis that progresses despite adequate rest, physical therapy, and other drug treatment. In addition, auranofin is an orally effective compound containing 29% gold used for the management of active severe rheumatoid arthritis. These gold compounds can temporarily arrest the progression of bone destruction in involved joints, but there is no substantial evidence that they can induce remission of rheumatoid arthritis. Gold compounds are potentially highly toxic substances, so persons receiving them must be carefully and continually observed for adverse reactions.

Injections are normally given at weekly or longer intervals for prolonged periods of time, occasionally with rest periods if remission has occurred. Because of the long course of therapy, the need for repeated injections, and the necessity of periodic laboratory tests to detect toxicity, patient compliance with this form of therapy is often poor. The oral gold preparation appears to be nearly as effective as the injectable drugs, with the advantage of a lower incidence of adverse reactions and better patient compliance.

Auranofin
(Ridaura)

Aurothioglucose
(Solganal)

Gold Sodium Thiomalate
(Myochrysine)

MECHANISM AND ACTIONS

Gold is capable of suppressing the symptoms of arthritis and possibly slowing progression of the disease, but it does not cure the underlying pathologic condition. Although the mechanism of action of gold is not completely known, several actions are thought to contribute to its beneficial effects. Gold can inhibit lysosomal activity in macrophages, decrease the phagocytic action of macrophages, reduce histamine release from mast cells, interfere with tryptophan binding to plasma proteins, block formation of glucosamine-6-phosphate in connective tissue and inactivate the first component of complement. The importance of the above actions to the effectiveness of gold in treating rheumatoid arthritis, however, remain to be fully determined.

USES
1. Adjunctive treatment of active adult or juvenile rheumatoid arthritis, where there has been an insufficient response to other less toxic drugs. The greatest benefit is obtained if the drugs are given in the early active stage of the disease. Gold cannot repair damage caused by a previously active disease condition.

ADMINISTRATION AND DOSAGE
The injectable forms of gold are available in concentrations of 10 mg/ml, 25 mg/ml, and 50 mg/ml. The oral preparation is used as 3-mg capsules. Recommended dosages for the various preparations are as follows:

Intramuscular
(Preferred site is intragluteal.)

Aurothioglucose
Adults—Weekly IM injections; first week, 10 mg; second and third weeks, 25 mg; thereafter, 50 mg/week. If improvement is noted, continue with 50-mg injections at 2-week to 4-week intervals as necessary. If no improvement is noted after admin-

(*Text continues on p. 431.*)

Table 23-3
Nonsteroidal Anti-Inflammatory Drugs

Drug	Preparations	Usual Dosage Range	Clinical Considerations
fenoprofen (Nalfon)	Capsules—200 mg, 300 mg Tablets—600 mg	Arthritis—300 mg to 600 mg four times/day (maximum 3200 mg/day) Mild–Moderate Pain—200 mg every 4 h to 6 h	Administer 30 min before or 2 h after meals unless GI distress occurs, then give with milk. Perform periodic auditory function tests during chronic therapy; do not use in persons with impaired hearing. Not recommended in children under age 14, or in patients with significantly impaired renal function. Periodic liver function tests are advised because drug can elevate serum transaminase, LDH, and alkaline phosphatase. Drowsiness and headache are common, and urinary toxicity is more likely than with other NSAIDs.
flurbiprofen (Ocufen)	Ophthalmic solution—0.03%	1 drop every ½ h beginning 2 h before surgery	Inhibits miosis that occurs during ocular surgery by blocking the constrictive effect of prostaglandins on the iris sphincter. Does *not* interfere with miotic effect of cholinergic drugs or alter intraocular pressure. Transient burning and stinging can occur. Do not use in patients with epithelial herpes simplex keratitis. Wound healing may be delayed.
ibuprofen (Advil, Haltran, Ibuprin, Medipren, Midol-200, Motrin, Nuprin, Pamprin-IB, Rufen, Trendar)	Tablets—200 mg, 300 mg, 400 mg, 600 mg, 800 mg	Arthritis—300 mg to 800 mg three to four times/day (maximum 3200 mg/day) Mild–Moderate Pain—400 mg every 4 h to 6 h Dysmenorrhea—400 mg every 4 h OTC for aches, pain, fever—200 mg every 4 h to 6 h to a maximum of 1200 mg/day	Available OTC (200-mg tablets) and for prescription-only use (all other strengths). Not to be used more than 10 days for pain or 3 days for fever. Slightly more effective than aspirin as an anti-inflammatory drug, and for relief of dysmenorrhea. Minimal interaction with oral anticoagulants. If blurred or diminished vision occurs, discontinue drug. Perform periodic ophthalmologic examination.

(continued)

Table 23-3 (continued)
Nonsteroidal Anti-Inflammatory Drugs

Drug	Preparations	Usual Dosage Range	Clinical Considerations
ketoprofen (Orudis)	Capsules—50 mg, 75 mg	Arthritis—75 mg three times/day or 50 mg four times/day (maximum 300 mg/day) Mild-moderate pain, Dysmenorrhea—50 mg three to four times/day	Principally indicated for rheumatoid arthritis and osteoarthritis. Recurrent peptic ulcers have occurred during prolonged use. Dyspepsia, GI distress, and headache are quite common. Initial dose should be reduced ⅓ to ½ in elderly patients with impaired renal function. Drug is dialyzable in cases of poisoning with renal failure.
meclofenamate (Meclomen)	Capsules—50 mg, 100 mg	200 mg to 400 mg/day in three to four divided doses	Not recommended in children under age 14. Should not be used as initial therapy for rheumatoid arthritis or osteoarthritis, due to high incidence of diarrhea (10%–30%), vomiting (10%–12%), and other GI disorders (10%). Also associated with frequent headache, dizziness, and rash. Take with meals, milk, or antacids. Periodic hemoglobin/hematocrit determinations are recommended during extended therapy.
mefenamic acid (Ponstel)	Capsules—250 mg	Acute pain—Initially, 500 mg; then 250 mg every 6 h for a maximum of 7 days Dysmenorrhea—Initially 500 mg; then 250 mg every 6 h for 2 to 4 days	Short-acting drug used to relieve moderate pain of brief duration and to treat symptoms of primary dysmenorrhea. Diarrhea occurs frequently, and may neccesitate discontinuation of therapy. Administer with food and do not exceed 1-week treatment. Maximum duration for dysmenorrhea is 3 to 4 days. Do not use in patients with a history of renal impairment or chronic inflammation or ulceration of the GI tract. Discontinue drug if skin petechiae, dark stools, or hematemesis are noted.

(continued)

Table 23-3 (continued)
Nonsteroidal Anti-Inflammatory Drugs

Drug	Preparations	Usual Dosage Range	Clinical Considerations
mefenamic acid (Ponstel) (*continued*)			Contraindicated in children under age 14. CNS response may vary. Warn patient of possible dizziness, decreased alertness. Over-dosage has resulted in muscle twitching and grand mal seizures.
naproxen (Naprosyn)	Tablets—250 mg, 375 mg, 500 mg Oral suspension—125 mg/5 ml	Arthritis—250 mg to 375 mg twice a day (maximum 1000 mg/day)	Prolonged half-life (13 h) in the body allows twice-a-day administration, which may aid patient compliance. Sodium salt is more quickly absorbed, giving a faster onset of action; duration of action is equal to base, however. Drug may have to be used for up to 1 month to obtain a significant clinical response. Readily crosses placental barrier and is excreted in significant concentrations in breast milk.
naproxen sodium (Anaprox)	Tablets—275 mg, 550 mg (equivalent to 250 mg or 500 mg naproxen base)	Mild–Moderate Pain—550 mg (sodium salt) initially, then 275 mg every 6 h to 8 h Acute Gout—750 mg to 825 mg followed by 250 mg to 275 mg every 8 h until attack has subsided	
piroxicam (Feldene)	Capsules—10 mg, 20 mg	Initially, 20 mg once daily. Maintenance dosage is 10 mg to 20 mg once daily	Long-acting drug used once daily in rheumatoid and osteoarthritis. Steady-state plasma levels are generally attained within 1 to 2 weeks. Antacids do not affect plasma levels, but aspirin can reduce blood levels of piroxicam to 80% of normal. GI side-effects are experienced by 20% of patients. Not recommended for use in children.
sulindac (Clinoril)	Tablets—150 mg, 200 mg	150 mg to 200 mg twice a day (maximum 400 mg/day)	Long-acting drug used twice a day. Useful in rheumatoid, osteo- and gouty arthritis; spondylitis, and acute painful shoulder. May allow a gradual reduction in corticosteroid dosage if used concurrently. Liver function test abnormalities can occur. Not indicated in children. High incidence (10%) of GI pain and other symptoms. Administer with food.

(continued)

Table 23-3 (continued)
Nonsteroidal Anti-Inflammatory Drugs

Drug	Preparations	Usual Dosage Range	Clinical Considerations
suprofen (Suprol)	Capsules—200 mg	Mild–Moderate Pain, Dysmenorrhea—200 mg every 4 h–6 h (maximum 800 mg/day)	More effective as an analgesic than an anti-inflammatory agent. Incidence of GI and CNS side-effects increases at higher doses. Diarrhea, skin rash, nausea, dyspepsia, drowsiness, and headache are most frequent effects. *Not* considered as initial treatment for any indication because flank pain sometimes accompanied by renal function abnormalities may occur. Patients should be adequately hydrated because significant uricosuria can occur.
tolmetin (Tolectin)	Tablets—200 mg Capsules—400 mg	*Adults*—Initially, 400 mg three times/day. Maintenance doses are 600 mg to 1800 mg/day in three or four divided doses. *Children* (older than 2 yr)—20 mg/kg/day in three to four divided doses (maximum 30 mg/kg/day)	May be used in juvenile rheumatoid arthritis in children over age 2. Minimal interaction with oral anticoagulants. If GI intolerance occurs, give with food, milk, or antacids other than sodium bicarbonate. Sodium and water retention can occur; caution in cardiac patients. Headache and nausea are frequently observed side-effects.

istration of a total of 1 g, reevaluate need for gold therapy. Cessation of treatment depends on individual response.

Children (6 years–12 years)—One fourth the adult dose. Maximum 25 mg/week to children under age 12.

Gold Sodium Thiomalate

Adults—Weekly injections; first week, 10 mg; second week, 25 mg; thereafter, 25 mg to 50 mg/week until clinical improvement or toxicity occurs. Injections of 25 mg to 50 mg may be given every 3 to 4 weeks if clinical improvement is maintained. If improvement is not observed with a total dose of 1 g, dose may be temporarily increased by 10-mg increments every 1 to 4 weeks, although the danger of adverse effects is also increased.

Children—1 mg/kg, not to exceed 50 mg on a single injection. Schedule is the same as adults.

Oral

Auranofin

Six mg a day, either as a single or two divided doses. If response is not adequate after 6 months, increase to 9 mg/day (3 mg three times/day).

FATE

The comparative pharmacokinetics of the various gold compounds are outlined in Table 23-4. Gold is well distributed in the body, and major sites of localization include bone marrow, liver, skin, and bone. Arthritic joints appear to concentrate more gold than noninvolved joints. No definite correla-

Table 23-4
Comparative Properties of Injectable vs Oral Gold Preparations

Drug	Gold Content	Peak Effect	Protein Binding	Serum Half-Life	Excretion
Injectable					
aurothioglucose	50%	4–6 h	95%–100%	5–25 days*	70% urine/30% feces
gold sodium thiomalate	50%	2–6 h	95%–100%	3–27 days*	70% urine/30% feces
Oral					
auranofin	29%	1–2 h	50%–60%	20–30 days	15% urine/85% feces

* Half-life increases with repeated dosage; up to 40 days after 3 to 5 doses and up to 175 days after 10 doses.

tion exists between plasma concentrations of gold and efficacy or safety.

SIDE-EFFECTS/ADVERSE REACTIONS
Adverse reactions to gold therapy can occur during treatment or for several months after treatment has been stopped. The incidence of untoward reactions is apparently unrelated to the plasma level of drug, but may be associated with the cumulative amount of drug in the body.

Between one fourth and one half of all patients receiving gold compounds experience some untoward reactions. The most common side-effects are dermatitis, stomatitis, pruritus, erythema, metallic taste, flushing, dizziness, sweating, and proteinuria. Diarrhea occurs in over 50% of patients receiving gold orally.

Many other adverse reactions have occurred in patients receiving gold, and they are listed below by organ system.

Dermatologic—Papular, vesicular, or exfoliative dermatitis; alopecia, chrysiasis (grayish blue skin pigmentation)
Mucous membrane—Gingivitis, pharyngitis, gastritis, colitis, upper respiratory tract inflammation, vaginitis
Hematologic—Blood dyscrasias (rare)
CV—Syncope, bradycardia
GI—Nausea, vomiting, colic, abdominal cramping, ulcerative enterocolitis (especially with oral preparation)
Renal—Glomerulitis, hematuria, tubular necrosis, nephritis
Allergic—Angioedema, difficulty in swallowing or breathing, anaphylactic shock
Other—Iritis, corneal ulcers (rare), hepatitis, acute yellow atrophy, peripheral neuritis, pulmonary fibrosis, synovial destruction, encephalitis, EEG abnormalities

Minor side-effects such as dermatitis, stomatitis, and proteinuria generally disappear with cessation of therapy. Other adverse reactions may persist for weeks or months due to drug cumulation, and may require other forms of drug therapy, such as corticosteroids, for control.

Laboratory signs of gold toxicity include leukopenia (less than 4000 WBC/mm^3), fall in hemoglobin, proteinuria, platelet count less than 100,000/mm^3, and a granulocyte count less than 1500/mm^3. Close monitoring of laboratory values is essential to ensure safe and effective therapy.

Gold therapy may be reinstituted at a reduced dosage schedule following resolution of mild side-effects, but should *not* be resumed after severe adverse or allergic reactions.

CONTRAINDICATIONS AND PRECAUTIONS
Gold salts are contraindicated in patients with uncontrolled diabetes, renal or hepatic disease, severe hypertension, cardiac failure, systemic lupus, blood dyscrasias, colitis, eczema, and urticaria. Other contraindications include pregnancy, lactation, severe debilitation, and patients who have recently undergone radiation therapy. *Cautious use of gold* should be undertaken in patients with a history of allergies, compromised coronary or cerebral circulation, or moderate hypertension. Use of aurothioglucose is not recommended in children under age 6.

INTERACTIONS
1. The incidence of blood dyscrasias and hematologic toxicity may be increased by concurrent use of pyrazolones, penicillamine, antimalarial drugs (*e.g.*, hydroxychloroquine), immunosuppressants (*e.g.*, azathioprine), or cytotoxic drugs.

2. Corticosteroids can reduce the effectiveness and increase the toxicity of gold salts.

NURSING CONSIDERATIONS

What attracts arthritic patients to this form of therapy, despite its toxicity, is the promise of long-term relief of symptoms. The patient receiving gold therapy must be willing to learn and closely monitor himself for signs of toxicity which can occur months after the treatment is given.

The patient receiving gold therapy should be relatively free of debilitating symptoms and should have a complete laboratory work-up before commencing treatment. This should include a complete blood count with white cell count, erythrocyte, platelet and hemoglobin levels particularly noted, and a urinalysis. The patient should be taught to watch for early signs of toxicity, which include mouth sores, pruritus, gastrointestinal upset, dermatitis, bleeding gums, petechiae, fever, chills, sore throat, weakness, and dysphagia. Any of these symptoms should be reported to the physician immediately. Routine lab studies should also be done at frequent intervals. The patient needs to understand the importance of keeping these appointments. Changing laboratory values that may occur include a decreased hemoglobin, decreased white cell count, and platelet levels below $100,000/mm^3$; proteinuria or hematuria are also possible. The patient must be closely followed even after treatment is completed because toxicity can occur several months later. Mild toxicity will respond to discontinuation of the drug. If severe toxicity occurs the treatment may include corticosteroids and dimercaprol (BAL).

When administering gold salts the vial must be well shaken and the liquid must be a pale yellow. Do not use if discolored. Inject deep into the gluteal muscle with the patient in a side-lying position with the upper knee flexed. The patient should remain recumbent about 20 minutes to reduce the possibility of dizziness from the medication.

Miscellaneous Anti-Inflammatory Agents

Severe active forms of rheumatoid arthritis refractory to more conventional pharmacotherapy (e.g., salicylates, nonsteroidal anti-inflammatory drugs, corticosteroids) can be treated by other drugs that have been shown to produce symptomatic improvement in joint function.

Hydroxychloroquine (Plaquenil) is a 4-amino-quinoline which is used primarily for treating malaria and has also been employed for many years in the treatment of chronic rheumatoid arthritis and systemic lupus erythematosus. Hydroxychloroquine is preferred to its close structural analogue chloroquine (Aralen) because it is *slightly* less toxic, although by no means should it be viewed as an innocuous drug. The antiarthritic mechanism of action of the 4-aminoquinolines is not precisely known, but they may stabilize lysosomal membranes, inhibit nucleic acid synthesis, interfere with replication of viruses, and suppress formation of antigens that cause hypersensitivity reactions.

Initial dosage is 200 mg two to three times/day. Several weeks are required to attain an optimal therapeutic effect, at which point the dosage can be reduced to 200 to 400 mg/day. If objective improvement is not observed within 6 months, the drug should be discontinued. Salicylates, NSAIDs, and corticosteroids can be given in conjunction with hydroxychloroquine, often allowing a reduced dosage of all drugs and lowered toxicity.

Untoward ophthalmic reactions involving the cornea, retina, and ciliary body have been associated with hydroxychloroquine. Periodic ophthalmic examinations are essential during prolonged therapy.

A complete discussion of the 4-aminoquinolines, chloroquine and hydroxychloroquine, may be found in Chapter 70.

Penicillamine

(Cuprimine, Depen)

Penicillamine is a chelating agent which has been successfully used to remove excess copper in patients with Wilson's disease and to increase cystine excretion in cystinuria. It is also approved for the treatment of severe forms of rheumatoid arthritis. Because of its potential to elicit serious adverse effects, however, its use should be restricted to those patients with progressive rheumatoid disease that is unresponsive to other less toxic anti-inflammatory agents.

MECHANISM AND ACTIONS

Although the precise mechanism by which penicillamine relieves symptoms of arthritis is unclear, several actions probably contribute to its effectiveness. The drug may inhibit lysosomal enzyme release in connective tissue, interfere with synthesis of DNA, collagen, and perhaps mucopolysaccharides, suppress T-cell activity, and lower the titer of IgM rheumatoid factor. Other actions that may be involved are inhibition of lymphocyte transformation and reduction of circulating immune complexes.

Penicillamine is capable of combining with copper, thus removing excess amounts of the substance from patients with Wilson's disease (see Disease Brief). The drug also reduces cystine excretion in cystinuria, probably by forming a substance more soluble and hence more readily excretable than cystine.

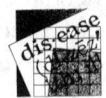

DISEASE BRIEF

■ Wilson's Disease

Wilson's disease or hepatolenticular degeneration is characterized by degenerative changes in the brain, especially the basal ganglia, and cirrhosis of the liver. It occurs primarily between 10 and 30 years of age and is manifested initially as tremor and incoordination. Later symptoms include rigidity, uncontrollable movements, dysphagia, and mental deterioration. A characteristic ocular sign of the disease is the presence of Kayser-Fleischer rings (golden-brown or brownish-green pigment rings) behind the border of the cornea. The primary biochemical disturbance in Wilson's disease is increased copper absorption, resulting in accumulation of the substance in the brain, liver, and many other bodily tissues, where it gradually disturbs normal functioning. Excretion of copper is also increased, and renal damage may ensue due to the increased copper levels. Treatment is directed toward reducing total body copper content and includes a high-protein, low-copper diet and administration of the copper-chelating drug, penicillamine.

USES

1. Treatment of severe, active rheumatoid arthritis resistant to other conventional forms of therapy, including rest, exercise, salicylates, nonsteroidal anti-inflammatory drugs, and corticosteroids
2. Promotion of copper excretion in patients with Wilson's disease (hepatolenticular degeneration)
3. Promotion of cystine excretion in patients with cystinuria, when conventional measures, such as alkalinization of the urine, increased fluid intake, and methionine restriction, are inadequate to reduce recurrent kidney stone formation
4. Investigational uses include treatment of primary biliary cirrhosis and scleroderma.

ADMINISTRATION AND DOSAGE

Penicillamine is used orally as capsules (Cuprimine) containing 125 mg or 250 mg or tablets (Depen Titratable Tablets) containing 250 mg.

Rheumatoid Arthritis

Initially, 125 to 250 mg/day is given for 4 weeks. Dosage may be increased at 4-week to 12-week intervals by 125- to 250-mg/day-increments depending on response and tolerance. If no substantial improvement occurs after 3 months to 4 months of therapy with 1000 to 1500 mg/day, discontinue the drug. Many patients will respond to 500 to 750 mg/day. Up to 500 mg/day can be given as a single dose. Larger amounts should be administered in divided doses. If remission persists for 6 months or more, consider reducing the dosage by 125-mg/day-increments at 3-month intervals.

Wilson's Disease

Initially, 1 g/day (250 mg four times/day) in both adults and children. Increase as necessary based on urinary copper analyses, to a maximum of 2 g/day.

Cystinuria

Adults: 1 to 4 g/day in divided doses (usually 2 g/day)
Children: 30 mg/kg/day in divided doses

FATE

Penicillamine is well-absorbed on an empty stomach. Oral absorption is significantly reduced by food, antacids, and iron (see under Interactions). Peak plasma levels occur in 1 hour to 2 hours. Serum half-life averages 2 hours. Up to several months may be required to obtain a significant clinical response. The drug is rapidly excreted in the urine, almost completely within 24 hours.

SIDE-EFFECTS/ADVERSE REACTIONS
Over 50% of patients receiving penicillamine experience untoward reactions. Skin and mucous membrane reactions, such as rash, stomatitis, pruritus, and loss of taste, are commonly encountered, as are epigastric pain, nausea, anorexia, and proteinuria. A variety of other adverse effects have been associated with penicillamine, as indicated below.

GI—Vomiting, diarrhea, oral ulceration, activation of peptic ulcer

Hematologic—Leukopenia, thrombocytopenia, bone marrow depression, agranulocytosis, aplastic anemia

Allergic—Arthralgia, lymphadenopathy, pemphigoid reaction, urticaria, exfoliative dermatitis, synovitis

Renal/hepatic—Hematuria, hepatic dysfunction, increased serum alkaline phosphatase and LDH, cholestatic jaundice, pancreatitis, colitis, glomerulonephritis (Goodpasture's syndrome)

CNS—Tinnitus, optic neuritis

Other—Thrombophlebitis, myasthenia-like reaction, hyperpyrexia, polymyositis, systemic lupus-like syndrome, mammary hyperplasia, epidermal necrolysis, skin friability and excessive wrinkling, alveolitis, obliterative bronchiolitis

CONTRAINDICATIONS AND PRECAUTIONS
Penicillamine is contraindicated in patients with renal insufficiency or those with a history of blood dyscrasias or penicillin hypersensitivity. The drug is also not recommended during pregnancy or in very young children. *Caution* should be exercised when administering the drug to patients with a history of allergies or respiratory diseases.

INTERACTIONS
1. The absorption of penicillamine can be significantly decreased by the presence of food, antacids, or iron salts.
2. Penicillamine can lower serum levels of digoxin.
3. The risk of renal and hematologic toxicity with penicillamine is increased by concurrent use of gold salts, antimalarial drugs, pyrazolones, or cytotoxic agents.
4. Penicillamine increases pyridoxine (vitamin B_6) requirements.

NURSING CONSIDERATIONS
Baseline urine and blood counts should be drawn prior to initiation of therapy. The patient should be alert and independent enough to monitor himself for side-effects and keep laboratory appointments so blood and urine samples can be evaluated. The patient must also be willing to go through 3-month trials on each dose of the drug, knowing that frequent dosage changing increases the incidence of untoward reactions.

The high incidence of drug toxicity means the nurse must carefully monitor the patient receiving penicillamine and teach him which side-effects to report, and how to deal with the other ones as they occur.

The patient needs to watch for early signs of blood dyscrasias: fever, chills, sore throat, bruising, and abnormal bleeding. The physician should be notified immediately and blood studies done.

The patient can also develop an allergy to penicillamine over time and should be alert for fever, intense pruritus, and rash. If noted early on, the physician will probably try to reduce rather than eliminate the dose and treat with antihistamines.

Another sign patients need to watch for and report is myasthenia-like muscle weakness. This can be a frightening symptom which will disappear when the drug is withdrawn.

This drug should always be taken on an empty stomach, at least 1 hour before any other drug, food, antacid, or milk.

Patients need to protect their skin, especially around elbows, knees, and buttocks, while taking this drug because skin friability can occur. Use of elbow, knee, and heel pads and sheepskin mats may decrease the amount of friction rub on those parts when the patient is in bed. Elbow and knee pads may be worn around the house if the patient is prone to bumping into things.

Antigout Drugs

Gout is an acute metabolic disorder resulting from an excess of uric acid in the blood (hyperuricemia) due to either overproduction or faulty elimination. When the solubility of uric acid salts in body fluids is exceded, crystals of monosodium urate begin to precipitate out and can be deposited in joints, skin, kidney, and other tissues. Acute gout can occur in any joint, although classically there is involvement of the great toe, characterized by pain (podalgia), swelling, tenderness, and other signs of inflammation. At the inflammatory site, there is local infiltration of granulocytes which phagocytize the urate crystals. The resulting breakdown of granulocytic cells liberates lactic acid and other acidic metabolic products, which lower the regional pH, thus favoring *further precipitation* of urate crystals. Thus, the acute phase of gout is cyclical and self-perpetuating. This process is schematically illustrated in Figure 23-1.

Hyperuricemia may be an endogenous, primary disorder, as seen in gout, or it can occur secondary to diseases (*e.g.,* leukemia, polycythemia vera, psoriasis, multiple myeloma), renal damage, use of drugs (*e.g.,* diuretics, cytotoxic agents) or during starvation diets. Primary hyperuricemia can result in deposition of urate crystals, leading to the major manifestations of gout, namely inflamed joints and kidney stones.

The pharmacotherapy of gout, therefore, involves lowering the serum levels of uric acid to prevent attacks, and providing relief of the symptoms of an acute attack. Drugs used as antigout agents may be classified as one of the following:
1. Anti-inflammatory agents—Relieve the pain and inflammation associated with an acute attack of gout
2. Hypouricemic (uricosuric) agents—Reduce the blood levels of uric acid on a chronic basis

The drugs that may be used to relieve the symptoms of an acute attack are indomethacin, phenylbutazone, naproxen, sulindac, and colchicine. The first four have been discussed previously in this chapter because they are also used to control symptoms of rheumatoid arthritis and osteoarthritis. Colchicine will be reviewed in detail in this section.

Hypouricemic agents are drugs that either interfere with the synthesis of uric acid (*e.g.,* allopurinol) or promote the urinary excretion of uric acid by blocking its renal tubular reabsorption (*e.g.,* probenecid, sulfinpyrazone). These drugs will also be discussed in this section.

Colchicine

Colchicine, an alkaloid obtained from *Colchicum autumnale,* is capable of dramatically relieving pain and inflammation associated with acute attacks of gouty arthritis within 12 hours to 24

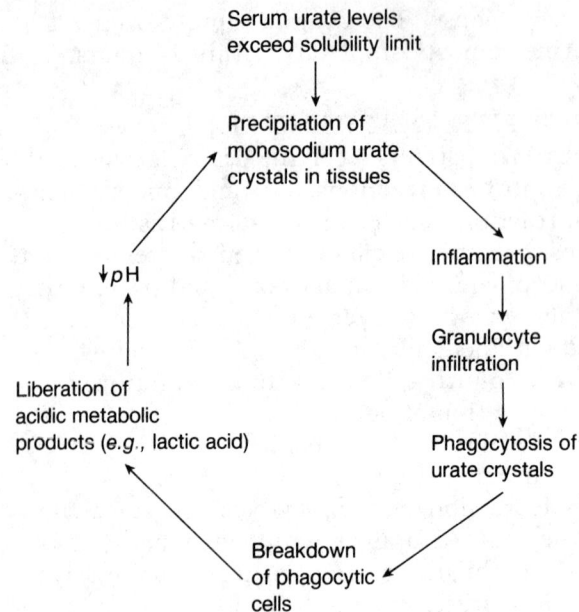

Figure 23-1. Sequence of events occurring during an attack of gout.

hours. It is also useful but somewhat less effective in the treatment of chondrocalcinosis (pseudogout). Colchicine is nonanalgesic and nonuricosuric, and is specific for the symptoms of gout, being effective in up to 90% of patients if given at the first sign of an attack. Although once it was exclusively the drug of choice, colchicine has now been largely supplanted by indomethacin, sulindac, or phenylbutazone, principally because of its high incidence of GI side-effects, especially diarrhea.

Colchicine has been used on a chronic basis in reduced dosage to reduce the frequency and lessen the severity of acute attacks of gout, although long-term therapy with colchicine is not generally advocated.

A fixed combination of colchicine and the uricosuric agent probenecid is available (Colbenemid, Proben) for treatment of chronic gouty arthritis complicated by frequent, acute attacks of gout. Gastric intolerance is common with this form of therapy.

MECHANISM AND ACTIONS
The anti-inflammatory activity of colchicine is comprised of several mechanisms. The drug reduces lactic acid production by leukocytes (thereby decreasing uric acid deposition) and impairs phagocytic breakdown of white blood cell membranes and subsequent release of tissue-damaging en-

zymes. Colchicine also binds to microtubular cellular proteins, thereby arresting mitosis at metaphase and interfering with movement of mobile cells (*e.g.*, leukocytes). These actions interrupt the cycle of urate crystal deposition and inflammation that serves to perpetuate an acute attack of gout.

USES
1. Relief of pain and inflammation of acute gout and pseudogout (no effect on nongouty arthritis or on uric acid metabolism)
2. Limit the destruction of joint cartilage and reduce the incidence of acute attacks (*not* an approved indication
3. Other experimental uses include symptomatic treatment of leukemia, adenocarcinoma, sarcoid arthritis, mycosis fungoides, acute calcium-dependent tendinitis, and familial Mediterranean fever.

ADMINISTRATION AND DOSAGE
Colchicine is available as tablets (0.5 mg, 0.6 mg) and injection solution (1 mg/2 ml). The drug is primarily given orally, although it may be used IV in the acute stages of a gouty arthritis attack. To relieve or abort an acute attack of gout, 1 mg to 1.2 mg is given orally with milk or food, followed by 0.5 mg to 1.2 mg every 1 hour to 2 hours until the pain is relieved or diarrhea occurs. The total amount of drug needed to treat an acute attack is usually 4 mg to 8 mg. Alternately, 1 mg to 2 mg may be administered IV, followed by 0.5 mg every 6 hours until the desired response is obtained. The maximum IV dose should not exceed 4 mg/24 h. Colchicine should not be given IM or SC. It is extremely irritating to tissue. IV extravasation can cause pain and tissue necrosis.

For prevention of gouty attacks, 0.5 to 0.6 mg/day may be administered orally for 3 days or 4 days out of each week. Higher doses (up to 1.8 mg/day) may be necessary in severe cases. This dose should be used 3 days pre- and postoperatively on any patient suffering from gout because surgery can precipitate a gouty attack.

FATE
Colchicine is rapidly absorbed orally and has a relatively short plasma half-life. It is partially metabolized in the liver; both metabolites and unchanged drug are recycled into the GI tract through the bile and intestinal secretions. Colchicine is mainly eliminated in the feces, with 10% to 20% excreted in the urine. The drug may persist for up to 9 days in leukocytes after a single IV dose.

SIDE-EFFECTS/ADVERSE REACTIONS
GI side-effects are quite common with colchicine, especially in high doses. Diarrhea (often of a severe, prolonged nature), abdominal pain, nausea, and vomiting are the most prominent symptoms. Other reported adverse reactions are muscle weakness, vascular damage, alopecia, hematuria, oliguria, dermatitis, peripheral neuritis, purpura, and azoospermia. Prolonged use has resulted in agranulocytosis, and bone marrow depression with aplastic anemia.

Acute overdose may be characterized by vomiting, diarrhea (profuse and/or bloody); burning in the throat, stomach, or skin; hematuria, shock due to extensive vascular damage, marked muscle weakness, delirium, and convulsions.

CONTRAINDICATIONS AND PRECAUTIONS
Use of colchicine is contraindicated in the presence of serious GI, renal, hepatic, or cardiac disorders and blood dyscrasias. IV administration should not be undertaken in persons with peripheral vascular damage. Administration should be undertaken with *caution* in elderly or debilitated patients, in pregnant women, nursing mothers, and children.

INTERACTIONS
1. The effects of colchicine are enhanced by alkalinizing agents (*e.g.*, sodium bicarbonate) and inhibited by acidifying agents (*e.g.*, ascorbic acid).
2. Colchicine may increase the response to CNS depressants and sympathomimetics.
3. Prolonged use of colchicine may reduce GI absorption of vitamin B_{12}.

NURSING CONSIDERATIONS
Because colchicine is used, for the most part, to treat acute gouty attacks, nursing care centers around the patient's needs at a time he is very uncomfortable. The earlier the drug therapy is begun the more effective it will be, so the patient needs to learn to report his symptoms as soon as observed. The oral route is preferred unless GI upset and toxicity are a problem. Be aware, however, with IV use that the chance of overdose is greater. Nausea, vomiting, diarrhea, and abdominal discomfort must be reported immediately because these are

early signs of toxicity which will subside once the drug is discontinued.

The patient on colchicine should force fluids of 2000 to 3000 ml/day to promote water excretion and reduce the formation of uric acid kidney stones.

Probenecid
(Benemid, Probalan)

MECHANISM
Probenecid is a uricosuric agent that enhances the renal excretion of uric acid by blocking its active tubular reabsorption. The drug has no analgesic or anti-inflammatory action, and thus is of no value in treating acute attacks. Probenecid also inhibits renal tubular secretion of penicillins and cephalosporins, and is often used to increase the plasma level of penicillins by two to four times, thus enhancing their effects.

USES
1. Treatment of hyperuricemia associated with gout and gouty arthritis (Most beneficial for gouty arthritis in patients with reduced uric acid excretion (800 mg/day) on an unrestricted diet)
2. Adjuvant to therapy with penicillins and cephalosporins, to elevate and prolong antibiotic plasma levels

ADMINISTRATION AND DOSAGE
Probenecid is given orally as 0.5-g tablets. Therapy should not be initiated until an acute gouty attack has subsided. The initial dose is 0.25 g twice daily for 1 week, followed by 0.5 g twice a day thereafter. Maximum daily dose is 2 g/day. When acute attacks have subsided for at least 6 months and serum uric acid levels are within the normal range, daily dosage may be decreased by 0.5 g every 6 months.

To enhance penicillin or cephalosporin therapy, 2 g/day is given to adults in divided doses. Children (2–14 years of age) receive 40 mg/kg/day in four divided doses, except those over 50 kg, who receive the adult dosage.

Probenecid may also be given as a single 1-g dose with 4.8 million units of penicillin or 3.5 g ampicillin for treatment of gonorrhea.

Probenecid is also available in fixed combination with colchicine (500 mg/0.5 mg) as Colabid, Colbenemid, or Proben-C for treatment of *chronic*

gouty arthritis complicated by frequent recurring attacks. Initial dosage is one tablet for 1 week, followed by one tablet twice a day. Therapy is continued until serum urate levels have remained normal for at least 6 months and no acute attacks have occurred during that time, at which point dosage may be slowly reduced.

FATE
Oral absorption is good and peak plasma levels are attained within 2 hours to 4 hours. Probenecid is highly protein bound and exhibits a serum half-life of 8 hours to 10 hours. The drug is metabolized in the liver and excreted in the urine, primarily as metabolites with some unchanged drug. Urinary excretion may be increased by alkalinization of the urine.

SIDE-EFFECTS/ADVERSE REACTIONS
GI irritation may occur with use of probenecid, as well as nausea, mild skin rash, headache, and a temporary worsening of symptoms for the first few days of treatment. Other reported untoward reactions are diarrhea, urinary frequency, hypersensitivity reactions (*e.g.*, pruritus, dermatitis, urticaria, fever), flushing, dizziness, sore gums, and hemolytic anemia. Hepatic necrosis, aplastic anemia, and nephrotic syndrome are rare.

CONTRAINDICATIONS AND PRECAUTIONS
Probenecid should not be given to patients with blood dyscrasias, uric acid kidney stones, severe renal impairment, or to children under 2 years of age. *Cautious use* is necessary in persons with peptic ulcers, acute intermittent porphyria, and glucose-6-phosphatase deficiency.

INTERACTIONS
1. Probenecid prolongs the action of penicillins and cephalosporins and may enhance the action of methotrexate, clofibrate, oral anticoagulants, oral hypoglycemics, naproxen, indomethacin, sulfinpyrazone, sulfonamides, and thiazide diuretics by reducing their renal excretion.
2. Salicylates can antagonize the uricosuric effect of probenecid, especially in small analgesic doses.
3. Xanthines (*e.g.*, caffeine, theophylline) and diuretics may antagonize the uricosuric effect of probenecid by elevating serum urate levels.

NURSING CONSIDERATIONS

Probenecid is not appropriately started during an acute gouty attack because it may worsen symptoms. However, if an attack occurs while the patient is taking probenecid the medication will be continued. Colchicine or indomethacin will be added to the treatment. Probenecid must be continued because acute withdrawal will drastically increase uric acid levels. To avoid confusion, encourage the patient to contact the physician whenever an attack occurs.

The patient can take probenecid with milk or meals to minimize the gastrointestinal upset. Fluid intake up to 3000 ml/day should also be encouraged. Sodium bicarbonate or potassium citrate may be prescribed to alkalinize the urine and retard the formation of uric acid kidney stones.

Although there is no firm evidence that excessive dietary intake of purines is a primary cause of gout, high-purine foods such as liver, meat extracts, peas, meat soups, broth, and alcohol should be prudently restricted during early stages of therapy, at least until uric acid levels have stabilized.

Sulfinpyrazone
(Anturane, Aprazone)

A pyrazolone derivative with relatively weak anti-inflammatory action, sulfinpyrazone is indicated primarily for the maintenance therapy of hyperuricemia. It rapidly reduces serum urate levels to normal, thereby preventing formation of new deposits in tissues. The anti-inflammatory action of sulfinpyrazone is minimal and it is not intended for relief of an acute attack. The drug also inhibits platelet aggregation, and some studies suggest that it is effective in reducing the incidence of cardiac death in patients with recent myocardial infarction. This latter effect may result from an inhibition of thromboxane A_2 synthesis in platelets, protection of the vascular endothelium from injury, and diminished release of ADP and possibly serotonin.

MECHANISM AND ACTIONS

Sulfinpyrazone inhibits the active renal tubular reabsorption of uric acid, thereby increasing its urinary excretion and reducing serum urate levels. Very small doses may interfere with active tubular *secretion* of uric acid (transport from blood to renal tubule), thereby causing retention of serum urates.

USES

1. Maintenance therapy in hyperuricemia, to reduce the incidence and severity of acute attacks of gouty arthritis
2. Prevention of cerebrovascular and ischemic heart disease and transient ischemic attacks, and reduction in fatalities following myocardial infarction

ADMINISTRATION AND DOSAGE

Sulfinpyrazone is used orally as 100-mg tablets or 200-mg capsules. The initial dose in hyperuricemia is 200 to 400 mg/day in two divided doses. Dosage may be increased gradually to a maximum of 800 mg/day. Treatment should be uninterrupted, even during an acute attack, which can be managed by concurrent use of colchicine, indomethacin, or phenylbutazone.

To decrease platelet aggregation, a dose of 200 mg four times a day has been recommended.

FATE

Sulfinpyrazone is well-absorbed after oral administration; effects are noted within 30 minutes to 60 minutes, and persist for 4 hours to 8 hours. The drug is highly protein bound (98%–99%) and excreted almost completely unchanged in the urine.

SIDE-EFFECTS/ADVERSE REACTIONS

The most commonly observed side-effects are upper GI distress, such as nausea, epigastric pain, burning, and dyspepsia. Less frequently noted adverse reactions are rash, reversible renal dysfunction, dizziness, tinnitus, fever, and occasionally blood dyscrasias. Acute attacks of gout may be precipitated during the early stages of sulfinpyrazone therapy.

CONTRAINDICATIONS AND PRECAUTIONS

Active peptic ulcer and GI inflammation are contraindications to use of sulfinpyrazone. The drug should be used *cautiously* in patients with impaired renal function or unexplained GI pain and during pregnancy. Because sulfinpyrazone can precipitate acute gouty arthritis or urolithiasis in the initial stages of therapy, adequate fluid intake and alkalinization of the urine are recommended, and use of colchicine during the initial days of treatment is often recommended.

INTERACTIONS

1. Sulfinpyrazone may potentiate the effects of anticoagulants, sulfonylurea hypoglycemic

agents, sulfonamides, penicillins, insulin, allopurinol, indomethacin, and nitrofurantoin.

2. The uricosuric effects of sulfinpyrazone may be reduced by salicylates (low doses) and xanthines (e.g., caffeine, theophylline).

3. Serum urate levels may be elevated by diuretics, alcohol, diazoxide, and mecamylamine, possibly necessitating higher sulfinpyrazone dosage.

4. The incidence of blood dyscrasias may be increased with combined use of sulfinpyrazone and colchicine, other pyrazolones, or indomethacin.

NURSING CONSIDERATIONS
(See Nursing Considerations for probenecid.)

Allopurinol
(Lopurin, Zurinol, Zyloprim)

Allopurinol reduces the plasma levels of uric acid by a mechanism unlike that of the previously discussed uricosuric drugs probenecid and sulfinpyrazone. Allopurinol is a potent inhibitor of the synthesis of uric acid from the purine breakdown products hypoxanthine and xanthine. It is the drug of choice for controlling hyperuricemia resulting from overproduction of uric acid and is especially effective in preventing development of uric acid stones.

MECHANISM AND ACTIONS
Allopurinol competitively inhibits the action of xanthine oxidase, the enzyme responsible for converting the natural purine hypoxanthine into xanthine and subsequently into uric acid. Xanthine oxidase converts allopurinol into oxypurinol (alloxanthine), which is also an inhibitor of xanthine oxidase, with a long duration of action. With allopurinol, substantial reductions occur in both serum and urinary levels of uric acid. The synthesis of other vital purines is not compromised. Allopurinol possesses no analgesic, anti-inflammatory, or uricosuric activity. The drug is effective in lowering uric acid levels even in the presence of marked renal damage.

USES
1. Treatment of gout, either primary or secondary to the hyperuricemia associated with blood dyscrasias and their treatment

2. Treatment of primary or secondary uric acid nephropathy

3. Treatment of recurrent uric acid stone formation

4. Prevention of urate deposition and uric acid nephropathy in patients receiving cancer chemotherapy or radiation for leukemia and other malignancies (usually given with colchicine or a uricosuric drug at the outset of therapy to prevent acute attacks of gouty arthritis; see under Side-Effects/Adverse Reactions)

ADMINISTRATION AND DOSAGE
Allopurinol is administered orally as 100-mg and 300-mg tablets. A high fluid intake (yielding at least 2 liters/day urinary output) and alkalinization of the urine are highly desired when allopurinol is given.

To control chronic gout and hyperuricemia, adults receive 200 to 600 mg/day depending on the severity of the symptoms. Doses above 300 mg/day should be administered in divided doses. Children with hyperuricemia secondary to malignancy can be given 300 mg/day if over 6 years of age, and half that amount if less than 6 years of age.

For preventing uric acid nephropathy during antineoplastic therapy, a dosage of 600 to 800 mg/day for two to three days is recommended together with a very high fluid intake.

Dosage should be reduced in patients with impaired renal clearance. If the creatinine clearance is 10 to 20 ml/min, daily allopurinol dosage should be 200 mg; if creatinine clearance is less than 10 ml/min, the daily dose should not exceed 100 mg.

FATE
Oral absorption is nearly complete. Peak plasma levels occur in 2 hours to 6 hours. The half-life of allopurinol is dependent on both its renal excretion, which is fairly rapid, and on its oxidation to oxypurinol, an active metabolite with a long half-life (18–30 hours). Distribution is extensive except for the CNS. Small amounts of the unchanged drug may be excreted in the urine and feces.

SIDE-EFFECTS/ADVERSE REACTIONS
Skin rash, usually of a maculopapular nature, accompanied by pruritus is the most frequently noted side-effect. Acute attacks of gouty arthritis may occur early in the course of therapy with allopurinol, because urate crystals are mobilized from tissues when plasma urate levels are decreased. This is

followed by recrystallization in the plasma and precipitation in joints. Colchicine can be given during the initial period of allopurinol therapy to minimize these acute attacks.

A number of other adverse reactions have been observed with use of allopurinol and while they are not common, their seriousness mandates close supervision of the patient.

Hypersensitivity—Fever, chills, malaise, nausea, muscle pain, eosinophilia, leukopenia, reversible acute interstitial nephritis

Dermatologic—Exfoliative, urticarial, or purpuric skin lesions; erythema multiforme; toxic epidermal necrolysis; alopecia; dermatitis

Hematologic—Blood dyscrasias, bone marrow depression, vasculitis, necrotizing angiitis

GI—Vomiting, diarrhea, abdominal pain

Other—Peripheral neuritis, cataract formation, hepatotoxicity, drowsiness, vertigo

CONTRAINDICATIONS AND PRECAUTIONS

The drug is contraindicated in children, except for those with hyperuricemia secondary to a malignancy, and in nursing mothers. *Cautious use* of allopurinol is indicated in patients with liver or kidney disease, and during pregnancy. Because skin rash may be followed by more serious dermatologic disorders (see above), the drug must be discontinued at the first sign of rash.

INTERACTIONS

1. Allopurinol slows the enzymatic inactivation of mercaptopurine and azathioprine, and the doses of these antineoplastic drugs should be reduced to one fourth the original dose. In addition, the drug is a nonspecific enzyme inhibitor, and therefore can potentially reduce the metabolism of a wide range of drugs (*e.g.*, anticoagulants) dependent on hepatic metabolism for clearance.
2. The effects of allopurinol may be reduced by thiazide and loop diuretics, salicylates, sulfinpyrazone, probenecid, and xanthines. Thiazides can also increase the incidence of hypersensitivity reactions.
3. Allopurinol may increase iron absorption and hepatic iron stores. Do not administer oral iron to patients taking allopurinol or use the two drugs together.
4. An increased incidence of skin rash may occur with combinations of ampicillin, or amoxicillin, together with allopurinol.
5. Allopurinol may increase serum levels of theophylline.

NURSING CONSIDERATIONS

Although the mechanism of action is different, most of the nursing considerations are the same as those for probenecid with one notable exception. When a patient is being transferred from a uricosuric agent to allopurinol, the dosage of the uricosuric agent must be gradually reduced while the dose of allopurinol is gradually increased to avoid an acute gouty attack from increased uric acid levels. The physician's prescription plan must be closely followed. A drug calendar may be a useful tool to facilitate memory of the dosage adjustments.

Allopurinol administration sometimes results in hypersensitivity, the early manifestation of which is skin rash. Patients need to watch for such signs and notify the physician immediately.

CASE STUDY 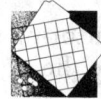 **Treatment of Arthritis**

Mary Ivars, 26 years old, has had rheumatoid arthritis for 10 years. The initial attack, which occurred early in adolescence, has affected primarily the joints of her hands with some effect to the ankles and knees. For the most part, Mary has managed her discomfort and stiffness with aspirin, taking doses that average approximately 3.9 g/day. After a rheumatic flare-up for which she was treated with steroids, Mary finds she is unable to obtain relief from aspirin even at higher doses, which are also causing side-effects.

The physician decides to try indomethacin at 150 mg/day. As the nurse involved in Mary's care, it is your responsibility to help her plan the management of her treatment regimen.

Discussion Questions

1. Mary states her pain and stiffness are greater in the morning and at bedtime. How should her dosage schedule be arranged? When should she take the medication?
2. Mary knows most of the side-effects of aspirin. How are these different from indomethacin? What should she watch for? What should she do if they occur?
3. Can Mary take aspirin with indomethacin? What anti-inflammatory drugs are safe with indomethacin? Which are contraindicated?

REVIEW QUESTIONS

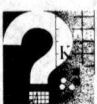

1. Briefly describe the mechanisms involved in the (a) analgesic, (b) antipyretic, and (c) anti-inflammatory action of the salicylates.
2. How does aspirin prevent platelet aggregation? Why is dosage a critical factor in the anti-aggregatory action of aspirin? Why is inhibition of platelet aggregation not seen to a significant extent with other salicylates?
3. What is salicylism?
4. Why do urinary alkalinizers, such as sodium bicarbonate, decrease excretion of aspirin?
5. How can aspirin and acetaminophen be used as effective non-narcotic pain relief? What role do they have as adjuncts to narcotics in pain relief?
6. List the advantages of acetaminophen over aspirin.
7. How does acetaminophen overdosage lead to liver damage? What is the nurse's role in acetaminophen overdose?
8. What are the principal adverse reactions associated with the use of (a) phenylbutazone and (b) indomethacin?
9. Give the major indications for the nonsteroidal anti-inflammatory drugs.
10. List the principal advantages of the nonsteroidal drugs over aspirin as anti-inflammatory agents.
11. Which nonsteroidal anti-inflammatory drugs can be used for (a) acute gouty arthritis and (b) juvenile rheumatoid arthritis?
12. Briefly outline the mechanism of action of gold compounds in relieving the symptoms of rheumatoid arthritis.
13. What is the nurse's role in monitoring the patient who has received gold therapy? What are the signs of toxicity? How should they be treated?
14. What are the major dangers associated with gold therapy for arthritis?
15. In what diseases can penicillamine be used effectively? What are the principal untoward reactions with penicillamine?
16. Outline the sequence of events occuring during an attack of acute gouty arthritis.
17. Describe the actions of colchicine in treating the symptoms of acute gout.

18. How do the uricosuric drugs (*e.g.*, probenecid, sulfinpyrazone) differ from allopurinol in treating hyperuricemia?
19. Why should the nurse stress the importance of forcing fluids to the patient receiving antigout drug therapy? What other dietary information should be provided?

BIBLIOGRAPHY

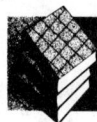

Beaver WT: Analgesic efficacy of dextropropoxyphene and dextropropoxyphene-containing combinations: A review. Human Toxicol 3:1915, 1984

Bloomfield SS: Analgesic management of mild to moderate pain. Rational Drug Therap 19(9):1, 1985

Bunch TW, O'Duffy JD: Disease-modifying drugs for progressive rheumatoid arthritis. Mayo Clin Proc 55:161, 1980

Chan WY: Prostaglandins and nonsteroidal anti-inflammatory drugs in dysmenorrhea. Annu Rev Pharmacol Toxicol 23:131, 1983

Clark WG: Mechanisms of antipyretic action. Gen Pharmacol 10:71, 1979

Clive DM, Stoff JS: Renal syndromes associated with nonsteroidal anti-inflammatory drugs. N Engl J Med 310:563, 1984

Cooper SA: New peripherally-acting oral analgesic agents. Annu Rev Pharmacol Toxicol 23:617, 1983

Hart FD, Huskisson EC: Non-steroidal anti-inflammatory drugs. Current status and rational therapeutic use. Drugs 27:232, 1984

Huskisson EC (ed): Anti-rheumatic Drugs. New York, Praeger Publishers, 1983

Koch-Weser J: Drug therapy: Acetaminophen. N Engl J Med 295:1297, 1979

Larsen GL, Henson PM: Mediators of inflammation. Annu Rev Immunol 1:335, 1983

Lewis JR: Evaluation of new analgesics. JAMA 245:1465, 1980

Lyle WH: Penicillamine. Clin Rheum Dis 5:569, 1979

Markenson JA: Antiarthritic drugs. A comparative overview. Drug Therapy II:45, 1981

Moncada S, Vane JR: Mode of action of aspirin-like drugs. Adv Intern Med 24:1, 1979

Rainsford KD, Velo G (eds): Side Effects of Antiinflammatory/ Analgesic Drugs. New York, Raven Press, 1984

Simkin PA: Management of gout. Ann Intern Med 90:812, 1979

Simon LS, Mills JA: Drug therapy: Nonsteroidal anti-inflammatory drugs (2 parts). N Engl J Med 302:1179, 1237, 1980

Spruck M: Gold therapy for rheumatoid arthritis. Am J Nurs 79:1246, 1979

Symposium for Rational Pharmacotherapy: The non-steroidal antiinflammatory drugs (NSAID's). Drug Intell Clin Pharm 18:34, 1984

Toxicity of nonsteroidal anti-inflammatory drug. Med Lett Drugs Ther 25:15, 1983

Vane J, Botting R: Inflammation and the mechanism of action of anti-inflammatory drugs. FASEB Journal 1(2):89, 1987

Sedative–Hypnotics: Barbiturates

Barbiturates
 Amobarbital, Aprobarbital,
 Butabarbital,
 Mephobarbital,
 Metharbital,
 Methohexital,
 Pentobarbital,
 Phenobarbital,
 Secobarbital,
 Talbutal, Thiamylal,
 Thiopental

24

Many different drugs are capable of causing CNS depression, and one such group of agents is commonly referred to as sedative–hypnotics. These drugs have the ability to calm the anxious patient by inducing a sense of quietude and relaxation, and in sufficient amounts they are able to induce sleep. Compounds possessing these actions are generally classified into two broad categories: (1) barbiturates—derivatives of barbituric acid, and (2) nonbarbiturates—a group of drugs structurally unrelated to barbituric acid but possessing pharmacologic actions in many instances quite similar to those of barbiturates. This chapter and the next chapter will deal with the barbiturate and nonbarbiturate sedative–hypnotics, respectively.

With increasing doses, sedative–hypnotic drugs can evoke a range of central effects, from mild sedation through hypnosis (i.e., sleep) and complete loss of consciousness (i.e., anesthesia) to severe depression of all CNS function (i.e., coma). As illustrated in Figure 24-1, however, the dose–response curves for the individual drugs vary significantly. For example, the dosage increment between the sedative and anesthetic doses or the hypnotic and toxic doses of one drug (e.g., drug X) may be considerably smaller than the corresponding dosage increment for another drug (e.g., drug Z). The steep slope of drug X indicates that marked CNS depression can occur at a dose only slightly higher than the effective hypnotic dose. Drug X, therefore, has a narrow safety margin. Conversely, the more shallow dose–response curves of drugs Y and Z suggest a greater margin of safety because there is a wider separation between the hypnotic dose and the toxic dose than with drug X. The rela-

tive safety of the various sedative–hypnotic drugs will be addressed as they are discussed throughout this and the next chapter.

Small doses of the sedative–hypnotic drugs can produce a state of drowsiness which may calm the anxious patient. Although some barbiturates and nonbarbiturates have been employed on occasion for the relief of simple anxiety states, their use for this particular clinical application has been almost completely supplanted by the benzodiazepine antianxiety drugs discussed in Chapter 28. The principal advantage of benzodiazepines over barbiturates is a significantly greater margin of safety of the former. Referring to Figure 24-1, drug Z might represent a benzodiazepine, while drug X might typify a barbiturate. Benzodiazepines are now also being widely employed for relief of simple insomnia, and benzodiazepine hypnotics (see Chap. 25), because of their greater safety margin, have become the most frequently prescribed hypnotics in clinical medicine. Nevertheless, barbiturates still occupy a deservedly important place in present-day therapeutics, and their pharmacology will now be reviewed.

Barbiturates

Amobarbital, Aprobarbital, Butabarbital, Mephobarbital, Metharbital, Methohexital, Pentobarbital, Phenobarbital, Secobarbital, Talbutal, Thiamylal, Thiopental

The barbiturates, most of which are structural derivatives of malonylurea (barbituric acid), were among the earliest effective groups of hypnotic drugs. The first barbiturate was introduced into medicine around the turn of the twentieth century, and there are now approximately ten barbiturates available for clinical use. They have traditionally been classified, based on their duration of action, as ultrashort-, short-, intermediate-, or long-acting compounds, as indicated in Table 24-1. While convenient, this classification is somewhat misleading, especially in attempting to distinguish between short- and intermediate-acting drugs, whose duration of action can be identical in many instances. The only clear delineation between groups of barbiturates occurs with the ultrashort-acting drugs.

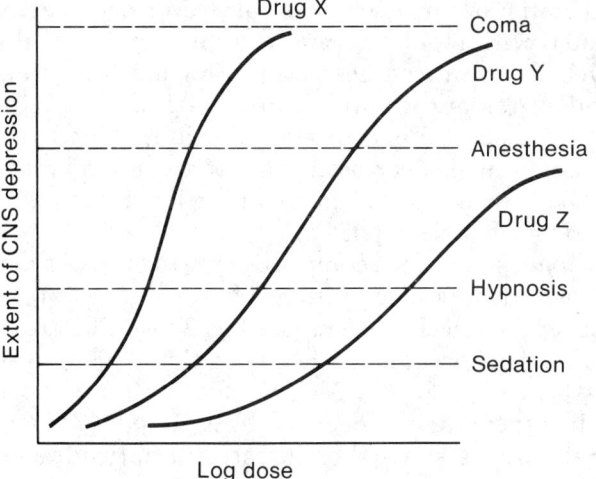

Figure 24-1. Representative dose–response curves for several types of sedative-hypnotic drugs.

Table 24-1
Classification of Barbiturates

Drug	Onset (min)	Peak Effect (h)	Elimination Half-Life (h)
Ultrashort-Acting	0–1	*	3–8
methohexital thiamylal thiopental			
Short-Acting	10–15	3–4	18–42
pentobarbital secobarbital			
Intermediate-Acting	45–60	6–8	15–40†
amobarbital aprobarbital butabarbital talbutal			
Long-Acting	60–90	10–12	60–120‡
mephobarbital metharbital phenobarbital			

* Peak effect for the ultrashort-acting barbiturates is usually within 3–5 min.
† Values for amobarbital, aprobarbital, and talbutal. Half-life for butabarbital is 3–5 days.
‡ Values are for phenobarbital *only*.

These agents, condensation products of thiourea and malonic acid, are highly lipid-soluble drugs that have an almost immediate onset of action following IV administration and a very brief duration of action. Ultrashort-acting barbiturates are primarily used as intravenous general anesthetics and are reviewed in Chapter 21. The remaining barbiturates, while exhibiting some minor differences in pharmacokinetics (see Fate under general discussion) possess essentially identical pharmacologic and toxicologic profiles, and their major actions are reviewed below.

PHARMACOLOGIC ACTIONS

The various barbiturates are capable of exerting a myriad of pharmacologic effects, such as sedation, hypnosis, anesthesia, antiepileptic or anticonvulsant activity, respiratory depression, and enzyme induction. In addition, they can significantly alter behavior and personality, especially with chronic use, and they have a considerable potential for habituation and dependence.

Sedation

In low doses, many of the orally administered barbiturates produce a mild degree of drowsiness, frequently accompanied by decreased motor activity and a sense of emotional well-being. Their sedative action results primarily from a nonspecific CNS depressive effect, probably involving the reticular activating system (RAS) originating in the brain stem. The RAS provides diffuse stimulation to higher brain centers in response to incoming sensory signals (*e.g.*, light, sound, touch). The level of sensory awareness of higher brain centers is in large part governed by the activity of the RAS, and depression of RAS functioning by barbiturates results in reduced alertness and blunted reactions to environmental stimuli. The use of barbiturates as daytime antianxiety agents has largely disappeared, because they are less effective, are potentially more toxic and more habituating than the benzodiazepines, and elicit a significant degree of drowsiness in many instances.

Hypnosis

The principal indication for most barbiturates is the relief of temporary insomnia, and all barbiturates will induce sleep when used in sufficient doses. Normal sleep consists of two major phases, REM (rapid eye movement) and non-REM sleep, which occur cyclically over an interval of approximately 80 minutes to 90 minutes (see Fig. 24-2). REM sleep accounts for about 20% to 25% of total sleep time, and it is during REM sleep that most dreaming occurs. The phase of REM sleep is associated with rapid back and forth movement of the eyeballs, increased heart rate, irregular breathing, and other autonomic manifestations (*e.g.*, increased secretions, penile erection). However, muscle tone is decreased and it is frequently more difficult to awaken a person during REM sleep than during other sleep phases.

Non-REM sleep comprises 75% to 80% of sleep time and progresses through four stages (1–4) as the level of sleep deepens (see Fig. 24-2). The greatest proportion of non-REM sleep time (50%–55%) is spent in stage 2, with only about 20% of sleep being spent in the deeper stages 3 and 4, where brain waves show their greatest amplitude and slowest frequency. The deeper phases of sleep occupy more of the early sleep cycles, whereas lighter sleep and REM sleep are more evident in the later

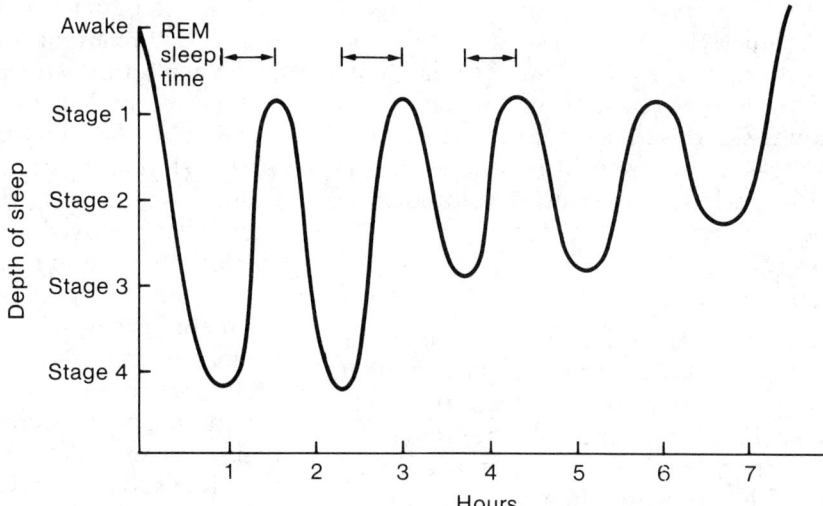

Figure 24-2. *Normal sleep cycles and stages of sleep.*

sleep cycles. Children spend more time than adults in deep sleep, whereas elderly persons may spend relatively little time in deep sleep.

Sleep induced by barbiturates resembles normal stage 2 sleep in many ways: there is reduction in heart rate, blood pressure, respiratory rate, body temperature, basal metabolic rate, CNS activity, and muscle tone. With a barbiturate, the latency of sleep onset is reduced (*i.e.*, sleep occurs more quickly), the duration of stage 2 sleep is increased, slow wave sleep time is reduced, and, perhaps most significantly, REM sleep time is shortened. The first two effects described above are primarily responsible for the clinical efficacy of barbiturates in relieving insomnia. The effect on REM sleep, however, may be responsible for the personality changes (*e.g.*, irritability, anxiety, suspicion) that are sometimes observed in chronic barbiturate users. Individuals deprived of REM sleep by being awakened each time they begin to dream quickly become more irritable, have difficulty concentrating on tasks, show signs of confusion and anxiety, and withdraw from interaction with others. Because dreaming may provide an outlet for resolution of emotional conflicts or for fulfilling wishes or desires, deprivation of normal REM sleep resulting from barbiturate use may very likely lead to behavioral changes.

Of equal importance is the observation that patients deprived of REM sleep by barbiturates will exhibit an *increase* in REM sleep time when the drug is withdrawn. This so-called rebound REM can result in nightmares and poor quality of sleep and may lead to recurrence of insomnia and a desire to resume the drug-taking habit. In order to minimize the problem of rebound REM, the drug

should be discontinued gradually, and the patient should be informed that unpleasant dreams and disturbed sleep may occur during the withdrawal stage but will ameliorate with time. Alternately, the barbiturate hypnotic can be replaced by a drug with less of an effect on REM sleep, such as a benzodiazepine (see Chap. 25).

It has been demonstrated that barbiturates generally lose their hypnotic effectiveness within 2 weeks. Therefore, *persistent* insomnia should not be treated with hypnotic drugs; rather, nondrug intervention should be sought, based on a careful assessment of the underlying cause of the insomnia. Chronic use of barbiturates in the insomniac will invariably result in tolerance, and continued use of the drugs is almost certain to lead to dependence. This aspect of barbiturate usage is considered later in the chapter.

Whenever possible, the pharmacokinetic properties of the chosen barbiturate should be matched to the type of insomnia. Thus, patients who have difficulty initially falling asleep but who seldom experience nocturnal awakening are candidates for short-acting barbiturates (*e.g.*, secobarbital, pentobarbital) which have a rapid onset and a relatively brief duration of action. Patients who complain of frequent nighttime awakenings, on the other hand, may benefit more from one of the intermediate-acting drugs possessing a slightly longer duration of action.

It is quite clear that barbiturates are only indicated for *short-term* relief of insomnia. Whenever possible, a short-acting derivative should be given to minimize the possibility of "hangover" effects such as daytime drowsiness, psychomotor impairment, and depression. Patients should be closely supervised to ensure that the proper dosage is taken and adjunctive measures, such as avoidance of stimulants, proper exercise, and regular hours for retiring, should be encouraged. Under no conditions should the dose be increased when effectiveness wanes. At that point the drug should be gradually discontinued to avoid development of dependence.

Analgesia

In subanesthetic doses, barbiturates do not significantly elevate the pain threshold. In fact, patients experiencing pain who are given a barbiturate without an analgesic frequently become agitated or delirious. Further, barbiturates are much less effective in inducing sleep when administered to persons in pain. In contrast, barbiturates can act synergistically with potent analgesics, often reducing the analgesic requirement by one half. It is therefore imperative that persons in pain be adequately dosed with an effective analgesic in addition to a barbiturate.

Anesthesia

As illustrated in Figure 24-1, sufficiently high doses of barbiturates depress the CNS to such an extent that an anesthetic state is attained. While most barbiturates have the ability to induce anesthesia when used in large doses, the suitability of a compound for induction of anesthesia is dependent on the pharmacokinetic properties that determine onset and duration of action, as well as distribution to the brain. Thus, the highly lipid-soluble, rapid-acting derivatives (methohexital, thiamylal, thiopental) that are administered IV are most suitable as anesthetics and are widely used for induction of the anesthetic state. These drugs quickly equilibrate into the brain, because it receives a substantial blood flow, and induce a rapid loss of consciousness. Due to their high lipid solubility, they are also quickly redistributed to other fatty depots in the body. This accounts for their brief duration of action. Although their CNS concentration falls rapidly, they may persist in other adipose tissue stores for extended periods of time, being more slowly released from these fatty tissue sites.

Anticonvulsant Activity

All barbiturates have the ability to reduce convulsive seizures when given in amounts sufficient to depress the motor cortex. These doses usually result in overall CNS depression, however, and clinically effective anticonvulsant doses of barbiturates

are associated with a significant degree of drowsiness and psychomotor impairment.

When administered IV, barbiturates can control convulsive seizure activity associated with tetanus, eclampsia, meningitis, status epilepticus as well as strychnine or local anesthetic poisoning. In general, short-acting derivatives (see Table 24-1) should be employed, and the drugs should be given by slow IV injection with careful patient monitoring. Phenobarbital sodium has been used IV or IM as an emergency anticonvulsant, but caution is indicated when it is given IV. Due to its weakly lipophilic nature, 15 minutes or more may be required for the drug to reach peak concentration in the brain. Therefore, following the initial dose, no further drug should be given for at least 15 minutes in order to accurately assess the effect of the drug and to minimize the danger of overdosage. Conversely, the onset of action following IV pentobarbital sodium is almost immediate. Although barbiturates are effective in reducing acute convulsive seizures, their use in this regard has diminished with the availability of other equally effective and less hazardous compounds, such as diazepam.

The three long-acting derivatives, metharbital, mephobarbital, and phenobarbital, are indicated for chronic therapy of several forms of epilepsy, especially generalized tonic–clonic (*i.e.*, grand mal) and cortical focal seizures. These drugs appear to have a selective anticonvulsant activity not present with other barbiturates at doses that only minimally affect the reticular activating system; cortical awareness is therefore not compromised significantly, and normal mentation is maintained. The antiepileptic activity of phenobarbital and related drugs is due to several actions, including elevation of the threshold for afterdischarges, and limitation of the spread of seizure activity. (The anticonvulsant action of barbiturates is considered in detail in Chap. 30.)

Respiratory Depression

Barbiturates exert a dose-dependent respiratory depression. The degree of depression noted with hypnotic doses in healthy persons is approximately that seen during normal sleep; however, significant impairment of respiratory function can occur even with therapeutic doses in patients with compromised respiratory function, and large doses can severely depress the medullary respiratory center.

Enzyme Induction

Barbiturates, especially phenobarbital, can accelerate the functioning of hepatic microsomal enzymes, a process known as *enzyme induction*. This may result in increased metabolism, and hence decreased effectiveness, of many other drugs (see under Interactions). Not only is the rate of metabolism of other drugs increased, but also that of endogenous substances such as cholesterol, steroid hormones, bile salts, and vitamin K. In addition, many barbiturates themselves are metabolized by liver microsomal enzymes. Thus, these drugs accelerate their own rate of metabolism, and this is one of the mechanisms responsible for the rapid development of tolerance to barbiturates.

A number of other drugs can also induce hepatic enzymes and can limit the effectiveness of barbiturates. (Enzyme induction as a determinant of drug interactions is discussed in Chap. 5, where a list of enzyme inducers is also found.)

OVERDOSAGE

Toxic doses of barbiturates vary considerably, and can be as low as 2 g. Acute barbiturate overdosage is characterized by marked respiratory depression, progressing to Cheyne–Stokes respiration, lowered body temperature, tachycardia, hypotension, oliguria, and eventually circulatory collapse and coma. Complications, such as pneumonia, arrhythmias, pulmonary edema, and congestive heart failure, can ensue. Treatment is essentially supportive. An adequate airway must be established with respiratory assistance and oxygen if necessary. Fluid replacement should be undertaken if needed and emergency drugs should be available in case respiratory or cardiac failure takes place. Emesis may be induced in a conscious patient; otherwise, gastric lavage with activated charcoal can be employed. Forced diuresis may increase excretion of phenobarbital in patients with normal renal function, especially if the urine is rendered alkaline. Hemodialysis may be used in cases of severe barbiturate intoxication.

DEPENDENCE AND ABUSE

Barbiturates are habit-forming and both psychologic as well as physical dependence can occur, especially with prolonged use of high doses. The rapid development of tolerance to these drugs, due to hepatic enzyme induction as well as neuronal cellular adaptation to the continual presence of the drug, leads to the need for increasing doses to maintain the desired pharmacologic effect. However, tolerance to a fatal dosage does *not* increase more than twofold. Psychologic dependence, or the need to have the drug to maintain an optimal state of well-being, can range from a minimal craving to

intense compulsion. A tendency to continually escalate the dose is common. Ultimately, physical dependence develops, at which point the drug is *necessary* for the maintenance of homeostasis, and even temporary abstinence results in withdrawal symptoms. With the short-acting barbiturates, approximately 1 month of continual use can result in physical dependence.

Withdrawal from barbiturates must be accomplished gradually, because sudden cessation can result in severe symptoms and even death. Minor withdrawal symptoms include anorexia, muscle twitching and weakness, orthostatic hypotension, and tremors. More serious manifestations are confusion, delirium, cardiovascular collapse, and psychotic reactions. Generally, withdrawal symptoms seen with long-acting barbiturates are slower to develop and less severe than with shorter-acting drugs. Major withdrawal symptoms can last up to 5 days, and the intensity gradually diminishes over 1 to 2 weeks. (The problem of barbiturate dependence is considered further in Chap. 85.)

Successful treatment of barbiturate dependence depends largely on providing a means for very *gradual* diminution in barbiturate dosage, which is often accomplished by substituting phenobarbital for the other barbiturate the patient has been taking. Substitution is made at a dosage ratio of 30 mg phenobarbital for every 100 mg to 200 mg of other barbiturate, divided into four daily doses. The total daily dose is then lowered by 30 mg/day as long as no complications arise.

The barbiturates will be considered as a group, with specific information pertaining to individual drugs presented in Table 24-2. The ultrashort-acting barbiturates used for induction of anesthesia are discussed with other general anesthetics in Chapter 21.

MECHANISM AND ACTIONS

The mechanisms by which barbiturates depress CNS function are incompletely understood. The drugs can depress the sensory cortex, reduce motor activity, and, in sufficient amounts, impair respiratory and vasomotor function in the brain stem. Various central sites are sensitive to the action of barbiturates depending on the concentration of drug present. The most sensitive area of the CNS to the action of these drugs is the midbrain reticular formation. Barbiturates appear to elevate the threshold for electrical stimulation of this area, depressing the firing rate of neurons and thus decreasing the diffuse cortical activation normally elicited by the tonic activity of the reticular forma-

(*Text continues on p. 453.*)

Table 24-2
Barbiturates

Drug	Preparations	Usual Dosage Range	Clinical Considerations
Ultrashort-Acting (See Table 21-3.)			
Short-Acting			
pentobarbital (Nembutal)	Capsules—50 mg, 100 mg Elixir—20 mg/5 ml Suppositories—30 mg, 60 mg, 120 mg, 200 mg Injection—50 mg/ml	*Oral:* Sedation—(Adults) 20 mg three to four times/day (Children) 2 mg/kg to 6 mg/kg/day in divided doses Hypnosis— Adults—100 mg *Rectal:* Adults—120 mg to 200 mg Children—30 mg to 120 mg based on age and weight *IM:* Adults—150 mg to 200 mg Children—25 mg to 80 mg *IV:* Adults—100 mg initially: repeat at 50-mg to 100-mg increments to a maximum of 500 mg	Used for preoperative sedation, for minor diagnostic or surgical procedures, and for emergency control of convulsions; hypnotic effects show rapid tolerance; parenteral solution is highly alkaline; avoid extravasation because necrosis can occur; do not give more than 5 ml at one IM site; administer slowly IV, and wait at least 1 min before giving subsequent injections; potent respiratory depressant; can produce bronchospasm, hypotension, and apnea if injection is too rapid; IM injections should be made deep into large muscle mass (*e.g.,* gluteus) (Schedule II)
secobarbital (Seconal)	Capsules—50 mg, 100 mg Tablets—100 mg Injection—50 mg/ml Rectal injection—50 mg/ml	*Oral:* Preoperative sedation—(Adults) 200 mg to 300 mg 1 h–2 h before surgery (Children) 50 mg to 100 mg 1 h–2 h before surgery Hypnosis— Adult—100 mg *Rectal:* Adults—120 mg to 200 mg Children—4 mg/kg to 5 mg/kg based on age and weight *IM:* Hypnosis— Adults—100 mg to 200 mg Children—3 mg/kg to 5 mg/kg *IV (Convulsions)*—5.5 mg/kg at a rate of 50 mg/15 sec; repeat every 3 h to 4 h as needed *IV (Anesthesia)*—50 mg/15 sec by slow IV injection until effect is attained (maximum 250 mg)	Used for insomnia, to provide basal hypnosis for anesthesia, in the emergency control of convulsions, and for dental and minor surgical procedures; tolerance develops quickly (within 2 weeks) to the hypnotic effect; aqueous solutions for injection must be freshly prepared with sterile water for injection. Make sure drug dissolves within 30 min because it is very unstable; injectable form is also available in a more stable aqueous polyethylene glycol vehicle that should be refrigerated; use of this latter vehicle is contraindicated in patients with renal dysfunction or insufficiency because it is very irritating to the kidneys; give slowly IV and monitor patient continually. Inject

(continued)

Table 24-2 (continued)
Barbiturates

Drug	Preparations	Usual Dosage Range	Clinical Considerations
Short-Acting (continued)			
secobarbital (Seconal) (continued)			deep IM to avoid tissue necrosis or nerve damage. (Schedule II) Also available in three fixed combinations with amobarbital (25 mg/25 mg, 50 mg/50 mg, 100 mg/100 mg as Tuinal (also Schedule II)
Intermediate-Acting			
amobarbital (Amytal)	Tablets—30 mg, 100 mg Capsules—65 mg, 200 mg (sodium salt) Powder for injection—250 mg, 500 mg powder with diluent	*Oral:* Sedation—30 mg to 50 mg two to three times/day Hypnosis—100 mg to 200 mg Preoperative—200 mg 1 h to 2 h before surgery Labor—200 mg to 400 mg initially; repeat at 1-h to 3-h intervals to a maximum of 1 g. *IM and IV:* Individualized based on condition, age and weight; usual adult range is 65 mg to 500 mg by deep IM injection or slow IV injection	Used as sedative, hypnotic, preanesthetic medication, anticonvulsant, and for the management of catatonic or manic reactions; prepare solutions with sterile water, and use within 30 min after opening vial; do not use if solution is not clear; inject deeply IM or slow IV (1 ml/min maximum IV rate). Available in fixed combination with secobarbital (see above) as Tuinal (Schedule II)
aprobarbital (Alurate)	Elixir—40 mg/5 ml	Sedation—40 mg three times/day Hypnosis—40 mg to 160 mg depending on severity	Only used orally for daytime sedation or relief of insomnia (Schedule III)
butabarbital (Barbased, Butalan, Buticaps, Butisol, Sarisol)	Tablets—15 mg, 30 mg, 50 mg, 100 mg Capsules—15 mg, 30 mg Elixir—30 mg/5 ml, 33.3 mg/5 ml	Sedation: Adults—15 mg to 30 mg three to four times/day Children—7.5 mg to 30 mg/day Preoperative sedation—50 mg to 100 mg 60 min to 90 min before surgery Hypnosis: Adults—50 mg to 100 mg Children—based on age and weight	Used as mild sedative, for insomnia, and preoperatively; similar to phenobarbital in most respects (Schedule III)
talbutal (Lotusate)	Tablets—120 mg	120 mg 15 min to 30 min before bedtime	Infrequently used for relief of insomnia (Schedule III)
Long-Acting			
mephobarbital (Mebaral)	Tablets—32 mg, 50 mg, 100 mg	Sedation: Adults—32 mg to 100 mg three to four times/day Children—16 mg to 32 mg three to four times/day	Used for daytime sedation in various anxiety states, and primarily as adjunctive treatment of grand mal and petit mal epi-

(continued)

Table 24-2 (continued)
Barbiturates

Drug	Preparations	Usual Dosage Range	Clinical Considerations
Long-Acting (continued)			
mephobarbital (Mebaral) (continued)		Epilepsy: Adults—400 mg to 600 mg/day Children—16 mg to 64 mg three to four times/day depending on age	lepsy (see Chap. 30); similar to phenobarbital in most respects but very weak hypnotic, and produces minimal drowsiness; dosage alterations should be made gradually in epileptic states, to avoid precipitation of convulsions (Schedule IV)
metharbital (Gemonil)	Tablets—100 mg	Epilepsy: Adults—initially 100 mg one to three times/day; increase to optimal level Children—5 mg to 15 mg/kg/day based on age and weight	Used in various forms of epilepsy (grand mal and petit mal, myclonic, and mixed seizures), either alone or more frequently combined with other drugs; not as effective as phenobarbital and produces more sedation (see Chap. 30) (Schedule III)
phenobarbital (various manufacturers)	Tablets—8 mg, 16 mg, 32 mg, 65 mg, 100 mg Capsules—16 mg Elixir—15 mg/ml, 20 mg/5 ml Injection—30 mg/ml, 60 mg/ml, 65 mg/ml, 130 mg/ml Powder for injection—120 mg/vial	*Oral:* Sedation— (Adults) 16 mg to 32 mg two to four times/day (Children) 1 mg to 3 mg/kg/day Hypnosis— (Adults) 100 mg to 320 mg Epilepsy— (Adults) 100 mg to 300 mg/day (Children) 3 mg to 5 mg/kg/day *IV:* Convulsions— (Adults) 300 mg to 800 mg initially, then 120 mg to 240 mg every 20 min, as needed (maximum 2 g/24 h) (Children) 20 mg/kg initially, then 6 mg/kg every 20 min as needed *IM:* Preoperative and postoperative— (Adults) 32 mg to 200 mg (Children) 8 mg to 100 mg	Widely used for sedation and in grand mal and focal seizures, either alone or combined with other antiepileptic drugs; used IV in acute convulsive states (see Chap. 30); solutions should be freshly prepared with sterile water for injection, and used within 30 min after preparation; do not use if solution is not clear after 5 min of mixing; some injectable forms contain alcohol and propylene glycol and are more stable than aqueous solutions; drug has a long half-life (2 days–5 days), and too frequent dosing can cause cumulation toxicity (Schedule IV)

tion by way of the reticular activating system. Neuronal activity in other areas such as the limbic system and hypothalamus is also reduced by barbiturate drugs. Biochemical actions responsible for the reduced neuronal activity may include a synaptic blocking action and decreased sensitivity of postsynaptic receptor sites. Facilitation of GABA (gamma-aminobutyric acid) activity, a substance functioning as an inhibitory transmitter, may likewise contribute to the reduced synaptic transmission, although the precise nature of this barbiturate–GABA interaction remains to be established. (The role of GABA in the actions of the benzodiazepine antianxiety drugs is more clearly delineated, and is discussed in Chap. 28.)

USES

1. Daytime sedative for the relief of anxiety, tension, and nervousness (infrequent use, generally replaced by benzodiazepines—see Chap. 28)
2. Short-term treatment of insomnia (2 weeks maximum)
3. Control of acute convulsive states (IV, IM)
4. Treatment of various forms of epilepsy (see Chap. 30)
5. Pre- and postoperative sedation
6. Induction anesthesia and brief, minor surgical procedures (ultrashort- and short-acting drugs)
7. Aid in psychoanalysis (narcoanalysis and narcotherapy)
8. Management of catatonic and manic reactions (IV, IM)

ADMINISTRATION AND DOSAGE

With the exception of the ultrashort-acting drugs used for induction anesthesia, barbiturates are generally administered orally unless this route is not feasible (*e.g.*, unconsciousness, vomiting) or impractical (*e.g.*, acute convulsive states). Dosage should be reduced in elderly or debilitated patients (because they may be more sensitive to the effects of barbiturates) and in patients with renal or hepatic damage. Dosing information for each individual barbiturate drug is given in Table 24-2.

FATE

Barbiturates are absorbed to varying degrees from the GI tract, rectum, and from IM injection sites depending on a number of factors, such as pH, presence of food, and the chemical form of the drug (acid or sodium salt). The presence of food decreases absorption *rate* but does not affect the overall extent of absorption. Soluble sodium salts are absorbed more rapidly than intact acid molecules, especially on an empty stomach, due to their more rapid dissolution rate. The onset of action, time to peak effect, and elimination half-life of the individual drugs are given in Table 24-1. Barbiturates are widely distributed in the body and attain high concentrations in the brain, liver, and kidneys, the more lipid-soluble derivatives (*e.g.*, thiopental, methohexital, thiamylal) penetrating body tissues more rapidly than the less lipid-soluble drugs. Plasma protein binding is variable, but in general, is greatest for the highly lipid-soluble agents. Onset of activity is dependent primarily on lipid solubility. For example, phenobarbital has low lipid solubility and a slow onset of action, whereas secobarbital is more lipid-soluble and hence more rapid acting. However, lipid-soluble drugs are quickly redistributed from active CNS sites to fatty tissue stores, from where the drug may be slowly released. Because the pharmacologic effects often disappear before the drug is totally eliminated from the body, too frequent dosing can result in cumulation toxicity. Most drugs are metabolized in the liver and excreted in the urine, principally as metabolites, except for aprobarbital and phenobarbital, of which up to 50 percent of a dose is excreted unchanged in the urine.

SIDE-EFFECTS/ADVERSE REACTIONS

Drowsiness is the most common side-effect and can occur at rather small doses in many patients. Impaired motor coordination and altered judgment are also seen frequently, especially at elevated dosage levels. "Hangover" effects are rather common with the use of the longer-acting derivatives, and the ability to safely operate machinery may be compromised. Chronic use of barbiturates, especially in large amounts, can lead to serious complications, and dependence is a common problem with steady use of these drugs. A number of other adverse reactions have occurred in persons taking barbiturates and are listed below according to their likelihood of occurring following either oral or parenteral use of the drugs.

Oral—Skin rash, vertigo, lethargy, agitation, confusion, ataxia, residual sedation, dizziness, nausea, diarrhea, bradycardia, hypotension, hypoventilation, hypersensitivity reactions (fever, urticaria, hives, serum sickness), muscle and joint pain, and rarely, exfoliative dermatitis, Stevens–Johnson syndrome, and blood dyscrasias. Paradoxical excitation is occasionally seen, especially in children and older people. Prolonged use may lead to tolerance, habituation, and addiction.

IV—See under Oral; in addition, respiratory depression, coughing, hiccups, laryngospasm, bronchospasm, apnea, syncope, pain at injection site, thrombophlebitis, and tissue necrosis.

Overdose can result in respiratory depression, hypothermia, depressed reflexes, anuria, rapid pulse, pulmonary edema, anoxia, cyanotic skin, stupor, and coma.

CONTRAINDICATIONS AND PRECAUTIONS

Barbiturates are contraindicated in patients with a history of manifest or latent porphyria or marked impairment of liver function. They are also contraindicated in the presence of severe respiratory disease accompanied by dyspnea, airway obstruction, or cor pulmonale, and large doses should not be given to patients with nephritis. Secobarbital sodium is also contraindicated in the presence of acute or chronic pain (agitation and hyperalgesia can occur) and during obstetric delivery.

There are a number of conditions that demand *cautious use* of barbiturates: fever, diabetes, hyperthyroidism, renal or cardiac impairment, severe anemia, and alcoholism. In addition, caution must be exercised when giving barbiturates to pregnant women (danger of fetal damage or bleeding), nursing mothers, elderly or debilitated persons, and children. Pediatric and geriatric patients may experience irritability, excitability, restlessness, and confusion when receiving a barbiturate.

IV administration of a barbiturate must be done slowly to prevent development of hypotension, laryngospasm, and extreme respiratory depression. Extravasation must also be avoided during IV administration, because parenteral solutions are highly alkaline and tissue necrosis is likely to occur.

INTERACTIONS

(*Note:* Most reports of interactions occurring with barbiturates involve *phenobarbital.*)

1. Barbiturates may potentiate the CNS and respiratory-depressant effects of alcohol, narcotic analgesics, other sedative–hypnotics, phenothiazine and other antipsychotic drugs, antihistamines, anesthetics, antidepressants, antianxiety agents, centrally acting muscle relaxants, and reserpine.
2. Barbiturates can increase the activity of liver metabolic enzymes and therefore may decrease the effects of drugs metabolized by those enzymes, such as oral anticoagulants, corticosteroids, diphenhydramine, digitalis glycosides, quinidine, methyldopa, lidocaine, griseofulvin, estrogens, progestins, androgens, pyrazolones, tricyclic antidepressants, and tetracyclines.
3. The effects of barbiturates may be increased by drugs that can impair their metabolism, such as MAO inhibitors, chloramphenicol, and valproic acid, as well as by sulfonamides, acidifying agents, anticholinesterase drugs, and disulfiram.
4. Barbiturates may inhibit GI absorption of griseofulvin.
5. Concurrent administration of barbiturates and furosemide can produce or aggravate orthostatic hypotension.
6. The efficacy of oral contraceptives may be reduced by prolonged use of barbiturates, especially phenobarbital.

■ *Nursing Process: Initiating Treatment with Barbiturates*

□ ASSESSMENT

□ *Subjective Data*

A brief sleep history from any patient about to be treated with hypnotic–sedatives is always helpful, but particularly so with barbiturates. The nurse can ask how many hours the person sleeps, when insomnia occurs, what measures the person takes to get to sleep or go back to sleep, and what he perceives to be a restful sleep. Sometimes a person's perception of restful sleep is based on what he considers the norm for other people or on his sleep pattern at a younger age. Discussions about why he is seeking sleeping medication may indicate faulty perceptions and once identified may reduce or eliminate the need for drug therapy.

A general drug history must also be obtained. Use of antihistamines, tranquilizers, alcohol, or street drugs can result in synergistic and dangerous interactions with barbiturates.

Medical history should focus on presence of renal, respiratory, or cardiovascular disease, as well as diabetes, hyperthyroidism, or blood disorders, especially porphyria and anemia.

□ *Objective Data*

Physical assessment of cardiovascular and respiratory systems is essential. Neurologic examination should focus on memory and mental functioning. Laboratory evaluation should rule out pregnancy as well as renal or hepatic dysfunction. A complete blood count should be drawn to ascertain hemoglobin level and adequacy of functions.

□ NURSING DIAGNOSES
Actual nursing diagnoses for patients receiving barbiturate sedative–hypnotics may include:
> Knowledge deficit related to action, administration, and side-effects of the drug
> Sleep-pattern disturbance related to the drug's effect on REM sleep

Potential nursing diagnoses are based primarily on the drug's common side-effects and may include:
> Potential for injury related to impaired motor coordination and altered judgment which may occur
> Alteration in thought processes related to changes in REM sleep and drowsiness may also occur if dependence develops

Other potential nursing diagnoses if habituation occurs may include:
> Anxiety
> Impaired individual coping
> Sensory–perceptual alterations

□ PLAN
The nursing care goals for the patient beginning treatment with barbiturates are:
1. To provide short-term sleep assistance through drug therapy with minimal side-effects
2. To provide an environment which enhances sleep
3. To help the patient develop nondrug sleep-inducing methods to facilitate relaxation

□ INTERVENTION
A study by Perry and Wu (1984) indicates that the prescription patterns of physicians ordering sleeping medications and the administration patterns of nurses giving these p.r.n. medications may need close evaluation. In this study, there was little difference reported in satisfaction with sleep between patients who had received hypnotics and those who had not. In addition, neither physicians nor nurses adequately recorded the rationale for giving a sleeping medication to a patient or whether the desired therapeutic response was achieved. The implication for nursing is the need for a serious review of the administration of hypnotics to promote sleep in institutions and to look at other measures which may cause sleep disturbance, such as nightly procedures, rounds, and methods of delivering care to patients while others are asleep.

Administration of sleeping medications, whether at home or in an institution, will always be enhanced by nondrug methods to promote sleep. These methods may include warm baths, back rubs, quiet atmosphere with few environmental disturbances, elimination of caffeine-containing beverages at night, daily exercise, avoidance of naps, establishing a regular time for retiring and awakening, use of a mild analgesic for aches and pains more prevalent in the evening, and the use of yoga, meditation, or muscle-relaxing strategies to relax the body.

Time of administration may also be important, particularly in elderly persons who are prone to the "hangover" effect of barbiturates in the morning. It may be appropriate with this age group to give the medication earlier than the traditional 10 PM or 11 PM "HS dose" frequently assigned in institutions to allow extra time for the medication to achieve its effect and for subsequent slowing of metabolism. The elderly person may then be less likely to be awake at a time when he prefers to be asleep and more likely to be alert during the day.

Whenever the medication is given, safety concerns must be met. For the patient in the hospital, instructions should be given to remain in bed and the side rails put up. People at home should be encouraged not to get up in the dark because the drug can make them drowsy and dizzy even when they awaken. In addition, those on home therapy should keep the medication in a medicine cabinet or cupboard away from the bedside to avoid overdosing. Drowsiness may cause a person to forget he took a dose and mistakenly repeat it if the medication is close at hand.

The nurse and patient also need to recognize that barbiturates are not effective in achieving pain relief. In fact, the drugs can cause paradoxical excitation in the patient in pain. Therefore, pain medication, if needed, should be spaced so that relief and relaxation are achieved before the barbiturate is administered. At the same time, the nurse must be aware that some analgesics, particularly narcotics, are potentiated by barbiturates, so careful dosing is necessary to avoid toxic, additive effects.

□ EVALUATION
In general, barbiturate sedative–hypnotics are not the long-term treatment of choice for the patient with insomnia. They are best used for short periods of time such as the night before surgery or during the acute phase of recovery from a major illness.

The nurse needs to evaluate the development of tolerance in any patient receiving these medications for more than 3 weeks and to report symptoms to the physician so a strategy for withdrawal can be developed.

■ Nursing Process: Patients Withdrawing from Barbiturates

□ ASSESSMENT
A plan for systematic withdrawal from barbiturates is outlined above under Dependence and Abuse. Systematic withdrawal is always indicated if the nurse begins to observe the patient complaining that the drug, in the dose prescribed, no longer helps, if the patient frequently asks for more than one dose per night, or if signs of withdrawal such as tremulousness appear during the day. In addition, if the patient begins to develop side-effects from the drug, particularly hematologic manifestations such as sore throat, fever, superficial bleeding, bruising, or jaundice, the drug should be gradually withdrawn.

□ NURSING DIAGNOSES
Actual nursing diagnoses for the patient withdrawing from a barbiturate sedative–hypnotic will include:
Sleep-pattern disturbance
Anxiety
Ineffective individual coping—may occur at times
Noncompliance with the withdrawal regimen if the patient can obtain the drug
Alteration in thought processes related to hallucinations and nightmares which frequently occur during withdrawal
Potential nursing diagnoses if withdrawal is sudden may include:
Alteration in cardiac output: decreased
Impaired gas exchange
Potential for violence: directed at self or others if a psychotic reaction occurs

□ PLAN
The nursing care goals for the patient withdrawing from barbiturates are:
1. To develop and implement a treatment plan with the patient to provide alternate methods of sleep induction while the barbiturates are being withdrawn
2. To provide support to the patient and manage manipulative behavior while withdrawal symptoms are occurring

3. To attempt to avoid making the drug available to the patient during withdrawal

□ INTERVENTION
The patient withdrawing from barbiturates needs tremendous emotional support and encouragement during the 1 to 2 weeks in which symptoms will occur. Intervention should include careful administration of the prescribed substituted drugs to facilitate withdrawal. All nurses administering the medications should be aware of the treatment plan so they do not use the drugs as a bargaining tool with the patient or forget to give them at the times prescribed. The patient should also be aware of what the treatment plan is so he knows what to expect and when to expect it. Strategies need to be developed to handle manipulation by the patient who will try to bargain for the withdrawn medication. Careful consideration should be made of nighttime strategies to decrease the night nurse's frustration with the patient who has difficulty sleeping. An empathetic attitude and use of some of the sleep-promoting strategies mentioned earlier are much more beneficial than ignoring the complaints of the patient who cannot sleep during withdrawal. In addition, the night nurse or family member must remember that this is the most difficult time for the patient partly because it is the time of day associated with the drug-taking behavior and partly because of the nightmares and hallucinations which frequently accompany withdrawal.

The nurse and family should also be aware that relapses are frequent if the patient can obtain the drug. Efforts should be made to avoid making the drug available—in the hospital by refusing to seek another order, in the home by discarding the barbiturate before the withdrawal regimen begins.

□ EVALUATION
As the physical need for the barbiturate diminishes, alternate sleep-inducing strategies should be evaluated including the use of nonbarbiturate drugs, if indicated. The goal is to return the patient to nondrug-induced sleep although this may take months to accomplish. If self-dosing from multiple prescriptions resulted in the withdrawal, the nurse can review with the patient and family the prescription patterns of the care givers, and steps can be taken to avoid future duplication. While this may be beneficial, the nurse and family must recognize that the patient who relapses into abuse of barbiturates will use the method of seeking prescriptions from multiple care givers to obtain the drug. (See Chap. 85 for further discussion.)

CASE STUDY

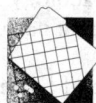

Donna O'Neill, a 30-year-old woman, is scheduled for outpatient oral surgery for removal of two wisdom teeth. Donna is to be admitted at 6 AM to the Day Stay Center of her local hospital. When meeting with her oral surgeon preoperatively, she tells him she is extremely afraid of dentists and is terrified of the surgery. She has already had several restless nights, nightmares, and was unable to sleep the last two nights. The surgeon prescribes Seconal 50 mg PO for the next two nights until the day of surgery.

Discussion Questions

1. What should Donna be told about this drug and home medication?
2. Should Donna drive herself to the hospital the day of surgery after taking Seconal the night before?
3. What other strategies might the nurse suggest to Donna to enhance sleep prior to the anxiety-producing event of surgery?

REVIEW QUESTIONS

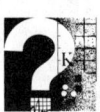

1. What are the principal advantages of benzodiazepines over barbiturates as sedatives?
2. How are the barbiturate drugs usually classified?
3. Which group of barbiturates is used as induction anesthetics? Which group is used as antiepileptics?
4. List the major pharmacologic actions of the barbiturates.
5. Briefly describe the sites and mechanisms of the CNS-depressant action of the barbiturates.
6. How does barbiturate-induced sleep differ from normal sleep? What are the clinical and behavioral implications of these differences?
7. Give the principal symptoms of barbiturate overdosage.
8. What is meant by "enzyme induction"? How is this phenomenon related to development of tolerance to barbiturates?
9. How may dependence on barbiturates be treated? What nursing interventions should be included?
10. What are the major contraindications to barbiturate usage?
11. What are the major components of a sleep history? How will such information assist the care giver administering sleep medication?
12. How can the nurse reduce the "hangover" effect of barbiturates, particularly in elderly persons?
13. What are the nondrug strategies the nurse can try or teach the patient to try to induce sleep?
14. What instructions would you give to the patient and family when barbiturates are prescribed for home use?

BIBLIOGRAPHY

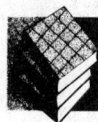

Dittmar S, Dulski T: Early evening administration of sleep medication to the hospitalized aged. Nursing Research 26:200, 1977
Harris E: Sedative-hypnotic drugs. Am J Nurs 81:1329, 1981
Hartmann E: Drugs for insomnia. Rational Drug Therapy 11:1, 1977
Ho IK, Harris RA: Mechanism of action of barbiturates. Annu Rev Pharmacol Toxicol 21:83, 1981

Kales A, Soldatos DR, Bixler EO, Kales JD: Rebound insomnia and
    rebound anxiety: A review. Pharmacology 26:121, 1983
Koch-Weser J, Greenblatt DJ: The archaic barbiturate hypnotics. N
    Engl J Med 291:790, 1974
Perry SW, Wu A: Rationale for the use of hypnotic agents in a general
    hospital. Ann Intern Med 100:441, 1984
Richter JA, Holman JR: Barbiturates: Their *in-vivo* effects and
    potential biochemical mechanisms. Prog Neurobiol 18:275, 1982
Rickels K: Clinical trials of hypnotics. J Clin Psychopharmacol 3:133,
    1983
Solomon F, White CC, Parron DL, Mendelson WB: Sleeping pills,
    insomnia and medical practice. N Engl J Med 300:803, 1979
Todd B: Drugs and the elderly: Why are some drugs withdrawn
    slowly? Geriatric Nursing 4:393, 1983
Todd B: Drugs and the elderly: Precautions with hypnotics. Geriatric
    Nursing 3:343, 1982

Sedative–Hypnotics: Nonbarbiturates

Acetylcarbromal

Benzodiazepine Hypnotics
Flurazepam, Temazepam,
Triazolam
Chloral Hydrate

Ethchlorvynol
Ethinamate
Glutethimide
Methyprylon
Paraldehyde
Propriomazine

25

A diverse group of chemicals share the ability to depress the functioning of the CNS and are commonly referred to as sedatives or hypnotics. One group of these drugs is the barbiturates, reviewed in Chapter 24. This chapter will consider a number of structurally dissimilar drugs that possess many of the properties of the barbiturates and are used for many of the same indications.

The terminology used to describe these other sedative–hypnotic drugs is quite vague. Here, they will be termed *nonbarbiturate sedative–hypnotics*, reflecting their chemical differences from the barbiturates more so than their pharmacologic differences. Many of these drugs were developed in an attempt to dissociate the undesirable properties of the barbiturates (e.g., respiratory depression, enzyme induction, habituation) from their desirable qualities (e.g., relief of insomnia, anticonvulsive activity). These attempts have been largely unsuccessful and most clinically available nonbarbiturate sedative–hypnotics share many common properties with barbiturates. However, one group, the benzodiazepine hypnotics, exhibit several advantages over barbiturates, such as absence of enzyme induction, little effect on REM sleep, and lowered abuse potential, and have become the most widely prescribed hypnotics in clinical medicine.

The nonbarbiturate sedative–hypnotics also include several compounds of simple chemical structure, such as chloral hydrate, ethchlorvynol, and paraldehyde. These agents are somewhat less effective than other sedative–hypnotics, and they are infrequently used today.

Confusion occasionally arises as to whether certain other drugs employed primarily for relief of anxiety should be grouped with nonbarbiturate sedative–hypnotics. Specifically, the benzodiazepine antianxiety agents, of which the prototype is diazepam (Valium), are widely used for relief of simple anxiety states. They are generally not classified with other sedative–hypnotic drugs because of their more favorable pharmacologic profile and their greater safety margin. Table 25-1 compares some important properties of nonbarbiturate sedative–hypnotics and benzodiazepine antianxiety agents. While useful as a general guide, it is important to recognize, however, that the information in Table 25-1 is based on the actions of these agents at recommended doses for short periods of time (i.e., 1–2 weeks). The differences cited in Table 25-1 become less distinct when the antianxiety drugs are used in large doses or for prolonged periods of time. Moreover, certain nonbarbiturate sedative–hypnotics, such as chloral hydrate and paraldehyde, are less sedating and less addicting than other agents like glutethimide or methyprylon and thus do not evidence as sharp a contrast with the benzodiazepine antianxiety drugs.

As previously noted, classification of nonbarbiturate sedative–hypnotics is difficult, owing to the variety of chemical structures possessed by these agents. However, they all share a common action—the ability to depress the CNS in a dose-related fashion. The mechanism of this action, however, is not completely understood in all cases. Several older drugs (e.g., acetylcarbromal, chloral hydrate, paraldehyde), once frequently used, have been rendered essentially obsolete by development

Table 25-1
Comparison Between Nonbarbiturate Sedative–Hypnotics and Benzodiazepine Antianxiety Drugs

	Nonbarbiturate Sedative–Hypnotics	Benzodiazepine Antianxiety Agents
Major indications	Insomnia	Stress, tension, psychoneuroses
Sedative/Hypnotic ratio	Low	High
Drowsiness, psychomotor impairment, and confusion	Moderate to severe	Mild
Dependence liability	High	Low to high (depending on dose, pattern of use, and emotional state of client)
Central skeletal muscle-relaxing effect	No	Yes

of more effective and somewhat safer agents, and these older drugs are addressed only briefly in this chapter. A detailed account, however, is given of those drugs currently used on a frequent basis.

In addition to the nonbarbiturate sedative–hypnotics to be reviewed in the chapter, several antihistamines may be considered as sedative–hypnotics because they are found in various over-the-counter sleep aids, where they provide a degree of drowsiness to assist the user in falling asleep. The recommended doses are 25 mg to 50 mg diphenhydramine (*e.g.,* Compoz, Nytol, Sleep-Eze, Sominex, Twilite), and 25 mg doxylamine (*e.g.,* Unisom). Maximum recommended dosages are 100 mg/24 h. Use of antihistamine-containing sleep aids is recommended for short periods of time only (7 days–10 days) as psychological dependence can occur with continuous usage. These preparations should not be given to children, pregnant women, or patients with asthma, prostate enlargement, or glaucoma.

Owing to the heterogeneity among the various nonbarbiturate sedative–hypnotics with regard to their potency, pharmacologic actions, incidence and severity of adverse effects, and dependence liability, the various drugs will be considered individually, with the exception of the benzodiazepine hypnotics, which will be reviewed together.

Acetylcarbromal

(Paxarel)

Acetylcarbromal is a short-acting, orally effective sedative–hypnotic which is infrequently used for the relief of anxiety, insomnia, premenstrual tension, and other manifestations of emotional stress. The drug acts by releasing free bromide, an ion with a CNS-depressant action, and, therefore, use of excessive amounts can lead to bromide intoxication. Large doses may cause excessive drowsiness, and other CNS depressants, including alcohol, should be avoided during acetylcarbromal therapy. Chronic administration may be habit-forming, and dizziness, irritability, motor incoordination, skin rash, GI disturbances, and impaired thoughts and memory may occur due to increased bromide levels. Overdosage may be treated by gastric lavage and forced diuresis. Chloride loading (at least 6 g/day sodium chloride) may enhance bromide excretion, but is contraindicated in patients with cardiovascular disease. The adult dosage of acetylcarbromal is 250 mg two to three times a day. The drug should be avoided in children.

Benzodiazepine Hypnotics

Flurazepam

(Dalmane)

Temazepam

(Restoril)

Triazolam

(Halcion)

The majority of benzodiazepines in clinical practice are used for the relief of anxiety states and are reviewed in detail in Chapter 28. Several benzodiazepine drugs, by virtue of their rapid absorption and clinical profile of action, are employed primarily for the short-term management of insomnia and are termed the benzodiazepine hypnotics. While all of the benzodiazepine drugs can theoretically relieve simple insomnia, the three drugs listed above are generally used solely for this indication and are seldom employed as daytime sedatives. While the following discussion pertains specifically to the benzodiazepine hypnotics, refer to Chapter 28 for an expanded review of benzodiazepine pharmacology in general.

The benzodiazepine hypnotics and the barbiturates are probably equally effective for the short-term treatment of insomnia. In contrast to the barbiturates as well as many other nonbarbiturate sedative–hypnotics, however, the benzodiazepine hypnotics display a greater safety margin (*i.e.,* shallower dose–response curve—see Fig. 3-2). Other potential advantages of the benzodiazepines over the barbiturates and most other nonbarbiturate hypnotics are their lack of significant effects on reducing REM sleep time (although they can suppress stages 3 and 4 of sleep) and their absence of enzyme-inducing effects. Thus, the benzodiazepines are the preferred hypnotics in most patients. Often, however, there is a false sense of security with benzodiazepine hypnotics, and although they are less likely than barbiturates to lead to physical dependence, the incidence of psychologic dependence on benzodiazepines is growing as their usage increases. An additional complication observed with those benzodiazepines, such as flurazepam, that form psychoactive metabolites is the accumulation of these long-lived active metabolites in the body and the consequent danger of "hangover" effects such as impaired visual/motor coordination, lethargy, and daytime drowsiness. Ingestion of alcohol or use of other CNS depressants during the day can greatly potentiate these "hangover" effects, occasionally to the point of serious impairment of psychomotor performance. An increased likelihood of adverse effects with benzodiazepine hypnotics is also seen in older people and in the presence of impaired renal or hepatic function.

As suggested above, the benzodiazepine hypnotic drugs differ with respect to their pharmacokinetic properties and the more important of the differences are presented in Table 25-2. Flurazepam exhibits the fastest onset of action, but is converted to N-desalkyl-flurazepam, an active metabolite with a long half-life. Temazepam and triazolam do not have quite as rapid an onset of action, but are not metabolized to active intermediates, hence the danger of cumulation toxicity is reduced. However, the extremely short duration of action of triazolam can result in nocturnal awakenings.

Following withdrawal of the drug after a period of continuous use, rebound insomnia can occur. In general, this insomnia occurs more frequently and is somewhat more intense with the shorter-acting benzodiazepines; conversely, rebound insomnia may be delayed 1 to 2 weeks following cessation of flurazepam therapy, because the active metabolite is slow to be eliminated.

MECHANISM AND ACTIONS
(Refer to the discussion of benzodiazepines in Chap. 28 for a more detailed description of the mechanism of action of these drugs.)

The primary mechanism of action of benzodiazepines is facilitation of the action of the inhibitory neurotransmitter gamma-aminobutyric acid (GABA). The precise means by which these drugs potentiate the action of GABA is not entirely known, but may involve increased membrane permeability to chloride, leading to membrane hyperpolarization. Also, the binding of GABA to its receptors may be enhanced by the ability of benzodiazepines to antagonize a protein that can inhibit the GABA–receptor interaction. The principal loci of action in the CNS appear to be the limbic system, thalamus, and midbrain reticular formation; unlike the barbiturates, these drugs do not exert a significant effect on higher cortical areas.

Clinical effects include hypnosis (decreased sleep latency and increased total sleep time), skeletal muscle relaxation, and an anticonvulsive action. REM sleep time is largely unaltered, and there is no microsomal enzyme induction. Tolerance can occur and although the degree of dependence is probably less than with barbiturates, the increasing use of benzodiazepine hypnotics has resulted in a surge in reported cases of benzodiazepine dependence. Severe overdosage is unlikely to be fatal unless ingestion of other depressant drugs has also occurred.

USES
1. Short-term (i.e., maximum 4 weeks) treatment of insomnia

ADMINISTRATION AND DOSAGE
See Table 25-3.

FATE
The oral absorption of all three drugs is good; sleep usually occurs within 15 minutes to 45 minutes. Peak plasma levels are attained at 30 minutes to 60 minutes with flurazepam, 2 hours to 3 hours with temazepam, and 1 hour to 1.5 hours with triazolam. Flurazepam is converted to an active metabolite with a half-life of 50 hours to 100 hours; thus, it has the longest duration of action and can elicit a prolonged "hangover" effect. Temazepam exhibits a plasma half-life of 8 hours to 12 hours and is metabolized to inactive compounds in the liver. Triazolam is also converted to inactive metabolites and has a plasma half-life of only 2 hours to 4

Table 25-2
Characteristics of Benzodiazepine Hypnotics

Drug	Onset of Sleep (min)	Elimination Half-Life (h)	Protein Binding (%)	Active Metabolites
flurazepam	15–20	50–100*	97	Yes
temazepam	30–45	8–12	98	No
triazolam	15–30	2–4	90	No

* Reflects half-life of active metabolite.

Table 25-3
Benzodiazepine Hypnotics

Drug	Preparations	Usual Dosage Range	Clinical Considerations
flurazepam (Dalmane, Durepam)	Capsules—15 mg, 30 mg	15 mg to 30 mg at bedtime (15 mg in elderly or debilitated patients)	Longest-acting benzodiazepine hypnotic; major metabolite is N-desalkylflurazepam, which is an active hypnotic with prolonged half-life (50 h–100 h); daytime carry-over effects can include decreased alertness, impaired coordination, confusion, and subtle personality changes; maximum hypnotic effectiveness may not be achieved for several nights; residual effects can persist for days following discontinuation of therapy; not recommended in children under age 15; do not discontinue drug abruptly after prolonged usage
temazepam (Razepam, Restoril)	Capsules—15 mg, 30 mg	15 mg to 30 mg at bedtime (15 mg in elderly or debilitated patients)	Intermediate-acting benzodiazepine (plasma half-life of 8 h–16 h); no accumulation of metabolites; hangover effects are minimal and early morning wakening is reduced; use in children under age 18 is not recommended; transient sleep disturbances can occur for several nights following discontinuation of therapy
triazolam (Halcion)	Tablets—0.125 mg, 0.25 mg, 0.5 mg	0.25 mg to 0.5 mg at bedtime (0.125 mg–0.25 mg in elderly or debilitated patients)	Short-acting hypnotic (plasma half-life is 2–4 h); metabolites are inactive; elicits few daytime hangover effects, but may lead to increased wakefulness during the last third of the night; not recommended for children under age 18

hours; therefore, it is very short-acting and early morning awakening has occurred. All three drugs are excreted largely in the urine.

SIDE-EFFECTS/ADVERSE REACTIONS
Hypnotic doses of the benzodiazepines frequently cause daytime drowsiness, especially when taken over a period of time. Other commonly observed side-effects with these drugs are lightheadedness, headache, dizziness, ataxia, and slight motor incoordination. Drugs with long half-lives or active metabolites tend to produce daytime "hangover" upon repeated administration, and this may interfere with performance of normal motor skills, such as driving. Concomitant use of alcohol creates a serious potential interaction that can result in profound CNS depression, with attendant psychomotor impairment.

Serious adverse reactions are relatively rare with occasional use of any of the benzodiazepine hypnotics. Among the adverse effects which have been reported are disorientation, confusion, slurred speech, weakness, memory impairment, and depression. Occasionally, paradoxical reactions are observed, such as nervousness, irritability, tachycardia, sweating, and nightmares. Gastrointestinal reactions are infrequent, but may include nausea, heartburn, vomiting, or diarrhea.

Overdosage generally results in somnolence, confusion, impaired coordination, and possibly coma. Treatment is supportive, and fatalities are rare if the benzodiazepine was the sole agent ingested.

As alluded to previously, the potential for habituation and abuse with the benzodiazepine hypnotics is probably greatly underestimated, and these drugs can easily become psychologically addicting. Withdrawal symptoms similar to those noted with barbiturates and alcohol have occurred following abrupt discontinuance of the drug after daily administration for as little as 3 to 4 weeks, but are seen much more frequently after extended periods of administration. Withdrawal symptoms range from a mild dysphoria to muscle cramping, sweating, tremors, vomiting, and convulsions.

CONTRAINDICATIONS AND PRECAUTIONS

Benzodiazepines are contraindicated in pregnant women because fetal damage has been reported with use of the drugs in early pregnancy, and neonatal CNS depression has occurred when the drugs were taken during the last weeks of pregnancy. *Cautious use* of these drugs is warranted in patients with renal or hepatic disease, depression, or a history of drug habituation. In addition, the drugs should be used cautiously in the elderly or debilitated patient.

INTERACTIONS

1. An additive CNS-depressive effect can occur when benzodiazepines are used concurrently with other CNS depressants, such as alcohol, barbiturates, and antihistamines.
2. Concurrent use of antacids may delay the oral absorption of the benzodiazepines.

NURSING CONSIDERATIONS

Refer to general nursing considerations for barbiturates (Chap. 24); most information is similar. In addition, the nurse needs to be aware that withdrawal from these hypnotics must be gradual, and symptoms and nursing care may be similar to that of the patient withdrawing from barbiturates. On the other hand, if the dose of the drug has been low and the course of therapy relatively short, a brief period of insomnia, nervousness, and irritability may be all that occurs.

The benzodiazepines, particularly flurazepam (Dalmane), are frequently prescribed for elderly patients. Like the other hypnotics this drug has the potential to produce the "hangover" effect in this age group. Careful consideration of dose, time of administration, and long-term use may reduce this side-effect.

Chloral Hydrate
(Aquachloral Supprettes, Noctec)

Chloral hydrate is a derivative of chloral (2,2,2-trichloroacetaldehyde) and is used as a mild sedative–hypnotic. It is converted in the body to tri-chloroethanol, which is considered to be the active metabolite.

MECHANISM AND ACTIONS

Within minutes following oral absorption, chloral hydrate is metabolized to trichloroethanol, which exerts a depressant effect on the CNS with minimal involvement of lower brain centers regulating blood pressure and respiration. The drug appears to have negligible effects on REM sleep when used in recommended doses, and "hangover" effects are minimal.

USES

1. Treatment of insomnia
2. Preoperative and postoperative sedation, as an adjunct to other drugs such as analgesics, opiates, and so forth

ADMINISTRATION AND DOSAGE

Chloral hydrate is available as capsules (250 mg, 500 mg), syrup (250 mg/5 ml, 500 mg/5 ml), and suppositories (324 mg, 500 mg, 648 mg). Capsules are given with a *full* glass of water and should not be chewed or broken. The syrup of elixir is administered well-diluted in water, juice, or soda to minimize gastric irritation. The hypnotic dose in adults is 500 mg to 1 g 30 minutes before bedtime, while children may be given 50 mg/kg up to 1 g in a single dose. One half the hypnotic dose has been employed as a mild sedative, but the drug is infrequently used in this manner.

FATE

Chloral hydrate is rapidly absorbed and quickly converted to trichloroethanol, which displays a half-life of 4 hours to 12 hours. Effects are usually seen within 30 minutes to 60 minutes and persist for 4 hours to 8 hours. Trichloroethanol is converted in the liver and kidney to trichloroacetic acid, which is highly protein bound (75%–85%) and slowly excreted in the urine, approximately 40% of a dose within 24 hours.

SIDE-EFFECTS/ADVERSE REACTIONS

Gastric upset is the most frequently encountered side-effect with chloral hydrate. In addition, an unpleasant taste has often been associated with its oral use. Other adverse reactions include excessive drowsiness, lightheadedness, motor incoordination, and allergic skin reactions such as erythema, urticaria and eczematoid dermatitis. Rarely, the drug has caused leukopenia, eosinophilia, and a variety of CNS effects, such as delirium, dizziness, confusion, nightmares, and hallucinations. Chronic use can lead to gastritis, severe skin eruptions, renal damage, and, of course, habituation and dependence. Psychologic dependence can develop within 2 weeks with continued use, and some addicts have required huge doses of chloral hydrate (up to 12 g/day). Sudden withdrawal usually results in extreme CNS excitation.

Symptoms of overdosage resemble those of the barbiturates (see Chap. 24). Treatment is symptomatic and includes gastric lavage, respiratory assistance, and maintenance of blood pressure and electrolyte balance.

CONTRAINDICATIONS AND PRECAUTIONS

Chloral hydrate is contraindicated in the presence of hepatic or renal impairment, gastritis, severe cardiac disease, and a history of allergies. It is also contraindicated in women in labor and in the neonate, because trichloroacetic acid, a metabolite, can free bilirubin from plasma albumin-binding sites, possibly leading to kernicterus, a serious neurologic condition resulting from deposition of bilirubin in cells of the gray matter of the neonate's brain. *Cautious use* of chloral hydrate is warranted in patients with arrhythmias, asthma, or a history of drug dependence, and in pregnant women.

INTERACTIONS

1. Effects of other CNS depressants may be potentiated by chloral hydrate.
2. Following conversion to trichloroacetic acid, chloral hydrate may potentiate the action of acidic, protein-bound drugs (*e.g.*, anticoagulants, salicylates, oral hypoglycemics) by displacing them from protein-binding sites.
3. Effects of chloral hydrate can be potentiated by MAO inhibitors and phenothiazines.
4. Use of IV furosemide with chloral hydrate may result in sweating, tachycardia, and hypertension due to a hypermetabolic state resulting from competition by both drugs for thyroid hormone–binding sites and subsequent increase in plasma levels of free thyroid hormones.

NURSING CONSIDERATIONS

Refer to Nursing Process for barbiturates (Chap. 24); most information is similar including treatment of overdose and care for the patient suffering withdrawal symptoms.

In addition, the main nursing administration technique is to attempt to reduce the gastrointestinal upset associated with this drug. Capsules should never be opened. If the patient cannot swallow the capsule, a liquid formulation is usually available. It can be diluted in juice or given with a snack or milk to reduce the gastrointestinal side-effects.

Ethchlorvynol

(Placidyl)

MECHANISM AND ACTIONS

Ethchlorvynol is a relatively short-acting sedative–hypnotic which also possesses anticonvulsant and muscle-relaxing action. Although its mechanism of action is not completely established, ethchlorvynol elicits an EEG pattern similar to that observed with barbiturates. The clinical picture seen with ethchlorvynol use also closely parallels that with barbiturates: sleep latency is shortened, REM sleep time is decreased, and total sleep time is increased. Upon cessation of treatment, rebound REM can occur. The safety margin with ethchlorvynol is approximately the same as with barbiturates, and habituation and psychologic dependence are frequent with prolonged use.

USES

1. Short-term treatment of insomnia (most effective in patients having difficulty falling asleep rather than having frequent awakenings)

ADMINISTRATION AND DOSAGE

Ethchlorvynol is given orally, as capsules (200 mg, 500 mg, 750 mg). The usual single dose is 500 mg to 750 mg at bedtime. Up to 1 g has been used in severe insomnia. A supplemental dose of 100 mg to 200 mg may be administered if awakening occurs after the original bedtime dose. The drug is not recommended for children. The duration of therapy should not exceed 2 weeks.

FATE

The drug is rapidly absorbed orally, and peak blood levels occur within 1 hour to 1.5 hours. Sleep generally ensues within 20 minutes to 30 minutes after administration and lasts for approximately 5 hours. Distribution within the body is extensive, and the drug localizes in adipose tissue. Plasma half-life of the parent compound is 10 hours to 20 hours. Extensive hepatic metabolism occurs, and both the unchanged drug and major metabolite undergo enterohepatic circulation. Approximately one-third of a dose is excreted in the urine within 24 hours.

466   III: Drugs Acting on the Nervous System

SIDE-EFFECTS/ADVERSE REACTIONS
The most common side-effects are dizziness, facial numbness, blurred vision, and a mint-like aftertaste. Mild hangover has occurred in a number of instances as well, and giddiness and ataxia are noted if absorption is particularly rapid. Other adverse reactions associated with ethchlorvynol include vomiting and gastric upset, hypotension, fainting, skin rash, urticaria, excitement, muscle weakness, profound hypnosis, hysteria, and, rarely, thrombocytopenia and cholestatic jaundice.

Acute intoxication is a medical emergency and is characterized by hypotension, hypothermia, bradycardia, respiratory depression, and coma. Treatment is supportive and symptomatic, and is similar to that described for barbiturates.

Withdrawal symptoms can occur following cessation of prolonged use, and resemble those of barbiturate or alcohol withdrawal. Dosage should be tapered gradually, or phenobarbital may be substituted for ethchlorvynol in the dependent person.

CONTRAINDICATIONS AND PRECAUTIONS
Contraindications to ethchlorvynol use include porphyria and early pregnancy. The drug is not recommended for use in children. Ethchlorvynol should be used *cautiously* in patients with impaired renal or hepatic function and in persons in severe pain, because delirium and excitement can occur. The drug should also be used with caution during the final trimester of pregnancy and in nursing mothers. Due to its potential for habituation, extreme caution must be exercised in prescribing ethchlorvynol to persons with a history of drug abuse.

INTERACTIONS
1. Additive depressant effects may occur if ethchlorvynol is used with other CNS depressants or MAO inhibitors.
2. The drug may reduce the effects of oral anticoagulants by causing a decreased prothrombin time response.
3. Delirium can occur if ethchlorvynol is used in combination with tricyclic antidepressants.

NURSING CONSIDERATIONS
Refer to Nursing Process for initiating treatment with barbiturates and patients withdrawing from barbiturates (Chap. 24); much of the information is similar.

In addition, the nurse needs to remember this drug has a high addiction potential, a narrow margin for safe dosing, and overdosing is extremely difficult to treat, particularly if the patient has combined overdose with CNS depressants such as alcohol, narcotics, or barbiturates.

Ethchlorvynol is rapidly absorbed in the GI tract and can be better controlled if given with food or milk to slow absorption. Symptoms of too rapid absorption are giddiness and ataxia.

Ethinamate
(Valmid)

Ethinamate is a urethane derivative possessing a nonspecific CNS depressant action. It may be employed as a short-acting hypnotic, but it has no significant advantage over barbiturates or other nonbarbiturate hypnotics, and there has been some question as to its effectiveness. Onset of sleep occurs within 20 minutes to 30 minutes, but effects persist for only about 4 hours, thus nocturnal awakening is common. The hypnotic effect is transient, and the drug rapidly becomes ineffective within 7 to 10 days. However, chronic use can lead to psychologic and in some cases physical dependence, and the abstinence syndrome is similar to that seen with barbiturates. Ethinamate is infrequently used today and of minimal clinical interest.

Glutethimide
(Doriden, Doriglute)

Glutethimide is a piperidine derivative which is promoted as an alternative hypnotic to barbiturates, but is considered to be much less desirable because it is potentially more hazardous and no more effective. It possesses no advantages over other hypnotic drugs, and its use should be discouraged.

MECHANISM AND ACTIONS
The pharmacology of glutethimide closely resembles that of the barbiturates, although the precise mechanism of action has not been established. REM sleep is suppressed, and rebound REM occurs when the drug is discontinued. Glutethimide has strong anticholinergic action, manifested by mydriasis, decreased salivary secretions, and reduced intestinal motility. There is minimal respiratory depression at recommended doses, but the drug can stimulate hepatic microsomal enzyme activity. It is physically addicting and has become a popular drug of abuse.

USES
1. Short-term relief of insomnia (maximum of 7 days)

ADMINISTRATION AND DOSAGE
The drug is administered orally as tablets (250 mg, 500 mg) or capsules (500 mg) and is only recommended for adults. The usual dose is 250 mg to 500 mg at bedtime. Repeat doses in the same night should be avoided.

FATE
Oral absorption is erratic, and peak plasma concentrations can occur anywhere from 1 hour to 6 hours after administration. The onset of hypnosis is usually within 30 minutes, and sleep lasts 4 hours to 8 hours. Approximately 50% of the drug in plasma is protein bound. The drug has a high lipid/water partition coefficient and quickly redistributes to adipose tissue sites. Glutethimide is largely metabolized in the liver, where it is conjugated with glucuronic acid. The metabolites undergo enterohepatic recirculation and are excreted in the urine. The plasma half-life ranges from 5 hours to 20 hours.

SIDE-EFFECTS/ADVERSE REACTIONS
Osteomalacia can occur with long-term use. Commonly encountered short-term effects are dizziness, skin rash, blurred vision, and hangover. Serious adverse reactions are relatively rare with occasional use of therapeutic doses, but can range from nausea, vomiting, hypotension, and urticaria, to exfoliative dermatitis, porphyria, paradoxical excitation, and blood dyscrasias. Both psychologic and physical dependence are likely to occur with chronic use, and prolonged administration of glutethimide can result in tonic muscle spasms, tremors, convulsions, irritability, confusion, memory impairment, ataxia, and delirium. Withdrawal of the drug following chronic use must be gradual.

Symptoms of acute intoxication closely resemble those of the barbiturates (see Chap. 24); tonic muscle spasms and convulsions have occurred during glutethimide overdose. A dose of 5 g is sufficient to produce severe intoxication in some patients, and the lethal dose is between 10 g and 20 g. Perhaps due to irregular absorption or to significant storage of the drug by fatty tissue, the degree of CNS depression following an overdosage can vary cyclically. Treatment of overdosage consists of gastric lavage with 1:1 mixture of castor oil and water, respiratory support, careful monitoring of vital signs with ECG, and maintenance of blood pressure. Forced diuresis and urinary alkalinization are not recommended. Dialysis or hemoperfusion should be considered in severe coma or other life-threatening situations (e.g., circulatory collapse, uremia, heart failure). Recognize, however, that as drug is removed from the bloodstream, more drug may be released from adipose storage sites into the bloodstream, and may prolong the symptoms of overdosage. Close monitoring of patients is therefore essential during treatment of withdrawal.

CONTRAINDICATIONS AND PRECAUTIONS
The only absolute contraindication for glutethimide is porphyria, although the drug probably should be avoided in pregnant women, children, and known or suspected drug abusers. Because glutethimide is a strong anticholinergic, *caution* should be exercised when the drug is given to patients with glaucoma, prostatic hypertrophy, bladder obstruction, or arrhythmias. Elderly or debilitated patients should be given reduced doses initially, because paradoxical excitation has occurred.

INTERACTIONS
1. Effects of other CNS depressants (e.g., alcohol, barbiturates) may be enhanced by glutethimide.
2. Glutethimide induces liver microsomal enzyme activity, so effects of anticoagulants, antihistamines, corticosteroids, griseofulvin, meprobamate, phenytoin, and other drugs metabolized by these enzymes may be reduced.
3. Glutethimide may exert an additive anticholinergic effect with tricyclic antidepressants, and other anticholinergic drugs.

NURSING CONSIDERATIONS
Refer to Nursing Process for initiating treatment with barbiturates and for patients withdrawing from barbiturates (Chap. 24); much of the information is similar.

In addition, the nurse needs to remember this drug has a high addiction potential and a narrow margin for safe dosing, and that overdose is extremely difficult to treat, particularly if the patient has combined overdose with CNS depressants such as alcohol, narcotics, or barbiturates. A common street combination is glutethimide and codeine, sometimes called a "load," "packet," or "threes and eights." The problem of treating glutethimide overdose is the development of intermittent coma which is related to the irregular absorption of the drug into the bloodstream. Early gastric evacuation by gastric lavage, emesis if the patient is awake, and administration of activated charcoal will decrease absorption. Measures, including cardiac and respiratory support, may be ineffective if the patient is in poor medical condition, or if the length of time between ingestion and treatment is such that a large portion of the drug has been absorbed. There is no specific antidote.

The patient receiving glutethimide should have adequate GI motility and renal function because the drug will slow normal function of these organ systems. The patient receiving this drug should be encouraged to increase fluids and roughage in his diet to counteract these effects.

Methyprylon

(Noludar)

Methyprylon, like glutethimide, is a piperidine and shares many of the same pharmacologic and toxicologic properties. In general, the drug has no particular advantage over barbiturates, but unlike glutethimide, it is highly water-soluble and therefore probably safer in the event of an overdosage.

MECHANISM AND ACTIONS

The mechanism of action of methyprylon is not completely established, but the drug probably functions similar to the barbiturates; for example, the firing threshold for brain stem neurons is elevated. REM sleep is reduced, rebound REM occurs following discontinuation, and hepatic microsomal enzyme activity is accelerated.

USES
1. Short-term treatment of insomnia (7 day maximum)

ADMINISTRATION AND DOSAGE
Methyprylon is available as tablets (50 mg, 200 mg) and capsules (300 mg). It is administered orally in a dose of 200 mg to 400 mg at bedtime. Children over age 12 may be given 50 mg to 200 mg depending on size and weight.

FATE
Sleep is usually induced within 30 minutes to 45 minutes following an oral dose; the duration of action ranges from 5 hours to 8 hours. Plasma half-life is about 4 hours. It is extensively metabolized in the liver and excreted in the urine, as both free and conjugated metabolites.

SIDE-EFFECTS/ADVERSE REACTIONS
Side-effects are usually infrequent; morning drowsiness, dizziness, and mild gastric upset are reported most often. Other untoward reactions occurring with methyprylon are vomiting, diarrhea, esophagitis, headache, skin rash, paradoxical excitation, and, rarely, neutropenia and thrombocytopenia. Chronic use leads to tolerance, habituation, and dependence. Withdrawal symptoms resemble those seen with barbiturates such as insomnia, confusion, tremors, convulsions, and delirium.

Acute overdosage is marked by symptoms that closely resemble those seen with barbiturate overdosage (see Chap. 24). Treatment includes gastric lavage, vasopressors, respiratory assistance, and hemodialysis. During recovery, CNS excitation can occur, and convulsions have been reported.

CONTRAINDICATIONS AND PRECAUTIONS
Use of methyprylon is contraindicated in children under age 12 and in patients with porphyria. The drug should be given *cautiously* to patients with liver or kidney dysfunction or severe pain, to known or suspected drug abusers, and to pregnant or nursing women.

INTERACTIONS
(See under Glutethimide.)

NURSING CONSIDERATIONS
Refer to Nursing Process for initiating treatment with barbiturates and for patients withdrawing from barbiturates (Chap. 24); much of the information is similar, including the potential for hematologic toxicity.

In addition, the nurse needs to remember that this drug has a high addiction potential but that overdose is somewhat more easily treated than glutethimide overdose.

Paraldehyde

(Paral)

Paraldehyde is a polymer of acetaldehyde which elicits a nonselective, reversible CNS depression. It is a rapid-acting hypnotic which is primarily (but infrequently) used IM or IV in a hospital setting for the emergency treatment of convulsive states, as outlined below.

MECHANISM AND ACTIONS

Paraldehyde is a general CNS depressant, although it has only slight effects on respiration or blood pressure in ordinary therapeutic doses. The drug has no analgesic properties and may actually elicit CNS excitation in the presence of severe pain. Large doses are effective in abolishing convulsions and delirium.

USES

1. Mild sedative and hypnotic
2. Emergency treatment of convulsive episodes associated with tetanus, eclampsia, status epilepticus, and poisoning by convulsive drugs
3. Induction of sleep to facilitate EEG study, especially in children

ADMINISTRATION AND DOSAGE

Paraldehyde is available as a liquid for oral or rectal administration and as an IM or IV injection each containing 1 g/ml.

Recommended doses are:

Adults

Oral: 4 ml to 8 ml in milk or fruit juice to mask taste and odor

Rectal: 10 ml to 20 ml with one to two parts of olive oil or isotonic sodium chloride to minimize rectal irritation

IM, IV:

Hypnosis: 10 ml IM in two divided doses or 10 ml IV, diluted with 200 ml 0.9% sodium chloride injection at a rate not exceeding 1 ml/min

Sedation: 2 ml to 5 ml IM or 5 ml IV diluted with at least 100 ml of 0.9% sodium chloride injection at a rate not exceeding 1 ml/min

Children

Hypnosis: 0.3 ml/kg IM

Sedation: 0.15 ml/kg IM

FATE

Paraldehyde is rapidly absorbed after oral administration and produces sleep within 10 minutes to 15 minutes which lasts 8 hours to 10 hours. Onset is slower with rectal administration. Plasma half-life ranges from 4 hours to 10 hours. Approximately 75% of the drug is metabolized by the liver, much of the remainder being exhaled unchanged by the lungs. In hepatic insufficiency, elimination is slowed and a greater proportion is exhaled in the expired air.

SIDE-EFFECTS/ADVERSE REACTIONS

The most noticeable side-effects with oral paraldehyde are a disagreeable taste and a strong aromatic odor. Oral or rectal mucosal irritation are also seen frequently, and GI upset is common. Other adverse reactions include skin rash, redness, swelling or pain at injection site; nerve damage; bradycardia; dyspnea; and metabolic acidosis with prolonged use. IV administration may cause coughing, an early sign of pulmonary toxicity. Prolonged use may result in addiction which resembles alcoholism, and withdrawal may produce delirium tremens and hallucinations.

Overdosage is infrequent, inasmuch as the drug is primarily used in a controlled hospital setting. Symptoms of overdose include rapid, labored breathing, hypotension, pulmonary edema, gastritis, and right-side heart dilatation. Death is usually the result of respiratory failure. Treatment is largely symptomatic; metabolic acidosis is corrected by IV administration of sodium bicarbonate or sodium lactate.

CONTRAINDICATIONS AND PRECAUTIONS

Paraldehyde is contraindicated in patients with bronchopulmonary disease (because a significant fraction of the drug is eliminated by the lungs), hepatic insufficiency, and severe GI ulceration. *Cautious use* of paraldehyde is warranted in the presence of severe pain or coughing and in pregnant women or nursing mothers. Do not give for prolonged periods of time, especially to persons with a history of drug abuse.

INTERACTIONS

1. The effects of other CNS depressants may be potentiated by paraldehyde.
2. Paraldehyde may antagonize the antibacterial activity of sulfonamides by increasing their rate of metabolism, which may result in crystalluria.
3. Tolbutamide (Orinase) may potentiate the hypnotic action of paraldehyde.
4. Disulfiram (Antabuse) used with paraldehyde may decrease its metabolism, resulting in a toxic reaction due to excessive blood levels of acetaldehyde and paraldehyde.

NURSING CONSIDERATIONS

See Nursing Process for initiating treatment with barbiturates and for patients withdrawing from barbiturates (Chap. 24); much of the information is similar.

Administration of paraldehyde should incorporate the following considerations:

1. Parenteral doses should be drawn up in a glass syringe because paraldehyde is incompatible

with most plastics. Give IM injections deep because the drug can cause tissue necrosis and nerve damage or paralysis.
2. Oral doses should be well chilled in milk or juice to mask the taste.
3. Rectal doses should be given as an oil retention enema combined with olive or cottonseed oil to reduce mucosal irritation.
4. If the nurse notes reconstituted paraldehyde to be brownish in color or have the odor of acetic acid (vinegar), the drug must be discarded; these are signs of decompensation.
5. The patient's room must be well ventilated during administration of paraldehyde to decrease the chance that people entering the room will develop side-effects from the aromatic drug. Staff working with the patient may develop eye, nose, or throat irritation if fumes of paraldehyde are inhaled in sufficient quantities. Much of the drug is eliminated by the lungs so patients receiving paraldehyde will have a characteristic odor to their breath.

Propriomazine

(Largon)

Propriomazine is a phenothiazine derivative possessing sedative, antihistamine and antiemetic effects. It is occasionally used IV or IM in a hospital setting as a sedative for the relief of apprehension either prior to or during surgery, and as a adjunct to analgesics during labor. Peak effects occur within 15 minutes to 30 minutes following IV injection, and within 30 minutes to 60 minutes with IM administration. Effects persist 4 hours to 6 hours with a single injection. Mild elevations in blood pressure and heart rate have been noted, and dizziness, confusion, and restlessness have occurred. An occasional hypotensive reaction has occurred and may be treated with norepinephrine; the use of epinephrine is not recommended, because propiomazine may reverse the pressor action of epinephrine.

IV injection can cause thrombophlebitis, and therefore should be made only into undamaged vessels, and care should be taken to avoid extravasation. Subcutaneous injection is likely to cause tissue irritation, and intra-arterial administration can result in vascular spasm. Because propiomazine can markedly enhance the action of other CNS depressants (e.g., barbiturates, narcotics), their dosage should be reduced by one third to one half when used concurrently with propiomazine. Dosage generally ranges from 20 mg to 40 mg and is frequently combined with 50 mg of meperidine (Demerol). For sedation during surgery with local or spinal anesthetics, a dosage of 10 mg to 20 mg is sufficient. Children have been given 0.25 mg to 0.5 mg per pound for pre- or postsurgical sedation.

REVIEW QUESTIONS

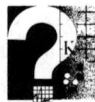

1. Outline the principal differences between the nonbarbiturate sedative–hypnotic drugs and the benzodiazepine antianxiety agents.
2. What are the major advantages of the benzodiazepine hypnotics (e.g., flurazepam) over the barbiturates?
3. What type of drug is found in the various over-the-counter sleep aids?
4. Which benzodiazepine hypnotic is the longest acting? The shortest acting? What problem is commonly associated with use of a very short-acting hypnotic?
5. Briefly describe the mechanism of action of the benzodiazepine hypnotics.
6. What is the active metabolite of chloral hydrate? Oral use of chloral hydrate is frequently associated with what side-effect?
7. What disadvantages does glutethimide have relative to the barbiturates? Why is overdose with glutethimide so difficult to treat?
8. What measures can be taken in the event of overdosage with methyprylon?
9. List several indications for paraldehyde. Give several approved means of administration.
10. What cautions must be observed when using any of the nonbarbiturate sedative–hypnotic drugs?

BIBLIOGRAPHY

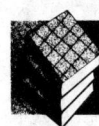

Bliwise D, Seidel W, Karacan I, Mitler M, Roth T, Zorick F, Dement W: Daytime sleepiness as a criterion in hypnotic medication trials: Comparison of triazolam and flurazepam. Sleep 6:156, 1983

Chartier D: Glutethimide and codeine overdose. J Emerg Nurs 9:307, 1983

Greenblatt DJ, Divoll M, Aberneth Dr, Shady RI: Benzodiazepine hypnotics: Kinetic and therapeutic options. Sleep 5:518, 1982

Harris B: Sedative-hypnotic drugs. Am J Nurs 81(7):1329, 1981

Kales A, Kales J: Sleep laboratory studies of hypnotic drugs: Efficacy and withdrawal effects. J Clin Psychopharmacol 3:140, 1983

Lader M, Petursson H: Long-term effects of benzodiazepines. Neuropharmacology 22:527, 1983

Simon C: Benzodiazepine hypnotics for insomnia. Am J Nurs 83(9):1330, 1983

Wincer MZ: Insomnia and the new benzodiazepines. Clin Pharmacokinet 1:425, 1982

Alcohols

26

The generic term *alcohol* refers to a hydroxy derivative of an aliphatic hydrocarbon produced by fermenting sugars and yeasts. Alcohols have long been used for a variety of purposes, such as foods, solvents, anesthetics, and in many industrial procedures; however, the clinical applications of alcohols are limited. The greatest use of alcoholic substances, especially ethyl alcohol, occurs in social situations, and the misuse of alcohol in this regard is one of the most extensive and serious problems in health care today. This aspect of alcohol use is addressed later in the chapter.

Although several alcohols, such as isopropyl, methyl, and butyl, are employed in various therapeutic or industrial ways, the most commonly used alcohol is ethanol (ethyl alcohol), and the discussion on alcohols presented here will focus primarily on this agent.

Pharmacokinetics of Ethanol

Ethanol, or ethyl alcohol (CH_3CH_2OH), is a water-soluble molecule that is extensively and rapidly absorbed from the stomach and small intestine. Vapors of ethanol can also be readily absorbed through the lungs. Gastric absorption is slowed by the presence of food or milk, while absorption from the intestines is quite rapid and largely independent of the presence of other substances. Absorption of alcohol through the intact skin is negligible.

When ingested in the fasting state, peak blood levels of alcohol are attained within 30 minutes to 40 minutes, and alcohol is rather uniformly distributed throughout the body. Alcohol gains ready access to the fetal circulation when ingested by pregnant women.

Over 90% of the alcohol that is consumed is completely oxidized in the liver, the remainder being eliminated through the lungs and in small amounts in the urine. Unlike most other substances, the rate of oxidation of alcohol follows *zero-order kinetics.* That is, it proceeds at a fairly constant rate irrespective of time and the concentration of drug. The *average* rate at which alcohol is metabolized is approximately 10 ml/hour, but this rate can vary from individual to individual depending on body weight, the presence of liver dysfunction, or metabolizing enzyme alterations. This *constant* rate of metabolism restricts the amount of alcohol a person can consume within a given period of time without causing an accumulation of alcohol in the body. For example, it would require about 1 hour to metabolize completely the alcohol contained in 10 oz to 12 oz of beer, 3 oz to 4 oz of wine, or 1 oz of a typical whiskey.

The principal pathway of alcohol metabolism is the oxidation of ethanol to acetaldehyde by the enzyme alcohol dehydrogenase, a zinc-containing enzyme located primarily in the liver. Alcohol can also be metabolized to acetaldehyde by another hepatic enzyme system, the mixed-function oxidases found on the smooth endoplasmic reticulum. This latter system appears to play a significant role in alcohol metabolism when alcohol concentrations are elevated for prolonged periods of time, as in the chronic alcoholic. The activity of this hepatic mixed-function oxidase system (sometimes referred to as the *microsomal enzyme system*) can be accelerated with prolonged exposure to alcohol, a process termed *enzyme induction,* which has been discussed in connection with barbiturates in Chapter 24. Thus, chronic ingestion of alcohol can facilitate the metabolism of the many drugs that depend on the mixed-function oxidase system in the liver for their clearance. Conversely, other hepatic enzyme inducers, such as barbiturates or phenytoin, can accelerate the metabolic clearance of alcohol by the liver.

The acetaldehyde that is formed from alcohol is then converted by aldehyde dehydrogenase to acetyl coenzyme A, which is subsequently oxidized to CO_2 and water in the citric acid cycle or utilized in other metabolic reactions in the body.

In general, the clinical effects of alcohol vary directly with the blood concentration, since the central nervous system (CNS) level of alcohol closely parallels that of the blood. The various behavioral signs and symptoms associated with increasing blood levels of alcohol are outlined in Table 26-1. In nontolerant individuals blood levels to approximately 0.1% are usually not associated with overt signs of impaired performance. As the blood alcohol level rises, there is a corresponding decrease in alertness, reaction time, and psychomotor performance until at approximately 0.4% the person loses consciousness and the vital signs begin to deteriorate. Levels in excess of 0.5% are usually fatal although higher levels have been reported in grossly tolerant alcoholics.

Many states have set limits on the blood alcohol level below which it is considered legally safe for a person to operate an automobile, and these limits generally are in the 0.1% to 0.15% range.

Table 26-1
Relationship Between Blood Alcohol Level and Clinical
Behavior in Nontolerant Persons

Blood Alcohol Level (%)	Corresponding Urinary Level (%)	Clinical Manifestations
0–0.1	0–0.14	No overt signs; slightly lowered inhibitions; may be some decrease in alertness; slightly impaired performance in special tests of learned motor skills
0.1–0.2	0.14–0.28	Slowed reaction time; slight muscular incoordination; emotional instability; impaired motor function; decreased caution
0.2–0.3	0.28–0.42	Slurred speech; staggering gait; loss of pain sensation; increased confusion; impaired ability to concentrate
0.3–0.4	0.42–0.54	Extreme muscle incoordination; lack of response to external stimuli; stupor; hypothermia; blunted reflexes; possible unconsciousness
0.4–0.5	0.54–0.66	Anesthesia; total unconsciousness; circulatory collapse; absent reflexes; coma; possible death
0.5 and above		Death

Pharmacologic Properties of Alcohol

Local Actions

When applied topically, alcohol has a number of local effects. It can cool the skin through evaporation; act as an astringent (alcohol precipitates protoplasm), counterirritant, or rubefacient (local effects include erythema and mild burning); help prevent bedsores and decubitus ulcers in bedridden persons (alcohol hardens and cleanses the skin); and serve as a general antibacterial agent. The use of alcohol for a back rub or to prevent decubitus ulcers must be undertaken cautiously, especially in the elderly, in view of the drying effect that the substance exhibits. Back rubs are now frequently given using a moisturizing lotion rather than alcohol.

Ethyl alcohol, when applied topically, is bactericidal to most common pathogens, primarily due to its ability to precipitate bacterial proteins and dissolve membrane lipids. Concentrations of 70% ethanol will kill up to 90% of surface bacteria within 2 minutes if the area is kept constantly moist. Conversely, a single brief swabbing of an area with ethanol, which then quickly evaporates, is much less effective in eradicating surface bacteria.

A brief exposure to alcohol rarely is damaging to the skin. However, prolonged contact of skin with alcohol can cause extreme drying and scaling. The drug should not be applied to open wounds or severely abraded surfaces since it may increase the degree of irritation and form a coagulation barrier under which bacteria may proliferate.

Topical alcohol has limited effectiveness against viral particles or spores (*e.g.*, fungi) and therefore its application to the skin prior to needle insertion or minor incisions is probably of limited clinical benefit.

Isopropyl alcohol, in concentrations above 70%, is slightly more germicidal than ethyl alcohol, but it is also more irritating and more drying. It also produces vasodilation, which may result in a greater likelihood of bleeding following puncture or incision. When injected into the region of a nerve, ethyl alcohol can cause neuritis and nerve degeneration; such a procedure has been employed to elicit prolonged or even permanent loss of sensation in treating severe pain, such as trigeminal neuralgia.

Systemic Actions

CENTRAL NERVOUS SYSTEM

Alcohol is a continuous and primary depressant of CNS function. The "stimulation" that frequently is noted with the initial consumption of alcohol is the result of a depression of the inhibitory control function of lower centers on higher cortical activity. Progressive depressant effects of alcohol range from sedation and decreased anxiety to ataxia, slurred speech, altered judgment, and erratic behavior (see Table 26-1). Mood swings are often violent and uncontrolled. Alcohol impairs performance of psychomotor tasks and progressively dulls the sensorium. In addition, limited "tolerance" to the acute CNS effects of the drug develops in chronic users.

Chronic ingestion of alcohol may lead to serious neurologic disorders ranging from memory loss, reduced perceptual activity, emotional lability, and sleep disorders to psychotic behavior. Peripheral nerve injury that may begin with paresthesias of the extremities is a well-established consequence of chronic alcohol intake. Nutritional and vitamin deficiencies that commonly occur in the chronic alcoholic may be responsible for such serious conditions as the Wernicke–Korsakoff syndrome (see Disease Brief) and polyneuritis.

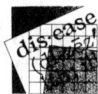

DISEASE BRIEF

- ### Wernicke–Korsakoff Syndrome

Wernicke–Korsakoff syndrome is a disorder of the CNS apparently caused by a deficiency of vitamin B$_1$ (thiamine) and associated with the chronic abuse of alcohol. It is characterized by impaired ocular motility, ataxia, reduced mentation, and sensorimotor polyneuropathy. Initially, many symptoms (tremor, confusion, agitation, altered sensory perception, autonomic hyperactivity) resemble those of alcohol withdrawal and may make early diagnosis difficult. Progressive forms of the disease lead to a condition sometimes referred to as *Korsakoff's psychosis*, a state of seriously impaired memory function that renders the affected person incapable of anything but simple tasks. Ability to learn new material is greatly reduced.

The ocular manifestations, with the exception of nystagmus, generally improve quickly with vitamin B$_1$ replacement therapy, whereas ataxia responds more slowly. Korsakoff's psychosis does not appear to improve significantly once it is well established.

CARDIOVASCULAR

In moderate amounts, alcohol causes vasodilation, especially of the cutaneous vessels, probably due to a mild depression of central vasomotor function. Myocardial contractility is reduced by consumption of alcohol, and excessive ingestion can lead to myocardial lesions that can gradually reduce myocardial function, resulting in congestive heart failure. The cardiotoxic effects of alcohol are probably due in part to accompanying nutritional deficiencies and to the presence of acetaldehyde. Prolonged consumption of alcohol is associated with a higher than normal blood pressure and may be a definite risk factor for hypertension. The effects of alcohol on plasma lipoproteins are variable. Elevated triglyceride levels are frequently noted in chronic alcohol users; however, small to moderate amounts of alcohol can elevate the levels of high-density lipoproteins (HDL), which may serve a protective function by aiding in the clearance of cholesterol. The ability of small amounts of alcohol to protect against coronary artery and cerebrovascular disease is the subject of considerable debate. Prolonged consumption of alcohol may lead to disturbances in rhythm of the heart, and sudden withdrawal of alcohol can result in serious arrhythmias, seizures, and possibly death.

MUSCULOSKELETAL

Increasing amounts of alcohol can significantly impair psychomotor performance and blunt reflex motor activity. Damage to skeletal musculature is frequently noted with chronic alcohol use. Ethanol is a smooth muscle relaxant in moderate amounts, and its myometrial relaxant action has been used for the suppression of premature labor, although this application is largely obsolete with the availability of other, more effective, safer uterine relaxants.

GASTROINTESTINAL/HEPATIC

The effects of alcohol on the gastrointestinal (GI) tract depend on many factors, such as the concentration of alcohol, amount of food present, the state of digestive function, the degree of alcohol tolerance, and so forth. Small amounts of alcohol generally stimulate secretion of gastric juice and hydrochloric acid. As the concentration of alcohol in the ingested beverage increases, gastric secretion is progressively inhibited and the activity of pepsin is depressed. High concentrations of alcohol, especially with prolonged consumption, usually result in inflammation of the mucosa and the development of gastritis. The presence of food in the stomach tends to lessen the acute irritative effects of alcohol but probably has little effect on the long-term ulcerative action. GI bleeding associated with ulcerative lesions can lead to blood loss and anemia. Impaired absorption of nutrients and vitamins, especially the water-soluble ones, is responsible for a number of clinical abnormalities seen with prolonged alcohol intake. Chronic alcohol consumption also increases the risk of pancreatitis.

Occasional acute use of alcohol does not appreciably alter hepatic function. Continued consumption of alcohol causes serious long-term complications, however, and impaired liver function is a common finding in the chronic alcohol user. Alcoholic liver disease is usually insidious in onset and generally progresses to a significant degree without overt clinical symptoms. Accumulation of fat in hepatic parenchymal cells may be benign at first, but eventually can progress to hepatitis and ultimately to cirrhosis. Although malnutrition and vitamin deficiencies may *contribute* to alcoholic liver damage, it is the presence of alcohol itself that is *primarily* responsible for the pathologic changes.

ENDOCRINE

Chronic consumption of alcohol has been implicated as the cause of a number of endocrine abnormalities. Gynecomastia and testicular atrophy have been noted in alcoholics, and fluid and electrolyte disorders have occurred, leading in some cases to edema, effusions, and ascites. Impotence and sterility are potential consequences of prolonged alcohol consumption, and decreased sexual responsiveness in both men and women has been attributed to alcohol use.

OTHER

Alcohol has a diuretic effect, which is essentially proportional to the blood alcohol level. This action is presumably due to inhibition of the release of the antidiuretic hormone, although the increased fluid intake is doubtless a contributing factor.

Chronic ingestion of alcohol increases the risk of certain types of cancers, notably oropharyngeal, laryngeal, esophageal, hepatic, and possibly pancreatic.

Excessive consumption of alcohol during pregnancy, especially during the first trimester, can lead to fetal abnormalities, the so-called *fetal alcohol syndrome.* A myriad of congenital abnormalities have been associated with maternal alcohol abuse, chief among them being blunted growth, facial malformations (shortened palpebral fissures, flattened and elongated middle upper lip, and ear anomalies), valvular heart defects, poor motor coordination, deficient mental function, and hydrocephalus. Consumption of even *moderate* amounts of alcohol during pregnancy should be avoided.

Tolerance and Dependence

Chronic alcohol consumption produces tolerance and eventually dependence. Tolerance to alcohol with repeated use is a complex process, probably involving several mechanisms such as accelerated metabolism and central neuronal receptor adaptation to the continued presence of alcohol. On reduction in the amount consumed or sudden cessation of all alcohol intake, a characteristic withdrawal syndrome is likely to develop, and may begin within 6 hours to 8 hours after the last drink. Depending on the duration of alcohol use and the amount consumed, withdrawal symptoms may range from mild to severe. In general, there is a progression of withdrawal through several stages, as follows:

Stage I: Early onset of nausea, vomiting, sweating, hyperactivity, tremors, sleeplessness, tachycardia, hypertension

Stage II: Increased severity of above symptoms *plus* auditory or visual hallucinations and seizures (grand mal, nonfocal)

Stage III: Delirium tremens (DTs), profound confusion, disorientation, extreme autonomic hyperactivity

In instances where chronic intake is very high, simply *reducing the rate* of consumption can elicit a withdrawal syndrome.

With continued use of alcohol, higher blood levels may be necessary to produce a state of intoxication. Although chronic alcoholics may be able to perform tasks at blood levels of alcohol two to three times higher than occasional indulgers, there is *no* marked increase in the lethal dosage threshold, even in heavy alcohol users. In addition, the CNS-depressant effects of alcohol are additive to those of other CNS-depressant drugs, and severe intoxication, with respiratory and cardiovascular depression, can occur quite readily with use of CNS-depressant drugs in the alcoholic.

Further consideration is given to the problem of alcohol abuse in Chapter 85.

Therapeutic Uses

External

Alcoholic preparations are used in a number of ways externally, some of which have been mentioned earlier in the chapter. Application of alcohol to the skin has a cooling effect with evaporation, and alcohol sponges are sometimes used to lower fever. Alcohol solutions can be used as rubbing agents to prevent decubitus ulcers in bedridden patients, although such use is currently discouraged, and as skin disinfectants prior to injection, blood sampling, and other invasive needle procedures. Alcohol is used as a solvent for many substances, and alcoholic solutions of drugs (*i.e.*, elixirs) are still commonly used in pharmacotherapy.

Local

Injection of dehydrated alcohol into the vicinity of nerves or ganglia has been used for the relief of chronic, intractable pain, such as that associated with trigeminal neuralgia or inoperable carcinoma. Although usually not a treatment of choice, alcohol injection may provide pain relief where other more conventional methods have failed.

Systemic

Ingestion of alcohol has limited therapeutic application, although it has long been used in one form or another by the lay public as a sedative, hypnotic, analgesic, antipyretic, and even as a stomachic to improve the appetite. Although chronic use of substantial amounts of alcohol should obviously be discouraged, ingestion of small amounts (*i.e.*, 1 oz–2 oz/day) has been advocated by some as having a favorable benefit-to-risk ratio in terms of decreasing the likelihood of cardiovascular problems and increasing the level of cholesterol-clearing, high-density lipoproteins (see Chap. 37). However, systemic use of alcohol can result in an increased incidence of interactions between ethanol and other drugs that can lead to a variety of undesirable effects such as increased CNS depression, GI bleeding, dizziness, and hypertension. A listing of drugs that can interact with alcohol and the resultant effects is presented in Table 26-2.

Methanol

Methyl alcohol, or methanol, is derived from the distillation of wood products and is therefore also known as *wood alcohol*. It is used as an industrial solvent, gasoline additive, substrate for bacterial protein synthesis, and to denature (*i.e.*, to make unfit to drink) commercially available ethyl alcohol products such as rubbing alcohol. Methanol is purely of toxicologic interest, and its accidental ingestion or absorption through the skin can result in serious toxicity.

Methanol is rapidly absorbed from the GI tract and is widely distributed in body tissues. It is largely metabolized to formaldehyde and subsequently to formic acid, and this oxidative conversion, like that of ethanol, proceeds independently of the blood concentration. However, methanol is metabolized only about one sixth as rapidly as ethanol. Since both ethanol and methanol are metabolized by the same enzymes and since ethanol has a higher affinity for this enzyme than methanol, ethanol can reduce the formation of the toxic metabo-

Table 26-2
Alcohol–Drug Interactions

Drug	Effects of Concurrent Use of Alcohol
Anticoagulants	Increased likelihood of bleeding
Anticonvulsants	Decreased anticonvulsive effectiveness
Antidepressants	Decreased antidepressant action; increased blood pressure
Antihistamines	Increased sedation/drowsiness
Antihypertensives	Increased blood pressure lowering action or reduced drug effectiveness in chronic alcohol users
Diuretics	Increased hypotension, increased diuresis
CNS stimulants (e.g., caffeine, diet pills)	Reduced stimulatory effect
Hypoglycemics (antidiabetics)	Interference with control of diabetic state; increased hypoglycemia
Narcotic analgesics	Increased drowsiness, respiratory depression, and motor impairment
Sedative/hypnotics	Increased CNS depression
Salicylates/other anti-inflammatory agents	Increased GI distress and bleeding
Vitamins	Decreased utilization of most vitamins

lites formaldehyde and formic acid. It is frequently used for this purpose as treatment for acute methanol poisoning.

The manifestations of methanol poisoning are due primarily to acidosis resulting from production of formic acid and to a direct toxic action of formaldehyde, especially on retinal cells. Symptoms may not appear for 24 hours to 36 hours, although they have been noted as early as 6 hours to 8 hours following ingestion. Principal symptoms include vomiting, upper abdominal pain, dyspnea, cyanosis, restlessness, and blurred vision. Extreme bradycardia is noted with severe intoxication, and delirium may be marked. Blindness frequently results from the toxic effect of formaldehyde on the retina, and ingestion of as little as 5 ml has resulted in loss of vision. Convulsions can occur and coma usually develops fairly rapidly, but death may not occur for some time.

Treatment of methanol intoxication is primarily directed at correcting the acidosis with alkali and retarding the oxidation of methanol to formaldehyde by administration of ethanol. The slow oxidation of methanol requires that appropriate therapy be continued for several days to prevent relapse and possible death.

Patient and Community Education About Alcohol

Over 5 million people in the United States abuse alcohol. The problems brought on by drinking result in symptoms that cause many of these people to seek medical and psychologic assistance. Therefore, most people the nurse meets who are alcoholics will not complain of alcoholism as their disease but of other symptoms. When asked, they may deny or understate their use of the drug. Therefore, careful assessments need to be made in order to uncover those people in need of assistance. Nursing care needs to focus on three levels with regard to alcohol as a drug: prevention of abuse by educating target populations, treatment of the patient going through alcohol withdrawal, and rehabilitation of the alcohol abuser through counseling and referral.

The nurse has multiple opportunities in her practice and community to give people information about alcohol. All age groups, ethnic groups, and socioeconomic levels have victims of the disease, so many populations can be targeted, but several are at high risk and bear special consideration.

Women and men of childbearing age are an important population to receive information about the effects of alcohol on the unborn child. Although the drinking habits of the pregnant woman will directly affect the baby, education directed at men can help them influence the drinking patterns of their partners and may be an effective strategy. Couples who are planning a pregnancy or who are not using birth control need this information before conception takes place since the effects of alcohol on the fetus are most damaging early in the pregnancy.

The manifestations of fetal alcohol syndrome were listed earlier in this chapter. Some of the effects on the fetus, such as intrauterine growth retardation, problems in motor coordination, and increased rate of stillbirth can occur with as few as 2 drinks per day. A drink consists of 1 oz of distilled liquor, 4 oz to 5 oz of wine, or 12 oz of beer

(McCarthy, 1983). The risk sharply increases if the woman has occasional episodes of drinking about 5 drinks or regularly consumes 6 or more drinks daily.

The most important action a nurse can take to open the door to discussion is to ask the pregnant woman about alcohol consumption early in the pregnancy. Although the abuser may understate the quantity of alcohol she drinks, information provided may help her recognize the drug's effect on the unborn child. Having easy-to-read literature or audiovisual material may provide more information without being judgmental. Such information is readily available from the local chapters of the March of Dimes or by writing to the National Institute on Alcohol Abuse and Alcoholism (NIAAA) 5600 Fishers Lane, Rockville, MD 20857.

A second target population for alcohol education is the teenager. This age group tends to use the drug as part of the effort to grow up. Experimentation with alcohol may be related to peer influences, the drinking patterns of parents, or the need to try "the forbidden." Education should be aimed, nonjudgmentally, at the effects of alcohol on the body, with particular attention to response times since many teenagers drink and drive. Other information should deal with handling peer pressure and drinking situations. Recent media advertising has focused strongly on dealing with peer pressure. Parents associations in local high schools have begun to send letters of agreement for parents of teenagers to sign stating that they do not allow adolescents to drink at parties in their homes and that they will be home if their teenager is giving a party. Lists of such parents are then made available to all parents in the schools. Such community action for dealing with peer situations is useful and needs further encouragement.

Teenagers also need information on the dangers of alcohol in combination with other drugs. The drugs most frequently combined with alcohol are marijuana, amphetamines, cocaine, barbiturates, hallucinogens, and tranquilizers. These combinations can produce accidental overdoses resulting in brain damage or death. These combinations are particularly deadly when the adolescent then attempts to drive. Yet, studies show that many adolescents have an unrealistic sense of their ability to combine alcohol, drugs, and driving, so education must focus on the effects of such combinations.

A third target population for alcohol information is the diabetic. There has been much controversy about whether or not diabetics can safely consume alcohol. Obviously, the patient himself will make the final choice but the nurse can provide valuable information to assist him in decision-making.

In general, the patient taking oral sulfonylurea drugs such as chlorpropamide or tolbutamide is not able to drink since these drugs in combination with alcohol will produce a hypersensitivity reaction similar to that seen with disulfiram and alcohol. However, the uncomplicated diabetic controlled by insulin or diet can safely take an occasional drink if certain parameters are followed. First, consumption should occur only with food, not on an empty stomach. Second, a drink (1 oz of liquor, 12 oz of beer, or 4 oz of wine) should be treated as approximately 2 fat exchanges in a calculated diabetic exchange diet (Criegler-Meringola and Ryan, 1984). The diabetic should choose alcoholic beverages that are lowest in carbohydrates. These include distilled spirits such as whiskey, gin, or vodka; dry wines; and light beer. Mixers must also be considered for their carbohydrate content. Acceptable mixers include club soda, water, and diet drinks. While this information is useful, the diabetic needs a clear understanding of the limitations of these parameters and should review them with his physician. Any diabetic with gastrointestinal, heart, liver, or kidney problems should avoid alcohol.

The last target population is the patient on multiple drug therapies. Alcohol adversely interacts with many prescription and over-the-counter medications. Any patient starting a new drug therapy needs information on the effects of combining alcohol with that drug.

■ *Nursing Process*

□ *ASSESSMENT*

□ *Subjective Data*

The traditional signs associated with alcohol withdrawal, hallucinations, bizarre behavior, and delirium tremens (DTs), are late withdrawal signs and difficult to treat. If the nurse assesses the patient going through withdrawal earlier in the syndrome, the symptoms can be more successfully and safely treated. See the section on Tolerance and Dependence, earlier in this chapter, for stages.

Assessment of these patients can be difficult because many of the symptoms they describe seem unrelated to alcohol. Some clues to watch for are persons who come in for treatment but refuse admission even when it is clearly indicated; become hostile or defensive when asked about drinking pattern in a social history; or understate drinking but describe a social life including many parties and social affairs. These patients may also have vague complaints such as nervousness or sleeplessness, or they may appear hyperactive. They will rarely associate the symptoms with alcohol use. Another useful sign is a history of frequent falls or accidents and multiple scars and bruises that the patient has difficulty explaining. Patients in whom the diagnosis of alcohol withdrawal is frequently missed are the elderly whose mental status may be unknown and the early postoperative patient emerging from general anesthesia.

Other diagnoses may be missed if the patient is clearly drunk. The symptoms of disorientation and lethargy seen in the alcoholic patient may mask more serious neurologic deficits, for instance, those that may have occurred with a fall.

Nurses frequently stereotype the alcoholic as male, young or middle-aged, black, or unemployed ("the bum"). Such characteristics lead one to assume a well-dressed, white, elderly woman could not be a problem drinker when it is quite possible she is an alcoholic. The best strategy for the nurse to use is to ask several open-ended questions about drinking and look for some of the above-stated clues before deciding whether or not alcohol is a problem for the patient.

OBJECTIVE DATA
A physical assessment may reveal liver enlargement but may also show no abnormalities. Neurologic impairment may be apparent if the patient is intoxicated. However, in the patient with high tolerance, gait and coordination may seem within normal limits.

Laboratory evaluation of blood alcohol levels can confirm consumption. However, state laws vary on whether the patient must give consent before samples for blood levels are drawn in cases where a motor vehicle violation has occurred. Institutional policy should clearly outline the method for obtaining a blood alcohol level under these circumstances.

□ NURSING DIAGNOSES
Nursing diagnoses for the patient withdrawing from alcohol may include

Anxiety

Alteration in bowel elimination: diarrhea related to autonomic hyperactivity

Alteration in cardiac output: decreased as a result of tachycardia, hypertension

Ineffective individual coping related to control of life by drug

Potential fluid volume deficit related to nausea, vomiting, diaphoresis

Potential impaired gas exchange related to seizures

Functional incontinence (if seizures occur)

Noncompliance with alcohol withdrawal if able to gain access to the drug

Self-care deficit may be complete if the patient becomes confused or disoriented

Sensory–perceptual alterations related to visual and auditory hallucinations

Sleep pattern disturbance

Alteration in thought processes

Potential for violence directed at self or others related to confusion and disorientation

□ PLAN
The nursing care goals should focus on

1. Safe administration of benzodiazepine therapy to facilitate withdrawal
2. Protection of the patient from injury during the acute phase
3. Monitoring for side-effects and responding as necessary
4. Assisting the patient to accept help and treatment once the acute phase has passed (See Considerations for Alcoholic Rehabilitation, below.)

□ INTERVENTION
To avoid or minimize the late stage of alcohol withdrawal, once symptoms are identified, benzodiazepine therapy should begin as quickly as possible. Initial therapy may include an intravenous (IV) dose of one of the longer-acting benzodiazepines such as Librium and an intramuscular (IM) dose of thiamine. The regimen should go on for 5 to 6 days beginning with Librium doses of 25 mg to 100 mg either IM or by mouth every 3 hours to 4 hours on the first day and gradually decreasing the dose on each consecutive day. Treatment should not be ordered "prn" as is frequently done since some nurses will fail to administer the dose if the patient is quiet or not hallucinating. Failure to maintain the tranquilizer blood level may result in later escalation of the hallucinations and hyperactivity associated with withdrawal and endanger the patient. If the regimen is ordered prn, the nurse should establish with the physician the circumstances under which the medication is to be held and make an effort to have the order changed to a routine regimen.

In addition to the benzodiazines and thiamine, the patient will generally be started on multiple vitamins and folic acid to try to improve nutritional status. Initially he may also need sleeping medication to help him relax. However, once the initial detoxification regimen is completed, efforts should be made to avoid giving these patients any CNS drugs such as tranquilizers, sedatives, or analgesics even though the patients may request them. Alcoholics tend to want, subconsciously, to substitute other drugs for the missing alcohol and may try many manipulative tactics to get them. However, the goal of detoxification is to assist this patient to recognize that chemicals, particularly alcohol, are not an appropriate method for dealing with stress.

While the patient is going through the detoxification drug regimen the nurse should provide supportive care. The patient will need continuous reorientation, support, and guidance when dealing with hallucinations, limited stimulation to help him control his environment, and protection in a safe environment. The nurse uses active listening techniques and gentle touch to help the patient through this traumatic withdrawal. Vital signs should be taken every 15 minutes through the acute stages of withdrawal when the chance of seizures, hypertension, and tachycardia may be life threatening. Monitoring can be decreased to every 4 hours once the patient is stabilized. Skin turgor and mucous membranes should be checked to determine the presence of dehydration. Fluid and electrolyte replacement should be initiated if volume and electrolyte levels are low. Intake and output should also be monitored.

□ EVALUATION

The outcome criteria for judging successful withdrawal are that the patient becomes calmer, alert, reoriented to the environment, and suffers minimal damage to organ systems. However, once the patient is reoriented, he may quickly forget the withdrawal experience (or may have no memory of it at all). Discussion about rehabilitation needs to begin immediately.

Considerations for Alcoholic Rehabilitation

Alcohol counseling may be a frustrating experience for the beginner since many alcoholics refuse to acknowledge their problem even after a frightening withdrawal experience. It is easy for the nurse to get discouraged, begin to feel any intervention is a waste of time, and fail to make any referrals for such patients. To minimize this frustration, nurses, especially as students, should gain experience in dealing with alcoholics and participate in resource groups such as Alcoholics Anonymous or Al-Anon. The nurse's own attitude, as much as anything else, will influence her interaction with the alcoholic. Nurses who are realistic in their expectations will be less frustrated by the resistance many alcoholics offer and are frequently more successful in getting the alcoholic to seek help.

Some useful strategies for initiating dialogue about alcohol use include giving hope, presenting a positive view of how help can be obtained, using empathetic listening to focus on the problems as the patient sees them, and concentrating on the drinking problem rather than on other emotional problems. It may help to have a significant other present who knows the consequences of the person's drinking. This makes it harder for the patient to deny the effects. The nurse who initiates a dialogue encouraging the alcoholic to seek help must know of and be able to tap available resources to get the referral system started if the patient agrees to treatment. The nurse cannot rely on informing the patient of the resources; she must actively seek to get him enrolled.

Another aspect of rehabilitation and counseling concerns nurses who deal with colleagues impaired by alcohol. Again, the nurse must be aware of the available resources for such colleagues and be willing to assist the person to get the needed help once confronted. In addition to local Alcoholics Anonymous and mental health centers, resources may include employee assistance programs at the job, the state nurses' association, the state board of nursing, or local groups such as Nurses Care, Inc.

The first step is to identify the impaired colleague. The alcoholic nurse may be irritable with patients and staff; withdrawn; have frequent mood swings; prefer isolation as manifested by wanting to work nights or avoiding staff gatherings; offer elaborate excuses for behavior such as being late; have blackouts or complete memory loss for unit events or conversations; do the minimum amount of work necessary; have difficulty meeting deadlines; and chart illogically and sloppily (Miller, 1984). After identification, the nurse must be confronted with this behavior. Nurses tend to want to cover up for impaired colleagues and protect them from disciplinary action. What is needed, however, is to be comfortable and caring enough to offer to help the person overcome the problem and break the "conspiracy of silence" that protects these professionals and keeps them from seeking help. Supervisors need to state clearly what the consequences are of failure to get help and colleagues may need to be willing to accompany the impaired nurse in getting started. The problem is much greater than we perceive; in recent years, however, available resources have expanded greatly. There is less reason now than ever before to accept and cover up for the impaired nurse, and the benefit is improved work conditions for everyone and safer care for the patients.

Alcohol Deterrent

Disulfiram

(Antabuse)

Disulfiram is an antioxidant that blocks the oxidative metabolism of ethyl alcohol at the acetaldehyde stage. Ingestion of even small amounts of ethanol in the presence of disulfiram results in a 5- to 10-fold increase in blood acetaldehyde levels, which elicits a range of unpleasant symptoms known as the *disulfiram reaction* or *mal rouge.* Thus, disulfiram is employed for the management of properly motivated chronic alcoholics who desire to be placed in a situation of enforced sobriety. The threat of illness with consumption of alcohol is the prime deterrent with this drug. The drug is slowly absorbed and excreted, and the effects persist for up to 2 weeks after the last dose has been taken. Users must be made aware of the consequences of ingesting even small amounts of alcohol in any form whatsoever (*e.g.*, cough syrups, mouthwashes, cold preparations, food sauces, vinegars). Also, application of alcohol-containing liniments or lotions (rubbing alcohol, colognes, toilet waters, aftershaves) should be avoided, because the alcohol may be absorbed systemically. The disulfiram–alcohol reaction consists of flushing, nausea, sweating, thirst, throbbing in the head, dyspnea, palpitations, chest pain, tachycardia, hypotension, weakness, vertigo, blurred vision, confusion, and syncope. With large amounts of alcohol, serious adverse reactions can occur, including arrhythmias, congestive heart failure, respiratory depression, convulsions, and even death. The intensity of the reaction is dependent on the amounts of disulfiram and alcohol ingested. Symptoms are usually fully developed at a blood alcohol level of 50 mg/dl, and unconsciousness occurs at 125 mg/dl to 150 mg/dl.

MECHANISM AND ACTIONS
Disulfiram blocks conversion of acetaldehyde to acetic acid by inhibiting the enzyme aldehyde dehydrogenase. Thus, levels of acetaldehyde, a toxic intermediate, are increased. In the absence of alcohol, disulfiram produces virtually no effects.

USES
1. Adjunctive treatment of chronic alcoholism in conjunction with proper motivation and behavioral therapy

ADMINISTRATION AND DOSAGE
The drug is given orally in a single daily dose of 500 mg, usually for 1 to 2 weeks. Once the patient is fully recovered, a maintenance dose of 125 mg to 500 mg a day may be used until such time as the patient feels no further compulsion to drink.

FATE
Disulfiram is rapidly and completely absorbed from the GI tract. Optimal effects appear within 8 hours to 12 hours and may persist for up to 2 weeks following withdrawal of medication since the drug is highly lipid soluble and localizes in fatty tissue initially. The elimination rate is quite slow and the drug is excreted in the urine.

SIDE-EFFECTS/ADVERSE REACTIONS
The most frequently encountered side-effect in the absence of alcohol is drowsiness, which is usually transient. Other adverse effects attributed to disulfiram include headache, restlessness, fatigue, impotence, metallic taste, skin eruptions, optic or peripheral neuritis, tremor, arthropathy, and occasional psychotic reactions. The reactions observed in a person who consumes alcohol while taking disulfiram are listed above.

CONTRAINDICATIONS AND PRECAUTIONS
Absolute contraindications to disulfiram use are severe myocardial disease, coronary occlusion, psychoses, and pregnancy. Patients who have *recently* received alcohol or alcohol-containing products should also not be given disulfiram. *Cautious* use of disulfiram is warranted in persons with epilepsy, diabetes, hypothyroidism, cirrhosis, nephritis, or cerebral damage.

INTERACTIONS

1. Disulfiram may potentiate the effects of diazepam, chlordiazepoxide, oral anticoagulants, and phenytoin.
2. Disulfiram plus isoniazid can result in coordination difficulties and behavioral changes.
3. Paraldehyde is partially metabolized to acetaldehyde and can produce toxic reactions in the presence of disulfiram.
4. Metronidazole given together with disulfiram can elicit psychotic reactions.

NURSING CONSIDERATIONS

Disulfiram is successfully used in situations where the patient has developed a recognition and understanding of his alcoholism as a disease process and sees the use of drug therapy as a means of forcing himself to remain sober. Such a patient is generally very motivated to eliminate drinking from his social habits and is usually positive at the beginning of the therapy.

The patient starting on disulfiram needs to know the drug will exert its effect for 5 to 9 days after the last dose. This knowledge assures the patient of some protection against temptation even if he occasionally forgets to take the medication. It also enables the person to "plan a drunk" if he deliberately stops taking the medication. Such actions can be discussed in the treatment program to help the patient gain some perspective on his conscious and unconscious behavior.

In general, disulfiram therapy helps the alcoholic make a daily decision not to drink. The therapy is most useful in helping recovering alcoholics get through the compulsion period when they are least able to handle drinking situations.

In addition to emphasizing the effects of the disulfiram–alcohol interaction, the nurse also needs to review with this patient where hidden alcohol occurs in foods, drugs, and other forms mentioned earlier in this section. The worst hidden culprits are in liquid medications, including vitamins and analgesics, and in dental products, particularly cold sore and toothache remedies.

Successful use of disulfiram can be measured by the patient's abstinence from alcohol even in threatening social situations and evidence that he followed the regimen as prescribed. Even when a patient lapses in the drug therapy, his return helps staff to work on why he chose to drink again and helps give the patient a second chance.

CASE STUDY

Cora Simon, a 78-year-old widow who lives alone, is brought to the emergency room by ambulance accompanied by a neighbor who found her on the floor of her apartment. Cora is drowsy but arousable. Radiographs show she has a fracture of the right tibia and fibula. The physician decides to do an open reduction of the leg, and surgery is performed under general anesthesia. Cora is easily aroused in the early postoperative period but about 12 hours after returning from the recovery room she becomes very restless, diaphoretic, and anxious. Her blood pressure and pulse are slightly elevated. Several hours later nausea and vomiting are noted and Cora seems to be disoriented and having some auditory hallucinations. The nursing staff have called the physician twice, and on examining the patient he feels she is either slightly senile or having a reaction to the anesthesia. When Cora has a seizure the next day the diagnosis of alcohol withdrawal is made.

Discussion Questions

1. What symptoms in Cora's clinical picture were clues to the development of early alcohol withdrawal?
2. What information could have been obtained in the emergency room or postoperative unit to learn more about this patient's drinking history? Would it have been logical, given the information known, to pursue such information?
3. What should the treatment plan be for Cora at this point?
4. How can the nurse use these experiences to help Cora

recognize her problem? When would be the most appropriate time to begin such intervention?

5. What resources need to be assessed before planning a treatment plan for Cora?

6. What are some of the differences between helping the elderly to stop drinking and helping younger populations stop drinking?

REVIEW QUESTIONS

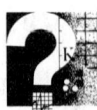

1. Briefly describe the metabolism of ethyl alcohol. What is meant by the term *zero-order kinetics* in relation to alcohol metabolism?

2. What is responsible for the apparent "stimulatory" effect observed initially with alcohol intake?

3. What is the generally accepted blood alcohol level under which it is considered legally safe to operate an automobile?

4. List several effects of alcoholic solutions applied *topically*.

5. Give the major toxic effects of chronic alcohol consumption on the (1) CNS, (2) GI tract, (3) liver, and (4) cardiovascular system.

6. For what may local injection of dehydrated alcohol be used?

7. What are the principal signs of methanol poisoning?

8. How does disulfiram (Antabuse) function as an alcohol deterrant?

9. List the stages of alcohol withdrawal in chronic users. In which patients should nurses be alert to potential alcohol withdrawal when alcoholism is not the primary diagnosis?

10. What should be the treatment and nursing care plan for the patient who is going through alcohol withdrawal?

11. How would you plan provision of alcohol information in a prenatal clinic?

12. What are some effective strategies to inform teenagers about the effects of alcohol?

13. Plan assessment and intervention strategies for the diabetic who wishes to have an occasional drink.

14. What local resources are available in your community or hospital for alcoholics and their significant others?

15. What state and local resources are available for nurses who are alcoholics? Are there employee assistance programs? How are referrals made?

BIBLIOGRAPHY

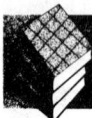

Brien JF, Loomis CW: Pharmacology of acetaldehyde. Can J Physiol Pharmacol 61:1, 1983

Criegler-Meringola D, Ryan D: The diabetic who takes a drink. Diabetes Educator 9:27, 1984

DiCicco-Bloom B, Space S, Zahourek RP: The homebound alcoholic. Am J Nurs 86:167, 1986

King KS: Three strikes against her: Female, old, and . . . drunk. Journal of Gerontological Nursing 10:30, 1984

Klatsky AR, Friedman JD, Siegelaub AB: Alcohol and mortality: A ten year Kaiser Permanente experience. Ann Intern Med 95:139, 1981

Majchrowicz E, Noble ED (eds): Biochemistry and Pharmacology of Ethanol, vol 1. New York, Plenum Press, 1979

McCarthy PA: Fetal alcohol syndrome and other alcohol related birth defects. Nurse Pract 8:33, 1983

Miller B: The confrontation process with impaired nurses. N.J. Nurse 14:6, 1984

Rector C, Foster ME: Assessment and care of the patient experiencing alcohol withdrawal syndrome. Critical Care Nurse 4:64, 1984

Reed JS, Liskow BI: Current medical treatment of alcohol withdrawal. Ration Drug Ther 21(2):1, 1987

Reisman B, Shrader RW: Effect of nurses' attitudes toward alcoholism on their referral rate for treatment. Occupational Health Nursing 32:273, 1984

Slawson M, Slawson S: When alcohol is contraindicated, don't forget . . . the hidden alcohol in drugs. RN 46:54, 1984

Spickard WA, Tucker PJ: An approach to alcoholism in a university medical center complex. JAMA 252:1894, 1984

Svitiik B: Helping the alcoholic patient on the road to recovery. Journal of Emergency Nursing 1:199, 1981

Wechsler H: Alcohol and other drug use and automobile safety: A survey of Boston area teenagers. J Sch Health 54:201, 1984

Antipsychotic Drugs

27

The antipsychotic drugs, represented by several chemically distinct but pharmacologically quite similar groups of compounds, are capable of improving the mood and calming the disturbed behavior of psychotic patients without causing marked sedation or habituation. Although the term *tranquilizer* has been used to describe these drugs, it is a misnomer because these agents fundamentally are not central nervous system (CNS) depressants. Rather, they appear to act principally at lower brain centers to improve the disturbed thought processes of the psychotic individual and therefore create a more favorable mental state for other forms of psychotherapy. In fact, the development of effective antipsychotic drugs revolutionized the institutional practice of psychiatry and saved countless thousands of patients from lives of confinement in locked psychiatric wards.

Antipsychotic drugs had their origin quite serendipitously. Chlorpromazine, a phenothiazine compound, was initially introduced in the early 1950s as an antihistamine and antiemetic. Observations that use of this drug in mentally disturbed persons produced an amelioration of some symptoms led to the subsequent licensing of chlorpromazine as an antipsychotic drug. The success of chlorpromazine has spawned a large number of imitators and today the physician is able to choose from nearly 20 compounds having the ability to modify the disturbed behavior of the psychotic individual.

Characteristics of Psychoses

The term *psychosis* denotes a variety of mental and emotional disorders in which mental function is impaired to the extent that the individual is unable to function socially in an acceptable manner. Symptoms are variable, depending on the etiology and the environment, and can include hostility, agitation, delusions, disordered thought processes, hallucinations, social withdrawal, lack of self-care, and paranoid ideation. *Schizophrenia* is probably the most common type of psychosis, characterized by a marked disturbance in normal thought processes, progressive social withdrawal, auditory hallucinations, and frequently by delusions. The possible influence of genetic predisposition on development of schizophrenia is a topic of considerable debate. While antipsychotic drug therapy does not cure schizophrenia, proper drug therapy together with psychotherapy frequently improves

the condition to such an extent that the individual can return to a productive life.

Other forms of psychosis include *organic psychoses*, which can result from brain damage due to tumors, trauma, infections, or strokes; *nonorganic psychoses* (affective disorders), such as depression or manic–depressive disorders; and *toxic psychoses*, which may occur following drug overdosage or drug withdrawal. These latter psychoses are less successfully managed by antipsychotic drugs than is schizophrenia.

Neurohormonal Correlates

Although the precise biochemical abnormalities responsible for the altered mentation of psychotic behavior are still not completely known, evidence has accumulated implicating dopamine as a major neurohormone controlling behavior and thought processes. More specifically, it is believed that many psychotic symptoms have their origin as a result of overactivity of dopaminergic pathways in the CNS, particularly in the so-called mesolimbic–frontal dopaminergic system. Implication of dopamine as a principal neurotransmitter governing emotional lability and regulated thought processes is based on several experimental and clinical observations: (1) most clinically effective antipsychotic drugs block postsynaptic dopamine receptors; (2) dopaminergic agonists, such as levodopa, can elicit schizophrenic behavior in high enough doses; and (3) drugs that enhance central dopaminergic function, such as the amphetamines, can produce a state closely resembling paranoid schizophrenia in overdosage. Of course, a disease as complex as schizophrenia doubtless is associated with multiple anatomic or biochemical deficits of central neuronal function, and altered functioning of no *one* substance can completely explain the myriad symptoms.

Classification of Antipsychotic Drugs

Structurally, the principal antipsychotic drugs can be divided into five groups, as shown in Table 27-1. In addition, several other drugs that affect central neuronal functioning in different ways will be discussed in this chapter. They are *lithium*, used in the control of manic–depressive psychoses; *pimozide*, used to control the erratic behavior of Gilles de la

Tourette's syndrome; *droperidol*, a unique tranquilizer; and *methotrimeprazine*, an analgesic.

The *phenothiazines* constitute the largest and most widely used group of antipsychotic drugs. Based on their structural configuration, they are divided into three groups: (1) aliphatics, (2) piperazines, and (3) piperidines. These groups differ in certain respects, as outlined in Table 27-1. The piperazines are the most potent phenothiazine derivatives and have the highest incidence of extrapyramidal side-effects (*i.e.*, involuntary motor movements—see Adverse Effects of Antipsychotic Drugs, below), whereas the aliphatics and piperidines in general possess the greatest sedative and hypotensive action. Antiemetic potency generally parallels antipsychotic potency, the only major exception being thioridazine, which is a potent antipsychotic essentially devoid of antiemetic activity.

The aliphatics exhibit the greatest anticholinergic activity among the phenothiazines, whereas the piperazines are only weak anticholinergics. Anticholinergic activity results in a wide range of annoying side-effects (xerostomia, blurred vision, urinary hesitancy) but also may reduce the incidence of extrapyramidal reactions.

Thioxanthene derivatives are chemically and pharmacologically similar to the phenothiazines, so the two classes can be used interchangeably. Clinical evidence of an antidepressant action for the thioxanthenes suggests that these agents might be more beneficial than phenothiazines in certain types of withdrawn, retarded, or apathetic psychotic states.

Haloperidol, a *butyrophenone derivative*, is a potent antipsychotic agent providing an alternative to the phenothiazines possibly in psychotic states

Table 27-1
Comparison of Effects of Antipsychotic Drugs

	Approximate Potency Relative to Chlorpromazine	Relative Incidence of Side-Effects			
		Extrapyramidal Symptoms	Sedation	Hypotension	Anticholinergic
Phenothiazines					
Aliphatics					
chlorpromazine	1	++	+++	+++	++
promazine	0.5	++	++	++	+++
triflupromazine	4	++	+++	++	+++
Piperazines					
acetophenazine	5	+++	++	+	++
fluphenazine	50	+++	+	+	+
perphenazine	12	+++	+	+	++
prochlorperazine	10	+++	++	+	+
trifluoperazine	25	+++	+	+	+
Piperidines					
mesoridazine	2	+	+++	++	++
thioridazine	1	+	+++	+++	+++
Thioxanthenes					
chlorprothixene	1	++	+++	+++	++
thiothixene	25	+++	+	++	+
Butyrophenone					
haloperidol	50	+++	+	+	+
Indolone					
molindone	5	+++	++	++	++
Dibenzoxazepine					
loxapine	5	+++	++	++	+

Key: +++, frequent; ++, occasional; +, infrequent

characterized by agitation, aggressiveness, or hostility. Its toxicity is quite high compared to that of the piperazine group of phenothiazines, but it is only a weak anticholinergic, and is not associated with a significant degree of orthostatic hypotension. This latter property makes it useful in many older patients.

Newer drugs used to control psychotic symptoms are chemically unrelated to other antipsychotic drugs, but are pharmacologically and toxicologically similar. Molindone and loxapine may provide alternatives to the other antipsychotics in unresponsive or intolerant patients but have no distinct advantages over any of the older compounds, except in a somewhat lower incidence of certain side-effects.

A comparison of the potencies and incidence of common side-effects among the various classes of antipsychotic drugs is presented in Table 27-1. Although distinct quantitative differences in milligram potency and toxicologic properties are evident among the different groups, no significant qualitative differences exist regarding the effectiveness of each drug; that is, when the drugs are used in therapeutically equivalent doses, their clinical efficacy is essentially equal. Choice of an antipsychotic drug, therefore, is based largely on the desire to minimize particular types of side-effects in different psychotic populations (e.g., reduced sedative effects in persons operating machinery, or reduced hypotensive effects in older patients).

Pharmacologic Effects

The pharmacologic actions of the antipsychotic agents are quite complex. In addition to their behavior-modifying effects, the agents have a range of other central and peripheral effects, the extent of which differs among the various chemical groups. An outline of the principal pharmacologic actions of the antipsychotic drugs is presented in Table 27-2.

Table 27-2
Pharmacologic Effects of Antipsychotic Drugs

Central Nervous System

Antipsychotic effect—Reduced agitation, emotional quieting, decreased paranoid ideation, and lessening of hallucinations and disturbed thought processes
Antiemetic effect—Decreased sensitivity of chemoreceptor trigger zone (CTZ) in medulla to activation by drugs or toxins and direct depression of brain stem vomiting center in large doses
Impaired temperature regulation—Hypothermia caused by increased heat loss and decreased compensatory heat production
Endocrine effects—Inhibition of follicle-stimulating hormone and luteinizing hormone release, and increased release of lactogenic hormone (prolactin), resulting in abnormal lactation. Hormonal effects are due to the blocking action of antipsychotic drugs on dopamine receptors either in the hypothalamic–pituitary pathway or on anterior pituitary cells themselves.
Motor effects—Increased involuntary muscle activity (e.g., tremors, dyskinesias, akathisias) caused by dopamine blockade in motor-integrating areas of the CNS

Peripheral Nervous System

Antiadrenergic effects—Blockage of central and peripheral alpha receptors, decreasing sympathetic outflow from the vasomotor center and vascular sympathetic tone, leading to orthostatic hypotension and reflex tachycardia
Anticholinergic/antihistamine effects—Blockade of cholinergic (largely muscarinic) and histaminergic activity

Other

Antiarrhythmic effects—Quinidine-like depressant action on the myocardium, and local anesthetic action
Diuretic effect—Depression of antidiuretic hormone release, and inhibition of water and electrolyte reabsorption (weak effect)

As indicated earlier, a primary action of these agents is to block dopaminergic transmission in the CNS. This dopamine-blocking action probably is responsible for both the therapeutic effects of the drugs as well as several of the adverse effects.

Antipsychotic

Blockade of postsynaptic dopamine receptor sites in the mesolimbic system (i.e., septum, nucleus accumbens, thalamus, hypothalamus, amygdala) appears to reduce the primary symptoms of schizophrenia (e.g., agitation, paranoid ideation, hallucinations, social isolation). The lessening in disturbed thought processes and the improvement in social interactive behaviors are vital for creating a mental state that is more receptive to other forms of psychotherapy and greatly aids the clinician in effectively communicating with the psychotic patient.

Not all schizophrenic patients show improvement with antipsychotic drugs and not all dopamine antagonists are effective antipsychotic drugs. Thus, while certainly contributory, dopamine blockade is probably not the *sole* action of the clinically effective antipsychotic drugs in reducing psychotic behavior.

Antiemetic

The dopamine-blocking action of antipsychotic drugs is also responsible for the antiemetic effect of the drugs. The purported site of action in this instance is the chemoreceptor trigger zone (CTZ) in the medulla, which is partially under dopaminergic control. Dopamine blockade in the CTZ reduces the activating effect of drugs, toxins, and other substances on this medullary relay center, which in turn decreases the activation of the vomiting center. Large doses of antipsychotic drugs may also directly inhibit the functioning of the vomiting center itself.

Endocrine

A third major site of dopamine receptor blockade in the CNS, namely the hypothalamic–pituitary axis, is responsible for several endocrine disturbances characteristic of antipsychotic drug ther-apy. Antagonism of dopamine activity in the tuberoinfundibular pathway releases prolactin (luteotropic hormone, LTH) from tonic inhibitory control by way of prolactin inhibitory factor in the hypothalamus. Thus, increased prolactin secretion occurs, resulting in abnormal lactation. Conversely, the release of follicle-stimulating hormone (FSH) and luteinizing hormone (LH) appears to be inhibited by dopamine receptor blockade, and there have been reports of amenorrhea, infertility, and impotence in persons receiving antipsychotic drugs.

Motor

Motor-integrating pathways in the CNS, such as the nigrostriatal system, are largely dopamine mediated, and dopamine is believed to function as an inhibitory neurotransmitter. Antagonism of dopamine receptors in the striatum by antipsychotic drugs leads to the development of a series of involuntary motor movements, termed *extrapyramidal reactions.* Proper functioning of striatal motor-integrating centers depends on a balance between the action of dopamine, an inhibitory transmitter, and acetylcholine, an excitatory transmitter. Loss of dopaminergic activity subsequent to receptor blockade allows cholinergic activity to proceed unchecked, giving rise to a series of disordered motor movements. These movements, which are described in greater detail below, generally appear early in the course of therapy and can be minimized by careful attention to dosage and use of a centrally acting anticholinergic.

Prolonged administration of antipsychotic drugs may result in a different type of involuntary muscle activity centered in the area of the face and mouth. Termed *oropharyngeal* or *tardive dyskinesia,* this phenomenon generally appears later in the course of therapy and is believed to be due to slowly developing receptor supersensitivity as a consequence of long-term blockade. As is discussed below, it is difficult to treat and every effort should be made to delay or prevent its onset.

Cardiovascular

Antipsychotic drugs elicit varying degrees of hypotension, primarily of the orthostatic type, and this is frequently associated with reflex tachycardia. Tolerance to the hypotensive action of antipsychotic drugs may develop within several weeks, but it is not always complete even with prolonged use. The mechanism responsible for this orthostatic hypotension is probably an alpha-adrenergic blocking effect, both centrally (at the level of the brain stem vasomotor centers) and peripherally, which leads to decreased sympathetic outflow from brain stem cardiovascular-regulating centers and reduced peripheral sympathetic vascular tone.

Electrocardiographic changes are noted to a significant degree with some antipsychotic drugs. Abnormalities observed most often are prolongation of the Q-T interval, blunting of the T wave (especially with thioridazine), and depression of the S-T segment. The clinical significance of these changes is unclear, and they are usually readily reversible on cessation of the drug. On the other hand, chlorpromazine and possibly other antipsychotic drugs may have an antiarrhythmic effect, which can result from a quinidine-like depressant or local anesthetic action on the myocardium.

Other

Evidence has accumulated indicating that many antipsychotic drugs have the ability to block serotonin and histamine-1 receptors, which may contribute to the sedative action of these drugs. As indicated in Table 27-1, the clinically useful antipsychotic agents possess varying degrees of cholinergic blocking effects as well. A significant anticholinergic action may reduce the incidence and severity of extrapyramidal reactions associated with a particular antipsychotic drug (see Adverse Effects of Antipsychotic Drugs, below), but also leads to a number of common side-effects, such as dry mouth, blurred vision, urinary hesitancy, and constipation. A marked central anticholinergic action has also been implicated as a possible cause of a toxic–confusional state sometimes noted with high doses of antipsychotic drugs.

Altered electroencephalographic (EEG) patterns have been observed during therapy with antipsychotic drugs, manifested chiefly as slowing and increased synchronization (i.e., decreased pattern variability). A lowered seizure threshold has occurred with some antipsychotic drugs, especially the aliphatic phenothiazines, and precipitation of seizure activity has been reported.

A weak diuretic effect has been seen with some antipsychotics (e.g., chlorpromazine), perhaps due to increased secretion of antidiuretic hormone

(ADH) or impaired reabsorption of water and electrolytes by the renal tubules.

Adverse Effects

The antipsychotic drugs have a considerable margin of safety, and deaths from overdosage are relatively rare. However, use of these drugs is frequently associated with a wide range of untoward reactions, from innocuous but annoying side-effects such as constipation, urinary hesitancy, drowsiness, nasal stuffiness, and weight gain to serious cardiovascular, endocrine, and especially neuromuscular complications. Many of the untoward reactions experienced with antipsychotic drugs are merely extensions of their pharmacologic actions and have been discussed briefly above. The likelihood of antipsychotic drugs to cause a particular adverse effect is variable, and the relative frequency of some important adverse effects among the individual drugs is shown in Table 27-1. The following discussion will consider the major types of adverse reactions seen with antipsychotic drug use.

Neurologic

Several types of involuntary muscle activities are frequently seen with antipsychotic drug use, and these neurologic disturbances are generally referred to as *extrapyramidal reactions*. Some of these neurologic disturbances, such as parkinsonian-like syndrome, akathisia, and acute dystonic reactions, appear in the early stages of drug therapy (i.e., 1 week–4 weeks). Blockade of dopamine receptors in the basal ganglia (caudate, putamen, globus pallidus, and related nuclei), a motor-integrating center in the CNS, is believed to underlie many of the extrapyramidal reactions noted with the antipsychotic drugs.

The *parkinsonian-like* syndrome is characterized by akinesia (slowed movement), rigidity, and tremor at rest. It can be treated with typical anticholinergic antiparkinsonian drugs (see Chap. 31), but is often self-limiting and may respond simply to a reduction in the dosage of the antipsychotic drug.

Akathisia, or extreme motor restlessness, may be mistaken for agitation in some patients. The individual feels compelled to be in constant movement, and this syndrome usually responds best to a dosage reduction; antiparkinsonian drugs are of limited benefit. *Acute dystonic reactions* may be manifested as grimacing, difficulty in speech or swallowing, oculogyric crisis (upward rotation of the eyeballs), muscle spasms of the neck or throat, and extensor rigidity of the back muscles. The reactions can be mistaken for hysteria or seizures. Antiparkinsonian drugs are quite effective in relieving these acute dystonic reactions, and diphenhydramine (Benadryl) is considered by many to be the drug of choice.

In contrast to these early-appearing neurologic disturbances, *tardive dyskinesia* is a slowly developing syndrome that is seen in a significant number of patients on chronic antipsychotic drug therapy. Tardive dyskinesia is most prevalent in older females, although it can occur at any age in either sex. Estimates of its frequency range from 10% to 50% of chronically treated patients. The syndrome is primarily orofacial in nature and is characterized by chewing motions, protrusion of the tongue, puffing of the cheeks, and puckering of the mouth. Occasionally, purposeless movements of the extremities are noted as well. Early recognition is important, since this syndrome is very difficult to treat once it is fully developed and may persist even after the antipsychotic drug has been discontinued. It is proposed that these neurologic manifestations result from a gradually developing *supersensitivity* of central dopamine receptor sites as a consequence of prolonged blockade by the antipsychotic drug. Thus, preventing the onset of tardive dyskinesia by using the minimal amount of drug necessary and observing "drug-free holidays" during the course of chronic treatment is the preferred approach. Many therapies have been suggested for reducing the symptoms once they have developed, but to date, results have been disappointing. Some measures that may be successful in ameliorating tardive dyskinesia include eliminating antiparkinsonian, anticholinergic drugs from the regimen; gradual discontinuation of the antipsychotic drug; and use of sedatives (*e.g.*, diazepam), beta-blockers (*e.g.*, propranolol), and drugs that can serve as precursors of acetylcholine (*e.g.*, lecithin, choline), thereby increasing its availability in those brain areas where dopamine activity has become dominant.

Autonomic/Cardiovascular

Most antipsychotic drugs possess some cholinergic blocking action, and while this action may reduce the incidence of extrapyramidal reactions seen with a particular drug, it can result in a variety of annoying side-effects, such as blurred vision, dry mouth, urinary hesitancy, and constipation. In addition, drugs with a strong anticholinergic action, like thioridazine or the aliphatic phenothiazines, may disturb the normal rhythm of the heart, can lead to impotence or failure to ejaculate, and have been linked to development of a toxic-confusional state in high doses.

Orthostatic hypotension occurs to varying degrees with use of antipsychotic drugs, and may be related to blockade of peripheral alpha-adrenergic receptors. Increased pulse rate has also been linked to antipsychotic drug therapy.

Endocrine

The principal endocrine abnormalities seen with antipsychotic drugs are amenorrhea, galactorrhea, gynecomastia in males, and altered libido. These changes are presumably the result of interference with the normal regulatory function of dopamine on the release of pituitary hormones through the tuberoinfundibular pathway. Other possible endocrine-related effects of antipsychotic drugs are weight gain and, as previously mentioned, impotence and infertility.

Other

Many other untoward reactions have been reported in patients receiving antipsychotic drugs and are reviewed in the general discussion of these drugs that follows. Much variation exists among the different drugs in the incidence of other untoward reactions and generalities should be avoided. The aliphatic phenothiazines, such as the prototype drug chlorpromazine, have been associated with such adverse effects as corneal deposits, jaundice, and agranulocytosis but the incidence of these reactions is relatively rare. Dermatologic reactions, such as urticaria, rash, pruritus, and photosensitization, are possible with most antipsychotic drugs, and long-term use has resulted in cases of abnormal pigmentation.

The following discussion deals with the pharmacology of the antipsychotic drugs as a group. Information specific to each individual drug is found in Table 27-3, along with pertinent dosage information.

(*Text continues on p. 500.*)

Table 27-3
Antipsychotic Drugs

Drug	Preparations	Usual Dosage Range	Clinical Considerations
Phenothiazines			
Aliphatics chlorpromazine (Thorazine and various other manufacturers)	Tablets—10 mg, 25 mg, 50 mg, 100 mg, 200 mg Sustained-release capsules —30 mg, 75 mg, 150 mg, 200 mg, 300 mg Syrup—10 mg/5 ml Concentrate—30 mg/ml, 100 mg/ml Suppositories—25 mg, 100 mg Injection—25 mg/ml	*Adults* *Psychoses* Oral—Initially 50 mg–100 mg/day; increase until desired effect occurs; usual maintenance range is 300 mg–400 mg/day IM—Initially 25 mg; increase gradually up to 400 mg every 4 h–6 h until patient is quiet and cooperative; substitute oral dosage when possible *Nausea/vomiting* Oral—10 mg–25 mg every 4 h–6 h IM—25 mg–50 mg every 3 h–4 h Rectal—50 mg–100 mg every 6 h–8 h *Preoperative sedation* Oral—25 mg–50 mg IM—12.5 mg–25 mg *Porphyria* Oral–25 mg–50 mg three to four times/day IM—25 mg three to four times/day *Tetanus* IM, IV—25 mg–50 mg three to four times/day *Hiccups* Oral—25 mg–50 mg three to four times/day IM—25 mg–50 mg IV—25 mg–50 mg diluted in 500 ml–1000 ml saline by infusion *Children* Oral—0.25 mg/lb two to four times/day Rectal—0.5 mg/lb every 6 h–8 h IM—0.125 mg–0.25 mg/lb every 6 h–8 h IV—0.25 mg/lb	Used in acute and chronic psychoses, manic phase of manic–depressive psychoses, for pre- and postoperative sedation, intractable hiccups, acute intermittent porphyria, tetanus, and control of severe nausea and vomiting resulting from drugs, surgery, or toxins; plasma levels following IM injection are several times higher than following oral administration; duration of action ranges from 3 h–6 h; high incidence of drowsiness, dizziness, hypotension, and other side-effects, especially during first few weeks of therapy and in older patients; thus, extent of use has declined; IV solution should be diluted to 1 mg/ml in saline and administered at a rate of 1 mg/min; doses in excess of 1000 mg/day for prolonged periods are not recommended.
promazine (Prozine, Sparine)	Tablets—25 mg, 50 mg, 100 mg Syrup—10 mg/5 ml Injection—25 mg/ml, 50 mg/ml	*Adults* Initially—50 mg–150 mg IM Maintenance—10 mg–200 mg every 4 h–6 h orally or IM as required *Children* (over 12 yr) 10 mg–25 mg every 4 h–6 h	Used primarily for management of psychotic disorders; the preferred parenteral route is IM; IV administration is recommended only in hospitalized patients; when used IV, injections

(continued)

Table 27-3 (continued)
Antipsychotic Drugs

Drug	Preparations	Usual Dosage Range	Clinical Considerations
Phenothiazines (continued) *Aliphatics* (continued)			
promazine (Prozine, Sparine) (continued)			should be given slowly in diluted solutions (25 mg/ml or less); concentrate for oral use should be diluted in fruit juice or other flavored vehicle (2 tsp of diluent for every 25 mg of drug); it is less potent and equally toxic compared to chlorpromazine.
triflupromazine (Vesprin)	Injection—10 mg/ml, 20 mg/ml	*Adults* *Psychoses* IM—60 mg–150 mg/day *Nausea/vomiting* IM—5 mg–15 mg every 4 hours IV—1 mg–3 mg *Children (over 2 yr):* *Psychoses* IM—0.2 mg–0.25 mg/kg (maximum 10 mg) *Nausea/vomiting* 0.2 mg–0.25 mg/kg IM (maximum 10 mg)	Effective in psychotic disorders (other than psychotic depression) and for control of nausea and vomiting; sedation and extrapyramidal reactions are common with parenteral use and in the elderly and debilitated; it has been used as an adjunct for pre- and postoperative management.
Piperazines acetophenazine (Tindal)	Tablets—20 mg	*Adults* 20 mg three times/day (80 mg–120 mg/day in hospitalized patients) *Children* 0.8 mg–1.6 mg/kg/day	Used for management of psychotic disorders. In patients with insomnia, last tablet should be taken 1 hour before bedtime.
fluphenazine (Permitil, Prolixin)	Tablets—1 mg, 2.5 mg, 5 mg, 10 mg Elixir—2.5 mg/5 ml Concentrate—5 mg/ml Injection HCl—2.5 mg/ml Enanthate—25 mg/ml Decanoate—25 mg/ml	Oral Initially—2.5 mg–10 mg/day (maximum 20 mg) Maintenance—1 mg–5 mg/day IM HCl—1.25 mg two to four times/day (range 2.5 mg–10 mg/day in divided doses) Enanthate/decanoate (esters in a sesame oil vehicle)—12.5 mg–25 mg every 2 weeks to 3 weeks (may also be given SC): range—12.5 mg–100 mg at 1-week to 3-week intervals	Used for control of psychotic manifestations; oral dosage forms and HCl injection are rapid acting and can be used initially to stabilize patient; enanthate and decanoate salts are released slowly from tissue sites and thus have a prolonged effect (1 wk–4 wk); indicated for maintenance therapy in patients who cannot be relied on to follow a regular oral dosage schedule; if given cautiously in low doses, may be useful in patients who are hypersensitive to other phenothiazines; very potent drug with high incidence of extrapyramidal reactions and mental depression; decan- *(continued)*

Table 27-3 (continued)
Antipsychotic Drugs

Drug	Preparations	Usual Dosage Range	Clinical Considerations
Phenothiazines (continued)			
Piperazines (continued)			
fluphenazine (Permitil, Prolixin) (continued)			oate may have a lower incidence of extrapyramidal side-effects than other dosage forms; monitor renal function and blood picture periodically in patients on long-term therapy; protect solutions from light, and use dry syringe and needle for injection because moisture may cloud the solution; avoid use of antacids with oral dosage forms, because GI absorption is impaired; due to prolonged effects of enanthate and decanoate salts, advise patients to report appearance of side-effects immediately; not indicated in children.
perphenazine (Trilafon)	Tablets—2 mg, 4 mg, 8 mg, 16 mg Repeat-action tablets—8 mg Concentrate—16 mg/5 ml Injection—5 mg/ml	Oral *Psychoses*—8 mg–16 mg two to four times/day (maximum 64 mg/day) initially; reduce to 4 mg–8 mg three times/day for maintenance *Anxiety and tension states*—2 mg–4 mg three times/day *Nausea and vomiting*—8 mg–16 mg/day in divided doses IM—Initially 5 mg–10 mg; repeat every 6 h (maximum 30 mg/day); switch to oral therapy as soon as possible IV—severe vomiting only—1 mg/minute infusion of an 0.5 mg/ml dilution (maximum 5 mg)	Effective in psychoses and in the control of severe nausea and vomiting due to surgery or other acute situations; may also be effective in the management of anxiety and tension due to severe neuroses and for control of intractable hiccups; do not use in children under age 12; repeat-action tablets are given twice a day; high incidence of extrapyramidal reactions; transient hypotension can occur, especially if given IV; keep patient recumbent, and monitor pulse and pressure; oral concentrate should be diluted (2 oz diluent/5 ml concentrate) with fruit juice, milk, carbonated beverage, or other liquid (tea is not recommended).
prochlorperazine (Chlorpazine, Compazine)	Tablets—5 mg, 10 mg, 25 mg Capsules—(sustained-release) 10 mg, 15 mg, 30 mg Syrup—5 mg/5 ml Suppositories—2.5 mg, 5 mg, 25 mg Injection—5 mg/ml	*Adults* *Psychoses* Oral—10 mg three to four times/day, increased gradually until maximum effect (usually 100 mg–150 mg/day) IM—10 mg–20 mg ini-	Used for control of psychotic manifestations in adults and children over 2 years and for relief of nausea and vomiting; widely used pre- and postoperatively; do not use in short-term vomiting in

(continued)

Table 27-3 (continued)
Antipsychotic Drugs

Drug	Preparations	Usual Dosage Range	Clinical Considerations
Phenothiazines (continued) *Piperazines* (continued)			
prochlorperazine (Chlorpazine, Compazine) (continued)		tially; repeat in 2 h–4 h (switch to oral form as soon as possible) *Nausea/vomiting* Oral—5 mg–10 mg three to four times/day Rectal—25 mg twice/day IM—5 mg–10 mg; repeat every 3 h–4 h to a maximum of 40 mg/day IV (severe vomiting)—5 mg–10 mg IV injection or 20 mg added to 1 liter of IV infusion 15 min–30 min before induction of anesthesia *Children* (over 2 yr and 20 lb): *Psychoses* Oral/rectal—2.5 mg two to three times/day IM—0.06 mg/lb *Nausea/vomiting* Oral/rectal—2.5 mg–5 mg one to two times/day based on weight IM—0.06 mg/lb	children or for vomiting of unknown cause; discontinue if signs of restlessness or excitement occur; inject deeply IM (avoid SC use), and do not mix solution with other agents in same syringe; do not confuse 2.5-mg child suppository with 25-mg adult suppository; use cautiously in the elderly or debilitated and in children who are dehydrated or who have an acute illness because extrapyramidal reactions are common; monitor blood pressure during IV use, because hypotension is likely to occur; supervise ambulation following parenteral use.
trifluoperazine (Stelazine, Suprazine)	Tablets—1 mg, 2 mg, 5 mg, 10 mg Concentrate—10 mg/ml Injection—2 mg/ml	*Adults* Oral—Initially 2 mg–5 mg twice/day (maximum 40 mg/day); maintenance—1 mg–2 mg twice/day IM—1 mg–2 mg every 4 h–6 h (maximum 10 mg/ day) *Children* (over 6 yr) Oral—1 mg one to two times/day (maximum 15 mg/day in older children) IM—1 mg one to two times/day	Indicated for treatment of psychotic disorders and for controlling manifestations of severe psychoneuroses; very potent agent with high incidence of extrapyramidal reactions; maximum response may be delayed 2 weeks to 3 weeks; increase dosage very slowly in elderly or debilitated patients; prolonged action of the drug allows once-a-day dosage in many less severe cases; dilute concentrate in 60 ml of appropriate vehicle (liquid or semisolid) to aid palatability; do not give IM injections more frequently than every 4 h because of danger of cumulation.
Piperidines mesoridazine (Serentil)	Tablets—10 mg, 25 mg, 50 mg, 100 mg Concentrate—25 mg/ml Injection—25 mg/ml	*Psychoses* Oral—Initially 25 mg–50 mg three times/day (range 100 mg–400 mg/day)	Used for treatment of schizophrenia, chronic brain syndrome, and psychoneuroses, and as ad-

(continued)

Table 27-3 (continued)
Antipsychotic Drugs

Drug	Preparations	Usual Dosage Range	Clinical Considerations
Phenothiazines (continued) *Piperidines* (continued)			
mesoridazine (Serentil) (continued)		IM—25 mg; repeat in 30 min–60 min if necessary (range 25 mg–200 mg/day) *Neuroses* Oral—10 mg three times/day (range 30 mg–150 mg/day) *Alcoholism* 25 mg twice/day (range 50 mg–200 mg/day)	junctive therapy in acute and chronic alcoholism; weak antiemetic; low incidence of extrapyramidal reactions but very sedating; may reduce hyperactive behavior associated with mental deficient states; not recommended in children under 12; concentrate should be diluted prior to use.
thioridazine (Mellaril, Millazine)	Tablets—10 mg, 15 mg, 25 mg, 50 mg, 100 mg, 150 mg, 200 mg Concentrate—30 mg/ml, 100 mg/ml Suspension—25 mg/5 ml, 100 mg/5 ml	*Adults* *Psychoses* Initially—50 mg–100 mg three times/day; maintenance—200 mg–800 mg/day in two to four divided doses *Depressive neuroses* Initially—25 mg three times/day, maintenance—20 mg–200 mg/day in three to four divided doses *Children* (over 2 yr): 0.5 mg–3.0 mg/kg/day depending on severity of condition	Indicated for psychotic disorders and short-term treatment of depressive neuroses; possibly useful in hyperactive or aggressive children, alcohol withdrawal, intractable pain, and senility; low incidence of extrapyramidal reactions and no antiemetic action, but strong anticholinergic effect and highly sedating; abnormal ECG readings have been noted, especially at high doses; may be potentially cardiotoxic; frequently produces dryness of the mouth, constipation, urinary retention, and impotence in early stages of therapy; discontinue drug or reduce dosage if visual changes (reduced or brownish vision, impaired night vision) occur; periodic blood and liver function tests should be performed during prolonged therapy; dilute oral concentrate immediately prior to use with fruit juice or water.
Thioxanthenes			
chlorprothixene (Taractan)	Tablets—10 mg, 25 mg, 50 mg, 100 mg Concentrate—20 mg/ml Injection—12.5 mg/ml	*Adults* Oral—Initially 25 mg–50 mg three to four times/day; increase to optimal level (maximum 600 mg/day) IM—25 mg–50 mg three to four times/day; substitute	Effective in acute and chronic schizophrenia; produces significant sedation and orthostatic hypotension; when used IM, keep patient recumbent during administration; do not give IM in children *(continued)*

Table 27-3 (continued)
Antipsychotic Drugs

Drug	Preparations	Usual Dosage Range	Clinical Considerations
Thioxanthenes (continued)			
chlorprothixene (Taractan) (continued)		oral therapy as soon as possible *Children* Oral—10 mg–25 mg three to four times/day IM—Over 12 yr, same as adult dose	under age 12, or orally in children under age 6; anticholinergic side-effects are prominent.
thiothixene (Navane)	Capsules—1 mg, 2 mg, 5 mg, 10 mg, 20 mg Concentrate—5 mg/ml Injection—2 mg/ml, 5 mg/ml	Oral—Initially 2 mg–5 mg two to three times/day; maintenance 20 mg–60 mg/day in divided doses IM—4 mg two to four times/day (usual range 16 mg–20 mg/day)	Used for management of acute and chronic schizophrenia; not for use in children under age 12; high incidence of extrapyramidal reactions and drowsiness in early stages of therapy; therapeutic effects may take several weeks to develop with oral administration; do not withdraw drug abruptly because delirium can occur; dosage may need to be adjusted when switching from IM to oral administration.
Butyrophenone			
haloperidol (Haldol)	Tablets—0.5 mg, 1 mg, 2 mg, 5 mg, 10 mg, 20 mg Concentrate—2 mg/ml Injection—5 mg/ml Depot injection—(decanoate) 50 mg/ml	*Adults* Oral—0.5 mg–5 mg two to three times/day depending on symptoms (maximum 100 mg/day) IM—2 mg–5 mg (up to 30 mg if necessary); repeat at 4-h to 8-h intervals as needed Depot injection—10×–15× daily oral dose IM every 4 weeks *Children* (3 yr–12 yr) 0.5 mg/day initially in two to three divided doses; increase at 0.5 mg increments every 5 to 7 days until desired effect (range is 0.05 mg/kg/day–0.15 mg/kg/day)	Indicated in psychotic disorders, manic phase of manic–depressive psychoses, and for management of tics and vocal utterances of Gilles de la Tourette's disease; very potent antipsychotic with high incidence of extrapyramidal reactions; strong antiemetic; less sedation and hypotension than with many other similar drugs; do not use in children under age 3 or in parkinsonian patients (drug is a potent dopamine-blocking agent); use cautiously in epileptic individuals because drug may lower convulsive threshold; when used for manic episodes, be alert for reversal to severe depression, which may invite suicidal attempts; concomitant use with lithium may elicit dyskinesias, parkinsonian-like symptoms, or dementia; *(continued)*

Table 27-3 (continued)
Antipsychotic Drugs

Drug	Preparations	Usual Dosage Range	Clinical Considerations
Butyrophenone (continued)			
haloperidol (Haldol) (continued)			observe patients closely, and provide emotional support as necessary; perform periodic liver function and blood studies; depot injection is for chronic psychotic patients; it is given IM only and is not recommended in children.
Indolone			
molindone (Moban)	Tablets—5 mg, 10 mg, 25 mg, 50 mg, 100 mg Concentrate—20 mg/ml	Initially—50 mg–75 mg/day Maintenance—5 mg–25 mg three to four times/day depending on symptoms (maximum 225 mg/day)	Used for control of schizophrenia; not recommended in children under 12; provides an alternative drug to the phenothiazines and thioxanthenes in unresponsive patients, although actions are essentially identical to other classes of antipsychotics; high degree of initial drowsiness; resumption of menses in previously amenorrheal women has been reported; no ophthalmologic complications have occurred; tablet contains calcium, which may interfere with GI absorption of phenytoin and tetracyclines.
Dibenzoxazepine			
loxapine (Loxitane)	Capsules—5 mg, 10 mg, 25 mg, 50 mg Concentrate—25 mg/ml Injection—50 mg/ml	Oral—Initially 10 mg twice/day; increase to optimal levels (usually 60 mg–100 mg/day) (maximum 250 mg/day) IM—12.5 mg–50 mg every 4 h–6 hours to control acutely agitated patients	Indicated for manifestations of schizophrenia; elicits strong sedation in early therapy, lowers convulsive threshold, produces hypotension, and is an anticholinergic of moderate potency; has antiemetic activity and may produce ocular toxicity; not recommended in children under age 16; produces frequent extrapyramidal reactions, usually parkinsonian-like in nature; no endocrine abnormalities have been reported; concentrate should be mixed with orange or grapefruit juice before administration.

Primary Antipsychotic Drugs

Phenothiazines, Thioxanthenes, Haloperidol, Molindone, and Loxapine

MECHANISM AND ACTIONS
The mechanism of action of antipsychotic drugs is complex and not completely understood; they act primarily at several subcortical brain sites, including the limbic system, hypothalamus, and brain stem. Among the known effects of the drugs are reduction of intraneuronal levels of cyclic adenosine monophosphate (AMP) in brain regions associated with emotion and behavior and decreased cortical sensory input from ascending spinal tracts by way of collateral nerves to the reticular formation. The principal biochemical effect of the antipsychotic drugs is a competitive antagonism at dopamine receptor sites. Other biochemical mechanisms of action include increased dopamine turnover, inhibition of neuronal uptake of norepinephrine and serotonin, and suppression of acetylcholine release. No appreciable direct cortical depression is evident. The drugs produce varying degrees of sedation, antiemesis, hypothermia, and altered pituitary hormone release in addition to an antipsychotic action. Peripheral actions responsible for many of the observed side-effects include antiadrenergic (alpha-blocking effect) and anticholinergic activity, as well as some degree of antiserotonergic, local anesthetic, and a quinidine-like cardiac depressant effect. These latter effects vary in degree among the different drugs.

USES
See Table 27-3 for specific indications of each drug.
1. Management of acute and chronic psychoses, either organic or drug-induced
2. Control of the manic phase of manic–depressive psychoses (lithium)
3. Relief of severe nausea and vomiting (especially prochlorperazine)
4. Control of intractable hiccups
5. Relief of anxiety, apprehension, and agitation associated with a variety of somatic disorders, or prior to surgery
6. Facilitation of alcohol withdrawal
7. Adjunctive treatment of tetanus and acute intermittent porphyria
8. Control of aggressiveness in disturbed children
9. Control of tics and vocal utterances of Gilles de la Tourette's disease (haloperidol, pimozide)

ADMINISTRATION AND DOSAGE
See Table 27-3.

FATE
Most drugs are well absorbed orally and parenterally and have a rather large volume of distribution in the body owing to their high lipid solubility and extensive protein binding. Onset of action depends on dosage form and route of administration; observable clinical effects may not occur for several weeks after initiation of therapy. Plasma half-lives are generally short (10 hours–24 hours) but clinical effects are prolonged and in many instances are due to active metabolites. Metabolism occurs in the liver, and drugs and metabolites are excreted both in the urine and feces by way of the enterohepatic circulation.

SIDE-EFFECTS/ADVERSE REACTIONS
See also the general discussion of adverse effects, above.

Side-effects commonly seen early in the course of therapy include drowsiness, dizziness, weakness, and, in those drugs having a strong anticholinergic component, dry mouth, blurred vision, nasal stuffiness, constipation, and urinary hesitancy. A number of other adverse reactions involving many body systems have occurred with use of some antipsychotics, although the incidence varies widely among the various drugs. Among the adverse reactions reported with antipsychotic drug therapy are

CNS—Hyperpyrexia (see Neuroleptic Malignant Syndrome, below), lowering of convulsive threshold, hyperactivity, confusion, bizarre dreams, insomnia, depression, cerebral edema

Neuromuscular—Extrapyramidal reactions, akathisia (motor restlessness), dystonias (muscle spasms of the face or throat, difficulty in speech or swallowing, extensor rigidity of the back muscles, upward rotation of the eyeballs), pseudoparkinsonism, tardive dyskinesia (involuntary orofacial movements such as chewing, protrusion of the tongue, puffing of the cheeks, and puckering of the mouth), hyperreflexia

Cardiovascular—Tachycardia, fainting, electrocardiographic changes, cardiac arrest (rare)

Hematologic—Blood dyscrasias
(agranulocytosis, leukopenia, leukocytosis,
anemias, thrombocytopenic purpura,
pancytopenia)
Hypersensitivity—Urticaria, itching, eczema,
photosensitivity, contact dermatitis,
angioneurotic edema, anaphylactic reaction,
exfoliative dermatitis, cholestatic jaundice
Endocrine—Abnormal lactation, breast
engorgement, gynecomastia, changes in
libido, amenorrhea, glycosuria and
hyperglycemia, increased appetite
Autonomic—Fecal impaction, adynamic ileus,
urinary retention, enuresis, incontinence,
impotence
Ocular—Ptosis, photophobia, pigmentary
retinopathy, lens opacities
Respiratory—Laryngospasm, bronchospasm,
dyspnea
Other—Skin pigmentation, polydipsia,
aggravation of peptic ulcers, fever, systemic
lupus-like reaction, psychotic flare-up

CONTRAINDICATIONS AND PRECAUTIONS

Antipsychotic drugs are contraindicated in the presence of jaundice, liver damage, coronary disease, parkinsonism, cerebral arteriosclerosis, subcortical brain damage, blood dyscrasias, bone marrow depression, severe hypo- or hypertension, chronic alcoholism, circulatory collapse, and in comatose or severely depressed states. *Cautious* use of the drugs is mandated in patients with epilepsy, diabetes, glaucoma, prostatic hypertrophy, severe hypertension, ulcers, cardiovascular disease, chronic respiratory disorders, liver or kidney impairment, and in children under age 6, pregnant or nursing mothers, and persons exposed to extreme heat. Caution is also indicated in patients who may be exposed to phosphorus insecticides, since altered metabolism can result.

INTERACTIONS

1. Antipsychotic drugs may potentiate the effects of other CNS depressants (*e.g.*, alcohol, barbiturates, general anesthetics, antianxiety agents, narcotic analgesics).
2. Additive anticholinergic effects may be observed with concomitant use of antipsychotic drugs and other agents having anticholinergic activity (*e.g.*, antihistamines, tricyclic antidepressants, antiparkinsonian drugs).
3. Effects of antipsychotics may be enhanced by estrogens, progestins, anticholinesterases (such as neostigmine, ambenonium, and many pesticides and insecticides), furazolidone, and MAO inhibitors.
4. The hypotensive action of antipsychotic drugs can be increased by antihypertensives, epinephrine, thiazide diuretics, and tricyclic antidepressants.
5. Antipsychotic drugs may decrease the effectiveness of amphetamines, oral anticoagulants, heparin, anticonvulsants (lowering of seizure threshold), oral hypoglycemics, levodopa, and other antiparkinsonian drugs.
6. The hypoglycemic effect of insulin may be potentiated by antipsychotics.
7. Oral absorption of antipsychotic agents can be impaired by antacids and antidiarrheal preparations.
8. Lithium and other antipsychotic drugs may exert additive hyperglycemic effects.
9. The combination of antipsychotic drugs and griseofulvin may precipitate acute porphyria.
10. Narcotic analgesics may increase the respiratory-depressant action of the antipsychotics.
11. Antipsychotics can reduce the effectiveness of guanethidine by interfering with its neuronal uptake.
12. Antipsychotic drugs can potentiate muscle relaxants and other drugs that have a neuromuscular respiratory-depressant effect (*e.g.*, polypeptides, aminoglycosides), possibly resulting in prolonged apnea.
13. Additive cardiac depressant effects may occur with quinidine and antipsychotic drugs.
14. Antipsychotic-induced extrapyramidal effects can be intensified by anticholinergic antiparkinsonian drugs and piperazine, and can be reduced by diphenhydramine.
15. Concurrent administration of phenothiazines and phenytoin may result in elevated phenytoin levels and increased toxic effects. Plasma levels of propranolol and possibly other beta blockers may likewise be elevated by phenothiazines.

■ Nursing Process

Treatment with antipsychotic drugs is a double-edged sword. On one side is the chance to reduce or eliminate psychotic symptoms effectively; on the other side is the problem of coping with side-effects that may alter the quality of life. Effective nursing care can help the patient achieve a balance between symptoms and side-effects first, during the acute phase of treatment, and later through long-term follow-up.

■ Acute Care

□ ASSESSMENT

□ Subjective Data
The person with acute psychotic symptoms will be a poor historian. History-taking may be improved by using a significant other as an added and perhaps more accurate resource. The nurse should learn if any drugs or alcohol have been used in the past few days, since combining antipsychotics with CNS depressants can lead to cardiac or respiratory arrest. A history of antipsychotic drug treatment should be identified because this may influence the patient's perception of such treatment, and recent use of these drugs will complicate treatment.

□ Objective Data
Baseline physical assessment is essential because side-effects from the drugs can affect many systems. Again, active psychosis will make examination difficult but certain parameters must be evaluated. Neurologic status should be checked with emphasis on motor strength and looking for evidence of head injury or increased intracranial pressure. Temperature should be recorded, blood pressure should be checked to be certain no hypo- or hypertension exists, and an electrocardiogram performed to check for cardiac arrhythmias. Recording the extent and severity of the patient's psychotic behavior is also important to establish a baseline against which to measure the effectiveness of the drugs.

Laboratory evaluation may include blood alcohol or barbiturate levels if abuse is suspected, renal and hepatic function studies, and a complete blood count with differential. Creatine phosphokinase (CPK) values and white blood cell (WBC) count should be noted because of their use in diagnosing neuroleptic malignant syndrome (NMS), which will be discussed later in this section.

□ NURSING DIAGNOSES
During the acute phase of treatment the nursing diagnoses for the patient may include
  Potential hyperthermia related to development of NMS
  Potential alteration in cardiac output: decreased related to possible arrhythmias and hypotension

  Potential fluid volume deficit related to diaphoresis and increased metabolic rate during the psychotic episode
  Functional incontinence related to sedation produced by the drug
  Potential alteration in nutrition: less than body requirements related to drug-induced sedation
  Self-care deficit related to sedation
  Potential impairment of skin integrity related to the need for restraints during the acute psychotic phase and to sedation produced by the drug
  Alteration in thought processes related to the disease, which may be improved by the drug but may still be altered
  Potential alteration in tissue perfusion related to drug-induced hypotension

□ PLAN
The nursing care goals for the patient in the acute phase of treatment with antipsychotic drugs should include
1. Safe, rapid administration of appropriate drugs to produce sedation and reduce or eliminate symptoms
2. Close monitoring of side-effects and rapid response to physiologic changes
3. Monitoring for the development of NMS

□ INTERVENTION
Administration of the antipsychotics either by rapid administration, sometimes called *rapid neuroleptization*, or by routine methods will be determined by the physician based on the patient's symptoms. The individual who is acutely psychotic and either a danger to himself or to others is most likely to receive rapid treatment.

The choice of drug will depend on a variety of factors. If the patient is unable to cooperate, initial treatment will be limited to those drugs that can be administered in parenteral form. Aside from this, past successes with certain drugs, cost to patient and family, and side-effect potential all will influence drug choice. Low-potency antipsychotics such as chlorpromazine cause more hypotension and sedation but fewer extrapyramidal symptoms. High-potency drugs such as fluphenazine and haloperidol are more likely to result in extrapyramidal symptoms. Planning acute-care treatment with these points in mind may reduce the need to switch drugs frequently when attempting to stabilize the patient for long-term care.

In most acute cases, drugs will be administered

intramuscularly. The solution should be given separately from all other medications and administered deep into muscle to prevent pain. A site-rotation sheet should be used to decrease the chance of tissue injury from multiple injections.

Before the initial test dose and before each subsequent dose, pulse, blood pressure, and mental status must be ascertained and recorded. After the initial test dose is given the patient is observed for sedation, hypotension, and allergic response. If no problems occur, the medication will be administered every 30 minutes to 60 minutes until the psychotic symptoms diminish or the patient becomes sedated. A flowsheet may be useful in documenting drug administration, behavior patterns, vital signs, and level of consciousness during this critical period. Sedation, hypotension, or change in heart rate or rhythm should be reported immediately and future drug doses held until the physician can evaluate the patient.

□ EVALUATION
The nurse can judge, along with the physician, the effectiveness of the drugs by observing changes in the patient's psychotic symptoms, level of consciousness, and absence of side-effects. Once initial sedation has been achieved, the nurse will begin planning long-term care with the patient and his significant others.

■ Neuroleptic Malignant Syndrome

A syndrome of symptoms related to antipsychotic drug therapy may occur in susceptible patients hours to weeks after initial therapy. To date, no predisposition to this syndrome has been identified. Although it occurs in a small number of patients receiving these drugs (about 1%), the mortality rate ranges from 20% to 30%.

The syndrome is characterized by severe muscle rigidity, temperature elevation of up to 108°F, diaphoresis, alterations in consciousness ranging from confusion to delirium, tachycardia, dyspnea, and either hyper- or hypotension. Laboratory values will generally show an increase in WBC count and CPK.

Diagnosis of the syndrome may be difficult because many of the symptoms mimic the symptoms of the disease itself, as well as some of the isolated side-effects usually seen in patients on long-term antipsychotic drug therapy. The syndrome has been misdiagnosed as a drug allergy, heat stroke, and malignant hyperthermia in a postoperative pa-

tient. The best diagnostic tool is an accurate history of the onset of symptoms and a drug history. Any of the antipsychotics can cause the syndrome but fluphenazine and haloperidol have been most frequently associated with NMS.

Treatment and nursing management must be rapid and preparations made to deal with potential respiratory and cardiac arrest. The drug should be immediately discontinued and efforts made to reduce the temperature elevation through use of a hypothermia blanket, antipyretics, and antibiotics. Bromocriptine mesylate (Parlodel), a dopamine agonist (see Chap. 31), and dantrolene, a skeletal muscle relaxant (see Chap. 19), are among the drugs that have been tried to reverse the symptoms caused by the antipsychotic drug. Anticholinergics, tranquilizers, and the antiparkinsonian drug amantadine have also been used. Symptoms usually begin to diminish within 48 hours after the drug is stopped but gradual improvement may take as long as 20 days.

Until the symptoms of rigidity, diaphoresis, and incontinence resulting from altered consciousness are resolved, the nurse must attempt to prevent skin breakdown. Frequent range of motion, position changes, and skin care are important. The patient may also need an indwelling catheter.

The potential development of NMS warrants close monitoring of patients on antipsychotic drugs throughout therapy. All inpatients should have routine vital signs and periodic evaluations of the electrocardiogram and CPK and WBC counts. Any temperature elevation should be thoroughly reviewed to rule out the presence of an infection versus the development of NMS. Outpatients and their families should report promptly any fever lasting more than 24 hours, changes in muscle tone and mobility, or changes in mental alertness.

■ Long-Term Care

□ ASSESSMENT
Once the acute phase of treatment has been completed and the patient stabilized, more information is needed to guide the long-term treatment plan. As with many chronic illnesses, psychoses may be treated with medications for several years or for the rest of the patient's life. The nurse needs to know whether or not the patient is motivated to take the drug and what his perception is of taking a drug for a long time. Family support systems should be reviewed and the patient's ability to remember the dosage schedule should be observed.

The nurse must also find out how the patient will pay for the drugs because some drugs, such as the high-potency antipsychotics, are much more expensive than the low-potency ones. All of these factors will affect compliance.

Responsiveness to the prescribed drug must also be assessed. Some patients respond better to one type of antipsychotic than to others. Therefore, patients may be asked to make changes in their dosage schedules or types of medication to find the best regimen, one that best controls the symptoms with the least side-effects. Unfortunately, changes in life patterns are very stressful for these patients and may reduce compliance rates. In addition, three to six weeks may pass before the drug's effectiveness can be fully evaluated. For most patients care will occur on an outpatient basis. The nurse will have to work hard to assess these patients through frequent follow-up.

□ NURSING DIAGNOSES

Actual nursing diagnoses for the patient taking antipsychotic drugs may include

   Knowledge deficit related to the action, dose, and side-effects of the drug

   Anxiety related to concerns about the drug's ability to control symptoms and about the dangerous side-effects that may occur

Potential nursing diagnoses may include the following (refer also to Neuroleptic Malignant Syndrome, above, for NMS side-effects):

   Activity intolerance related to the development of parkinsonian side-effects

   Alteration in bowel elimination: constipation, a drug side-effect

   Alteration in cardiac output: decreased related to orthostatic hypotension and development of tachycardia or arrhythmias

   Ineffective family coping: compromised, related to change in patient's level of independence as a result of drug therapy

   Noncompliance related to multiple factors (see text)

   Alteration in nutrition: potential for more than body requirements related to appetite-stimulating effect of drug

   Alteration in oral mucous membranes related to dry mouth

   Self-care deficit related to stiffness and tremor from drug side-effects

   Sexual dysfunction related to problems with orgasm or ejaculation

   Impairment of skin integrity related to rash and photosensitivity

   Urinary retention related to drug side-effect

□ PLAN

Nursing care goals should focus on helping the patient to do the following:

1. Establish a safe, effective drug regimen
2. Learn to take the drug correctly
3. Understand the need for drug therapy and handle compliance issues
4. Learn to monitor, manage, and report side-effects as appropriate

The nurse must also plan within institutional guidelines and state laws how to handle the patient who refuses treatment.

□ INTERVENTION

The goal in establishing a dosage schedule is to provide the maximum benefit for the patient while minimizing the interference in his life by side-effects. For many patients, once-a-day dosages are best and scheduling the dose around bedtime minimizes problems with hypotension and sedation.

In handling the regimen the patient needs to know what to do if he forgets to take a dose. If on a divided-dose schedule, he should add the missed dose to the next one. If on a once-a-day schedule, he should *not* double up the next time because this could cause toxicity.

The nurse needs to deal early on with the myths of treatment with antipsychotic drugs. Some patients and their families or friends feel that these drugs are addictive, that the patient who takes a larger dose of them is "crazier" than the patient on the lower dose. They may feel that if the patient works very hard at counseling he can be medication free. Clear information about these drugs and regard for the patient's views are crucial to compliance.

In addition, stabilization of psychoses by medication may bring some "normalcy" to the patient–family relationship for the first time. The independence and responsibility the patient now has may be more disruptive to the family system and more difficult to cope with than the psychotic behavior that they knew well. The nurse should initiate family discussions on changes in family life due to the therapy. In some families this change is too disruptive; the patient may be encouraged by his family to stop taking the drug so the familiar relationship can resume. Early family conferences help the nurse to determine the nature of family supports and how they will affect the patient's compliance.

The extrapyramidal symptoms (EPS) mentioned earlier, such as parkinsonian-like syndrome, akathisia, dystonia, and tardive dyskinesia, are very debilitating and can be mistaken for symptoms of the disease itself. For example, the flattened affect or sluggish gait associated with schizophrenia may in fact be symptoms of parkinsonian syndrome. The nurse must learn to recognize the difference and teach patients and families to do the same. The easiest way to test the difference is to perform basic motor strength tests. The Abnormal Involuntary Movement Scale (AIMS) form is a useful guide (see Fig. 27-1). On an outpatient basis these tests should be performed on each visit. In addition, the patient and his family can be taught to watch for the most visible signs: tremors of the tongue or of the hands at rest.

Photosensitivity is another disturbing side-effect. Patients need to be encouraged to stay out of the sun as much as possible and to wear sunscreens, protective clothing, they have decreased tolerance to alcohol and should be encouraged to limit alcohol to occasional use and limit the amount to 1 or 2 drinks.

Anticholinergic side-effects such as constipation and mouth dryness can usually be managed. Constipation can be relieved by adequate roughage and fluids with occasional use of stool softeners or laxatives as necessary. Adequate fluid intake as well as sucking on hard candy will help relieve dry mouth. Other symptoms such as sedation, nasal congestion, and blurring of vision are usually temporary and will subside quickly. The patient should

---

Patient Identification   Date

Rated by

Either before or after completing the examination procedure, observe the patient unobtrusively at rest (e.g., in waiting room).

The chair to be used in this examination should be a hard, firm one without arms.

After observing the patient, he may be rated on a scale of 0 (none), 1 (minimal), 2 (mild), 3 (moderate), and 4 (severe) according to the severity of symptoms.

Ask the patient whether there is anything in his/her mouth (i.e., gum, candy, etc.), and if there is, to remove it.

Ask patient about the current condition of his/her teeth. Ask patient if he/she wears dentures. Do teeth or dentures bother patient now?

Ask patient whether he/she notices any movement in mouth, face, hands, or feet. If yes, ask to describe and to what extent they currently bother patient or interfere with his/her activities.

0 1 2 3 4   Have patient sit in chair with hands on knees, legs slightly apart, and feet flat on floor. (Look at entire body for movements while in this position.)

0 1 2 3 4   Ask patient to sit with hands hanging unsupported. If male, between legs, if female and wearing a dress, hanging over knees. (Observe hands and other body areas.)

0 1 2 3 4   Ask patient to open mouth. (Observe tongue at rest within mouth.) Do this twice.

0 1 2 3 4   Ask patient to protrude tongue. (Observe abnormalities of tongue movement.) Do this twice.

0 1 2 3 4   Ask the patient to tap thumb, with each finger, as rapidly as possible for 10–15 seconds; separately with right hand, then with left hand. (Observe facial and leg movements.)

0 1 2 3 4   Flex and extend patient's left and right arms. (One at a time.)

0 1 2 3 4   Ask patient to stand up. (Observe in profile. Observe all body areas again, hips included.)

0 1 2 3 4   *Ask patient to extend both arms outstretched in front with palms down. (Observe trunk, legs, and mouth.)

0 1 2 3 4   *Have patient walk a few paces, turn, and walk back to chair. (Observe hands and gait.) Do this twice.

* Activated movements

Figure 27-1. The Abnormal Involuntary Movement Scale (AIMS) provides a simple method to determine tardive dyskinesia symptoms.

report any increase in symptoms as well as those symptoms that do not subside.

Urinary retention is another anticholinergic drug effect. The patient should be told to monitor changes in frequency or quantity of urine voided. Bladder palpation can be done on each visit. If this problem develops, a change in medication may be necessary.

The patient on antipsychotic drugs may experience weight gain from an increased appetite. The patient should be told to monitor weight, or it should be evaluated on each clinic visit. Calorie intake control should be encouraged.

Sexual dysfunction may also occur, leading to problems in orgasm for both sexes and ejaculatory problems in men. This side-effect may go unreported but may be a reason for noncompliance with the therapy. The nurse needs to ask open-ended questions in a nonthreatening atmosphere to encourage the patient to share sexual concerns. A change in drug or in dose may alleviate the problem but alternate strategies for sexual expression may need to be discussed if dysfunction is not resolved.

Orthostatic hypotension may be an early side-effect that subsides or, occasionally, may be severe. The patient may be able to control it by rising slowly from sitting or lying positions, moving around rather than standing still, and, if necessary, wearing elastic stockings to facilitate venous return.

Undesirable side-effects are the main reason patients give for altering or eliminating their prescribed dose of antipsychotic drug. The other main reason is that the therapy may lead to a state of well-being that the patient associates with being cured, and subsequently to the belief that he no longer needs the drug. One or more relapses are usually enough to convince such a patient of his lifelong need. The nurse can facilitate this awareness by having the patient relate how he felt after stopping the drug. He may report loss of concentration, anxiety, withdrawal, change in appetite, or other symptoms. Acknowledging the relationship between his relapse and discontinuation of the drug may help him comply in the future.

However, some patients will refuse to return to a medication regimen that causes undesired side-effects, or they may request permission to discontinue taking the drug. Both situations cause concern for the patient's well-being, and they bring up legal and ethical issues as well, particularly if the patient is hospitalized. The laws on whether a patient can be forced to take medication against his will vary from state to state. They relate to whether the admission to a facility was voluntary or invol-

untary, whether an emergency exists, the potential for adverse side-effects, and the outcomes of prior judicial involvement. Guided by the state laws, a facility should set up a mechanism for dealing with the patient who refuses antipsychotic drugs. The patient's decision must be weighed against his behavior. Depending on patterns, the demand could be seen as a first positive step toward making decisions in a patient with low self-esteem or it could be an attempt at "self-abuse." In one facility, if the physician or nurse working with the patient is comfortable with the refusal, he or she reports it and the treatment is stopped. If not comfortable with the patient's decision, the issue is taken to the treatment team where a decision is made after a clinical evaluation of the patient is completed. If the patient's decision is accepted, treatment is stopped and the patient carefully observed for escalating symptoms.

Health teams can well empathize with patients who want to discontinue the drug since patients report severe limitations in quality of life, such as feeling stiff all the time or feeling like they are hooked on heroin or living under water. One way to help is to offer these patients drug-free holidays, specific time periods during which they do not have to take any drugs. If carefully monitored, some patients are able to return to drug therapy before a serious relapse occurs. Other patients may have learned enough about coping to avoid returning to the drugs at all and still others will learn during the holiday that the drug therapy is essential to having an independent life. The holiday can be a useful tool in long-term therapy.

□ *EVALUATION*

The parameters against which a nurse can evaluate the effectiveness of antipsychotic drug therapy are the therapeutic effectiveness in terms of life-style and independence; the development and management of side-effects, which is a continuing struggle; and the patient's ability to manage, maintain, and stay with the prescribed regimen.

Other Psychotherapeutic Drugs

Lithium

(Cibalith-S, Eskalith, Lithane, Lithobid, Lithonate, Lithotabs)

Lithium is an alkali medication available as either the carbonate or citrate salt. It is used to treat patients with manic–depressive psychoses, the so-called bipolar affective disorders. Lithium is capable of calming the agitated patient and "smoothing out" the wide swings in mood between mania and depression. Although the biochemical disturbances responsible for episodes of manic–depressive psychoses are not fully delineated, this disorder appears to have a strong genetic component, and excessive adrenergic activity in the CNS is believed to be partly responsible for the extreme mood swings. When the episodes of mania are mild or infrequent, lithium *alone* may be sufficient to control the manifestations of bipolar affective disorders, preventing both the manic *and* the depressive episodes. More severe disorders generally require use of an antipsychotic or antidepressant drug, at least until the erratic behavior has been controlled, at which point lithium may be continued alone for maintenance therapy. Chronic use of lithium in patients with classic bipolar affective disorders is widely accepted and control of symptoms is attained in nearly 75% of the patients receiving prophylactic lithium therapy. Although lithium should not be used alone to treat acute endogenous depression, it may be effective in minimizing the frequency of *recurrent* endogenous depression having a cyclic pattern, especially in combination with a tricyclic antidepressant.

The therapeutic index (*i.e.*, safety margin) of lithium is rather small and its toxicity is directly related to its serum levels. Therefore, repeated and accurate serum lithium levels should be determined in all patients receiving the drug. A daily lithium dose of 0.5 mEq/kg (300 mg lithium carbonate = 8.1 mEq lithium) will generally produce the desired therapeutic serum level (1.0 mEq–1.5 mEq/liter) within 5 days to 7 days if kidney function is normal. Serum lithium levels therefore should be obtained initially about 5 days after beginning therapy, at which time steady-state plasma levels should be present. Blood samples are taken 8 hours to 12 hours following the last dose. Dosage changes are then made if necessary based on both serum levels of lithium *and* careful clinical evaluation of the patient's behavior. Serum levels should be obtained twice weekly during the acute dosing phase and until the patient's condition has stabilized. Maintenance serum levels during prophylactic lithium use are usually in the range of 0.5 mEq to 1.0 mEq/liter, although many factors can influence the optimal serum level of lithium, such as other illnesses, introduction of a new drug, reduced renal function, or a change in fluid and salt intake. During maintenance therapy, serum levels should be measured approximately every 2 months if there

are no significant changes in the patient's condition.

MECHANISM AND ACTIONS

The specific mechanism for control of mania is unknown although lithium has effects on neurotransmitter function, cell membranes, and electrolyte balance. The drug can alter sodium transport at the nerve ending, thereby changing the electrophysiologic characteristics of nerve cells. It promotes neuronal uptake of norepinephrine and serotonin, thereby causing their more rapid inactivation, and may also reduce norepinephrine release and inhibit catecholamine-activated cyclic AMP formation.

Lithium produces minimal sedation and does not appear to block adrenergic or cholinergic receptor function. It may displace calcium in cell membranes, rendering them more permeable, and the entry of choline into cells is enhanced by lithium.

USES

1. Control of symptoms of acute mania (*i.e.*, motor hyperactivity, talkativeness, restlessness, poor judgment, grandiose ideation, aggressiveness, and possibly hostility
2. Prophylaxis of recurrent manic–depressive episodes in patients with classic bipolar affective disorder
3. Adjunctive therapy of psychoses associated with excitement
4. Investigational uses include management of violent, aggressive behavior in prisoners, prophylaxis of cluster headache and frequent, cyclic migraine attacks, and improvement of the neutrophil count in patients with chronic neutropenia or cancer chemotherapy-induced neutropenia.

ADMINISTRATION AND DOSAGE

Lithium is administered orally as either the carbonate salt in capsules (300 mg), tablets (300 mg), or slow-release tablets (300 mg, 450 mg) or the citrate salt as a syrup. A dose of 300 mg of lithium carbonate is equivalent to 8.12 mEq of lithium.

In acute mania, the recommended dosage is 600 mg three times/day (900 mg twice a day for sustained-release products) to produce the desired serum lithium level of 1 mEq to 1.5 mEq/liter, generally within 5 days to 7 days. Dosage may then be adjusted until the serum level and clinical condition of the patient have stabilized.

Recurrence of manic–depressive episodes may be minimized by a maintenance dose of approximately 300 mg three to four times a day to provide a serum level of between 0.6 mEq and 1.2 mEq/liter. Elderly patients frequently exhibit toxicity at relatively low serum levels, and dosage must be carefully titrated.

FATE

Lithium is rapidly absorbed orally; peak serum levels occur in 1 hour to 2 hours, although optimal clinical response may take a week or longer to develop. The drug is widely distributed in the body; very little is protein bound. Lithium crosses the blood-brain barrier. Excretion occurs through the kidneys (half-life about 24 hours), the rate being directly proportional to the plasma concentration; excretion is diminished by low sodium levels, for example, those resulting from diminished salt intake or concomitant diuretic therapy. The plasma half-life is approximately 20 hours to 24 hours but may be up to 36 hours in the elderly.

SIDE-EFFECTS/ADVERSE REACTIONS

There are numerous side-effects and adverse reactions associated with lithium therapy, the majority of which are seldom encountered at serum levels of less than 1.5 mEq/liter, although individual variability in drug response is considerable. Initial therapy is frequently accompanied by thirst, polyuria, and fine hand tremor, as well as nausea, fatigue, and occasional muscle weakness. Most of these side-effects subside with continued therapy although the polyuria and tremor may persist. Propranolol (Inderal) has been shown to alleviate the fine hand tremor caused by lithium.

Myriad other untoward reactions have occurred during lithium treatment. Some are related to the serum level but others appear independent of the lithium level in the plasma. These adverse reactions are grouped below according to the organ system involved.

Neuromuscular—Lack of coordination, ataxia, muscle hyperirritability and twitching, choreiform movements, clonic movements, extrapyramidal-like symptoms, coarse hand tremor

CNS—Drowsiness, dizziness, restlessness, confusion, hallucinations, slurred speech, tinnitus, incontinence, psychomotor retardation, epileptic-like seizures, stupor, coma

Autonomic—Dry mouth, blurred vision

Cardiovascular—Hypotension, arrhythmias, bradycardia, edema, circulatory collapse

Gastrointestinal—Anorexia, vomiting, diarrhea, abdominal pain, gastritis, flatulence, salivary gland swelling

Urinary—Albuminuria, glycosuria, oliguria, diabetes insipidus, decreased glomerular function, chronic interstitial nephritis

Dermatologic—Rash, pruritus, thinning of hair, folliculitis, alopecia, topical anesthesia, acneiform eruptions, cutaneous ulceration

Other—Hypothyroidism, transient hyperglycemia, excessive weight gain, leukocytosis, blurred vision, scotomas, flattening and inversion of the T wave, worsening of psoriasis

Treatment of lithium overdosage is supportive in nature, and the removal of the ion from the body can be hastened by gastric lavage, osmotic diuretics, and hemodialysis. Lithium intoxication can occur secondary to changes in the patient's status, such as diminishing renal function, reduced salt intake, or use of diuretics. Periodic serum lithium determinations aid in maintaining the desired serum concentration and should be an integral part of the treatment protocol.

CONTRAINDICATIONS AND PRECAUTIONS

Use of lithium is seldom absolutely contraindicated if the patient's condition is sufficiently severe. Relative contraindications, that is, conditions in which the likelihood of lithium toxicity is greatly increased, include significant renal or cardiovascular disease, dehydration, sodium depletion, diuretic therapy, severe debilitation, organic brain syndrome, early pregnancy, and age of less than 12 years. Lithium should be used cautiously in the presence of thyroid disease and epilepsy, in the elderly, and in nursing mothers.

INTERACTIONS

1. The effects of lithium may be decreased by acetazolamide and other urinary alkalizing agents (e.g., sodium bicarbonate, antacids), aminophylline, caffeine, excess sodium chloride, and urea, all substances that increase its excretion.

2. Toxic effects of lithium may be intensified by use of diuretics (sodium loss), methyldopa, antipsychotic drugs, phenytoin, carbamazepine, mazindol, tetracycline, indomethacin, and probably other nonsteroidal anti-inflammatory agents.

3. Combinations of lithium and haloperidol may produce severe encephalopathic symptoms such as parkinsonism, dyskinesias, and dementia.

4. Profound hypothermia may occur with simultaneous use of benzodiazepines (*e.g.*, Valium, Librium) and lithium.
5. Lithium may reduce the pressor effects of sympathomimetic drugs.
6. Lithium may prolong the effects of neuromuscular blocking agents.

■ Nursing Process

Lithium differs from the other antipsychotics in that it causes few extrapyramidal side-effects. Its therapeutic index, however, is extremely narrow, so small deviations in dosage range can result in severe drug toxicity. Many of the safety considerations noted earlier in the general discussion on antipsychotics also apply to lithium but several specific nursing concerns will be mentioned here.

□ ASSESSMENT
The best candidate for lithium therapy is the individual who is highly motivated toward compliance. The nurse can assess motivation early in the treatment program while the patient receiving lithium is being evaluated with blood levels done every other day to establish therapeutic serum level. Clinical response should occur within 7 days to 10 days. If no response occurs within 3 weeks, lithium is not the correct treatment for the patient.

During the initial drug evaluation period the nurse can monitor the individual's willingness to submit to the frequent blood work, maintain regular clinic appointments, and follow the drug administration schedule exactly as prescribed. A strong support system will help the patient and is usually an asset, but much of the success will depend on the individual's desire to follow the regimen.

□ NURSING DIAGNOSES
Actual nursing diagnoses for the patient taking lithium may include
Knowledge deficit related to action, dose, and side-effects of the drug
Anxiety about drug effectiveness and dangerous side-effects
Potential nursing diagnoses include
Noncompliance usually related to side-effects
Activity intolerance related to tremors
Alteration in bowel elimination: diarrhea, a drug side-effect but if severe may signal toxicity
Fluid volume deficit related to polyuria
Alteration in nutrition: potential for more

than body requirements, a drug-related appetite-stimulating effect

□ PLAN
The nursing care goals are the same as for the patient on other antipsychotic drugs. The patient must learn to take the medication as prescribed, monitor and respond to side-effects, report signs of toxicity, and prevent recurrent mania. The patient must also understand the need for continuous follow-up with health-care providers, and be assisted in managing the effects of the drug on quality of life.

□ INTERVENTION
Lithium's numerous side-effects are listed above. Some can be managed in the same way as those described under the other antipsychotic drugs. Drowsiness will recede as the therapy progresses. If patients know this they may be better able to deal with the symptoms until it subsides. Others, such as neurologic changes, vomiting, and dizziness, may signal serious problems or toxicity and should be reported immediately.

The chance of toxicity can be reduced by encouraging fluid intake of between 2500 ml to 3000 ml per day, which will keep circulating fluid volume adequate. Fever, dehydration, profuse sweating, and diarrhea are all dangerous to the patient taking lithium since such changes result in hemoconcentration and can cause drug toxicity. For these reasons, lithium therapy must be carefully monitored in the elderly, whose diminished renal function increases the chance of problems. Patients should be told to report any illness.

Mania can also recur during the therapy if the patient self-regulates the dose, frequently forgets the medication, or becomes resistant to the therapy. Early in the treatment the nurse can review with the patient, but particularly with the significant others, what the signs of mania were for him. These symptoms should be noted somewhere for easy reference so all will remember what to watch for. A return of such symptoms should be reported immediately.

Blood levels will be checked monthly and an interview will be done to find out how the patient feels. Both strategies are geared to catch early any signs of toxicity or changing dosage needs. Initially the dose of lithium will be high. As the mania diminishes, so does the need for lithium, and the dose should be reduced.

Lithium therapy is a long-term treatment and poses the same problems for the patient as any other chronic illness. He must remember to take the medication. This may be accomplished by timing the taking of the drug with regular events such as mealtime or bedtime. Unlike some other medications, however, if a dose is missed it should be skipped. Doubling doses can result in toxicity.

Long-term lithium therapy can result in compliance problems. For further discussion on these, see the general discussion on antipsychotics earlier in this chapter.

□ *EVALUATION*

Lithium may take away the manic symptoms that interfere with a person's life but does not remove the person's problems. To evaluate the effectiveness of lithium the nurse needs to look at how the patient copes with life problems before and during drug treatment and the management of side-effects, the confines of the regimen, and the occasional relapses that occur.

Pimozide
(Orap)

Pimozide is a potent, centrally acting dopamine receptor antagonist that is used to suppress severe motor and phonic tics in patients with Gilles de la Tourette's syndrome. This disorder is characterized by unpredictable and spontaneous outbursts of foul language, barking sounds, and other motor abnormalities. Some cases have been successfully managed by haloperidol, another dopamine antagonist, but the majority of severe cases are resistant to other modes of drug therapy, and pimozide appears to be effective in treating many of these resistant cases.

Since pimozide is a strong dopamine receptor antagonist, its prolonged use is associated with a high frequency of tardive dyskinesias (see discussion earlier in the chapter). Dosage must therefore be kept as low as possible and periodic "drug holidays" should be used to minimize the likelihood of tardive dyskinesias developing. Extrapyramidal reactions are frequent occurrences, often during the first few days of treatment. Their severity and frequency are dose-related, and they are usually reversible with dosage reduction. Many other untoward reactions have occurred in patients receiving pimozide, most of which are also seen with antipsychotic drug use. Refer to Adverse Reactions of Antipsychotic Drugs, earlier in this chapter, for a complete listing of potential adverse effects.

Sudden death has occurred in some patients taking high doses of pimozide for conditions other than Tourette's disorder. These deaths are thought to be due to a prolongation of the Q-T interval, predisposing the person to ventricular arrhythmias. Electrocardiographic recordings should be obtained prior to drug administration and at periodic intervals during therapy. Prolongation of the Q-T interval more than 25% above the predrug baseline reading is considered valid reason for stopping the drug.

The drug must be given with caution to patients with impaired renal or hepatic function, during pregnancy and nursing, and to persons whose condition may be aggravated by the anticholinergic activity of pimozide. Pimozide is *contraindicated* for controlling tics and vocal utterances associated with conditions other than Gilles de la Tourette's syndrome and in patients with a history of Q-T interval disturbances or cardiac arrhythmias.

Pimozide may lower the convulsive threshold and may therefore interfere with the action of anticonvulsants, and it can potentiate the effects of other CNS depressants.

The initial dose of pimozide (tablets) is 1 mg to 2 mg daily in divided doses. Dosage may be gradually increased every other day until an optimal effect is noted. Usual maintenance doses are 10 mg/day or less; doses in excess of 20 mg/day are not recommended. Periodic attempts should be made to reduce the dose to see if the tics persist.

NURSING CONSIDERATIONS

Nursing concerns should center on ensuring that baseline measurements are taken to test cardiac status. Each patient should have an electrocardiogram (ECG) and cardiac enzymes drawn before treatment is initiated. If therapy is prolonged, ECGs should be repeated at regular intervals since there is evidence that reversible cardiac changes may occur during treatment with pimozide.

The advantage of pimozide is that the therapeutic dose usually causes less sedation and mental dulling than haloperidol. However, the nurse should watch for the development of extrapyramidal side-effects since the drug may need to be titrated downward. This can sometimes be done without causing a return of symptoms.

Droperidol
(Inapsine)

A butyrophenone producing tranquilization, sedation, and mild peripheral vascular dilation, droperidol has a strong antiemetic effect and can potentiate the action of other CNS depressants. It also has a peripheral alpha-adrenergic blocking action and can reduce the pressor effect of epinephrine and reduce the incidence of epinephrine-induced arrhythmias. Droperidol is principally used in combination with a narcotic analgesic (fentanyl) as Innovar (see Chap. 21) for the production of neuroleptanalgesia, which is a state of quietude, reduced motor activity, and indifference to pain. Alone, droperidol is given to provide tranquilization and reduce nausea and vomiting during surgical and diagnostic procedures, and as an adjunct to general and regional anesthesia. It has also been employed as an intravenous antiemetic during cancer chemotherapy.

Mild hypotension and tachycardia are common side-effects and usually subside spontaneously. Hypotension secondary to hypovolemia is managed with appropriate parenteral fluid therapy. Postsurgical drowsiness is also a frequent occurrence with use of droperidol, especially when given as an adjunct to general anesthesia. Extrapyramidal reactions occur in approximately 1% of patients. Other untoward reactions reported include dizziness, shivering, bronchospasm, and postoperative hallucinations. When used in combination with fentanyl, respiratory depression, muscle rigidity, and elevated blood pressure have been noted.

Recommended doses for the various indications for droperidol are as follows:

Adults

Premedication—2.5 mg to 10 mg IM 30 minutes to 60 minutes preoperatively

Adjunct to general anesthesia—2.5 mg/20 lb to 25 lb IV during induction

Maintenance—1.25 mg to 2.5 mg IV

Diagnostic procedures (without a general anesthetic)—2.5 mg to 10 mg IM 30 minutes to 60 minutes before procedure, then 1.25 mg to 2.5 mg IV as needed

Children (2 years–12 years)—1 mg to 1.5 mg/ 20 lb to 25 lb for premedication or induction of anesthesia

Onset of action IV or IM is generally within 10 minutes, and peak effects occur in about 30 minutes. Sedative effects persist 2 hours to 4 hours, whereas the altered state of consciousness may last for up to 12 hours. The drug should be given cautiously to patients with liver or kidney dysfunction, and to elderly or debilitated persons.

NURSING CONSIDERATIONS

Postoperative care of the patient who receives droperidol, especially as Innovar, should include several measures. In the early postoperative period, doses of narcotics or other CNS depressants should be reduced for 8 hours to 12 hours since an additive effect can occur. Even at reduced doses, adminis-

tration of such medications can cause respiratory depression. Because respiratory depression can occur without the administration of narcotics, careful postoperative evaluation should be made hourly, particularly in the elderly or in very young children. Drowsiness is also very common so extra care should be taken getting the patient out of bed the first few times.

Extrapyramidal side-effects can occur as late as 1 to 2 days after administration. The nurse needs to watch for tremors and stiffness and to report them quickly. The side-effects can be treated with an antiparkinsonian agent until they subside.

Methotrimeprazine

(Levoprome)

Methotrimeprazine is a phenothiazine derivative having a profound CNS-depressant effect. Its action is characterized by sedation, reduced motor activity, increased pain threshold, and amnesia. It also exhibits antihistaminic, anticholinergic, and antiadrenergic activity. Analgesia is comparable to that elicited by morphine but is *not* accompanied by signs of dependence or addiction, even with prolonged use. It rarely produces respiratory depression and does not alter the cough reflex. A high incidence of orthostatic hypotension and sedation somewhat limits its usefulness, but most other phenothiazine-related side-effects (*e.g.*, extrapyramidal symptoms) occur less frequently than with other antipsychotic drugs.

The primary indication for its use is for relief of moderate to marked pain in nonambulatory patients. Additional uses include obstetric analgesia where respiratory depression is to be avoided and as a preanesthetic agent to produce somnolence and relief of anxiety and apprehension.

The principal side-effect of methotrimeprazine is orthostatic hypotension, accompanied by weakness and fainting. Blood pressure begins to fall within 10 minutes to 20 minutes following intramuscular administration and generally persists for 4 hours to 6 hours. This effect can be avoided by keeping the patient supine for at least 6 hours following injection. The orthostatic hypotensive effect generally diminishes with continued administration. Other adverse effects include disorientation, weakness, urinary hesitancy, xerostomia, nasal congestion, pain and inflammation at the injection site, and agranulocytosis and jaundice with prolonged high-dose therapy.

Use of methotrimeprazine is contraindicated in the presence of severe myocardial, renal, or hepatic disease, significant hypotension, and in patients receiving antihypertensive drugs or CNS depressants, since additive effects can occur. Methotrimeprazine is given by deep intramuscular injection into a large muscle mass. Intravenous and subcutaneous administration should be avoided. Usual dosage ranges are as follows:

Analgesia—10 mg to 20 mg IM every 4 hours to 6 hours (5 mg–10 mg in elderly patients)

Obstetric analgesia—15 mg to 20 mg IM; repeat as needed

Preanesthetic sedation—10 mg to 20 mg IM 1 hour to 3 hours before surgery, often with atropine or scopolamine in reduced doses

Postoperative analgesia—2.5 mg to 7.5 mg IM every 4 hours to 6 hours as needed

Since methotrimeprazine is a phenothiazine derivative, refer to the discussion of antipsychotic drugs earlier in the chapter for additional information on potential adverse effects as well as drug interactions and nursing considerations.

CASE STUDY

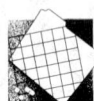

Jonathan Olsen is a 16-year-old white male who is brought to the crisis intervention center by his family after he has refused to eat or come out of his room for over a week. His family reports that his withdrawal began soon after his father, an alcoholic, was admitted for emergency surgery due to bleeding ulcers. Prior to this, Jonathan was reported by his mother to be a "good boy," always doing well in school, always obedient, and a great help to her with her two younger children, ages 11 and 8.

When the nurse begins to interview Jonathan she observes him to be curled on the floor in the farthest corner of the room. He begins to remove his shoes and starts throwing them at her yelling, "Get out, get out, let me out, I know you're trying to get me." The psychiatrist and security team are called when attempts to calm Jonathan verbally fail. While the team restrains Jonathan, the nurse gives him chlorpromazine, 50 mg IM, as ordered and attempts unsuccessfully to get some vital signs. Jonathan is admitted to the psychiatric inpatient unit of the facility. He continues to be extremely agitated and is given 5 more 50-mg doses of chlorpromazine before he becomes sedated.

Discussion Questions

1. What data could the nurse collect from Jonathan's mother on his physical health to determine whether he could safely receive phenothiazines?
2. Design a flowsheet that could be used to monitor Jonathan's status during the rapid tranquilization with chlorpromazine.
3. What data should be collected from Jonathan when he is more alert, and from his family, to determine appropriate treatment once the acute anxiety passes?

REVIEW QUESTIONS

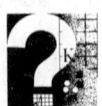

1. Describe the symptoms of schizophrenia.
2. Briefly explain the purported role of dopamine in psychotic behavior.
3. What are the major groups of antipsychotic drugs?
4. Outline the principal CNS effects of antipsychotic drugs.
5. What are the mechanisms responsible for the (1) antiemetic, (2) hypotensive, and (3) galactorrhea-inducing effects of antipsychotic drugs?

6. How do extrapyramidal reactions (EPRs) differ from tardive dyskinesias?
7. Why are antipsychotic drugs with *strong* anticholinergic activity generally associated with a *low* incidence of EPRs?
8. Briefly describe (1) akathisia and (2) dystonic reactions.
9. Outline the major biochemical mechanisms of action of antipsychotic drug use.
10. List the important adverse reactions seen with antipsychotic drugs.
11. What essential data should be collected before initiating any antipsychotic drug therapy?
12. What is the nurse's responsibility during rapid induction of neuroleptanalgesia with antipsychotic drugs?
13. How will perceptions of long-term drug therapy affect the patient taking antipsychotics?
14. What is AIMS and how can it be helpful in caring for the patient taking an antipsychotic drug?
15. What should an individual do if he misses a dose of an antipsychotic drug? If he misses a dose of lithium?
16. What are the patient's rights in refusing antipsychotic drug therapy in your state? What is the policy for handling refusal in the facility where you work?
17. What are the indications for lithium? How does this drug affect catecholamine activity?
18. What are the common side-effects of lithium therapy?
19. Why must serum levels of lithium be controlled so rigidly?
20. Who is the best candidate for lithium therapy?
21. What data can be collected to determine whether a patient will derive maximum benefit from lithium?
22. What can the nurse teach a patient taking lithium that will reduce his chance of developing toxicity?
23. For what is pimozide (Orap) indicated? How does it act?
24. What are the major dangers associated with pimozide?
25. What baseline data should be known before administering pimozide?
26. Droperidol (Inapsine) is used for what purposes? For what indication is it combined with a narcotic analgesic?
27. What pharmacologic actions are possessed by methotrimeprazine (Levoprome)?
28. What is the principal disadvantage to use of methotrimeprazine?

BIBLIOGRAPHY

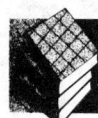

Cahill C, Arana GW: Navigating neuroleptic malignant syndrome. Am J Nurs 86:671, 1986
Carlsson A: Antipsychotic drugs, neurotransmitters and schizophrenia. Am J Psychiatry 135:164, 1978
Cole R: Patient's right to refuse antipsychotic drugs. Law, Medicine & Health 4:19, 1981
Dellefield K, Miller J: Psychotropic drugs and the elderly patient. Nurs Clin North Am 17(6):303, 1982
Diamond R: Drugs and the quality of life: The patient's point of view. J Clin Psychiatry 46:29, 1985
Ehrensing RH: Tardive dyskinesia. Arch Intern Med 138:1261, 1978
Harris E: Antipsychotic medications. Am J Nurs 81:1316, 1981

Harris E: Lithium. Am J Nurs 81:1310, 1981

Jeste DR, Wyatt RJ: Understanding and Treating Tardive Dyskinesia. New York, Guilford Press, 1982

Keltner NL, McIntyre CW: Neuroleptic malignant syndrome. J Neurosurg Nurs 17:363, 1985

Mansch TC: Current concepts in psychiatry: Schizophrenic disorders. N Engl J Med 305:1628, 1981

Ressler KA, Waletzky JP: Clinical use of antipsychotics. Am J Psychiatry 138:202, 1981

Rivera-Calimlin L, Hershey L: Neuroleptic concentrations and clinical response. Annu Rev Pharmacol Toxicol 24:361, 1984

Rosel-Greif VL: Drug induced dyskinesias. Am J Nurs 82:66, 1982

Shapiro AK, Shapiro E: Controlled study of pimozide vs placebo in Tourette's syndrome. J Am Acad Child Psychiatry 23:161, 1984

Snyder SH: Dopamine receptors, neuroleptics and schizophrenia. Am J Psychiatry 138:460, 1981

Tarsy D, Baldessarini RJ: The pathophysiologic basis of tardive dyskinesia. Biol Psychiatry 12:431, 1977

Tosteson DC: Lithium and mania. Sci Am 239:164, 1981

Youssef FA: Compliance with therapeutic regimens: A follow-up study for patients with affective disorders. J Adv Nurs 8:513, 1983

Antianxiety Drugs

Benzodiazepines
    Alprazolam,
        Chlordiazepoxide,
        Clorazepate,
        Diazepam,
        Halazepam,
        Lorazepam,
        Midazolam,
        Oxazepam, Prazepam

Carbamates
    Meprobamate

Miscellaneous Antianxiety Drugs
    Buspirone
    Hydroxyzine
    Chlormezanone

28

Throughout history, man has sought relief from stress, tension, and anxiety through the use of mind-altering substances. Perhaps the most widely used such substance is alcohol, which is the subject of Chapter 26. Other chemicals used for the relief of anxiety and tension have included bromides, paraldehyde, chloral hydrate, and barbiturates, but none of these substances approach the ideal antianxiety agent in terms of efficacy and safety. The continuing quest for the "perfect" anxiety-relieving drug led to the development, in the late 1950s, of chlordiazepoxide, the first of the so-called benzodiazepine anxiolytic drugs, which have now become the most widely used of all the antianxiety agents currently available. In addition to the benzodiazepines now in clinical use, several other chemically distinct substances are also occasionally prescribed for the relief of simple anxiety. These nonbenzodiazepine antianxiety drugs include meprobamate, buspirone, chlormezanone, and hydroxyzine. As mentioned above, certain barbiturates, especially phenobarbital and butabarbital, were used previously for the chronic management of stress and tension states, but this practice has largely disappeared with the availability of the more effective and less hazardous benzodiazepines.

The antianxiety drugs are sometimes referred to as *minor tranquilizers* (a largely unsatisfactory term) to distinguish them from the more potent and more toxic antipsychotic drugs, or *major tranquilizers* (also an inappropriate term) from which they exhibit several significant differences (Table 28-1). In contrast to the antipsychotic agents, the occurrence of serious adverse reactions with the antianxiety drugs is rather low when they are administered in normal therapeutic doses. Moreover, except for buspirone, their central skeletal muscle relaxant action is an action not seen with antipsychotic drugs and may contribute to their effectiveness in treating emotional disorders compounded by excessive muscular tension or spasm. However, again with the exception of buspirone, their prolonged use is invariably associated with development of tolerance, and a significant potential for habituation and abuse exists with these compounds, whereas it is highly unlikely with the more potent antipsychotic drugs.

Most antianxiety agents also have clinically significant anticonvulsant activity when administered intravenously, and can effectively control acute convulsive states such as status epilepticus or those associated with acute alcohol withdrawal. Moreover, their use is not accompanied by extrapyramidal or autonomic side-effects.

Pharmacologically, the antianxiety agents, especially when used in high doses, resemble the barbiturates in many ways, and possess an ability to cause central nervous system (CNS) depression that is largely dependent on the level of drug in the body. Their principal advantage relative to the barbiturates, however, is their significantly higher sedative-to-hypnotic ratio. In other words, the margin between the calming, tension-relieving dose and the hypnotic, sleep-inducing dose is much greater with the antianxiety agents than with the barbiturates. Refer to Figure 24-1, where curve X might represent a barbiturate while curve Z represents a benzodiazepine antianxiety drug. The antianxiety drugs are said to have a *shallow* dose–response curve, and the difference between the sedative and hypnotic or anesthetic doses is quite large. Conversely, the rather "steep" dose–response curve of the barbiturates is reflected in the very small difference between the sedative and the

Table 28-1
Comparison of Antipsychotic Drugs and Antianxiety Drugs

Drugs	Major Indications	Incidence of Major Adverse Reactions	Skeletal Muscle Relaxant Effect	Anticonvulsive Activity	Dependence Liability
Antipsychotic drugs	Psychoses	+++	−	−	−
Antianxiety drugs	Psychoneuroses, psychosomatic disorders (anxiety, stress, tension)	+	++	++	+++

Key: +++, high; ++, moderate; +, low; −, not significant

anesthetic dose. Thus, the antianxiety drugs are less likely than barbiturates to result in severe CNS depression, even at large doses. Their primary use, therefore, is to provide a degree of relief from emotional symptoms (such as agitation, anxiety, muscle tension, and motor hyperactivity) associated with psychoneurotic and psychosomatic disorders. They are rarely satisfactory alone for controlling severely disturbed psychotic patients, although they have been employed in conjunction with antipsychotic drugs in treating acute psychotic episodes.

The currently available antianxiety agents can be conveniently classified into one of three groups:
1. Benzodiazepines
2. Carbamates
3. Miscellaneous (buspirone, chlormezanone, hydroxyzine)

Benzodiazepines

Alprazolam, Chlordiazepoxide, Clorazepate, Diazepam, Halazepam, Lorazepam, Midazolam, Oxazepam, Prazepam

The benzodiazepines are the most commonly prescribed antianxiety agents. Much of their popularity is due to their demonstrated effectiveness at dose levels that are not associated with excessive drowsiness, a high risk of untoward reactions, or development of physical dependence, which are characteristic of chronic barbiturate consumption. The benzodiazepines discussed in this chapter are indicated *primarily* for the relief of situational anxiety, with the exception of midazolam, a short-acting benzodiazepine used parenterally for preoperative and perioperative sedation and to supplement general anesthesia. Other benzodiazepines have somewhat different indications and are discussed elsewhere in the book. Flurazepam (Dalmane), triazolam (Halcion), and temazepam (Restoril) are effective nonbarbiturate hypnotics used to relieve insomnia and have been reviewed in Chapter 25. Clonazepam (Klonopin) is used in certain forms of epilepsy and is discussed in Chapter 30.

MECHANISM AND ACTIONS
The benzodiazepines appear to act at several subcortical brain sites, most notably the limbic system and the reticular formation. Higher cortical function is largely unaffected by therapeutic doses of these drugs, and ataxia and sedation generally occur only with amounts in excess of those needed for the relief of anxiety states. Benzodiazepines are believed to potentiate the action of gamma-aminobutyric acid (GABA), an inhibitory neurotransmitter in the CNS, possibly by enhancing the binding of GABA to its receptor sites. A direct GABA-mimetic action at the receptor site has also been proposed for the benzodiazepines. Potentiation of GABA function underlies the reduced neuronal activity in the limbic and reticular systems of the brain, thereby reducing the level of emotional reactivity without significant cortical depression. In addition, enhancement of GABA activity in the spinal cord appears to play a major role in the skeletal muscle relaxant action of the benzodiazepines, as GABA probably functions as an inhibitor in spinal motor reflex pathways. The seizure threshold is elevated by benzodiazepines, resulting in a clinically significant anticonvulsant action for certain derivatives. Again, potentiation of GABA activity in brain areas controlling gross motor function probably contributes to the usefulness of certain benzodiazepines in treating acute convulsive episodes. A major factor in the previously mentioned wide safety margin of benzodiazepine drugs is the fact that even in large amounts, these agents, unlike the barbiturates, do not appear significantly to depress the respiratory or vasomotor centers in the medulla. Thus, even with massive overdosage, fatalities with benzodiazepines are rare. High doses of these drugs, however, can markedly increase the CNS-depressant effects of alcohol and other depressants of central function. Deaths have occurred in patients using benzodiazepines in combination with heavy alcohol consumption and such practice should be strongly discouraged.

The effectiveness of benzodiazepines in relieving symptoms of anxiety over *prolonged periods* has not been conclusively established; these drugs should not be used for longer than 3 months to 4 months unless careful patient reassessment establishes a *definite* need for continued treatment. Prolonged administration of benzodiazepines will often lead to dependence, and true physical addiction has been reported, most often following chronic use of high doses. Withdrawal symptoms can occur on cessation of therapy and are more likely to be present if the drug is short acting, has been used for longer than 4 months to 6 months, and is abruptly discontinued. Thus, dosage should be gradually tapered when discontinuing therapy.

Dependence on benzodiazepines ranges from a psychologic need for the drug in order to function productively to a true physiologic dependence on the presence of the drug to avoid a withdrawal syndrome. The degree of dependence is frequently greater in the emotionally labile person, and these patients should be given benzodiazepines with extreme caution. Most types of situational anxiety, such as that associated with loss of a loved one, loss or change of employment, stressful social situations, or change in marital status, are largely self-limiting and should not require prolonged use of antianxiety drugs. Patients requesting sustained benzodiazepine prescribing must be carefully evaluated, and alternate methods for coping with their anxiety should be proposed.

USES

1. Symptomatic relief of anxiety, tension, and irritability associated with neuroses, depression, psychoneuroses, and psychosomatic disorders (short-term use only—maximum 4 months)
2. Symptomatic relief of the symptoms of acute alcohol withdrawal (chlordiazepoxide, clorazepate, diazepam, oxazepam)
3. Preoperative sedation
4. Relief of muscle hypertonicity associated with anxiety or tension states
5. Adjunctive therapy in the management of epileptic states (clorazepate, diazepam)
6. Control of acute (e.g., status epilepticus) or severe recurrent convulsive seizure states (diazepam or lorazepam IV)
7. Adjunctive treatment prior to cardioversion or endoscopic procedures to lessen anxiety and reduce recall (diazepam or lorazepam IV, IM)
8. Control of nocturnal enuresis and "night terrors" (experimental use only)

ADMINISTRATION AND DOSAGE
See Table 28-2.

FATE
See Table 28-3 for an outline of benzodiazepine pharmacokinetics.

Benzodiazepines are generally well absorbed orally although rates differ widely, reflecting the variability in onset of action following a single dose (Table 28-3). Intramuscular absorption of lorazepam is rapid and complete, but that of chlordiazepoxide and diazepam is erratic. The onset of action ranges from 30 minutes to 60 minutes orally (diazepam has the quickest onset of action) and 15 minutes to 30 minutes intramuscularly. The drugs are quite lipid soluble and distribute widely throughout the body. Protein binding is high (80%–99%). Most drugs (except oxazepam and lorazepam) have long elimination half-lives, since their metabolites are clinically active as well (see Table 28-3). Prazepam and clorazepate are inactive as parent compounds, but are metabolized to desmethyldiazepam, an active metabolite. The drugs are excreted as both unchanged drug and metabolites, largely through the kidney; elimination may occur in two stages; a rapid (within several hours) phase followed by a slower (within days) phase. Danger of accumulation exists with chronic use, especially of those derivatives having active metabolites. Since oxazepam and lorazepam exhibit one-step inactivation, they are preferred in elderly patients or in patients with liver disease.

Although the clinical efficacy of one benzodiazepine does not differ appreciably from another, rapidly absorbed benzodiazepines such as diazepam are frequently perceived to be more effective by some patients due primarily to the quicker onset of action.

SIDE-EFFECTS/ADVERSE REACTIONS
Transient drowsiness is frequently encountered during the first few days of therapy and appears to be more common in the elderly or debilitated patient. Ataxia, confusion, fatigue, and lethargy can also occur in the initial phase of therapy.

Other adverse reactions are less commonly observed during short-term therapy but their incidence may increase with prolonged administration. Adverse effects noted during benzodiazepine therapy are grouped below according to the organ system involved.

CNS—Confusion, disorientation, agitation, slurred speech, headache, syncope, vertigo, depression, hyporeactivity, stupor, weakness, rigidity, extrapyramidal symptoms, tremor; paradoxical excitement (hostility, rage, muscle spasticity, irritability, vivid dreams, euphoria, insomnia, hallucinations) can occur, especially in psychotic patients.

Gastrointestinal/urinary—Dry mouth, constipation, nausea, anorexia, vomiting, salivation, urinary retention, incontinence

Cardiovascular/hematologic—Bradycardia, hypotension, palpitations, edema and weight gain, cardiovascular collapse, agranulocytosis, neutropenia

Hypersensitivity—Skin rash, urticaria, fever, angioneurotic edema, bronchial spasm

(Text continues on p. 522.)

Table 28-2
Benzodiazepines

Drug	Preparations	Usual Dosage Range	Clinical Considerations
alprazolam (Xanax)	Tablets—0.25 mg, 0.5 mg, 1.0 mg	Initially, 0.25 mg–0.5 mg three times/day; maximum total doses is 4 mg/day Elderly—0.25 mg two to three times/day	Metabolized to benzophenone, which is inactive, and alpha hydroxyalprazolam, which is approximately one-half as active as alprazolam; has a short half-life (12 h–15 h) and relatively brief duration of action; possesses some antidepressant activity, particularly at higher doses; drowsiness and light-headedness are common during early stages of therapy (Schedule IV).
chlordiazepoxide (Libritabs, Librium, Lipoxide, Mitran, Reposans-10)	Capsules—5 mg, 10 mg, 25 mg Tablets—5 mg, 10 mg, 25 mg Powder for injection—100 mg/5 ml	*Oral* Adults Anxiety—5 mg–10 mg three to four times/day up to 25 mg four times/day Alcohol withdrawal—50 mg–100 mg up to 300 mg/day Children (over 6 yr)—5 mg–10 mg two to four times/day as needed *Parenteral* Adults—50 mg–100 mg IM or IV Children (over 12 yr)—25 mg–50 mg IM or IV	Less potent than diazepam and has less anticonvulsive activity; excreted slowly by the kidneys, so danger of accumulation exists; prepare IM solution immediately before administration and discard unused portion; do not use IM diluent if hazy or opalescent; IM solution should not be given IV because of air bubbles that form in solution; inject slowly and deeply IM; IV solution can be prepared with sterile water or saline; give IV injection slowly over 1 minute; do not inject IV solution IM because pain is common; do not add to IV infusion, because solution is unstable and quickly deteriorates; sterilization by heating should not be attempted; available in combination with amitriptyline as Limbitrol for treatment of anxious depressions (Schedule IV).
clorazepate (Tranxene)	Capsules—3.75 mg, 7.5 mg, 15 mg Tablets—3.75 mg, 7.5 mg, 15 mg Long acting tablets—11.25 mg, 22.5 mg	Anxiety—15 mg–60 mg daily in divided doses or 11.25 mg–22.5 mg once a day Elderly—7.5 mg–15 mg/day Adjunct to anticonvulsants Adults: 7.5 mg three times/day initially; increase gradually	Fairly rapid onset (about 60 min) and long duration (up to 24 h) of action; active metabolite is desmethyl-diazepam; single daily dose is usually given at bedtime; recommended in children only as adjunct to other anti-

(continued)

Table 28-2 (continued)
Benzodiazepines

Drug	Preparations	Usual Dosage Range	Clinical Considerations
clorazepate (Tranxene) (continued)		Children: 7.5 mg twice a day; increase gradually Alcohol withdrawal Day 1: 30 mg initially, then 30 mg–60 mg in divided doses Day 2: 45 mg–90 mg in divided doses Day 3: 22.5 mg–45 mg in divided doses Day 4: 15 mg–30 mg in divided doses	convulsant drugs; effects parallel those of diazepam (Schedule IV).
diazepam (Valium, Valrelease, Vazepam, Zetran)	Tablets—2 mg, 5 mg, 10 mg Capsules (sustained release) —15 mg Injection—5 mg/ml Oral solution—1 mg/ml, 5 mg/ml	*Oral* Adults Anxiety—2 mg–10 mg two to four times/day or 15 mg–30 mg sustained-release capsules Alcohol withdrawal—10 mg three to four times/day initially, followed by 5 mg three to four times/day Adjunct in muscle spasm and convulsive states—2 mg–10 mg two to four times/day or 15 mg–30 mg once daily Children (over 6 months)— 1 mg–2.5 mg three to four times/day; may increase gradually as required *Parenteral* Adults Psychoneuroses—2 mg–10 mg IM or IV every 3 h–4 h as necessary depending on severity of symptoms Alcohol withdrawal—5 mg–10 mg IM or IV; repeat every 3 h–4 h Preoperative and minor surgical procedures (e.g., endoscopy)—5 mg–10 mg IM or IV 10 min to 20 min prior to procedure Status epilepticus–convulsive states—5 mg–10 mg IV; repeat at 10-min to 15-min intervals to a maximum of 30 mg Cardioversion—5 mg–15 mg IV 5 min to 10 min before procedure Children Tetanus—2 mg–10 mg IM or slow IV every 3 h–4 h	Effects occur within 20 min to 30 min with oral administration, 15 min to 30 min IM, and immediately IV; when using IV, inject slowly (5 mg/min) and avoid small veins to reduce danger of thrombophlebitis and local swelling and irritation; do not mix or dilute with other solutions or add to IV fluids; IM injection should be made deeply and slowly into a large muscle, such as the gluteus; when used to control convulsions, be prepared to readminister drug if seizures recur, as duration of action with IV use is rather short; use cautiously in patients with chronic lung disease or unstable cardiovascular status; facilities for respiratory assistance should be present when drug is given parenterally; use of diazepam for endoscopic procedures has been associated with coughing, dyspnea, hyperventilation, laryngospasm, and pain in the throat and chest; use a topical anesthetic, and have countermeasures available (e.g., respiratory assistance); reduce dose of narcotic analgesic by one third when used with diazepam (Schedule IV).

(continued)

Table 28-2 (continued)
Benzodiazepines

Drug	Preparations	Usual Dosage Range	Clinical Considerations
diazepam (Valium, Valrelease, Vazepam, Zetran) (continued)		Status epilepticus Under 5 years: 0.2 mg–0.5 mg by slow IV every 2 min to 5 min Over 5 years: 1 mg every 2 min to 5 min	
halazepam (Paxipam)	Tablets—20 mg, 40 mg	20 mg–40 mg three to four times/day Elderly—20 mg one to two times/day	Long-acting benzodiazepine; maximum plasma levels are attained in 1 h–3 h; highly protein-bound; do not use in children under 18 (Schedule IV).
lorazepam (Alzapam, Ativan)	Tablets—0.5 mg, 1 mg, 2 mg Injection—2 mg/ml, 4 mg/ml	*Oral* Anxiety—1 mg–2 mg two to three times/day Insomnia—2 mg–4 mg at bedtime *IM* Preoperative medication—0.05 mg/kg 2 h before procedure (maximum 4 mg) *IV* Acute anxiety—2 mg–4 mg	Short-acting drug used for anxiety, preanesthetic medication, and temporary relief of insomnia; not recommended in children under 12 years of age; dosage must be individually titrated; increase dose gradually to minimize adverse effects; elderly or debilitated persons should receive an initial dose of 1 mg–2 mg/day; less danger of accumulation than with other phenothiazine derivatives because no active metabolites are formed; inject IM deep into muscle mass; dilute in appropriate diluent for IV administration; do not use if discolored (Schedule IV).
oxazepam (Serax)	Capsules—10 mg, 15 mg, 30 mg Tablets—15 mg	Adults—10 mg–30 mg three to four times/day Elderly or debilitated—10 mg three to four times/day	Slow onset and short duration of action; not recommended in children under 12 years of age; paradoxical excitation may occur in first 2 weeks of therapy; reduce dose until symptoms subside (Schedule IV).
prazepam (Centrax)	Tablets—10 mg Capsules—5 mg, 10 mg, 20 mg	Adults—20 mg–60 mg/day in divided doses Elderly—10 mg–15 mg/day	Slow onset and prolonged duration of action; not indicated in patients under 18 years of age; can be used as a single daily dose (20 mg–40 mg) at bedtime; it is similar to diazepam in actions and toxicity (Schedule IV).

Table 28-3
Benzodiazepine Pharmacokinetics

Drug	Usual Daily Dosage Range	Oral Onset of Action	Peak Plasma Levels (h)	Activity of Metabolites	Elimination Half-life (h)
alprazolam (Xanax)	0.75 mg–3.0 mg	Fast	1–2	Active*	12–15
chlordiazepoxide (Librium)	15 mg–100 mg	Moderate	0.5–4	Active	5–30
clorazepate (Tranxene)	15 mg–60 mg	Fast	1–2	Active	30–90
diazepam (Valium)	4 mg–40 mg	Very fast	0.5–1.5	Active	20–50
halazepam (Paxipam)	60 mg–160 mg	Fast	1–3	Active	12–15
lorazepam (Ativan)	2 mg–8 mg	Moderate	1–4	Inactive	10–15
oxazepam (Serax)	30 mg–120 mg	Slow	1–4	Inactive	5–15
prazepam (Centrax)	20 mg–60 mg	Slow	2–6	Active	30–100

* Alprazolam has two metabolites, one of which is inactive, the other being approximately one half as active as the parent compound.

Other—Changes in libido, menstrual irregularities, nasal congestion, hiccups, difficulty swallowing, blurred vision, diplopia, nystagmus, hepatic dysfunction (jaundice), thrombophlebitis on IV injection, pain or burning on IM injection

Overdosage with benzodiazepines alone is seldom fatal, and most fatalities are the result of multiple drug ingestion. Symptoms of benzodiazepine overdosage include drowsiness, confusion, ataxia, and hypotension but rarely is there significant circulatory or respiratory depression. Treatment is usually supportive, and can include intravenous fluids, pressor agents, osmotic diuretics, and occasionally intravenous physostigmine to reverse symptoms of central anticholinergic overdosage.

CONTRAINDICATIONS AND PRECAUTIONS

Principal contraindications to the use of benzodiazepines are the presence of psychoses, narrow-angle glaucoma, and shock. In addition, benzodiazepines should not be given to pregnant women, since fetal malformations have occurred with their use, nor should they be administered to nursing mothers, because they are readily excreted in breast milk.

Cautious use should be undertaken in patients with a history of or tendency toward alcohol or drug abuse, patients with impaired liver or kidney function, and in elderly, very young, or debilitated patients. Injectable benzodiazepines must be used with great care in elderly or very ill patients or those with limited pulmonary reserve because apnea and cardiac arrest can occur. Caution is also required in the presence of acute alcoholism and in patients with extreme muscle weakness. Intra-arterial injection can lead to arteriospasm and possible gangrene. Persons on long-term or high-dose therapy should be cautioned against abrupt discontinuation of therapy, as withdrawal symptoms can occur.

INTERACTIONS

1. Benzodiazepines may enhance the CNS-depressant effects of alcohol, barbiturates, antihistamines, phenothiazines, opiates, and other CNS-depressant drugs, and such combinations should be avoided.
2. The effects of phenytoin may be potentiated by benzodiazepines.
3. An increased muscle-relaxant effect can occur with combinations of benzodiazepines and other centrally and peripherally acting muscle relaxants.
4. The effects of levodopa may be antagonized by benzodiazepines.
5. The effects of benzodiazepines may be lessened in individuals who smoke.
6. Antacids or food may slow oral absorption of some benzodiazepines, especially chlordiazepoxide and diazepam.
7. The half-life of some benzodiazepines, but *not* lorazepam or oxazepam, can be prolonged by cimetidine or disulfiram as a result of impaired hepatic metabolism.
8. Oral contraceptives and valproic acid have been shown to reduce the metabolism of diazepam and possibly chlordiazepoxide.

■ Nursing Process

See Chapter 26 for use of chlordiazepoxide in alcohol withdrawal and Chapter 30 for use of diazepam in status epileptics.

☐ *ASSESSMENT*

☐ *Subjective Data*

Benzodiazepines are among the most commonly prescribed drugs in the United States. Repeated media coverage about abuse and inappropriate prescription of these agents has also heightened consumer awareness about the risks and dangers of such drugs. The nurse needs to investigate what a person knows about the prescribed antianxiety agent, what his perception is of what the drug will do, and what fears or preconceived notions he may have about the drugs. Such information will help in teaching the patient about the risks and benefits of a benzodiazepine.

The nurse should assess habituation potential since benzodiazepines can be habit-forming. The person who is known to abuse other drugs or alcohol is at high risk for abusing antianxiety agents. Such persons may continue to increase the dose when the prescribed dose fails to achieve the desired outcome. This may happen to anyone who has an unrealistic view of what the drug can do to alleviate anxiety and to improve coping. Discussions about habituation will help the nurse understand the patient's pattern of drug taking. A thorough drug history may facilitate this process.

☐ *Objective Data*

Liver and kidney function should be tested to determine whether the patient can eliminate drug metabolites. Baseline neurologic assessment of motor and sensory function is useful in monitoring the development of side-effects. Psychiatric assessment of the type and level of anxiety to be treated will also provide a basis for comparison as drug therapy continues.

☐ *NURSING DIAGNOSES*

Actual nursing diagnoses may include
> Knowledge deficit related to drug action, correct dose and time of administration, and side-effects
> Anxiety related to drug effectiveness in anxiety-producing situations

Potential nursing diagnoses include
> Potential for injury: trauma, related to drowsiness, lethargy, and ataxia sometimes noted early in therapy (especially in the elderly)
> Alteration in thought processes related to confusion (especially in the elderly)

☐ *PLAN*

The nursing care goals should focus on safe administration in acute care (see also Chaps. 26 and 30) as well as the development of a teaching plan aimed at helping the patient to learn the following:

1. Appropriate dose and times of drug taking
2. How to monitor and manage side-effects
3. Symptoms of overdosage or toxic reaction
4. How to withdraw from the drug, under supervision

☐ *INTERVENTION*

Explanation of how to take the drug will depend on the prescription selected. Initially, a benzodiazepine may be ordered on a tid or qid schedule and later reduced to a prn (as needed) prescription. Either pattern poses concerns for the patient as to when and where to take the drug. Many patients want to take the drug prior to approaching an anxiety-producing situation rather than on a routine basis. This may be helpful to the patient but can pose problems if the anxiety situations exceed a safe dosage range of medication for a day. Patients need to know the safe limits of the prescribed drug. They may need counseling to avoid overdependence on the drug.

Patients become psychologically dependent on benzodiazepines when they use the drug to cope with anxiety-producing or stress-producing situations. This is not necessarily a negative phenomenon. The person who is terrified of airplanes but is able to board a plane and complete a trip with the aid of Valium has successfully used the drug to help overcome his fear. His psychologic dependency may soon reach the stage where he needs only to have the drug in his pocket "just in case" when he boards a plane. On the other hand, an agoraphobic who gradually needs more and more of the drug to find the courage to leave her home is also psychologically dependent on the drug but the drug is not working. In addition, by increasing the dosage, she is increasing the risk of toxicity and a physiologic dependence, which will result in painful and dangerous symptoms when the drug is withdrawn. The nurse can explore with patients how the drug is used to determine the pattern of administration and what dangers may be developing. Self-dosing beyond certain limits should be discouraged.

Common side-effects such as drowsiness, fatigue, and lethargy are usually transient, subside within the first few days of treatment, and are more frequent in the elderly. The patient should be warned to avoid driving, operating machinery, or engaging in any hazardous activity until his response to the drug is known. The physician should be notified if such symptoms do not subside or if gait problems or confusion develops. The drug dose may need to be decreased or the drug discontinued.

Patients need to know what symptoms will occur with excessive drug use. These include ataxia, dizziness, and slurred speech. All the patient's significant others need to know such signs and that they must be reported immediately to avert more dangerous signs of toxicity. Supportive care for overdose is outlined above under Side-Effects/Adverse Reactions.

Patients must also remember not to withdraw suddenly from the drug by themselves. Some patients will try to do this when things are going well and they want to be drug-free or if they begin to develop fears of dependency. Anyone who has been on an average adult daily dose for over 6 months needs to withdraw from the drug slowly by decreasing the dose by one eighth every 2 weeks. Faster reduction may result in harmful reactions such as vomiting, cramping, sweating, sleep difficulties, and even convulsions or delirium. The patient who wants to withdraw from the drug needs to explore his reasons. Drug-free "holidays" of one day a week may be useful to help a patient try to eliminate the drug "crutch" from his life. These can be gradually increased if successful. As the drug-free days increase, both the patient and his clinical caretakers need to watch for return of symptoms and methods of dealing with life stresses. An increase in anxiety and loss of coping mean serious consideration must be given to the value of drug withdrawal. Sometimes non-drug intervention strategies such as relaxation and distraction techniques can be useful in helping patients cope with life problems. They should be part of the treatment plan since the drug alone can never solve the problem.

The elderly need careful monitoring on benzodiazepine treatment because their reduced liver and kidney function makes them more susceptible to the development of side-effects and toxicity. In addition, elderly patients tend to use benzodiazepines for situational crises, sleep problems, and depression commonly associated with the loneliness of old age. Discovery of frequent use may indicate the need to teach such a person to use non-drug strategies rather than pills. Benzodiazepines tend to make the elderly patient drowsy and less interested in interacting. Consequently a dangerous cycle can develop, starting with depression, then drug taking, then social withdrawal and more depression.

□ *EVALUATION*

Successful use of the benzodiazepines can be best determined by comparing pretreatment psycho-logic profiles with current life and coping strategies. In addition, the nurse can review with the individual knowledge of side-effects and withdrawal symptoms. A review of drug-taking strategies and the frequency of refill requests will let the health team know when, where, and how the patient is using the benzodiazepine.

Midazolam

(Versed)

MECHANISM AND ACTIONS

Midazolam is a short-acting benzodiazepine used parenterally for preoperative and perioperative sedation and as a supplement to nitrous oxide anesthesia for short surgical procedures. Its actions resemble those of the other benzodiazepines and its onset of sedative action is very rapid following injection. There is a slight to moderate decrease in mean arterial pressure, cardiac output, stroke volume, and systemic vascular resistance.

USES

1. Preoperative sedation and to reduce recall of perioperative events (IM)
2. Production of sedation prior to short diagnostic or endoscopic procedures (alone *or* with a narcotic drug) (IV)
3. Induction of general anesthesia, before administration of other anesthetic agents (IV)
4. Supplementation of nitrous oxide/oxygen anesthesia for short surgical procedures (IV)

ADMINISTRATION AND DOSAGE

Midazolam is available as an injectable solution containing 1 mg/ml and 5 mg/ml. The drug may be given either intramuscularly deep into a large muscle mass, or by slow intravenous injection (rapid IV injection may result in significant respiratory depression). The following dosage schedules are recommended:

Preoperative/perioperative sedation. 0.07 mg/kg to 0.08 mg/kg IM 1 hour before surgery

Endoscopic or cardiovascular procedures: 0.1 mg/kg to 0.15 mg/kg IV (up to 0.2 mg/kg); dosage should be reduced if narcotic premedication is used or if given to patients over 60 years of age.

Induction of general anesthesia: 0.3 mg/kg to 0.35 mg/kg initially (IV); increments of 25% of the initial dose may be given if needed after 2 to 3 minutes. If patient has received narcotic premedication, the recommended dose is 0.15 mg/kg to 0.3 mg/kg IV.

FATE
Peak plasma levels occur within 45 minutes after intramuscular administration. Midazolam is approximately 97% protein bound. The onset of sedative effects after intramuscular administration is 15 minutes, while following intravenous injection, onset occurs within 3 to 5 minutes. When given intravenously, induction of anesthesia occurs within 2 to 3 minutes. Awakening from general anesthesia usually occurs within 2 hours, but may require up to 6 hours.

SIDE-EFFECTS/ADVERSE REACTIONS
Commonly encountered side-effects with midazolam include decreased respiratory rate and tidal volume, hiccups, nausea, vomiting, pain and tenderness on injection, and apnea following rapid intravenous injection. Other adverse reactions associated with midazolam administration include headache, muscle stiffness, and redness and induration at intramuscular injection sites.

Following intravenous administration, a variety of untoward reactions have occurred in a small percentage of patients; these include

CNS—Sedation, headache, confusion, dizziness, amnesia, nervousness, agitation, anxiety, delirium, insomnia, nightmares, tremor, involuntary movements, ataxia, paresthesias, slurred speech, blurred vision, and tonic/clonic movements

Cardiovascular—Premature ventricular contractions, tachycardia, bigeminy, hematoma at IM injection site

Respiratory—Bronchospasm, laryngospasm, dyspnea, hyperventilation, wheezing, tachypnea

Dermatologic—Swelling or feeling of burning or warmth at injection site, rash, pruritus, urticaria

Other—Salivation, retching, yawning, lethargy, weakness, chills, toothache

Symptoms of overdosage are characteristic of other benzodiazepines and include somnolence, sedation, confusion, impaired coordination, reduced reflexes, and respiratory distress. Treatment is supportive.

CONTRAINDICATIONS AND PRECAUTIONS
Midazolam is contraindicated in patients with acute narrow-angle glaucoma, and in patients in shock, those with acute alcohol intoxication, or those with significantly depressed vital signs or in coma. It is not recommended in pregnant or nursing mothers nor for obstetric use, since neonatal depression can easily occur. The safety of midazolam in children under 18 years of age has not been established. The drug must be given cautiously to patients with respiratory disease, hypotension, congestive heart failure, or renal dysfunction, and to elderly patients.

INTERACTIONS
1. The duration or degree of respiratory depression may be enhanced by concurrent use of other respiratory depressants, such as barbiturates, narcotics, or alcohol.
2. The dosage of induction or inhalational anesthetics may need to be reduced if midazolam is used preoperatively.
3. The hypnotic effects of midazolam may be accentuated by preanesthetic use of narcotics, barbiturates, or other sedative agents.

NURSING CONSIDERATIONS
Refer to the general nursing considerations for benzodiazepines, above. However, since midazolam is primarily used on an acute basis, the risk of dependence is minimal.

Carbamates

The carbamate class of antianxiety drugs is presently represented by only one agent, meprobamate. Although the pharmacologic actions of meprobamate resemble those of the benzodiazepines in many respects, this drug is probably closer to the barbiturates than to the benzodiazepines with regard to its degree of CNS depression, especially with large doses, and in its potential to cause habituation and abuse. As a simple antianxiety drug, meprobamate has no significant advantages over the benzodiazepines, while being potentially more toxic and addicting. Thus, the clinical use of meprobamate should be reserved to those *few* situations in which the benzodiazepines are not appropriate for the management of anxiety states.

Meprobamate
(Equanil, Miltown, and various other manufacturers)

MECHANISM AND ACTIONS
Meprobamate acts at several levels of the CNS, including the limbic system, thalamus, and spinal cord. It does not appear to possess a specific depressant action on the reticular-activating system, but it is mildly to moderately tranquilizing and exhibits anticonvulsant and skeletal muscle relaxing activity. Unlike the benzodiazepines, meprobamate does not interact with the inhibitory neuro-

transmitter GABA but it does appear to inhibit multineuronal spinal reflexes. During meprobamate therapy, rapid eye movement (REM) sleep time is reduced, as it is with barbiturates, and hepatic enzyme induction occurs with prolonged administration. High doses over extended periods of time can lead to significant respiratory and cardiovascular depression. Habituation and dependence, including true physical addiction, can result from chronic meprobamate use, and the incidence of meprobamate dependence is quite high among regular users.

USES
1. *Short-term* relief of anxiety and tension associated with neuroses and psychosomatic disorders (*alternate drug only* to the less hazardous benzodiazepines)

ADMINISTRATION AND DOSAGE
Meprobamate is given orally as tablets (200 mg, 400 mg, 600 mg), capsules (400 mg), or sustained-release capsules (200 mg, 400 mg). The adult dosage range is 1200 mg to 1600 mg a day in three or four divided doses to a maximum of 2400 mg/day. Children (6 years–12 years) may be given 100 mg to 200 mg two to three times a day, although the drug is probably best avoided in young children.

FATE
Oral absorption of meprobamate is rapid and effects are noted within 30 minutes to 60 minutes. Peak plasma concentrations are attained within 1 hour to 3 hours, and the plasma half-life usually ranges from 6 hours to 18 hours, but during prolonged administration it can be as high as 48 hours. The drug is rather uniformly distributed throughout the body and readily crosses the placental barrier. The extent of plasma protein binding is minimal (10%–20%). Meprobamate is extensively metabolized by the liver and is excreted primarily in the urine (90%) with some appearing in the feces. The drug can induce liver microsomal enzymes.

SIDE EFFECTS/ADVERSE REACTIONS
The most frequently occurring side-effects with meprobamate are drowsiness and ataxia, the incidence and severity of which are largely proportional to the dose. Many other untoward reactions have been reported in conjunction with meprobamate use, and these are listed below:

CNS—Dizziness, vertigo, slurred speech, weakness, paresthesias, headache, depression, confusion, paradoxic excitation, euphoria, hyperactivity

Hypersensitivity—Pruritus, urticaria, fever, edema, petechiae, ecchymoses, adenopathy; *less commonly*, bronchospasm, oliguria, anuria, stomatitis, angioedema, anaphylaxis, exfoliative dermatitis, erythema multiforme

Hematologic—Leukopenia, agranulocytosis, thrombocytopenic purpura, aplastic anemia, pancytopenia

Cardiovascular—Hypotension, flushing, syncope, palpitations, tachycardia, arrhythmias

Gastrointestinal—Nausea, vomiting, diarrhea, dry mouth, glossitis

Other—Exacerbation of porphyria, increased incidence of grand mal attacks, pain at IM injection site

Acute overdosage is characterized by lethargy, stupor, ataxia, vasomotor and respiratory collapse, arrhythmias, profound hypotension, shock, and possibly death. Fatalities have occurred with doses as low as 12 g, but survival has been reported with ingestion of amounts up to 40 g.

Treatment is essentially symptomatic and supportive. Gastric lavage is of value only if carried out shortly after ingestion due to the rapid drug absorption. Plasma expanders may be necessary but fluid overload must be avoided since pulmonary edema has occurred. Meprobamate is dialyzable.

CONTRAINDICATIONS AND PRECAUTIONS
Meprobamate is contraindicated in acute intermittent porphyria. In addition, there is probably little justification for its use in pregnant or nursing mothers, in children under age 6, or in known or suspected drug addicts. The drug must be used *cautiously* in the presence of impaired renal or hepatic function, epilepsy (may precipitate seizures), and in elderly or debilitated patients. Persons performing tasks requiring alertess should be extremely careful when taking meprobamate, since drowsiness, dizziness, and blurred vision are common occurrences. Abrupt discontinuation of meprobamate after prolonged or high-dose therapy can precipate a withdrawal syndrome marked by anxiety, vomiting, ataxia, tremors, muscle twitching, confusion, hallucinations, and, in some cases, convulsions. Following prolonged administration, dosage should be gradually reduced over 1 week to 2 weeks rather than stopped abruptly.

INTERACTIONS
1. Additive depressant effects can occur between meprobamate and other CNS depressants (*e.g.,*

alcohol, barbiturates, phenothiazines, tricyclic antidepressants).

2. Meprobamate may augment the metabolism of oral anticoagulants and steroid hormones, thereby reducing their pharmacologic effects.

NURSING CONSIDERATIONS
See the discussion of nursing considerations under benzodiazepines. This drug should also be withdrawn gradually after long-term use since severe symptoms can occur. Reduction of dose should occur over a 1-week to 2-week period. Warn the patient that sudden withdrawal can precipitate vomiting, tremors, muscle twitching, hyperactivity, confusion, and possibly convulsions.

Miscellaneous Antianxiety Drugs

Buspirone
(BuSpar)

MECHANISM AND ACTIONS
Buspirone is a chemically unique antianxiety agent that is pharmacologically distinct from other sedative or anxiolytic drugs. The mechanism of action of buspirone is not completely established but the drug appears to have an affinity for certain serotonin and dopamine receptors. Unlike the benzodiazepines, however, buspirone does *not* interact the GABA nor bind to benzodiazepine receptor sites. Studies have indicated that buspirone lacks the muscle-relaxant and anticonvulsant actions of the benzodiazepines, and does not exhibit the significant sedative effect of other anxiolytic drugs. There is no evidence that tolerance develops to buspirone and it does not appear to cause psychologic or physical dependence. The drug is not classified as a controlled substance. Buspirone has not been demonstrated to increase alcohol-induced impairment of motor or mental function as is frequently noted with other antianxiety agents.

USES
1. Short-term management of anxiety disorders (Efficacy for longer than 3 weeks–4 weeks has not been conclusively demonstrated although patients have been given the drug for several months with no obvious untoward effects.)

ADMINISTRATION AND DOSAGE
Buspirone is used as 5-mg or 10-mg tablets. The initial adult dose is 5 mg three times a day. Dosage may be increased by 5 mg/day at 2-day to 3-day intervals as needed to a maximum of 60 mg/day. The usual maintenance dosage range is 20 mg/day to 30 mg/day in divided doses.

FATE
Oral absorption is rapid and peak plasma levels occur within 45 minutes to 90 minutes. First-pass hepatic metabolism is extensive. Approximately 95% of buspirone is protein bound in the plasma. The drug is metabolized by the liver, mainly to inactive hydroxylated metabolites, which are excreted largely in the urine (30%–65%), with lesser amounts in the feces (20%–40%). The elimination half-life is about 2 hours to 3 hours.

SIDE-EFFECTS/ADVERSE REACTIONS
The most common side-effects occurring during buspirone therapy are dizziness, nausea, headache, nervousness, lightheadedness, fatigue, excitement, and insomnia. Other less frequently reported side-effects include dry mouth, diarrhea, nonspecific chest pain, tachycardia, palpitations, drowsiness, dream disturbances, impaired concentration, confusion, depression, tinnitus, sore throat, blurred vision, nasal congestion, muscle aching, paresthesias, incoordination, mild tremor, weakness, and sweating.

A variety of other adverse effects have been reported on occasion in patients receiving buspirone; they are listed by organ system below:

CNS—Dysphoria, loss of interest, akathisia, fearfulness, hallucinations, seizures, slurred speech, cold intolerance, and suicidal ideation

Gastrointestinal—Anorexia, salivation, irritable colon, rectal bleeding

Genitourinary—Urinary hesitancy, menstrual irregularities, dysuria

Dermatologic—Rash, edema, pruritus, flushing, easy bruising, dry skin, hair loss

Musculoskeletal—Muscle cramps, arthralgia, muscle spasm

Respiratory—Hyperventilation, shortness of breath, chest congestion

Neurologic—Involuntary movements, slowed reaction time

Other—Altered taste or smell sensation, conjunctivitis, itching of the eyes, altered libido, increased SGOT and SGPT, weight gain, fever

Overdosage can result in vomiting, drowsiness, dizziness, gastric distress, and miosis. No deaths have occurred with doses as high as 375 mg. Treatment is supportive.

CONTRAINDICATIONS AND PRECAUTIONS

Buspirone administration should be undertaken with *caution* in patients with liver or kidney impairment, parkinsonism (due to the drug's dopamine receptor interaction), and in pregnant and nursing mothers. Safety for use in children under 18 has not been established. Buspirone has no antipsychotic activity. Although drowsiness is less likely with buspirone than with other antianxiety drugs, patients should be cautioned about driving or performing other hazardous activities until the effects of the drug are known.

Because the drug can bind to dopamine receptors, the potential exists for buspirone to cause changes in motor or neurologic function related to dopamine receptor activity. Patients should be told to watch for signs of abnormal motor activity (*e.g.*, restlessness, repetitive movements, dystonia) and to report them immediately).

INTERACTIONS

1. Buspirone can displace digoxin from protein-binding sites possibly potentiating its effects and toxicity.
2. Buspirone may have additional CNS-depressive effects when given together with other depressants, such as hypnotics, narcotics, and alcohol, although the likelihood of a clinically significant interaction is minimal.

NURSING CONSIDERATIONS

Refer to the nursing considerations for benzodiazepines, above. However, buspirone is significantly different from benzodiazepines in its pharmacology, and it does not exhibit tolerance nor a potential for dependence. Patients should be cautioned, however, to limit drug use to several weeks whenever possible.

Hydroxyzine

(Atarax, Vistaril, and various other manufacturers)

Hydroxyzine is an antihistamine that exhibits a mild CNS-depressant action, apparently exerted at subcortical brain levels. It also possesses a number of other pharmacologic actions, including anticholinergic, antihistaminic, bronchodilator, analgesic, antispasmodic, antiemetic, and mild antisecretory and skeletal muscle relaxant activity. The drug displays a good safety margin, and adverse reactions are usually minimal at recommended doses; thus, it is often used in children as a mild sedative preoperatively and for relief of itching.

MECHANISM AND ACTIONS

The precise mechanism by which hydroxyzine exerts its effects has not been completely established. It suppresses neuronal activity in subcortical brain areas but does not appear to depress cortical function. Interference with the action of histamine, acetylcholine, and possibly serotonin may contribute to its antispasmodic and bronchodilator activity.

USES

1. Symptomatic treatment of psychoneurotic states characterized by anxiety, tension, hostility, and motor hyperactivity
2. Relieve symptoms of anxiety associated with organic disturbances such as digestive disorders, allergic conditions, senility, menopause, alcoholism, and behavioral problems, especially in children
3. Management of pruritus associated with urticaria, dermatoses, and other histamine-mediated conditions
4. Adjunctive preoperative and prepartum therapy to help reduce anxiety and lessen narcotic analgesic requirements (oral or IM)
5. Adjunctive treatment of alcohol withdrawal or delirium tremens (IM)

ADMINISTRATION AND DOSAGE

Hydroxyzine may be used orally as tablets (10 mg, 25 mg, 50 mg, 100 mg), capsules (25 mg, 50 mg, 100 mg), or liquid (10 mg/5 ml, 25 mg/5 ml), and as an intramuscular injection (25 mg/ml, 50 mg/ml). The drug should never be injected subcutaneously, intravenously, or intra-arterially. The following are recommended dosage ranges for both oral and intramuscular administration.

Oral
Relief of anxiety
  Adults: 50 mg to 100 mg four times/day
  Children: 50 mg to 100 mg/day in divided doses
Relief of pruritus
  Adults: 25 mg three to four times/day
  Children: 50 mg to 100 mg/day in divided doses
Preoperative sedation
  Adults: 50 mg to 100 mg
  Children: 0.6 mg/kg

Intramuscular
Acute alcoholism
  50 mg to 100 mg every 4 hours to 6 hours as needed

Nausea/vomiting
    Adults: 25 mg to 100 mg
    Children: 1.1 mg/kg
Preoperative/postoperative
    Adults: 25 mg to 100 mg
    Children: 1.1 mg/kg

FATE

Hydroxyzine is rapidly absorbed both orally and parenterally. Effects are usually noted within 15 minutes to 30 minutes and peak plasma levels occur in 2 hours to 4 hours. Metabolism occurs primarily in the liver and excretion is mainly by the biliary/fecal route, with some drug appearing in the urine. Elimination half-life is approximately 3 hours.

SIDE-EFFECTS/ADVERSE REACTIONS

Transient drowsiness and dry mouth are the most frequently reported side-effects and generally disappear after a few days. Other adverse reactions attributable to hydroxyzine include hypersensitivity reactions (skin eruptions, urticaria, dyspnea, chest tightness), involuntary motor activity, and dizziness.

Overdosage is primarily characterized by oversedation and hypotension. General supportive care is recommended. Unlike the benzodiazepines and meprobamate, dependence does not appear to be a significant problem with chronic use of hydroxyzine, although prolonged administration should be avoided if possible.

CONTRAINDICATIONS AND PRECAUTIONS

Hydroxyzine is contraindicated in early pregnancy, since a potential for fetal damage exists. The drug should also be avoided in nursing mothers. *Cautious* administration is necessary in persons performing hazardous tasks and in persons with a history of drug abuse because of the sedative action of hydroxyzine.

INTERACTIONS

1. Hydroxyzine can potentiate the action of other CNS depressants, such as alcohol, narcotics, or barbiturates.

NURSING CONSIDERATIONS

This drug is most frequently used in combination with barbiturates or narcotics as a preoperative medication to reduce anxiety and dry secretions. These combinations will have additive effects so dosages of the controlled substances must be reduced in order to avoid respiratory depression.

Administration of hydroxyzine by intramuscular route must be deep since it is very irritating to tissue. The best site is the gluteus muscle in an adult or the midlateral thigh in a child. Sites should be rotated when injections are repeated.

Hydroxyzine causes mouth dryness, which can be alleviated with increased fluids and hard candy. It also causes transient drowsiness significant to anyone who must be alert in order to operate machinery. Such individuals should avoid or limit their use of dangerous machinery until the effect of the drug on them is known.

Chlormezanone

(Trancopal)

Chlormezanone is an infrequently used antianxiety drug for the treatment of mild anxiety and tension states. Its usual dosage range is 100 mg to 200 mg three to four times/day for adults, and 50 mg to 100 mg three to four times/day in children 5 years to 12 years of age. The onset of action is within 15 minutes to 30 minutes, and effects persist for up to 6 hours. Adverse reactions can include dizziness, rash, drowsiness, dryness of the mouth, muscle weakness, edema, and depression.

The warnings, precautions, and nursing considerations discussed previously in connection with the benzodiazepines generally pertain to the use of chlormezanone as well. The drug has no particular advantage over the other antianxiety agents and is simply an alternative drug.

CASE STUDY

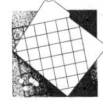

Mrs. Elma Isaacs, 77, lost her husband and son within the same year. She also sold her home and moved to a senior citizen apartment in a town where she knew no one. Almost immediately after moving, she became fearful of leaving the apartment. At her daughter's urging, she visited her family physician. She reported to him that she liked her apartment and enjoyed having her neighbors visit, but hated to go out unless her daughter took her. She also reported having trouble falling asleep and periods of weeping when she thought about her husband's death. After some discussion and Mrs. Isaacs' request for something to make her feel better, the physician prescribed Valium 5 mg PO tid or prn for 2 months.

The office nurse called Mrs. Isaacs 3 weeks later to see how she was doing. Mrs. Isaacs told the nurse she was attending a Bible study group held at her neighbor's apartment once a week and was feeling much better.

Three weeks after the nurse's follow-up call, Mrs. Isaacs called the office for a prescription renewal for Valium. The doctor asked her to make an appointment to come in instead.

Discussion Questions

1. What information do you need to collect from Mrs. Isaacs about her drug-taking pattern? How would you approach your concerns with this patient?
2. Is Valium an appropriate long-term treatment for Mrs. Isaacs? What do you need to know in order to determine that? What other intervention strategies could be used?
3. What strategies could be used to help Mrs. Isaacs be more aware of when she takes Valium?

REVIEW QUESTIONS

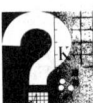

1. Outline the major differences between antianxiety drugs and antipsychotic drugs.
2. List several advantages of benzodiazepines over barbiturates for the relief of simple anxiety states.
3. What is the significance of a "shallow" dose–response curve?
4. Briefly describe the mechanism of action of the benzodiazepines.
5. Give six uses for the benzodiazepines.
6. Which benzodiazepine has the quickest onset of action when given orally? Which benzodiazepines are *not* converted to active metabolites? Which benzodiazepine also exhibits significant antidepressant activity?
7. What blood studies should be performed before benzodiazepines are prescribed?
8. What is the difference between psychologic and physiologic dependence on a benzodiazepine? How can the psychologic dependence be therapeutic to patients?
9. How can a nurse teach a patient to take a benzodiazepine safely on an as-needed basis?
10. How should a patient be withdrawn from long-term benzodiazepine therapy? What are the symptoms of withdrawal?
11. Why do the elderly need extra monitoring when a benzodiazepine is prescribed?
12. How does meprobamate differ pharmacologically from the benzodiazepines?
13. Outline the various pharmacologic effects exhibited by hydroxyzine.

14. Give the principal uses for hydroxyzine.
15. When hydroxyzine is prescribed by the intramuscular route, how should it be administered?
16. Are antianxiety drugs required for all types of anxiety states? Briefly explain.

BIBLIOGRAPHY

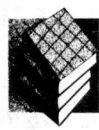

Bellantuono C, Reggi V, Tognoni G, Garatini S: Benzodiazepines: Clinical pharmacology and therapeutic use. Drugs 19:195, 1980

Bellantuono C, Reggi V, Tognoni G, Garatini S: Diazepam: The question of long term therapy and withdrawal reactions. Drug Therapy (special supplement) Proceeding of a symposium at Georgetown University, April 26, 1980

Burrows GD, Norman TR, Davies B (eds): Antianxiety Agents. Amsterdam, Elsevier, 1984

Dement W, Seidel W, Carskadon M: Daytime alertness, insomnia and benzodiazepines. Sleep 5(1):S28, 1982

Goldberg HL: Benzodiazepine and nonbenzodiazepine anxiolytics. Psychopathology, 17:(Suppl 1)45, 1984

Greenblatt DJ, Shader RI, Abernethy DR: Current status of benzodiazepines (2 parts). N Engl J Med 309:354, 410, 1983

Kastenholz KV, Crismon ML: Buspirone: A novel nonbenzodiazepine anxiolytic. Clin Pharmacol Ther 3:600, 1984

Lader M: Clinical pharmacology of benzodiazepines. Ann Rev Med 38:19, 1987

Lader M: Rational use of anxiolytic drugs. Ration Drug Ther 21(9):1, 1987

Lader M, Petursson H: Long-term effects of benzodiazepines. Neuropharmacology 22:527, 1983

Meyer BR: Benzodiazepines in the elderly. Med Clin North Am 66:1017, 1982

Miller CA: PRN drugs . . . to give or not to give. Geriatric Nursing Jan/Feb:37, 1982

Olsen RW: Gaba-benzodiazepine-barbiturate receptor interactions. J Neurochem 37:1, 1981

Owen RT, Tyrer P: Benzodiazepine dependence. Drugs 25:385, 1983

Rosenbaum JF: The drug treatment of anxiety. N Engl J Med 306:401, 1982

Schopf J: Withdrawal phenomena after long-term administration of benzodiazepines: A review of recent investigations. Journal of Pharmacopsychiatry 16:1, 1983

Skolnick P, Paul SM: The mechanism of action of the benzodiazepines. Med Res Rev 1:3, 1981

Tallman JF, Paul SM, Skolnick P, Gallager DW: Receptors for the age of anxiety: Pharmacology of the benzodiazepines. Science 207:274, 1980

Trimble MR (ed): Benzodiazepines Divided: A Multidisciplinary Review. New York, John Wiley & Sons, 1983

Wincor MZ: Insomnia and the new benzodiazepines. Clin Pharm 1:425, 1982

Antidepressants

*Biochemical Theories of
    Depression*

*Classification of Antidepressant
    Drugs*

Tricyclic Antidepressants
    Amitriptyline, Amoxapine,
        Desipramine,
        Doxepin, Imipramine,
        Maprotiline,
        Nortriptyline,
        Protriptyline,
        Trimipramine

Monoamine Oxidase Inhibitors
    Isocarboxazid, Phenelzine,
        Tranylcypromine

Miscellaneous Antidepressants
    Trazodone

29

Antidepressants are drugs that can alleviate many of the symptoms associated with a broad range of somatic disorders collectively known as *depression*. Drug treatment of depression is a confusing and somewhat controversial area of pharmacotherapy. The rather high "placebo" response rate in certain types of depressions—the apparent clinical benefit without active drug—suggests that great reliance should not be placed solely on drug therapy to the exclusion of other forms of treatment, including psychotherapy, environmental changes, and electroconvulsive therapy.

Nevertheless, in some types of depressions, significant therapeutic benefit has been obtained with many antidepressant drugs. Optimal clinical responses depend mainly on an accurate diagnosis of the depressive etiology, and it is here that much controversy still exists. One useful, though certainly not universally accepted, classification of depressions, based primarily on their etiology, categorizes them as follows:

1. *Endogenous depression*
   - Characterized by anhedonia (absence of pleasure), sleep disturbances, motor retardation, loss of libido, anorexia, emotional withdrawal, and inability to cope with stress
   - Comprises approximately 25% of all depressions; may occur at any age
   - Tends to recur repeatedly
   - May be genetically determined (*i.e.*, family history)
   - Does not appear to have an external precipitating factor
   - Imbalances in central neurohormonal function are likely present
   - Usually responds quite well to antidepressant drugs
2. *Anxious neurotic depression*
   - Marked by anxiety, "overreactiveness" to loss or disappointment, and signs of irritability, hostility, and sometimes helplessness
   - Frequently occurs together with endogenous depression
   - May respond to conventional antidepressants but more frequently benefited by antianxiety or antipsychotic drugs
3. *Situational, reactive depression*
   - Characterized by profound sorrow, tension, guilt, vague bodily symptoms (muscular fatigue, headache, gastrointestinal disturbances)
   - Generally precipitated by a stressful or grief-producing life event, such as death of a loved one, serious illness, loss of employment, or aging; may also result from use of certain drugs (beta-blockers, reserpine, methyldopa, hormones)
   - Comprises the majority of clinical depressions (50%–60%)
   - Frequently self-limiting and spontaneous remission often follows resolution of precipitating adverse life event
   - Antidepressant drugs are variably effective but often are not required.
4. *Manic–depressive depression*
   - Marked by excessive and sometimes violent mood swings between mania and depression on a regularly recurring basis (*bipolar* affective disorder)
   - Comprises approximately 10% of all clinically evident depressions
   - Lithium is usually the drug of choice, although antidepressants are used concurrently in some cases.

Severe depressions, in which agitation is a predominant feature or in which risk of suicide is high, are often best treated initially with electroconvulsive therapy (ECT). Rapid and dramatic improvement is frequently noted in *severely* depressed persons following ECT, making these patients more amenable to subsequent drug therapy. Concurrent use of oral antidepressants during ECT may increase the hazards, and such therapy should be avoided. Patients receiving oral antidepressants who are to undergo ECT generally should have the drugs discontinued for 24 hours to 48 hours prior to the ECT.

Biochemical Theories of Depression

Depressive symptomatology cannot be ascribed to any one particular neurochemical deficit in the brain. Reduced availability of the amine neurohormones norepinephrine and serotonin, however, is generally believed to underlie most types of endogenous depressions. This is termed the *amine hypothesis* and has been proposed to explain the development of depression. While certainly oversimplistic in many aspects, it suggests that reduced functional levels of norepinephrine and serotonin at central synapses (perhaps due to impaired synthesis or decreased neuronal release) occur in most depressive states. As a result, postsynaptic receptor activity may increase over time, and this receptor supersensitivity may be an essential development in endogenous depression. Clinically effective antidepressant drugs facilitate the action of central neurohormones by several different mechanisms, and thereby appear to restore normal receptor function. This action will be explored in detail below.

Classification of Antidepressant Drugs

A variety of chemical compounds possess antidepressant activity; however, no one group of drugs represent the ideal antidepressants in terms of efficacy as well as safety. The clinically useful antidepressant drugs can be categorized into one of the following groups:
1. *Tricyclic antidepressants* (e.g., imipramine, amitriptyline)
2. *Monoamine oxidase inhibitors* (e.g., isocarboxazid, tranylcypromine)
3. *Amphetamines and other central nervous system stimulants* (e.g., dextroamphetamine, methylphenidate)
4. *Miscellaneous* (e.g., trazodone)

The *tricyclic antidepressants* are the most widely used drugs for the treatment of endogenous depression and will be reviewed in detail below. Structurally dissimilar but pharmacologically comparable drugs, such as trazodone, are also considered here. They are sometimes referred to as "second-generation" antidepressants and their side-effect profile is somewhat different from that of the more classical drugs. *Monoamine oxidase inhibitors* were the first clinically effective group of antidepressants to be introduced into clinical medicine, but their lower clinical effectiveness relative to the tricyclics and their greater potential to elicit untoward reactions have largely relegated these drugs to alternative status in treating severe depressions not managed successfully by the tricyclic drugs. The monoamine oxidase (MAO) inhibitors will be discussed in this chapter. Finally, several central nervous system (CNS) stimulants, most of which are amphetamine derivatives, have been utilized in some instances of mild depressive states, but their lack of potency in more severe depressions and especially their potential for abuse have rendered their use in true depression essentially obsolete. They have other recognized indications, however, and will be reviewed in Chapter 32.

Successful outpatient treatment of depression is a difficult task at best and requires accurate diagnosis, critical dosage adjustment, and careful

observation of the patient for untoward reactions. The available antidepressant drugs are both effective and potentially hazardous substances; they must be prescribed and monitored with care and attention. Moreover, depressed patients need emotional support perhaps as much as they need the proper drugs, and lack of support can negate the beneficial effects of any antidepressant drug.

Tricyclic Antidepressants

Amitriptyline, Amoxapine, Desipramine, Doxepin, Imipramine, Maprotiline, Nortriptyline, Protriptyline, Trimipramine

Tricyclic antidepressants are so named because of their characteristic three-ring nuclear structure. Some newer compounds (e.g., maprotiline) possess a four-ring nuclear structure but are similar in most respects to the tricyclic drugs. The discussion that follows uses the term *tricyclic* as a matter of convention; however, the information refers to the tetracyclic compounds as well. Differences among the various drugs are noted throughout the discussion where appropriate.

The currently available tricyclic antidepressants are structurally analogous to the phenothiazine antipsychotic agents, and there are many similarities in the pharmacologic and toxicologic spectrum of action of these two classes of drugs (e.g., sedation, anticholinergic action, orthostatic hypotension). Tricyclics possess a specific blocking action on the uptake of biogenic amines (e.g., norepinephrine, serotonin) at the nerve ending. Uptake of these biogenic amines following their release from the presynaptic nerve endings represents the major means by which their synaptic action is terminated (see Fig. 15-2). Blockade of this reuptake mechanism by tricyclic drugs thus prolongs and potentiates the action of these biogenic amines at the synaptic junction, resulting in a longer postsynaptic receptor activation. This effect accounts for at least a part of the drugs' antidepressant action. Selective differences exist among the different tricyclic drugs in their relative potency for blocking norepinephrine versus serotonin uptake. These differences are outlined in Table 29-1 and may account for the varying degrees of effectiveness among tricyclics observed in differ-

Table 29-1
Pharmacologic Characteristics and Major Side-Effects of Tricyclic Antidepressants

	Blockade of Amine Pump		Side-Effects		
	Norepinephrine	Serotonin	Sedation	Anticholinergic Action	Orthostatic Hypotension
amitriptyline	+	+++	+++	+++	++
amoxapine	++	++	++	+	+
desipramine	+++	+	+	+	+
doxepin	−	+	+++	++	++
imipramine	++	+++	++	++	+++
maprotiline*	++	0	++	+	+
nortriptyline	++	++	++	++	+
protriptyline	−	−	0	+++	++
trimipramine	−	−	+++	++	++

* Tetracyclic derivative
Key: +++, strong effect; ++, moderate effect; +, weak effect; 0, no significant effect; −, variable, inconsistent effect (studies are inconclusive)

ent depressed populations although there appears to be *no* consistent relationship between amine-uptake blocking action and clinical antidepressant efficacy. As noted earlier, endogenous depressions are often characterized by either a predominant norepinephrine or serotonin deficiency. Patients with a norepinephrine deficiency, as determined by low urinary levels of 3-methoxy-4-hydroxy phenylglycol (MHPG), the major norepinephrine metabolite, may respond well to tricyclics that block norepinephrine uptake to a significant extent (*i.e.,* desipramine, nortriptyline, imipramine). Conversely, low urinary levels of 5-hydroxyindoleacetic acid (5-HIAA), the serotonin metabolite, suggest a relative serotonergic deficiency, and tricyclics with strong serotonin-uptake blocking activity (*i.e.,* amitriptyline) appear to be the logical drugs of choice in this situation.

It is important to realize that blockade of biogenic amine uptake into nerve endings is not the sole mechanism of the antidepressant action of the tricyclics. In fact, clinical observations suggest it may not even be the principal mechanism of action. It is well known that the therapeutic benefit—the relief of depressive symptoms—of most tricyclics is evident only after several weeks of continual therapy, whereas the blocking effect of these drugs on amine uptake occurs almost immediately. Therefore, it is difficult to correlate the latency of clinical action with the immediacy of the biochemical action. Tricyclics also have been shown to exert a blocking action at presynaptic alpha-adrenergic receptors (alpha-2 sites) regulating norepinephrine release. Presynaptic alpha-blockade results in in-

creased norepinephrine release, because normal activation of these receptors is responsible for inhibiting release of norepinephrine through a negative feedback effect. The combined effects of reuptake inhibition and increased presynaptic neurohormone release by way of alpha-2 antagonism lead to a persistent occupation of postsynaptic receptor sites, which eventually become fewer in number and less sensitive to their respective neurohormones. Loss of receptor population, termed *down-regulation*, is slow in developing when a patient is started on a tricyclic antidepressant, and the time course of the receptors' down-regulation closely corresponds to the onset of antidepressant activity. Therefore, it may play a major role in the therapeutic efficacy of the tricyclic antidepressants.

Tricyclic compounds have a sedative action, can exert a central and peripheral anticholinergic action, and may induce orthostatic hypotension, especially in the elderly. Although these various side-effects have been noted with most of the derivatives, the frequency of occurrence and degree of effect vary considerably among the different drugs, as outlined in Table 29-1. Again, however, there appears to be no *consistent* relationship between the differential amine-uptake blocking action of these drugs and the severity of side-effects, such as sedation or hypotension. In addition to the side-effects noted above, tricyclic antidepressants are associated with a wide range of other untoward reactions, and these are listed under Side-Effects/Adverse Reactions, below. Specific mention should be made of the potential for these drugs to elicit electrocardiographic (ECG) abnormalities, especially in high doses. Because of the danger of prolonged conduction time, sinus tachycardia, and other cardiac arrhythmias, tricyclic antidepressants must be used with caution in patients with heart disease.

Although it would seem that tricyclics with prominent sedative activity would be most useful in depressive states characterized by anxiety or agitation, whereas a drug such as protriptyline, which is largely nonsedating, might be preferred in retarded or apathetic depressions, this differential applicability remains to be proven clinically.

Differences in selectivity of amine-uptake blockade and degree of side-effects notwithstanding, the overall profile of all tricyclic antidepressants is remarkably similar. In fact, recommended dosage ranges for all these drugs, except protriptyline, are nearly identical. These drugs will therefore be reviewed as a group. Selective differences among the drugs are presented in Table 29-2.

MECHANISM AND ACTIONS
Tricyclic antidepressants inhibit neuronal uptake of biogenic amines (norepinephrine, serotonin) into presynaptic endings, blocking a major mechanism for their inactivation, thereby potentiating their effects. They also exert a blocking effect at presynaptic alpha-adrenergic receptor sites (alpha-2 receptors), which results in increased release of neurotransmitters from the nerve ending. The increased receptor activation that results at postsynaptic adrenergic and serotonergic receptor sites gradually decreases their number and sensitivity, and the clinical efficacy of these agents is now thought to be primarily the result of the down-regulation of beta-adrenergic receptors in the CNS. Alterations in the responsiveness of central serotonin receptors through a similar action may likewise play a role in the therapeutic effectiveness of some tricyclic antidepressants. These drugs also possess anticholinergic and antihistaminic action, and produce peripheral vasodilation and orthostatic hypotension.

USES
1. Relief of the symptoms of depression (endogenous depression is most responsive)
2. Control of anxiety and sleep disturbances associated with depressive states (*especially* doxepin and amoxapine)
3. Treatment of depression in patients with manic–depressive disorders (*especially* maprotiline and doxepin)
4. Treatment of childhood enuresis (especially imipramine)

5. Investigational uses include enhanced control of pain (in combination with narcotic analgesics), prevention of migraine and cluster headaches (especially amitriptyline), treatment of obstructive sleep apnea (protriptyline), symptomatic management of peptic ulcer disease (doxepin, trimipramine), and treatment of attention-deficit disorders (desipramine).

ADMINISTRATION AND DOSAGE
See Table 29-2.

FATE
See Table 29-3.

Tricyclic antidepressants are generally well absorbed orally, but undergo significant first-pass inactivation. Peak plasma concentrations are usually attained within 2 hours to 4 hours. The drugs are highly protein bound (75%–95%), highly lipid soluble, and widely distributed throughout the body, including the CNS. Due to differences in extent of first-pass metabolism, there are wide interpatient variations in steady-state plasma levels, and dosage levels must be individualized. The plasma half-life is long for most drugs (Table 29-3), and permits single daily dosing for most drugs once steady-state levels have been attained. Metabolism occurs in the liver at variable rates, and many tricyclic drugs are metabolized to pharmacologically active derivatives (*e.g.*, imipramine to desipramine; amitriptyline to nortriptyline). Excretion is primarily in the urine, largely as metabolites. The therapeutic plasma range (*i.e.*, "therapeutic window") for the different drugs is also given in Table 29-3, but the correlation between plasma levels and therapeutic effectiveness remains to be definitely established.

SIDE-EFFECTS/ADVERSE REACTIONS
The most frequently occurring side-effects with the majority of tricyclic antidepressants are sedation (except with protriptyline), anticholinergic effects (such as dry mouth, blurred vision, constipation, and urinary hesitancy), headache (transient), tachycardia, muscle twitching, and weight gain. Children receiving tricyclic drugs for enuresis commonly experience nervousness, sleep disturbances, tiredness, and gastrointestinal upset on initiation of therapy but these effects usually disappear with continued therapy.

Use of tricyclic antidepressants can result in a wide range of other adverse reactions, which are listed below. Not all of the following untoward effects have been noted with *every* tricyclic antidepressant but the possibility of their occurrence

(*Text continues on p. 540.*)

Table 29-2
Tricyclic Antidepressants

Drug	Preparations	Usual Dosage Range	Clinical Considerations
amitriptyline (Amitril, Elavil, Emitrip, Endep, Enovil)	Tablets—10 mg, 25 mg, 50 mg, 75 mg, 100 mg, 150 mg Injection—10 mg/ml	*Oral* Initially—75 mg–150 mg/day Maintenance—50 mg–100 mg/day in divided doses or at bedtime *IM* 20 mg–30 mg four times/day initially; replace with oral form as soon as possible	Most effective in endogenous depressions, especially those accompanied by anxiety, or in patients over age 50; investigational uses include prevention of migraine headaches and control of chronic pain, especially in combination with potent narcotics; sedative effect is prominent, especially early in therapy; give drug at bedtime to minimize daytime drowsiness.
amoxapine (Asendin)	Tablets—25 mg, 50 mg, 100 mg, 150 mg	50 mg two to three times/day initially; increase to 100 mg two to three times/day on the third day if necessary (Elderly patients should receive 25 mg two to three times/day initially, with gradual increases as tolerated) Once effective dose is established, may be given in a single bedtime dose not to exceed 300 mg	Used in a wide range of depressions; exhibits a moderate sedative action; clinical effects are usually observed within 7 days; may be used on a once-daily basis at bedtime; highly bound (90%) to plasma proteins, so interactions with other protein-bound drugs can occur; serum half-life is 8 h–12 h, but converted to an active metabolite with a half-life of 30 h; do not use in children under age 16; most frequent adverse reactions (10%–15%) are sedation, dry mouth, and constipation.
desipramine (Norpramin, Pertofrane)	Tablets—10 mg, 25 mg, 50 mg, 75 mg, 100 mg, 150 mg Capsules—25 mg, 50 mg	25 mg–50 mg three to four times/day (maximum 300 mg/day) 25 mg–100 mg/day in geriatric patients to a maximum of 150 mg/day	Active metabolite of imipramine, with essentially the same uses and adverse effects; not recommended in children; slightly lower incidence of sedation and anticholinergic action than imipramine; increased psychomotor activity may occur in first few weeks of therapy; orthostatic hypotension is common early in treatment and may necessitate dosage reduction; caution against rapid position changes; improvement is usually apparent within 1 week to 2 weeks.

(continued)

Table 29-2 (continued)
Tricyclic Antidepressants

Drug	Preparations	Usual Dosage Range	Clinical Considerations
doxepin (Adapin, Sinequan)	Capsules—10 mg, 25 mg, 50 mg, 75 mg, 100 mg, 150 mg Oral concentrate—10 mg/ml	25 mg–50 mg three times/day (maximum 300 mg/day) *Alternately*, up to 150 mg once daily at bedtime	Indicated for relief of depression and anxiety associated with psychotic or psychoneurotic disorders; antianxiety effects occur within several days, but antidepressant action requires several weeks; do not use in children under age 12; sedation is marked during initial stage of treatment; effects of alcohol may be enhanced; dilute oral concentrate with 4 oz of water, juice, or milk prior to administration.
imipramine (Janimine, Tipramine, Tofranil)	Tablets—10 mg, 25 mg, 50 mg Long-acting capsules (pamoate salt)—75 mg, 100 mg, 125 mg, 150 mg Injection—25 mg/2 ml	*Depression* Oral Initially—75 mg–150 mg/day in divided doses (maximum—300 mg/day) Maintenance—50 mg–150 mg once daily at bedtime IM 100 mg/day in divided doses *Enuresis* Initially—25 mg–50 mg/night, orally to a maximum of 75 mg Alternately, 25 mg in mid-afternoon and 25 mg at bedtime	Used for relief of symptoms of endogenous depressions and for reducing enuresis in children age 6 and older; decreases time spent in deep phases of sleep associated with bedwetting; may be administered in a single dose (Tofranil-PM) for depression; do not use the PM (pamoate salt) dosage form in enuresis; see also Nursing Process.
maprotiline (Ludiomil)	Tablets—25 mg, 50 mg, 75 mg	Initially—75 mg/day in single or divided doses; adjust to desired maintenance range, usually 75 mg–225 mg/day (maximum 300 mg/day) Elderly patient—50 mg/day–75 mg/day	A tetracyclic antidepressant with a slightly lower incidence of cardiovascular reactions and fewer anticholinergic side-effects than most tricyclic compounds; may have a rapid response (within 1 week) in some patients; used in manic–depressive disorders; most common side-effects are dry mouth and drowsiness; not indicated in children under age 18; reduce dosage in elderly patients, and during prolonged maintenance therapy.
nortriptyline (Aventyl, Pamelor)	Capsules—10 mg, 25 mg, 50 mg, 75 mg Liquid—10 mg/5 ml	25 mg three to four times/day (maximum 150 mg/day) 30 mg–50 mg/day in geriatric patients	Primarily effective in endogenous depressions; not recommended in children under age 12; drug is a metabolite of

(continued)

Table 29-2 (continued)
Tricyclic Antidepressants

Drug	Preparations	Usual Dosage Range	Clinical Considerations
nortriptyline (Aventyl, Pamelor) (continued)			amitriptyline and is similar to imipramine in most of its pharmacologic effects.
protriptyline (Vivactil)	Tablets—5 mg, 10 mg	5 mg–10 mg three to four times/day (maximum 60 mg/day) 5 mg three times/day in geriatric patients	Most effective in endogenous depressions in withdrawn and anergic patients; use is associated with minimal sedation but drug has more CNS-stimulatory and anticholinergic action than other tricyclics; orthostatic hypotension and tachycardia can occur frequently; use with caution in cardiac patients or in those with insomnia; not recommended in children under age 12; last dose should be taken not later than mid-afternoon, to avoid excessive stimulation at bedtime.
trimipramine (Surmontil)	Capsules—25 mg, 50 mg, 100 mg	Initially—75 mg–150 mg/day in divided doses Maintenance—50 mg–150 mg/day at bedtime 50 mg–100 mg/day in geriatric patients	Possesses significant sedative action; similar to amitriptyline in most respects; it is not recommended in children.

Table 29-3
Pharmacokinetics of Tricyclic Antidepressants

Drug	Plasma Half-Life (h)	Therapeutic Plasma Levels (ng/ml)	Protein Binding (%)	Latency to Attain Steady-State Plasma Levels (days)
amitriptyline	30–45	100–250	85–95	5–10
amoxapine	8–12	200–400	90	2–8
desipramine	12–60	150–300	75–90	2–10
doxepin	8–30	100–250	NA*	2–8
imipramine	6–20	200–300	75–90	2–5
maprotiline†	20–30	200–300	NA	5–10
nortriptyline	20–30	50–150	90–95	4–20
proptriptyline	60–120	100–200	90–95	8–10
trimipramine	8–30	150–200	NA	2–6

* Not available
† Tetracyclic derivative

should be recognized whenever one of these drugs is prescribed.

CNS—Anxiety, restlessness, agitation, irritability, fever, insomnia, nightmares, disorientation, confusion, delusions, hypomania, hallucinations, dizziness, tinnitus, numbness and tingling in extremities, ataxia, tremors, extrapyramidal symptoms, paresthesias, seizures

Cardiovascular—Orthostatic hypotension, arrhythmias, palpitations, congestive heart failure, infarction, heart block, stroke. ECG changes include prolongation of the P-R and Q-T intervals, reduction of the T wave, and formation of a prominent U wave.

Allergic—Skin rash, pruritus, urticaria, petechiae, photosensitization, edema, fever

Gastrointestinal—Nausea, anorexia, vomiting, diarrhea, cramping, epigastric distress, stomatitis

Endocrine—Galactorrhea, gynecomastia, testicular and breast swelling, altered libido, delayed ejaculation or impotence, altered blood sugar levels

Hematologic—Blood dyscrasias (agranulocytosis, eosinophilia, leukopenia, thrombocytopenia), bone marrow depression

Other—Altered liver function (including jaundice), alopecia, parotid gland enlargement, flushing, sweating, chills, nocturia, nasal congestion, lacrimation, increased appetite

Abrupt discontinuation of drug after prolonged therapy may produce a withdrawal syndrome characterized by nausea, vertigo, headache, nightmares, and malaise. Cessation of chronic therapy may also be associated with restlessness, irritability, sleep disturbances, and rarely hypomania.

Overdosage is characterized by CNS signs, such as confusion, agitation, hyperreflexia, seizures, and hallucinations; autonomic effects, such as dilated pupils, flushing, and hyperpyrexia; and cardiovascular complications, such as tachycardia, arrhythmias, pulmonary edema, hypotension, and possibly ventricular fibrillation. Treatment is directed toward removal of unabsorbed drug by lavage, maintaining respiratory function, providing necessary supportive therapy (fluids, oxygen, electrolytes), minimizing external stimulation, and vigorously treating arrhythmias, hypotension, and CNS disturbances. Physostigmine, 1 mg to 3 mg IV, may be used to reverse the anticholinergic effects, but caution must be exercised since profound bradycardia,

asystole, and seizures may occur. ECG activity must be closely monitored for at least 72 hours because relapse can occur following restoration of cardiac function.

CONTRAINDICATIONS AND PRECAUTIONS

Tricyclic antidepressants are contraindicated during the acute recovery phase of a myocardial infarction and in patients with narrow-angle glaucoma. They should not be given concomitantly with a MAO inhibitor. *Cautious* use of these drugs is necessary in the presence of renal or hepatic impairment, urinary retention, cardiovascular disease, hyperthyroidism, or psychoses. They should also be used cautiously in patients with a history of seizure disorders and in pregnant or nursing mothers. Other than for treating enuresis, tricyclics are *not* recommended in children under age 12.

INTERACTIONS

1. Tricyclics may enhance the effects of other CNS depressants (*e.g.,* alcohol, barbiturates, benzodiazepines, hypnotics, phenothiazines); catecholamines; other adrenergic drugs (*e.g.,* ephedrine, amphetamine); anticholinergics; narcotic analgesics; thyroid drugs; disulfiram; anticoagulants; vasodilators; and centrally acting muscle relaxants.
2. Tricyclics may antagonize the action of antihypertensives (*e.g.,* guanethidine, clonidine); beta-blockers; anticonvulsants (increase incidence of seizures); phenylbutazone; and cholinergic drugs.
3. The effects of tricyclics may be potentiated by phenothiazines, methylphenidate, cimetidine, amphetamines, furazolidone, acetazolamide, MAO inhibitors, and urinary alkalizers (*e.g.,* sodium bicarbonate).
4. Tricyclics should not be administered within 14 days of MAO inhibitors because hypertension, hyperpyrexia, and convulsions can occur.
5. Reserpine and tricyclic antidepressants can result in a stimulating effect, possibly leading to mania.
6. Therapeutic effects of tricyclics may be reduced by barbiturates (due to enzyme induction) and urinary acidifiers such as ammonium chloride and ascorbic acid (due to decreased renal tubular reabsorption), and oral contraceptives.
7. Increased cardiovascular toxic effects may be seen with thyroid drugs, quinidine, or procain-

amide in combination with tricyclic antidepressants.

■ *Nursing Process*

□ ASSESSMENT

□ *Subjective Data*
A thorough drug history needs to be taken. Tricyclic antidepressants interact with many other drugs; the interview should focus on the use of prescription drugs, over-the-counter medications, and street drugs. By using memory joggers for the prescription drugs listed above under Interactions and asking about the frequency of use of drugs for colds, nasal congestion, and coughing, the nurse can be fairly sure that the patient will remember most, if not all, the drugs he has taken. As part of this process the nurse can then introduce the discussion of street drug and alcohol use. Since these drugs in combination with tricyclics can be potentially fatal, abusers of such drugs are at high risk. They need to be identified before treatment begins.

The nurse also needs to explore the patient's perception of long-term therapy since tricyclics take several weeks to act on depressive symptoms. Discussions about the risks (side-effects) versus benefits (diminution of depression) of the drug, how to manage a regimen consistently, and the availability of support systems will help the nurse determine how to assist the patient through the transition period. Such discussions need to emphasize the importance of prescribed psychotherapy and clinical follow-up as equally important parts of the total care so the patient has a realistic understanding of the process.

Last, the nurse needs to assess the patient's thoughts of suicide. Some evidence suggests that as the tricyclic drugs lessen symptoms of depression, the patient with thoughts of suicide may be spurred to action. The suicidal patient needs to be even more carefully evaluated and followed since the therapy may introduce a new kind of instability that can threaten his existence.

□ *Objective Data*
A complete physical assessment is necessary with a focus on neurologic status and cardiovascular function. The patient should be weighed and extremities palpated for evidence of edema. An ECG should be included since development of cardiac arrhythmias is a major side-effect of tricyclic antidepressants.

Laboratory evaluation is intended to provide a baseline for future blood studies and reflects potential side-effects. Hepatic, renal and hematologic function blood studies, thyroid levels, blood sugar levels, and acid–base levels are appropriate.

□ NURSING DIAGNOSES
Actual nursing diagnoses include
  Knowledge deficit related to the action, dose, and side-effects of the drug
  Anxiety about the drug's effectiveness and long-term side-effects
Potential nursing diagnosis may include
  Alteration in bowel function: constipation
  Alteration in cardiac output: decreased related to drug-induced hypotension and arrhythmias
  Potential for injury: trauma related to sedation and dizziness
  Noncompliance with the regimen usually related to side-effects
  Alteration in oral mucous membrane related to dry mouth
  Sensory–perceptual alteration in vision: blurring
  Urinary retention
  Potential for violence: self-directed related to reemergence of suicidal thoughts

□ PLAN
The nursing care goals should focus on teaching the patient
  1. How to take the drug safely as prescribed
  2. The importance of therapy along with drug treatment
  3. How to manage common side-effects
  4. Which side-effects to report
  5. Symptoms of overdosage
  6. How to withdraw from the drug, when appropriate

□ INTERVENTION
Initially, the drug will be given in divided doses as the physician establishes an appropriate therapeutic blood level and modifies the dosage accordingly. The problem during this period is that early side-effects are more apparent and therefore more difficult to manage and accept. Pulse and blood pressure should be monitored several times a day and an ECG done biweekly until the dose is established and the patient's cardiovascular response is known. The nurse helps the patient achieve success by maintaining frequent contact to review side-effects and their management.

As therapy progresses, most medications can be given once a day. Selecting the time of day depends on whether the drug exerts a sedating effect, as it does in most patients, or a stimulating effect, as occasionally happens. The patient who reports the drug to be producing a stimulating effect should be carefully monitored for increased anxiety, mania, or returning depression, which may indicate the drug is not working. Unless this is done, the patient may continue to receive inappropriate treatment or even an inappropriate increase in dosage when the drug should actually be discontinued. If the patient shows no improvement in 8 weeks on a tricyclic drug, alternate therapy should be chosen. Careful monitoring by the patient, family, and health team will discover problems promptly.

Most of the side-effects can be detected by periodic blood studies so the patient should be encouraged to keep his clinic appointments. He will be monitored for liver and kidney function, evidence of blood dyscrasias, and development of arrhythmias, weight gain, or edema. He should be told to report any changes in his health status immediately.

Anticholinergic side-effects such as orthostatic hypotension, constipation, and mouth dryness can be handled as symptoms appear. They are usually transient and most bothersome early in the therapy. They are particularly troublesome to elderly patients and may persist throughout therapy in this population. Strategies need to be developed to help elderly patients cope with dizziness and protect themselves from injury if they must continue the drug. Eating hard candy, frequent mouth care, and extra fluids may help the patient manage dry mouth. Constipation can be treated with increased dietary fiber and fluids. Bulk laxatives and stool softeners may be added, as necessary.

Problems in sexual performance may not be reported even if they are experienced. The nurse needs to open the door to this subject by asking open-ended questions. Depression frequently leads to loss of libido and performance problems. The tricyclics can cause ejaculatory difficulties and further loss of libido. If sexual activity is important to the patient and he perceives the drug is causing problems in this area, he may abandon its use without ever discussing his reasons unless the nurse or physician creates an opportunity for him. The side-effect may be transient or dose-related, so such discussion can help reduce the risk of compliance problems.

Tricyclics can also cause sun sensitivity. Patients should be reminded to keep skin covered and to wear sun-block lotion and dark glasses when outdoors.

As depression abates during therapy, suicidal tendencies may emerge in susceptible patients and the risk is that such a patient will combine the tricyclic drug with alcohol or other central nervous system drugs in an attempt to kill himself. The combination can be fatal. Overdose by tricyclics is a serious emergency, since severe cardiac arrhythmias that are difficult to control, respiratory arrest, convulsions, severe hypotension, and hyperpyrexia are all possible consequences. Prevention by providing good support and follow-up is the best solution. Treatment of overdose is symptom related and will include gastric lavage to remove as much of the drug as possible.

On the positive side, as the person begins to feel well again, he may feel less need for the drug. The nurse needs to remind him that withdrawal from tricyclics should occur only under supervision and be done gradually. Drug-free holidays can be used to test the patient's ability to cope with life stresses once gradual reduction has begun.

□ **EVALUATION**
Evaluation may include patient reports of mood elevation; improved sleep, appetite, and coping; and a feeling of increased self-worth. Other gauges include the ability to manage side-effects and incorporate drug therapy into daily activities. However, drug therapy alone does not accomplish these things and must be evaluated in relation to the individual's participation in the other aspects of his prescribed therapy. Nursing Care Plan 29-1 summarizes the nursing process for the patient taking tricyclic antidepressants.

□ *Childhood Enuresis*
Imipramine has been shown to be effective in treating enuresis in children over age 6. Before treatment is prescribed the child's sleep patterns and the family dynamics in dealing with the child's "failure" to learn control need to be reviewed. Drug therapy will help control the symptom, bedwetting, but will not correct the problem if the underlying cause is not treated. More often than not, enuresis returns when the drug is discontinued because the underlying problems have not changed.

Careful monitoring of side-effects, especially sleep disturbances and nervousness, is very important because they may exacerbate the already difficult situation and lead to further problems.

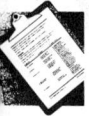

Nursing Care Plan 29-1
The Patient Receiving Tricyclic Antidepressants

Assessment

Subjective Data

1. Medication history: Refer to Interactions section to formulate pertinent inquiries
   a. Ask about OTC and street drug use because problems may be severe if patient attempts to overdose
   b. Allergies/hypersensitivity to these drugs
2. Medical history
   a. Check for preexisting conditions that may precipitate adverse reactions, including cardiovascular disease, narrow-angle glaucoma, renal or hepatic dysfunction, hyperthyroidism, seizure disorders
   b. Current pregnancy or lactation
   c. History of the development of symptoms that led client to seek treatment
3. Compliance issues/personal history
   a. Explore client/family perception of illness and treatment, motivation to get well, feelings about long-term therapy
   b. Explore suicidal thought

Objective Data

1. Physical assessment
   a. Vital signs
   b. Cardiovascular status: presence of arrhythmias, presence of peripheral edema
   c. Weight
   d. Neurologic status: mental acuity, memory, peripheral sensation
2. Laboratory/diagnostic data
   a. ECG as baseline
   b. Renal and hepatic function studies
   c. CBC with differential
   d. Thyroid function
   e. Fasting blood sugar
   f. Acid–base levels

Nursing Diagnosis	Expected Client Outcome	Intervention
Knowledge deficit related to drug effect, dosage schedule, how to monitor potential side-effects, potential adverse drug interactions, and the need to withdraw from the drug only under supervision	Will verbalize knowledge of drug effect, correct dosage schedule, how to monitor potential side-effects, which drugs to avoid and the need to withdraw from the drug under supervision	Administer or teach patient to take drug as prescribed, usually in divided doses initially to establish a therapeutic blood level, and then once a day. Monitor patient for sedation or excitation. If drug produces sedation, dose should be taken at night; if excitation occurs, drug should be taken in the morning. Teach patient to monitor common side-effects as described below and follow preventive strategies given. Encourage patient to return for follow-up laboratory evaluations as ordered to enable physician to detect early any liver dysfunction, blood dyscrasias, etc. Teach patient to read labels on all drugs and to avoid taking any new drug without first contacting the physician.

(continued)

Nursing Care Plan 29-1 (continued)
The Patient Receiving Tricyclic Antidepressants

Nursing Diagnosis	Expected Client Outcome	Intervention
		Teach the patient not to abruptly withdraw from the drug. Gradual dosage reduction under supervised care is necessary to avoid adverse side-effects.
Potential alteration in cardiac output: decreased, related to drug-induced arrhythmias	Arrhythmias will be avoided or detected early	Monitor vital signs at least every 4 h during initial treatment phase. Teach patient to report dizziness (possible hypotension) or palpitations immediately.
		Ensure ECGs are performed as ordered; usually biweekly during initial phase until cardiac response is known.
Potential alteration in comfort: GI upset related to drug effect	Gastrointestinal distress will be avoided or controlled	Encourage patient to take drug with food or milk.
		Encourage smaller, more frequent meals until symptoms subside.
		Encourage early reporting if symptoms persist.
Potential alteration in bowel elimination: constipation related to drug effect	Will maintain a regular bowel schedule	Encourage increasing fluids, fiber, and roughage food intake throughout drug therapy.
		Administer laxatives, as prescribed. Encourage patient to avoid regular use.
Potential alteration in oral mucous membrane	Will obtain relief from dry mouth	Encourage frequent mouth care, sucking on hard candy, increased fluid intake.
		Encourage patient to report immediately any breakdown in mucous membrane.
Potential alteration in nutrition: more than body requirements, related to drug effect	Will maintain weight within normal range for size and age	Encourage patient to weigh self daily and report immediately any sudden weight gain.
		Encourage monitoring intake and following a balanced diet.
		Encourage exercise and distractive activity to focus attention away from food.
Potential for injury related to drowsiness	Will avoid injury	Keep side rails up on bedridden patients to avoid falls.
		Assist patient in ambulation until effects of drug are known.
		Caution outpatients to avoid driving, climbing, operating machinery until drug effects are known.
		Be prepared for paradoxical or exaggerated reactions in elderly or children. Dosage adjustment may be necessary.

(continued)

Nursing Diagnosis	Expected Client Outcome	Intervention
Potential for violence: self-directed related to suicidal tendencies	Will learn to cope with life stresses	Assess suicidal tendencies in all patients beginning treatment. Look for cues such as high level of anxiety, formulation of a realistic plan to carry out the act, perception of life stressors as overwhelming, depression, irritability, return to use of alcohol or street drugs. Alert significant others that suicide attempt may occur when drug begins to reduce depression sufficiently for the patient to acquire energy to act. Maintain close contact and follow-up with high-risk clients. Increase psychotherapy as needed. Formulate strategies to abort plan if enacted.

Monoamine Oxidase Inhibitors

Isocarboxazid, Phenelzine, Tranylcypromine

Drugs that form stable complexes with the enzyme monoamine oxidase (MAO), thus inhibiting its enzymatic activity, have been employed for many years as antidepressants. MAO is an enzyme system that catalyzes the deamination, or inactivation, of several naturally occurring biogenic amines, most notably norepinephrine, epinephrine, and serotonin, in numerous body tissues, especially the liver, kidney, intestines, and nerve endings. It is found within the mitochondria of cells comprising these tissues, and its principal role in neuronal transmission is the regulation of intracellular neurotransmitter levels. Inhibition of MAO in nerve endings leads to the accumulation of these neurotransmitters in the presynaptic nerve ending, thus increasing the amount of free neurotransmitter available for release after the arrival of a nerve impulse. By blocking a major means for intraneuronal breakdown of biogenic amine neurohormones, MAO inhibitors enhance the synaptic actions of these neurohormones, resulting in increased postsynaptic receptor activation. As discussed under tricyclic antidepressants above, continued postsynaptic receptor stimulation ultimately reduces the sensitivity and number of these receptor sites, a process termed *receptor down-regulation.* The amelioration of depressive symptomology is believed to be the result of this down-regulation of central aminergic receptor sites.

Although MAO inhibitors were the first clinically effective antidepressants to be introduced, their relatively low therapeutic effectiveness coupled with their potential to elicit serious adverse effects and interact with many other drugs and foods have restricted their usefulness in favor of the more effective and potentially less toxic tricyclic antidepressants. Today, MAO inhibitors are employed principally in patients refractive to or intolerant of the tricyclics. Their use must be carefully and continually monitored, and necessary precautions must be taken to avoid precipitation of serious adverse reactions and drug interactions.

Since MAO inhibitors interfere with the activity of enzymes responsible for inactivating many endogenous and exogenous amines, the effects of many aminergic drugs and biogenic amines contained in various foods may be markedly enhanced in the presence of an MAO inhibitor. Certain sympathomimetic amines, such as tyramine, which is found in many foods, can exert a potent pressor effect. Normally, tyramine is efficiently metabolized by MAO and does not exert adverse cardiovascular changes. In the presence of an MAO inhibitor, however, the pressor action of tyramine can be substantially potentiated and hypertensive crises have occurred with ingestion of tyramine-containing foods as well as foods containing other pressor substances normally metabolized by MAO (see Table 29-4) in persons taking an MAO inhibitor.

MAO inhibitors require several weeks of therapy for optimal antidepressant action to develop. Likewise, their effects may persist for up to 2 weeks following termination of therapy, because they irreversibly inhibit MAO, requiring the synthesis of new enzyme for the restoration of function. This prolonged duration of action makes it difficult to maintain a stable level of symptomatic improvement without the danger of serious toxicity. Moreover, when severe untoward reactions do occur, they may persist for a disturbingly long period of time. It is imperative, then, that both clinicians and patients be fully aware of the potential hazards associated with MAO inhibitor therapy.

MECHANISM AND ACTIONS
MAO inhibitors impair the normal enzymatic activity of the MAO enzyme system by forming stable, essentially irreversible complexes with the enzymes. Consequently, inactivation of biogenic amines such as norepinephrine and serotonin is impaired and their functional levels are elevated. Increased intraneuronal concentrations of these amine neurohormones result in a larger pool of neurohormone available for release and thus an enhanced postsynaptic action. The increased activity of norepinephrine, serotonin, and possibly other neurohormones at postjunctional receptor sites in the CNS is believed to underlie the effectiveness of MAO inhibitors in relieving depression. In addition, increased neurohormone availability in other body tissues is thought to underlie many of the toxic reactions elicited by these agents. These drugs also inhibit hepatic microsomal drug-metabolizing enzymes, thereby prolonging the action of many other drugs.

USES
1. Management of severe endogenous, exogenous (atypical), or reactive depressions resistant to treatment with tricyclic antidepressants, ECT, or other adjunctive psychotherapy
2. Control of the depressive phase of manic–depressive psychoses

ADMINISTRATION AND DOSAGE
See Table 29-5.

FATE
MAO inhibitors are readily absorbed orally; enzyme inhibition occurs rapidly, but clinical effects take several weeks to develop, except with tranylcypromine (10 days–14 days). Termination of drug effect following administration of the irreversible inhibitors (isocarboxazid, phenelzine) depends largely on regeneration of MAO enzyme, a process taking several weeks; tranylcypromine effects decline within 3 days to 5 days following discontinuation of therapy. The drugs are metabolized in the liver and excreted in the urine as metabolites and some unchanged drug.

SIDE-EFFECTS/ADVERSE REACTIONS
Side-effects noted with greatest frequency during MAO inhibitor therapy include orthostatic hypo-

---

Table 29-4
Foods and Drugs Containing Pressor
Amines to Be Avoided by Persons
Taking MAO Inhibitors

Tyramine-Containing Substances

High levels
  Fermented sausages (e.g., bologna, pepperoni, salami)
  Some cheeses (Boursault, Camembert, Cheddar, Emmenthaler, Stilton)
  Smoked or pickled fish, especially herring
  Yeast extracts (e.g., marmite, brewer's yeast)
  Chianti wine
  Caviar

Moderate levels
  Red wine
  Beef and chicken liver
  Avocado
  Canned figs
  Dried fish
  Cheeses (American, blue, Brie, mozzarella, parmesan, Roquefort)

Low levels
  Beer and ale (especially imported)
  Bananas
  Sour cream
  Soy sauce
  Yogurt

Phenethylamine-Containing Substances

Chocolate
Decongestant drugs
Anorexiants
Amphetamines

Other Pressor Substances

Fava beans (dopamine)
Coffee, tea, colas (caffeine)

Table 29-5
Monoamine Oxidase Inhibitors

Drug	Preparations	Usual Dosage Range	Clinical Considerations
isocarboxazid (Marplan)	Tablets—10 mg	Initially—30 mg/day; reduce to maintenance levels (usually 10 mg–20 mg/day) as soon as possible	Administer with meals to reduce gastric upset; adjust dosage critically, based on careful patient observation; note that although therapeutic effects may take several weeks to develop, toxic interactions can occur within hours; may be administered either as a single dose or in divided doses.
phenelzine (Nardil)	Tablets—15 mg	Initially—15 mg three times/day; reduce slowly to maintenance levels, usually 15 mg every 1 to 2 days	Effective in moderate to severe depressive states, especially accompanied by anxiety and agitation; do not exceed 75 mg a day.
tranylcypromine (Parnate)	Tablets—10 mg	Initially—20 mg–30 mg/day; reduce to 10 mg–20 mg/day as needed. With concurrent electroconvulsive therapy, 10 mg one to two times/day	Incidence of hypertensive reactions is higher with other MAO inhibitors; latency of therapeutic effect is generally shorter (3–5 days) than with other similar drugs; it is a structural analog of amphetamine and probably exerts a direct receptor activation as well as MAO inhibition; withdraw drug slowly, as original symptoms can recur on abrupt withdrawal.

tension, disturbances in cardiac rate and rhythm, dizziness, weakness, fatigue, jitteriness, hyperactivity, insomnia, headache, dry mouth, blurred vision, confusion, gastrointestinal disturbances, and hyperhidrosis. Minor skin reactions, edema, tremors, agitation, and anorexia have also been reported frequently. A range of other adverse reactions are associated with administration of MAO inhibitor drugs and include

CNS—Vertigo, hypomania, euphoria, chills, memory impairment, drowsiness, ataxia, delirium, hallucinations, convulsions
Autonomic/cardiovascular—Dysuria, incontinence, impotence, palpitations, weight gain
Hematologic/dermatologic—Leukopenia, hypochromic anemia, hepatocellular jaundice
Other—Peripheral neuritis, photosensitivity reactions, nystagmus, sodium retention, hypoglycemia, galactorrhea, glaucoma, optic damage

Overdose—Restlessness, tachycardia, hypotension, respiratory depression, confusion, incoherence, convulsions, shock

Symptoms of overdosage may include irritability, excitement, sweating, flushing, tachycardia, muscle fasciculations, grimacing, clonic movements, and exaggerated tendon reflexes. Severe overdosage is associated with convulsions, hypertension, hyperpyrexia, acidosis, respiratory arrest, and death. Treatment is symptomatic, and can include emesis, gastric lavage, respiratory support, maintenance of fluid and electrolyte balance, and support of cardiovascular and respiratory function. Massive overdosage may require hemodialysis and sodium bicarbonate to correct acidosis.

CONTRAINDICATIONS AND PRECAUTIONS
MAO inhibitors are contraindicated in patients with congestive heart failure, liver disease, pheochromocytoma, hyperthyroidism, hypertension, cardiovascular or cerebrovascular disease, and

a history of headache. They should not be used in patients over 60 years of age, in debilitated patients, and in children under 16 years of age. *Cautious* use of these agents is warranted in persons with epilepsy, diabetes, drug or alcohol addiction, chronic brain syndromes, impaired renal function, a history of anginal attacks, and in pregnant or nursing mothers.

INTERACTIONS

1. The effects of sympathomimetic drugs (*e.g.,* amphetamines, catecholamines, L-DOPA, ephedrine, phenylephrine, methylphenidate) may be potentiated by MAO inhibitors, resulting in severe hypertension, headache, and possibly cerebrovascular hemorrhage.
2. Hypertensive reactions can occur in patients taking MAO inhibitors who ingest foods containing tyramine, a pressor substance (see Table 29-4), as well as caffeine and chocolate, which also contain pressor substances.
3. Concurrent use of MAO inhibitors and tricyclic antidepressants (or within 10 days of each other) can result in marked hypertension, convulsions, fever, sweating, delirium, tremor, circulatory collapse, and coma, although some tricyclic antidepressants have been employed safely in conjunction with MAO inhibitors.
4. MAO inhibitors may increase the toxic effects of barbiturates and phenothiazines by decreasing their metabolism by the liver.
5. The effects of antihypertensive drugs may be potentiated by MAO inhibitors (leading to an increased likelihood of orthostatic hypotension). However, severe *hypertension* can occur with parenteral use of reserpine or guanethidine, due to release of large amounts of catecholamines.
6. Hypotension, respiratory arrest, shock, and coma can occur if MAO inhibitors are used in combination with CNS depressants such as alcohol, anesthetics, narcotics (especially meperidine), and sedative–hypnotics.
7. Increased hypoglycemic effects have occurred with combined use of MAO inhibitors and either insulin or oral hypoglycemics.
8. The muscle-relaxing action of succinylcholine may be increased because MAO inhibitors interfere with plasma pseudocholinesterase, the enzyme that inactivates succinylcholine.
9. MAO inhibitors reduce the convulsive seizure threshold and may reduce the efficacy of antiepileptic drugs.
10. The effects of anticholinergic, antihistamine, and antiparkinsonian drugs may be potentiated

by MAO inhibitors, which decrease their rate of metabolism.

■ *Nursing Process*

□ *ASSESSMENT*
Baseline medical data, careful history taking on drug use, perceptions of drug taking, and suicidal tendencies are assessed as for those patients beginning on tricyclic antidepressants. Several other parameters must also be included. Baseline vital signs, especially blood pressure in both sitting and standing positions, are important since MAO inhibitors can dramatically lower blood pressure. In addition, the patient being considered for this drug therapy should be competent to learn what foods and drugs to avoid in order to reduce the risk of hypertensive crisis or should have a strong support system who will guide him in this effort. Otherwise the risk of problems may out-weigh the benefit of treatment.

□ *NURSING DIAGNOSES*
Actual nursing diagnoses may include
  Knowledge deficit related to the action, dose, side-effects, and dietary restrictions of the drug
  Anxiety related to drug effectiveness and side-effects
Potential nursing diagnoses may include
  Alteration in bowel elimination: constipation
  Alteration in cardiac output: decreased related to postural hypotension, a drug side-effect, but may also be related to hypertensive crises as a result of tyramine ingestion
  Alteration in comfort: pain from headache
  Potential for injury: trauma, related to dizziness and sedation
  Noncompliance with the regimen usually related to side-effects or difficulty in managing the therapy
  Alteration in oral mucous membrane related to dry mouth
  Sensory–perceptual alteration in vision: blurring
  Sexual dysfunction
  Sleep pattern disturbance

□ *PLAN*
The nursing care goals should focus on helping the patient learn
1. To take the drug safely and correctly
2. To identify and manage common side-effects
3. The foods and drugs to avoid during therapy

4. The symptoms and management of a hypertensive crisis
5. The symptoms of drug overdose (described under Side-Effects/Adverse Reactions, above)
6. How to withdraw from the drug, if necessary

□ INTERVENTION

As with the tricyclics, this patient needs routine clinical follow-up to monitor side-effects. During clinic visits laboratory studies will be performed to evaluate liver, kidney, and cardiac function. At home the patient needs to watch for jaundice-like reactions such as yellowing skin and pruritus. The patient with cardiac disease needs to be treated with MAO inhibitors with great caution since the drug may mask anginal pain and eliminate the warning signs of ischemic attack.

Many of the side-effects of MAO inhibitors are the same as those of the tricyclic drugs and are discussed in detail in that section. These include the anticholinergic side-effects of dry mouth, sedation, constipation, and blurred vision, as well as sexual problems with orgasm and orthostatic hypotension resulting in dizziness and tachycardia.

The patient may also suffer insomnia from these drugs, which can be handled by completing the regimen before 4 PM each day. Even bid and tid schedules can be given following this format (i.e., 10 AM and 2 PM or 8 AM, 12 noon, 3 PM).

The most attention should be directed toward devising a method of helping the patient remember which foods and drugs to avoid to prevent hypertensive crises. Table 29-4 may be a useful tool. Chocolate, caffeine, and most over-the-counter cold remedies, cough medicines, and allergy-relief medications must also be avoided. Once the patient is comfortable with the basic list of foods and drugs to be avoided, he must learn to read package ingredients to find the hidden offending agents.

In addition, the patient needs to know the symptoms of impending hypertensive crises and what to do if they occur. Symptoms include headache, palpitations, neck stiffness, sweating, nausea, and photophobia. A method must be devised by which the patient will know he can get immediate help. Treatment of hypertensive crises requires a select list of antihypertensive drugs since some agents will actually worsen the condition (see Interactions, above).

The patient who reports an improved sense of well-being and wants to withdraw from an MAO inhibitor must understand the need to do so only under supervision. Rapid withdrawal may cause excitability, hallucinations, and severe depression. In addition, the drug will exert its MAO-inhibiting

effect for 2 weeks to 3 weeks after it has been discontinued. The patient must understand the need to continue diet and drug restrictions until the effect has passed.

As the feeling of depression subsides the patient with suicidal tendencies may try to take an overdose of the drug. Prevention by providing good support and follow-up is the best treatment since overdose is potentially fatal especially when the drug is combined with CNS depressants. Symptoms of overdose and its treatment are listed under Adverse Reactions, above.

□ EVALUATION

Successful therapy is signaled by change in affect, an improved feeling of self-worth, ability to cope with life stresses, management of side-effects, and avoidance of a hypertensive crisis. As with most therapies, successful drug taking does not ensure successful treatment. Participation in the total prescribed psychiatric program is essential.

Miscellaneous Antidepressants

Trazodone
(Desyrel, Trialodine)

Trazodone is an effective antidepressant chemically unrelated to tricyclics, tetracyclics, or MAO inhibitors. Its clinical efficacy is comparable to that of the tricyclics. However, its use is associated with minimal anticholinergic and cardiac conductive effects, although arrhythmogenic incidences have occurred with trazodone, particularly at high doses, and patients with cardiac disease must be closely monitored during trazodone therapy. Symptomatic improvement is often noted within 1 week, but some patients do not respond well to the drug.

MECHANISM AND ACTIONS
Trazodone selectively interferes with uptake of serotonin by nerve endings. It has minimal anticholinergic and cardiotoxic effects but is highly sedating.

USES
1. Treatment of endogenous depression, with or without accompanying anxiety

ADMINISTRATION AND DOSAGE
Trazodone is administered orally as tablets (50 mg, 100 mg, 150 mg). Dosage is initiated at 150 mg/day

in divided doses and may be increased by 50-mg/day increments every 3 days to 4 days until an optimal effect is noted. The maximum recommended dose in severely depressed patients is 600 mg/day. The lowest effective dose should be employed and a gradual reduction in dosage should be attempted once the desired response has been maintained. The 150-mg tablet is double scored (Desyrel Dividose) and may be divided to yield 50 mg, 75 mg, or 100 mg of drug.

FATE
Trazodone is well absorbed orally; peak plasma levels occur in 1 hour if taken on an empty stomach and within 2 hours if taken with food. A clinically significant therapeutic response is seen within 1 week in one third to one half of patients, and three fourths of all patients show a clinical response within 2 weeks. Metabolism occurs in the liver and the elimination half-life is approximately 4 hours to 8 hours.

SIDE-EFFECTS/ADVERSE REACTIONS
Side-effects seen with greatest frequency during trazodone therapy are drowsiness, lightheadedness, fatigue, dry mouth, constipation, and nasal congestion. Other adverse reactions reported with trazodone are

Cardiovascular—Hypotension, syncope, tachycardia, palpitations, sinus bradycardia, chest pain

CNS—Confusion, headache, insomnia, nervousness, disorientation, reduced concentration, malaise, blurred vision

Gastrointestinal—Nausea, vomiting, salivation, constipation

Neurologic—Incoordination, paresthesias, tremors

Other—Allergic skin conditions, myalgia, altered menses, priapism, tinnitus, weight gain, tired and itching eyes, sweating, dyspnea, decreased libido, anemia, leukopenia, neutropenia

CONTRAINDICATIONS AND PRECAUTIONS
While there are no absolute contraindications to trazodone, the drug is not recommended during the initial recovery phase of a myocardial infarction and during electroconvulsive therapy. Trazodone should be used *cautiously* in patients with arrhythmias or hypotension, in pregnant or nursing mothers, in children under age 18, and in patients concurrently receiving MAO inhibitors.

INTERACTIONS
1. Increased serum levels of digoxin and phenytoin have been reported with trazodone therapy.
2. Increased CNS depression can occur with concurrent use of trazodone and alcohol, barbiturates, and other CNS depressants.
3. Trazodone may enhance the hypotensive effects of most antihypertensive drugs; however, the effects of clonidine may be inhibited by trazodone.

The interactions listed under tricyclic antidepressants are *theoretically* possible with trazodone as well.

NURSING CONSIDERATIONS
Nursing considerations with this drug are essentially the same as those for the tricyclic antidepressants discussed earlier.

CASE STUDY
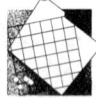

Christine Olender, age 34, was initially diagnosed with depression 3 years ago when she attempted suicide by taking an overdose of Fiorinal, a medication she used for migraine headaches. She had reported feeling worthless after being bypassed for a promotion. Prior to that incident she had been highly rated in her company and had received 3 promotions in 3 years. She was hospitalized, started in group therapy, and placed on amitriptyline hydrochloride (Elavil), 50 mg bid. She was subsequently discharged and was able to return to work. Elavil was eventually discontinued 8 months later.

Christine is brought to her psychiatrist by her mother who went to Christine's house after being unable to reach her for 2 days. Christine appears disheveled and withdrawn and expresses a wish to die. She has not been to work in 3 days and states she has not eaten or gotten out of bed. Mrs. Olender has already confirmed the absence with Christine's boss and states her daughter's bedroom appears as though Christine has not left it for days. Christine is admitted to a psychiatric facility. She is started on phenelzine (Nardil), 15 mg PO tid, and begins group therapy. Over the next 3 weeks the drug dosage is reduced to 15 mg PO daily as Christine begins to improve. Plans are being made for her discharge.

Discussion Questions

1. Phenelzine is an MAO inhibitor. What are the drug's side-effects, and how are some of them similar to Christine's initial symptoms?
2. Outline a drug teaching plan for this patient. Include information about dietary considerations.
3. Christine will live with her parents immediately after discharge. What should they know about diet, toxic reactions, and overdose?

REVIEW QUESTIONS

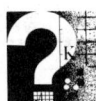

1. Briefly characterize the major types of depression.
2. What is the "amine hypothesis" of depression?
3. Outline the major mechanisms of action of the tricyclic antidepressants.
4. List the principal side-effects of the tricyclic antidepressants.
5. What are the major contraindications to the use of tricyclic antidepressants?
6. Which antidepressant drug is a *tetra*cyclic derivative?
7. What are the important differences between trazodone (Desyrel) and the tricyclic antidepressants?
8. How does the mechanism of action of the MAO inhibitors differ from that of the tricyclic antidepressants?
9. List several types of foods that must be avoided by patients receiving MAO inhibitors.
10. Give several contraindications to the use of MAO inhibitors.
11. Outline the questions you would use to assess the patient about to receive an antidepressant drug.
12. How would you determine which side-effects to cover when teaching a patient about tricyclic antidepressants? About MAO inhibitors?
13. How would you approach a parent seeking treatment for a child with a "bedwetting problem."
14. Devise a basic teaching plan for the patient receiving an MAO inhibitor.
15. What emergency equipment and drugs should be available when a patient is suspected of having overdosed on a tricyclic antidepressant? On an MAO inhibitor?

BIBLIOGRAPHY

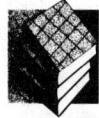

Baldessarini RJ: Biochemical Aspects of Depression. Washington, DC, American Psychiatric Press, 1983

Baldessarini RJ: Treatment of depression by altering monoamine metabolism: Precursors and metabolic inhibitors. Psychopharmacol Bull 20:224, 1984

Bloom PE, Baetge G, Deyo S, et al: Chemical and physiological aspects

of the actions of lithium and antidepressant drugs.
Neuropharmacology 22:359, 1983

Cassem N: Cardiovascular effects of antidepressants. J Clin Psychiatry 43:22, 1982

Cavenar JO (ed): Psychiatry. Philadelphia, JB Lippincott, 1985

Davidson J: When and how to use MAO-inhibitors. Drug Ther 13:197, 1983

DeGennaro MD, Hymen R, Crannell AM, Mansky PA: Antidepressant drug therapy. Am J Nurs 81:1304, 1981

Donlon PT: Cardiac effects of antidepressants. Geriatrics 37:53, 1982

Feighner JP: The new generation of antidepressants. J Clin Psychiatry 44(11):49, 1983

Fink M: Convulsive and drug therapies of depression. Annu Rev Med 32:405, 1981

Garver DL, Davis IM: Biogenic amine hypothesis of affective disorders. Life Sci 24:383, 1979

Glassman AH, Bigger JT: Cardiovascular effects of therapeutic doses of tricyclic antidepressants. Arch Gen Psychiatry 38:815, 1981

Goodwin FK: The impact of tricyclic antidepressants and lithium on the course of recurrent affective disorder. McLean Hosp J 8:1, 1983

Harris B: Drugs and depression. Am J Nurs 86:292, 1986

Hollister LE: Second generation antidepressants. Ration Drug Ther 16:1, 1982

Karusu TB: Psychotherapy and pharmacotherapy. Am J Psychiatry 139:67, 1982

Prien RF (ed): Antidepressant drug therapy: the role of the new antidepressants. Psychopharmacol Bull 20:209, 1984

Rawls WN: Trazodone. Drug Intell Clin Pharm 16:7, 1982

Richelson E: Pharmacology of antidepressants in use in the United States. J Clin Psychiatry 43:4, 1982

Shaw DM: The practical management of affective disorders. Br J Psychiatry 130:432, 1977

Antiepileptics–Anticonvulsants

Anticonvulsant Barbiturates
   Mephobarbital,
      Metharbital,
      Phenobarbital

Primidone

Hydantoins
   Ethotoin, Mephenytoin,
      Phenytoin

Oxazolidinediones
   Paramethadione,
      Trimethadione

Succinimides
   Ethosuximide,
      Methsuximide,
      Phensuximide

Carbamazepine

Valproic Acid Derivatives
   Valproic Acid
   Valproate Sodium
   Divalproex Sodium

Benzodiazepine Antiepileptics
   Clonazepam
   Diazepam
   Clorazepate

Phenacemide

Acetazolamide

Magnesium Sulfate

30

Epilepsy is a chronic disorder of the central nervous system (CNS) that is estimated to afflict approximately 0.5% to 1% of the population. The term is used to describe a number of conditions having in common the occurrence of sudden, recurring discharges from abnormally functioning brain cells, leading to the appearance of motor, sensory, and autonomic manifestations. Such abnormal brain discharges are termed *seizures*. Attempts have been made to classify the various epilepsies according to the type of seizure manifestation (*e.g.*, tonic–clonic convulsions, localized involuntary muscle activity, akinetic–atonic behavior); a simplified classification of the most common epilepsies is presented in Table 30-1.

Seizures can be broadly categorized into either *generalized* or *partial* (*i.e.*, localized) types. Among the more common generalized seizures are (1)

Table 30-1
Seizure Classification and Management

Seizure Type	Usual Age at Onset	Characteristics	Effective Drugs
Generalized			
Tonic–clonic (grand mal)	Any age (usually before 20)	Tonic rigidity of extremities, followed by massive clonic jerking for several minutes. Urinary incontinence is common. Lassitude and stupor ensue.	phenytoin phenobarbital primidone carbamazepine
Simple absence (petit mal)	3 yr–10 yr	Sudden loss of consciousness lasting up to 30 sec but usually of much shorter duration. Can occur hundreds of times a day. Characteristic 3/sec spike-wave EEG pattern. May be accompanied by some clonic jerking of the eyelids or extremities and autonomic manifestations but frequently no motor activity is evident. Rare in the adult.	ethosuximide trimethadione clonazepam valproic acid
Myoclonic jerking	5 yr–20 yr	Sudden, violent contractions of the extremities, with or without loss of consciousness. Occur most often after awakening or before retiring, often in combination with other seizure types.	phenobarbital clonazepam valproic acid
Atonic/akinetic	1 yr–5 yr	Sudden loss of muscle tone, usually lasting 10 sec–60 sec. Sagging of the head and dropping to ground are noted. EEG shows a slow spike-wave pattern. Most often due to an organic brain abnormality.	diazepam clonazepam
Infantile spasms (hypsarrhythmia)	Under 1 yr	Brief, recurrent myoclonic jerks with abrupt flexion or extension of the limbs or whole body. Most patients are mentally retarded. High-voltage, slow waves are predominant in the EEG, but asynchronous spiking can occur.	diazepam clonazepam phenobarbital corticotropin
Partial			
Elementary (focal) seizures	Any age	Manifestations are variable depending on site of the lesion. Convulsions may be confined to a single limb or muscle group (jacksonian seizures). No impairment of consciousness. Sensory disturbances are also noted. EEG shows spiking at the site of the focus.	primidone clorazepate carbamazepine (?) valproic acid (?)
Complex, partial seizures (psychomotor epilepsy)	Any age	Confused behavior, with involuntary, purposeless, repetitive motor activity. Usually accompanied by autonomic manifestations and loss of consciousness. Seizures last several minutes, but patients have no recall of the attack. Bizarre actions are sometimes seen. EEG spiking is present in the temporal lobe. Control is difficult.	carbamazepine primidone phenytoin phenacemide

tonic–clonic convulsions, frequently referred to as *grand mal epilepsy;* (2) simple absence seizures, also known as *petit mal epilepsy;* (3) myoclonic jerking; (4) atonic–akinetic; and (5) infantile spasms. Generalized seizures are bilateral and symmetric and do not appear to have a specific locus of onset in the CNS. Both convulsive as well as nonconvulsive types have been described. Partial seizures are those that originate in a specific part of the brain and may be subdivided according to the degree of total body involvement into (1) elementary or simple seizures, in which there is minimal spread of the discharge and limited involvement of the extremities, and (2) complex seizures, in which the discharge becomes more widespread and complex motor or behavioral aberrations are noted. These latter seizures arise primarily in the temporal lobe and are therefore sometimes referred to as *temporal lobe* or *psychomotor* epilepsy. Partial motor seizures, however, can lead to generalized seizure activity as the discharge spreads across the brain. For example, rhythmic clonic movement in one area (*e.g.,* leg, fingers, foot) often is followed by an orderly spread of abnormal activity to adjacent muscle groups, eventually resulting in a generalized convulsive seizure. This type of "progressive" seizure is frequently termed a *jacksonian seizure.* The brief discussion of seizure types given here, together with the information presented in Table 30-1, should provide sufficient information to enable the reader to understand the actions of the antiepileptic drugs discussed below. A more detailed review of seizure disorders may be found in several of the articles listed in the Bibliography at the end of the chapter.

Although the precise etiology of most forms of epilepsy is difficult to define, most seizures appear to result from an uncontrolled discharge at an area of abnormally functioning CNS tissue, termed the *focal lesion* or *seizure focus.* This focus may be continually or sporadically active. Discharges from this focus may be spontaneous or can be initiated by a variety of stimuli, including trauma, infections, anoxia, neoplasms, neurologic toxins, electrolyte or acid–base changes, metabolic or nutritional alterations, and so on. Once the focus becomes activated, the neuronal discharges may remain localized in a discrete area around the focus or they may spread to adjacent or distant parts of the CNS, resulting in either partial or generalized symptoms, respectively. Eventually, the frequency of neuronal discharge slows, the neuronal refractory period is lengthened, and the synchronous focal discharge ceases. Termination of seizure activity may be due to many factors, including inhibitory feedback mechanisms, local cerebral anoxia, decreased energy reserves, or accumulation of toxic metabolites.

The manifestations of seizure activity, as outlined above, can vary widely depending on the site of the principal focal lesion in the brain as well as the extent of spread of the abnormal discharges. The majority of epilepsies are believed to be idiopathic; that is, the cause cannot be accurately determined. Others, however, occur secondary to other disease states, and these latter forms of epilepsy can often be well controlled by proper treatment of the underlying disease state. Idiopathic epilepsy, however, must be treated symptomatically, and the goal of antiepileptic drug therapy, therefore, is to minimize, or perhaps totally abolish, seizure activity. Recognize, however, that the primary lesion in most instances is not altered.

Anticonvulsant drugs are effective in controlling the various manifestations of the epilepsies, but critical dosage regulation is of paramount importance for optimal seizure control. Drugs and doses must be individualized according to a particular patient's needs. Some antiepileptic drugs are not only ineffective in specific types of seizure disorders, they may actually worsen certain aspects of these conditions. Successful therapy, therefore, depends on accurate diagnosis, careful selection of drugs, and critical adjustment of dosage.

Therapy usually is initiated with a single agent selected on the basis of the type of seizure present. Dosage of this drug is then increased, as necessary, until seizures are controlled or toxicity is noted. Frequently, *complete* control of most seizure types requires addition of a second and often a third drug. Frequent dosage alterations or too-rapid shifting among anticonvulsant drugs should be avoided. The essential requirement of any antiepileptic drug is that it control the seizures without causing undue sedation and with minimal adverse drug effects. While many agents possess significant anticonvulsant activity at doses associated with disabling side-effects, the clinically useful antiepileptic drugs provide adequate control of most seizure types without subjecting the patient to frequent and debilitating adverse reactions. As stated above, the drugs do not cure the affliction, but they do allow the epileptic patient to function in a productive manner.

Stabilization of epileptic patients is a difficult task, and once attained, patients should be advised of the dangers inherent in altering the prescribed drug regimen or in subjecting themselves to physical and emotional stresses that might compromise their stable conditions. Patients should be taught to observe their conditions and to report any unusual symptoms that occur during therapy, because these may indicate early manifestations of serious toxicity. Drugs should be discontinued gradually whenever necessary, and changes in medication should be accomplished slowly over several weeks. Abrupt discontinuance or alteration in drug therapy can precipitate status epilepticus, a series of rapid, repetitive seizures that may be fatal unless terminated quickly. Intravenous diazepam (Valium) is considered the drug of choice for treating status epilepticus (see Chap. 28).

A variety of drugs are available for treating epilepsies, and they are listed in Table 30-2 along with their principal indications. Some of the drugs shown in the table, such as phenobarbital, clorazepate, and diazepam, have other indications as well,

and have been discussed in previous chapters; only their use in controlling epileptic seizures will be addressed here. The remaining antiepileptic drugs listed in Table 30-2 will be reviewed in detail below.

■ Nursing Process

The person labeled an epileptic, or one who is identified as seizure-prone, needs extensive nursing care regardless of the type of medication prescribed. Such persons face societal attitudes about their condition that range from fear to outright shunning. In the past, epileptics have been sterilized, institutionalized, and prohibited from marriage due to misconceptions about the disease.

Table 30-2
Antiepileptic Drugs: Major Indications and Principal Adverse Effects

Drug	Indications	Principal Adverse Effects

barbiturates
  mephobarbital
  metharbital
  phenobarbital
	All forms of epilepsy	Sedation, dizziness, drowsiness, nausea, skin rash

hydantoins
  ethotoin
  mephenytoin
  phenytoin
	Grand mal, complex partial (psychomotor) seizures. In addition, mephenytoin is used in elementary focal and jacksonian seizures.	Ataxia, confusion, slurred speech, diplopia, nystagmus, skin rash, gingival hyperplasia, epigastric distress, anemia (megaloblastic)

succinimides
  ethosuximide
  methsuximide
  phensuximide
	Petit mal (absence) seizures	Nausea, gastric upset, anorexia, drowsiness, fatigue, dizziness, minor behavioral disturbances, skin eruptions

oxazolidinediones
  paramethadione
  trimethadione
	Petit mal (absence) seizures (alternate drugs only)	Gastric distress, nausea, drowsiness, skin rash, visual disturbances (e.g., photophobia, hemeralopia), blood dyscrasias

benzodiazepines
  clonazepam
  clorazepate
  diazepam
	Petit mal (absence) seizures; myoclonic seizures; akinetic seizures	Ataxia, drowsiness, blurred vision, behavioral changes

primidone	Grand mal, complex partial (psychomotor) seizures; elementary focal seizures	Ataxia, drowsiness, dizziness, skin rash, gastrointestinal distress
carbamazepine	Grand mal, complex partial (psychomotor seizures; mixed seizures)	Drowsiness, gastrointestinal upset, impaired coordination, muscle/joint pain, skin rash, blood dyscrasias, visual disturbances
phenacemide	Complex, partial (psychomotor) seizures refractory to other drugs	Gastrointestinal disturbances, skin rash, drowsiness, weakness, headache, personality changes, hepatotoxicity, blood dyscrasias
valproic acid	Petit mal (absence) seizures; multiple seizures (alternate therapy); investigational uses include tonic/clonic, myoclonic, atonic, complex partial, and infantile spasm seizures	Nausea, indigestion, sedation, diarrhea, transient hair loss, hepatotoxicity, altered platelet aggregation

Many states, even now, require an epileptic to show evidence that he has been seizure-free for between 6 months and 5 years before being permitted a driver's license. Many epileptics are denied employment, overtly because their potential for seizures makes it hazardous for them to operate certain machinery. Covertly, the employer may be looking for an easy way to avoid hiring someone he considers handicapped.

As a result of societal beliefs about seizures, most epileptics try to keep their illness a secret from as much of the world as possible. For some, the required drug therapy seems an admission of illness; this sometimes results in compliance problems, leading to an increase in seizures. For others, the medication may be perceived as the only method they have to be a "normal" human being. Nursing care plans must consider these perceptions.

Seizure disorders occur in a wide range of age groups and are linked with other chronic problems. Therefore, the nurse can better plan care for all patients on anticonvulsant drug therapy if she applies certain general guidelines. Specific information about each drug will be listed in the discussion of that drug, but for most drugs the general principles given here apply.

☐ ASSESSMENT

☐ Subjective Data

The nurse needs to explore with the patient and family what their general perceptions are of the seizure disorder and what their expectations are of drug therapy. Many will be looking for the "magic cure," the chance that the drugs will enable them to appear "normal," and they will be surprised and dismayed to learn that finding the right drug combination may take weeks and may not completely eliminate the seizures. The nurse gives reality-based information during the assessment and throughout care to focus on what the drugs can and cannot do.

In dealing with children and their parents, the nurse must be creative when exploring perceptions. Children may be assessed through therapeutic play experiences; it is important to learn how they see themselves. Parents must be given an opportunity to express their fears about the illness and how to cope with the child's behavior. If the child is school-age, it may be appropriate to get some feedback from the child's teacher. All of these people will play an important role in getting the child to cooperate with the drug regimen and cope with seizure activity.

In addition to understanding perceptions, the nurse needs to obtain a thorough drug history, including use of over-the-counter and street drugs. The antiepileptics interact with many drugs but are particularly dangerous when combined with CNS depressants, including alcohol. A complete medical history should also be obtained.

☐ Objective Data

A complete physical assessment should be performed focusing on neurologic evaluation. Diagnostic testing may include an electroencephalogram (EEG) and laboratory evaluation of renal and hepatic function.

☐ NURSING DIAGNOSES

Actual nursing diagnoses for a patient taking antiepileptic medication may include

> Knowledge deficit related to the action, dose, and side-effects of the drug
> Anxiety about the inability of the drug to reduce or eliminate symptoms

Potential nursing diagnoses vary depending on the drug and route, since side-effects and adverse reactions are significantly greater with intravenous administration. For all patients *noncompliance* with the regimen is a potential problem. The reader is advised to check the side-effects/adverse reactions section on each drug for clues on appropriate diagnoses for the patient receiving that drug.

☐ PLAN

The nursing care goals should focus on management of administration and side-effects in the acute-care setting (see specific drugs) and planning a teaching program with the patient that teaches him (1) safe, accurate administration; (2) incorporation of drug therapy into daily activities; (3) monitoring and management of side-effects and adverse reactions; and (4) inclusion of information for the pregnant patient who must continue drug therapy.

☐ INTERVENTION

The main problem during drug therapy is the recurrence of seizures. The patient who has seizures needs to know that the relationship between drug therapy and seizure activity is dynamic; seizure activity may occur in spite of consistent drug-taking behavior. Factors that may make a patient more seizure-prone include growth spurts; hormonal changes such as menstruation, pregnancy, or menopause; illness or fever; changes in electrolyte balance from illness or exercise; lack of sleep; emotional stress; and poor nutrition. In such cases, dosage of medication may need to be altered and patients must learn to seek help whenever necessary. Another factor that may cause changes in therapeutic blood levels is a change in the drug formulation. This can occur if the patient changes pharmacies or the pharmacy changes drug companies. Patients must learn to be their own advocates to ensure they get the proper medication.

The health team and patient must be aware of the factors beyond the patient's control that may result in subtherapeutic drug levels. However, the most frequent cause of problems is that the patient forgets to take the medication. The nurse can provide the motivation to remember by teaching the patient that the blood levels taken on clinic visits are fairly accurate measures of whether he has been taking the drug as prescribed and that seizure activity tends to occur when drug doses are missed.

Successful therapy is usually a matter of remembering to take the drugs and finding the best time of day in order to minimize the side-effects. Drug calendars, daily pill boxes, and planning to take the pill during a special daily ritual such as a meal or after brushing teeth may serve as important memory joggers. The support of significant others is also helpful. Finding the best time of day may be another problem. Most patients prefer to take medicine as infrequently as possible. Hydantoin, phenobarbital, and ethosuximide can be taken in 1 or 2 divided doses, but most of the other drugs discussed in this chapter must be taken at intervals spread throughout the day. If the patient cannot use a once-a-day formulation, the nurse may need to work with him to find ways to decrease the visibility of the problem and minimize the limitations created by side-effects.

While most patients want to minimize the visibility of their problem, it is important that they always carry identification that lists their current drug therapy. The best method is for them to wear a Medic-Alert bracelet but a drug history card is helpful. Significant others should also know the regimen. Pregnancy causes tremendous hormonal changes that can adversely influence seizure activity. In addition, most antiepileptic drugs are potentially damaging to the fetus. Hydantoin is associated with cleft palate deformities, valproic acid with an increased incidence of spina bifida, and oxazolidinediones with multiple fetal malformations. The risk of damage to the fetus from anoxia due to a seizure or status epilepticus must be measured against the potential for deformities from

drug therapy. The pregnant patient needs thorough counseling and close monitoring throughout the pregnancy.

□ EVALUATION
General parameters that measure effective drug therapy with antiepileptics include maintenance of therapeutic blood levels, decreased incidence of seizures or side-effects, and the patient's ability to cope with the stresses and stigma of a chronic illness.

Anticonvulsant Barbiturates

Mephobarbital, Metharbital, Phenobarbital

Although all barbiturates can abolish seizure activity at doses sufficient to produce anesthesia, only three barbiturates, phenobarbital, metharbital, and mephobarbital, appear to be particularly suited for chronic treatment of epilepsy. They are effective antiepileptics at subhypnotic doses, exert a prolonged action, and tend to be reasonably well tolerated during extended drug therapy. Phenobarbital is the most commonly used of the above three drugs. There are some claims that mephobarbital produces fewer side-effects than phenobarbital, although these are based on largely anecdotal data.

MECHANISM AND ACTIONS
The antiepileptic activity of the barbiturates is probably the result of several mechanisms. The excitability of nerve cells is reduced as a consequence of an increased firing threshold; decreased neuronal excitability limits the spread of the abnormal discharge. The active transport of ions across neuronal membranes is impaired, which may also lower their firing rate. The role of gamma-aminobutyric acid (GABA), an inhibitory neurotransmitter, in barbiturate action is presently unclear, although potentiation of GABA-ergic activity has been associated with barbiturate-induced hypnosis and may play a role in the antiepileptic activity of these drugs as well.

USES
1. Treatment of generalized tonic–clonic seizures (grand mal); used alone in infants and young children, and most often in combination with phenytoin in adults

2. Treatment of generalized myoclonic jerks and cortical focal seizures
3. Treatment of complex absence seizures with autonomic manifestations
4. Adjunctive treatment of infantile spasms (effectiveness is not conclusively established)
5. Control of status epilepticus (IV phenobarbital)

ADMINISTRATION AND DOSAGE
See Table 30-3.

FATE
The antiepileptic barbiturates are generally well absorbed orally, especially from an empty stomach. The onset of action following oral administration ranges from 30 minutes to 2 hours, and effects persist for approximately 8 hours to 12 hours. The drugs are widely distributed in the body and are metabolized primarily by the hepatic microsomal enzyme system. Both metabolic products as well as some unchanged drug are excreted in the urine.

SIDE-EFFECTS/ADVERSE REACTIONS
Drowsiness, lethargy, and dizziness are the most frequently noted side-effects with the barbiturates used in the treatment of epilepsy. Other less common adverse reactions seen with barbiturate use are nausea, vomiting, diarrhea, bradycardia, hypotension, hypoventilation, bronchospasm, laryngospasm, respiratory depression, apnea, skin rash, angioedema, urticaria, fever, agitation, confusion, ataxia, nervousness, insomnia, nightmares, hallucinations, and altered behavior. Barbiturates may produce excitability, aggression, and hyperkinetic behavior in children. Blood dyscrasias are rare, as is exfoliative dermatitis and osteomalacia. Intravenous injection can lead to thrombophlebitis, and subcutaneous administration has resulted in pain, tenderness, and necrosis. Chronic *phenobarbital* therapy has been associated with fever, headache, megaloblastic anemia, and liver damage.

CONTRAINDICATIONS AND PRECAUTIONS
Antiepileptic barbiturates are contraindicated in patients with latent or manifest prophyria or severe respiratory disease or obstruction. These drugs must be used *cautiously* in persons with severe liver impairment or kidney dysfunction, status asthmaticus, hyperthyroidism, uremia, diabetes, or shock, and in elderly or debilitated patients and pregnant or nursing mothers. When injecting phenobarbital intravenously, go slowly, since rapid intravenous administration can result in hypotension, apnea, laryngospasm, and respiratory depression. Avoid extravasation, since solutions are highly alkaline and tissue necrosis can occur. Do not discontinue these drugs abruptly, because status epilepticus has resulted from sudden termination of therapy, and may represent a symptom resulting from withdrawal following chronic use of the drug.

INTERACTIONS
Most of the following interactions have been noted with *phenobarbital*; it is likely, however, that they can occur with the other barbiturates as well.
1. Concurrent use of other CNS depressants (*e.g.*, alcohol, narcotics, phenothiazines, sedative–hypnotics, antihistamines, and so on) with barbiturates can result in marked depression of CNS function.
2. Barbiturates may decrease the effects of the following drugs by hepatic microsomal enzyme induction: anticoagulants, antidepressants, digoxin, corticosteroids, doxycycline, estrogens, lidocaine, methyldopa, phenytoin, progestins, pyrazolones, quinidine, tetracyclines.
3. Phenobarbital interferes with the oral absorption of griseofulvin.
4. Chloramphenicol and valproic acid can inhibit the metabolism of phenobarbital.
5. Concurrent use of ether, other inhaled general anesthetics, or skeletal muscle relaxants together with barbiturates may produce additive respiratory depression.
6. Monoamine oxidase inhibitors may prolong the effects of barbiturates.
7. Use of furosemide and barbiturates can elicit or aggravate orthostatic hypotension.

NURSING CONSIDERATIONS
See also Nursing Process, earlier in this chapter.

Phenobarbital is frequently used for children and the elderly since it has fewer side-effects than many other antiepileptic drugs.

The most frequent side-effect in children is drowsiness and may occur only when the dose of the drug is changed. It is usually transient but may affect school work, appetite, and play. Phenobarbital may also cause paradoxical excitement in children, resulting in hyperactivity or problems in playing with toys or friends. It may cause the child to have trouble staying asleep, to develop behavior problems, and to become depressed. Parents need to be taught to watch for these signs, particularly the onset of depression, since that may signal the need to change the drug. Nursing care can focus on

Table 30-3
Anticonvulsant Barbiturates

Drug	Preparations	Usual Dosage Range	Clinical Considerations
mephobarbital (Mebaral)	Tablets—32 mg, 50 mg, 100 mg	Adults: 400 mg–600 mg/day Children (over 5 yr): 32 mg–64 mg three to four times/day; (under 5 yr) 16 mg–32 mg three to four times/day	Similar to phenobarbital in most respects, producing somewhat less sedation; may be used alternately or concurrently with phenobarbital at one-half the recommended doses; largely converted to phenobarbital within 24 h; may be used as a single daily dose at bedtime for nocturnal seizures; withdraw slowly when necessary, and reduce dose of other antiepileptics when added to the regimen (Schedule IV).
metharbital (Gemonil)	Tablets—100 mg	Adults: Initially 100 mg one to three times/day; adjust to optimal level Children: 5 mg–15 mg/kg/day	Less effective than phenobarbital and possesses somewhat greater sedative action; usually used in combination with other antiepileptic drugs for grand mal, petit mal, myclonic, or mixed seizures (Schedule III).
phenobarbital (various manufacturers)	Tablets—8 mg, 16 mg, 32 mg, 65 mg, 100 mg Capsules—16 mg Elixir—15 mg/ml, 20 mg/5 ml Injection—30 mg/ml, 60 mg/ml, 65 mg/ml, 130 mg/ml	*Oral* Adults: 50 mg–100 mg two to three times/day Children: Initially 3 mg–5 mg/kg/day for 7 to 10 days; adjust to blood level of 10 mcg/ml to 15 mcg/ml *IM, IV* Adults: 200 mg–300 mg; repeat in 6 h *or* 300 mg–800 mg initially, then 120 mg–240 mg every 20 min as needed. Children (IV): 20 mg/kg initially, then 6 mg/kg every 20 min as needed	Very effective alone for treatment of grand mal (especially in children) and as part of the drug regimen in most other forms of epilepsy; also used IV or IM for status epilepticus and other acute convulsive states; following IV injection, 15 min or more may be required to attain peak CNS concentration. Thus, give drug intermittently, even though convulsions persist; continuous injection can result in excessive CNS levels of drug after convulsions have ceased, possibly leading to respiratory depression. Solutions should be prepared in sterile water for injection and should not be used if not completely clear after 5 min of mixing. Inject drug within 30 min after preparation of solution. Drowsiness is common in early stages of therapy but diminishes with continued use. Frequency of IV administration is determined by patient's response. Discontinue drug as soon as desired response is obtained (Schedule IV).

helping parents recognize changes, acknowledging the difficulty in distinguishing them from the child's normal behavior, and developing strategies for handling them during long-term drug therapy.

The elderly frequently have the same side-effects as children taking phenobarbital. They may become extremely drowsy or excited especially early in therapy and some may suffer gait changes. This age group should have supervision and some protection, especially early in treatment, to ensure a safe environment and support if they need it.

All patients should be taught to maintain adequate vitamin D levels since long-term therapy with barbiturates may alter serum calcium levels. In addition to having samples drawn for periodic serum calcium blood levels, patients can protect themselves by getting plenty of sunshine, eating foods fortified with vitamin D, and taking a supplement if necessary.

The barbiturates are CNS depressants and are dangerous when combined with any other depressants, including alcohol, since the potential for respiratory depression and arrest is high. Therefore, known alcoholics and drug addicts are poor-risk patients for treatment with phenobarbital.

Overdose and withdrawal from barbiturates are discussed in Chapter 24. Early symptoms of overdose include respiratory depression, ataxia, slurred speech, and difficulty in arousing the patient. Such symptoms are sometimes mistaken for the onset of a seizure and the only way to be certain is to have a barbiturate blood level drawn. In the interim, the patient should be closely monitored and emergency equipment for respiratory support should be on hand.

Phenobarbital is sometimes used intravenously in the treatment of status epilepticus especially in children. Continuous monitoring of the patient is in order in such a case and should include protection from injury, frequent vital signs, if possible, especially respiratory rate and recording of the frequency of medication administration. A flowsheet may be used to keep records accurate. The danger of acute overdose of phenobarbital is high during episodes of status epilepticus since the drug may need to be repeated until seizure activity ceases.

Primidone

(Myidone, Mysoline)

MECHANISM AND ACTIONS

Primidone, or 2-desoxyphenobarbital, possesses anticonvulsant activity itself and is metabolized to phenobarbital and phenylethylmalonamide (PEMA), both of which also exhibit clinically significant anticonvulsive activity.

The mechanism of primidone's anticonvulsant action has not been established. In part, its effects are due to its conversion to phenobarbital, but it also possesses an anticonvulsant action similar to that of phenytoin (see below).

USES
1. Treatment of grand mal, complex partial (*i.e.*, psychomotor), and elementary (focal) seizures, either alone or in combination with other anticonvulsants
2. Treatment of benign, familial tremor (investigational use only)

ADMINISTRATION AND DOSAGE
Primidone is administered orally as tablets (50 mg, 250 mg) or suspension (250 mg/5 ml). The clinically effective serum level of primidone is between 5 mcg and 12 mcg/ml. Adults and children over 8 years are started on 100 mg to 125 mg at bedtime for 3 days, then gradually increased to 250 mg three to four times a day by day 10, which is the usual maintenance dose. The 250-mg dose may be given up to six times a day if necessary.

Children under 8 years are given 50 mg/day initially, then gradually increased to a maintenance level of 125 mg to 250 mg three times a day.

FATE
Oral absorption is rather slow but complete. Peak serum levels usually are attained within 3 hours, but considerable variation has been reported. Protein binding is virtually zero. Primidone is converted to PEMA, the principal metabolite, and to phenobarbital (approximately 15%–25%). Plasma half-lives are 4 hours to 12 hours for primidone, 24 hours to 48 hours for PEMA, and 2 days to 6 days for phenobarbital. Excretion is by way of the kidney, but clearance is slow and metabolites accumulate with chronic use of primidone.

SIDE-EFFECTS/ADVERSE REACTIONS
The most frequently encountered side-effects are lethargy, ataxia, and vertigo. Other untoward reactions reported with primidone are nausea, anorexia, fatigue, irritability, drowsiness, diplopia, nystagmus, impotence, skin eruption, emotional disturbances, and rarely megaloblastic anemia and blood dyscrasias. Since phenobarbital is one of the metabolites, the adverse reactions listed under the

antiepileptic barbiturates, above, are theoretically possible with primidone as well.

CONTRAINDICATIONS AND PRECAUTIONS

Latent or manifest porphyria is a contraindication to use of primidone. Patients should be urged to exert *caution* when driving or operating machinery, since dizziness and drowsiness can occur. Cautious use is also warranted in pregnant or nursing mothers. Therapy should be discontinued gradually to avoid precipitation of status epilepticus.

INTERACTIONS

1. Concurrent administration of phenytoin may increase the toxic effects of primidone by altering its metabolism.
2. Primidone can decrease plasma levels of carbamazepine.
3. Isoniazid may inhibit the metabolism of primidone to active metabolites.

In addition, the interactions listed for phenobarbital, above, are theoretically possible with primidone, since primidone is converted in part to phenobarbital.

NURSING CONSIDERATIONS

See also Nursing Process, earlier in this chapter.

One of the metabolites of primidone is phenobarbital. Therefore, most of the same nursing considerations apply to this drug and the nurse needs to remember that the patient who is allergic to phenobarbital will probably not tolerate primidone.

In addition, a dangerous side-effect of primidone is the development of blood dyscrasias. Patients need to watch for and report early warning signs such as swollen lymph glands, fever, sore throat, bruising, or generalized weakness. Primidone can also cause folic acid depletion so patients should be encouraged to take a supplement and get additional sources of vitamin B_6 in their diets.

Children and elderly patients may develop extreme sedation or excitability from primidone. Children may also become more aggressive or irritable. The nurse may need to work with parents to develop strategies for dealing with these behavior changes in order to cope with long-term therapy.

Hydantoins

Ethotoin, Mephenytoin, Phenytoin

Antiepileptic agents in the hydantoin group generally are the most effective drugs for the treatment of grand mal seizures and can be used in the control of psychomotor epilepsy as well. These drugs, unlike barbiturates, are not CNS depressants and do not appreciably interfere with normal sensory function. There are three currently marketed hydantoins, of which phenytoin is the most frequently prescribed. They are reviewed here as a group, then listed individually in Table 30-4.

MECHANISM AND ACTIONS

The hydantoins inhibit the spread of seizure activity to neurons surrounding a seizure focus. The primary site of action appears to be the motor cortex. Hydantoin administration results in stabilization of neuronal membranes (*i.e.*, increased threshold of excitability) and reduction in the duration of after-discharge. Possibly by increasing Na^+–K^+ adenosine triphosphatase (ATPase) activity, sodium efflux from neuronal cells is stimulated, blocking post-tetanic potentiation, which may prevent focal seizure activity from spreading to adjacent cortical areas. Increased release or activity of GABA, an inhibitory neurotransmitter, has been postulated as a possible mechanism of action as well.

USES

1. Control of grand mal seizures (may be used alone or combined with primidone, phenobarbital, or carbamazepine)
2. Treatment of complex, partial (psychomotor) seizures
3. Adjunctive treatment of trigeminal neuralgia or management of alcohol withdrawal syndrome
4. Control of status epilepticus and seizures occurring during neurosurgery (intravenous phenytoin)
5. Treatment of elementary (focal) or jacksonian seizures (mephenytoin only)
6. Termination of digitalis-induced cardiac arrhythmias (intravenous phenytoin—investigational use only)

ADMINISTRATION AND DOSAGE

See Table 30-4.

FATE

This discussion applies to phenytoin, the only hydantoin whose pharmacokinetics have been extensively studied.

Phenytoin is slowly absorbed from the small intestine; the rate and extent of phenytoin absorption vary widely among the different available preparations, the sodium salt being the best absorbed. Bioavailability also differs markedly

Table 30-4
Hydantoins

Drug	Preparations	Usual Dosage Range	Clinical Considerations
ethotoin (Peganone)	Tablets—250 mg, 500 mg	Adults: 250 mg four times/day initially; increase to optimal levels usually 2 g–3 g/day) Children: 750 mg/day initially; maintenance 500 mg–1000 mg/day based on age and weight	Administer with food, and begin therapy at small dose levels; compatible with most other anticonvulsants (dosage must be adjusted) except phenacemide (danger of paranoid reactions); less effective than phenytoin, but somewhat less toxic as well; not used as an antiarrhythmic.
mephenytoin (Mesantoin)	Tablets—100 mg	Adults: Initial dose 50 mg–100 mg/day; increase gradually to optimal levels (usual range 200 mg–600 mg/day) Children: 100 mg–400 mg/day based on age, weight, and severity of seizures	Most toxic of the hydantoins; reserved for patients refractory to less toxic anticonvulsants; may be useful in jacksonian seizures; possesses a strong sedative action; blood counts should be performed every 2 weeks to 4 weeks; more rapidly absorbed than other hydantoins with an onset of action in 30 minutes.
phenytoin (Dilantin Infatabs, Dilantin-30 Pediatric, Dilantin-125) phenytoin sodium, extended (Dilantin Kapseals) phenytoin sodium, prompt (Diphenylan) phenytoin sodium, parenteral (Dilantin)	Chewable tablets—50 mg Suspension—30 mg, 125 mg/5 ml Capsules—30 mg, 100 mg Capsules—30 mg, 100 mg Injection—50 mg/ml	*Oral* Adults: Initially, 100 mg three times/day; usual range is 300 mg–400 mg/day Children: Initially 5 mg/kg/day in two or three divided doses Usual maintenance range is 4 mg–8 mg/kg/day in children under 6 yr *Parenteral* IV Status epilepticus—150 mg–250 mg; repeat in 30 min with 100 mg–150 mg if necessary (Children—250 mg/m² body surface area) Arrhythmias—100 mg every 5 min until arrhythmia is abolished (maximum 1000 mg) IM Neurosurgery—100 mg–200 mg every 4 hours during surgery and postoperative period (maximum 1000 mg/day)	Extended phenytoin sodium capsules (Dilantin) can be used on a more convenient once-daily basis when seizure control has been established with divided doses initially due to their slower dissolution rate; do not administer IM in status epilepticus, because sufficient plasma levels cannot be attained due to erratic absorption; an IM dose 50% greater than the oral dose is necessary to maintain stable plasma levels; clinically effective serum level is 10 mcg–20 mcg/ml; margin between the effective and toxic IV dose is very small; administer slowly, and carefully monitor vital signs; flush catheter after each injection with sterile saline; avoid continuous infusions; do not exceed IV infusion rate of 50 mg/min; effective against digitalis-induced arrhythmias (see Chap. 34); phenytoin is also available in combination with phenobarbital (Dilantin-Pb capsules).

(20%–90%) among products of different manufacturers. Oral phenytoin sodium extended (Dilantin) dissolves slowly and attains peak plasma levels in 4 hours to 12 hours. Phenytoin sodium prompt (other clinically available preparations) can achieve peak serum levels in 2 hours to 3 hours although much variation occurs. The drug is erratically absorbed following intramuscular injection; peak blood levels occur at varying times up to 24 hours and are significantly lower than blood levels obtained with oral or intravenous administration. Phenytoin is highly bound (85%–95%) to plasma proteins. It is metabolized in the liver and excreted largely as conjugated metabolites in the urine. The elimination half-life is dose dependent and ranges from 8 hours to 60 hours (average hours 20–30 hours). Steady-state plasma levels are usually attained within 7 days to 10 days.

SIDE-EFFECTS/ADVERSE REACTIONS

Sluggishness, ataxia, slurred speech, nystagmus, and confusion are the most frequently encountered side-effects with the hydantoins. Less frequently, dizziness, insomnia, nervousness, fatigue, and irritability are noted. Other untoward reactions that have occurred with use of hydantoins are listed by organ system below:

Gastrointestinal—Nausea, vomiting, diarrhea, abdominal pain, dysphagia
CNS—Headache, depression, tremors, behavioral disturbances
Dermatologic—Skin rashes (morbilliform, maculopapular, scarlatiniform), urticaria, keratosis, hirsutism, lupus erythematosus, exfoliative dermatitis (rare)
Hematopoietic—Blood dyscrasias, anemias (especially megaloblastic), lymphadenopathy, bone marrow depression
Other—Gingival hyperplasia (20%–30% incidence, especially children), periodontal infection, polyarthropathy, hepatitis, liver damage, alopecia, hyperglycemia, edema, chest pain, numbness, photophobia, pulmonary fibrosis, osteomalacia

Intravenous administration of phenytoin has also resulted in hyperkinesia, hypotension, cardiac arrhythmias, and cardiovascular collapse.

CONTRAINDICATIONS AND PRECAUTIONS

Hydantoins are contraindicated in the presence of severe hepatic dysfunction, hematologic disorders, and incomplete heart block. Intravenous phenytoin should not be given to persons with sinus bradycardia, sinoatrial block, second- or third-degree heart block, and Adams-Stokes syndrome. These drugs must be given with *caution* to patients with hypotension, myocardial insufficiency, hyperglycemia, anemia, osteoporosis, or acute intermittent porphyria, and to pregnant or nursing mothers. Abrupt withdrawal of the drug may result in status epilepticus; discontinue therapy slowly.

INTERACTIONS

Most interactions given below are documented for phenytoin but can occur with other hydantoins as well.

1. Phenytoin may increase the effects of warfarin, antihypertensives, thyroid hormones, sedatives, lithium, hypnotics, propranolol, and methotrexate.
2. Phenytoin may diminish the effects of corticosteroids, cyclosporine, dicumarol, methadone, oral contraceptives, disopyramide, quinidine, digitoxin, estrogens, haloperidol, and tetracyclines (by increasing their liver metabolism).
3. The effects of phenytoin can be increased by drugs that (1) *inhibit its metabolism* (e.g., allopurinol, cimetidine, diazepam, disulfiram, acute ethanol ingestion, isoniazid, phenacemide, phenylbutazone, succinimides, sulfonamides, trimethoprim, and valproic acid) or (2) *displace the drug from protein-binding sites* (e.g., salicylates and anti-inflammatory drugs, valproic acid).
4. The effects of phenytoin can be reduced by drugs that (1) *increase its metabolism* (e.g., barbiturates, carbamazepine, diazoxide, chronic ethanol ingestion, folic acid, and theophylline), (2) retard its oral absorption (e.g., antacids, antineoplastics, calcium, charcoal) and (3) by various other drugs such as influenza virus vaccine, loxapine, nitrofurantoin, and pyridoxine.
5. Tricyclic antidepressants may precipitate seizures, so phenytoin dosage should be adjusted accordingly. Valproic acid and phenytoin may result in breakthrough seizures.
6. Phenytoin can impair the absorption of furosemide.
7. Concomitant administration of phenytoin and dopamine may lead to hypotension and bradycardia.
8. The effects of primidone may be altered by phenytoin administration, due to changes in the metabolism of primidone.

NURSING CONSIDERATIONS

See also Nursing Process, earlier in this chapter.
While many patients find that hydantoins help them achieve best control over their seizures, these

drugs have a price. Side-effects are dangerous and the potential for toxic overdose is high since the therapeutic index is narrow. Since there is no antidote, treatment of overdose is symptomatic and may be complicated by the development of cardiac arrhythmias and subsequently cardiac arrest. Therefore, patients must learn which symptoms signal the need for immediate medical attention. They should report changes in behavior such as nervousness or irritability, photophobia, or feeling of change in heartbeat as well as any dermatologic changes. Many patients on long-term hydantoin therapy develop a sense of something being wrong when they become toxic. Patients should be encouraged to follow these instincts and seek help immediately.

Some patients develop nystagmus as a transient side-effect of the drug. If the symptom persists or is accompanied by diplopia, trouble reading, confusion, or ataxia it also signals the development of toxicity and should be reported immediately. Another adverse reaction that should be immediately reported is the development of blood dyscrasias. Early symptoms may include swollen lymph glands, fever, sore throat, or malaise.

Hydantoin may also result in folic acid deficiency leading to anemia, neuropathies, and changes in mental status. As a precautionary measure patients may be advised to take a supplement. If they do so, hydantoin blood levels must be closely monitored since folic acid enhances hydantoin metabolism and may result in the need to adjust the drug dosage.

Phenytoin, and to some extent the other hydantoins, may lead to vitamin D deficiency resulting in a loss of bone mass. To minimize the risk, which is especially high in children, patients should be encouraged to take a supplement, get out in the sunshine, get regular exercise, and have periodic serum calcium levels drawn.

Children may have different side-effects than adults. Phenytoin may cause exceptional drowsiness in some children while in others there will be no effect. Children are also more prone to the development of gingival hyperplasia. Good oral hygiene, regular gum massage, frequent brushing, and frequent dental care will ensure that the problem is managed as well as possible.

Hydantoins should be used with extreme caution in elderly patients whose renal and liver function may be insufficient to metabolize the drug. This age group is very prone to toxicity and should be carefully monitored. Patients who are very forgetful or who have few family supports are poorrisk candidates for treatment with these drugs.

The diabetic who has seizures must also be carefully monitored since the hydantoins may inhibit insulin release, causing the patient to develop hyperglycemia. A hyperglycemia-induced seizure must be treated by glucose, not an antiepileptic. The nurse must work closely with the diabetic patient attempting to cope with both of these illnesses.

Another side-effect of hydantoins is brown or reddish-brown urine. While the nurse may consider this innocuous, a patient may be panic stricken if he sees "blood" in his urine. In this case, foreknowledge can allay much anxiety.

Dilantin is the only form of hydantoin approved for once-a-day dosing. All other formulations must be taken between two and four times daily. Many patients will prefer the once-a-day schedule but some will not be able to tolerate the dose and will quickly become toxic. Therefore, it is essential that any patient starting the Dilantin protocol be aware of the early warning symptoms and be willing to have blood levels closely monitored during the early weeks of therapy.

Patients who receive phenytoin through a feeding tube also need special consideration since research has shown an increased difficulty in achieving and maintaining blood levels when this route is used. Although some have advocated stopping feedings before and after drug administration and adequate tube flushing, the only effective method seems to be close monitoring of blood levels and subsequent increases in dose as necessary (Ozuna et al, 1984). Since most patients receiving phenytoin through a feeding tube have altered levels of consciousness, they are unlikely to report developing symptoms of toxicity. Therefore, the nurse must watch for vomiting, diarrhea, tremors, rashes, and the early signs of blood dyscrasias to prevent toxic overdose in these patients.

Intravenous phenytoin is used in the treatment of status epilepticus and for cardiac arrhythmias (see Chap. 34). Blood pressure should be closely monitored with this route of administration since hypotension is an early sign of toxicity but may be difficult to obtain if the patient is rigid or thrashing. Other early signs of toxicity may include nystagmus and decreased respiratory rate. Changes in mental acuity, ataxia, and slurring of speech may not be observable during a status epilepticus episode. Emergency drugs and equipment should be available to respond to potential respiratory or cardiac arrest. Nursing Care Plan 30-1 summarizes the nursing process for the patient taking oral phenytoin.

(Text continues on p. 568.)

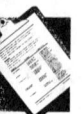

Assessment

Subjective Data

1. Medication history
   a. Refer to Interactions section to formulate pertinent questions
   b. Current IV drugs that may be physically incompatible with phenytoin
   c. Allergies/hypersensitivity
   d. Use of alcohol, street drugs that will interfere with drug effectiveness
2. Medical history
   a. Check for preexisting conditions that contraindicate use or warrant cautious use (see Contraindications and Precautions section) or that could increase the likelihood of toxicity, necessitating an alteration in dosage
   b. Determine characteristics of seizures requiring treatment, *e.g.*, type of seizure, etiology, frequency, duration, precipitating factors, presence of aura
3. Personal history/compliance issues
   a. Knowledge of condition, perception of illness, ability or willingness to cooperate with a long-term regimen
   b. Financial and personal resources and support systems
   c. Past compliance with drug therapy

Objective Data

1. Physical assessment
   a. Neurologic status: orientation, level of consciousness, pupil size, vision, motor function, coordination, memory, mental acuity
   b. Vital signs
   c. Presence of seizure-related injuries, motor limitations that may interfere with self-medication
   d. Cardiovascular status
2. Laboratory/diagnostic data
   a. Serum level of previous anticonvulsant, if applicable
   b. Renal and hepatic function studies
   c. CBC with differential
   d. EEG or other neurologic function studies

Nursing Diagnosis	Expected Client Outcome	Intervention
Knowledge deficit related to drug effect, frequency of administration, potential side-effects, and potential drug interactions	Will verbalize knowledge of drug effect, potential side-effects, and drugs to avoid while taking phenytoin	Administer or teach patient to take divided doses during dosage adjustment period until adequate serum level to control seizures is achieved.
		Teach the need to maintain dosage schedule and to notify physician if unable to take drug because of illness. Once-a-day dosing may be used for a stable patient able to tolerate it.
		Teach the patient drugs (including alcohol) to avoid, because many interfere with phenytoin absorption. Encourage patient to contact physician before taking any new drug.
		Explain how drug reduces seizure activity, but that it may not completely eliminate seizures.
		Teach patient to monitor common side-effects and early symptoms of adverse reactions as described below, and follow preventive strategies given.

(continued)

Nursing Diagnosis	Expected Client Outcome	Intervention
Anxiety related to presence of seizures and drug's ability to control them	Will verbalize feelings about self-concept, concerns about future seizures	Encourage discussion about seizures and self-concept. Maintain a dialogue to build trust over time and discuss situations as they arise.
		Give patient realistic information about drug therapy.
		Keep patient informed of serum drug levels. Get realistic therapy goals to help patient achieve success.
Potential alteration in oral mucous membrane, related to drug-induced gingival hyperplasia	Gingival hyperplasia will be prevented or controlled	Encourage good oral hygiene after each meal, regular dental care, regular gum massage.
Potential alteration in comfort: GI distress related to drug effect	Will prevent or obtain relief from common GI symptoms	Encourage patient to take drug with meals or food to decrease GI symptoms.
		If symptoms persist, dose may need to be divided through the day. Physician must be notified if changes are needed.
Potential for injury related to seizures from inadequate dose or from overdosage resulting in ataxia, confusion	Serum phenytoin levels will remain within therapeutic limits (10–20 mcg/ml)	Encourage patient to keep appointments for serum drug level determinations as a way of checking drug effectiveness.
		Teach necessity of precautions, *i.e.*, not driving or swimming until degree of drug control is known.
		Teach patient to notify physician at first sign of increase in seizure activity and if early symptoms of drug toxicity develop, *e.g.*, nystagmus, ataxia, confusion. Dosage adjustment is necessary.
		Encourage patient to wear a Medic-Alert appliance and to notify all caregivers that he takes phenytoin.
		Teach patient not to discontinue drug abruptly, but to seek supervision. Withdrawal must be gradual and safety precautions must be increased because seizure activity may increase.
Potential disturbance in self-concept related to changes in body image	Will verbalize concerns about body image and develop strategies for handling stigma	Discuss patient's concerns about looking "different" and what he perceives as most stigmatizing.
		Help patient learn to feel comfortable with disclosure about condition to others as appropriate and to develop strategies to improve self-image.
		Provide or help design a supportive network the patient can rely on in times of stress.

(continued)

Nursing Diagnosis	Expected Client Outcome	Intervention
Potential noncompliance with drug regimen related to chronicity of condition	Will consult with health team before making a decision to discontinue drug therapy	Teach patient the importance of supervised withdrawal for safety reasons.
		Attempt to establish a climate of trust so patient feels comfortable expressing need to stop drug therapy without taking action alone.
		Recognize patient will make the final decision; the health team can only serve as a support.

Oxazolidinediones

Paramethadione, Trimethadione

The oxazolidinediones are effective drugs for the control of simple absence (petit mal) seizures, but they elicit a rather high incidence of untoward reactions. They are largely reserved for patients intolerant of or unresponsive to other less toxic agents and are rarely used today. The two currently available drugs, trimethadione and paramethadione, differ only slightly in their pharmacologic properties; thus, they are reviewed together, and are then listed separately in Table 30-5.

MECHANISM AND ACTIONS
The antiepileptic action of the oxazolidinediones is complex and only incompletely understood. The drugs prolong the recovery period of postsynaptic neurons in those CNS systems (primarily thalamocortical) where repetitive discharges produce absence attacks through a negative feedback mechanism. Other central effects of the oxazolidinediones include elevating the threshold for seizure discharge in the thalamus and interference with the propagation of seizure activity from a cortical focus to the thalamus. They possess little sedative or hypnotic action but may exert a mild analgesic effect. The role of the inhibitory neurotransmitter GABA in the action of these agents remains to be established.

USES
1. Treatment of simple absence seizures (*i.e.,* petit mal) refractory to treatment with other antiepileptic drugs

ADMINISTRATION AND DOSAGE
See Table 30-5.

FATE
These drugs are readily absorbed from the gastrointestinal tract, and peak plasma concentrations occur in 30 minutes to 60 minutes. Distribution is extensive in the body and the drugs are not protein bound. Both paramethadione and trimethadione are metabolized in the liver to an active metabolite, which is slowly excreted by the kidneys. The plasma half-life of the parent compounds is 12 hours to 24 hours, whereas the active metabolite has a half-life of 6 days to 12 days.

SIDE-EFFECTS/ADVERSE REACTIONS
The side-effects noted with greatest frequency with the oxazolidinediones are drowsiness, gastrointestinal distress, hiccups, and photophobia. Many other adverse effects have occurred with use of these drugs, and these include

Gastrointestinal—Nausea, vomiting, abdominal pain, anorexia

CNS—Vertigo, irritability, personality changes, headache, paresthesias, precipitation of grand mal seizures

Ocular—Diplopia, scotomata, hemeralopia (day blindness), retinal hemorrhage

Hematologic—Epistaxis, mucosal bleeding (*e.g.,* gums, vagina), blood dyscrasias (especially neutropenia), changes in blood pressure

Dermatologic—Skin rash (acneiform, morbilliform), exfoliative dermatitis, erythema multiforme

Table 30-5
Oxazolidinediones

Drug	Preparations	Usual Dosage Range	Clinical Considerations
paramethadione (Paradione)	Capsules—150 mg, 300 mg Solution—300 mg/ml	Adults: 300 mg–600 mg three to four times/day (initial dose 900 mg/day; increase by 300 mg/wk to above range) Children: 300 mg–900 mg/day in three to four divided doses	Less effective but slightly less toxic than trimethadione; no myasthenic-like reactions have occurred, but sedation is common; oral solution contains 65% alcohol and should be diluted with water before administration to children.
trimethadione (Tridione)	Chewable tablets—150 mg Capsules—300 mg Solution—40 mg/ml	Adults: Initially 300 mg three times/day; usual maintenance dose 900 mg–2400 mg/day in divided doses Children: 300 mg–900 mg/day in three to four divided doses	Plasma level of dimethadione, the active metabolite of trimethadione may be used as a dosage guide; this level should be maintained about 700 mcg/ml for optimal control of petit mal attacks in patients receiving trimethadione; alkalization of the urine will increase excretion of this metabolite.

Other—Albuminuria, alopecia, lymphadenopathy, systemic lupus-like reaction, myasthenia gravis-like reaction, nephrosis, hepatitis

In addition, fetal malformations have occurred during therapy with oxazolidinediones, and these drugs should not be used during pregnancy.

CONTRAINDICATIONS AND PRECAUTIONS

Since other equally effective and safer antiepileptics are available, oxazolidinediones should not be used in persons with hepatic or renal impairment, blood dyscrasias or other hematologic abnormalities, diseases of the retina or optic nerve, or myasthenia gravis, and in pregnant women. The drugs should be used *cautiously* in nursing mothers and in persons with acute intermittent porphyria. On discontinuation of therapy, the dosage should be slowly tapered, since abrupt termination may result in precipitation of absence seizures or status epilepticus. Oxazolidinediones should be withdrawn at the first sign of skin rash, jaundice, proteinuria, impaired vision, lymph node enlargement, or indications of a developing blood dyscrasia, such as mucosal ulceration, unexplained fever, abnormal bruising or bleeding, and sore throat.

INTERACTIONS
1. CNS depression induced by oxazolidinediones may be augmented by other depressants, oral anticoagulants, and p-aminosalicylic acid.

NURSING CONSIDERATIONS
See also Nursing Process, earlier in this chapter.

Oxazolidinediones are rarely used today since many safer drugs are available. The patient who is prescribed one of these drugs must be closely monitored for the adverse reactions listed above. Frequent blood studies should be drawn to watch for the development of hematologic abnormalities. The patient should learn to report the development of sedation or of glaring or blurring of vision, which may indicate retinal damage.

These drugs can also cause tonic–clonic seizures, especially in patients who have a mixed type of seizure activity, another reason for close monitoring.

Oxazolidinediones should only be used in patients who can be relied on to follow the prescribed dosing schedule closely and who will report clearly any untoward reactions.

Succinimides

Ethosuximide, Methsuximide, Phensuximide

Although no more effective than the oxazolidinediones in the treatment of simple absence (petit mal) seizures, the succinimides remain the drugs of choice for these conditions primarily because of their reduced toxicity compared to the other alternative drugs (oxazolidinediones, valproic acid, clonazepam). Because they may increase the frequency of grand mal attacks, however, their use in mixed seizure patterns must be accompanied by other antiepileptics capable of controlling tonic–clonic seizures. Three succinimides are currently available, offering little in the way of significant differences among them although methsuximide is

considered to be slightly more toxic. They are discussed as a group, then listed individually in Table 30-6.

MECHANISM AND ACTIONS

The precise mechanism of action of the succinimides remains to be definitely established. In laboratory tests, their effects generally resemble those of the oxazolidinediones, and they are known to suppress the three-per-second spike-wave EEG pattern characteristic of absence seizures. Evidence suggests they may have a depressant effect on the motor cortex, and possibly elevate the firing threshold of cortical neurons. In addition, the succinimides have been reported to depress inhibitory mechanisms descending from the reticular system.

USES
1. Treatment of simple absence seizures (petit mal)
2. Adjunctive treatment of psychomotor epilepsy and minor motor seizures (methsuximide only —investigational use)

Table 30-6
Succinimides

Drug	Preparations	Usual Dosage Range	Clinical Considerations
ethosuximide (Zarontin)	Capsules—250 mg Syrup—250 mg/5 ml	Adults: Initially 500 mg/day; increase by 250 mg every 4 to 7 days until control is achieved (maximum 1500 mg/day) Children: 250 mg/day, increased slowly to optimal level	Inform patient that drug may color urine pink to reddish-brown; appearance of frequent gastrointestinal distress, dizziness, ataxia, or other neurologic disorders signifies need for dosage adjustment; administer with meals to reduce gastrointestinal upset; long half-life; therefore, do not exceed recommended dosage as danger of accumulation exists.
methsuximide (Celontin)	Capsules—150 mg, 300 mg	Initially 300 mg/day for 1 week; may increase by 300 mg weekly to a maximum of 1200 mg	Equally effective in petit mal as ethosuximide but somewhat more toxic, especially to the CNS (*e.g.*, severe depression, confusion); may be useful in certain cases of psychomotor epilepsy.
phensuximide (Milontin)	Capsules—500 mg	Adults: 500 mg–1000 mg two to three times/day (range 1 g–3 g/day) Children: 600 mg–1200 mg two to three times/day	Slightly less effective and less toxic than other succinimides; may color urine reddish-brown.

ADMINISTRATION AND DOSAGE
See Table 30-6.

FATE
Oral absorption is complete and peak serum levels occur within 3 hours to 6 hours with ethosuximide and 1 hour to 4 hours with the other drugs. The drugs are metabolized by the liver and excreted in the urine as both unchanged drug and inactive metabolites.

SIDE-EFFECTS/ADVERSE REACTIONS
Gastrointestinal side-effects are the most frequently encountered untoward reactions and may include nausea, gastric upset, cramping, diarrhea, epigastric or abdominal pain, and anorexia. Drowsiness, ataxia, or dizziness is also noted on occasion. Other adverse reactions associated with use of the succinimides include

CNS—Irritability, nervousness, euphoria, aggressiveness, hyperactivity, confusion, lethargy, fatigue, depression, sleep disturbances, night terrors, inability to concentrate, hiccups, insomnia

Ocular—Blurred vision, myopia, photophobia, periorbital edema

Hematologic—Blood dyscrasias

Dermatologic—Urticaria, erythematous rashes, erythema multiforme, systemic lupus erythematosus, Stevens-Johnson syndrome (see Chap. 6)

Genitourinary—Urinary frequency, hematuria, albuminuria, renal damage (rare)

Other—Alopecia, vaginal bleeding, hyperemia, swelling of the tongue, muscular weakness, hirsutism

CONTRAINDICATIONS AND PRECAUTIONS
Extreme *caution* should be exercised when administering these drugs to persons with liver or renal impairment or acute intermittent porphyria. These drugs can *increase* the frequency of grand mal seizures in some patients and should not be used alone in mixed seizure types. Succinimides may need to be gradually withdrawn on the appearance of depression, aggressiveness, or other unusual behavioral alterations.

INTERACTIONS
1. Absorption of ethosuximide may be reduced by amphetamine.
2. Increased libido may result if ethosuximide is combined with other anticonvulsants.

NURSING CONSIDERATIONS
See also Nursing Process, earlier in this chapter.

Aside from drowsiness, these drugs usually cause few side-effects in children. However, the child's level of alertness may cause problems in school, at play, and at rest so parents need to be taught how to help the child make adjustments until the side-effect abates.

The major concern with the succinimides is the potential for the development of toxicity. Early warning signs may be dizziness, skin rash, fever, blurred vision, joint pain, bleeding, or bruising. The drug must be gradually withdrawn since rapid withdrawal will precipitate seizures so early reporting is essential.

Carbamazepine
(Epitol, Tegretol)

Carbamazepine is structurally related to the tricyclic antidepressants, and has been successfully employed to treat the pain of trigeminal neuralgia (tic douloureux). It has an antiepileptic spectrum of action similar to that of phenytoin but is a highly toxic agent usually restricted to the treatment of grand mal and psychomotor seizures in patients not responding satisfactorily to other less toxic drugs.

MECHANISM AND ACTIONS
The mechanism of action of carbamazepine is complex and incompletely understood. The drug has been postulated to increase latency, decrease responsivity, and suppress after-discharges in polysynaptic pathways associated with cortical and limbic function. It may also reduce post-tetanic potentiation. Carbamazepine has anticholinergic, antidepressant, and muscle-relaxing actions as well.

USES
1. Treatment of psychomotor seizures (alone or with primidone or phenytoin)
2. Treatment of grand mal seizures (with phenytoin)
3. Adjunctive treatment of mixed seizures or complex partial seizures
4. Relief of pain associated with trigeminal neuralgia
5. *Experimental uses* include treatment of neurogenic diabetes insipidus, alcohol withdrawal syndrome, and certain psychiatric disorders, such as bipolar depressive illness and schizoaffective disorders

ADMINISTRATION AND DOSAGE
Carbamazepine is used orally as regular tablets (200 mg) and chewable tablets (100 mg). Recommended dosage ranges are as follows:

Epilepsy

Adults and children over 12 years: Initially 200 mg twice a day; increase by 200 mg/day in divided doses until optimal response is achieved; maximum 1200 mg/day; usual maintenance level is 800 mg to 1200 mg daily.

Children 6 years to 12 years: Initially 100 mg twice a day; increase by 100 mg/day until optimal response is achieved; usual maintenance level is 400 mg to 800 mg daily.

Trigeminal neuralgia

Initially 100 mg twice a day; increase by 100 mg/12 hours to a maximum of 1200 mg/day if necessary; usual maintenance range is 400 mg to 800 mg/day.

FATE
Oral absorption is slow but complete; peak plasma levels are usually attained in 4 hours to 6 hours. Effective serum levels are 4 mcg to 12 mcg/ml. The drug is approximately 75% protein bound and is distributed primarily to highly perfused tissues. The serum half-life is quite long initially (25 hours–50 hours) but decreases to 12 hours to 20 hours with repeated doses. Carbamazepine is metabolized in the liver (epoxide metabolite has anticonvulsant activity), and excreted as several metabolites and some unchanged drug through the kidney. It may induce its own metabolism.

SIDE-EFFECTS/ADVERSE REACTIONS

■ WARNING
Serious and sometimes fatal blood dyscrasias (aplastic anemia, agranulocytosis, leukopenia, thrombocytopenia) have occurred with carbamazepine. Early detection is vital, because in some patients, aplastic anemia is irreversible. Obtain complete pretreatment blood counts and repeat tests weekly during the first three months and monthly thereafter. Discontinue drug at the first sign of any significant abnormalities and advise patients of the early toxic signs of potential blood dyscrasias (e.g., sore throat, fever, mouth ulcers, abnormal bruising, or petechial hemorrhaging).

The most common side-effects seen with carbamazepine therapy are dizziness, ataxia, nausea, diplopia, and blurred vision. In addition to the potential blood dyscrasias noted above, an extensive range of adverse reactions are associated with carbamazepine therapy. These are listed below by organ system:

CNS—Confusion, incoordination, speech disturbance, involuntary movements, dysphasia, visual hallucinations, tinnitus, depression, peripheral neuritis, paresthesias, nystagmus

Dermatologic—Rash, sweating, urticaria, photosensitivity reactions, alopecia, exfoliative dermatitis, purpura, erythema multiforme, abnormal pigmentation

Hematologic—Blood dyscrasias (aplastic anemia, leukopenia, agranulocytosis, eosinophilia, leukocytosis, thrombocytopenia)

Genitourinary—Urinary frequency, albuminuria, glycosuria, urinary retention, oliguria, impotence

Gastrointestinal—Diarrhea, vomiting, abdominal pain, anorexia, xerostomia, glossitis

Cardiovascular—Hypotension, syncope, arrhythmias, aggravation of coronary artery disease and hypertension, thrombophlebitis, atrioventricular block, congestive heart failure

Other—Abnormal liver function, jaundice, hepatitis, hepatic cellular necrosis, muscle aching, osteomalacia, fever, chills, lenticular opacities, adenopathy

Overdosage is generally marked by neuromuscular disturbances, tachycardia, hypotension, irregular respiration, tremor, convulsions, vomiting, and urinary retention. Prompt removal of the drug from the body by lavage and forced diuresis is essential to minimize fatalities. Treatment is symptomatic and may include respiratory assistance, plasma expansion, control of convulsions, and maintenance of kidney function.

CONTRAINDICATIONS AND PRECAUTIONS
Carbamazepine is contraindicated in persons with a history of bone marrow depression or blood dyscrasias, and in combined use with monoamine oxidase (MAO) inhibitors. The drug should be given with caution to patients with renal, hepatic, or cardiac disease; hypertension; glaucoma; psychotic disorders; and to pregnant or nursing mothers. The

safety for use of the drug in children under 6 years of age has not been established.

Patients should be cautioned to notify the physician immediately if any of the following occur, since they may indicate developing toxicity: abnormal bruising, fever, sore throat, mucosal ulceration, abdominal pain, pale stools, darkened urine, CNS disturbances, impotence, or swelling of the hands or feet.

INTERACTIONS
1. Carbamazepine may accelerate the metabolism and therefore decrease the effects of itself as well as other anticonvulsants (phenobarbital, phenytoin, primidone), oral anticoagulants, and doxycycline.
2. Concurrent use of carbamazepine with MAO inhibitors or tricyclic antidepressants is not recommended because toxicity may be increased.
3. Carbamazepine is highly protein bound and therefore may potentiate other protein-bound drugs (*e.g.*, salicylates, oral hypoglycemics, anticoagulants, anti-inflammatory agents) by displacing them from protein-binding sites.
4. Cimetidine, isoniazid, erythromycin, and propoxyphene can elevate serum levels of carbamazepine, leading to increased toxicity.
5. Carbamazepine can result in breakthrough bleeding in women taking oral contraceptives.
6. Increased CNS toxicity can occur with combined use of carbamazepine and lithium.
7. Carbamazepine can enhance the antidiuretic effects of vasopressin, lypression, or desmopressin.

NURSING CONSIDERATIONS
See also Nursing Process, earlier in this chapter.

Adequate pretreatment data collection is essential to minimize the risk of side-effects and adverse reactions. The nurse should ensure that platelet and reticulocyte count, serum iron level, liver function studies, and blood urea nitrogen are drawn and that a complete ocular examination is done before drug therapy begins. As mentioned in the warning on this drug, adequate follow-up testing must be done regularly. Consequently, patients must be motivated to follow the treatment plan closely and seek regular follow-up care. Otherwise they are at risk of developing serious side-effects and consideration should be given on whether to treat them with carbamazepine.

Side-effects in children are rare and are more likely to occur in those who have other CNS prob-

lems, such as the mentally retarded. Elderly patients are much more prone to behavioral disturbances and confusion than other patients and should be closely monitored to reduce the chance of accidents or falls.

Withdrawal from carbamazepine should always be done by gradual dosage reduction under supervision. Rapid withdrawal can result in status epilepticus.

Valproic Acid Derivatives

Valproic Acid
(Depakene)

Valproate Sodium
(Depakene, Myproic Acid)

Divalproex Sodium
(Depakote)

Although chemically unrelated to other anticonvulsants, valproic acid, its sodium salt, and a stable compound composed of equal parts valproic acid and valproate sodium (*i.e.*, divalproex sodium) generally provide improved seizure control when added to the drug regimen of refractory patients with multiple seizure types. They are most effective against simple and complex absence seizures, but may also be useful against a variety of generalized as well as localized seizures. Divalproex is an enteric-coated dosage form and has a slightly lower incidence of gastrointestinal side-effects than the other dosage forms, but a similar pharmacologic profile. The major danger associated with use of valproic acid is hepatotoxicity, and liver function must be closely monitored during and for some time following drug therapy.

MECHANISM AND ACTIONS
The mechanism of action of valproic acid has not been definitely established but its action appears to be associated with an elevation in the functional levels of gamma-aminobutyric acid (GABA), an inhibitory neurotransmitter in the CNS. This action may result from inhibition of the enzyme gamma-transaminase, which blocks conversion of GABA to succinic semialdehyde. The metabolic acidosis resulting from valproic acid administration may also have a protective effect against certain seizures. Valproic acid exhibits a prolactin-inhibitory

effect, which likewise may be related to potentiation of GABA.

USES

1. Treatment of simple and complex absence seizures, including petit mal (alone or in combination with other anticonvulsants)
2. Adjunct in the treatment of multiple seizure types
3. *Investigational uses* include management of grand mal seizures, myoclonic seizures, complex and elementary partial seizures, infantile spasms, and prevention of recurrent febrile seizures (alone or in combination with other antiepileptic drugs).

ADMINISTRATION AND DOSAGE

Valproic acid is available as capsules (250 mg), syrup (250 mg valproic acid as valproate sodium per 5 ml), and enteric-coated tablets (125 mg, 250 mg, 500 mg valproic acid as divalproex sodium). Dosage is expressed as valproic acid equivalents. The recommended initial dose is 15 mg/kg/day, which may be increased by 5 mg to 10 mg/kg/day at 1-week intervals until seizures are controlled or side-effects occur. The maximum daily dose is 60 mg/kg. Dosages greater than 250 mg/day should be given in divided doses.

FATE

Valproic acid and valproate sodium are rapidly absorbed orally; divalproex is enteric coated and absorption is delayed 1 hour, but is uniform and consistent. Peak serum levels occur within 30 minutes to 60 minutes with valproate sodium and within 1 hour to 4 hours with the other dosage forms. The drug is widely distributed and highly (90%) protein-bound. Valproic acid is primarily metabolized in the liver and is excreted in the urine, almost entirely as conjugated metabolites. The serum half-life ranges from 6 hours to 16 hours but may be increased in neonates, young children, and patients with hepatitis or cirrhosis.

SIDE-EFFECTS/ADVERSE REACTIONS

■ *WARNING*
Fatal hepatic failure has occurred in patients receiving valproic acid, usually during the first 6 months of treatment. Frequent liver function tests are required, especially during the initial months of therapy, and the drug should be discontinued immediately at the first sign of hepatic dysfunction.

Initially, the most frequently observed side-effects are nausea, vomiting, and indigestion. These are usually transient and seldom require discontinuation of therapy. Other side-effects occasionally noted at the onset of therapy include sedation, diarrhea, abdominal cramping, and minor elevations in serum transaminases (SGOT, SGPT) and LDH.

In addition to the hepatotoxicity noted above, a number of other adverse reactions have occurred in patients receiving valproic acid; however, because the drug is usually given in combination with other antiepileptic medications, the following adverse effects cannot be ascribed *solely* to valproic acid: lenticular opacities, nystagmus, visual disturbances, diplopia, dizziness, incoordination, tremor, dysarthria, skin rash, petechiae, alopecia, depression, aggression, hyperactivity, behavioral disturbances, altered bleeding time (drug inhibits platelet aggregation), muscle weakness, irregular menses, amenorrhea, acute pancreatitis, and blood dyscrasias (rare).

CONTRAINDICATIONS AND PRECAUTIONS

Valproic acid is contraindicated in patients with hepatic disease. The drug should be used *cautiously* in the presence of renal dysfunction and bleeding disorders (increased bleeding tendency), and in pregnant or nursing mothers.

INTERACTIONS

1. Valproic acid may potentiate the depressant effects of other CNS-depressant drugs (*e.g.,* barbiturates, narcotics, alcohol).
2. Serum phenobarbital levels may be elevated by concomitant use of valproic acid.
3. Simultaneous use of valproic acid and clonazepam may induce absence seizures (although this combination has provided excellent control of some absence seizure states). Combinations of valproic acid and phenytoin may result in breakthrough seizures.
4. Valproic acid interferes with platelet aggregation and therefore may increase the bleeding tendency with anticoagulants, dipyridamole, salicylates, and other inhibitors of platelet aggregation.
5. Valproic acid may alter the response to phenytoin, and breakthrough seizures have occurred with this combination.

NURSING CONSIDERATIONS

See also Nursing Process, earlier in this chapter.
To minimize the potential for hepatic side-ef-

fects, patients should have pretreatment and periodic liver function studies. A complete ocular examination should also be performed. Patients should be taught to report any seizures, weakness, or bleeding.

Valproic acid is very irritating to mucous membranes. To decrease the nausea, vomiting, and loss of appetite associated with the drug, patients should plan to take it with food. Capsules and tablets should never be chewed since they will irritate the mouth and throat on contact. Anyone who has trouble swallowing the drug should be offered the option of the syrup form.

Valproic acid has a fairly narrow therapeutic index. Therefore, patients should never double up when a dose is missed. Doing so may increase the potential for toxicity.

Nurses and patients should also be aware that the drug produces a ketone-containing metabolite that will interfere with urine tests for ketone bodies. Alternate testing methods must be found when necessary.

Benzodiazepine Antiepileptics

Clonazepam
(Klonopin)

Several benzodiazepines (see Chap. 28) have been successfully employed in treating various epileptic states, and clonazepam probably enjoys the widest use in this regard. It is a long-acting drug that is useful primarily against absence seizures, especially the akinetic and myoclonic variants. Sedation is quite common, and prolonged use can lead to varying degrees of dependence and result in the appearance of withdrawal symptoms on discontinuation of therapy. Tolerance develops with continued use of clonazepam, limiting its usefulness for chronic therapy.

MECHANISM AND ACTIONS
The precise mechanism of action of clonazepam in alleviating absence seizures is not well established. It may potentiate inhibitory mechanisms in subcortical brain structures, and has been shown to suppress the spike-wave discharge characteristic of absence seizures, and to decrease the frequency, duration, amplitude, and spread of minor motor seizure discharges.

USES
1. Treatment of petit mal variant (Lennox-Gastaut syndrome)
2. Treatment of myoclonic and akinetic seizures
3. Treatment of simple absence seizures refractory to succinimides (may be used alone or as an adjunct; some evidence of benefit in psychomotor and focal seizures in combination with other drugs)

ADMINISTRATION AND DOSAGE
Clonazepam is administered orally as 0.5-mg, 1-mg, or 2-mg tablets. In adults, the initial dose is 0.5 mg three times/day. This may be increased in 0.5-mg to 1-mg increments every 3 days until an optimal effect is noted. The maximum dose is 20 mg/day. Children should receive between 0.01 mg and 0.03 mg/kg/day in 2 or 3 divided doses. Dosage may be increased by 0.25 mg to 0.5 mg every third day until an optimal effect is observed. The usual maintenance dose is 0.1 mg to 0.2 mg/kg/day.

FATE
The onset of action following oral administration is 30 minutes to 60 minutes; maximum plasma levels occur in 1 hour to 2 hours. Effects persist 6 hours to 12 hours. The half-life of the parent compound varies from 20 hours to 40 hours. Clonazepam is metabolized in the liver and primarily excreted in the urine.

SIDE-EFFECTS/ADVERSE REACTIONS
The most commonly observed side-effects are drowsiness (50%), ataxia (30%), and behavioral problems (25%). These may ameliorate with time. Other adverse reactions reported in patients receiving clonazepam are

CNS—Confusion, insomnia, depression, hysteria, headache, hypotonia, involuntary movements, slurred speech, tremor, vertigo, nystagmus, hallucinations, psychosis

Gastrointestinal—Anorexia, constipation, dry mouth, coated tongue, gastritis, nausea, sore gums, hepatomegaly

Respiratory—Rhinorrhea, shortness of breath, hypersecretion

Dermatologic—Rash, ankle edema, hirsutism or hair loss

Urinary—Dysuria, enuresis, nocturia, urinary retention

Other—Palpitations, muscle weakness, fever, lymphadenopathy, dehydration, blood dyscrasias (rare), diplopia, abnormal eye movements, increased salivation

See also Chapter 28 for additional possible adverse reactions.

CONTRAINDICATIONS AND PRECAUTIONS

Clonazepam is contraindicated in patients with significant liver disease and acute narrow-angle glaucoma. The drug should be administered with *caution* in the presence of renal dysfunction or chronic respiratory diseases (drug can increase secretions), to persons evidencing behavioral disturbances or drug addiction, and to young children and pregnant or nursing mothers. Clonazepam should not be given alone in the presence of mixed seizures, since it may worsen tonic–clonic seizures or precipitate grand mal convulsions. The drug should not be discontinued abruptly because marked worsening of certain seizures has occurred.

INTERACTIONS

1. The CNS-depressive effects of clonazepam may be enhanced by other drugs having a depressant action (*e.g.,* alcohol, narcotics, sedatives, phenothiazines, barbiturates, and so forth).
2. Phenytoin, phenobarbital, and carbamazepine can reduce serum clonazepam levels.
3. Combined use of clonazepam and valproic acid may elicit absence seizures and increase the risk of drowsiness

NURSING CONSIDERATIONS

See also Nursing Process, earlier in this chapter.

The patient on clonazepam must learn to cope with two major side-effects, drowsiness and tolerance. Drowsiness may be transient but patients need to exercise caution to protect themselves from falls or injury. Level of alertness should be firmly established before the patient attempts to operate an automobile or any other machinery. Elderly patients may have more trouble than other patients with this side-effect.

All patients on long-term therapy have the potential to develop tolerance. The first sign of it may be increased seizure activity. Dosage adjustments may correct the problem, but if the drug is no longer effective it must be gradually withdrawn. Rapid withdrawal may result in seizures or status epilepticus.

Children receiving clonazepam must also be observed for personality changes and behavioral problems. Such symptoms may indicate the need

for a dosage adjustment or gradual withdrawal from the drug.

Diazepam
(Valium)

Diazepam is a benzodiazepine widely used for control of simple anxiety states (see Chap. 28). It is also useful orally as an adjunct in the management of convulsive disorders, especially minor motor seizures, but it rarely is effective alone. Its principal indication is parenterally (IV) for the treatment of status epilepticus and other severe recurrent convulsive seizures. Diazepam may also be used for convulsions accompanying acute alcohol withdrawal. The drug is discussed fully in Chapter 28; thus, only those aspects relating to its use as an antiepileptic will be reviewed here.

Although the mechanism of the antiepileptic action of diazepam remains to be precisely elucidated, it is known to suppress polysynaptic neuronal activity in the spinal cord and mesencephalic reticular formation. The drug also facilitates the action of GABA, an inhibitory neurotransmitter, in the CNS, although the contribution of this effect to the clinical antiepileptic action of diazepam is unknown.

Diazepam is administered intravenously for the control of status epilepticus and other acute convulsive states, including those associated with acute alcohol withdrawal. Orally, the drug is sometimes used adjunctively with other antiepileptic drugs for controlling minor motor seizures.

Oral adult dosage ranges from 2 mg to 10 mg two to four times a day, whereas children may be given 1 mg to 2.5 mg three to four times a day. IV doses are 5 mg to 10 mg in the adult, to be repeated as needed at 10-minute to 15-minute intervals to a maximum of 30 mg. Children receive 0.2 mg to 1 mg every 2 minutes to 5 minutes depending on age and body weight.

Refer to the discussion of benzodiazepines in Chapter 28 for a complete review of the side-effects, adverse reactions, contraindications, and interactions associated with diazepam. The principal limiting factors in the use of benzodiazepines for epilepsy are their often pronounced sedative action and the frequent development of tolerance with chronic administration.

NURSING CONSIDERATIONS

Diazepam is primarily used for the treatment of status epilepticus and acute alcohol withdrawal seizures, both emergency situations. In such cases, the physician will probably be administering large intermittent doses of diazepam until the seizure activity ceases or respiratory depression occurs. Nursing care should focus on frequent monitoring of vital signs, constant bedside attention, and protection of the patient from injury as much as possible. Resuscitative equipment and drugs should be immediately available since the chance of arrest is high. Use of a vital sign observation flowsheet to chart care and frequency of medication administration is helpful in maintaining an accurate record of the sequence of events during the acute episode.

Although the route of choice for diazepam in treating status epilepticus is slow intravenous injection, the drug can cause severe thrombosis, swelling, or phlebitis. A large vein should always be used in such an episode and the drug should be administered no faster than 5 mg per minute. If no large veins can be found and the patient is already in status, consideration should be given to administering diazepam deep IM although this is not the preferred route.

Clorazepate
(Tranxene)

Clorazepate is a benzodiazepine antianxiety agent that has been used adjunctively in the management of partial seizures. The initial dose is 7.5 mg three times a day in adults and twice a day in children 9 to 12 years of age. Dosage may be increased in 7.5-mg increments once a week to the level providing optimal control. Drowsiness and dizziness can occur and patients should be cautioned against driving until the effects of the drug are known. Concurrent use of alcohol or other CNS depressants should be avoided. Refer to Chapter 28 for a complete discussion of benzodiazepines.

NURSING CONSIDERATIONS
See Nursing Considerations for clonazepam, above.

Phenacemide
(Phenurone)

Phenacemide is a structural analog of the hydantoins useful in severe epileptic states, especially mixed forms of psychomotor seizures refractory to other medications. It is generally employed as a last resort, however, because of its extreme toxicity.

The exact mechanism of action of phenacemide is unknown; however, it has been demonstrated to elevate the threshold for experimental electroshock seizures in animals.

Recommended doses in adults are 250 mg to 500 mg orally three times a day, initially. The usual maintenance range is 2 g to 3 g a day. Children (5 years–10 years) should receive one half of the adult dose. Phenacemide is available in 500-mg tablets.

Phenacemide can produce serious untoward reactions. Most frequently encountered adverse effects are psychic changes (*e.g.,* psychosis, depression), gastrointestinal disturbances, skin rash, drowsiness, dizziness, weakness, and headache. In addition, phenacemide administration has been associated with insomnia, paresthesias, fatigue, fever, muscle pain, palpitations, increased serum creatinine, hepatitis (occasionally fatal), blood dyscrasias (*e.g.,* leukopenia, aplastic anemia), and bone marrow depression. The drug is contraindicated in persons with personality disorders and in pregnant women. Cautious use is warranted in patients with a history of allergy or renal dysfunction, and in nursing mothers. Concomitant use of other antiepileptics, especially ethotoin, can increase the incidence of untoward reactions.

NURSING CONSIDERATIONS
To minimize gastrointestinal disturbances, this drug should be administered with food. Patients should also be taught to watch for and report any early warning symptoms of toxicity. These include skin rash, depression, apathy, paranoia, pruritus, sore throat, and fever.

Phenacemide should always be gradually withdrawn to decrease the chance of seizures.

Acetazolamide
(Ak Zol, Dazamide, Diamox)

Acetazolamide is an inhibitor of the enzyme carbonic anhydrase and has been used as an adjunct in the control of certain seizures, especially simple absence and other nonlocalized seizure states. The drug is also occasionally employed as a mild diuretic, for treatment of chronic open-angle glaucoma (as it reduces formation of aqueous humor), and for the relief of mild migraine headaches. Acetazolamide has been used experimentally for prophylactic treatment of acute mountain sickness produced at high altitudes.

The mechanism of its antiepileptic action is not

completely established, but appears to result from reduced formation of H^+ and HCO_3^- ions, and accumulation of CO_2, which may retard abnormal or excessive discharges from central neurons. A mild acidosis develops following acetazolamide administration, which may also contribute to the observed decrease in seizure activity.

The usefulness of acetazolamide in treating epileptic seizures is greatly limited by the rapid onset of tolerance, with return of seizure activity often within a few weeks. The drug is available as tablets (125 mg, 250 mg), sustained-release capsules (500 mg), and injectable solution (500 mg/vial). The sustained-release dosage form is not recommended for use as an antiepileptic. When given in combination with other anticonvulsants, the starting dose is 250 mg/day. The usual maintenance dosage range is 375 mg to 1000 mg a day.

The most frequently encountered side-effects are paresthesias of the face and extremities. Other untoward reactions observed with acetazolamide include polyuria, glycosuria, drowsiness, confusion, myopia, urticaria, rash, hepatic dysfunction, and flaccid paralysis. The drug is contraindicated in patients with sulfonamide allergy, since the drug is a sulfonamide derivative, and also in the presence of acidosis, hypokalemia, kidney or liver dysfunction, adrenal insufficiency, and early pregnancy. The drug should be used with caution in diabetic patients, since it may increase blood glucose levels resulting in the need to alter antidiabetic drug requirements.

Magnesium Sulfate

Magnesium, in the form of magnesium sulfate, is an effective anticonvulsant in seizures associated with the toxemia of pregnancy and other clinical situations characterized by abnormally low levels of plasma magnesium. The drug may be used intravenously or intramuscularly, depending on the speed of action desired, although intravenous use is significantly more hazardous. Other clinical applications for magnesium sulfate are its use orally as a cathartic, topically as an antipruritic, and parenterally to control uterine tetany, paroxysmal atrial tachycardia, hypertension, and cerebral edema. It has also been employed as an adjunct in hyperalimentation and for replacement therapy in acute magnesium deficiency.

Magnesium controls convulsions by interfering with neuromuscular transmission, possibly by blocking release of acetylcholine from motor nerve endings. It also exerts a depressant effect on the CNS. The principal uses of magnesium are to control the seizures of severe preeclampsia or eclampsia and in treating convulsions associated with abnormally low levels of magnesium. In addition, it may be effective in controlling hypertension, encephalopathy, and convulsions in children with acute nephritis. Magnesium has also been used experimentally to inhibit premature labor, although it is not considered a drug of first choice.

Dosage is individualized and administration is terminated as soon as the desired effect is obtained. Adult intramuscular doses range from 1 g to 5 g of a 25% to 50% solution, up to five times a day as necessary. With intravenous injection, 1 g to 4 g of a 10% to 20% solution may be given at a rate not exceeding 1.5 ml/minute; alternately, 4 g in 250 ml of a 5% dextrose solution may be infused at a rate not to exceed 3 ml/minute. Pediatric intramuscular doses range from 20 mg to 40 mg/kg in a 20% solution. With repeated administration, knee jerk reflexes should be tested before every dose; if the reflex is absent, magnesium should *not* be administered. The onset of action is immediate with intravenous injection and within 1 hour with intramuscular administration.

Side-effects include flushing (common), sweating, hypotension, sedation, confusion, hypothermia, flaccid paralysis, depressed reflexes, cardiac and respiratory depression, and circulatory collapse. Hypocalcemia with tetany has been reported secondary to magnesium sulfate administration. The drug must be given cautiously to persons with renal impairment and is contraindicated in the presence of heart block and myocardial insufficiency. Additive CNS-depressant effects can occur when magnesium is given together with narcotics, barbiturates, anesthetics, and other sedative–hypnotic drugs. Magnesium may potentiate the muscle-relaxing action of neuromuscular blocking agents. The drug is available for injection as solutions of 10%, 12.5%, 25%, and 50% concentrations.

NURSING CONSIDERATIONS
The antidote to magnesium sulfate-induced respiratory depression is calcium, so an intravenous formulation should be on hand whenever magnesium is administered.

To reduce the chance of toxic overdose, the nurse should closely monitor blood pressure, pulse, and urine output. The drug should be discontinued if urine output falls below 100 ml/4 hours or if the patient develops thirst, a feeling of warmth, confusion, depressed deep tendon reflexes, or muscle weakness, since these are all signs of impending toxicity.

CASE STUDY

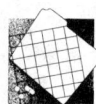

Casey Donahue, aged 2, is seen by her pediatrician after having a febrile convulsion. This is the third episode related to high fever she has had in 6 months. He prescribes phenobarbital, 60 mg daily. Mrs. Donahue asks the nurse why Casey has to take the medication daily since the only time she has had a seizure is when her fever rises to 103°F.

Discussion Questions

1. What information can the nurse give Mrs. Donahue about the way phenobarbital works? What effects can she expect the drug to have on Casey?
2. What would be the best way to encourage Casey to take the medication considering her age?
3. What strategies could the nurse employ to allay Mrs. Donahue's fears and improve the chance of compliance?

REVIEW QUESTIONS

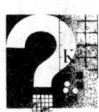

1. Briefly describe the following types of epilepsy: (1) grand mal, (2) petit mal, (3) psychomotor seizures, (4) status epilepticus.
2. How can the nurse deal with a patient who expects antiepileptic drugs to provide the "magic cure" for his seizures? What reality-based information can she give to provide him with hope?
3. What areas of a child's life should be assessed in planning care for the child and his family when he must take antiepileptic medication?
4. What body changes may make an individual more prone to seizures?
5. Describe several strategies a nurse might use to promote compliance in a patient taking antiepileptic drugs?
6. What kind of monitoring should an epileptic woman receive when she becomes pregnant?
7. What are the principal indications for the antiepileptic barbiturates? List their major adverse reactions.
8. What side-effects of barbiturates occur most frequently in children? How can the nurse help parents to cope with these side-effects?
9. How can patients receiving barbiturates ensure that they maintain adequate vitamin D levels?
10. Describe the mechanism of action of the hydantoins (*e.g.*, phenytoin) in treating epilepsy.
11. Give the primary adverse reactions associated with use of hydantoins.
12. Describe nursing goals for a patient who is prescribed a once-a-day dose of phenytoin (Dilantin).
13. How should phenytoin be administered to a patient with a feeding tube?
14. What are the indications for the oxazolidinediones? What are their major adverse reactions?
15. List the antiepileptic drugs useful in (1) grand mal, (2) petit mal, and (3) psychomotor seizures.
16. What are the principal uses for carbamazepine (Tegretol)? What are the major dangers associated with its use?
17. Describe the mechanism of action of valproic acid and its derivatives. List the adverse effects observed with its use.

18. What precautions should be taken before giving valproic acid as a tablet to a child?
19. Which benzodiazepines are principally used as antiepileptic drugs? What are the disadvantages associated with their use?
20. Outline nursing care goals for the first 30 minutes of care for a patient who is brought to the emergency room in status epilepticus.
21. Give the indications for acetazolamide (Diamox).
22. What are the uses for magnesium sulfate? List the important adverse reactions associated with this drug.
23. What drug should be on hand when a patient is receiving magnesium sulfate? What monitoring is essential during magnesium sulfate administration?

BIBLIOGRAPHY

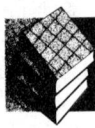

Bocchese JD, Merker A: Seizure disorders in the neonate. Critical Care Nurse 3:42, 1983

Browne TR, Feldman RG: Epilepsy: Diagnosis and Management. Boston, Little, Brown & Co, 1983

Coulter DL: The treatable epilepsies. N Engl J Med 309:1456, 1983

Dalessio DJ: Current concepts: Seizure disorders and pregnancy. N Engl J Med 312:559, 1985

Delgado-Escueta AV, Treiman DM, Walsh GO: The treatable epilepsies, Parts I and II. N Engl J Med 308:1508, 1576, 1983

Drugs for Epilepsy. Med Lett Drugs Ther 25:81, 1983

Ferrari M et al: Psychologic and behavioral disturbance among epileptic children treated with barbiturate anti-convulsants. Am J Psychiatry 140:112, 1983

Frey HH, Janz D (eds): Antiepileptic drugs. In Handbook of Experimental Pharmacology, Vol. 74. Berlin, Springer-Verlag, 1985

Glaser GH, Penry JK, Woodbury DM (eds): Antiepileptic Drugs: Mechanisms of Action. New York, Raven Press, 1980

Hachinski V: Management of a first seizure. Arch Neurol 43:1290, 1986

Jobe PC, Dailey JW, Laird HE (eds): Epilepsy: Neurotransmitter abnormalities as determinants of seizure susceptibility and severity. Fed Proc 43:2503, 1984

Johnston D: Valproic acid: Update on its mechanism of action. Epilepsia 25(1):51, 1984

Norman S, Brown T: Seizure disorders: Nursing management. Am J Nurs 81:990, 1981

Ozuna J et al: Effect of enteral tube feeding on serum phenytoin levels. J Neurosurg Nurs 16:289, 1984

Parrish MA: A comparison of behavioral side effects related to commonly used anticonvulsants. Pediatric Nursing 10:149, 1984

Pedley TA, Meldrum BS (eds): Recent Advances in Epilepsy. New York, Churchill Livingstone, 1983

Penry JK, Porter RJ: Epilepsy: Mechanisms and therapy. Med Clin North Am 63:801, 1979

Piepho RW, Lorenzo AS: Therapeutic management of seizure disorders. U.S. Pharmacist Sept:36, 1979

Reynolds EH, Shorvou SD: Single drug or combination therapy for epilepsy. Drugs 21:374, 1981

Sasso SC: Phenytoin for seizure disorders. Maternal Child Nursing 9:279, 1984

Solomon GE, Kutt H, Plum F: Clinical Management of Seizures: A Guide for the Physician, 2nd ed. Philadelphia, WB Saunders, 1983

Spero L: Epilepsy. Lancet 2:1319, 1982

Woodbury DM, Penry JK, Pippender CE (eds): Antiepileptic Drugs. New York, Raven Press, 1983

Antiparkinsonian Drugs

Dopaminergic Agents
    Levodopa
    Levodopa/Carbidopa
    Amantadine
    Bromocriptine

Anticholinergic–
    Antihistaminic Agents

31

Parkinson's disease, or paralysis agitans, is a chronic progressive disorder of the central nervous system (CNS), the etiology of which is largely unknown in the majority of cases. The term *parkinsonism* is used to describe the symptom complex that may result from either the normal course of the disease itself or from administration of certain groups of drugs (*e.g.*, phenothiazines) that produce similar symptoms. However, the term is frequently applied to both disorders interchangeably. Although the symptoms vary depending on the stage of the disease—which becomes progressively more disabling—the three cardinal manifestations of Parkinson's disease are the following:

1. *Akinesia (bradykinesia)*—A lack of or difficulty in initiating voluntary muscle movement; advanced disease states are characterized by "frozen" muscles, resulting in mask-like facial expression; impairment of postural reflexes; and inability to care for oneself adequately. Spontaneous movements are sluggish, but once initiated, it may be difficult for patients to stop their progress, and they frequently stagger and fall.
2. *Rigidity*—Usually of the "plastic" type; the affected area usually can be moved without great difficulty but often remains fixed once again in its new position; it is often referred to as *cogwheel* or *ratchet* resistance to passive movement.
3. *Tremor*—Coarse (3 cycles/sec–7 cycles/sec), repetitive muscle activity, usually worse when the person is at rest; commonly manifested as a "pill-rolling" motion of the hands and a bobbing of the head; distal extremities are more commonly involved than proximal muscles.

Besides the principal symptoms of the disease, afflicted patients may show disturbances in gait or posture, impaired speech, muscular weakness, and autonomic hyperactivity such as salivation and seborrhea. The symptoms are usually insidious in onset and a mild tremor at rest is often the initial sign. As the disease progresses, symptoms become more frequent and severe and common functions such as walking, eating, and writing become increasingly more difficult. Advanced stages are frequently characterized by autonomic *insufficiency*, resulting in severe orthostatic hypotension, which may be exacerbated by the anticholinergic drugs that are sometimes used in treating the disease.

Onset of Parkinson's disease usually occurs in middle age, and during the early stages symptoms frequently are much worse on one side of the body. Diagnosis is largely symptomatic, although definite biochemical changes are present in the CNS.

The most characteristic pathologic feature of parkinsonism is a degeneration of dopaminergic neurons having their cell bodies in the *substantia nigra* in the midbrain. Because motor-regulatory areas such as the *corpus striatum* receive their dopamine supply from the substantia nigra, degeneration of these nigral–striatal neurons decreases the functional amount of dopamine available to the nuclei of the corpus striatum (*i.e.*, caudate nucleus, putamen). This upsets the normal balance between the inhibitory transmitter dopamine and the excitatory transmitter acetylcholine in these brain regions, resulting in an excitatory predominance on lower motor centers by the intact cholinergic pathways.

The above is probably an oversimplification of the extremely complex interaction of neurohormones on central motor-integrating pathways. Although striatal dopamine deficiency provides a common basis for the various manifestations of parkinsonism, the only true symptom resulting from low striatal dopamine is *akinesia*. As such, akinesia is the abnormality most benefited by dopamine-replacement therapy. Other symptoms probably reflect the effects of the abnormal neurotransmitter ratio triggered by the dopamine deficit and involve alterations in more complex pathways among central motor-regulatory structures. Therefore, tremor and rigidity are less well controlled by supplemental dopamine and may respond better to both dopamine replacement and cholinergic antagonism.

Drug therapy of parkinsonism is directed either toward augmentation of central dopaminergic function or reduction of central cholinergic activity. Drugs effective in the control of Parkinson's disease may be grouped as follows:

1. Dopaminergic agents
   a. Dopamine precursor (*e.g.*, levodopa)
   b. Dopamine-releasing agent (*e.g.*, amantadine)
   c. Dopamine receptor agonist (*e.g.*, bromocriptine)
2. Anticholinergic/antihistaminergic agents (*e.g.*, benztropine, ethopropazine)

In addition to proper drug treatment, which of course is not curative but simply palliative, adjunctive therapy for parkinsonism should include physical therapy to delay disability and emotional support to help lessen feelings of helplessness and inadequacy as the disease inexorably progresses and limits the patient's activities.

The initial response to drug therapy is often dramatic and parkinsonian patients frequently show marked improvement in their ability to function in a more coordinated manner soon after treatment is begun. Posture, balance, and gait are all improved, and there is frequently a significant reduction in salivation, drooling, sweating, and seborrhea. Approximately one third of patients benefit greatly from the drugs used for treatment, another one third show mild to moderate improvement in most symptoms, while the remaining one third either do not evidence clinically significant benefit or cannot tolerate the drugs.

Symptoms resembling those of Parkinson's disease can be elicited by use of certain drugs that act to interfere with central dopaminergic function. This condition, known as *drug-induced parkinsonism*, can result from administration of antipsychotic drugs (dopamine receptor blockers) or reserpine (depletes neuronal dopamine stores) and may be treated by most of the same drugs used to control Parkinson's disease.

A somewhat different type of drug-induced parkinsonism has been reported among drug abusers. Attempts by certain clandestine laboratories to synthesize a meperidine-like narcotic drug have resulted in the formation of certain by-products, one of which is 1-methyl-4-phenyl-1,2,5,6-tetrahydropyridine (MPTP). When this substance was accidentally injected along with the meperidine analog, individuals developed severe parkinsonism within two weeks. Subsequent investigation demonstrated that MPTP is a neurotoxin that can selectively destroy dopaminergic neurons in the substantia nigra, leading to the development of classical parkinsonism, which is irreversible and requires antiparkinsonian drug therapy. MPTP is now being evaluated in the laboratory as a model for Parkinson's disease and may assist researchers in developing newer and better antiparkinsonian drugs. It is unfortunate that this potential scientific breakthrough was attained at the expense of human suffering.

Dopaminergic Agents

Three types of drugs are available that can enhance dopaminergic functioning in the motor-regulatory centers of the CNS. Levodopa (L-DOPA), the levorotatory isomer of dihydroxyphenylalanine, is the metabolic precursor of dopamine (see Fig. 15-1) and its use results in increased concentrations of dopamine in the corpus striatum. It is used rather than dopamine itself because L-DOPA readily passes the blood–brain barrier, whereas dopamine does not and therefore does not reach sufficient levels in the CNS following systemic administra-

tion. L-DOPA is used either alone or in a fixed-ratio combination with carbidopa, the latter being an inhibitor of peripheral dopa decarboxylase, the enzyme responsible for converting dopa to dopamine. Peripheral inhibition of this enzyme by carbidopa allows a greater fraction of intact L-DOPA to penetrate the CNS, thereby increasing the amount of dopamine formed in central motor areas. Thus, much smaller doses of L-DOPA may be employed when given with carbidopa as compared to when given alone, thereby reducing the incidence of side-effects.

In addition to being available in two fixed dosage ratios with L-DOPA (1:4, 1:10), carbidopa is also marketed alone in 25-mg tablets (Lodosyn) that allow the clinician to titrate more carefully the dosage ratio to obtain better symptom control. Carbidopa is only indicated for use with L-DOPA because carbidopa has no therapeutic effect of its own in parkinsonism.

Another drug employed to potentiate the effects of dopamine in the CNS is amantadine. Originally developed as an antiviral prophylactic agent against the Asian (A) influenza strain, amantadine was demonstrated to have a beneficial action in certain parkinsonian patients to whom it was administered. It apparently increases the release of dopamine from presynaptic nerve endings. Therefore, its effectiveness is limited to those patients having functional stores of dopamine present in striatal brain areas.

The third type of dopaminergic drug is bromocriptine, a dopamine receptor agonist. It finds its principal clinical application in cases of parkinsonism refractory to conventional therapy as an adjunct to levodopa/carbidopa treatment. Bromocriptine can provide additional therapeutic benefit in those patients whose condition has begun to deteriorate and may allow a reduction in levodopa dosage, thus reducing the incidence of side-effects associated with prolonged levodopa therapy. However, patients unresponsive to levodopa are not likely to benefit from bromocriptine.

Levodopa
(Dopar, Larodopa)

Levodopa/Carbidopa
(Sinemet)

Because the symptoms of Parkinson's disease are related to a deficiency of striatal dopamine, replacement therapy with exogenous dopamine seemed a logical therapeutic alternative. However, dopamine itself fails to cross the blood–brain barrier in adequate amounts and is not effective as such in treating the disease. Its metabolic precursor, levodopa, however, does penetrate the CNS and is converted to dopamine in the brain, thus supplying the deficient neurohormone. Unfortunately, the enzyme that converts dopa into dopamine, aromatic l-amino acid decarboxylase or dopa decarboxylase, is found not only in the CNS, but in the plasma as well. Thus, a significant fraction of an oral dose of L-DOPA is metabolized to dopamine in the plasma before it can penetrate the blood–brain barrier, and much of its central effectiveness is lost. As a result, very large amounts of L-DOPA are required to provide a clinically effective level of dopamine in the brain, and these large doses are often associated with many untoward reactions. In an attempt to overcome this problem, levodopa is available in fixed combination (4:1, 10:1) with carbidopa.

Carbidopa competes for the enzyme dopa decarboxylase, thereby retarding the peripheral conversion of L-DOPA to dopamine. This allows a greater fraction of the administered L-DOPA dose to pass the blood–brain barrier, resulting in higher dopamine levels in central motor-regulatory centers. Carbidopa itself does not cross the blood–brain barrier and therefore does not interfere with conversion of L-DOPA to dopamine in the CNS. Levodopa dosage requirements are reduced approximately 75% by combination with carbidopa, because plasma levels and plasma half-life are increased. Consequently, much less dopamine is formed peripherally than with the use of L-DOPA alone, resulting in a lower incidence of many systemic side-effects, especially nausea, vomiting, and cardiovascular disturbances. However, adverse CNS effects (e.g., dyskinesias) may occur sooner and at lower doses of L-DOPA when combined with carbidopa than when given alone, because more levodopa is reaching the brain to be converted there to dopamine. Carbidopa also prevents the antagonism of L-DOPA by vitamin B_6 (pyridoxine) (see Interactions, below).

The pharmacologic and toxicologic properties of carbidopa/levodopa are similar to those of levodopa in most respects. However, the fixed ratio combinations allow use of lower doses of L-DOPA, provide a smoother response, and permit more rapid dosage adjustments than can be obtained with L-DOPA alone. Untoward reactions, contraindications, and drug interactions observed with carbidopa/levodopa are essentially the same as those noted with levodopa itself, although blood levels of urea nitrogen, uric acid, and creatinine are lower during carbidopa/levodopa administration than during treatment with levodopa alone.

MECHANISM AND ACTIONS

Levodopa is a precursor of dopamine that readily passes the blood–brain barrier, then is decarboxylated to dopamine. Addition of carbidopa to levodopa prevents much of the *peripheral* decarboxylation of levodopa, allowing a much greater fraction of the dose to enter the CNS. Increased formation of dopamine in motor-regulatory areas of the CNS, such as the basal ganglia, restores the depleted dopamine levels and improves the symptoms of Parkinson's disease. Levodopa is most effective in relieving akinesia and bradykinesia, somewhat less efficacious in controlling rigidity, and seldom of significant benefit in reducing tremor. The response to levodopa is greatest at the outset of therapy but diminishes gradually over 2 to 5 years, at which time it is usually necessary to initiate therapy with other antiparkinsonian drugs, such as anticholinergics, amantadine, or bromocriptine.

USES

1. Treatment of Parkinson's disease, whether idiopathic, postencephalitic, or arteriosclerotic
2. Control of symptoms of drug-induced extrapyramidal disorders
3. Relief of pain associated with herpes zoster (investigational use)

ADMINISTRATION AND DOSAGE

Levodopa Alone

Levodopa is available in tablets and capsules (100 mg, 250 mg, 500 mg). The initial levodopa dosage is 0.5 g to 1 g daily in two or more divided doses. Doses are increased gradually in increments of 0.75 g/day every 3 to 7 days to a maximum of 8 g/day. Optimal clinical response may not be obtained for up to 6 months. Dosage is highly individualized and must be reassessed frequently.

Levodopa/Carbidopa

The dosage of levodopa/carbidopa, like that of levodopa itself, is highly individualized. Tablets are available in a fixed ratio of either 10 mg carbidopa/100 mg levodopa, 25 mg carbidopa/100 mg levodopa, or 25 mg carbidopa/250 mg levodopa. Dosage schedules are as follows:

Patients not receiving levodopa—Initially, 1 tablet (10/100 or 25/100) three times/day; increase by 1 tablet daily until 6 tablets/day. If more L-DOPA is necessary, substitute 1 tablet (25/250) three to four times/day; increase by ½ to 1 tablet/day to a maximum of 8 tablets (25/250) per day.

Patients receiving levodopa—(Discontinue L-DOPA for at least 8 h.) Initially, 1 tablet (25/250) three to four times/day in patient previously requiring 1500 mg or more of levodopa alone per day. Otherwise, 1 tablet (10/100) three to four times/day. Adjust by ½ to 1 tablet a day until control is obtained.

Patients should be closely observed for development of involuntary movements or blepharospasm, since these are often early indications that the dosage may be excessive. Carbidopa (Lodosyn) is also available alone as 25-mg tablets to be used only with L-DOPA. Individual dosing of the two drugs allows separate titration of each agent and may result in better control of the symptoms and a lower incidence of side-effects than with use of the fixed-dosage combinations. Although most parkinsonian patients can be managed adequately with the carbidopa/levodopa combination (Sinemet), certain patients may require individual titration of each drug, especially when nausea and vomiting are prominent.

FATE

Levodopa is well absorbed from the intestinal tract; peak plasma levels occur in 0.5 hour to 2 hours. Significant amounts are metabolized to dopamine in the stomach, intestines, and liver when used alone, and a relatively small fraction of the administered dose reaches the CNS unchanged (1%–2%). The plasma half-life ranges from 1 hour to 3 hours. Dopamine metabolites are rapidly and almost completely excreted in the urine. Carbidopa inhibits the decarboxylation of peripheral levodopa, but does not cross the blood–brain barrier and therefore does not interfere with the conversion of dopa to dopamine in the CNS. Concurrent use of carbidopa with levodopa reduces the required dose of levodopa by 70% to 80%, and increases its plasma half-life.

SIDE-EFFECTS/ADVERSE REACTIONS

Side-effects noted with greatest frequency during levodopa administration are nausea, vomiting, anorexia, orthostatic hypotension, salivation, dry mouth, dysphagia, ataxia, headache, confusion, dizziness, weakness, fatigue, hand tremor, insomnia, anxiety, euphoria, choreiform and other involuntary movements (*i.e.*, dyskinesias), nightmares, and agitation. Use of carbidopa with levodopa may reduce the incidence of peripheral side-effects but can exacerbate the centrally mediated side-effects. Dyskinesias occur in a majority of patients receiving long-term L-DOPA therapy and tend to develop with smaller doses as treatment continues. Control is difficult but most patients will tolerate dyskinetic episodes in order to gain better control of parkinsonian symptoms.

Other adverse reactions attributable to levodopa include

Gastrointestinal—Diarrhea, gastrointestinal bleeding, ulceration

Cardiovascular—Palpitations, tachycardia, arrhythmias, phlebitis, hemolytic anemia

Neurologic/psychiatric—Bradykinetic episodes ("on–off" phenomenon, *i.e.*, sudden loss of symptom control lasting minutes to hours), muscle twitching, grinding of the teeth, convulsions, paranoid ideation, psychotic reactions, depression, dementia

Ocular—Spasmodic winking (blepharospasm), diplopia, blurred vision

Other—Urinary retention, bitter taste, skin rash, sweating, flushing, hot flashes, edema, alopecia, leukopenia

Levodopa may elevate blood urea nitrogen (BUN), serum glutamic-oxaloacetic transaminase (SGOT), serum glutamic-pyruvic transaminase (SGPT), lactate dehydrogenase (LDH), bilirubin, alkaline phosphatase, and protein-bound iodine (PBI), and may reduce white blood count, hemoglobin, and hematocrit.

CONTRAINDICATIONS AND PRECAUTIONS

Contraindications to use of levodopa include narrow-angle glaucoma, acute psychoses, undiagnosed skin lesions or history of melanoma (as drug can activate a malignant melanoma), and concomitant use of monoamine oxidase inhibitors. The drug must be used *cautiously* in patients with severe cardiovascular, pulmonary, renal, hepatic, or endocrine disease; peptic ulcer; chronic wide-angle glaucoma; bronchial asthma; diabetes; psychiatric disturbances (including depression); a history of myocardial infarction with residual arrhythmias; and also in pregnant or lactating women. Safety for use in children under 12 years has not been determined.

INTERACTIONS

1. Effects of levodopa may be decreased by antipsychotics, phenytoin, papaverine, pyridoxine, reserpine, phenylbutazone, and benzodiazepines (*e.g.*, diazepam).
2. Levodopa may enhance the hypotensive effect of methyldopa, guanethidine, diuretics, and possibly other antihypertensive drugs.

3. Therapeutic effects of L-DOPA may be potentiated by propranolol, methyldopa, and anticholinergics.
4. Cardiovascular effects of sympathomimetic drugs such as amphetamines, ephedrine, and epinephrine can be increased by levodopa.
5. Diabetic control with oral hypoglycemic drugs may be adversely affected by L-DOPA.
6. Concomitant use of L-DOPA and tricyclic antidepressants or monoamine oxidase inhibitors can result in tachycardia and hypertension.

■ *Nursing Process*

□ ASSESSMENT

□ *Subjective Data*
A medication history is essential, especially if the patient has a history of hypertension, cardiovascular disease, or diabetes, since many of the drugs used in treatment of these problems adversely interact with antiparkinsonian agents. In addition, the patient with a history of severe cardiac arrhythmias, glaucoma, pulmonary disease, melanoma, psychoses, or disorders of renal, hepatic, or endocrine function may be a poor candidate for treatment.

The nurse should interview the patient and family to review with them their perceptions of drug therapy. Most patients expect to see rapid results and will be disappointed when they learn that it may take 2 or 3 weeks before the drug achieves a noticeable degree of effectiveness. Although most patients are highly motivated to comply with drug therapy once they see motor improvement, they may need tremendous initial support to reach that point. A strong support system can improve successful therapy and will be essential when limitations in motor skills later decrease self-care ability.

□ *Objective Data*
To determine baseline capabilities and to judge the drug's effectiveness, the physical assessment should focus on neuromuscular, ocular, and cardiac function and blood pressure.

The nurse needs to ascertain the patient's current ability to perform activities of daily living. Parameters for review include the patient's ability to dress himself, to write his name, to get up from a chair, and to negotiate 180-degree turns during ambulation. Losses of these abilities during the course of drug therapy may indicate a lessening of drug effectiveness, a progression of the disease, or the development of drug toxicity.

Laboratory tests should include renal, liver, and cardiac studies and a baseline electrocardiogram.

□ NURSING DIAGNOSES
Actual nursing diagnoses may include
Knowledge deficit related to the action, administration, and side-effects of the drug
Impaired physical mobility related to tremors, which will gradually improve with drug treatment but may deteriorate if drug toxicity develops
Potential nursing diagnoses may include
Alteration in bowel elimination: diarrhea
Alteration in cardiac output: decreased, related to orthostatic hypotension
Alteration in comfort: headache or gastrointestinal upset
Potential fluid volume deficit related to diuresis
Potential for injury: trauma related to changes in balance and coordination
Self-care deficit: variable, related to ability of the drug to maintain function (changes may be related to loss of drug effectiveness)
Altered sexuality patterns
Sleep pattern disturbance
Alteration in thought processes related to mental deterioration (a sign that the drug dose must be adjusted)

□ PLAN
The nursing care goals may focus on
1. Facilitating dosage adjustment during the initial treatment phase to help the patient cope with common side-effects
2. Teaching the patient safe drug-taking techniques, how to manage his diet and control common side-effects, and the signs of drug toxicity.

□ INTERVENTION
Dosage adjustment is important to avoid adverse effects of levodopa or carbidopa and the drugs should therefore be increased in small doses. Early in treatment many patients experience gastrointestinal upset. This can be lessened by having the patient take the drug with meals, by giving antacids before meals, by allowing the patient to keep crackers with him to reduce nausea, and by giving milk prior to a between-meal dose.

Overweight patients treated with levodopa should be encouraged to lose weight since the extra fat they carry makes dosage regulation difficult and absorption irregular. Parkinsonism patients requiring a multiple vitamin supplement should be encouraged to avoid the type containing the vitamin B_6, pyridoxine, which tends to counteract the desired effects of levodopa. However, eliminating pyridoxine from the diet completely is harmful and should be discouraged. If the carbidopa formulation is used, this will not be a problem. Alcohol, in large amounts, will also antagonize the action of levodopa. However, for some patients, an occasional drink will ease rigidity. Patients should limit drinks to 1 to 2 per day and never drink alone. High-protein diets have also been found to interfere with the effectiveness of levodopa. Patients should learn to decrease their intake of high-protein foods and spread protein intake throughout the day, perhaps by eating smaller, more frequent meals. Such eating habits also tend to decrease the problem of nausea. Caffeine should also be limited since it may be related to the development of dyskinesias by speeding drug absorption. The nurse should work with the family, patient, and dietitian to set up a plan that the patient can follow.

Since levodopa also acts as a diuretic, fluids should be encouraged and the patient's weight monitored. In addition, urine may be noted to be pink or bright red, which turns black upon exposure to air. The color change is due to the metabolites of dopamine and the patient should be informed that it is a harmless side-effect.

After long-term therapy, an "on–off" effect may occur at various times, whereby the patient has worsening of symptoms. Most studies claim little can be done to eliminate this phenomenon; however, splitting the dose into 1-hour and 2-hour intervals and watching protein intake may help reduce the occurrence. Family should be aware of this problem so they do not begin to believe the patient is "faking" when he is unable to perform a task as before.

The best method to monitor changes in side-effects of the drugs is to use a flowsheet. Several good ones exist for the parkinsonian patient (see Hahn, 1982) and the reader is also referred to the Abnormal Involuntary Movement Scale (AIMS) in Chapter 27, which monitors dyskinesia development. Flowsheets provide memory joggers to the care giver and a consistent approach to track side-effects of drug therapy. This is especially important for the patient with Parkinson's disease since response to therapy can vary greatly over time. Neuromuscular function can vary and be directly related to the drug's effectiveness. The nurse should note the frequency with which the patient falls or comes close to falling; the development of freezing or hesitation, whereby a patient becomes "glued" to one spot; and the amount of extremity flexibility.

Changes in mentation can occur as a result of medication or progression of the disease. The nurse and family need to watch for signs of mental deterioration, which may indicate that the patient will forget to take medications, leading to a worsening of symptoms. Hallucinations, depression, and sleep changes may also occur and signal the need for dosage adjustments.

Another difficult side-effect of levodopa and carbidopa is orthostatic hypotension. It is usually a transient symptom occurring early in therapy. Elastic stockings may help venous return and reduce the dizziness that occurs when the patient rises quickly. Patients should be reminded to rise slowly from a lying or sitting position and be encouraged to sit down until the dizzy feeling passes since loss of balance and falls can result. If orthostatic hypotension persists or returns over the course of treatment, it may be a signal of toxicity development.

The patient may also experience an increase in sexual drive on drug therapy. These feelings may have been depressed by the disease; patients may not understand the change and may make seemingly inappropriate suggestions to care givers. The nurse who recognizes these expressions can allay the patient's anxiety by allowing verbalization and giving information; she can also provide the hospitalized patient and significant other with opportunities for privacy, if appropriate. Labeling such patients as a "dirty old man" or a "dirty old woman" loses an important opportunity to help patients understand how treatment is affecting them.

The main early signs of drug toxicity are blepharospasm (eye winking), dyskinesia (especially chewing movements), increasing or returning development of orthostatic hypotension, and the development of premature ventricular contractions (sensation of the heart skipping beats). The patient and family need to be aware that they should contact the physician if any of these symptoms occur and seek medical attention at once. The arrhythmias can be fatal, especially when they occur in a patient receiving Sinemet, and should be treated immediately. Drug dosage may need to be adjusted or a medication change may be indicated.

□ EVALUATION

Parameters for evaluation may include functional abilities, mentation, and management of side-effects. Unfortunately, changes cannot always be prevented through drug therapy so the nurse must also evaluate how the patient and significant others cope with a progressive chronic illness.

Amantadine
(Symadine, Symmetrel)

Amantadine is a synthetic antiviral agent useful for prophylaxis against and symptomatic management of influenza A virus strains (see Chap. 74). The drug was subsequently found to benefit some patients with Parkinson's disease and thus is also used as adjunctive therapy in some parkinsonian patients.

MECHANISM AND ACTIONS
While the exact mechanism of action of amantadine is incompletely understood, the drug is believed to act in part by releasing dopamine from dopaminergic nerve terminals in the corpus striatum as well as other sites in the CNS and by blocking neuronal reuptake of dopamine. Its effectiveness, therefore, is greatly reduced in the absence of functional dopaminergic nerve endings. Amantadine is less effective than levodopa in managing Parkinson's disease but is slightly more efficacious than anticholinergics, although its efficacy diminishes with continued use. The drug is usually given with levodopa when control of parkinsonian symptoms is deteriorating.

Amantadine is also an effective antiviral drug and this aspect is discussed in Chapter 74.

USES
1. Adjunctive treatment of parkinsonism and drug-induced extrapyramidal reactions (usually in combination with levodopa)
2. Prophylaxis against influenza A virus strains, especially in high-risk patients (see Chap. 74)
3. Symptomatic management of respiratory disease caused by influenza A virus (see Chap. 74)

ADMINISTRATION AND DOSAGE
Amantadine is available as capsules (100 mg) and syrup (50 mg/5 ml). In treating Parkinson's disease in patients receiving other antiparkinsonian drugs, an initial dose of 100 mg daily is recommended. After several weeks of therapy, dosage may be increased to 100 mg twice a day, and, if necessary, to a maximum of 400 mg/day under close supervision. When used alone, the recommended dose is 100 mg twice a day.

Doses of 100 mg twice a day are used to control drug-induced extrapyramidal reactions, and up to 300 mg may be given in divided doses.

Patients with reduced kidney function should be given smaller or less frequent doses, according to the degree of creatinine clearance.

FATE
Amantadine is well absorbed orally and peak plasma levels occur in 2 hours to 4 hours. The drug is widely distributed and readily crosses the blood–brain barrier. The elimination half-life in patients with normal renal function is approximately 15 hours to 20 hours, but can increase to days or weeks when kidney function is impaired. A small fraction (10%) of the dose is metabolized, but most of the drug is excreted unchanged in the urine; excretion is enhanced in an acidic urine.

SIDE-EFFECTS/ADVERSE REACTIONS
Side-effects seen most frequently with amantadine are irritability, anxiety, nausea, anorexia, dizziness, ataxia, mild depression, constipation, urinary retention, orthostatic hypotension, peripheral edema, and skin mottling (livedo reticularis). Less commonly noted adverse reactions include vomiting, headache, weakness, insomnia, tremors, confusion, dyspnea, skin rash, dermatitis, congestive heart failure, psychotic reactions, leukopenia, neutropenia, visual disturbances, oculogyric episodes, and hallucinations.

The neurologic side-effects generally can be attenuated by reducing the dosage. Accidental overdosage may result in a toxic psychosis due to increased brain dopamine levels. Treatment is supportive and physostigmine (see Chap. 13) can be used to control the neurologic manifestations.

CONTRAINDICATIONS AND PRECAUTIONS
There are no absolute contraindications to amantadine, although the drug should be used with *caution* in patients with congestive heart failure, epilepsy (may increase seizure activity), renal dysfunction, peripheral edema, dermatitis, or history of psychotic disturbances, and in pregnant or nursing mothers. Caution is also warranted in elderly patients, since renal function is frequently reduced and cumulation of the drug can occur.

The drug should be discontinued slowly and other medications increased gradually, since abrupt termination has resulted in *sudden* deterioration of the patient's condition.

INTERACTIONS
1. Amantadine may increase the incidence of side-effects with anticholinergics.
2. Excessive CNS stimulation may occur with

amantadine and other stimulants, such as amphetamines, ephedrine, or caffeine.

3. Decreased urinary excretion has occurred when amantadine has been given together with a thiazide plus a potassium-sparing diuretic.

NURSING CONSIDERATIONS

Amantadine is occasionally used in early Parkinson's disease. However, it has a large number of side-effects and should be used with caution. Dizziness and drowsiness may be severe, limiting the patient's ability to function well early in therapy. Despite this, the patient may suffer from insomnia if he takes the dose too close to bedtime; experimentation in dosage times may be necessary to minimize the limitations of these and other symptoms.

Skin mottling may occur, particularly in the lower extremities, when the patient is exposed to cold. The effect appears early in therapy and may disappear when the drug is discontinued or the dosage is reduced. The patient should be taught to test for sensation to temperature and touch and to report any significant loss of feeling.

The patient should also be aware that the therapeutic effectiveness of amantadine may diminish abruptly and is very unpredictable. Any rapid increase in parkinsonian symptoms should be reported immediately. Although drug effectiveness may be restored by increasing the dose or by briefly discontinuing the drug and then restarting it, such changes should be closely monitored and undertaken only when the patient is under careful supervision.

Bromocriptine

(Parlodel)

Bromocriptine is a dopamine receptor agonist that directly stimulates postsynaptic dopamine receptors in the corpus striatum and other CNS areas. It is used orally as adjunctive therapy to provide additional therapeutic benefits in patients currently maintained on L-DOPA who are beginning to show signs of deterioration in their condition. Due to the progressive degenerative nature of parkinsonism, even persons receiving maximum doses of L-DOPA in combination with carbidopa are eventually susceptible to breakthrough effects. These are sometimes referred to as "late L-DOPA failures." Examples of such conditions are return of tremor or rigidity, "end-of-dose" failure (appearance of akinesia between dosing), and "on–off" phenomena (abrupt loss of mobility). Bromocriptine may

delay the onset of late L-DOPA failure and may also ameliorate the symptoms (*e.g.*, dyskinesia) that result from excessive L-DOPA levels by allowing a dosage reduction.

In addition to its use as an antiparkinsonian agent, bromocriptine is also indicated for treatment of amenorrhea and galactorrhea associated with hyperprolactinemia, for prevention of postpartum lactation, and to treat selected cases of female infertility associated with excessive secretion of prolactin.

MECHANISM AND ACTIONS

Bromocriptine functions as a direct receptor agonist at dopaminergic sites in the CNS. Its effects in parkinsonism are the result of increased dopamine receptor activation in the corpus striatum. Bromocriptine may provide increased control of parkinsonian symptoms in patients whose condition has begun to deteriorate after prolonged levodopa therapy (*i.e.*, patients experiencing end-of-dose levodopa failure or increasing incidence of "on–off" phenomena). However, patients unresponsive to levodopa are generally poor candidates for bromocriptine. Continued efficacy of bromocriptine for more than 2 years has not been established. Bromocriptine activates dopamine receptors in the tuberoinfundibular dopaminergic system of the pituitary, resulting in secretion of prolactin inhibitory factor (PIF) from the hypothalamus. Secretion of PIF blocks release of prolactin from the anterior pituitary.

USES

1. Adjunctive treatment of Parkinson's disease (usually in combination with levodopa/carbidopa) or drug-induced parkinsonian-like symptoms (may provide increased symptom control and reduce the incidence of levodopa-induced side-effects by permitting use of a smaller dose)
2. Treatment of amenorrhea/galactorrhea associated with hyperprolactinemia (*not* indicated in patients with normal prolactin levels)
3. Treatment of female infertility associated with hyperprolactinemia
4. Prevention of postpartum lactation
5. Reduce plasma growth hormone levels in patients with acromegaly

ADMINISTRATION AND DOSAGE

Bromocriptine is available as tablets (2.5 mg) and capsules (5 mg). For treatment of Parkinson's disease, initial dosage is one half of a 2.5-mg tablet twice daily, in conjunction with carbidopa/levodopa at their previously employed doses, unless increased side-effects necessitate a dosage reduction. Bromocriptine dosage may be increased by 2.5-mg increments every 2 weeks to 4 weeks until satisfactory control has been attained.

Recommended doses for the other uses of bromocriptine are as follows:

Amenorrhea/galactorrhea: 2.5 mg two to three times a day; not to exceed 6 months

Prevention of lactation: 2.5 mg two to three times a day for 14 days to 21 days

Treatment of infertility: initially 2.5 mg once daily; increase to two or three times a day within the first week

Acromegaly: 1.25 mg to 2.5 mg daily for 3 days; increase slowly every 3 days to 7 days as tolerated; usual therapeutic range is 20 mg to 30 mg daily to a maximum of 100 mg daily.

FATE
Approximately one fourth of an oral dose is absorbed from the gastrointestinal tract. The drug is highly protein bound (90%–95%). Bromocriptine is metabolized in the liver and excreted almost entirely through the bile into the feces. Less than 5% of the dose is eliminated in the urine.

SIDE-EFFECTS/ADVERSE REACTIONS
Side-effects encountered most frequently with bromocriptine include nausea and vomiting, headache, dizziness, drowsiness, fatigue, lightheadedness, confusion, visual disturbances, nasal congestion, vertigo, shortness of breath, abdominal discomfort, diarrhea, abnormal involuntary movements, insomnia, depression, and hypotension.

Other less commonly noted untoward reactions are nervousness, nightmares, blepharospasm, anxiety, anorexia, dry mouth, dysphagia, foot and ankle edema, skin mottling, paresthesia, skin rash, urinary frequency, and epileptiform seizures. In addition, signs and symptoms of ergotism have occurred, such as numbness and tingling in the extremities, cold feet, muscle cramping, and Raynaud's syndrome.

Elevations in BUN, SGOT, SGPT, creatine phosphokinase (CPK), alkaline phosphatase, and serum uric acid have been noted but are usually of a transient nature.

CONTRAINDICATIONS AND PRECAUTIONS
Use of bromocriptine is contraindicated in patients with severe ischemic heart disease or peripheral vascular disease, in pregnant or nursing mothers, and in any person sensitive to the ergot alkaloids, since bromocriptine is an ergot derivative. *Cautious* use of bromocriptine is mandated in the presence of severe hypotension, epilepsy, psychoses, cardiac arrhythmias, and impaired hepatic or renal function. Safety and efficacy of bromocriptine in children under 15 years of age have not been established.

INTERACTIONS
1. Bromocriptine can potentiate the hypotensive action of other blood pressure–lowering drugs.
2. Antipsychotic drugs that are dopamine antagonists may antagonize the action of bromocriptine.

NURSING CONSIDERATIONS
The normal treatment dose of bromocriptine for the patient with Parkinson's disease is ten times the dose given when the drug is used to improve fertility. Therefore, it may restore fertility to a woman who has been amenorrheal for years. Such patients should be made aware of the potential for pregnancy and be encouraged to use an effective method of birth control. Pregnancy tests should be part of routine clinical testing during follow-up if the patient is of childbearing age.

Since the dose is high, side-effects may be severe. Dizziness and hypotension may limit the patient's ability to manage his own care, especially early in therapy. Care should be taken to ensure the patient's safety in his environment. Support of significant others in assisting the patient is important.

Anticholinergic–Antihistaminic Agents

The first drugs used for the treatment of Parkinson's disease were the belladonna alkaloids, especially atropine and scopolamine, and for many years these were the only effective drugs available for treatment of this disease. These agents, although still occasionally employed, have been supplanted largely by a group of synthetic drugs having more selective central anticholinergic (and in some instances antihistaminergic) activity.

The centrally acting anticholinergics may be used in all forms of Parkinson's disease, although they are generally less effective than levodopa in most patients.

These agents are useful on their own in patients with mild symptoms, and the centrally acting anticholinergics appear to be most effective in relieving rigidity and occasional tremor. They are most commonly prescribed in combination with levodopa to obtain more efficient control of the condition than either drug alone is capable of providing. The usefulness of these compounds is mainly limited by their side-effects, which, although not usually serious, are frequent and annoying (*e.g.*, blurred vision, constipation, dizziness, dysuria). Moreover, large doses are associated with development of CNS toxicity resembling atropine intoxication and characterized by confusion, ataxia, delirium, and hallucinations.

In addition to their use in parkinsonism, these drugs are also widely employed to control the extrapyramidal manifestations (akinesia, dystonias, akathisia, tremor) characteristic of treatment with the antipsychotic agents.

The anticholinergic/antihistaminergic drugs used in Parkinson's disease are pharmacologically and toxicologically similar, and are reviewed as a group. Most of the individual drugs have been mentioned previously, either in Chapter 14 (anticholinergics) or Chapter 18 (antihistamines). They are listed again here in Table 31-1, where specific information is provided relating to their use in parkinsonism and extrapyramidal disorders.

MECHANISM AND ACTIONS
The centrally acting anticholinergics exhibit a postsynaptic blocking effect on central cholinergic excitatory pathways that normally exert increasing effect, since dopaminergic inhibition is reduced due to lack of functional dopamine. These drugs can also retard reuptake of dopamine into presynaptic nerve endings, thereby blocking its inactivation. Some agents may also have a direct relaxing effect on smooth muscle. Peripheral anticholinergic effects, such as constipation, urinary retention, and tachycardia, are frequently noted, especially at large doses and may limit the amount of drug that can be given.

USES
1. Sole or adjunctive therapy in all forms of Parkinson's disease (drugs are most effective in relieving rigidity)
2. Prevention and relief of extrapyramidal reactions resulting from antipsychotic drug therapy

ADMINISTRATION AND DOSAGE
See Table 31-1.

FATE
The drugs are generally well absorbed orally and display an onset of action within 30 minutes to 60 minutes. The duration of effect is variable, and averages 4 hours to 6 hours (except for sustained-release dosage forms, which produce effects for up to 12 hours). Most of the drugs are excreted largely by the kidney both as intact drug and as metabolites.

SIDE-EFFECTS/ADVERSE REACTIONS
Commonly encountered side-effects with the anticholinergic drugs used in Parkinson's disease include dry mouth, blurred vision, dizziness, nausea, urinary hesitancy, and drowsiness. A variety of other untoward reactions have been associated with these drugs especially with large doses or prolonged therapy. These are listed by organ system below:

CNS—Confusion, nervousness, agitation, fever, excitement, lightheadedness, memory loss, delusions, delirium, euphoria, hallucinations, paranoia, psychotic behavior
Cardiovascular—Tachycardia, palpitations, hypotension, flushing
Gastrointestinal—Vomiting, epigastric distress, constipation, paralytic ileus
Ophthalmic—Mydriasis, diplopia, increased intraocular tension
Renal—Urinary retention, dysuria
Other—Muscle weakness and cramping, paresthesias, decreased sweating, impotence

Severe overdosage may result in circulatory collapse, respiratory depression, cardiac arrest, toxic psychosis, and a plethora of less intense symptoms listed above. Treatment is largely symptomatic and supportive. Physostigmine (Antilirium) can reverse most cardiovascular and CNS effects in a dose of 1 mg to 3 mg IM or IV given *slowly* over 2 minutes to 3 minutes (rapid IV injection of physostigmine can result in convulsions).

CONTRAINDICATIONS AND PRECAUTIONS
Anticholinergic drugs are contraindicated in persons with glaucoma (especially angle-closure types), pyloric or duodenal obstruction, peptic ulcers, prostatic hypertrophy or bladder neck obstruction, and myasthenia gravis. These drugs should be given with *caution* to persons with tachycardia, cardiac arrhythmias, hypertension, urinary hesitancy, obstructive disorders of the urinary or gastrointestinal tracts, liver or kidney disorders, depression, psychoses, or unexplained muscle weakness. Cautious use is also advocated in pregnant or nursing mothers, elderly or debilitated patients, alcoholics, persons who are constantly exposed to hot environments, and children. Also,

Table 31-1
Anticholinergic–Antihistaminergic Drugs Used for Parkinsonism

Drug	Preparations	Usual Dosage Range	Clinical Considerations
benztropine (Cogentin)	Tablets—0.5 mg, 1 mg, 2 mg Injection—1 mg/ml	*Parkinsonism* 1 mg–2 mg/day (range 0.5 mg–6 mg) *Extrapyramidal reactions* 1 mg–4 mg one to two times/day *Acute dystonic reactions* 1 mg–2 mg IM or IV, followed by 1 mg–2 mg PO two times/day	IM injection used for rapid response (acute dystonic reactions) (onset 15 min); do not use in children under 3; effects are cumulative and may take several days to develop; usually not effective against tremor; large doses may cause weakness and transient muscle paralysis.
biperiden (Akineton)	Tablets—2 mg Injection—5 mg/ml	*Parkinsonism* 2 mg three to four times/day *Extrapyramidal reactions* Oral—2 mg one to three times/day IM, IV—2 mg; may repeat every 30 min to a total of four doses	Most effective against akinesia and rigidity; effectively reduces salivation and seborrhea; may produce mood elevation or temporary euphoria, especially parenterally; IV injection can cause hypotension and incoordination
diphenhydramine (Benadryl and others; see Chap. 18)	Capsules—25 mg, 50 mg Tablets—50 mg Elixir—12.5 mg/5 ml Syrup—12.5 mg, 13.3 mg/5 ml Injection—10 mg, 50 mg/ml	Oral—25 mg–50 mg three to four times/day IV, IM—10 mg–50 mg (maximum 400 mg/day)	Effective in mild parkinsonism and extrapyramidal reactions (especially dystonias); often combined with other anticholinergics or L-DOPA; see Chapter 18 for adverse effects, contraindications, and interactions; may be better tolerated by elderly patients than other anticholinergics; sedative action may be beneficial in patients with insomnia.
ethopropazine (Parsidol)	Tablets—10 mg, 50 mg	Initially 50 mg one to two times/day; increase gradually to a maximum of 600 mg/day in severe cases	A phenothiazine derivative with significant anticholinergic activity; effectively controls most symptoms including tremor; does not potentiate other CNS depressants; high incidence of side-effects and poorly tolerated by many older patients; used for treatment of extrapyramidal reactions, even though it is a phenothiazine itself; see Chapter 27 for potential adverse effects and drug interactions.

(continued)

Table 31-1 (continued)
Anticholinergic–Antihistaminergic Drugs Used for Parkinsonism

Drug	Preparations	Usual Dosage Range	Clinical Considerations
orphenadrine hydrochloride (Disipal)	Tablets—50 mg	*Parkinsonism* 50 mg three times/day (maximum 250 mg/day)	Antihistamine that is also a centrally acting muscle relaxant; relieves rigidity and controls autonomic manifestations as well; minimal drowsiness, but high incidence of other atropine-like side-effects; use with chlorpromazine has resulted in hypoglycemic coma; may decrease the effects of barbiturates, phenylbutazone, and griseofulvin; also available as the citrate for treatment of musculoskeletal disorders (see Chap. 19).
procyclidine (Kemadrin)	Tablets—5 mg	*Parkinsonism* Initially, 2.5 mg three times/day; increase gradually to a maximum of 20 mg/day *Extrapyramidal reactions* Initially, 2.5 mg three times/day (usual range 10 mg–20 mg/day)	Anticholinergic and smooth muscle antispasmodic; most effective against rigidity; controls excessive salivation as well; may temporarily worsen tremor as rigidity is relieved; be alert for confusion, agitation, and behavioral changes, which are common in the elderly with hypotension; similar to trihexyphenidyl.
trihexyphenidyl (Aphen, Artane, Trihexane, Trihexidyl, Trihexy)	Tablets—2 mg, 5 mg Capsules—5 mg (sustained release) Elixir—2 mg/5 ml	*Parkinsonism* Initially 1 mg–2 mg/ increase by 2-mg increments every 3 to 5 days to a maximum of 15 mg/day Usual range 6 mg–10 mg/day, in three to four divided doses or 5 mg sustained-release once or twice a day *Extrapyramidal Reactions* Initially 1 mg; increase by 1 mg every few hours until control is obtained Usual range 5 mg–15 mg/day in divided doses	Anticholinergic and smooth muscle relaxant; do not use sustained-release capsules for initial therapy because they do not allow enough flexibility in dosage regulation; major effect is on rigidity, although most symptoms improve to some extent; effects may be potentiated by monoamine oxidase inhibitors.

anticholinergic drugs should be used cautiously in patients receiving chronic antipsychotic drug treatment, since they may aggravate the symptoms of tardive dyskinesias (see Chap. 27).

INTERACTIONS

1. Combined use with other drugs having an anticholinergic action (e.g., phenothiazines, antihistamines, tricyclic antidepressants) may result in an increased incidence of toxicity.
2. Anticholinergic drugs may potentiate the sedative action of other CNS depressants (e.g., alcohol, barbiturates, narcotics).
3. Certain centrally acting anticholinergic drugs can impair the antipsychotic effectiveness of phenothiazines and haloperidol by increasing their rate of gastrointestinal metabolism.
4. Oral absorption of levodopa can be reduced by anticholinergic drugs, since they delay gastric emptying, thus increasing the gastric degradation of levodopa. However, the reduced gastrointestinal motility may increase absorption of slowly dissolving preparations, such as digoxin.

NURSING CONSIDERATIONS

See also Chapters 14 and 18.

The main objectives in caring for patients receiving these drugs for symptom control of Parkinson's disease are correct administration and management of side-effects.

Dosage of these drugs must be frequently adjusted to minimize side-effects. Drugs may be gradually added and others gradually tapered off in order to reduce symptoms. Therefore, patients being treated with either anticholinergic or antihistaminic agents must be closely monitored and be able to comply with frequent changes in medications, time schedules, and numbers of pills. A Parkinson's patient who is having mentation problems or who lacks adequate family supports may be an inappropriate candidate for treatment with anticholinergic or antihistaminic agents. None of these drugs should be abruptly discontinued. Doing so may result in the development of severe tremor and rigidity that will completely immobilize the patient.

Patients may suffer from mouth dryness or gastric upset from these drugs. Both symptoms are alleviated by food and fluids and may be transient. However, several serious side-effects can occur and the patient must be aware of these and able to take action. Diminished urinary output and paralytic ileus should be watched for and should be reported immediately. The patient should be instructed to note the frequency and volume of urination; the significance of regular bowel movements and alertness to the development of abdominal distention should also be stressed.

Impaired sweating is another serious problem, especially in hot weather. The patient who has this symptom should be encouraged to avoid exerting himself and consideration should be given to reducing the drug dosage.

CASE STUDY

Mr. Barrett, a 62-year-old retired executive, is receiving levodopa, 500 mg tid, for Parkinson's disease. He is hospitalized because of an increase in symptoms. When first admitted he seemed constantly about to fall as he shuffled forward. His hands moved in a continuous tremor when at rest, as a result of which he was unable to write or feed himself. Although his wife hovered over him constantly and tried to help, he frequently refused to eat, which upset her even more. In an attempt to alleviate his symptoms a decision was made to switch Mr. Barrett to Sinemet, 25/250 mg, tid.

Discussion Questions

1. How should the levodopa be discontinued and the Sinemet started?
2. What data should be collected before the drugs are changed?
3. How could the nurse use a flowsheet in Mr. Barrett's care?
4. What family goals should the nurse attempt to establish with this couple to improve care?

REVIEW QUESTIONS

1. What are the three cardinal manifestations of Parkinson's disease? Briefly describe each one.
2. What is the principal central biochemical deficit in Parkinson's disease? Why does this occur?
3. What are the advantages of Sinemet (carbidopa/levodopa) over levodopa therapy?
4. List the most common side-effects encountered during levodopa therapy.
5. In what other conditions might the use of levodopa be contraindicated?
6. What data should be gathered before initiating levodopa or levedopa/carbidopa therapy?
7. What dietary teaching goals should the nurse establish for the patient receiving levodopa?
8. How can the nurse use a flowsheet in monitoring parkinsonism drug therapy?
9. What are the symptoms of early levodopa toxicity?
10. What are the indications for use of amantadine (Symmetrel)?
11. How does amantadine (Symmetrel) relieve the symptoms of Parkinson's disease?
12. What facts about amantadine should be considered when teaching a patient to use this drug safely?
13. Give the principal used for bromocriptine (Parlodel). What is its mechanism of action?
14. Give a teaching goal for a menopausal woman about to receive bromocriptine for Parkinson's symptoms.
15. Briefly describe how centrally acting anticholinergics can relieve some of the symptoms of Parkinson's disease.
16. In which conditions would centrally acting anticholinergic drugs be contraindicated?
17. What major side-effects of anticholinergic–antihistaminic drugs should be reported immediately?

BIBLIOGRAPHY

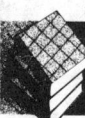

Calne DB: Progress in Parkinson's disease. N Engl J Med 310:523, 1984
Calne DB, Langston JW: The etiology of Parkinson's disease. Lancet 2:1457, 1983
Campanella G, Roy M, Barbeau A: Drugs affecting movement disorders. Ann Rev Pharmacol Toxicol 27:113, 1987
Duvoisin R: Parkinson's disease: A review. U.S. Pharmacist 4:63, 1979
Fahn S, Calne DB: Considerations in the management of parkinsonism. Neurology 31:371, 1981
Garrett E: Parkinsonism: Forgotten considerations in medical treatment and nursing care. J Neurosurg Nurs 14:13, 1982
Hahn K: Management of Parkinson's disease. Nurse Pract January:13, 1982
Hoehn MM: Bromocriptine and its use in parkinsonism. J Am Geriatr Soc 24:251, 1981
Langston JW, Ballard P, Tetrud JW, Irwin I: Chronic parkinsonism in humans due to a product of meperidine-analog synthesis. Science 219:979, 1983

Leff SE, Creese I: Dopamine receptor re-explained. Trends Pharmacol
    Sci 4:463, 1983
Nutt JG, Woodward WR, Hammerstad JP, et al: The "on–off"
    phenomenon in Parkinson's disease. N Engl J Med 310:483, 1984
Parkes JD: Adverse effects of antiparkinsonian drugs. Drugs 21:341,
    1981
Quinn NP: Antiparkinsonian drugs today. Drugs 28:236, 1984
Seeman P: Brain dopamine receptors. Pharmacol Rev 32:229, 1981
Symposium: Current concepts and controversies in Parkinson's
    disease. Can J Neurol Sci 11(Suppl 1):89, 1984
Todd B: Drugs and the elderly: Therapy for Parkinson's disease.
    Geriatric Nursing 6(2):117, 1985
Vance ML, Evans WS, Thorner MO: Bromocriptine. Ann Intern Med
    100:78, 1984
Young RR: Step therapy for Parkinson's disease. Patient Care 14:24,
    1980

Central Nervous System Stimulants

Caffeine
Caffeine and Dextrose
Caffeine and Sodium
    Benzoate, Citrated
    Caffeine

Amphetamines

Amphetamine,
    Amphetamine
    Complex,
    Dextroamphetamine,
    Methamphetamine

Anorexiants

Benzphetamine,
    Diethylpropion,
    Fenfluramine,
    Mazindol,
    Phendimetrazine,
    Phenmetrazine,
    Phentermine,
    Phenylpropanol-
    amine
Methylphenidate
Pemoline

32

Although a large number of pharmacologic agents can have a stimulating effect on the central nervous system (CNS), the number of drugs actually employed clinically for this purpose is quite small. Principal reasons for the limited therapeutic applications of CNS stimulants are the lack of specificity, which leads to many undesirable side-effects and their significant potential for abuse. A useful classification of the therapeutically effective CNS stimulants is as follows:

· Respiratory stimulants (analeptics)
  (e.g., doxapram)
· Caffeine
· Amphetamines
  (e.g., dextroamphetamine, methamphetamine)
· Anorexiants
  (e.g., phentermine, diethylpropion,
  phenylpropanolamine)
· Methylphenidate
· Pemoline

Drugs classified as respiratory stimulants, or analeptics, are believed to act at the level of the brain stem and peripheral carotid chemoreceptors and are used primarily as physiologic antagonists of respiratory depression due to overdosage with CNS depressants. Because these agents principally affect respiratory function, they are discussed with other drugs acting on the respiratory system in Section VII of this book.

The remaining CNS stimulants will be considered in this chapter.

Caffeine
(Caffedrine, Dexitac, Nodoz, Tirend, Vivarin)

Caffeine and Dextrose
(Quick-Pep)

Caffeine and Sodium Benzoate, Citrated Caffeine

Caffeine is the most widely used CNS stimulant, largely because it is consumed in coffee, tea, soda, and many over-the-counter analgesic drug combinations (Table 32-1).

Caffeine is a xanthine derivative possessing relatively weak CNS-stimulant, smooth-muscle relaxant, vasodilatory, diuretic, and myocardial stimulant actions. It also constricts cerebral arteries, enhances the contraction of skeletal muscles, and augments gastric acid secretion. In small amounts, it is a weak cortical stimulant which aids in maintaining mental alertness and allaying fatigue. In-

Table 32-1
Representative Caffeine Concentrations in Selected Sources

	Caffeine (mg)
Beverages	
Coffee	
Brewed	100–150/cup
Instant	85–100/cup
Decaffeinated	2–4/cup
Tea	60–75/cup
Cocoa	5–40/cup
Cola drinks	3–5/oz
Over-the-Counter Analgesics	
Anacin	32/tablet
Cope	32/tablet
Midol	32/tablet
Vanquish	33/tablet
Excedrin	65/tablet

creasing amounts, however, can result in restlessness, irritability, insomnia, and possibly anxiety, hyperventilation, and tremors. It is also employed parenterally as a central stimulant and may relieve the pain of vascular headaches by virtue of its constricting action on cerebral blood vessels. It is often combined with ergotamine, a powerful vasoconstrictor, for treating migraine attacks.

MECHANISM AND ACTIONS
Caffeine appears to competitively block receptors for adenosine, a naturally occurring substance which normally depresses neuronal firing in the CNS, thereby permitting these neurons to fire more readily. It also increases the concentration of cyclic AMP in tissues by inhibiting the phosphodiesterase enzyme which inactivates cyclic AMP, and can increase release of calcium from the sarcoplasmic reticulum, improving skeletal muscle tone. Caffeine can stimulate all levels of the CNS when used in sufficient amounts.

USES
1. Allay fatigue and increase sensory awareness (orally)
2. Treatment of mild to moderate respiratory depression caused by overdosage with CNS depressants such as morphine or alcohol (parenterally, caffeine and sodium benzoate)
3. Relief of pain associated with vascular headaches or spinal puncture (orally or parenterally, often with ergotamine—see Chap. 18)

4. Adjunct in analgesic preparations (see Table 32-1)
5. Investigational uses include treatment of neonatal apnea (IV), and control of atopic dermatitis (30% caffeine in hydrocortisone cream, or hydrophilic base).

ADMINISTRATION AND DOSAGE
Caffeine is available as various strength tablets (100 mg, 200 mg) and timed-release capsules (200 mg, 250 mg). In addition, some preparations also contain dextrose or citric acid. An injection solution (250 mg/ml) containing equal parts of caffeine and sodium benzoate is also available. The recommended dosage ranges are as follows:

Oral—100 mg to 200 mg every 4 hours *or* 200 mg to 250 mg sustained-release capsules every 4 hours to 6 hours. Oral administration of caffeine is not recommended in children.

IM—Adults receive 200 mg to 500 mg, repeated as needed every 4 hours. Infants and young children are given 8 mg/kg, with a maximum single dose of 500 mg.

Caffeine may be given IV in certain situations, such as an excited or comatose alcoholic patient or to alleviate headaches following spinal puncture, although this route is not generally recommended.

FATE
Caffeine is well absorbed orally and following IM injection and peak plasma levels usually occur within 30 minutes to 45 minutes. Plasma protein binding is minimal. The drug readily crosses the blood–brain barrier and placental barrier. The plasma half-life ranges from 3 hours to 6 hours. Caffeine is metabolized in the liver and excreted largely in the urine as metabolites and some unchanged drug.

SIDE-EFFECTS/ADVERSE REACTIONS
The most frequently encountered side-effects with small amounts of caffeine are nervousness, restlessness, insomnia, and some degree of gastric irritation. Larger amounts can lead to the development of tinnitus, headache, tremor, scotoma, excitement, tachycardia, arrhythmias, hypotension, nausea, vomiting, diarrhea, and diuresis.

An anxiety neurosis-like syndrome has been associated with large doses of caffeine, marked by muscle twitching, palpitations, flushing, irritability, tachypnea, GI distress, tremulousness, and sensory disturbances.

Abrupt cessation of caffeine after regular consumption of 500 mg/day or more can result in headache, anxiety, and increased muscle tension. Overdosage is characterized by dyspnea, delirium, insomnia, diuresis, arrhythmias, and possibly seizures. The acute lethal dose ranges from 5 g to 10 g. Treatment is symptomatic and supportive and might include sedatives and anticonvulsants.

CONTRAINDICATIONS AND PRECAUTIONS
There are no absolute contraindications to caffeine. The drug should be used *cautiously* in the presence of gastric ulcers, diabetes (drug may increase blood glucose), respiratory depression (too vigorous therapy can further depress respiration), and following a myocardial infarction. Caffeine should be discontinued if palpitations, tachycardia, or dizziness occur.

INTERACTIONS
1. Caffeine may cause hypertensive reactions in combination with MAO-inhibitors.
2. Caffeine can increase CNS stimulation due to propoxyphene overdosage, resulting in convulsions.
3. Increased effects of caffeine can occur in combination with oral contraceptives or cimetidine, because they may inhibit caffeine metabolism.
4. Smoking may increase the elimination of caffeine.

■ *Nursing Process*

□ ASSESSMENT
As part of every drug history the nurse needs to learn how much caffeine a person consumes daily. Many people do not realize the effects caffeine-containing beverages can have and will not relate anxiety or GI distress to overindulgence in caffeine until they recognize how much caffeine they consume. Many children, including those termed "hyperactive," also consume large quantities of caffeine through cocoa, chocolate, and soda. A drug history can help focus on this habit and initiate a plan to reduce consumption, if necessary.

□ NURSING DIAGNOSES
Actual nursing diagnoses for the patient consuming caffeine include:

Knowledge deficit about the drug's effects on the body

Anxiety, especially if consumption is high
Alteration in comfort: headache, if
    consumption is too high

□ PLAN
The goal for any individual suffering symptoms of
overconsumption of caffeine is to reduce intake
and minimize side-effects.

□ INTERVENTION
The nurse can help begin the process of eliminating
or reducing caffeine by helping the person to recognize caffeine-containing products (see Table 32-1).
Cold remedies and indigestion aids may also contain caffeine. Patients should read product labels
before using any over-the-counter medicines.

Once the beverages have been identified, the
person still must cope with breaking the "drinking" habit. The nurse can help devise substitutes
for the caffeine beverage such as noncaffeinated
soda, tea, or coffee and to focus on times of day
that the desire is greatest so changes can be made in
activity if possible.

When caffeine is administered therapeutically
(to treat headache from spinal puncture, for example), the nurse needs to remember to have a short-
acting barbiturate on hand to counteract CNS stimulation if it occurs. Caffeine should never be given
in doses greater than 1000 mg, because increased
respiratory depression may occur.

□ EVALUATION
Breaking the caffeine habit is difficult for most
people even when it is desirable. Objective measures of evaluation include the amount of caffeine
consumed and the presence of side-effects. Other
parameters may be the individual's reports of
changes in alertness, mental outlook, and activity
level.

Amphetamines

Amphetamine, Amphetamine Complex, Dextroamphetamine, Methamphetamine

The amphetamines are synethetic sympathomimetic amines with marked CNS-stimulatory action. Over the short term, they increase alertness
and concentration, elevate mood, and stimulate

motor activity. Amphetamines can induce varying
degrees of euphoria depending on the dose as well
as the personality of the user. Major peripheral effects of the compounds include elevation of blood
pressure, relaxation of bronchiolar smooth muscle,
contraction of the urinary sphincter, and mydriasis.

Although the initial effects of amphetamines
are generally pleasant, tolerance does occur to the
mood-elevating action of these compounds, and
prolonged oral use of amphetamines can lead to
irritability, insomnia, and dizziness. Increased
alertness gradually gives way to jitteriness, easy
distractibility, and confusion. The stimulation resulting from amphetamine usage is invariably followed by an equally intense depression, usually accompanied by fatigue and listlessness. The desire
to overcome this poststimulatory depression often
leads to repetitive amphetamine dosing, and in the
emotionally unstable person, can evolve into a vicious circle culminating in habituation and addiction. Large, repeated doses of amphetamines can
bring about a behavioral state that is difficult to
distinguish clinically from paranoid schizophrenia,
and is marked by delirium, usual and auditory hallucinations, and disturbed ideation. This paranoid-
like state can also occur when these agents are
abused parenterally (IV) as "spree drugs"; users are
given to violent outbursts which can endanger
themselves and others (see Chap. 85 for a discussion of amphetamine abuse), and this situation is
an extreme medical emergency.

Approved clinical indications for amphetamines are few and are listed below; use of these
drugs must be undertaken cautiously, and patients
must be closely observed. Chronic administration
should be avoided if possible, because the danger of
habituation is considerable. The amphetamines are
discussed as a group, and then are listed individually in Table 32-2.

MECHANISM AND ACTIONS
Amphetamines promote release of catecholamines
from presynaptic nerve terminals and prevent their
re-uptake into these nerve endings. The net effect
is potentiation of endogenous catecholamine (i.e.,
norepinephrine, dopamine) activity. In addition,
the drugs exert a direct-activating effect on adrenergic (e.g., alpha, beta) receptor sites and interfere
with the functioning of monoamine oxidase
(MAO), an enzyme responsible for intracellular
breakdown of monoamines such as norepinephrine, dopamine, and serotonin. The CNS stimulant
effect of amphetamines is thought to be due to an

action on the cortex and possibly also the reticular formation. The anorexiant (appetite suppressant) effect, on the other hand, appears to be the result in part of stimulation of a beta-receptor-mediated satiety system in the lateral hypothalamus. Elevated mood is also believed to contribute to the anorectic action by lessening the desire to eat. The usefulness of amphetamines in treating attention deficit disorder in children has been related to their ability to potentiate catecholamine activity in the CNS, and possibly increase stimulus discrimination as a result of increased activity of the reticular activating system.

USES

1. Short-term (*i.e.*, 4 weeks–8 weeks) adjunct in the treatment of obesity, as an aid to a total weight control program (potential benefit does *not* outweigh inherent risks—see below)
   Caution: Tolerance develops quickly, cardiovascular side-effects can occur, and habituation is common with prolonged use.
2. Treatment of narcolepsy (see Disease Brief: Narcolepsy)
3. Treatment of attention deficit disorder in children (see Disease Brief: Attention Deficit Disorder)

DISEASE BRIEF

■ Narcolepsy

Narcolepsy is a neurologic disorder characterized by excessive sleepiness and associated, in most cases, with one or more of auxiliary symptoms such as cataplexy, sleep paralysis, and hypnagogic hallucinations. "Sleep attacks" may last from several seconds to 30 minutes and usually occur during periods of boredom, monotony, or sedentary situations, but can happen under most circumstances, including emotional outbursts. *Cataplexy* consists of sudden loss of muscle tone, either partial or complete, is generally of brief duration, and is triggered by strong emotions (*e.g.*, anger, surprise). *Sleep paralysis* is loss of muscle tone and subsequent inability to move which occurs in the interim between sleep and waking. *Hypnagogic* hallucinations are vivid auditory or visual disturbances which also occur between the sleeping and waking state. Symptoms usually develop during childhood and tend to persist for a lifetime. REM (*i.e.*, rapid eye movement) sleep phases are frequently disordered and disturbed nocturnal sleep is seen in approximately one-half of narcoleptic patients.

ADMINISTRATION AND DOSAGE
See Table 32-2.

FATE
Oral absorption is complete, and the drugs are widely distributed in the body. They attain high concentrations in the CNS. Effects are seen within 30 minutes to 60 minutes and may persist for up to 24 hours to 36 hours, depending on rate of elimination in the urine. Urinary excretion of the unchanged drug is *p*H-dependent, and plasma half-life increases by approximately 7 hours for every 1 unit increase in the urinary *p*H.

SIDE-EFFECTS/ADVERSE REACTIONS
Side-effects noted with greatest frequency during acute amphetamine usage are nervousness, palpi-tations, tachycardia, and insomnia. A number of other adverse reactions have been reported during treatment with the amphetamines including:

CNS—Dizziness, euphoria or dysphoria, headache, chills, tremor; large doses may cause confusion, hallucinations, panic, aggressiveness, and psychotic episodes.

Cardiovascular—Hypertension, arrhythmias

GI—Nausea, vomiting, diarrhea, anorexia and weight loss, cramping

Other—Impotence, urticaria, delayed or difficult urination; large doses can cause dyspnea, anginal pain, syncope, convulsions, and coma

Amphetamines have been frequently abused, and extreme psychological dependence has occurred. Dosage may be increased many times above that recommended, and serious personality dis-

Table 32-2
Amphetamines

Drug	Preparations	Usual Dosage Range	Clinical Considerations
amphetamine sulfate	Tablets—5 mg, 10 mg	*Narcolepsy:* 5 mg to 60 mg/day in divided doses *Attention deficit disorder:* 3 years to 5 years—2.5 mg/day; increase by 2.5 mg/week until optimal response Over 6 years—5 mg one to two times/day; increase by 5 mg/week until optimal response *Obesity:* 5 mg to 30 mg/day in divided doses 30–60 min before meals	Note development of insomnia or anorexia, and reduce dose; give first dose on awakening and last dose 4–6 h before bedtime if possible; attempt to provide drug-free periods in children with attention deficit disorder, especially during periods of reduced stress (*e.g.*, summer vacations, holidays); be aware that response is more variable in children than in adults, and observe more closely (Schedule II)
amphetamine complex (Biphetamine)	Capsules—12½ mg, 20 mg (contain 6.25 mg and 10 mg each of dextroamphetamine and amphetamine, respectively)	*Obesity:* 1 capsule daily in the morning	Indicated for short-term adjunctive treatment of exogenous obesity; high potential for abuse; should be prescribed cautiously and patient's consumption monitored carefully; may also be used as once-a-day therapy in attention deficit disorder in children *after* appropriate daily dosage has been determined using dextroamphetamine alone (Schedule II) (*continued*)

orders can result from amphetamine abuse. Tolerance to amphetamines can be extreme, and a daily intake of 1 g to 2 g has been noted in some highly dependent individuals. Abrupt cessation following prolonged high dosage can result in extreme fatigue and depression.

Overdosage is characterized by a progression of central stimulatory effects from restlessness, irritability, and tremor through sweating, flushing, hyperreflexia, confusion, and hypertension to delirium, tachypnea, arrhythmias, and convulsions. Extreme depression and fatigue may follow the central stimulation. Overdosage is rarely fatal and is treated symptomatically. External stimulation should be minimized and diazepam or haloperidol may be administered to control hyperactivity and psychotic symptoms, respectively. Acidification of

the urine with ammonium chloride will hasten excretion.

CONTRAINDICATIONS AND PRECAUTIONS

Amphetamines are contraindicated in symptomatic cardiovascular disease, moderate to severe hypertension, arteriosclerosis, hyperthyroidism, glaucoma, and agitated states. They should not be given to patients with a history of drug abuse or within 14 days of administration of an MAO-inhibitor, because hypertensive crisis can result. Amphetamines are not recommended in children under age 12, except for treatment of attention deficit disorder, in which they can be given to children over 3 years of age. *Cautious use* of these drugs is warranted in patients with mild hypertension or

Table 32-2 (continued)
Amphetamines

Drug	Preparations	Usual Dosage Range	Clinical Considerations
dextroamphetamine sulfate (Dexedrine, Ferndex, Oxydess II, Spancap #1)	Tablets—5 mg, 10 mg Capsules—15 mg Capsules—(sustained-release) 5 mg, 10 mg, 15 mg Elixir—5 mg/5 ml	*Narcolepsy:* 5 mg to 60 mg/day in divided doses *Obesity:* 5 mg to 10 mg one to three times/day *Attention deficit disorder:* (Over 3 yr)—2.5 mg to 5 mg/day; increase gradually to optimal effect (maximum 40 mg/day)	More potent CNS stimulant than amphetamine, but exerts less of an effect on the cardiovascular and peripheral nervous systems; give last dose at least 6 h before bedtime; tolerance usually develops within several weeks; possesses the same pharmacologic properties and hazards as amphetamine, and should be used sparingly and cautiously (Schedule II)
methamphetamine (Desoxyn)	Tablets—5 mg, 10 mg Long-acting tablets—5 mg, 10 mg, 15 mg	*Obesity:* 5 mg three times/day (long-acting—1 tablet daily) *Attention deficit disorder:* (Over 6 yr)—Initially 5 mg one to two times/day; increase by 5 mg/week to optimal level (usual range 20 mg to 25 mg/day)	CNS effects slightly greater than amphetamine; do not use long-acting tablets to initiate dosage; give 30 minutes before meals and last dose at least 6 h before bedtime; large doses may result in cardiac stimulation; tolerance develops quickly, so drug has high abuse potential; commonly called speed among abusers; has caused severe psychotic reactions following repeated injections of dissolved tablets (Schedule II)

arrhythmias and in pregnant women or nursing mothers.

INTERACTIONS
1. Amphetamines may reduce the antihypertensive effects of guanethidine, methyldopa, hydralazine, and possibly other antihypertensive drugs.
2. Effects of amphetamines can be potentiated by acetazolamide, cocaine, furazolidone, propoxyphene, tricyclic antidepressants, MAO-inhibitors, and by sodium bicarbonate and other substances that alkalinize the urine.
3. The effects of amphetamines may be antagonized by urinary acidifying agents (ascorbic acid, methenamine, reserpine, glutamic acid, fruit juices), barbiturates (due to increased rates of metabolism), lithium, haloperidol, and phenothiazines.
4. Amphetamines may delay the effects of phenytoin, ethosuximide, and other anticonvulsants by impairing their GI absorption.
5. Insulin requirements in diabetes may be altered by amphetamines.

■ Nursing Process for Children Requiring CNS Stimulants for Attention Deficit Disorder (ADD)

☐ *ASSESSMENT*

☐ *Subjective Data*
The use of stimulants in treating "hyperactive" children has received considerable media attention

DISEASE BRIEF

■ Attention Deficit Disorder

Attention deficit disorder (ADD) is a behavioral/cognitive disorder of childhood characterized by an increased level of motor activity, impaired coordination, short attention span, easy distractibility, impulsive behavior, and learning disability. Synonyms for this disorder include hyperkinetic syndrome and minimal brain dysfunction with hyperactivity. Affected children display extreme restlessness when required to remain still (e.g., in school or church) and tend to perform poorly in school because of their short attention span. In addition, some children appear to have a neurologic deficit which impairs their auditory and visual perception and their ability to process didactic information. The precise etiology of ADD remains a mystery. The altered behavior has been ascribed to a deficiency in catecholamine action in the CNS, which might result in reduced inhibition of higher cortical function by lower brain centers. The easy distractibility may thus be due to the child's inability to "screen out" excessive stimuli. Behavioral control can be realized in many of these children by use of a CNS stimulant, such as amphetamine, methylphenidate, or pemoline, although such treatment has its opponents due to the potential long-term adverse effects of these drugs.

because several research studies indicated that hundreds of thousands of children were being given these drugs. Therefore, parents and teachers may have some opinions about the usefulness of these drugs and concerns about the long-term effects of such drug therapy. Any fears and concerns should be discussed prior to initiation of drug therapy so that all have a well-informed, reality-based orientation.

Information should also be collected on the development of the behavior problem that led to the recommendation of drug treatment. The nurse needs to know the teacher's as well as the parents' observations because many times the problem appears only when the child is in a confined learning situation. Other important data include information on family, home, or school stressors and the types of behavior modification or learning disability programs used to counteract the child's problem. Drug therapy can only be seen as an adjunct to these other programs and not the "magic cure" for a behavior disorder.

Renal and hepatic function studies should be collected and a complete history and physical performed. All of these drugs have systemic side-effects which should be closely monitored throughout treatment.

□ NURSING DIAGNOSES

Actual nursing diagnoses for the patient and his family beginning therapy with CNS stimulants may include:

Knowledge deficit about the action, dose, and side-effects of the drug

Alteration in family process related to escalating concerns over the child's behavior at home and at school

Impaired social interactions resulting from behavior problems

Potential nursing diagnoses related to side-effects may include:

Alteration in comfort: gastrointestinal distress

Alteration in nutrition: less than body requirements related to anorexia

Sleep pattern disturbances

□ PLAN

The nurse must try to form a communication quartet among the parents/child, the teacher, the physician, and the nurse in order to provide optimum care. Although the parents and child will make some observations about the drug treatment, the teacher may actually provide the most accurate perceptions about drug effectiveness in terms of learning and attention span. This information must be conveyed to the physician so appropriate dosage adjustments can be made. Therefore, the nurse must include the teacher and the family in the teaching plan. All should know what to expect from effective drug therapy, what side-effects to watch for, and the best method for communicating with one another.

Stated goals might then include:

1. Establishing a regular forum for communica-

tion among parents, child, teacher, and physician

2. Teaching the parents, child, and teacher the correct drug dose and possible side-effects
3. Assisting the teacher, school nurse, and parents to develop a flowsheet to monitor positive behavior changes as well as side-effects
4. Planning drug-free holidays to measure child's ability to manage without the drug

□ INTERVENTION

Parents and teacher should observe the child's attention span, degree of restlessness, social and emotional behavior, work accuracy, and work output as measures of the drug's effectiveness. The teacher and school nurse will keep a flowsheet to record observations that will be useful to the physician in making dosage changes. The goal is to keep the drug dose as low as possible while improving school performance and social interaction.

Drug-free holidays should also be planned to see how the child does without the drugs. As the child learns to focus attention on school and achieves more success he may need the drug less and less. Stimulant therapy is not intended to be long term and should be frequently reevaluated. Supervised holidays allow parents, child, teacher, and nurse the opportunity to look at achievement of these goals.

The most bothersome side-effects of CNS stimulants are gastric upset, anorexia, and insomnia. Gastric upset can be minimized by giving the child the medication with food and making provisions for him to have small frequent meals. Such actions can usually decrease the loss of appetite as well. However, the child's weight should be carefully monitored, and changes should be reported.

Insomnia may be lessened with dosage adjustments or by making sure the child takes the prescribed dose early enough in the day so the drug's effect will be minimal around bedtime.

All concerned should learn to watch for adverse effects of these drugs including the development of tolerance, which may manifest itself in recurrence of previous behavior patterns. Other adverse effects such as restlessness, irritability, or reports by the child of "my heart feels funny" should be reported immediately.

□ EVALUATION

Parameters used to determine drug effectiveness include attention span, degree of restlessness, social and emotional behavior, work accuracy, and work output. However, it is important for the nurse, parents, and teacher to recognize that improvement may not be absolute but a matter of degree over previous behavior. Drug therapy should never be viewed as the sole cause (or lack) of behavior change but as part of a total therapeutic regimen, which may consist of therapy, family counseling, and behavior modification and learning techniques. Nursing Care Plan 32-1 summarizes the nursing process for the child receiving CNS stimulants.

■ Nursing Process for Other Patients Receiving CNS Stimulants

(See also Nursing Process for Children Requiring CNS Stimulants for ADD.)

□ ASSESSMENT

A drug history should be obtained to help discern whether the patient has the potential for abusing amphetamines. This is less of a problem in the patient being treated for narcolepsy or attention deficit disorder. However, the obese patient, particularly one who reports having been to many doctors and on many diets, is a high-risk candidate who may, in fact, already be an amphetamine abuser.

A complete history and physical should be performed with particular focus on cardiovascular status. A lying and standing blood pressure should be taken, and an ECG should be performed. Anyone with a history of hypertension or cardiovascular problems should not receive amphetamines.

□ NURSING DIAGNOSES

Actual nursing diagnoses for patients taking amphetamines include:

Knowledge deficit related to action, dose and side-effects of the drug

Potential nursing diagnoses related to drug side-effects may include:

Alteration in comfort: gastrointestinal distress
Alteration in nutrition: less than body requirements
Sleep pattern disturbance

□ PLAN

The goal for the patient with narcolepsy is to reduce or eliminate the dangerous symptoms and to help him become productive. For obese patients, the goal is to use the drug as an appetite suppressant in conjunction with a rigidly maintained di-

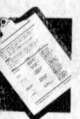

Assessment

Subjective Data

1. Medication history
   a. Refer to Interactions section to formulate pertinent questions
   b. Consider the child's intake of caffeinated beverages as well

2. Medical history
   a. Description of symptoms, course of problem that led child/parent to seek treatment
   b. Check for preexisting conditions that may precipitate adverse drug reactions, such as cardiovascular disease, behavioral problems, renal or hepatic dysfunction, glaucoma, diabetes mellitus, neurologic disease

3. Family/personal history
   a. Perceptions of the problem: methods of managing the child's behavior disorder
   b. Financial, personal resources, family network of support

Objective Data

1. Physical assessment highlighting
   a. Vital signs
   b. Height and weight
   c. Neurologic function: reflexes, motor function, mental acuity, developmental level for age

2. Laboratory Data
   a. Renal and hepatic function studies
   b. CBC with differential

Nursing Diagnosis	*Expected Client Outcome*	*Intervention*
Knowledge deficit related to drug effect on performance, effect of food on behavior, correct administration, and potential side-effects	Will verbalize knowledge of drug's action, correct administration, and common side-effects Will maintain a flowsheet to monitor child's progress	Ensure prescribed dose is correct for the age and weight of the child. Teach family that drug may improve school performance and decrease motor hyperactivity, but may also make child listless. Balance must be achieved. Teach the family and teacher to monitor common side-effects as described below and follow preventive strategies given. Meet with family and teacher to outline guidelines for monitoring child's progress. Monitor hepatic and renal function through laboratory data and blood pressure during visits. Establish a flowsheet for family/teacher to periodically monitor the following to detect side-effects and evaluate progress: · Pulse, respiration · food intake · height and weight · school performance · social interactions · sleep disturbances · neurologic changes

(continued)

Nursing Diagnosis	Expected Client Outcome	Intervention
Potential alteration in nutrition: less than body requirements, related to gastric upset or anorexia from drug, which may influence growth	Will maintain normal weight and growth pattern for age	Teach parents to monitor child's intake to ensure child gets enough calories, protein, fats, and complex carbohydrates to meet nutritional needs, and to limit caffeine and refined carbohydrates. Encourage healthy snacks and small, frequent meals if child is anorexic. Encourage child to take drug with food. Monitor height and weight monthly.
Potential sleep pattern disturbance related to drug effect	Will obtain adequate sleep time during therapy	Teach parent to administer drug early in the day to avoid sleep disturbances. Persistent night wakening should be reported to physician. Dosage adjustment may be necessary.
Potential alteration in social interactions with family, teacher, and peers related to effect	Will engage in positive interactions with others	Teach family that improvements may be mild or noticeable. Ability to interact is based on the child's social network, the responses he has received in the past, and perceptions of others based on previous interactions. Change occurs gradually.
Potential alteration in cardiac output: decreased, related to drug-induced dysrhythmias	Will prevent or report early cardiac changes	Monitor pulse and BP weekly through school nurse, if possible. Teach family to listen to child's complaints of fatigue, restlessness, or heart beating fast and report these immediately. Drug dose may need to be reduced or discontinued.

etary and behavior modification regimen. As with other drugs, knowledge of side-effects is also important.

□ **INTERVENTION**

The obese patient needs to understand that amphetamines are intended for short-term use to assist appetite suppression. The nurse should help the patient focus on achieving weight loss through diet, behavior changes, and exercise and not through drug ingestion. This patient should be carefully monitored for the development of tolerance to the drug. If it occurs, the drug should be discontinued and restarted several weeks later, if necessary. Increasing the dose is not appropriate because the potential for habituation and addiction increases rapidly with larger doses.

A patient taking amphetamines should be taught to avoid tyramine-containing foods to avoid excessive rise in blood pressure. Such foods include cheese, beer, Chianti, liver, salted fish, broad beans, and avocados.

Amphetamines should be gradually withdrawn after prolonged therapy because abrupt cessation can cause a psychotic depressive reaction. Withdrawal should occur under supervision, in an environment where the patient can receive adequate rest and reduced stimulation.

□ **EVALUATION**

For the patient suffering from narcolepsy, the decrease in "sleep attacks" will indicate whether the drug has been effective. Weight loss may be one parameter to measure the drug's effectiveness in the obese patient. However, the nurse should caution the patient that drug therapy alone cannot produce prolonged weight loss.

For a discussion of nursing considerations in abuse of amphetamines, see Chapter 85.

Anorexiants

Benzphetamine, Diethylpropion, Fenfluramine, Mazindol, Phendimetrazine, Phenmetrazine, Phentermine, Phenylpropanolamine

A group of indirect-acting sympathomimetic amines have been employed as alternates to amphetamine in the treatment of exogenous obesity. These agents, termed *anorexiants*, *anorectics*, or *anorexigenics*, are mostly structural analogues of amphetamine and possess essentially the same spectrum of pharmacologic and toxicologic actions. With the exception of fenfluramine, which produces CNS depression, all these drugs evoke varying degrees of stimulation which appear to be a major component of their anorectic action. They are primarily indicated for the temporary, adjunctive management of obesity in conjunction with a carefully supervised program of caloric restriction and proper exercise. Although none of these agents is superior to amphetamine in effectiveness, some do have less potential for habituation and may cause fewer adverse cardiovascular, central, and gastrointestinal side-effects. Thus, they may be preferable for short-term therapy. It is important to recognize, however, that all of these drugs can become habituating with continued use. Because their therapeutic benefit is restricted to a few weeks at best, because of developing tolerance, there is significant danger in their prolonged consumption, and their usage should be accorded the same degree of caution as the use of amphetamines.

The above-mentioned drugs used as diet aids are available by prescription only. However, two other agents used as diet aids are available over the counter. Phenylpropanolamine, a sympathomimetic commonly prescribed as a decongestant is also employed orally as an over-the-counter diet aid, either alone or in combination with various vitamins or a grapefruit extract. A weak CNS stimulant, phenylpropanolamine is recommended for the short-term management of obesity, although its efficacy is subject to considerable doubt. Moreover, because it stimulates alpha-adrenergic receptors and releases norepinephrine, it can significantly elevate blood pressure and should not be taken by anyone with even mild hypertension. Severe hypertensive episodes have occurred during concomitant administration of phenylpropanolamine and propranolol or indomethacin.

Benzocaine, a local anesthetic, is also used in the form of candy or gum to decrease taste sensation as an adjunct to weight reduction in a calorie-restricted regimen.

Because the anorexiant drugs are quite similar in their pharmacologic effects, they will be discussed as a group. However, there are considerable differences among certain of these drugs in their potential to cause habituation and in their side-effects. Their likelihood to result in habituation is largely reflected in their classification into different schedules of controlled substances (see Chap. 7). Thus, phenmetrazine, a strongly habituating agent, is a Schedule II drug, whereas the less habituating compounds, diethylpropion, fenfluramine, mazindol, and phentermine, are classified as Schedule IV drugs. Benzphetamine and phendimetrazine are grouped in Schedule III. Other differences among the anorexiants are outlined in Table 32-3.

MECHANISM AND ACTIONS
The ability of the anorexiant drugs to suppress the appetite is probably the result of effects similar to those of amphetamine. A direct stimulant action on the hypothalamic satiety center has been postulated as a mechanism for the anorexiant effect of these drugs, although their general CNS stimulatory action to improve mood and willingness to adhere to a diet is probably as important. Interaction with central neurohormones (norepinephrine, dopamine, serotonin) may also contribute to the clinical effects of these drugs. While most anorexiants possess a central excitatory action, fenfluramine is a depressant of central function, and drowsiness has been reported; increased brain glucose utilization may contribute to this latter effect. All drugs can elevate blood pressure.

USES
1. Short-term (8 weeks–12 weeks) management of obesity, as an adjunct to caloric restriction (*Caution:* The limited benefit observed with anorexiant drugs probably does *not* outweigh the inherent risk. These drugs should be used with extreme caution.)

2. Fenfluramine has been used investigationally to treat autistic children with elevated serotonin levels.

ADMINISTRATION AND DOSAGE
See Table 32-3.

FATE
Most anorexiants are quickly and completely absorbed orally, and the onset of action occurs usually within 1 hour. Effects generally persist 4 hours to 6 hours; sustained-release formulations may have a prolonged action (12 hours–18 hours). Tolerance develops within several weeks, and effectiveness gradually declines. The drugs are metabolized by the liver and excreted both as unchanged drug and metabolites by the kidney.

SIDE-EFFECTS/ADVERSE REACTIONS
Common side-effects of anorexiant drugs include nervousness, irritability, insomnia, palpitations, and tachycardia. A variety of other adverse reactions have been associated with these agents and are noted below:

Cardiovascular—Dyspnea, hypertension, precordial pain, arrhythmias, syncope

CNS–Anxiety, dizziness, headache, euphoria, tremors, confusion, incoordination; occasionally depression (especially fenfluramine), dysphoria, dysarthria (In addition, fenfluramine may cause drowsiness and impotence. Abrupt withdrawal of fenfluramine after prolonged use has resulted in ataxia, tremor, visual hallucinations, loss of sense of reality, depression, and suicidal tendencies.)

GI—Nausea, vomiting, unpleasant taste, cramping, constipation, glossitis, stomatitis, dry mouth

Genitourinary—Dysuria, polyuria, diuresis, cystitis, impotence, menstrual irregularities, changes in libido, gynecomastia

Other—Rash, urticaria, erythema, mydriasis, blurred vision, muscle pain, chills, flushing, fever, sweating, alopecia, blood dyscrasias (rare)

Overdosage is manifested by CNS excitation, tachycardia, arrhythmias, vomiting, diarrhea, and abdominal cramping, followed eventually by depression and fatigue. Treatment is symptomatic and supportive. Sedatives (*e.g.,* diazepam) and antipsychotics (*e.g.,* haloperidol) may be given if necessary.

CONTRAINDICATIONS AND PRECAUTIONS
Refer to the previous discussion of amphetamines for contraindications to the anorexiants. In addition, benzphetamine is contraindicated during pregnancy; fetal abnormalities have occurred. The anorexiant drugs should be used with *caution* in patients with diabetes, epilepsy, anxiety neuroses, and mild hypertension, in pregnant women or nursing mothers, and in persons engaged in potentially hazardous activities because dizziness, drowsiness, and impaired coordination have occurred. Fenfluramine should not be administered to alcoholics because psychiatric symptoms (such as depression, paranoia, or psychoses) can occur.

The drugs should not be administered for longer than 8 weeks to 12 weeks because their efficacy diminishes but the risk of habituation increases with prolonged use. Upon discontinuation, fatigue and depression may ensue.

INTERACTIONS
See under Amphetamines. In addition:
1. Fenfluramine may augment the effects of other CNS depressants (*e.g.,* alcohol, narcotics, barbiturates) and may potentiate the action of antihypertensive drugs.
2. Anorexiants may reduce diabetic drug requirements by increasing glucose uptake by skeletal muscle cells, possibly necessitating a dosage adjustment.
3. Concurrent use of anorexiants with general anesthetics may increase the risk of cardiac arrhythmias.
4. Mazindol may potentiate the pressor effects of exogenous catecholamines and increase the risk of lithium toxicity.

NURSING CONSIDERATIONS
See also Nursing Process for Amphetamines. Because these drugs are used primarily for treatment of obesity, the same principles apply.

The nurse is most likely to come in contact with young women who have had adverse reactions to over-the-counter diet products containing phenylpropanolamine. These reactions may range from anxiety attacks to hypertensive crises and convulsions depending on the amount of drug taken. The OTC diet aids containing this drug can be powerful CNS stimulants when dosing exceeds recommended ranges. Most patients will have overdosed in an attempt to lose weight faster. The nurse needs to explore the reasons for this attempt. The social "norm" of being thin, peer pressure to

Table 32-3
Anorexiant Drugs

Drug	Preparations	Usual Dosage Range	Clinical Considerations
benzocaine (Ayds, Slim-Line)	Candy—5 mg Gum—6 mg	6 mg to 15 mg just prior to food consumption (maximum 45 mg/day)	An anesthetic used as gum or candy to decrease taste sensation as an adjunct to weight reduction. Decreases ability of taste receptors to detect sweetness.
benzphetamine (Didrex)	Tablets—25 mg, 50 mg	Initially 25 mg to 50 mg/day; increase as necessary (usual range 50 mg to 150 mg/day)	Usually given as single daily dose, midmorning or midafternoon. Contraindicated during pregnancy. (Schedule III)
diethylpropion (Tenuate, Tepanil)	Tablets—25 mg Tablets (sustained-release)—75 mg	25 mg three times/day 1 h before meals and in midevening if needed, or 75 mg daily in the morning	Less effective but somewhat less hazardous than amphetamines; caution in epileptics because drug has been shown to increase convulsions; may alter ECG (T-wave changes) (Schedule IV)
fenfluramine (Pondimin)	Tablets—20 mg	Initially 20 mg three times/day before meals; increase by 20 mg/week to a maximum of 120 mg/day	Differs from other anorexiants because it often produces CNS depression; thus, may be more useful than other anorexiants for persons who eat heavily at night. May enhance glucose uptake by skeletal muscles; use cautiously in depression and diabetes; diarrhea is often noted early in therapy; reduce dose or discontinue if severe; do not discontinue abruptly because severe depression can ensue; avoid use in alcoholics because psychiatric symptoms can develop; may potentiate effects of both CNS stimulants and CNS depressants. (Schedule IV)
mazindol (Mazanor, Sanorex)	Tablets—1 mg, 2 mg	1 mg three times/day before meals or 2 mg daily before lunch	Take with food if necessary, to reduce GI discomfort; may alter diabetic drug requirements by lowering blood glucose levels; elicits CNS and cardiovascular stimulation, and appears to alter mood by an action on the limbic system. (Schedule IV)

(continued)

Table 32-3 (continued)
Anorexiant Drugs

Drug	Preparations	Usual Dosage Range	Clinical Considerations
phendimetrazine (various manufacturers)	Tablets—35 mg Capsules—35 mg Sustained-release capsules —105 mg	35 mg two to three times/ day 1 h before meals, or 105 mg once a day	Similar to amphetamine in action but somewhat less potent (Schedule III)
phenmetrazine (Preludin)	Tablets—25 mg Tablets (sustained-release) —75 mg	25 mg two to three times/ day 1 h before meals, or 75 mg daily in the morning	Blood pressure may be elevated by drug; monitor pressure periodically; congenital malformations have occurred but a causal relationship has not been proven; sustained-release forms are no more effective than regular tablets and may be more hazardous if taken in excess; more intense CNS stimulation than most other anorexiants, and greater incidence of abuse. (Schedule II)
phentermine (Ionamin and various other manufacturers)	Tablets—8 mg, 15 mg, 30 mg Tablets (long-acting)—37.5 mg Capsules—8 mg, 15 mg, 18.75 mg, 30 mg Capsules (long-acting)—15 mg, 30 mg, 37.5 mg	8 mg three times/day before meals or 15 mg to 37.5 mg daily in the morning	Less potent stimulant of CNS and cardiovascular activity than amphetamine; available as a resin-complex capsule (15 mg, 30 mg) providing prolonged action (10 h–15 h); do not use resin complex if patient has diarrhea because effectiveness is lost. (Schedule IV)
phenylpropanolamine (Acutrim, Dexatrim, Diadax, Prolamine and various other manufacturers)	Tablets—25 mg Capsules—37.5 mg Tablets (timed-release)—75 mg Capsules (timed-release)— 50 mg, 75 mg	25 mg three times/day or 50 mg to 75 mg once daily in the morning	Over-the-counter diet aid possessing weak central stimulatory action. Can activate peripheral alpha and beta receptors, resulting in vasoconstriction and cardiac stimulation. Use must be closely supervised as blood pressure elevations have occurred. Discontinue drug if tachycardia, dizziness, nervousness, or insomnia occur. Do not exceed recommended dose.

reduce weight, exclusion from activities because of weight, or stressors at home, school, or in personal relationships may be the cause of an adolescent's desire to diet. Intervention should be aimed at dealing with the causes, assessing whether there is an actual need to diet, and, if so, helping the adolescent learn the behaviors that will lead to successful weight loss without drugs.

Methylphenidate

(Ritalin)

Methylphenidate is a CNS stimulant with a pharmacologic profile of action similar to that of amphetamine, but having a more marked effect on mental rather than physical or motor activities at normal doses. Methylphenidate shares the same potential for habituation and psychological addiction as the amphetamines, although its central excitatory effects may be slightly less intense. In usual therapeutic dosage, it does not significantly elevate the blood pressure, heart rate, or respiratory rate; however, in large doses, signs of generalized CNS excitation can occur (e.g., tremors, tachycardia, hyperpyrexia, confusion). It is most widely used as an adjunct in the therapy of attention deficit disorder in children, in whom its effectiveness equals that of the amphetamines. Methylphenidate is a Schedule II controlled drug.

MECHANISM AND ACTIONS
The mechanism of action of methylphenidate is not fully understood but is probably similar to that of amphetamine. Its stimulatory action appears to be exerted primarily at the level of the cortex. Release of catecholamines from presynaptic nerve endings may also contribute to the drug's actions.

USES
1. Adjunctive therapy of attention deficit disorder in children
2. Treatment of narcolepsy
3. Relief of mild depression and apathetic or withdrawn senile behavior ("possibly effective")

ADMINISTRATION AND DOSAGE
Methylphenidate is used orally as 5-mg, 10-mg, or 20-mg tablets and a 20-mg sustained-release tablet. Adult dosage is 20 mg to 30 mg a day, taken in two or three divided doses, 30 minutes to 45 minutes before meals. The maximal dose is considered to be 60 mg/day. In children over 6 years of age, 5 mg may be given initially twice a day, before breakfast and lunch. Dosage may be increased by 5 mg to 10 mg a week to a maximum of 60 mg/day. If improvement is not observed within 1 month after dosage adjustment, the drug should be discontinued. During prolonged therapy, periodic discontinuation of therapy should be attempted to assess the patient's condition. Drug treatment is not intended to be indefinite.

Evidence suggests that limiting the dosage to 0.3 mg/kg in children is as effective as higher doses with a reduced incidence of side-effects (Brown et al., 1984).

FATE
The drug is rapidly and well absorbed from the GI tract and is distributed throughout the body, including the CNS. The onset of action occurs in 30 minutes to 60 minutes, and peak blood levels are achieved in 1 hour to 3 hours. Effects persist up to 6 hours with oral administration. Approximately 80% of a dose is metabolized and excreted in the urine.

SIDE-EFFECTS/ADVERSE REACTIONS
Nervousness and insomnia are the most commonly encountered side-effects of methylphenidate. In children receiving the drug for attention deficit disorder, anorexia, weight loss, and tachycardia are also observed frequently. Other adverse reactions noted during methylphenidate therapy are listed below.

CNS—Dizziness, drowsiness, headache, dyskinesia, agitation, toxic psychoses, chorea, Tourette's syndrome

Cardiovascular—Palpitations, blood pressure changes, tachycardia, anginal attacks, arrhythmias

Allergic—Skin rash, fever, urticaria, arthralgia, erythema multiforme, necrotizing vasculitis, exfoliative dermatitis

GI—Anorexia, nausea, abdominal pain

Other—Visual disturbances, alopecia, anemia, leukopenia

Prolonged use in children can result in suppression of growth and exacerbation of behavioral and thought disorders.

CONTRAINDICATIONS AND PRECAUTIONS
Contraindications to methylphenidate use include the presence of marked anxiety, tension or agita-

tion, glaucoma, history of seizure disorders, motor tics, and severe depression. The drug should not be given to children under age 6. *Cautious use* is warranted in patients with hypertension, a history of drug or alcohol dependence, and in pregnant women and nursing mothers. Periodic blood counts should be performed during therapy, and patients receiving methylphenidate should be cautioned that dizziness, blurred vision, and impaired coordination can occur and may interfere with driving or other tasks requiring alertness.

INTERACTIONS

1. Methylphenidate may increase the effects of oral anticoagulants, anticonvulsants, tricyclic antidepressants, and phenylbutazone by inhibiting their metabolism.
2. Hypertensive reactions may occur with combinations of methylphenidate and vasopressors, MAO-inhibitors, and furazolidone.
3. Methylphenidate decreases the antihypertensive action of guanethidine.
4. The effects of methylphenidate can be antagonized by phenothiazines and propoxyphene.

NURSING CONSIDERATIONS
See Nursing Process for Children Requiring CNS Stimulants for ADD.

Pemoline
(Cylert)

A chemically unique CNS stimulant having minimal sympathomimetic effects, pemoline is otherwise pharmacologically comparable to amphetamine and methylphenidate. It appears to have a lower abuse potential than most other CNS stimulants and is classified as a Schedule IV controlled substance.

MECHANISM AND ACTIONS
The exact mechanism of action of pemoline is unknown. The drug may increase dopaminergic function in the CNS and exert a direct action on the cortex. Principal effects seen with pemoline are increased alertness, enhanced motor activity, and mild euphoria. Pemoline displays a gradual onset of action and clinical effects may not be evident until the third or fourth week of administration.

USES
1. Adjunctive therapy of attention deficit disorder in children

2. Treatment of narcolepsy and excessive sleepiness (investigational use only)

ADMINISTRATION AND DOSAGE
Pemoline is used orally as tablets (18.75 mg, 37.5 mg, 75 mg) or chewable tablets (37.5 mg). The recommended starting dose is 37.5 mg/day as a single morning dose. Increments of 18.75 mg/week may be given until the desired response is obtained. The maximum dose is considered to be 112.5 mg/day.

FATE
Pemoline is well absorbed from the GI tract, with peak blood levels occurring in 2 hours to 4 hours. The plasma half-life is approximately 12 hours. Pemoline is metabolized by the liver and excreted in the urine both as unchanged drug (45%) and various conjugated metabolites. The drug has a gradual onset of action, and clinical effects may not be evident for 3 weeks to 4 weeks.

SIDE-EFFECTS/ADVERSE REACTIONS
The most frequent side-effects early in treatment are insomnia and anorexia with weight loss. Other adverse reactions noted include nausea, abdominal pain, skin rash, dyskinesias of the tongue, lips, face and extremities, nystagmus, dizziness, drowsiness, headache, irritability, depression, seizures, hallucinations, and Tourette's syndrome.

Elevated levels of SGOT, SGPT, and serum LDH have occurred and are reversible on drug withdrawal. There have been a few reports of jaundice.

Overdose can result in agitation, tachycardia, dyskinetic movements, hyperreflexia, and irregular respiration. Management is primarily symptomatic and supportive.

CONTRAINDICATIONS AND PRECAUTIONS
Use in children under 6 years of age is not recommended. Pemoline must be given with *caution* to patients with impaired liver or kidney function, a history of drug abuse, and during pregnancy. Chronic administration can result in growth inhibition, and long-term effects in children have not been definitely established.

INTERACTIONS
1. Pemoline may enhance the effects of other CNS stimulants.

NURSING CONSIDERATIONS
See Nursing Process for Children Requiring CNS Stimulants for ADD.

CASE STUDIES

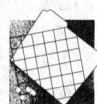

I. Connie Mannas is a 35-year-old housewife who is about 30 pounds overweight for her height and frame. She has come to your neighborhood clinic because she has heard you are working with a nutritionist and a physician to try to help people lose weight. She states she has been to many doctors but no one has been able to help her. She is anxious to see the doctor and wants to know if you or the doctor can give her something to curb her appetite. Connie seems restless, gestures constantly when speaking, and complains of difficulty sleeping and a constant headache. Her heart rate is 130/minute.

Discussion Questions

1. What other data do you need to evaluate this patient?
2. Develop a care plan to assist Connie to decrease her possible dependence on drugs to reduce weight and to control obesity.

II. Timmy Brown, age 7, has been repeatedly reported to the principal for disturbing other students during class. The principal and teacher are both concerned about Timmy's seeming hyperactivity, but Mrs. Brown thinks the problem is the teacher. Mrs. Brown finally agrees to an evaluation by the school physician, and a referral is made to Timmy's pediatrician. After consultation, a decision is made to put Timmy on Ritalin.

Discussion Questions

1. Develop a teaching plan that includes information for the parents, Timmy, the teacher, and the school nurse about administration and side-effects of this drug.
2. You are the school nurse. What information should the family and teacher have about this drug? What factors may contribute to Timmy's hyperactivity? How should these factors be assessed?
3. Design a care plan to deal with this problem, including the concerns for Timmy, his family, and his interactions at school.

REVIEW QUESTIONS

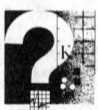

1. List the major pharmacologic effects of caffeine.
2. In large amounts, caffeine may result in development of what symptoms?
3. How can a nurse help patients eliminate their "caffeine" habit?
4. Describe the principal (a) central and (b) peripheral actions of amphetamines.
5. What are the mechanisms responsible for the anorectic effects of amphetamines?
6. What are the principal uses for amphetamines?
7. Describe the symptoms of amphetamine overdosage. How is overdosage treated?

8. What foods should a patient avoid when taking amphetamines?
9. How do the anorexiant drugs differ from amphetamine itself?
10. Name an over-the-counter diet aid. What kind of drug is it, and what are its major pharmacologic actions?
11. Which anorexiant induces CNS depression? How may this property be used to clinical advantage?
12. List the approved indications for methylphenidate. In what conditions is it contraindicated?
13. What is the mechanism of action of pemoline? List its common side-effects.
14. Why is a communication quartet between nurse, physician, family, and teacher important in the drug therapy for attention deficit disorder (ADD)?
15. What parameters may indicate drug effectiveness for the child with ADD?

BIBLIOGRAPHY

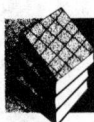

Algozzine B, Algozzine K: Some practical considerations of hyperactivity and drugs. J Sch Health 48:479, 1978

Brown RT et al: How much stimulant medication is appropriate for hyperactive school children? J Sch Health 54(3):128, 1984

Hallal JC: Caffeine: Is it hazardous to your patient's health? Am J Nurs 86:422, 1986

Ludwikowski KL: PPA: An innocent over-the-counter drug? Pediatr Nurs 10(6):387, 1984

Piepho RW, Gourley DR, Hill JW: Minimal brain dysfunction. J Am Pharmaceut Assoc 17(8):500, 1977

Soldatos CR, Vales A, Cadieux RJ: Treatment of sleep disorders II: Narcolepsy. Ration Drug Ther 17(3):1, 1983

Steiner JF, Fowler RM: Attention deficit disorder. US Pharmacist 7(12):30, 1982

Tan TL, Handford HA, Soldatos CR: Current therapy of eating disorders II: Obesity. Ration Drug Ther 18(2):1, 1984

Tesar GE: The role of stimulants in general medicine. Drug Therapy 12:1986, 1982

Weiss G: Controversial issues of the pharmacotherapy of the hyperactive child. Am J Psychiatry 26:385, 1981

Wender PH, Reimherr FW, Wood DR: Attention deficit disorder in adults. Arch Gen Psychiatry 38:449, 1981

Zarcone V: Narcolepsy. N Engl J Med 288:1156, 1973

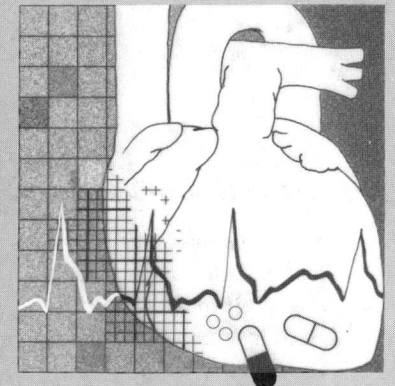

Drugs Acting on the Blood and Cardiovascular System

IV

Cardiotonic Drugs

33

Drugs that have a cardiotonic action are capable of increasing the tone of cardiac muscle, thus improving its functional capability. The term has traditionally been applied to a group of drugs known as the digitalis glycosides, although newer drugs that exhibit similar properties are now available. Cardiotonic drugs are primarily indicated for the treatment of congestive heart failure, because they have the ability to improve the force of contraction of the failing heart.

In order to more fully understand the pharmacology of cardiotonic drugs, a brief review of the anatomy and physiology of the heart will first be presented.

The Heart

The human heart is a four-chambered, highly muscular organ lying within the mediastinum enclosed by a double-layered pericardium (Fig. 33-1). The heart wall is composed of three layers: an outer thin transparent epicardium (visceral pericardium); a thick middle muscular myocardium; and an inner serous lining, or endocardium. In addition to lining the chambers of the heart, the endocardium covers the valves of the heart and is continuous with the endothelium of the blood vessels.

The thin-walled superior chambers, or atria, function primarily as reservoirs for blood returning to the heart. The right atrium receives systemic venous blood from the superior and inferior venae cavae and coronary venous blood chiefly through the coronary sinus. The left atrium receives oxygenated blood from the lungs by way of four pulmonary veins. Because no true valves separate the great veins near the heart from the atrial chambers, elevations in right atrial pressure are reflected backward into the systemic venous circulation, while elevations in left atrial pressure lead to pulmonary congestion.

The inferior chambers or ventricles are thick walled, being formed by three indistinct layers of muscle arranged in a complex spiral fashion. During contraction, the myocardium of each ventricle generates a force sufficient to overcome the existing pressure in the receiving artery. The right ventricle ejects its contents into the pulmonary artery, while the left ventricle pumps oxygenated blood into the aorta. Because the pulmonary circulation functions at a considerably lower pressure than the systemic circulation, the thickness of the right ventricular wall is approximately one-third that of the left, reflecting the lighter workload of the right ventricle.

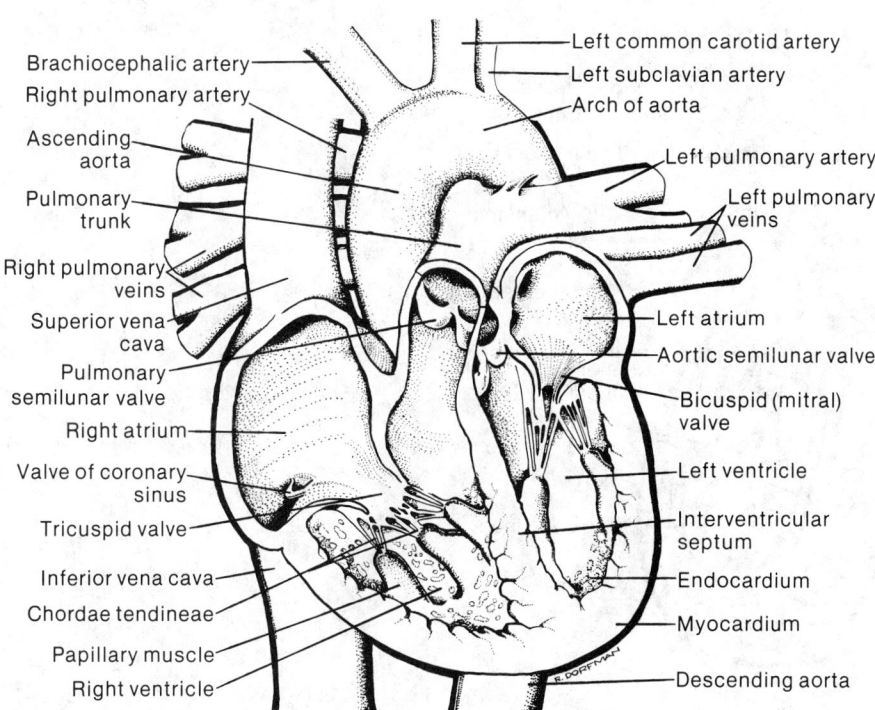

Figure 33-1. *The human heart contains four chambers and is enclosed by a double-layered pericardium.*

619

Unidirectional blood flow through the heart is maintained by two types of valves; the atrioventricular (AV) valves and the semilunar valves. The AV valves separate the atria from the ventricles. Each valve is composed of leaflets of cusps that attach to the papillary muscles of the ventricles by way of chordae tendinae. A tricuspid valve separates the right atrium from the right ventricle, while a bicuspid or mitral valve is found between the left atrium and left ventricle.

The semilunar valves consist of three symmetrical cuplike cusps secured onto a fibrous ring. The pulmonic valve is situated between the right ventricle and the pulmonary artery, while the aortic valve is located between the left ventricle and the aorta. Immediately above the free margins of the aortic valve are the sinuses of Valsalva and the openings of the coronary arteries.

The Conduction System

The muscle fibers of the myocardium exhibit the physiologic properties of excitability, conductivity, contractility, and autorhythmicity. The heart spontaneously and rhythmically generates impulses which are distributed along specialized conduction pathways to all parts of the myocardium, permitting synchronous contraction of the ventricular myocardium. Like all excitable tissues, the myocardium exhibits a refractory period following a contractile event. During such times of decreased reactivity, the myocardium is unresponsive to a second stimulus.

The rhythmic synchronized activity of the heart is maintained by a spontaneously active, highly specialized conduction system illustrated in Figure 33-2.

The cardiac impulse normally originates in the sinoatrial (SA) node, a small mass of specialized myocardial tissue located in the posterior wall of the right atrium, below the opening of the superior vena cava. This nodal tissue undergoes spontaneous depolarization, the frequency of which establishes the heart rate.

A second specialized mass of conduction tissue, the atrioventricular (AV) node, lies in the posterior right side of the interatrial septum near the opening of the coronary sinus. The AV node is continuous with a tract of conducting tissue termed the atrioventricular (AV) bundle or the bundle of His. Descending along the interventricular septum, the AV bundle divides into right and left bundle branches that descend along opposite sides of the

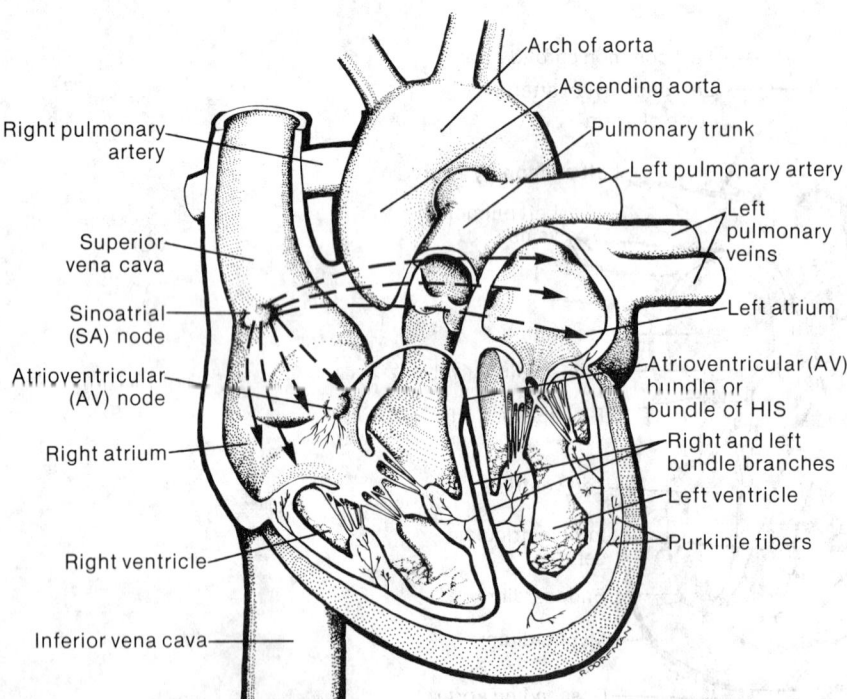

Figure 33-2. *A highly specialized conduction system maintains the rhythmic synchronized activity of the heart.*

interventricular septum and ultimately terminate in an extensive network of fine branches known as Purkinje fibers.

The spread of the cardiac impulse over the Purkinje fibers is extremely rapid, thereby ensuring virtually simultaneous excitation of the entire ventricular myocardium. Adjacent myocardial cells approximate at specialized junctions of low resistance, called intercalated discs. These intercalated discs facilitate the rapid spread of excitation from cell to cell, thereby allowing the heart to function as a synctium.

The SA node initiates a wave of depolarization which spreads rapidly throughout the atria. Upon reaching the AV node, the impulse is delayed briefly (0.08 seconds–0.12 seconds) before entering the ventricle to allow completion of atrial contraction. Excessive delay or failure of impulse conduction at the AV node results in heart block. Following the normally brief delay at the AV node, the cardiac impulse then proceeds along the bundle of His and its right and left bundle branches to the rapidly depolarizing fibers of the Purkinje network. The impulse sweeps through the ventricular myocardium from the endocardial (inner) to the epicardial (outer) surface. Muscular contraction follows the path of electrical depolarization.

While all parts of the conduction system can rhythmically discharge cardia action potentials, the cells of the SA node intrinsically depolarize at the highest frequency (60–100 times per minute), thereby setting the pace or rhythm of the heart. Hence the SA node is commonly termed the cardiac pacemaker. The discharge rate of the SA node may be affected extrinsically by the autonomic nervous system, as well as by certain hormones, drugs, and even temperature changes. If the SA node fails to generate rhythmic cardiac impulses, or if its frequency of depolarization becomes too slow, other sites, such as the AV node or AV bundle, may assume a pacemaker role.

Disturbances of normal cardiac rhythm, termed arrhythmias, result from altered myocardial electrophysiology. Cardiac arrhythmias may result from abnormal sites of impulse formation (ectopic foci), abnormal rates of impulse formation, or abnormal rates or routes of impulse conduction (see Chap. 34). A shortened myocardial refractory period may also contribute to the development of cardiac arrhythmias. Predisposing factors such as cardiac ischemia, electrolyte imbalance, excessive autonomic stimulation, and drug toxicity can cause changes in the electrophysiologic properties of the myocardium, which can result in the appearance of arrhythmias.

The Electrocardiogram

The electrocardiogram (ECG or EKG) is a graphic record of the electrical activity of the heart. A typical ECG (lead II tracing) is shown in Figure 33-3. The P wave depicts atrial depolarization, the QRS complex depicts ventricular depolarization, and the T wave depicts ventricular repolarization.

The P–R interval (normally 0.12 seconds–0.20 seconds) indicates conduction time through the atria and includes the delay at the AV node. Abnormal prolongation of the P–R interval, called first-degree heart block, indicates an abnormality of conductivity within the AV node.

The Q–T interval encompasses both ventricular depolarization and repolarization. The Q–T interval may be prolonged by some antiarrhythmic drugs such as quinidine.

The shape of the T wave can be altered by a variety of factors. For example, the T wave may be flattened or inverted by digitalis overdosage while hyperkalemia causes peaking and elevation of the T wave. To a skilled reader, the ECG offers valu-

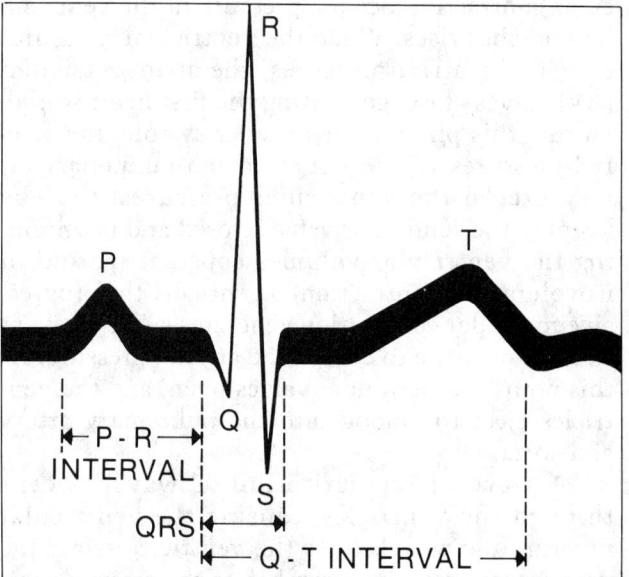

Figure 33-3. A typical electrocardiogram includes the following features: the P wave (depicting atrial depolarization), the QRS complex (depicting ventricular depolarization), and the T wave (depicting ventricular repolarization).

able information about cardiac rhythm (atrial and ventricular rates), conduction rate, chamber hypertrophy, presence of ischemia or infarction, ionic imbalance, and drug effects.

Cardiac Cycle

The cardiac cycle consists of an orderly sequence of interdependent electrical and mechanical events associated with one complete cycle of contraction (systole) and relaxation (diastole) of the heart. Electrical excitation of the heart precedes muscular contraction.

During diastole, the atrial and ventricular chambers are relaxed and the semilunar valves are closed. Blood that has entered the atria through the great veins flows passively from the atria to the ventricles through the open atrioventricular (AV) valves. The period of slow ventricular filling is termed diatasis, and it occurs in mid-diastole. During late diastole, a wave of depolarization (P waves) sweeps through the atria, leading to contraction of the atrial musculature. Atrial contraction (atrial systole) contributes approximately 30% to the ventricular blood volume.

Ventricular contraction follows the wave of depolarization through the ventricular conduction system and myocardium (QRS complex). As muscular contraction occurs, pressure in the ventricular chamber rises. When the ventricular pressures exceed the atrial pressures, the atrioventricular (AV) valves close, generating the first heart sound. During this phase of ventricular systole, the arterial pressures within the aorta and pulmonary artery exceed the ventricular pressures, thereby keeping the semilunar valves closed and maintaining the ventricular volumes constant (period of isovolumetric contraction). Eventually the progressive muscular contraction generates sufficient ventricular pressure to exceed the arterial pressure. At this point the semilunar valves open, and the ventricles eject the blood into the pulmonary artery and aorta.

A wave of repolarization (T wave) sweeps through the ventricles, causing the ventricular myocardium to relax. As the ventricles relax, the ventricular pressures drop below the arterial pressures of the pulmonary artery and aorta, causing the semilunar valves to close and generating the second heart sound.

With continued ventricular relaxation, the ventricular pressures fall below the atrial pressures, causing the atrioventricular (AV) valves to open. The venous blood that has been accumulating in the atria during ventricular systole now rapidly flows through the open atrioventricular valves into the ventricles. At rest, approximately 70% of ventricular filling takes place during this period of early diastole.

Cardiac Output

The work of the heart may be expressed in terms of cardiac output, that is, the volume of blood ejected from each ventricle in 1 minute. Cardiac output is the product of stroke volume and heart rate. The cardiac output of a resting adult falls in the range of 4.5 L to 5 L per minute; however, during exercise an average adult may achieve a cardiac output of 15 L to 20 L per minute.

Multiple factors contribute to the control of cardiac output. The stroke volume (the volume of blood ejected from a ventricle during a single contraction) is equal to the difference between the end-diastolic and end-systolic volumes. The end-diastolic volume represents the degree of ventricular filling, and it is determined by factors such as ventricular filling time, atrial contraction, myocardial distensibility, and the effective filling pressure. Normally, the bulk of ventricular filling occurs during early diastole, so that ventricular filling time is inversely related to the heart rate. At very rapid heart rates, the ventricular filling time is substantially reduced under these conditions, atrial contraction may contribute a greater proportion of the ventricular volume than at normal rates.

The effective filling pressure is directly related to the venous return, which is determined largely by the circulating blood volume and venous tone. Venous return to the heart is enhanced by the thoracicoabdominal pump and by skeletal muscle contraction. The pressure within the thorax is negative with respect to atmospheric pressure, whereas the pressure within the abdominal cavity is slightly positive. This pressure gradient, which becomes even greater during inspiration, favors the return of blood from the abdomen to the thorax. According to Starling's law of the heart, there is, within physiologic limits, a direct relationship between myocardial fiber length and the force of ventricular contraction. The degree of stretch of myocardial fibers before contraction is termed preload, and it is determined largely by the end-diastolic ventricular volume.

Increased preload will, within physiologic limits, increase the force of ventricular contraction and thereby increase the stroke volume. Excessive stretching of myocardial fibers will, however, ultimately lead to cardiac failure.

The end-systolic volume is primarily determined by the afterload and the contractility of the myocardium. The term afterload refers to the amount of tension that a ventricle must develop during systole in order to open the semilunar valve and to eject blood into the receiving artery. Afterload is a function of arterial pressure and ventricular size. As the size of a ventricle increases, the ventricle must develop a greater tension in order to generate a given pressure. Therefore, a dilated ventricle would have to develop a greater tension than a normal ventricle to generate the same systolic pressure.

Elevations in arterial pressure will also increase resistance to the outflow of blood from a ventricle, thereby necessitating an increase in ventricular tension. Chronic or excessive increases in afterload will adversely affect the cardiac output by elevating end-systolic volume, thereby reducing stroke volume.

The contractility of the myocardium is affected by a multitude of factors, including the metabolic state of the myocardium, physical and mechanical factors (Starling's law of the heart), nervous activity, hormones, and pharmacologic agents.

Factors that enhance the contractility of the myocardium are said to have a *positive inotropic effect* on the heart. Sympathetic stimulation, epinephrine, and isoproterenol, for example, enhance the contractile force of the myocardium and thereby increase the stroke volume and cardiac output. Cardiac output may also be altered by changes in heart rate.

Heart rate is responsive to extrinsic control by the autonomic nervous system. The sinoatrial (SA) and atrioventricular (AV) nodes are richly innervated by sympathetic and parasympathetic nerve fibers. The atria receive some innervation from each division of the autonomic nervous system, while the ventricles are innervated principally by sympathetic fibers. Sympathetic stimulation, through the release of norepinephrine from adrenergic nerve terminals, accelerates the heart rate and speed of cardiac impulse conduction. Sympathetic activation also can markedly enhance the force of myocardial contractility.

Parasympathetic nerves to the heart are anatomically vagal and functionally cardioinhibitory.

Vagal stimulation through mediation of the neurotransmitter acetylcholine produces a notable decrease in heart rate and speed of impulse conduction, and a slight reduction of cardiac contractility.

Congestive Heart Failure

Congestive heart failure (CHF) is a pathophysiologic state in which the heart is unable to pump enough oxygenated blood to supply the metabolic needs of the body's organs. Principal causes of CHF are hypertension, coronary artery disease, and valvular heart disease. Failure to eject a sufficient quantity of blood from the ventricles results in venous engorgement and leads to fluid leakage from the venous capillaries. Fluid accumulation in the tissues is responsible for many of the signs and symptoms of cardiac failure.

Heart failure may be *acute* or *chronic.* Acute heart failure is usually due to a myocardial infarction or, on rare occasions, a ruptured heart valve. Chronic heart failure is a gradually evolving loss of cardiac reserve.

Heart failure may be either *left-sided* or *right-sided.* Failure of the left ventricle is observed much more frequently than failure of the right ventricle and results in blood backing up into the pulmonary vessels. Right-sided failure results in systemic venous congestion and most often occurs secondary to uncorrected left ventricular failure, although it can also occur as a result of an increased pressure load on the right ventricle.

When the heart begins to fail, several compensatory mechanisms (Fig. 33-4) are brought into play to maintain an adequate cardiac output and perfusion of vital organs. Although this compensation may be successful for a period of time, and patients may not show signs and symptoms of deteriorating cardiac function for months or even years, eventually these compensatory mechanisms can no longer overcome the progressive loss of cardiac function. Once the compensatory mechanisms are no longer sufficient, the clinical signs and symptoms of heart failure become evident. It is unfortunate that many of the compensatory changes that served to delay the onset of symptomatic heart failure become counterproductive once ventricular function begins to deteriorate. For example, retention of sodium and water results in fluid overload, placing an additional burden on the failing heart. The increased heart rate does not allow for adequate ventricular filling, and cardiac output is thus reduced

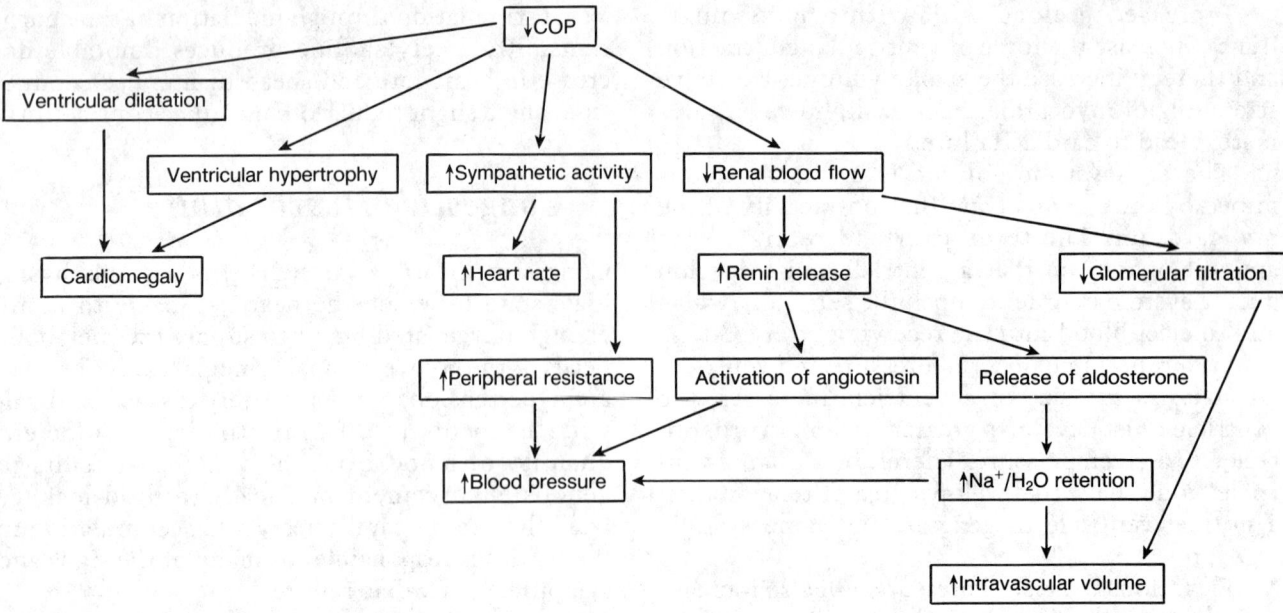

Figure 33-4. *Compensatory changes in congestive heart failure.*

further. Moreover, tachycardia increases the cardiac oxygen demand, decreasing the efficiency of the myocardium.

CLINICAL SIGNS AND SYMPTOMS OF HEART FAILURE

The clinical manifestations of progressive heart failure develop once the compensatory mechanisms become insufficient to overcome the deteriorating status of myocardial function. This phase is referred to as cardiac *decompensation.* Individual patient's signs and symptoms may vary, depending on the degree of decompensation, the speed with which cardiac function deteriorated (*i.e.,* acute vs chronic heart failure), and the heart chamber(s) involved (*i.e.,* left- vs right-sided failure). The clinical signs may be detected both by physical examination and laboratory testing (*e.g.,* x-rays). Table 33-1 lists the major symptoms associated with both left-sided and right-sided heart failure.

Left-sided failure is characterized primarily by cough, orthopnea (shortness of breath when lying down), dyspnea (feeling of breathlessness both at rest and upon exertion), tachypnea (rapid shallow breathing), wheezing, and rales (abnormal lung sounds). X-ray findings include an enlarged left ventricle and pulmonary venous distention. When the heart becomes excessively dilated, rapid ventricular filling causes blood to "splash" against the ventricle wall, creating a third heart sound termed

the S_3 gallop, heard soon after the second heart sound.

Right-sided heart failure can be characterized by a multiplicity of signs, most common of which are anorexia, nausea, bloating, nocturia, right

---

Table 33-1
Signs and Symptoms of Congestive Heart Failure

Left-sided	Right-sided
Cough	Anorexia
Hoarseness	Bloating
* Dyspnea	Nausea
At rest	* Nocturia
Exertional	Right upper abdominal
Paroxysmal nocturnal	pain
* Orthopnea	Peripheral edema
* Tachypnea	Proteinuria
* Cardiomegaly	Cyanosis
* Pulmonary rales	Daytime oliguria
Wheezing	* Hepatomegaly
* S_3 gallop rhythm	* Hepatojugular reflex
Hemoptysis	* Jugular venous
Cyanosis	distention
Pleural effusion	Splenomegaly
Cheyne-Stokes	Malabsorption
respiration	syndrome
	* Venous engorgement

* Most characteristic signs and symptoms.

upper abdominal pain (reflecting visceral and hepatic engorgement), and edema of the ankles and legs. Jugular vein distention is noted in cases of severe peripheral congestion. Other clinical and laboratory signs are listed in Table 33-1.

Treatment of congestive heart failure is first directed toward removing or ameliorating the cause if possible. Thus, valvular dysfunction should be surgically corrected and any underlying disease state (*e.g.*, thyrotoxicosis, pericarditis, anemia) should be treated. If correctable disease is not present, other nonpharmacologic measures are an important component of therapy. These include bedrest to decrease the workload on the heart and promote diuresis, sodium restriction, weight loss, and wearing of elastic stockings.

Pharmacologic intervention plays a major role in the management of congestive heart failure. A number of different strategies and different kinds of drugs have been employed successfully in the treatment of heart failure, including the cardiotonic (digitalis) glycosides, diuretics, vasodilators, and positive inotropic agents. Table 33-2 outlines the various measures that can be used in the management of congestive heart failure.

This chapter will focus primarily on the digi-

Table 33-2
Management of Congestive Heart Failure

Correction of Underlying Disease

1. Antihypertensives
2. Antithyroid drugs
3. Antianemic drugs
4. Repair of valvular dysfunction

Nonpharmacologic

1. Bedrest
2. Weight loss
3. Limited activity
4. Sodium restriction

Pharmacologic

1. Diuretics
2. Digitalis glycosides
3. Vasodilators
4. Positive inotropic agents (amrinone, milrinone)

talis drugs and the positive inotropic agents, such as amrinone. (Diuretics are discussed in Chap. 41, and the vasodilators are reviewed in Chaps. 35 and 36.)

Cardioactive Glycosides

The cardioactive glycosides encompass a group of both naturally occurring and semisynthetic steroidal compounds having qualitatively similar effects on cardiac function. Most of the commonly used drugs are derived from the leaves of either *Digitalis purpurea* or *Digitalis lanata*, both species of the foxglove plant. Because digitalis is the name of the principal botanic source of most of these agents, they are frequently referred to collectively as the *digitalis glycosides*.

While all the digitalis glycosides have similar pharmacologic effects on the heart, they differ with respect to onset and duration of action (due to differences in absorption, biotransformation, and extent of protein binding) as well as mode of administration. The drugs can be divided arbitrarily into three groups according to their routes of administration: oral only, parenteral only, and both oral and parenteral. The major characteristics of the

currently available digitalis glycosides, grouped according to their methods of administration, are listed in Table 33-3.

Digitalis Glycosides

Deslanoside, Digitalis Leaf, Digitoxin, Digoxin

The digitalis glycosides have long been employed in the management of congestive heart failure and for treating certain types of rhythm disorders. Although these drugs are quite effective in improving cardiac function, they are potentially hazardous substances and exhibit a rather narrow safety margin. Approximately 10% to 20% of patients taking any of the digitalis drugs will develop signs of tox-

Table 33-3
Characteristics of Digitalis Glycosides

	Onset		Maximum Effect		Plasma Half-Life	Extent of GI Absorption	Protein Binding
	IV	PO	IV	PO			
Parenteral							
deslanoside	10 min–30 min		60 min–90 min		30 h–36 h		20%–30%
Oral/Parenteral							
digitoxin	30 min–90 min	2 h–3 h	6 h–8 h	6 h–12 h	5–7 days	90%–100%	95%–97%
digoxin	10 min–30 min	1 h–2 h	2 h–4 h	4 h–8 h	32 h–40 h	60%–90%	20%–30%
Oral							
digitalis leaf		3 h–4 h		12 h–24 h	5–7 days	40%	Significant

icity, the most serious of which are disturbances in cardiac rhythm. A discussion of digitalis toxicity can be found later in this chapter.

Because the pharmacology of the various digitalis glycosides is similar, they will be reviewed as a group. Characteristics of the individual drugs are then given in Table 33-4. Throughout the discussion, the generic term digitalis will be used to refer to the group of drugs as a whole.

MECHANISM AND ACTIONS

The pharmacologic actions of the digitalis drugs are complex and in many cases dependent on the blood level of drug. The major cardiovascular effects of these agents are summarized in Table 33-5 (see p. 630) and will be reviewed below.

Force of Contraction

The principal action of the digitalis drugs responsible for their effectiveness in treating congestive heart failure (CHF) is their ability to increase the force of contraction of the heart. This effect is termed a positive inotropic action. Myocardial contractility is increased in both normal and failing hearts; consequently, there is significant improvement in cardiovascular performance and an associated decrease in the size of the ventricles. Although there is some increase in oxygen demand because of increased contractility, this is more than compensated for by the reduced oxygen demand that occurs as ventricular size is reduced. Therefore, in the failing heart, there is an overall increase in efficiency (work performed/energy required) as a result of this positive inotropic effect.

The mechanism by which the digitalis drugs increase the force of contraction of the heart is complex and incompletely understood. Most of the evidence indicates that increased intracellular calcium levels are responsible for facilitating the interaction of actin and myosin filaments to develop increased muscle tension. Activation of the actomyosin system occurs when calcium binds to the associated troponin–tropomyosin complex. Several theories have been proposed as to why digitalis drugs increase free calcium levels in myocardial cells. One theory is that these drugs inhibit the Na^+–K^+ ATPase enzyme found in cell membranes, thus reducing the energy available for the operation of the sodium–potassium pump. Because the pump functions to remove sodium from the cells following depolarization in exchange for potassium, inhibition of this pumping mechanism may lead to increased transmembrane exchange of sodium for calcium. Thus, calcium ions would enter myocardial cells at a greater rate, increasing the level of free calcium and enhancing the contractile mechanism. Increased release of calcium from intracellular binding sites on the sarcoplasmic reticulum may also result in improved contractility. A schematic outline of the mechanism of the inotropic action of the digitalis drugs is presented in Figure 33-5 (see p. 631).

Cardiac Output

The positive inotropic action of the digitalis agents results in an increased cardiac output, leading to improved pulmonary and systemic circulation and reduced edema. Increased output also *decreases* intraventricular volume and thus can reduce the size of the dilated heart chambers and lower oxygen demand. Improved cardiac output also diminishes reflex sympathetic activity, and decreased heart rate and venous tone are observed. Slowed heart rate, in turn, allows more time for the ventricles to fill during diastole, resulting in further increased stroke volume and consequently improved cardiac output.

Heart Rate

The heart rate is slowed by the digitalis drugs, although the degree of slowing is variable dependent on the underlying rate. That is, slowing is more dramatic when the initial rate is rapid, such as observed with tachycardia of congestive heart failure or atrial fibrillation. Because of their bradycardic action, the digitalis glycosides are said to possess a *negative chronotropic effect.* Several mechanisms contribute to the slowing of heart rate with these drugs. Digitalis reduces the rate of firing of SA nodal pacemaker cells, presumably by stimulating medullary vagal nuclei and increasing the sensitivity of pacemaker cells to acetylcholine, the vagal neurohormone. In addition, as discussed below, digitalis glycosides slow AV nodal conduction and prolong the AV refractory period, two other actions which also contribute to slowed ventricular rate.

It is important to note that although digitalis is used to treat atrial and nodal tachycardia and atrial fibrillation, the drug does *not* directly affect the atria. The slowing is manifested on the ventricles, which have been driven by the excessive atrial firing to beat too rapidly. The primary action of the cardiotonic glycosides is to stabilize the rapid, irregular ventricular rate, thus restoring efficient ventricular operation. Atrial fibrillation is *sometimes* converted to normal sinus rhythm by digitalis, but more often restoration of atrial function is accomplished by cardioversion or administration of an antiarrhythmic drug such as quinidine or procainamide.

Conduction Velocity/Refractory Period

Conduction velocity is decreased in both the AV node and to a lesser degree in the Purkinje system and ventricular muscle in a dose-dependent manner. In normal amounts, the drugs exert no significant effect on conduction velocity on the atrial musculature. Both the rate of rise and the amplitude of the action potential in AV nodal cells are reduced by digitalis.

The refractory period in AV nodal cells is prolonged with digitalis, again in a dose-dependent manner, whereas the refractory period of atrial, ventricular, and Purkinje cells is either shortened or unchanged.

The progressive slowing of conduction velocity and prolongation of the refractory period in the AV node seen with increasing drug concentrations results in the development of increased degrees of AV block.

The progressive AV block seen with increasing dosage can lead to a major manifestation of digitalis toxicity—disturbances in cardiac rhythm. The arrythmias that develop following toxic doses of these drugs also are attributable to a greatly lengthened AV refractory period, suppression of normal pacemaker activity, and increased ventricular automaticity. Many factors can predispose the heart to digitalis-induced arrhythmias, the most important being hypokalemia (reduced serum potassium levels), hypercalcemia (elevated serum calcium levels), catecholamine depletion, concurrent use of quinidine, systemic alkalosis, and renal or hepatic impairment. Decreased AV conduction velocity also contributes to the reduced heart rate seen with digitalis, and a rate below 60 beats/minute usually indicates that a reduction in dosage is necessary. The arrhythmogenic action of digitalis glycosides will be considered later in this chapter.

Excitability

Small doses of digitalis drugs do not markedly alter the excitability of the heart. Large doses can decrease the excitability of the SA node, but may increase the excitability of other areas of the heart, resulting in the development of ectopic foci and disordered cardiac rhythm.

Other

The digitalis drugs also have important actions on the kidney, although they are of an indirect nature. Diuresis is frequently observed in the patient with congestive heart failure given digitalis. This diuretic effect is thought to be secondary to the cardiodynamic effects of these drugs. That is, increased cardiac output improves renal blood flow and glomerular filtration leading to increased excretion of sodium and water. Tubular retention of sodium appears to be reduced as well, perhaps due in part to a redistribution of intrarenal blood flow, but primarily to a deactivation of the renin-angiotensin-aldosterone mechanism as a consequence of the improved renal hemodynamics. Renin release is diminished when blood volume through the renal vessels increases, and the secretion of aldosterone from the adrenal gland is subsequently slowed. (The renin-angiotensin-aldosterone mechanism is outlined in Chap. 35.)

Table 33-4
Cardioactive Glycosides

Drug	Preparations	Usual Dosage Range		Clinical Considerations
		Digitalizing	*Maintenance*	
deslanoside (Cedi-lanid-D)	Injection—0.2 mg/ml	IV—1.6 mg as one injection or in 0.8-mg portions IM—0.8 mg at each of two sites		Rapid-acting glycoside used in emergency treatment of acute pulmonary edema or supraventricular arrhythmia; maintenance therapy with an oral glycoside may be instituted within 12 h after deslanoside; injection should be over 5 min
digitalis leaf	Tablets—100 mg Capsules—100 mg	1.2 g total dose in several equal parts administered every 6 h	100 mg to 200 mg/day (range 30 mg–400 mg daily)	Extract of leaves of *Digitalis purpurea*, consisting mainly of gitalin, gitoxin, and digitoxin, the latter component primarily responsible for the therapeutic action of the mixture. Rarely used.
digitoxin (Cystodigin, Purodigin)	Tablets—0.05 mg, 0.1 mg, 0.15 mg, 0.2 mg	Rapid—0.6 mg initially, followed by 0.4 mg, then 0.2 mg at intervals of 4 h–6 h Slow—0.2 mg twice a day for 4 days	0.05 mg to 0.3 mg/day (usual-0.1 mg/day) Children—one-tenth digitalizing dose	Long-acting, potent glycoside mainly employed for maintenance rather than digitalizing therapy; slow onset and extremely long half-life make digitalization difficult; danger of accumulation toxicity is high with this drug; do not give full digitalizing doses to patients receiving other digitalis glycosides within the preceding 3 weeks. *(continued)*

USES

1. Treatment of congestive heart failure, especially low-output failure associated with depressed left ventricular function. Digitalis is most effective in treating congestive heart failure due to coronary heart disease, hypertensive heart disease, aortic stenosis or insufficiency, or mitral insufficiency. It is somewhat less effective in treating heart failure due to cardiomyopathy or cor pulmonale, and of relatively little value in patients with "high-output" congestive heart failure, such as that resulting from hyperthyroidism, infection, anemia, bronchopulmonary insufficiency or arteriove-

Table 33-4 (continued)
Cardioactive Glycosides

Drug	Preparations	Usual Dosage Range		Clinical Considerations
		Digitalizing	*Maintenance*	
digoxin (Lanoxin, Lanoxicaps)	Tablets—0.125 mg, 0.25 mg, 0.5 mg Capsules—0.05 mg, 0.1 mg, 0.2 mg Elixir—(pediatric) 0.05 mg/ml Injection—0.1, 0.25 mg/ml	*Oral:* Adults Rapid—0.5 mg–0.75 mg initially, followed by 0.25 mg–0.5 mg every 6 h–8 h to a total of 1 mg–1.5 mg Slow—0.125 mg–0.25 mg daily for 7 days Children Newborn—40 mcg/kg–60 mcg/kg 1 month–2 years—60 mcg/kg–80 mcg/kg 2 years–10 years—40 mcg/kg–60 mcg/kg *IV:* Adults—0.25 mg–0.5 mg initially, then 0.25 mg every 4 h–6 h to a total of 1 mg Children—25 mcg/kg–50 mcg/kg in divided doses	*Oral/IV:* Adults—0.125 mg to 0.5 mg/day (average 0.25 mg/day) Children—20% to 30% of the total digitalizing dose daily	Widely used for both rapid digitalization and maintenance therapy; little danger of accumulation because drug is rapidly excreted; capsules have greater bioavailability than tablets; therefore, 0.2-mg capsule is equivalent to 0.25-mg tablet and 0.1-mg capsule is equivalent to 0.125-mg tablet; drug can be given IM but absorption is erratic; do not give full digitalizing dose if patient has received a more slowly excreted cardiac glycoside within the last 2 weeks; administration with food slows rate of absorption but does not affect the total amount absorbed; closely monitor patients with renal insufficiency because drug is primarily excreted unchanged through the kidney; dosage may need to be decreased in patients receiving quinidine and various other drugs (see under Interactions). Administer by IV injection over 5 min or longer to prevent side-effects.

Table 33-5
Cardiovascular Actions of Digitalis Glycosides

1. Force of contraction—↑
2. Cardiac output—↑
3. Heart rate—↓
4. Conduction velocity
   AV conduction system—↓ (dose-dependent)
   Cardiac muscle—0(↑)
5. Refractory period
   AV conduction system—↑ (dose-dependent)
   Cardiac muscle—↓
6. Excitability of myocardium
   Small doses—0(↑)
   Large doses—↓
7. Blood pressure
   Venous—↓
   Systolic—slight↑
   Diastolic—slight↓
8. ECG
   P–R interval—prolonged
   Q–T interval—shortened
   S–T segment—depressed
   T wave—decreased or inverted
9. Diuretic action
   Renal blood flow and glomerular filtration—↑
   Aldosterone release (depression of renin-
      angiotensin mechanism)—↓
   Sodium reabsorption in renal tubules—↓

0, no effect; ↑, increased or prolonged; ↓, decreased or shortened; 0(↑), 0(↓), slight increase or decrease

nous fistula. Digitalis is also not beneficial in patients with mitral stenosis with normal sinus rhythm. *Note:* Patients with angina and a normal size heart may have their pains *exacerbated* by digitalis.

2. Treatment of certain cardiac arrhythmias, including atrial fibrillation, atrial flutter, and paroxysmal atrial tachycardia, especially where the ventricular rate is elevated. *Note:* Digitalis is not indicated in sinus tachycardia or premature systoles *in the absence of heart failure.*

3. Treatment of cardiogenic shock, especially if accompanied by pulmonary edema

ADMINISTRATION AND DOSAGE

The term *digitalization* has traditionally been applied to the use of loading doses of the digitalis drugs to achieve the desired plasma concentration of drug. Following administration, digitalis glycosides are distributed widely in the body, into both inactive reservoir (binding) sites and active recep-

tor sites in the myocardium. Therefore, it is necessary to administer sufficient drug to saturate the reservoir of nonspecific binding sites in order to achieve the desired effect at the active myocardial receptor sites. In acute congestive failure, large loading doses of drug may be administered *rapidly* to achieve the desired effect quickly. This process carries the risk of serious toxicity if the loading dose is excessive or if electrolyte disturbances (*e.g.,* hypokalemia) are present. Therefore, in less acute conditions, the patient should be loaded (digitalized) more slowly to reduce the risk of potential toxicity. Such slow loading can often be effectively accomplished by simply administering the small recommended maintenance doses from the beginning of therapy. Over time, reservoir saturation will occur. For example, most patients with chronic congestive heart failure begun on 0.125 mg/day to 0.25 mg/day of digoxin will achieve therapeutic plasma levels in 6 to 7 days with little risk of sudden cardiotoxicity. This method is especially useful for elderly patients who may become toxic if loading doses are used.

The maintenance dose is the amount of drug sufficient to replace the amount of drug eliminated between dosing, and therefore maintain a steady state plasma level of the drug. Maintenance doses, therefore, are smaller than rapid-loading doses (but often identical to slow-loading doses as indicated above) and must be individualized based on the patient's condition and the type of digitalis preparation used (long- or short-acting). Periodic clinical assessment is necessary to ensure that the optimal maintenance dose of the cardiac glycoside is being used, and that adverse reactions are kept at a minimum. Because there is often a difference between the rapid digitalizing and maintenance doses of some agents, both dosage ranges are given for each digitalis glycoside in Table 33-5.

Because the digitalis glycosides possess rather narrow safety margins, serum drug levels should be monitored closely. Although the *precise* relationship between serum levels and development of symptoms of intoxication varies from person to person, general guidelines are available. The normal therapeutic plasma level for digoxin is 0.5 to 2.0 ng/ml, and toxic effects are common above 2.5 ng/ml. With digitoxin, therapeutic plasma levels range from 14 to 26 ng/ml, with toxicity becoming prominant above 35 ng/ml.

Renal insufficiency can slow elimination of all digitalis glycosides (except digitoxin), and dosage must be adjusted downward accordingly. Digitoxin

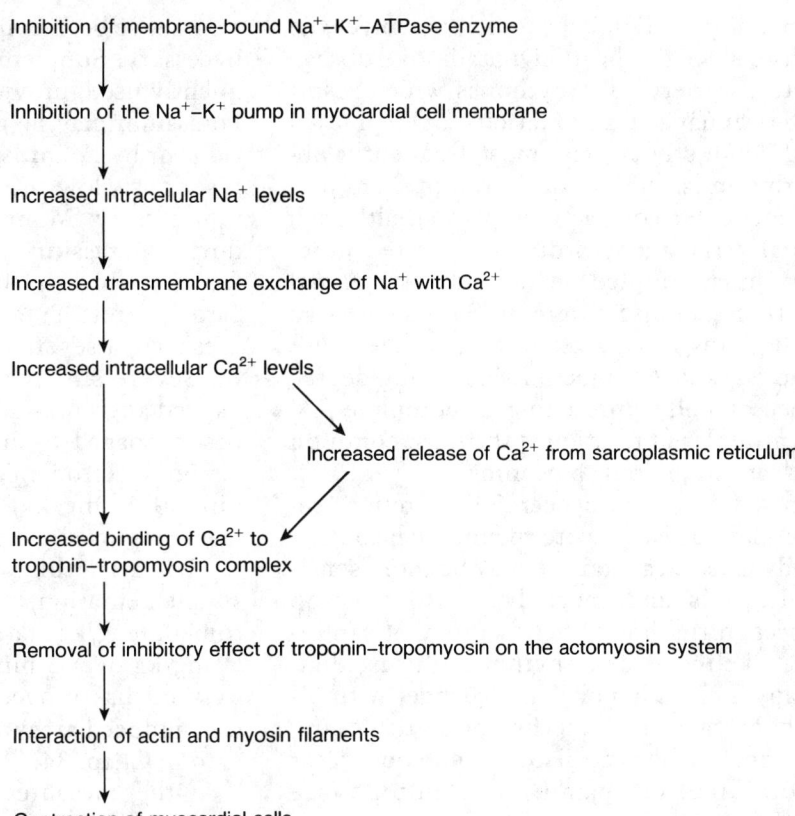

Inhibition of membrane-bound Na⁺–K⁺–ATPase enzyme

Inhibition of the Na⁺–K⁺ pump in myocardial cell membrane

Increased intracellular Na⁺ levels

Increased transmembrane exchange of Na⁺ with Ca²⁺

Increased intracellular Ca²⁺ levels

Increased release of Ca²⁺ from sarcoplasmic reticulum

Increased binding of Ca²⁺ to troponin–tropomyosin complex

Removal of inhibitory effect of troponin–tropomyosin on the actomyosin system

Interaction of actin and myosin filaments

Contraction of myocardial cells

Figure 33-5. Proposed mechanism of the inotropic action of the digitalis glycosides.

may be preferred, for this reason, in patients with significant renal impairment because it is largely metabolized in the liver. Renal clearance of digitalis glycosides may also be significantly reduced in elderly patients, and lower doses may be required.

FATE
The variations among the digitalis glycosides with respect to their pharmacokinetic properties are outlined in Table 33-3. Only digitoxin is highly lipid-soluble and almost completely absorbed orally. The extent of oral digoxin absorption ranges from 60% to 90% depending on dosage form (elixir or fluid-filled capsules or tablet) and the presence of food in the gut (decreases the rate but not the extent of absorption). The digitalis glycosides are widely distributed in the body, and high concentrations are found in the myocardium, intestine, liver, and kidneys. Digoxin crosses the blood–brain barrier, whereas penetration of digitoxin is poor. Digitoxin is highly (95%–97%) protein bound; digoxin is bound only 20%–30%. Digoxin and deslanoside are excreted by the kidneys largely as the unchanged drugs; approximately 30% of digoxin and 15% of digitoxin undergo enterohepatic recy-

cling. Digitoxin is largely inactivated by the liver (50%–70%) with the remainder being eliminated unchanged in the urine and feces. Plasma half-life is 32 hours to 40 hours for digoxin and 5 to 7 days for digitoxin.

SIDE-EFFECTS/ADVERSE REACTIONS
Digitalis can cause a variety of both cardiac and noncardiac toxic effects. In some cases, untoward reactions are noted in the early stages of therapy, and this most often indicates that the dosage is excessive. However, adverse reactions frequently develop upon prolonged therapy with doses that were initially well tolerated. The most characteristic *noncardiac* adverse reactions are anorexia, nausea, vomiting, diarrhea, drowsiness, headache, weakness, anxiety, precordial or facial pain, visual disturbances (greenish-yellow vision, blurring, "snowflakes") and mental depression. Occurrence of any of these symptoms must be viewed as an indication of possible impending digitalis toxicity, and the clinician should be notified immediately. More severe toxicity is marked by confusion, disorientation, seizures, EEG abnormalities, and delirium.

The major type of digitalis toxicity involves the drugs' actions on the heart. Digitalis overdosage can lead to a variety of arrhythmias which result from either enhanced automaticity or depressed AV nodal conductivity. The most frequently observed arrhythmias are unifocal or multiform premature ventricular contractions (PVCs), although paroxysmal atrial tachycardia, accelerated junctional rhythms, coupled beats, and paroxysmal nodal rhythms are also common. Following large doses of digitalis, excessive slowing of the pulse may be noted, and AV block of increasing degree occurs, occasionally proceeding to complete AV block. Ventricular fibrillation is the most common cause of death in digitalis poisoning.

Patients with acute myocardial infarction, severe pulmonary disease, acute rheumatic heart disease, or advanced heart failure may be more sensitive to digitalis and more likely to develop disturbances in rhythm. Other factors that can increase the likelihood of arrhythmias during digitalis therapy include hypokalemia (danger with diuretics), hypercalcemia, catecholamine depletion, alkalosis, renal or hepatic disease, and concurrent use of quinidine, verapamil, or nifedipine (see under Interactions).

Arrhythmias may occur even in the absence of other indications of digitalis toxicity, especially in patients with advanced heart failure, rheumatic carditis, and severe pulmonary disease. Therefore, noncardiac toxicity will not always serve as a warning of impending cardiac toxicity. Ventricular premature beats are a frequent initial toxic manifestation. In children, nausea, vomiting, diarrhea, neurologic and visual disturbances are *rarely* seen as initial signs of digitalis toxicity; atrial arrhythmias are most often the first indication of drug overdosage, and children must be closely monitored during digitalis therapy.

Less commonly encountered adverse reactions with digitalis drugs are pruritus, urticaria, fever, facial edema, joint pain, gynecomastia, eosinophilia, thrombocytopenia, and thromboembolic episodes.

Treatment of Digitalis Toxicity

In many cases of digitalis toxicity, discontinuation of the drug is sufficient to abolish the signs and symptoms of noncardiac toxicity especially if the plasma levels are not too high and if the drug is relatively short-acting (*e.g.*, digoxin).

With more severe toxic manifestations, such as arrhythmias, or if longer acting drugs such as digi-

toxin have been employed, other treatment may be necessary. Supplemental potassium salts are frequently used, provided renal function is adequate. Potassium may be given orally in less acute situations or by IV infusion when the serum potassium is seriously low and rapid control of the arrhythmia is necessary. Monitoring of the ECG is essential during potassium infusion to prevent potassium toxicity which itself can result in heart block and cardiac arrest. Potassium should not be used in the presence of severe heart block or renal failure.

Severe slowing of the heart rate due to advanced digitalis-induced heart block is probably best managed by insertion of a temporary transvenous electronic pacemaker. Alternately, IV atropine (0.01 mg/kg) or possibly isoproterenol has been employed to increase the heart rate.

For arrhythmias unresponsive to potassium supplementation, administration of either phenytoin (0.5 mg/kg at a rate of 50 mg/min) or lidocaine (1 mg/kg over 5 minutes followed by 10–50 mcg/kg/min) has proved effective in controlling digitalis-induced arrhythmias. These drugs are considered in Chap. 34.

Other measures that may be beneficial in treating digitalis overdosage include use of drugs such as cholestyramine, colestipol, or activated charcoal to bind unabsorbed digitalis drug in the intestines, preventing its enterohepatic recirculation and accelerating its excretion. A new approach to treating digitalis poisoning involves use of antigen-binding globulin fragments (Fab fragments) which combine in equimolar quantities with the digitalis glycosides (see below). Administration of Fab fragments has rapidly and completely reversed all signs and symptoms of digitalis overdosage and resulted in total recovery in over 80% of the cases treated.

CONTRAINDICATIONS AND PRECAUTIONS

Digitalis glycosides are contraindicated in the presence of ventricular tachycardia or fibrillation, severe myocarditis, hypersensitive carotid sinus syndrome, and signs and symptoms of digitalis toxicity (see under Side-Effects/Adverse Reactions). These agents should probably not be used in the presence of hypertrophic cardiomyopathy unless cardiac failure is severe. The drugs should be used *cautiously* in patients with Wolff-Parkinson-White syndrome (danger of fatal arrhythmias), Adams-Stokes syndrome, acute myocardial infarction, severe pulmonary disease, advanced heart failure, myxedema, incomplete AV block, chronic constrictive pericarditis, or hypertrophic subaortic stenosis. *Cautious use* is also indicated in the presence of hypoxia, hypomagnesemia, hypokalemia, hypercalcemia, renal or hepatic insufficiency, obesity, and in elderly, debilitated, pregnant, or nursing patients (drug enters breast milk).

Because many of the symptoms of congestive heart failure, such as anorexia, nausea, vomiting, and arrhythmias, may also be indications of digitalis intoxication, it is important to ascertain the cause of the symptoms (*i.e.*, disease-induced vs drug-induced) in order to effect proper management.

INTERACTIONS

1. Absorption of digitalis drugs may be reduced by antacids, cholestyramine resin, colestipol, laxatives, metoclopramide, neomycin, sulfasalazine, and combination chemotherapeutic regimens.
2. The effects of digitalis drugs can be reduced by agents that increase their metabolism, such as anticonvulsants, antihistamines, barbiturates, oral hypoglycemics, and phenylbutazone.
3. Toxic effects of cardiac glycosides (especially arrhythmias) may be increased by concurrent use of adrenergics, amphotericin, calcium salts, corticosteroids, diuretics (except potassium-sparing drugs), glucose, insulin, magnesium, pancuronium, reserpine, succinylcholine, and thyroid preparations.
4. Marked bradycardia may develop if digitalis drugs are given in combination with carbamazepine, guanethidine, phenytoin, propranolol, and reserpine.
5. Digitalis drugs may decrease the effects of oral anticoagulants and heparin.
6. Quinidine, nifedipine, and verapamil can increase serum levels of digoxin, possibly by displacement from tissue-binding sites or reduced renal clearance.
7. Increased plasma levels of digitalis drugs can also result from combined use with potassium-sparing diuretics, anticholinergics, tetracyclines, erythromycin, and hydroxychloroquine.
8. Digoxin serum levels may be reduced by penicillamine.

CARDIOACTIVE GLYCOSIDES AND THE ELDERLY PATIENT

The average older American, aged 70 or above, has three chronic diseases, at least one of which is probably cardiovascular in nature. As a result, elderly adults receive digitalis drugs more frequently than any other age group. Unfortunately, these same patients have a variety of body system changes which make them more susceptible to the drug's actions and consequently to the development of toxicity.

Normal physiologic changes in the elderly include reduced cardiac output, lowered contractile strength and efficiency of heart muscle, decreased body muscle mass, decreased body water, and reduced renal and liver function. These changes result in major differences in the way the elderly patient utilizes a normal dose of a digitalis drug.

Decreased cardiovascular efficiency will lengthen the time it takes for the drug to reach the cell site, leading to a slower digitalization. As a result, the elderly patient tolerates slower digitalization with lower doses much better than a rapid process.

Renal and liver function changes may increase the drug's half-life to almost twice its normal time from 30 to 40 hours to as much as 70 hours. Therefore the active drug will be in the body for much longer periods of time. Utilizing this principle, some patients on long-term digitalis therapy may be able to have drug-free holidays every week. For example, a patient on digoxin 0.125 mg PO daily might take the drug Sunday through Friday and skip a dose on Saturday every week.

Changes in body weight, water, and muscle mass occur slowly but may mean that the individual started and maintained on a dose of digoxin at age 50 will become toxic with that same dose at age 75. In fact, all the normal physiologic changes of aging increase the chance that the elderly person *will* develop digitalis toxicity over time unless carefully monitored. For this reason, any care plan developed for the elderly person taking a digitalis drug should consider the age, specific differences, and the increased risk of toxicity.

CARDIOACTIVE GLYCOSIDES AND THE PEDIATRIC PATIENT

Digoxin elixir is frequently the drug of choice in the treatment of children with congestive heart failure resulting from congenital anomalies, cardiac surgery, or pathologic murmurs. The age range of children who can receive this drug is wide, and long-term studies have demonstrated few harmful side-effects. However, the danger of drug toxicity is extremely high in children for a variety of reasons. Liver and kidney function are immature in the infant and toddler resulting in a slowed ability to metabolize and excrete digoxin. Fluid and electrolyte balance are more easily disrupted because of the child's high fluid volume. Consequently, toxicity resulting from low potassium levels may occur quickly, such as during an episode of flu-related diarrhea. In addition, periods of rapid growth will necessitate regular changes in digoxin dose to accommodate the increased load placed on the heart. Doses may have to be reduced again after the growth spurt subsides. Lastly, children of similar height and weight may vary in their responses to a similar dose; therefore, each child must be closely monitored throughout therapy.

Parents will usually express concern over the care of a child who requires such a dangerous medication. The nurse can help allay such fears by providing clear information on dosage and side-effects and by helping the parent to learn to give the dose exactly as prescribed. To ensure accuracy, some families prefer to use a tuberculin syringe instead of the drug medicine dropper to draw up the medication. The parents also need time to learn how to get the child to take the dose. (See Chap. 9 for strategies of administration for different age groups.)

■ Nursing Process for the Patient Receiving Cardiac Glycosides

□ ASSESSMENT

□ Subjective Data
A medication history is required. Digitalis preparations interact with many drugs including other heart medications and several over-the-counter preparations. Notable offenders include antacids and some allergy and cold relief medications.

A thorough history of the illness leading to use of digoxin is important. The nurse needs to find out how the illness has affected the patient's activity. Heart disease may affect the individual's ability to move about, walk or play, sleep, and do self-care activities. Changes in these parameters can later be used to measure drug effectiveness. A history of other illnesses, such as hypothyroidism, chronic respiratory disease, and renal or liver disease, may require drug dosage adjustments. Knowledge of such problems may decrease the chance of later drug toxicity. A diet history may also be done if sodium restriction is anticipated.

The nurse also needs to assess the willingness of the patient and family to participate in the drug regimen. Drug toxicity increases in a patient who is forgetful or ambivalent about taking the drug. Because the safety margin for digoxin is narrow, following the regimen is essential.

□ Objective Data
A complete physical assessment with careful attention to cardiovascular status is important. Apical pulse should be auscultated while the radial pulse is palpated before each dose of digoxin is given. If a difference between them is noted, each should be counted separately and the smaller number subtracted from the larger. The difference between them is called the pulse deficit. Any number greater than 10 indicates serious problems in perfusion may occur as a result of dangerous arrhythmias. This assessment parameter is important, initially, for baseline information and is also useful throughout care to monitor digitalization and later to watch for signs of toxicity. In addition, heart rate and rhythmicity should be noted and blood pressure should be taken.

To provide a baseline of information about fluid volume the patient should be weighed. Extremities and sacral area should be palpated for evidence of edema and a notation made if pitting is present. Intake and output ratios should be carefully monitored throughout therapy. Respiratory assessment is also important. Degree of breathing difficulty, rate and evidence of cough or abnormal breath sounds (rales) should be recorded. Patients should be observed for jugular venous distention.

Diagnostic data may include a complete ECG as well as more sophisticated tests such as ultrasound and measurements of cardiac output. Laboratory tests should include electrolyte studies of potassium, magnesium, and calcium because low levels of all of these predispose the patient to digitalis toxicity. Renal and hepatic function studies are also important. Patients who may have received a digitalis drug recently may require a serum drug level to assist in determining the initial dose of a digitalis preparation.

□ NURSING DIAGNOSES
Actual nursing diagnoses for the patient beginning therapy with cardiac glycoside may include:
   Knowledge deficit related to the drug, its administration, and side-effects
   Anxiety related to concerns about the drug's ability to improve exercise tolerance and reduce symptoms
Potential nursing diagnoses related to side-effects and the *early* warning signs of toxicity may include:
   Alteration in cardiac output related to arrhythmia
   Alteration in comfort related to

gastrointestinal distress and potentially
leading to electrolyte imbalance
Sensory perceptual alterations in vision
related to color changes and halos (not
easily identified in children)

□ *PLAN*

For the patient beginning drug therapy the goals
may be:

1. To successfully digitalize the patient to achieve
   therapeutic drug levels
2. To monitor body responses to the drug in order
   to identify early signs of toxicity

For the patient on long-term drug therapy at
home the goals may be to teach the patient:

1. The action of digoxin and its effect on the patient's problem
2. Safe drug-taking techniques
3. Symptoms of side-effects, how to prevent and
   manage them, and which ones to report
4. The need for follow-up clinic visits and laboratory evaluations
5. How to restrict sodium intake
6. How to self-monitor for signs and symptoms
   of congestive heart failure

□ *INTERVENTION*

Early in therapy the clinician will not know the
exact dose of digitalis preparation needed to
achieve therapeutic levels so careful monitoring is
essential. A flow sheet may be useful for serum
drug levels, ECG results, blood pressure, and pulse
as well as signs and symptoms of adverse responses. Vital signs ought to be taken at least four
times a day when the slow-loading method is employed and more frequently if rapid digitalization
is necessary. Serum levels should be drawn about 6
hours after each daily dose to ensure that drug
equilibrium has been achieved between the serum
and tissue (reservoir sites). Patients who are receiving rapid digitalization should have continuous
ECG monitoring. A therapeutic digoxin level is 0.8
to 2 ng/ml in adults. Drug levels are considered
toxic at greater than 2.5 ng/ml.

Once the patient has been digitalized, plans
may be made for discharge. Formulations of digitalis drugs may vary between manufacturers so patients need to know which one they are taking.
Once a particular formulation is selected, efforts
should be made not to change it to reduce the
chance of toxicity. This can become a problem if
the patient changes pharmacies or is admitted to a
nursing home or another hospital.

Because digitalis has such a narrow safety margin, patients must find a reliable method by which
to remember to take the drug and learn to take it
the same time every day. Drug calendars, weekly
pill boxes, and other memory joggers may help. Patients must also be advised not to "double up"
when they miss a dose. They must clearly understand that, while digitalis is a "heart medicine," it
is not intended to relieve anginal pain and should
not be taken if pain occurs. Patients have been
treated for digitalis toxicity because they wrongly
assumed the drug was to be taken the same way as
nitroglycerin, at the onset of pain.

Gastric distress, a common side-effect of digoxin, can usually be eliminated by taking the drug
with food. If the symptom is not alleviated, patients should not take antacids because these drugs
will interfere with digitalis absorption. Instead, the
symptoms should be reported because persistent
gastric upset, especially nausea and diarrhea, may
be an early warning sign of toxicity.

Arrhythmias or bradycardia are one of the early
warning signs of digitalis toxicity in all age groups.
As a result, most acute care facilities have a written
policy that digoxin be held and the physician notified if the pulse rate is less than 60 or irregular. The
patient or family should learn a pulse-taking technique before discharge to monitor this side-effect
at home. In teaching this skill, the nurse must emphasize the following points:

- Use a watch with a second hand or a digital
  clock with a stop-watch type mechanism.
- Use an anatomical site where the pulse is
  strong such as the radial, carotid, or femoral
  artery.
- Record the rate in the same place each day
  (*i.e.*, on a calendar) so pulse range is known.
- Call the physician if the rate is less than 50,
  greater than 100, or difficult to count because
  of irregularity in rhythm.

Most patients can be taught to be more aware
of their heart beat and to find it even if they cannot
count it. Such awareness will help them recognize
changes which should always be reported.

The symptoms of digitalis toxicity vary among
different age groups. Infants and young children
may exhibit arrhythmias such as supraventricular
tachycardia, AV block, or sinus bradycardia, vomiting and poor feeding. The elderly adult may develop confusion and depression symptoms which
are frequently mistaken as "signs of old age."
Consequently, the nurse must be alert to mental
changes in a previously alert older patient. Arrhythmias may not develop in the older patient

until late in the toxicity syndrome when they become difficult to treat. Other classic symptoms of toxicity seen in adults include changes in color vision and appearance of halos around lights, bradycardia, arrhythmias, and nausea or vomiting.

A simple way to detect digoxin toxicity is to monitor potassium levels, serum digoxin levels, and renal function. Consequently, it is important that the patient keep follow-up appointments as outlined by his care giver.

The patient also needs to know that illness might affect the drug level. Vomiting or diarrhea can result in electrolyte imbalances or decreased drug absorption leading to either drug toxicity or acute congestive failure. The physician should be notified any time a patient on digitalis becomes ill.

The patient in congestive heart failure is usually taught to limit sodium intake to reduce water retention. If the patient is overweight, weight loss will be encouraged to reduce the workload on the heart. Frequently, the patient will also be treated with diuretics (see Chap. 41) to facilitate loss of water retention edema. These drugs deplete the body of potassium, an important electrolyte for digitalis utilization. Therefore, the patient may need a potassium supplement and certainly needs to eat foods high in potassium, such as bananas, orange juice, and apricots. If this combination of drugs is used, the patient also needs to learn the early signs of hypokalemia—drowsiness, muscle weakness, anorexia—and that he must contact the physician immediately if they occur.

If digitalis toxicity develops or is suspected, the drug must be immediately discontinued and the physician notified. Care will center around management of arrhythmias, monitoring of ECG, and accelerating drug excretion. Treatment was outlined specifically earlier in this chapter.

□ EVALUATION
Most patients early in digitalis therapy report an improved sense of well-being. They may notice weight loss, less extremity edema, better urine output, easier breathing, and improved activity tolerance. All of these, in addition to a slowed heart rate, are objective parameters against which to measure the drug's effectiveness. In addition, the nurse can review the number of pills left in a prescription on clinic visits, the serum drug levels, and the patient's report of drug side-effects to determine compliance. However, it is important to remember that digitalis toxicity can occur because the drug accumulates in the body, so periodic blood studies and consistent follow-up are extremely im-

portant. Nursing Care Plan 33-1 summarizes the nursing process for the patient receiving cardiotonic glycosides.

Digoxin Immune Fab-Ovine
(Digibind)

Digoxin immune Fab consists of antigen-binding fragments (Fab) derived from antidigoxin antibodies produced in immunized sheep. The antibodies are papain-digested, and digoxin-specific Fab fragments are then isolated and purified. The preparation contains 40 mg/vial of lypophilized powder for reconstitution. Each vial binds approximately 0.6 mg of digoxin (or digitoxin).

Digoxin immune Fab is used to treat potentially life-threatening digoxin (or digitoxin) intoxication. In most instances, improvement in signs and symptoms of intoxication are noted within 1 hour. The drug is administered IV over 30 minutes, but may be given as a bolus injection if cardiac arrest is imminent. Dosage guidelines are provided with the drug packaging and vary with the amount of digoxin (or digitoxin) to be neutralized. If this value is not readily obtainable, administration of 20 vials (800 mg) is usually adequate to treat most life-threatening intoxications in adults and children. Larger doses have a more rapid onset of action than smaller doses but are associated with a greater likelihood of febrile or allergic reactions. Hypokalemia may also occur, and withdrawal of the effects of digoxin may result in reduced cardiac output and worsening of congestive heart failure.

Amrinone
(Inocor)

Amrinone is the first of a new class of positive inotropic agents that are structurally and mechanistically unlike the digitalis glycosides. Amrinone and its close structural analogue milrinone increase myocardial contractility and exert a peripheral vasodilatory action and can provide additional symptomatic relief of congestive heart failure in patients not satisfactorily controlled by conventional therapy (i.e., digitalis drugs, diuretics, vasodilators). Due to its potential to cause thrombocytopenia, however, amrinone is not considered a first-line drug.

MECHANISM AND ACTIONS
The precise mechanism responsible for the positive inotropic action of amrinone is not completely es-

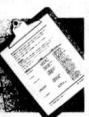

Nursing Care Plan 33-1
The Patient Receiving Cardiotonic Glycosides

Assessment

Subjective Data

1. Medication history
   a. Refer to Interactions section to formulate pertinent questions. Multiple potentially adverse interactions exist.
   b. Current use of digitalis or use within the last 3 weeks must be noted
   c. Allergies/hypersensitivity

2. Medical history
   a. Refer to Contraindications and Precautions section for disorders that should be highlighted
   b. Check for preexisting conditions that may precipitate adverse reactions, such as severe cardiac trauma, myocardiopathy, constrictive pericarditis, intermittent complete heart block, severe respiratory disease, myxedema, fluid or electrolyte imbalance, renal or hepatic dysfunction
   c. Current pregnancy or lactation
   d. Progress of symptoms that led patient to seek treatment

3. Personal history/compliance issues
   a. Patient's understanding of his condition; current symptoms
   b. Personal resources to manage treatment
   c. Financial resources and supportive network

Objective Data

1. Physical assessment highlighting
   a. Cardiovascular status: heart rate, rhythm, pulse deficit, blood pressure, cardiac output (L/min), urinary output, and presence of edema
   b. Respiratory status: rate, breath sounds, presence of cyanosis
   c. Neurologic status: mental acuity, psychomotor function
   d. Height and weight (especially in children)

2. Laboratory/diagnostic data
   a. ECG
   b. Arterial blood gases
   c. Serum electrolytes
   d. Renal and hepatic function studies
   e. Serum digitalis levels if patient has received drug within 3 weeks

Nursing Diagnosis	Expected Client Outcome	Intervention
Knowledge deficit related to drug action, correct administration, potential side-effects, and potential adverse drug interactions	Will verbalize knowledge of reasons for taking drug, how to take it, how to monitor pulse rate, signs of improvement from drug, the relationship of diet and exercise, symptoms of toxicity, and what drugs to avoid	Teach the patient the action of digitalis, how it slows and strengthens the heart rate. Encourage patient to take the drug at the same time every day. Teach the patient to take heart rate for 1 minute, and record number on a flow sheet (calendar) for reference before each dose. If rate is below 60 beats/min in adults or 100 beats/min in young children, physician should be notified *before* dose is taken. Monitor and teach patient to observe the signs of drug effectiveness such as low heart rate, low respiratory rate, low weight, low edema, increased exercise tolerance, and improved mental status.

(continued)

Nursing Care Plan 33-1 (continued)
The Patient Receiving Cardiotonic Glycosides

Nursing Diagnosis	Expected Client Outcome	Intervention
Knowledge deficit related to drug action, correct administration, potential side-effects, and potential adverse drug interactions (continued)		Encourage sodium restriction in diet.
		Compile a list of drugs patient should avoid. Encourage patient to contact physician before taking any new drug.
		Teach patient the early symptoms of drug toxicity as described below and to contact the physician immediately if any should occur.
		Encourage increase in exercise as tolerated and as prescribed.
		Keep drug out of reach of children. Store securely to prevent accidental poisoning.
Potential alteration in cardiac output: decreased, related to dysrhythmias from drug toxicity	Normal sinus rhythm is maintained and serum drug level remains within normal limits	Monitor ECG during digitalization process. Encourage patient to have follow-up ECGs and serum drug level determinations as prescribed.
		Encourage patient to monitor and report any decrease in heart rate immediately. The most common drug-induced dysrhythmia in adults and children is sinus bradycardia. Adults may also exhibit PVCs; children may develop sinus arrest.
		Emergency equipment and drugs should be on hand, such as lidocaine, atropine, defibrillator, and emergency pacing equipment to provide life support if cardiac arrest occurs.
	Serum potassium level will remain within normal limits	Be aware that dysrhythmias are more likely if potassium level drops below normal. Encourage patient to eat potassium-rich foods, take K^+ supplement as prescribed, and have follow-up serum K^+ levels determined as prescribed.
Potential alteration in comfort: GI distress related to drug toxicity	Gastrointestinal symptoms are absent and serum drug level remains within normal limits	Teach patients to report early anorexia, nausea, vomiting, or abdominal discomfort, which are early warning signs of toxicity.
		Report poor feeding in babies or young children because this may be the only early warning sign.
Potential sensory–perceptual alterations: changes in vision and perception as well as confusion related to drug toxicity	Vision, mental acuity will remain normal	Teach patient to report any vision changes, blurred vision, changes in color vision, feeling of isolation, or confusion because these are early signs of toxicity and may be the first ones seen in the elderly.

(continued)

Nursing Diagnosis	Expected Client Outcome	Intervention
Potential sensory–perceptual alterations: changes in vision and perception as well as confusion related to drug toxicity (continued)		Serum drug level should be drawn, drug dose withheld, and physician notified immediately.
Anxiety related to diagnosis and effect on life	Will verbalize concerns and help establish realistic goals	Provide information to keep patient/family informed of progress.
		Help patient/family establish realistic goals on diet, weight, exercise based on condition and effect of drug.
		Help patient establish a network of support through family, friends, or a support group to help cope with life stresses that result from a chronic illness.

tablished. The drug is *not* a beta-adrenergic agonist, nor does it inhibit the activity of Na^+–K^+ ATPase, as do the digitalis glycosides. It appears to inhibit myocardial cell phosphodiesterase, the enzyme responsible for inactivating cyclic AMP, thus increasing cellular levels of cyclic AMP which facilitate the contractions of myocardial muscle cells. Amrinone also exhibits a relaxant effect on vascular smooth muscle, thereby reducing both preload and afterload (see review of cardiac physiology at the beginning of this chapter). Increased inward calcium flux during the action potential has also been postulated as a contributory mechanism for amrinone. Effects noted following amrinone administration include enhanced myocardial contractility *even after full doses of digitalis*, increased cardiac output, reduced ventricular filling pressure and pulmonary capillary wedge pressure, increased left ventricular ejection fraction, and improved exercise capacity. There is little change in heart rate or arterial pressure.

USES

1. Short-term management of congestive heart failure in patients who have not responded adequately to digitalis drugs, diuretics, and vasodilators

ADMINISTRATION AND DOSAGE

Amrinone is currently available for IV administration only. The drug is marketed as 20-ml ampules containing 5 mg/ml as the lactate salt. It may be given as supplied or diluted in normal saline (*not* dextrose-containing solutions) to a concentration of 1 to 3 mg/ml.

The initial dose is 0.75 mg/kg by IV bolus over 2 to 3 minutes, followed by a maintenance infusion of 5 mcg/kg/min to 10 mcg/kg/min to a total daily dose of 10 mg/kg (including bolus). An additional bolus injection may be given 30 minutes after the initial bolus, if needed. Plasma concentrations with this dosing schedule are approximately 3 mcg/ml.

FATE

Following IV administration, the peak effect, as measured by increased cardiac output, occurs within 10 minutes. The duration of action is largely dose-dependent and ranges from 30 minutes to 2 hours. Amrinone is variably protein-bound (10%–50%). The drug is metabolized by conjugative pathways and is primarily excreted in the urine as both unchanged drug and metabolites. The mean elimination half-life is 3.5 hours, although patients with congestive heart failure show considerable interpatient variation in half-life (3 hours–15 hours).

SIDE-EFFECTS/ADVERSE REACTIONS

The most important untoward reactions with IV amrinone are arrhythmias (3%) and thrombocytopenia (2.5%) especially with prolonged therapy. Other adverse effects associated with amrinone therapy are nausea, vomiting, anorexia, abdominal pain, hepatotoxicity, hypotension, fever, chest pain, burning at injection site, and hypersensitivity. Alterations in liver enzyme values have occurred during therapy and asymptomatic platelet count reductions (less than 150,000/mm³) may be noted. If liver enzymes are elevated or platelet count is reduced *together* with clinical symptoms,

Table 33-6
Vasodilators Useful in Congestive Heart Failure

Drug	Administration/Dosage	Remarks
hydralazine (Apresoline)	Oral—50 mg–100 mg every 6 h to a maximum of 2400 mg/day	Major effect is on arterial resistance vessels. Causes marked reduction of systemic and pulmonary vascular resistance and significant increase in cardiac output in patients with CHF. May improve renal flow. Beneficial effect in mitral insufficiency and reduced left ventricular function. See Chapter 35.
minoxidil (Loniten)	Oral—10 mg–40 mg daily in divided doses	Similar to hydralazine in action. Potent arteriolar vasodilator. Not approved for treatment of congestive heart failure. Sodium/water retention is a common problem. See Chapter 35.
phentolamine (Regitine)	IV—0.2 mg/min–2.0 mg/min by slow infusion	Alpha-adrenergic blocker with predominant dilatory effect on arteriolar-resistance vessels. Decreases arterial impedance and improves cardiac output. Effects begin within 15 min after start of infusion and persist for 45 min–60 min after termination. Reflex tachycardia limits its usefulness. See Chapter 16.
nitroglycerin	IV—10 mcg/min by slow infusion; increase by 10 mcg/min every 5 min until desired effect. Average dose is 50 mcg/min–100 mcg/min Ointment—1–4 inches applied every 4 h–6 h	Nitroglycerin and isosorbide are nitrates that can markedly reduce left ventricular filling pressure by dilating venous capacitance vessels. IV nitroglycerin is useful in acute situations (e.g., following myocardial infarction) while topical nitroglycerin and oral or sublingual isosorbide are used in chronic congestive heart failure. Improvement in cardiac output is generally slight. Headache is a common side-effect early in therapy, but reflex tachycardia is infrequent. See Chapter 36.
isosorbide (Isordil)	Oral—20 mg–80 mg four times a day Sublingual—5 mg–20 mg every 3 h–4 h	
captopril (Capoten)	Oral—Initially: 12.5–25 mg 3 times/day; usual maintenance range is 75 mg/day	Oral antihypertensives that act to inhibit the activation of angiotensin and the formation of aldosterone. In congestive heart failure, left ventricular filling pressure is reduced, mean
enalapril (Vasotec)	Oral—5 mg–20 mg twice a day	
lisinopril (Prinivil, Zestril)	Oral—20 mg–40 mg once a day	

(continued)

the drug should be discontinued. If these changes occur *in the absence* of clinical symptoms, consider the benefit-to-risk ratio in deciding whether to discontinue therapy.

CONTRAINDICATIONS AND PRECAUTIONS

There are no known absolute contraindications to amrinone. *Cautious use* is mandated in patients with aortic or pulmonic valvular disease, hypertrophic subaortic stenosis, arrhythmias, thrombocytopenia, hypotension, and following an acute myocardial infarction or vigorous diuretic therapy. Safety for use in pregnant or nursing women and in children has not been established.

INTERACTIONS

1. Additive hypotensive effects may occur with concurrent use of disopyramide.

Table 33-6 (continued)
Vasodilators Useful in Congestive Heart Failure

Drug	Administration/Dosage	Remarks
captopril (Capoten) enalapril (Vasotec) lisinopril (Prinivil, Zestril) (continued)		arterial pressure is lowered, and cardiac output is increased. Heart rate remains essentially unchanged. Drug appears most useful in cases where systemic vascular resistance is quite high. See Chapter 35.
nitroprusside (Nipride, Nitropress)	IV—Initially, 10 mcg/min by slow infusion. Increase by 5 mcg/min every 5 min until desired effect. Maximum recommended dose is 400 mcg/min.	Potent vasodilator of both arterial and venous vessels used for rapid reduction of systemic vascular resistance in *acute* congestive heart failure. Decreases arterial impedance and increases venous pooling. Cardiac output is slightly increased but arterial blood pressure is relatively unaffected because increased stroke volume counterbalances decreased peripheral resistance. Effects occur within 2 min–5 min after beginning infusion and cease quickly on termination of infusion. Abrupt discontinuation of infusion must be avoided because rebound hemodynamic changes can occur (increased blood pressure, increased ventricular filling pressure, reduced cardiac output). See Chapter 35.
prazosin (Minipress)	Oral—0.5 mg–1.0 mg initially. Increase gradually to desired response. Average dosage range is 2 mg–7 mg four times a day.	An alpha-adrenergic blocker exhibiting a balanced vasodilator effect on arterial resistance and venous capacitance vessels. Reduces systemic resistance, decreases left ventricular filling pressure, increases cardiac output and improves exercise tolerance and ventricular function. Useful in long-term management of congestive heart failure. Tolerance occurs in many patients and may necessitate a temporary change in drugs, such as to nitrates plus hydralazine. See Chapter 35.

NURSING CONSIDERATIONS

If amrinone is given as a bolus in a peripheral IV, it should be diluted with normal saline because the drug is extremely irritating; in a central line, irritation is not a problem. Amrinone should not be given through the same IV line as other drugs because the danger of precipitation secondary to physical incompatibility is extremely high, especially with furosemide.

The patient should be instructed to report any untoward symptoms such as chest pain or gastrointestinal distress. An additional danger, the development of thrombocytopenia, must be closely monitored. Platelet counts should be performed regularly and any level below 100,000/mm^3 reported immediately. The patient should also be observed for any signs of unusual bleeding such as petechiae, purpura, hematuria, or melena. A periodic ECG should also be performed to monitor arrhythmias.

Vasodilators

Although diuretics and digitalis glycosides are generally considered the mainstays in the treatment of most forms of congestive heart failure, a significant number of cases are refractory to these drugs. In such instances, use of a vasodilator frequently can significantly improve hemodynamic performance. Drugs eliciting vasodilation that are used in congestive heart failure can be categorized based on their principal sites of action as

- *Arteriodilators* (hydralazine, minoxidil, phentolamine)
- *Venodilators* (isosorbide, nitroglycerin)
- *Combined Arterio-Venodilators* (captopril, enalapril, nitroprusside, prazosin)

These drugs all have other indications, predominately as antihypertensive or antianginal agents, and will be reviewed in detail in the appropriate chapter of this book. An overview of their applicability in the treatment of congestive heart failure is presented in Table 33-6. Choice of an agent is usually determined by the patient's signs and symptoms. Thus, for heart failure associated with high ventricular filling pressures and symptoms of pulmonary congestion such as dyspnea, venodilators such as nitrates are quite beneficial in lowering the filling pressure by decreasing venous return through increasing venous capacitance. Reduced left ventricular output generally is benefited most by an arteriodilator, which lowers resistance to ventricular ejection (*i.e.*, afterload). Many forms of congestive heart failure, however, are characterized by both increased ventricular filling *and* reduced cardiac output and are probably best managed by the combined arterio-venodilators.

Although vasodilators have generally been viewed as *adjunctive* therapy in managing congestive heart failure, there is increasing support for their application as first line drugs in certain types of heart failure, particularly where sinus rhythm is normal or the left ventricle is small, in which case digitalis may not be an appropriate choice.

CASE STUDY

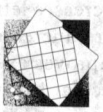

Roy Evert, aged 62, recently retired from the railroad and lives with his wife of 40 years in their two-story home. Mr. Evert has a 20-year history of hypertension; he is currently being treated with methyldopa, 750 mg daily, and hydrochlorothiazide, 50 mg daily. In the past 4 years he has had three episodes of hypertensive crisis for which he was admitted to the hospital. These episodes usually occurred when he forgot to take his medication for a period of time.

Mr. Evert is about 35 lb overweight and has gained 15 lb since retiring 5 months ago. He states he enjoys his wife's cooking too much to worry about losing weight.

Mrs. Evert brings her husband to the hypertension clinic. He complains of swelling of his hands and feet and states he can hardly climb the stairs to bed at night without getting short of breath. Once in bed he must sleep propped on three pillows to breathe comfortably and even that is not always helpful. He came to the clinic after a particularly restless night. He swears he had not missed a dose of his medication since he retired. Mrs. Evert verifies this.

Mr. Evert's blood pressure is 160/120, his pulse is 110 and irregular, his skin moist, his color pale, and respirations are 40. He is admitted to the hospital with a diagnosis of congestive heart failure.

In addition to bedrest and oxygen, the physician decides to treat Mr. Evert with digoxin, 0.25 mg PO daily, and furosemide, 40 mg PO bid, in addition to the methyldopa he was taking at home.

Discussion Questions

1. Is Mr. Evert's dose of digoxin considered a "digitalizing dose"? Why do you think the physician ordered this dose? Would you question it?
2. What factors in Mr. Evert's history predisposed him to the development of congestive heart failure?
3. What should be the major nursing goals in caring for Mr. Evert in the early course of his drug therapy?
4. What are the major teaching goals the nurse should set to prepare the Evert couple for discharge?
5. What changes may the Everts need to make in their lives to accommodate Mr. Evert's new illness?

REVIEW QUESTIONS

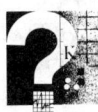

1. Describe the location of the various valves in the heart.
2. Trace the path through the heart of an impulse generated by the SA node.
3. Briefly outline the "cardiac cycle."
4. Distinguish between the terms "preload" and "afterload."
5. What is meant by the terms (a) inotropic and (b) chronotropic?
6. What is meant by the term congestive heart failure?
7. Outline the compensatory changes in the body in response to a failing heart.
8. Briefly distinguish symptomatically between right-sided and left-sided heart failure.
9. List the principal pharmacologic treatments for congestive heart failure.
10. What are the major differences between digoxin and digitoxin?
11. Describe the mechanism by which digitalis glycosides increase the force of contraction of the heart.
12. What factors contribute to the slowing of the heart rate seen with digitalis drugs?
13. What normal physiologic changes in elderly patients influence the action of digitalis in the body? What changes in dose and drug should be made to accommodate these changes?
14. What is pulse deficit? How can the nurse assess for it? What should the nurse do with the information in terms of digitalis therapy?
15. In what types of congestive heart failure are the digitalis drugs most effective?
16. Should digitalis drugs be given in large loading doses initially in most patients? Why or why not?
17. What nursing measures should be initiated for the patient going through the digitalization process?
18. How can the nurse help the patient to remember to take digitalis at home?
19. What are the principal adverse reactions seen with excessive doses of digitalis?

20. What adverse effects of digitalis is the elderly patient most likely to exhibit? What are the early symptoms of toxicity in the infant?
21. What factors can increase the likelihood of arrhythmias developing with the digitalis glycosides?
22. What is believed to be the mechanism of action of amrinone in treating congestive heart failure?
23. List the major adverse reactions associated with amrinone therapy.
24. List the vasodilators most commonly used as adjunctive therapy in congestive heart failure.
25. What are the principal hemodynamic actions of those vasodilators that are primarily (a) arteriodilators and (b) venodilators?

BIBLIOGRAPHY

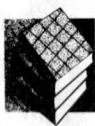

Aronow WS: Treatment of congestive heart failure, Parts I and II. Ration Drug Ther 16(9) and 16(10):1982

Assex ME, Miller G: Defining the role of vasodilator therapy in chronic CHF. Modern Medicine 54(9):37, 1986

Bristol JA, Evans DB: Agents for the treatment of heart failure. Med Res Rev 3:259, 1983

Cavenaugh AL, Mancini RE: Drug interactions and digitalis toxicity. Am J Nurs 80:2170, 1980

Colucci WS, Wright MD, Braunwald E: New positive inotropic agents in the treatment of congestive heart failure. N Engl J Med 314(6):349, 1986

Conn J: Physiologic basis of vasodilator therapy for heart failure. Am J Med 71:135, 1981

Farah AF, Alousi AA, Schwarz RP: Positive inotropic agents. Ann Rev Pharmacol Toxicol 24:275, 1984

Franciosa JA: Intravenous amrinone: An advance or a wrong step? Ann Intern Med 102:399, 1985

Franciosa JA: Treating CHF: How to get the most from drug therapy. Mod Med 54(1):36, 1986

Hoffman BF: The pharmacology of cardiac glycosides. In Rosen MR, Hoffman BF (eds): Cardiac Therapy, p 387. Boston, Martinus Nijhoff, 1983

McCall D, O'Rourke RA: Congestive heart failure. I. Biochemistry, pathophysiology, and neurohumoral mechanisms. Mod Concepts Cardiovasc Dis 54:55, 1985

McCauley K, Burke KG: Your detailed guide to drugs for C.H.F. Nursing 84 14(5):47, 1984

Moree N: New drugs: Hands on experience. Am J Nurs 85:252, 1985.

Parmley WW: Pathophysiology of congestive heart failure. Am J Cardiol 55:9A, 1985

Potempa K, Roberts KV: Cardiovascular drugs and the older adult. Nurs Clin North Am 17:263, 1982

Rajda MJ, Belock S: Drug reduction works. J Gerontol Nurs 10:19, 1984

Schwartz AB, Chatterjee K: Vasodilator therapy in chronic congestive heart failure. Drugs 26:148, 1983

Ward A, Brogden RN, Heel RC: Amrinone: A preliminary review of its pharmacologic properties and therapeutic use. Drugs 26:468, 1983

Willerson JT: What is wrong with the failing heart? N Engl J Med 307:243, 1982

Antiarrhythmic Drugs

34

Antiarrhythmic drugs are used to prevent and treat disorders of cardiac rhythm. Cardiac arrhythmias may be defined as any deviation from the normal rate and rhythm of the heart. Depending on the type of arrhythmia present, various hemodynamic complications can ensue, cardiac output may be reduced, and serious rhythm alterations may be lethal.

In order to understand the actions of the drugs used to control abnormal cardiac rhythm, it is necessary first to review the normal physiology of cardiac conduction and then consider the electrophysiologic disturbances that lead to the development of arrhythmias.

The conductile system of the heart is reviewed in Chapter 33 and outlined schematically in Figure 33-2. A typical electrocardiogram (ECG) depicting the electrical activity of the heart is presented in Figure 33-3. The orderly progression of electrical events through the heart is essential for efficient operation and coordinated contraction of the heart chambers. Impulses arise at the sinoatrial (SA) node, the normal pacemaker, and spread quickly across the atria. They transit through the atrioventricular (AV) node and are then conducted by way of the Purkinje system into ventricular muscle, where they trigger the contractions. These contractions propel blood throughout the systemic and pulmonary circulation. Deviations from the orderly propagation and conduction of impulses through this cardiac conductile system result in a decrement in cardiac function and reduced flow of oxygenated blood to the body organs. Irregularities in rate and rhythm of the heart markedly impair its ability to function and are a cause of eventual development of cardiac failure. A brief review of the etiology of cardiac arrhythmias follows.

Mechanisms of Cardiac Arrhythmias

Although many factors can precipitate a disturbance in cardiac rhythm (Table 34-1), all cardiac arrhythmias may be broadly classified as resulting from (1) disorders of impulse formation, (2) disorders of impulse conduction, or (3) a combination of both.

Disorders of Impulse Formation

Alterations in the rate of SA nodal discharge are manifested as changes in the automaticity (*i.e.*,

Table 34-1
Factors That May Precipitate Cardiac Arrhythmias

Electrolyte imbalances
  Hypokalemia
  Hypocalcemia
Acid–base disturbances
Ischemia/hypoxia
Excessive adrenergic activity
Hyperthyroidism
Myocardial infarction
Pericarditis
Cardiomyopathy
Pulmonary emboli
Drug toxicity, for example
  Digitalis
  Tricyclic antidepressants
  Beta-adrenergic agonists
  Thrombolytic drugs

ability to generate an impulse spontaneously) of the heart. Decreased automaticity results in sinus bradycardia, whereas increased automaticity leads to sinus tachycardia. These disturbances frequently are the result of drug toxicity or excessive sympathetic activation and can usually be controlled by eliminating the offending agent.

The SA node usually depolarizes more rapidly than other excitable tissue in the heart and attains threshold potential first. Thus, the SA node controls the heart rate and generally functions as the pacemaker. When the SA nodal rate slows excessively, however, other excitable cardiac tissue may reach threshold potential earlier than the SA node and generate an abnormal impulse. Such an area of impulse generation is termed an *ectopic focus*, and this area can discharge at either a regular or an irregular rate, thus creating an arrhythmia. Ectopic pacemakers can be stimulated by hypokalemia, ischemia, or hypoxia, and may arise in atrial, nodal, Purkinje, or ventricular muscle sites.

Disorders of Impulse Conduction

Alterations in both the rate of impulse conduction as well as the pathway can result in a variety of arrhythmias. Conduction of an impulse through the AV node may be abnormally delayed or in some cases totally blocked, and this situation is termed *heart block*. In *first-degree* heart block, impulses originating in the SA node are slowed in their passage through the AV node, and this may result in a slowing of the heart rate. This is reflected by a prolongation of the PR interval on the ECG. *Second-degree* heart block is noted when some of the atrial beats fail to reach the ventricles completely. Ventricular rate may be slow and the ECG shows more atrial waves than ventricular responses. Often there is a regular character to the arrhythmia (e.g. every third impulse is blocked). In *third-degree* block, the AV node conducts no atrial impulses at all, and the atria and ventricles beat independently. The ability of the ventricles to establish a spontaneous rhythm is referred to as *ventricular escape.* The inherent ventricular rate is approximately 25 to 40 beats per minute and is often too slow to maintain effective cardiac output. Conduction may also be impaired in one of the branches of the bundle of His below the AV node, in which case the condition is termed a *bundle branch block;* however, this condition is not usually categorized as an arrhythmia.

A more commonly encountered conduction abnormality is *reentry excitation,* in which an impulse reenters an area of the heart more than once,

before being extinguished, thus causing repetitive firing. The reentry phenomenon is outlined in Figure 34-1. In order for reentry excitation to occur, there must be an obstacle to the passage of the impulse in the normal conductile pathway, which is generally an area of damage. This area is capable of conducting an impulse in *one* direction only (i.e., unidirectional block). Normally, an impulse passing along a Purkinje fiber spreads to two branches and activates the ventricular muscle in the region. Upon entry into the connecting branch, the two branched impulses collide and are extinguished (Fig. 34-1, *A*). However, in the presence of a unidirectional block in one branch, the impulse travels down the undamaged branch, again to excite the ventricular wall, but is *not* extinguished by an impulse traveling in the opposite direction. Thus, the impulse from the ventricular tissue reenters the damaged area from the opposite direction and recycles repetitively provided the tissue ahead of the impulse is not in a refractory state (Fig. 34-1, *B*). This "circus movement" of an impulse results in a

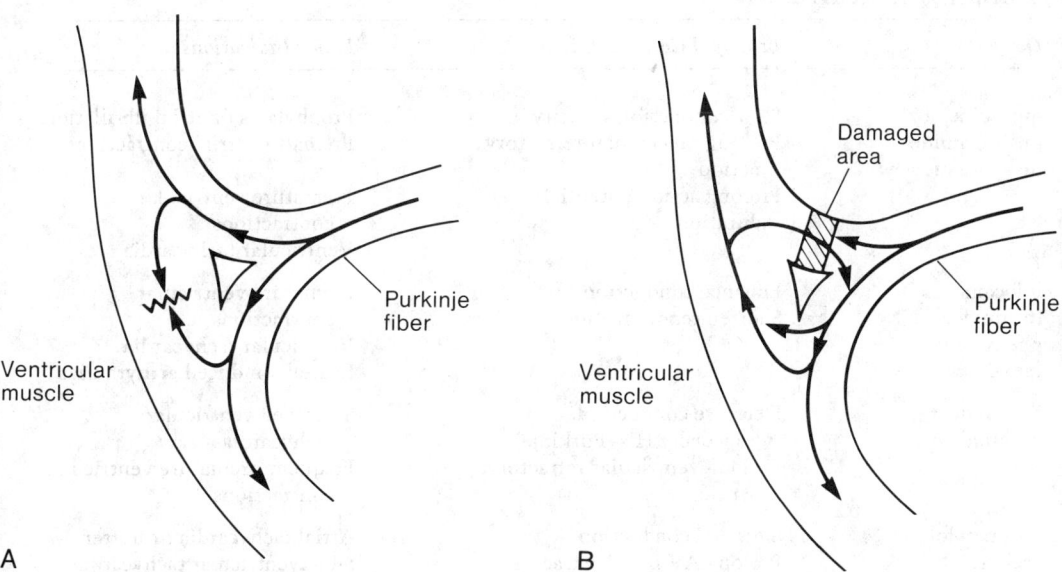

A   B

Figure 34-1.   Mechanism of reentry excitation. Normal conduction of an impulse from the Purkinje fiber to the ventricular wall is illustrated in A. The impulse bifurcates as it enters the ventricular wall, and after exciting the muscle, the impulses "collide" and extinguish each other. When the Purkinje fiber impulse encounters an area of damage in one branch (e.g., due to ischemia), there is a "unidirectional" block, and conduction of the impulse is inhibited as it encounters the damaged area (B). Conversely, the impulse traveling in the other branch reaches the ventricular wall intact and excites the ventricular tissue. In addition, the strong wave of ventricular depolarization is able to traverse the damaged area in a retrograde fashion (i.e., reentry) as indicated in B. Provided the tissue on the other side of the damaged area is excitable (no longer refractory), a repetitive recycling of the impulse may be established and a reentry arrhythmia can be generated.

disturbance in normal rhythm and, depending on the precise location of the block, can lead to a variety of different arrhythmias.

Classification of Antiarrhythmic Drugs

Antiarrhythmic drugs possess the capability of modifying the electrophysiologic properties of cardiac cell membranes, but differ somewhat with respect to their actions on specific properties of cardiac electrophysiology. Most drugs depress automaticity in ectopic foci and can terminate the activity of ectopic pacemakers. Conduction velocity may either be increased or decreased and the effective refractory period of cardiac cells may either be lengthened or shortened. Effects on SA nodal rate are variable, and their action on depo-

larized tissue is usually greater than on normal polarized tissue.

Although the electrophysiologic properties of antiarrhythmic drugs are quite complex, attempts have been made to classify these drugs based on their primary mechanisms of action. Table 34-2 outlines the various groups of antiarrhythmic drugs categorized according to their principal actions on the heart. It must be noted that drugs within a particular group (e.g., group IA) generally share similar electrophysiologic effects but can differ significantly in other respects. Thus, one member of the group may be effective for a particular indication while other members may not. Pharmacokinetic and electrophysiologic differences among the individual antiarrhythmic drugs are outlined in Table 34-3. Selection of an appropriate antiarrhythmic agent depends not only on the type of arrhythmia present but also on the characteristics of the drugs themselves—their onset, dura-

Table 34-2
Classification of Antiarrhythmic Drugs

Group	Drugs	Principal Cardiac Actions	Major Indications
IA	quinidine procainamide disopyramide	Slow conduction velocity Prolong myocardial refractory period Prolong action potential duration	Prophylaxis of atrial fibrillation Premature atrial contractions Premature ventricular contractions Ventricular tachycardia
IB	lidocaine tocainide phenytoin* mexiletine	Enhance conduction Shorten repolarization	Premature ventricular contractions Ventricular tachycardia Digitalis-induced arrhythmias
IC	flecainide encainide	Decrease conduction (especially His–Purkinje) Prolong ventricular refractory period	Sustained ventricular tachycardia Frequent premature ventricular contractions
II	propranolol acebutolol	Slow AV conduction Prolong AV nodal refractory period Decrease automaticity of SA node	Atrial tachycardia or flutter Supraventricular tachycardia Exercise-induced arrhythmias
III	bretylium amiodarone	Prolong refractory period Increase action potential duration	Life-threatening ventricular arrhythmias (not responding to other treatment)
IV	verapamil	Prolong AV nodal refractory period Decrease sinus node automaticity	Supraventricular tachyarrhythmias Control of rapid ventricular rate in atrial fibrillation

* Phenytoin is not approved for treatment of arrhythmias, but is used for digitalis-induced arrhythmias.

Table 34-3
Pharmacokinetic and Electrophysiologic Properties of Antiarrhythmic Drugs

Drug	Pharmacokinetics				Electrophysiology							
					Automaticity		Conduction Velocity		Refractory Period			
	Onset (min)	Duration (h)	Plasma Half-Life (h)	% Protein Binding	SA Node	Ectopic Pacemakers	AV Node	Purkinje Fibers	AV	Purkinje	Ventricle	Heart Rate
quinidine	30	6–10	6–7	70–90	↕	↓	↕	↓	↑	↑	↑	↕
procainamide	30	3–5	3–5	15–25	↕	↓	↕	↓	↑	↑	↑	↕
disopyramide	30	5–7	4–8	30–60	↕	↓	↑	↓	↑	↑	↑	↕
lidocaine	1–3*	0.2	1–2	40–80	0	↓	↑	↑	↕	↕	↕	0
phenytoin	30–60	24	24–36	90–95	↕	↓	↑	↑	↕	↕	↕	↕
tocainide	30–60	4–8	10–15	10–20	↕	↓	0	0	↓	↕	↓	0
mexiletine	30–60	4–8	10–12	50–60					↕	↑	↑	
encainide	30–60	8–12	1–2	75–85			↓	↓	↑	↑		
flecainide	30–60	8–12	12–24	40–50			↓	↓	0	↑	↑	0
propranolol	30	3–6	2–4	90–95	↓	↓	↓	↓	↑	0	0	↓
acebutolol	30	12–16	3–4	25–30	↓	↓	↓	↓	↑	0	0	↓
bretylium	1–3*	6–8	6–10	10	↑	↑	0	↑	↕	↑	↑	0
amiodarone	†	†	1–4 days	95					↑	↑	↑	
verapamil	30	6–8	4–8	90	↓	↓	↓	0	↑	0	0	↓

Key: ↑ increase; ↓ decrease; 0 no significant effect; ↕ variable effect.
* Onset reflects time after IV administration.
† Onset may take several weeks and effects persist from weeks to months, even after drug is discontinued.

tion, type, and incidence of side-effects, in addition to other factors.

Drugs used in treating arrhythmias alter the heart's basic electrical properties, including excitability, conduction velocity, refractory period, and automaticity. These, then, are potentially dangerous drugs, and their use has resulted in serious toxicity on occasion. Because not all arrhythmias require drug therapy, careful diagnosis of the type of disordered rhythm present is essential for effective and safe management of these conditions. Since the overall pharmacology and toxicology of the different drugs vary to a considerable degree, they will be discussed individually in this chapter.

■ Nursing Process

□ ASSESSMENT

□ Subjective Data
Certain general guidelines can be applied in the care of all patient's receiving antiarrhythmic drugs. These drugs are used in the treatment of arrhythmias that threaten life. Each patient will perceive that concept differently but most will be very

aware that their heart is not working properly. To many people, the heart represents life so its dysfunction usually brings thoughts of death that may or may not be expressed. The patient with arrhythmias may have actually suffered sudden cardiac arrest and been successfully resuscitated or he may have come very close to cardiac arrest but received treatment before the actual event occurred. In either case, or in the event that the arrhythmia is discovered before severe symptoms occur, the patient faces his own mortality and may see drug therapy as his lifeline. Therefore, the nurse can use discussions about drug therapy and patient teaching to explore perceptions and fears of the patient and his significant others.

Many patients with arrhythmias suffer from long-standing sleep disturbances. The mechanism of the disturbances is not clearly understood but arrhythmias may interfere with rapid-eye-movement (REM) sleep. Therefore, a sleep–rest assessment should also be performed since loss of sleep increases stress, which may, in turn, increase or worsen the arrhythmia and interfere with successful therapy. The patient should be asked if he has difficulty falling asleep or staying asleep and if he feels constantly tired. He may appear tired, have dark circles under his eyes, yawn frequently, or appear nervous. Incorporating this information into the care plan may facilitate drug therapy.

☐ *Objective Data*

In many cases, the luxury of a detailed assessment will be absent if the patient is brought to the emergency room with a life-threatening arrhythmia. An ECG and rhythm strip as well as vital signs may be the only information the health-care team has on which to base treatment.

If time and condition permit, certain baseline data should be collected before antiarrhythmia therapy begins. Laboratory data should include hepatic and renal function studies since the therapeutic dose of most of these drugs will be lower if impairment exists in these systems. Blood electrolytes will also be valuable since imbalances must be corrected in order to provide heart tissue with an environment conducive to responding to the drugs administered.

Cardiovascular assessment may include an ECG and Holter monitoring to evaluate the relationship between a patient's activities and his symptoms and arrhythmias. An exercise tolerance test may be performed in some patients, and in others programmed stimulation of the heart may be conducted in a cardiac catheterization laboratory to attempt to induce the arrhythmia and then discover which drugs it best responds to. Although the nurse may not actually administer these tests, she will provide support to the patient in answering questions and discussing his fears. Many patients will be frightened by the prospect of developing severe symptoms during a test and will want much reassurance about how such an event would be treated.

☐ *NURSING DIAGNOSES*

Actual nursing diagnoses for patients receiving antiarrhythmia drugs may include

   Knowledge deficit about the action, dose, and
      side-effects of the drug
   Alteration in cardiac output: decreased related
      to resultant hypotension from the drug
   Anxiety related to condition and fear of
      impending death

Potential nursing diagnoses may include

   Alteration in respiratory function ranging
      from dyspnea to respiratory arrest as a side-
      effect of the drug
   Sleep-pattern disturbance, which may have
      started prior to treatment and continue
      throughout therapy

Antiarrhythmic drugs produce a wide variety of side-effects, which are discussed under each drug group. Additional nursing diagnoses might be used in planning nursing care for patients who exhibit such problems.

☐ *PLAN*

Nursing care for the patient on antiarrhythmic drugs can be planned using short-term (acute-care) and long-term (extended-care) goals.

Short-term goals focus on

1. Emergency initial patient management aimed at providing adequate monitoring, careful administration, and having available appropriate equipment for handling emergencies
2. Providing the patient with a restful environment
3. Providing the patient with an opportunity to discuss fears in order to facilitate therapy

Long-term goals focus on home care and patient/family teaching, and include

1. Information about the arrhythmia
2. What the drug does and how to take it correctly to achieve desired results
3. How to deal with side-effects and recognize adverse effects (discussed under each drug)
4. What to do in case of an emergency

☐ *INTERVENTION*

☐ *Acute Care*

The patient having an arrhythmia will be immediately placed on a cardiac monitor. While antiarrhythmic drugs are being administered the nurse must observe the monitor for signs of cardiac toxicity. Signs of toxicity include QRS widening, dropped beats, prolongation of the PR interval, heart block (second or third degree), and an increase in the ventricular rate especially when an atrial tachycardia is being treated. Most of the antiarrhythmic drugs will reverse the arrhythmia within minutes of being administered intravenously. If this does not occur, toxicity should be suspected. In any event, if any of these symptoms occur, the drug should be either slowed or stopped and the physician notified immediately. Emergency and intravenous administration of most antiarrhythmic agents is usually determined by hospital protocols. Most times the drugs are administered in the emergency room or intensive-care unit by physicians or by nurses who have taken special courses in arrhythmia management. All of the drugs mentioned in this chapter can lead to cardiac toxicity and cardiopulmonary arrest, so their administration, particularly early on when the heart tissue is irritable, is potentially hazardous.

The drugs are usually ordered with a titration schedule; that is, the physician orders the drug as a milligrams/minute dosage with criteria for increasing or decreasing the rate of infusion. Criteria might include heart rate, number of irregular beats per minute, or development of certain side-effects such as hypotension or nausea. Since the accuracy of dosage is critical, the drug should be administered through an infusion pump.

A primary intravenous line should be inserted with the antiarrhythmic drug infused as a secondary (piggyback) line so that it can be discontinued without interfering with the IV.

Most of these drugs also produce severe hypotension. Therefore, vital signs should be closely monitored, especially during initial administration, and the patient kept supine, if possible. If blood pressure falls more than 15 mm Hg or if ventricular rate slows significantly without development of regular AV conduction, the drug should be discontinued and the physician notified immediately.

Cardiopulmonary resuscitative equipment and emergency drugs should be close at hand. Drugs that should be available include vasopressors such as dopamine to manage hypotension; atropine to manage bradycardia; any drugs known to be antidotes for the drugs being used; a variety of antiarrhythmic agents such as lidocaine to manage a change in arrhythmia; and electrolyte solutions such as sodium bicarbonate or calcium gluconate to manage electrolyte imbalances.

Emergency laboratory work-ups should include arterial blood gases, electrolyte levels, and drug serum levels to provide continuous information about how the patient is responding to the drug or drugs being administered.

In short, during emergency management of an arrhythmia, much of the nursing care will focus on stabilizing the patient's condition. However, the nurse must also remember that this event will be extremely frightening for the patient who will be aware of the drastic changes the drugs are producing in his body. Attempts should be made to provide him with verbal support, explanations of events as they occur, and a hand to hold to help reduce fear as much as possible and provide him with the sense that he is a human being and not an object on which the health team is performing a series of operations.

Once the arrhythmia has been stabilized, the patient should be placed in an environment where stimuli can be reduced and the arousal of the patient minimized to enhance sleep and rest. If the patient has trouble sleeping, medication may be necessary, but a better long-term therapy is to teach him relaxation techniques he can use at home. He may also need to discuss what things go through his mind as he is trying to sleep to enable him to reduce the mental distractors. Many patients are afraid their heart will stop and they will die in their sleep. If the patient expresses this fear, some psychological counseling may be needed. As the antiarrhythmic agent begins to work and the patient feels better, some of these fears may lessen. But dealing with them will better enable the patient to cope with his illness since there is no guarantee the arrhythmia won't return.

□ *Long-Term Goals*
Some patients will have a sense that something is wrong when they develop an arrhythmia. The nurse can use these sensations to help the patient recognize the symptoms of his arrhythmia, and these are the symptoms that should be reported in addition to side-effects specific for the drug he is taking. He should be taught how to take his own pulse, if possible, to help him identify changes in the rate or rhythm that must be reported. He may be taught self-administration of atropine or lidocaine if the arrhythmia responds favorably to one of these drugs and administration is essential during an emergency.

□ *Dealing With an Emergency Situation*
The patient who suffered a cardiac arrest or who came close to cardiac arrest will be very fearful of a recurrence of that event. The family who were present, and who probably felt extremely helpless, will be equally fearful. Therefore, any teaching plan the nurse provides should include a step-by-step emergency plan for the patient and his significant others. Everyone should know the signs and symptoms to watch for and how to reach emergency help. This may be the local first aid squad, an emergency hot-line number to the cardiac intensive-care unit, or a combination of resources. Family members may wish to learn cardiopulmonary resuscitation (CPR) and may be encouraged to do so if they are able. The goal is to attempt to help the patient and family to feel that they have some control over the situation if the arrhythmia should recur or worsen.

□ *EVALUATION*
There are several outcome criteria against which to judge the success of antiarrhythmic therapy. The arrhythmia may disappear or decrease in severity as evidenced on an ECG; the patient may report an improved sense of well-being and activity tolerance. The patient's sleeping pattern may improve. All of these will indicate the medication is working. If the patient also begins to cope with his illness and its limitations, then the medication regimen will be facilitating a more important outcome, an improved quality of life.

Group IA Antiarrhythmic Drugs

Quinidine

(Cardioquin, Cin-Quin, Duraquin, Quinaglute, Quinatime, Quinidex Extentabs, Quinora, Quin-Release)

Quinidine is an alkaloid obtained from the bark of the cinchona tree and is an isomer of quinine, with which it shares many pharmacologic properties (*e.g.,* antipyretic, oxytocic, antimalarial). Quinidine, however, exerts its principal action on the heart and is primarily used as an oral antiarrhythmic agent although its use has declined in recent years due to its less favorable benefit-to-risk ratio as compared to other available drugs.

MECHANISM AND ACTIONS
Quinidine decreases sodium influx through activated sodium channels in cardiac cell membranes during depolarization and potassium efflux during repolarization. Myocardial excitability is reduced, and automaticity of cardiac pacemaker cells and especially of ectopic foci is suppressed. Quinidine slows conduction velocity and prolongs the effective refractory period of the myocardium, thereby increasing conduction time and preventing reentry excitation (see above under Mechanisms of Cardiac Arrhythmias). By slowing impulse conduction through healthy cardiac tissue or lengthening the time the tissue is refractive, circling impulses responsible for the generation of reentry arrhythmias arrive at an area of refractory (*i.e.,* unresponsive) tissue and are extinguished. Quinidine also possesses an anticholinergic action, and can reduce vagal tone and accelerate conduction through the AV junction by this anticholinergic action. If the anticholinergic action is prominent, the ventricular

rate can increase significantly and compromise the effectiveness of quinidine in treating certain arrhythmias, as increased ventricular rate can occur.

USES
1. Treatment of the following arrhythmias
   a. Paroxysmal supraventricular tachycardia
   b. Atrial flutter and fibrillation (following digitalis to control AV nodal conduction)
   c. Premature atrial and ventricular contractions
   d. Paroxysmal AV junctional rhythm
   e. Paroxysmal ventricular tachycardia not associated with complete heart block
2. Maintenance therapy after electrical conversion of atrial flutter or fibrillation

ADMINISTRATION AND DOSAGE
Quinidine is available as three salts containing the following percentages of active drug: sulfate (83%), gluconate (62%), and polygalacturonate (60%). Administration is generally by the oral route; the drug has occasionally been given IM or IV in emergency situations, but is considered more hazardous than lidocaine or procainamide by these latter routes. The drug is used orally as tablets (100 mg, 200 mg, 300 mg) or capsules (200 mg, 300 mg) as well as sustained-release tablets (300 mg, 324 mg, 330 mg), and occasionally by injection as the sulfate (200 mg/ml) or gluconate (80 mg/ml) salts. Dosage is adjusted to maintain the plasma level of quinidine between 2 mcg and 6 mcg/ml, and is generally in the range of 10 mg/kg/day to 20 mg/kg/day in four to six divided doses. Recommended dosages for the principal indications of quinidine are as follows:
Paroxysmal supraventricular tachycardia—400 mg to 600 mg every 2 hours to 3 hours until paroxysm is terminated
Premature atrial and ventricular contractions—200 mg to 300 mg three to four times/day
Atrial fibrillation—200 mg every 2 hours to 3 hours for 5 to 8 doses; increase gradually until sinus rhythm is restored (maximal daily dose is 3 g-4 g)
Maintenance—200 mg to 300 mg three to four times/day (sustained-release forms—1 to 2 tablets two to three times/day)
IM—600 mg gluconate salt initially, then 400 mg every 2 hours as needed
IV—200 mg to 750 mg gluconate salt or equivalent by slow IV infusion of a dilute

(800 mg gluconate/50 ml 5% glucose)
solution at a rate of 1 ml (16 mg) per minute

FATE

Oral absorption is usually rapid and complete. Peak effects with the sulfate and gluconate salts occur in 1 hour to 3 hours and activity persists for 6 hours to 8 hours (slightly longer with sustained-release dosage forms). Quinidine is 70% to 90% bound to plasma proteins. The drug is largely metabolized in the liver to inactive metabolites, although approximately 20% to 25% of a dose is excreted unchanged in the urine. Elimination half-life ranges from 4 hours to 10 hours (average 6 hours to 7 hours), but may be prolonged in elderly patients and patients with hepatic insufficiency or congestive heart failure. Urinary excretion is enhanced in an acidic urine.

SIDE-EFFECTS/ADVERSE REACTIONS

The most frequently encountered side-effects with quinidine are nausea, diarrhea, and abdominal distress, and may require discontinuation of therapy in up to one third of patients. Sustained-release dosage forms may be slightly better tolerated in some individuals. Large doses result in a syndrome termed *cinchonism*, characterized by headache, tinnitus, dizziness, lightheadedness, blurred vision, and tremor. These effects can be eliminated by a dosage reduction.

Cardiotoxic effects can occur with use of quinidine and can include ventricular ectopic beats, ventricular tachycardia and fibrillation, widening of the QRS complex, and cardiac asystole. These effects are more likely to develop when there is considerable myocardial damage.

Drug administration should be terminated if there is an increase of more than 25% in the duration of the QRS complex, if the P wave disappears, or if heart rate decreases to below 120 beats/minute. Heart block and cardiac standstill have been reported with large doses. Hypotension has also been associated with quinidine, particularly when given IV.

Hepatic toxicity, including granulomatous hepatitis, unexplained fever, and elevation of hepatic enzymes, can occur, particularly in the initial stages of therapy. It appears to be a hypersensitivity reaction to quinidine, and cessation of therapy usually results in disappearance of toxicity.

Other adverse reactions reported with use of quinidine include

Gastrointestinal—Vomiting, cramping

Central nervous system—Fever, impaired hearing, altered color perception, photophobia, diplopia, scotomas, excitement, confusion, delirium, syncope

Cardiovascular—Severe bradycardia, atrial flutter and fibrillation, arterial embolism

Hematologic/dermatologic—Acute hemolytic anemia, thrombocytopenic purpura, leukopenia, agranulocytosis (rare), flushing, urticaria, angioedema, pruritus, sweating

Other—Arthralgia, dyspnea, respiratory depression, asthmatic episodes

IV use—Sweating, nervousness, vomiting, cramping, urge to urinate or defecate

Occasionally, a sudden loss of consciousness can occur with use of quinidine (*i.e.*, "quinidine syncope") and is usually the result of ventricular fibrillation on long-term therapy. The syndrome does not appear to be related to dose or plasma level but is frequently associated with prolonged QT intervals on the ECG.

CONTRAINDICATIONS AND PRECAUTIONS

Quinidine is contraindicated in the presence of intraventricular conduction defects characterized by marked QRS widening, AV conduction defects or complete AV block, ectopic impulses and rhythms due to escape mechanisms, thrombocytopenic purpura, myasthenia gravis, and acute rheumatic fever. Also, quinidine should not be used in patients with cardiac enlargement caused by congestive heart failure, renal dysfunction with azotemia or tubular acidosis, and a hypersensitivity to quinidine marked by febrile reactions, skin eruptions, or thrombocytopenia. A single tablet of quinidine may be given as a test dose prior to initiation of therapy to determine the presence of hypersensitivity. The drug should be given *cautiously* to patients with incomplete heart block, digitalis intoxication, congestive heart failure, hypotension, respiratory disorders, potassium imbalance (*e.g.*, diuretic therapy), and impaired renal or hepatic function. Safety and efficacy of quinidine in pregnant or nursing mothers and in children have not been established.

INTERACTIONS

1. Quinidine may increase the effects of oral anticoagulants, antihypertensives, neuromuscular blocking agents, anticholinergics, digitalis, and other antiarrhythmics.
2. Blood levels of quinidine can be elevated and its action prolonged by substances that alkalin-

ize the urine (*e.g.*, sodium bicarbonate, ant-acids, carbonic anhydrase inhibitors), thereby retarding quinidine excretion.
3. Effects of cholinergic drugs (*e.g.*, neostigmine, edrophonium) may be antagonized by quinidine.
4. Additive cardiac-depressant effects may occur with use of propranolol or phenothiazines with quinidine.
5. Administration of phenytoin, rifampin, or phenobarbital may reduce the serum half-life of quinidine because of enzyme induction.
6. Quinidine may elevate blood levels of digoxin (and probably digitoxin) by reducing its tissue binding or by retarding its renal clearance.
7. Cimetidine may increase the pharmacologic effects of quinidine.
8. Concurrent use of nifedipine and quinidine can result in decreased serum levels of quinidine.

NURSING CONSIDERATIONS
See also Nursing Process, earlier in this chapter.

Quinidine is a troublesome drug, with many serious side-effects, and has been largely replaced by less hazardous medications. A thorough history should be obtained before the drug is given since many contraindications and precautions surround its use. In addition, a thorough drug history should be obtained, especially if the patient has been treated with other cardiac drugs.

ECG monitoring is essential during initial therapy and for the duration of therapy when IM or IV routes are used (rarely done now). Outpatients should have periodic ECGs as well as liver enzyme studies since hepatic toxicity is a serious drug side-effect.

When quinidine is administered orally, the major side-effects are gastric distress and diarrhea. Both are usually transient and can be minimized by taking the drug with food. However, the patient should be cautioned to minimize consumption of citrus juices, vegetables, and milk products since these foods will slow quinidine excretion by changing urine *p*H, resulting in increased quinidine blood levels and potential toxicity.

The main toxic symptoms with quinidine that the patient should learn are the symptoms of cinchonism mentioned earlier under Side-Effects/Adverse Reactions and any sensations of dizziness, faintness, or of "the heart not beating right," which may indicate a worsening of arrhythmias. Both symptoms should be reported immediately.

Procainamide
(Promine, Pronestyl)

Procainamide Sustained-Release
(Procan-SR, Pronestyl-SR, Procamide SR, Rhythmin)

MECHANISM AND ACTIONS
Procainamide is the amide of the local anesthetic procaine and is used in the treatment of a variety of arrhythmias. It is similar in many respects to quinidine but is shorter acting and, like quinidine, has the potential for serious toxicity with chronic oral administration.

The pharmacologic actions of procainamide are essentially identical to those of quinidine described above. Cardiac excitability is reduced (and therefore weaker ectopic impulses are screened out); conduction is slowed in the atria, bundle of His, and ventricles; and the atrial refractory period is lengthened, more so than that of the ventricles. Cardiac output and force of contraction are relatively unaffected. The drug possesses a degree of anticholinergic activity and can increase heart rate due to a vagolytic action, but this effect is somewhat less marked than that observed with quinidine. Procainamide has a mild peripheral vasodilatory action and can produce a fall in blood pressure, especially after IV administration. Large doses can result in progressive AV block and development of ventricular extrasystoles. The most characteristic ECG changes with increasing doses are widening of the QRS complex and prolongation of the PR and QT intervals (see Fig. 33-3, Chap. 33).

USES
1. Treatment of premature ventricular contractions (PVCs), ventricular tachycardia, paroxysmal atrial tachycardia, and atrial fibrillation
2. Treatment of arrhythmias associated with surgery, general anesthesia, or myocardial infarction (IV administration)

ADMINISTRATION AND DOSAGE
Procainamide is available as tablets and capsules (250 mg, 375 mg, 500 mg), sustained-release tablets (250 mg, 500 mg, 750 mg, 1000 mg), and for injection (100-mg/ml, 500-mg/ml vials). Sustained-release formulations are *not* recommended for initial therapy, but may be substituted for regular tablets or capsules when patients have been stabilized. Recommended doses for the various routes of administration are given below.

Oral

Ventricular tachycardia—Initially, 1-g loading dose, then 50 mg/kg/day in divided doses every 3 hours (every 6 hours with sustained-release tablets)

Atrial fibrillation and paroxysmal atrial tachycardia—Initially, 1.25 g, followed in 1 hour by 0.75 g; then, 0.5 g to 1 g every 2 hours until arrhythmia is interrupted; maintenance dose, 0.5 g to 1 g every 4 hours to 6 hours

Parenteral

IM—Initially, 50 mg/kg/day in divided doses every 3 hours to 6 hours; switch to oral therapy as soon as possible (for arrhythmias during anesthesia or surgery, 0.1 g–0.5 g IM). *Deep* IM injection is recommended.

IV injection—100 mg every 5 minutes by slow IV injection (25 mg–50 mg/minute) to a maximum of 500 mg; usual serum level is 4 mcg/ml to 8 mcg/ml; continuous ECG monitoring must be performed.

IV infusion (extreme emergencies only)—20 mg to 25 mg/minute of a diluted solution over 30 minutes to a maximum of 600 mg with continual ECG monitoring; if necessary, change to a second infusion (2 mg–6 mg/minute) for maintenance. Therapeutic plasma levels are 4 mcg/ml to 8 mcg/ml.

FATE

Oral absorption is rapid and nearly complete. Onset of action is almost immediate following IM or IV injection and within 30 minutes following oral administration. Steady-state plasma levels are attained within 15 hours to 30 hours. Effects of a single dose persist for only 3 hours to 4 hours (up to 6 hours with sustained-release formulations). Plasma protein binding ranges from 15% to 25%. The drug is hydrolyzed in the liver, between 7% and 35% being converted to n-acetylprocainamide (NAPA), a cardioactive metabolite with a 6-hour half-life. The remainder, approximately 40% to 70% of the drug, is excreted in the urine unchanged, as is NAPA. Half-lives of procainamide and NAPA are prolonged in patients with congestive heart failure or impaired renal function, necessitating a dosage reduction of up to 50% in some cases.

SIDE-EFFECTS/ADVERSE REACTIONS

Anorexia, nausea, and occasionally vomiting can occur with procainamide but the incidence is much less than that observed with quinidine. IV administration frequently results in a fall in blood pressure.

Cardiac toxicity is seen to approximately the same degree with procainamide as with quinidine. Premature ventricular contractions, ventricular tachycardia, and ventricular fibrillation have occurred with procainamide, and heart block has been precipitated, especially with IV use.

Chronic maintenance therapy has resulted in development of a systemic lupus erythematosus (LE) syndrome, characterized by arthralgia, arthritis, and pleuritic pain, and less commonly by fever, myalgia, skin lesions, and pericarditis. Although 60% to 70% of patients receiving procainamide show an increased antinuclear antibody (ANA) titer within 1 month to 12 months, only 20% to 30% of these develop signs and symptoms of LE. A rising titer *or* appearance of clinical signs of lupus indicates a need for discontinuation of the drug and symptoms are generally reversible. Failure to attain remission of all symptoms may require use of steroid therapy.

Agranulocytosis has occurred during procainamide therapy, frequently accompanied by flu-like symptoms. The incidence appears to be higher with sustained-release forms of the drug. Patients receiving chronic procainamide should be instructed to report the development of early signs of agranulocytosis such as sore throat, unexplained fever, mucosal ulceration, and upper respiratory distress. Routine blood counts are necessary at regular intervals during therapy, and the drug should be discontinued if symptoms appear or a granulocyte depression is noted.

Other adverse reactions reported during procainamide treatment include urticaria, pruritus, angioedema, maculopapular rash, hepatomegaly, granulomatous hepatitis, hemolytic anemia, weakness, depression, confusion, convulsions, psychotic behavior, and thrombocytopenia.

IV administration can lead to flushing, severe hypotension, ventricular fibrillation, and ventricular asystole.

CONTRAINDICATIONS AND PRECAUTIONS

Procainamide is contraindicated in second-degree or third-degree heart block and myasthenia gravis and in patients allergic to procaine and related local anesthetics. The drug is administered with *caution* to persons with impaired liver or kidney function, myocardial damage, or conduction disturbances. Safety for use in either pregnant or nursing mothers has not been established.

INTERACTIONS

1. Procainamide may potentiate the muscle-relaxing action of neuromuscular blocking agents and those antibiotics (especially aminoglycosides) having a skeletal muscle relaxant effect.
2. Additive effects on the heart may occur with combinations of procainamide and other antiarrhythmic or digitalis-like drugs.
3. Procainamide may increase the hypotensive effects of antihypertensives and diuretics.
4. Effects of procainamide can be potentiated by agents that alkalinize the urine and reduce urinary excretion, such as acetazolamide, sodium lactate, and sodium bicarbonate.
5. The action of cholinesterase inhibitors in treating myasthenia gravis can be antagonized by procainamide.
6. Concurrent use of cimetidine and procainamide can reduce the renal clearance of procainamide and its active metabolite NAPA.

NURSING CONSIDERATIONS

See also Nursing Process, earlier in this chapter.

When procainamide is administered orally, the main side-effects are gastric distress and hypotension. The drug can be administered with meals to reduce gastrointestinal symptoms. Patients who suffer lightheadedness and dizziness should be cautioned about driving or operating hazardous machinery until they are more stabilized on the drug.

All patients on long-term procainamide therapy should have periodic hematology studies and antinuclear antibody tests. They should know the symptoms of agranulocytosis and lupus reaction and be told to report any symptoms immediately. Serum drug levels should be drawn at regular intervals and the patient should learn to take his pulse daily since changes in these parameters may indicate early drug toxicity.

Disopyramide

(Napamide, Norpace, Norpace CR)

MECHANISM AND ACTIONS

Disopyramide is a type IA antiarrhythmic drug that resembles both quinidine and procainamide in many of its actions on the heart. It is primarily used for the control of chronic ventricular arrhythmias.

Disopyramide decreases the rate of spontaneous diastolic depolarization of myocardial cells, prolongs the action potential duration of normal cardiac cells, and lengthens the refractory period. Ectopic pacemaker activity is decreased. AV nodal conduction and AV refractory period are not significantly altered, nor is conduction time in His–Purkinje fibers slowed. Disopyramide possesses some anticholinergic activity and exerts a negative inotropic effect (decreased force of contraction), which is most evident in patients with reduced left ventricular function (*e.g.,* in congestive heart failure). Cardiac performance in persons with normal left ventricular function is largely unimpaired. Peripheral vascular resistance is elevated approximately 20%.

USES

1. Suppression and prevention of recurrence of the following arrhythmias:
   a. Unifocal premature (ectopic) ventricular contractions
   b. Premature (ectopic) ventricular contractions of multifocal origin
   c. Paired premature ventricular contractions
   d. Episodes of ventricular tachycardia
2. Investigational uses include conversion of atrial arrhythmias to sinus rhythm and control of ventricular arrhythmias in emergency situations (IV).

ADMINISTRATION AND DOSAGE

Disopyramide is only available for oral administration as regular and controlled-release capsules, in doses of 100 mg and 150 mg each. To achieve the desired plasma concentration rapidly, an oral loading dose of 200 mg to 300 mg can be given (lower dosage for patients with mild hepatic or renal dysfunction or for patients weighing less than 110 lb). The normal adult dosage range is 400 mg to 800 mg a day in divided doses every 6 hours (regular capsules) or every 8 hours (controlled-release capsules). In patients with cardiomyopathy or cardiac decompensation, *no* loading dose is given and dosage is limited to 100 mg every 6 hours. When transferring from the immediate-release form to the controlled-release form, begin the controlled-release form 6 hours after the last dose of the immediate-acting form. The controlled-release form should not be used for initial loading doses.

Children's doses are based on age as follows and given in divided doses every 6 hours:

1 year to 4 years—10 mg/kg to 20 mg/kg/day
4 years to 12 years—10 mg/kg to 15 mg/kg/day
12 years to 18 years—6 mg/kg to 15 mg/kg/day

FATE

The drug is rapidly and almost completely absorbed. Onset of action is 30 minutes, and effects persist for 4 hours to 6 hours. Peak plasma levels occur within 1 hour to 3 hours. Plasma protein binding is concentration dependant and ranges from 20% to 60% (normal range 25%–30%). Approximately 50% of a dose is excreted as unchanged drug in the urine, and most of the remainder as metabolites. Plasma half-life ranges from 4 hours to 10 hours, but may be markedly lengthened in patients with impaired renal function or following a myocardial infarction. Renal excretion is independent of urinary pH.

SIDE-EFFECTS/ADVERSE REACTIONS

Although the overall incidence of serious toxicity with disopyramide is less than that observed with either quinidine or procainamide, the drug possesses significant anticholinergic activity, which is responsible for the frequent development of dry mouth, urinary hesitancy, constipation, and blurred vision. In addition, nausea, gastrointestinal (GI) pain, fatigue, headache, malaise, and muscle weakness can occur in many patients given disopyramide, although not as frequently as it with quinidine. The major cardiovascular toxicity with disopyramide is its potential to impair cardiac contractility (i.e., a negative inotropic effect), thus reducing cardiac output and left ventricular performance. This action is generally of minimal clinical significance when left ventricular function is normal, but can be of major consequence in persons with preexisting ventricular decompensation, and severe myocardial depression has occurred in some patients.

Other adverse reactions seen with disopyramide are listed below:

Cardiovascular—Hypotension, congestive heart failure, edema, cardiac conduction disturbances, QRS widening, AV block, chest pain, dyspnea

Central nervous system—Dizziness, nervousness, insomnia, depression

Dermatologic/hematologic—Rash, pruritus, dermatoses, decreased hemoglobin, thrombocytopenia, agranulocytosis (rare)

Other—Urinary retention, anorexia, diarrhea, vomiting, elevated liver enzymes, impotence, elevated creatinine, reversible cholestatic jaundice, elevated cholesterol, triglycerides and blood urea nitrogen, hypokalemia, hypoglycemia, anaphylactoid reaction

CONTRAINDICATIONS AND PRECAUTIONS

Disopyramide is contraindicated in cardiogenic shock, second-degree or third-degree heart block, uncompensated congestive heart failure, or hypotension. Loading doses should not be given to patients with myocarditis or other cardiomyopathies. The drug must be given *cautiously* to persons with sick sinus syndrome, bundle branch block, Wolff-Parkinson-White syndrome, first-degree heart block, urinary retention, prostatic hypertrophy, renal impairment, glaucoma, hypoglycemia, hepatic dysfunction, hypokalemia (correct potassium deficit first), and to pregnant or nursing mothers. *Concomitant* use of disopyramide and another type IA antiarrhythmic drug (quinidine, procainamide) or propranolol should be reserved for life-threatening arrhythmias unresponsive to a single agent.

INTERACTIONS

1. The cardiodepressive effects of disopyramide may be enhanced by concurrent use of other antiarrhythmic drugs, beta-adrenergic blockers, and certain calcium channel blockers (*e.g.*, verapamil).
2. Plasma levels of disopyramide can be increased by the presence of other protein-bound drugs (*e.g.*, sulfonamides, anti-inflammatory agents, oral anticoagulants, oral hypoglycemics).
3. Therapeutic effects of disopyramide may be reduced by the presence of hypokalemia (*e.g.*, diuretic therapy).
4. Effects of cholinesterase inhibitors in relieving myasthenia gravis may be impaired by disopyramide.
5. Plasma levels of disopyramide may be lowered by the presence of enzyme inducers, such as phenytoin, barbiturates, rifampin, glutethimide, and primidone.

NURSING CONSIDERATIONS

See also Nursing Process, earlier in this chapter.

A drug history should be obtained before a patient begins taking disopyramide especially if he has been treated with other cardiac drugs, many of which interact with disopyramide. In addition, use of over-the-counter cold and allergy remedies should be discouraged since anticholinergic side-effects may be increased with such a combination.

If possible, the patient should learn to take his own pulse to monitor the drug effect. If the heart rate falls below 60 beats/minute (80 beats/minute in children) or goes higher than 120 beats/minute, the drug should not be taken and the physician notified.

Multiple side-effects occur with disopyramide use. The patient must monitor his weight closely and report rapid increases as well as the development of swelling of hands or feet, dyspnea, or decreases in urinary output, symptoms of congestive heart failure. Lightheadedness and dizziness can occur because the drug has a hypotensive effect. Patients should be cautioned about climbing stairs, operating machinery, or driving until stabilized on the drug. They should be taught to rise slowly from a sitting or supine position to minimize the effects of postural hypotension. Anticholinergic side-effects such as dry mouth can be alleviated by chewing gum, sucking on hard candy, or frequently rinsing the mouth. Disopyramide can also result in sun sensitivity. Patients should be warned to use sun block, hat, sunglasses, and protective clothing when outdoors.

Group IB Antiarrhythmic Drugs

Lidocaine

(Lidopen, Xylocaine)

Lidocaine is a local anesthetic (see Chap. 20) that is primarily used IV for the control of acute ventricular arrhythmias. Its margin of safety is considerably greater than that of the type IA antiarrhythmic drugs.

MECHANISM AND ACTIONS

Lidocaine exerts multiple actions on cardiac electrophysiology. The drug decreases automaticity of ectopic pacemaker cells, slowing spontaneous firing, shortens the duration of the action potential in Purkinje fibers; and decreases the effective refractory period in both Purkinje fibers and ventricular muscle cells. The electrical stimulation threshold of the ventricles during diastole is elevated, an action that screens out weaker ectopic impulses. Lidocaine has little effect on conduction velocity in the AV or His–Purkinje systems, and does not alter the atrial refractory period. In normal therapeutic doses, there is no change in myocardial contractility, systemic arterial pressure, or autonomic tone. Lidocaine appears to suppress electrical activity in depolarized arrhythmogenic tissue without significantly interfering with electrical activity of normal tissue. Thus, it is quite effective in treating ar-

rhythmias associated with depolarization, such as those associated with myocardial ischemia or digitalis toxicity, but is relatively ineffective against arrhythmias associated with normally polarized tissues, such as atrial flutter or fibrillation.

USES
1. Management of acute ventricular arrhythmias such as those resulting from myocardial infarction, cardiac surgery, or catheterization, and digitalis intoxication (IV administration)
2. Emergency control of arrhythmias where IV administration is impractical, such as in a mobile emergency unit (IM administration)

ADMINISTRATION AND DOSAGE
Lidocaine is available for IM administration as a 10% solution; for direct IV administration as 1% and 2% solutions; for IV admixture as 4%, 10%, and 20% solutions; and for IV infusion as 0.2%, 0.4%, and 0.8% solutions.

Intravenous
A loading dose is given initially by IV bolus injection (1 mg/kg at a rate of 25 mg–50 mg/minute), which produces a brief therapeutic effect (10 minutes–20 minutes). If the initial injection does not produce the desired effect, a second bolus of one-third to one-half the initial dose may be given in 5 minutes. No more than 300 mg should be given in one hour.

Plasma levels are then maintained by IV infusion at a rate of 1 mg/minute to 4 mg/minute (reduce infusion dose in patients with congestive heart failure or liver disease or in patients over age 60). The infusion should be terminated as soon as the cardiac rhythm has stabilized or at the earliest signs of toxicity. Infusions are not recommended for longer than 24 hours. (In children, the initial bolus dosage is 1 mg/kg, followed by an infusion of 20 mcg/kg/minute to 50 mcg/kg/minute.)

Intramuscular
IM administration of lidocaine is occasionally used in emergency situations when facilities for IV administration are unavailable. Deltoid sites are preferred. The dose is 300 mg of a 10% solution in an average-size adult; if necessary, an additional injection may be given in 60 minutes to 90 minutes. Patients should be switched to IV therapy as soon as possible.

FATE
Lidocaine is not effective orally, since it undergoes extensive first-pass hepatic inactivation. Following

IV injection, onset of action is almost immediate, and effects persist 10 minutes to 20 minutes. With IM injection, effects are noted within 5 minutes to 15 minutes and persist for 60 minutes to 120 minutes. The elimination half-life ranges from 1 hour to 2 hours, but the initial distribution-phase half-life is only 5 minutes to 10 minutes, accounting for the short duration of action of IV administered drug. Lidocaine is widely distributed and variably (40%–80%) protein bound. The drug undergoes extensive biotransformation in the liver (90%), and the metabolites are largely eliminated in the urine.

SIDE-EFFECTS/ADVERSE REACTIONS

The most common side-effects with lidocaine are neurologic, and paresthesias, coldness or numbness in the extremities, drowsiness, lightheadedness, slurred speech, and mild tremor occur frequently. The incidence of other adverse reactions is largely dependent on the plasma level (therapeutic levels are 1.5 mcg/ml–6 mcg/ml), and significant cardiovascular and central nervous system toxicity can occur with plasma levels above 7 mcg/ml. Central nervous system toxicity includes tinnitus, blurred vision, impaired hearing, anxiety, vomiting, muscle twitching, tremor, euphoria, convulsions, and, in large amounts, respiratory depression and cardiovascular collapse. Hypotension and bradycardia can occur even with therapeutic plasma levels. Other adverse reactions noted during lidocaine administration are hypersensitivity reactions (urticaria, cutaneous lesions, edema, and anaphylactoid reactions), fever, thrombophlebitis, and pain at IM injection sites.

Use of certain local anesthetics has been associated with the rare development of malignant hyperthermia, which is frequently fatal if not treated quickly and vigorously. Patients receiving lidocaine should be observed for the initial signs of this condition, such as spasm of the jaw muscles, rigidity, tachycardia, and hyperpyrexia.

Plasma levels above 8 mcg/ml can result in *serious* overdosage toxicity marked by seizures, decreased cardiac output, respiratory depression, and hypotension. The drug should be discontinued and resuscitative measures and supportive treatment should be initiated. Among the procedures undertaken are IV fluids, vasopressors, anticonvulsants, and ventilatory assistance.

CONTRAINDICATIONS AND PRECAUTIONS

Lidocaine is contraindicated in patients with Adams-Stokes syndrome, Wolff-Parkinson-White syndrome, or severe SA, AV, or intraventricular conduction block, and in persons hypersensitive to local anesthetics. *Cautious* use of the drug is especially warranted in patients with congestive heart failure, since reduced distribution and clearance can result in markedly elevated blood levels and increased risk of toxicity. The drug must also be used cautiously in patients with reduced cardiac output, severe respiratory depression, hypovolemia, heart block, shock, sinus bradycardia, myasthenia gravis, and renal or hepatic dysfunction. In addition, caution is necessary in pregnant or nursing women, in children, and in elderly patients.

INTERACTIONS

1. Cardiac depression may increase if lidocaine is used along with other antiarrhythmic drugs, especially phenytoin or propranolol.
2. Concurrent administration of procainamide may result in additive neurologic effects.
3. The muscle-relaxant effects of neuromuscular blocking agents (*e.g.*, succinylcholine, aminoglycosides) and other skeletal muscle relaxants may be increased by lidocaine.
4. Lidocaine inhibits the antibacterial action of sulfonamides.
5. Barbiturates (especially phenobarbital) may decrease the action of lidocaine through enzyme induction.
6. Serum lidocaine levels can be elevated by cimetidine and beta blocking agents, presumably due to decreased metabolic clearance.

NURSING CONSIDERATIONS

See also Nursing Process, earlier in this chapter.

Central nervous system toxicity can develop with rapid IV infusion of lidocaine. To reduce the chance of toxicity the drug should be given as a bolus over a period ranging from 30 seconds to 1 minute. This should be immediately followed by an IV drip, which must be closely monitored. Micro-drip tubing or an infusion pump should be used. Early warning signs of central nervous system toxicity include drowsiness, slurred speech, hearing loss, and fine tremors. If toxicity develops the drug should be stopped, the physician notified, and the patient closely monitored for convulsions. Diazepam or barbiturates should be on hand in case convulsions develop.

Once a lidocaine drip has been initiated, it should be gradually titrated down while an oral antiarrhythmic agent is started when the patient is capable of taking oral medications. The recommended titration time is 8 hours to 24 hours to reduce the chance of arrhythmia recurrence before an oral drug serum level has been reached.

Tocainide

(Tonocard)

MECHANISM AND ACTIONS

Tocainide, a close structural analog of lidocaine, is resistant to gastric acid and relatively unaffected by first-pass hepatic metabolism. Thus, the drug is effective orally and may be used for treating ventricular arrhythmias.

The mechanism of action of tocainide is similar to that of lidocaine. The drug decreases myocardial cell excitability, reduces automaticity, and decreases the effective refractory period of the Purkinje fibers and ventricular muscle cells. Sinus node function is largely unaltered and conduction times are not changed appreciably. Tocainide does not elicit significant changes in heart rate, blood pressure, or myocardial contractility, although a slight degree of depression of left ventricular function is noted, usually without appreciable change in the cardiac output in well-compensated patients. A slight increase in vascular resistance and pulmonary arterial pressure may occur.

USES

1. Treatment of symptomatic ventricular arrhythmias, such as premature ventricular contractions, ventricular tachycardia, and unifocal or multifocal couplets

ADMINISTRATION AND DOSAGE

Tocainide is available as tablets (400 mg, 600 mg). The initial dose is 400 mg every 8 hours and the usual maintenance range is 1200 mg to 1800 mg/day in two or three divided doses. The maximum recommended dose is 2400 mg/day. Dosage may have to be reduced in patients with renal or hepatic impairment.

FATE

Oral absorption is rapid and complete, and peak serum levels are attained in 0.5 hour to 3 hours. Food delays the rate but not the extent of absorption. Only 10% to 20% of a dose is protein bound. The drug is inactivated in the liver and is excreted in the urine as metabolites as well as unchanged drug (30%–50%). Elimination half-life is approximately 12 hours to 15 hours, and is increased in the presence of severe renal dysfunction. The pharmacokinetics of the drug are not appreciably altered in patients with a myocardial infarction.

SIDE-EFFECTS/ADVERSE REACTIONS

Side-effects occurring most often with tocainide therapy are lightheadedness, dizziness, nausea, paresthesias, numbness, mild tremor, and giddiness. Other adverse reactions noted during tocainide therapy are the following:

Central nervous system—Nervousness, visual disturbances, tinnitus, headache, drowsiness, nystagmus, ataxia, anxiety, incoordination, confusion, disorientation, altered mood, hallucinations

Cardiovascular—Bradycardia, hypotension, palpitations, chest pain, ventricular arrhythmias, congestive heart failure, AV or bundle branch block, cardiomegaly

Gastrointestinal—Anorexia, loose stools, diarrhea, vomiting, abdominal pain, dysphagia

Other—Sweating, rash, skin lesions, arthralgia; rarely, blood dyscrasias, lupus-like syndrome, pulmonary fibrosis and edema, and pneumonia

CONTRAINDICATIONS AND PRECAUTIONS

Tocainide is contraindicated in the presence of second-degree or third-degree heart block and in patients hypersensitive to amide-type local anesthetics. The drug should be given *cautiously* to persons with heart failure or reduced cardiac reserve, conduction disturbances, atrial arrhythmias (since ventricular rate may accelerate), pulmonary dysfunction, hypokalemia, or severe liver or kidney disease, and to pregnant or nursing mothers and children.

INTERACTIONS

1. Concurrent use of tocainide with other drugs having a negative inotropic action (e.g., beta blockers, verapamil, disopyramide) may further depress left ventricular function.

NURSING CONSIDERATIONS

See also Nursing Process, earlier in this chapter.

Patients who develop gastrointestinal or initial neurologic side-effects such as dizziness on divided doses every 12 hours may tolerate the therapy better if the drug is given every 8 hours instead and is taken with a fair-sized meal. Bedtime doses should be given with snacks. Most side-effects are transient in nature but if symptoms persist the physician should be notified. Neurologic side-effects are usually the early warning signs of toxicity. A rare but frightening side-effect to watch for is the onset of nightmares, which indicates the need to change to another drug.

Phenytoin
(Dilantin, Diphenylan)

Phenytoin is an antiepileptic drug (see Chap. 30) that has also been employed in the treatment of certain arrhythmias, particularly those arising from overdosage with digitalis drugs. The drug has been discussed fully in Chapter 30, and only those aspects of its pharmacology pertaining to its use in treating arrhythmias will be discussed here.

MECHANISM AND ACTIONS
The electrophysiologic effects of phenytoin in the heart are similar to those of lidocaine. The drug depresses ectopic pacemaker automaticity and shortens the action potential duration and effective refractory period in Purkinje fibers. Therapeutic levels of phenytoin have little or no effect on SA nodal firing rate and, in general, do not alter atrial function. When given to digitalized patients, AV nodal refractory period is usually shortened considerably. Conduction velocity through the AV node and Purkinje system is either unchanged or slightly increased. Phenytoin can abolish premature atrial or ventricular beats without furthering the degree of conduction block in depressed cardiac tissue as is frequently observed with some other antiarrhythmic drugs.

USES
Phenytoin, although not approved as an antiarrhythmic, has been used successfully to abolish paroxysmal atrial tachycardia and especially ventricular ectopic rhythms with AV block associated with digitalis drug overdosage. Conversely, it is much less effective against recurrent ventricular arrhythmias due to chronic ischemic heart disease, and is relatively ineffective in treating common atrial arrhythmias.

ADMINISTRATION AND DOSAGE
Phenytoin is available for injection as a solution (50 mg/ml) and as oral tablets (50 mg), capsules (30 mg, 100 mg), and suspension (30 mg/5 ml, 125 mg/5 ml). The drug may be administered either IV or orally, depending on the need for immediate action. In acute situations, 100 mg is given by IV injection every 5 minutes to 10 minutes until the arrhythmia is abolished or until adverse effects are noted. The rate of injection should not exceed 50 mg/minute and the maximum dose is considered to be 1000 mg. Intermittent and continuous infusion should be avoided since the drug rapidly precipitates when added to solution. Oral administration is usually initiated with a loading dose of 15 mg/kg the first day in divided doses, then 7.5 mg/kg the second and third days, followed by 4 mg/kg to 6 mg/kg a day thereafter. The desired serum level is 10 mcg/ml to 20 mcg/ml.

FATE
Oral absorption is slow and erratic, while tissue distribution is rapid with IV administration. The drug is highly protein bound (85%–95%). Metabolism occurs in the liver at a relatively slow rate and conjugated metabolites are eliminated in the urine. See Chapter 30 for a complete discussion of the pharmacokinetics of phenytoin.

SIDE-EFFECTS/ADVERSE REACTIONS
The most common untoward reactions noted when phenytoin is employed in the acute treatment of arrhythmias are drowsiness, nystagmus, diplopia, ataxia, and nausea. These effects are dose related and their appearance usually signifies that the plasma level is near the upper limit (*i.e.*, approaching toxic levels). A variety of other adverse reactions are associated with chronic use of phenytoin and are listed under the discussion of phenytoin in Chapter 30.

CONTRAINDICATIONS AND PRECAUTIONS
Phenytoin should not be employed to treat arrhythmias in patients with advanced heart block, as it can lead to complete heart block. *Cautious* use of phenytoin is necessary in the presence of severe bradycardia and in pregnant or nursing mothers. The drug should not be administered IM (erratic absorption) nor by *rapid* IV injection (danger of hypotension, ventricular fibrillation, and cardiac arrest). Emergency resuscitative equipment and drugs should be on hand.

Mexiletine
(Mexitil)

MECHANISM AND ACTIONS
Mexiletine is an orally effective antiarrhythmic that is similar to lidocaine and tocainide in its actions. It reduces the rate of rise of phase 0 of the action potential, decreases the effective refractory period in Purkinje fibers, and shortens the action potential duration. Mexiletine has minimal effects on impulse generation or propagation, cardiac output, force of contraction, pulse rate, blood pressure, and peripheral vascular resistance. The QRS duration and QT interval are relatively unaffected.

USES

1. Management of symptomatic ventricular arrhythmias, such as multifocal premature ventricular contractions, couplets, and ventricular tachycardia

ADMINISTRATION AND DOSAGE

Mexiletine is used orally as capsules (150 mg, 200 mg, 250 mg). The initial dose is usually 200 mg every 8 hours, with gradual adjustments in 50-mg to 100-mg increments as needed. When rapid control of ventricular arrhythmias is required, an initial loading dose of 400 mg may be given, followed by 200 mg in 8 hours. Up to 400 mg may be given every 8 hours if necessary, although the severity of central nervous system side-effects increases with increasing dosage.

FATE

Oral absorption is good and peak serum levels occur in 2 hours to 3 hours. The effective plasma range is 0.5 mcg/ml to 2 mcg/ml and can be maintained with two to three times daily dosing. Mexiletine is 50% to 60% protein bound. The drug is metabolized in the liver and metabolites are excreted in the urine together with approximately 10% unchanged drug. Elimination half-life is 10 hours to 12 hours with normal liver function, but may be prolonged up to 25 hours to 30 hours in patients with liver impairment.

SIDE-EFFECTS/ADVERSE REACTIONS

Most frequent side-effects occurring during mexiletine therapy are gastrointestinal distress, tremor, lightheadedness, dizziness, impaired coordination, palpitations, chest pain, nervousness, and headache. Among the other adverse reactions associated with mexiletine therapy are the following:

Gastrointestinal—Diarrhea, loss of appetite, abdominal pain, dysphagia, gastrointestinal bleeding, peptic ulcer, altered taste, oral mucosal ulceration

Central nervous system—Confusion, short-term memory loss, depression, hallucinations, convulsions, psychotic behavior

Cardiovascular—Anginal-like pain, premature ventricular contractions, bradycardia, hypotension, syncope, edema, conduction disturbances, atrial arrhythmias

Other—Rash, arthralgia, fever, urinary hesitancy, hiccoughs, dyspnea, sweating, hair loss, decreased libido/impotence, systemic lupus-like syndrome, blood dyscrasias, abnormal liver function tests, positive ANA titer

Mexiletine can *worsen* arrhythmias, especially in more seriously ill patients.

CONTRAINDICATIONS AND PRECAUTIONS

Mexiletine is contraindicated in cardiogenic shock and second-degree or third-degree heart block. The drug must be given cautiously to persons with sinus node dysfunction, conduction abnormalities, hypotension, congestive heart failure, liver or kidney dysfunction, or a history of convulsive disorders, and to pregnant or nursing women and to children.

INTERACTIONS

1. Phenytoin, phenobarbital, rifampin, and other hepatic enzyme inducers may lower mexiletine plasma levels.
2. Cimetidine can reduce mexiletine clearance and increase its plasma levels.
3. Drugs that alkalinize the urine may slow mexiletine excretion, while acidifying agents can enhance its rate of excretion.

NURSING CONSIDERATIONS

See also Nursing Process, earlier in this chapter.

Initial and periodic assessments of blood pressure and ECG are essential with this drug, since symptoms of toxicity can develop. Periodic liver enzymes should also be drawn, since hepatic toxicity is known to occur. The drug should be used with extreme caution in patients with liver disease.

Drug side-effects may be disabling. They can occur with normal doses and are a frequent cause of noncompliance. Nausea, vomiting, and central nervous system effects such as tremors, dizziness, and incoordination may respond to taking the drug with food or with antacids to slow absorption time. Dose reduction may also help. However, the patient should limit driving or operating any hazardous machinery until response is known. Patients should learn to rise slowly from a sitting or lying position to minimize the drug's hypotensive effects.

Group IC Antiarrhythmic Drugs

Flecainide

(Tambocor)

MECHANISM AND ACTIONS

Flecainide is an orally effective class IC antiarrhythmic drug that possesses membrane-stabilizing activity and has local anesthetic-like properties.

The drug produces decreased conduction in all parts of the heart, with the greatest effect noted in the His–Purkinje system. Ventricular refractory period is prolonged. Flecainide suppresses single and multiple premature ventricular contractions and can decrease the recurrence of ventricular tachycardia. Alterations in heart rate and blood pressure are minimal. A negative inotropic effect has been observed following single doses but there is no consistent reduction in contractile force with continued therapy. Flecainide can cause new arrhythmias or worsen existing ones, and its use is associated with a wide range of untoward reactions.

USES
1. Treatment of life-threatening ventricular arrhythmias (*e.g.*, sustained ventricular tachycardia)
2. Treatment of symptomatic ventricular tachycardia and frequent premature ventricular beats where the benefits outweigh the risks (see below)

ADMINISTRATION AND DOSAGE
Flecainide is available as 100-mg tablets. Dosage is titrated individually based on symptoms. The effective plasma levels range between 0.2 mcg/ml and 1.0 mcg/ml, taken as the trough value. Higher trough levels are associated with a significant increase in toxicity. Recommended doses for the different indications are as follows:

Sustained ventricular tachycardia—Initially, 100 mg every 12 hours. Increase in 50-mg increments twice daily *every 4 days only* (maximal effect requires several days to develop) until an optimal effect is noted. Maximum dose is 400 mg/day, while most patients are controlled at 300 mg/day.

Symptomatic nonsustained ventricular tachycardia or premature ventricular complexes—Initially, 100 mg every 12 hours. Increase in 50-mg increments twice a day *every 4 days only* (see above) until desired control is achieved. Most patients will respond at 400 mg/day; however, dosage may be increased cautiously to 600 mg/day if patient is still symptomatic at 400 mg/day.

Once arrhythmia is controlled, dosage may be reduced gradually if possible to minimize side-effects or effects on conduction.

FATE
Oral absorption is complete and peak plasma levels are attained in about 3 hours. Steady-state plasma levels occur within 3 days to 5 days, and the plasma half-life ranges from 12 hours to 24 hours. Cumulation rarely occurs during chronic therapy. Plasma protein binding is approximately 40%. About one third of an oral dose is eliminated unchanged in the urine. The remainder is metabolized in the liver and conjugated metabolites are excreted in the urine. Renal impairment increases the drug's half-life.

SIDE-EFFECTS/ADVERSE REACTIONS

■ WARNING
Flecainide can initiate or worsen arrhythmias. The likelihood of this effect is related to the dose and the degree of underlying cardiac disease. Therapy with flecainide should be initiated in the hospital and patients monitored closely. The drug also exhibits a negative inotropic effect and may cause or worsen congestive heart failure, particularly in patients with cardiomyopathy, preexisting heart failure, or low ejection fractions.

The most commonly encountered side-effects during flecainide therapy are lightheadedness, faintness, dizziness, visual disturbances, dyspnea, headache, nausea, fatigue, palpitations, exacerbation of arrhythmias (see Nursing Alert), tremors, and constipation.

Other less frequently encountered adverse effects include the following:

Cardiovascular—Sinus bradycardia, sinus arrest, second-degree or third-degree heart block, anginal-like symptoms, hypotension

Central nervous system—Flushing, sweating, tinnitus, paresthesias, ataxia, somnolence, anxiety, depression, weakness, speech disorders, stupor, amnesia, euphoria, convulsions, morbid dreams

Gastrointestinal—Diarrhea, vomiting, anorexia, dyspepsia, dry mouth, altered taste

Ocular—Blurred vision, diplopia, photophobia, eye pain, nystagmus

Other—Decreased libido, impotence, polyuria, skin rash, urticaria, pruritus, exfoliative dermatitis, fever, swollen lips or tongue, bronchospasm, arthralgia, myalgia, leukopenia, thrombocytopenia

Large doses may significantly lengthen the PR interval; increase the QRS duration, QT interval, and amplitude of the T wave; and reduce heart rate and contractile force. Conduction disturbances, hypotension, respiratory failure, and asystole have resulted from overdosage.

CONTRAINDICATIONS AND PRECAUTIONS

Contraindications to use of flecainide are preexisting second-degree or third-degree heart block, bundle branch block (unless a pacemaker is present), and cardiogenic shock. The drug must be given very *cautiously* to patients with congestive heart failure, sick sinus syndrome, myocardial dysfunction, renal impairment, electrolyte imbalances (hypokalemia or hyperkalemia can alter the effects of flecainide), or liver disease. Cautious use must also be undertaken in patients with pacemakers or pacing electrodes and in pregnant or nursing mothers. Safety and efficacy for use in children under 18 have not been established.

INTERACTIONS

1. Concurrent use of flecainide with propranolol (and probably other beta blockers), verapamil, or disopyramide can result in additive negative inotropic effects.
2. Acidification of the urine can increase the renal elimination of flecainide, whereas alkalinization reduces the rate of excretion.
3. Plasma levels of flecainide and propranolol may both be increased when the two drugs are given together.

NURSING CONSIDERATIONS

See also Nursing Process, earlier in this chapter.

Baseline assessment of ECG and cardiovascular function is essential since many cardiovascular side-effects can occur. Renal functions should also be assessed since decreased kidney function will greatly increase the amount of time flecainide remains active, thus increasing the chance of toxicity. Initial weight determination and examination for evidence of peripheral edema are also essential and should be reevaluated throughout therapy since congestive heart failure may develop. The patient should be alerted to report immediately any rapid weight gain, puffiness of hands or feet, or dyspnea on exertion. Most drug side-effects will develop within 1 week to 2 weeks after initial therapy.

Drug effectiveness is enhanced by maintenance of consistent blood levels. Therefore, the drug should be given every 12 hours instead of twice a day (bid). Periodic plasma drug levels should also be drawn.

Encainide
(Enkaid)

MECHANISM AND ACTIONS

Encainide blocks the sodium channel of the Purkinje fibers and the myocardium and slows phase 0 depolarization in a dose-dependent fashion. It also increases the ratio of the effective refractive period to action potential duration. Encainide decreases intracardiac conduction in all parts of the heart. Peripheral blood pressure is largely unaffected.

USES

1. Treatment of life-threatening arrhythmias, such as sustained ventricular tachycardia
2. Treatment of symptomatic nonsustained ventricular tachycardia and frequent premature ventricular complexes where the benefits of treatment outweigh the risks

ADMINISTRATION AND DOSAGE

Encainide is used as capsules containing either 25 mg, 35 mg, or 50 mg. The initial dose in adults is 25 mg every 8 hours. Dosage may be increased to 35 mg every 8 hours after 3 to 5 days if necessary and eventually to 50 mg every 8 hours if the desired therapeutic response has not been attained. The maximum recommended dose for life-threatening arrhythmias is 75 mg 4 times a day. Use of loading doses is *not* recommended.

FATE

Oral absorption is complete and peak plasma levels are attained within 30 to 90 minutes. Plasma protein binding is 75–85%. Encainide has two active metabolites that are eliminated more slowly than the parent compound (4 to 8 hr *vs.* 1 to 2 hr). Steady state plasma levels are attained within 3 to 5 days. The major route of elimination is *via* the kidney.

SIDE-EFFECTS/ADVERSE REACTIONS

The most often encountered side-effects with encainide are dizziness, blurred vision, headache, and initiation or worsening of ventricular arrhythmias, which may occur in up to 10% of patients. Other adverse reactions reported with encainide are the following:

Cardiovascular—Palpitations, tachycardia, syncope, peripheral edema, prolonged QRS interval, congestive heart failure

Central nervous system—nervousness, somnolence, tremor, anorexia, insomnia

Gastrointestinal—abdominal pain, constipation, nausea, vomiting, dry mouth

Other—dyspnea, coughing, skin rash,

tinnitus, altered taste, paresthesia, lower extremity pain, chest pain

Overdosage can result in hypotension, bradycardia, asystole, convulsions, and death. Acute overdosage should be treated by gastric lavage, activated charcoal, and usual supportive measures.

CONTRAINDICATIONS AND PRECAUTIONS

Encainide is contraindicated in patients with preexisting second- or third-degree heart block, right bundle branch block (unless a pacemaker is present), or cardiogenic shock. The drug should be used with extreme *caution* in persons with congestive heart failure, electrolyte disturbances, sick-sinus syndrome, renal or hepatic impairment, and in pregnant or nursing women.

INTERACTIONS

1. Concurrent use of cimetidine can increase the plasma levels of encainide.

NURSING CONSIDERATIONS

See nursing considerations for flecainide.

Group II Antiarrhythmic Drugs

Propranolol
(Inderal)

Acebutolol
(Sectral)

Propranolol and acebutolol are beta-adrenergic blocking agents that have been employed in treating a variety of arrhythmias, particularly exercise-induced arrhythmias or those associated with excessive sympathetic stimulation or circulating catecholamine levels. The beta blockers are used for a number of disease states, and they are reviewed in detail as a group in Chapter 16. The following discussion is limited to their usefulness in treating arrhythmias.

MECHANISM AND ACTIONS

The beta blockers competitively antagonize the action of adrenergic agents at beta receptor sites. Specifically, on the heart, sinus rate is slowed, AV conduction is depressed, force of contraction is reduced, and automaticity of the SA node and ectopic pacemakers is decreased. AV nodal refractory period is lengthened and reentry excitation is reduced.

USES

Propranolol is effective in controlling the following arrhythmias: Exercise-induced ventricular tachycardia, supraventricular tachyarrhythmias (atrial fibrillation, atrial flutter, paroxysmal atrial tachycardia), tachyarrhythmias of digitalis intoxication, tachycardias due to thyrotoxicosis or excessive catecholamine activity during anesthesia, and persistent premature ventricular extrasystoles not controlled by other measures.

Acebutolol currently is indicated *only* for management of ventricular premature beats.

ADMINISTRATION AND DOSAGE

Propranolol
The usual oral dose is 10 mg to 30 mg three to four times a day. IV propranolol is generally reserved for life-threatening arrhythmias or those occurring under anesthesia. The usual IV dose is 1 mg to 3 mg at a rate of 1 mg/minute. If necessary, a second dose can be given in 2 minutes, but no further drug should be given for at least 4 hours.

Acebutolol
The initial oral dose is 200 mg twice a day. Dosage is then increased gradually until the desired response is obtained. Usual dosage range is 600 mg to 1200 mg a day.

FATE

See Chapter 16 for a discussion of the fate of orally administered beta blockers. Following IV administration of propranolol, effects are noted within 1 minute to 2 minutes and persist for up to 6 hours.

SIDE-EFFECTS/ADVERSE REACTIONS

Refer to Chapter 16 for a complete discussion of the adverse effects associated with beta blockers. When propranolol is given IV for the emergency control of arrhythmias, significant hypotension or left ventricular failure can occur. In addition, AV block, severe bradycardia, and asystole have been reported following administration of propranolol.

NURSING CONSIDERATIONS

See also Nursing Process, earlier in this chapter.

The beta blockers interact with many drugs, particularly other drugs used in cardiovascular disease. Therefore, the nurse needs to obtain a detailed drug history since many of these drug interactions can be life threatening. Extreme caution should be used when administering propranolol to any patient on digitalis drugs, antiarrhythmic agents, or drugs for hypertension.

During intravenous administration the patient should be kept supine and blood pressure and ECG monitored continuously since hypotension, AV block, severe bradycardia, and asystole can occur.

Reflex peripheral vasoconstriction can result when the beta blockers are administered. The problem occurs more frequently in patients with a history of peripheral vascular disease. Consequently, the patient receiving a beta blocker should be monitored for the development of cold extremities and intermittent claudication. If these occur, the physician should be notified since decreased circulation in the already impaired individual can lead to extensive tissue damage. All patients should also be monitored for symptoms of cardiac failure and bronchospasm.

Beta blockers should always be withdrawn gradually. Abrupt withdrawal can result in rapid rebound hypertension or exacerbation of angina pectoris. Vital signs should be closely monitored during any withdrawal process.

Group III Antiarrhythmic Drugs

Bretylium
(Bretylol)

Bretylium was originally introduced into clinical medicine as an antihypertensive agent and subsequently was found to have antiarrhythmic activity. It is now used exclusively as an alternate drug for the emergency control of serious ventricular arrhythmias.

MECHANISM AND ACTIONS
The mechanism of action of bretylium is complex and incompletely understood. The drug can prolong the effective refractory period and action potential duration of Purkinje fibers and ventricular muscle cells. The ventricular fibrillation threshold is considerably increased. Minimal effects are noted on sinus node or His–Purkinje automaticity (although initial increases have been noted), conduction velocity in Purkinje fibers or ventricular muscle cells, or atrial refractory period.

The drug initially releases norepinephrine from adrenergic nerve terminals, resulting in tachycar-

dia, increased peripheral vascular resistance, and possibly a transient *worsening* of certain arrhythmias. Subsequently, release of norepinephrine is *blocked* in response to nerve stimulation, although catecholamine stores do not appear to be depleted.

USES
1. Control of life-threatening ventricular arrhythmias that have not responded to first-line antiarrhythmic drugs, such as lidocaine or procainamide

The use of bretylium is limited to emergency rooms and intensive-care or coronary-care facilities with appropriate monitoring devices. Severe, refractive ventricular arrhythmias have responded in dramatic fashion to bretylium, but due to its adverse effects (see below), it is not considered a first-line drug.

ADMINISTRATION AND DOSAGE
Bretylium is available as an injection (50 mg/ml) that may be given undiluted (IV or IM) or as a diluted solution by IV infusion. Doses are as follows:

Acute
Ventricular fibrillation or life-threatening ventricular tachycardia
　　IV—5 mg/kg (undiluted) by rapid injection; may repeat at 10 mg/kg every 15 minutes to 30 minutes to a total dose of 30 mg/kg
Other ventricular arrhythmias
　　IV—5 mg/kg to 10 mg/kg of a diluted solution by IV infusion over 10 minutes to 30 minutes. Repeat at 1-hour to 2-hour intervals if arrhythmia persists.
　　Dilution—10 ml (500 mg) diluted to a minimum of 50 ml with dextrose or sodium chloride injection
　　IM (do not dilute)—5 mg/kg to 10 mg/kg; may repeat in 1 hour to 2 hours, then every 6 hours to 8 hours thereafter (maximum injection volume is 5 ml at any one site)

Maintenance
5 mg/kg to 10 mg/kg of diluted solution infused over 10 minutes to 30 minutes every 6 hours, or 1 mg/kg to 2 mg/kg of diluted solution by constant infusion

FATE
The onset of antifibrillatory action following IV injection is within minutes, while suppression of ventricular tachycardia and other ventricular ar-

rhythmias may require 0.5 hour to 2 hours. Peak plasma concentrations occur within 1 hour following IM injection but maximal therapeutic effects (*i.e.*, suppression of premature ventricular beats) do not occur for 6 hours to 9 hours. Elimination half-life ranges from 5 hours to 10 hours and is increased in the presence of renal insufficiency. The drug is excreted intact by the kidneys; approximately 70% to 80% of an IM dose is eliminated during the first 24 hours.

SIDE-EFFECTS/ADVERSE REACTIONS

The most frequent adverse effect with bretylium is hypotension, both orthostatic (most common) and supine, and is marked by dizziness, lightheadedness, faintness, and vertigo. Dopamine may be used to treat significant hypotension. Patients *must* be kept supine during administration and until tolerance to the hypotensive effect has developed, which can take up to several days. Nausea and vomiting are frequently noted on too-rapid IV injection or infusion. During chronic therapy, parotid pain is often observed. Other adverse reactions include bradycardia, substernal pain, and, during the initial period of administration, transitory tachycardia, hypertension, and increased arrhythmias.

Other untoward reactions seen with bretylium use for which a definite cause-and-effect relationship has not been established are diarrhea, flushing, hyperthermia, dyspnea, anxiety, abdominal pain, erythematous rash, diaphoresis, confusion, nasal congestion, and renal dysfunction.

CONTRAINDICATIONS AND PRECAUTIONS

There are no absolute contraindications to use of bretylium in treating life-threatening ventricular arrhythmias; use in less serious arrhythmias is contraindicated in severe pulmonary hypertension or in aortic stenosis and in patients with fixed cardiac output. The drug should be used *cautiously* during pregnancy and in children and dosage may need to be reduced in patients with reduced renal function. Oral antiarrhythmic maintenance therapy with another drug should be initiated as soon as possible.

INTERACTIONS

1. Bretylium may increase digitalis toxicity by releasing norepinephrine initially. Do not give concurrently with digitalis drugs.
2. Peripheral vasodilation occurring in patients already receiving procainamide or quinidine may be increased by bretylium.

NURSING CONSIDERATIONS

See also Nursing Process, earlier in this chapter.

Since bretylium is considered an emergency drug it is used for a short period of time, and must be closely monitored for adverse reactions. The IV route is preferred, however, since the drug produces severe hypotension; the patient must be kept supine throughout most of the therapy. In addition, if bretylium is administered too quickly, severe, projectile vomiting can occur. The nurse must be prepared to prevent aspiration if this occurs. As a result of these side-effects, bretylium should be administered slowly by an intravenous drip whenever possible. An infusion pump should be used to prevent accidental overdosage.

Bretylium will usually be slowly discontinued over a 3-day to 5-day period, while an oral antiarrhythmic agent is administered. The patient should be closely monitored for return of arrhythmias since, in most cases, bretylium was initiated when the arrhythmias failed to respond to other drugs.

Amiodarone

(Cordarone)

Amiodarone is an orally effective class III antiarrhythmic that is reserved for life-threatening ventricular arrhythmias not responding to other agents. The drug is highly toxic and should only be used by clinicians thoroughly familiar with its actions.

MECHANISM AND ACTIONS

Amiodarone prolongs myocardial cell action potential duration (APD) and refractory period. It possesses both an alpha-adrenergic and a beta-adrenergic blocking action. Vascular smooth muscle is relaxed and peripheral vascular resistance is reduced. Automaticity of cardiac cells is decreased, but amiodarone can cause marked sinus bradycardia and has resulted in heart block and sinus arrest. Electrocardiographic changes include increased PR and QT intervals, appearance of U waves, and altered T wave contour.

USES

1. Treatment of life-threatening recurrent ventricular arrhythmias (ventricular fibrillation, hemodynamically unstable ventricular tachy-

cardia) that do not respond to other antiar-rhythmics

ADMINISTRATION AND DOSAGE

Amiodarone is used as 200-mg tablets. Loading doses of 800 mg to 1600 mg/day in divided doses are required for 1 week to 3 weeks (occasionally longer) until the desired therapeutic response occurs. When arrhythmia control is attained, dosage is reduced to 600 mg to 800 mg/day in divided doses for approximately one month, then to 400 mg/day as a single daily dose or in two divided doses if GI intolerance occurs.

In order to minimize the untoward reactions to amiodarone, the drug should always be given at the lowest effective dose, and dosage adjustments require careful patient monitoring as the drug has a long and variable half-life.

FATE

Oral absorption is slow and variable. Peak plasma concentrations are attained within 3 hours to 7 hours, but the onset of clinical effects requires several days to several weeks, even with loading doses. The drug is widely distributed throughout the body and accumulates in fatty tissue and highly perfused organs. Plasma protein binding is approximately 95%. Elimination of the drug is through hepatic excretion into the bile of both the unchanged drug and metabolites. Renal excretion is negligible. The plasma half-life is extremely variable, and ranges from 24 days to 120 days for the parent compound (average 40 days to 50 days) and 50 days to 70 days for the metabolite. The effects of the drug persist for weeks or months after the drug is discontinued. There is no precise relationship between plasma level and clinical effectiveness; however, concentrations below 1 mg/liter are usually ineffective and levels above 2.5 mg/liter are probably unnecessary.

SIDE-EFFECTS/ADVERSE REACTIONS

■ WARNING

Amiodarone is a highly toxic drug. Fatalities have occurred as a result of pulmonary toxicity (e.g., interstitial pneumonitis, alveolitis), liver disease, arrhythmias, heart block, and sinus bradycardia. Due to its slow onset and very prolonged duration of action, even after drug discontinuation, patients must be monitored very closely during therapy and for several months follow-ing termination of therapy. Drug treatment should be initiated in a hospital setting and prolonged hospitalization may be required in unstable patients.

A wide range of adverse effects have been noted in patients receiving amiodarone. The most common side-effects are corneal microdeposits, nausea and vomiting (relative incidence 20%–30%), photosensitivity, fatigue, tremor, incoordination, ataxia, dizziness, paresthesias and peripheral neuropathy, constipation, anorexia, pulmonary inflammation or fibrosis, visual disturbances, and abnormal liver function tests (relative incidence 5%–10%).

Other reported untoward reactions are listed below:

Central nervous system—Insomnia, headache, sleep disturbances, decreased libido, photophobia

Cardiovascular—Bradycardia, congestive heart failure, SA node dysfunction, hypotension, conduction abnormalities, arrhythmias (most often exacerbation of existing arrhythmias)

Dermatologic—Solar dermatitis, blue skin discoloration, rash, alopecia, spontaneous ecchymosis

Other—Abdominal pain, dryness of the eyes, hepatic disease, hepatitis, abnormal taste and smell, salivation, edema, altered thyroid function, coagulation abnormalities

CONTRAINDICATIONS AND PRECAUTIONS

Amiodarone is contraindicated in marked sinus bradycardia, second-degree and third-degree heart block, and syncope due to episodes of bradycardia. The drug must be administered cautiously to patients with reduced hepatic function, thyroid abnormalities (drug increases levels of T_4 and reduces levels of T_3; see Chap. 52), electrolyte disturbances, coagulation difficulties, or pulmonary disease, and to pregnant or nursing mothers. Corneal microdeposits occur in the majority of patients and may result in the appearance of halos or blurred vision. They are reversible on drug discontinuation and are not a cause for stopping therapy if asymptomatic. The risk of photosensitivity is increased in patients of fair complexion and those with excessive sun exposure. Elevated hepatic enzymes are common but are asymptomatic in most cases; significant elevations or the appearance of clinical symptoms of liver dysfunction may require termination of therapy.

Amiodarone should be discontinued if patients develop pulmonary infiltrates or fibrosis, paroxysmal ventricular tachycardia, congestive heart failure, or symptoms of hepatic dysfunction.

INTERACTIONS
1. Amiodarone can increase serum levels of digoxin, quinidine, procainamide, and phenytoin if given concurrently. Dosage reductions of one third to one half may be necessary for these drugs.
2. Beta blockers and calcium-channel blockers (especially verapamil) may result in potentiation of bradycardia and increase the risk of AV block or sinus arrest when given together with amiodarone.
3. Amiodarone may increase the hypoprothrombinemic effects of warfarin, leading to serious bleeding.

NURSING CONSIDERATIONS
See also Nursing Process, earlier in this chapter.

Amiodarone has a wide range of debilitating side-effects; consequently it is usually used as a last resort when other drugs have failed. Nursing care should focus on frequent monitoring and response to side-effects as they develop.

Corneal deposits may develop since the drug is excreted in part through the lacrimal ducts, depositing small crystals. A complete ocular examination with a slit-lamp evaluation should be performed initially and periodically during therapy. Artificial tears are instilled four to six times per day to facilitate excretion of crystals. However, the patient should be told to report blurring of vision, development of light halos, especially at night, or changes in visual activity.

Gastrointestinal side-effects such as nausea and vomiting may be transient and may be relieved by administration of the drug with food. However, absorption is slow so food may only prolong the upset. Constipation can be dealt with by increasing liquids and fiber content. Laxatives should be avoided if possible since drug absorption may be impaired.

Neurologic side-effects can occur, including headaches and peripheral neuropathies especially in the glove and stocking dermatomes of the hands and feet. The patient should be periodically assessed for gait, sensation, and fine motor coordination, and told to report any numbness or tingling in hands, feet, arms, or legs.

A blue–gray discoloration of the skin may occur and is seen most often in fair-skinned females. It is reversible as the drug is withdrawn but the drug should be used cautiously in any patient with known dermatologic disease. Photosensitivity also occurs. Patients should be told to use sunscreens and protective clothing and to minimize time spent in direct sunlight.

Hyperthyroidism is another drug side-effect. Periodic thyroid function studies, especially T_3 and T_4, should be completed and patients should report immediately any feeling of heart rate increase, increased perspiration, increased appetite with weight loss, or difficulty sleeping.

Patients taking the drug are more susceptible to congestive heart failure, pulmonary changes, and liver toxicity. Baseline hepatic function, arterial blood gases, and cardiopulmonary assessment should be performed and reviewed periodically. The patient should be weighed daily and output should be measured. Dyspnea, rales, edema, lip cyanosis, or neck vein distention should be reported immediately as should any changes in laboratory values.

Unfortunately, amiodarone has a long half-life so excretion of the drug is very slow. Toxic side-effects may take days to weeks to resolve even when the drug is discontinued. Consequently, supportive care must be given.

Group IV Antiarrhythmic Drugs

Verapamil
(Calan, Isoptin)

Verapamil is a calcium channel blocker that together with the other calcium channel blockers diltiazem and nifedipine is used orally for the treatment of angina (this application is reviewed in Chap. 36). Verapamil is also used orally for the control of mild to moderate hypertension (see Chap. 35). In addition, verapamil is indicated for the treatment of supraventricular tachyarrhythmias because it has a much greater effect on SA and AV nodal function than do the other calcium blockers (see Table 36-3, Chap. 36). Its use as an antiarrhythmic is discussed below.

MECHANISM AND ACTIONS
Verapamil inhibits influx of calcium ions through slow membrane channels (*i.e.*, calcium channels)

into cells of the cardiac conductile system. AV conduction is slowed and the effective refractory period of the SA and AV nodes is prolonged, thus reducing elevated ventricular rate, interrupting AV nodal impulse reentry (see Fig. 34-1), and restoring normal sinus rhythm in supraventricular tachycardias. Automaticity of the SA node is suppressed. Verapamil also decreases myocardial contractility and reduces aortic impedance to left ventricular ejection (i.e., afterload). Systemic arterial pressure may be transiently lowered, and left ventricular filling pressure is slightly elevated.

USES
(Antiarrhythmic applications only)
1. Treatment of supraventricular tachyarrhythmias, such as paroxysmal atrial tachycardia and those associated with Wolff-Parkinson-White syndrome
2. Temporary control of excessive ventricular rate in patients with atrial flutter or atrial fibrillation

ADMINISTRATION AND DOSAGE
Verapamil is available as tablets (80 mg, 120 mg) for use in chronic treatment of angina (see Chap. 36), sustained-release tablets (240 mg) for use in hypertension (see Chap. 35), and as an undiluted IV injection solution (5 mg/2 ml) for the treatment of arrhythmias. The drug is given by slow IV injection under close monitoring of cardiac function.
Recommended dosage ranges are as follows:
Adults: Initially, 5 mg to 10 mg over 2 minutes to 3 minutes; repeat with 10 mg 30 minutes after first dose if initial response is inadequate.
Children: Age 0 to 1 year—0.75 mg to 2 mg over 2 minutes; 1 year to 15 years—2 mg to 5 mg over 2 minutes; may repeat initial dose in 30 minutes, if necessary

FATE
Effects are usually noted within 2 minutes to 5 minutes of injection. Duration of action of a single injection is 30 minutes to 45 minutes. Elimination half-life is 3 hours to 8 hours. Verapamil is rapidly metabolized in the liver and metabolites are excreted in the urine (70%) and feces (15%–20%). It is highly protein bound (90%).

SIDE-EFFECTS/ADVERSE REACTIONS
In general, adverse effects with IV administration of verapamil are infrequent. Transient hypotension, dizziness, and bradycardia can occur with therapeutic doses, but are more likely with excessive doses. Other adverse reactions seen occasionally during IV administration are tachycardia, headache, vertigo, fatigue, sweating, muscle weakness, marked hypotension, depression, AV block, congestive heart failure, and asystole.

Depressed AV conduction and myocardial contractility can result in marked bradycardia and greatly decreased left ventricular function. Congestive heart failure can be exacerbated or precipitated by verapamil, especially if used in combination with beta blockers or other drugs with similar actions on the heart. When given IV to patients with Wolff-Parkinson-White syndrome or atrial fibrillation, verapamil can increase the ventricular rate.

A variety of side-effects are associated with the oral administration of verapamil and the other calcium channel blockers, and these are listed in Chapter 36.

CONTRAINDICATIONS AND PRECAUTIONS
IV verapamil is contraindicated in the presence of second-degree or third-degree heart block, severe congestive heart failure or left ventricular dysfunction, cardiogenic shock, sick sinus syndrome, and severe hypotension (90 mm Hg systolic). IV verapamil should not be given concurrently (within 2 hours to 3 hours) with an IV beta blocker, since excessive depression of AV conduction and myocardial contractility can result (see Interactions, below). Verapamil must be used cautiously in patients with hypertrophic cardiomyopathy and renal or hepatic dysfunction.

INTERACTIONS
1. Verapamil may be potentiated by other strongly protein-bound drugs, such as oral anticoagulants, anti-inflammatory drugs, and sulfonamides.
2. The desired effects of verapamil may be reduced by administration of supplemental calcium.
3. The depressant action of verapamil on the myocardium and AV node can be enhanced by simultaneous use of an IV beta-blocking drug or disopyramide.
4. Excessive bradycardia or AV block can occur if verapamil is given together with a digitalis drug. Chronic verapamil therapy increases serum digoxin levels.

5. Verapamil can enhance the blood-pressure-lowering action of antihypertensive drugs.

NURSING CONSIDERATIONS

See also Nursing Process, earlier in this chapter, and Chapter 36.

Since verapamil can result in marked bradycardia, atropine, temporary pacing equipment, and cardioversion equipment should be kept on hand. In addition, the drug can potentiate a variety of cardiovascular effects when given with other cardiovascular drugs. Vital signs and cardiac monitoring are essential during initial therapy. Monitor ECG for onset of increasing AV block, bradycardia, bundle branch block, or increasing ventricular rate. Also observe for signs of cardiac failure.

The drug should be given on an empty stomach to enhance absorption. Verapamil can cause constipation, a severe problem for the cardiac patient. Roughage foods, adequate fluids, and administration of a stool softener may reduce the occurrence of constipation.

CASE STUDY

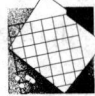

See case study at the end of Chapter 36.

REVIEW QUESTIONS

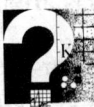

1. Briefly describe the basic mechanisms responsible for most cardiac arrhythmias.
2. List some external factors that can precipitate an arrhythmia.
3. Distinguish between first-degree, second-degree, and third-degree heart block.
4. Outline the major groups of antiarrhythmic drugs, and give their principal actions on the heart.
5. What data will be obtained before initiating emergency treatment of an arrhythmia? What other baseline data will be collected over the course of therapy?
6. What perceptions of drug therapy might the nurse expect in a patient who has suffered a cardiac arrest?
7. Outline treatment goals for emergency care of a patient with a life-threatening arrhythmia.
8. Outline a patient teaching plan for a patient going home on an antiarrhythmic drug.
9. What are the signs of cardiac toxicity in a patient being treated with an antiarrhythmic agent?
10. What are some of the symptoms a patient with an altered rest/sleep pattern might exhibit? Is he likely to relate these to his changed heart pattern?
11. What outcome criteria can the nurse use to measure the success of antiarrhythmic drug therapy?
12. What are the common side-effects associated with quinidine therapy? What is meant by "quinidine syncope"?
13. In what conditions would use of quinidine be contraindicated?
14. Give the major advantages *and* disadvantages of procainamide relative to quinidine.
15. What are the *early signs* of a developing (1) lupus-like syndrome and (2) agranulocytosis sometimes seen with chronic use of procainamide?

16. Give the major adverse effects expected with use of disopyramide. With what other drugs must disopyramide be used with caution?
17. In which other conditions is the use of disopyramide contraindicated?
18. Briefly describe the principal actions of lidocaine on the heart.
19. Describe the proper dosing procedure for lidocaine.
20. What are the most commonly occurring side-effects during lidocaine administration?
21. How does tocainide resemble lidocaine? How does it differ from lidocaine?
22. What types of arrhythmias respond best to phenytoin? What are the most common untoward reactions seen with IV injection of phenytoin?
23. What are the indications for mexiletine? List the common side-effects associated with its use.
24. Give the major uses for flecainide.
25. What is the principal danger associated with flecainide?
26. What cardiac effects of the beta blockers underlie their usefulness in treating arrhythmias?
27. Against what type of arrhythmias are beta blockers most effective?
28. What is the principal indication for bretylium? How does the drug affect norepinephrine in adrenergic nerve endings?
29. What is the major disadvantage to the use of bretylium? What measures must be taken during its administration?
30. Briefly describe the actions of amiodarone and give its principal indication.
31. What are the most serious untoward reactions associated with amiodarone?
32. Why is toxicity sometimes difficult to manage with amiodarone?
33. Briefly describe the mechanism of action of verapamil. List the major indications for IV verapamil.
34. In what conditions is verapamil contraindicated?
35. What drug or drugs would you recommend for the following arrhythmias?
    a. Atrial fibrillation
    b. Supraventricular tachycardia
    c. Premature ventricular contractions
    d. Premature atrial contractions
    e. Life-threatening sustained ventricular tachycardia

BIBLIOGRAPHY

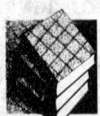

Advances in antiarrhythmic drug therapy—Changing concepts (Proceedings of a symposium). Fed Proc 45(8):2184, 1986

Cantwell R et al: Think fast: What do you know about cardiac drugs for a code? Nursing 82 12:34, October, 1982

Federman J: Antiarrhythmic drug therapy. Mayo Clin Proc 54:531, 1979

Garfein OB (ed): Clinical pharmacology of cardiac antiarrhythmic agents. Ann NY Acad Sci 432:1, 1984

Greenspon AJ, Vlasses PH, Ferguson RK: Amiodarone: A new drug for the treatment of cardiac arrhythmias. Ration Drug Ther 18(8):1, 1984

Hoffman BF, Rosen MR: Cellular mechanisms of cardiac arrhythmias. Circ Res 49:1, 1981

Keefe DL, Kates RE, Harrison DC: New antiarrhythmic drugs: Their place in therapy. Drugs 22:363, 1981

Kienzle MG et al: Antiarrhythmic drug therapy for sustained ventricular tachycardia. Heart Lung 13(6):614, 1984

Pratt CM, Delclos G, Wierman AM et al: The changing baseline of complex ventricular arrhythmias: A new consideration in assessing long-term antiarrhythmic drug therapy. N Engl J Med 313:1444, 1985

Roberts WC: Symposium on the management of ventricular dysrhythmias. Am J Cardiol 54:1A, 1984

Rosen MR, Wit AL: Electropharmacology of antiarrhythmic drugs. Am Heart J 106:829, 1983

Rossi L: Nursing care for survivors of sudden cardiac death. Nurs Clin North Am 19(3):411, 1984

Ruskin JN: Arrhythmias: Are you selecting the right drug. Mod Med 54(11):54, 1986

Scherer P: New drugs of 1985 in theory and in practice. Am J Nurs 86:406, 1986

Sjogren ER: Tonocard. Crit Care Nurs 3(6):12, Nov/Dec, 1983

Smith A: Amiodarone: Clinical considerations. Focus on Critical Care 11(5):30, 1984

Stanford J, Felner J, Arensberg D: Antiarrhythmic drug therapy. Am J Nurs 80(10):1288, 1980

Stone KS, Scordo KA: Understanding the calcium channel blockers. Heart Lung 13(5):563, 1984

Treatment of cardiac arrhythmias. Med Lett Drugs Ther 25:21, 1983

Wilson H: Drug therapy for cardiac arrhythmias. American Druggist p 137, April, 1985

Woosley RL, Echt DS, Roden DM: Treatment of ventricular arrhythmias in the failing heart: Pharmacologic and clinical considerations. Ration Drug Ther 19(10):1, 1985

Woosley RL: Mexiletine and tocainide: A profile of two lidocaine analogs. Ration Drug Ther, 21(3):1, 1987

Antihypertensive Drugs

35

Hypertension, an abnormally elevated blood pressure, is one of the most prevalent diseases in the world, and although the number of Americans afflicted is impossible to determine with any degree of accuracy, it is estimated to be between 30 million and 50 million. Unfortunately, this disease is frequently asymptomatic for many years, although organ damage is progressive and it is often not until *significant* organ dysfunction has occurred that clinical signs become evident. Thus, hypertension has been termed the "silent killer," and early detection and treatment of elevated blood pressure can markedly reduce morbidity and prolong life. Sustained, untreated hypertension results in damage to blood vessels in the major organs (*e.g.*, liver, kidney, brain, heart) and can lead to the development of coronary artery disease, congestive heart failure, myocardial infarction, renal failure, and stroke.

The risk of vascular damage is largely related to the *degree* of blood pressure elevation, although even "mild" hypertension can significantly increase long-term pathology associated with end-organ damage. In addition, the risk of organ damage due to elevated arterial pressure is increased by a number of additional factors, including obesity, excessive salt intake, smoking, hyperlipidemia, diabetes, and stressful life-style. Males and blacks tend to develop cardiovascular complications as a result of elevated blood pressure more often and sooner than females (especially premenopausal) and whites. Genetic predisposition to hypertension is an often debated point, but a family history of hypertension, stroke, or coronary artery disease should prompt careful evaluation of the need for controlling blood pressure.

Before discussing the etiology and diagnosis of hypertension, a brief review of the mechanisms involved in the regulation of arterial pressure will be presented.

Arterial Blood Pressure

The arterial blood pressure serves as the driving force for blood flow through the vascular system. The magnitude of arterial blood pressure changes throughout the cardiac cycle. The maximum pressure (systolic pressure) occurs at the peak of ventricular contraction or systole. The magnitude of systolic pressure may be altered by changes in cardiac output or arterial distensibility. An increase in stroke volume, and hence cardiac output, will elevate systolic pressure, as will a reduction in arterial distensibility such as that occurring in arteriosclerosis.

The lowest pressure (diastolic pressure) occurs during diastole, just before ventricular contraction. Changes in peripheral resistance alter the level of diastolic pressure.

The difference between the systolic and diastolic pressures is termed pulse pressure. Pulse pressure is directly related to the stroke volume and is inversely related to the heart rate and peripheral resistance.

The mean arterial pressure is generally assumed to equal the diastolic pressure plus one-third of the pulse pressure. At rapid heart rates, the times spent in systole and diastole are more nearly equal, and mean arterial pressure equals approximately one-half of the sum of systolic and diastolic pressures.

The mean arterial pressure equals the product of cardiac output and peripheral vascular resistance (*i.e.*, MAP = CO × PVR). Any factor or condition that alters either or both of these variables will therefore affect the blood pressure.

The arterial blood pressure is constantly and carefully regulated by normal physiologic processes to provide a driving force sufficient to distribute blood to all body tissues without imposing an excessive load on the heart and blood vessels. Several control mechanisms exist for the continuous and precise regulation and integration of cardiovascular functions.

Within the medulla of the brain stem are cardiovascular (cardiac and vasomotor) control centers which receive and integrate input from various sensory receptors. Homeostatically, the most important of these are the pressure-sensitive baroreceptors located in the carotid sinus and aortic arch. Associated with the baroreceptors are branches of the glossopharyngeal (IX) and vagus (X) nerves, which serve as "buffer" nerves for the physiologic regulation and maintenance of systemic arterial pressure.

In response to blood pressure changes detected by the baroreceptors, afferent (sensory) impulses travel along the glossopharyngeal (sinus) and vagus (aortic) nerves to the cardiovascular integrating centers of the medulla. Activation of autonomic sympathetic and parasympathetic efferent nerves to the heart and blood vessels produces appropriate changes in cardiac output and peripheral resistance for the homeostatic restoration of blood pressure.

Efferent responses to an elevated blood pressure include the following: (1) a slowing of the heart (bradycardia) resulting from increased parasympathetic and decreased sympathetic activity, (2) reduced myocardial contractility caused by decreased sympathetic discharge, and (3) vasodilation resulting from decreased sympathetic tone. The reduction in cardiac output (resulting from a decreased heart rate and stroke volume) and the decreased peripheral vascular resistance restore the blood pressure toward normal.

The activity of the medullary cardiovascular integrating centers may also be influenced by afferent impulses from higher brain centers such as the hypothalamus and cerebral cortex. It is through such afferent input that emotional responses, for example, fear or rage, alter blood pressure.

A peripheral mechanism operative in the control of blood pressure is the renin-angiotensin-aldosterone system, which is outlined in Figure 35-1. Renin is released from renal juxtaglomerular cells (see Fig. 41-3) in response to a number of stimuli, including hypotension, reduced renal perfusion pressure, and beta-adrenergic stimulation. Renin acts on the plasma protein angiotensinogen to form the decapeptide angiotensin I, which is then converted by endothelial cell and plasma enzymes into the physiologically active angiotensin II. Angiotensin II is a potent vasopressor which acts through several mechanisms, but primarily by direct stimulation of vascular smooth muscle, to produce intense vasoconstriction and increased peripheral resistance. Angiotensin II also stimulates release of aldosterone from the adrenal cortex. Aldosterone stimulates renal tubular reabsorption of sodium, thereby promoting water reabsorption and increasing blood volume. The increased blood volume and the increased peripheral resistance both contribute to the elevation of blood pressure.

The contribution of the renin-angiotensin-aldosterone system to hypertension, other than those cases resulting from renal dysfunction or renovascular stenosis, has yet to be definitively established. Although it does not appear that abnormalities of this system are a consistent factor in the development of most forms of hypertension, a number of different compounds that reduce the formation of angiotensin II are very effective antihypertensive drugs under a wide variety of circumstances. In addition, several currently used antihypertensives reduce the release of renin,

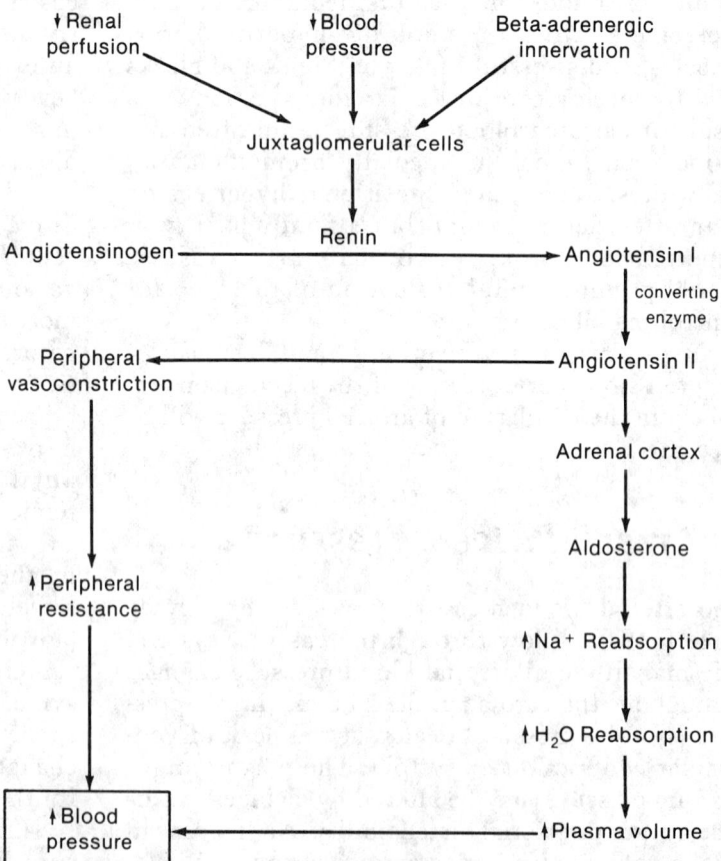

Figure 35-1.   *Renin–angiotensin–aldosterone mechanism for blood pressure regulation. See text for explanation.*

presumably because of a beta-blocking action, and this action may contribute to their efficacy in reducing blood pressure.

Hypertension

Blood pressure is reported as a ratio of the systolic pressure to diastolic pressure stated in terms of mm of mercury (*e.g.*, 120 mm Hg/85 mm Hg or simply 120/85). The criteria for defining hypertension as established by the American Heart Association are based on these values, obtained during *several* consecutive readings over a period of time. Blood pressure may be *transiently* elevated due to a number of exogenous factors, such as stress, trauma, infection, or excessive physical activity. These short-lived changes in arterial pressure have a relatively minor impact on long-term morbidity and generally do not require drug treatment. However, *consistent* increases in blood pressure obtained repeatedly during the resting state are likely to indicate a persistently elevated arterial pressure, and depending on the magnitude of the changes and the presence of other risk factors, may or may not necessitate drug therapy.

A generally (although not universally) accepted classification of hypertension based on differences in both systolic and diastolic readings is presented in Table 35-1. The diastolic reading is usually viewed as the primary determinant of the degree of hypertension, while the systolic pressure is often utilized to further refine the categorization when

Table 35-1
General Categories of Hypertension*

Pressure (mm Hg)	Category
Diastolic	
Less than 85	Normal
85–90	High normal
91–105	Mild
106–115	Moderate
Greater than 115	Severe
Systolic (when diastolic is less than 90)	
Less than 140	Normal
140–160	Borderline systolic
Greater than 160	Isolated systolic

* Values given are for adults; lower values have been advocated for younger children.

the diastolic is "borderline." Consistent diastolic pressures between 85 and 90 are viewed as high normal and seldom require specific treatment, while pressure between 90 and 100 may be termed borderline, in that the decision to employ drug treatment for pressure at this level is frequently based on the presence of end-organ damage or other risk factors. Borderline hypertension can often be controlled by weight reduction, salt limitation, cessation of smoking or a change in lifestyle, but drug therapy should seriously be considered in borderline hypertension in *high-risk patients*, for example young, black males or those with evidence of end-organ damage or a strong family history of cardiovascular disease. Diastolic pressures above 100 or systolic pressures above 160 when diastolic readings are borderline are definite indications for drug treatment.

Etiology and Diagnosis of Hypertension

In the majority of hypertensive patients (90%–95%), the pathophysiological changes responsible for the elevations in blood pressure are not identifiable, and these patients are said to have *essential* (or *primary*) hypertension.

A number of different causes have been proposed to account for the blood pressure elevations in patients with essential hypertension, including increased sympathetic functioning, elevated angiotensin/aldosterone levels, adrenal gland hyperactivity, increased vascular responsiveness, and genetic predisposition. Nevertheless, definite cause–effect relationships cannot be identified in the overwhelming majority of these hypertensive patients. On the other hand, a small percentage of people with elevated arterial blood pressure demonstrate specific etiologic factors, such as chronic kidney disease (*e.g.*, glomerulonephritis), renal arteriolar stenosis (congenital or arteriosclerotic), coarctation of the aorta, hyperaldosteronism, pheochromocytoma (tumor of adrenal medullary tissue), or use of certain drugs (*e.g.*, oral contraceptives, corticosteroids, thyroid hormones). These *secondary* types of hypertension are usually amenable to definitive treatment (*i.e.*, surgery, removal of offending drug), and specific antihypertensive drug therapy is seldom warranted.

Because most hypertensive patients evidence no overt symptoms from which a diagnosis can easily be made, the major criterion on which a definitive diagnosis of hypertension is made is a repeated, reproducible elevation in the diastolic (and occasionally systolic) blood pressure in a resting patient above the level generally recognized as indicative of hypertension (see Table 35-1). In general, hypertension can be considered as present when at least three consecutive diastolic pressure readings, obtained during three separate trials, are all above 90 mm Hg. Further tests may then be valuable for accurately assessing the extent of organ damage (e.g., papilledema, constriction of arterioles in the fundus of the eye, cardiac enlargement, elevated BUN or serum creatinine) and determining the need for appropriate drug therapy.

Judicious use of one or more of the available antihypertensive agents can provide excellent control of blood pressure for extended periods of time. The agents can also markedly delay the onset of vascular damage and can significantly prolong the life of the hypertensive patient. Drug therapy, however, is only one aspect of a complete therapeutic regimen that should also include proper rest, exercise, reduced caloric and salt intake, cessation of smoking, limitation of alcohol consumption, and avoidance of stressful situations.

Drug Therapy of Hypertension

Drug therapy of hypertension is directed toward reducing elevated arterial pressure, which is believed to be the primary cause of vascular degeneration and other complications that impair health and reduce life expectancy. Because the etiology of most cases of hypertension is unknown, treatment is essentially palliative—that is, directed at lowering the elevated systolic and diastolic pressures.

As previously noted, however, there is considerable difference of opinion as to what degree of mild hypertension requires drug treatment. Although most antihypertensive drugs can effectively reduce mildly elevated blood pressure, their use is associated with a number of side-effects. Thus, the decision whether to utilize a drug to control borderline or mild hypertension must be made with the recognition that drug-induced untoward reactions, such as elevated plasma lipids, increased serum uric acid levels, hypokalemia, depression, impotence, and many others, can adversely affect the benefit-to-risk ratio. It is therefore essential to critically balance the potential risk of drug toxicity against the risk of continued elevation of arterial pressure, the latter being heavily dependent on the

degree of blood pressure elevation, as well as the patient profile.

Drug selection is made based on several factors, such as the degree of hypertension being treated, the presence of other disease states (e.g., reserpine is contraindicated in active hepatic disease), the presence of other drugs (e.g., antidepressants reduce guanethidine's effectiveness), and a patient's acceptance of the mild yet often inescapable side-effects of many agents. Although many antihypertensive drugs have more than one site or mechanism of action, they can be conveniently grouped according to their principal sites of action, recognizing, however, that these may not be the only active sites for many of the compounds. Such a grouping is presented in Table 35-2.

The generally accepted method for selecting the appropriate antihypertensive drug is the *stepped-care approach*, a systematic method advocated by the Joint National Committee on Detec-

Table 35-2
Antihypertensive Drugs—Principal Sites of Action

I. CNS
   A. Cardiovascular centers (hypothalamus, medulla)
      1. clonidine/guanabenz/guanfacine
      2. methyldopa
      3. beta-adrenergic blockers (e.g., propranolol)
II. Sympathetic ganglia
   A. Ganglionic blocking agents (e.g., trimethaphan)
III. Adrenergic nerve endings
   A. alpha-adrenergic blockers (e.g., phentolamine, prazosin)
   B. beta-adrenergic blockers (e.g., propranolol)
   C. alpha-beta adrenergic blocker (e.g., labetalol)
   D. reserpine and rauwolfia derivatives
   E. guanethidine/guanadrel
   F. metyrosine
   G. pargyline
IV. Vascular smooth muscle
   A. hydralazine
   B. diazoxide
   C. minoxidil
   D. nitroprusside
   E. diuretics
   F. calcium channel blockers (e.g., verapamil)
V. Kidney and afferent arteriole
   A. diuretics
   B. beta-adrenergic blockers (e.g., propranolol)
VI. Renin-angiotensin system
   A. captopril/enalapril/lisinopril

tion, Evaluation and Treatment of High Blood Pressure. This approach consists of a number of sequential prescribing steps, beginning with a single agent in increasing dosage, then adding or substituting other agents in gradually increasing doses until the therapeutic goal is attained, side-effects become intolerable, or maximum dosage is reached. Despite some minor disagreements on the placement of certain drugs into a particular "step," the stepped-care approach, outlined in Table 35-3, provides a logical plan for treating all degrees of hypertension.

Mild hypertension is usually treated initially with a thiazide diuretic (step 1), although beta-blockers have been recommended as suitable alternatives, especially in younger patients with a high pulse pressure (*i.e.*, systolic minus diastolic) and rapid heart beat, and in patients with arrhythmias, angina, or hyperuricemia. In addition, certain

Table 35-3
Stepped-Care Approach to Treating Hypertension

Step 1 (Mild Hypertension)

Diuretics
    thiazides/sulfonamides (most frequently used)
    high-ceiling (loop) drugs
    potassium-sparing drugs
Beta-blockers

Step 2 (Mild to Moderate Hypertension)

beta-blockers
labetalol
clonidine/guanabenz/guanfacine
methyldopa
prazosin/terazosin
calcium-channel blockers (verapamil)
captopril/enalapril/lisinopril
rauwolfia alkaloids (*e.g.*, reserpine)

Step 3 (Moderate Hypertension)

captopril/enalapril/lisinopril
hydralazine

Step 4 (Severe Hypertension)

guanethidine/guanadrel
minoxidil

Hypertensive Emergencies

diazoxide
nitroprusside
trimethaphan

drugs listed in step 2 have been used as *initial* drugs in mild hypertension and may provide a more favorable benefit-to-risk profile than diuretics or beta-blockers.

Adrenergic inhibitors (*e.g.*, clonidine, guanabenz, guanfacine, prazosin, methyldopa) are usually added next (step 2), when maximally tolerated doses of diuretics or beta-blockers fail to provide sufficient control. A diuretic is most often continued in lower doses. Significant differences in mechanisms and side-effects among the antiadrenergic drugs, however, mandate that careful drug selection be made to optimize the therapeutic benefit. Several different step-2 drugs should be tried before adding a third drug. Other drugs being utilized in mild hypertension are angiotensin-converting enzyme inhibitors. In low doses, they are quite effective in controlling blood pressure with minimal side-effects. Calcium channel blockers (see Chap. 36) are also now being used successfully in the control of mild hypertension and represent alternatives in the management of mild to moderate hypertension.

Direct-acting vasodilators, such as hydralazine, are considered step-3 drugs and may provide additional therapeutic benefit in moderate degrees of hypertension refractory to combinations of step-1 and step-2 drugs. Captopril is also considered as an alternative in the management of refractory hypertension.

Severe hypertension may not be controlled by the three-step combination antihypertensive regimen. In these instances, additional drugs may be needed, or the extremely potent step-4 drugs, guanethidine or minoxidil, may be substituted for the other drugs. However, these latter agents are associated with severe side-effects and many drug interactions, and patients must be carefully monitored.

Hypertensive emergencies may be managed by IV sodium nitroprusside or diazoxide, both vascular smooth muscle relaxants, or trimethaphan, a ganglionic blocking agent. Pheochromocytoma, a catecholamine-secreting tumor of chromaffin tissue (*e.g.*, adrenal medulla), leads to marked elevations in blood pressure. Metyrosine or possibly phentolamine can be used to reduce the excessively high blood pressure in pheochromocytoma.

Most of the clinically useful antihypertensive drugs are discussed in this chapter according to the stepped-care concept. Several classes of antihypertensive agents have other indications as well and have been reviewed in previous chapters (*e.g.*, alpha- and beta-adrenergic blocking agents, ganglionic blocking agents). Only those aspects relating to their antihypertensive action will be mentioned here. Likewise, diuretics, perhaps the most widely used group of drugs in mild hypertension, are reviewed in detail in Chapter 41, and calcium channel blockers which are more commonly employed as anti-anginal agents, are discussed in Chapter 36, and only a brief mention made here of their antihypertensive effects.

■ Nursing Process for Antihypertensive Drugs

□ ASSESSMENT

□ Subjective Data

A drug history is useful for several reasons. The hypertensive patient may "doctor shop" if he has difficulty following a prescribed regimen or control is not easily achieved. Consequently, he may be taking several different drugs for hypertension or have taken them in the recent past. The more complete the drug history the safer the treatment plan can be. The patient should also be asked about over-the-counter (OTC) drugs and alcohol consumption. Many OTC drugs, especially those used for sinus or cold symptoms, can trigger rebound hypertension when combined with antihypertensive drugs. Conversely the use of alcohol or other CNS depressants with these same drugs can result in severe hypotension. The nurse can use interview time to review with the patient the need to consult with his physician before using any medication. It may also provide an opportunity to begin to identify alcohol use or abuse and the potential problems which may result as a consequence.

A medical history is equally important but may seem perplexing to the beginner because there may be no symptoms of disease beyond an elevated blood pressure. The clinician needs to uncover evidence of family predisposition to cardiovascular, renal, or hepatic disease and presence of risk factors such as obesity, smoking, diabetes, or hyperlipedemia. In addition, if the patient is a black male, the risk of developing severe cardiovascular complications from hypertension is extremely high. The nurse can utilize this data to explain to the patient the dangers of the disease.

If the patient has been hypertensive for a number of years, the course of symptoms and drug treatment or life-style modifications should be re-corded, especially if blood pressure control has been difficult to achieve. Compliance issues should be discussed within this framework to determine the patient's perception of previous treatment plans and his role in following them.

□ Objective Data

A complete physical assessment is essential on initiation of any antihypertensive drug regimen. Special attention should be given to cardiovascular status and renal function.

Initial blood pressure readings should be taken in both arms with the patient in each of three positions: sitting, standing, and lying. All six readings should be recorded. Subsequent readings throughout therapy should be taken in the same arm and position. The patient should rest for at least 10 minutes prior to any reading.

Antihypertensive drugs, which work on the renin-angiotensin system in the kidney, will affect sodium and water retention. Consequently the patient should be weighed prior to initiation of therapy. This is especially important when initiating a step-2 regimen in which a diuretic and antihypertensive agent are employed. Intake and output should be monitored both to establish a baseline and throughout therapy to monitor fluid retention. Extremities should be examined and lungs auscultated because fluid retention will manifest as peripheral edema and rales.

Laboratory evaluation will vary depending on the drug used. Many of the antihypertensive drugs display a variety of hematologic side-effects; consequently a complete blood count with differential is usually ordered. In addition, electrolyte studies are essential with every treatment regimen, especially when a diuretic is included in the therapy. Acid–base studies and renal and liver function studies may also be ordered.

□ NURSING DIAGNOSES

Actual nursing diagnoses for any patient taking an antihypertensive drug include

> Knowledge deficit related to the drug's action, administration, and side-effects
> Alteration in cardiac output: decreased due to vasoconstriction

Potential nursing diagnoses vary with specific drug regimens. Common ones which the nurse may find with many patients include

> Noncompliance with the prescribed regimen. (The reasons are complex and are discussed under Intervention)
> Alteration in fluid volume: excess either

because of sodium retention or
cardiovascular dysfunction
Potential for injury: trauma; related to
postural hypotension and dizziness
Sensory-perceptual alteration in vision: also
related to dizziness
Sexual dysfunction related to drug side-effects
Alteration in thought processes: depression
related to adjustment to drug

□ *PLAN*
Nursing care goals for the patient taking antihypertensive medications may include helping the patient:
1. To learn correct drug taking and to accept the
   drug therapy as necessary to maintain a blood
   pressure within normal limits (see Table 35-1)
2. To recognize and manage common side-effects
   and report disturbing ones or adverse reactions

□ *INTERVENTION*
Achieving blood pressure control through drug
therapy is not easy. A patient may be controlled for
years with diet and diuretics and then suddenly
may require an antihypertensive drug as well. The
efficacy and side-effects of many drugs vary widely
among patients. Dosage adjustments may be required before control is initially achieved, and then
may have to be adjusted again as blood levels stabilize. Because the cost of many antihypertensives is
high, if the dose or type of drug must be changed
frequently the cost may be prohibitive to some patients. In addition, when changes are frequently
necessary the patient has to relearn the new regimen and incorporate it into his life over and over
again.

Many of the antihypertensive drugs also cause
uncomfortable side-effects which are sometimes
dose-related. Some of them may interfere with sexual relations, job performance, and ability to care
for oneself, at least initially. Between problems in
establishing an effective regimen, high cost of therapy, and uncomfortable side-effects it is no wonder
patients with hypertension are more frequently
noncompliant with their drug therapy than any
other group of patients. In addition, the fact that
hypertension has no initial symptoms complicates
a patient's acceptance of the necessity of therapy.

The nurse can do a great deal to foster compliance in the hypertensive patient. Studies have
shown that the extra time given by nurses and
nurse practitioners in counseling these patients actually improves compliance. Nursing interventions

that use contracting to help patients reach specific
goals and use, as rewards, such things as assistance
with getting through the system and additional
time with the nurse, have been very successful.
Teaching and support are valued by the hypertensive patient who must frequently manage a complex regimen. Another valuable nursing intervention is follow-up. The patient who receives an
appointment card or phone call may feel the health
team cares about him and is more likely to return
for appointments than those who don't receive the
same attention. Nonetheless, compliance is a personal decision and many times the patient will stop
drug therapy because of side-effects. Orthostatic
hypotension, sexuality changes, lethargy and fatigue, and fluid retention are the most frequent
reasons patients stop taking antihypertensives.

Orthostatic hypotension may be transient and
may occur during initial therapy or when doses are
being adjusted. The patient might benefit by taking
the drug with food (except captopril) to slow absorption or at bedtime when the effects of the drug
will be minimized during sleep. He can be taught to
rise slowly from supine or sitting positions and to
avoid squatting or standing in one position for any
length of time. Saunas and hot showers should be
avoided. If the problem persists, a dosage adjustment may be in order. The side-effect may subside
at a lower dose.

Sexual concerns will vary depending on the
drug and the length of time the patient has been
taking it. Amenorrhea, impotence, and failure to
ejaculate are among the problems caused by antihypertensives. Many patients, especially older
ones, may be reluctant to discuss these problems
unless directly asked. Because our society holds
certain myths about the sexually active older adult,
the nurse must be aware that sexual activity has no
age limit in order to effectively provide care.
Open-ended questions about sexuality may begin
the dialogue. Frequently, a change in dosage or
drug may alleviate the problem. If dosage or drug
change does not work, a discussion about alternative methods for sexual satisfaction may be appropriate. Helping the patient cope with this side-effect is very important because it is frequently the
cause of noncompliance when unresolved.

Many patients experience lethargy, fatigue, and
sometimes mental depression secondary to antihypertensives. Patients need to know these symptoms
will usually subside as the body adjusts to the drug.
If symptoms become intolerable or the family notices increased withdrawal, the physician should be
notified and a change in dose or drug made.

(Text continues on p. 684.)

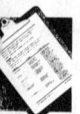

Assessment

Subjective Data

1. Medication history
   a. Refer to Interactions section to formulate pertinent questions
   b. Previous antihypertensive therapy; problems encountered
   c. Allergies/hypersensitivity

2. Medical history
   a. Refer to Contraindications and Precautions section to identify disorders that may complicate antihypertensive therapy
   b. Check for preexisting conditions that may require dosage modification, including hepatic dysfunction, angina, pheochromocytoma, renal dysfunction, endocrine disorders, pregnancy
   c. History of complications of hypertension, *i.e.*, CVA, heart disease, renal disease

3. Personal history/compliance issues
   a. Perception of illness, understanding of current therapy, compliance with past regimens
   b. Ability to manage self-care, report symptoms, and monitor BP at home if necessary
   c. Personal and financial resources; supportive network

Objective Data

1. Physical assessment highlighting
   a. Blood pressure: both arms; lying, sitting, and standing
   b. Cardiovascular status: heart rate, rhythm, peripheral pulses, presence of edema, signs of CHF
   c. Neurovascular status: mental acuity, memory, orientation, sensation, motor function

2. Laboratory data
   a. Renal and hepatic function studies
   b. CBC with differential
   c. Serum electrolytes

Nursing Diagnosis	Expected Client Outcome	Intervention
Knowledge deficit related to drug action, correct administration, potential side-effects, adverse drug interactions, the need for supervised withdrawal and clinical follow-up	Will verbalize understanding of drug action, correct administration, and potential side-effects	Explain what high blood pressure is and what it will do to the body without treatment.
		Explain what drugs, diet, and other therapy can do to control hypertension, emphasizing long-term nature of the treatment.
		Explain the importance of taking the dose as directed to obtain maximum benefit, and that it is essential to contact the physician if unable to take the drug because of illness. Methyldopa should never be abruptly discontinued.
		Teach patient to monitor common side-effects and early symptoms of adverse reactions as described below and follow preventive and reactive strategies given. Teach home BP monitoring if possible.
		Teach the patient to seek physician's advice before taking any new drug, including OTC medications.

(continued)

Nursing Care Plan 35-1 (continued)
The Patient Receiving Methyldopa

Nursing Diagnosis	Expected Client Outcome	Intervention
Knowledge deficit related to drug action, correct administration, potential side-effects, adverse drug interactions, the need for supervised withdrawal and clinical follow-up (*continued*)	Will seek clinical follow-up as recommended	Emphasize the importance of supervision to monitor the achievement of goals (*e.g.,* weight loss), to monitor serum drug levels, to discuss side-effects or other problems that the patient finds difficult to manage, to monitor any changes in hepatic, renal, or hematologic function.
Anxiety related to disease process, long-term drug therapy, and drug side-effects	Will verbalize concerns and set realistic treatment goals	Attempt to build a climate of trust so the patient feels comfortable discussing problems.
		Acknowledge that side-effects may develop, but they can usually be controlled by dosage reduction or changing to a different drug.
		Set realistic goals with the patient and measure progress to help the patient build confidence.
		Teach the patient relaxation techniques to decrease stress and anxiety.
		Set up a network for long-term support to deal with stresses of treatment as they arise.
Potential for injury: trauma related to postural hypotension	Will achieve blood pressure goals as set by physician that are within the range normal for the patient's age and with minimal postural changes	Obtain sitting, lying, and standing BP prior to each drug dose during initial treatment phase.
		Obtain BP 2 h following dose to check drug effect.
		Encourage patient to rise slowly from supine position, sit for 1 minute, then stand slowly; also, to avoid standing in one position for too long.
		Keep side rails up on bedridden patients to avoid falls if episode is acute.
		Caution patient to avoid driving, climbing, operating machinery until drug effects are known.
		Persistent problems should be reported to physician.
Potential alteration in cardiac output: decreased, related to hypotension	Will maintain normal sinus rhythm	Follow safety precautions to avoid hypotension as indicated above.
		Teach patient to monitor pulse and to report at once any decrease in heart rate, anginal pain, weakness, or peripheral edema. Dosage reduction may be required.
Potential alteration in bowel elimination: diarrhea	Will maintain normal bowel schedule and normal stool consistency	Encourage patient to report any persistent nausea, vomiting, or diar-

(continued)

Nursing Care Plan 35-1 (continued)
The Patient Receiving Methyldopa

Nursing Diagnosis	Expected Client Outcome	Intervention
Potential alteration in bowel elimination: diarrhea (continued)		rhea. Drug dose may need reduction, or drug may need to be discontinued.
Potential alteration in oral mucous membrane	Will maintain intact oral mucous membrane	Encourage frequent mouth care and oral hygiene. Encourage the patient to report tongue swelling or oral lesions, which may force drug discontinuation.
Potential for infection related to decreased WBC count	WBC and platelet counts will remain within normal limits	Encourage patient to keep follow-up laboratory appointments. Ensure periodic CBC is performed to monitor changes in WBC and platelets.
		Teach patient to report any sore throat, fever, or weakness immediately.
Potential alteration in fluid volume: excess	Weight and urinary output will remain within normal limits	Monitor urinary output, I/O ratio, and weight daily during initial period of dosage adjustment.
		Teach patient to report any rapid weight gain, edema, or shortness of breath. A diuretic may be needed if fluid retention develops.
Potential sexual dysfunction: impotence related to drug effect	Will discuss sexual concerns before discontinuing the drug	Encourage patient to report any sexual concerns by asking direct questions when appropriate.
		Report any problems to physician, because dosage can be reduced or drug changed. Sexual dysfunction can lead to noncompliance.
Potential alteration in thought processes: depression related to drug effect	Will report changes in mental status early	Encourage family to monitor patient for withdrawal from social interactions, isolation, and change in outlook, and to report such changes immediately.

Fluid retention is another uncomfortable side-effect. The patient should learn to regularly weigh himself and record how frequently he urinates each day. He should also be taught to monitor any increase in heart rate or difficulty in breathing. These are all early signs of fluid retention which should be brought to the physician's attention immediately.

The patient on antihypertensives must also be aware of the fragility of his fluid balance. When fluid is lost through perspiration, vomiting, or diarrhea, the effects of the drug may change. The patient needs to be careful in warm weather and to notify the physician if illness occurs, especially if

he is unable to take the medication. Nursing Care Plan 35-1 summarizes the nursing process for a patient receiving methyldopa, a commonly used antihypertensive medication.

□ *EVALUATION*

Outcome criteria against which to measure the success of antihypertensive therapy include achievement of goal blood pressure readings; returns to clinic for follow-up; and no evidence of fluid retention or other side-effects. The patient and nurse may also measure success by the patient's ability to manage and cope with side-effects and changes in the regimen.

ANTIHYPERTENSIVE DRUG THERAPY AND ELDERLY PATIENTS

Patients over age 65 are more susceptible to orthostatic hypotension, mental confusion, and electrolyte imbalances, such as hypokalemia and hyponatremia, and should, therefore, be more closely monitored. Drugs must be carefully titrated in this age group and changed more slowly (over a period of weeks) because normal age-related cardiovascular changes include decreased blood volume and decreased baroreceptor reflex activity. Because titration may mean changes in prescriptions, it is less costly to provide prescriptions for smaller quantities of pills until the effects of the drug are known. Patients who are stabilized may also benefit from the use of combination drugs, which decrease the number of pills they must remember to take.

Step-1 Drugs

Diuretics
(See Chapter 41.)

Beta-Adrenergic Blocking Agents

Acebutolol, Atenolol, Metoprolol, Nadolol, Pindolol, Propranolol, Timolol

Diuretics are still recognized as initial drugs of choice for mild hypertension *in the majority of patients*, and their overall safety record is quite good, especially when electrolyte levels are controlled. However, serious untoward reactions such as arrhythmias (some fatal), and increases in serum triglycerides, blood viscosity, and platelet aggregation have been associated with use of diuretics, particularly in large doses or in patients with cardiac abnormalities. These have prompted a reevaluation of the relative role of diuretics vs beta-blockers as initial therapy in treating mild, uncomplicated hypertension.

Due to these concerns, there is increasing support for the use of beta-blockers as initial drugs for mild hypertension, although it must be recognized that these drugs are capable of causing untoward reactions as well, such as bradycardia, congestive heart failure, and bronchoconstriction. While the choice of a diuretic vs a beta-blocker as a step-1 antihypertensive drug is still largely a matter of physician preference, there are definite cautions that must be observed when making this choice. Diuretics are generally preferred in patients with congestive heart failure, sinus bradycardia, and asthma, while beta-blockers are a logical choice in patients with cardiac arrhythmias, tachycardia, angina, hyperuricemia, and coagulation disorders.

Beta-blockers have numerous clinical indications and are considered in detail in Chapter 16. Most of the available beta-blockers are approved for use in treating hypertension and that particular indication is discussed below.

MECHANISM AND ACTIONS

Beta-blockers are effective in lowering both standing and supine blood pressure, either alone or in combination with other blood pressure-lowering drugs. Although the precise mechanisms of action responsible for the blood pressure-lowering effects of beta-blockers have not been completely elucidated, several actions of these drugs probably contribute to their antihypertensive effect. By competitively blocking beta-adrenergic receptor sites in various body tissues, these agents can decrease cardiac output, reduce release of renin from the juxtaglomerular cells of the kidney (thus decreasing production of angiotensin and secretion of aldosterone), and impede outflow of sympathetic (i.e., vasoconstrictor and cardioaccelerator) impulses from brain stem vasomotor control centers to peripheral organs. In addition, beta-blockers may retard release of norepinephrine from adrenergic nerve endings by blockade of presynaptic beta receptors. No *one* of the above actions, however, can account completely for antihypertensive efficacy of all the beta-blockers. For example, plasma renin activity is markedly reduced by some drugs (e.g., propranolol, metoprolol) but not to a great extent by others (e.g., pindolol), yet their antihypertensive efficacy is equivalent. Likewise, some drugs are highly lipophilic (propranolol, metoprolol) and attain high concentrations in the CNS, whereas others are only slightly lipid soluble (atenolol, acebutolol) and probably do not pass the blood–brain barrier to a significant extent. Despite these differences, however, their ability to lower blood pressure is comparable.

As indicated in Table 16-1, certain drugs (acebutolol, atenolol, metoprolol) are *relatively selective* in blocking beta$_1$ receptor sites at normal doses. This selectivity is of no apparent advantage in the clinical antihypertensive activity of beta-blockers but may result in a reduced likelihood for beta$_1$ selective drugs to elicit bronchoconstriction, an effect mediated by blockade of beta$_2$ receptors in bronchiolar smooth muscle. However, receptor selectivity is only relative, and as doses are increased, the beta$_1$ selective agents can also interact with beta$_2$ sites. Thus, patients with a history of bronchospastic diseases must be observed very carefully for changes in respiratory function even if they are receiving a "beta$_1$ selective" agent.

Comparisons among the various beta-blocking agents with regard to many of their pharmacologic and pharmacokinetic properties can be found in Table 16-1. Complete prescribing information, including available preparations, recommended dosage ranges for treating hypertension, and nursing considerations, is given in Table 16-3.

Step-2 Drugs

Labetalol

(Normodyne, Trandate)

MECHANISM AND ACTIONS

Labetalol is a unique adrenergic blocking agent which combines an alpha$_1$ blocking action with a nonspecific beta-blocking action at both beta$_1$ and beta$_2$ receptor sites. The ratio of alpha to beta blockade with oral administration is approximately 1:3. Blood pressure is lowered by labetalol, standing pressure more so than supine (due to the alpha$_1$ blocking action); however, changes in heart rate are minimal. Exercise-induced increases in heart rate and blood pressure are blunted, and elevated plasma renin levels are reduced. Cardiac output and renal function are relatively unaffected, as are AV conduction time and refractory period. Labetalol also appears to possess some intrinsic beta$_2$ agonistic activity, although the clinical significance of this action is not known. Postural hypotension can occur.

USES

1. Treatment of mild to moderate hypertension, either alone or combined with other antihypertensive agents, especially diuretics
2. Emergency control of blood pressure in severe hypertension (IV administration)

ADMINISTRATION AND DOSAGE

Labetalol is available for oral use as tablets (100 mg, 200 mg, 300 mg) and for IV injection (5 mg/ml). Orally, 100 mg is administered twice a day as an initial dose. Dosage may be increased in increments of 100 mg twice a day every 2 to 3 days until the desired effect is obtained. The usual oral maintenance dose is 200 mg to 400 mg twice a day, although up to 2400 mg/day has been used in severe hypertension.

For acute control of elevated blood pressure, 20 mg is injected IV over 2 minutes. Additional injections of 40 mg to 80 mg can be given every 10 minutes thereafter until the desired supine blood pressure is attained or a total of 300 mg has been administered. Alternately, 2 mg/min (2 ml/min of diluted injection solution) can be infused IV until the desired blood pressure response has been attained. The usual IV dosage range is 50 mg to 200 mg. Labetalol is compatible with and stable in 5% dextrose, 0.9% sodium chloride, dextrose and sodium chloride mixtures, Ringer's solution, and lactated Ringer's solution. It is *not* compatible with 5% sodium bicarbonate injection.

FATE

Oral labetalol is completely absorbed, and peak plasma levels occur within 1 hour to 2 hours. Maximum effects with a single oral dose are noted within 2 hours to 4 hours, and effects persist 8 hours to 12 hours. There is extensive first-pass hepatic metabolism, and the drug is approximately 50% protein bound.

The maximum effect following IV injection occurs within 5 minutes and persists for up to 12 hours to 15 hours following discontinuation. The drug is partially metabolized in the liver and excreted both in the urine and feces and by way of the bile as conjugated metabolites as well as unchanged drug. The elimination half-life following oral and IV administration is 6 hours and 5.5 hours, respectively.

SIDE-EFFECTS/ADVERSE REACTIONS
Labetalol is generally well tolerated, and side-effects with oral administration are usually mild and transient at recommended doses. Among the side-effects sometimes associated with its use are fatigue, dizziness, rash, and tingling of the scalp and skin. Because the drug possesses both alpha$_1$- and nonselective beta-blocking activity, its use can result in any of the adverse reactions seen with the use of other alpha$_1$- and beta-blocking agents. Refer to Chapter 16 for a complete listing of the adverse reactions that may result from blockade of these adrenergic receptor sites.

Oral use of labetalol has resulted in an elevation in the titer of antinuclear antibodies and symptoms of systemic lupus erythematosus. Careful observation of patients during prolonged therapy for early signs of a developing lupus-like reaction (arthralgia, dyspnea) is important.

CONTRAINDICATIONS AND PRECAUTIONS
Labetalol use is contraindicated in patients with bronchial asthma, cardiac failure, 2nd or 3rd degree heart block, severe bradycardia, or cardiogenic shock. The drug should be given with *caution* to persons with bronchitis, emphysema, diabetes mellitus, hepatic dysfunction, and to children, pregnant women, or nursing mothers.

INTERACTIONS
1. Labetalol can reduce the bronchodilator effects of beta-adrenergic agonists.
2. The incidence of tremor with combined use of labetalol and tricyclic antidepressants is significantly higher than with use of labetalol alone.
3. Cimetidine can increase the plasma levels of labetalol.

4. Labetalol reduces the reflex tachycardia seen with direct-acting vasodilators.

NURSING CONSIDERATIONS
(See also Nursing Process for Antihypertensive Drugs.)

Although many of the nursing considerations are the same as for beta-blockers, labetalol has some important differences. The drug is less likely to slow heart rate, an advantage for cardiac patients, or to cause fatigue or nightmares, problems usually encountered with other beta-blockers. One early side-effect, nausea, is usually transient and can be alleviated by taking the drug with food. Another, retrograde ejaculation, may not be reported by a patient because he will not be impotent but may be a reason he stops taking the medication. Sexuality discussions during clinic visits may uncover this problem and help the patient deal with it.

The patient on long-term therapy should be told to report any symptoms of a lupus-like reaction, such as joint pain, stiffness, or dyspnea. Periodic laboratory evaluation of antinuclear antibody titer should be completed.

Labetalol can be combined with diuretics as in a step-2 regimen. In such a combination it may be necessary to titrate labetalol to a lower dose. The first sign of this need may be a drop in blood pressure or a complaint of increasing postural hypotension. Many patients will tolerate a lower dose well, and some studies indicate that at least a third of patients taking this drug will continue to be controlled on lower doses.

Clonidine
(Catapres)

Guanabenz
(Wytensin)

Guanfacine
(Tenex)

Clonidine, guanabenz, and guanfacine are similar, orally active antiadrenergic agents that are indicated in the treatment of mild to moderate hypertension. In addition, clonidine is available in the form of an adhesive patch (see below). These drugs are centrally acting antihypertensive drugs with a very low incidence of serious toxicity; principal side-effects are drowsiness and dry mouth.

MECHANISM AND ACTIONS

Clonidine, guanabenz, and guanfacine are alpha₂ adrenergic agonists that inhibit the outflow of sympathetic vasoconstrictor and cardioaccelerator impulses from brain stem cardiovascular control centers (see Fig. 35-2). Blood pressure is reduced in the supine position to essentially the same extent as in the standing position, thus orthostatic effects are infrequent. Heart rate is slowed somewhat, but renal blood flow is unchanged. Cardiac output decreases initially but gradually returns to pretreatment levels with continued usage, while peripheral resistance may not decline initially but gradually decreases. Transient vasoconstriction may occur because the drugs initially can stimulate *peripheral* alpha-adrenergic receptors. Although this effect is usually clinically insignificant, a paradoxical rise in blood pressure has occurred in some patients receiving these drugs.

USES

1. Treatment of mild to moderate hypertension, either alone or in combination with a diuretic or other antihypertensive drug
2. Investigational uses for *clonidine* include prophylaxis of migraine, treatment of episodes of menopausal flushing, symptomatic management of opiate detoxification, and treatment of Gilles de la Tourette Syndrome.

ADMINISTRATION AND DOSAGE

Clonidine is available as 0.1-mg, 0.2-mg, and 0.3-mg tablets alone and in fixed combination with 15 mg of chlorthalidone as Combipres. It is also available as a transdermal patch (Catapres-TTS) in three strengths (1, 2, and 3) which deliver 0.1 mg, 0.2 mg, and 0.3 mg per day, respectively (see separate discussion below). Guanabenz is used as either 4-mg, 8-mg, or 16-mg tablets, and guanfacine is available as 1-mg tablets. Dosage recommendations for each drug are as follows:

Clonidine

Initially 0.1 mg orally twice a day; increase by 0.1 mg to 0.2 mg/day to desired response; usual range is 0.2 mg to 0.8 mg/day in divided doses; maximum 2.4 mg/day; may be effective as a single daily dose

Opiate withdrawal: 10 mcg/kg to 17 mcg/kg/day in divided doses (experimental use only)

Gilles de la Tourette Syndrome: 0.05 mg to 0.6 mg/day (experimental use only)

Transdermal Patch: Apply to skin once

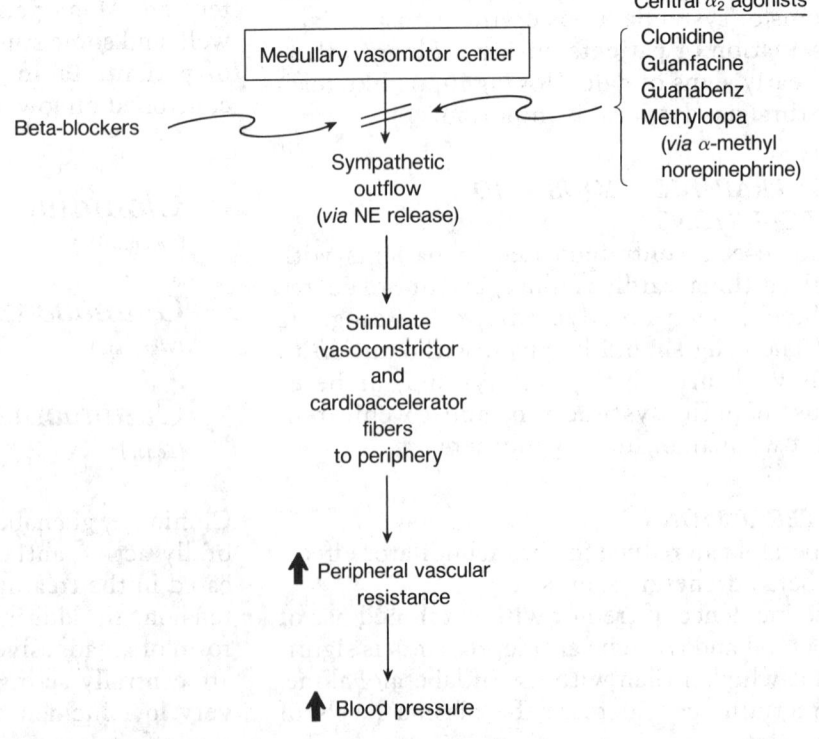

Figure 35-2. Central adrenergic control of blood pressure. Sympathetic outflow from brain stem centers controlling cardiovascular function, perhaps mediated by release of NE from adrenergic nerve endings, increases peripheral vascular resistance and elevates blood pressure. Activation of alpha₂ receptors in these medullary vasomotor areas reduces sympathetic outflow and lowers peripheral arterial tone. A similar action may result from inhibition of beta receptors in these same regions.

every 7 days; start with 0.1-mg system and increase by 0.1-mg increments as needed (see below).

Guanabenz
Initially, 4 mg orally twice a day; increase in increments of 4 mg to 8 mg/day every 1 week to 2 weeks; maximum dose is 32 mg a day in divided doses.

Guanfacine
Initially, 1 mg daily at bedtime with a thiazide diuretic; may increase up to 3 mg daily if necessary

FATE
Onset of action for these drugs is approximately 30 minutes to 60 minutes following oral administration. Maximum effects occur within 2 hours to 4 hours. The plasma half-life is 12 hours to 16 hours for clonidine and 6 hours to 8 hours for guanabenz. The drugs are largely metabolized in the liver and excreted in both the urine and feces as metabolites and some unchanged drug.

SIDE-EFFECTS/ADVERSE REACTIONS
Dry mouth and drowsiness are the most frequently reported side-effects with these agents and in some cases can be quite severe. Other commonly encountered side-effects are dizziness, headache, fatigue, weakness, and constipation. A number of other adverse effects have occurred during therapy with clonidine, guanfacine, and guanabenz and are listed below:

GI—Anorexia, nausea, vomiting, parotid pain, liver function test abnormalities
CNS—Insomnia, nervousness, anxiety, depression, vivid dreams or nightmares
Dermatologic—Rash, angioedema, urticaria, hives, hair loss, pruritus
Cardiovascular—Raynaud's phenomenon (pallor, cyanosis, pain in extremities), palpitation, flushing, congestive heart failure (rare)
Other—Weight gain, hyperglycemia, gynecomastia, urinary retention, impotence, itching or burning of eyes, pallor, dryness or nasal mucosa, muscle aching

CONTRAINDICATIONS AND PRECAUTIONS
There are no absolute contraindications to use of these agents. They should, however, be used *cautiously* in patients with coronary insufficiency, ce-

rebrovascular disease, chronic renal failure, thromboangiitis obliterans, or a history of depression. Caution is also warranted following a recent myocardial infarction and in pregnant women and young children.

Patients receiving these drugs should be cautioned against discontinuing therapy abruptly because rebound hypertension can occur, possibly leading to severe headache and agitation. Periodic eye examinations are recommended during prolonged therapy; retinal degeneration has been reported in laboratory studies.

INTERACTIONS
1. Clonidine, guanfacine, and guanabenz may intensify the CNS-depressant effects of alcohol, barbiturates, narcotics, and other depressants.
2. Effects of clonidine, guanfacine, and guanabenz may be antagonized by tricyclic antidepressants (except doxepin) and tolazoline.
3. Excessive bradycardia can occur when clonidine, guanfacine, or guanabenz is used in combination with digitalis agents, propranolol, or guanethidine.

Clonidine Transdermal Therapeutic System
(Catapres–TTS)

The clonidine transdermal therapeutic system is a drug-impregnated patch and adhesive overlay which is applied to the skin at 7-day intervals. Three different strengths are available (1, 2, and 3), which are claimed to deliver 0.1 mg, 0.2 mg, and 0.3 mg of drug per day for 7 days. Good contact between the patch and skin must be maintained to ensure adequate absorption of the drug through the intact skin. Local erythema is occasionally noted at the site of application, and rash and localized vesiculation has occurred. Other side-effects are similar to those described for oral administration above. Although compliance may be improved by once weekly administration, the transdermal application of clonidine does not represent a significant advantage in the majority of patients.

NURSING CONSIDERATIONS
(See also Nursing Process for Antihypertensive Drugs.)
Nursing considerations for clonidine, guanfacine, and guanabenz center on their various side-effects. Patients must be advised that these drugs

can evoke depressive episodes, particularly in patients with a history of mental depression. Change in affect, loss of appetite, complaints of fatigue or energy loss should be reported. These agents may also produce urinary hesitancy. Patients should be taught to be aware of their urination patterns and to report any changes noted.

Drowsiness from these drugs may be transient. One way to deal with the problem is to have the patient take most of the daily dose at bedtime, when the effect will be most beneficial. Postural hypotension may result in dizziness, which may be a *continuing* problem. The patient should be made aware of this possibility and should plan activities accordingly.

These agents can cause a transient elevation in blood glucose in the diabetic patient. During the initial period of dosage adjustment, blood glucose should be frequently monitored, and changes should be made in insulin or antidiabetic drugs as necessary.

Tolerance to these drugs can develop in long-term therapy, the first sign of which may be an increase in blood pressure. As a result, patients on these drugs should be reevaluated regularly. A dose change or addition of other drugs may be necessary to maintain lowered blood pressure. Conversely, the drugs should always be gradually withdrawn because abrupt withdrawal can result in rebound hypertension, headache, and mental confusion.

Methyldopa
(Aldomet)

MECHANISM AND ACTIONS
Methyldopa is converted by the action of the enzyme aromatic-amino acid-decarboxylase (dopa-decarboxylase) to alpha-methyl norepinephrine, a potent alpha$_2$ receptor agonist. Like clonidine, guanfacine, and guanabenz, alpha-methyl norepinephrine decreases brain stem sympathetic outflow, resulting in lowered peripheral vascular resistance. Standing blood pressure and, to a lesser extent, supine pressure, are reduced, and orthostatic effects are infrequent. Cardiac output and heart rate are minimally altered in younger patients but can decrease in older patients. Renin secretion is reduced, although the contribution of this effect to the antihypertensive action of the drug is probably unimportant. Fluid retention and weight gain can occur, possibly negating the blood pressure-lowering action of the drug over time.

USES
1. Alternative treatment of sustained mild to moderate hypertension, either alone or combined with other agents
2. Treatment of acute hypertensive crisis (IV infusion of methyldopate HCL)
   Note: Due to the relatively slow onset of action, methyldopa is generally not used in acute hypertensive emergencies.

ADMINISTRATION AND DOSAGE
Methyldopa is available as tablets (125 mg, 250 mg, 500 mg), oral suspension (250 mg/5 ml), and as the methyldopate ester hydrochloride for IV infusion (250 mg/5 ml). It is also marketed in fixed combinations with the diuretics hydrochlorothiazide (Aldoril) or chlorothiazide (Aldoclor). Recommended dosage ranges are as follows:
   Oral
      Adults—Initially 250 mg two to three times/day; adjust dosage by increments at intervals of not less than 2 days until desired response occurs; usual maintenance dosage is 500 mg to 2000 mg/day in two to four divided doses (maximum 3 g/day)
      Children—10 mg/kg/day in two to four divided doses adjusted to desired level; maximum dose is 65 mg/kg or 3 g daily.
   IV infusion (infrequently used)
      Adults—250 mg to 500 mg at 6-hour intervals (dose is added to 100 ml 5% dextrose injection and infused over 30 minutes to 60 minutes); maximum dose is 1 g every 6 hours.
      Children—20 mg to 40 mg/kg in divided doses every 6 hours; maximum dose is 3 g/day

Because the drug is excreted largely unchanged by the kidney (see under Fate), smaller doses may be necessary in persons with renal dysfunction. Similarly, older patients may need reduced amounts to minimize the danger of syncope (see under Side-Effects).

FATE
Absorption of methyldopa from the GI tract is variable and ranges from 10% to 60%. Peak plasma levels occur within 2 hours to 4 hours; however, maximal antihypertensive effects require 2 days to 3 days to develop after oral dosing. Blood pressure begins to decline within 4 hours to 6 hours after IV administration, and effects persist for up to 16

hours to 18 hours. The elimination half-life is about 2 hours, but antihypertensive activity persists for up to 24 hours following oral administration. Much of the drug is eliminated unchanged in the urine, although some hepatic metabolism occurs.

SIDE-EFFECTS/ADVERSE REACTIONS
The most commonly encountered side-effects with methyldopa, especially during the initial stages of therapy, are drowsiness, weakness, nasal stuffiness, and headache. Less frequently noted untoward reactions are:

Cardiovascular—Bradycardia, anginal pain, orthostatic hypotension, edema, myocarditis, paradoxical pressor response with IV use

CNS—Dizziness, paresthesias, parkinsonian-like symptoms, involuntary movements of the extremities (choreoathetoid movements), psychoses, depression, nightmares, memory impairment

GI—Nausea, vomiting, constipation, "black" tongue, abdominal distention, pancreatitis, sialadenitis

Hematologic—Positive Coombs' test (see below), hemolytic anemia, leukopenia, thrombocytopenia, granulocytopenia

Hepatic—Jaundice, liver dysfunction

Other—Fever, myalgia, arthralgia, dermatoses, rash, breast enlargement, gynecomastia, lactation, impotence, decreased libido, galactorrhea, amenorrhea

Laboratory test variations—Abnormal liver function tests; positive tests for antinuclear antibody, LE (*i.e.*, lupus erythematosus) cells, and rheumatoid factor; rise in BUN; falsely high urinary catecholamines

With prolonged therapy, approximately 10% to 20% of patients receiving methyldopa develop a positive direct Coombs' test, indicating the presence of proteins (*e.g.*, IgG gamma globulins) on red blood cell surfaces. While this condition may make crossmatching of blood difficult, it is not in itself an indication for discontinuing therapy. However, in a small percentage (less than 15%) of patients with a positive direct Coombs' test, hemolytic anemia may develop. It is therefore important to perform baseline and periodic blood counts during methyldopa therapy, and if a Coombs' positive hemolytic anemia is detected, the drug must be discontinued immediately. The hemolytic anemia and positive Coombs' test are generally reversible, although the positive Coombs' test may not revert to normal for weeks or even months.

Liver dysfunction has occurred in some patients receiving methyldopa, possibly representing a hypersensitivity reaction. Fever has developed within the first few weeks of therapy and may be associated with abnormalities in one or more liver function tests. Jaundice has been noted within 2 to 3 months after initiating treatment. Regular determinations of liver function must be performed, and the drug must be discontinued if unexplained fever or signs of liver dysfunction appear.

CONTRAINDICATIONS AND PRECAUTIONS
Contraindications to the use of methyldopa include active liver disease and blood dyscrasias. The drug must be given with *caution* to persons with chronic liver dysfunction, angina, pheochromocytoma, renal impairment, endocrine disorders, and to pregnant women or nursing mothers.

INTERACTIONS
1. Additive hypotensive effects can occur with methyldopa and anesthetics, alcohol, diuretics and other antihypertensive drugs, narcotics, methotrimeprazine, levodopa, quinidine, and vasodilators.
2. The hypotensive action of methyldopa can be antagonized by amphetamines, catecholamines (except levodopa), tricyclic antidepressants, MAO-inhibitors, phenothiazianes, sympathomimetics, and vasopressors.
3. Methyldopa can potentiate the hypoglycemic action of tolbutamide by impairing its metabolism.
4. Elevated serum lithium levels can occur with methyldopa.
5. Psychiatric disturbances and extreme sedation can result from combined use of methyldopa and haloperidol.
6. Phenoxybenzamine and methyldopa together have resulted in reversible urinary incontinence.
7. Paradoxical hypertension has occurred rarely with the combination of methyldopa and propranolol.
8. The effects of methyldopa may be potentiated by fenfluramine and verapamil.

NURSING CONSIDERATIONS
(See also Nursing Process for Antihypertensive Drugs.)

Because drowsiness and sedation are the most common side-effects during initial therapy, the patient should be warned to limit or avoid driving or operating any potentially hazardous machinery until he is aware of the effect of the drug on his body. Although methyldopa is generally less likely than most drugs to produce orthostatic hypotension, this side-effect may occur in the elderly who should be warned of the problem.

In long-term therapy, methyldopa may produce impotence with the result that a patient may decide to stop taking the drug. Good clinic follow-up with an opportunity to discuss sexual concerns may uncover the problem before the patient gives up therapy. Dosage adjustments or a change of medication may alleviate impotence.

The patient should also be aware that methyldopa produces a by-product which darkens urine. This effect is not harmful but may be frightening to the uninformed patient who might believe he has blood in his urine.

Prazosin
(Minipress)

MECHANISM AND ACTIONS
Prazosin is a selective alpha$_1$ adrenergic receptor antagonist that dilates both resistance (i.e., arterioles) and capacitance (i.e., veins) vessels. Blood pressure is lowered in both the supine and standing position, and effects are most pronounced on the diastolic pressure. Unlike nonselective alpha blockers and direct-acting vasodilators, reflex tachycardia does not occur to a significant extent. Cardiac output and renal blood flow are largely unaffected. The drug can cause sodium and water retention and increased plasma volume, which may reduce its blood pressure-lowering effect when given alone; diuretics are frequently prescribed together with prazosin for this reason. Postural hypotension can occur, especially with large doses. In patients with congestive heart failure, prazosin reduces both left ventricular end diastolic volume (i.e., preload) and aortic impedance to left ventricular ejection (i.e., afterload). In addition, cardiac output is improved and pulmonary congestion is relieved.

USES
1. Treatment of mild to moderate hypertension, either alone or with a diuretic or other antihypertensive agent

2. Adjunctive treatment of severe, refractive congestive heart failure
3. Management of vasospasm in Raynaud's disease (investigational use only)

ADMINISTRATION AND DOSAGE
Prazosin is used as capsules containing 1 mg, 2 mg, or 5 mg, either alone or in combination with 0.5 mg polythiazide as Minizide. The initial dose is 1 mg two to three times a day, which can be increased in small increments until an optimal effect is attained. The usual maintenance dosage range is 6 mg/day to 15 mg/day in two or three divided doses. Doses above 20 mg/day usually do not result in greater efficacy.

FATE
Oral absorption is generally good and is not significantly affected by the presence of food. Peak plasma concentrations are noted in 1 hour to 3 hours. The plasma half-life is 2 hours to 3 hours, but the antihypertensive effects persist for up to 10 hours. The drug is highly protein-bound (92%–97%). Prazosin is extensively metabolized by the liver and excreted largely by way of the bile and the feces (90%) with smaller amounts in the urine (10%). The metabolites appear to be active. Elimination is slowed in patients with congestive heart failure and chronic renal failure.

SIDE-EFFECTS/ADVERSE REACTIONS
Side-effects noted with greatest frequency during initial prazosin therapy are dizziness, headache, drowsiness, weakness, palpitations and nausea; these effects are usually transient and disappear with continued therapy. Occasionally, a sudden loss of consciousness, believed to be due to an excessive postural hypotensive effect, has occurred immediately following the first dose of prazosin. This has been termed the "first dose effect" and is noted most often when the initial dose is 2 mg or higher or when a too-large increment in dosage is given. The occurrence of this phenomenon can be minimized by limiting the initial dosage to 1 mg and making any subsequent dosage increases minimal.

Other adverse effects that have been associated with prazosin somewhat less frequently are:
GI—Vomiting, constipation, abdominal pain
Cardiovascular—Tachycardia, angina, syncope, edema, orthostatic hypotension
CNS—Nervousness, paresthesias, vertigo, depression

Other—Urinary frequency or incontinence, impotence, rash, pruritus, dyspnea, blurred vision, tinnitus, dry mouth, nasal congestion, epistaxis, diaphoresis, arthralgia, leukopenia, drug-induced lupus-like syndrome (rare)

CONTRAINDICATIONS AND PRECAUTIONS
There are no absolute contraindications to use of prazosin. Safety for use in pregnant women and children has not been established. Patients should be cautioned against driving or performing other hazardous duties during the early stages of therapy because dizziness or drowsiness can occur.

INTERACTIONS
1. Enhanced hypotensive effects can occur in combination with other antihypertensive drugs, especially propranolol.
2. The effects of prazosin may be potentiated by other highly protein-bound drugs.

NURSING CONSIDERATIONS
(See also Nursing Process for Antihypertensive Drugs.)

To minimize the danger of "first dose syncope," prazosin should be initially administered under supervision and the patient should remain recumbent for about 2 hours after the first dose. Syncope can occur within 30 to 90 minutes of this dose but can also recur when a dose change is made or when other antihypertensives are added to the regimen. In addition, orthostatic hypotension and syncope may last for several days. Consequently, blood pressure should be closely monitored as the patient adjusts to the drug. The patient should have a close support system if he is discharged early and must be cautioned against driving or engaging in any hazardous activity during the first few days. Taking the drug at bedtime may minimize the effects of orthostatic hypotension.

Urinary side-effects may occur and can be embarrassing unless the patient is warned about the possibility of enuresis and urgency.

Tolerance to prazosin can develop within a few months. Increases in dosage beyond 20 mg/day are not usually effective, and another drug must be substituted to achieve the continued antihypertensive effect. In addition, the drug is usually difficult to titrate and may not be appropriate for patients who are poorly motivated, forgetful, or who have few supports.

Verapamil
(Calan, Isoptin)

Verapamil is a calcium-channel blocker useful in the chronic management of angina (see Chap. 36) and in the control of supraventricular arrhythmias (see Chap. 34). It is also indicated for control of mild to moderate hypertension and in addition to 40-mg and 80-mg regular tablets, it is also available as sustained-release tablets (240 mg), which are administered once daily. Verapamil relaxes vascular smooth muscle, thus decreasing peripheral vascular resistance. Its use may be associated with fewer side-effects than many other step-2 drugs such as depression, impotence, and elevated serum uric acids or triglycerides. However, constipation occurs frequently, and verapamil can also cause dizziness, nausea, and edema. Due to its negative inotropic action and its ability to slow AV conduction, its use is contraindicated in left ventricular dysfunction, cardiogenic shock, sick sinus syndrome, and second- or third-degree AV block. Recommended dosage in treating hypertension is 240 mg once daily although some patients may require twice daily dosing to adequately control their pressure. (Refer to the complete monograph on the calcium channel blockers in Chap. 36 and to Table 36-4 for additional information on verapamil.)

Angiotensin-Converting Enzyme Inhibitors

Captopril
(Capoten)

Enalapril
(Vasotec)

Lisinopril
(Prinivil, Zestril)

Angiotensin-converting enzyme (ACE) inhibitors are orally effective antihypertensive drugs which are used either alone or in combination with other antihypertensive agents in treating mild to moderate hypertension. These drugs (especially captopril) may also be used at higher doses for controlling more severe resistant forms of hypertension, although at these elevated dose levels serious toxicity such as blood dyscrasias or renal damage can occur. This high-dose therapy should be reserved for patients who fail to respond to other drug combinations. In addition, these agents may be used as alternative drugs in managing congestive heart failure (see Chap. 33).

MECHANISM AND ACTIONS

These drugs inhibit an enzyme (angiotensin-converting enzyme; ACE) that hydrolyzes the inactive angiotensin I to the active angiotensin II in the plasma and lungs. (See Fig. 35-1). Inhibition of ACE reduces the formation of the pressor substance angiotensin II and decreases the angiotensin-mediated secretion of aldosterone from the adrenal cortex. Peripheral vascular resistance is lowered, and salt and water retention is reduced. Plasma renin activity increases due to loss of negative feedback, and serum potassium may rise due to absence of aldosterone activity. There is either no change or an increase in cardiac output, and renal blood flow is increased. Both supine and standing blood pressure are lowered to approximately the same extent. Orthostatic hypotension is rare, and reflex tachycardia seldom occurs.

Inhibition of the converting enzyme by these drugs also appears to decrease the inactivation of bradykinin, a potent endogenous vasodilator, an action that may also contribute to its blood pressure-lowering effect. An increased synthesis of prostaglandin E, which may result in peripheral vasodilation, has been proposed as an additional action, possibly resulting from the increased levels of bradykinin.

The reduction in blood pressure is gradual and progressive, and several weeks of therapy may be required to achieve maximal therapeutic benefit.

In patients with congestive heart failure, these agents decrease systemic vascular resistance (i.e., afterload) and pulmonary capillary wedge pressure and increase cardiac output.

USES

1. Treatment of all degrees of hypertension, either alone or combined with other drugs, especially diuretics, as blood pressure-lowering effects are additive
   a. *Small doses* may be used in mild hypertension in patients with normal renal function, especially where other step-1 or step-2 drugs are inappropriate or ineffective.
   b. *Large doses* of captopril may be used in moderate to severe forms of hypertension in patients who fail to respond to or cannot tolerate other multiple drug regimens (risk of toxicity is significantly increased).
2. Adjunctive treatment of refractory congestive heart failure, usually combined with digoxin and a diuretic
3. Symptomatic treatment of rheumatoid arthritis (investigational use for captopril)

ADMINISTRATION AND DOSAGE

Captopril

Captopril is used orally as tablets (12.5 mg, 25 mg, 37.5 mg, 50 mg, 100 mg). The initial dosage for *mild to moderate hypertension* is 12.5 mg to 25 mg two to three times/day. Dosage may be increased gradually to 50 mg two to three times/day; if blood pressure is not adequately controlled at this dosage, small doses of a thiazide diuretic may be added and gradually increased as necessary.

In treating *moderate to severe hypertension*, the initial dose is 25 mg three times a day. Dosage may be increased to 50 mg three times a day, then in 50-mg increments until the desired effect is attained or toxicity occurs. The drug is usually given with a thiazide diuretic. The usual maintenance dosage range for moderate hypertension is 50 mg to 150 mg two to three times a day, with a maximum daily dose of 450 mg in very severe hypertension.

For adjunctive therapy of *congestive heart failure*, 12.5 mg to 25 mg is administered three times a day. Increases of 25 mg may be made weekly until an optimal effect is noted. The usual dosage range is 50 mg to 100 mg three times a day in combination with digoxin and a diuretic.

Smaller, less frequent dosing may be necessary in patients with impaired renal function or in hypovolemic or hyponatremic patients.

Enalapril

Enalapril is available as tablets (5 mg, 10 mg, 20 mg), and the initial dose (in patients not taking diuretics) is 5 mg once daily. Dosage increases can be made gradually as needed. The usual dosage range is 10 mg to 40 mg daily in a single or two divided doses. If the patient is already receiving a diuretic, begin at 2.5 mg to avoid the development of excessive hypotension.

Lisinopril

Initially, 10 mg to 20 mg once daily. Increase gradually until desired response. Usual dosage range is 20 mg to 40 mg daily.

FATE

All drugs are adequately absorbed orally, although the presence of food can reduce absorption of captopril by 30% to 40%. The maximal blood pressure-lowering effect is achieved within 60 minutes to 90 minutes with captopril and within 4 hours to 6 hours with enalapril and lisinopril. However, optimal clinical antihypertensive effects may require several weeks to develop. Approximately 25% to 30% of captopril in the plasma is protein-bound. Following absorption, enalapril is converted to enalaprilat, a more potent ACE-inhibitor. The elimination half-life of captopril is less than 2 hours but may be up to 12 hours for enalaprilat. Approximately 95% of a dose of captopril and enalapril is eliminated within 24 hours, in both the urine and the feces. Lisinopril is not metabolized and is excreted unchanged in the urine.

SIDE-EFFECTS/ADVERSE REACTIONS

The most common side-effects with captopril are loss of taste sensation, rash, and pruritus. Commonly reported side-effects with enalapril are headache, dizziness, and fatigue. Lisinopril can cause GI upset, light headedness, and loss of energy.

Adverse reactions noted on occasion with all three drugs include:

CNS—Insomnia, paresthesias, headache, dizziness, fatigue

GI—Nausea, vomiting, diarrhea, abdominal pain, altered taste sensation

CV—Chest pain, hypotension, palpitations

Other—Cough, dyspnea, pruritus, rash, angioedema

In addition, certain untoward reactions are most often associated with one of the two drugs as indicated below:

Captopril

GI irritation, constipation, peptic ulcer, malaise, dry mouth, lymphadenopathy, tachycardia, angina, Raynaud's syndrome, congestive heart failure, photosensitivity, alopecia, oncholysis, exfoliative dermatitis, proteinuria, polyuria, oliguria, renal insufficiency, renal failure, neutropenia, agranulocytosis, thrombocytopenia, hemolytic anemia

Enalapril

Decreased hemoglobin and hematocrit, hyperhidrosis, hyperkalemia, syncope, dyspepsia, elevated liver enzymes or serum bilirubin, nervousness, somnolence, muscle cramping, impotence

CONTRAINDICATIONS AND PRECAUTIONS

■ WARNING

Excessive hypotension has occurred following ACE-inhibitor administration, especially in severely salt or volume-depleted patients, such as those with severe congestive heart failure who are receiving diuretics. Excessive perspiration, vomiting, diarrhea, or dehydration may increase the likelihood of extreme hypotension. Extreme caution must be used when initiating therapy with these agents in patients who are receiving other blood pressure-lowering drugs such as diuretics or adrenergic inhibitors.

While there are no absolute contraindications to these drugs, large doses should be given with extreme *caution*, if at all, to patients with severe renal dysfunction. Caution must also be exercised when administering ACE-inhibitors to persons with systemic lupus-like symptoms (increased risk of neutropenia), reduced white cell counts, valvular stenosis, diabetes mellitus (increased risk of hypercalemia), to persons about to undergo general anesthesia and to pregnant women, nursing mothers, or children under 15 years of age.

INTERACTIONS

1. The hypotensive effects of ACE-inhibitors may be increased by diuretics, adrenergic-blocking agents, other antihypertensive drugs, nifedipine, and by severe salt or fluid restriction.
2. Serum potassium levels can be elevated by concurrent use of ACE-inhibitors and potassium-sparing diuretics or potassium supplements.
3. Vasodilators (*e.g.*, nitrites) may be potentiated by these agents and should be discontinued before beginning therapy with ACE-inhibitors.
4. The antihypertensive efficacy of captopril can be reduced by indomethacin and possibly by aspirin and other salicylates.

NURSING CONSIDERATIONS

(See also Nursing Process for Antihypertensive Drugs.)

Adequate baseline data are essential to determine appropriateness of using ACE-inhibitors. The patient should have urinary proteins evaluated and have a complete blood count with differential. The white blood cell count should be within normal limits. Over the course of therapy these laboratory values should be monitored and the drug discontinued if abnormalities occur. In addition, the patient should be taught to report any signs of infection such as fever or a sore throat.

Sodium restriction may result in hypotension during initial therapy with these drugs. Consequently, the patient starting this drug should continue with moderate salt intake. As a result of this effect, any condition leading to increased perspiration or dehydration, such as extreme exercise, exposure to heat, diarrhea, or vomiting, may also result in a further reduction of blood pressure.

One of the disadvantages of these agents is their possible additive effects with many diuretics and antihypertensives. Caution must be used when changing drugs, and blood pressure should be closely monitored while changes are made. If possible, other antihypertensives should be discontinued for at least a week before these drugs are initiated. Another disadvantage is that these drugs must be gradually titrated to achieve full therapeutic benefit, a course which may take several weeks of careful monitoring. As a result, the drugs may not be appropriate for the patient who is poorly motivated, forgetful, or is without support systems.

Captopril must be taken on an empty stomach for best absorption. Captopril is taken either 1 hour before or 2 hours after a meal. The drug should be taken with water. Patients also complain that it frequently alters taste perception, a side-effect that may continue throughout therapy.

Absorption of enalapril and lisinopril is unaffected by food.

Rauwolfia Derivatives

Alseroxylon, Deserpidine, Rauwolfia Whole Root, Rescinnamine, Reserpine

The rauwolfia derivatives are a group of products derived from the *Rauwolfia* family of plants, comprising whole root rauwolfia, an extraction of alkaloids (alseroxylon), and the refined alkaloids deserpidine, rescinnamine, and reserpine (see Table 35-4). Although once widely used, reserpine and the other rauwolfia alkaloids are seldom employed today for treating hypertension, because they are no more effective than many other currently available antihypertensive drugs and have the potential to elicit a wide range of troublesome side-effects.

MECHANISM AND ACTIONS
These rauwolfia compounds have the ability to lower blood pressure by gradually depleting the stores of neurohormones (primarily norepinephrine) in nerve endings by blocking their uptake into vesicular storage sites. They also exert a CNS depressant effect and their tranquilizing and sedative actions are probably the result of depletion of amines (*e.g.*, norepinephrine, serotonin) from nerve endings in the brain. Both the hypotensive and depressant effects can persist for some time following withdrawal of these drugs. Prolactin levels can be elevated by reserpine, leading to pseudolactation and gynecomastia (see under Side-Effects/Adverse Reactions).

USES
1. Treatment of mild to moderate essential hypertension, usually combined with other antihypertensive medications (infrequent use)
2. Management of psychotic behavior, primarily in patients intolerant of other antipsychotic drugs (except alseroxylon and rescinnamine)

ADMINISTRATION AND DOSAGE
See Table 35-4.

FATE
The onset of action is slow following oral administration. Several days are necessary to deplete existing norepinephrine stores in nerve endings. Maximum antihypertensive activity may take up to several weeks to develop and may persist for as long as several weeks following discontinuation of therapy. The drugs are extensively metabolized and excreted primarily in the urine.

SIDE EFFECTS/ADVERSE REACTIONS
Side-effects occurring most often with the rauwolfia alkaloids are drowsiness, abdominal cramping, diarrhea, mental depression, nasal congestion, bradycardia, and increased gastric acid secretion. A number of other adverse reactions can occur during therapy with the rauwolfia alkaloids and these are listed below:

GI—Nausea, vomiting, abdominal pain, hypersecretion, bleeding
CNS—Nervousness, anxiety, nightmares, extrapyramidal symptoms
Cardiovascular—Palpitations, arrhythmias,

Table 35-4
Rauwolfia Alkaloids

Drug	Preparations	Usual Dosage Range	Clinical Considerations
alseroxylon (Rauwiloid)	Tablets—2 mg	Initially 2 mg–4 mg/day Usual maintenance dose is 2 mg/day	Mixture of alkaloids derived from rauwolfia; used for treatment of mild essential hypertension; serious mental depression can occur at high doses
deserpidine (Harmonyl)	Tablets—0.25 mg	Hypertension—initially 0.75 mg–1 mg/day; maintenance dose 0.25 mg/day Psychoses—initially 0.5 mg/day; usual range is 0.1–1 mg/day	An alkaloid derived from rauwolfia; used for treatment of mild essential hypertension and for relief of symptoms in agitated psychotic states; do not make dosage adjustments more frequently than every 10 to 14 days because effects of the drug are slow to develop
rauwolfia whole root (Raudixin and various other manufacturers)	Tablets—50 mg, 100 mg	Usual starting dose is 200 mg–400 mg/day in divided doses Maintenance dose is 50 mg–300 mg/day in a single or two divided doses	Powdered whole root of Rauwolfia serpentina, which contains several alkaloids, including reserpine; used in mild essential hypertension, and for relief of symptoms in agitated psychotic states; usually administered with food or milk to minimize GI upset; rarely used today
rescinnamine (Moderil)	Tablets—0.25 mg, 0.5 mg	Initially 0.5 mg twice a day Usual maintenance dose is 0.25 mg–0.5 mg daily	Alkaloid derived from the rauwolfia plant; used in mild essential hypertension and may be effective as an adjunct to other antihypertensive medications in more severe forms of hypertension; lower incidence of sedation and bradycardia reported with rescinnamine than with reserpine
reserpine (Serpasil and various other manufacturers)	Tablets—0.1 mg, 0.25 mg, 1 mg	Oral: Hypertension—initially 0.5 mg/day; reduce slowly to 0.1 mg–0.25 mg/day Psychiatric disorders—0.1 mg–1 mg/day adjusted to patient's response	An alkaloid derived from rauwolfia; used orally for treating mild hypertension and for relief of symptoms of agitated psychotic states; oral doses higher than 0.25 mg/day may cause severe depression; combined with other antihypertensive drugs (e.g., diuretics, hydralazine) for treatment of more severe forms of hypertension

angina-like symptoms, orthostatic hypotension, syncope, cutaneous vasodilation, and flushing

Ocular—Uveitis, glaucoma, optic atrophy

Other—Rash, pruritus, dryness of mouth, epistaxis, headache, dysuria, impotence, breast engorgement, pseudolactation, gynecomastia, asthma, dyspnea, muscle aching, weight gain, menstrual irregularities

CONTRAINDICATIONS AND PRECAUTIONS

Reserpine and the other rauwolfia alkaloids are contraindicated in patients with mental depression, active peptic ulcer, breast cancer, ulcerative colitis, pheochromocytoma, bronchial asthma, and in patients receiving electroconvulsive therapy or MAO-inhibitor drugs. These agents must be given with *caution* to patients with arrhythmias, epilepsy, bronchitis, gallstones, renal or hepatic dysfunction, and to pregnant women or nursing mothers. Safety and efficacy for use in children have not been established.

Prolonged use of rauwolfia alkaloids can result in increased adrenergic postsynaptic receptor sensitivity consequent to the depletion of presynaptic neurohormonal stores. Subsequent administration of agents containing sympathomimetic amines, such as decongestants, cold preparations, or adrenergic bronchodilators under such circumstances can result in excessive elevation of blood pressure. Thus, use of other drugs containing sympathomimetic drugs, including over-the-counter cough and cold remedies together with reserpine should be carefully controlled.

While there is no conclusive evidence that reserpine increases the risk of breast cancer in females, a few epidemiologic studies have suggested a slightly higher risk in women who have used reserpine. It is probably prudent to avoid reserpine in females, as other alternative therapy is readily available today.

INTERACTIONS

1. Enhanced hypotensive effects may be seen when rauwolfia derivatives are combined with anesthetics, barbiturates, diuretics and other antihypertensive drugs, methotrimeprazine, phenothiazines, quinidine, propranolol, and vasodilators.

2. Cardiac arrhythmias can occur if reserpine is given with digitalis or quinidine; reserpine combined with theophylline can result in tachycardia.

3. CNS-depressant effects of other agents (*e.g.*, alcohol, barbiturates, narcotics, antihistamines, phenothiazines) may be enhanced by reserpine.

4. Rauwolfia derivatives may decrease the effects of anticholinergics (antisecretory action), anticonvulsants, indirect-acting sympathomimetics (*e.g.*, ephedrine, amphetamine), levodopa, morphine, salicylates, vasopressors (*e.g.*, metaraminol, mephentermine).

5. If used with tricyclic antidepressants, rauwolfia derivatives can be antagonized and excitation and mania can occur.

6. Excitation and hypertension can initially result from combined used of rauwolfia drugs and MAO-inhibitors, but prolonged therapy can lead to severe depression and markedly increased GI activity.

NURSING CONSIDERATIONS

(See also Nursing Process for Antihypertensive Drugs.)

The patient receiving one of the rauwolfia drugs should be carefully monitored because the effects of the drug may persist several weeks after the drug is discontinued. In addition, full therapeutic benefit will take several weeks to achieve. Consequently, this drug may not be appropriate for the patient who is unable to follow a regimen closely and consistently.

To alleviate gastrointestinal distress, rauwolfia compounds may be administered with milk or food. The patient should also learn to weigh himself daily and to report any rapid weight changes immediately. The patient and his family need to be aware that drug-induced depression can occur. At the first signs of despondency, insomnia, anorexia, or change in affect the physician should be notified and the drug discontinued. Such depression can last for several weeks after the drug is stopped and has been known to lead to suicide.

Rauwolfia compounds should be discontinued several weeks before surgery to avoid severe hypotension during anesthesia due to the drug's CNS depressant effect. The patient should also be cautioned against drinking alcoholic beverages, because the same hypotensive effect can occur.

Step-3 Drugs

Hydralazine
(Alazine, Apresoline)

MECHANISM AND ACTIONS
Hydralazine dilates peripheral arterioles through a direct relaxant effect on arteriolar smooth muscle. There is little effect on venous capacitance vessels. Diastolic pressure is usually lowered more than the systolic pressure, and there may be a slight increase in renal and cerebral blood flow. Reflex tachycardia is common. In congestive heart failure, the drug reduces arteriolar impedance, thus improving cardiac output.

USES
1. Management of moderate forms of hypertension, sometimes alone but more commonly in combination with other antihypertensive medications
2. Short-term treatment of severe essential hypertension (IV or IM)
3. Adjunctive treatment of congestive heart failure, severe aortic insufficiency and following valve replacement

ADMINISTRATION AND DOSAGE
Hydralazine may be given orally as 10-mg, 25-mg, 50-mg, or 100-mg tablets or by IV or IM injection (20 mg/ml). It is also available in several fixed combinations with diuretics and/or reserpine (*e.g.,* Apresazide, Hydral, Ser-Ap-Es).

Orally, the initial dose is 10 mg four times/day for 2 to 4 days. This may be increased to 25 mg four times/day for the balance of the first week, then to 50 mg four times/day if necessary. Maintenance dosage should be adjusted to the lowest effective level, and the drug may be given twice a day in some patients. Tolerance develops during chronic therapy and may necessitate higher doses.

Children can be given 0.75 mg/kg to 3 mg/kg daily orally in two or three divided doses.

Parenteral (IM, IV) use of hydralazine is indicated in the hospitalized patient when the drug cannot be given orally; however, IV injection is the preferred route. The initial dose is usually 5 mg to 10 mg; dosage may be titrated upward as dictated by the response; repeat doses are given at 30-min-

ute intervals in acute situations. Too-rapid increases in dosage can result in a precipitous drop in blood pressure. Parenteral children's doses are 0.1 mg/kg to 0.2 mg/kg every 4 hours to 6 hours as needed.

FATE
The drug is well absorbed orally but undergoes extensive first-pass metabolism. Peak blood levels occur within 1 hour. Protein binding is high (88%–90%), and elimination half-life can range from 2 hours to 8 hours; hypotensive effects last for 6 hours to 8 hours. Onset of action following IM injection is 10 minutes to 15 minutes, and effects persist for 3 hours to 4 hours. Hydralazine is metabolized in the liver, and metabolites are excreted largely in the feces, with small amounts of unchanged drug appearing in the urine.

SIDE-EFFECTS/ADVERSE REACTIONS
The most common side-effects with hydralazine are headache, nausea, diarrhea, tachycardia, palpitations, and sweating. Other less frequently noted untoward reactions include anorexia, vomiting, rash, urticaria, pruritus, nasal congestion, flushing, muscle cramping, peripheral neuritis, dizziness, lacrimation, delayed micturition, impotence, lymphadenopathy, and rarely blood dyscrasias, psychotic reactions, hepatitis, and obstructive jaundice.

Large doses (*i.e.,* greater than 400 mg/day), particularly with chronic use, can result in a clinical picture resembling acute systemic lupus erythematosus (fever, myalgia, arthralgia, dermatoses, anemia, splenomegaly). Appearance of these signs mandates discontinuation of the drug. Symptoms usually regress upon cessation of therapy, but residual effects may linger for months or even years.

CONTRAINDICATIONS AND PRECAUTIONS
Hydralazine is contraindicated in the presence of coronary artery disease (due to the reflex myocardial stimulation seen with the drug), and rheumatic heart disease (drug can increase pulmonary artery pressure). It must be given *cautiously* to persons with renal impairment, cerebral vascular disease, peripheral neuritis, and to pregnant women or nursing mothers.

INTERACTIONS

1. The hypotensive action of hydralazine can be antagonized by amphetamines, ephedrine, and other sympathomimetic agents, and the incidence of tachycardia and anginal pain may be increased.
2. Additive hypotensive effects can occur with combined use of hydralazine and anesthetics, antidepressants, other antihypertensives, diuretics, quinidine, and procainamide.

NURSING CONSIDERATIONS

(See also Nursing Process for Antihypertensive Drugs.)

In addition to previously mentioned laboratory data, the patient receiving hydralazine should have a complete blood count, LE cell preparation, and antinuclear antibody titer drawn. This blood work should be done at regular intervals throughout therapy because the drug can cause a lupus-like reaction. The patient should watch for early warning signs such as fever, myalgia, and arthralgia, which must be reported immediately. The drug will be discontinued.

Hydralazine can produce significant and debilitating orthostatic hypotension. The patient needs to learn to change positions slowly, avoid prolonged standing or squatting, and limit driving or operation of hazardous machinery until his response to the drug is known. Headaches and palpitations may occur early in treatment, but the patient should be reassured that they usually disappear. However, a change in mental alertness, in mood or affect, or in social interaction should be immediately reported because such symptoms may be the early warning signs of cerebral ischemia or drug psychosis, both serious side-effects of hydralazine.

Hydralazine may result in a peripheral neuritis which causes paresthesia, numbness, and tingling. This neuritis may respond to pyridoxine (vitamin B_6), but if it persists, hydralazine should be discontinued.

The patient should be taught to weigh himself regularly and monitor urinary output. Urinary retention and edema can occur and should be reported immediately.

Hydralazine must be gradually discontinued to avoid rebound hypertension.

The drug should be taken with meals to enhance absorption.

Hydralazine may be the drug of choice for the third trimester pregnant patient with preeclampsia with a rising blood pressure over 160/110 and urine proteins of 2+ or greater. The drug is thought to lower blood pressure sufficiently to prevent organ damage to the mother while avoiding compromise to the fetus. The drug is administered in an IV bolus (see under Administration and Dosage) until the baby can be delivered. Fetal monitoring is essential throughout therapy.

In addition, nursing care for any patient receiving parenteral administration of hydralazine should include vital signs every 2 to 5 minutes, hourly monitoring of urinary output, and observation for signs of reduced cerebral blood flow such as a change in mental status, extremity weakness or numbness, and slurred speech.

Step-4 Drugs

Guanadrel
(Hylorel)

Guanethidine
(Ismelin)

Guanadrel and guanethidine are two antihypertensive drugs with similar pharmacologic and toxicologic properties. Yet, guanadrel is generally classified as a step-2 drug, whereas guanethidine is largely viewed as a step-4 drug. Although both drugs are effective in the treatment of severe, refractive hypertension, guanadrel has been employed successfully in treating mild to moderate hypertension. It should, however, be reserved for patients who have not responded to other step-2 drugs.

MECHANISM AND ACTIONS

These drugs accumulate in peripheral adrenergic nerve endings, where they inhibit norepinephrine release in response to nerve stimulation. A gradual depletion of norepinephrine stores in the nerve endings ensues, resulting in a prolonged reduction in heart rate and peripheral vascular resistance. Venous return is diminished, cardiac output is reduced, and plasma renin activity is decreased. Blood pressure reduction is greater in the standing than prone position, and orthostatic effects are common and can result in significant dizziness and weakness. Renal blood flow is reduced relative to blood flow to the heart and brain, thus sodium and water retention is significant. Sensitivity of adrenergic receptors to circulating norepinephrine is enhanced due to impaired neuronal uptake.

USES

1. Treatment of moderate to severe hypertension, not adequately controlled by other antihypertensive drugs. (Although guanadrel has been used for milder degrees of hypertension, it should be viewed as an alternative drug, at best, to other step-2 antihypertensive drugs.)
2. Treatment of renal hypertension, including that secondary to renal artery stenosis and pyelonephritis

ADMINISTRATION AND DOSAGE

Both guanadrel and guanethidine are available as tablets (10 mg, 25 mg). Recommended doses for both drugs are quite similar and are given below:

Guanadrel
  Initially 10 mg/day; increase gradually until optimal effect is seen; usual dosage range is 20 mg to 75 mg in twice daily doses

Guanethidine
  Ambulatory patients: initially 10 mg/day; increase gradually every 5 to 7 days to achieve optimal response; usual dose is 25 mg to 50 mg/day in a single dose
  Hospitalized patients: initially 10 mg to 50 mg, depending on other antihypertensive drugs being used; increase by 10 mg to 25 mg every 2 to 4 days until desired response is obtained
  Children: initially, 0.2 mg/kg/24 hours as a single oral dose; increase by 0.2 mg/kg/24 hours every 7 to 10 days; maximum dose is 3 mg/kg/24 hours

Tolerance may occur during prolonged therapy, necessitating a dosage increase. Orthostatic hypotension may develop during dosage elevations.

FATE

Guanethidine is poorly but consistently absorbed orally. The peak effect occurs within 8 hours of a single dose. Half-life is 5 days, so drug accumulates slowly. It is partially metabolized by the liver and excreted as active drug and inactive metabolites, primarily by the kidney. Guanadrel is rapidly absorbed orally and attains peak plasma concentration in 1.5 hours to 2 hours. Effects are noted within 2 hours, and maximal blood pressure decreases occur within 4 hours to 6 hours. The drug is excreted primarily in the urine, approximately 40% as unchanged drug.

SIDE-EFFECTS/ADVERSE REACTIONS

Frequently occurring side-effects with both guanethidine and guanadrel are fatigue, headache, faintness, drowsiness, nocturia, urinary urgency, increased bowel movements, diarrhea, shortness of breath on exertion, palpitations, bradycardia, fluid retention, and ejaculation disturbances.

Other less commonly noted adverse reactions are dyspnea, nasal congestion, nausea, vomiting, paresthesias, incontinence, dermatitis, anorexia, constipation, leg cramps, hair loss, blurred vision, asthma, chest pains, myalgia, tremor, depression, cardiac irregularities, and, rarely, anemia, thrombocytopenia, and leukopenia.

Excessive dosage can lead to dizziness, blurred vision, bradycardia, and syncope, due to extreme postural hypotension. Patient should be kept supine until these symptoms ameliorate.

CONTRAINDICATIONS AND PRECAUTIONS

These drugs are contraindicated in patients with pheochromocytoma or congestive heart failure *not* due to hypertension, and they should not be given concurrently with or within 1 week of MAO-inhibitors.

Cautious use of guanethidine and guanadrel is necessary in persons with fever (dosage should be reduced), bronchial asthma, renal disease, coronary insufficiency, recent myocardial infarction, cerebral vascular disease, colitis, peptic ulcer, and during pregnancy.

Orthostatic hypotension is a frequent occurrence, especially during periods of dosage adjustment and can be accentuated by hot weather, alcohol, or strenuous exercise.

Withdrawal of these drugs 2 weeks prior to administration of general anesthesia is recommended to reduce the possibility of vascular collapse and cardiac arrest. If emergency surgery is necessary, anesthetic agents should be given cautiously in reduced doses.

INTERACTIONS

1. The antihypertensive effects of guanethidine and guanadrel may be antagonized by amphetamines, antidepressants, antihistamines, antipsychotics (e.g., phenothiazines, thioxanthenes, haloperidol), cocaine, diethylpropion, ephedrine, MAO-inhibitors, methylphenidate, oral contraceptives, and sympathomimetic agents.
2. Enhanced hypotensive effects may be observed when guanethidine or guanadrel is given in combination with alcohol, diuretics, hydralazine, levodopa, methotrimeprazine, propranolol, quinidine, reserpine, and vasodilator drugs.
3. Excessive bradycardia can occur if guanethidine or guanadrel is used in combination with digitalis drugs.
4. Guanethidine or guanadrel may impair the hyposecretory effect of anticholinergics.
5. Guanethidine or guanadrel may exert an additive hypoglycemic effect with insulin or oral antidiabetic drugs.
6. Increased responses to direct-acting adrenergic agents (e.g., catecholamines, phenylephrine, metaraminol) may occur with guanethidine or guanadrel, as they block neuronal uptake of the sympathomimetic agents.

NURSING CONSIDERATIONS

(See also Nursing Process for Antihypertensive Drugs.)

Adequate baseline data must be obtained before starting a patient on guanethidine or guanadrel. Liver and kidney function tests as well as a complete blood count should be evaluated initially and periodically throughout therapy. A weight should be obtained and extremities and lungs evaluated for signs of edema because fluid retention can occur with these drugs. A drug history must also be obtained. Specific questions should be asked about the patient's use of over-the-counter drugs for sinus or cold symptoms, which in combination with these agents can cause severe hypertension, and the use of street drugs and alcohol, which can result in severe hypotension. The patient must clearly understand the dangers of using any other drugs with guanethidine or guanadrel.

Side-effects of these drugs are frequently the cause of drug discontinuation with or without supervision. The patient should be cautioned to seek assistance if side-effects become unmanageable because abrupt discontinuation of the drug can result in severe rebound hypertension.

Guanethidine and guanadrel can cause severe postural hypotension, which is worsened by alcohol, heat, hot showers, and exercise. The patient must respond to dizziness by sitting or lying down and should inform the care giver if fainting or dizziness does not abate as therapy continues. In the extreme, the side-effect can lead to myocardial or cerebral ischemia.

Side-effects of the drugs respond slowly to dose changes, and improvement may take as long as 3 to 5 days. Consequently, during any period of dosage adjustment blood pressure should be closely monitored. Wide variations between blood pressure readings of a patient in sitting, standing, or supine positions should be reported. If possible, the patient on either of these drugs should obtain a device for self-blood pressure monitoring.

Diarrhea is another side-effect of these drugs which may warrant serious attention. If diarrhea cannot be controlled, valuable fluids and electrolytes are lost, which will alter drug absorption. This symptom should be reported immediately because the drug may have to be discontinued.

Guanethidine and guanadrel may cause ejaculatory inhibition which may result in the patient discontinuing therapy. The nurse may need to ask some direct open-ended questions to find out if the patient is having difficulty. With counseling, the patient may agree to continue therapy or request a change in drug. Without counseling, the patient may make an erroneous decision to discontinue therapy, which could have serious consequences.

The patient on guanethidine or guanadrel should combine therapy with adequate sodium restriction to avoid water retention. Even with dietary restrictions, the patient may still need diuretics.

Minoxidil

(Loniten, Minodyl)

MECHANISM AND ACTIONS

Minoxidil dilates arteriolar resistance vessels with minimal effects on venous capacitance vessels. The drug appears to reduce calcium uptake through the cell membrane, thus reducing arteriolar tone and lowering peripheral vascular resistance. Minoxidil does not exert a CNS action nor interfere with vasomotor reflexes; thus, orthostatic effects are rare. Renal blood flow is maintained. Reflex responses to minoxidil include tachycardia, increased renin secretion, and augmented salt and water retention. Blood pressure is substantially reduced, but due to the potential of minoxidil to elicit serious untoward reactions, the drug is reserved for treatment of severe hypertension not controlled by other antihypertensive drugs.

USES
1. Treatment of severe hypertension not manageable by maximum doses of a diuretic plus two other antihypertensive drugs; usually given together with a diuretic and beta-blocker, to minimize fluid retention and reflex tachycardia, respectively. Methyldopa and clonidine have also been used concurrently.
2. Treatment of alopecia areata and androgenic alopecia (male pattern baldness) (unlabeled use of minoxidil as a topical lotion or ointment—based on the ability of the drug to cause hypertrichosis—see under Side-Effects/Adverse Reactions)

ADMINISTRATION AND DOSAGE
Minoxidil is administered orally as tablets (2.5 mg, 10 mg) at the following recommended doses:
Adults: Initially 5 mg/day as a single dose; increase step-wise up to 40 mg/day in divided doses, or until optimal control is attained; usual range is 10 mg to 40 mg/day (maximum is 100 mg/day)
Children (under 12): Initially, 0.2 mg/kg/day as a single dose; increase in 50%- to 100%-increments until optimal control is attained; usual range is 0.25 mg/kg to 1.0 mg/kg/day (maximum is 50 mg/day)
Dosage adjustments should be made at intervals of at least 3 days. The drug may be given either once or twice a day depending on degree of blood pressure control.

FATE
Minoxidil is almost completely absorbed orally, and plasma levels reach maximum within 1 hour. The blood pressure-lowering effects are maximal in 2 hours to 3 hours and persist for over 24 hours. The drug does not bind to plasma proteins. The average plasma half-life is 4 hours. Approximately 90% of a dose is metabolized in the liver, and excretion is largely by way of the kidney.

SIDE-EFFECTS/ADVERSE REACTIONS
The most commonly encountered side-effect during minoxidil treatment is hypertrichosis, an elongation and thickening of fine body hair, beginning in the facial region and later extending to the back, arms, legs, and scalp. It usually develops within 3 to 6 weeks, and occurs in up to 80% of patients. No endocrine abnormalities have been associated with this condition.

Hair growth ceases upon discontinuation of the drug but up to 6 months may be required for previous hair growth to disappear. Other frequently encountered side-effects are changes in the amplitude and direction of the T waves (without evidence of cardiac dysfunction), temporary edema, sweating, and headache. Tachycardia is common when beta-blockers are not used concurrently but is rare when adequate doses of beta-blocking agents are administered with minoxidil.

Minoxidil has produced cardiac lesions in experimental animals, but human pathologic findings have not substantiated this effect in humans. However, the possibility of such damage must be considered, especially with prolonged therapy. Pericardial effusion, occasionally with tamponade, has occurred in about 3% of patients receiving minoxidil, especially when renal function is compromised. Echocardiographic studies are diagnostic, and treatment may involve vigorous diuretic therapy, dialysis, or surgery. Anginal symptoms can be precipitated or worsened by reflex sympathetic activity associated with minoxidil. Beta-blockers will minimize this possibility.

Other adverse reactions observed in minoxidil-treated patients include nausea, vomiting, fatigue, breast tenderness, skin darkening, allergic rash, *temporary* decreases in hematocrit, hemoglobin, and erythrocyte counts, and increases in serum creatinine and alkaline phosphatase.

Too rapid decline in blood pressure following minoxidil can lead to syncope, myocardial infarction, and ischemia of many body organs. Cautious therapy is indicated to minimize the danger of sudden blood pressure declines.

CONTRAINDICATIONS AND PRECAUTIONS
Contraindications to use of minoxidil include pheochromocytoma, acute myocardial infarction, and dissecting aortic aneurysm. *Caution* is required when administering minoxidil to persons with cardiac disease, edema, renal or hepatic insufficiency, and to pregnant women or nursing mothers.

INTERACTIONS
1. Minoxidil may markedly worsen the degree of orthostatic hypotension caused by guanethidine, guanadrel, or ganglionic blocking agents.

NURSING CONSIDERATIONS
(See also Nursing Process for Antihypertensive Drugs.)

Baseline data which should be collected prior to initiating minoxidil therapy include a complete blood count, kidney function studies including creatinine and BUN levels, and liver function studies including alkaline phosphatase. Blood levels of the drug should be monitored throughout therapy because elevations can occur. In addition, an ECG should be done periodically to monitor changes in the S–T segment as a result of the drug.

Physical assessment should include a complete cardiovascular examination including heart size and notation of any discrepancy between apical and radial pulses. (See Chap. 33 for a description.)

Minoxidil is usually prescribed when a patient fails to respond adequately to guanethidine or when the addition of guanethidine to a medical regimen·is inappropriate. The best approach to drug change is to discontinue the guanethidine first and then add minoxidil, but for patients with severe hypertension this may be hazardous. In such a case, the patient should be hospitalized while the therapy is being changed because minoxidil and guanethidine in combination can result in a severe hypotension, which has been known to cause a myocardial infarction (MI) or cerebrovascular accident (CVA). The nurse should monitor blood pressure and heart rate very carefully during this period and provide a protective environment which will decrease the chance of a patient injuring himself as a result of dizziness from blood pressure variations.

Because minoxidil is most often used in combination with a diuretic and a beta-blocker, the patient receiving this drug should be very carefully followed. If possible, the patient or his family should learn to monitor his own blood pressure and to keep records of sitting, standing, and supine blood pressures. In addition to wide and sudden changes in blood pressure, he should learn to report any increase in pulse of 20 beats or more over normal, rapid weight gain, swelling in his extremities, dyspnea, dizziness, or chest pain. All of these symptoms indicate the need for a dosage adjustment. Consequently, minoxidil is best prescribed for the patient who has good supports and is motivated to learn to monitor his own pulse, blood pressure, and weight throughout the course of therapy.

The patient should be warned about the possibility of increased hair growth and darkening of body hair, a side-effect of the drug currently being tested for treatment of baldness.

The drug should be used with extreme caution in patients with renal insufficiency or angina. Such patients should be told to report immediately any increase in angina pain, dyspnea, or weakness because pericardial effusion and tamponade can occur (see under Side-Effects/Adverse Reactions).

Drugs for Hypertensive Emergencies

Hypertensive emergencies, or marked elevations in blood pressure, require immediate treatment to avoid serious and often life-threatening complications. A number of drugs are available to lower blood pressure rapidly , and they are commonly administered IV, frequently with or following a diuretic. Among the drugs indicated for hypertensive emergencies that have been discussed previously are trimethaphan, a ganglionic blocking agent (reviewed in Chap. 17), and methyldopa and hydralazine, two orally effective antihypertensive drugs, discussed in this chapter, that can be given IV in acute hypertension.

The two most frequently used drugs for hypertensive emergencies, however, are nitroprusside sodium and diazoxide parenteral, which are reviewed below.

A hypertensive crisis may occur as a result of poor medication control, noncompliance with antihypertensive therapy, or in a patient previously undetected as a hypertensive. A nonhypertensive patient may develop a hypertensive emergency as a result of brain trauma or tumor, pregnancy, or drug abuse. Regardless of cause, rapid action is required, and close monitoring by the nurse is essential.

If possible, a brief history of the symptoms leading to the crisis and a drug history should be obtained. Such data can facilitate drug and treatment choices. Electrolytes and renal function studies should be drawn.

Administration of emergency antihypertensive medications is by IV bolus or infusion; subsequently, changes in symptoms will be rapid and dramatic. Any IV infusion should be monitored by an infusion pump with an infiltration alarm.

If possible, an arterial line should be inserted to accurately measure blood pressure. Blood pressure and heart rate should be assessed every 2 to 3 minutes while hypertension is being brought under control. Assessment of cerebral perfusion is also essential. Changes in mental status, speech, or weakness or numbness of extremities must be immediately reported. Urinary output should be monitored hourly because decreases may be the first sign of renal ischemia. Continuous cardiac monitoring is also essential. The patient should be closely observed for chest pain and arrhythmias, signs of myocardial ischemia.

See specific drugs for further discussion.

Nitroprusside Sodium
(Nipride, Nitropress)

Nitroprusside sodium is a rapid and short-acting blood pressure-lowering agent given by IV infusion. In addition to its use in controlling acute hypertensive emergencies, nitroprusside is also effective in treating symptoms of severe congestive heart failure.

MECHANISM AND ACTIONS
Nitroprusside has a direct short-lived relaxant effect of both arteriolar and venular smooth muscle, resulting in reduced systemic vascular resistance. Reflex tachycardia is sometimes noted but is generally mild, and cardiac output may be slightly reduced. Renin activity may be increased due to a drop in renal perfusion pressure. The hypotensive action of nitroprusside develops rapidly and persists for only several minutes following discontinuation of the infusion, allowing precise titration of the dose to attain the optimal therapeutic benefit.

In the presence of left ventricular failure, nitroprusside can reduce both afterload (aortic resistance) and preload (ventricular filling pressure), improve cardiac output, and reduce pulmonary capillary wedge pressure. Heart rate is essentially unchanged.

USES
1. Emergency treatment of hypertensive crises (*Note:* Oral antihypertensive medication should be initiated while blood pressure is being controlled by IV nitroprusside.)
2. Production of controlled hypotension during surgery or anesthesia
3. Adjunctive therapy of severe, refractory congestive heart failure, treatment of lactic acidosis due to reduced peripheral perfusion, and attenuation of the vasoconstrictor effects of norepinephrine and dopamine

ADMINISTRATION AND DOSAGE
Nitroprusside is available as a powder for injection (50 mg/vial) to be diluted and infused *slowly* IV. The contents of the 50-mg vial are dissolved in 2 ml to 3 ml of 5% dextrose in water, then diluted in 250 ml to 1000 ml of 5% dextrose in water and immediately wrapped in foil or other opaque substance. Nitroprusside is administered by infusion pump, microdrip regulator, or other device allowing precise measurement of the flow rate.

In patients not receiving other antihypertensive drugs, the average dose is 3 mcg/kg/min (range 0.5–10 μg/kg/min). If blood pressure is not adequately reduced within 10 minutes, discontinue administration and employ alternative therapy.

FATE
Nitroprusside has an immediate onset of action (30 seconds–60 seconds), and effects are maximum within 1 minute to 2 minutes. Upon termination of the infusion, blood pressure can return to pretreatment levels within several minutes. Nitroprusside decomposes to cyanide in the blood, which either reacts with methemoglobin to form cyanmethemoglobin or is converted in the liver and kidney to thiocyanate, which is slowly cleared by the kidney, and has a half-life of 4 days in patients with normal renal function. In patients with impaired renal function, prolonged infusion or excessive doses can cause cyanide toxicity (see under Side-Effects/Adverse Reactions).

SIDE-EFFECTS/ADVERSE REACTIONS
Side-effects noted most often are generally the result of too rapid infusion or excessive dosage and include nausea, sweating, headache, restlessness, muscle twitching, dizziness, palpitations, and abdominal or substernal discomfort.

Accumulation of thiocyanate (see under Fate) can result in tinnitus, blurred vision, delirium, weak pulse, shallow breathing, dyspnea, ataxia, diminished reflexes, convulsions, dilated pupils, pink skin color, and loss of consciousness. Hypothyroidism has occurred with prolonged therapy, and methemoglobinemia has been reported. Nitroprusside may have antiplatelet activity.

CONTRAINDICATIONS AND PRECAUTIONS

Nitroprusside should not be used to treat compensatory hypertension (*e.g.*, coarctation of the aorta, arteriovenous shunt) or in patients with inadequate cerebral circulation. *Cautious* administration of nitroprusside is warranted in patients with hypothyroidism, renal or hepatic impairment, and anemia or hypovolemia and in elderly or poor surgical risk patients.

INTERACTIONS

1. Enhanced hypotension can occur if nitroprusside is given to patients receiving other antihypertensive medications, circulatory depressants, and volatile liquid anesthetics.
2. Tolbutamide may decrease the effects of nitroprusside.

NURSING CONSIDERATIONS

(See also Nursing Process for Antihypertensive Drugs.)

Renal function must be assessed by history and laboratory evaluation prior to drug administration. Drug toxicity from nitroprusside is more pronounced in the patient with impaired renal function.

Nitroprusside must be mixed with dextrose and water and infused as a secondary (or piggyback) solution into an IV line. The site should be carefully monitored for irritation or extravasation because the drug is extremely irritating to tissue. No other drugs should be administered through this line while nitroprusside is running. The IV should be controlled by an infusion pump which has been primed and checked before insertion into the patient because even minor adjustments in the rate can result in rapid variations in blood pressure. The solution will be pale tan in color, but clear. Any darkening or cloudiness indicates decomposition of the drug, and the solution should be discarded. The solution must be shielded from light by a paper bag or aluminum foil (provided by manufacturer) around the container. It is not necessary to cover the tubing. Nitroprusside should be discarded after 4 hours from preparation time, and a fresh solution should be hung.

The dosage of nitroprusside will be titrated against arterial blood pressure. The physician must order a blood pressure goal which the nurse will use in regulating the infusion rate. The patient should be kept in bed until pressure is stabilized.

Hourly outputs should be obtained while nitroprusside is administered and renal function should be evaluated. Because nitroprusside is metabolized to cyanide and then to thiocyanate, thiocyanate blood levels should be done if the drug is continued more than 24 hours. The patient should be closely monitored for cyanide intoxication (see symptoms under Side-Effects/Adverse Reactions) and treated with sodium nitrite and sodium thiosulfate if symptoms appear. Consequently, these drugs should be on hand whenever nitroprusside is administered.

Diazoxide, Parenteral
(Hyperstat IV)

Diazoxide is a rapid-acting antihypertensive which is administered by IV injection for controlling severe hypertension. It is longer acting than nitroprusside sodium and thus does not permit precise moment-to-moment control of the pressure. Diazoxide is also available in capsules as Proglycem for treatment of hypoglycemia caused by excessive secretion of insulin (*e.g.*, islet cell carcinoma). This latter application is considered in Chapter 54.

MECHANISM AND ACTIONS

Diazoxide exerts a direct relaxant effect on arteriolar smooth muscle without significantly affecting venular smooth muscle. Reflex increases in heart rate, stroke volume, and cardiac output occur as pressure is lowered. Coronary and cerebral blood flow are maintained, and renal blood flow may increase following an initial decline. Diazoxide causes sodium retention, and transient hyperglycemia is seen in the majority of patients due to inhibition of insulin secretion.

USES

1. Treatment of acute hypertensive emergencies and severe hypertension where rapid reduction of diastolic pressure is required (IV injection)
2. Management of hypoglycemia caused by hyperinsulinism (oral diazoxide—see Chap. 54)

ADMINISTRATION AND DOSAGE

Diazoxide is available for IV injection as ampules containing 300 mg/20 ml. The drug is injected IV undiluted over 30 seconds or less with the patient in the supine position. One mg/kg to 3 mg/kg (to a maximum of 150 mg per injection) is given rapidly and may be repeated at 5-minute to 15-minute intervals until a satisfactory response has been attained. Blood pressure can then be maintained with repeated administration at 4 hour to 24 hour intervals until a regimen of oral antihypertensive drug therapy is initiated. Diazoxide should not be used for longer than 10 days and never administered by infusion. If repeated administration becomes necessary, a diuretic should be given to minimize the danger of sodium and water retention.

FATE

Following IV injection, blood pressure decreases within 2 to 5 minutes to its maximum extent, then increases rapidly over the next 10 minutes to 30 minutes, followed by a slower increase over 2 hours to 12 hours. Diazoxide is extensively bound to plasma protein (90%), and the plasma half-life ranges from 20 hours to 36 hours. The response to successive injections is frequently greater than the initial response.

SIDE-EFFECTS/ADVERSE REACTIONS

Hypotension, nausea, vomiting, dizziness, and weakness are seen most frequently when doses of 300 mg are administered; smaller doses (*e.g.,* 150 mg) are less likely to cause these common untoward reactions. Additional adverse reactions noted during diazoxide administration include:

Cardiovascular—Hypotension, dizziness, myocardial and cerebral ischemia, palpitations, arrhythmias, sweating, flushing, supraventricular tachycardia
CNS—(Secondary to blood flow changes in the brain) confusion, headache, lightheadedness, somnolence, hearing impairment, euphoria, convulsions, paralysis
GI—Abdominal pain, nausea, vomiting, anorexia, parotid swelling, salivation, dry mouth, constipation or diarrhea, ileus
Dermatologic/hypersensitivity—Rash, fever, leukopenia
Respiratory—Cough, dyspnea, choking sensation
Other—Pancreatitis, weakness, lacrimation, cellulitis, pain along injected vein, back pain, nocturia, hyperuricemia

Transient hyperglycemia is frequently encountered with diazoxide, especially after repeated injections. While seldom clinically significant in the nondiabetic, marked elevations in blood glucose can occur in the noninsulin-dependent diabetic receiving oral hypoglycemic drugs. Diazoxide has induced subendocardial necrosis and necrosis of papillary muscles in dogs; however, the clinical significance of this finding is unknown.

CONTRAINDICATIONS AND PRECAUTIONS

Diazoxide parenteral should not be used in treating compensatory hypertension due to aortic coarctation, arteriovenous shunt, or dissecting aortic aneurysm or in treating pheochromocytoma. *Cautious use* of diazoxide must be undertaken in patients with impaired cerebral or coronary circulation, hyperglycemia, congestive heart failure, and in pregnant women or nursing mothers.

INTERACTIONS

1. Combined use of diuretics with diazoxide may intensify its hyperglycemic, hyperuricemic, and hypertensive effects.
2. Diazoxide may potentiate the action of other highly protein-bound drugs (*e.g.,* oral anticoagulants, anti-inflammatory agents, sulfonamides, phenytoin, quinidine, propranolol) by displacing them from binding sites.
3. Chlorpromazine and furosemide may potentiate the hyperglycemic effect of diazoxide.
4. An increased hypotensive response can occur when diazoxide is used along with other antihypertensive drugs such as vasodilators (*e.g.,* nitrites, hydralazine), catecholamine-depleting drugs (*e.g.,* reserpine), beta-blockers, or centrally acting agents.
5. The hepatic metabolism of hydantoins (*e.g.,* phenytoin) may be accelerated by diazoxide.
6. Diazoxide may reduce the effectiveness of oral hypoglycemic agents by blunting insulin secretion.

NURSING CONSIDERATIONS

(See Nursing Process for Antihypertensive Drugs.)
Baseline data should include a complete blood count, blood glucose, electrolytes, and uric acid levels. The patient should be weighed, if possible, and intake and output monitored closely throughout drug therapy because sodium and water retention is a major problem.

Diazoxide causes severe initial hypotension which resolves slowly as the body adjusts to the drug. Therefore, the patient should be kept supine for at least 30 minutes after administration. Unfortunately, diazoxide also causes nausea and vomiting. The nurse should be aware of the danger of aspiration, especially in the patient whose mental status is altered by the hypertensive crisis, and should have suction equipment and oxygen readily available. The patient should be within view at all times until stabilized.

Blood pressure should be closely monitored throughout therapy and should follow the expected changes described under Fate. An appropriate guideline would be to take blood pressure readings every 2 minutes for the first 10 minutes, every 5 minutes for the next hour, every hour for the next 2 hours, and then drop to an every 2- to 4-hour sched-

ule gradually over the next 12 hours. The cycle of monitoring should be repeated with each injection. Blood pressure should be taken sitting, standing, and supine before a patient is allowed out of bed. Assistance should be provided until the extent of dizziness from position change is known.

Fluid retention may occur in patients with a history of congestive heart failure or renal insufficiency. Close monitoring of urine output, peripheral and sacral edema, and lung sounds can alert the nurse to early development of this symptom. Cardiac monitoring may also be necessary because diazoxide can cause arrhythmias.

Miscellaneous Antihypertensive Drugs

Phenoxybenzamine
(Dibenzyline)

Phenoxybenzamine is an orally effective, long-acting nonselective (i.e., alpha$_1$ and alpha$_2$) alpha-adrenergic blocking agent indicated for the control of episodes of hypertension and sweating associated with pheochromocytoma. Phenoxybenzamine produces a "chemical sympathectomy," interrupting impulse transmission through alpha-adrenergic receptor sites, which results in reduced blood pressure and increased blood flow to the skin, mucosa, and abdominal organs. In addition to its use in pheochromocytoma, it has been shown to be effective in certain disorders of the bladder, in which micturition is impaired. (Phenoxybenzamine is discussed in detail in Chap. 16.)

The initial dose is 10 mg/day orally, which is increased by 10 mg every 4 days until the desired blood pressure lowering is attained. The usual dosage range is 20 mg to 60 mg a day. At least 2 weeks are generally required to attain significant improvement, and possibly several more weeks are required for full benefits.

Principal adverse reactions with phenoxybenzamine are nasal congestion, orthostatic hypotension, miosis, tachycardia, and impaired ejaculation. These effects are due to adrenergic blockade and generally disappear with time. Phenoxybenzamine should be used with caution in patients with coro-

nary or cerebral vascular insufficiency or renal damage.

Phentolamine
(Regitine)

Phentolamine is a nonselective alpha-adrenergic blocking agent used by injection to control hypertensive episodes that might occur in patients with pheochromocytoma during surgery for removal of the chromaffin tumor. The drug has also been employed to prevent the dermal necrosis and sloughing that can occur upon extravasation during IV infusion of epinephrine, norepinephine, or dopamine solutions. Treatment of rebound hypertension during withdrawal of antihypertensive medications has also been accomplished by injection of phentolamine.

Phentolamine has an immediate onset and short duration of action. In addition to its alpha-blocking action, the drug has a direct relaxant effect on vascular smooth muscle.

The usual dosage for reducing blood pressure is 5 mg IM or IV; a dose of 1 mg may be used in children. For treatment of dermal necrosis and sloughing resulting from extravasation of infusion solutions, 5 mg to 10 mg in 10 ml of saline is injected into the area of extravasation. Alternately, 10 mg may be added to each liter of infusion solution containing norepinephrine. The pressor effect of norepinephrine is not affected by this procedure.

Tachycardia and cardiac arrhythmias may occur with use of phentolamine. Other adverse effects include weakness, dizziness, flushing, orthostatic hypotension, nasal stuffiness, vomiting, and diarrhea.

Phentolamine has been employed to diagnose pheochromocytoma, based on a rather sharp drop in blood pressure (more than 35 mm systolic and 25 mm diastolic) within 2 minutes after injection. This test is not a procedure of choice, however, and should be reserved for cases in which additional confirmation is required following performance of conventional urinary catecholamine assays.

Mecamylamine
(Inversine)

Mecamylamine is a potent, orally effective ganglionic blocking agent which exerts a considerable orthostatic hypotensive effect. Due primarily to its many side-effects, it is only used for the control of severe hypertension in patients not responding to a combination of other antihypertensive drugs. Initial dosage is 2.5 mg twice a day, which may be adjusted in increments of 2.5 mg at intervals of at least 2 days until a desired response is attained. The average dose is 25 mg/day in two to four divided doses. (Mecamylamine is reviewed in detail in Chap. 17.)

Metyrosine
(Demser)

Metyrosine, or alpha-methyltyrosine, is a competitive inhibitor of the enzyme tyrosine hydroxylase which catalyzes the conversion of tyrosine to dopa, the first step in the subsequent synthesis of dopamine, norepinephrine, and epinephrine. Because this is the *rate-limiting step*, inhibition of tyrosine hydroxylase results in decreased levels of catecholamines in the CNS and periphery. The drug is indicated for the management of patients with pheochromocytoma, either as preoperative preparation or for control of excessive blood pressure when surgery is contraindicated. Metyrosine is not recommended for the control of essential hypertension.

Initial dosage is 250 mg orally, four times a day. Dosage may be increased by 250 mg to 500 mg every day to a maximum of 4 g/day in divided doses. Preoperative preparation for surgery should be accomplished by giving optimally effective doses (usually 2 g–3 g a day) for at least 5 to 7 days.

Patients not adequately controlled by metyrosine may also be given phenoxybenzamine.

The drug is well absorbed orally and is recovered largely in the urine as unchanged drug. Because metyrosine inhibits catecholamine synthesis, central and peripheral sympathetic activity is impaired, resulting in a variety of adverse effects. The most common side-effect is sedation, which can be moderate to severe during the first few days of therapy. Other frequently occurring untoward reactions are diarrhea (occasionally severe), drooling, mild tremor, and speech difficulty. Less common adverse reactions with metyrosine include anxiety, confusion, depression, hallucinations, dry mouth, nausea, abdominal pain, impotence, ejaculation disturbances, galactorrhea, dysuria, crystalluria, hematuria, and hypersensitivity reactions, (rash, urticaria, pharyngeal edema).

A sufficient daily intake of water to achieve a urinary volume of at least 2000 ml per day is important to minimize the risk of crystalluria. Additive sedative effects can occur if metyrosine is taken in combination with alcohol or other CNS depressants.

Pargyline
(Eutonyl)

Pargyline is an infrequently used oral antihypertensive drug which exerts predominantly an orthostatic effect. It is an MAO-inhibitor (see Chap. 29), but the exact mechanism of its hypotensive action is unknown. Pargyline has been used in the treatment of moderate to severe hypertension, usually in combination with diuretics or other antihypertensive drugs. Initial dosage is 25 mg in a single daily dose. Dosage may be increased by 10 mg/week until the desired response is obtained. The usual maintenance range is 25 mg to 50 mg a day. The drug has a slow onset of action, and a therapeutic response may not occur for several weeks. Similarly, effects may persist for several weeks following discontinuation of the drug.

Commonly noted side-effects are dry mouth, insomnia, nervousness, weakness, palpitations, dizziness, dizziness, sweating, muscle twitching, blurred vision, fluid retention, and mild constipation. Because the drug is an MAO-inhibitor, all of the adverse reactions listed for the other MAO-inhibitors in Chapter 29 are theoretically possible with pargyline. Refer to the discussion of MAO-inhibitors in Chapter 29 for contraindications, precautions, and potential interactions.

CASE STUDY

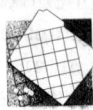

Fred Samuels, age 62, has a 10-year history of hypertension. He is currently maintained on methyldopa (Aldomet) 500 mg bid and has been on this medication 6 months. On a routine clinic visit his blood pressure is 138/80 sitting and 134/78 standing. The clinic nurse, Ms. James, asks Mr. Samuels how he is doing on the medication. He complains of occasional headaches and says he's doing fine. However, when Ms. James accompanies Mr. Samuels to the examining room he asks to see the doctor privately.

When Mr. Samuels returns, Ms. James notices he looks a little distraught and she asks if she might talk to him to review some of his care. The following dialogue takes place:

Ms. James: "Did the doctor answer your questions, Mr. Samuels?"

Mr. Samuels: "Yes."

Ms. James: "I sense you're a little unhappy. Do you want to talk about it?"

Mr. Samuels: "Uh . . . no . . . it's ok."

Ms. James: "Were your questions about your sex life?"

Mr. Samuels: "Uh, yes! How did you know that?"

Ms. James: "What did the doctor say?"

Mr. Samuels: "He said I have to make a choice, sex or the drug."

Ms. James: "And what are you going to choose."

Mr. Samuels: "I'd rather have a good sex life. My wife is only 42."

Discussion Questions

1. What would you do at this point in the conversation?
2. What options does Mr. Samuels have? How can you help him remain compliant?

REVIEW QUESTIONS

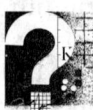

1. Distinguish between the terms systolic, diastolic, and pulse in regard to blood pressure.
2. Briefly discuss the role of *renin* in control of blood pressure.
3. What are the accepted guidelines for classifying hypertension as mild, moderate, or severe?
4. List the principal sites of action of antihypertensive drugs.
5. What is the stepped-care approach to the treatment of hypertension?
6. Give two examples of (a) step-1, (b) step-2, (c) step-3, and (d) step-4 antihypertensive drugs.
7. What baseline laboratory data should be collected before a patient receives any antihypertensive medication?
8. What should be included in a drug history for the patient starting antihypertensive drug therapy?
9. What strategies can the nurse use to improve drug compliance of hypertensive patients?
10. How can the nurse help a patient deal with orthostatic hypotension, changes in sexual function, or fluid retention?
11. What physiologic changes in elderly patients make dosage adjustments of antihypertensive medications more difficult?

12. In what situations might a beta-blocker be preferred over a diuretic as a step-1 antihypertensive drug?
13. How do beta-blockers lower blood pressure?
14. What is unique about the mechanism of action of labetalol? For what is the drug used?
15. Briefly describe the actions of clonidine, guanfacine, and guanabenz. What are the most common side-effects associated with their use?
16. What is the significance of a positive direct Coombs' test as seen with methyldopa? What are the common side-effects noted with this drug?
17. List the principal indications for prazosin. What is the "first dose" prazosin effect?
18. Describe the mechanism of action of reserpine in lowering blood pressure. Why are the rauwolfia alkaloids infrequently used in treating hypertension?
19. Discuss the mechanism responsible for the blood pressure-lowering action of captopril, enalapril, and lisinopril. Why are these drugs suitable for treatment of *all degrees* of hypertension? Explain.
20. What serious adverse reaction has occurred with high doses of hydralazine? What are the early signs?
21. In what situations is hydralazine contraindicated?
22. Why is hydralazine a drug used in preeclampsia? What are the nursing responsibilities for the pregnant patient receiving this drug?
23. How does guanethidine or guanadrel reduce blood pressure? What is the major danger with use of these agents?
24. Give the major indication for minoxidil. What side-effect is noted in most patients receiving the drug? Mention an investigational use for minoxidil.
25. How do the actions of nitroprusside differ from diazoxide parenteral in treating hypertensive emergencies?
26. Why should use of nitroprusside be undertaken cautiously in persons with impaired renal function?
27. What are the specific techniques the nurse must follow when administering a nitroprusside drip?
28. What are the principal indications for (a) metyrosine, (b) phentolamine, and (c) pargyline?

BIBLIOGRAPHY

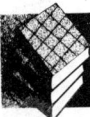

Alexander JK: Managing the elderly patient with hypertension. Mod Med 55(1):58, 1987

Caris TN: Hypertension in older patients: What drugs to use and when. Geriatrics 37:38, 1982

Cressman MD, Clifford RW: Controversies in hypertension: Mild hypertension, isolated systolic hypertension and the choice of a step one drug. Clin Cardiol 6:1, 1983

Dollery CT: Hypertension and new antihypertensive drugs: Clinical perspectives. Fed Prod 42:207, 1983

Drayer JI, Weber MA: The impact of antihypertensives on cardiovascular risks. Drug Therapy 13(4):116, 1983

Ferguson RK, Vlasses PH, Riley LJ: Captopril and enalapril: Angiotensin converting enzyme (ACE) inhibitors. Ration Drug Ther 18:1, 1984

Finnerty FA: Step-down treatment of mild systemic hypertension. Am J Cardiol 53:1304, 1984

Freis ED: Should mild hypertension be treated? N Engl J Med 307:306, 1982

Frolich ED, Cooper RA, Lewis RJ: Review of the overall experience of captopril in hypertension. Arch Intern Med 144:1441, 1984

Hypertension Detection and Follow-up Program Cooperative Group: The effect of treatment on mortality in mild hypertension. N Engl J Med 307:1976, 1982

Johnson CI, Arnolda L, Hiwatari M: Angiotensin-converting enzyme inhibitors in the treatment of hypertension. Drugs 27:271, 1984

Johnson GP, Johanson BC: Beta blockers. Am J Nurs 83:1034, 1983

Kaplan NM: New approaches to the therapy of mild hypertension. Am J Cardiol 51:621, 1983

Kelley M, Mongiello R: Hypertension in pregnancy: Labor, delivery and postpartum. Am J Nurs 83:813, 1983

Kirschenbaum HL, Rosenberg JM: Emergency antihypertensives. RN 46:53, 1983

New antihypertensive drugs—A symposium. Fed Proc 42:153, 1983

Reichgott M et al: The nurse practitioner's role in complex patient management: Hypertension. J Natl Med Assoc 75:1197, 1983

Spivack C, Ocken S, Frishman WH: Calcium antagonists: Clinical use in the treatment of systemic hypertension. Drugs 25:154, 1983

Vidt DG, Bravo EL, Fovad FM: Captopril. N Engl J Med 306:214, 1982

Westfall TC, Meldrum MJ: Alterations in the release of norepinephrine at the vascular neuroeffector junction in hypertension. Annu Rev Pharmacol Toxicol 25:621, 1985

Antianginal Agents and Vasodilators

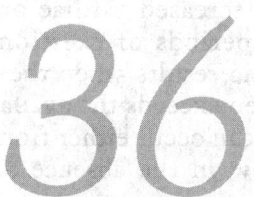

Drugs that can improve blood flow through circulatory vessels by increasing their functional diameter are termed vasodilators. These agents are usually effective in reducing the incidence and severity of exertional pain in patients with ischemic coronary artery disease (e.g., angina) but are generally of limited clinical usefulness for improving circulation in peripheral vascular diseases. The drugs discussed in this chapter are divided into those principally used for the treatment of angina pectoris and those usually indicated for the treatment of peripheral and cerebrovascular insufficiency.

Antianginal Agents

Angina pectoris (ischemic coronary artery disease) is a leading cause of death in the United States and most other western countries. Drugs useful in the treatment of angina pectoris act to correct the imbalance between the myocardial oxygen demand and the supply of available oxygen. In order to better understand the action of antianginal drugs, a brief review of normal coronary circulation and the pathophysiology of angina will first be presented.

Coronary Circulation

The myocardium is richly vascularized, its blood supply coming by way of the coronary circulation. The coronary vessels course around the heart in two external anatomical grooves: the atrioventricular groove and the interventricular groove.

The coronary arteries arise from the ascending aorta immediately above the free margins of the aortic semilunar valve. They form a crown around the heart and provide branches to supply the atrial and ventricular myocardium.

The right coronary artery, with its marginal and posterior interventricular branches, supplies the right atrium, right ventricle, and a portion of the left ventricle. The left coronary artery and its major branches, the circumflex and anterior interventricular, supply the left atrium, left ventricle, and part of the right ventricle. Anastomoses between arterial branches exist and serve as potential routes for collateral circulation if gradual occlusion of a vessel occurs. Coronary veins accompany the coronary arteries. The most significant myocardial venous return occurs by way of the coronary sinus, which opens into the right atrium near the orifice of the inferior vena cava.

Blood flow through the coronary arteries occurs primarily during ventricular relaxation (diastole) because contraction of cardiac muscle during ventricular contraction (systole) compresses the arteries and impedes arterial flow. The reduced time in diastole that occurs at rapid heart rates can markedly decrease coronary arterial perfusion, a potentially critical situation in coronary patients.

Coronary perfusion is primarily controlled by local metabolites and is minimally affected by autonomic nervous system activity. Coronary vessels dilate in response to increased acidity (reduced pH), increased carbon dioxide, and diminished oxygen availability in the blood.

If a coronary artery is partially occluded by a plaque or embolus, the vasodilation that automatically occurs distal to the block may provide sufficient blood flow to meet the needs of a resting heart. However, during exercise or emotional stress, such vasodilation may not be sufficient to meet the increased demand on the heart, and ischemia may result. The characteristic substernal thoracic pain, which occasionally radiates along the medial aspect of the left arm, and results from moderate inadequacy of coronary perfusion, is termed angina pectoris.

Pathophysiology of Angina

Angina pectoris is a condition characterized by intermittent substernal (chest) pain, often of a "crushing" nature, which may remain localized in the sternal region or may radiate to other areas of the body (e.g., the left shoulder or left arm). The pain is the symptomatic manifestation of ischemia (reduced blood supply) in the area of the myocardium, leading to decreased cardiac oxygenation, especially during periods of exertion or stress. Myocardial ischemia results when the demand of the tissue for oxygen exceeds the available supply. Such an imbalance can occur either from a reduced coronary blood flow in the absence of increased myocardial demand, or from an excessive oxygen demand relative to the capacity of the coronary vasculature to deliver sufficient blood flow.

Several types of angina can be described based on the etiology of the myocardial ischemia and the severity of the symptoms:

1. *Classic, stable angina.* Occurs when there is a disproportionate increase in myocardial oxygen demand due to exercise, emotional stress, or simply increased physical exertion; sometimes termed "exertional angina" or "angina of effort"; attacks of pain are usually transient and often cease spontaneously when the person rests.
2. *Classic, unstable angina.* Chest pain occurs even at rest, and ischemia is probably severe; coronary blood flow is significantly impaired, and person is at high risk for a myocardial infarction.
3. *Vasospastic (Prinzmetal's variant) angina.* Ischemia is result of temporary coronary artery vasospasm; pain may develop either during activity or at rest and may be prolonged; can lead to sudden death due to arrhythmias or infarction.

Determinants of Myocardial Oxygen Supply

Myocardial oxygen supply is primarily a function of coronary blood flow. Extraction of oxygen from the blood supplying the myocardium is nearly maximal, even at rest, and the oxygen content of blood cannot be increased significantly under normal conditions. Therefore, increased myocardial oxygen demands can usually *only* be met by improving coronary blood flow. However, if the increased oxygen demand becomes excessive, as during extreme exertion or stress, the coronary vasculature may not be able to supply a sufficient volume of blood to provide the needed oxygen, especially if some of the coronary vessels are occluded or stenosed. In addition, ischemia itself is an effective stimulus for vasodilation, and the major coronary vessels are therefore probably reflexly dilated to begin with in most instances.

Determinants of Myocardial Oxygen Demand

Myocardial oxygen demand can increase when there are increases in heart rate, force of contrac-

tion, arterial blood pressure, and left ventricular volume. Unlike skeletal muscle, cardiac muscle cannot accumulate an oxygen debt, that is, the heart cannot store oxygen for future use. The myocardium is constantly in need of oxygen and is able to extract over 75% of the available oxygen even under conditions of no stress. When increased demands are made on the heart, the myocardium requires greater amounts of oxygen, which as explained above, must be met by an increased coronary blood flow. Because augmented coronary perfusion is not always possible, an imbalance between oxygen demand and oxygen supply is created, and symptoms of angina result.

Treatment of Angina

Treatment of patients with angina is directed at improving the myocardial oxygen demand-to-supply ratio, that is, to provide sufficient oxygen to meet the demands of the myocardium. Thus, two avenues of therapy may be utilized. First, oxygen supply can be increased by improving coronary blood flow with use of coronary vasodilators. Secondly, myocardial oxygen demand can be curtailed by reducing the workload on the heart. Although *both* approaches are theoretically feasible, drug-induced dilation of coronary blood vessels probably only plays a minor role in the treatment of most forms of angina, inasmuch as the ischemia is usually the result of *occluded* vessels rather than *constricted* vessels.

As indicated above, a reflex vasodilation is probably already present secondary to the impaired coronary perfusion.

The principal effect of most antianginal drugs, therefore, is to lower myocardial oxygen demand by reducing the workload of the heart. Actions of antianginal drugs that can accomplish the latter effect include decreasing venous return, lowering arteriolar resistance to ventricular ejection, and reducing the heart rate and force of contraction.

Drug therapy of angina may be viewed as twofold: namely, to provide relief of pain during an *acute* anginal attack, and to decrease the overall frequency and severity of chronic attacks by improving the oxygen supply-to-demand ratio. Treatment of an acute anginal attack is usually accomplished by sublingual administration of one of the rapid-acting nitrites or nitrates (*e.g.*, nitroglycerin, isosorbide dinitrate), which have a quick onset and a relatively short duration of action. Prophylaxis against anginal episodes can be conferred by use of longer acting, orally effective nitrates (*e.g.*, pentaerythritol, erythrityl), topical nitroglycerin, beta-adrenergic blockers, calcium-channel blockers, and possibly dipyridamole. These various drugs are all reviewed in detail in this chapter.

In addition to drug therapy of angina, non-pharmacologic methods of treatment may include bedrest, cessation of smoking, weight loss, avoidance of stressful situations, and coronary bypass surgery.

Nitrites/Nitrates

Amyl Nitrite, Erythrityl Tetranitrate, Isosorbide Dinitrate, Nitroglycerin, Pentaerythritol Tetranitrate

The nitrites and nitrates are the prototype drugs for the treatment of angina. Depending on drug and dosage form, they may be used to relieve the pain and distress of an acute attack of angina as well as to provide a degree of protection against frequent or severe anginal episodes.

While the efficacy of the rapid-acting agents such as sublingual nitroglycerin or isosorbide in aborting an acute anginal attack is unquestioned, controversy surrounds the use of the long-acting nitrates as prophylactic drugs. Although clinical evidence suggests that these long-acting agents may improve exercise tolerance in some anginal patients, there are conflicting data on their efficacy in reducing the frequency and severity of recurring attacks. Long-acting nitrates are quickly transported to the liver following ingestion, being rapidly and almost completely metabolized in most cases before attaining significant plasma concentrations. Cross-tolerance has been noted between the long-acting and rapid-acting nitrates. This condition may prove hazardous if a rapid-acting drug is administered in a crisis situation, only to exhibit greatly reduced effectiveness because of the increased tolerance. Currently, use of the long-acting nitrates is rated as only "possibly effective" for the prophylaxis of angina, and their use remains largely a matter of physician preference.

Another method for administering chronic nitroglycerin is the transdermal infusion system (Deponit, Nitrodisc, Nitro-Dur, Transderm-Nitro). A small adhesive bandage containing nitroglycerin in a specialized medium (e.g., solid polymer, gel-like matrix) or encased in a semipermeable membrane

is applied to a nonhairy skin area once a day and is claimed to provide constant absorption of drug over a 24-hour period, perhaps improving clinical efficacy and reducing untoward reactions. However, the initial enthusiasm for this transdermal dosage form has waned in view of questions raised concerning the effectiveness of these preparations over a full 24 hours and the fairly rapid tolerance that appears to develop to this mode of administration.

An alternative means of topical application of nitroglycerin is use of nitroglycerin ointment, which also depends on transdermal absorption of the drug. Blood levels may remain fairly stable over 4 hours to 6 hours with the ointment, but it is frequently irritating to the skin and stains easily. This preparation is discussed below.

The nitrites/nitrates will be discussed as a group, followed by a listing of individual drugs and dosage forms in Table 36-1.

MECHANISM AND ACTIONS

The major actions of nitrites/nitrates in angina are outlined in Figure 36-1. These drugs exert a direct relaxing effect on vascular smooth muscle, resulting in generalized vasodilation throughout the peripheral vascular system. Venous effects generally predominate, resulting in pooling of blood in the great veins and reduced venous return, which lowers the left ventricular end-diastolic pressure (LVEDP), also known as the preload. Decreased venous return also leads to reduced cardiac output and lowered myocardial oxygen demand. Decline in LVEDP results in improved blood flow to deeper (subendocardial) layers of the myocardium, which may be oxygen starved.

Relaxation of arteriolar smooth muscle lowers systemic vascular resistance and aortic impedance to left ventricular ejection (afterload), also reducing the workload on the heart. Pulmonary vascular pressures are reduced, and heart size is decreased.

Although total coronary blood flow is probably not significantly increased by nitrites/nitrates, the drugs may cause a shunting or redistribution of flow to ischemic areas by dilation of collateral channels.

Most nonvascular smooth muscle is transiently relaxed, and reflex tachycardia due to a drop in blood pressure can occur.

USES
1. Relief of pain of acute anginal attacks (rapid-acting drugs only)

Table 36-1
Onset and Duration of Nitrite and Nitrate Preparations

Drug	Dosage Form	Onset	Duration
amyl nitrite	Inhalant	0.5 min	3–5 min
nitroglycerin	Sublingual	1–2 min	30–45 min
	Oral (sustained-release)	30–45 min	3–6 h
	Ointment	30–60 min	2–8 h
	Translingual spray	1–2 min	30–45 min
	Transmucosal tablet	2–3 min	4–5 h
	Transdermal patch	30–60 min	16–24 h
	IV	1–2 min	5–10 min
isosorbide	Sublingual/chewable	2–4 min	1–2 h
	Oral	20–30 min	3–6 h
	Oral (sustained-release)	60–120 min	6–10 h
erythrityl	Sublingual/chewable	3–10 min	3–4 h
	Oral	30–45 min	4–6 h
pentaerythritol	Oral	30–45 min	4–6 h
	Oral (sustained-release)	30–60 min	6–10 h

2. Prevention of anginal episodes, and reduction in frequency and severity of acute attacks (long-acting nitrates, transdermal nitroglycerin, sustained-release forms of nitroglycerin)
3. Reduce cardiac workload in patients with myocardial infarction or congestive heart failure
4. Production of controlled hypotension during surgery and control of blood pressure in perioperative hypertension (IV nitroglycerin)

ADMINISTRATION AND DOSAGE
See Table 36-2.

FATE
The onset and duration of action of the various nitrite/nitrate preparations and dosage forms are given in Table 36-1. Plasma protein binding of nitroglycerin is approximately 60%. Nitrites/nitrates are rapidly metabolized in the liver. Following oral administration, there is extensive first-pass hepatic

(Text continues on p. 722.)

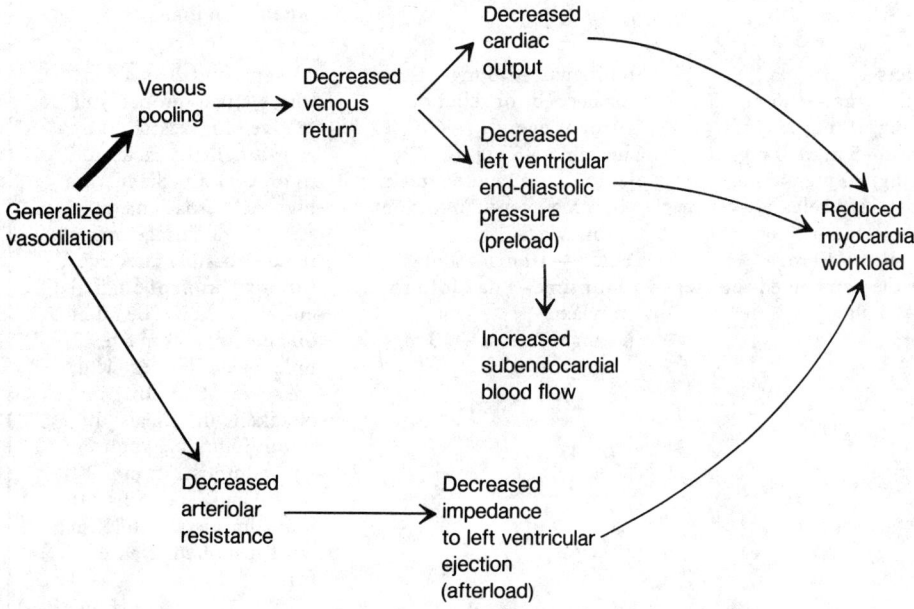

Figure 36-1. Mechanisms of action of nitrites/nitrates in treating angina.

Table 36-2
Nitrites and Nitrates

Drug	Preparations	Usual Dosage Range	Clinical Considerations
amyl nitrite	Inhalation ampules—0.18 ml, 0.3 ml	0.18 ml–0.3 ml inhaled as required (2–6 inhalations from crushed ampules; may repeat in 3 min–5 min if necessary)	Available as thin ampules in a woven fabric cover; ampule is wrapped in gauze or cloth, crushed between fingers, and contents inhaled; drug has a strong, fruity odor; volatile and highly flammable; tachycardia often occurs for a brief period following inhalation; has been employed to relieve renal and gallbladder colic, but infrequently used now due to odor, cost, and inconvenience; excessive doses may cause methemoglobinemia (see adverse reactions); drug is abused as a sexual stimulant.
erythrityl tetranitrate (Cardilate)	Tablets Oral—5 mg, 10 mg Chewable—10 mg Sublingual—5 mg, 10 mg	Sublingual—5 mg–10 mg three times/day or prior to stressful episodes Oral—10 mg–15 mg three times/day; additional dose at bedtime if nocturnal attacks are frequent	Comparable onset but longer duration (4 h) of action than nitroglycerin; primarily used for prophylaxis in patients with frequent, recurrent anginal pain and reduced exercise tolerance; vascular headaches are common early in therapy; less frequent with oral than sublingual administration; GI disturbances are noted with high oral doses.
isosorbide dinitrate (Isordil, Sorbitrate, and various other manufacturers)	Tablets Sublingual—2.5 mg, 5 mg, 10 mg Oral—5 mg, 10 mg, 20 mg, 30 mg, 40 mg Sustained-release—40 mg Chewable—5 mg, 10 mg Capsules—40 mg Capsules (sustained-release)—40 mg	Sublingual—2.5 mg–10 mg as needed for relief of pain or every 2 h–6 h Chewable—5 mg initially for relief of acute attack, or 5 mg every 2 h–3 h for prophylaxis Tablets—10 mg–20 mg four times a day for prophylaxis Sustained release—40 mg every 6 h–12 h	Sublingual and chewable forms rated "probably effective" for treatment of acute anginal attacks and to prevent attacks in high-risk situations (e.g., stress); oral dosage forms rated "possibly effective" for prevention of anginal episodes; should be taken on an empty stomach, unless vascular headaches are severe; then drug may be taken with meals; duration following sublingual administration is 1 h–2 h, and up to 6 h with oral administration (12 h with sustained-release forms)

(continued)

Table 36-2 (continued)
Nitrites and Nitrates

Drug	Preparations	Usual Dosage Range	Clinical Considerations
nitroglycerin, sublingual (Nitrostat and various other manufacturers)	Tablets—0.15 mg, 0.3 mg, 0.4 mg, 0.6 mg	0.3 mg–0.6 mg under the tongue or in the buccal pouch at first indication of acute anginal attack; repeat as needed up to three tablets	Very effective in relieving pain of acute anginal episodes and for preventing attacks when taken immediately prior to a stressful event; onset is almost immediate, and effects persist 10 min–15 min; keep bottles tightly capped, store in cool and dry place, and, if possible, only a week's supply of tablets should be carried at any one time; remainder should be kept in tightly closed amber stock bottle; discard unused tablets remaining in stock bottle 6 months after opening.
nitroglycerin, translingual (Nitrolingual)	Oral spray—0.4 mg per metered dose (200 doses/cannister)	One to two sprays onto oral mucosa; no more than three sprays within 15 min	Oral spray used for relief of an acute attack of angina or prophylactically 5 min–10 min before engaging in strenuous activities. If chest pain persists after three sprays, prompt medical attention is needed; spray should *not* be inhaled.
nitroglycerin, transmucosal (Nitrogard)	Controlled-release buccal tablets—1 mg, 2 mg, 3 mg	One tablet placed in buccal pouch every 3 h–5 h while awake	Tablets are placed between lip and gum above incisors or between cheek and gum and adhere to the mucosa; drug is slowly absorbed over several hours; used for chronic management of angina; caution must be exercised in drinking and eating; if tablet is accidentally swallowed, insert a new tablet as most of the drug that is swallowed is metabolized upon first pass through the liver
nitroglycerin injection (Nitrostat IV, Nitrol IV, Nitro-Bid IV, Tridil)	Injection—0.5 mg/ml, 0.8 mg/ml, 5 mg/ml, 10 mg/ml	Initially 5 mcg/min by IV infusion; increase gradually in 5-mcg/minute increments every 3 min–5 min up to 20 mcg/min; if no response, further increases should be made in increments of 10 mcg/	Used to reduce the incidence of myocardial ischemic injury resulting from an acute myocardial infarction; to control hypertension associated with certain surgical procedures; to provide "con-*(continued)*

Table 36-2 (continued)
Nitrites and Nitrates

Drug	Preparations	Usual Dosage Range	Clinical Considerations
nitroglycerin injection (Nitrostat IV, Nitrol IV, Nitro-Bid IV, Tridil) (continued)		min, then 20 mcg/min until an effect is noted	trolled hypotension" during surgery; and to treat acute angina pectoris in patients not responding to other means of therapy; dilute and store solutions only in glass containers because nitroglycerin can be absorbed by plastic; some preparations contain alcohol; use caution with intracoronary injections; to discontinue, gradually decrease dose 5 mcg/min every 5 min and monitor blood pressure; see Nursing Process for Patients Receiving Intravenous Nitroglycerin.
nitroglycerin topical ointment (Nitro-Bid, Nitrol, Nitrong, Nitrostat)	Ointment—2%	Initially, half-inch strip of ointment every 4 h–8 h; apply by spreading a thin, uniform layer on a 6-×-6-inch area of skin; do not rub in; increase by half-inch-increments with each succeeding dose until the optimal response is obtained; usual dose is 1–2 inches every 8 h although up to 4–5 inches every 4 h have been administered.	Effective prevention of anginal attacks, especially at night. Begin with half-inch of ointment/dose, and increase by half-inch every succeeding dose until vascular headache occurs, then decrease slightly; ointment is measured by squeezing a ribbon onto calibrated measuring tapes provided; rotate sites of application to minimize dermal inflammation and sensitization; area should be covered with plastic wrap to protect clothing; equally effective when applied to any skin area; gradually reduce dosage and frequency of application upon termination of drug, to prevent sudden withdrawal reaction; 1 inch of ointment contains approximately 15 mg nitroglycerin.
nitroglycerin sustained-release (Nitro-Bid, Nitrospan, Nitrostat SR, and various other manufacturers)	Sustained-release tablets—2.6 mg, 6.5 mg, 9.0 mg Sustained-release capsules—2.5 mg, 6.5 mg, 9.0 mg	Initially, 2.5 mg every 6 h–8 h; increase stepwise in 2.5-mg increments two to four times a day until side-effects limit the	Rated only "possibly effective" for prophylaxis of anginal attacks. Drug should be taken on an empty stomach, and tab- *(continued)*

Table 36-2 (continued)
Nitrites and Nitrates

Drug	Preparations	Usual Dosage Range	Clinical Considerations
nitroglycerin sustained-release (Nitro-Bid, Nitrospan, Nitrostat SR, and various other manufacturers) (continued)		dose. Doses as high as 27 mg have been given four times/day	lets or capsules should be swallowed whole; blood pressure should be monitored at initiation of therapy and with each dosage change.
Nitroglycerin transdermal systems (Deponit, Nitrocine, Nitro-disc, Nitro-Dur, NTS, Transderm-Nitro)	*Adhesive pads providing stated release rates* Deponit—5 mg/24 h, 10 mg/24 h Nitrocine—5 mg/24 h, 10 mg/24 h, 15 mg/24 h Nitrodisc—5 mg/24 h; 7.5 mg/24 h; 10 mg/24 h Nitro-Dur—2.5 mg/24 h; 5 mg/24 h; 7.5 mg/24 h; 10 mg/24 h; 15 mg/24 h NTS—5 mg/24 h, 15 mg/24 h Transderm-Nitro—2.5 mg/24 h; 5 mg/24 h; 10 mg/24 h; 15 mg/24 h	Apply one patch to a non-hairy skin area once every 24 h.	Transdermal patch system provides for continuous drug absorption over approximately 24 h although absorption rates and hence nitroglycerin plasma levels can vary significantly; dosage is stated in amount of drug absorbed over 24 h; total nitroglycerin content in patch is much larger than the quantity actually absorbed; patch must be in complete contact with skin to be effective; any tears or breaks in the patch system will change the rate of absorption; rotate application sites to minimize undue skin irritation; dosage is individualized and titrated to clinical response and tolerance of side-effects (e.g., headache, hypotension); terminate usage gradually over 4 weeks to 6 weeks to prevent sudden withdrawal reactions; not intended for treatment of acute anginal attacks.
pentaerythritol tetranitrate (Peritrate, and various other manufacturers)	Tablets—10 mg, 20 mg, 40 mg, 80 mg Sustained-release tablets—80 mg Sustained-release capsules—30 mg, 45 mg, 60 mg, 80 mg	Initially 10 mg–20 mg three to four times/day; increase gradually to a maximum 40 mg four times/day; maintenance 40 mg to 80 mg sustained-release forms once every 12 h	Rated "possibly effective" for prophylactic treatment of angina, observe for development of skin rash or persistent headaches and caution patient that prolonged use may reduce effectiveness of rapid-acting drugs; also available in combination with phenobarbital, although this is a poor combination and should not be used.

metabolism, although hepatic enzyme activity can be saturated by large oral doses of these drugs. Two dinitroglycerol metabolites have some vasodilator activity and longer plasma half-life than the parent compounds. Metabolites are excreted in the urine.

SIDE-EFFECTS/ADVERSE REACTIONS
Headache, flushing, dizziness, and palpitations are the most frequently encountered side-effects following administration of the nitrites/nitrates, and these reactions are especially common with larger doses. A burning sensation is commonly noted under the tongue with use of sublingual tablets. *Topical* application of nitroglycerin, especially in ointment form, has resulted in localized allergic reactions such as pruritus, contact dermatitis, eczematous eruptions, and erythematous or vesicular lesions.

Other adverse reactions associated with use of nitrites/nitrates include nausea, vomiting, incontinence, abdominal pain, restlessness, vertigo, weakness, confusion, tachycardia, orthostatic hypotension, fainting, muscle twitching, perspiration, pallor, cold sweat, exfoliative dermatitis (rare), and anaphylactoid reactions.

High doses of nitrites/nitrates may result in development of methemoglobinemia which, if severe, can lead to cyanosis, acidosis, convulsions, and cardiovascular collapse.

CONTRAINDICATIONS AND PRECAUTIONS
Nitrites/nitrates are contraindicated in patients with head trauma or cerebral hemorrhage because they can increase intracranial pressure. Other contraindications include severe anemia, marked hypotension, and the early postinfarction stage. In addition, IV nitroglycerin should not be given to persons with hypovolemia, inadequate cerebral circulation, constrictive pericarditis, and pericardial tamponade.

Nitrites and nitrates should be used cautiously in patients with hypotension, glaucoma, severe hepatic or renal disease, and in pregnant women or nursing mothers. Sustained-release preparations must be given with caution to persons with GI hypermotility or malabsorption syndrome because proper drug absorption may be impaired.

INTERACTIONS
1. The hypotensive effects of nitrites and nitrates may be enhanced by alcohol, beta-blockers, calcium-channel blockers, antihypertensives, narcotics, tricyclic antidepressants, and phenothiazines.
2. Nitrates can potentiate the effects of antihistamines and anticholinergic drugs.
3. Cross-tolerance can occur among all nitrites and nitrates.
4. Nitrites and nitrates can antagonize the pressor actions of sympathomimetic drugs.

■ Nursing Process for Patients Taking Nitrites/Nitrates

The following discussion focuses on the care a patient should receive when taking antianginal drugs by PO, SL, or topical route. Special considerations for IV nitroglycerin are discussed at the end of this section.

□ ASSESSMENT

□ Subjective Data
Before teaching a patient how to use any formulation of nitrite/nitrate the nurse needs some specific information. A history of the symptoms of angina is essential because many episodes are triggered by certain events such as mealtimes, confrontations at work, exercise, and, occasionally, sexual intercourse. By exploring the pattern of anginal pain the nurse and patient can better plan drug taking according to daily activities. The nurse must also discover the patient's perception of how the drug works and what he expects to accomplish. Sometimes, the cardiac patient has an unrealistic expectation about drug therapy, wrongly assuming medication will cure his symptoms. Such an attitude may influence his participation in care.

A drug history is essential because many patients take other cardiac drugs which may enhance the hypotension frequent with nitrites and nitrates. Use of alcohol and over-the-counter (OTC) drugs for colds or allergy should also be explored because many adverse interactions can occur with these compounds. The patient should be told to limit alcohol intake to an occasional drink and to contact the care giver before taking any new medication, including OTC drugs. A clear understanding must be established about the difference between administration of nitrites/nitrates and other cardiovascular medications, especially if the patient is taking sublingual tablets. Several patients have been treated for digitalis toxicity because they took digitalis at the onset of chest pain. Likewise, if the patient is switching from a sublingual to an oral form of the drug he should also be clear on the change in method to avoid problems of hypotension.

□ *Objective Data*

A complete physical assessment is essential for any patient being treated for angina. Cardiovascular assessment will be extensive, and baseline vital signs are essential. The rate, rhythm, and force of pulse should be taken, and discrepancy between apical and peripheral pulses should be noted. Blood pressure should be taken in the sitting position after the patient has been resting for 10 minutes to 15 minutes because this method will give the best indicator of venous return which is most affected by the drug.

Laboratory evaluation should include a complete blood count to test for anemia which may contraindicate drug use and renal and hepatic function studies because patients with significant changes in these organ systems need to be treated with caution.

□ *NURSING DIAGNOSES*

Actual nursing diagnoses for the patient on nitrites/nitrates include:

Knowledge deficit related to action, dose, time of drug taking, and side-effects of the drug

Alteration in cardiopulmonary tissue perfusion related to drug effect

Potential nursing diagnoses may include:

Alteration in comfort: headache related to vasodilation from the drug

Potential for injury: trauma, related to dizziness from hypotensive effects

Impaired tissue integrity related to skin irritation (topical formulation).

□ *PLAN*

Nursing care goals should focus on:

1. Teaching the patient correct drug-taking techniques depending on method of administration
2. Helping the patient develop a drug-taking pattern that relieves anginal pain
3. Teaching the patient common side-effects, how to manage them, and when to contact the care giver.

□ *INTERVENTION*

See Table 36-2 for administration guidelines.

Dose and appropriate drug taking vary. The nurse should be clear about the physician's prescription before initiating any teaching and should ensure the patient can manage the regimen as prescribed. Patients should be told never to chew sublingual or buccal tablets. A return demonstration of ointment application should be performed so the nurse and patient are assured that the patient can read the application paper, accurately measure out the prescribed dose, and correctly apply it. The nurse should also ensure the patient will be able to open and remove the small sublingual tablets from the bottle. Nitrites/nitrates can be difficult to hold in an arthritic hand. The medication should never be placed in a bottle with a childproof cap.

Initially, blood pressure and pulse must be closely monitored until a suitable dose range has been established. Vital signs should be taken before the drug is administered and then during the drug's expected peak (see Table 36-1). A drop in blood pressure of 10 mm Hg or a 10-beat increase in resting heart rate is considered clinically appropriate; beyond that the drug dose probably needs to be adjusted downward, and the physician should be notified.

Nitrites/nitrates given on a regular dosage schedule must be gradually withdrawn to prevent rebound ischemic pain. Patients must be taught not to discontinue the drug without supervision. However, in all cases, if a dose is missed there should be no attempt to "catch up" by taking an extra dose.

These drugs may be administered in combination with other vasodilators such as the beta-blocker, propranolol, to achieve an additive effect when angina is difficult to control. When the patient is using two drugs he should be taught a method of administration which will provide peak effects at the same time. For example, if pain occurs during exercise the patient might plan to begin his exercise about 1 hour to 1½ hours after taking the beta-blocker and then take the nitrate about 10 minutes to 15 minutes before commencing his walk.

When nitroglycerin is to be used during an angina attack a family or support person should know where the medication is and how to use it in case the patient needs assistance. Symptoms and time of drug taking during an attack should be noted. Such information can help the patient or family member remember the number of doses taken and will assist the physician in evaluating the course of pain development.

The nitrites/nitrates have few toxic effects, and most persistent side-effects can be managed by lowering the dose. The three main problems associated with the drug are dizziness, headache, and, in the case of the topical formulations, contact dermatitis.

Some patients report dizziness regardless of dose. To reduce dizziness the patient should sit for about 10 minutes after taking the medication. If dizziness occurs he should sit with his head between his knees or lie down and elevate his feet for 15 minutes to 20 minutes. Both methods will promote venous return. Resting will also decrease the workload of the heart.

Most headaches that result from nitrites/nitrates will subside within 15 minutes to 20 minutes. A mild analgesic may be taken if necessary. Headaches that persist should be reported to the physician because a reduction in drug dosage may be necessary.

Contact dermatitis from ointments or patches can be avoided if the patient and nurse learn to rotate administration sites with every dose. This may be a problem for the patient with heavy body hair; however, if several sites are shaved for drug use it will be less bothersome. The disadvantage of site rotation is that occasionally the old patch or cover is left in place when the new one is applied. To avoid this the teaching plan should include, as the first step, the removal of the old patch and cleansing of skin before applying the new one.

□ *EVALUATION*
Outcome criteria against which to measure success include control of pain, increased activity tolerance, and ability to manage the administration schedule with minimal headache or dizziness.

■ *Nursing Process for Patients Receiving Intravenous Nitroglycerin*

□ *ASSESSMENT*
Nitroglycerin is generally used in emergency situations where decisions must be rapidly made. A brief history of the illness and symptoms should be obtained as well as presence of renal or hepatic disease because patients with altered function may need a lower dose of the drug.

Physical assessment should include a complete physical focusing on cardiovascular status. Prior to initial infusion of nitroglycerin an arterial line should be inserted to provide continuous arterial blood pressure readings. A central venous line

should also be inserted and positioned so that pulmonary wedge pressure (PWP) can be monitored. Heart rate should be obtained, but the patient should be placed on a continuous ECG monitor.

□ *NURSING DIAGNOSES*
Actual nursing diagnoses may include:
    Knowledge deficit about the action of the
        drug and how it will affect him
    Anxiety about his condition
    Alteration in cardiac putput: decreased,
        related to drug effect
Potential nursing diagnoses may vary depending on the development of side-effects but can include:
    Alteration in comfort: headache, nausea
    Alteration in tissue perfusion of any major
        organ related to decrease in blood pressure
    Alteration in patterns of urinary elimination
        related to decreased renal perfusion

□ *PLAN*
Nursing care goals, aside from pain relief in severe angina, may include:
1. Maintaining blood pressure at goals set by physicians through drug infusion
2. Safe administration of infusion
3. Monitoring and responding to symptoms of side-effects

□ *INTERVENTION*
Intravenous nitroglycerin comes in a variety of preparations and is usually premixed by a pharmacist before being delivered to a critical care area for administration. Dosage is usually ordered in micrograms per milliliter (mcg/ml), and the nurse should be familiar with the dosage concentration. See Table 36-2 for a titration schedule for increasing and decreasing doses. Vital signs should be monitored every 1 minute to 2 minutes until the physician-ordered goals for blood pressure and heart rate are met. Titration of the drug is aimed at achieving the set goal without side-effects.

Nitroglycerin should be given by IV infusion, not by injection. The solution should be diluted in 5% dextrose and water or normal saline and set up as a secondary line (or piggyback) to a main IV site. Microdrip tubing or an infusion pump should be used; inline filters should be avoided. Most manufacturers warn against use of any but their own intravenous tubing because the drug is thought to absorb into most plastics. Usually the effects of this absorption are minimal if the drug is correctly titrated.

The major side-effects of intravenous nitroglycerin are sudden fall in blood pressure, chest pain, shortness of breath, and decreased urine output, all of which must be reported immediately. Usually the infusion rate must be slowed to alleviate symptoms. Nausea and vomiting may occur, and suction equipment should be available to prevent aspiration if the patient is not alert. The patient receiving intravenous nitroglycerin must be closely monitored throughout drug administration and, if possible, should not be left alone.

□ *EVALUATION*
Outcome criteria indicative of drug success include relief of pain, lowered blood pressure, and absence of side-effects. Nursing Care Plan 36-1 summarizes the nursing process for the patient receiving intravenous nitroglycerin.

Beta-Adrenergic Blockers

The beta-adrenergic blocking agents approved for use in the treatment of angina include atenolol, propranolol, and nadolol. They are particularly suited for patients who experience frequent or severe acute attacks at rest because they can markedly reduce the myocardial oxygen demand. The principal hemodynamic actions of the beta-blockers responsible for this effect include a decreased heart rate, blood pressure, and myocardial contractility, all of which reduce cardiac workload. Decreased heart rate may also result in lengthened diastolic perfusion time, leading to increased coronary blood flow. Although beta-blockers may cause a slight increase in the end-diastolic pressure due to the slowed heart rate, this potentially undesirable action can readily be offset by concurrent use of one of the nitrates. Conversely, the reflex tachycardia frequently seen with nitrates is attenuated by beta-blockers. Therefore, combined nitrate–beta-blocker therapy is frequently more advantageous than use of either drug alone.

The beta-blockers are discussed in detail in Chapter 16, and only those aspects of the use of propranolol, nadolol, and atenolol in angina will be considered here.

Propranolol
(Inderal)

Propranolol is a nonselective beta-blocker used for the management of moderate to severe angina (*i.e.,*
frequent or intense acute attacks, occurring both during exertion and at rest). The drug is administered orally, usually in combination with sublingual nitrates as needed. Initial dose is 10 mg to 20 mg three to four times/day; dosage may be increased gradually to optimal levels, which are usually in the range of 80 mg to 160 mg a day. Sustained-release capsules (60 mg, 80 mg, 120 mg, 160 mg) may be given once daily when patients have been stabilized on the drug. However, sustained-release preparations are *not* recommended for *initial* treatment.

Patients receiving propranolol for angina should be reevaluated periodically as to the necessity for dosage adjustment as their condition changes. Refer to Chapter 16 for side-effects, adverse reactions, contraindications, and precautions associated with beta-blockers. When therapy is to be discontinued, dosage should be tapered gradually rather than the drug stopped abruptly; sudden cessation of therapy has resulted in marked worsening of angina and occasionally precipitation of a myocardial infarction. Continuation of therapy in the absence of decreased pain and improved work capacity is not recommended.

Nadolol
(Corgard)

The actions of nadolol are virtually identical to those of propranolol in reducing myocardial oxygen consumption. The drug possesses a rather long half-life and is used on a once-a-day dosing schedule. Initial dosage is 40 mg, which may be increased by 40-mg to 80-mg increments every 3 to 7 days until an optimal clinical response is attained. The usual maintenance dose of nadolol in angina ranges from 80 mg to 240 mg a day. The drug is reviewed in detail in Chapter 16.

Atenolol
(Tenormin)

Atenolol is a long-acting cardioselective beta-blocker with actions in angina similar to those of propranolol. The dose is usually 50 mg once daily. Atenolol is excreted unchanged by the kidney and may be preferred in patients with liver dysfunction. Conversely, caution is necessary when the drug is given to persons with renal impairment. The drug is considered in detail in Chapter 16.

(*Text continues on p. 728.*)

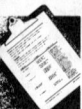

Nursing Care Plan 36-1
The Patient Receiving Intravenous Nitroglycerin

Assessment

Subjective Data

1. Medication history
   a. Refer to Interactions section to formulate pertinent questions.
   b. Identify drugs the patient is receiving that will require an alteration in nitroglycerin dosage or that will be potentiated by nitroglycerin.
   c. Identify physical incompatibilities. IV nitroglycerin cannot be combined with other drugs.
   d. Allergies/hypersensitivity to nitrates

2. Medical history
   a. Presence of conditions that contraindicate use, including head trauma, cerebral hemorrhage, severe anemia, severe hypotension, early post acute MI, inadequate cerebral circulation, constrictive pericarditis, pericardial tamponade
   b. Pre-existing conditions that may warrant dosage adjustment or more frequent monitoring: hypotension, glaucoma, severe renal or hepatic disease, any circulatory insufficiency that would increase with drug-induced hypotension, pregnancy, or lactation

3. Determine patient's understanding of condition, symptoms, and outcome.

Objective Data

1. Physical assessment: complete, but highlighting
   a. Cardiovascular status: arterial blood pressure (direct or indirect), pulmonary artery wedge pressure (PAWP), heart rate, peripheral pulses, presence of edema, presence of rales, urinary output, weight
   b. Cerebrovascular status: mental acuity, ability to communicate

2. Laboratory/diagnostic data
   a. ECG: continuous monitoring
   b. Renal and hepatic function studies
   c. Cardiac enzymes (LDH, fractionated CPK)
   d. Serum electrolytes

Nursing Diagnosis	Expected Client Outcome	Intervention
Alteration in cardiac output: decreased related to drug effect	Arterial blood pressure (ABP) and PAWP will remain within the target goals set in the physician's order	Initiate drug administration in micrograms per minute as prescribed in accordance with manufacturer's instructions. Usual order is to start with 5 mcg/min, then increase dose in 5 mcg/min increments every 3–5 minutes until pressure goals are reached or adverse reaction is noted.
		Use 5% Dextrose in water in highly concentrated solution to reduce sodium and water intake.
		Use glass solution bottle and manufacturer's tubing to reduce drug absorption into plastic.
		Monitor ABP and PAWP every 1–2 minutes during drug titration.
		Monitor drug effectiveness including: ABP and PAWP within normal limits; symptoms of CHF resolve (low rates, low PAWP, low periph-

(continued)

726

Nursing Diagnosis	Expected Client Outcome	Intervention
Alteration in cardiac output: decreased related to drug effect (*continued*)		eral edema, high urinary output, low hepatomegaly).
		When desired pressures are reached or symptoms subside, maintain current dosage/infusion rate.
		Be prepared to manage drug side-effects as necessary.
Alteration in comfort: anginal pain, nausea, vomiting, headache	Pain, gastrointestinal symptoms will be relieved	Question patient about pain relief as drug takes effect. Notify physician if pain is unremitting.
		Provide mild analgesics for headache. Decrease environmental stimuli as much as possible.
		Be prepared to prevent aspiration through suctioning if patient is not alert and vomiting occurs. Anti-emetics may be prescribed.
Potential alteration in tissue perfusion related to decreased arterial pressure	Arterial BP remains within normal limits	Monitor patient closely for low BP, angina, confusion, dysrhythmias—all signs of alteration in tissue perfusion.
		Reduce infusion rate as ordered; pressure should rise within 3–5 minutes, the duration of drug action.
		Have methoxamine or phenylephrine on hand to increase BP if necessary.
Knowledge deficit related to drug action, the need for intensive monitoring	Will verbalize understanding of how drug works and why monitoring is essential	Explain how drug will enhance heart function and decrease pain.
		Explain how monitoring devices help determine dose and prevent side-effects.
		Tell patient what symptoms to report.
Anxiety related to condition which patient may perceive as life-threatening	Will verbalize fears and reduce anxiety	Give explanations of each action taken.
		Encourage verbalization about condition, feeling, fears, stressors.
		Encourage questions, including those of family.
		Encourage and assist patient to perform relaxation techniques that will enhance drug effect.
Potential for injury related to dizziness	Will use safety precautions	Keep side rails up to prevent falls
		Monitor BP closely; dizziness is usually related to fall in BP.
		Tell patient to remain in bed. Assist any patient who must get out of bed.

Calcium-Channel Blockers

Diltiazem, Nifedipine, Verapamil

Most types of smooth muscle and cardiac muscle cells are dependent on transmembrane calcium influx for maintenance of normal resting tone and for activation. This influx occurs subsequent to the rapid influx of sodium noted during the initial depolarization phase and proceeds at a much slower rate by way of membrane channels which are relatively selective for calcium. These so-called slow membrane channels are blocked by a group of drugs known as calcium-channel blockers. The entry of extracellular calcium into smooth muscle cells and myocardial cells is inhibited by these agents, resulting in vasodilation, bradycardia, decreased force of contraction, and reduced AV nodal conduction.

These actions of calcium-channel blocking drugs form the basis for their use in angina and for treating certain types of cardiac arrhythmias. Although all of the currently available calcium-channel blockers can interfere with movement of calcium ions across membranes, considerable differences exist among the drugs with regard to their pharmacokinetic and pharmacologic properties. These differential hemodynamic actions appear to be due in part to differences in binding affinity at sites along the calcium channel as well as to differences in their effects on vascular smooth muscle vs

cardiac muscle. A comparison of the major properties of the available calcium-channel blockers is presented in Table 36-3.

All of the drugs produce marked vasodilation of the coronary vasculature, but there is significant variation in their ability to dilate peripheral vessels, nifedipine causing the greatest degree of peripheral vasodilation; verapamil and diltiazem are somewhat less active. Heart rate is slowed by diltiazem, and possibly by verapamil, although this slowing with verapamil is offset to some extent by reflex sympathetic stimulation. Conversely, a reflex tachycardia is usually noted with nifedipine. SA and AV nodal tissue is markedly affected by verapamil, and the drug decreases SA nodal automaticity, AV conduction, and myocardial contractility. AV conduction and SA nodal activity are depressed to a lesser extent by diltiazem and are relatively unaffected by nifedipine. Because nifedipine is a more potent arteriodilator than diltiazem or verapamil, blood pressure is decreased to a greater extent with nifedipine than with the other calcium-channel blockers. However, as noted, reflex tachycardia occurs more frequently with nifedipine than with the other drugs.

MECHANISM AND ACTIONS
Calcium-channel blockers inhibit the influx of extracellular calcium ions into cardiac muscle and smooth muscle cells through specific "slow calcium channels." Antianginal effects include dilation of coronary arteries and arterioles and preven-

Table 36-3
Pharmacokinetic and Pharmacologic Properties of Calcium-Channel Blockers

	Diltiazem	Nifedipine	Verapamil
Pharmacokinetics			
Onset of action (min)	15–30	20	30 (2–5 IV)
Peak effect (h)	0.5–1	1–2	2–4 (0.2 IV)
Half-life (h)	3–6	2–4	4–8
Protein binding (%)	70–80	90–98	85–90
Pharmacologic Effects			
Coronary vasodilation	↑↑↑	↑↑↑	↑↑↑
Peripheral vasodilation	↑	↑↑↑	↑↑
rrPreload	0	0	0
Afterload	↓	↓↓↓	↓↓
Heart rate	0 (↓)	↑ (reflex)	↑ or ↓
Contractility	↓	0 (↓)	↓↓
AV nodal conduction	↓↓	0 (↓)	↓↓↓
SA nodal automaticity	↓	0	↓↓

↑↑↑ or ↓↓↓ = marked effect; ↑↑ or ↓↓ = moderate effect; ↑ or ↓ = minimal effect; 0 (↓) or 0 (↑) = variable effect; 0 = no effect

tion of coronary artery spasm. Dilation of peripheral arterioles also occurs to varying degrees, reducing total resistance against which the heart must work; thus, there is a corresponding reduction in myocardial energy consumption and oxygen demand. Verapamil and, to a lesser extent, diltiazem markedly decrease calcium influx into cardiac contractile and conductile cells of the SA node and AV node. This latter action slows AV conduction, prolongs effective AV refractory period, and interrupts reentry of impulses at the AV node, thus restoring normal sinus rhythm. Verapamil may also exert some blocking action at alpha-adrenergic receptor sites.

Because arteriolar smooth muscle appears to be more sensitive than venular smooth muscle, orthostatic hypotension is relatively rare, although blood pressure is usually reduced. Verapamil may be employed in the treatment of mild to moderate hypertension. Cardiac contractility and cardiac output are reduced in a dose-dependent fashion, and these effects are most prominent with verapamil. Contraction of skeletal muscle is not significantly affected by calcium-channel blockers, because the source of utilizable calcium for skeletal muscle contraction is predominately *intra*cellular. Non-vascular smooth muscle (*i.e.*, bronchiolar, gastrointestinal, uterine) is also relaxed by calcium-channel blockers, and these drugs are being investigated for potential application in treating asthma, dysmenorrhea, and premature labor among other conditions.

USES

1. Management of all forms of angina (chronic stable, unstable, or vasospastic). The relative efficacy of calcium-channel blockers vs nitrates or beta-blockers on chronic, stable angina remains to be established; the combination of a calcium-channel blocker with a beta-blocker appears to be more effective than either drug alone.
2. Treatment of supraventricular tachyarrhythmias and control of rapid ventricular rate in atrial flutter or atrial fibrillation (IV verapamil —see Chap. 34)
3. Control of mild to moderate hypertension (verapamil)
4. Investigational uses include treatment of bronchial asthma, migraine prophylaxis, and Raynaud's phenomenon.

ADMINISTRATION AND DOSAGE
See Table 36-4.

FATE
See Table 36-3.

All drugs are well absorbed orally, but diltiazem and verapamil undergo extensive first-pass hepatic metabolism; onset of action is within 30 minutes, and effects persist for 4 hours to 6 hours. All drugs are significantly protein-bound. Hepatic metabolism is extensive, and excretion of metabolites proceeds largely by way of the kidney, except for diltiazem, which is eliminated primarily in the feces.

SIDE-EFFECTS/ADVERSE REACTIONS
In general, side-effects are noted most frequently with nifedipine but are usually not serious and rarely require discontinuation of therapy. Those side-effects noted most often are nausea, dizziness, flushing, hypotension, lightheadedness, peripheral edema, headache, and weakness. Constipation also occurs frequently with verapamil.

Many other adverse reactions have been reported with use of calcium-channel blockers; however, the incidence of most of the following effects is relatively rare:

Cardiovascular—Palpitations, bradycardia, myocardial infarction, heart failure (see below); in addition, third-degree AV block has occurred with verapamil.
Respiratory—Dyspnea, cough, wheezing, chest congestion, pulmonary edema
GI—Heartburn, diarrhea, cramping, flatulence, sore throat
CNS—Fatigue, tremor, nervousness, confusion, mood changes, blurred vision, insomnia
Musculoskeletal—Muscle cramping, joint stiffness, inflammation
Other—Hair loss, menstrual irregularities, claudication, dermatitis, urticaria, fever, sweating, chills, impotence

Verapamil is the most likely of the group to result in depressed cardiac functioning, because it markedly slows AV conduction and reduces myocardial contractility. Symptoms of congestive heart failure have developed during verapamil therapy and varying degrees of AV block have been reported. Concurrent use of beta-blockers can worsen the cardiac depressant actions of verapamil.

CONTRAINDICATIONS AND PRECAUTIONS
Verapamil and diltiazem are contraindicated in the presence of severe left-ventricular dysfunction, sick sinus syndrome, second- or third-degree heart block, and systolic pressure less than 90 mm Hg. In

Table 36-4
Calcium-Channel Blockers

Drug	Preparations	Usual Dosage Range	Clinical Considerations
diltiazem (Cardizem)	Tablets—30 mg, 60 mg, 90 mg, 120 mg	Initially 30 mg four times/day; increase gradually at 1- to 2-day intervals to achieve optimal response; maximum dose is 360 mg/day in divided doses	Potent coronary vasodilator with little or no negative inotropic effect; weak peripheral vasodilation results in a modest fall in blood pressure; heart rate is slightly reduced; slows AV conduction and may have additive bradycardiac effects with beta-blockers or digitalis; incidence of adverse reactions is very low; nausea, headache, and peripheral edema are occasionally reported; hyperbilirubinemia and elevated serum transaminases have occurred but are reversible upon cessation of therapy; not recommended for use in children
nifedipine (Adalat, Procardia)	Capsules—10 mg, 20 mg	Initially 10 mg three times/day; increase slowly until optimal effect is noted; usual dosage range is 10 mg–20 mg three times/day; maximum recommended dose is 180 mg/day	Orally effective calcium-channel blocker used in chronic, stable angina as well as vasospastic angina; does not alter conduction system of the heart as does verapamil and is of no use in arrhythmias; elicits a marked reduction in peripheral arteriolar resistance coupled with minimal increase in heart rate; discontinue drug gradually if necessary
verapamil (Calan, Isoptin)	Tablets—40 mg, 80 mg, 120 mg; Sustained-release tablets—240 mg; Injection—5 mg/2 ml	*Oral* Angina—Initially 80 mg–120 mg three to four times/day; increase at daily or weekly intervals until optimal effect is attained; usual dosage range is 320 mg–480 mg daily. Hypertension—240-mg sustained-release tablet once daily; may give up to 240 mg twice a day if necessary. *IV* Supraventricular arrhythmias (see Chap. 34)	Orally effective calcium-channel blocker used in angina, and for relief of mild to moderate hypertension; also administered IV for treatment of supraventricular tachyarrhythmias (see Chap. 34); significantly reduces SA nodal automaticity and AV conduction and decreases force of contraction; high oral doses are necessary due to extensive first-pass metabolism; use with caution in patients with left-ventricular dysfunction.

addition, verapamil should not be given to patients in cardiogenic shock or with severe congestive heart failure. IV verapamil should not be given together with IV beta-blockers, because both may depress myocardial contractility and slow AV conduction. Nifedipine has no absolute contraindications, although it probably should not be given in the presence of severe hypotension.

The calcium-channel blockers must be given with *caution* to patients with pulmonary edema, reduced left ventricular function (except nifedipine), impaired renal and hepatic function, mild to moderate hypotension, sinus bradycardia, and to pregnant women and nursing mothers.

INTERACTIONS

1. Calcium-channel blockers and beta-blockers together may be beneficial in some patients with chronic, stable angina, but can also increase the likelihood of congestive heart failure or severe hypotension and may worsen existing angina, especially when given IV in patients with left ventricular dysfunction or conduction defects.
2. Verapamil and nifedipine can elevate serum levels of digoxin and digitoxin if used concurrently, possibly leading to digitalis toxicity.
3. Calcium-channel blockers may have an additive antihypertensive effect if administered together with other antihypertensive drugs.
4. Actions of calcium-channel blockers may be enhanced by concomitant use of other highly protein-bound drugs (*e.g.*, anticoagulants, anti-inflammatory agents, sulfonamides, barbiturates).
5. The effectiveness of verapamil may be reduced by combined use with calcium and vitamin D.
6. Nifedipine may decrease serum quinidine levels in patients with diminished left ventricular function.
7. Cimetidine may increase the effects of calcium channel blockers, perhaps due to reduced first-pass hepatic metabolism.

■ Nursing Process

□ ASSESSMENT

□ Subjective Data
A complete medical history and specific information about the development of cardiovascular symptoms are essential. A drug history should also be obtained because these drugs interact with many other cardiovascular drugs.

□ Objective Data
Physical assessment should be complete with special attention to pulse, blood pressure, weight, and palpation of extremities for signs of edema. Diagnostic tests should include an ECG and renal and hepatic function blood studies.

□ NURSING DIAGNOSES
Actual nursing diagnoses for calcium-channel blockers may include:

Anxiety related to failure of other therapies and fear this one will fail too
Knowledge deficit related to the action, dose, and side-effects of the drug

Potential nursing diagnoses are usually related to side-effects and may include:

Alteration in bowel elimination: constipation
Alteration in cardiac output: decreased related to hypotension
Alteration in comfort: increased anginal pain
Alteration in fluid volume: excess related to the development of congestive heart failure

□ PLAN
Nursing care goals should focus on (1) relieving ischemic pain, (2) management of side-effects during initial therapy, (3) helping the patient learn correct drug taking for home management, and (4) teaching the patient how to monitor for side-effects.

□ INTERVENTION
Dosage will be adjusted to achieve maximum relief with minimal side-effects. See Table 36-4 for a range in schedules for different drugs.

The major side-effects of calcium-channel blockers are hypotension, increased anginal pain during initial therapy, development of congestive heart failure, and constipation. Hypotension and increased anginal pain are most likely to occur when the drug reaches its peak level (see Table 36-3). Consequently blood pressure and cardiac monitoring should be performed most frequently early after the drug is administered. For example, vital signs and patient monitoring should be most frequent in the first half hour after the initial dose of diltiazem but should be spaced over a 4-hour period with verapamil. If blood pressure falls more than 10 mm Hg, the physician should be notified because a dose change may be in order. Cardiac changes are also likely in this period, especially with verapamil. The patient should be attached to a cardiac monitor, and periodic strips should be reviewed for changes in the PR interval and arrhythmia development.

Congestive heart failure occurs more slowly. Consequently, the patient should be taught to watch for weight increase, edema of hands and feet, dyspnea or difficulty sleeping flat, irregular heart beat, and to report these changes immediately.

The patient should be told to note any change in the frequency or intensity of anginal pain. While duration and precipitating events should be recorded, the physician should be notified because such symptoms must be monitored.

Dizziness may also be a transient side-effect of the calcium-channel blockers. The patient should exercise caution in driving or using machinery early in therapy until his response to the drug is known. If dizziness occurs the patient should sit or lie down for about 15 minutes or until the feeling passes, then rise slowly. Persistence of the symptom should be reported.

Constipation may occur with long-term use. The patient can be encouraged to increase fluid intake and eat a diet high in fiber. Stool softeners or bulk laxatives can be used if necessary.

These drugs (except nifedipine) can result in rebound ischemia if abruptly withdrawn. Intravenous forms should be gradually titrated and oral forms gradually discontinued if necessary. The patient must understand the need for gradual withdrawal and notify the physician if he must discontinue the drug or stops taking the drug because of nausea and vomiting.

□ EVALUATION
The outcome criteria against which to measure the drug's effectiveness include control of anginal pain, improved activity tolerance, and management of side-effects.

Dipyridamole
(Persantine, Pyridamole)

MECHANISM AND ACTIONS
Dipyridamole is an orally effective coronary vasodilator. It acts predominately on the small resistance vessels of the coronary bed to increase coronary blood flow. Dipyridamole inhibits the activity on adenosine deaminase, thereby increasing functional levels of adenosine and other vasodilatory nucleotides. It also appears to block the action of phosphodiesterase, resulting in elevated levels of cyclic AMP, another coronary vasodilator. Increased cyclic AMP also reduces platelet aggregation. Synthesis of prostacyclin is increased by dipyridamole, resulting in further vasodilation and impaired platelet aggregation. Blood pressure is relatively unchanged, and systemic blood flow is largely unaffected. A mild positive inotropic action has also been reported.

Dipyridamole either alone or in combination with aspirin has been used to prevent transient ischemic attacks and protect against further thromboembolic complications following stroke. The efficacy of this application remains to be definitely established, although data appear to indicate that such therapy may be beneficial in certain patients.

USES
1. Adjunct to coumarin anticoagulants (see Chap. 39) in preventing postoperative thromboembolic complications of cardiac valve replacement.
2. Investigational uses include prevention of thrombotic complications associated with cerebrovascular or ischemic heart diseases, prevention of myocardial reinfarction and mortality following infarction, and prevention of coronary bypass graft occlusion.

ADMINISTRATION AND DOSAGE
Dipyridamole is administered orally as tablets (25 mg, 50 mg, 75 mg). The average dose is 75 mg four times a day, as an adjunct to the usual coumarin anticoagulant dose.

FATE
Oral absorption is good, although bioavailability is variable (25%–75%). Peak plasma concentrations occur within 2 hours to 3 hours, although, as noted above, therapeutic effects may not be evident for weeks to months. Protein binding is extensive (90%–97%). The drug is metabolized in the liver and excreted in the feces by enterohepatic recirculation.

SIDE-EFFECTS/ADVERSE REACTIONS
Dipyridamole is very well tolerated by the majority of patients, and side effects are rare. GI distress, headache, flushing, weakness, nausea, dizziness, and skin rash have occurred but seldom require discontinuation of therapy.

CONTRAINDICATIONS AND PRECAUTIONS
There are no absolute contraindications to dipyridamole. The drug should be used cautiously in patients with hypotension.

INTERACTIONS
1. Dipyridamole can enhance the effects of oral anticoagulants and heparin.

Peripheral Vasodilators

Peripheral vasodilator drugs have been employed in an attempt to improve blood flow to areas that have been deprived of sufficient perfusion because of vascular obstruction (*i.e.*, thromboembolism, atherosclerosis) or arterial vasospasm.

Vasodilator drugs may increase blood flow through circulatory vessels by either a direct action (smooth muscle relaxing) or an indirect action (interference with sympathetic nerve supply). Although these agents may improve blood flow to limbs and body organs in the *normal* person, their efficacy in relieving the ischemia of peripheral vascular disease is severely limited. It is unlikely that any peripheral vasodilator can markedly increase blood flow distal to an occlusion. Moreover, regulatory mechanisms on cerebral and skeletal vascular beds elicit compensatory vasodilation in response to ischemia; thus vasodilator drugs probably increase blood flow primarily to *nonischemic* areas. Therefore, minimal therapeutic benefit should be expected from the treatment of peripheral vascular diseases with the currently available peripheral vasodilators. Despite this fact, peripheral vasodilators continue to be frequently prescribed for symptomatic treatment of chronic occlusive vascular disease, at a significant cost to the public. Their use in treating cerebrovascular insufficiency in the elderly patient is particularly hazardous, inasmuch as these drugs can elicit a significant degree of hypotension, which can actually result in *reduced* cerebral perfusion, negating any potential benefit derived from dilation of cerebral vessels. Peripheral circulation should be closely monitored when any of these drugs is used. In addition, reflex tachycardia can occur with use of these peripheral vasodilators, which may prove dangerous in the patient with cardiac disease. Lastly, increased intraocular pressure may occur. Patients taking the drug should be warned to immediately report any vision change or eye pain.

Cyclandelate

(Cyclan, Cyclospasmol)

Cyclandelate is a direct-acting vascular smooth muscle relaxant that exhibits no significant sympathomimetic or adrenergic blocking action. It is rated only "possibly effective" for treatment of ischemic peripheral and cerebrovascular disease (*e.g.*, intermittent claudication, arteriosclerosis obliterans, Raynaud's phenomenon, thrombophlebitis, nocturnal leg cramps). Cyclandelate is available as tablets (100 mg, 200 mg) and capsules (200 mg, 400 mg). Initial dosage is 400 mg three to four times a day, which is gradually reduced to the usual maintenance dosage of 400 mg/day to 800 mg/day in two to four divided doses. Side-effects include flushing, headache, weakness, sweating, dizziness, tachycardia, and GI distress. Most of these are transient; GI distress can be minimized by taking the drug with meals. The drug must be used cautiously in patients with glaucoma, severe coronary artery or cerebral vascular disease, and bleeding tendencies (prolonged bleeding time has been noted at high doses). Clinical benefit, if any, is slow to develop.

Isoxsuprine

(Vasodilan, Voxsuprine)

Isoxsuprine is a peripheral vasodilator that can increase resting blood flow in skeletal muscle. The drug possesses several actions, namely a beta-adrenergic agonistic, alpha-adrenergic antagonistic, and direct vascular smooth muscle relaxant effect. Because its vasodilatory actions are *not* blocked by beta-blocking agents, it is doubtful whether its beta-agonistic properties contribute to its vasodilatory action. Isoxsuprine can also increase heart rate, myocardial contractility, and cardiac output, and can relax uterine smooth muscle, probably due to a beta-activating action. High doses may inhibit platelet aggregation. It is rated only "possibly effective" for the relief of symptoms associated with cerebral and peripheral vascular insufficiency. In addition, isoxsuprine has been employed IM to inhibit premature labor and to prevent threatened abortion, although these latter indications are considered experimental and more selective agents, such as ritodrine (see Chap. 15) are preferred. Oral dosage is 10 mg to 20 mg three to four times a day. When given IM, 5 mg to 10 mg may be administered two to three times a day. The drug should not be given IV because the likelihood of side-effects is greatly increased. Flushing, palpitations, nausea, dizziness, skin rash, tachycardia, abdominal distress, hypotension, and nervousness have been reported with the use of isoxsuprine. (A further discussion of isoxsuprine is found in Chap. 15.)

Nylidrin

(Adrin, Arlidin)

The vasodilatory action of nylidrin appears to be the result of both a beta-adrenergic agonistic action and a direct relaxant effect on vascular smooth muscle. Heart rate and cardiac output are increased, and blood pressure may be lowered. Nylidrin is rated "possibly effective" in treating peripheral vascular diseases, such as arteriosclerosis obliterans, diabetic vascular disease, Raynaud's disease, or acroparesthesia. It has also been used in treating circulatory disturbances of the inner ear, such as cochlear cell, macular or ampullar ischemia, or labyrinthine artery spasm. Oral dosage is 3 mg to 12 mg three to four times a day. Side-effects include nausea, nervousness, weakness, dizziness, tremor, palpitations, and postural hypotension. Nylidrin is contraindicated in myocardial infarction, paroxysmal tachycardia, progressive angina pectoris, and thyrotoxicosis. (Additional information on nylidrin is presented in Chap. 15.)

Papaverine

(Cerespan, Pavabid, Paverolan, and others)

Ethaverine

(Ethaquin, Ethatab, Ethavex-100)

Papaverine and its closely related analogue ethaverine exert a direct, nonspecific relaxant effect on smooth muscle. Vasodilatory effects are noted on the coronary, cerebral, pulmonary, and systemic blood vessels. The drugs may elevate the levels of cyclic AMP in vascular smooth muscle. Cerebral blood flow may be increased due to decreased cerebral vascular resistance; however, blood pressure may decline, offsetting the beneficial effect of reduced cerebral vascular resistance. Papaverine and ethaverine have been used orally for relieving cerebral, myocardial, and peripheral ischemia resulting from vascular spasm, although their clinical effectiveness has not been conclusively demonstrated. They have also been employed as smooth muscle spasmolytics for treatment of various spastic states of GI, urinary, ureteral, or biliary smooth muscles.

Papaverine is available as tablets (30 mg, 60 mg, 100 mg, 200 mg, 300 mg), sustained-release capsules (150 mg, 300 mg), and injection solution (30 mg/ml). Oral dosage is 100 mg to 300 mg three to five times a day or 150 mg sustained-release preparation every 12 hours. IV or IM dosage ranges from 30 mg to 120 mg every 3 hours. For immediate effect, the IV route is recommended, and administration may be by *slow* injection or intermittent infusion. Absorption from sustained-release preparations is highly variable, and plasma levels may be very low following this mode of administration.

Ethaverine is used as tablets (100 mg) or capsules (100 mg). Recommended dosage is 100 mg to 200 mg three times a day.

Side-effects associated with these drugs include nausea, abdominal distress, flushing, sweating, headache, fatigue, skin rash, diarrhea, dizziness, tachycardia, and anorexia. Hepatic hypersensitivity can also occur and may be manifested as eosinophilia, jaundice, and elevated serum transaminases and alkaline phosphatase. IV administration of papaverine can lead to increased blood pressure, respiratory rate and heart rate, and profound sedation. Large doses of these agents can suppress AV nodal conduction and may lead to arrhythmias. The drugs are contraindicated in severe liver disease, complete AV block, and serious arrhythmias, and must be used with caution in patients with glaucoma (increases intraocular pressure), myocardial depression, or impaired liver function.

Nursing care should focus on monitoring for arrhythmias. Atropine should be kept on hand for bradycardia as well as antiarrhythmias useful in treatment of symptoms of AV block.

Intraocular pressure may increase during drug use. The patient should be told to immediately report any change in vision, eye pain, or scleral redness.

Ergoloid Mesylates

(Deapril-ST, Gerimal, Hydergine, Hydroloid-G, Niloric)

Ergoloid mesylates contains equal parts of three dihydrogenated ergotoxine alkaloids, namely dihydroergocornine, dihydroergocristine, and dihydroergocryptine. The compound is used to provide symptomatic relief of those signs and symptoms associated with a decline in mental acuity and capacity in the elderly, such as confusion and forgetfulness and lessened self-care, sociability, and appetite. A degree of improvement in the above parameters is observed within 8 weeks to 12 weeks and may be the result of improved cerebral circulation. Although the precise mechanism by which ergoloid mesylates is able to improve mentation is not known, it is believed the drug can increase brain metabolic activity, thereby improving cerebral blood flow. Vasodilation of cerebral vessels may also play a role, albeit minor, in the action of the drug. Blood pressure may decline, reducing cerebral perfusion, and orthostatic effects have been noted.

Ergoloid mesylates is available as oral tablets (1 mg), sublingual tablets (0.5 mg, 1 mg), liquid capsules (1 mg), and liquid (1 mg/ml). The drug is erratically absorbed orally and undergoes extensive first-pass hepatic metabolism. Thus, the preferred route of administration is sublingual, although this may be difficult in elderly or senile patients. Rec-

ommended starting dosage is 1 mg three times a day. Onset of clinical response is gradual, and results may not be evident for 3 weeks to 4 weeks. Doses up to 12 mg/day have been used for extended periods of time.

Side-effects are generally mild and include GI upset, nausea, sublingual irritation, lightheadedness, nasal stuffiness, blurred vision, skin rash, and orthostatic hypotension. Ergoloid mesylates should not be used in persons with acute or chronic psychosis, or in persons with a history of acute intermittent porphyria. In view of the cost of ergoloid mesylates therapy, it is imperative that clinical benefit be evident to justify continuing therapy, and such benefit may require up to 6 months to adequately assess.

CASE STUDY

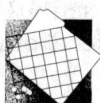

Howard Bennett, age 62, suffered his first myocardial infarction at age 58. He began to have anginal pain soon after he recovered. The pain occurred primarily on exertion (a long walk) but occasionally happened after meals. Initially, the pain was controlled by sublingual nitroglycerin (Nitrostat) 0.3 mg at onset of pain. Later, when higher doses of Nitrostat failed to provide relief, Mr. Bennett was started on propranalol, and the dose was gradually increased to 20 mg qid. He continued to take Nitrostat before meals, exercise, or stressful situations.

Mr. Bennett is brought to the Emergency Room today by his wife. He is complaining of severe chest pain, is short of breath, and is diaphoretic. His wife tells the nurse her husband was sitting reading the morning paper when the pain struck. He took three nitroglycerin tablets with no relief, he has had one dose of propranalol today.

An ECG is performed and shows no change from Mr. Bennett's previous strips. He is given nifedipine, 10 mg PO and within 15 minutes he states the pain is beginning to lessen. Within 30 minutes the pain has subsided. Mr. Bennett is admitted for observation but during his stay shows no evidence of another myocardial infarction. The physician decides to start Mr. Bennett on nifedipine 10 mg tid and continue the propranolol.

Discussion Questions

1. Will Mr. Bennett continue to need nitroglycerin when the new drug begins to work?
2. How should administration of the calcium-channel blocker and beta-blocker be spaced for optimum relief? What should the patient be taught about this combination?
3. What teaching goals should the nurse establish for this patient regarding his drug regimen?
4. How will Mr. Bennett use drug therapy now to manage his anginal pain?

REVIEW QUESTIONS

1. What factors can lead to coronary artery dilation?
2. Describe the principal types of angina.
3. List several ways in which antianginal drugs reduce myocardial oxygen demand.
4. Briefly outline the mechanisms of action of the nitrates in treating angina.
5. List the various dosage forms of *nitroglycerin*. Which are used for relief of acute anginal attacks?
6. Give the most common side-effects of the nitrates.
7. How is the dosage of the transdermal nitroglycerin patch stated? What cautions should be observed when using these patches?
8. How is the therapeutic dose of a nitrite/nitrate determined?
9. How much nitroglycerin should a patient take before seeking help during an angina attack?
10. What administration techniques should be followed when giving intravenous nitroglycerin?
11. Why are pain patterns important in teaching a patient about appropriate self-administration of "p.r.n." nitroglycerin?
12. Which beta-blockers are approved for use in angina? What is their principal mechanism of action?
13. List the major hemodynamic effects of the calcium-channel blockers.
14. What are the approved indications for calcium-channel blockers? List several investigational uses for this group of drugs.
15. How frequently should vital signs/cardiac monitoring be performed during initial therapy with calcium-channel blockers? Why does the time frame vary among drugs?
16. Briefly describe the mechanism of action of dipyridamole. What are its approved and investigational indications?
17. Why are most peripheral vasodilators ineffective in improving blood flow to ischemic areas?
18. What are the principal indications of ergoloid mesylates? Which usage form is preferred and why?

BIBLIOGRAPHY

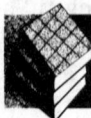

Anders Vedin J, Wilhelmsson CF: Beta receptor blocking agents with secondary prevention of coronary heart disease. Annu Rev Pharmacol Toxicol 23:29, 1983

Baumwald E: Mechanism of action of calcium-channel blocking agents. N Engl J Med 307:1618, 1982

Butler JD, Harrison L: Keeping pace with calcium channel blockers. Nursing 83 13(7):38, 1983

Cauvin C, Loutzenhiser R, Van Breeman C: Mechanisms of calcium antagonist-induced vasodilation. Annu Rev Pharmacol Toxicol 23:373, 1983

Flaim SF, Zelis R (eds): Calcium Blockers. Baltimore, Urban and Schwarzenberg, 1982

Hansen MS, Woods SL: Nitroglycerin ointment: Where and how to apply it. Am J Nurs 80:1122, 1980

Herlihy B et al: A nursing care plan for the patient receiving calcium antagonists. Crit Care Nurse 4(1):38, 1984

Hoffman JE, Buckberg GD: The myocardial supply:demand ratio: A critical review. Am J Cardiol 41:327, 1978

Mar DD: New topical nitroglycerin preparations. Am J Nursing 82:462, 1982

McGourty JC, Silas JH, Solomon SA: Tolerability of combined treatment with verapamil and beta-blockers in angina resistant to monotherapy. Postgrad Med J 61:229, 1985

Meyer JS: Calcium channel blockers in the prophylactic treatment of vascular headache. Ann Intern Med 102:395, 1985

Oates JA, Wood AJJ: Dipyridamole. N Engl J Med 316(20):1247, 1987

Opie LH (ed): Calcium Antagonists and Cardiovascular Disease, Vol. 6: Perspectives in Cardiovascular Research. New York, Raven Press, 1984

Piepho RW: The calcium antagonists: Mechanisms of action and pharmacologic effects. Drug Therapy 13:69, 1983

Purcell JA, Holder CK: Intravenous nitroglycerin. Am J Nurs 82:254, 1982

Roberts R: Intravenous nitroglycerin in acute myocardial infarction. Am J Med 74 (Suppl):45, 1983

Roberts R (ed): Second North American Conference on Nitroglycerin Therapy: Perspectives and mechanisms. Am J Med 76:1, 1984

Rossi LP, Antman EM: Calcium channel blockers: New treatment for cardiovascular disease. Am J Nurs 83:382, 1983

Schneck DW: Calcium-entry blockers: A review of their basic and clinical pharmacology and therapeutic applications. Ration Drug Ther 19(5):1, 1985

Schroeder JS: Calcium and beta blockers in ischemic heart disease: When to use which. Mod Medicine 26:94, 1982

Shub C, Ulietstra RE, McGoon MD: Selection of optimal drug therapy for the patient with angina pectoris. Mayo Clin Prac 60:539, 1985

Snyder SH, Reynolds IJ: Calcium-antagonist drugs: Receptor interactions that clarify therapeutic effects. N Engl J Med 313:995, 1985

Strauss WE, Parisi AF: Superiority of combined diltiazem and propranolol therapy for angina pectoris. Circulation 71(5):951, 1985

Zelis R, Flaim SF: Calcium blocking drugs for angina pectoris. Annu Rev Med 33:465, 1982

Prophylaxis of Atherosclerosis: Hypolipemic Drugs

Bile Acid Sequestering Resins
    Cholestyramine
    Colestipol
    Clofibrate

Dextrothyroxine
Gemfibrozil
Lovastatin
Nicotinic Acid (Niacin)
Probucol

37

Atherosclerosis is a condition characterized by deposition of lipid (fatty) material within the walls of the arterial system, resulting in a gradual occlusion of blood flow. It is a major cause of death in the United States and in many other countries in the world. Clinical consequences of this lipid deposition include the development of ischemic heart disease, cerebrovascular disease (including stroke), peripheral ischemia, and renovascular hypertension. The presence of generalized atherosclerosis greatly increases the risk of mortality from one or more of these conditions.

Although the basic mechanisms involved in the development of the atherosclerotic process are quite complex and still somewhat uncertain, there appears to be a metabolic disturbance in the synthesis, transport, and utilization of lipids; this, in combination with damage to the smooth vascular endothelial lining, results in the adherence and eventual buildup of fatty deposits within the lining of the vessel walls.

Lipids do not circulate freely in the bloodstream, but rather are bound to plasma proteins (albumin, globulins). These complexes are termed lipoproteins and contain varying proportions of high-density proteins and low-density lipids. The four major types of lipoproteins, and a brief description of their characteristics are listed below.

· Chylomicrons—Largest and lightest of the lipoproteins, formed in the intestine during absorption of dietary fat; composed mainly (80%–90%) of triglycerides, and impart a cloudiness to plasma; normally cleared rapidly from the blood, their presence in plasma taken from a fasting patient suggests an inability to handle dietary fats
· Very low-density lipoproteins (VLDL)—Pre-beta-lipoproteins containing large amounts (50%–60%) of triglycerides that were synthesized in the liver; major means by which endogenous triglycerides are carried from the liver to the plasma
· Low-density lipoproteins (LDL)—Beta-lipoproteins derived partly from breakdown of VLDL, containing about 50% to 60% cholesterol, 25% protein, and very little triglycerides; most of the circulating serum cholesterol is transported in this form, and elevated plasma levels of LDL indicate excessive cholesterol levels and suggest that the patient is at high risk for developing atherosclerosis.
· High-density lipoproteins (HDL)—Alpha-lipoproteins, the smallest and most dense

(heaviest) of the lipoproteins, containing approximately 50% protein, 25% cholesterol, and very small amounts of triglycerides; believed to play an important role in clearing cholesterol from body tissues, and may protect against development of atherosclerosis by blocking uptake of LDL cholesterol by vascular smooth muscle cells.

Approximately one-fourth of all adults have elevated levels of one or more of their plasma lipids or lipoproteins, which may reflect improper diet, excessive alcohol consumption, secondary disease (such as hypothyroidism or diabetes), or an inherited trait. Measurements of serum cholesterol and triglycerides can easily be done and are a common component of laboratory blood studies. However, a more accurate and useful classification of patients having defects in lipid metabolism or transport is based on the types of *lipoproteins* that are elevated in the plasma. This grouping allows precise diagnosis and treatment of each patient's condition. The term *hyperlipoproteinemia* is used to indicate an increase in one or more of the classes of lipoproteins. Table 37-1 lists the types of hyperlipoproteinemias that are currently recognized, with a brief description of each type and the most effective treatment of each subgroup.

It has not been *conclusively* established whether lowering serum lipids or cholesterol has a beneficial effect on morbidity or mortality associated with atherosclerosis. However, it appears as if elevated plasma cholesterol or LDL is a major risk factor for development of atherosclerosis, and results of a recent multicenter, randomized clinical study strongly suggested that reductions in plasma concentrations of LDL-cholesterol can significantly reduce the risk of coronary artery disease.

Several therapeutic strategies may be employed in the treatment of hyperlipoproteinemias. The cornerstone of therapy still lies in diet modification and weight reduction. Reduced consumption of cholesterol and saturated animal fats is recommended for all types of hyperlipoproteinemias. Protein intake is either maintained or increased in most instances. Other risk factors should be eliminated as well, such as cessation of smoking, curtailment or abstinence from alcohol, treatment of elevated blood pressure, and maintenance of an adequate program of exercise and physical fitness.

Drug therapy of hyperlipoproteinemia involves the use of agents that can lower plasma concentrations of lipoproteins, either by blocking their production or enhancing their removal from the plasma. These drugs, termed hypolipemic or hypo-

Table 37-1
Classification of Hyperlipoproteinemias

Type	Descriptive Name	Characteristic Features	Treatment	
			Diet	Drugs
I	Fat-induced (exogenous)	Relatively rare; increase in plasma chylomicrons containing large amounts of triglycerides of dietary origin; frequently seen in infancy, and marked by abdominal pain and pancreatitis; does not lead to atherosclerosis	Low fat, no alcohol; no restrictions on proteins, carbohydrates, or cholesterol	None effective
IIa	Familial hypercholesterolemia	High levels of LDL; normal VLDL; slight elevation of triglycerides; fairly common, and a definite risk for development of atherosclerosis and coronary heart disease	Low cholesterol; low saturated fats; increased intake of poly-unsaturated fats	cholestyramine colestipol dextrothyroxine lovastatin probucol
IIb	Combined hyperlipoproteinemia	Elevated LDL and VLDL; presence of hypercholesterolemia and hypertriglyceridemia; lipid deposits (xanthomas) occur in feet, elbows, knees	See IIa	cholestyramine colestipol dextrothyroxine lovastatin nicotinic acid probucol
III	Broad beta-lipoproteinemia	Elevated LDL and VLDL, cholesterol, and triglycerides are elevated; relatively uncommon but associated with atherosclerosis; recessively inherited disorder	Weight reduction; low cholesterol, low saturated fats; maintain high protein	clofibrate dextrothyroxine nicotinic acid
IV	Carbohydrate-induced (endogenous)	Marked elevation of VLDL; triglycerides are increased, but LDL and cholesterol are normal or slightly elevated; HDL is reduced; most common type; definite risk for atherosclerosis and coronary heart disease	Weight reduction; low carbohydrate; low cholesterol; low alcohol; maintain protein intake	clofibrate (?) gemfibrozil nicotinic acid
V	Mixed hyperlipemia	Elevated VLDL and triglycerides; chylomicrons are increased; HDL is reduced; relatively uncommon type *not* generally associated with atherosclerosis or heart disease; xanthomas, hyperuricemia and pancreatitis can occur	Low fat; high protein, low carbohydrate; no alcohol	clofibrate (?) gemfibrozil (?) nicotinic acid

lipidemic agents are widely employed in a significant percentage of the population with hyperlipoproteinemia. However, in view of the potential for many hypolipemic drugs to cause untoward reactions, dietary changes should always be undertaken initially before drug therapy is instituted. Only if diet alone is ineffective in controlling the plasma lipid picture or if the degree of hyperlipidemia is severe should drugs be employed, and then only upon careful diagnosis of the type of hyperlipoproteinemia present. To date, drug therapy is entirely prophylactic—that is, hypolipemic agents can reduce the rate and extent of fatty deposition within arterial walls by lowering plasma lipid concentrations, but they do not dissolve or remove existing lipid deposits. Diet control is, of course, an essential adjunct to drug treatment and must be continued throughout the period of drug therapy to obtain maximal therapeutic benefit. A variety of different drugs are available for the treatment of the various types of hyperlipoproteinemias and owing to the many differences among them, they will be discussed individually below.

Bile Acid Sequestering Resins

Cholestyramine

Colestipol

Cholestyramine and colestipol are anion-exchange resins which combine with bile acids in the intestines, preventing their reabsorption and therefore increasing their excretion in the feces. They are effective plasma cholesterol-lowering drugs, and cholestyramine is also used for relieving pruritus associated with partial biliary obstruction. They are discussed together here, then listed individually in Table 37-2.

MECHANISM AND ACTIONS
The bile acid sequestering resins form an insoluble complex with bile acids in the intestine because they are not absorbed from the GI tract. The increased fecal loss of bile acids leads to an increased oxidation of cholesterol to bile acids, resulting in lowered plasma levels of both cholesterol and low-density lipoproteins (LDL). Serum triglyceride levels may increase slightly or remain essentially unchanged. The decline in serum cholesterol occurs within 1 month; however, cholesterol levels

may eventually begin to rise, even with continued drug usage. The drugs can interfere with the GI absorption of many drugs, vitamins, and other substances if taken concurrently (see under Interactions).

USES
1. Adjunctive treatment of primary type II hyperlipoproteinemia
2. Relief of pruritus associated with partial biliary obstruction (cholestyramine only)
3. Investigational uses for cholestyramine include treatment of antibiotic-induced pseudomembranous colitis due to *Clostridium difficile* and treatment of poisoning with the pesticide chlordecone (Kepone).

ADMINISTRATION AND DOSAGE
See Table 37-2.

FATE
Cholestyramine and colestipol are not absorbed from the GI tract, nor are they hydrolyzed by digestive enzymes. The drugs are excreted in the feces as insoluble bile acid complexes.

SIDE-EFFECTS/ADVERSE REACTIONS
Constipation is the most frequently encountered side-effect and may be severe. Laxatives, stool softeners, and high fluid intake may be helpful in minimizing the severity. Other common side-effects include abdominal discomfort, belching, flatulence, nausea, and anorexia. Less frequently observed adverse reactions with the bile acid sequestering resins are vomiting; steatorrhea; fecal impaction; vitamin-K deficiency with bleeding tendencies; vitamin A, D, and E deficiencies; rash and irritation of the skin, tongue, and perianal region; and osteoporosis.

A wide variety of other adverse reactions have been reported in persons taking these drugs, but their relationship to the drugs themselves is unclear. They include rectal bleeding, peptic ulceration, dysphagia, pancreatitis, diverticulitis, cholecystitis, ecchymoses, anemia, urticaria, dermatitis, muscle and joint aching, anxiety, vertigo, fatigue, tinnitus, drowsiness, paresthesia, hematuria, dysuria, uveitis, edema, swollen glands, dyspnea, and elevation in SGOT and alkaline phosphatase.

CONTRAINDICATIONS AND PRECAUTIONS
Complete biliary obstruction is the lone absolute contraindication to use of cholestyramine and co-

Table 37-2
Bile Acid Sequestering Resins

Drug	Preparations	Usual Dosage Range	Clinical Considerations
cholestyramine (Questran)	Powder—4 g resin/9 g powder	Initially 4 g resin two to three times/day before meals; adjust to patient's needs (range 16 g–24 g/day) No dosage schedule for children; if used, start with very small doses and observe for hypochloremic acidosis	Place drug on surface of 4 oz–6 oz liquid; allow to stand 1 min–2 min without stirring, then gently twirl container or stir slowly to obtain a uniform suspension; rinse glass with fluid to ensure taking entire dose; may also be mixed with soups or pulpy fruits (e.g., applesauce); relief of pruritus may take 1 week–2 weeks to become evident; decline in serum cholesterol is usually apparent by 1 month
colestipol (Colestid)	Water-insoluble beads—5-g packets or 500-g bottles	15 g–30 g/day in divided doses two to four times/day	Add prescribed amount of drug to at least 3 oz of liquid, and stir until completely mixed (does not dissolve); May also be added to cereals, soups, or pulpy fruits; does not have the disagreeable odor or taste of cholestyramine

lestipol. The drugs should be administered *cautiously* to patients with constipation, bleeding tendencies, anemia, systemic acidosis (prolonged drug use can lead to hypochloremic acidosis) and hypothyroidism and to pregnant women and children.

INTERACTIONS
1. Bile acid sequestering resins may interfere with oral absorption of a wide range of drugs, including anticoagulants, cephalexin, clindamycin, corticosteroids, digitalis drugs, folic acid, iron preparations, penicillin G, phenobarbital, phenylbutazone, thiazide diuretics, thyroid drugs, tetracyclines, trimethoprim, and vitamins A, D, E, and K.
2. Concurrent use of cholestyramine and iopanoic acid can result in abnormal cholecystography, because cholestyramine has a fair affinity for iopanoic acid.

NURSING CONSIDERATIONS
See Nursing Process for Patients Starting Hypolipemic Drugs.

Clofibrate
(Atromid-S)

Clofibrate primarily lowers serum triglyceride and VLDL levels and is indicated for Type III hyperlipoproteinemia. Due to its potential to cause serious toxicity, however, clofibrate should be reserved for those patients with *significant* hyperlipidemia who have not responded adequately to diet, weight reduction, and perhaps other less toxic drugs.

MECHANISM AND ACTIONS
The mechanism of action of clofibrate has not been definitely established. The drug lowers elevated triglyceride and VLDL levels, possibly by increasing breakdown of free fatty acids in the liver by action of lipoprotein lipase. It also appears to decrease release of VLDL from liver to plasma, and interfere with binding of free fatty acids to albumin. Clofibrate may slightly reduce plasma cholesterol and LDL, presumably by inhibiting cholesterol biosynthesis and increasing biliary and fecal excretion of cholesterol. A platelet-inhibiting effect is also noted with clofibrate.

USES

1. Adjunctive treatment of type III hyperlipoproteinemia that does not respond adequately to diet
2. Adjunctive treatment of types IV and V hyperlipoproteinemia characterized by very high serum triglyceride levels and a risk of pancreatitis

ADMINISTRATION AND DOSAGE

Clofibrate is administered as 500-mg capsules. The usual dose is 2 g/day in divided doses, usually four times a day.

FATE

Following administration, clofibrate is hydrolyzed to p-chlorophenoxyisobutyric acid (CPIB), the active form of the drug, which is slowly but completely absorbed. Peak CPIB plasma levels occur in 3 hours to 6 hours. The plasma half-life ranges from 6 hours to 24 hours, but is much longer (up to 100 hours) in patients with renal impairment. CPIB is highly protein-bound (90%–95%). It is largely metabolized in the liver and excreted in the urine as a conjugated metabolite (50%–75%), as well as unchanged CPIB (10%–20%).

SIDE-EFFECTS/ADVERSE REACTIONS

■ WARNING

Clofibrate has produced benign and malignant GI tumors in rats at five to eight times the human dose. The drug also has the potential to elicit hepatic tumors in humans, produce cholelithiasis (twice the risk of nonusers), and evoke a wide range of other untoward reactions. Due to these characteristics, coupled with the lack of substantial evidence for a beneficial effect for clofibrate on cardiovascular mortality, it should be reserved for those patients with significant hyperlipidemia and a high risk of coronary heart disease who have not responded adequately to diet, weight loss, and other less toxic drugs.

Common side-effects with clofibrate are nausea, dyspepsia, abdominal distress, and flatulence. Among the other adverse reactions linked to use of clofibrate are

GI—Diarrhea, vomiting, gastritis, stomatitis, increased gallstones, (see *Warning* above), hepatomegaly

Cardiovascular—Arrhythmias, swelling, and phlebitis at site of xanthoma, angina, thromboembolic complications

Dermatologic—Rash, urticaria, pruritus, alopecia, dry skin, dry hair

Hematologic—Leukopenia, anemia, eosinophilia

Neurologic—Drowsiness, weakness, dizziness, headache

Other—Myalgia and flu-like symptoms (possibly due to increased plasma levels of creatine phosphokinase), arthralgia, impotence, decreased libido, dysuria, hematuria, decreased urinary output, weight gain, polyphagia, abnormal liver function tests, hepatic tumors

CONTRAINDICATIONS AND PRECAUTIONS

Clofibrate is contraindicated in the presence of significant hepatic or renal dysfunction, in primary biliary cirrhosis, and in pregnant women or nursing mothers. The drug must be given with *caution* to patients with peptic ulcer, cardiac arrhythmias, gout, and to persons receiving oral anticoagulants or oral hypoglycemic drugs (see under Interactions).

INTERACTIONS

1. Clofibrate may enhance the effects of oral anticoagulants, antidiabetics, cholinesterase inhibitors, furosemide, and thyroxine.
2. Oral contraceptives, other estrogens, and rifampin can decrease the action of clofibrate through enzyme induction.
3. The effects of clofibrate may be enhanced by acidifying agents, neomycin, probenecid, and thyroxine.

NURSING CONSIDERATIONS

See Nursing Process for Patients Starting Hypolipemic Drugs.

Dextrothyroxine

(Choloxin)

Dextrothyroxine is a synthetic analogue of the thyroid hormone levothyroxine that was developed in an attempt to retain the desirable lipid-lowering actions of the thyroid hormones while eliminating the calorigenic and cardiac-stimulating effects. This separation has not been completely accomplished, however, and dextrothyroxine has a limited therapeutic application in treating selected hyperlipoproteinemias in patients with no organic heart disease.

MECHANISM AND ACTIONS

Dextrothyroxine increases catabolism and excretion of cholesterol by way of the bile into the feces. Serum cholesterol and LDL levels are reduced, however there are no consistent effects on triglyceride or VLDL levels. Dextrothyroxine may also increase the number of receptors for LDL on cell membranes.

USES

1. Adjunctive treatment for reduction of elevated cholesterol and LDL levels in type II (and possibly type III) euthyroid patients with no evidence of organic heart disease
2. Treatment of hypothyroidism in patients with cardiac disease who cannot tolerate other thyroid drugs

ADMINISTRATION AND DOSAGE

Dextrothyroxine is available as tablets of 1 mg, 2 mg, 4 mg, and 6 mg. The initial adult dose is 1 mg to 2 mg a day. Increases of 1 mg to 2 mg at intervals of not less than 1 month may be made until the optimal dosage is attained. The usual maintenance dose is 4 mg to 8 mg a day. Children are given an initial dose of 0.05 mg/kg/day, which may be increased in increments of 0.05 mg/kg at monthly intervals to a maximum of 4 mg/day. If signs and symptoms of cardiac disease occur, the drug should be discontinued.

FATE

The drug is adequately absorbed from the GI tract. Plasma protein binding is minimal. Metabolism occurs in the liver, and the drug is rapidly excreted in the urine as both metabolites and unchanged drug.

SIDE-EFFECTS/ADVERSE REACTIONS

Most side-effects with dextrothyroxine are due to increased metabolic activity and are seen more frequently at higher doses and in persons with organic heart disease. Among the more common side-effects are nervousness, sweating, flushing, palpitations, and dyspepsia. Other untoward reactions noted during dextrothyroxine therapy include:

Cardiovascular—Angina, arrhythmias, myocardial damage, increased heart size
CNS—Insomnia, tremors, headache, hyperthermia, dizziness, visual disturbances, tinnitus, paresthesia, psychic changes
GI—Vomiting, diarrhea, anorexia
Other—Hair loss, weight loss, diuresis, menstrual irregularities, altered libido, hoarseness, muscle pain, skin rash, gallstones, hyperglycemia, elevated protein-bound iodine (PBI), worsening of peripheral vascular disease

CONTRAINDICATIONS AND PRECAUTIONS

Dextrothyroxine is contraindicated in patients with organic heart disease (angina, arrhythmias, myocardial infarction, congestive heart failure, rheumatic heart disease), hypertension (other than mild, labile forms), liver or kidney disease, and in pregnant women or nursing mothers. Dextrothyroxine should be discontinued at least 2 weeks prior to elective surgery because the drug can increase the likelihood of cardiac arrhythmias during anesthesia or surgery.

Cautious use of dextrothyroxine is warranted in obese patients and in patients with diabetes. The drug should be withdrawn if signs of iodism (*i.e.*, excessive use of iodine-containing compounds) appear, such as rash, pruritus, coryza, or conjunctivitis. In the patient with diabetes, blood glucose levels should be monitored regularly, and symptoms of hyperglycemia should be reported. Dosage adjustments may be needed (increase the antidiabetic drugs or decrease dextrothyroxine).

INTERACTIONS

1. Dextrothyroxine may potentiate the effects of oral anticoagulants.
2. Toxic actions of digitalis preparations may be enhanced by dextrothyroxine.
3. Dextrothyroxine can reduce the effects of oral hypoglycemics or insulin (by increasing blood sugar levels).
4. Increased response to injections of epinephrine or norepinephrine (*e.g.*, episodes of coronary insufficiency) may occur in the presence of dextrothyroxine.
5. The GI absorption of dextrothyroxine may be reduced by cholestyramine and colestipol.
6. Concurrent use of dextrothyroxine and tricyclic antidepressants may result in CNS excitation and tachycardia.

NURSING CONSIDERATIONS

See Nursing Process for Patients Starting Hypolipemic Drugs.

Gemfibrozil
(Lopid)

Gemfibrozil is a structural analogue of clofibrate that shares many of the pharmacologic and toxicologic properties of the latter drug.

MECHANISM AND ACTIONS
The precise mechanism of action of gemfibrozil has not been elucidated; however, the drug has been demonstrated to lower elevated serum triglycerides, primarily the VLDL fraction and less frequently the LDL fraction. It may also increase the high-density lipoprotein fraction, an action also considered to be beneficial in atherosclerosis. The biochemical mechanisms of action may include inhibition of peripheral lipolysis, reduction of liver triglyceride production, and impairment in the synthesis of VLDL carrier apoprotein. Gemfibrozil may also reduce incorporation of long-chain fatty acids into newly formed triglycerides and accelerate removal of cholesterol from the liver.

USES
1. Treatment of type IV and V hyperlipoproteinemia in patients with high serum triglyceride levels and a definite risk of pancreatitis in patients who do not respond adequately to dietary therapy

ADMINISTRATION AND DOSAGE
Gemfibrozil is administered as 300-mg capsules. Recommended dosage is 1200 mg a day in two divided doses, 30 minutes before meals. The useful dosage range is 900 mg/day to 1500 mg/day.

FATE
Gemfibrozil is well absorbed from the GI tract, and peak serum levels occur within 1 hour to 2 hours. The plasma half-life is 1 hour to 2 hours, but the elimination half-life is considerably longer owing to significant enterohepatic circulation. The drug is excreted largely unchanged (70%) in the urine, with small amounts also eliminated in the feces.

SIDE-EFFECTS/ADVERSE REACTIONS

■ WARNING
Due to pharmacologic similarities between gemfibrozil and clofibrate, the serious adverse effects reported in patients receiving clofibrate must be considered a possibility in patients receiving gemfibrozil as well.

Refer to the discussion of clofibrate for details.

Most frequently noted side-effects with gemfibrozil are abdominal pain, nausea, and diarrhea. Dizziness, blurred vision, flatulence, and vomiting have also been reported often. Many other adverse reactions have been observed in persons receiving gemfibrozil, and they are listed below, although a definite causal relationship has not been established in each instance.

GI—Constipation, dry mouth, gas pain, anorexia
CNS—Headache, vertigo, insomnia, tinnitus, paresthesias
Musculoskeletal—Arthralgia, back pain, myalgia, muscle cramping, swollen joints
Skin—Rash, dermatitis, pruritis, urticaria
Hepatic—Liver function abnormalities (increased SGOT, SGPT, LDH, CPK, alkaline phosphatase)
Other—Anemia, eosinophilia, leukopenia, malaise, syncope, cholelithiasis

CONTRAINDICATIONS AND PRECAUTIONS
Gemfibrozil is contraindicated in patients with severe hepatic or renal dysfunction, gallbladder disease, and biliary cirrhosis. *Cautious use* of gemfibrozil must be undertaken in persons with cardiac arrhythmias, diabetes (drug has a mild hyperglycemic effect) and in persons with altered liver function values. Pregnant women and nursing mothers must also exercise caution, because gemfibrozil has been demonstrated to be tumorigenic in male rats at one to ten times the human dose.

INTERACTIONS
1. Gemfibrozil may enhance the effects of oral anticoagulants.

NURSING CONSIDERATIONS
See also Nursing Process for Patients Starting Hypolipemic Drugs.

Gemfibrozil has been associated with the development of gallbladder disease and liver dysfunction, including benign liver nodules and liver carcinoma in animals. The benefit-to-risk ratio must be seriously considered before this drug is prescribed, and the patient must be monitored closely throughout therapy. If the drug has produced no significant response in lipid levels within 3 months it should be withdrawn.

Lovastatin

(Mevacor)

Lovastatin is a cholesterol-lowering agent isolated from a strain of *Aspergillus terreus*. Compared to many other hypolipemic drugs, it is quite well-tolerated in the majority of patients.

MECHANISM AND ACTIONS
Following oral ingestion, lovastatin, an inactive lactone, is hydrolyzed to a beta-hydroxy acid form, which is a potent inhibitor of HMG-CoA reductase, an enzyme that catalyzes the conversion of HMG-CoA to mevalonate, an early and *rate-limiting* step in the biosynthesis of cholesterol. Both normal and elevated LDL cholesterol levels are lowered. Lovastatin reduces the concentration of circulating LDL particles, increases HDL cholesterol levels, and reduces VLDL cholesterol and plasma triglycerides. However, the drug does not appear to adversely affect steroidogenesis.

USES
1. Adjunct to diet for reducing elevated total and LDL cholesterol levels in patients with primary hypercholesterolemia (types IIa and IIb)
2. Reduction of elevated LDL cholesterol levels in patients with combined hypercholesterolemia and hypertriglyceridemia

ADMINISTRATION AND DOSAGE
Lovastatin is available as 20-mg tablets. The recommended starting dose is 20 mg once a day with the evening meal. Dosage adjustments should be made at 4-week intervals until the desired effect is noted. The usual dosage range is 20 mg to 80 mg a day in single or divided doses.

FATE
Less than one third of an oral dose is absorbed, and the drug undergoes extensive first-pass hepatic metabolism, such that less than 5% of an oral dose reaches the systemic circulation as active drug or metabolite. The maximum therapeutic response occurs witin 4 weeks to 6 weeks and is maintained by single daily dosing in the evening. Both lovastatin and its beta-hydroxy acid metabolite are highly protein-bound in the plasma (95%). Excretion is largely in the feces by way of the bile (about 85%) with some drug and metabolite (10% to 15%) appearing in the urine.

SIDE-EFFECTS/ADVERSE REACTIONS
The most frequently encountered side-effects during lovastatin therapy are headache, abdominal pain/cramping, flatulence, diarrhea, nausea, rash, and pruritus. Lovastatin may elevate creatine phosphokinase in approximately 10% of patients, but these increases are usually transient and mild. However, myalgia and muscle tenderness may indicate myositis in patients with markedly elevated CPK. Persistent increases in serum transaminases have occurred in about 2% of patients receiving lovastatin for at least 1 year. Other adverse reactions reported during lovastatin therapy include dizziness, blurred vision, and peripheral neuropathy.

CONTRAINDICATIONS AND PRECAUTIONS
Use of lovastatin is contraindicated in the presence of acute liver disease, persistent elevation of serum transaminases, pregnancy, or lactation. The drug must be used with extreme *caution* in patients at risk for developing renal failure, such as those with severe acute infections, hypotension, trauma, or severe metabolic, endocrine, or electrolyte disturbances. The drug should also be given cautiously to patients with uncontrolled seizures, chronic liver dysfunction, or skeletal muscle disorders.

NURSING CONSIDERATIONS
See Nursing Process for Patients Starting Hypolipemic Drugs.

Nicotinic Acid (Niacin)

Nicotinic acid is a water-soluble vitamin (vitamin B_3) that is discussed more fully in Chapter 76. It can lower VLDL and LDL levels and increase HDL levels and may be used as adjunctive therapy in certain types of hyperlipoproteinemias.

MECHANISM AND ACTIONS
Nicotinic acid (but *not* its conversion product nicotinamide) reduces lipolysis and release of free fatty acids from adipose tissue. Decreased free fatty acid levels lead to reduced hepatic VLDL and triglyceride synthesis. LDL formation is also decreased, while HDL levels may be elevated. Nicotinic acid accelerates the removal of chylomicron triglycerides by increasing the activity of lipoprotein lipase. Hepatic cholesterol synthesis may also be inhibited. Plasma free fatty acid and triglyceride levels fall within hours after oral dose, whereas several days may be required for cholesterol levels to decline.

USES

1. Adjunctive therapy in patients with elevated cholesterol or triglycerides who do not respond adequately to diet and weight loss
2. Correction of nicotinic acid deficiency (see Chap. 76)

ADMINISTRATION AND DOSAGE

Nicotinic acid is available as tablets, timed-release capsules, elixir, and injection. For treatment of hyperlipidemia, the drug is given orally in a dosage of 1 g to 2 g, one to three times a day. The maximum recommended dose is 8 g/day.

FATE

Nicotinic acid is readily absorbed orally. Peak serum concentrations occur within 1 hour. Plasma elimination half-life is approximately 45 minutes to 60 minutes. The drug is partially metabolized by the liver and excreted as both metabolites and unchanged drug by the kidney.

SIDE-EFFECTS/ADVERSE REACTIONS

The commonly encountered side-effects with nicotinic acid are flushing, sensation of warmth, itching, tingling in the extremities, and GI distress. These effects are transient and disappear with time. Other adverse reactions reported with nicotinic acid include headache, dizziness, diarrhea, palpitations, hypotension, skin rash, epigastric pain, gouty arthritis, hyperuricemia, jaundice, peptic ulceration, toxic amblyopia, increased sebaceous gland activity, and impaired liver function.

CONTRAINDICATIONS AND PRECAUTIONS

Contraindications to use of nicotinic acid are hepatic dysfunction, active peptic ulcer, severe hypotension, gastritis, and overt hemorrhaging. Nicotinic acid must be given *cautiously* to patients with allergic disorders, glaucoma, gallbladder disease, diabetes, gout, a history of jaundice, and to pregnant women or nursing mothers.

INTERACTIONS

1. Nicotinic acid may enhance the blood pressure-lowering effects of antihypertensive medications.
2. Nicotinic acid may antagonize the effects of antidiabetic drugs by elevating blood glucose levels.

NURSING CONSIDERATIONS

See also Nursing Process for Patients Starting Hypolipemic Drugs.

Hepatic function studies and blood glucose levels should be drawn throughout therapy to monitor for liver dysfunction and hyperglycemia. Uric acid levels should also be drawn periodically in patients susceptible to gout.

Hypotension may be severe with this drug. Patients should be closely monitored for this side-effect and should avoid driving, climbing, or any hazardous activity until the effect on them is known. If hypotension occurs, the physician should be notified and the dosage reduced.

Nicotinic acid is very irritating to the GI tract and may be better tolerated if taken with food. There is some evidence that reduction of serum lipids can be enhanced if the tablets are chewed rather than swallowed whole and ingested with large quantities of cold water.

Probucol

(Lorelco)

MECHANISM AND ACTIONS

Probucol lowers serum cholesterol with relatively little effect on serum triglycerides or VLDL. It may inhibit hepatic synthesis of cholesterol at an early stage and impair GI absorption of cholesterol. There is increased excretion of fecal bile acids. Cholesterol is reduced not only in the LDL fraction, which is desirable, but also apparently in some HDL fractions, which may be detrimental.

USES

1. Treatment of elevated serum cholesterol in patients with primary hypercholesterolemia (type II hyperlipoproteinemia) who have not responded to diet and weight reduction (*not* indicated where hypertriglyceridemia is the predominant factor)

ADMINISTRATION AND DOSAGE

Probucol is administered as 250-mg tablets. The usual dose is 500 mg twice a day, given with meals.

FATE

GI absorption is variable and limited. Peak blood levels are higher when the drug is administered with food. The drug accumulates slowly in adipose tissue and may persist for up to 6 months at these sites. The major route of elimination is the feces by way of the bile.

SIDE-EFFECTS/ADVERSE REACTIONS

Diarrhea is the most common side-effect with probucol, followed by flatulence, abdominal pain, nausea, headache, paresthesias, dizziness, and eosinophilia. Other less frequently encountered adverse reactions are vomiting, decreased hemoglobin, rash, pruritus, insomnia, impotence, blurred vision, tinnitus, impaired taste, anorexia, indigestion, GI bleeding, petechiae, nocturia, angioedema, palpitations, syncope, chest pain, thrombocytopenia, peripheral neuritis, and elevated serum transaminases, bilirubin, alkaline phosphatase, uric acid, glucose, and creatine phosphokinase.

CONTRAINDICATIONS AND PRECAUTIONS

Probucol is contraindicated in patients with cardiac arrhythmias and in pregnant women or nursing mothers.

NURSING CONSIDERATIONS

See Nursing Process for Patients Starting Hypolipemic Drugs.

Several other drugs have the capacity to lower elevated serum lipid levels, but are largely unsuitable for the treatment of hyperlipoproteinemia, primarily because of their high incidence of untoward reactions and the availability of more effective and less toxic agents. Neomycin sulfate reduces plasma cholesterol by blocking its gastric absorption and lowers LDL levels as well, especially when given in combination with cholestyramine resin. However, neomycin is highly toxic (GI distress, ototoxicity, kidney damage) and is only employed in type II hyperlipoproteinemia that is resistant to other forms of therapy.

Estrogens effectively lower cholesterol and LDL levels but may elevate triglycerides and VLDL. They are obviously unsuited for use in males because of their feminizing action, and they can result in thromboembolic disorders, abdominal pain, and pancreatitis in women. Administration of norethindrone acetate, a progestin, has decreased VLDL levels in some women with type V hyperlipoproteinemia. However, this agent has significant estrogenic activity and is therefore associated with many of the same adverse effects as the estrogens themselves.

Finally, although heparin can increase the conversion of triglycerides to free fatty acids, resulting in degradation of chylomicrons to soluble, dispersible complexes, heparin is of no clinical use as a hypolipemic drug because of its potential to cause hemorrhage and its need to be administered parenterally.

■ Nursing Process for Patients Starting Hypolipemic Drugs

□ ASSESSMENT

□ Subjective Data

The patient who is a candidate for these drugs may have no symptoms of any disease, but, by history and some physical findings, may be in danger of developing cardiovascular problems. Consequently, from the outset, the health-care team must recognize that they can provide the information and therapy to assist this individual to reduce his risk factors, but only the patient can decide whether he will adhere to them. At the point where hypolipemic drugs are employed other attempts should already have been tried. Therefore, initial discussion should focus on what dietary adjustments have been made and that they must continue, whether an exercise program has been initiated, and, if appropriate, what steps have been taken to reduce or eliminate alcohol and smoking. The patient should begin to relate the connection between changed health habits which must continue for life, drug administration, and his risk factors for cardiovascular disease. If he denies their existence, the probability for compliance is low.

Other information is also necessary for the nurse. A drug history should be taken. Many of the hypolipemic drugs will interfere with absorption of many drugs so administration patterns will have to be planned to avoid this. Cost factors should also be discussed early in the therapy. Many of these drugs are extremely expensive. Therapy may cost hundreds of dollars per month. The patient should be aware of this before he gets to the pharmacy, and plans should be made for how the costs can be defrayed through insurance, drug plans, or other assistance.

The patient's bowel habits should also be reviewed because many of the drugs cause major gastrointestinal side-effects and these can be minimized by careful planning.

□ Objective Data

Laboratory work-up is essential for baseline information about the patient. Lipid series should be performed as well as liver function studies and blood clotting times. A baseline ECG may be ordered to assess cardiac status because cardiac changes may be further compromised by use of dextrothyroxine, gemfibrozil, and clofibrate. In women of childbearing age, a pregnancy test should also be done because most of these drugs can cause fetal damage. The drugs should not be administered to anyone who is trying to conceive and should be stopped several months before conception is attempted. Effective birth control measures should be advised throughout therapy.

☐ *NURSING DIAGNOSES*

Actual nursing diagnoses for patients using hypolipemic drugs may include:

    Knowledge deficit related to the action, administration, and side-effects of the drug

    Alteration in tissue perfusion related to arteriosclerosis which may improve as drug therapy becomes effective

Potential nursing diagnoses may include:

    Alteration in bowel elimination: diarrhea or constipation

    Alteration in nutrition: less than body requirements related to interference with vitamin A, D, E, and K absorption

    Noncompliance with the regimen usually related to side-effects but also may be related to lack of symptoms, cost, or a variety of other factors.

☐ *PLAN*

Nursing care goals should focus on helping the patient:

1. To view drug therapy as a part of a total life strategy to reduce his risk of atherosclerosis
2. To incorporate correct self-medication into his daily routine
3. To learn to manage common side-effects and to report serious changes
4. To seek regular follow-up care to monitor positive changes in cholesterol and triglycerides as well as to ensure hepatic and hematologic dysfunction do not occur

☐ *INTERVENTION*

Frequently, compliance is an issue with the patient who is prescribed hypolipemic drugs. The health-care team may face a challenge in convincing the patient of the need for expensive, aggressive therapy especially if the individual is young and symptom-free. In addition, changes in laboratory values may take weeks to months to accomplish. Strategies to enhance participation may include group support meetings, participation in a health fitness program such as those sponsored by local YMCAs

and other health groups, incentives from employers for individuals who reduce cardiac risks, and contractual arrangements between the health-care team and the patient. Many other strategies can be used, but the patient at high risk for atherosclerosis must take an active part in his care. It may be appropriate for him to keep records of his laboratory results over time to measure improvement.

All of the hypolipemic drugs can interfere with the absorption of many other drugs. Therefore, administration should be timed so that any other drug is taken either 1 hour before or 4 hours after the hypolipemic. Hypolipemics also interfere with the absorption of fat-soluble vitamins A, D, E, and K. Consequently, anyone on long-term therapy should be advised to supplement vitamins A, D, E, and K which should be ordered by the physician as appropriate. In addition, the patient should be told to report any bleeding around the gums or increase in bruising which would indicate a vitamin-K deficiency.

Many patients can alleviate the nausea and diarrhea from these drugs by taking them with meals and by eating smaller quantities of food more frequently than three times a day. If constipation is a problem, the patient should be encouraged to increase dietary bulk by including grains, fiber, and raw fruits and vegetables and to increase fluid intake. If these measures do not help, or if the patient has a history of constipation prior to drug therapy, a prescription for stool softeners may be needed.

The patient needs to recognize the importance of follow-up care, especially the need for laboratory tests to monitor progress and the need to watch for side-effects. Periodic liver function studies, clotting times, and prothrombin levels should be performed. The patient receiving dextrothyroxine or nicotinic acid and the diabetic patient should also have frequent serum glucose levels drawn because these drugs may produce hypoglycemia. Protein-bound iodine (PBI) may also be monitored in the patient receiving dextrothyroxine, but elevations in this level indicate the occurrence of drug absorption and transport *not* the development of hypermetabolism due to hyperthyroidism.

☐ *EVALUATION*

The main outcome criterion against which to judge therapeutic success is lowered serum lipids, especially cholesterol and triglycerides. These laboratory studies should be performed at regular intervals to help the patient see his progress. However, many of the drugs take weeks to months to achieve results so the patient must understand the long-term nature of the therapy. Other parameters such as weight loss, increased exercise tolerance, successful cessation of smoking, alcohol, and improved handling of life stress are important adjuncts and must also be rewarded. Drug therapy is only one part of a series of life changes necessary to reduce risk of arteriosclerosis.

CASE STUDY

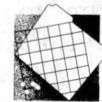

Harrison Mitchell, age 38, is the head of industrial design for a Fortune 500 company, the youngest man to hold that position in the history of his firm. Mr. Mitchell is seen by the company physician for a required semiannual executive physical examination. During the initial interview, Mr. Mitchell reveals that he smokes about two packs of cigarettes a day and states he has no time for exercise. He lists cards (poker, bridge) and chess as the pastimes he uses for relaxation. His family history includes the following: father died at age 46 from a stroke; mother died at age 50 from a heart attack; one older brother, currently 43, had a "mild" heart attack last year. Mr. Mitchell is about 25 lb overweight and admits he's a little concerned about his family history. But he states he does not dwell on it because he is too busy with his job.

Routine lab work shows Mr. Mitchell has elevated serum lipids with cholesterol at 300 mg/dl and triglycerides at 175 mg/dl. The company physician recommends a low-cholesterol, low-fat diet, exercise, and attendance at the company-sponsored Smoke-Enders program. Mr. Mitchell seems motivated to comply.

Six weeks later, Mr. Mitchell reports back for an update. He has quit smoking but has gained 7 lb. Serum lipids are unchanged, and Mr. Mitchell admits he has not been as careful with his meals as the diet suggested. He asks that his wife be included in further counseling. The nurse sets up an appointment with the couple and suggests that Mr. Mitchell also enroll in the company's fitness program for more frequent monitoring. Mr. Mitchell agrees.

Two months later, Mr. Mitchell has lost 10 lb, has begun an exercise routine, and claims to be eating much better. Serum lipids are still unchanged, however, and the decision is made to start him on cholestyramine 4 g tid.

Discussion Questions

1. Mr. Mitchell has already made some major changes in his life-style to accommodate his cardiac risk factors. How is he likely to view the proposed drug therapy? How can the nurse help him to develop a positive outlook about its potential?
2. What laboratory data should be collected before starting Mr. Mitchell on cholestyramine?
3. What strategies can the nurse provide to assist Mr. Mitchell in planning meals which will reduce cholestyramine's side-effects? What dietary supplements might be included?
4. What are the major side-effects Mr. Mitchell should watch for?
5. How will Mr. Mitchell know if the drug is working? What will be his motivation to continue therapy for an extended period?

REVIEW QUESTIONS

1. Briefly describe the four major types of lipoproteins.
2. What are the principal characteristics of the following types of hyperlipoproteinemias:
   (a) type IIa   (b) type III   (c) type IV
3. What are the preferred drugs for treating the following types of hyperlipoproteinemias:
   (a) type IV   (b) type IIb   (c) type III   (d) type I
4. How do the bile sequestering resins lower plasma levels of cholesterol?
5. What is the most common side-effect noted with cholestyramine?
6. What types of plasma lipids are reduced by clofibrate?
7. Briefly describe the major hazards associated with use of clofibrate.
8. For what types of hyperlipoproteinemias is dextrothyroxine indicated?
9. List the most frequently noted side-effects with dextrothyroxine. What blood studies monitor some of these side-effects?
10. What are the indications for gemfibrozil? What other hypolipemic drug has similar actions?
11. In what conditions is gemfibrozil contraindicated?
12. How does lovastatin lower serum cholesterol?
13. What laboratory tests should be performed regularly in patients taking lovastatin?
14. Describe the effects of nicotinic acid on the various types of lipoproteins.
15. Outline the major actions of probucol on plasma lipids. What are the common side-effects associated with its use?
16. List several drugs that can lower elevated serum lipids but which are *not* used as hypolipemic agents due to the potential adverse consequences.
17. What baseline data must be collected before initiating drug therapy with any hypolipemic agents?
18. What dietary considerations are important during hypolipemic drug therapy?
19. What are some potential interventions for dealing with constipation as a result of drug therapy?

BIBLIOGRAPHY

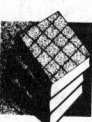

Blum CB, Levy RI: Rational drug therapy of the hyperlipoprotein-emias: Parts I and II, Ration Drug Ther 20(9); 20(10):1, 1986.

Connor WE, Connor SL: The dietary treatment of hyperlipidemia. Med Clin North Am 66:485, 1982

Dujovne CA, Block JE: Drug treatment of hyperlipidemia. Ration Drug Ther 18(6):1, 1984

Havel RJ: Approach to the patient with hyperlipidemia, Med Clin North Am 66:323, 1982

Havel RJ, Kane JP: Therapy of hyperlipidemic states. Annu Rev Med 33:417, 1982

Heel RC, Brogden RN, Pakes GE, Speight TM, Avery GS: Colestipol: A review of its pharmacological properties and therapeutic efficacy in patients with hypercholesterolemia. Drugs 19:161, 1980

Kane JP, Malloy HJ: Treatment of hypercholesterolemia. Med Clin North Am 66:537, 1982

Krauss R: Regulation of HDL levels. Med Clin North Am 66:417, 1982

Nursing update: Antilipemics. Nursing '84 14:57, 1984

Samuel P: Effects of gemfibrozil on serum lipids. Am J Med 74:23, 1983

Antianemic Drugs

38

The term *anemia* describes a group of clinical conditions characterized by a reduction in the number of erythrocytes (red blood cells) or in the hemoglobin concentration within erythrocytes, or both. Because oxygen is transported in the bloodstream primarily in combination with hemoglobin contained within the red blood cells, either condition will result in an impaired oxygen-carrying capacity of the blood and therefore inadequate tissue oxygenation.

Red cells are formed continually in the bone marrow by a complicated process known as *erythropoiesis*. Their synthesis requires many nutrients, of which the most important are iron, folic acid, and vitamin B_{12} (cyanocobalamin). These substances are usually present in sufficient amounts in the diet; if they are adequately absorbed from the gastrointestinal (GI) tract, erythrocyte formation and hemoglobin synthesis proceed normally. However, when the diet is deficient in any of these nutrients, when their GI absorption is impaired, or when they are destroyed too rapidly, symptoms of anemia develop. Anemia may also result from extreme loss or destruction of red blood cells due to such conditions as trauma, hemorrhage, or excessive menstruation, thereby increasing the nutritional requirements above the level that can be supplied by diet alone.

Although anemias can occur in a number of ways, such as through deficiency or impaired availability of dietary factors, excessive destruction or loss of red blood cells (*e.g.*, hemorrhage), or loss of bone marrow cells, most anemias are the result of inadequate availability of iron, folic acid, or vitamin B_{12}, and so they are considered deficiency anemias. Correction of the deficiency has proven highly successful in treating these conditions, if an accurate diagnosis of the type of anemia as well as any underlying causative factor (*e.g.*, ulcers, malignancy) has been made.

Microscopically, anemias may be categorized according to cell size and intensity of pigmentation.

Of the deficiency anemias, those that result from lack of iron and thus reduced synthesis of hemoglobin are characterized by fewer than normal erythrocytes, which are frequently smaller (microcytic) and paler (hypochromic) than usual because they contain less hemoglobin. These anemias are referred to as *microcytic* or *hypochromic* and are often marked by symptoms such as fatigue, weakness, dizziness, anorexia, and headache. Other hypochromic microcytic anemias result from failure to incorporate adequate iron into the develop-

ing cells, although an actual nutritional deficiency may not be present.

Anemias that occur because of insufficient levels of folic acid or vitamin B_{12} (*i.e.*, dietary deficiency, reduced absorption) are characterized by the presence of large, immature red cells (megaloblasts) in the bone marrow and blood, as well as enlarged erythrocytes (macrocytes) that may contain abnormally *high* levels of hemoglobin. These anemias are labeled *megaloblastic*, *macrocytic*, or *hyperchromic*.

Other types of anemias include *acute hemorrhagic anemia; aplastic anemia*, which is due to bone marrow damage; and *hemolytic anemia*, which is due to destruction of circulating red cells. The latter two anemias are usually the result of drug toxicity and are discussed in Chapter 6.

It should be noted that hypochromic and hyperchromic anemias seldom occur together, underlining the importance of accurate diagnosis for proper replacement therapy. Likewise, carefully differentiating those anemias caused by nutritional iron deficiency from those caused by failure of iron incorporation into red blood cells is essential, because supplemental iron in the latter case is not only ineffective but can result in iron overload (hemochromatosis) and subsequent toxicity. The "shotgun" approach of combining many factors (*e.g.*, iron, B_{12}, folic acid) in treating anemias has no place in clinical medicine, and should never be used in lieu of careful diagnosis and selective replacement of the deficient factor, as well as correction of any underlying pathologic disorder.

The antianemic drugs to be discussed in this chapter include the iron preparations, folic acid, and vitamin B_{12}. In addition to these agents, therapy may also include other drugs and measures to correct any underlying abnormality that may be responsible for the anemia. Self-medication with any of the antianemic drugs should be strongly discouraged, because the apparent beneficial effects gained by treating oneself often may mask the symptoms of a more serious underlying disorder (*e.g.*, internal bleeding, neurologic dysfunction).

Body Iron

Iron is an essential mineral that is widely distributed in the body. Approximately 70% of the total body iron content is in the form of hemoglobin in the red blood cells. Between 10% to 20% of body iron is contained in a storage form, as either ferritin or hemosiderin (see below). Myoglobin, a muscle protein, contains about 10% of the total iron in the body, and the remainder is distributed primarily among other enzymes.

The average diet supplies between 15 mg and 20 mg of elemental iron a day. Since much of the iron in red blood cells is reutilizable, only a very small amount of iron must be absorbed from the diet to maintain sufficient body iron concentrations. Normal (*i.e., non* iron-deficient) persons absorb only about 5% to 10% of the iron available in the diet or between 0.5 mg and 1.0 mg a day, which is an adequate amount to meet the needs of most individuals. However, iron absorption is increased in the presence of lowered body iron stores or increased iron requirements, such as during menstruation, pregnancy, periods of rapid growth, or disease.

Iron is primarily absorbed from the duodenum and upper jejunum by an active transport mechanism. Absorption can be increased by the presence of hydrochloric acid and vitamin C, and reduced by the presence of chelators or complexing agents in the intestines. The ferrous form of iron (*i.e.,* Fe^{+2}) is much more efficiently absorbed than the ferric form (*i.e.,* Fe^{+3}), and the presence of hydrochloric acid favors conversion of ferric iron to ferrous iron in the lumen of the intestine. Once in the gastric mucosal cell, the newly absorbed iron can be converted back to the ferric state and combined with *transferrin*, a beta-globulin that transports iron from the mucosal cell to the bone marrow cells. Transferrin also transports iron in the plasma from storage sites in the liver and spleen to erythroid cells in the bone marrow.

Absorbed iron can also be converted to *ferritin* or *hemosiderin*, two storage forms of iron, which are found in the liver, spleen, and bone marrow. Ferritin is also present in intestinal mucosal cells and in plasma. Iron stored as either ferritin or hemosiderin can readily be mobilized for use in synthesizing hemoglobin.

Although *small* quantities of iron are excreted in the feces (from loss of intestinal mucosal cells), urine, and sweat, generally no more than 1 mg of iron is lost daily. It is evident, then, that regulation of body iron levels must be accomplished by critical adjustment of the *rate* and *extent* of *absorption.* Factors regulating iron absorption include the amount of storage iron present, especially as ferritin in intestinal mucosal cells, and the rate of synthesis of red blood cells. For example, in iron-deficiency states, levels of transferrin are elevated and ferritin levels are decreased, conditions that promote increased absorption of iron from the intestinal tract.

Indications for Supplemental Iron

The primary use of supplemental iron is the prevention or treatment of iron-deficiency anemia. The most common cause of iron deficiency in adults is blood loss. Heavy or abnormally frequent menstruation is a major cause of temporary iron deficiency, and up to four times the normal loss of iron can occur during menses. Women who display signs of anemia should be evaluated for excessive iron loss during menstruation. Blood loss can also result from GI bleeding, which may be unrecognized (*i.e.,* occult) for long periods of time. Occult GI bleeding must always be considered as a cause of unexplained iron-deficiency anemia, and careful evaluation is necessary to rule out a more serious underlying disorder, such as GI carcinoma or peptic ulcers.

Iron-deficiency states can also occur in infants (especially premature infants), in young children during periods of rapid growth, and in pregnant and lactating women. Supplemental iron is frequently given during these periods in the growth and reproductive cycle to meet the increased need.

Oral Iron Preparations

Ferrous Fumarate, Ferrous Gluconate, Ferrous Sulfate, Polysaccharide–Iron Complex

Various preparations containing iron (capsules, tablets, liquids, injections) are used as replacement therapy in iron-deficiency anemias. The oral forms of therapy are preferred; parenteral administration of iron is largely restricted to those persons who cannot tolerate oral iron because of its gastric irritative action, those who do not absorb sufficient iron from the GI tract, or those who are noncompliant. Oral iron is available in either the bivalent (ferrous) or trivalent (ferric) forms; bivalent iron is more widely used because it is better absorbed and somewhat less irritating than the trivalent form. An acid environment favors reduction of trivalent to bivalent iron, which increases absorption. GI distress can be reduced by using one of the iron complexes or sustained-release forms, but the absorption of elemental iron may be retarded with use of these specialized dosage forms, because much of their iron content may be released beyond the major iron-absorptive sites in the duodenum and jejunum.

The oral iron preparations are essentially alike in terms of their pharmacologic action, because they all release elemental iron, and therefore are reviewed as a group. Individual salts and dosage forms are listed in Table 38-1. The parenteral iron preparation, iron dextran, is also discussed in detail.

MECHANISM AND ACTIONS
Iron is an essential component of hemoglobin, since it forms the nucleus of the iron–porphyrin ring heme, which is combined with globin chains to form hemoglobin. Oxygen is transported from the lungs to other body tissues bound to hemoglobin in a reversible state. Thus, iron is necessary to provide a sufficient quantity of hemoglobin to supply the oxygen needs of body tissues.

USES
1. Prevention and treatment of iron-deficiency anemias
2. Prophylactic therapy during periods of increased iron requirements (*e.g.,* pregnancy, rapid growth, and sustained hemorrhaging)

ADMINISTRATION AND DOSAGE
See Table 38-1.

Table 38-1
Oral Iron Preparations

Drug	Preparations	Usual Dosage Range	Clinical Considerations
ferrous fumarate (Femiron, Feostat, Fumasorb, Fumerin, Hemocyte, Ircon, Palmiron, Span-FF)	Tablets—63 mg, 195 mg, 200 mg, 300 mg, 324 mg, 325 mg Chewable tablets—100 mg Suspension—100 mg/5 ml Drops—45 mg/0.6 ml Controlled-release capsules—325 mg	Adults—200 mg–300 mg 1 to 3 times/day Children (under 6)—100 mg–300 mg/day in divided doses	Contains 33% elemental iron; essentially similar to ferrous sulfate in most respects, with slightly lower incidence of some GI side-effects; available in combination with docusate as timed-release capsules (Ferocyl, Ferro-Sequels)
ferrous gluconate (Fergon, Ferralet, Simron)	Tablets—300 mg, 320 mg, 325 mg Capsules—86 mg, 325 mg, 435 mg Elixir—300 mg/5 ml	Adults—300 mg–650 mg 3 times/day Children (6 yr–12 yr)—300 mg 1 to 3 times/day Children (under 6 yr)—100 mg–300 mg/day in divided doses	Contains 11.6% elemental iron; somewhat better tolerated and better utilized than other forms of iron; lower incidence of GI distress
ferrous sulfate (Feosol, Fer-In-Sol, Fer-Iron, Ferralyn, Fero-Gradumet, Ferospace, Mol-Iron, Slow FE)	Tablets—195 mg, 200 mg, 300 mg, 325 mg Timed-release capsules—150 mg, 160 mg, 250 mg Timed-release tablets—160 mg, 525 mg Syrup—90 mg/5 ml Elixir—220 mg/5 ml Drops—75 mg/0.6 ml, 125 mg/ml	Adults—300 mg–1200 mg/day in divided doses Children (6 yr–12 yr)—120 mg–600 mg/day in divided doses Children (under 6 yr)—300 mg/day in divided doses	Contains 20% elemental iron; most widely used form of oral iron; best absorbed and least expensive; high degree of GI irritation that can be minimized by using sustained-release forms; available in combination with magnesium–aluminum hydroxide as Fermalox
polysaccharide–iron complex (Hytinic, Niferex, Nu-Iron)	Tablets—50 mg iron Capsules—150 mg iron Elixir—100 mg iron/5 ml	Adults—50 mg–300 mg/day in divided doses as required Children—50 mg–100 mg/day	Water-soluble complex of elemental iron and a low-molecular-weight polysaccharide; fewer GI side-effects than with other forms of iron, no teeth staining, and no metallic aftertaste; fairly expensive

FATE

Absorption occurs primarily from the duodenum and jejunum. Only 5% to 10% of a dose is absorbed when body iron stores are normal; up to 20% may be absorbed in iron-deficient persons. Ferrous iron (*i.e.*, Fe^{+2}) is much more efficiently absorbed than ferric iron (*i.e.*, Fe^{+3}). Bivalent iron is then converted to trivalent iron in gastric mucosal cells and then either combined with transferrin for transport to bone marrow cells or converted to ferritin or hemosiderin and stored either in gastric mucosal cells, liver, spleen, or bone marrow. Excretion of iron is minimal (generally less than 1 mg a day) and occurs mainly in feces through sloughing of iron-containing intestinal mucosal cells. Very small amounts of iron may also be eliminated in the urine and sweat.

SIDE-EFFECTS/ADVERSE REACTIONS

Oral iron preparations may cause GI irritation, nausea, constipation, and darkened stools. Iron-containing liquids can temporarily stain the teeth. Large amounts of iron may result in vomiting, diarrhea, lethargy, weak pulse, tachycardia, hypotension, stomach and intestinal erosion, convulsions, and shock.

CONTRAINDICATIONS AND PRECAUTIONS

Iron supplementation is contraindicated in persons with peptic ulcer, ulcerative colitis, regional enteritis, hemochromatosis, hemosiderosis, or hemolytic anemia. Persons with normal iron levels should not take supplemental iron chronically.

INTERACTIONS

1. Intestinal absorption of iron may be impaired by antacids (especially those containing magnesium trisilicate), cholestyramine, or pancreatic extracts, as well as by ingestion of eggs, milk, coffee, or tea.
2. Oral iron retards absorption of tetracyclines and penicillamine.
3. Effectiveness of iron may be impaired by vitamin E, hydroxyurea, and oral contraceptives.
4. Vitamin C may facilitate iron absorption by maintaining it in the ferrous state.
5. Chloramphenicol can delay clearance of iron from the plasma and its incorporation into red blood cells.
6. Allopurinol may interfere with the action of an enzyme that controls iron absorption, leading to excessive absorption.

■ Nursing Process

☐ ASSESSMENT

☐ Subjective Data

A brief drug history is appropriate to determine if the individual takes a vitamin supplement. Self-dosing with vitamins containing iron in addition to prescribed iron may produce toxicity. The patient should be aware of the potential danger and advised to take an alternate vitamin if desired. A drug history can also reveal if the patient is currently taking any drugs that are potentially iron depleting, such as quinidine, sulfonamides, or anti-inflammatory agents, or agents that may impair iron absorption such as antacids.

☐ Objective Data

A hemoglobin, hematocrit, and reticulocyte blood count should be performed in order to establish the need for iron supplement. In some people, it may be appropriate to obtain ferritin levels in order to determine the amount of stored iron ready for use by the body. Some physicians consider this level a more reliable test than hemoglobin in determining iron needs.

☐ NURSING DIAGNOSES

Actual nursing diagnoses for the patient taking an iron compound include
    Knowledge deficit related to the action, administration, and side-effects of the drug
Potential nursing diagnoses may include
    Alteration in bowel function: constipation
    Alteration in nutrition: less than body requirements related to poor iron absorption

☐ PLAN

Nursing care goals focus on helping the patient
1. Improve his blood picture and decrease symptoms of iron deficiency through correct drug-taking techniques
2. Minimize drug side-effects

☐ INTERVENTION

The patient's blood picture will improve if adequate iron can be absorbed. Several dietary strategies can facilitate this process. Since ascorbic acid (vitamin C) enhances iron absorption some patients will do well by taking the drug with a citrus juice or by taking an iron preparation that has ascorbic acid as an added ingredient. Taking iron on an empty stomach also facilitates rapid absorption. The patient should be advised not to take the drug with calcium-containing foods or drugs that will bind to it and decrease absorption. Even with a well-absorbed iron supplement, the patient needs to include iron-rich foods in his diet. These include liver, dark molasses, egg yolk, whole grains, legumes, dark green leafy vegetables, raisins, prunes, brewer's yeast, and nuts.

Unfortunately, in some patients rapid absorption of iron results in nausea, vomiting, and abdominal cramping. If this occurs, the patient should be advised to take the drug with meals but continue to avoid mixing iron with calcium foods. If the gastrointestinal symptoms do not subside, another form of iron compound should be tried.

Constipation is another bothersome side-effect of iron. If the patient consumes the iron-rich foods listed earlier he will add needed bulk and suffer fewer problems. He should also drink at least 6 glasses of water a day. If constipation continues to be a problem a mild vegetable-base laxative or stool softener can be used. However, these should be avoided if possible since they tend to decrease drug absorption.

Blood levels should be drawn intermittently to monitor progress. If hemoglobin levels do not rise after several weeks, ferritin levels may need to be drawn. If ferritin levels are normal (women 20 ng–120 ng/ml; men 30 ng–200 ng/ml) the iron is working. Hemoglobin and hematocrit may not rise, especially in cases of hemodilution, such as during pregnancy, until delivery occurs.

Iron compounds can stain teeth. Adults should take liquid forms through a straw and rinse the mouth immediately after ingestion. Infants should be given iron drops in the buccal pouch of the mouth. Their teeth can be wiped with a moist cloth to prevent staining. Iron will also cause green or black stools. Any patient receiving the compound should know this so he is not fearful that he has blood in his stool.

□ EVALUATION
Useful outcome criteria may be an improved blood picture, although as mentioned earlier this may not change during pregnancy. The patient may also report an increase in energy, increased exercise tolerance, and alertness.

■ NURSING ALERT
Keep iron tablets out of reach of children. Ingestion can result in fatal toxicity. If you suspect a child of ingesting iron tablets, seek help immediately.

Parenteral Iron Preparation

Iron Dextran
(Imferon and Various Other Manufacturers)

Iron dextran is a complex of ferric hydroxide with dextran in physiologic saline containing 50 mg of iron per milliliter of solution. It is used either IV or IM for treating iron-deficiency anemias in patients intolerant of or resistant to oral iron preparations.

MECHANISM AND ACTIONS
Hydrolysis of the iron–dextran complex following phagocytosis by reticuloendothelial cells of liver, spleen, and bone marrow releases ferric iron, which combines with transferrin and is transported to the bone marrow to be used in the synthesis of hemoglobin. Some of the iron is rapidly returned to the plasma and made available for erythropoiesis. Most of the iron, however, remains confined within the reticuloendothelial cells and is gradually converted to a utilizable form of iron.

USES
1. Treatment of iron-deficiency anemias in patients where oral iron administration is ineffective or poorly tolerated

ADMINISTRATION AND DOSAGE
Iron dextran is available as an injection solution containing 50 mg of elemental iron per milliliter.

To determine the approximate quantity of iron needed to restore the hemoglobin to normal, the following formula may be used:

$$0.3 \times \text{wt (lb)} \times \left(100 - \frac{\text{Hb (g\%)} \times 100}{14.8}\right) = \text{mg iron}$$

A more practical rule is 250 mg iron for each gram of hemoglobin below normal. *Recommended* procedures for administration are as follows:

IM—Test dose of 25 mg (*i.e.*, 0.5 ml) on first day to test for allergic reactions; if no evidence of hypersensitivity within 1 hour to 2 hours, the remainder of the first day's dose can be given. Each day's dose should not exceed 25 mg iron for infants under 10 lb, 50 mg iron for children under 20 lb, 100 mg iron for patients under 110 lb, and 250 mg iron for other patients until the calculated total dose has been given.

Clinical considerations for IM administration —For adults, intramuscular injections of iron dextran should be given in the upper outer quadrant of the buttocks using a large-gauge needle (19–20 gauge; 2–3 inches long) and the Z-track method of injection (see Chap. 8). No more than 5 ml should be injected in each injection site and buttock sites should be rotated with each dose. Injection of this medication is very painful and can cause abscess formation. Periodic assessment should be done, watching for pain and swelling. An injection should *never* be given in a site that feels hard or lumpy or that causes pain. If the buttock site is no longer usable, an alternate route of drug administration must be sought.

IV infusion—Dilute the calculated iron dose in 200 ml to 250 ml of normal saline. Administer a test dose of 25 mg over 5 minutes; if no adverse effects occur, infuse the rest of the dose over 1 hour to 2 hours.

Clinical considerations for IV administration —Use only single-dose vials when administering iron dextran intravenously since multiple-dose vials (for IM administration) contain a phenol preservative. Do not mix other drugs with iron dextran in the same IV line.

Note: IV infusion of iron dextran is *not* an FDA-approved method of administration, but it is widely used because it eliminates the need for multiple IM injections, pain and skin staining at the IM injection site, danger of abscess formation, and the possibility of poor absorption from muscle. It is used in patients who have poor IM absorptive capacity or uncontrolled bleeding, or where prolonged therapy is indicated.

■ *WARNING*
Oral iron should be discontinued prior to IM or IV administration of iron dextran to prevent iron overload.

FATE
The elemental iron in iron dextran is slowly but well absorbed from IM injection sites (60% within 2 days–3 days and 90% within 1 week–2 weeks). The iron is distributed through the reticuloendothelial system and slowly excreted in urine, bile, and feces.

SIDE-EFFECTS/ADVERSE REACTIONS
IM administration frequently results in soreness or tenderness at the site of injection. Too-rapid IV injection is often associated with flushing and dizziness. This can be minimized by keeping the patient recumbent for 30 minutes to 60 minutes after the drug is given. Local phlebitis at the injection site and lymphadenopathy have also occurred with IV administration. A variety of hypersensitivity reactions can occur with iron dextran administration, including rash, itching, fever, sweating, urticaria, dyspnea, myalgia, arthralgia, and anaphylactic shock. Other adverse effects reported with use of iron dextran are headache, backache, malaise, paresthesia, shivering, vomiting, hypotension, convulsions, and leukocytosis.

CONTRAINDICATIONS AND PRECAUTIONS
Iron dextran is contraindicated in anemias other than iron-deficiency anemias. It should be used with extreme *caution* in patients with liver dysfunction, rheumatoid arthritis, a history of allergies, or bronchial asthma, and in pregnant women or women of childbearing potential. Vials of iron dextran for IM use contain 0.5% phenol, a preservative, and should not be used for IV administration.

INTERACTIONS
1. Chloramphenicol may delay or reduce the response to iron dextran.

Vitamin B₁₂ and Folic Acid

Vitamin B_{12} and folic acid are two vitamins essential for normal deoxyribonucleic acid (DNA) synthesis. A deficiency of either can result in impaired DNA synthesis, inhibition of normal cell division, and anemia.

Vitamin B₁₂

Cyanocobalamin, Crystalline
(Betalin 12, Redisol, Rubramin PC, and Others)

Cyanocobalamin (vitamin B_{12}) is a cobalt-containing substance essential for normal growth, cell reproduction, hematopoiesis, and nucleoprotein and myelin synthesis. It is a biologically potent compound, so only minute amounts (1 mcg–2 mcg) are necessary in the daily diet to supply the normal body needs. Since the average diet supplies between 5 mcg to 15 mcg of vitamin B_{12} per day, the most common cause of vitamin B_{12} deficiency is insufficient GI absorption, due primarily to reduced availability of calcium and the intrinsic factor, a glycoprotein secreted by the gastric mucosal cells that is necessary for adequate absorption of B_{12}. This condition is referred to as *pernicious anemia* and is characterized hematologically by megaloblasts in the bone marrow and macrocytes in the plasma. The patient feels fatigued, and frequently there are GI and neurologic complications. Symptoms are usually readily reversed by supplemental injections of crystalline cyanocobalamin.

Cyanocobalamin is available over the counter for oral use as tablets and by prescription for IM or SC injection. Tablets containing less than 500 mcg are not intended for treatment of pernicious anemia, but should only be used as nutritional supplements (see Chap. 76).

MECHANISM AND ACTIONS
Cyanocobalamin activates folic acid coenzymes necessary for the synthesis of red blood cells, and facilitates the maturation of megaloblasts into normal erythrocytes. In vitamin B_{12} deficiency states, cyanocobalamin improves GI function; relieves neurologic symptoms such as numbness, tingling, and incoordination; and arrests further neurologic damage.

USES
1. Treatment of vitamin B_{12} deficiency states caused by impaired GI absorption (*e.g.*, pernicious anemia, GI dysfunction or surgery, tapeworm infestation, sprue)
2. Prevention of vitamin B_{12} deficiency resulting from increased requirements (*e.g.*, pregnancy, hemorrhage, malignancy, or thyroid, liver, or renal disease) or inadequate dietary intake (*e.g.*, poverty, famine, alcoholism, vegetarian diet)
3. Performance of the vitamin B_{12} absorption test (Schilling test)
4. Treatment of nutritional vitamin B_{12} deficiency (oral doses of less than 500 mcg; see Chap. 76)

ADMINISTRATION AND DOSAGE
For treating vitamin B_{12} deficiency states, cyanocobalamin is used orally as tablets (500 mcg, 1000 mcg) or by intramuscular or subcutaneous injection (30 mcg/ml, 100 mcg/ml, 1000 mcg/ml). The route of administration and duration of therapy are dependent on the cause and severity of the deficiency state.

Initial therapy in most deficiency states is 30 mcg to 100 mcg daily IM or SC for 5 days to 10 days, then on alternate days for 7 doses, then every 3 days to 4 days for 2 weeks to 3 weeks. This is followed by 100 mcg to 200 mcg monthly. More seriously ill patients may require considerably higher doses (*e.g.*, 1000 mcg/day) or more frequent administration (*e.g.*, every week for 6 months). Folic acid should be given in conjunction with vitamin B_{12} unless body levels are sufficient.

Although injection is the preferred route of administration in most cases of vitamin B_{12} deficiency, oral doses of 1000 mcg daily may be used in patients unwilling to have the injection or intolerant of the injection, provided the intestinal absorptive mechanism is not seriously impaired.

Although the safety and efficacy of vitamin B_{12} for use in children have not been established, amounts in the range of 0.5 mcg to 3 mcg a day have been recommended as safe when required.

Diminished absorptive capacity of vitamin B_{12} may be ascertained by the Schilling test. A dose of 1000 mcg is given IM 2 hours after an oral dose of radioactive cobalt–B_{12} (0.5 mcg–1 mcg). Urine is collected for 24 hours and radioactivity is measured; impaired absorption is indicated by less than 5% urinary excretion of vitamin B_{12} (normal is 10%–30%).

Again, it should be stressed that oral doses of vitamin B_{12} less than 500 mcg are *not* indicated for treatment of vitamin B_{12} deficiency states, but should only be used as nutritional supplements. Refer to Chapter 76 for a review of vitamin B_{12} as a supplement to normal nutritional needs.

FATE
Intestinal absorption of vitamin B_{12} is dependent on the availability of sufficient intrinsic factor and calcium. Intrinsic factor is a glycoprotein secreted by the parietal cells of the gastric mucosa and combines with vitamin B_{12} liberated from dietary sources in the intestines.

The vitamin B_{12}–intrinsic factor complex is transported through cells of the distal ileum by a specific receptor-mediated transport system. Absorption from intramuscular or subcutaneous sites is rapid and the plasma level peaks within 1 hour. Once absorbed, vitamin B_{12} is transported bound to a plasma glycoprotein, transcobalamin II. Vitamin B_{12} is stored mainly in the liver and slowly released as needed for cellular metabolism. The average adult stores 2500 mg to 5000 mg in the liver; therefore, a deficiency state only develops after considerable time in the absence of supplemental B_{12}. Only trace amounts (2 mcg–5 mcg) are normally lost in the urine and feces; however, when administered in large doses, 50% to 98% of the dose appears in the urine within 48 hours, mostly within the first 8 hours.

SIDE-EFFECTS/ADVERSE REACTIONS

Vitamin B_{12} injections are occasionally associated with diarrhea, itching, and flushing. Other adverse reactions that have occurred during parenteral administration of vitamin B_{12} include urticaria, pain at the injection site, hypokalemia, peripheral vascular thrombosis, pulmonary edema, congestive heart failure, polycythemia vera, optic nerve atrophy, and anaphylactic shock.

CONTRAINDICATIONS AND PRECAUTIONS

Vitamin B_{12} should not be given to persons with cobalt hypersensitivity or optic nerve atrophy. The response to vitamin B_{12} may be blunted in persons with infections, uremia, iron or folic acid deficiency, or bone marrow depression. Potassium levels must be monitored, since conversion of megaloblastic anemia to normal can increase erythrocyte potassium requirements, lowering serum potassium. Polycythemia vera can be "unmasked" by vitamin B_{12} treatment, since vitamin B_{12} deficiency suppresses signs of polycythemia. Folic acid (see below) is *not* a substitute for vitamin B_{12}, since folic acid may prevent anemia but will *not* arrest progression of neurologic deficit.

INTERACTIONS

1. GI absorption of vitamin B_{12} may be impaired by alcohol, p-aminosalicylic acid, colchicine, neomycin, and potassium chloride.
2. Chloramphenicol may impair the beneficial therapeutic response to vitamin B_{12}, since it can suppress erythrocyte maturation in bone marrow cells.

NURSING CONSIDERATIONS

Oral vitamin B_{12} should be taken with meals since food stimulates production of the intrinsic factor and enhances absorption. However, the patient should be cautioned *not* to take the drug with citrus fruits or juices because ascorbic acid will adversely affect vitamin B_{12} stability.

The patient with pernicious anemia needs to understand that he will need to take vitamin B_{12} for life and will need periodic medical follow-up to monitor his progress even when he is feeling well. His need for the drug may change over time, especially if he develops an infection. This should be reported immediately. In addition, he should also report fatigue or increase in neurologic or GI symptoms as this may indicate a need for more of the drug.

Since vitamin B_{12} can result in hypokalemia as the erythrocyte count increases, the patient should be taught the signs of this problem (muscle weakness, cramping, fatigue, or palpitations) and be told to seek help immediately should they occur. He can help prevent the problem by including potassium-rich foods such as bananas, apricots, and oranges in his diet, but, again, he must avoid taking citrus with vitamin B_{12}.

Hydroxocobalamin, Crystalline
(AlphaRedisol and Others)

Hydroxocobalamin is a structural analog of cyanocobalamin in which a hydroxyl radical replaces the cyano radical. It functions similarly to cyanocobalamin in promoting hematopoiesis but is more slowly absorbed than cyanocobalamin, resulting in a more sustained rise in serum cobalamin levels and less urinary excretion of cobalamin following each injection. In addition, hydroxocobalamin may be taken up by the liver in larger quantities than cyanocobalamin.

Hydroxocobalamin is used for the same indications as cyanocobalamin and is preferred by some because it remains in the circulation longer. In addition, hydroxocobalamin has been utilized to treat cyanide toxicity, such as that associated with excessive doses of sodium nitroprusside (see Chap. 35). It can combine with cyanide to yield cyanocobalamin, which is nontoxic and readily excreted in the urine.

The drug is available as an injection containing 1000 mcg/ml. The recommended IM dosage of hydroxocobalamin is 30 mcg/day for 5 days to 10 days, followed by 100 mcg to 200 mcg once a month. Children may be given up to 5 mg over several weeks in doses of 100 mcg, then 30 mcg to 50 mcg once a month. Folic acid may be given concurrently early in treatment if necessary.

Side-effects are similar to those reported above for cyanocobalamin. Mild pain and irritation occur frequently at the injection site.

Folic Acid
(Folvite)

Folic acid, otherwise known as pteroylglutamic acid, folate, or vitamin B_9, is a member of the B-complex vitamin group and is essential for synthesis of nucleoproteins and maintenance of normal erythrocyte production. Folic acid stimulates production of red and white blood cells as well as platelets in megaloblastic anemias.

Dietary folic acid is present in foods predominantly as reduced folate polyglutamate. It undergoes a series of metabolic biotransformations in the GI tract prior to absorption and is then ultimately converted to tetrahydrofolic acid, which functions as a coenzyme in many reactions, especially the synthesis of purine and pyrimidine precursors of nucleic acids. Since folic acid is available in many different foods (e.g., vegetables, milk, eggs, liver), deficiencies rarely occur. Most likely causes of deficiency are malnutrition, greatly increased demands (e.g., repeated pregnancy), and malabsorption syndromes such as sprue or celiac disease. Patients lacking sufficient folic acid usually develop a megaloblastic anemia similar to that observed in pernicious anemia, although the incidence of neurologic damage is much less than the damage observed in cases of vitamin B_{12} deficiency. Oral or parenteral administration of folic acid readily corrects the anemia, both symptomatically and hematologically, and improvement can be maintained with very small daily doses of folic acid.

MECHANISM AND ACTIONS
Folic acid is converted to tetrahydrofolic acid, which is essential for normal synthesis of purines and pyrimidines, and ultimately nucleic acids. A deficiency of folic acid impairs production of bone marrow blood cell precursors. Symptoms of folic acid deficiency resemble those of vitamin B_{12} deficiency, except that neurologic abnormalities are usually *not* present in folic acid–deficient states.

USES
1. Treatment of megaloblastic anemia due to a deficiency of folic acid, for example, those due to sprue, malnutrition, alcoholism, pregnancy, infancy, or childhood

ADMINISTRATION AND DOSAGE
Folic acid is available as tablets (0.1 mg, 0.4 mg, 0.8 mg, 1 mg) and injection (5 mg/ml, 10 mg/ml). The drug is usually given orally (except in the presence of severe malabsorption) but may be administered intramuscularly, subcutaneously, or intravenously if the disease is severe or GI absorption is severely compromised.

The initial oral dosage can be up to 1 mg/day until the clinical symptoms have subsided and the blood picture returns to normal. The recommended oral maintenance dosages are as follow:

Adults/children over 4—0.4 mg/day
Children under 4—0.1 mg to 0.3 mg/day
Infants—0.1 mg/day
Pregnant/lactating women—0.8 mg/day

IV injection may be given over 1 minute using a 100-mcg/ml solution (5 mg folic acid [1 ml] in 49 ml of sterile water for injection). IV infusion can also be performed using most fluids; however, folic acid should not be mixed with calcium or a heavy metal salt.

FATE
Folic acid is well absorbed orally and widely distributed in the body. It is stored in the liver and is excreted in both the urine and feces. Serum levels fall within a few days when intake is reduced, and megaloblastic anemia can develop within a few months after intake ceases. Folic acid is excreted in breast milk.

SIDE-EFFECTS/ADVERSE REACTIONS
Side-effects are infrequent, especially with oral use. Allergic reactions, GI distress, irritability, and depression have been reported in persons taking folic acid. Flushing has occurred following IV injection and anaphylactic reactions have been reported.

CONTRAINDICATIONS AND PRECAUTIONS
Folic acid should not be used in pernicious, aplastic, or normocytic anemias. Doses greater than 0.1 mg/day may mask the signs of pernicious anemia. Suspected pernicious anemia should be ruled out prior to folic acid therapy by the Schilling test and vitamin B_{12} plasma level determination. Although the hematologic picture in pernicious anemia may improve with folic acid therapy, irreversible neurologic damage can ensue. The effectiveness of folic acid can be reduced by alcoholism, antimetabolite drug therapy, and a deficiency of vitamins B_6, B_{12}, C, and E.

INTERACTIONS
1. The effects of folic acid may be decreased by para-aminosalicylic acid, chloramphenicol, oral contraceptives, phenytoin, primidone, and sulfasalazine.
2. Folic acid may reduce phenytoin blood levels by increasing its metabolic clearance, requiring an increase in dosage.
3. Trimethoprim, triamterene, and pyrimethamine may interfere with utilization of folic acid by causing a deficiency in dihydrofolate reductase activity.

Leucovorin Calcium

(Wellcovorin)

Leucovorin (folinic acid) is a formyl reduction product of folic acid that may be used IM to treat folate-deficient megaloblastic anemia when oral folic acid therapy is not feasible. The drug is also indicated for "leucovorin rescue," that is, to minimize the cellular toxicity resulting from large doses of methotrexate used in certain neoplastic diseases. Leucovorin prevents severe methotrexate-induced toxicity by preferentially protecting or "rescuing" normal cells from the action of folic acid antagonists such as methotrexate without interfering with the desired oncolytic action of the drug. This cellular protective function is considered further in Chapter 75.

Leucovorin is available as tablets (5 mg, 25 mg), powder for oral solution (1 mg/ml after reconstitution), solution for injection (3 mg/ml, 5 mg/ml), and powder for injection (10 mg/ml after reconstitution). In treating megaloblastic anemia, leucovorin is administered IM in a dose of 1 mg/day. It should not be used in anemias secondary to a vitamin B_{12} deficiency, because the hematologic picture may improve, while the neurologic deficit continues to accrue. Allergic reactions represent the principal group of adverse reactions. Potential drug interactions are those listed above for folic acid.

REVIEW QUESTIONS

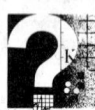

1. List several occurrences that can result in development of anemia.
2. Distinguish between anemias that result from lack of iron and those that result from lack of folic acid or vitamin B_{12}.
3. In what forms is iron found in the body?
4. Briefly outline the mechanisms involved in the absorption of iron from the GI tract.
5. What is the major process that regulates body levels of iron? Explain.
6. List several reasons for development of an iron-deficiency state.
7. In what forms is iron used orally?
8. What laboratory values can be used to determine the effectiveness of iron therapy?
9. What dietary guidelines should a patient be given when iron is prescribed? Name several that will enhance absorption and minimize gastrointestinal distress.
10. List the steps necessary to administer iron dextran safely intramuscularly and intravenously.
11. What are the major untoward reactions associated with injection of iron dextran?
12. What is pernicious anemia?
13. What substances are necessary for adequate intestinal absorption of vitamin B_{12}?
14. Why might hydroxocobalamin be preferred over cyanocobalamin?
15. How do symptoms of folic acid deficiency differ from those of vitamin B_{12} deficiency?
16. Why is folic acid contraindicated in pernicious anemia due to vitamin B_{12} deficiency?
17. What are the indications for leucovorin calcium?
18. What should patients be taught about self-medication with any of the drugs listed in this chapter?

BIBLIOGRAPHY

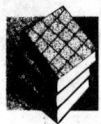

Callander ST: Treatment of iron deficiency. Clin Haematol 11:327, 1982

Chanarin I (ed): The Megaloblastic Anemias. Oxford, Blackwell Scientific Publications, 1979

Cook JD: Clinical evaluation of iron deficiency. Semin Hematol 19(1):6, 1982

Cooper BA: Megaloblastic anemia. Drug Ther 14(4):65, 1984

Hallberg L: Bioavailability of dietary iron in man. Annu Rev Nutr 1:123, 1981

Hoffbrand AV, Wickremasinghe RG: Megaloblastic anemia. In Hoffbrand AV (ed): Recent Advances in Hematology, p 25. Edinburgh, Churchill-Livingstone, 1982

Huebers H, Huebers E, Csiba E et al: The significance of transferrin for intestinal iron absorption. Blood 61:283, 1983

Lee GR: The anemia of chronic disease. Semin Hematol 20:61, 1983

Pollit E, Leibel RL (eds): Iron Deficiency: Brain Biochemistry and Behavior. New York, Raven Press, 1982

Siegel RS, Lessin LS: The hemolytic anemias: Guidelines to rational management. Drug Ther 14(4):87, 1984

Anticoagulants

39

Drugs capable of inhibiting the clotting process of blood are known as *anticoagulants*. Clotting of blood normally serves a protective function against excessive blood loss following an insult or injury. However, abnormalities in the hemostatic mechanisms can lead to development of intravascular thrombi, that is, blood clots within the blood vessels that may reduce or obstruct normal vascular flow. Fragmentation of thrombi may result in the formation of emboli, that is, clot fragments that can travel through the vessels and become lodged in smaller arteries or veins, obstructing blood flow to tissues and organs. These conditions, termed *thromboembolic disorders*, are responsible for considerable morbidity and mortality, and prevention of thromboembolic episodes is a major indication for anticoagulant drugs.

Hemostasis, that is, prevention of bleeding, is an extremely complex process involving reactions of the vasculature, blood proteins, and platelets. A brief review of the hemostatic process will be presented prior to the discussion of anticoagulant drug therapy. The following presentation of blood-clotting mechanisms is not intended to be an in-depth treatise of this complex phenomenon. Interested readers should consult more specific references for a detailed account of hemostatic mechanisms.

Basic Concepts of Hemostatic Mechanisms

While flowing freely through the vascular system, blood remains in the liquid state but may begin to solidify (clot) upon encountering a disturbance to flow, such as an injury or obstruction. Hemostasis is achieved through several mechanisms, involving the vessel, platelets, and blood proteins.

Immediately upon injury to a blood vessel, reflex vasoconstriction occurs, which limits the loss of blood from the ruptured vessel, although this vasoconstriction is probably of little consequence in the hemostatic response. More importantly, blood vessel injury results in an interruption in the continuity of the smooth endothelial lining of the vessel, and blood is exposed to the collagen under the epithelial lining. Platelets begin to adhere to the exposed collagen and undergo a "release reaction" in which adenosine diphosphate (ADP) is secreted. This facilitates further adhesion of more platelets. Other substances, including serotonin, are also released and act as local vasoconstrictors. Arachi-

donic acid, which is formed from membrane phospholipids by phospholipase (see Fig. 82-1), is subsequently converted to two prostaglandin endoperoxides, PGG_2 and PGH_2. In the platelet, the endoperoxides give rise to thromboxane A_2, a potent vasoconstrictor and activator of platelet aggregation. Thus, further aggregation of platelets ensues, and eventually a platelet plug forms at the site of injury. The various events occurring in response to blood vessel injury are outlined in Figure 39-1.

While the platelet plug may temporarily stop bleeding at a site of injury, it must be reinforced by fibrin to provide a firm, stable clot. This latter process involves a series of reactions commonly referred to as *blood coagulation*, and requires the presence of a number of blood proteins known as *coagulation factors*. The coagulation factors, which are listed in Table 39-1, function in either of two distinct pathways, the intrinsic clotting pathway and the extrinsic clotting pathway. The intrinsic pathway is so named because all of the coagulation proteins are present in the blood itself. The reactions are relatively slow, and several minutes are required to produce a clot. The extrinsic pathway is triggered by clotting factors derived from injured cells in tissues. It is a much more rapidly acting system, and can result in formation of a blood clot within seconds. The interaction of the intrinsic and extrinsic pathways to produce a fibrin clot is shown schematically in Figure 39-2 and is reviewed below.

Intrinsic Pathway

The first event that occurs when blood comes into contact with exposed collagen or platelet phospholipids is the activation of the Hageman factor (factor XII). Factor XII_a (*i.e.*, activated Hageman factor, indicated by the subscript a) then activates factor XI (plasma thromboplastin antecedent; PTA), which, in combination with calcium, activates factor IX (Christmas factor). In conjunction with calcium and platelet phospholipid (released from damaged platelets), activated factor IX_a interacts with factor VIII (antihemophilic factor) to accelerate the activation of factor X (Stuart-Prower factor). This step is termed the *final common pathway* since it is the point at which the intrinsic and extrinsic pathways converge (see Fig. 39-2). Activated factor X_a, in conjunction with calcium, platelet phospholipids, and factor V (proaccelerin), forms a complex known as the *prothrombin activator*,

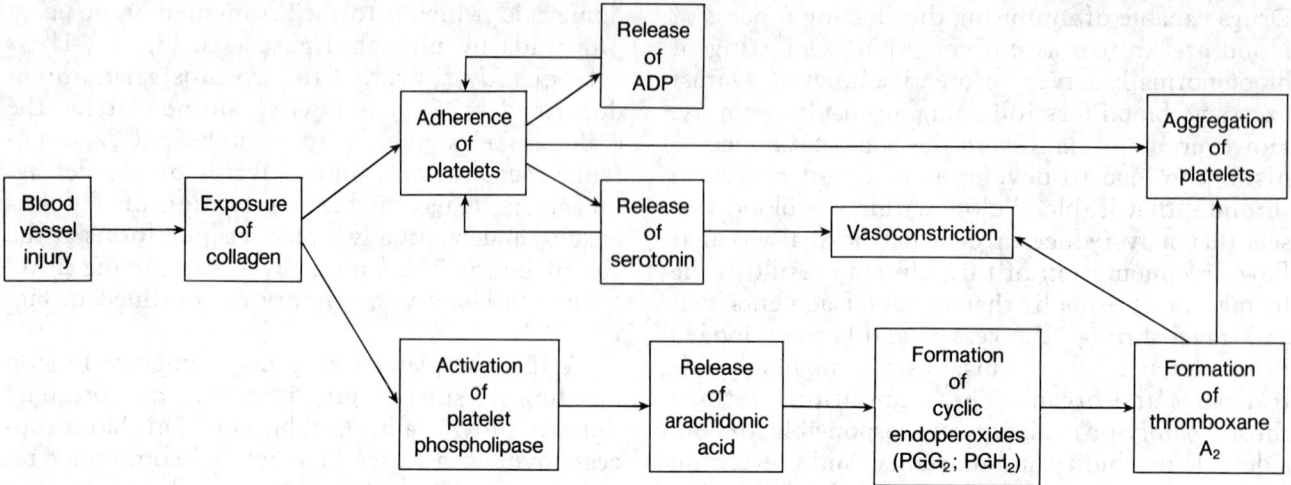

Figure 39-1. *Series of events resulting in aggregation of platelets in response to blood vessel injury.*

Table 39-1
Blood Coagulation Factors

Factor	Name	Function
I	Fibrinogen	Precursor of fibrin
II	Prothrombin	Precursor of thrombin
III	Thromboplastin	Triggers extrinsic coagulation pathway
IV	Calcium	Essential for several reactions in coagulation pathways
V	Proaccelerin	Accelerates conversion of prothrombin to thrombin
VII	Proconvertin	Accelerates the extrinsic coagulation pathway
VIII	Antihemophilic factor	Accelerates activation of factor X
IX	Christmas factor (plasma thromboplastin component; PTC)	Accelerates activation of factor X
X	Stuart-Prower factor	Accelerates conversion of prothrombin to thrombin
XI	Plasma thromboplastin antecedent (PTA)	Accelerates activation of factor IX
XII	Hageman factor	Triggers intrinsic coagulation pathway—activates factor XI
XIII	Fibrin stabilizing factor	Strengthens fibrin clot when activated by thrombin and calcium

which converts prothrombin to thrombin. Thrombin then enzymatically converts fibrinogen into soluble fibrin, which is ultimately transformed into a stable fibrin clot by the action of factor XIII (fibrin-stabilizing factor), which is activated by thrombin and calcium.

Extrinsic Pathway

Upon injury, tissue cells release a lipoprotein substance known as *tissue thromboplastin* (factor III), which triggers the rapid extrinsic coagulation pathway by combining with factor VII (proconver-

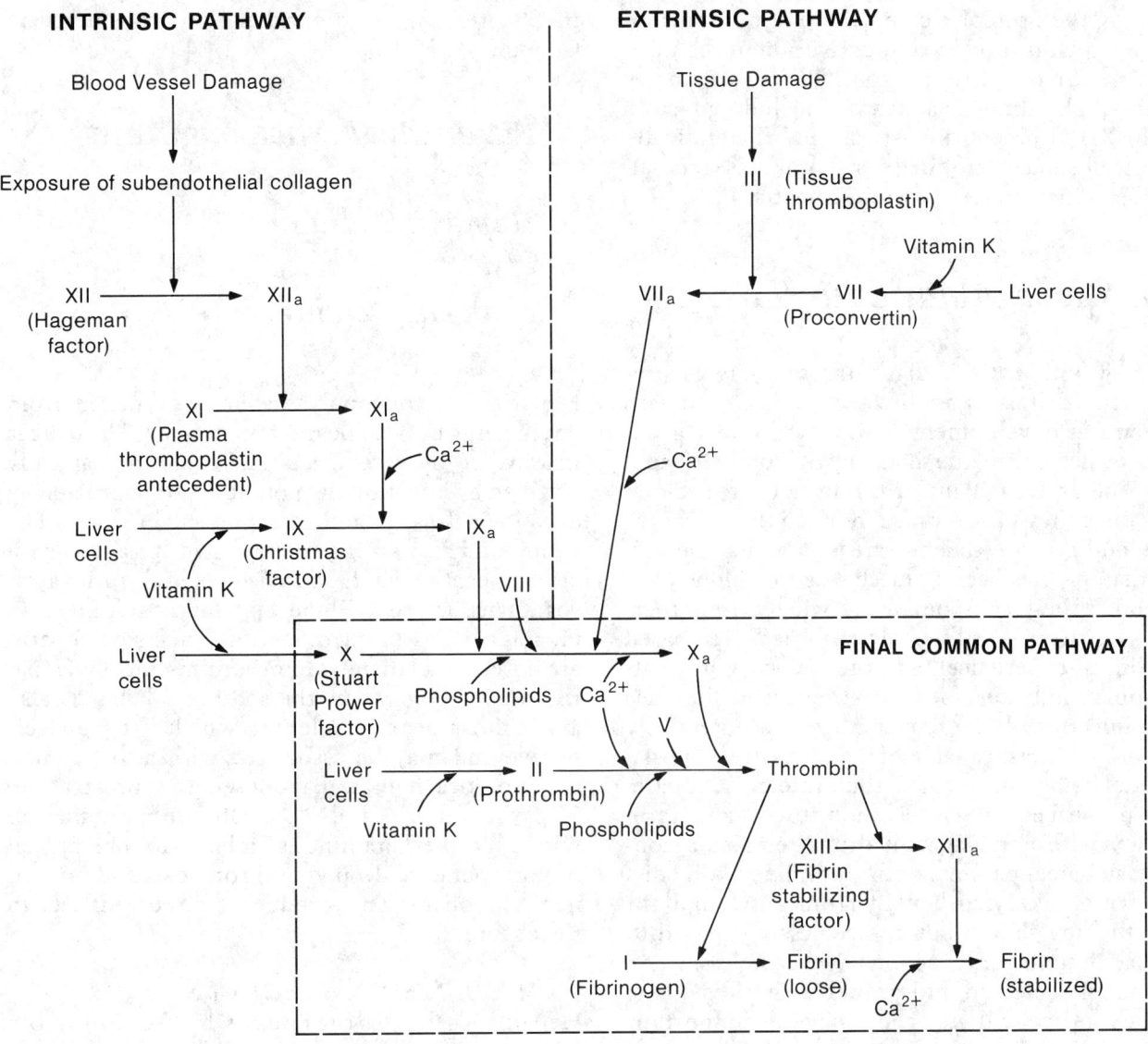

Figure 39-2. Coagulation pathways involved in hemostasis.

tin) and calcium to activate factor X (Stuart-Prower factor), at which point the extrinsic and intrinsic pathways converge into the final common pathway, as described above. The sudden initiation of the extrinsic pathway can significantly shorten the time required for clot formation. Both systems function simultaneously and a deficiency in *either* pathway can lead to a coagulation disorder.

Inhibitory Mechanisms

The normal hemostatic mechanism requires inhibitory control to prevent overactivity of the clotting system, spontaneous clot formation, and subse-

quent obstruction of the circulatory system. There are a number of physiologic inhibitors of hemostasis, of which the principal one is antithrombin III (heparin cofactor), a plasma protein synthesized by the liver. Antithrombin III inactivates thrombin, factor IX_a, factor X_a, factor XI_a, and factor XII_a, and its activity is optimal in the presence of heparin. Other inhibitors of hemostasis include alpha$_2$-macroglobulin, alpha$_2$-plasmin inhibitor, alpha-antitrypsin, and C_1 esterase inhibitor.

In addition to these inhibitors, the fibrinolytic system serves to counterbalance the deposition of fibrin and formation of the fibrin clot. The fibrinolytic process is capable of lysing (degrading) fibrin, resulting in clot dissolution. This process is trig-

gered by the proteolytic enzyme plasmin (fibrinolysin), which is produced by activation of the inactive precursor plasminogen. There are many
potential plasminogen activators, including factors
XI_a or XII_a, epinephrine, stress, and the clinically
useful substances urokinase, streptokinase, and alteplase, which are discussed in Chapter 40.

Anticoagulant Drug Therapy

Therapy with anticoagulant drugs is largely prophylactic, that is, it is directed primarily toward
preventing development of intravascular thromboses by decreasing the tendency of blood to coagu-
late. The anticoagulant drugs do not affect blood
clots once they have formed, nor can they improve
the blood flow to ischemic areas in which the vascular supply has been reduced due to a blood clot.
Although these compounds are widely used, therapy with them is still largely empirical (i.e., based
on clinical experience), and their efficacy in treating some conditions for which they are utilized has
been questioned. Moreover, they are potentially
dangerous drugs, capable of causing severe, possibly fatal hemorrhaging, and therefore must be carefully prescribed and closely monitored. Long-term
therapy with anticoagulant drugs remains a controversial area; patients with thromboembolic disorders not likely to benefit from anticoagulant
drug therapy should not be needlessly exposed to
the risk of untoward reactions. Nevertheless, when
judiciously selected and properly employed, the
various anticoagulant agents have an important
place in clinical therapy, and can markedly reduce
the incidence of vascular clotting, thus improving
the quality of life and preventing death.

There are many valid indications for anticoagulant drugs, and these are listed under Uses in the
discussions that follow. Both parenteral and oral
agents are available. Heparin is the sole available
parenteral agent, while the oral anticoagulant
group encompasses several drugs, characterized as
either coumarin or indandione derivatives. Following a separate discussion of heparin, the oral anticoagulants are discussed as a group, followed by a
listing of individual drugs. Both protamine sulfate,
a heparin antagonist, and vitamin K and its derivatives, which are antagonists of the oral anticoagulant drugs, are discussed in this chapter. Other
drugs have been demonstrated to interfere with
platelet aggregation and are discussed elsewhere in
this text. Aspirin and sulfinpyrazone are reviewed

in Chapter 23, and dipyridamole is considered in
Chapter 36.

Parenteral Anticoagulants

Heparin Sodium
(Liquaemin)

Heparin Calcium
(Calciparine)

Heparin is a mucopolysaccharide extracted from
bovine lung or porcine intestinal tissue. The drug is
inactivated by gastric acid and therefore can only
be given by injection. Its potency is standardized by
a biological assay and is expressed in units. The
compound is a strong organic acid, possessing an
electronegative charge that is essential for its anticoagulant activity. Blood clotting is inhibited in
vivo as well as in vitro, and the effects of heparin
are noted immediately upon administration. Heparin is usually given as the sodium salt but is also
available as heparin calcium, which is equally effective and may be associated with a lower incidence of local hematoma following administration.
Heparin sodium is also available in combination
with dihydroergotamine as Embolex for prevention
of postoperative deep vein thrombosis and pulmonary embolism. This product is discussed later in
the chapter.

MECHANISM AND ACTIONS
Heparin accelerates the rate at which antithrombin
III, an $alpha_2$ globulin produced by the liver, inactivates factors IX, X, XI, and XII, thus inhibiting
the synthesis of thrombin. Conversion of fibrinogen to fibrin is blocked, and activation of the fibrin-stabilizing factor (XIII) is also impaired, preventing development of a stable fibrin clot. The
rate-limiting step in the coagulation cascade (see
Fig. 39-2) is activation of factor X. This is inhibited
by lower doses of heparin than those needed to
neutralize thrombin. Thus, prophylactic therapy
may be accomplished with much lower doses than
those necessary to neutralize the action of thrombin and prevent further coagulation once the coagulation process has begun. Platelet adhesiveness
may also be reduced. However, the drug has no
fibrinolytic action.

Heparin does not appear significantly to alter
the concentration of clotting factors in the plasma.
Clotting time is usually prolonged following full

therapeutic doses, but may not be appreciably lengthened with small doses. Bleeding time is usually unchanged.

Heparin can increase the release of lipoprotein lipase, which serves to clear the plasma of circulating lipids; however, the drug is of no use as a hypolipemic agent due to its toxicity and need for parenteral administration.

USES

1. Prophylaxis and treatment of venous thromboses, pulmonary embolism, and atrial fibrillation with embolization
2. Prevention of postoperative deep venous thrombosis and pulmonary embolism in patients undergoing major (abdominothoracic, cardiac, arterial) surgery (low-dose regimen)
3. Prevention of cerebral thrombosis in evolving stroke
4. Diagnosis and treatment of acute and chronic consumption coagulopathies (disseminated intravascular coagulation)
5. Prevention of peripheral venous thrombosis following acute myocardial infarction
6. Anticoagulant in blood transfusion, dialysis procedures, blood samples for laboratory procedures, and extracorporeal circulation

ADMINISTRATION AND DOSAGE

Heparin may be used by deep subcutaneous or intermittent IV injection or by IV infusion. When given subcutaneously or by IV infusion, an initial IV bolus dose is generally employed. IM injections should be avoided, since there is a higher risk of hematoma and local irritative reactions with this route.

Heparin sodium is available in multiple-dose vials (1000 U/ml–40,000 U/ml), single-dose ampules (1000 U/ml–40,000 U/ml), and unit-dose syringes (1000 U/dose–20,000 U/dose). The drug is also available as heparin sodium lock flush solution (10 U/ml, 100 U/ml), to maintain the patency of indwelling IV catheters in intermittent IV therapy or blood sampling. Heparin calcium is used as injection solution containing 5,000 U/dose, 12,500 U/dose, and 20,000 U/dose.

The dosage is based on the patient's coagulation test results, determined just prior to each injection. Dosage is adequate when whole blood clotting time is 2.5 to 3 times the control value or the activated partial thromboplastin time (APTT) is 1.5 to 2.0 times the control value.

Although dosage must be individualized, rec-

ommended guideline doses for an average size (*i.e.,* 150-lb) patient are as follows:

General anticoagulation
  SC—10,000 U to 20,000 U initially (preceded by an IV loading dose of 5,000 U), then 8,000 U to 20,000 U every 8 hours to 12 hours
  IV injection—10,000 U initially, then 5,000 U to 10,000 U every 4 hours to 6 hours (may be given undiluted or in 50 ml to 100 ml of isotonic sodium chloride)
  IV infusion—5,000 U by IV injection initially, then 20,000 U to 40,000 U/day in 1,000 ml of isotonic sodium chloride solution
  Pediatric—50 units/kg IV drip initially, followed by 100 U/kg IV every 4 hours or 20,000 U/m^2/24 hours by continuous IV infusion

■ WARNING
Heparin should not be mixed in IV line with barbiturates, cephalothin, diphenhydramine, erythromycin, gentamicin, narcotics, procainamide, prochlorperazine, or promazine. (See Appendix.) IV lines should be flushed with normal saline prior to and following injection or infusion of these drugs.

Prophylaxis of postoperative thromboembolism
  SC—5,000 U 2 hours before surgery and 5,000 U every 8 hours to 12 hours for 7 days following surgery or until patient is fully ambulatory (see Contraindications and Precautions). *Note:* Higher doses may be necessary in febrile states.
Heart/blood vessel surgery
  IV—150 U/kg to 400 U/kg depending on length of surgery
Blood transfusion—Prepare 7,500 U/100 ml sterile sodium chloride injection; then add 6 ml to 8 ml of dilution to each 100 ml whole blood.
Laboratory samples—70 U to 150 U/10 ml to 20 ml whole blood sample

FATE
Heparin is quickly inactivated by gastric acid and therefore is not effective orally. An IV bolus injection results in an immediate anticoagulant effect. Following subcutaneous administration, peak plasma levels are attained within 2 hours to 4 hours

and therapeutic effects are maintained for 8 hours to 12 hours. Heparin is widely distributed in the plasma and is highly protein bound (95%). Clearance from the plasma is rapid, the average plasma half-life being 60 minutes to 90 minutes, although the half-life is dose dependent and may be significantly prolonged at higher doses. Heparin is partially metabolized by the liver and excreted in the urine as both metabolites and unchanged drug (20%–50%). Clearance is reduced in patients with renal disease.

SIDE-EFFECTS/ADVERSE REACTIONS

A frequent complication of heparin therapy is bleeding, especially if the dose is excessive or an underlying lesion is present. Other common side-effects include hypersensitivity reactions such as chills, fever, and urticaria, and elevations in serum glutamic-oxaloacetic transaminase (SGOT) and serum glutamic-pyruvic transaminase (SGPT) levels. Administration of a small test dose (e.g., 1000 U) may be advisable prior to initiating full therapy in persons with a history of allergic reactions.

Less commonly encountered adverse reactions include local erythema; pain or ulceration at injection sites; rhinitis; lacrimation; headache; diarrhea; vomiting; anaphylactic reaction; chest pain; elevated blood pressure; arthralgia; vasospastic conditions resulting in cyanosis, cold extremities, or tachypnea; alopecia; osteoporosis; suppression of renal function; and thrombocytopenia.

Thrombocytopenia may occur in up to one third of patients receiving heparin and is of two types. Early thrombocytopenia develops within 2 days to 3 days after initiating therapy, is usually mild, and is seldom of clinical consequence. It appears to be due to a direct action of heparin on platelets and may remain stable or even reverse even if heparin is continued. Delayed thrombocytopenia occurs 6 days to 12 days after initiation of therapy, probably reflects the presence of an immunoglobulin that induces platelet aggregation, and may be associated with hemorrhage and paradoxical thromboembolic episodes due to irreversible aggregation of platelets, the so called white-clot syndrome. This condition may lead to skin necrosis, gangrene, pulmonary embolism, myocardial infarction, or stroke. If significant thrombocytopenia develops during heparin therapy, the drug should be discontinued and oral anticoagulants substituted. Most instances of delayed thrombocytopenia are attributable to heparin prepared from bovine lung rather than porcine intestine.

CONTRAINDICATIONS AND PRECAUTIONS

Heparin is contraindicated in patients with severe thrombocytopenia or uncontrollable bleeding (except when due to disseminated intravascular coagulation) and in patients in whom suitable blood coagulation tests cannot be performed. Heparin should be given with extreme caution in the presence of disease states in which there is increased danger of bleeding:

Cardiovascular—Severe hypertension, arterial sclerosis, dissecting aneurysm, subacute bacterial endocarditis, hemophilia, thrombocytopenia

Central Nervous System—Intracranial hemorrhage, during and following spinal tap or surgery involving the brain, eye, or spinal cord

Gastrointestinal—Ulcerative lesions, diverticulitis, tube drainage

Other—Menstruation, threatened abortion, hepatic or renal disease, biliary dysfunction

Cautious use is also warranted in persons with a history of allergies and those receiving acid–citrate–dextrose (A.C.D.)-converted blood, since heparin activity persists for several weeks without diminution in such patients.

INTERACTIONS

1. An increased risk of bleeding is present when heparin is used in combination with other drugs that can interfere with platelet aggregation, such as salicylates; phenylbutazone; indomethacin and other nonsteroidal anti-inflammatory drugs; dipyridamole; valproic acid; and hydroxychloroquine.
2. Heparin can antagonize the action of ACTH, insulin, and corticosteroids.
3. The action of heparin may be partially reduced by antihistamines, hydroxyzine, digitalis, tetracyclines, and phenothiazines, although the mechanism of this interaction is not established.
4. Heparin may elevate the plasma levels of diazepam.

■ Nursing Process

□ ASSESSMENT

□ Subjective Data

A brief history should be obtained focusing on potential sources of bleeding including gastric ulcers or other gastrointestinal problems, prolonged menses, and disease states in which the danger of bleeding is increased, such as hypertension, thrombocytopenia, or hemophilia.

Any allergies to beef or pork should be noted since heparin is derived from these sources. The patient should also be asked if he has ever received heparin, and if so, what was his reaction to it. Previous sensitivity to the drug contraindicates its use. Further drug history information should be obtained including use of aspirin or other nonsteroidal anti-inflammatory drugs, steroids, and antihistamines frequently found in cold or allergy medications. See Interactions, above, for further drugs.

☐ *Objective Data*
Complete blood work should be done including a platelet count and partial thromboplastin time (PTT) or its activated form (APTT). These should be recorded in a prominent place on the patient's chart and used as a baseline for comparing future values while the patient is receiving the drug.

☐ *NURSING DIAGNOSES*
Actual nursing diagnoses may include
  Knowledge deficit related to action, administration, and side-effects of the drug
  Fear related to multiple abdominal injections (if subcutaneous route of administration is used)

Potential nursing diagnoses may include
  Potential fluid volume deficit related to diuresis (long-term therapy)
  Potential for injury: trauma related to increased capillary fragility and decreased clotting
  Alteration in tissue perfusion related to potential for hemorrhage

☐ *PLAN*
The nursing care goal is to provide safe administration of the drug in order to establish therapeutic anticoagulation with a minimum of side-effects.

☐ *INTERVENTION*
Prior to initial dosage of heparin the physician should establish what the desired therapeutic PTT range should be. The nurse should record this goal next to the drug administration record and compare each subsequent PTT result to it before administering heparin. If the laboratory value drops, more heparin may be needed; if it increases above the desired range, the dose may need to be lowered. In either case the physician needs to be notified *before* the dose is given in order to ensure the patient's safety.

The preferred technique for administration of subcutaneous heparin is given here.

Preferred Injection Technique for Administration of Subcutaneous Heparin

1. *Site Selection.* Use the fatty subcutaneous tissue of the abdominal wall, at least 2 inches away from the umbilicus and above the iliac crest. Secondary sites are the plane of the abdomen lateral to and slightly above the umbilicus or the lateral plane of the upper thigh. Avoid any scar tissue. See Figure 39-3.
2. *Skin Preparation:* Gently wipe area with an alcohol swab and allow to dry. Avoid vigorous rubbing.
3. *Handling of Skin:* Gently hold a roll of skin between thumb and forefinger. Roll should be approximately 1 inch across. Avoid pinching skin.
4. *Injection:* Use appropriate syringe with a ½″ to ⅝″ 25-gauge needle attached. Quickly insert needle at a 90-degree angle into the skin roll. Inject heparin, then withdraw needle at the same degree inserted. Release skin roll.
5. *Postinjection Skin Care:* Gently press alcohol swab over site for several seconds. Do not rub.

Current research indicates that in terms of skin bruising there are no clear advantages to techniques such as pulling back the plunger of the syringe, releasing the skin roll prior to injection, or injecting a small amount of air at the end of the injection to minimize solution leakage. Careful

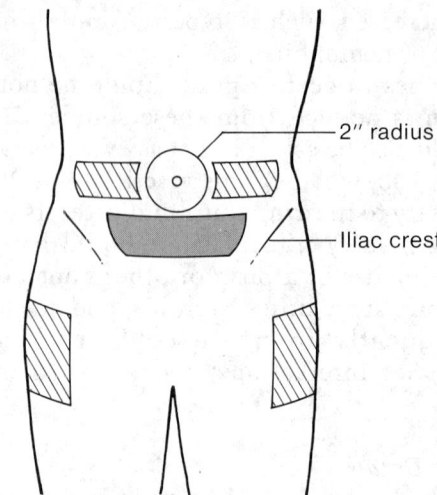

Figure 39-3. *Injection sites for heparin administration.*

▨ Preferred injection sites

▧ Secondary injection sites

manipulation of skin and site rotation seem to be the only factors that can help (Fig. 39-3). However, the nurse should be particularly cautious when administering heparin to the elderly, particularly elderly women, who seem to be more prone to bruising from the drug. Administration by way of intravenous heparin lock may be most appropriate for this age group. Occasionally, a patient will be extremely squeamish about abdominal injections and may refuse the medication out of fear of pain. At least one patient has said he was afraid the needle would act like a knife. Frequently, once the patient allows one injection to be given the fear can

be dissipated since abdominal injections are actually less painful than most extremity injections. However, for the patient who cannot overcome such a fear, an intravenous heparin lock may be an appropriate alternative.

Heparin can be administered intravenously in two ways. A continuous infusion can be started in an IV line, which should be monitored by an infusion pump.

The suggested technique for another method, intravenous injection through a heparin lock, is described here

---

Suggested Technique for Medication Administration by Heparin Lock

1. *Site Selection:* Insert heparin lock in a hand or arm vein away from the wrist or elbow joints. Choose a site where extremity movement will not cause pain at the catheter insertion site and where the chance of the catheter becoming dislodged is minimal.
2. *Needle Entry:* All needles are inserted through the rubber port at the end of the lock. Prior to insertion of *any needle* the port must be swabbed with iodophor or alcohol, according to institutional policy.
3. *Administration Technique*
   a. *Check the lock for patency:* Fill a syringe with sterile normal saline. Amount depends on age of patient, size of heparin lock, and institutional guidelines. The range is 0.5 ml to 1.5 ml. Insert needle of syringe into rubber port. Aspirate plunger to check for blood-tinged return. Slowly inject normal saline to flush the line.
   b. *Administer the medication:* Insert a syringe containing heparin or other medication and inject at the rate recommended by policy, medication literature, or pharmacy guidelines.
   c. *Flush the line:* When medication administration has been completed, re-
   (continued)

Suggested Technique for Medication Administration by Heparin Lock (continued)

move the needle or tubing. Insert another needle and syringe containing sterile normal saline and inject the prescribed amount to flush the line of all medication.

d. *Inject heparin solution:* Insert a syringe containing heparin lock flush solution. Solution will contain between 1 U heparin/ml to 10 U heparin/ml. Amount and strength will be determined by institutional policy and patient's age. Injecting this solution is critical to maintain the patency of the lock for future use.

The drug is administered on a scheduled basis through an IV site that is kept patent by heparinized saline solution. IV locks are also used for administration of other drugs such as antibiotics and antineoplastic agents (see Chaps. 59 and 75).

The most frequent, dangerous side-effect of heparin is bleeding, which may be secondary to a heparin overdose or to the presence of a lesion susceptible to bleeding such as a gastric ulcer. The patient should be told to report any unusual bruises; color changes in urine or feces; hematemesis; vaginal, gum, or nose bleeding; petechiae; and severe headaches; or lower back pain, which might indicate abdominal bleeding. Care givers should closely monitor venipuncture and arterial puncture sites for oozing or swelling while the lines are in place. Any puncture site should have a pressure dressing applied following removal of a needle or catheter. Care should be taken when removing urinary catheters to monitor for bleeding.

The best prevention of bleeding is close monitoring of the PTT time to maintain a therapeutic range of anticoagulation. Protamine sulfate should be on hand at all times as a drug antidote should bleeding occur. It is discussed later in this chapter.

A second dangerous side-effect, thrombocytopenia, may result in white-clot syndrome, mentioned earlier. Platelet counts should be closely monitored every 2 days to 3 days during heparin therapy and the patient should be examined for bruising and petechiae. He should be told to report chest pain or extremity pain immediately. To minimize the risk of white-clot syndrome, whenever appropriate the patient should be started on oral anticoagulants as quickly as possible.

Prolonged heparin therapy may also cause alopecia, which is usually temporary, and diuresis, which may produce hypokalemia that necessitates potassium supplements.

When the decision is made to start the patient on oral anticoagulants a baseline prothrombin time

(PT or Pro-Time) should be drawn. This should be done at least 5 hours after the last IV dose and 24 hours after the last subcutaneous dose of heparin to ensure accuracy of the laboratory value. Heparin may be withdrawn when prothrombin activity is within desired range (usually 1½ to 2 times the control value) following oral anticoagulant therapy. Administration of an oral anticoagulant usually overlaps heparin for 3 to 5 days.

□ *EVALUATION*
The outcome criteria for heparin therapy would be a therapeutic PTT 1½ to 2½ times normal and successful anticoagulation without bleeding or thrombocytopenia.

Heparin Sodium and Dihydroergotamine Mesylate
(Embolex)

Dihydroergotamine (DHE) possesses alpha-adrenergic blocking activity and a direct stimulating effect on vascular smooth muscle, primarily of the capacitance vessels with little or no effect on precapillary sphincters or arterial resistance vessels. It appears to protect against thrombotic episodes by accelerating venous return, thereby reducing venostasis. The combination of heparin and DHE is indicated for the prevention of postoperative deep vein thrombosis and pulmonary embolism in patients over 40 years of age undergoing major abdominothoracic or pelvic surgery. When compared to either heparin or DHE alone, the combination reduced the incidence of postoperative deep vein thrombosis approximately 50% and 30%, respectively.

Embolex is available as an injection containing 5000 units heparin and 0.5 mg DHE mesylate with 7.46 mg lidocaine per 0.7-ml ampule. One ampule is given by deep subcutaneous injection 2 hours prior to surgery and every 12 hours thereafter for 5 days to 7 days.

Refer to the previous discussion of heparin for a review of the adverse effects associated with its use, since they apply to this preparation as well. In addition, DHE itself can result in a number of untoward reactions, primarily as a result of its vasospastic properties. These effects are usually manifested as numbness and coldness of the extremities, muscle pain and weakness, precordial distress, and anginal-like pain. Other adverse effects related to DHE include tachycardia, nausea, vomiting, localized itching and edema, headache, and leg cramps.

The combination of heparin and DHE should be used cautiously in patients with bleeding tendencies (see heparin discussion, above), peripheral vascular diseases, coronary artery insufficiency, hypertension, or impaired renal or hepatic function, and in patients taking anticoagulants or platelet-inhibiting drugs (see Interactions, above, in the discussion on heparin). DHE possesses oxytocic properties and should not be given to pregnant women.

NURSING CONSIDERATIONS
See also Nursing Process, above.

In addition, this drug combination can produce vasospastic effects. The patient should be closely monitored for changes in the temperature and sensation of extremities, blanching of skin, or complaints of numbness, pain, or tingling.

In the immediate postoperative period the patient should be monitored for nausea and vomiting. Suction equipment and position change should be used to prevent aspiration.

Heparin Antagonist

Protamine Sulfate

Protamine sulfate is a mixture of proteins exhibiting a strongly positive charge that is capable of chemically combining with heparin, producing a stable salt, and thereby neutralizing the anticoagulant action of heparin. However, it may exert an anticoagulant effect when administered alone or when dosage exceeds that required to neutralize heparin.

It is used to treat heparin overdosage in those situations where a rapid reversal of heparin's anticoagulant action is desired, as, for example, if bleeding occurs following prophylactic heparin during surgery.

Protamine sulfate is available as an injection solution (10 mg/ml) that may either be given undi-

luted or diluted in 5% dextrose in water or normal saline. The drug is administered by slow IV injection, not exceeding 50 mg in a 10-minute period. One milligram neutralizes approximately 90 units of heparin derived from lung tissue, or 115 units of heparin derived from intestinal mucosa; therefore, the dose of protamine is based on the amount of heparin used and the time elapsed since the last dose of heparin. Protamine's effects occur almost immediately and persist for approximately 2 hours. Since heparin is cleared rapidly from the circulation, the required dose of protamine decreases the later it is given following heparin. For example, if protamine is administered 30 minutes after heparin, the dose required is only about one-half the usual dose. No more than 100 mg of protamine should be given over a short period, since larger doses may exert an anticoagulant effect. Blood coagulation studies such as heparin titration or plasma prothrombin time should be performed before repeat doses are given. Too-rapid injection of protamine can lead to severe hypotension, bradycardia, dyspnea, and anaphylaxis. In addition, since protamine is derived from a fish source, hypersensitivity reactions can occur. The most frequently encountered side-effects are flushing and a feeling of warmth. Protamine sulfate may be inactivated by blood, and when it is used to neutralize large doses of heparin, a "heparin rebound" can occur. Additional injections of protamine sulfate may overcome the heparin-rebound effect.

NURSING CONSIDERATIONS
Monitor heart rate and blood pressure immediately after injection and then every 2 minutes to 3 minutes until the patient is stable since severe hypotension and bradycardia can occur. The patient should remain flat in bed and vasopressors should be on hand in case they are needed.

Oral Anticoagulants

Coumarins

Dicumarol, Warfarin

Indandione

Anisindione

There are two chemical classes of anticoagulants available for oral use, the coumarins and the indandiones. Unlike heparin, these drugs are only effective *in vivo*. They will be discussed as a group, then listed individually in Table 39-2.

MECHANISM AND ACTIONS

Oral anticoagulants depress the hepatic synthesis of vitamin K–dependent clotting factors II, VII, IX, and X by inhibiting vitamin K-2, 3-epoxide reductase enzymes. Factor VII is the first to be depleted, since it has the shortest half-life (6 hours), followed sequentially by factors IX, X, and II, which have longer half-lives (24 hours, 40 hours, 60 hours, respectively). Thus, initial prolongation of prothrombin time occurs within 8 hours to 12 hours due to depletion of factor VII, but maximal anticoagulant activity requires several days to develop, since the other clotting factors are more slowly depleted. These drugs exert no effect on established thrombus, but may prevent further extension of the formed clot, thereby preventing secondary thromboembolic complications.

USES

1. Prophylaxis and treatment of venous thrombosis and its extension
2. Treatment of atrial fibrillation with embolism
3. Prophylaxis and treatment of pulmonary embolism
4. Adjunctive treatment of coronary occlusion
5. Prophylaxis in patients with prosthetic heart valves
6. Reduce risk of recurrent myocardial infarction (investigational use)
7. Prevention of recurrent transient ischemic attacks (investigational use)

ADMINISTRATION AND DOSAGE

See Table 39-2. (Dosage is individualized and adjusted to maintain the one-stage prothrombin time at 1.5 to 2.5 times the control value.)

FATE

Oral absorption is usually rapid and complete, except for dicumarol. Peak anticoagulation activity

Table 39-2
Oral Anticoagulants

Drug	Preparations	Usual Dosage Range	Clinical Considerations
Coumarins			
dicumarol	Tablets—25 mg, 50 mg	200 mg–300 mg first day; 25 mg–200 mg/day thereafter, depending on prothrombin time	Slowly and incompletely absorbed orally; peak effect in 3 days to 5 days and effects can last up to 10 days; be alert for accumulation toxicity (especially bleeding), because drug is long acting; poorly water soluble; half-life increases with increasing dose.
warfarin sodium (Carfin, Coumadin, Panwarfin, Sofarin)	Tablets—2 mg, 2.5 mg, 5 mg, 7.5 mg, 10 mg Injection—50 mg/vial with 2 mg diluent	Initially—10 mg–15 mg/ day (up to 60 mg/day) orally; thereafter, adjust based on prothrombin time Usual maintenance—2 mg–15 mg/day (may be given IM or IV for one dose if necessary)	Well absorbed orally; peak effect in 1 day to 3 days, and duration of 3 days to 5 days; most widely used oral anticoagulant, giving most uniform response; reduce dose by one half in elderly or debilitated patients; do not use injectable solution if precipitate is present.
Indandione			
anisindione (Miradon)	Tablets—50 mg	300 mg first day, 200 mg second day, 100 mg third day; then 25 mg–250 mg daily for maintenance	Indandione derivative infrequently used as oral anticoagulant. Peak effects occur with 2 days to 3 days and persist for 1 day to 3 days. Dermatitis is the most common side-effect. May turn urine red–orange.

occurs within 2 days to 3 days (except for dicu-marol, which is 3 days–5 days). Effects of a single dose persist for 2 days to 5 days with warfarin, and 2 days to 10 days with dicumarol. Anisindione is short acting (1 day–2 days). All drugs are highly (99%) but rather weakly bound to plasma proteins, and can therefore easily be displaced by other highly protein-bound drugs. The oral anticoagu-lants are metabolized by hepatic microsomal en-zymes and are excreted as inactive metabolites in the urine and feces.

SIDE-EFFECTS/ADVERSE REACTIONS

Bleeding episodes are the most frequently occur-ring side-effects of oral anticoagulant drug therapy. Manifestations may include bleeding gums, pete-chiae, hematuria, nosebleed, or bleeding from wounds or ulcerative lesions.

Excessive uterine bleeding can occur (although menstrual flow is usually normal), and ovarian, lu-teal, and adrenal hemorrhages have been reported, the latter condition being associated with acute adrenal insufficiency. Other adverse effects of oral anticoagulants include nausea, vomiting, anorexia, diarrhea, cramping, jaundice, alopecia, urticaria, dermatitis, fever, nephropathy, eosinophilia, agranulocytosis, leukopenia, hepatitis, and delayed hypersensitivity reactions (especially with anisin-dione) that can range from mild (erythema, derma-titis, fever) to life-threatening (exfoliative derma-titis, acute tubular necrosis, anuria, paralytic ileus).

Oral anticoagulants may cause red–orange dis-coloration of alkaline urine, and interfere with some laboratory tests.

CONTRAINDICATIONS AND PRECAUTIONS

There are a number of contraindications to the oral anticoagulants, including hemorrhagic tendencies; hemophilia; thrombocytopenic purpura; recent or contemplated surgery (especially eye or central nervous system surgery); active bleeding; ulcera-tive, traumatic, or surgical wounds; visceral carci-noma; diverticulitis; colitis; aneurysm; pericardial effusion; acute nephritis; suspicion of cerebrovas-cular hemorrhage; pregnancy, eclampsia, or pre-eclampsia; threatened abortion; uncontrolled hy-pertension; hepatic insufficiency; polyarthritis; polycythemia vera; subacute bacterial endocarditis; ascorbic acid (vitamin C) deficiency; spinal punc-ture; continuous gastrointestinal drainage; and re-gional block anesthesia.

Cautious use of oral anticoagulants is necessary in the presence of congestive heart failure, mild

liver or kidney dysfunction, alcoholism, steator-rhea, tuberculosis, history of ulcerative disease, diabetes, allergic disorders, poor nutritional states, collagen disease, pancreatic disorders, vitamin K deficiency, thyrotoxicosis, hypothyroidism, x-ray therapy, edema, and hyperlipidemia, since the anti-coagulant effects of these drugs may be altered. In infections, where anti-infective therapy is em-ployed, altered intestinal flora may interfere with vitamin K production, resulting in enhanced anti-coagulation (see Interactions, below). Oral antico-agulants must be used cautiously in potentially noncompliant patients, such as psychotic, senile, or emotionally unstable individuals or alcoholics or drug abusers.

INTERACTIONS

■ WARNING

Oral anticoagulants have a great potential to interact with a wide range of other drugs. Clinically important drug interactions are listed below; however, all patients receiv-ing oral anticoagulants along with other medication must be closely monitored.

1. The hypoprothrombinemic effect of oral anti-coagulants may be enhanced by drugs that de-crease vitamin K levels (antibiotics, cholestyr-amine, mineral oil); drugs that displace the anticoagulants from their protein-binding sites (clofibrate, chloral hydrate, diazoxide, nali-dixic acid, phenylbutazone, salicylates, sulfon-amides, oral hypoglycemics); drugs that inhibit the metabolism of anticoagulants (alcohol, al-lopurinol, chloramphenicol, cimetidine, co-tri-moxazole, disulfiram, methylphenidate, met-ronidazole, phenylbutazone, propoxyphene, sulfinpyrazone); and also by acetaminophen, anabolic steroids, erythromycin, gemfibrozil, ketoconazole, glucagon, danazol, quinidine, sulindac, and thyroid drugs.

2. Increased incidence of hemorrhage can occur with combined use of oral anticoagulants and inhibitors of platelet aggregation (dipyrida-mole, indomethacin, pyrazolones, salicylates), inhibitors of procoagulant factors (antimeta-bolites, alkylating agents, quinidine, salicy-lates), or ulcerogenic drugs (corticosteroids, in-domethacin, pyrazolones, potassium salts, salicylates).

3. A decreased anticoagulant effect may be ob-served if oral anticoagulants are used in the presence of enzyme inducers (barbiturates,

carbamazepine, ethchlorvynol, glutethimide, griseofulvin, phenytoin, rifampin); activators of procoagulant factors (estrogens, oral contraceptives, vitamin K); and drugs that can decrease gastrointestinal absorption (aluminum hydroxide, cholestyramine, colestipol).
4. Oral anticoagulants may potentiate the action of phenytoin and the oral hypoglycemic drugs by inhibiting their liver metabolism.
5. Concurrent use of oral anticoagulants with streptokinase and urokinase increases the risk of bleeding.

■ Nursing Process

□ ASSESSMENT

□ Subjective Data
A thorough drug history must be obtained before administering any oral anticoagulants since these drugs interact with a vast number of prescription and over-the-counter medications. The patient must be aware of the potential for dangerous interactions and be taught early on that he should take no medication, including vitamin preparations, without first checking with the health team.

The patient must also be assessed for his ability to follow through with the prescribed regimen. Oral anticoagulants must be taken on a rigid, regular schedule. The patient who is forgetful or known to abuse alcohol or drugs, or who is without strong emotional supports may be a poor candidate for this drug regimen. Improper use of anticoagulants can cause fatal hemorrhage.

□ Objective Data
Laboratory data should also be collected to provide a baseline. A complete blood count, liver function studies, and a prothrombin time (PT) should be drawn before therapy begins.

□ NURSING DIAGNOSES
Actual nursing diagnoses may include
  Knowledge deficit related to the action, dose, and side-effects of the drug
Potential nursing diagnoses may include
  Noncompliance with the regimen based on lack of motivation or lack of understanding about the need to use the medication and the complexity of the therapy
  Potential for injury: trauma related to increased susceptibility for bruising and bleeding

Alteration in tissue perfusion related to potential for hemorrhage

□ PLAN
The nursing care goals should focus on helping the patient learn
1. To correctly administer the drug
2. To seek follow-up care as directed
3. To monitor for the development of side-effects that should be immediately reported
4. To incorporate anticoagulant therapy and its constraints into daily living

□ INTERVENTION
Oral anticoagulants are usually started while the patient is still on heparin. The patient will remain on both drugs for 3 days to 5 days until laboratory values of PT are within therapeutic range. During the time the patient is on both heparin and oral agents the PT blood sample should be drawn just prior to a dose of heparin, that is, 5 hours after the last IV dose or 24 hours after the last subcutaneous dose. Table 39-2 lists both the initial and maintenance doses of the oral drugs used to achieve a therapeutic PT.

Success in drug therapy will depend on the patient's ability to follow the dosage schedule strictly, have laboratory work drawn and evaluated regularly, and maintain an even life-style. When teaching home administration the nurse should focus on helping the patient to establish a regular, consistent time of day when the anticoagulant is taken in order to maintain the therapeutic blood level needed. The patient must also be aware of the importance of PT determinations in order to maintain a safe dosage level. PTs may be drawn daily during initial stages of therapy, dosage-adjustment periods, or when other changes occur such as illness, addition of other drugs, or changes in climate. Once a maintenance blood level is obtained, the PT can be drawn at 1-week to 4-week intervals. The patient should keep a record of each PT level and the date it was drawn.

The patient must also understand that anticoagulant therapy must be withdrawn gradually, over a 3-week to 4-week period. PT will gradually return to normal in 2 days to 10 days so the patient must continue to follow the same guidelines as during drug administration until the anticoagulant is completely cleared from the body.

The patient taking oral anticoagulants will benefit from having written information on the dose, administration, and side-effects of the drug as well as what to do in an emergency. A drug card may facilitate collecting all of this information (see Chap. 6).

The most serious side-effect of oral anticoagulants is bleeding. The patient should report immediately any signs of abnormal bleeding such as oozing from shaving nicks, hematuria, nosebleeds, bleeding gums after toothbrushing, petechiae or ecchymoses, tarry stools or frank rectal bleeding, hematemesis, or excessive menses. Dosage adjustment is usually warranted but the patient must not attempt this without health-care supervision. The patient needs to be assured that a drug antidote, vitamin K, can stop the bleeding but that it must be administered by a member of the health-care team; therefore, early reporting is essential.

The patient on oral anticoagulants should wear a Medic-Alert bracelet or carry some identification that states the drug and dose he is taking. He should also be told to remind any dentist or other physician that he is taking the drug and to remind laboratory personnel who will need to apply prolonged pressure to any venipuncture site. While hospitalized this patient should be clearly identified on the medication administration record or with a bedside sign so injections of all types are minimized.

Since vitamin K is the antidote for oral anticoagulants, it should be kept on all units where the drug is given. Patients need to limit foods rich in the vitamin while taking the drug. These include green leafy vegetables, cabbage, cauliflower, fish, and liver.

Two other serious side-effects are agranulocytosis and hepatitis. The patient can be taught symptoms to watch for and be told to report them at once. Early symptoms of agranulocytosis are fever, chills, sore throat, and mucosal ulceration. Symptoms of hepatitis are itching, darkened urine, and jaundice.

The indandione oral anticoagulants may cause a red-orange discoloration of urine. This can be differentiated from hematuria by a simple laboratory test with a chemical-impregnated stick that tests for blood. The patient should report any urine color change and have the urine tested. Discoloration can be minimized by acidifying the urine, and the patient can facilitate this by increasing intake of citrus fruits and juices.

The risks versus the benefits of oral anticoagulant therapy should be carefully weighed when considering administration to a pregnant woman. The drug crosses the placenta and has resulted in fetal hemorrhage and congenital malformation. If the drug must be given postpartum the infant should be given formula since oral anticoagulants will be present in breast milk.

□ **EVALUATION**

The outcome criteria against which to judge drug effectiveness are a prothrombin time 1½ to 2 times normal (or institution-set therapeutic range) and absence of bleeding or hematologic or hepatic changes.

Oral Anticoagulant Antagonist

Vitamin K

Vitamin K is effective as an antidote to overdosage with the oral anticoagulant drugs. Three types of vitamin K preparations are available: (1) phytonadione (vitamin K_1), a fat-soluble derivative resembling naturally occurring vitamin K; (2) menadione (vitamin K_3), another synthetic fat-soluble derivative that is less effective than vitamin K_1 as an antidote to oral anticoagulants; and (3) menadiol (vitamin K_4), a synthetic water-soluble analog to menadione that is converted to menadione *in vivo* but is only about half as potent. Phytonadione is the preferred drug for treatment of anticoagulant-induced prothrombin deficiency because the other derivatives (K_3 and K_4) are less potent, less dependable, less rapid acting, and shorter acting than K_1.

The complete pharmacology of the various vitamin K preparations is reviewed in detail in Chapter 77. The present discussion is limited to the use of these preparations solely for the treatment of oral anticoagulant overdosage. Thus, only phytonadione (vitamin K_1), the preferred antidote, is reviewed at this time.

Phytonadione (K_1)
(Aquamephyton, Konakion, Mephyton)

MECHANISM AND ACTIONS
Vitamin K promotes the hepatic synthesis of blood clotting factors II (prothrombin), VII (proconvertin), IX (plasma thromboplastin component), and X (Stuart factor). The mechanism of the action is not established.

USES
1. Treatment of anticoagulant-induced prothrombin deficiency (oral or parenteral vitamin K_1)

2. Treatment of hypoprothrombinemia second-ary to antibacterial therapy, obstructive jaundice, biliary fistulas, or salicylate administration (oral or parenteral vitamin K_1)
3. Prophylaxis and therapy of newborn hemorrhagic disease (parenteral vitamin K_1)
4. Treatment of hypoprothrombinemia secondary to malabsorption or impaired synthesis of vitamin K such as can occur in ulcerative colitis, obstructive jaundice, celiac disease, intestinal resection, or regional enteritis (parenteral vitamin K_1)

ADMINISTRATION AND DOSAGE

Phytonadione is available as 5-mg tablets (Mephyton), an aqueous colloidal solution (2 mg/ml, 10 mg/ml for subcutaneous or IM use) (Aquamephyton), and an aqueous dispersion (2 mg/ml, 10 mg/ml) *for IM use only* (Konakion).

For treating anticoagulant-induced prothrombin deficiency, recommended doses are as follows:

Oral—2.5 mg to 10 mg (maximum 50 mg) initially; repeat in 12 hours to 24 hours as determined by prothrombin time or clinical response.

Subcutaneous, IM—0.5 mg to 10 mg (maximum 25 mg) initially; repeat in 6 hours to 8 hours as needed.

IV (*emergency only*; see Side-Effects/Adverse Reactions)—0.5 mg to 10 mg at a rate of 1 mg/minute

Dilute injection with sodium chloride or dextrose solution and administer very slowly by IV injection or short-term infusion. Protect container from light during use.

Doses for other indications of vitamin K are listed in Table 77-3, Chapter 77.

FATE

Oral phytonadione requires the presence of bile salts in the gastrointestinal tract for its absorption. Effects occur within 6 hours to 10 hours. The effects of parenteral phytonadione occur within 1 hour to 2 hours and bleeding is usually controlled within 3 hours to 6 hours. Prothrombin levels are normalized within 12 hours to 15 hours. Metabolism is rapid and tissue accumulation is minimal.

SIDE-EFFECTS/ADVERSE REACTIONS

Gastric upset, nausea, and headache have occurred with oral administration. Transient flushing sensations and pain, swelling, or tenderness at the injection site have been reported with parenteral use. Occasional allergic reactions ranging from rash, urticaria, and dermatitis to bronchospasm, dyspnea, and anaphylaxis have been reported with use of vitamin K. Other adverse reactions include cramping, chills, fever, weakness, dizziness, profuse sweating, hypotension, and cyanosis.

■ *WARNING*
Severe anaphylactic reactions have occurred following IV injection of Aquamephyton (an aqueous colloidal solution of vitamin K_1), resulting in shock, cardiac arrest, and respiratory arrest. Therefore, the IV route should be used only when other routes are not feasible and with full consideration of all risks.

CONTRAINDICATIONS AND PRECAUTIONS

There are no absolute contraindications to use of vitamin K_1. Hypoprothrombinemia due to hepatocellular disease is *not* corrected by vitamin K, and large doses may further impair liver function in such conditions. Excessive dosage with vitamin K may result in an increase in thromboembolic episodes; dosage should be kept as low as possible and prothrombin time checked regularly. *Cautious* use of vitamin K is warranted during pregnancy, since it readily crosses the placenta.

INTERACTIONS

1. Concurrent administration of phytonadione with mineral oil or cholestyramine may result in impaired vitamin K absorption.
2. When large doses of phytonadione are used, temporary resistance to oral anticoagulants may be encountered. If anticoagulant therapy becomes necessary, heparin may be required.
3. Oral antibiotics, quinidine, and salicylates may interfere with vitamin K activity.

NURSING CONSIDERATIONS

The danger of anaphylaxis is greatest within the first few minutes after injection; therefore, the patient should be observed for dyspnea, and heart rate and blood pressure should be closely monitored until the drug takes effect.

Hemorheologic Agent

Pentoxifylline
(Trental)

Pentoxifylline is a xanthine derivative, structurally related to caffeine and theophylline. It is termed a hemorheologic agent, inasmuch as it lowers blood viscosity and improves the flexibility of red blood cells. Therefore, in patients with impaired blood flow in microcirculatory areas, pentoxifylline can increase oxygenation of tissues supplied by these occluded vessels by improving microcirculatory blood flow. It is primarily used in the treatment of intermittent claudication resulting from chronic occlusive arterial disease of the limbs.

MECHANISM AND ACTIONS

Pentoxifylline improves regional blood flow by reducing blood viscosity and enhancing red blood cell flexibility. The drug increases cellular ATP content by stabilizing cellular membranes, thereby reducing the tendency of red blood cells to aggregate and thus lowering blood viscosity. In addition, pentoxifylline stimulates formation and release of prostacyclin (PGI_2) and blocks degradation of cyclic AMP, which reduces formation of thromboxane A_2. Increased prostacyclin and reduced thromboxane levels decrease platelet aggregation and promote vasodilation. Blood fibrinogen concentration is lowered by pentoxifylline, which results in increased blood fibrinolytic activity. The net result of the above actions is increased tissue oxygenation, which reduces the local ischemia and resultant pain associated with impaired regional circulation.

USES

1. Symptomatic treatment of intermittent claudication due to chronic occlusive arterial disease
2. Symptomatic treatment of cerebrovascular insufficiency (investigational use)

ADMINISTRATION AND DOSAGE

Pentoxifylline is available as controlled-release tablets containing 400 mg. Recommended dosage is 400 mg three times daily with meals for at least 8 weeks. If gastrointestinal or central nervous system side-effects are bothersome, dosage may be decreased to 400 mg twice a day.

FATE

Following oral administration, peak plasma levels occur within 2 hours to 4 hours and remain constant thereafter. Plasma half-life ranges from 0.5 hour to 1.5 hours. Therapeutic effects, however, generally are not seen for 4 weeks to 8 weeks. The drug is metabolized in the liver and excreted primarily in the urine.

SIDE-EFFECTS/ADVERSE REACTIONS

The most frequently encountered side-effects with pentoxifylline are dyspepsia, dizziness, and nausea. Other untoward reactions observed in less than 1% of patients receiving the drug are vomiting, dry mouth, anorexia, constipation, headache, anxiety, mild tremor, nasal congestion, epistaxis, flu-like symptoms, pruritus, rash, urticaria, brittle fingernails, blurred vision, conjunctivitis, scotomata, bad taste in mouth, earache, salivation, malaise, sore throat, dyspnea, hypotension, edema, swollen glands, and leukopenia.

CONTRAINDICATIONS AND PRECAUTIONS

Pentoxifylline should not be used in persons sensitive to methylxanthines, such as caffeine or theophylline. Safety and efficacy in children under 18 years of age have not been established. The drug should be given with *caution* to patients with angina, arrhythmias, or severe hypotension, and to pregnant or nursing mothers.

NURSING CONSIDERATIONS

The main nursing responsibility is to teach the patient correct administration in order to minimize side-effects. He should take this drug with meals to reduce the likelihood of dizziness and gastrointestinal side-effects. However, if nausea, headache, or dizziness persists, he should contact the physician. In most cases dosage reduction will eliminate the problem.

The patient should be told not to expect results from the drug for several weeks. Gradually he may begin to notice a lessening of pain and increased ability to walk further. These are the outcomes sought with drug therapy.

Although unlikely, patients should be warned not to donate blood while on pentoxifylline since blood coagulation will be altered. For the same reason the patient treated with this drug and anticoagulants may need a smaller dose of the latter and should be carefully watched for bleeding. Instruct the patient to notify his physician if anginal symptoms worsen.

CASE STUDY

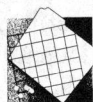

Joan Starkowski, age 48, sees her physician with a complaint of persistent pain in the right leg for 3 days. Mrs. Starkowski is a beautician who stands for 8 to 10 hours a day while at work, and the pain in her leg is becoming disabling. She has also been recently started on estrogen therapy for menopausal symptoms of "hot flashes."

On examination, the doctor finds her right leg to be warm, mottled, and slightly larger than the left. She has a positive Homans' sign (pain on dorsiflexion of the foot).

Mrs. Starkowski is admitted to the hospital with a diagnosis of thrombophlebitis. Her care includes bedrest, antiembolic stockings, and heparin, 5000 U subcutaneously every 8 hours. After 4 injections of heparin into her abdomen, Mrs. Starkowski is badly bruised and refuses the next dose.

Discussion Questions

1. What are your nursing responsibilities in this case? What are the options for administration of heparin?
2. How long before Mrs. Starkowski could be started on oral anticoagulants? Outline a hypothetical drug regimen. What blood studies should be performed? What blood levels should be achieved?
3. Mrs. Starkowski will be going home on Coumadin. What information should she have about this drug? Devise a teaching plan.

REVIEW QUESTIONS

1. Briefly describe the platelet "release reaction."
2. What role do prostaglandins play in platelet aggregation?
3. How do the intrinsic and extrinsic coagulation pathways differ?
4. What is meant by the "final common pathway" in blood coagulation?
5. What is the function of plasma antithrombin III?
6. Briefly describe the mechanism of action of heparin.
7. What are the preferred routes of administration for heparin? On what laboratory parameter is the dose of heparin based?
8. Distinguish between "early" and "delayed" thrombocytopenia occasionally observed with heparin.
9. In which disease states must heparin be administered with caution?
10. How can the nurse minimize the chance of bruising from repeated subcutaneous heparin injections? Which patients are the best candidates for heparin lock devices?
11. How does protamine function as a heparin antagonist? What is the danger of overdosage with protamine?
12. What is the mechanism of action of oral anticoagulants? Why is there a delay in the onset of their action?
13. On what laboratory parameter is the dosage of oral anticoagulants based?
14. Give several general ways in which oral anticoagulants can interact with other drugs.

15. Who are the best candidates for oral anticoagulants? How can the nurse attempt to determine if the patient will successfully comply with the prescribed regimen?
16. What drug is used as an oral anticoagulant antidote? What are the principal side-effects associated with its use?
17. What are the major indications for pentoxifylline? What is its mechanism of action?
18. What are the nursing responsibilities in teaching a patient who is taking pentoxifylline?

BIBLIOGRAPHY

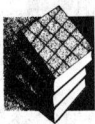

Baker DE, Campbell RK: Pentoxifylline: A new agent for intermittent claudication. Drug Intell Clin Pharm 19:345, May, 1984

Bjork I, Lindahl U: Mechanism of the anticoagulant action of heparin. Mol Cell Biochem 48:161, 1982

Bouchier-Hayes D: Drugs in the treatment of thromboembolic diseases. Ir Med J 76:101 and 155, 1983

Buckler P, Douglas AS: Antithrombotic treatment. Br Med J 287:196, 1983

Chamberlain SL: Low dose heparin therapy. Am J Nurs 80:115, 1980

Cipolle RJ, Rodrold RA, Seifert R et al: Heparin-associated thrombocytopenia: A prospective evaluation of 211 patients. Ther Drug Monit 5:205, 1983

Furie B: Using oral anticoagulants effectively. Drug Ther 9:108, 1979

Jacques LB: Heparin: A unique misunderstood drug. Trends in Pharmacological Science 3:289, 1982

Loeliger EA, Lewis SM: Progress in laboratory control of oral anticoagulants. Lancet 2:318, 1982

Miller P, Yardley S: White clot syndrome: A complication of heparin therapy. Am J Nurs 85:1051, 1985

Nelson PH, Moser KM, Stoner C, Moser KS: Risk of complications during intravenous heparin therapy. West J Med 136:189, 1982

Pepper G: New drug for intermittent claudication. Nurse Pract 10(5):54, May, 1985

Salem HH: Current status of anticoagulants. Drug Ther 13:57, 1983

Serlin MJ, Breckenridge AM: Drug interactions with warfarin. Drugs 25:610, 1983

Thomas DP: Heparin. Clin Haematol 10:443, 1981

Vanbree NS, Hollerback AD, Brooks GP: Clinical evaluation of three techniques for administering low-dose heparin. Nurs Res 33(1):15, 1984

Weykei D: Current status of anticoagulant therapy. Am J Med 72:659, 1982

Thrombolytic and Hemostatic Drugs

40

Drugs possessing the ability to degrade blood clots or to accelerate the endogenous dissolution process are termed *thrombolytic agents.* Drugs used to control bleeding through a variety of mechanisms are referred to as *hemostatic agents.* Before discussing the clinically available thrombolytic and hemostatic drugs, a brief review of the function of the fibrinolytic system will be presented.

Fibrinolysis

The critical balance between clot formation and clot lysis is controlled by the action of both activators and inhibitors of these processes. Clot formation is reviewed in detail in Chapter 39. The breakdown of blood clots, or fibrinolysis, is similar in that it also involves a sequential activation of factors from inactive precursors. The process is initiated by the activation of plasminogen (or profibrinolysin), an inactive plasma protein, to form plasmin (or fibrinolysin), the active fibrinolytic enzyme. A variety of substances found in the blood and tissues, as well as several exogenous substances, can serve as plasminogen activators. Once formed, plasmin is capable of degrading fibrin, fibrinogen, and other plasma proteins, with the subsequent production of fibrin degradation products (FDPs). These FDPs appear to have an anticoagulant effect and may result in significant bleeding if present in excess. The activation of plasminogen to plasmin is most efficient when plasminogen is bound to fibrin, since bound plasmin is apparently less susceptible to inactivation, and the affinity of fibrin-bound plasminogen for endogenous activators is greater than that of free plasminogen. The fibrinolytic system is schematically represented in Figure 40-1.

Attenuation of plasmin activity can be brought into effect in several ways, including direct inactivation of plasmin by an alpha$_2$ plasmin inhibitor, inhibition of circulating proteases by alpha$_2$-macroglobulin, and inhibition of plasminogen activators and interference with the binding of plasmin to fibrin, as observed with aminocaproic acid.

Thrombolytic Drugs

Thrombolytic, or fibrinolytic, drugs are capable of facilitating the dissolution of blood clots and are used in the treatment of various thromboembolic disorders. Unlike heparin and the oral anticoagulants, which function to *prevent* clot formation or extension, thrombolytic agents can actually break down and dissolve previously formed fibrin clots.

The currently available thrombolytic drugs are enzymes, one derived from beta-hemolytic streptococci (streptokinase), another from human kidney cells (urokinase), and a third produced in tissue

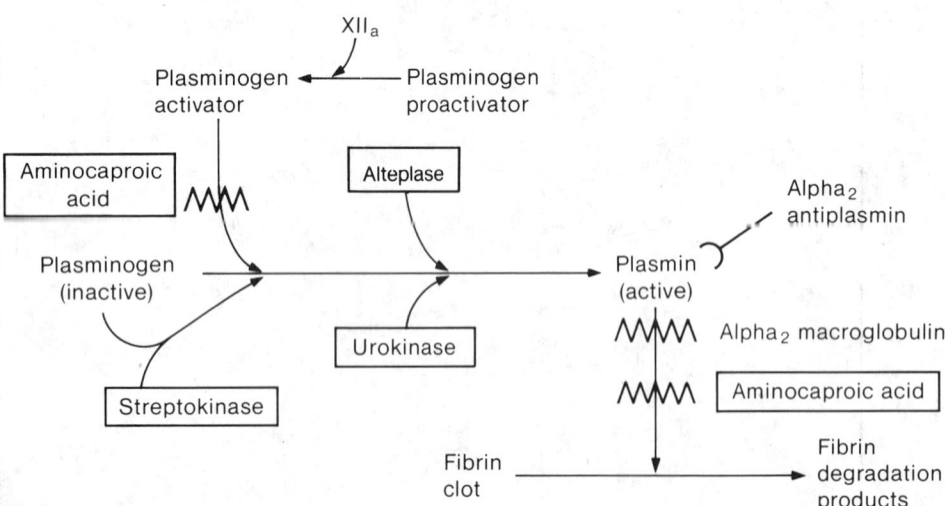

Figure 40-1. Mechanisms of fibrinolysis. Drugs are boxed to differentiate them from naturally occurring substances. Note: factor XII$_a$ is a common factor in clot formation and clot lysis.

culture by recombinant-DNA techniques (alteplase). Although they are quite often beneficial and sometimes life-saving, they are potentially dangerous agents, associated with definite risk of hemorrhage, which is often difficult to manage. Thrombolytic drugs should be administered only by persons trained and experienced in their use. Their clinical effectiveness is subject to some debate, and it is imperative that the potential benefit be carefully weighed against the considerable risk before prescribing these agents to treat thromboembolic conditions. However, thrombolytic therapy appears to be a potentially valuable form of therapy in such life-threatening diseases as pulmonary emboli and myocardial infarction, and critical patient selection and intensive patient management can greatly enhance the safety and efficacy of these drugs.

As mentioned, the risk of bleeding is considerable with thrombolytic drugs, especially at sites of invasive procedures. In addition, streptokinase and urokinase create a *generalized* lytic condition, in which normally occurring protective hemostatic thrombi are dissolved as well as the desired intravascular thrombi. The danger of systemic thrombus lysis can be reduced by intracoronary perfusion of these agents, but this is obviously a more difficult and hazardous technique.

Streptokinase and urokinase are considered together, since they are quite similar in their actions. Alteplase is a more clot-selective thrombolytic agent and is reviewed separately below.

Streptokinase

(Kabikinase, Streptase)

Urokinase

(Abbokinase)

MECHANISM AND ACTIONS

Both of these enzymatic drugs convert plasminogen to the fibrinolytic enzyme plasmin, which degrades fibrin clots, fibrinogen, and other plasma proteins. Urokinase activates plasminogen directly by cleaving peptide bonds at two different sites. Streptokinase works indirectly by first combining with plasminogen to form an activator complex, exposing the plasminogen-activating site. Plasminogen is then cleaved as described above for urokinase. Further, the streptokinase–plasminogen complex can be converted to a streptokinase–plasmin complex, which is also able to cleave plasmin-

ogen. Thrombin time is usually decreased to less than two times normal following administration of both drugs and there is an increase in the amount of circulating fibrin degradation products, which can exert anticoagulant activity.

USES
1. Lysis of acute, massive pulmonary emboli (streptokinase, urokinase)
2. Lysis of acute coronary artery thrombi associated with evolving myocardial infarction (streptokinase, urokinase) (*Note:* Most effective when given within 6 hours of onset of symptoms)
3. Lysis of acute, extensive thrombi of deep veins (streptokinase)
4. Clearance of occluded arteriovenous cannulas (streptokinase)
5. Restoration of patency of IV and central venous catheters obstructed by clotted blood (urokinase)

ADMINISTRATION AND DOSAGE

Streptokinase
Streptokinase is available as powder for injection, containing 250,000 U, 600,000 U, or 750,000 U per vial. It may be administered either by IV infusion or by a coronary catheter. Recommended doses are as follows:

Venous thrombosis and pulmonary or arterial embolism—Initially 250,000 U IV over a 30-minute period to neutralize anti-streptokinase antibodies present in most patients, then 100,000 U/hour over 72 hours for venous thrombosis, or 100,000 U/hour over 24 hours to 72 hours for pulmonary embolism or arterial thrombosis

Reconstitute contents of each vial with 5 ml sodium chloride injection or 5% dextrose injection, directed to the side of the vial rather than directly into the solution. The vial is rolled or tilted gently to reconstitute the drug but should *not* be shaken. The contents are then diluted further to a total volume of 45 ml. The solution may be filtered through a 0.22-μ filter. Solution containing large amounts of flocculation should be discarded.

Arteriovenous cannula occlusion—Infuse by pump at a constant rate, 250,000 U/2 ml IV solution, into each occluded limb of cannula over a 30-minute period, then clamp off for 2 hours; aspirate contents of infusion cannula, flush with saline, and reconnect cannula.

Reconstitute contents of 250,000 U/vial with 2 ml sodium chloride injection or 5% dextrose injection.

Myocardial infarction

IV—250,000 U initially, followed by 100,000 U/hour for 24 hours; alternately, 500,000 U to 1,500,000 U in a single IV infusion over 1 hour

Intracoronary—10,000 U to 20,000 U initially, followed by 2000 U to 4000 U/ minute until lysis occurs, then 2000 U/ minute for 1 hour

Urokinase

Urokinase is available as powder for injection (250,000 U/vial) and powder for reconstitution (5,000 U/ml) in 1-ml vials for opening occluded IV catheters. When being prepared for systemic use, the powder is reconstituted by adding 5.2 ml of sterile water for injection to the vial, rolling it gently to aid mixing (*do not shake*), then diluting with either normal saline or 5% dextrose injection to the desired concentration before infusing. The drug should be mixed immediately before infusing since the solution contains no preservatives. An initial priming dose of 4400 U/kg is given over 10 minutes at a rate of 1.5 ml/minute, followed by continuous infusion of 4400 U/kg/hour at a rate of 15 ml/hour for 12 hours. The tubing is then flushed with normal saline injection or 5% dextrose injection at the same rate. Approximately 3 hours to 4 hours following urokinase therapy, a continuous heparin IV infusion should be initiated.

For lysis of coronary artery thrombi, following a bolus dose of heparin (2500 U–10,000 U), urokinase is infused into the occluded artery at a rate of 4 ml/minute (6000 U/minute) for up to 2 hours. Therapy should be continued until the artery is maximally opened.

FATE

Plasminogen is activated almost immediately on infusion of either enzyme. The metabolism of these drugs is poorly understood. Plasma half-life of streptokinase is 15 minutes to 20 minutes initially, while antistreptokinase antibodies are present. Following saturation of antibodies with a loading dose, half-life is prolonged up to 90 minutes. Serum half-life of urokinase is less than 20

minutes, but it is prolonged in the presence of impaired liver function. Excretion is by way of the urine and bile.

SIDE-EFFECTS/ADVERSE REACTIONS

Minor bleeding episodes may occur, frequently at sites of venipuncture or other invaded areas. Superficial bleeding is generally controlled by prolonged direct pressure. Excessive handling of patients can result in easy bruising. Mild allergic reactions (itching, flushing, urticaria) may also occur, especially with streptokinase; since urokinase is a protein of human origin, allergic reactions are less common. Fever is much more common in patients receiving streptokinase (30%) than in patients given urokinase (2%–3%). Symptomatic treatment is usually sufficient. Nausea, headache, and musculoskeletal pain have been reported especially with streptokinase.

Severe allergic reactions (anaphylaxis, angioneurotic edema, dyspnea, and bronchospasm) are also possible, most often with streptokinase. Internal bleeding (cerebral, gastrointestinal, urinary, retroperitoneal) has resulted in several fatalities, and if serious bleeding occurs, the infusion should be discontinued. Use of aminocaproic acid as an antidote is not approved, but a loading dose of 5 g over 30 minutes to 60 minutes, followed by infusion of 1 g/hour has been reported to be effective in controlling serious bleeding.

CONTRAINDICATIONS AND PRECAUTIONS

Thrombolytic therapy is contraindicated in the presence of active internal bleeding, recent cerebrovascular accident, intracranial or intraspinal surgery, and intracranial neoplasm. A *cautious* approach to thrombolytic therapy is mandated in the following situations: recent or imminent surgery or obstetric delivery, ulcerative wounds, trauma with internal injuries, malignancies, urinary or gastrointestinal lesions (*e.g.*, colitis, diverticulitis), severe hypertension, diabetic retinopathy, hepatic or renal disease, hemorrhagic disorders, chronic lung disease, rheumatic heart disease, mitral stenosis, subacute bacterial endocarditis, history of allergic reactions, pregnancy, and immediate postpartum period, and in children or persons over 75 years of age.

INTERACTIONS

1. Drugs that alter platelet function (*e.g.*, salicylates, dipyridamole, indomethacin, phenylbutazone) or coagulation (*e.g.*, heparin, warfarin)

may increase the risk of hemorrhage with streptokinase.

Alteplase, Recombinant

(Activase)

MECHANISM AND ACTIONS
Alteplase is a tissue plasminogen activator (tPA) manufactured by recombinant DNA technique using complementary DNA for natural tissue-type plasminogen activator obtained from a human melanoma cell line. When administered systemically, alteplase binds to fibrin in a thrombus and converts the enmeshed plasminogen to plasmin. Unlike the other thrombolytic enzymes, it produces only limited conversion of plasminogen in the absence of fibrin, and therefore is associated with a much reduced likelihood of inducing a systemic lytic state.

USES
1. Management of acute myocardial infarction, to lyse thrombi obstructing coronary arteries and improve ventricular function

ADMINISTRATION AND DOSAGE
Alteplase is available as a powder for injection containing either 20 mg (11.6 million units) or 50 mg (29 million units) per vial with diluent. The drug is given by IV infusion only and should be administered as soon as possible after the onset of symptoms, preferably no later than 4 hours to 6 hours. The recommended dose is 100 mg, given as 60 mg in the first hour (6 mg–10 mg as a bolus in the first 1 to 2 minutes), 20 mg over the second hour, and 20 mg over the third hour. Heparin is usually given concomitantly for at least 48 hours, and aspirin or dipyridamole may be administered orally either during or following heparin administration. Doses of 150 mg or larger have been associated with an increased incidence of intracranial bleeding and should be avoided.

FATE
Alteplase is cleared quickly from the plasma by the liver; more than one-half the dose is cleared within 5 minutes and over 75% of a dose is cleared within 10 minutes.

SIDE-EFFECTS/ADVERSE REACTIONS
The principal adverse effect associated with altepase administration is bleeding, which may be categorized into two types. *Internal* bleeding involving the GI tract and genitourinary system occurs at approximately a 5% incidence, whereas retroperitoneal, gingival, and nosebleeds occur in less than 1% of patients. Conversely, *superficial* bleeding at invasive sites (*e.g.*, arterial punctures, venous cutdowns, recent surgical procedures) is more common, and invasive procedures should be avoided if at all possible for 24 hours to 48 hours following drug administration. Other side-effects reported during alteplase treatment include mild hypersensitivity reactions, and occasional nausea, vomiting, and hypotension.

CONTRAINDICATIONS AND PRECAUTIONS
Contraindications to use of alteplase include active internal bleeding, history of cerebrovascular accident, recent intracranial or intraspinal surgery, intracranial neoplasm, arteriovenous aneurysm, and severe uncontrolled hypertension. Many *cautions* to alteplase administration exist, and include recent major surgery, trauma, or GI bleeding; blood pressure above 180/110; pericarditis or bacterial endocarditis; hemostatic defects; mitral stenosis; liver dysfunction; hemorrhagic ophthalmic conditions; pregnancy; concurrent use of oral anticoagulants; advanced age. Reperfusion of occluded coronary arteries may result in development of arrhythmias. IM injections should be avoided during therapy, and handling of the patient should be minimized. If bleeding occurs that cannot be controlled by pressure, alteplase and concurrent heparin therapy should be terminated.

INTERACTIONS
1. Drugs that alter platelet function (aspirin, dipyridamole, sulfinpyrazone) can increase the risk of bleeding with alteplase.

■ Nursing Process

Thrombolytic agents are potentially hazardous drugs that require constant supervision and consistent monitoring. The circumstances under which they are generally given, to the patient with a myocardial infarction or pulmonary emboli, are fraught with pain, fear, and extreme discomfort for the patient and his family. Administration of these drugs may be the responsibility of the physician in most facilities but the nurse caring for the patient must know the intricacies of the therapy to provide safe monitoring. If possible, the nurse should be present when the physician explains the therapy and its hazards to the patient so she can better answer later questions and lend support.

☐ *ASSESSMENT*

☐ *Subjective Data*
The patient must be carefully screened, through history taking, for any evidence of problems that may increase bleeding tendencies. A history of bleeding disorder; hypertension; gastrointestinal ulcers or bleeding within the past six months; and surgery, biopsy, invasive procedures, or delivery of a child within 10 days of drug therapy are all contraindications for drug treatment since the risk of hemorrhage is high. The patient must also be questioned about any recent streptococcal infections since the presence of streptococcus antibodies will render the patient resistant to the drug.

A drug history should also be obtained. Chronic use of aspirin or nonsteroidal anti-inflammatory agents (*i.e.*, arthritis drugs) as well as recent administration of anticoagulants increases the risk of hemorrhage.

☐ *Objective Data*
A complete physical assessment should be performed with special emphasis on the cardiovascular system and respiratory system depending on the rationale for drug therapy. Essential baseline values include temperature; pulse, including all peripheral pulses; respiration; blood pressure; cardiac sounds; and breath sounds. The patient to receive urokinase should be weighed since dosage is based on that value.

Laboratory data should be collected before administering any thrombolytic medications. A complete blood count, platelet count, and coagulation studies (including thrombin time, prothrombin time, partial thromboplastin time, fibrinogen, and fibrin degradation products) should be obtained to provide baseline data against which to measure drug effectiveness. Liver and cardiac enzymes and renal function studies are also necessary and the patient should be typed and crossmatched for blood as a precaution. In addition, a streptokinase resistance test (the ability of the drug to dissolve 10 ml–15 ml of a clotted blood sample) will indicate whether the patient is resistant to the drugs as a result of past streptococcal infection. If this level exceeds 1,000,000 units, the drug should probably not be administered.

If the drug is to be given for coronary thrombus an electrocardiogram should be performed. Evidence of ST wave depression and additional Q waves indicates ischemia, which may benefit from thrombolytic therapy. Therapy is considered most successful if the patient has had unremitting chest pain for less than 3 hours to 4 hours.

If the drug is to be administered because of pulmonary emboli a pulmonary arteriogram and arterial blood gases will be performed.

☐ *NURSING DIAGNOSES*
Actual nursing diagnoses may include
Knowledge deficit related to the action and effects of the drug on the body
Fear of bodily injury and of the effects of the drug
Alteration in tissue perfusion related to thrombus formation
and either
Alteration in cardiac output: decreased related to thrombus formation
or
Alteration in respiratory function related to thrombus formation
Potential nursing diagnoses include
Potential fluid volume deficit related to hemorrhage
Hyperthermia related to drug side-effect
Potential for injury: trauma related to ineffective clotting (may occur at *any* internal or external body site)
Alteration in respiratory function related to anaphylaxis
Impaired tissue integrity related to impaired clotting

☐ *PLAN*
Nursing care goals for the patient receiving thrombolytic agents aim to
1. Reduce the anxiety associated with the procedures surrounding accurate drug administration
2. Monitor the patient closely for improvement and side-effects
3. Be prepared to deal with major side-effects promptly
4. Establish teaching goals for the patient who will be placed on long-term anticoagulant therapy after thrombolytic agents have been administered (see Chap. 39)

☐ *INTERVENTION*
Multiple venipuncture sites will be necessary during streptokinase therapy. As many as four intravenous lines may be needed in addition to the femoral

artery site used in the intracoronary administration. All sites should be started before the thrombolytic is administered and closely monitored throughout treatment for signs of bleeding. If possible, one site should be reserved for the intermittent blood samples needed during therapy to ensure appropriate dosages without the danger of multiple punctures.

Dosage calculation and drug mixing are very specific and vary depending on the manufacturer. Package inserts and institutional criteria should be closely followed when mixing and administering the drug. Intravenous administration should be monitored by an infusion pump to ensure accuracy of dosage per hour. Changes in dosage should be based on thrombin time and fibrinogen levels as well as by the patient's response to the drug.

Several drugs should be on hand and may be used prophylactically to counteract potential side-effects. In addition to standard emergency drugs the patient may be given antihistamines or steroids to counteract anaphylaxis; an antiarrhythmic such as lidocaine, intravenous nitroglycerin, or nifedipine to counteract angina; aminocaproic acid and typed and crossmatched blood to facilitate hemostasis if hemorrhage occurs; and analgesics or tranquilizers for chest pain or anxiety surrounding the event.

To reduce anxiety, the patient and his family need to be told what is actually happening throughout antithrombolytic therapy. If streptokinase is administered by the intracoronary route the entire procedure may take 2 hours to 5 hours and will occur in a cardiac catheterization laboratory. Because of the length of time, the patient may think he is actually having open heart surgery and must be assured of the difference. If the drugs are administered intravenously the procedure will be done in a coronary care unit. In either case, the patient must understand that the drug therapy does not reverse but attempts to limit tissue damage from the blood clot.

After drug treatment is completed the patient will be unable to achieve hemostasis for several hours. Consequently, an arterial sheath or pressure dressing may be necessary to control site bleeding. Dressings should be checked every hour and reinforced as necessary but should not be removed unless frank hemorrhage is noted since clot formation should not be disturbed.

Bleeding is the major side-effect of thrombolytic therapy. Thrombin times should be drawn intermittently throughout therapy, and if the value falls below one-half of normal, the physician

should be notified and the drug discontinued. Blood pressure should be monitored every 2 hours; hypotension is an early sign of hemorrhage. Other clinical signs of serious bleeding that bear monitoring include hematuria, ecchymosis, epistaxis, gum bleeding, chest pain, dyspnea, abdominal pain or tenderness, vaginal bleeding, and melena or frank blood in the stools. Signs of an intracerebral bleed include headache and changes in vision or mental alertness.

Internal bleeding can occur if the patient is turned or handled too firmly or if a pressure point develops from infrequent position changes. The patient should be placed on a mattress that provides even weight support and should be turned gently and frequently. Invasive procedures such as insertion of nasogastric or urinary catheter tubes, endotracheal intubation, or suctioning should be minimized to decrease the chance of internal bleeding. If suctioning must be done, a low vacuum setting (below 110 mm Hg) should be used.

If serious bleeding occurs the physician should be notified and the drug discontinued. Whole blood, dextran, or aminocaproic acid may be administered as appropriate.

Another serious side-effect, especially of streptokinase, is allergic reactions. Mild ones manifested mainly by fever, a common side-effect, may be controlled by antihistamines or antipyretics (acetaminophen, not aspirin), but if asthmatic symptoms or blood pressure changes occur the physician should be notified and the drug discontinued. Epinephrine and corticosteroids should be on hand to manage any serious allergic reactions.

Arrhythmias may develop, especially when reperfusion occurs in the intracoronary administration of streptokinase. The patient should be continuously monitored and carefully watched for ventricular problems. Lidocaine is the drug of choice but several antiarrhythmics should be on hand as alternates if necessary.

Although the thrombolytic agents may dissolve a primary clot, the lysis of this clot may result in thrombosis at other sites. The patient must be closely monitored for evidence of chest pain or extremity color changes, pallor, cyanosis, swelling, or pain. Peripheral pulses should be evaluated frequently and any change promptly reported.

At the end of thrombolytic therapy, heparin will be given for about 2 days to 3 days to achieve a prothrombin time 2 to 3 times normal. During that time oral anticoagulants will be started and the patient may also receive aspirin or dipyridamole to enhance anticoagulation. Oral therapy will continue 2 months to 3 months; the patient must learn to follow the prescribed schedule carefully (see Chap. 39).

□ *EVALUATION*
Outcome criteria against which to measure success of therapy is relief of symptoms caused by thrombosis, a change in the arteriogram if the patient has suffered a myocardial infarction or pulmonary emboli, and successful management of any side-effects that may occur.

Hemostatic Drugs

Hemostatic drugs enhance coagulation and may be used to control bleeding in a variety of situations. Certain *systemically* administered agents such as antihemophilic factor, anti-inhibitor coagulant complex, or factor IX complex are employed to elevate or replenish one or more coagulation factors that may be deficient because of a hereditary or acquired defect. Aminocaproic acid, another systemically acting hemostatic, is used to treat excessive systemic bleeding resulting from hyperfibrinolytic conditions. *Topically* applied hemostatics in the form of sponges, pads, pellets, powders, and so on are primarily used to control continual oozing or mild bleeding from capillaries and other small blood vessels (*e.g.,* following surgery), or in the treatment of decubitus or chronic leg ulcers. These various hemostatic drugs are reviewed below. Vitamin K may also be employed to control certain types of bleeding, and is discussed with the other fat-soluble vitamin in Chapter 77. The use of vitamin K_1 as an oral anticoagulant antidote is considered in Chapter 39.

Systemic Hemostatics

Aminocaproic Acid
(Amicar)

MECHANISM AND ACTIONS
Aminocaproic acid blocks fibrinolysis by inhibiting plasminogen activators and by interfering with the binding of plasmin to fibrin (see Fig. 40-1).

USES
1. Treatment of severe bleeding resulting from systemic hyperfibrinolysis, such as that associated with heart surgery, hematologic disorders, abruptio placentae, cirrhosis of the liver, or neoplastic disorders
2. Treatment of urinary hyperfibrinolysis, such as that associated with severe trauma, shock, prostatectomy, nephrectomy, or renal malignancies
3. Treatment of overdosage with fibrinolytic drugs (*e.g.,* streptokinase, urokinase)
4. Prevention of recurrence of subarachnoid hemorrhage, abort or prevent attacks of hereditary angioneurotic edema, and decrease need for platelet transfusion in cases of megakaryocytic thrombocytopenia (investigational uses only)

ADMINISTRATION AND DOSAGE
Aminocaproic acid is available as tablets (500 mg), syrup (250 mg/ml), and for injection (250 mg/ml).

The plasma level necessary for inhibition of fibrinolysis is approximately 0.13 mg/ml. An initial dose of 5 g (orally or IV) followed by 1 g to 1.25 g hourly will generally achieve and maintain such a plasma level.

When given IV, a slow infusion is recommended. Rapid IV injection can lead to hypotension, bradycardia, and arrhythmias. For infusion, 4 g to 5 g is diluted in 250 ml of appropriate diluent (*e.g.,* sterile water for injection, 5% dextrose, normal saline, or Ringer's solution) and administered during the first hour, followed by 1 g/hour in 50 ml of diluent for 8 hours or until bleeding ceases. The maximum recommended dose is 30 g/24 hours.

FATE
The drug is rapidly absorbed orally, and peak plasma levels occur within 2 hours. The duration of action is relatively short (less than 3 hours with IV injection). The drug is widely distributed, and the majority of a dose is recovered unmetabolized in the urine.

SIDE-EFFECTS/ADVERSE REACTIONS
Common side-effects with aminocaproic acid are nausea, cramping, diarrhea, and malaise. Other untoward reactions reported include hypotension, dizziness, tinnitus, headache, visual and auditory disturbances, delirium, nasal stuffiness, skin rash, menstrual cramping, reversible acute renal failure, thrombophlebitis, and myopathy, characterized by weakness, elevated serum creatinine phosphokinase and serum glutamic-oxaloacetic transaminase (SGOT), and occasional acute rhabdomyolysis. An isolated report of cardiac and hepatic lesions has

appeared. A teratogenic potential has been demonstrated, and the drug may impair fertility.

CONTRAINDICATIONS AND PRECAUTIONS
Aminocaproic acid is contraindicated in patients with evidence of active intravascular clotting (*e.g.,* disseminated intravascular coagulation; DIC), and in the presence of hematuria of upper urinary tract origin. The drug must be given *cautiously* to persons with cardiac, hepatic, or renal disease and to pregnant women or to children.

INTERACTIONS
1. Oral contraceptives or other estrogens may increase the danger of increased coagulation.
2. Serum potassium levels can be elevated by aminocaproic acid.

■ *Nursing Process*

□ ASSESSMENT

□ *Subjective Data*
A drug history should be obtained to determine if the patient is using estrogens or oral contraceptives since these will interfere with the action of the drug and result in hypercoagulability.

□ *Objective Data*
Several laboratory values should be obtained in order to determine the appropriateness of therapy with aminocaproic acid. If platelet count and euglobulin lysis time are abnormal the condition is considered primary fibrinolysis and treatment with aminocaproic acid is warranted. If euglobulin lysis time is normal the condition is more likely to be DIC and use of aminocaproic acid would be inappropriate.

□ *NURSING DIAGNOSES*
Actual nursing diagnoses may include
    Knowledge deficit about the action and effects
      of the drug
    Fear related to bleeding and the sensation of
      something being wrong
Potential diagnoses may include
    Alteration in cardiac output related to
      hypotension and arrhythmias
    Alteration in comfort related to
      gastrointestinal distress or pain

□ PLAN
The nursing care goals focus on correct administration of the drug to achieve a therapeutic plasma level and minimize the dangerous side-effects.

□ INTERVENTION
When the drug is given orally, the patient may be required to swallow as many as 10 pills since Amicar comes only in 500-mg tablets. For some patients this may be impossible to do; the syrup formulation may then be an appropriate alternative.

When loading doses are given intravenously the nurse's primary responsibility is to monitor the patient for side-effects. Frequent vital signs and continuous electrocardiographic monitoring are essential since the main side-effects are arrhythmias and hypotension. These occur more frequently if the drug has been administered too rapidly but may occur at any time during the therapy. An infusion pump should be used to control dosage accuracy. Appropriate emergency medications should be on hand to counteract these problems and the patient's activity should be limited to ensure his safety. The IV site should be closely observed for swelling and pain, and the site should be removed at the first sign of infiltration. Drug extravasation can cause tissue damage.

Thromboembolic complications can occur as a result of hemostatic drug administration. The nurse must closely monitor the patient for signs of clot formation such as chest pain; changes in color, temperature, or pain in any extremity; dyspnea; abdominal pain; changes in neurologic signs; or changes in peripheral pulses. These must be reported immediately since the drug may need to be discontinued. Alternate therapy may be needed.

Gastrointestinal side-effects are usually dose related and transient in nature. Since it may not be possible to reduce the drug until a therapeutic plasma level has been achieved the use of antiemetics or antidiarrheals may be necessary for the patient's comfort.

If bleeding continues to be severe, emergency treatment may be instituted while aminocaproic acid is being given. Fresh whole blood or fibrinogen may be infused to provide clotting factors to the faulty system. The patient must then be more carefully monitored for potential fluid overload or thromboembolic complications.

The pregnant patient with abruptio placentae needs careful consideration. Aminocaproic acid can be damaging to the fetus. However, the drug may be given when the benefits to the mother outweigh the risks to the fetus. In either case, the mother faces a loss of the unborn child and needs tremendous emotional support.

☐ EVALUATION
Outcome criteria against which to measure success of drug therapy would be a therapeutic plasma level of 0.13 mg/ml or higher, cessation of bleeding, and successful prevention or management of side-effects.

Tranexamic Acid
(Cyklokapron)

MECHANISM AND ACTIONS
Tranexamic acid is a competitive inhibitor of plasminogen activation and may directly interfere with the action of plasmin at high concentrations. Thrombin time is prolonged, but the drug has no effect on platelet aggregation or coagulation time.

USES
1. Reduce or prevent hemorrhage and reduce the need for replacement therapy during and following tooth extraction in hemophilia patients (short term use, 3 to 8 days)

ADMINISTRATION AND DOSAGE
Tranexamic acid is used as either tablets (500 mg) or injection (100 mg/ml). One day prior to dental surgery, 25 mg/kg is given orally 3 to 4 times/day. Alternately, the above dose can be given IV if oral medication cannot be taken, or 10 mg/kg is given IV immediately prior to surgery. Following surgery, 25 mg/kg is administered 3 to 4 times a day for up to 8 days. Reduced doses are necessary in patients with impaired renal function (based on serum creatinine levels).

FATE
Absorption following oral administration is 25% to 50% of the dose. Peak plasma levels occur in 2 hours to 3 hours and effective concentrations persist in the plasma for up to 8 hours. Protein binding is insignificant. Urinary excretion is the major route of elimination, and greater than 95% of a dose is excreted unchanged in the urine.

SIDE-EFFECTS/ADVERSE REACTIONS
Nausea, vomiting, and diarrhea occur occasionally with oral administration but usually disappear quickly. Too-rapid IV injection can elicit hypoten-

sion. Visual abnormalities have been reported and appear to depend on length of therapy.

CONTRAINDICATIONS AND PRECAUTIONS
Tranexamic acid is contraindicated in patients with subarachnoid hemorrhage and acquired defective color vision, as this may interfere with detection of toxicity (altered color vision is an early indication of visual toxicity). A cautious approach to therapy must be undertaken in patients with renal insufficiency and in pregnant or nursing women.

NURSING CONSIDERATIONS
See Nursing Process above.

Antihemophilic Factor
(H.T. Factorate, Hemofil T, Koate-HS, Koate-HT, Monoclate)

Antihemophilic factor (AHF) is a protein found in plasma (factor VIII) that is an essential component of the intrinsic pathway of blood coagulation. A congenital lack of AHF results in the development of classical hemophilia (hemophilia A), a disease in which afflicted persons are subject to serious bleeding, even from minor wounds. AHF is a commercially lyophilized or dried extract of human plasma containing a concentrated form of factor VIII.

MECHANISM AND ACTIONS
Administration of AHF replaces deficient endogenous factor VIII and can temporarily arrest the coagulation defect in patients with classical hemophilia. Factor VIII functions as part of the intrinsic clotting pathway, ultimately leading to the conversion of prothrombin to thrombin.

USES
1. Treatment of classical hemophilia A, in which there is a demonstrated deficiency of the plasma clotting factor VIII, in order to correct or prevent bleeding or permit the performance of surgical procedures
Note: AHF is not effective in controlling bleeding in persons with von Willebrand's disease (pseudohemophilia), since factor VIII is only one of the factors deficient in this disease, the others being Willebrand factor and factor VIII antigen.

ADMINISTRATION AND DOSAGE
Antihemophilic factor is available as a stable lyophilized concentrate in single-dose vials with diluent

or as a stable dried preparation in concentrated form in either single-dose or multiple-dose vials with diluent. One AHF unit is the activity present in 1 ml of normal pooled human plasma less than 1 hour old. It is administered by IV injection only, using plastic syringes, since the solution may adhere to the surface of glass syringes. Dosage is individualized based on patient's weight, severity of bleeding, presence of factor VIII inhibitors, and the desired level of factor VIII. Therapy should be based on factor VIII level assays. The following average doses are recommended:

Prophylaxis of spontaneous hemorrhage—10 U/kg as a single dose; do not repeat in mild cases unless further bleeding occurs.

Moderate hemorrhage/minor surgery—15 U/kg to 25 U/kg initially, followed by 10 U/kg to 15 U/kg every 8 hours to 12 hours as needed.

Severe hemorrhage—40 U/kg to 50 U/kg initially, followed by 20 U/kg every 8 hours to 12 hours

Refer to the dosage instructions included with the package for complete directions. Doses less than 34 U/ml may be given at a rate of 10 ml to 20 ml over 3 minutes; doses greater than 34 U/ml should be given at a maximum rate of 2 ml/minute. If a significant increase in pulse rate occurs, the rate of administration should be decreased.

FATE
Upon infusion, there is an almost instantaneous rise in coagulant level, followed by a rapid decrease in activity. Plasma half-life following the initial dose ranges from 8 hours to 24 hours, and increases with subsequent doses.

SIDE-EFFECTS/ADVERSE REACTIONS
Allergic reactions, such as pruritus, urticaria, erythema, and fever, may occur but usually disappear within 30 minutes. Other adverse reactions reported include nausea, vomiting, headache, chills, tachycardia, hypotension, backache, somnolence, lethargy, and visual disturbances. Massive doses have resulted in acute hemolytic anemia, increased bleeding tendency, and hyperfibrinogenemia.

CONTRAINDICATIONS AND PRECAUTIONS
There are no absolute contraindications to use of AHF although safety for use during pregnancy has not been established. Since AHF is prepared from human plasma, the risk of transmitting hepatitis

and acquired immunodeficiency syndrome (AIDS) during infusion exists, and although more data are required to confirm or refute the risk potential, this risk should be recognized and the patient made aware of it prior to AHF administration. Donor screening tests to detect antibodies to AIDS should be used to screen donated blood.

Approximately 5% to 10% of hemophilia A patients have inhibitors to factor VIII. In these patients, the response to AHF may be markedly reduced or absent; such patients may be candidates for anti-inhibitor coagulant complex (see below). Large or frequent doses of AHF in patients with blood types A, B, or AB may result in intravascular hemolysis and anemia; appropriate blood monitoring is necessary during extended or high-dose therapy.

NURSING CONSIDERATIONS
AHF is extremely expensive and usually in limited supply in most facilities. Therefore, the nurse's primary responsibility is to ensure the factor is correctly reconstituted and given in a timely fashion in order to avoid precipitation, gel formation, or bacterial contamination. In addition to the package instructions the nurse should be aware of the following:

1. The drug should be stored between 2°C and 8°C until *reconstituted.* After reconstitution it should *not* be refrigerated.
2. During reconstitution the drug vial should be gently rotated, *not* shaken. To facilitate reconstitution, the concentrate and diluent can be brought to room temperature. If gel formation occurs during reconstitution the pharmacy or blood bank should be notified. The factor should not be used.
3. Once the AHF has been reconstituted it should be administered within 3 hours to minimize the risk of bacterial contamination.

Since AHF is given by IV push method *only,* facility policy may dictate which personnel are authorized to give the drug. The nurse giving this drug for the first time should confirm hospital policy before administering it.

Anti-inhibitor Coagulant Complex
(Autoplex, Feiba VH Immuno)

Anti-inhibitor coagulant complex is prepared from pooled human plasma and consists of a concentrate of activated and precursor clotting factors and factors of the kinin-generating system. It is standardized based on its ability to correct the clotting time of hemophilic plasma containing inhibitors to factor VIII.

MECHANISM AND ACTIONS
Anti-inhibitor coagulant complex provides necessary clotting factors to arrest bleeding in patients with hemophilia A, who possess significant levels of factor VIII inhibitors and who are therefore unresponsive to AHF.

USES
1. Treatment of symptoms of hemophilia in patients with significant levels of factor VIII inhibitors (i.e., greater than 10 Bethesda units) who are bleeding or about to undergo surgery. (Patients with factor VIII inhibitor levels between 2 and 10 Bethesda units may be treated with either AHF [see previous discussion] or anti-inhibitor coagulant complex.)

ADMINISTRATION AND DOSAGE
Anti-inhibitor coagulant complex is available as a dried coagulant complex in multiple-dose vials with diluent. Each bottle is labeled with the units of factor VIII correctional activity that it contains. One unit of factor VIII correctional activity is the quantity of activated complex, which upon addition to an equal volume of factor VIII deficient or inhibitor plasma will correct the clotting time to a normal 35 seconds. The drug is administered by IV infusion only. The usual recommended dose is 25 to 100 factor VIII correctional units per kilogram, depending on the severity of the hemorrhage. If no improvement is observed, the dosage may be repeated within 6 hours to 12 hours. The rate of infusion may be as fast as 10 ml/minute, but should be reduced if headache, flushing, or changes in pulse rate or pressure occur.

SIDE-EFFECTS/ADVERSE REACTIONS
Allergic reactions, manifested by fever, chills, urticaria, rash, or hypotension, may occur on administration. Severe anaphylactoid reactions have been reported as well. Other untoward effects include headaches, flushing, and tachycardia, especially with too-rapid infusion. Hypercoagulability can occur and may be characterized by dyspnea, chest pain, cough, and changes in blood pressure and heart rate. If these signs are noted, the drug should

be discontinued and the patient given proper supportive therapy.

CONTRAINDICATIONS AND PRECAUTIONS
Anti-inhibitor coagulant complex is contraindicated in states of fibrinolysis and DIC. The preparation is to be used cautiously in patients with liver disease or a history of allergies, in small children, and during pregnancy. Since this product is obtained from large pools of human plasma, there is a risk of transmitting hepatitis and possibly AIDS. While quite small, this risk should nevertheless be recognized.

INTERACTIONS
1. The possibility of hypercoagulability states is increased with concomitant use of anti-inhibitor coagulant complex and aminocaproic acid.

NURSING CONSIDERATIONS
Prothrombin time should be closely monitored in all patients receiving this infusion. Postinfusion prothrombin time should be at least two thirds of the preinfusion value if reinfusion is ordered. The nurse should keep the physician apprised of laboratory values and seek clarification before readministering the drug.

The main serious side-effect of anti-inhibitor coagulant complex is an allergic reaction. Emergency drugs such as epinephrine, antihistamines, and corticosteroids should be on hand to treat respiratory symptoms or generalized edema if it occurs.

The patient should be instructed to report the onset of chest pain, shortness of breath, or coughing. These may herald the onset of hypercoagulability.

Blood pressure and heart rate should be monitored frequently, especially during the initial phase of drug administration.

Factor IX Complex—Human
(Konyne, Profilnine, Proplex)

Factor IX complex is a stable, dried, purified concentrate that causes an increase in blood levels of factors II, VII, IX, and X. A deficiency of factor IX complex results in a hemorrhagic condition termed hemophilia B (Christmas disease). Acquired deficiencies of factor II can occur also, and are almost always associated with deficiencies of factors VII, IX, and X as well.

MECHANISM AND ACTIONS

Factor IX complex raises factor IX plasma levels and restores hemostasis in patients with factor IX deficiency. It provides replacement therapy for congenital or acquired deficiencies of one or more of the above-named clotting factors that can result in increased bleeding tendencies.

USES

1. Treatment of factor IX deficiency (hemophilia B or Christmas disease) to prevent or control bleeding episodes (not a substitute for fresh-frozen plasma in patients with *mild* factor IX deficiency)
2. Control of bleeding episodes in patients with factor VIII inhibitors (Proplex)
3. Reversal of oral anticoagulant-induced hemorrhaging

ADMINISTRATION AND DOSAGE

Factor IX complex is available as a dried plasma fraction of coagulant factors II, VII, IX, and X in single-dose bottles with diluent. Dosage is highly individualized depending on circumstances and patient status, that is, severity of bleeding, degree of factor deficiency, and desired level of factor IX. Dosage is measured in units (1 unit is the activity present in 1 ml of normal plasma less than 1 hour old). Potency is adjusted based on factor IX, because the other factors (II, VII, X) are present in approximately the same amount.

Recommended IV dosage guidelines are as follows:

Treatment of bleeding in hemophilia A patients with inhibitors to factor VIII—75 U/kg; repeat in 12 hours if needed.
Reversal of coumarin effect—15 U/kg
Hemarthroses in hemophiliacs with factor VIII inhibitors—75 U/kg; repeat in 12 hours if necessary.
Prophylaxis in patients with congenital deficiency of procoagulant factors—10 U to 20 U/kg once or twice a week to prevent spontaneous bleeding

The infusion rate should not exceed 10 ml/minute.

SIDE-EFFECTS/ADVERSE REACTIONS

Too-rapid infusion or large doses can result in flushing, hypotension, and tachycardia, and, on occasion, chills, fever, headache, nausea, vomiting, somnolence, and urticaria. Thrombosis and DIC have been reported.

CONTRAINDICATIONS AND PRECAUTIONS

Factor IX complex is contraindicated in patients with liver disease in which there are signs of intravascular coagulation or fibrinolysis. The drug should not be used in patients undergoing elective surgery, since the risk of thrombosis in the postoperative period is substantial. Factor IX complex should *not* be used in cases where fresh-frozen plasma is satisfactory. The risk of transmitting viral hepatitis and AIDS is present, and although minimal, should be considered. Indiscriminate prophylactic use in patients *not* demonstrating a specific clotting factor deficiency is discouraged. If signs of intravascular coagulation occur (*e.g.*, cough, chest pain, respiratory distress, altered pulse and pressure), discontinue infusion promptly.

NURSING CONSIDERATIONS

Baseline coagulation assays of factors II, VII, IX, and X should be performed before treatment is initiated. Periodic assessment of these factors will be done throughout drug administration in order to evaluate the effectiveness of the drug. The nurse may want to establish a flow sheet so all data will be collected in one place and can be easily reviewed for individualized dosing.

Reconstitution of factor IX complex follows the same guidelines given for antihemophilic factor.

The main side-effects of the drug are dose dependent and can be controlled by slowing the infusion rate. Use an infusion pump to control rate and minimize the development of side-effects. However, the nurse should monitor the patient closely for chest pain, extremity pain or discoloration, and changes in peripheral pulses since thrombosis can occur.

Topical Hemostatics

A variety of substances are available for topical application for controlling minor bleeding episodes and reducing oozing and leakage from small blood vessels that may occur as a result of trauma or surgery. These topical hemostatics are rarely effective in controlling extensive hemorrhaging. Many of these products are employed during or following surgery to retard blood loss through capillary and small vessel leakage. Most of the products are slowly absorbable and therefore provide a temporary framework on which platelets can adhere.

Others are of a gelatin composition, which can absorb many times its weight in blood and which adheres to the damaged site, slowing further blood loss. The clinically available topical hemostatic products are discussed below.

Absorbable Gelatin Film

(Gelfilm)

Absorbable gelatin film is a nonantigenic substance with the appearance and texture of cellophane. When moistened, it acquires a rubbery consistency and then can be cut and molded to fit a particular area. It is employed to reduce local bleeding and facilitate healing in various types of ocular, thoracic, and neurologic surgery. The product is immersed in sterile saline, soaked until pliable, cut to the desired size and shape, and applied to the desired surface. The rate of absorption after implantation is variable, depending on the size of implant and the area involved, and ranges from 1 month to 6 months. Tissue reactions are rare and the likelihood of developing adhesions is minimal. Absorbable gelatin film should *not* be implanted into grossly contaminated or infected surgical wounds, since the rate of absorption is greatly accelerated and effectiveness may be compromised.

Absorbable Gelatin Powder

(Gelfoam)

When applied locally, absorbable gelatin powder promotes growth of granulation tissue and facilitates healing of ulcers (such as leg ulcers) and other slow-healing wounds. It may be made into a paste by addition of small amounts of sterile saline, which can then be applied to the surface of cancellous bone to arrest bleeding. Chronic leg ulcers or decubitus ulcers may be packed with the sterile powder and covered with a dressing to accelerate healing. The product is completely absorbed from the application site within 4 weeks to 6 weeks without excessive scar tissue formation. When applied to surface bleeding sites (nose, skin, rectum, vagina), it liquefies within 2 days to 5 days. The powder should not be used in the presence of infection, nor to control postpartum bleeding or menorrhagia. It should never be utilized to close skin incisions because it may interfere with the healing of skin edges. Since the powder can form a focus for abscess formation, patients should be closely observed during the healing process.

Absorbable Gelatin Sponge

(Gelfoam)

Absorbable gelatin sponge is a pliable, nonantigenic sponge capable of absorbing many times its weight in whole blood. It is prepared from specially treated, purified gelatin solution. The product is completely absorbed in 4 weeks to 6 weeks when implanted into tissues, and liquefies within several days when applied to actively bleeding areas.

Absorbable gelatin sponge is used to assist hemostasis during surgical procedures when control of bleeding by conventional means such as ligature is ineffective or impractical. It is available as sponges of various sizes, dental packs for use during oral or dental surgery, and prostatectomy cones for use with the Foley bag catheter in prostatic surgery. The sponges are cut to a desired size and applied either dry or saturated with sodium chloride injection to the desired area. The sponge is held in place with moderate pressure for 10 seconds to 15 seconds, then allowed to remain in contact with the bleeding site. The wound may be closed over the sponge. Dental packs are inserted into a cavity or socket either dry or in a moistened state.

Care should be taken to avoid *over*packing closed tissue spaces, since the sponge can expand by absorbing fluid and may impact on neighboring structures. The sponges should not be used in the presence of infection, and should not be employed to control postpartum bleeding or menorrhagia. The sponge can become a focus for abscess formation or fibrous tissue deposition, and patients should be observed for such possibilities during the healing process.

Microfibrillar Collagen Hemostat

(Avitene)

Microfibrillar collagen hemostat is a dry, fibrous, water-insoluble preparation of purified bovine corium collagen. When applied to the source of bleeding, it attracts platelets, which adhere to the fibrils of the preparation, triggering further platelet aggregation into thrombi. It also stimulates a mild, chronic inflammatory response and does not interfere with bone regeneration or healing.

The product is used *dry* and is applied directly to the source of bleeding as an adjunct to hemostasis. The surface to be treated is compressed with a dry sponge for several minutes, then the dry product is applied, followed again by pressure with a dry sponge for several minutes. Gloved fingers should not be used to apply pressure, since the product adheres to wet gloves, instruments, or tissue. Excess material can then be teased away.

Microfibrillar collagen hemostat can seal over exit sites for deeper hemorrhage, resulting in hematoma formation. Application of the product can lead to abscess formation, wound dehiscence, and development of adhesions. In addition, allergic reactions have been reported. Contact of the product with nonbleeding internal surfaces should be avoided, because it is very tenacious and can result in local inflammatory reactions and adhesions. Use in contaminated wounds may enhance the development of infection. It is contraindicated on bone surfaces to which prosthetic appliances are to be attached, because it may reduce the adhesiveness of materials used on such appliances. It is also contraindicated in closure of skin incisions.

This product cannot be resterilized; it is inactivated by autoclaving.

Negatol

(Negatan)

Negatol is a colloidal solution (45%) obtained by reacting a metacresol sulfonic acid with formaldehyde. It is a highly acidic compound that has a coagulant effect on proteins. Negatol exerts an astringent and hemostatic action and can precipitate cervical mucus. It is used to control minor bleeding from the vagina, cervix, and vulvae. Initially, a 1:10 dilution is applied with an applicator. If no effect is noted, increasing concentrations may be employed. Negatol should *not* be used as a douche. Untoward reactions include irritation, burning, and erythema at the site of application. Local hypersensitivity reactions have also been reported. Contact with eyes or abraded skin should be avoided.

Oxidized Cellulose

(Novocell, Oxycel, Surgicel)

Oxidation of cellulose by nitrogen dioxide results in formation of an absorbable hemostatic product of known acidity. Upon contact with blood, oxidized cellulose swells into a dark brown, tenacious adhesive mass that conforms and adheres to the bleeding surface. After 24 hours to 48 hours it becomes gelatinous and can be removed without causing further bleeding. If left intact, it is slowly absorbed. It does not alter the normal clotting mechanism, but produces an artificial clot within minutes of contact. In addition to its hemostatic action, oxidized cellulose is bactericidal against a range of gram-positive as well as gram-negative organisms.

Oxidized cellulose is available as pads and strips of various sizes and pellets for dental implantation. The desired-size pad is placed on the bleeding site or held firmly against the tissues until hemostasis is achieved. Dental pellets are applied to the tooth socket or wound with pressure. Undissolved portions may be removed in several days. Oxidized cellulose is not intended for use as a packing or wadding, especially in rigid cavities, since swelling may result in impaired function or tissue necrosis. It should not be used to control hemorrhage from large arteries and is largely ineffective on nonhemorrhagic serous oozing, as it does not react with body fluids other than blood. Packing or implantation into fractures or laminectomies may interfere with bone regeneration or cause cyst formation. Although oxidized cellulose may be left *in situ*, wherever possible it should be removed by forceps or irrigation once hemostasis has occurred. Adverse reactions to oxidized cellulose include stinging, burning, headache, and sneezing with nasal application; foreign body reactions; encapsulation of fluid; and urinary or intestinal obstruction due to adhesion formation. Oxidized cellulose should not be closed in a contaminated wound without drainage. Due to its low *p*H, it will destroy other hemostatics and anti-infectives that are added to it.

This product cannot be resterilized; autoclaving causes physical breakdown. Opened, unused product should be discarded.

Thrombin, Topical

(Thrombinar, Thrombostat)

Topical thrombin is a powder derived from bovine sources from which a solution is prepared that is used to reduce oozing and minor bleeding from capillaries and small venules. The solution may also be used as a soak for absorbable gelatin sponge. The speed with which thrombin clots blood is dependent on its concentration. Solutions are prepared in sterile distilled water or isotonic saline, and concentrations range from 100 U/ml to 2000 U/ml, depending on extent and severity of bleeding. The area is usually sprayed or flooded with solution; the most effective hemostasis occurs when thrombin mixes freely with blood on the surface. Alternately, dried powder from the vial may be placed directly on the area, or absorbable gelatin sponge may be soaked in thrombin solution and then applied to the area of bleeding. Treated surfaces should not be sponged, to avoid dislodging clots. Thrombin should *never* be given parenterally or allowed to enter large vessels, since intravascular coagulation may result. Side-effects are rare; allergic reactions have been noted on occasion when thrombin is used to control epistaxis. Solutions are relatively unstable and should be used within 4 hours after preparation if no preservatives are added.

Avoid adding the solution to any wound in which acids, alkalis, heat, or heavy metals are used because these will reduce thrombin activity.

CASE STUDY

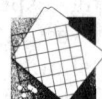

Mr. John Edwards comes to the emergency room complaining of chest pain and shortness of breath. Mr. Edwards, age 58, suffered a myocardial infarction 3 years ago. He states the present pain was not relieved by sublingual nitroglycerin and he decided to seek help. Mr. Edwards' electrocardiogram shows ST wave depression. An IV is started and blood is drawn. He is given morphine sulfate, 10 mg subcutaneously, with little relief. Oxygen is started and the patient is admitted to coronary care. When the laboratory results of cardiac enzyme studies come back elevated and Mr. Edwards' pain is not relieved by intravenous morphine, the decision is made to start a streptokinase infusion of 250,000 units. The drug is to be given over a 30-minute period.

Discussion Questions

1. What other laboratory data should be obtained before streptokinase is administered?
2. How should the nurse explain the action of streptokinase to Mr. Edwards?
3. What side-effects might occur while streptokinase is being infused? What drugs should be available in case of emergency?
4. What will be the long-term drug therapy for Mr. Edwards once streptokinase administration is completed? Why is anticoagulation important?

REVIEW QUESTIONS

1. What substances can serve as fibrinogen activators?
2. What is the principal action of streptokinase? How does its mechanism differ from that of urokinase?
3. How does tissue plasminogen activator (t-PA) differ from streptokinase or urokinase?
4. What are the major adverse reactions associated with streptokinase therapy? What drugs should be available to deal with them?
5. What assessment parameters should be completed before the decision is made to administer streptokinase?
6. What are some of the misconceptions a patient or family may have about thrombolytic therapy? How should the nurse deal with these?

7. Why should all venipunctures be completed before thrombolytic therapy begins?
8. How can the nurse assess the effectiveness of a pressure dressing used for hemostasis following thrombolytic therapy?
9. What emergency drugs should be available during administration of streptokinase?
10. In which situations is thrombolytic therapy contraindicated?
11. How does aminocaproic acid function as a hemostatic?
12. What are the dangers associated with *rapid* IV injection of aminocaproic acid?
13. What laboratory data should be obtained prior to aminocaproic acid administration?
14. Under what conditions might anti-inhibitor coagulant complex be preferred to antihemophilic factor?
15. What procedure should the nurse follow when reconstituting antihemophilic factor (AHF) or factor IX complex?
16. What is the composition of factor IX complex? What is the term given to the disease resulting from a deficiency of factor IX complex?
17. List the principal indications for topical hemostatic therapy.
18. What are the dangers associated with the use of absorbable gelatin preparations as topical hemostatics?
19. From what is microfibrillar collagen hemostat obtained? What adverse effects can occur with its application?
20. What properties does oxidized cellulose possess? Why should it not be used as a "packing" substance in closed body cavities?
21. Why should topical thrombin never be allowed to enter major blood vessels?

BIBLIOGRAPHY

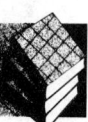

Anderson JL et al: A randomized trial of intracoronary streptokinase in the treatment of acute myocardial infarction. N Engl J Med 308:1312, 1983

Arnesen H, Hoiseth A, Ly B: Streptokinase or heparin in the treatment of deep vein thrombosis. Acta Med Scand 211:65, 1982

Bouman CC: Intracoronary thrombolysis and percutaneous transluminal coronary angioplasty. Nurs Clin North Am 19(3):397, 1984

Gever LN: Stopping bleeding with aminocaproic acid. Nursing 84 14(9):8, 1984

Koch-Weser J: Thrombolytic therapy. N Engl J Med 306:1268, 1982

Laffel GL, Braunwald E: Thrombolytic therapy: A new strategy for the treatment of acute myocardial infarction. N Engl J Med 311:710 and 770, 1984

Nissen MB: Streptokinase therapy in acute myocardial infarction. Heart Lung 13:223, 1984

Shafer K, Jaffe AS: Thrombolytic therapy: Current and potential uses. Drug Ther 13:95, 1983

Sherry S: Tissue plasminogen activator (t-PA): Will it fulfill its promise? N Engl J Med 313:1014, 1985

Sherry S, Gustafson E: The current and future use of thrombolytic therapy. Annu Rev Pharmacol Toxicol 25:413, 1985

Sherry S: Thrombolytic agents for acute evolving myocardial infarction: Comparative effects. Ration Drug Ther 21(1):1, 1987

Spann JF, Sherry S: Coronary thrombolysis for evolving myocardial infarction. Drugs 28:465, 1984

Taylor GJ et al: Intravenous versus intracoronary streptokinase therapy for acute myocardial infarction in community hospitals. Am J Cardiol 54:256, 1984

TIMI Study Group: The thrombolysis in myocardial infarction (TIMI Trial): Phase I findings. N Engl J Med 321:932, 1985

Totly WG et al: Low-dose intravascular fibrinolytic therapy. Radiology 143:59, 1982

Van de Werf F et al: Coronary thrombolysis with tissue-type plasminogen activator in patients with evolving myocardial infarction. N Engl J Med 310:609, 1984

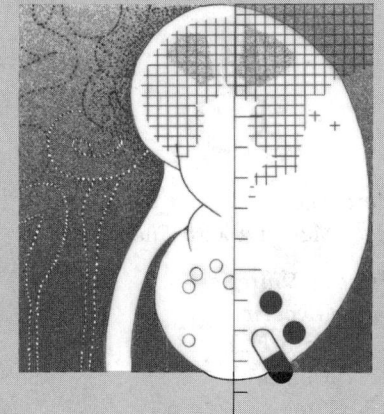

Drugs Affecting
Renal Function

V

Diuretics

41

A diuretic is an agent capable of increasing the volume of urine and promoting a net loss of body water. The retention of excess fluid by the body depends in large measure on the retention of sodium. Therefore, the effectiveness of a diuretic is primarily related to its ability to increase the excretion of sodium, which is accomplished in most cases by interfering with the reabsorption of sodium ions in the tubules of the kidney. Loss of sodium is accompanied by excretion of an osmotically equivalent quantity of water, which is derived from body fluids removed from the tissues. In order to better understand the actions of diuretic drugs, the anatomy and physiology of the kidney will be reviewed first.

Renal Function—A Review

The kidneys play a major role in the maintenance of homeostasis by regulating the volume and composition of the extracellular body fluid. In addition to controlling the water, electrolyte, and solute concentrations of the extracellular fluid, the kidneys selectively excrete drugs, hormones, and by-products of metabolism. The kidneys also partici-

pate in the maintenance of acid–base balance, renin and angiotensin production, and vitamin D metabolism.

Gross Anatomy of the Kidney

The kidneys are paired, bean-shaped organs located retroperitoneally on each side of the vertebral column at the level of the 12th thoracic to the 3rd lumbar vertebrae. The right kidney is placed slightly lower than the left because of displacement by the liver.

Each kidney is invested with a fibrous capsule that is interrupted medially at the hilus for passage of blood vessels, lymphatics, nerves, and a ureter.

A frontal section of the kidney reveals an outer granular cortex located deep to the capsule and an inner medulla composed of several striated pyramids (Fig. 41-1). Interspersed among the pyramids are columns of cortical tissues known as the renal columns of Bertin.

The apex of each renal pyramid forms a papilla, which projects into a cup-like minor calix. Several minor calices unite to form major calices, and the latter merge to form the renal pelvis. The renal

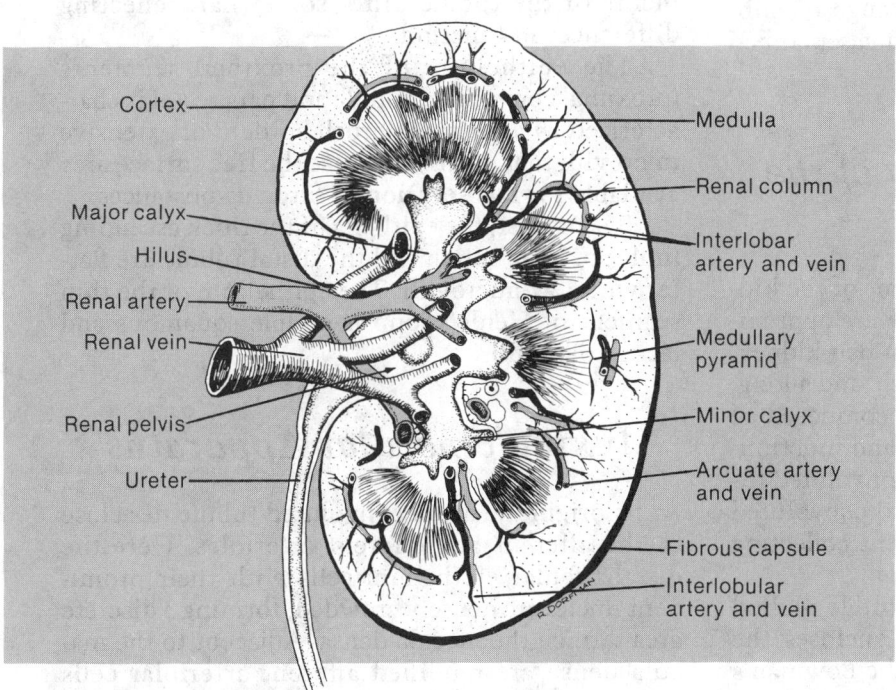

Figure 41-1. Frontal section of a human kidney. (Malseed RT: Pharmacology: Drug Therapy and Nursing Considerations, 2nd ed, p 346. Philadelphia, JB Lippincott, 1985)

pelvis is continuous with the ureter, which drains its contents into the urinary bladder.

Renal Blood Supply

Paired renal arteries arise from the abdominal aorta, branching as they enter the hilus. These branches divide into interlobar arteries, which pass between the medullary pyramids. At the corticomedullary junction the vessels form the arcuate arteries, which arch over the bases of the pyramids. Branching from the arcuate arteries are numerous interlobular arteries, which penetrate the cortical substance and give rise to afferent arterioles supplying individual nephron units.

Each afferent arteriole terminates in a tuft of capillaries, the glomerulus, which rejoin to form the efferent arteriole. Efferent arterioles terminate in peritubular capillaries, which surround the renal tubules. The peritubular capillaries eventually converge into venules that carry the blood into a series of veins corresponding in name and in course to the arteries described above.

A series of long, straight peritubular capillaries termed vasa recta course through the medulla, turning sharply at various levels. The vasa recta participate in countercurrent exchange of substances between the renal tubules and vascular bed as detailed later in this chapter.

Microscopic Anatomy of the Kidney

The basic anatomic and functional unit of the kidney is the nephron (Fig. 41-2). There are approximately 1 million nephrons in each human kidney. A nephron consists of a renal corpuscle and a long, often tortuously coiled renal tubule composed of the following anatomically modified and functionally distinct segments: the proximal convoluted tubule, the loop of Henle, and the distal convoluted tubule, which empties into a confluent collecting tubule.

Each nephron originates as a double-walled cup, the Bowman's capsule, which encloses the glomerular capillaries. Collectively, the Bowman's capsule and the glomerulus are termed the renal (malpighian) corpuscle. The epithelium of the Bowman's capsule is simple squamous, with the inner (visceral) layer containing modified cells called podocytes. The podocytes exhibit numerous foot-like extensions called pedicels, which contact the basement membrane of the glomerular capillaries.

The podocyte layer (visceral epithelium) of the Bowman's capsule together with the basement membrane and fenestrated endothelium of the glomerulus form a functional filtration membrane.

The outer (parietal) layer of the Bowman's capsule becomes continuous with the epithelium of the proximal convoluted tubule. The proximal convoluted tubule then straightens and plunges toward the medulla, forming the thick descending segment (pars recta) of the loop of Henle.

The loop of Henle is a U-shaped structure composed of a thick descending segment (pars recta), a thin segment, and a thick ascending segment. The thick ascending segment becomes continuous with the distal convoluted tubule at a modified site, the macula densa, where the tubular cells and their prominent nuclei are densely crowded.

The distal tubule coils in the area of the renal cortex before joining a collecting tubule. The latter descends into the medulla as part of a renal pyramid and empties through the papilla into a minor calix.

Histologically, the proximal and distal segments of the tubule differ somewhat, reflecting differences in function.

The epithelium of the proximal segments (proximal convoluted tubule and pars recta) is characterized by a luminal "brush border" of extensive microvilli that greatly increase the free surface area available for reabsorption of filtered substances.

By contrast, the epithelia of the thick ascending limb of Henle's loop and the distal tubule are flatter with few microvilli. The epithelium of the thin segment of Henle's loop is simple squamous and lacks microvilli.

Juxtaglomerular Apparatus

At its origin the distal convoluted tubule lies close to the afferent and efferent arterioles. Here the distal tubular epithelium cells with their prominent nuclei are densely crowded, forming a discrete area termed the macula densa. Adjacent to the macula densa are modified afferent arteriolar cells called juxtaglomerular cells, which contain granules of the proteolytic enzyme renin. Collectively the juxtaglomerular cells and the macula densa are termed the juxtaglomerular apparatus (Fig. 41-3).

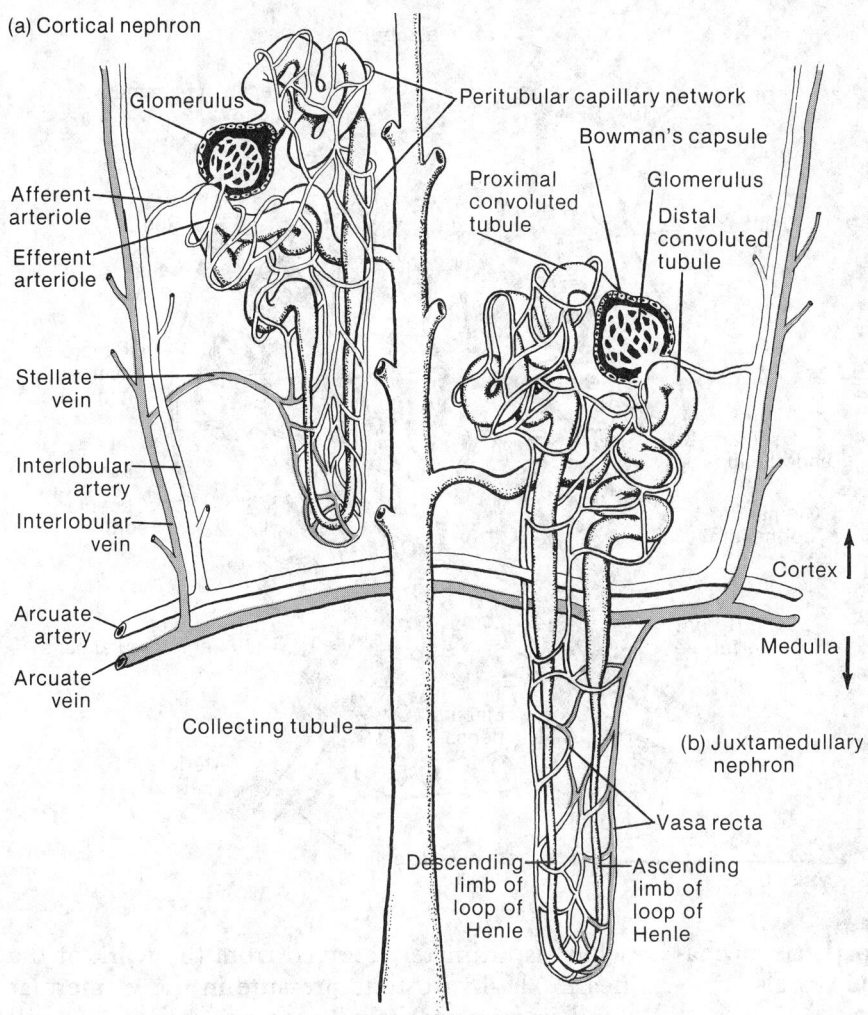

Figure 41-2. *Diagram of two nephrons and their blood supply. One nephron (left) has a short loop of Henle; the other nephron (right) has a long loop of Henle and a more extensive blood supply. (Malseed RT: Pharmacology: Drug Therapy and Nursing Considerations, 2nd ed, p 347. Philadelphia, JB Lippincott, 1985)*

The juxtaglomerular cells secrete renin in response to reduced renal perfusion (renal ischemia), hypotension, hyponatremia, hyperkalemia, and beta-adrenergic receptor stimulation.

By way of the macula densa, the nature of the tubular fluid in the distal tubule can also influence renin secretion by the juxtaglomerular cells.

Upon entering the blood, renin converts the plasma protein angiotensinogen into the decapeptide angiotensin I. Converting enzymes found largely in the lungs split a dipeptide from angiotensin I to form the physiologically active angiotensin II. Angiotensin II is a potent vasopressor substance that elevates blood pressure by promot-

ing intense peripheral vasoconstriction and by stimulating secretion of the sodium-retaining hormone aldosterone, as outlined in Figure 35-1.

Control of Renal Blood Flow

Sympathetic vasoconstrictor nerve fibers arising from thoracolumbar segments of the spinal cord innervate the kidneys. In an average adult at rest the kidneys receive 20% to 25% of the cardiac output. Pain, cold, fright, strenuous exercise, hemorrhage, deep anesthesia, and other stressors reduce

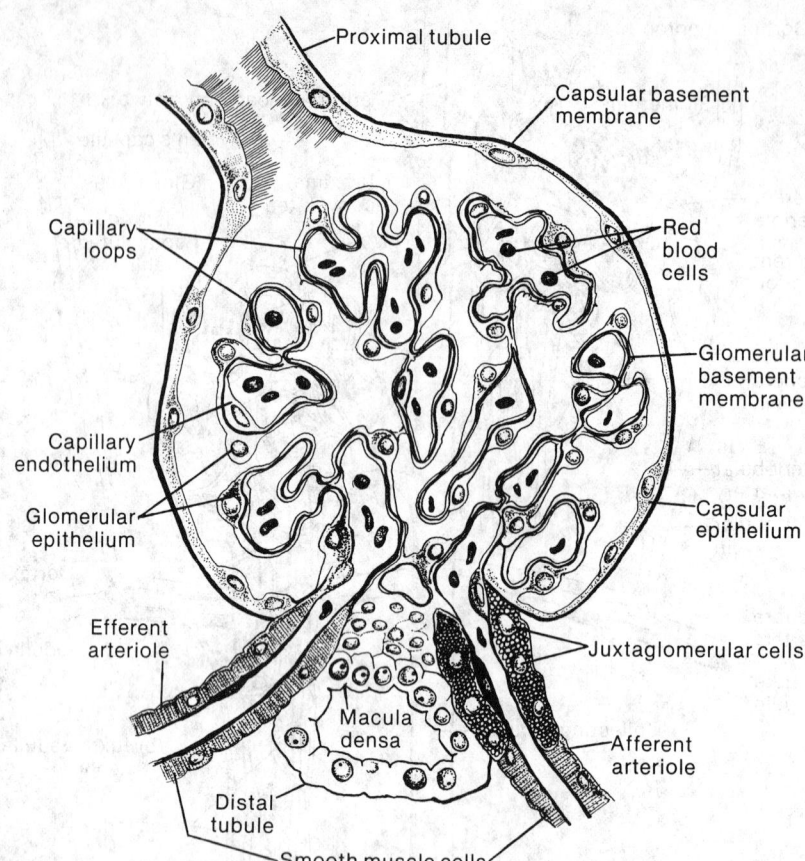

Figure 41-3. Semidiagrammatic drawing of a renal corpuscle. Note that the distal tubule appears to be attached to the afferent arteriole. Also depicted are the macula densa and the juxtaglomerular cells. The combined structure at the point of attachment is called the juxtaglomerular apparatus. (Malseed RT: Pharmacology: Drug Therapy and Nursing Considerations, 2nd ed, p 348. Philadelphia, JB Lippincott, 1985)

renal blood flow by activating sympathetic mechanisms for constriction of renal blood vessels.

Renal Physiology

The formation of urine by the nephrons involves three basic processes: glomerular filtration, renal tubular reabsorption, and renal tubular secretion.

Glomerular Filtration

Glomerular filtration is a process whereby approximately one fifth of the plasma flowing through the glomerulus is passively transferred into the Bowman's capsule. The glomerular filtration membrane described earlier acts as a sieve, allowing passage of small molecules while restricting transfer of large molecular weight substances such as proteins.

The driving force for filtration is the hydrostatic pressure within the glomerular capillaries,

which is ultimately derived from the work of the heart. The hydrostatic pressure in the glomerular capillaries is notably higher than that in other capillaries because the glomerulus is interposed between two arterioles.

Forces opposing filtration include the colloidal osmotic pressure of the plasma and the hydrostatic pressure of the Bowman's capsule. The colloidal osmotic pressure of the Bowman's capsule is close to zero because the glomerular filtrate is essentially protein-free.

The equation below shows how net filtration pressure can be calculated:

Net filtration pressure

= Glomerular capillary hydrostatic pressure

− [Plasma colloidal osmotic pressure

+ Capsular hydrostatic pressure]

(50 mm Hg) − (30 mm Hg + 10 mm Hg)

Therefore,

Net filtration pressure = 10 mm Hg

Approximately 125 ml of filtrate are formed each minute. The glomerular filtration rate remains remarkably stable within a rather wide range of blood pressure variation due to an intrinsic mechanism of autoregulation. Glomerular filtration may be affected by changes in plasma colloidal osmotic pressure, a force that opposes glomerular filtration. Decreases in plasma colloidal osmotic pressure will enhance filtration and vice versa.

The high rate of glomerular filtration (125 ml/min) yields a total of 180 L of plasma filtered each day. Yet the average volume of urine excreted in 1 day is less than 2 L. Hence, over 99% of the glomerular filtrate is reabsorbed during passage through the renal tubules.

Renal Tubular Reabsorption and Secretion

Renal tubular reabsorption involves the transport of filtered substances across the renal tubular epithelium from the tubular lumen to the blood of the peritubular capillaries.

Renal tubular secretion, on the other hand, involves transtubular movement of substances from the blood of the peritubular capillaries to the tubular lumen.

Substances may be reabsorbed or secreted passively by diffusion along existing chemical, electrical, or osmotic gradients. They may also be actively transported against electrical chemical gradients into or out of the tubular lumen by selective, carrier-mediated and energy-requiring transport systems. Each active renal transport system exhibits a transport maximum (T_m), which is the maximal rate at which a given substance can be carried across the renal tubular epithelium. For actively reabsorbed substances such as glucose, the plasma concentration of the substance that causes its transport maximum to be exceeded is termed the renal threshold.

Nutrients such as glucose and amino acids, and vitamins such as ascorbic acid are actively reabsorbed in the proximal tubule. Uric acid, an end product of purine metabolism, is both actively reabsorbed and actively secreted in the proximal tubule. Urea, the major end product of nitrogen metabolism, is formed chiefly in the liver in accordance with the rate of protein catabolism. Filtered urea is passively reabsorbed by the renal tubules to an extent determined by the rate of urine flow and degree of water reabsorption.

Creatinine, a product of muscle metabolism, and histamine, a vasoactive amine, are actively secreted in the proximal tubule.

Many organic compounds of medical importance are also actively secreted in the proximal tubule. Among these are the drugs and diagnostic agents listed in Table 41-1. Because renal tubular secretion supplements glomerular filtration and enhances the removal of substances from the

Table 41-1
Organic Compounds of Medical Importance Actively Secreted by the Proximal Tubule

Compound	Medical Use
Drugs	
acetazolamide (Diamox)	Carbonic anhydrase (CA) inhibitor
chlorothiazide (Diuril)	Diuretic
penicillin	Antibiotic
probenecid (Benemid)	Uricosuric agent
salicylates	Analgesic and anti-inflammatory agents
tolazoline (Priscoline)	Alpha-adrenergic blocking agent
Diagnostic Agents	
iodopyracet (Diodrast)	Urologic contrast medium
para-aminohippuric acid (PAH)	Measurement of renal plasma flow and tubular secretion
phenolsulfonphthalein (Phenol red or PSP)	Measurement of renal plasma flow

blood, impaired renal function may interfere with the excretion of therapeutic agents and may therefore require an adjustment (reduction) in drug dose.

Renal Handling of Ions and Water

The amount of sodium excreted is normally equivalent to the amount ingested, over a wide range of dietary sodium intake. Renal handling of sodium is of singular importance to the maintenance of extracellular fluid volume, because renal tubular reabsorption of sodium is the major driving force for the passive reabsorption of water. Also linked to the active reabsorption of sodium are the secretion of hydrogen and potassium and the reabsorption of chloride and bicarbonate in certain tubular segments. Chloride and bicarbonate reabsorption

are reciprocally related. If chloride reabsorption increases, bicarbonate reabsorption decreases, and vice versa, so that total anion concentration of the plasma remains constant.

The renal tubular handling of electrolytes is presented schematically in Figure 41-4.

The bulk (approximately 70%) of sodium reabsorption takes place actively in the proximal tubule. Chloride and bicarbonate passively follow the sodium out of the proximal tubule, accompanied by an osmotic equivalent of water so that tubular fluid osmolarity in this segment equals that of plasma. The reabsorption of water in this tubular segment is therefore termed obligatory.

In the descending loop of Henle, water is extracted by osmotic forces into the medullary interstitial space (see under Countercurrent Mechanism below), but this segment is relatively impermeable to sodium and chloride, although some solute (e.g., sodium chloride, urea) may enter the tubule at this point. As the tubular fluid enters the ascending

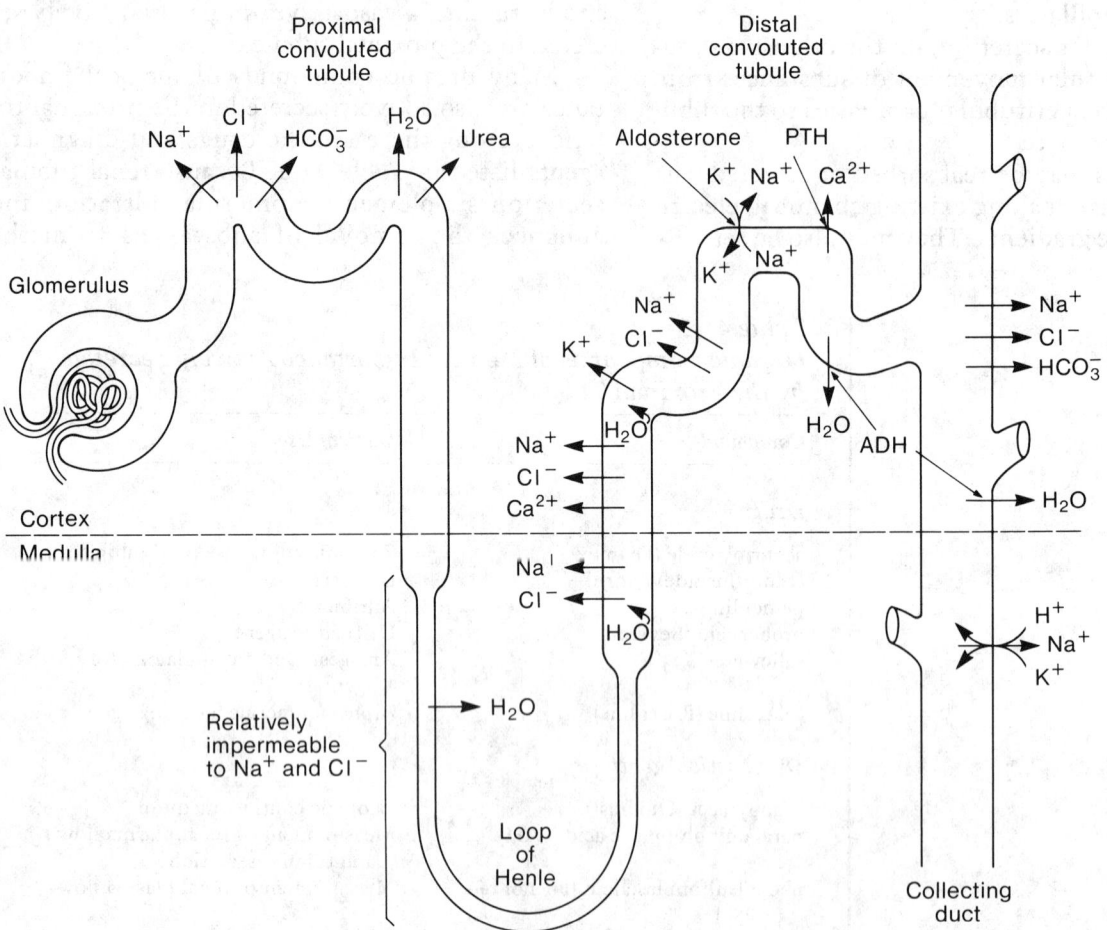

Figure 41-4.   Renal tubular handling of electrolytes and water.

limb of Henle's loop, chloride is actively pumped out of the thick ascending segment, followed passively by sodium. The water impermeability of the ascending limb of Henle's loop leads to a net loss of sodium chloride and thus hypo-osmolarity of the tubular fluid entering the distal tubule.

Active reabsorption of sodium resumes in the distal tubule and continues in the collecting tubules. Much of the reabsorbed sodium is accompanied by anion (chloride or bicarbonate). Other reabsorbed sodium ions are accompanied by movement *into* the tubules of hydrogen and potassium ions. The movements of sodium, potassium, and hydrogen are closely interrelated but apparently do *not* involve a *direct* exchange mechanism as was formerly believed. Aldosterone, an adrenal cortical hormone acts on the distal tubule to facilitate sodium reabsorption and potassium excretion, perhaps by increasing synthesis of distal tubular membrane proteins which then act to increase membrane permeability to these ions.

The *passive* reabsorption of water from the distal and collecting tubules is under the control of antidiuretic hormone (ADH). In the absence of ADH the epithelium of the distal and collecting tubules is essentially impermeable to water. The tubular fluid remains hypotonic, and urinary volume is high. In the presence of ADH the epithelium of these tubular segments becomes highly permeable to water, permitting the facultative reabsorption of water according to osmotic gradients established in the loop of Henle through the countercurrent mechanism.

Countercurrent Mechanism

The conservation of water and concentration of urine by the kidneys is made possible by the operation of a countercurrent mechanism. Within this mechanism the loops of Henle act as countercurrent multipliers that establish an osmotic gradient in the renal medulla, while the vasa recta (Fig. 41-2)

serve as countercurrent exchangers to maintain this gradient.

In the water-impermeable thick ascending limb of Henle's loop, chloride is actively transported out of the tubular fluid, followed passively by sodium, thus creating a hyperosmolarity in the medullary interstitium. The permeability of the epithelium in the descending limb of Henle's loop permits diffusion of water from the tubular fluid into the hyperosmolar medullary interstitium, and diffusion of sodium chloride and urea into the tubular fluid. Thus, a gradually increasing osmolarity of the tubular fluid and medullary interstitium is created as the turn in the loop of Henle is approached. ADH controls the final volume of urine available for excretion by promoting the facultative reabsorption of water from the collecting tubules passing through the medullary pyramids according to the osmotic gradient established by the countercurrent mechanism.

Renal Function in Acid–Base Regulation

The renal tubular epithelium participates in acid–base regulation by reabsorbing sodium bicarbonate and secreting hydrogen ions and ammonia. The hydrogen ions are derived from the dissociation of carbonic acid (H_2CO_3), which forms when carbon dioxide and water combined in the presence of the enzyme catalyst carbonic anhydrase. Hydrogen ions thus secreted into the tubular lumen combine chemically with phosphate buffers present in the tubular fluid to form monosodium phosphate (NaH_2PO_4).

Secreted hydrogen ions may also combine with the ammonia produced by the renal tubular epithelium from the deamination of amino acids such as glutamine. The secreted hydrogen ions and ammonia combine to form the ammonium ion (NH_4^+), which is excreted together with tubular anions such as chloride (Cl^-).

Classification of Diuretic Drugs

A large number of chemically dissimilar compounds have a diuretic action, and diuretic drugs are usually classified on the basis of their predominant sites and mechanisms of action. The major categories of diuretics reviewed in this chapter are listed in Table 41-2, along with their principal sites of action in the kidney and major electrolyte disturbances associated with each group.

The handling of electrolytes by the kidney involves a complex series of interrelated mechanisms (see Fig. 41-4). Drugs such as diuretics that affect the handling of one electrolyte (e.g., sodium) almost invariably alter the handling of other electrolytes as well (such as chloride, potassium, hydrogen, bicarbonate). Depending on the mechanism of action of the individual diuretic drugs, therefore, various electrolyte or acid–base balance disturbances, or both, can develop during diuretic therapy. These electrolyte imbalances are responsible for many of the disturbing and occasionally serious side-effects resulting from diuretic administration, and an understanding of the sites and mechanisms of action of the diuretics can aid in predicting the types of electrolyte changes expected with any one drug. The overall drug regimen can then be tailored to produce an optimal diuretic action with a mini-

mal degree of electrolyte-induced side-effects (e.g., combining a drug that produces potassium loss with a potassium-sparing drug).

It should be noted that the effectiveness and safety of diuretics are greatly compromised in the presence of kidney disease. Most diuretics are of little value in patients with significantly impaired renal function, and in many instances they can be quite hazardous. These drugs should be prescribed for patients with known or suspected kidney impairment only after consideration of the potential risks.

■ General Nursing Process for Diuretics

Regardless of the type of diuretic to be administered many of the nursing process concerns will be the same. Typical guidelines are presented below; details for each category are presented separately.

□ ASSESSMENT

□ Subjective Data
A complete data base is extremely important when planning diuretic therapy. The nurse needs to find

Table 41-2
Diuretic Drugs: Site of Action and Electrolyte Disturbances

Classes of Diuretics	Major Sites of Action	Electrolyte Disturbances
I. Carbonic anhydrase inhibitors (e.g., acetazolamide)	Proximal tubule and distal tubule	Hyponatremic acidosis Hyperchloremic acidosis Hypokalemia
II. Loop (high-ceiling) diuretics (e.g., furosemide)	Thick ascending loop of Henle and proximal and distal tubules	Hypokalemia Hypochloremic alkalosis Hyponatremia (excessive diuresis) Hypocalcemia
III. Mercurials (e.g., mersalyl)	Thick ascending loop of Henle and possibly proximal and distal tubule sites	Hypochloremic alkalosis Hypokalemia (mild) Hyponatremia (excessive diuresis)
IV. Osmotics (e.g., mannitol)	Proximal tubule, descending loop of Henle, and collecting tubule	Minimal
V. Potassium-sparing diuretics (e.g., triamterene)	Distal tubule and collecting duct	Hyperkalemia
VI. Thiazides/sulfonamides (e.g., hydrochlorothiazide, chlorthalidone, indapamide)	Distal tubule and possibly cortical ascending loop of Henle	Hypokalemia Hypochloremic alkalosis Hyponatremia Hypercalcemia

out why the patient is getting a diuretic and what he thinks the drug does for his body. Some patients think diuretics are prescribed to increase their urine but will not understand how the drug affects hypertension, glaucoma, or heart disease unless the relationship is made clear. Knowledge about the presence of other conditions is also important because gout, arthritis, and diabetes will influence the type and dose of diuretic prescribed.

A drug history is also essential. Diuretics interact with many drugs, and dosages or types may be influenced by the current medication the patient takes. Such information is especially important when dealing with an elderly client who may take many prescription and over-the-counter drugs and in whom adverse reactions to diuretics are more likely to occur.

□ *Objective Data*

Baseline laboratory data, including electrolyte, acid–base, hepatic, and renal function studies, should be gathered before therapy begins; these studies will need to be done periodically throughout the treatment course to monitor adverse drug responses.

A complete physical assessment should be performed with a focus on fluid volume changes. Diuretics affect body fluid volume considerably. In order to measure changes in fluid balance throughout therapy the patient should be weighed and examined for evidence of peripheral edema. Also, the patient should be questioned about weight gain in recent weeks, swelling of hands or feet, ring tightness, and frequency of urination. These parameters can then be reassessed during therapy to determine drug effectiveness.

□ *NURSING DIAGNOSES*

Actual nursing diagnoses for the patient taking diuretics may include:
Knowledge deficit related to action, administration, and side-effects of the drug
Alteration in fluid volume: excess
Potential nursing diagnoses based on common drug side-effects may include:
Alteration in comfort: gastrointestinal upset
Potential for injury: trauma related to dizziness from postural hypotension
Alteration in nutrition: potential for more than body requirements of sodium
Sensory-perceptual alterations in vision related to photosensitivity
Sexual dysfunction

□ *PLAN*

Nursing care goals should focus on safe administration and monitoring in the acute care setting and developing a teaching plan which helps the patient to
1. Learn to take the drug safely
2. Monitor the drug's effectiveness
3. Watch for and respond to side-effects
4. Limit sodium intake when necessary

□ *INTERVENTION*

Most diuretics should be taken early in the day to avoid nocturia. Diuresis will be greatest within several hours after administration and will gradually subside. The patient may need assistance in planning the most convenient administration time in order to avoid inconvenient bathroom stops. For example, the individual who works may choose to take the drug immediately before leaving for work so it does not reach peak levels until after his commute.

The patient can learn to judge whether the diuretic is working by weighing himself daily or at least three times a week. Any immediate gain or loss of 5 lb or more should be reported. In addition, he should note changes in swelling of fingers, hands, or feet, and sensations of puffiness or tightness or shortness of breath. A flow sheet may be a way to help remind him to do these things, will make reporting them easier, and can serve as a basis for follow-up teaching especially if he also records his salt intake on the same sheet. Fluid changes can also cause thirst, especially if diuresis is occurring rapidly. Encourage fluid intake of at least 1500 ml/day unless contraindicated by cardiovascular or renal function. Figure 41-5 shows an example of a flow sheet suitable for a patient on close monitoring of diuretic therapy.

One of the side-effects of most diuretics is gastrointestinal distress. This can be minimized by taking the drug with or immediately after a meal or with a glass of milk. This will slow but not inhibit drug absorption.

If nausea or vomiting persists or if the patient develops vomiting or diarrhea for over 24 hours from flu or other problems, the physician should be notified. Electrolyte imbalance could occur, resulting in dangerous decreases in chloride or potassium, a problem the patient on diuretics cannot afford.

Electrolyte imbalances can occur with diuretic therapy, and potassium depletion is the most common one with all but the potassium-sparing drugs. The patient needs to learn early symptoms of hy-

Guideline	Sunday	Monday	Tuesday	Wednesday	Thursday	Friday	Saturday
1. Drug/Time							
2. Weight Goal: 3×/week							
3. Edema—swelling in feet, puffy legs, or tightness of clothing?							
4. Breathing—easy or hard?							
5. Fluid Intake Goal: 1500 ml/day							
6. Sodium Intake Goal: 1000 mg/day Breakfast Lunch Dinner							

Figure 41-5. *A flow sheet for monitoring diuretic therapy.*

pokalemia, which include muscle cramping or weakness, dizziness, fatigue, and dyspnea, and know to report them immediately. Some patients may need to take potassium supplements, and these are often prescribed prophylactically (see Chap. 78). In others, supplementing the diet with potassium rich foods may be sufficient. Foods high in potassium include bananas, citrus fruits and juices, dates, apricots, raisins, fish, fowl, and cola beverages. In any case, the patient should have a potassium level drawn regularly as part of his ongoing care.

Some patients on diuretic therapy, such as the elderly and individuals taking anticholinergics, are more prone to hypokalemia than others. Hypokalemia is also more dangerous to patients taking digitalis because this drug acts in the presence of potassium to decrease cardiac workload. Digitalized patients are more prone to digitalis toxicity and subsequent arrhythmias if potassium levels fall below normal.

Diuretics may also cause problems for the diabetic patient because the drug can increase blood glucose levels. Blood sugar levels should be closely monitored, and doses of insulin or oral antidiabetic drugs should be adjusted. The patient should be more aware of the chance of developing hyperglycemia and should report symptoms immediately.

Another side-effect of diuretic therapy, orthostatic hypotension, can be a problem especially early in therapy. Until the patient adjusts to the fluid volume changes he should rise slowly from a sitting or standing position, sit immediately if dizziness occurs, and avoid driving or operating dangerous machinery until his response to the drug is known.

Many diuretics can result in sexual dysfunction ranging from loss of libido to premature ejaculation and impotence. These side-effects may go unreported but could be the cause of compliance failure. The nurse needs to establish a rapport with the patient, ask open-ended questions, and let the patient know he can talk about such a problem if necessary. The effect on sexual function may be transient or may be resolved by an alteration in dose or type of medication.

Photosensitivity is another side-effect which occurs with several diuretics and can be managed by consistent use of sunscreens, sunglasses, and protective clothing. Patients should be warned of the potential for severe sunburn in summer months or on snow-covered winter days when the sun is very bright.

The patient taking diuretics for hypertension needs to limit salt intake and to avoid processed foods such as soup, lunch meats, smoked meats, cheeses, Chinese food, salty snacks. He should learn to read labels on all food packages and avoid using table salt. A low-sodium diet (e.g., 1000 mg/day) should be ordered. A dietitian should then see the patient to provide comprehensive instruction and written information.

During episodes of excess diuresis this same patient could develop hyponatremia from most of the diuretics. Symptoms include thirst, lethargy, muscle weakness, and oliguria, and should be reported immediately. Follow-up electrolyte studies, including sodium level, will help detect problems.

□ EVALUATION

Outcome criteria against which to measure the success of drug therapy include slow, consistent weight loss of 1 to 2 lb per week in early therapy, lessening of edema in hands and feet, lowered blood pressure (if being treated), lowered intraocular pressure (if glaucoma is being treated), improved cardiac status, and stabilized electrolyte levels on follow-up.

Carbonic Anhydrase Inhibitors

Acetazolamide, Dichlorphenamide, Methazolamide

Carbonic anhydrase inhibitors are sulfonamide derivatives that competitively interfere with the activity of the enzyme carbonic anhydrase (CA), thus blocking the hydration of carbon dioxide (CO_2) to carbonic acid (H_2CO_3) and its subsequent ionization to yield hydrogen (H^+) and bicarbonate (HCO_3^-) ions. In addition to their mild diuretic action, these agents also reduce the synthesis of aqueous humor in the eye, as formation of bicarbonate is necessary for the production of aqueous humor. Therefore, they are also used for adjunctive treatment of glaucoma. Finally, due to their ability to produce an acidosis, they have been employed adjunctively in treating some forms of epilepsy (see Chap. 30). The CA inhibitors are reviewed as a group, followed by a listing of individual drugs in Table 41-3.

MECHANISM AND ACTIONS

Carbonic anhydrase inhibitors reduce the production of H^+ and HCO_3^- in renal tubules, thereby decreasing hydrogen-ion secretion by the renal tubule. Consequently, there is increased urinary excretion on NA^+, HCO_3^-, K^+, and water, resulting in an alkaline diuresis. The diuretic effect of carbonic anhydrase inhibitors is limited, because tolerance develops as serum bicarbonate levels decline, and prolonged treatment can lead to metabolic acidosis, resulting from loss of extracellular Na^+ and HCO_3^-.

In the eye, carbonic anhydrase inhibitors reduce the rate of aqueous humor formation, leading to a decrease in intraocular pressure. These drugs may also reduce the frequency of seizures (especially petit mal), possibly by lowering the pH of brain tissue.

USES

1. Adjunctive treatment of drug-induced edema or edema due to congestive heart failure refractory to single drug therapy (not indicated alone in edema)
2. Adjunctive treatment of chronic simple (open-angle) glaucoma and secondary glaucoma; also, preoperatively in acute angle-closure (narrow-angle) glaucoma
3. *Adjunctive* treatment of certain forms of epilepsy, especially petit mal
4. Prophylaxis or treatment of acute mountain sickness (*e.g.*, weakness, dizziness, nausea) at high altitudes (acetazolamide)
5. Treatment of hyperkalemic and hypokalemic periodic paralysis (investigational use)

ADMINISTRATION AND DOSAGE
See Table 41-3.

FATE
The drugs are readily absorbed orally; onset of action is usually within 1 hour to 2 hours (up to 4 hours with methazolamide). The peak effect occurs within 2 hours to 4 hours with acetazolamide and dichlorphenamide, 6 hours to 8 hours with methazolamide, and 8 hours to 12 hours with sustained-release dosage forms of acetazolamide. Effects may last up to 12 hours, except for the sustained-release preparations, which can exhibit a duration of action up to 24 hours. The drugs are excreted either in the unchanged form or as metabolites, some of which are active.

SIDE-EFFECTS/ADVERSE REACTIONS
The most frequently reported side-effects are paresthesias of the extremities, tongue, lips, mouth, or anus. A variety of other adverse reactions have been reported with carbonic anyhydrase inhibitors:

Table 41-3
Carbonic Anhydrase Inhibitors

Drug	Preparations	Usual Dosage Range	Clinical Considerations
acetazolamide (Ak-Zol, Da-zamide, Diamox)	Tablets—125 mg, 250 mg Sustained-release capsules—500 mg Injection—500 mg/vial (sodium salt)	Glaucoma—250 mg orally, one to four times/day depending on response Children—10 mg to 15 mg/kg/day in divided doses every 6 h–8 h Edema—250 mg to 375 mg orally, once daily in the morning for 1 day to 2 days; then skip a day Children—5 mg/kg once daily in the morning IV—500 mg initially; then 125 mg to 250 mg every 4 h as needed in acute situation (500 mg/5 ml sterile water for injection) Epilepsy—Adults and children—8 mg to 30 mg/kg/day in divided doses Acute mountain sickness—500 mg to 1000 mg daily in divided doses; initiate 24 h–48 h before ascent and continue as long as needed to control symptoms	Used for edema of congestive heart failure, minor and motor epilepsies, chronic open-angle glaucoma, and preoperatively in narrow-angle glaucoma; doses in excess of 1000 mg do not usually produce an increased effect. Sustained-release form may be used on a twice-daily basis. Reconstituted injection solution should be used within 24 h. Avoid IM administration if possible because alkaline solution is very painful upon injection.
dichlorphenamide (Daranide)	Tablets—50 mg	100 mg to 200 mg initially, followed by 100 mg every 12 h until desired response is achieved; maintenance 25 mg to 50 mg one to three times/day	Indicated as adjunctive treatment for open-angle glaucoma and preoperatively in narrow-angle glaucoma, together with miotics and osmotic diuretics
methazolamide (Neptazane)	Tablets—50 mg	50 mg to 100 mg two to three times/day	Adjunctive therapy for both open-angle and narrow-angle glaucoma, with miotics and osmotic diuretics; contra-indicated in severe or absolute glaucoma, hemorrhagic glaucoma, or that due to peripheral anterior synechiae; higher incidence of drowsiness than with other CA inhibitors

CNS—Confusion, myopia, tinnitus, malaise, drowsiness, vertigo, headache, xerostomia, depression, nervousness, weakness, flaccid paralysis, convulsions, tremor, ataxia
Dermatologic—Skin eruptions, urticaria, pruritus, melena, photosensitivity
Hepatic/renal—Hepatic insufficiency, pancreatitis, polyuria, dysuria, glycosuria, hematuria, urinary frequency, ureteral colic
Electrolyte—Hypokalemia, hyponatremia
GI—Anorexia, nausea, vomiting, constipation
Other—Myopia (transient), weight loss, fever, loss of taste or smell, acidosis, bone marrow depression, blood dyscrasias

Table 41-4 (continued)
Loop (High-Ceiling) Diuretics

Drug	Preparations	Usual Dosage Range	Clinical Considerations
furosemide (Lasix, SK-Furosemide)	Tablets—20 mg, 40 mg, 80 mg Oral solution—10 mg/ml, 40 mg/5 ml Injection—10 mg/ml	Oral: Adults Diuresis—20 mg to 80 mg as a single dose; may increase by 20-mg to 40-mg increments to a maximum of 600 mg/day Hypertension—40 mg twice a day; adjust according to response; usual maintenance dose 40 mg to 80 mg/day in a single or two divided doses Children Initially 2 mg/kg as a single dose; may increase by 1-mg/kg to 2-mg/kg increments to a maximum of 6 mg/kg day Parenteral: Adults 20 mg to 40 mg IV or IM as a single dose; may increase by 20-mg increments every 2 h–3 h until desired response is obtained Acute pulmonary edema—40 mg IV over 1 min–2 min; may increase to 80 mg IV after 1 h Children 1 mg/kg IV or IM; may increase by 1 mg/kg no sooner than 2 h after previous dose; maximum 6 mg/kg	Oral doses should be given on an intermittent schedule (e.g., 2 to 4 consecutive days/wk); parenteral therapy is indicated for emergency situations only and should be replaced by oral therapy as soon as possible; do not mix parenteral solutions with highly acidic preparations; use mixture within 24 h of preparation and do not use if solution is yellow; use cautiously in patients allergic to sulfonamides, because cross-reactions can occur; when adding drug to an existing antihypertensive regimen, reduce dose of other drugs by ½ to avoid excessive drop in blood pressure and titrate furosemide dosage to obtain optimal hypotensive effect; in patients with impaired renal function, use controlled IV infusion not to exceed 4 mg/min to minimize danger of azotemia or oliguria; drug can stimulate renal synthesis of prostaglandin E_2, which can complicate the neonatal respiratory distress syndrome; use normal saline, Ringer's, lactate, or dextrose 5% in water as diluents

USES

1. Treatment of refractory edema associated with congestive heart failure, hepatic cirrhosis, and renal disease
2. Relief of acute pulmonary edema (IV administration)
3. Adjunctive treatment of hypertension (furosemide orally)
4. Management of ascites due to malignancy, idiopathic edema, and lymphedema (ethacrynic acid)
5. Short-term management of pediatric patients with congenital heart disease or the nephrotic syndrome (ethacrynic acid)
6. Treatment of acute hypercalcemia (IV furosemide with normal saline infusion)

ADMINISTRATION AND DOSAGE
See Table 41-4.

FATE
Onset of diuresis following oral administration is 30 minutes to 60 minutes; peak effect occurs in 1

hour to 2 hours, and duration is 6 hours to 8 hours, except for bumetanide (3 hours–6 hours). IV injection produces a diuretic response within 5 minutes to 10 minutes, which then peaks within 15 minutes to 30 minutes and persists for 2 hours. Drugs are highly bound to plasma proteins (94%–98%) and are rapidly excreted in the urine, both as metabolites and unchanged drug. Approximately one-third of the dose is eliminated by way of the bile in the feces.

SIDE-EFFECTS/ADVERSE REACTIONS
The most frequently occurring side-effects of loop diuretics are abdominal discomfort and electrolyte imbalances with too vigorous therapy. Many other adverse reactions have been reported during loop diuretic therapy, although not every untoward reaction has been observed with each of the three available drugs. The various adverse effects associated with the individual drugs are listed below:

All drugs
  GI—Anorexia, nausea, vomiting, diarrhea, acute pancreatitis, jaundice
  CNS—Headache, blurred vision, tinnitus, hearing loss, weakness, vertigo
  CV—Orthostatic hypotension
  Electrolyte—Hypokalemia, hyponatremia, hypochloremic alkalosis, hypomagnesemia, hypocalcemia
  Other—Rash, pruritus, muscle spasm or cramping, hyperglycemia, hyperuricemia, azotemia, increased serum creatinine, agranulocytosis, thrombocytopenia

Bumetanide
  Dry mouth, arthritic pain, hives, premature ejaculation, ECG changes, chest pain, hyperventilation, breast tenderness

Ethacrynic acid
  GI bleeding, *profuse* watery diarrhea, fever, chills, dysphagia, hematuria, neutropenia, confusion, fatigue, hypovolemia, and nystagmus

Furosemide
  GI irritation, constipation, paresthesias, leukopenia, anemia, hives, photosensitivity, erythema multiforme, exfoliative dermatitis, necrotizing angiitis, urinary frequency, urinary bladder spasm, and thrombophlebitis

Overdosage may result in profound water loss, severe volume and electrolyte depletion, and possible circulatory collapse, with the danger of vascular embolism. A dose-related *reversible* ototoxic effect, manifested as tinnitus, hearing impairment, and rarely deafness, can occur. This effect is usually noted with overzealous therapy (*e.g.*, rapid IV injection of large doses) in patients with reduced renal function.

CONTRAINDICATIONS AND PRECAUTIONS
High ceiling diuretics are contraindicated in the presence of anuria, hepatic coma, and severe dehydration or electrolyte depletion. In addition, ethacrynic acid should not be used in infants or pregnant women. These diuretics should be administered *cautiously* to persons with hepatic cirrhosis, diabetes, gout or hyperuricemia, cardiogenic shock, hearing impairment, systemic lupus erythematosus, postural hypotension, and to the elderly. Persons receiving digitalis drugs or corticosteroids should be closely monitored for hypokalemia. The drugs must also be given with caution to pregnant women or nursing mothers.

INTERACTIONS
1. Loop diuretics may potentiate the blood pressure-lowering action of antihypertensive medications.
2. Loop diuretics may increase the toxicity of aminoglycoside antibiotics (ototoxicity), cephalosporins (nephrotoxicity), salicylates, lithium, and cardiac glycosides.
3. Increased orthostatic hypotension can occur with narcotics or barbiturates.
4. Increased potassium loss may occur when corticosteroids are given with loop diuretics.
5. Loop diuretics may reduce the effectiveness of uricosuric drugs by elevating serum uric acid levels.
6. Probenecid may reduce the diuretic effectiveness of bumetanide and furosemide.
7. Phenytoin, indomethacin, and possibly other nonsteroidal anti-inflammatory drugs may impair the action of loop diuretics.
8. Loop diuretics can antagonize the muscle-relaxing effects of the antidepolarizing neuromuscular-blocking drugs (*e.g.*, tubocurare, gallamine) but may potentiate the muscle-relaxing action of succinylcholine.
9. Increased requirements for oral antidiabetic drugs or insulin may occur in persons taking loop diuretics, which can elevate blood glucose levels.
10. Furosemide (and possibly bumetanide) can potentiate the pharmacologic effects of theophylline.
11. Ethacrynic acid may displace oral anticoagulants from their protein-binding sites.

NURSING CONSIDERATIONS
(See also General Nursing Process for Diuretics.)

A complete drug history should be obtained using the interactions listed above as a reference. Loop diuretics interact with many drugs and chemicals, some of which the patient is unlikely to report unless asked appropriate questions. These include alcohol, street drugs, OTC medications for arthritis, and imported licorice containing glycyrrhizin, which when taken in large amounts can result in severe hypokalemia.

Almost all patients taking loop diuretics should be started on a potassium supplement and encouraged to eat potassium-rich foods. However, these diuretics can also cause many electrolyte problems affecting calcium, sodium, and magnesium as well as potassium, resulting in metabolic acidosis. Periodic electrolyte values should be drawn throughout therapy to monitor any changes, but the patient should be taught to report immediately such early symptoms as hypoventilation, nausea, agitation, confusion, muscle weakness, and palpitations. Deficits will be corrected based on laboratory results, and drug dose may need to be changed. Serum electrolyte imbalances are most likely to occur in elderly patients, in young children, during intravenous drug therapy, and in patients with renal impairment.

Other early symptoms of overzealous therapy are abdominal discomfort and dizziness, which the patient may not relate to the diuretic unless informed of the possibility. These symptoms should also be immediately reported.

Loop diuretics also cause uric acid retention which can result in gout in a susceptible individual. The patient should be taught to report early any signs of joint swelling, tenderness, or pain. Serum uric acid levels should be monitored periodically, and elevations should be promptly treated.

Diuretics must be administered intravenously with extreme caution because electrolyte imbalances and blood volume depletion can occur rapidly, resulting in hypovolemia, hypotension, vascular collapse, and, possibly, cardiac arrest. The rate and frequency of drug administration outlined in Table 41-4 should be closely followed, and the patient should be given the smallest effective dose. Rapid injection should be avoided. Close and thorough monitoring of the patient is essential and should include serum sodium, potassium, calcium, and magnesium levels, BUN, and creatinine several times a day. Hourly urine outputs should be measured; guidelines are usually set for minimum and maximum output beyond which future doses

should be held until the physician is notified. Assessment of heart rate and rhythm and blood pressure will give clues about cardiovascular status; checking skin turgor and appearance of mucous membranes can help identify early signs of dehydration. Nursing Care Plan 41-1 summarizes the nursing process for the patient receiving oral furosemide.

Intravenous diuretic therapy also increases the risk of significant adverse reactions. The patient on ethacrynic acid should be closely observed for signs of gastrointestinal bleeding or diarrhea. The patient receiving furosemide should be told to report any ringing in the ears because tinnitus is an early sign of drug-induced ototoxicity. The patient on bumetanide should be monitored on a continuous ECG because arrhythmias may develop. These symptoms should be reported immediately, and further drug doses should be held until the physician evaluates the patient.

Mercurials

Mersalyl with Theophylline
(Theo-Syl-R)

The use of mercurial diuretics has declined dramatically in recent years with the availability of equally effective and safer diuretic drugs. Currently, only one mercurial diuretic, mersalyl with theophylline, is available, and it is used very infrequently. Mercurial diuretics are so named because they are complex organic compounds containing mercury in the divalent (mercuric) state. Mersalyl produces prompt and copious diuresis and is occasionally used in severe edematous states secondary to other conditions such as congestive heart failure, renal disease, or cirrhosis. Its principal disadvantage is that it must be administered parenterally for optimal effect and thus is of limited usefulness for ambulatory or out-of-hospital patients.

Mersalyl liberates free mercuric (Hg^{++}) ions in an acid environment, which inhibit enzymes that supply energy for tubular mechanisms involved in sodium reabsorption. Mersalyl also depresses the tubular secretion of potassium and thus elicits a lower degree of hypokalemia than most other potent diuretics. The preparation contains theophylline, which increases the absorption of the mercurial from the injection site and also assists in the removal of the potentially toxic mercury ions by the kidneys, reducing the danger of cumulation

(Text continues on p. 822.)

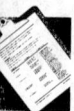

Nursing Care Plan 41-1
The Patient Receiving Oral Furosemide

Assessment

Subjective Data

1. Medication history
   a. Refer to Interactions section to formulate pertinent questions
   b. Previous diuretic therapy
   c. Allergies/hypersensitivities

2. Medical history
   a. Presence of conditions that contraindicate furosemide therapy
   b. Pre-existing conditions that may require modification in drug dosage such as cirrhosis, diabetes mellitus, hyperuricemia, cardiogenic shock, hearing impairment, systemic lupus erythematosus, postural hypotension, extremes in age
   c. Presence of urinary problems (*i.e.*, incontinence or retention)
   d. Current pregnancy or lactation

3. Personal history/compliance issues
   a. Understanding of condition and ability to manage self-care
   b. Personal and financial resources, supportive network

Objective Data

1. Physical assessment: complete, but highlighting
   a. Cardiovascular status: pulse, BP, CVP (if possible), peripheral pulses, presence of edema, evidence of adequate hydration
   b. Respiratory status: respiratory rate and effort, presence of rales, hypoxia
   c. Renal status: urinary output, weight, ability to void
   d. Hepatic status: liver size, abdominal girth, presence of jaundice

2. Laboratory/diagnostic data
   a. ECG
   b. Urinalysis, specific gravity
   c. BUN, serum creatinine, uric acid
   d. Serum electrolytes
   e. CBC with differential

Nursing Diagnosis	Expected Client Outcome	Intervention
Knowledge deficit related to drug action, correct administration, potential side-effects, the need for clinical follow up, and the need to use electrolyte supplements to prevent side-effects	Will verbalize understanding of drug action, correct administration, potential side-effects, and need for clinical follow-up	Explain how furosemide will eliminate fluid; onset of oral drug is 30–60 minutes after administration.
		Dose should be taken early in the day to minimize disruption of sleep from evening diuresis.
		Teach patient to plan administration so that immediate access to a bathroom is available for 1–2 hours after the drug is taken.
		Monitor and teach patient to monitor signs of drug effectiveness: high urinary output, low BP and low CVP, low respiratory rate and effort, low rales, low peripheral edema, low weight, low abdominal girth. Changes in these are also the early signs of drug failure.
	Serum sodium and potassium levels will remain within normal limits	Obtain pre-treatment electrolytes and monitor sodium and potassium levels throughout therapy.
		Administer and teach patient to take potassium supplements as ordered.

(continued)

Nursing Diagnosis	Expected Client Outcome	Intervention
Knowledge deficit related to drug action, correct administration, potential side-effects, the need for clinical follow up, and the need to use electrolyte supplements to prevent side-effects *(continued)*		Emphasize the need to include potassium-rich foods in diet (see text).
		Teach patient how to restrict sodium in diet.
		Teach patient to report immediately early symptoms of hypokalemia and hyponatremia (see text).
		Teach patient the importance of contacting the health team if vomiting, diarrhea, or other illness occurs which may disrupt electrolyte balance.
		Be aware that patients on high doses or who take other drugs which alter electrolytes (*e.g.,* digitalis, steroids) are at greater risk for electrolyte problems.
Potential fluid volume deficit related to diuresis from the drug	Normal hydration will be maintained.	Monitor and teach patient to monitor weight daily. Excessive weight loss or weight gain (5 lb either way) should be immediately reported.
		Monitor and teach patient to measure daily urine output and to keep a record of fluid intake so I/O ratio can be evaluated, especially early in treatment.
		Teach patient to report immediately signs of dehydration: low weight, skin turgor loss, weakness. In acute care also monitor for low BP, low CVP, low urine specific gravity, high BUN.
Potential for injury related to dizziness from drug-induced postural hypotension	Blood pressure will remain within normal limits with minimal postural effects.	Obtain sitting, standing, and lying BP frequently during dosage adjustment period and any time patient complains of dizziness. Wide variations in BP may require dosage adjustment.
		Encourage patient to rise slowly from supine position, sit for 1 minute, then stand slowly; and to avoid standing in one position for too long.
		Keep side rails up on bedridden patients to avoid falls if dizziness occurs.
		Caution patient to avoid driving, climbing stairs, or operating machinery until drug effects are known.
		Persistent problems should be reported.

(continued)

Nursing Diagnosis	Expected Client Outcome	Intervention
Potential for infection related to alteration in WBC count	WBC count will remain within normal limits	Monitor WBC count at regular intervals for patients on long-term therapy. Encourage patient to report any weakness, fever, or flu-like symptoms.
Potential alteration in tissue integrity related to hematologic changes or skin sensitivity to drug	Platelet level will remain within normal limits	Monitor platelet level at regular intervals for patients on long-term therapy. Teach patient to report immediately any bruising, petechiae, or bleeding.
	Skin and tissue will remain intact	Teach patient to check skin daily and to report immediately any rash, swelling, discoloration, or itching. Teach patient to use a sunscreen when in sun and to avoid direct exposure as much as possible.
Potential alteration in comfort; pain or GI distress related to drug side-effects	Will remain symptom-free	Teach patient to take drug with food to minimize GI distress. Teach patient to report immediately any nausea, vomiting, diarrhea, or abdominal pain.
Potential sensory-perceptual alteration: hearing related to drug-induced ototoxicity	Will maintain normal hearing	Monitor hearing at regular intervals in all patients on high-dose or long-term therapy. Teach patients to report immediately any ringing in the ears or dizziness.

and possible nephrotoxicity. Tolerance to the diuretic action of mersalyl develops over time, and patients become refractory with continued use.

Recommended dosage of mersalyl with theophylline, which contains 100 mg of mersalyl and 50 mg of theophylline per milliliter, is 1 ml to 2 ml daily or every other day IM or by *slow* IV injection if IM administration is unfeasible. Subcutaneous injection is painful and should be avoided. The diuretic response occurs within 1 hour to 2 hours, peaks within 4 hours to 8 hours and persists for 12 hours to 24 hours. Up to 95% of a dose is recovered in the urine within 24 hours.

A variety of untoward reactions can occur with mersalyl, including hypersensitivity reactions, nausea, vomiting, diarrhea, electrolyte disturbances, azotemia, hyperuricemia, thrombocytopenia, leukopenia, and agranulocytosis. Symptoms of mercury poisoning (*e.g.*, stomatitis, gingivitis, salivation, diarrhea, colitis, metallic taste) can occur, especially following too frequent administration or in patients with impaired renal function.

Dimercaprol (BAL) should be on hand as an antidote to prevent toxic effects in case an overdose is administered. The drug is rarely used today and is largely of historic interest.

Osmotic Diuretics

The term osmotic diuretic refers to any solute that is readily filtered by the kidney but poorly reabsorbed in the renal tubules. Consequently, the large amount of nonreabsorbed material increases the osmotic pressure of the tubular fluid, causing an osmotically equivalent amount of water to be carried through the tubule with it, eventually to be excreted. Sodium excretion is not significantly increased, however, by normal therapeutic doses of the osmotic diuretics. For this reason, as well as the fact that most of these diuretics must be administered IV in large doses, they are infrequently used for routine treatment of edema and are primarily indicated for the prevention of acute renal failure associated with a sharply reduced glomerular filtration rate.

Their osmotic effects are not confined to the kidney but extend to the bloodstream as well, where the presence of the drug in the circulation creates an increased plasma osmotic pressure which draws fluid from tissue spaces into the blood. This effect underlies their application in reducing elevated intraocular and intracranial pressures, actions important in treating cranial injuries and acute congestive glaucoma, and as an aid to neurosurgery.

There are four osmotic diuretics currently in clinical use, and they are discussed individually below. A comparison of their pharmacokinetic properties is presented in Table 41-5.

NURSING CONSIDERATIONS
(See also General Nursing Process for Diuretics.)

The main nursing responsibility for all of these drugs is to carefully monitor urinary output. Some patients may require bladder catheterization to manage the large volume of urine expected and to facilitate accurate measurements. If output drops below 30 ml/hour, extracellular fluid volume overload may be developing which can lead to congestive heart failure (CHF). The physician should be notified at once, and the patient should be observed for other signs of CHF such as shortness of breath, pallor, and increased heart rate. Renal function should also be closely monitored through periodic evaluations of BUN and creatinine levels.

Glycerin
(Glyrol, Osmoglyn)

Glycerin is a liquid preparation used orally for reducing intraocular pressure to treat acute attacks of glaucoma and prior to ophthalmic surgery for glaucoma or cataracts where preoperative reduction of intraocular pressure is desirable. The drug has been administered by the IV route to lower intracranial as well as intraocular pressure, but this is not an approved means of administration.

Oral dosage is 1 g to 1.5 g/kg 1 hour to 1½ hour before surgery. Adverse reactions include nausea, vomiting, diarrhea, headache, confusion, arrhythmias, and dehydration. *Cautious use* of glycerin is necessary in patients with diabetes, congestive heart disease, hypervolemia, confused mental states, and in elderly or senile persons. Safety and efficacy for use in pregnant women, nursing mothers, or in children have not been established.

Isosorbide
(Ismotic)

Isosorbide is available as an oral solution (45%) for reduction of intraocular pressure prior to or following surgery for glaucoma or cataracts or to temporarily interrupt an acute attack of glaucoma. Initial dosage is 1.5 g/kg two to four times a day; the usual dosage range is 1 g to 3 g/kg two to four times a day. The liquid preparation may be better tolerated if chilled. Side-effects include nausea, vomiting, headache, confusion, and less often diarrhea, thirst, dizziness, lightheadedness, lethargy, irritability, rash, hiccoughs, and hypernatremia. Isosor-

Table 41-5
Pharmacokinetic Properties of Osmotic Diuretics

Drug	Route of Administration	Onset (min)	Peak Effect (h)	Duration (h)	Elimination Half-Life (h)	Metabolism	Excretion
Glycerin	PO	15–30	0.5	4–6	0.5–1	80%–90% liver	Urine (metabolites)
Isosorbide	PO	15–30	1–1.5	4–6	6–8	0%	Urine (unchanged)
Mannitol	IV	30–60	1	6–8	0.5–2	5%–10% liver	Urine (mostly unchanged)
Urea	IV	30–60	1	4–6			Urine (unchanged)

bide should not be used in patients with acute pulmonary edema, hemorrhagic glaucoma, severe dehydration, or cardiac decompensation or anuria. Adequate fluid and electrolyte balance must be maintained with repeated administration.

Mannitol
(Osmitrol)

MECHANISM AND ACTIONS
Mannitol is a sugar which is given IV and is rapidly filtered by the kidney, but is *not* appreciably reabsorbed by the tubules. The resultant increased tubular osmotic pressure retains water in the tubules and increases urine volume. Plasma osmotic pressure is also elevated, which results in removal of fluid from extracellular tissue spaces.

USES
1. Prevention and treatment of the oliguric phase of acute renal failure before irreversible renal failure occurs
2. Treatment of cerebral edema and elevated intracranial pressure (*e.g.,* resulting from head injury or surgery)
3. Reduction of elevated intraocular pressure in acute congestive glaucoma
4. Treatment of acute chemical poisoning, by enhancing renal excretion of toxic substances
5. Measurement of glomerular filtration rate

ADMINISTRATION AND DOSAGE
Mannitol is available for injection as 5%, 10%, 15%, 20%, and 25% solution. Mannitol is administered by IV infusion *only*. The infusion rate is adjusted based on urinary output. Recommended doses for the various indications are as follows:
Prevention of acute renal failure—50 g to 100 g as a 5% to 25% solution
Reduction of intracranial pressure—1.5 g to 2 g/kg as a 15% to 25% solution over 30 minutes to 60 minutes
Reduction of intraocular pressure—1.5 g to 2 g/kg as a 15% to 25% solution over 30 minutes to 60 minutes
Acute chemical poisoning—100 g to 200 g as a 5% to 10% solution over 30 minutes to 60 minutes depending on fluid requirement and urinary output
Measurement of glomerular filtration rate—100 ml of 20% solution diluted with 180 ml of sodium chloride injection infused at a rate of 20 ml/minute

Test dose (patients with marked oliguria or inadequate renal function)—0.2 g/kg infused over 3 minutes to 5 minutes to produce a urine flow of at least 30 ml to 50 ml/h

Mannitol solution may crystallize, especially in concentrations greater than 15% and when exposed to low temperatures. Crystallization can be prevented by warming the solution in a hot water bath, then cooling to body temperature before administration.

FATE
See Table 41-5.

SIDE-EFFECTS/ADVERSE REACTIONS
Adverse reactions are generally infrequent during mannitol infusion, but may include dry mouth, thirst, headache, blurred vision, nausea, vomiting, diarrhea, dizziness, fever, chills, urticaria, rhinitis, marked diuresis with dehydration, urinary retention, acidosis, pulmonary congestion, skin necrosis, tachycardia, angina-like pain, and thrombophebitis.

CONTRAINDICATIONS AND PRECAUTIONS
Use of mannitol is contraindicated in patients with anuria, severe pulmonary edema or congestive heart failure, intracranial bleeding, severe dehydration, progressive renal disease after initiating mannitol therapy, and in children under 12 years of age. Mannitol must be used with caution in persons with renal dysfunction or electrolyte imbalances and in pregnant women.

NURSING CONSIDERATIONS
(See also Nursing Considerations for osmotic diuretics.)

Intravenous mannitol should be administered by an infusion pump with an infiltration alarm. The drug is very irritating to the tissue. If pain, inflammation, or signs of infiltration occur, the line must be removed and the physician notified. Careful monitoring of the infusion rate is also essential because too rapid infusion can lead to circulatory overload, water intoxication, and cardiac decompensation.

Mannitol crystallizes when 15% to 25% solutions are used. To reduce the chance of this development the vial should be warmed in water then cooled just prior to infusion. An in-line filter should be attached to the IV line.

Mannitol should not be administered with

blood unless 20 mEq Na has been added to the solution.

Urea
(Ureaphil)

Urea is an infrequently used osmotic diuretic which is filtered by the kidney but not reabsorbed, thereby increasing the rate and volume of urine flow. It also elevates plasma osmotic pressure, resulting in removal of fluid from extracellular tissue spaces. It may be given by *slow* IV infusion (1 g–1.5 g/kg of a 30% solution) at a rate not to exceed 4 ml/min to reduce intraocular and intracranial pressure. Children over age 2 may be given 0.5 g to 1.5 g/kg; younger children should receive 0.1 g/kg. The solution is very irritating and may cause tissue necrosis if extravasation occurs. An infusion pump with an infiltration alarm should be used. Adverse effects are generally minimal when the drug is infused slowly, but headache, nausea, vomiting, agitation, confusion, and syncope have been reported. Urea is contraindicated in patients with severely impaired renal function, marked dehydration, liver failure, and active intracranial bleeding. It should not be infused into veins of the lower extremities in elderly patients because phlebitis can occur. An isosmotic concentration of dextrose or invert sugar should be administered with urea to prevent hemolysis that can occur with pure solutions of urea. Urea is *strictly* an alternate drug and should not be used unless other osmotic diuretics are inappropriate.

Frequent renal function studies (BUN, creatinine) should be drawn to help determine if the kidneys are capable of diuresis and elimination of urea. If the patient does not diurese within 6 hours to 12 hours, the drug should be discontinued.

Potassium-Sparing Diuretics

Unlike most other major classes of diuretic drugs, the potassium-sparing diuretics do *not* cause a loss of potassium by way of the kidney, but rather act to conserve potassium by reducing its distal tubular secretion in conjunction with sodium reabsorption. These drugs are not potent diuretic drugs when used alone, and their use as single agents can result in significant *hyper*kalemia. Their principal application, therefore, is in combination with other oral diuretics (*e.g.*, thiazides, high-ceiling drugs) both to increase the excretion of sodium and water and, more importantly, to minimize the potassium loss normally induced by the more potent drugs. Because several important differences exist among the available potassium-sparing diuretics, they are reviewed individually.

Amiloride
(Midamor)

MECHANISM AND ACTIONS
Amiloride acts primarily on the distal tubule to inhibit active transport of sodium and potassium across tubular membranes. Inhibition of Na^+-K^+-ATP'ase enzyme may play a role in blocking transtubular transport of these ions. Amiloride possesses weak diuretic and blood pressure-lowering activity and does not significantly alter renal blood flow or glomerular filtration rate.

USES
1. Adjunctive treatment (with thiazide *or* loop diuretics) of congestive heart failure or hypertension to prevent hypokalemia or help restore depleted potassium levels

ADMINISTRATION AND DOSAGE
Amiloride is used orally as 5-mg tablets. The initial dose is 5 mg/day as a single dose. If necessary, dosage may be increased in 5-mg increments up to 20 mg/day in cases of severe, persistent hypokalemia. Amiloride is also available in fixed combination with hydrochlorothiazide (5 mg/50 mg) as Moduretic. Dosage is one or two tablets a day, with meals.

FATE
Following oral administration, the onset is within 2 hours, with a peak effect occurring within 6 hours to 10 hours. Effects persist for up to 24 hours. The drug is only slightly protein bound (20%–25%) and has a half-life of 6 hours to 9 hours. There are no

active metabolites, and over 50% of a dose is excreted unchanged in the urine.

SIDE-EFFECTS/ADVERSE REACTIONS
The most common side-effects with amiloride are nausea, anorexia, diarrhea, headache, and hyperkalemia (possibly manifested as paresthesias, muscle weakness, fatigue, and bradycardia). A number of other adverse reactions have occurred during amiloride therapy and are listed below:

GI—Vomiting, abdominal pain, dyspepsia, constipation, flatulence, dry mouth, GI bleeding

CNS—Dizziness, confusion, insomnia, tremors, depression, encephalopathy

Respiratory—Dyspnea, coughing

Musculoskeletal—Muscle cramping, weakness, pain in the joints, back, chest, neck, or shoulders

Other—Impotence, photosensitivity, polyuria, dysuria, arrhythmias, skin rash, pruritus, alopecia, visual disturbances, nasal congestion, tinnitus, increased intraocular pressure

When given alone, amiloride causes hyperkalemia in approximately 10% of patients, and the incidence is greater in persons with renal impairment or diabetes mellitus and in elderly persons. When given together with a thiazide diuretic, the incidence of hyperkalemia is less than 2%.

CONTRAINDICATIONS AND PRECAUTIONS
Use of amiloride is contraindicated in the presence of hyperkalemia (i.e., serum potassium greater than 5.5 mEq/L), anuria, acute or chronic renal insufficiency, diabetic nephropathy, and in conjunction with potassium supplements or other potassium-sparing diuretics. *Caution* must be observed when amiloride is used in patients with diabetes, respiratory or metabolic acidosis, renal impairment, cardiopulmonary disease, and in pregnant women, nursing mothers, children, and elderly or debilitated persons.

INTERACTIONS
1. Amiloride may increase lithium toxicity by reducing its renal clearance.
2. Hyperkalemia may be augmented by concomitant use of other potassium-sparing drugs (e.g., spironolactone, triamterene), potassium supplements, or captopril.
3. Amiloride can reduce the clinical effectiveness of digitalis drugs but also reduces the risk of toxicity resulting from hypokalemia.

Spironolactone
(Alatone, Aldactone)

MECHANISM AND ACTIONS
Spironolactone is a competitive antagonist of the naturally occurring hormone aldosterone at renal tubular sites involved in the exchange of sodium for potassium; aldosterone normally stimulates enzymes that supply energy for active sodium and potassium transport in the distal tubule. Inhibition of aldosterone results in excretion of sodium and retention of potassium. Spironolactone does not appear to elevate serum uric acid or alter carbohydrate metabolism, but it can interfere with testosterone synthesis, leading to increased estrogenic-to-androgenic activity ratio.

USES
1. Management of edema associated with congestive heart failure, primary aldosteronism, cirrhosis of the liver, and nephrotic syndrome
2. Treatment of essential hypertension, usually combined with other diuretics or antihypertensive drugs
3. Adjunctive therapy with other potent diuretics to minimize potassium loss
4. Diagnosis and treatment of primary aldosteronism
5. Treatment of hirsutism (investigational use only)

ADMINISTRATION AND DOSAGE
Spironolactone is available as 25-mg, 50-mg, and 100-mg tablets. Recommended doses for the various indications are as follows:

Edema—Adults: 25 mg to 200 mg/day in a single dose or divided doses; Children: 3.3 mg/kg in a single dose or divided doses

Hypertension—50 mg to 100 mg daily in a single dose or divided doses; maximum 200 mg/day

Diagnosis of aldosteronism—400 mg/day for 4 days; if serum potassium increases during this time, then falls when drug is stopped, a presumptive diagnosis of primary aldosteronism may be considered

Treatment of aldosteronism—100 mg to 400 mg/day

Hypokalemia—25 mg to 100 mg/day to prevent diuretic-induced potassium loss

Spironolactone is also available in fixed combination with hydrochlorothiazide (25 mg/25 mg or 50 mg/50 mg) for use as a diuretic and an antihypertensive under the trade names Alazide, Aldactazide, Spironozide, and Spirozide.

FATE

Although peak plasma levels occur within 3 hours to 4 hours following a single dose, the maximal diuretic effect is not observed for 2 to 3 days and may persist for several days. Protein binding is extensive (98%). The drug is metabolized in part to an active metabolite and excreted primarily in the urine.

SIDE-EFFECTS/ADVERSE REACTIONS

■ WARNING
Spironolactone has been shown to be a mammary and hepatic tumorigen in chronic toxicity studies in rats at significantly higher than recommended doses. Its use should be restricted to those indications outlined above for which other diuretic drugs are ineffective or inappropriate.

The following untoward reactions have occurred in patients receiving spironolactone:
GI—Cramping, diarrhea, thirst
CNS—Headache, drowsiness, lethargy, confusion, ataxia
Endocrine—Gynecomastia and breast tenderness (most often with chronic therapy—usually reversible when drug is discontinued), irregular menses, impotence, hirsutism, deepening of the voice, postmenopausal bleeding
Dermatologic—Urticaria, cutaneous eruptions
Other—Fever, metabolic acidosis

CONTRAINDICATIONS AND PRECAUTIONS

Contraindications to use of spironolactone include anuria, acute renal insufficiency, significantly impaired renal function, and hyperkalemia. Spironolactone should be given *cautiously* to persons with decreased renal function and to pregnant or nursing women. The drug should not be used in combination with other potassium-sparing diuretics or potassium supplements.

INTERACTIONS

1. Spironolactone potentiates the effects of other diuretics and antihypertensive drugs.
2. Salicylates may decrease the effectiveness of spironolactone.
3. Spironolactone may reduce the clinical effectiveness of digitalis drugs but also reduces the likelihood of digitalis-induced arrhythmias occurring as a result of hypokalemia.
4. The renal clearance of lithium may be reduced by spironolactone.
5. The effects of oral anticoagulants may be reduced due to hemoconcentration of clotting factors resulting from diuretic action.
6. Ammonium chloride and other acidifying agents can induce systemic acidosis when given in combination with spironolactone.
7. Hyperkalemia may result if potassium supplements, potassium-sparing diuretics, or captopril are used together with spironolactone, or if patients consume a potassium-rich diet.

Triamterene
(Dyrenium)

MECHANISM AND ACTIONS

Triamterene inhibits active reabsorption of sodium and secretion of potassium by distal tubular cells. It does not appear to interfere with aldosterone, but acts directly on the renal tubule.

USES

1. Treatment of edema associated with congestive heart failure, cirrhosis of the liver, or the nephrotic syndrome, and in steroid-induced or idiopathic edema
2. Adjunctive therapy of hypertension, in combination with other diuretics, for its added diuretic effect as well as its potassium-conserving effect

ADMINISTRATION AND DOSAGE

Triamterene is available as 50-mg and 100-mg capsules. When given alone, the initial dose is 100 mg twice a day (maximum 300 mg/day). The dosage should be reduced when triamterene is combined with another diuretic.

Triamterene is also available in fixed combination with hydrochlorothiazide as Dyazide (50 mg/25 mg) and Maxzide (75 mg/50 mg).

FATE

Following oral administration, the onset of action is 2 hours to 3 hours, and the peak diuretic effect occurs in 6 hours to 8 hours. Effects persist up to 16 hours. The drug is 50% to 70% protein bound and has a plasma half-life of 3 hours to 4 hours. The majority of a dose is metabolized in the liver and excreted in the urine.

SIDE-EFFECTS/ADVERSE REACTIONS

Triamterene may cause GI upset, weakness, headache, dry mouth, rash, and photosensitization. Other adverse reactions noted during therapy with triamterene include nausea, vomiting, hypotension, leg cramps, metallic taste, and rarely blood dyscrasias. Triamterene has been found in renal stones, and interstitial nephritis has been reported. Hyperkalemia can occur, especially in patients with renal insufficiency or those receiving potassium supplements.

CONTRAINDICATIONS AND PRECAUTIONS

Triamterene is contraindicated in patients with anuria, severe hepatic disease, hyperkalemia, and severe or progressive kidney dysfunction. It should not be given to patients receiving other potassium-sparing diuretics. Patients with a history of gouty arthritis or renal stone formation, impaired renal function, or hepatic cirrhosis should be given triamterene *cautiously*. Its use during pregnancy or nursing should be undertaken only when clearly indicated.

INTERACTIONS

1. Concurrent use of triamterene with other potassium-sparing diuretics, captopril, or potassium supplements can result in hyperkalemia.
2. Serum levels of digitalis glycosides may be increased by triamterene.
3. Acute renal failure has been reported when indomethacin was given with triamterene.
4. Triamterene may decrease the renal clearance of lithium, resulting in lithium toxicity.

NURSING CONSIDERATIONS FOR POTASSIUM-SPARING DIURETICS

(See also General Nursing Process for Diuretics.)

The most significant difference between the potassium-sparing diuretics and other diuretics is the possible development of *hyper*kalemia as a side-effect. Patients should be taught to report any early symptoms such as weakness, confusion, paresthesias, or a feeling of heart beat irregularities. In addition, the patient should have periodic potassium levels drawn, and the drug should be withheld if the level exceeds 5.5 mEq/L. He should also be aware to limit potassium-rich foods, such as bananas, citrus fruits, dates, raisins, apricots, and cola beverages, and not to take potassium supplements. This is especially important for the patient who has been receiving other types of diuretics where potassium supplementation is usually advised.

Thiazides/Sulfonamides

Bendroflumethiazide, Benzthiazide, Chlorothiazide, Chlorthalidone, Cyclothiazide, Hydrochlorothiazide, Hydroflumethiazide, Indapamide, Methyclothiazide, Metolazone, Polythiazide, Quinethazone, Trichlormethiazide

The largest group of orally effective diuretic drugs are the thiazides/sulfonamides. They are structurally related to the sulfonamide antibacterial drugs; however, they possess no anti-infective properties. Most of these sulfonamide diuretics are derived from a benzothiadiazine nucleus, and hence are commonly referred to as thiazide diuretics. A few other sulfonamide diuretics differ slightly in their chemical structure from the thiazides, although their pharmacologic and toxicologic properties are essentially similar, and these compounds are referred to as sulfonamide or thiazide-like diuretics. Structural differences notwithstanding, all of these drugs possess parallel dose-response curves, that is, there is essentially no difference among them in their clinical efficacy, and all drugs in this category possess similar sites and mechanisms of diuretic action. A comparison of the pharmacokinetic properties of the thiazide/sulfonamide diuretics is presented in Table 41-6.

The thiazide/sulfonamide diuretics are the most widely used drugs for the treatment of edematous states and for the control of mild to moderate hypertension. Because of the similarity of action among the various drugs in this class, they will be reviewed as a group. Individual drugs are then listed in Table 41-7.

MECHANISM AND ACTIONS

The thiazide/sulfonamide diuretics impair active sodium and chloride reabsorption in the early portion of the distal segment of the renal tubule and possibly also in the cortical thick ascending loop of Henle, resulting in excretion of these ions with an osmotically equivalent volume of water. They also possess weak carbonic anhydrase inhibitory activity, although the importance of this action to their diuretic effect is probably minimal. Potassium ex-

Table 41-6
Pharmacokinetic Properties of Thiazide/Sulfonamide Diuretics

Drug	Onset of Action (h)	Peak effect (h)	Duration (h)	Optimal Oral Dose (mg/day)
bendroflumethiazide	2	4	6–12	2.5–10
benthiazide	2	4–6	6–12	50–200
chlorothiazide	1–2	4	6–12	500–1000
chlorthalidone*	2	2–6	24–48	50–100
cyclothiazide	4–6	6–12	18–24	1–2
hydrochlorothiazide	2	4–6	6–12	25–100
hydroflumethiazide	2	4	6–12	25–100
indapamide*	1–2	2	18–36	2.5–5
methyclothiazide	2	6	18–24	2.5–10
metolazone*	1	2	12–24	2.5–10
polythiazide	2	6	24–48	1–4
quinethazone*	2	6	18–24	50–100
trichlormethiazide	2	6	18–24	2–4

* Sulfonamide derivatives.

cretion is augmented, bicarbonate excretion is slightly increased, whereas calcium excretion is reduced.

The exact antihypertensive mechanism of action of the thiazide/sulfonamide diuretics is not completely established but may be due to (1) reduction of plasma volume and sodium levels, (2) direct relaxation of arteriolar smooth muscle, and (3) decreased reactivity of vascular smooth muscle to endogenous pressor substances, possibly the result of alterations in sodium content within the muscle fibers.

Other actions of the thiazide/sulfonamide diuretics include interference with insulin release, possibly a result of hypokalemia and elevations in serum uric acid levels, due to decreased tubular secretion of uric acid. These drugs exert a paradoxical antidiuretic effect in diabetes insipidus, possibly by enhancing the action of antidiuretic hormone (ADH) as a consequence of sodium depletion.

USES
1. Treatment of edema associated with congestive heart failure, hepatic cirrhosis, renal dysfunction, and steroid or estrogen therapy
2. Management of all forms of hypertension, either alone (mild cases) or in combination with other antihypertensive drugs (moderate to severe cases)
3. Symptomatic treatment of diabetes insipidus to reduce polyuria

4. Prevent formation and recurrence of calcium stones in hypercalciuria, either alone or with amiloride or allopurinol (investigational use)

ADMINISTRATION AND DOSAGE
See Table 41-7.

FATE
See Table 41-6.

SIDE-EFFECTS/ADVERSE REACTIONS
Hypokalemia, marked by paresthesias, muscle cramping, weakness, and dizziness, can occur, especially if supplemental potassium is not given. Other adverse reactions noted during therapy with thiazide/sulfonamides include:
GI—Nausea, GI irritation, vomiting, anorexia, dry mouth, diarrhea, cramping, bloating, jaundice, pancreatitis, sialadenitis, hepatitis
Cardiovascular—Orthostatic hypotension, palpitation, irregular heartbeat, premature ventricular contractions, angina-like pain, hemoconcentration
CNS—Headache, vertigo, blurred vision, syncope, fatigue, drowsiness, restlessness, depression
Hypersensitivity—Rash, photosensitivity, fever, purpura, urticaria, vasculitis, Stevens-Johnson syndrome, dyspnea, pneumonitis, anaphylactic reactions
Hematologic—Blood dyscrasias (rare)

(Text continues on p. 832.)

Table 41-7
Thiazide/Sulfonamide Diuretics

Drug	Preparations	Usual Dosage Range	Clinical Considerations
bendroflumethiazide (Naturetin)	Tablets—5 mg, 10 mg	Edema—initially 5 mg to 20 mg/day; maintenance 2.5 mg to 5 mg/day Hypertension—initially, 5 mg to 20 mg/day; maintenance 2.5 mg to 15 mg/day	Short-acting preparation (6 h–12 h); low doses do not appreciably alter serum electrolyte levels; available in fixed combinations with rauwolfia (Rauzide) and nadolol (Corzide)
benzthiazide (Aquatag, Exna, Hydrex, Marazide, Proaqua)	Tablets—25 mg, 50 mg	Edema—initially 50 mg to 200 mg/day; maintenance 50 mg to 150 mg/day Hypertension—initially 50 mg to 100 mg/day; maintenance 50 mg two times/day	Maximal effect in 4 h–6 h, with a duration of 6 h–12 h. Drug is given twice a day after breakfast and lunch.
chlorothiazide (Diachlor, Diuril)	Tablets—250 mg, 500 mg Suspension—250 mg/5 ml Injection—500 mg/20 ml	Edema Adults—0.5 g to 2 g one to two times a day, 3 days to 5 days/week Children—22 mg/kg/day in two doses Hypertension—0.5 g to 2 g/day, adjusted to optimal response	Following oral administration, onset is within 2 h and duration is 6 h–12 h; IV solution is prepared by adding 18 ml sterile water to vial; do not administer with plasma or whole blood, nor give SC or IM; use IV only in emergency situations and avoid extravasation; IV injections are not recommended in children; solutions may be stored up to 24 h at room temperature; available with reserpine (Diupres) and methyldopa (Aldoclor) in oral form
chlorthalidone (Hygroton, Hylidone, Thalitone)	Tablets—25 mg, 50 mg, 100 mg	Edema—50 mg to 100 mg/day or 100 mg/day three times a week on alternate days Hypertension—initially 25 mg to 50 mg; adjust to optimal response; maximum 100 mg/day Children—3 mg/kg/day, three times/week	Sulfonamide diuretic; onset 2 h–3 h and duration 24 h–72 h; given by single daily dosage in the morning; effective hypotensive agent, often used as an initial therapy in mild hypertension; doses above 25 mg/day provide little additional blood pressure-lowering activity but are more likely to increase potassium loss; may elevate plasma levels of cholesterol, triglycerides, and LDL; available with clonidine (Combipres), reserpine (Regroton, Demi-Regroton), and atenolol (Tenoretic)

(continued)

Table 41-7 (continued)
Thiazide/Sulfonamide Diuretics

Drug	Preparations	Usual Dosage Range	Clinical Considerations
cyclothiazide (Anhydron)	Tablets—2 mg	Edema—1 mg to 2 mg/day; reduce to 1 mg to 2 mg two to three times a week as necessary Hypertension—2 mg once a day (maximum 6 mg once a day)	Slow onset (4 h–6 h) and prolonged duration of action (18 h–24 h); given in early morning to minimize sleep disturbance; rarely used product
hydrochlorothiazide (Esidrix, HydroDiuril, and various other manufacturers)	Tablets—25 mg, 50 mg, 100 mg Solution—50 mg/5 ml Intensol solution—100 mg/ml	Edema—initially 25 mg to 200 mg/day; maintenance 25 mg to 100 mg/day, usually on an intermittent schedule Hypertension—initially 50 mg to 100 mg/day; adjust to desired response; usual range 25 mg to 100 mg/day Children—2.2 mg/kg/day	Most widely used thiazide diuretic; onset 1 h–2 h and duration 6 h–12 h; excreted largely unchanged in the urine; available in fixed combination with many other antihypertensive drugs; oral absorption may be improved if taken with food
hydroflumethiazide (Diucardin, Saluron)	Tablets—50 mg	Edema—initially 50 mg to 100 mg/day; usual maintenance dose 25 mg to 200 mg/day on an intermittent schedule Hypertension—50 mg twice a day; adjusted to desired response	Rapid onset (1 h–2 h) and short duration (6 h–12 h); do not exceed 200 mg/day; available with reserpine (Salutensin)
indapamide (Lozol)	Tablets—2.5 mg	Initially, 2.5 mg/day as a single daily dose; may increase to 5 mg/day after 1 wk–4 wk if necessary	Indoline derivative used for hypertension and edema of congestive heart failure; increases serum uric acid an average of 1 mg/dl; doses greater than 5 mg/day do not provide additional therapeutic benefit but are associated with a greater degree of hypokalemia than smaller doses
methyclothiazide (Aquatensen, Enduron, Ethon)	Tablets—2.5 mg, 5 mg	Edema—2.5 mg to 10 mg once daily Hypertension—2.5 mg to 5 mg once daily	Onset in 2 h and duration lasts about 24 h; do not exceed 10 mg/day; available with reserpine (Diutensen-R), deserpidine (Enduronyl), pargyline (Eutron), and cryptenamine (Diutensen)
metolazone (Diulo, Microx, Zaroxolyn)	Tablets—2.5 mg, 5 mg, 10 mg	Edema—5 mg to 20 mg once daily Hypertension—2.5 mg to 5 mg once daily	Sulfonamide derivative with rapid onset (1 h) and moderate duration (12 h–24 h) of action; dosage should be in upper end of range in patients with congestive heart failure to ensure diuretic effect for full 24 h; not recommended in children; pro- *(continued)*

Table 41-7 (continued)
Thiazide/Sulfonamide Diuretics

Drug	Preparations	Usual Dosage Range	Clinical Considerations
metolazone (Diulo, Microx, Zaroxolyn) (continued)			found volume and electrolyte depletion can occur in combination with furosemide
polythiazide (Renese)	Tablets—1 mg, 2 mg, 4 mg	Edema—1 mg to 4 mg/day Hypertension—2 mg to 4 mg/day	Onset 1 h–2 h and duration 24 h–36 h; available with reserpine (Renese-R) and prazosin (Minizide)
quinethazone (Hydromox)	Tablets—50 mg	50 mg to 100 mg in a single daily morning dose; maximum 200 mg/day	Sulfonamide diuretic with an onset of 2 h and a duration of 18 h–24 h; available with reserpine (Hydromox-R)
trichlormethiazide (Aquazide, Diurese, Metahydrin, Naqua, Niazide, Trichlorex)	Tablets—2 mg, 4 mg	Edema—1 mg to 4 mg/day Hypertension—2 mg to 4 mg/day Children—0.07 mg/kg/day	Onset 2 h and duration up to 24 h; available with reserpine (Metatensin, Naquival)

Other—Muscle spasm, chills, rhinorrhea, flushing, impotence, hyperglycemia, hyperuricemia, acute gouty attacks, elevated BUN, hypercalcemia

Large doses of thiazide/sulfonamide diuretics may result in elevated plasma levels of cholesterol, triglycerides, and LDL cholesterol, and development of a systemic lupus erythematosus-like syndrome has occurred in some patients receiving these agents. The hypercalcemia produced by these drugs can aggravate manic-depressive episodes previously controlled by lithium.

CONTRAINDICATIONS AND PRECAUTIONS

Thiazide/sulfonamide diuretics are contraindicated in patients with anuria or renal decompensation and in patients with a history of sulfonamide hypersensitivity. IV use of these drugs is *not* recommended in infants and young children. Metolazone is also contraindicated in persons with hepatic coma or pre-coma.

Cautious use of thiazide/sulfonamide diuretics is recommended in persons with renal or hepatic disease, bronchial asthma, diabetes, gout, history of allergies, lupus erythematosus, advanced arteriosclerosis, or advanced heart disease, and in elderly or debilitated persons and pregnant women or nursing mothers. These drugs should also be given cautiously to patients receiving digitalis drugs or patients with a history of cardiac arrhythmias because hypokalemia can increase the likelihood of the development of arrhythmias.

INTERACTIONS

1. Thiazides potentiate the hypotensive action of other antihypertensive drugs and may increase the incidence of orthostatic hypotension due to alcohol, narcotics, barbiturates and other CNS depressants, phenothiazines, and tricyclic antidepressants.
2. The effects of oral anticoagulants, vasopressors, hypouricemic drugs, and oral antidiabetics may be antagonized by thiazide diuretics.
3. Hypokalemia may be intensified if thiazides are combined with corticosteroids.
4. Thiazide-induced hypokalemia may increase digitalis toxicity.
5. Indomethacin and the pyrazolones may reduce the diuretic efficacy of the thiazides.
6. Hypercalcemia can occur if thiazides are given with calcium carbonate or other calcium-containing products or vitamin D.
7. Thiazides can potentiate amphetamines, quinidine, and lithium by decreasing their excretion.
8. Prolonged relaxation of skeletal muscle (including respiratory) may occur if thiazides are given together with nondepolarizing muscle relaxants (*e.g.,* curare, gallamine, pancuronium, atracurium).
9. Oral absorption of thiazides may be impaired by cholestyramine and colestipol.
10. Concurrent use of diazoxide and thiazide/sulfonamide diuretics can increase the likelihood of hyperglycemia, hyperuricemia, and hypotension.

11. Severe and prolonged volume and electrolyte depletion can occur when loop diuretics are used together with thiazides.

NURSING CONSIDERATIONS
(See also General Nursing Process for Diuretics.)

When obtaining a drug history from a patient who will take a thiazide diuretic, refer to the drug interactions listed above. Thiazides interact with many drugs some of which the patient is unlikely to report unless directly questioned. These include alcohol, vitamin D, OTC preparations for arthritis, and street drugs. Thiazides, when taken with large amounts of imported licorice containing glycyrrhizin, can also result in severe hypokalemia. The patient who is taking thiazides should have them discontinued 48 hours before any surgery because the drug enhances the action of muscle relaxants and may reduce the effectiveness of vasopressor agents.

Thiazide diuretics can cause multiple electrolyte problems affecting calcium, potassium, sodium, and, in the elderly, magnesium. It can also result in metabolic alkalosis. Baseline serum electrolyte levels should be drawn during the initial phase of therapy and periodically thereafter. The patient should learn the early warning signs of these imbalances; hypoventilation, nausea, agitation, drowsiness, excessive thirst, muscle weakness, or cramping, and palpitations should be reported to the physician immediately. The elderly patient taking a thiazide and digoxin is especially at risk because imbalances in potassium and magnesium can rapidly lead to dangerous digitalis-induced arrhythmias. Any patient taking this drug combination should learn to take his pulse prior to each dose and report any rate less than 60 beats per minute to the physician before continuing the drug therapy.

The patient who is to start thiazide therapy should also have a blood lipid series drawn. Because thiazides appear to interfere with lipid metabolism, anyone who is a cardiac risk or has high serum lipids should be carefully evaluated to weigh the benefits of therapy against the risk of cardiovascular incident.

Thiazides also cause retention of uric acid which can result in gout in the susceptible individual. Teach the patient to watch for joint swelling, tenderness, or pain, and to report such symptoms immediately. Some patients may require prophylactic drug therapy to prevent high uric acid levels.

The diabetic patient should have blood glucose levels closely monitored during initial therapy because hyperglycemia may occur, especially if the patient takes oral antidiabetic drugs. Periodic blood glucose levels should be drawn throughout therapy, and drug doses should be altered accordingly.

CASE STUDY

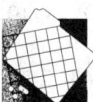

Irma Mathers, aged 75, is a type II diabetic who has been treated with diet therapy and glipizide (Glucotrol) 20 mg P.O. daily. Recently Mrs. Mathers complained of shortness of breath and swelling in her hands and feet. After a thorough physical examination, ECG, laboratory work-up, and echocardiogram, Mrs. Mathers was diagnosed as having mild left-sided congestive heart failure. She was placed on digoxin 0.125 mg P.O. daily and chlorothiazide (Diuril) 500 mg P.O. in the morning three times per week on Mondays, Wednesdays, and Fridays. As a precaution, she was also ordered a potassium supplement in effervescent tablets 20 mEq/tablet, one dose every day dissolved in juice or water.

Mrs. Mathers lives alone in a senior citizen apartment complex but sees her three daughters and two sons weekly. She is alert, oriented, and prior to this visit has independently managed her diabetic diet and dosage schedule for glipizide. Mrs. Bronowski, the eldest daughter, usually accompanies her mother to the physician's office and has volunteered to learn about the new drug regimen as well.

Discussion Question

Prepare a drug teaching plan for this patient and her family considering the following:

1. The actions and side-effects of each of the drugs (see Chaps. 33, 54, and 78 for additional information)
2. Potential drug interactions among the prescribed drugs
3. The need for dosage adjustments based on the patient's response
4. Incorporation of the total regimen into Mrs. Mather's daily routine
5. Memory joggers to help Mrs. Mathers adjust to the more complex regimen
6. Side-effects Mrs. Mathers and her family need to observe and the use of a flow sheet to facilitate this process (see Fig. 41-5 for an example)

REVIEW QUESTIONS

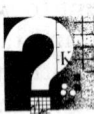

1. Briefly describe the blood supply of the kidneys.
2. What is the function of the juxtaglomerular apparatus?
3. Distinguish between renal tubular reabsorption and renal tubular secretion.
4. From which segment(s) of the renal tubule are the following substances reabsorbed: (a) K^+, (b) Na^+, (c) Ca^{++}, (d) HCO_3^-, and (e) water?
5. What laboratory studies should be obtained on any patient about to start diuretic therapy?
6. How can the nurse assess fluid volume in the patient receiving diuretics? How can the patient monitor this at home?
7. How do carbonic anhydrase inhibitors function as diuretics? What are their major indications?
8. What are the symptoms of metabolic acidosis associated with administration of carbonic anhydrase inhibitors?
9. Briefly outline the mechanism of action of the high-ceiling (loop) diuretics.
10. What are the principal electrolyte disturbances associated with use of high-ceiling (loop) diuretics? What symptoms can occur with overdosage of high-ceiling (loop) diuretics?
11. What are the symptoms of metabolic alkalosis associated with the administration of loop or thiazide diuretics?
12. How do mercurial diuretics promote diuresis? What are the major disadvantages to their use?
13. List the osmotic diuretics. How do they act to increase fluid loss?
14. What are the approved indications for IV mannitol?
15. What are the main nursing responsibilities when administering an osmotic diuretic?
16. Briefly describe the site and mechanism of action of the potassium-sparing diuretics.
17. What is the principal danger of potassium-sparing diuretics when used alone? In what conditions are potassium-sparing diuretics contraindicated?
18. List the major adverse effects associated with chronic use of spironolactone (Aldactone).

19. What is meant by the statement, "Thiazide/sulfonamide diuretics have parallel dose-response curves"?
20. What are the effects of thiazide/sulfonamide diuretics on (a) insulin release, (b) serum uric acid levels, (c) serum potassium levels and (d) serum calcium levels?
21. Describe the principal symptoms associated with hypokalemia. What foods are rich in potassium? Outline a strategy to help a patient taking a thiazide or loop diuretic to avoid hypokalemia?

BIBLIOGRAPHY

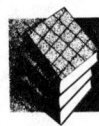

Beermann B, Groschinsky-Grind M: Clinical pharmacokinetics of diuretics. Clin Pharmacokinet 5:221, 1980

Brater DC: Pharmacodynamic considerations with use of diuretics. Annu Rev Pharmacol Toxicol 23:45, 1983

Cragoe EJ (ed): Diuretics: Chemistry, Pharmacology and Medicine. New York, John Wiley & Sons, 1983

Flamenbaum W, Friedman R: Pharmacology, therapeutic efficacy and adverse effects of bumetanide, a new "loop" diuretic. Pharmacotherap 2:213, 1982

Francisco LL, Ferris TF: The use and abuse of diuretics. Arch Intern Med 142:28, 1982

Freis ED: The cardiovascular risk of diuretic-induced hypokalemia and elevated cholesterol. Ration Drug Ther 20(3):1, 1986

Lamy P: Side effects of diuretics a danger for the aged. J Geront Nursing 11(6):44, June 1985

Madias NE, Zelman SJ: What are the metabolic complications of diuretic treatment? Geriatrics 37(2):93, 1983

Perez-Stable E, Caralis PV: Thiazide-induced disturbances in carbohydrate, lipid and potassium metabolism. Am Heart J 106:245, 1983

Rybak LP: Pathophysiology of furosemide ototoxicity. J Otolaryngol 11:127, 1982

Shoback DM, Williams GH: Potassium-sparing diuretics: Clinical pharmacology and therapeutic uses. Drug Therap 12(2):113, 1982

Symposium—Indapamide: A new indoline diuretic agent. Am Heart J 106:183, 1983

Warren SE, Blantz RC: Mannitol. Arch Intern Med 141:493, 1981

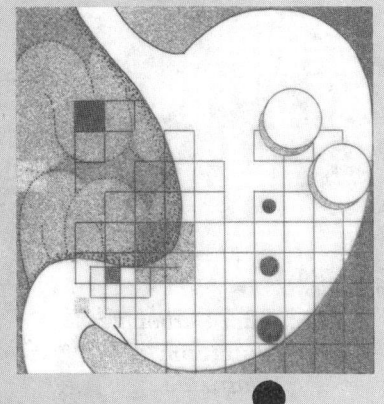

Drugs Affecting Gastrointestinal Function

VI

Antacids and Antiflatulents

42

The drugs reviewed in this chapter, antacids and antiflatulents, represent one of the most widely used group of medications for the treatment of upper GI disorders, ranging from mild indigestion and heartburn to peptic ulcer. It is estimated that nearly 10% of the population is subject to peptic ulcer disease, and this translates into many millions of dollars spent annually on antacids and other acid-reducing drugs. Before discussing the clinically useful antacids, however, a brief review of gastric secretory processes and the derangements responsible for the development of peptic ulcers will be presented.

Gastric Secretion

The mucosal lining of the stomach contains a number of different cell types which are capable of secreting various substances:

1. *Mucous cells*—Secrete an alkaline, viscous fluid (mucus) that coats and protects the epithelial lining of the stomach against irritation and erosion
2. *Parietal cells*—Secrete hydrochloric acid, which has several important functions, including conversion of pepsinogen into active pepsin, maintenance of optimal stomach pH for the activity of pepsin, denaturation of proteins, and destruction of certain bacteria
3. *Chief (zymogenic) cells*—Synthesize, store, and release pepsinogen, the inactive precursor of the proteolytic enzyme pepsin, which is then rapidly converted to pepsin in an acidic environment
4. *Gastrin-containing cells*—Secrete the hormone gastrin in response to numerous stimuli (caffeine, alcohol, protein digestion products, vagal activation); gastrin in turn stimulates the parietal and chief cells to secrete hydrochloric acid and pepsinogen, respectively.

Gastric secretion occurs in three phases, cephalic, gastric, and intestinal, and is controlled by neural and humoral mechanisms.

The cephalic phase, which occurs before food enters the stomach, may be initiated by the thought, sight, smell, or taste of food. This phase, which is mediated by the vagus nerve (and may therefore be abolished by vagotomy), elicits secretion of gastric juice high in acid and pepsin content.

The gastric phase of secretion, which is mediated by the hormone gastrin, takes place while food is present in the stomach. Gastrin is released from the pyloric antrum in response to mechanical distention or chemical stimulation (*e.g.*, protein digestion products, alcohol, caffeine). Gastrin release is the major stimulus to acid secretion.

During the intestinal phase, the arrival of chyme in the duodenum causes the stomach to secrete small amounts of gastric juice. This stimulation is hormonally mediated by an intestinal gastrin.

Peptic Ulcer Disease

Erosion of a localized area of the gastric or duodenal mucosa is referred to as a peptic ulcer. Mild ulceration may simply involve the outer mucosal lining, and the affected tissue may heal itself if the offending stimulus is removed. In other instances, however, the ulcerative lesion may extend more deeply into the underlying layers of connective tissue and muscles and result in more extensive bleeding and pain. The most serious situations involve complete erosion of a large blood vessel, which can cause serious bleeding or perforation of the stomach or intestinal wall, which can lead to peritonitis.

The pathogenesis of peptic ulcers is not completely understood, and no *one* factor or circumstance can be implicated in the development of an ulcer. While gastric hydrochloric acid and pepsin are capable of eroding mucosal tissue, ulcers do not always occur when acid/pepsin levels are elevated. Conversely, gastric ulcers can develop when acid secretion is normal. The degree of mucosal protection afforded by the secretion of mucus is a vital factor in the etiology of peptic ulcers. Other endogenous mucosal protectants, such as prostaglandin E, may likewise play a significant role in the development of an ulcer focus. The contribution of emotional or psychologic factors in ulcerogenesis is unknown, although anxiety and stress are strongly linked to ulcer development.

Peptic ulcers can be differentiated, based on location, into *gastric* and *duodenal* ulcers. *Gastric* ulcers usually occur in the lower fundal or antral region of the stomach and are linked to both excessive gastric hyperacidity *and* decreased tissue resistance. Most are located close to the pylorus. Gastric ulcers may remain asymptomatic for long periods or may manifest themselves as a gnawing, aching sensation or "hunger pangs." Episodes usually occur within 60 minutes after eating and are relieved by food or antacids. Gastric ulcers tend to be recurrent.

Duodenal ulcers are more common than gastric ulcers and most are located within the first 2 inches of the duodenum. Symptoms include a burning or aching feeling, "heartburn," cramping, and nausea. The distress occurs 45 minutes to 60 minutes after a meal, worsens during the day, and is often most intense between midnight and 2 AM. It is relieved by food, milk, antacids, and vomiting. Spontaneous exacerbations and remissions are common and appear to occur cyclically. Most people only require periodic management during periods of exacerbation.

Treatment of Peptic Ulcer

The aim in management of peptic ulcer disease is to relieve the pain and facilitate the healing of the lesion(s). These aims may be accomplished by decreasing the volume of secretion from the gastric glands, neutralizing the gastric acidity, and protecting the mucosa from the damaging effects of hydrochloric acid and pepsin. Pepsin is a proteolytic enzyme that is capable of digesting the mucosal lining of the stomach and duodenum, leading to the formation of a crater. This proteolytic activity of pepsin is optimal at a *p*H of 1 to 2 and is therefore increased in the presence of hydrochloric acid.

Several classes of drugs are now available for the management of peptic ulcer disease. The antacids, which are discussed below, have traditionally been employed to relieve the symptoms of ulcers and are effective in promoting healing when given in proper amounts. Anticholinergic drugs have long been given to reduce gastric secretions and while potentially useful in treating certain ulcer symptoms, they require the administration of large doses and are associated with a considerable degree of side-effects. (These drugs are discussed in Chap. 14.)

Newer agents that are proving highly effective in treating ulcer symptomatology are the histamine$_2$ receptor antagonists cimetidine, famotidine, and ranitidine, drugs that markedly reduce the secretion of gastric hydrochloric acid. (These H$_2$-antagonists are considered in detail in Chap. 18.) Gastroprotective agents that shield the mucosal surface from the damaging effects of acid and pepsin represent another new facet of ulcer management. One such agent is currently available (sucralfate) and is reviewed in this chapter. Other similar drugs are in various investigational stages, including a synthetic prostaglandin E analogue that exhibits both an acid-inhibitory and a cytoprotective action.

Antacid Therapy for Peptic Ulcer

The principal action of antacids in the treatment of peptic ulcers is to neutralize acidity, thus raising gastric *p*H. Increasing the *p*H results in progressive inhibition of the proteolytic activity of pepsin, thereby reducing its digestive action on the gastric mucosa. Consequently, antacids can reduce pain resulting from activation of mucosal nerve endings by excessive gastric acid as well as promote healing of damaged or ulcerated mucosa by protecting it from the destructive effects of pepsin.

The efficacy of antacids depends on many factors, most importantly their acid-neutralizing capacity (ANC), formulation, and dosage schedule. Among the various commercially available antacid preparations, there is nearly a 20-fold difference in acid-neutralizing capacity. Sodium bicarbonate and calcium carbonate possess the greatest neutralizing capacity, whereas aluminum phosphate and magnesium trisilicate are considerably weaker.

It is important to recognize, however, that the most potent preparation may not always be the most suitable in terms of potential toxicity (*e.g.*, diarrhea, constipation, hypercalcemia, systemic alkalosis), patient acceptance (*e.g.*, taste, consistency), sodium content (danger in cardiovascular conditions), or cost. For example, persons with conditions such as edema, hypertension, or congestive heart failure, which require low salt intake, should be given antacid preparations containing little or no sodium, such as Riopan Plus. Magnesium-containing antacids, on the other hand, may cause central nervous system (CNS) toxicity in patients with renal failure and may intensify chronic diarrhea, and thus should be avoided in these conditions. Antacids containing aluminum require cautious use in the presence of constipation or gastric outlet obstruction because they may further reduce gastric emptying. Preparations containing calcium carbonate or sodium bicarbonate are only indicated for short-term therapy, because their side-effects (e.g., systemic alkalosis, rebound hyperacidity, milk–alkali syndrome) are significantly enhanced during prolonged treatment.

Aluminum-containing antacids bind phosphate ions in the intestine, resulting in impaired absorption and accelerated elimination and the possible danger of hypophosphatemia. However, clinical advantage is taken of this property in the use of aluminum carbonate gel for prevention of phosphatic urinary stones or in the management of hyperphosphatemia associated with advanced renal failure.

Product formulation (suspension, tablet, powder) may also be a determining factor in the effectiveness and acceptance of antacids—liquid suspensions generally providing the best neutralizing action and greatest palatability. Dosage schedules should be based on the type and severity of the condition being treated; both the frequency and duration of therapy should be sufficient to provide maximum therapeutic benefit with minimal untoward reactions.

Antacid failure is frequently a result of poor selection, inadequate dosage, or improper administration, and can be eliminated in most cases by judicious choice of an agent appropriate for both the patient and the condition. Selection of an appropriate antacid regimen requires consideration of many factors, and persons should be cautioned against indiscriminate use of these widely available and easily obtainable products.

Antacids are usually administered as one of the many available combination products, inasmuch as these products generally provide good acid-neutralizing activity with a reduced incidence of side-effects when compared to the individual components themselves. A popular pairing of antacids is aluminum hydroxide and magnesium hydroxide, a mixture that significantly reduces the occurrence of the constipation and diarrhea frequently observed with aluminum (constipation) and magnesium (diarrhea) alone.

It is inevitable that comparisons are made between the effectiveness of antacid regimens and that of the histamine H_2-blockers in the treatment of gastric and duodenal ulcers (see Chap. 18). Although the efficacy of the H_2-blockers in relieving pain and promoting healing of duodenal ulcers is unquestioned, comparative studies with large-dose antacid regimens have demonstrated a nearly comparable level of effectiveness for the antacid products when used on a sufficiently frequent basis. Clinicians are prescribing both H_2-blockers and supplemental antacids, when necessary, and it appears as if such a combination provides, in most cases of gastric and duodenal ulcers, optimal therapeutic benefit with minimal untoward reactions. On the other hand, less serious gastric disorders such as heartburn, acid indigestion, and gastritis generally respond quite well to antacid therapy alone and do not require H_2-blockers unless the antacids do not provide sufficient relief.

Antacid drugs are discussed as a group, then listed individually in Table 42-1, in which the major uses and characteristics (including acid-neutralizing capacity [ANC], where established) of each drug are presented. Because most antacid preparations are combination products, the composition of the most commonly used combination products, including sodium content and ANC, is given in Table 42-2. Another antiulcer drug discussed in this chapter is sucralfate, a sulfated sucrose–aluminum hydroxide complex that appears to form a protective barrier over the ulcerated area. Finally, a review of simethicone, an antiflatulent drug used to relieve symptoms associated with excessive production of gas in the digestive tract, and charcoal, an adsorbent, are presented at the end of this chapter.

Antacids

Aluminum Carbonate, Aluminum Hydroxide, Aluminum Phosphate, Calcium Carbonate, Dihydroxyaluminum Sodium Carbonate, Magaldrate (Hydroxymagnesium Aluminate), Magnesium Hydroxide, Magnesium Oxide, Sodium Bicarbonate

MECHANISM AND ACTIONS

Antacids neutralize gastric acidity and usually elevate gastric and duodenal pH above 3 to 4; the proteolytic activity of pepsin on gastric mucosa is suppressed above pH 4 and totally abolished above pH 7 to 8. Acid neutralization also may increase lower esophageal sphincter tone. Antacids do not

(text continues on p. 844.)

Table 42-1
Antacids

Drug	Preparations	Sodium Content	Acid Neutralizing Capacity (mEq)	Usual Dosage Range	Clinical Considerations
aluminum carbonate gel, basic (Basaljel)	Suspension (equivalent to 400 mg aluminum hydroxide per 5 ml)	0.58 mg/ml	12	Antacid—2 capsules or tablets, 2 tsp of regular suspension or 1 tsp extra-strength suspension four to eight times/day Prevention of phosphate stones—2 capsules or tablets 1 h after meals and at bedtime or 1 tbsp suspension in water or juice 1 h after meals and at bedtime	Used as an antacid and for preventing development of urinary phosphate stones; exhibits strong phosphate binding capacity, increasing fecal and decreasing urinary phosphate excretion; periodic determinations of serum electrolytes, especially calcium and phosphate, should be performed; low-phosphate diet is recommended; excessive doses can lead to phosphate depletion (weakness, tremors, bone pain, demineralization); be alert for signs of urinary infection (fever, chills, dysuria); high fluid intake should be maintained
	Extra-strength suspension (equivalent to 1000 mg aluminum hydroxide per 5 ml)	4.6 mg/ml	22		
	Capsules and swallow tablets (equivalent to 500 mg of aluminum hydroxide)	2.8 mg/capsule	12		
		2.8 mg/tablet	13		
aluminum hydroxide gel (ALternaGEL, Alu-Cap, Alu-Tab, Amphojel, Dialume)	Suspension—320 mg/5 ml	less than 0.5 mg/ml	10	500–1800 mg three to six times/day between meals and at bedtime Hypophosphatemia in children—50–150 mg/kg/24 h in divided doses every 4 h–6 h	Antacid with moderate acid-neutralizing capacity; does not produce acid rebound or alkalosis; possesses phosphate-binding capacity although to a lesser degree than aluminum carbonate; constipation is a frequent side-effect; do not use for prolonged periods in patients with low serum phosphate or those on a low-sodium diet
	Concentrated suspension—600 mg/5 ml	less than 0.5 mg/ml	16		
	Capsules—475 mg, 500 mg	1 mg/capsule	10		
	Tablets—300 mg, 600 mg	300 mg–1.8 mg	8		
		600 mg–2.9 mg	16		
aluminum phosphate gel (Phosphal jel)	Suspension—233 mg/5 ml	1.4 mg/ml		15 ml–30 ml every 2 h between meals and at bedtime	No longer labeled for use as antacid; only used to reduce fecal excretion of phosphates.
calcium carbonate (Alka-Mints, Amitone, Chooz, Dicarbosil, Equilet, Mallamint, Tums)	Tablets—650 mg Chewable tablets—350 mg, 420 mg, 500 mg, 750 mg, 850 mg	Less than 2 mg/tablet	750-mg tab —15 500-mg tab —10 350-mg tab —7	0.5 g–1.5 g three to six times/day as needed	Very effective antacid, possessing high neutralizing capacity, rapid onset, and relatively prolonged duration of action; does not cause sys-

(continued)

Table 42-1 (continued)
Antacids

Drug	Preparations	Sodium Content	Acid Neutralizing Capacity (mEq)	Usual Dosage Range	Clinical Considerations
calcium carbonate (Alka-Mints, Amitone, Chooz, Dicarbosil, Equilet, Mallamint, Tums) *(continued)*					temic alkalosis, but is constipating and may elicit acid rebound and gastric hypersecretion; converted to calcium chloride by gastric acid, which may be absorbed in sufficient quantities to produce hypercalcemia with prolonged treatment; chronic use with foods high in vitamin D (*e.g.,* milk) may lead to milk–alkali syndrome (see under Side-Effects/Adverse Reactions). Contains 40% calcium. Use with caution in patient receiving thiazide diuretics, which may inhibit calcium excretion.
dihydroxy-aluminum sodium carbonate (Rolaids)	Chewable tablets—334 mg	53 mg/tablet	7–8	1 to 2 tablets three to six times/day as needed	Converted to aluminum hydroxide in the presence of gastric acid, releasing carbon dioxide; gives rapid but transient neutralizing effect; because of high sodium content, use with caution in sodium-restricted patients.
magaldrate (Lowsium, Riopan)	Suspension—540 mg/5 ml	less than 0.1 mg/5 ml	15	480 mg–1080 mg three to six times/day between meals and at bedtime	A chemical combination of magnesium and aluminum hydroxides equivalent to 28%–39% magnesium oxide and 17%–25% aluminum oxide; has somewhat lower neutralizing capacity than a physical mixture of the two ingredients; does not elicit acid rebound or systemic acidosis; has a low incidence of diarrhea and constipation, and very *(continued)*
	Tablets—480 mg	less than 0.1 mg/tablet or chewable tablet	13–14		
	Chewable tablets—480 mg				

Table 42-1 (continued)
Antacids

Drug	Preparations	Sodium Content	Acid Neutralizing Capacity (mEq)	Usual Dosage Range	Clinical Considerations
magaldrate (Lowsium, Riopan) (continued)					low sodium content; available with simethicone as Riopan Plus
magnesium hydroxide (Milk of Magnesia M.O.M.)	Tablets—325 mg Liquid—390 mg/5 ml	0.1 mg/5 ml	10–14	Antacid—5 ml–15 ml or 650 mg–1.3 g orally four times/day Cathartic: Adults—15 ml–30 ml Children—5 ml–30 ml	Used as an antacid in small doses or as a cathartic in slightly higher doses. Elicits prompt and sustained neutralization of gastric acid without marked acid rebound or systemic alkalosis. However, laxative action is commonly observed at higher doses; therefore drug is often combined with aluminum or calcium antacids. Also available as an emulsion containing mineral oil (Haley's MO). Laxative dose should be given at bedtime, followed by a full glass of water. (See Chap. 44.)
magnesium oxide (Mag-Ox 400, Maox, Par-Mag, Uro-Mag)	Tablets—400 mg, 420 mg Capsules—140 mg	NA	20–21	280 mg–1.5 g with water or milk four times/day	Slow-acting antacid with prolonged effects; high neutralizing capacity, but frequently elicits nau- (continued)

NA = Sodium content is not available.

appear to "coat" the mucosal barrier but can bind bile acids (especially the aluminum products), although the contribution of this latter action to the therapeutic effects of the drugs is unclear.

USES
1. Symptomatic treatment of GI symptoms associated with hyperacidity (*e.g.,* heartburn, acid indigestion)
2. Treatment of hyperacidity associated with gastritis, peptic ulcer, hiatal hernia, or esophagitis (facilitate healing in peptic ulcer but their effect in relieving pain is not substantiated)
3. Prophylaxis of GI bleeding or stress ulcers

4. Reduce phosphate absorption in hyperphosphatemia and chronic renal failure (investigational use for aluminum hydroxide and aluminum carbonate)

ADMINISTRATION AND DOSAGE
See Table 42-1.

FATE
Most preparations (except sodium bicarbonate) are not appreciably absorbed from the GI tract and are excreted largely in feces. Calcium and magnesium products can form chloride salts by reaction with

Table 42-1 (continued)
Antacids

Drug	Preparations	Sodium Content	Acid Neutralizing Capacity (mEq)	Usual Dosage Range	Clinical Considerations
magnesium oxide (Mag-Ox 400, Maox, Par-Mag, Uro-Mag) (continued)					sea and diarrhea; in large doses has been used as a cathartic; frequently used in powder form; available as light and heavy magnesium oxide; light is five times bulkier than heavy, but possesses greater neutralizing power due to larger surface area
sodium bicarbonate (Bell/ans, Soda Mint)	Tablets—325 mg, 520 mg, 650 mg	27%		0.3 g–2 g as needed one to four times/ day	Systemic, absorbable antacid, with a short duration of action; its use should be discouraged because it frequently elicits acid rebound, belching (due to liberated carbon dioxide), and gastric distention, and may result in systemic alkalosis; high sodium content precludes its use in patients with hypertension or cardiac or renal disease; large doses may cause phosphaturia

hydrochloric acid, which may be partly absorbed and require elimination by the kidneys. Food acts as a buffer to gastric acid for approximately 60 minutes, and the presence of food can prolong the action of antacids. Thus, antacids taken on an empty stomach have a duration of action of 30 minutes, whereas if they are taken 1 hour after meals, their duration is approximately 3 hours.

SIDE-EFFECTS/ADVERSE REACTIONS
The most frequently encountered side-effects with antacid products are diarrhea with magnesium-containing formulations and constipation with aluminum- and calcium-containing compounds. Other adverse reactions reported with the various antacid products are as follows:

Aluminum—Intestinal impaction, phosphate depletion (anorexia, weakness, impaired reflexes, depression, tremors, bone pain, osteomalacia)

Magnesium—Profound diarrhea, dehydration, hypermagnesemia (nausea, vomiting, impaired reflexes, hypotension, respiratory depression—high risk in patients with impaired renal function), bradyarrhythmias

Calcium carbonate—Rebound hyperacidity, milk–alkali syndrome (metabolic alkalosis, hypercalcemia, vomiting, confusion, headache, renal insufficiency), renal calculi, neurologic impairment, GI hemorrhage, fecal impaction

Sodium bicarbonate—Systemic alkalosis, sodium overload, milk–alkali syndrome, rebound hypersecretion

(text continues on p. 850.)

Table 42-2
Antacid Combinations

Brand Name	Dosage Form	Aluminum Hydroxide	Calcium Carbonate	Magnesium Oxide or Hydroxide
Algicon	Tablet	360 mg		
Alka-Seltzer	Tablet			
Alkets	Tablet		780 mg	65 mg
Almacone	Tablet	200 mg		200 mg
	Liquid	40 mg/ml		40 mg/ml
Almacone II	Liquid	80 mg/ml		80 mg/ml
Alma-Mag	Liquid	40 mg/ml		40 mg/ml
Aludrox	Tablet	233 mg		83 mg
	Liquid	61.4 mg/ml		20.6 mg/ml
Alumid	Liquid	45 mg/ml		40 mg/ml
Alumid Plus	Liquid	40 mg/ml		40 mg/ml
Bisodol	Tablet		194 mg	178 mg
	Powder			
Bromo Seltzer	Granules			
Camalox	Tablet	225 mg	250 mg	200 mg
	Liquid	45 mg/ml	50 mg/ml	40 mg/ml
Citro-carbonate	Effervescent powder			
Delcid	Liquid	120 mg/ml		133 mg/ml
Di-Gel	Tablet	282 mg (co-dried with magnesium carbonate)		85 mg
	Liquid	40 mg/ml		40 mg/ml
Di-Gel (Advanced Formula)	Tablet		280 mg	128 mg
ENO	Powder			
Gaviscon	Tablet	80 mg		
Gaviscon-2	Tablet	160 mg		
Gaviscon	Liquid	6.3 mg/ml		
Gelusil	Tablet	200 mg		200 mg
	Liquid	40 mg/ml		40 mg/ml

Simethicone	Other	Sodium Content	Acid Neutralizing Capacity (mEq)
	magnesium carbonate 320 mg	5 mg/tablet	17–18
	sodium bicarbonate 958 mg; citric acid 832 mg; potassium bicarbonate 312 mg	284 mg/tablet	10–11
	magnesium carbonate 130 mg		
20 mg			
4 mg/ml		0.15 mg/ml	10
6 mg/ml		0.3 mg/ml	20
5 mg/ml			
		1.4 mg/tablet	10
		0.46 mg/ml	12
4 mg/ml			
		0.3 mg/ml	
	sodium bicarbonate 129 mg/g; magnesium carbonate 95 mg/g	31 mg/g	15
	sodium bicarbonate 2.8 g/dose; citric acid 2.2 g/dose; acetaminophen 0.325 g/dose	0.75 g/dose	
		1 mg/tablet	18
		0.24 mg/ml	18
	sodium citrate 1.82 g and sodium bicarbonate 0.78 g per 3.9-g dose	700 mg/dose	
		3 mg/ml	42
25 mg		Less than 5 mg/tablet	9
4 mg/ml		1.0 mg/ml	11
20 mg			
	sodium tartrate 324 mg/g and sodium citrate 235 mg/g	104 mg/g	
	magnesium trisilicate 20 mg plus alginic acid and sodium bicarbonate	19 mg/tablet	0.5
	magnesium trisilicate 40 mg plus alginic acid and sodium bicarbonate	37 mg/tablet	
	magnesium carbonate 27.5 mg/ml	2.6 mg/ml	1
25 mg		0.8 mg/tablet	11
5 mg/ml		0.14 mg/ml	12

(continued)

Table 42-2 (continued)
Antacid Combinations

Brand Name	Dosage Form	Aluminum Hydroxide	Calcium Carbonate	Magnesium Oxide or Hydroxide
Gelusil-II	Tablet	400 mg		400 mg
	Liquid	80 mg/ml		80 mg/ml
Gelusil-M	Tablet	300 mg		200 mg
	Liquid	60 mg/ml		40 mg/ml
Glycate	Tablet		300 mg	
Kolantyl	Wafer	180 mg		170 mg
	Liquid	30 mg/ml		30 mg/ml
Lowsium Plus	Tablet			
	Liquid			
Maalox	Liquid	45 mg/ml		40 mg/ml
Maalox No. 1	Tablet	200 mg		200 mg
Maalox No. 2	Tablet	400 mg		400 mg
Maalox TC	Tablet	600 mg		300 mg
Maalox Plus	Tablet	200 mg		200 mg
	Liquid	45 mg/ml		40 mg/ml
Magnatril	Tablet	260 mg		130 mg
	Liquid	52 mg/ml		26 mg/ml
Marblen	Tablet		520 mg	
	Liquid		104 mg/ml	
Mylanta	Tablet	200 mg		200 mg
	Liquid	40 mg/ml		40 mg/ml
Mylanta II	Tablet	400 mg		400 mg
	Liquid	80 mg/ml		80 mg/ml
Remegel	Chewable squares			
Riopan Plus	Tablet			
	Liquid			
Rulox No. 1	Tablet	200 mg		200 mg
Rulox No. 2	Tablet	400 mg		400 mg
Rulox	Liquid	45 mg/ml		40 mg/ml
Silain-Gel	Liquid	56.4 mg/ml		57 mg/ml
Simeco	Liquid	75 mg/ml		60 mg/ml
TC	Liquid	120 mg/ml		60 mg/ml
Tempo	Tablet	133 mg	414 mg	81 mg
Titralac	Tablet		420 mg	
	Liquid		200 mg/ml	
Win-Gel	Tablet	180 mg		160 mg
	Liquid	36 mg/ml		32 mg/ml

Simethicone	Other	Sodium Content	Acid Neutralizing Capacity (mEq)
30 mg		2.1 mg/tablet	21
6 mg/ml		0.26 mg/ml	24
25 mg		1.3 mg/tablet	12–13
5 mg/ml		0.24 mg/ml	15
	glycine 150 mg		
		2 mg/tablet	10–11
		less than 1 mg/ml	10–11
20 mg	magaldrate 480 mg		
4 mg/ml	magaldrate 96 mg/ml		
		0.27 mg/ml	13–14
		0.7 mg/tablet	9–10
		1.4 mg/tablet	18
		0.5 mg/tablet	28
25 mg		0.8 mg/tablet	11–12
5 mg/ml		0.26 mg/ml	13–14
	magnesium trisilicate 455 mg		
	magnesium trisilicate 52 mg/ml		
	magnesium carbonate 400 mg	3.2 mg/tablet	18
	magnesium carbonate 80 mg/ml	0.6 mg/ml	18
20 mg		0.77 mg/tablet	11–12
4 mg/ml		0.14 mg/ml	12–13
40 mg		1.3 mg/tablet	23
8 mg/ml		0.23 mg/ml	25–26
	aluminum hydroxide/magnesium carbonate complex 476 mg	25 mg/square	13–14
20 mg	magaldrate 480 mg	0.1 mg/tablet	13–14
4 mg/ml	magaldrate 108 mg/ml	Less than 0.02 mg/ml	15
		0.16 mg/ml	12
5 mg/ml		0.96 mg/ml	15
6 mg/ml		2.4 mg/ml	22
		0.16 mg/ml	27–28
20 mg		2.5 mg/tablet	14
	glycine 150 mg	Less than 0.3 mg/tablet	7–8
	glycine 60 mg/ml	2.2 mg/ml	19
		2.5 mg/tablet	12
		0.5 mg/ml	11–12

CONTRAINDICATIONS AND PRECAUTIONS

Contraindications to the different antacid drugs depend on the individual formulations and are discussed under Clinical Considerations in Table 42-1. The sodium content of some products is considerable (see Tables 42-1 and 42-2), and formulations high in sodium should be avoided in patients with hypertension or congestive heart failure or persons on a low-sodium diet. Magnesium-containing antacids should be given *cautiously* to persons with renal insufficiency, and aluminum products must be used with caution in patients with gastric outlet obstruction, as they decrease smooth muscle contraction and delay gastric emptying. Absorbable antacids, such as sodium bicarbonate, can result in systemic alkalosis, especially if used in large amounts.

INTERACTIONS

■ WARNING
Due to the absorptive capacity of most antacids and their ability to alter gastric *p*H, other drugs should not be administered within 1 hour to 2 hours of antacid ingestion, if possible.

1. Antacids can impair the absorption of tetracyclines, anticholinergics, digoxin, digitoxin, phenothiazines, indomethacin, phenylbutazone, isoniazid, and possibly also phenytoin, oral anticoagulants, quinidine, oral iron products, propranolol, other antibiotics, barbiturates, and salicylates.
2. Systemic antacids can increase the excretion of acidic drugs, like salicylates or barbiturates, by raising the urinary *p*H.
3. Urinary excretion of basic drugs (*e.g.,* quinidine, theophylline, amphetamine) may be reduced by systemic antacids, resulting in increased toxicity.

■ Nursing Process

□ ASSESSMENT

□ Subjective Data
The patient who seeks medical treatment for peptic ulcer disease has probably been self-treating for weeks to months before seeking supervised care.

Consequently, the nurse needs to review the types of remedies used and the patient's perceptions of their value in relieving discomfort. Old habits are difficult to break; if they can be incorporated into the prescribed regimen, compliance may improve. Ask the patient to identify remedies used, when used, and to describe the relationship between self-dosing and pain, meals, drinking, or stressful situations. The patient with peptic ulcer disease might report using several remedies, especially before cocktails or a heavy meal or in anticipation of a stressful situation at home or at work. Milk is often used to "coat the stomach" if a meal is missed, other remedies are absent, or the patient intends to eat or drink something known to be aggravating. Such information can be used to illustrate the benefit of some remedies as well as the negative effects of others. Milk may actually increase acid secretion, and using multiple antacid products may decrease overall effectiveness.

Ask about eating habits such as the frequency of meals, including quantity and hours of the day. Late night eating and long periods between eating aggravate the pain in ulcer disease. Also ask about bowel habits and problems with diarrhea or constipation. Certain antacids cause diarrhea, while aluminum type antacids can result in constipation. Knowledge of the patient's bowel habits and tendency toward either of these conditions can help determine an appropriate antacid. In addition, find out if the patient has ever been told to restrict sodium intake before choosing an antacid because several brands are high in sodium content.

A drug history should also be obtained. Antacids can affect absorption of many drugs (see under Interactions), therefore, administration schedules may need alteration to ensure the effectiveness of all medications.

□ Objective Data
Laboratory data should include renal function, electrolyte studies, and a complete blood count, especially if bleeding is suspected. An upper GI series may also be done.

Physical assessment should include a cardiovascular assessment focusing on heart rate and blood pressure, both of which will fall if the patient is bleeding.

□ NURSING DIAGNOSES
Actual nursing diagnoses may include:
   Knowledge deficit related to action, dose, timing, and side-effects of the drug as well

as the interrelationship between diet and drug therapy

Alteration in comfort: epigastric pain

Potential nursing diagnoses may include:

Alteration in bowel function: diarrhea or constipation depending on type of antacid

Alteration in fluid volume: deficit or overload depending on the type of antacid used and the resultant electrolyte imbalance which may occur (see under Side-Effects/Adverse Reactions)

□ *PLAN*

The nursing care goals focus on helping the patient:

1. Learn to adhere to an administration schedule which maximizes drug benefit
2. Incorporate diet changes required by the disease process
3. Manage and minimize drug side-effects

□ *INTERVENTION*

In the acute care setting antacids may be given to prevent stress ulcers after major surgery or trauma or to a hospitalized patient with active peptic ulcer disease. Frequently, the drug must be given through a nasogastric tube. Prior to administration the nurse should ensure tube patency (see Chap. 8), administer the antacid, and flush the tube with at least 60 ml of water. If the tube is inadequately flushed the antacid will precipitate on the sides, making further drug administration impossible.

Appropriate administration is the key to successful treatment of peptic ulcers with antacids, and the dosage schedule should be incorporated into the patient's eating pattern for the day. Teaching should begin while the patient is hospitalized, and the patient should have the antacid at the bedside and keep a record of the doses taken throughout the day. Because foods act as a buffer to gastric acid for about 1 hour after ingestion, the antacid should always be taken 1 hour after meals. A dose should also be given at bedtime as most patients complain of pain at night, a time when the stomach may be completely empty. In addition, antacids may also be given 3 hours after meals to maintain acid neutralization. Therefore, a typical dosage schedule might be:

Breakfast   7–7:30 AM; antacid 8:30 AM, 11:30 AM

Lunch   12–12:30 PM; antacid 1:30 PM, 4:30 PM

Dinner   6–7 PM; antacid 8 PM, 11 PM

In the early stages of treatment the patient might also wish to take another dose through the night. If the meal schedule changes, then the antacid schedule should change and the patient must understand the rationale for the schedule so he can make appropriate adjustments. If the time between meals lengthens, encourage the patient to include a snack.

Another factor to consider in the administration schedule is the other medications a patient may take. Because antacids interact with so many drugs, advise the patient to plan to take other drugs 1 hour to 2 hours after taking the antacid. If a new drug from another provider is prescribed, the patient should inform him of the antacid therapy because several drugs are completely deactivated by this drug.

Antacids come in liquid, tablet, and capsule forms; the liquid is significantly more effective and should be recommended. However, because of convenience or distaste for liquids, tablets may be preferred. Encourage the patient to chew tablets well before swallowing. If liquids are used, the suspension should be thoroughly shaken before the dose is poured. Whatever formulation used, the drug should be followed by a small amount of water.

Eating habits can also affect antacid success. Smaller, more frequent meals may be better tolerated by this patient in the early stages of therapy and will result in less gastric acid secretion. Most patients can eat whatever they want as long as it doesn't cause pain, however, some physicians recommend abstinence from all caffeine-containing beverages (coffee and cola), alcohol, and hot, spicy foods. Such foods are known to increase gastric acidity and may diminish the effectiveness of the drug regimen. For patients taking calcium-based antacids, milk and other dairy products high in calcium (yogurt, cheese) may be restricted. The combination may increase the risk of hypercalcemia. Milk is thought to actually increase acid production.

The most common side-effects of antacids are constipation (with aluminum or calcium formulations) or diarrhea (with magnesium compounds). The patient must monitor changes in bowel function closely early in therapy and must report any changes. To offset these side-effects the drug formulation may be changed, an antidiarrheal agent or stool softener may be prescribed, or diet may be altered. For diarrhea, the addition of bananas, rice, applesauce, and tea may be effective (known as the BRAT regimen). Constipation may be relieved by increasing fluids and adding bulk and fiber foods to the diet.

The most significant side-effect of antacid therapy is electrolyte imbalance (see Side-Effects/Adverse Reactions for symptoms with specific drugs). Symptoms of disturbance may not occur for weeks, but each patient should know the warning signals for the drug he takes and what to do if they occur. In addition, follow-up care should always include electrolyte studies and any patient taking antacids for more than 2 months on a regular basis should also have renal function studies reevaluated.

□ EVALUATION

Outcome criteria on which to base the success of antacid therapy include patient reports of pain reduction or cessation, endoscopic examination indicating healing of ulcer and minimal or no side-effects from the drugs.

Sucralfate

(Carafate)

Sucralfate is a complex of sulfated sucrose and polyaluminum hydroxide used orally for the short-term treatment of duodenal ulcers. Because it is not absorbed from the GI tract, it is virtually free of systemic side-effects. It requires an acidic environment for optimal activity, so it should not be administered simultaneously with antacids or H_2-antagonists, because its effectiveness may be somewhat reduced.

MECHANISM AND ACTIONS

The precise antiulcer mechanism of action of sucralfate is not completely established. The drug exerts a local action in the GI tract and may form an ulcer-adherent complex with exudative material at the ulcer site, thus protecting the ulcerated area from further attack by acid, pepsin, and bile salts. It also appears to inhibit the activity of pepsin by approximately one-third. However, sucralfate does not neutralize gastric acid.

USES

1. Short-term treatment of duodenal ulcer (may be used up to 8 weeks at a time)
2. Unlabeled uses include treatment of gastric ulcers and prophylaxis of duodenal and gastric ulcers.

ADMINISTRATION AND DOSAGE

Sucralfate is available as 1-g tablets. The recommended adult dose is 1 g four times a day on an empty stomach at least 1 hour before or 2 hours after meals and at bedtime. Antacids may be used as needed for relief of pain but should not be taken within ½ hour of sucralfate. Therapy should be continued for 4 weeks to 8 weeks unless complete healing has been demonstrated by endoscopy.

FATE

Systemic absorption following oral administration is minimal (3%–5%). Most of a dose is eliminated in the feces.

SIDE-EFFECTS/ADVERSE REACTIONS

Adverse reactions are minimal, the most common complaint (2%–3%) being constipation. Other infrequently encountered side-effects include nausea, gastric upset, diarrhea, indigestion, dry mouth, rash, pruritus, sleepiness, and dizziness.

CONTRAINDICATIONS AND PRECAUTIONS

There are no absolute contraindications to sucralfate. Safety and efficacy in children have not been determined, and caution should be exercised in giving sucralfate to pregnant women or nursing mothers.

INTERACTIONS

1. Sucralfate may reduce GI absorption of tetracyclines, phenytoin, and cimetidine.
2. Sucralfate may interfere with the action of warfarin.

NURSING CONSIDERATIONS

Because the administration of sucralfate is best undertaken on an empty stomach, help the patient plan an administration schedule which allows enough time for this to occur. Antacids, which may also be prescribed, should not be given within ½ hour of sucralfate. This may further complicate planning a schedule. However, sucralfate will reduce pain as it begins to work so the patient may find less need for antacids as therapy progresses.

The main side-effect, constipation, may be managed by increasing fluids, bulk, and fiber foods in the diet. However, patients should be taught to carefully monitor their bowel patterns and seek help if dietary measures do not relieve the constipation.

Antiflatulents

Drugs used to reduce the symptoms resulting from excess production of gas in the GI tract are termed antiflatulents. Simethicone is a silicone derivative commonly found in combination with antacids (see Table 42-2), although it is available alone in tablet and liquid form. Charcoal is an adsorbent used as tablets or capsules for a variety of indications, including the relief of indigestion and bloating resulting from accumulation of intestinal gas.

Simethicone

(Gas-X, Mylicon, Phazyme, Silain)

Simethicone possesses a defoaming action which may help relieve flatulence by dispersing gas pockets trapped in the GI tract. It appears to alter the surface tension of gas bubbles, facilitating their coalescence. The gas may then be more easily expelled by belching or by flatus. Simethicone is used to relieve painful symptoms resulting from gas retention, such as associated with dyspepsia, spastic colon, diverticulitis, or postoperative atony. The drug is available as tablets (regular, chewable, enteric-coated), capsules, and drops. Recommended dosage is 40 mg to 125 mg four times a day after meals and at bedtime. If symptoms are not relieved within several days, a physician should be con-

sulted, as a more serious underlying condition may be present.

Charcoal

(Charcocaps)

Charcoal is an inert adsorbent that can adsorb toxins and gas onto the surface of its particles. It reduces the volume of intestinal gas and can provide temporary relief of indigestion, cramping, bloating, and flatulence. Other uses for charcoal are as an antidote in poisonings (see Appendix) and to prevent nonspecific pruritus associated with kidney dialysis treatment. The usual adult dosage to relieve intestinal gas is 520 mg to 975 mg after meals or at the onset of discomfort. Dosage may be repeated as needed to a maximum of 4 g/day. Charcoal is available as tablets (325 mg) or capsules (260 mg). Tablets should be chewed or dissolved in the mouth before swallowing. The drug should not be used for more than 3 days as it can adsorb nutrients, digestive enzymes, and other essential substances although conclusive evidence that charcoal alters the nutritional state of the individual is lacking.

CASE STUDY

George Panzer, age 32, is a corporate purchasing agent who handles multimillion dollar accounts. He was diagnosed with peptic ulcer disease 5 years ago when he complained of severe epigastric pain that was relieved by food. Initially, he was successfully treated with antacids, later with a course of cimetidine and antacids. He has been symptom-free for 18 months.

Today, Mr. Panzer, an admitted junk-food addict, complained of heartburn to his wife after he had a lunch of two fast-food hamburgers, french fries, cole slaw, and a large cola. He took 30 ml of Mylanta and lay down. About 3 hours later he awakened with abdominal cramping, slight epigastric pain, and had a bowel movement that seemed slightly darker than usual. He took 30 ml more Mylanta and a tablet of 300 mg cimetidine he had in the medicine cabinet and went back to bed.

At 2 AM, Mr. Panzer awoke, nauseated, and vomited bright red blood. His wife called the physician who advised bringing Mr. Panzer to the emergency room.

The physician admitted Mr. Panzer with a diagnosis of possible bleeding peptic ulcer. A nasogastric tube was inserted, and cold saline lavage was started. After three lavage treatments there was no further bleeding. An IV of 5D/NS was started and cimetidine 300 mg IVPB was ordered after 6 hours. Maalox 30 ml after 3 hours by nasogastric tube was also ordered.

Thirty-six hours later the nasogastric tube was removed. An endoscopic examination revealed a tiny duodenal perforation. Mr. Panzer was placed on a bland diet, Maalox 30 ml 1 hour and 4 hours after meals, HS and p.r.n. for pain. The IV was discontinued, and cimetidine 300 mg orally every 6 hours was started. The nurse was asked to make plans for the patient's discharge the following day.

Discussion Questions

1. During administration of Maalox via nasogastric tube, what measures should the nurse take to ensure the patient receives the full dose and the tube remains in the patient?
2. What data do the nurse need to help Mr. Panzer plan a home administration schedule of Maalox and cimetidine?
3. What does Mr. Panzer need to know to safely take both of these drugs? (See Chap. 18 for information on cimetidine.)
4. Mr. Panzer admits to frequent self-medication to relieve ulcer symptoms. Outline a basic teaching strategy with this in mind.

REVIEW QUESTIONS

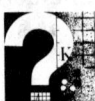

1. Describe the major secretory cells in the stomach.
2. What are the three phases of gastric secretion?
3. Briefly contrast the characteristics of gastric vs duodenal ulcers.
4. In what ways can the various antiulcer medications facilitate the healing of ulcers?
5. What is the effect of elevated gastric pH on pepsin activity?
6. What information is needed by the health-care team to determine the most appropriate antacid for a given patient and to plan an administration schedule?
7. What are the common side-effects of (a) aluminum-containing antacids, (b) magnesium-containing antacids, and (c) sodium bicarbonate?
8. What potential electrolyte disturbances occur with (a) aluminum-containing antacids, (b) magnesium-containing antacids, and (c) sodium bicarbonate? What symptoms should the patient learn to watch for?
9. Define ANC as it relates to antacids.
10. Should antacids be taken with food or on an empty stomach? Explain.
11. What should a patient know about the effectiveness of antacids in order to work out an at-home administration schedule?
12. What effects do systemic antacids (*e.g.*, sodium bicarbonate) have on renal excretion of basic drugs, such as quinidine or theophylline?
13. What are the *most common* ingredients in combination antacid products?
14. Briefly describe the action of sucralfate (Carafate). Why are side-effects minimal with this agent?
15. What type of drug is simethicone? What is its mechanism of action?

BIBLIOGRAPHY

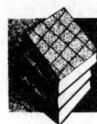

Garnett WR: Sucralfate—Alternative therapy for peptic ulcer disease. Clin Pharm 1:307, 1982

Halter F (ed): Antacids in the Eighties. Munich, Urban and Schwarzenberg, 1982

Ippoliti AF: Antacid therapy for duodenal and gastric ulcer: Experience in the United States. Scand J Gastroenterol 17(suppl 75):82, 1982

Lewis JH: Treatment of gastric ulcer: What is old and what is new? Arch Intern Med 143(2):204, 1983

Mar DD: Antacid therapy. Am J Nurs 81:788, 1981

Marks IN: Current therapy in peptic ulcer. Drugs 26(4):283, 1980

Morgan M: Control of intragastric pH and volume. Br J Anaesth 56:47, 1984

Peppercorn MA: Drug therapy of peptic ulcer disease. Compr Ther 9:47, 1983

Piper DW: Drugs for prevention of peptic ulcer recurrence. Drugs 26:439, 1983

Somerville KW, Langman MJ: Newer antisecretory agents for peptic ulcer. Drugs 25:315, 1983

Sucralfate for peptic ulcer—A reappraisal. Med Lett Drugs Ther 26:43, 1984

Todd B: Antiulcer preparations. Geriatric Nursing (March/April):122, 1983

Walan A: Antacids and anticholinergics in the treatment of duodenal ulcer. Clin Gastroenterol 13(2):473, 1984

Weinstein WW: Treating peptic ulcer: Are you using all your options? Mod Medicine 53(5):44, 1985

Wilson DE (ed): Symposium on peptic ulcer disease. Drug Therap 13(7):53, 1983

Digestants

43

Digestants are substances used as replacements for normally occurring digestive enzymes to facilitate the physiologic process of nutrient digestion in the gastrointestinal (GI) tract. Most substances ingested in the diet are structurally complex carbohydrates, fats, or proteins, which cannot be absorbed and utilized by the body in their natural states. During the process of digestion these complex organic constituents are chemically broken down into molecules that can be absorbed readily into body fluids. Specific digestive enzymes from the salivary glands, stomach, small intestine, and pancreas hydrolyze (1) complex carbohydrates into simple sugars; (2) fats into monoglycerides, fatty acids, and glycerol; and (3) proteins into amino acids.

The digestion of carbohydrates is initiated in the mouth by salivary amylase and is completed in the small intestine by pancreatic amylase and intestinal disaccharidases. Proteins are broken down by the combined actions of gastric, pancreatic, and intestinal proteolytic enzymes. Fats are emulsified by bile and are hydrolyzed mainly by pancreatic lipase. The major digestive enzymes are outlined in Table 43-1. The usefulness of most enzymes (e.g., amylase, lipase, protease, peptidase) as exogenous digestive aids is probably greatly overstated, inasmuch as symptoms of GI distress can rarely be attributed to an actual deficiency of endogenous digestive chemicals. Nevertheless, certain digestive substances such as hydrochloric acid, bile salts, and especially the pancreatic enzymes, pancreatin and pancrelipase, have proven valuable as replacement therapy in elderly or debilitated persons or in persons with conditions such as GI surgery, achlorhydria, chronic pancreatitis, or gastric carcinoma, in whom there exists a *definite lack* of one or more of these digestive substances. In such cases, however, the deficient chemicals must be replaced in sufficient amounts to restore digestive activity, and it should be recognized that many commercially available products contain amounts too small to provide the required quantity of digestant. Thus, empiric use of combination or "shotgun" digestive products has no place in rational pharmacotherapy. Moreover, the inclusion of anticholinergics, barbiturates, or antacids in these formulations merely increases the likelihood of untoward reactions without adding to the therapeutic benefit.

The digestive aids most frequently employed clinically may be grouped as follows:

1. Gastric acidifiers (e.g., glutamic acid hydrochloride)
2. Digestive enzymes (e.g., pepsin, pancreatin, pancrelipase)

3. Choleretics/hydrocholeretics (e.g., bile salts, dehydrochloric acid)

Gastric hydrochloric acid deficiency (achlorhydria) can occur in association with various pathologic conditions such as pernicious anemia or gastric carcinoma, as well as in the absence of observable disease. Dilute solutions (10%) of hydrochloric acid were previously used to aid digestion in patients with achlorhydria and to relieve complaints such as belching, nausea, and epigastric distress. Today, glutamic acid hydrochloride is used as a source of hydrochloric acid, because it is available in capsule and tablet form and offers a safer and more convenient mode of therapy. However, glutamic acid does not yield as much free acid as did hydrochloric acid.

Pepsin is a proteolytic enzyme activated by gastric acid, and thus is sometimes administered with glutamic acid to stimulate digestion. It is of doubtful benefit in most instances, because absolute lack of pepsin is relatively rare, except perhaps in gastric carcinoma and occasionally in pernicious anemia, and the acid deficiency is usually of far greater consequence. On the other hand, deficiency of pancreatic enzymes is a frequent occurrence, especially in cases of pancreatitis and duct obstruction, and of course following pancreatectomy. In these instances, replacement therapy with either pancreatin, a powdered concentrate of bovine or porcine pancreas containing amylase, lipase, and protease activity, or pancrelipase, a more concentrated mixture of pancreatic enzymes of porcine origin, is indicated.

Natural bile contains a series of organic acids secreted as sodium salts, which lower the surface tension of fat globules, breaking them into small droplets. Bile further aids fat digestion by stimulation of pancreatic secretions and activation of pancreatic lipase. Exogenous bile salts (e.g., ox bile extract) have occasionally been used as replacement therapy in patients with partial biliary obstruction or following removal of the gallbladder (cholecystectomy), but their effectiveness in this regard is subject to dispute. Bile salts also exhibit a choleretic action, that is, they stimulate the outflow of bile. Certain bile salts, especially the synthetic derivative dehydrochloric acid, markedly increase the output of a thin, watery bile, and are termed *hydrocholeretics.* Dehydrocholic acid is used to facilitate flushing and drainage of partially obstructed bile ducts, thereby minimizing infections and preventing biliary calculi from lodging in the duct.

In addition to the bile salts, a naturally occurring human bile acid, chenodeoxycholic acid, is available for treating selected patients with gall-

Table 43-1
Major Digestive Enzymes

Source	Enzyme	Activator	Substrate	Action
Salivary glands	Salivary amylase (ptyalin)		Starch, glygogen	Initiates digestion of carbohydrates, converting starch into dextrins and disaccharides
Gastric glands	Pepsin (pepsinogen*)	Hydrochloric acid	Proteins, polypeptides	Converts proteins and polypeptides into smaller polypeptides
Exocrine pancreas	Trypsin (trypsinogen*)	Enterokinase	Proteins, polypeptides	Converts proteins and polypeptides into smaller peptides and amino acids
	Chymotrypsin (chymotrypsinogen*)	Trypsin	Proteins, polypeptides	Converts proteins and polypeptides into smaller peptides and amino acids
	Carboxypeptidase (procarboxypeptidase*)	Trypsin	Polypeptides	Converts polypeptides into smaller peptides and amino acids
	Pancreatic amylase (amylopsin)	Chloride ion	Starch, glycogen, dextrins	Converts complex carbohydrates into disaccharides
	Pancreatic lipase (steapsin)	Emulsifying agents	Triglycerides	Converts fats into fatty acids and glycerol
	Ribonuclease		Ribonucleic acid	Converts ribonucleic acid into nucleotides
	Deoxyribonuclease		Deoxyribonucleic acid	Converts deoxyribonucleic acid into nucleotides
Intestinal mucosa	Enterokinase		Trypsinogen	Converts trypsinogen into the active proteolytic enzyme trypsin
	Aminopeptidase		Polypeptides	Converts polypeptides into smaller units
	Dipeptidase		Dipeptides	Completes protein digestion by converting dipeptides into absorbable amino acids
	Disaccharidase		Disaccharides	Converts disaccharides into absorbable monosaccharides
	Sucrase		Sucrose	Converts sucrose into glucose and fructose
	Lactase		Lactose	Converts lactose into glucose and galactose
	Maltase		Maltose	Converts maltose into glucose
	Intestinal lipase		Monoglycerides	Converts fats into fatty acids and glycerol
	Nuclease (nucleotidase)		Nucleotides	Converts nucleotides into nucleosides and phosphates

* Inactive form of the enzyme.

stones. Chenodeoxycholic acid (chenodiol) retards hepatic synthesis of cholesterol and cholic acid, possibly resulting in gradual dissolution of cholesterol gallstones in some patients. Another substance, monooctanoin, an esterified glycerol, may be used by continuous bile duct perfusion as a solubilizing agent for cholesterol-containing gallstones. Chenodeoxycholic acid and monooctanoin are also reviewed in this chapter.

It should be reemphasized that the majority of clinically available digestive products are multiple formulations containing digestive enzymes, bile extracts, or hydrochloric acid derivatives, frequently combined with anticholinergics, antiflatulents, antacids, or barbiturates. Not only is the content of these products often insufficient to provide the needed replacement in cases of deficiency states, but the digestants included in these formulations are frequently unnecessary and usually ineffective for the symptomatic treatment of simple digestive dysfunction, inasmuch as lack of endogenous digestive substances is only rarely the cause of GI distress.

A large number of combination products containing various proportions of digestive enzymes, bile extracts, hydrocholeretics, and acidifiers, as well as a myriad of other types of agents (e.g., anticholinergics, antacids, charcoal, barbiturates, simethicone), are available for symptomatic treatment of digestive disorders and for other GI dysfunctions. These combination products are rarely of clinical benefit, inasmuch as a GI disorder is seldom the result of an overall deficiency of several substances at one time. Specific deficiency states are more appropriately treated with the actual substance that is lacking rather than by employing a "shotgun" approach to therapy. Moreover, inclusion of many different drugs, especially barbiturates and anticholinergics, in a single preparation only serves to increase the likelihood of untoward reactions. Commercially available digestive combinations include Donnazyme, Entozyme, Festal, Festalan, and Kanulase.

Gastric Acidifier

Glutamic Acid Hydrochloride
(Acidulin)

Glutamic acid hydrochloride is a source of hydrochloric acid that aids digestion in conditions associated with reduced (hypoacidity) or absent (achlorhydria) gastric acid. It is used as a hydro-

chloride salt of glutamic acid in tablet or capsule form that releases hydrochloric acid in the stomach, thus minimizing the oral mucosal irritation and damage to dental enamel that was previously associated with administration of liquid forms of dilute hydrochloric acid.

MECHANISM AND ACTIONS
Glutamic acid hydrochloride provides a source of hydrochloric acid that lowers the pH of the stomach, thus facilitating conversion of pepsinogen to pepsin. The increased acidity provides optimal conditions for pepsin activity and may also stimulate pancreatic secretions and inhibit growth of putrefactive microorganisms in ingested food.

USES
1. Replacement therapy to assist digestion in hydrochloric acid deficiency states (e.g., gastritis, pernicious anemia, gastric carcinoma, primary achlorhydria, gastric resection)
2. Prevent growth of putrefactive microorganisms in ingested food

ADMINISTRATION AND DOSAGE
Glutamic acid is available as capsules containing 340 mg. A dose of 340 mg glutamic acid contains approximately 1.8 mEq of hydrochloric acid. The recommended dose is 1 to 3 capsules 3 times/day before meals.

SIDE-EFFECTS/ADVERSE REACTIONS
Side-effects are infrequent; gastric irritation may occur on occasion. Large doses may lead to systemic acidosis.

CONTRAINDICATIONS AND PRECAUTIONS
Glutamic acid is contraindicated in gastric hyperacidity or peptic ulcer. Capsules should not be permitted to become wet, since hydrochloric acid is released on contact with moisture.

Pancreatic Enzymes

Pancreatin
(Dizymes)

Pancrelipase
(Cotazym, Creon, Festal II, Ilozyme, Ku-Zyme-HP, Pancrease, Viokase)

Pancreatin and pancrelipase are pancreatic enzyme concentrates, derived from either a bovine or porcine source, containing lipase, protease, and amylase activity. Pancrelipase has greater lipase activity than pancreatin and may control steatorrhea in lower doses.

MECHANISM AND ACTIONS

Pancreatic enzyme preparations provide the enzymatic activity needed to help digest carbohydrates, fats, and proteins. Their effects are exerted primarily in the duodenum and upper jejunum. Although enteric coating of the tablets may reduce inactivation by gastric juices, the amount of enzymes delivered to the duodenum may also be reduced.

USES

1. Replacement therapy in pancreatic enzyme deficiency states, such as chronic pancreatitis or pancreatic insufficiency, steatorrhea of malabsorption syndrome, cystic fibrosis, postgastrectomy, or postpancreatectomy
2. Test for pancreatic function in pancreatic insufficiency due to chronic pancreatitis

ADMINISTRATION AND DOSAGE

Pancreatin

Pancreatin is available as tablets containing varying amounts of pancreatin, lipase, protease, and amylase. The recommended dosage is 1 to 3 tablets after meals (each milligram contains not less than 25 U amylase activity, 2 U lipase activity, and 25 U protease activity).

Pancrelipase

Pancrelipase is used as tablets, capsules, or powder containing varying amounts of lipase, protease, and amylase. Recommended dosage is 1 to 3 tablets or capsules or 0.7 g of powder before or during meals or snacks. (Each milligram contains not less than 100 U amylase activity, 24 U lipase activity, and 100 U amylase activity).

SIDE-EFFECTS/ADVERSE REACTIONS

Adverse effects noted with pancreatic enzymes include nausea, diarrhea, cramping, and GI distress. Very large doses have resulted in hyperuricemia and hyperuricosuria. Allergic reactions have been reported, especially if the finely powdered concentrates are inhaled or contact the skin.

CONTRAINDICATIONS AND PRECAUTIONS

Pancreatic enzymes are contraindicated in patients hypersensitive to beef or pork products. Safety of these products for use in pregnant or nursing mothers has not been established. Enteric-coated products should be swallowed whole and not chewed or crushed, as the enzymes may be released in the stomach and destroyed.

INTERACTIONS

1. Pancreatic enzymes may retard the absorption of oral iron.
2. Availability of pancreatin in the duodenum may be enhanced by histamine-2 antagonists (see Chap. 18).
3. Antacids containing magnesium hydroxide or calcium carbonate may reduce the effects of the enzymes.

NURSING CONSIDERATIONS

The main goal for the nurse is to teach the patient appropriate administration so he will get maximum benefit from the enzymes. The drugs should be taken during meals; enteric-coated capsules should be swallowed whole and powders or granules mixed with water or food. The patient should be encouraged to eat meals containing starch, protein, and fat to minimize indigestion.

One of the side-effects, diarrhea (refractive steatorrhea), occurs when fats have been incompletely digested. Antacids may be helpful in controlling this problem; however, they should not be given within 1 hour of the pancreatic enzymes.

Among certain religious groups, particularly the Moslem and Jewish faiths, ingestion of pork in any form is forbidden. Therefore, it is important the nurse establish the patient's religious affiliation prior to therapy initiation.

Bile Salts (Choleretics)

Ox Bile Extract

Ox Bile Extract With Iron
(Bilron)

MECHANISM AND ACTIONS

Bile is secreted by the liver, stored in the gallbladder, and released through the common bile duct into the duodenum, where it aids in the digestion and absorption of fats and fat-soluble vitamins. Bile salts are complex organic salts (e.g., sodium glycocholate and taurocholate) that function as detergents to lower the surface tension of fat globules, breaking them into smaller fat droplets that are more readily digested by lipases. In addition, bile salts, on absorption, can stimulate the outflow of bile from the liver (choleretic effect) and may exert a mild laxative action. Bile salts may aid digestion in conditions associated with a deficiency of natural bile, such as partial biliary obstruction or following cholecystectomy.

USES
1. Symptomatic treatment of uncomplicated constipation
2. Replacement therapy in bile deficiency states (e.g., partial biliary obstruction, cholecystectomy) (Note: Conclusive evidence for a beneficial effect of bile salts in bile deficiency states is lacking.)

ADMINISTRATION AND DOSAGE
Ox bile extract is used in the form of enteric-coated tablets (324 mg). Dosage is 1 or 2 tablets/day with meals, up to 6 tablets/day if necessary.

Ox bile extract with iron is available as capsules containing either 150 mg or 300 mg. The dose is 150 mg to 600 mg one to three times/day, during or after meals.

SIDE-EFFECTS/ADVERSE REACTIONS
Large doses may result in loose stools and abdominal cramping.

CONTRAINDICATIONS AND PRECAUTIONS
Bile salts are contraindicated in the presence of complete biliary obstruction or severe jaundice. Caution should be exercised in giving bile salts to patients with hepatic impairment or symptoms of appendicitis (abdominal pain, nausea, vomiting).

Hydrocholeretics

Dehydrocholic Acid
(Atrocholin, Cholan-DH, Decholin)

MECHANISM AND ACTIONS
Dehydrocholic acid, a semisynthetic derivative of cholic acid, is termed a hydrocholeretic agent because its principal pharmacologic action is to increase the volume of dilute, low-viscosity bile without markedly altering the amount of solid bile constituents. Hydrocholeretics are much less ef-

fective than natural bile salts or choleretics (such as ox bile extract) in emulsifying GI fats and in promoting fat absorption, and are therefore not used as a replacement for bile-deficiency states.

USES
1. Adjunctive treatment of chronic or recurrent biliary tract disorders (e.g., biliary dyskinesia, chronic partial biliary obstruction, noncalculous cholecystitis) to provide a flushing action
2. Assist prolonged drainage from biliary fistulas or T tubes
3. Postoperative management following cholecystectomy or surgery on the biliary tract to prevent occlusion or infection of the common bile duct (rarely used)
4. Temporary relief of constipation

ADMINISTRATION AND DOSAGE
Dehydrocholic acid is marketed as tablets containing 130 mg, 244 mg, or 250 mg. The usual dosage is 244 mg to 500 mg three times/day after meals. Concurrent administration of ox bile extract during dehydrocholic acid use may be necessary to ensure sufficient digestion and absorption of nutrients, especially in the presence of biliary fistula.

Dehydrocholic acid is also available in combination with homatropine (2.5 mg) plus phenobarbital (8 mg) as G.B.S. Recommended dose for this product is 1 to 2 tablets two to four times/day.

FATE
Dehydrocholic acid is absorbed from upper intestines, passes through the liver, and is recycled in the intestinal tract by the bile ducts before being excreted in the feces.

SIDE-EFFECTS/ADVERSE REACTIONS
Dehydrocholic acid is virtually free of side-effects; mild diarrhea may occur rarely.

CONTRAINDICATIONS AND PRECAUTIONS
Contraindications to use of dehydrocholic acid include jaundice, cholelithiasis, severe hepatitis, advanced cirrhosis, complete obstruction of the common or hepatic bile ducts or of the GI or urinary tracts, and in the presence of unexplained abdominal pain or vomiting. The drug should be given with caution to persons with prostatic hypertrophy, acute yellow atrophy of the liver, partial obstruction of the GI or urinary tracts, history of asthma or allergies, and in children under 6 years of age or in elderly persons.

Dehydrocholic acid should not be used as a diuretic or as an adjunct to diuretics.

Gallstone-Solubilizing Agents

Chenodeoxycholic Acid— Chenodiol
(Chenix)

When cholesterol is present in bile in concentrations that exceed the capacity of bile acids and lecithin to solubilize it, crystals can precipitate, and eventually coalesce into gallstones. Oral administration of chenodeoxycholic acid (chenodiol), a naturally occurring bile acid, can decrease the concentration of cholesterol in bile by inhibiting its hepatic synthesis. Thus, chronic treatment with chenodeoxycholic acid can, in some patients, result in gradual dissolution of noncalcified, radiolucent cholesterol gallstones. The drug is potentially hepatotoxic, and it is not appropriate therapy for all patients with gallstones. Therefore, careful selection and close monitoring of patients are essential to minimize complications and to offer the greatest chance for successful therapy.

MECHANISM AND ACTIONS
Chenodiol retards hepatic synthesis of cholesterol and cholic acid, resulting in a reduction in biliary cholesterol levels and gradual dissolution of radiolucent, noncalcified gallstones. The drug has *no* apparent effect on radiopaque, calcified gallstones or on bile pigment stones. The likelihood of stone dissolution decreases as the size and number of stones increase. Stones have recurred in approximately 50% of patients within 5 years. Retreatment with chenodiol has proved effective in dissolving newly reformed stones; however, the long-term toxic effects of repeated therapy remain to be established.

USES
1. Treatment of patients with radiolucent gallstones in well-opacified gallbladders, in whom surgery is not feasible due to age or presence of systemic disease (small, flotable stones are more likely to be dissolved than large, partially calcified stones)

ADMINISTRATION AND DOSAGE
Chenodiol is available as 250-mg tablets. The recommended dosage range is 13 mg/kg/day to 16 mg/kg/day in two divided doses, beginning with 250 mg twice a day for 2 weeks, then increasing by 250 mg/day each week until the recommended dosage is attained or the drug is no longer tolerated.

> ■ **WARNING**
> Doses *less than* 10 mg/kg/day are usually ineffective and may be associated with an *increased* risk of cholecystectomy.

FATE
Chenodiol is well absorbed orally but undergoes extensive first-pass hepatic clearance. It is conjugated by the liver and secreted in the bile. The drug is converted in the colon to lithocholic acid, which is excreted largely (80%) in the feces; the remainder is absorbed, and metabolized in the liver. In patients unable to form hepatic sulfate conjugates of lithocholic acid, liver toxicity can occur. Fecal bile acids are increased threefold to fourfold.

SIDE-EFFECTS/ADVERSE REACTIONS
Dose-related diarrhea is the most commonly seen side-effect during chenodiol therapy, occurring in between 30% and 50% of patients. Dose reduction may be required to reduce the incidence of diarrhea. Increased serum aminotransferase (SGPT) levels are noted in over 25% of persons receiving the drug; most are minor and transient and generally return to control levels within 6 months, even with continued administration. Less frequent adverse effects include nausea, vomiting, cramps, heartburn, dyspepsia, flatulence, anorexia, elevated serum cholesterol and low-density lipoprotein levels, and decreased white cell count.

CONTRAINDICATIONS AND PRECAUTIONS
Use of chenodiol is contraindicated in the presence of intrahepatic cholestasis, primary biliary cirrhosis, sclerosing cholangitis, radiopaque bile pigment stones, acute cholecystitis, gallstone pancreatitis, biliary GI fistula, and pregnancy. Chenodiol is a potential teratogen that should not be used in women who are or may become pregnant. Alert women to the possibility of fetal damage should they become pregnant while taking the drug.

Lithocholic acid, a metabolite of chenodeoxycholic acid formed in the colon, may be partially absorbed and subsequently transported to the liver, where it may be hepatotoxic in certain persons who fail to metabolize it adequately to a sulfated conjugate. Patients who develop chenodiol-induced elevations in serum aminotransferase may be more likely to form lithocholic acid.

INTERACTIONS
1. Bile acid sequestering agents (cholestyramine, colestipol) and aluminum-based antacids may reduce absorption of chenodeoxycholic acid.
2. Estrogens, oral contraceptives, clofibrate, and other lipid-lowering drugs may decrease the effectiveness of chenodeoxycholic acid by increasing biliary cholesterol secretion.

NURSING CONSIDERATIONS
Patients receiving this medication must be aware that the drug may not eliminate their gallstones and that the side-effects are dangerous. Patients must agree to regular follow-up to monitor potential problems. Liver enzymes (especially SGPT) and serum cholesterol should be drawn regularly at 3-month intervals. Oral cholecystogram or ultrasound should also be performed 6 months after therapy begins to evaluate drug effectiveness.

Monooctanoin
(Moctanin)

MECHANISM AND ACTIONS
Monooctanoin is a semisynthetic esterified glycerol that acts as a solubilizing agent for cholesterol gallstones in the biliary tract. Treatment with monooctanoin results in complete stone dissolution in about one third of patients, especially those with single stones. Another one third of patients show reduction in stone size, while approximately one-third of patients are not benefited.

USES
1. Solubilization of radiolucent gallstones in the biliary tract following cholecystectomy, when other means of removal are inappropriate

ADMINISTRATION AND DOSAGE
Monooctanoin is administered as a continuous perfusion through a catheter inserted into the common bile duct or through a T-tube or nasobiliary tube. The drug is perfused at a rate of 3 ml/hour to 5 ml/hour at a pressure of 10 cm of water to minimize biliary or GI irritation.

The solution should be warmed to between 60°F to 80°F before perfusion. Administration may be interrupted during meals. Perfusion may be continued for 7 days to 21 days; however, if after 10 days x-ray films or endoscopy indicates that stones are neither being reduced in size nor eliminated, the perfusion should be terminated.

FATE
Monooctanoin is readily hydrolyzed by pancreatic or other digestive lipases and the resultant fatty acids are either absorbed and metabolized or excreted intact.

SIDE-EFFECTS/ADVERSE REACTIONS
The most common adverse effects noted with monooctanoin are GI discomfort or pain (50%), nausea, vomiting, diarrhea, and fever. GI irritation appears to be closely related to rate of administration and perfusion pressure. Other untoward reactions seen during monooctanoin therapy are anorexia, indigestion, increased serum amylase, bile shock, leukopenia, pruritus, fatigue, chills, diaphoresis, headache, allergic reactions, metabolic acidosis, depression, and *rarely* acute pancreatitis, cholangitis, and hematemesis.

CONTRAINDICATIONS AND PRECAUTIONS
Monooctanoin is contraindicated in patients with jaundice, biliary tract infection or a history of recent jejunitis or duodenal ulcer. It must be used *cautiously* in pregnant or nursing women and in children.

NURSING CONSIDERATIONS
Therapy with monooctanoin may take up to 21 days and many patients will prefer to be at home during the treatment. The care goals for this patient may be to ensure the patient or a family member knows how to operate the infusion pump, how to check to make sure the appropriate amount of medication is being infused, and how to manage the side-effects that occur, especially since most of the GI side-effects are related to infusion rate and pressure.

The patient and family will need an instant referral source should questions arise. This may be formally established through the services of the hospital or equipment supplier or through a home health agency. Such support is vital during the therapy.

Side-effects are primarily related to GI irritation, which may be relieved by reducing the rate and pressure of the infusion. However, nutritional status should be routinely assessed since the side-effects may prevent the patient from eating anything substantial. Side-effects that are unremitting should be immediately reported to the physician.

REVIEW QUESTIONS

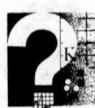

1. What is the function of (1) gastric hydrochloric acid, (2) pepsin, and (3) bile salts?
2. In what form is hydrochloric acid used clinically? In what conditions is its use contraindicated?
3. Pancreatic enzyme preparations contain what type of enzymatic activity? What are the most common side-effects associated with their use?
4. Briefly describe the action of bile salts in digestion.
5. What is the difference between a choleretic and a hydrocholeretic?
6. What are the principal indications for dehydrocholic acid?
7. In what way does chenodeoxycholic acid result in the dissolution of noncalcified cholesterol gallstones?
8. What are the major adverse reactions observed with chenodeoxycholic acid?
9. How must monooctanoin be administered to solubilize gallstones? What are its common side-effects?

BIBLIOGRAPHY

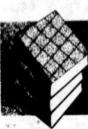

Hoffman AF: Gallstone dissolving drugs: New approach to an old disease. Drug Ther 12:57, 1982

Scherer P: New drugs of 1985 in theory and practice. Am J Nurs 86:407, 1986

Schoenfield LJ et al: Chenodiol (chenodeoxycholic acid) for dissolution of gallstones: The National Cooperative Gallstone Study. Ann Intern Med 95:257, 1981

Laxatives

44

A laxative is an agent that facilitates evacuation of the bowel. The valid indications for use of such drugs are few, and laxatives are frequently misused and abused by a large number of persons suffering from constipation, a condition characterized by a reduced frequency of fecal elimination.

A brief review of the mechanisms involved in stool formation will be presented prior to discussing the laxatives.

Stool Formation

Ingested foodstuffs are digested and nutrients are absorbed during transit through the gastrointestinal tract.

Muscular movements propel materials through the digestive tract, aid in the mechanical breakdown of food, promote mixing of luminal contents with mucus and digestive secretions, and facilitate absorption by renewing the absorptive surface.

The motor functions of the alimentary canal are of two basic types: mixing and propulsive. These movements are subject to intrinsic and extrinsic neural influences as well as to hormonal regulation.

The alimentary canal is extensively innervated by autonomic nerve fibers belonging to both the sympathetic and parasympathetic divisions. Autonomic elements are represented in the intrinsic nerve supply, the submucosal plexus (of Meissner), and more extensively in the myenteric plexus of Auerbach. The nerves maintain muscle tone and regulate the force and velocity of muscular contractions.

GI motility is generally increased by parasympathetic (vagal and sacral nerve) stimulation and inhibited by sympathetic activation. Only the sphincters respond in an opposite manner, being relaxed by parasympathetic stimulation and contracted by sympathetic stimulation.

During intestinal passage, fluid is continually absorbed, so that intestinal contents are gradually converted from a liquid state to a semisolid mass by the time they arrive at the transverse and descending colon. This mass is termed the feces and generally contains up to 75% water.

As the feces move into the rectum by a mass movement, that is, a strong peristaltic contraction occurring several times a day, the rectum is distended. Distention then activates a defecation reflex, in which the muscles of the descending and sigmoid colons contract, while the external and internal sphincters relax, and the fecal mass is expelled. However, the defecation reflex can be voluntarily inhibited, as the external anal sphincter is a skeletal muscle.

Constipation

The diagnosis of constipation is made difficult by the realization that there is a tremendous variation in the frequency of "normal" bowel movements, estimated to range from as low as three per week to as high as three per day. Given this inherent variability, constipation cannot be characterized strictly in terms of bowel frequency, but must be viewed in relation to previous bowel habits, presence of disease states, or to other drug therapy, diet, and other conditions.

Chronic simple constipation can be relieved frequently by proper diet, adequate fluid intake, and sufficient exercise, and does not usually require drug therapy. When indicated, laxative therapy should be short term (that is, 1 week to 2 weeks) and should be discontinued once bowel regularity has returned. Prolonged use of laxative drugs should be strongly discouraged because regular use of most laxatives can lead to dependence on the drug to achieve bowel movements rather than on the natural defecation reflex.

Persistent constipation is most often a result of improper diet, chronic disease states, prolonged laxative use, or a depressive state that can impair normal bowel function. As such, laxative drug therapy is usually ineffective and frequently harmful and should never be employed in lieu of determining and correcting the underlying cause of the dysfunction.

Acute constipation, on the other hand, is often amenable to drug therapy, especially in those individuals who do not have a history of bowel irregularities. Certain laxative products (e.g., stimulants, saline, or osmotics) are also indicated for rapid lower bowel evacuation in preparation for radiographic or endoscopic examination of the intestinal tract or in cases of poisoning with toxic substances.

There are a variety of laxative products available that function by a number of different mechanisms. The choice of a laxative product is dependent on many factors, including speed and intensity of evacuation desired (e.g., chronic, mild constipation versus preradiologic intestinal flushing), presence of other disease states (e.g., cardiac impairment, anorectal disorders), or need for sodium restriction.

A classification of laxatives based on their respective mechanisms of action is presented in the adjacent box. In general, bulk-producing agents

Classification of Laxatives

A. Bulk-Forming

methylcellulose
nondiastatic barley malt extract
polycarbophil
psyllium
Cellulose derivatives that swell in intestinal fluid, stimulating peristalsis by retaining water in the stool; considered the safest and most physiologic type of laxative; each dose should be taken with sufficient water to minimize risk of intestinal or esophageal obstruction; onset of action is usually 12 hours to 24 hours; major sites of action are small and large intestines.

B. Emollient/Fecal Softeners

docusate
Anionic surfactants, which increase the wetting efficiency of intestinal water, thus softening the fecal mass by facilitating mixture of aqueous and fatty substances; most useful in conditions in which straining is hazardous (e.g., heart disease, perianal disease, hypertension, hernia, rectal surgery); may require several days before an effect is seen; act primarily in the colon

C. Lubricants

mineral oil
Softens fecal matter by lubricating the intestinal mucosa, facilitating passage of the stool; may prevent absorption of fat-soluble vitamins and nutrients and delay gastric emptying; do not administer with meals; effects usually occur within 6 hours to 8 hours; site of action is the colon.

D. Saline/Osmotic

lactulose
magnesium citrate
magnesium hydroxide
magnesium sulfate
sodium biphosphate/sodium phosphate
Nonabsorbable cations (magnesium), anions (phosphate), or sugars (lactulose) that retain water in the intestinal lumen, thus mechanically stimulating peristalsis and altering stool consistency; may alter fluid and electrolyte balance; action is rapid (0.5 hours–2 hours) and should be used only for acute bowel evacuation, except for lactulose, which may be administered in chronic constipation; principal action is in small and large intestines.

E. Irritants/Stimulants

bisacodyl
cascara sagrada
castor oil
danthron
phenolphthalein
senna
Increase intestinal propulsion by either a direct irritant effect on the mucosa or an activation of sensory nerve endings in intestinal smooth muscle; may produce excessive catharsis, leading to fluid and electrolyte disturbances; prolonged use can result in habituation and laxative dependency; onset of action is generally 6 hours to 8 hours orally; major site of action is the colon

F. Miscellaneous

glycerin
Exerts a local irritant effect on colonic tissue and possesses a hyperosmolar action; onset of action is within ½ hour.

(e.g., methylcellulose) are considered the safest and most "physiologic" type of laxative and are the preferred agents for short-term treatment of most types of mild constipation. Emollients or fecal softeners are likewise relatively safe and are widely used in conditions in which hard or dry stools might prove painful or dangerous, such as after rectal or anal surgery, or in the presence of hemorrhoids and other conditions in which straining is undesirable (e.g., heart disease, hernias).

The various laxative products are discussed as a group, and are followed by a tabular listing of each product with specific comments. In addition, a polyethylene glycol-electrolyte solution used to cleanse the bowel prior to radiologic examination is reviewed at the end of the chapter. It should be noted that in addition to the products reviewed here, several of the bile salts (see Chap. 43) have also been employed for the symptomatic treatment of mild, uncomplicated constipation, although their efficacy has been questioned.

Laxatives

Bisacodyl, Cascara Sagrada, Castor Oil, Danthron, Docusate Calcium, Docusate Potassium, Docusate Sodium, Glycerin, Lactulose, Magnesium Citrate, Magnesium Hydroxide, Magnesium Sulfate, Methylcellulose, Mineral Oil, Nondiastatic Barley Malt, Phenolphthalein, Polycarbophil, Psyllium, Senna, Sodium Biphosphate, Sodium Phosphate

MECHANISM AND ACTIONS
The mechanisms of action of the various laxative drugs differ according to the type of drug and are outlined in the box entitled Classification of Laxatives.

USES
1. Short-term treatment of constipation
2. Evacuation of the lower intestinal tract in preparation for surgery or endoscopic or radiologic examination (especially saline and stimulant laxatives)
3. Removal of toxic substances from the lower intestinal tract
4. Prevention of straining where such action is painful or hazardous, as for example in anorectal disorders, hernia, cardiac disease (especially lubricants and fecal softeners)
5. Management of constipation associated with the irritable bowel syndrome (especially psyllium).

Note: Irritable bowel syndrome may be accompanied by diarrhea as well, in which case laxatives are inappropriate.

ADMINISTRATION AND DOSAGE
See Table 44-1.

FATE
Drugs are given either orally or rectally and the onset of action ranges from 10 minutes to 15 minutes with some suppositories or retention enemas; up to several days with some bulk-forming preparations (see box entitled Classification of Laxatives). Systemic absorption of most drugs is minimal in recommended amounts, and the drugs are excreted largely unchanged in the feces, although some drugs may be partially metabolized and excreted in the urine.

SIDE-EFFECTS/ADVERSE REACTIONS
The most frequently encountered side-effect during laxative therapy is excessive bowel activity, characterized by diarrhea, nausea, and cramping. Other adverse reactions include vomiting, perianal irritation, allergic reactions (e.g., facial swelling), electrolyte imbalances (especially with saline/osmotic drugs) resulting in weakness, dizziness, fainting, sweating and palpitations, and esophageal, intestinal or rectal obstruction (particularly with bulk laxatives). Chronic use of laxative products can lead to laxative dependence. Oral ingestion and subsequent aspiration of mineral oil can result in lipid pneumonitis, especially if the patient is reclining. Use of cascara, senna, or phenolphthalein may cause a yellow-brown discoloration of urine.

CONTRAINDICATIONS AND PRECAUTIONS
The use of laxatives in general is contraindicated in the presence of abdominal pain, nausea, vomiting, or other signs of acute appendicitis. Laxatives are also contraindicated in patients with diverticulitis, colitis, or regional enteritis; acute surgical abdo-

(Text continues on p. 876.)

Table 44-1
Laxatives

Drug	Preparations	Usual Dosage Range	Clinical Considerations
Bulk Forming			
methylcellulose (Citrucel, Cologel)	Liquid—450 mg/5 ml Powder—2 g/tbsp	Adults—5 ml to 20 ml three times a day or 1 tbsp of powder in 8 oz of water one to three times a day Children—1 tsp in 4 oz water 3 to 4 times a day	Used orally for constipation; also available in ophthalmic drops for relief of dry, irritated eyes and as an ocular lubricant for artificial eyes and contact lenses; oral doses should be taken with one or more glasses of water for each dose, and additional fluids are indicated throughout the day to prevent fecal impaction; sodium carboxymethylcellulose is available in capsule form with dioctyl sodium sulfosuccinate (Disoplex)
nondiastatic barley malt (Maltsupex)	Tablets—750 mg Liquid—16 g/tbsp Powder—16 g/tbsp	Tablets: Adults only—4 tablets with meals and at bedtime four times/day with liquid Powder/liquid: Adult—2 tbsp twice a day for 3 to 4 days; then 1 tbsp to 2 tbsp at bedtime Children—1 tbsp to 2 tbsp in milk one to two times a day Infants—½ tbsp to 1 tbsp in day's formula or 1 tsp to 2 tsp one to two times a day	Useful in treating functional constipation in infants and children, as well as in adults, including those with laxative dependence; also may provide relief from itching in pruritus ani; use with caution in diabetics, because preparations contain 14 g carbohydrates per tbsp and 0.6 g per tablet; mixes more easily with cold liquids when first stirred with a little hot water; available in combination with powdered psyllium seed (Syllamalt)
polycarbophil calcium (Equilactin, Fiber-Con, Mitrolan)	Chewable tablets—(equivalent to 500 mg polycarbophil)	Adults—1 g four times a day Children (6 yr–12 yr)—500 mg 1 to 3 times a day Children (3 yr–6 yr)—500 mg 1 to 2 times a day	A hydrophilic agent used for treating both diarrhea and constipation; claimed to restore a more normal moisture level and to provide bulk in the GI tract; as a bulk laxative, retains free water in the lumen of the intestine; a full glass of water or other liquid should be taken with each dose; discontinue use after 1 week if desired effects are not noted; also used for controlling simple diarrhea (see Chap. 45)

(continued)

Table 44-1 (continued)
Laxatives

Drug	Preparations	Usual Dosage Range	Clinical Considerations
Bulk Forming(continued)			
psyllium (Effersyllium, Konsyl, Metamucil, Mucilose, Perdiem, Serutan, and various other manufacturers)	Powder Granules Flakes Chewable tablets containing various amounts of psyllium hemicellulose, psyllium hydrophillic muciloid, or psyllium seed husk powder	1 or 2 rounded teaspoons, or 1 packet of powder in a glass of liquid one to three times a day (check package instructions for individual dosage recommendations)	Natural products derived from the blond psyllium seed (*Plantago ovata*); available in several dosage forms, many containing dextrose as a dispersing agent; contact with water in GI tract produces a bland, nonirritating bulk that aids peristalsis; sodium content is negligible, except in effervescent mixes containing sodium bicarbonate; drug should be taken with adequate water to prevent esophageal, gastric, intestinal, or rectal obstruction; each dose should be followed by a second full glass of water; do not attempt to swallow dry; available in combination with malt soup extract (Syllamalt)
Emollient/Fecal Softeners			
docusate calcium-dioctyl calcium sulfosuccinate (DC 240, Sulfolax, Surfak, Pro-Cal-Sof)	Capsules—50 mg, 240 mg	Adults—240 mg/day Children—50 mg to 150 mg/day	Similar in action to docusate sodium but does not contain sodium, which may be hazardous in patients with hypertension, congestive heart failure, edema, impaired renal function, or in persons on sodium-restricted diets; do not use in combination with mineral oil because drug may enhance systemic absorption of the oil. (See docusate sodium.) Combined with phenolphthalein as Doxidan capsules
docusate sodium-dioctyl sodium sulfosuccinate (Colace, Doxinate, DSS, Modane Soft, Regutol, and various other manufacturers)	Capsules—50 mg, 60 mg, 100 mg, 240 mg, 250 mg, 300 mg Tablets—50 mg, 100 mg Solution—50 mg/ml Syrup—50 mg/15 ml, 60 mg/15 ml Liquid—150 mg/15 ml	Adults—50 mg to 500 mg a day Children (6 yr–12 yr)—40 mg to 120 mg a day Children (3 yr–6 yr)—20 mg to 60 mg a day Larger doses may be given initially, then adjusted to optimal response	A surface-wetting agent that increases the wetting efficiency of intestinal water, thus facilitating the mixing of aqueous and fatty substances to soften the fecal mass for easier passage; effect on stools is apparent 1 day to 3 days

(continued)

Table 44-1 (continued)
Laxatives

Drug	Preparations	Usual Dosage Range	Clinical Considerations
Emollient/Fecal Softeners (continued)			
docusate sodium-dioctyl sodium sulfosuccinate (Colace, Doxinate, DSS, Modane Soft, Regutol, and various other manufacturers) (continued)			after first dose; does not exert a laxative action itself but is mainly used as adjunctive treatment in constipation associated with hard, dry stools or in patients who should avoid straining (e.g., with cardiac disease, hernia, anorectal disorders); combined with casanthranol (e.g., Peri-Colace), senna concentrate (e.g., Senokot S), phenophthalein (e.g., Correctol, Feen-a-Mint Pills), sodium carboxymethylcellulose (e.g., Disoplex), and various other laxatives; should not be used regularly by patients who must restrict sodium intake; may increase systemic absorption of mineral oil if given in combination
docusate potassium-dioctyl potassium sulfosuccinate (Dialose, Diocto-K, DSMC Plus, Kasof)	Capsules—100 mg, 240 mg	Adults—100 mg to 300 mg/day with a full glass of water Children (over 6)—100 mg at bedtime	See docusate sodium; may be used where sodium restriction is necessary; available in enema form with benzocaine and soft soap (Therevac Plus) and in capsules combined with casanthranol (Dialose Plus)
Lubricants			
Mineral oil (Agoral Plain, Fleet Mineral Oil Enema, Kondremul Plain, Milkinol, Neo-Cultol, Zymenol)	Liquid Jelly Suspension Emulsion Enema	Oral: Adults—15 ml to 30 ml at bedtime Children—5 ml to 20 ml at bedtime Rectal: Adults—60 ml to 120 ml Children—30 ml to 60 ml	Useful to maintain soft stools to avoid straining; coats fecal contents, preventing colonic absorption of water; probably not as effective or safe as emollients; may interfere with absorption of fat-soluble vitamins and nutrients; therefore, administer on an empty stomach; do not use with emollients; enema may avoid interference with nutrient absorption, but oil seepage from rectum can stain clothing. Use

(continued)

Table 44-1 (continued)
Laxatives

Drug	Preparations	Usual Dosage Range	Clinical Considerations
Lubricants (continued)			
Mineral oil (Agoral Plain, Fleet Mineral Oil Enema, Kondremul Plain, Milkinol, Neo-Cultol, Zymenol) (continued)			cautiously in the very old or debilitated or very young (under 2 yr) because danger of aspiration and possible development of lipid pneumonia is increased; emulsified preparations mask the objectionable consistency of plain oil and may be slightly more effective, but tend to increase systemic absorption of oil and are significantly more expensive; avoid prolonged or excessive use; available in combination with docusate sodium (Liqui-Doss), phenolphthalein (Agoral), cascara extract (Kondremul with Cascara), and magnesium hydroxide (Haley's M-O)
Saline/Osmotic			
lactulose (Cephulac, Chronulac)	Syrup—10 g/15 ml with several other sugars	Laxative (Chronulac)—15 ml to 30 ml/day to a maximum of 60 ml/day Portal-systemic encephalopathy (Cephulac)—30 ml to 45 ml three to four times a day May also be given to comatose patient by means of retention edema as 300 ml in 700 ml of water or saline for acute hepatic coma (see box entitled Suggested Technique for Administering Lactulose by Means of Retention Irrigation [Enema]). Dosage is adjusted to minimize diarrhea and may be repeated every 4 h–6 h	A complex sugar that is not hydrolyzed in the GI tract, but enters the colon unchanged, where it is broken down primarily to lactic acid by colonic bacteria; this elevates the osmotic pressure, increasing stool water content and softening the fecal matter; may require 24 h–48 h to produce a bowel movement; use cautiously in pregnant or nursing women, in elderly or debilitated patients, and in diabetics; initial doses may produce flatulence and cramping; may be mixed with fruit juice or milk to improve palatability; reduces blood ammonia levels by 25% to 50% and is also used for prevention and treatment of portal-systemic encepha- *(continued)*

Table 44-1 (continued)
Laxatives

Drug	Preparations	Usual Dosage Range	Clinical Considerations
Saline/Osmotic (continued)			
lactulose (Cephulac, Chronulac) (continued)			lopathy, including the stages of hepatic precoma and coma; may be administered chronically for this indication, and dosage is usually adjusted to produce two to three soft stools a day
magnesium citrate (Citrate of Magnesia, Citroma, Citro-Nesia)	Liquid	Adult—200 ml to 250 ml (one glassful) at bedtime Children—One-half glassful at bedtime	Chilling liquid improves the taste; do not use in patients with renal impairment; observe for signs of magnesium toxicity (thirst, drowsiness, dizziness); component of several evacuation kits (Evac-Q-Kwik, Tridrate Bowel Evacuation Kit)
magnesium hydroxide (Milk of Magnesia, M.O.M.)	Liquid—78 mg/ml Concentrated liquid—233 mg/ml Tablets—325 mg	Adults—15 ml to 30 ml of regular liquid or 10 ml to 20 ml of concentrated liquid at bedtime Children—One-quarter to one-half adult dose of regular liquid	Recommended for short-term use only because accumulation of magnesium ions can result in serious toxicity (CNS or neuromuscular depression, fluid and electrolyte imbalance); tablets are less effective than liquid as a laxative; concentrated liquid (233 mg/ml) is lemon flavored to improve palatability; do not use in patients with renal impairment; also used as an antacid (see Chap. 42); available in emulsion form containing mineral oil (Haley's M-O)
magnesium sulfate (Epsom Salt)	Granules	Adults—10 g to 15 g in a glass of water or fruit juice Children—5 g to 10 g in a glass of water	Administer in a flavored vehicle if necessary to mask the salty taste; effects are noted within several hours; infrequently used laxative
sodium phosphate and sodium biphosphate (Fleet Enema, Phospho-Soda)	Solution—1.8 g sodium phosphate and 4.8 g sodium biphosphate per 10 ml Enema—7 g sodium phosphate and 19 g sodium biphosphate per 118-ml dose	Oral: 20 ml to 30 ml in one-half glass of water (Children —5 ml–15 ml) Rectal: Adults—118 ml Children—60 ml	Indicated only for acute evacuation of the bowel (*e.g.*, prior to rectal or bowel examinations); high sodium content (4.4 g/dose); available in packaged forms with bisacodyl tablets, suppositories, or enema (Fleet Barium Enema Prep Kits)

(continued)

Table 44-1 (continued)
Laxatives

Drug	Preparations	Usual Dosage Range	Clinical Considerations
Stimulants			
bisacodyl (Bisco-Lax, Daco-dyl, Deficol, Dulcolax, Fleet Bisacodyl, Theralax)	Tablets—5 mg Suppositories—10 mg Enema—10 mg/30 ml	Oral: Adults—10 mg to 15 mg Children—5 mg to 10 mg Rectal (suppository): Adults— 10 mg following each bowel movement Children—5 mg Enema: 1 container (37.5 ml)	Increases peristalsis, probably by a direct effect on sensory nerve endings in colonic mucosa; used to relieve constipation and to evacuate the bowel before examination; onset of action is 6 h–10 h orally and 15 min–60 min after insertion of suppository; tablets should not be crushed or chewed, and milk or antacids should not be consumed within 1 h of the drug because they may prematurely dissolve the enteric coating on the tablet; rectal burning and itching may follow use of suppositories; no untoward systemic effects have been observed with either oral or rectal use; habituation can occur, with gradual loss of effectiveness
bisacodyl tannex (Clyso-drast)	Powder packets—1.5 mg bisacodyl and 2.5 g tannic acid per packet	Cleansing enema—2.5 g in 1 L warm water Barium enema—2.5 g to 5 g in 1 L barium suspension (maximum four packets in 72 h)	A nonabsorbable complex of bisacodyl and tannic acid used as a colonic evacuant; tannic acid is claimed to reduce intestinal secretions and, when used with barium suspension, to improve the adherence of barium to intestinal walls; contraindicated in pregnant women and in children under 10 years; tannic acid may be hepatotoxic if sufficient quantities are absorbed; use cautiously where multiple enemas are being administered and in elderly or debilitated patients
cascara sagrada	Tablets—325 mg Aromatic fluid extract	1 to 2 tablets, or 5 ml aromatic fluid extract at bedtime	Direct chemical irritant that increases propulsive movements in the colon; onset of action is 6–10 h; urine may be colored reddish to yellow brown, and rectal mucosa may become discolored; prolonged use should be

(continued)

Table 44-1 (continued)
Laxatives

Drug	Preparations	Usual Dosage Range	Clinical Considerations
Stimulants (continued)			
cascara sagrada (continued)			avoided because habituation can result; available with phenolphthalein (Caroid Laxative Tablets) or aloe (Nature's Remedy)
castor oil (Alphamul, Emulsoil, Fleet Castor Oil, Kellogg's Castor Oil, Neoloid, Purge)	Liquid or emulsion in various strengths	Adults—15 ml to 60 ml Children (over 2 yr)—5 ml to 15 ml Children (under 2 yr)—1 ml to 5 ml (depending on strength of emulsion)	Natural product that is broken down in small intestine to glycerol and ricinoleic acid, a local irritant; stimulates intestinal activity, resulting in production of liquid stools; primarily used for prompt evacuation of bowel before radiologic examination or in cases of poisoning; onset is 2 h–6 h; do not use in pregnant women or to treat infestation with fat-soluble vermifuge, because systemic absorption may be increased
danthron	Tablets—75 mg	75 mg to 150 mg with, or 1 h after, the evening meal	Synthetic irritant laxative that stimulates peristalsis in the large intestine; onset of action is approximately 6 h–10 h; administer in the evening for morning evacuation; do not use in nursing mothers (drug is excreted in breast milk); pink to brown discoloration of urine may occur; prolonged use may discolor rectal mucosa and produce liver damage
phenolphthalein (Alophen, Espotabs, Ex-Lax, Feen-A-Mint, Modane, and various other manufacturers)	Tablets—60 mg, 90 mg, 130 mg Chewable tablets—60 mg, 80 mg, 90 mg, 97.2 mg Wafers—64.8 mg Liquid—60 mg/5 ml, 65 mg/15 ml	60 mg to 194 mg at bedtime	Stimulant laxative similar to bisacodyl in most respects; onset of action is 6 h–8 h; bile must be present for drug to be absorbed; may color urine red to yellow-brown; effects may be prolonged for several days due to enterohepatic circulation; allergic skin reactions can occur; drug should be discontinued at first sign of rash; some preparations are fruit or chocolate flavored; keep out of reach

(continued)

Table 44-1 (continued)
Laxatives

Drug	Preparations	Usual Dosage Range	Clinical Considerations
Stimulants (continued)			
phenolphthalein (Alophen, Espotabs, Ex-Lax, Feen-A-Mint, Modane, and various other manufacturers) (continued)			of children because serious toxicity can result if large quantities are consumed; available in combination with docusate sodium (e.g., Colax, Correctol, Disolan, Ex-Lax Extra Gentle), docusate calcium (e.g., Doxidan), mineral oil (e.g., Agoral, Kondremul w/Phenolphthalein), and cascara (e.g., Caroid Laxative Tablets)
senna concentrate (Senexon, Senokot, Senolax) senna equivalent (Black Draught) senna extract (Senokot, x-Prep)	Tablets—187 mg, 217 mg Granules—326 mg/tsp Suppositories—652 mg Tablets—600 mg Granules—1.65 g/0.5 tsp Syrup—44 mg/ml Liquid—75 ml single dose bottle	Constipation: Adults—2 tablets, 1 tsp granules, or 1 suppository at bedtime Children—One-half adult dose Adults—2 tablets or ¼ tsp to ½ tsp granules with water Constipation: Adults—2 tablets or 5 ml to 15 ml syrup at bedtime Children—1.25 ml to 10 ml syrup at bedtime depending on age and weight Preradiographic bowel evacuation—75 ml taken between 2 PM and 4 PM on day before examination	Natural product prepared from species of *Cassia*, having a similar but more potent laxative action than cascara; concentrate may provide a more uniform effect than other preparations, with less colic; onset of action is usually 6 h–12 h, but may require 24 h in some cases; may impart a yellow brown to red color to the urine or feces
Hyperosmolar			
glycerin (Fleet Babylax, Sani-Supp)	Suppositories Liquid (4 ml/applicator)	1 suppository or 4 ml of liquid inserted high into the rectum	Produces dehydration of exposed mucosal tissue, leading to irritation and subsequent evacuation; laxative effect occurs within 25 min–30 min

men, fecal impaction, intestinal obstruction or perforation, acute hepatitis, or late pregnancy.

In addition, use of magnesium or potassium salts is contraindicated in patients with renal dysfunction, use of sodium salts is contraindicated in patients requiring sodium restriction, and use of emollients and mineral oil together is contraindicated.

Castor oil should not be used as a cathartic in treating infestations with fat-soluble worms because increased toxicity can occur as a result of increased absorption of the worms. Bisacodyl tannex should not be given in the presence of ulcerative lesions of the colon.

Laxatives must be given with *caution* to persons with rectal bleeding, young children (especially stimulants), or pregnant women (especially castor oil, mineral oil stimulants, or saline cathartics). Bulk-forming laxatives should be given with a large glass of water to minimize the likelihood of intestinal impaction; they should never be swallowed as dry powder.

INTERACTIONS

1. Systemic absorption of mineral oil or danthron can be enhanced by emollient (*i.e.*, fecal softening) laxatives.
2. Prolonged use of mineral oil may impair the GI absorption of fat-soluble vitamins (A, D, E, K) or nutrients.
3. Laxatives (particularly bulk-forming) may decrease absorption of other drugs present in the GI tract, either by chemically combining with them or by hastening their passage through the intestinal tract.
4. Antacids, other alkaline substances, or histamine H_2 antagonists may prematurely dissolve the enteric coating on bisacodyl tablets, decreasing the laxative action, and leading to gastric or duodenal stimulation.

■ Nursing Process

□ ASSESSMENT

Before administering laxatives, the nurse needs to determine if the patient has a history of constipation or if this is a new development. It is also important to learn about the person's dietary habits, fluid intake, activity level, drug history, and if the patient has had previous surgery for hemorrhoids, anal repair, or episiotomy, as all of these may affect bowel regularity. These parameters are relevant whether the individual is a confused elderly woman in a nursing home or a young man recovering from surgery because they will help determine an appropriate overall strategy.

The nurse needs to know why the patient thinks he's constipated. If a person is accustomed to having a bowel movement every day, he may think he's constipated even if he misses only 1 day. Hospitalized patients may worry about this without realizing that such experiences as remaining NPO for a period of time, having a cleansing enema, or having only liquids or low-residue foods for several days may significantly alter the bowel pattern without actually causing constipation. Therefore it is important to discuss these changes before seeking an order for a laxative.

□ NURSING DIAGNOSES

Actual nursing diagnoses for the patient receiving laxatives may include:

Knowledge deficit related to the action, dose, correct administration, and side-effects of the drug as well as dietary considerations

Anxiety related to the ability of the drug to relieve constipation or related to concern over the ability to control the defecation reflex once the drug has begun to take effect

Potential nursing diagnoses may include:

Alteration in bowel function: constipation and impaction related to misuse of bulk laxatives

Alteration in bowel function: diarrhea related to strength or dose of the drug used

Anxiety related to changes in bowel routine as a result of laxative use

Potential fluid volume deficit related to electrolyte imbalance from improper laxative use

Noncompliance with a changed regimen when the patient is a long-time laxative user

Sleep disturbance related to inaccurate timing of laxative administration

□ PLAN

Nursing care goals for the patient receiving laxatives vary depending on the purpose of the drug administration. For the patient having surgery or a diagnostic procedure, the goal is to completely evacuate the bowel to facilitate the therapy. For the person suffering from constipation as a result of surgery or drug therapy or for whom constipation is a new symptom the goal is to facilitate the return of normal bowel function through diet, activity, fluid intake, and drug therapy as necessary. This is also the goal for the individual with chronic constipation. However, if diet, activity, fluids, and drug therapy cannot be manipulated much as in the case of many debilitated elderly, then the goals are to achieve regular bowel movement with a mild laxative program to minimize the necessity and frequency of impaction removal enemas, and to monitor the patient closely to avoid untoward side-effects.

□ INTERVENTION

Specific administration techniques are mentioned under the clinical considerations for each drug listed in Table 44-1. In addition, a specific technique for administering lactulose by retention enema is explained in the adjacent box. In most cases, administration of a laxative should be based on when evacuation will be most convenient, for example, if a mild laxative is given at night the patient will be most likely to have a bowel movement the next morning. Sometimes when complete evacuation is required, the laxative should be given early enough in the previous day so as not to disturb the patient's sleep the night before the procedure. Frequently such harsh laxatives as magnesium citrate or bisacodyl are given too late in the

Suggested Technique for Administering Lactulose by Means of Retention Irrigation (Enema)

1. *Equipment needed:* Protective coverings for the bed, catheter with a 30-ml balloon tip, 30-ml syringe, enema bag with tubing and clamp, Y-connector, a straight piece of plastic connector tubing long enough to serve as a drainage tube; bedpan or bucket, two clamps large enough to clamp the drainage tube
2. *Solution:* 300 ml of lactulose in 700 ml warm water (adult dose). Concentration will vary depending on physician order and patient tolerance. The goal is to achieve two to three stools per day to remove sufficient ammonia and improve level of consciousness without producing diarrhea and electrolyte imbalance.
3. *Set-up:* See Figure 44-1. Connect equipment as shown. Cut the tip of the enema bag tubing to fit over one end of the Y-connector. Hang the solution no more than 20 inches above the anal opening. Run the solution completely through the enema tubing and reclamp before inserting the catheter. Clamp the drainage tube with two clamps.
4. *Patient position:* Place patient in left lateral position, knees flexed, if possible. Almost any position can be used, if necessary. If patient is completely comatose, use pillows for support or get assistance.
5. *Catheter insertion:* Test the balloon by inflating with air and deflate. Measure the catheter and mark it about 5 inches if it is not precalibrated. Catheter should be inserted about 4 inches beyond the anal sphincter in an adult. Lubricate the catheter tip and insert slowly. Inflate the catheter balloon with air.
6. *Irrigation:*
   a. Once the catheter is secured, unclamp the enema tubing and allow about 250 ml to 300 ml of solution to run *slowly* into the bowel. Amount will vary based on patient's tolerance and physician's order.
   b. Allow solution to remain in the bowel for prescribed time, usually 15 minutes to 20 minutes, by keeping drainage tube clamps closed. There may be some seepage around the catheter balloon.
   c. Unclamp drainage tubing and allow solution to drain into bedpan or bucket.
   d. Repeat the irrigation until all solution is used.

Note: If fecal contents are also expelled, tubing may have to be removed during drainage and reinserted for instillation.

day, and the patient finds he is awake most of the night instead of resting before the stressful procedure. Check the length of time between administration and expected defecation stimulus and gauge administration time accordingly.

The nurse should be aware that many bulk laxatives contain sugar, which may be a problem for the diabetic patient who uses them regularly. Bulk laxatives can also cause constipation and dangerous impaction if not taken with sufficient water. The patient who uses them should be encouraged to follow the dose with a full glass of water. These are the laxatives most routinely used by the elderly.

Stool softeners listed in Table 44-1 as emollient fecal softeners are not laxatives in the true sense of the word, that is, they do not stimulate defecation. They are used primarily to lubricate the stool sufficiently to facilitate its passage through the anal sphincter. As such they are ideal for the patient who has had rectal or anal surgery or when straining would be contraindicated such as the patient who has had a myocardial infarction or abdominal surgery. Stool softeners do not prevent constipation. Bowel activity should be monitored, and laxatives should be used as necessary.

One way to prevent laxative overuse is to closely monitor bowel activity on a flow sheet. This can be done at home or in a health-care facility. Then a plan can be enacted when bowel activity changes. This may include first, the addition of

extra fluids or natural laxatives such as bran, prunes, raw and cooked vegetables. If this doesn't work, then a mild laxative may be tried. In many nursing homes, a BM flow sheet helps the staff determine who may need help, and a protocol may be set up so a patient automatically receives certain medications if he has a small, hard bowel movement or none at all (see Aman, 1980). Such a strategy may also be useful for the patient who has overused laxatives in the past and may need help to reestablish his normal bowel pattern.

Laxatives are one of the most frequently used over-the-counter medications, yet they are not as safe as many people presume. Two serious side-effects can develop—electrolyte imbalance and loss of normal defecation reflex leading to laxative dependence.

Electrolyte balance can be upset if the laxative pulls fluid into the bowel from the interstitial space or if diarrhea results from too strong a dose of the drug. Symptoms are listed under Side-Effects/Adverse Reactions, and the patient should be told to report such effects immediately. The best strategy is to minimize laxative use as much as possible.

Laxative dependence is avoidable in most patients. The patient who becomes dependent is usually one who worries about the frequency of his bowel movements. If bowels do not move on schedule, he takes a laxative. This completely empties the bowel, which prevents the formation

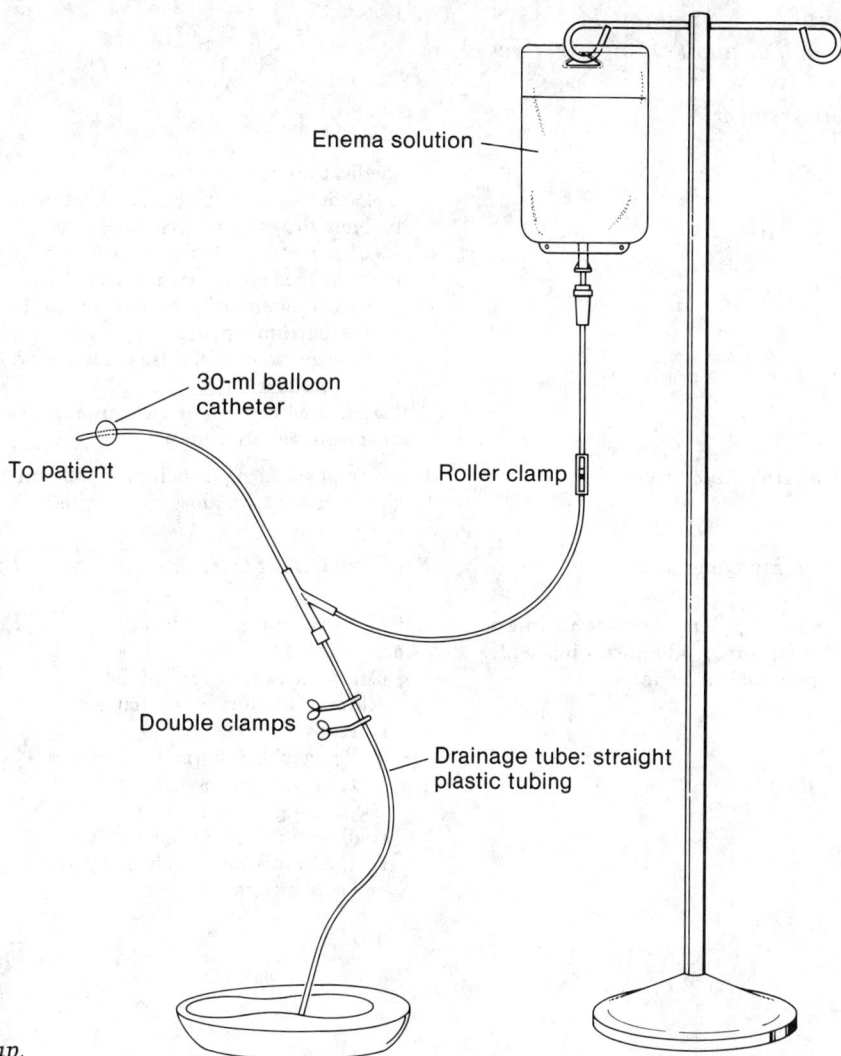

Enema solution

30-ml balloon
catheter

To patient

Roller clamp

Double clamps

Drainage tube: straight
plastic tubing

Figure 44-1. Retention enema set-up.

of sufficient mass the next day to stimulate the defecation reflex and worries the person more. He may then take a stronger laxative, and a vicious cycle is quickly established. To break the cycle the laxatives must be gradually withdrawn and the patient taught other strategies for managing his bowel routine. This may be very difficult to do especially if laxative use has been regular for many years. In the elderly person who refuses to give up laxatives, it may be more appropriate to find a milder drug coupled with more dietary fiber and fluids than to attempt to get the individual to totally abandon laxatives.

☐ *EVALUATION*
The outcome criteria by which the nurse can measure success of laxative therapy are that the patient has regular bowel movements or that the bowel is emptied as required for a procedure, that diarrhea

does not occur, that the patient is able to return to a normal bowel routine without continued drug use or that an acceptable bowel routine is established by using the mildest dose of drug possible in combination with activity, diet, and fluids. Nursing Care Plan 44-1 summarizes the nursing process for the patient receiving laxatives.

Polyethylene Glycol–Electrolyte Solution
(Co-Lyte, GoLYTELY)

Polyethylene glycol–electrolyte solution is prepared from powder to yield, following reconstitution, 4 L containing 17.6 mM/L of polyethylene glycol (PEG) 3350, 125 mM/L of sodium, 40 mM/L of sulfate, 35 mM/L of chloride, 20 mM/L of bicarbonate, and 10 mM/L of potassium. PEG 3350

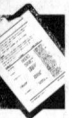

Assessment

Subjective Data	1. Medication history
	   a. Laxatives may decrease absorption of many oral drugs
	   b. Note drugs taken that have constipation as a side-effect.
	2. Medical history: Identify a history of symptoms or precipitating events that may have led to constipation, such as
	   a. Surgery: hemorrhoids, anal repair, NPO status
	   b. Postpartum: episiotomy
	   c. Changes in diet, fluids, activity, or routine especially during hospitalization
	3. Patient's perception of the symptoms as constipation in comparison to normal bowel routine

Objective Data	Focus on physical signs including abdominal firmness, decreased bowel sounds, headache, nausea, and loss of appetite.

Nursing Diagnoses	*Expected Client Outcome*	*Intervention*
Knowledge deficit: related to drug action, correct administration, and potential side-effects	Will verbalize the goal of laxative therapy · Complete evacuation will be achieved for surgery or diagnostic study. · Will reestablish normal bowel pattern without regular laxative use (if drug is used for constipation), and will learn the drug action, administration schedule, and side-effects.	Explain the goal of therapy to the patient. Many patients will be distressed about the frequency of evacuation required for surgery or diagnostic procedures. Time administration so that rest is uninterrupted. Preprocedure laxatives should be given in daytime so that most evacuation occurs before sleep. Regular laxatives should be given depending on expected peak action. Discuss the role of diet, activity, and fluid intake in facilitating normal bowel evacuation. Teach patient to monitor common side-effects as described below and follow preventive and reactive strategies given. Teach patient to avoid laxative use, especially bulk laxatives, around the time of other drug therapy.
Anxiety: related to the ability of the drug to relieve symptoms and ability to control defecation once the drug is taken	Will verbalize fears and help establish methods to manage any problems.	Discuss patient's regular bowel routine and what factors disrupt it. Attempt to provide privacy and decrease distracting stimuli so the patient can relax and allow the defecation reflex to work. Provide rapid, easy access to commode or bathroom.
Potential alteration in bowel function: either constipation or diarrhea related to drug misuse	Will reestablish a normal bowel pattern without regular laxative use.	Establish guidelines with the patient about progression of intervention prior to laxative use, *i.e.*, adding fiber for bulk to diet, increasing fluids, increasing activity (if possible), and then using drugs only if necessary.

(continued)

Nursing Diagnoses	Expected Client Outcome	Intervention
Potential alteration in bowel function: either constipation or diarrhea related to drug misuse (*continued*)		Establish realistic goals with the patient about what constitutes a "normal" bowel routine.
Potential fluid volume deficit related to electrolyte imbalance and dehydration from overly vigorous treatment with laxatives	Fluid volume and electrolyte levels will remain within normal limits.	Use a flow sheet to monitor progress. Teach the patient to report immediately any weakness, dizziness, fainting, sweating, palpitations, or abdominal cramping.
		Ensure laxative dose is appropriate for age and weight of patient. Use with extreme caution in any patient whose fluid or electrolyte status is compromised.

is a nonabsorbable substance which acts as an osmotic agent following oral ingestion, and can induce evacuation of the bowel within 3 hours to 4 hours. There is little net absorption or secretion of ions, however, due to the electrolyte composition of the solution, and large volumes may be administered without significant alterations in water or electrolyte balance.

The solution is used to cleanse the bowel prior to GI examination, and the patient should fast 3 hours to 4 hours prior to ingestion of the solution. Although administration is usually orally, the drug may be given by way of a nasogastric tube. The recommended dosing schedule is 240 ml every 10 minutes until 4 L are consumed. Each portion should be drunk rapidly. The first bowel movement should occur about 1 hour after administration is begun.

Polyethylene glycol-electrolyte solution is contraindicated in the presence of GI obstruction, gastric retention, or bowel perforation, and must be used cautiously in patients with impaired gag reflex. Side-effects are infrequent and transient, and may include nausea, bloating, cramps, and vomiting. Safety for use in pregnant women or in children has not been established. The reconstituted solution should be kept refrigerated and used within 24 hours.

CASE STUDY

Gloria Howard, age 42, has been on one diet after another for 10 years. She is about 25 lb overweight. After many unsuccessful attempts she starts a "natural health" plan recommended by a friend. The regimen consists of a daily milkshake with the health powder and the intake of 6 pills containing "natural ingredients." Her friend assures her she will feel great, have lots of energy, and lose weight.

After 3 weeks Gloria has lost 10 lb and is feeling well but wants to lose more. On the advice of the product counselor, she increases the milkshakes and pills to two times a day and decreases her meals to one per day.

About 10 days later Gloria develops nausea, diarrhea, weakness, and dizziness. She calls the doctor when she begins to feel palpitations. The physician takes a history and on examination finds her pulse is slightly irregular and she is somewhat dehydrated. He recommends that she stop taking the health food diet regimen and asks to see the labels on the preparations. Among the ingredients in the powder and pills he finds senna extract, methylcellulose, barley malt extract, psyllium granules, and mineral oil. He explains to Gloria that these are all laxatives and are probably the cause of her symptoms.

Gloria begins to feel better after 3 days of forcing fluids and eating small bland frequent meals but calls the physician's office complaining of fullness and constipation.

Discussion Questions

1. What has happened to Gloria's defecation reflex during the "natural health" diet?
2. What strategies can the nurse provide Gloria to help her through her withdrawal from laxative overuse?
3. What elements should be included in a teaching plan for this patient?

REVIEW QUESTIONS

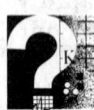

1. Can "constipation" be strictly defined? Why or why not?
2. What are the major classes of laxative drugs?
3. What is the principal mechanism of action of the (a) emollient laxatives, (b) osmotic laxatives, (c) bulk-forming laxatives, and (d) stimulant laxatives?
4. What information is needed to thoroughly assess a patient prior to administration of laxatives?
5. How should an emollient/fecal softener be incorporated into a bowel regimen? What is its main function?
6. What is the primary danger associated with chronic use of laxatives?
7. How can laxative abuse be prevented? Develop a strategy for helping a patient break a laxative overuse habit.
8. Laxatives are generally contraindicated in what conditions?
9. Give the major danger associated with use of (a) bulk-forming laxatives, (b) stimulant laxatives, and (c) mineral oil.
10. For what indications is lactulose used? What is its mechanism of action?
11. When should lactulose be administered by retention enema? How can the nurse provide comfort and privacy to the patient during this procedure?
12. What is the principal advantage of polyethylene glycol-electrolyte solution in cleansing the bowel prior to GI examination?

BIBLIOGRAPHY

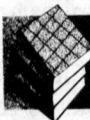

Aman RA: Treating the patient, not the constipation. Am J Nurs 80:1634, 1980

Binder HJ: Pharmacology of laxatives. Annu Rev Pharmacol Toxicol 17:355, 1977

Devroede G: Constipation: Mechanisms and management. In Sleisenger MH, Fortran JS (eds): Gastrointestinal Disease, 2nd ed, p 288. Philadelphia, WB Saunders, 1983

Donowitz M: Current concepts of laxative action: Mechanisms by
    which laxatives increase stool water. J Clin Gastroenterol 1:77,
    1979
Ewe K: Physiological basis of laxative action. Pharmacology 20(1):2,
    1980
Gever LN: Lactulose: A crucial element in treating hepatic
    encephalopathy. Nursing 82 12(8):76, 1982
Henderson V, Nite G: Principles and Practice of Nursing, 6th ed, pp
    1237–1239. New York, Macmillan Publishing, 1978
Thompson WG: Laxatives: Clinical pharmacology and rational use.
    Drugs 19(1):49, 1980

Antidiarrheal Drugs

45

Diarrhea, the passage of excessive, watery stools, is generally viewed as a symptom of an underlying pathologic condition rather than as a disease entity in itself. Distinction must be made, however, between acute and chronic diarrhea, because significant differences exist between the two conditions with respect to etiology, potential danger to the patient, and preferred treatment. Acute diarrhea, characterized by sudden onset of frequent, watery stools, often accompanied by fever, pain, vomiting, and weakness, may have several causes, including viral or bacterial infection, food or drug poisoning, or radiation exposure. The major danger of severe acute diarrhea is that it can quickly lead to dehydration and electrolyte imbalances, especially in pediatric patients. Fortunately, most episodes of acute diarrhea are self-limiting, that is, once the offending organisms, foods, or medications are removed, the symptoms soon subside.

Chronic diarrhea likewise has many possible causative factors, such as secondary disease states (e.g., ulcerative colitis, diverticulitis, irritable colon, hyperthyroidism, gastric carcinoma), surgery (such as subtotal gastrectomy, vagotomy, ileal resection), or presence of excessive amounts of hormones, bile acids, or other substances in the GI tract. Chronic diarrhea may also be of psychogenic origin, a most difficult type to treat.

Whatever the type of diarrhea, every effort should be made to determine and remove the underlying cause of the distress. For example, diarrhea resulting from the presence of an infectious organism may best be treated by use of an appropriate antibiotic. Likewise, drug-induced diarrhea can often be corrected by simply discontinuing the offending drug. Successful treatment of secondary disease states associated with diarrhea usually reduces or eliminates the accompanying episodes of diarrhea. In those instances in which the cause of the diarrhea is not readily apparent or cannot be successfully eliminated by other means, use of antidiarrheal drugs for symptomatic relief should be considered on a short-term basis. In no instance, however, should antidiarrheal agents be employed in lieu of attempts to eradicate the cause of the condition, nor should these drugs be administered over prolonged periods of time except in unusual circumstances, because many of the more effective antidiarrheals have the potential to elicit a wide range of side-effects in addition to becoming habituating.

The most effective antidiarrheal medications are the opiates (such as paregoric) and related opiate derivatives (e.g., diphenoxylate, loperamide), systemically acting agents that reduce intestinal hypermotility and slow peristalsis. Anticholinergics have also been used to reduce GI motility by impairing parasympathetic nerve stimulation to intestinal smooth muscle. Although they are possibly effective in some forms of diarrhea, the doses of anticholinergic drugs required to effectively slow peristalsis are quite high and usually result in a wide range of unacceptable side-effects. Anticholinergic drugs are reviewed in detail in Chapter 14 and are not discussed here.

Various locally active drugs have been employed for the symptomatic relief of diarrhea, frequently in combination form. Among the pharmacologic products used in this way are adsorbents (kaolin, pectin), astringents (zinc phenolsulfonate), antacids (aluminum hydroxide, bismuth salts), and bacterial cultures (Lactobacillus acidophilus). These substances are relatively safe for normal use, but there is insufficient clinical evidence to establish their effectiveness for the intended purpose. Nevertheless, they are available without prescription and are widely used by the general public. A warning appearing on every product states that they should not be used for longer than 2 days, nor in the presence of high fever, and they should only be given to children under 3 years upon physicians' orders. The composition of commonly-used antidiarrheal combination products is presented in Table 45-1 on page 891.

Treatment of most types of diarrhea, with the possible exception of severe acute diarrhea in infants and children, is usually best carried out conservatively. One of the locally acting drug combinations (such as kaolin and pectin) is usually satisfactory for the symptomatic management of mild, episodic diarrhea. More intense acute diarrhea may require addition of one of the opiate derivatives plus the ingestion of large amounts of fluids or possibly electrolyte solutions (e.g., Lytren, Pedialyte) (see Table 78-1) to prevent dehydration and electrolyte depletion. Persistent or recurrent diarrhea generally signifies an underlying pathologic condition that should be identified and corrected. Routine use of antidiarrheal drugs for extended periods should be confined to certain conditions (such as chronic inflammatory bowel disease, GI carcinoma, intestinal surgery, radiation therapy), only undertaken following careful examination, and closely supervised by a physician. Continuous self-use of antidiarrheal drug formulations by persons with mild, intermittent, or episodic diarrhea should be strongly discouraged, because the drugs may not only elicit untoward reactions, but can mask the symptoms of a more severe underlying disease.

A type of diarrhea frequently experienced by persons visiting foreign countries has been termed "travellers' diarrhea" and is generally the result of ingesting food or water contaminated by certain enterotoxins, such as those produced by strains of the pathogen *Escherichia coli*. Because vacations may be temporarily interrupted or even completely ruined by the abdominal cramping, nausea, vomiting, and diarrhea associated with this condition, methods for prevention of travellers' diarrhea have received consideration attention, although there is considerable difference of opinion as to their safety and efficacy. Among the more popular preventative measures are the use of antibiotics such as doxycycline (see Chap. 63) or trimethoprim-sulfamethoxazole (see Chap. 60) beginning on the day of departure and continuing for the duration of travel. Alternatively, large doses of bismuth subsalicylate (*e.g.*, Pepto-Bismol) have been advocated for both prevention *and* treatment of travellers' diarrhea. The principal danger of antibiotic treatment is the possibility of emergence of resistant strains of the causative pathogens with daily administration of the antibiotic. In addition, drug toxicity can occur, such as allergic reactions, or photosensitivity, and treatment of other infections, should they develop, may be rendered more difficult. Of course, potentially contaminated foods, such as fresh fruits or vegetables, tap water, raw shellfish, or any other possible source of disease, should be avoided. Fruits and vegetables should be peeled or washed in chlorinated water, and water should be drunk only if it has been boiled or is bottled. Ice can also be a source of infection if it is made from contaminated water.

■ Nursing Process

□ ASSESSMENT
Prior to administration of any antidiarrheal agent a history should be taken to determine the cause of the symptom because that may be the best way to determine treatment. The nurse needs to learn the frequency and consistency of the stools, whether any blood, mucus, or other material has been passed, and the presence of accompanying symptoms such as cramping, pain, or perirectal burning. Such symptoms may require additional drug therapy. If the patient is on tube feeding, stool consistency will be soft, unformed. Stools that are watery and occur more often than twice a day are considered diarrhea.

In children, especially small infants, it is important to estimate fluid loss and look for early symptoms of dehydration such as weak cry, poor skin turgor, and lethargy. In the younger child only a 5% loss of fluid through diarrhea or vomiting can result in serious dehydration, and action must be taken quickly to replace lost fluids and electrolytes.

□ NURSING DIAGNOSES
Actual nursing diagnosis for the patient taking an antidiarrheal is:

Knowledge deficit related to appropriate drug taking, dose, and side-effects.

Potential nursing diagnoses may include:

Alteration in comfort: acute abdominal pain from toxic megacolon, a drug side-effect

Alteration in cardiac output: decreased related to tachycardia, a sign of overdosage

Alteration in respiratory function: depression, a sign of drug overdose

Hyperthermia related to drug overdose

□ PLAN
Nursing care goals vary depending on the symptoms. A goal for the patient traveling to a foreign country may be to prevent diarrhea through a plan of antimicrobial therapy, dietary discretion, and antidiarrheal agent. For the patient with acute diarrhea the goal may be to attempt to eliminate the cause and treat the symptom for as short a time as possible to provide relief. For the patient with chronic diarrhea, the goal may be to incorporate use of antidiarrheal agents on a p.r.n. basis along with diet, activity, and other therapeutic measures aimed at reducing the symptoms of the problem.

□ INTERVENTION
Most antidiarrheal agents are over-the-counter preparations to which the public has ready access. There are several concepts the nurse can stress when given the opportunity to discuss the use of these products with the patient, which also apply to the prescription remedies. Patients should be encouraged to let diarrhea run its course if they suspect the cause is a viral infection or food poisoning. The toxin will be removed from the intestine, and the symptom will subside. In the interim, encourage the patient to rest, drink fluids, and eat bland foods. One suggested regimen called the BRAT routine is to eat *b*ananas, *r*ice, *a*pplesauce and *t*ea. If the cause of the diarrhea is related to drug therapy, the physician should be notified and a course decided. The patient should be discouraged from self-dosing because many of the OTC antidiarrheal products contain absorbents which may significantly alter drug absorption.

If a tube-fed patient must be given an antidiarrheal agent, the drug is usually administered in the tube feeding and is given on a regular schedule until the diarrhea is under control.

When using systemic antidiarrheal agents, several side-effects should also be monitored. The patient should be cautioned to watch for abdominal distention and pain, signs of possible toxic megacolon. The physician should be notified immediately and the drug discontinued. With diphenoxylate and loperamide the danger of respiratory depression and overdosage exists. Early warning signs include flushing, tachycardia, drying of the mucosa, and hyperthermia. Help should be sought immediately if any of these occur. In addition, the patient should be warned not to drink alcohol or use any other CNS depressants with these two drugs because the danger of overdosage increases with such combinations.

□ **EVALUATION**
The outcome criterion for success with antidiarrheal agents is control of the symptom without debilitating side-effects or habituation.

Systemic Antidiarrheals

The potent systemically active antidiarrheal drugs are reviewed individually, followed by a brief, general discussion of the principal locally acting antidiarrheal agents and a listing of commonly used antidiarrheal combination products in Table 45-1.

The systemic antidiarrheals comprise the opiates, principally camphorated tincture of opium (paregoric); anticholingerics, which are discussed in Chapter 14; and two derivatives of the opiate meperidine, namely diphenoxylate and loperamide. These latter two agents are claimed to have a lower incidence of CNS effects and reduced addiction liability compared to other opiates.

Diphenoxylate Hydrochloride With Atropine Sulfate
(Lomotil and various other manufacturers)

Diphenoxylate is a structural analogue of meperidine with a rather low risk of dependence at normal doses although typical opiate effects (such as euphoria) may occur with high doses. Prolonged ingestion can lead to habituation and physical dependence. Diphenoxylate is combined with a subtherapeutic amount of atropine to discourage deliberate abuse; excessive doses result in development of a variety of atropine-induced adverse effects that are distinctly unpleasant (see under Side-Effects/Adverse Reactions).

MECHANISM AND ACTIONS
Diphenoxylate slows intestinal motility, probably by a direct inhibitory action on circular and longitudinal GI smooth muscle and may exert an antisecretory action as well. It prolongs intestinal transit time, increases viscosity and density of intestinal contents, and reduces daily fecal volume. There is little or no analgesic effect.

USES
1. Control of diarrhea, either alone or in combination with locally-acting antidiarrheals

ADMINISTRATION AND DOSAGE
Diphenoxylate with atropine sulfate is available as tablets (2.5 mg/0.025 mg) or liquid (2.5 mg/0.025 mg per 5 ml). In adults, the recommended initial dosage is 5 mg four times a day (*i.e.*, 2 tablets or 10 ml liquid); dosage may be reduced as symptoms are controlled. If no effect is observed within 48 hours, the drug is not likely to be effective. Children (over 2 years) are given 0.3 mg to 0.4 mg/kg/day initially in divided doses. The liquid form should be used in children under age 12, and the average daily doses in the various age groups are as follows:
   2 years–5 years: 4 ml (2 mg) three times a day
   5 years–8 years: 4 ml (2 mg) four times a day
   8 years–12 years: 4 ml (2 mg) five times a day
   When administering the liquid preparation, use only the calibrated dropper provided with the bottle.

FATE
The drug is well absorbed when taken orally, and the onset of action is 30 minutes to 60 minutes. Diphenoxylate is quickly and extensively metabolized to diphenoxylic acid (difenoxin), the major active circulating metabolite. The plasma half-life

of the parent drug is 2 hours to 3 hours, while the elimination half-life of difenoxin is 12 hours to 15 hours. The drug and its metabolites are excreted in both the feces (approximately 50%) and the urine.

SIDE-EFFECTS/ADVERSE REACTIONS

Untoward reactions can result from either diphenoxylate or atropine, and the most frequently occurring side-effects are drowsiness and dry mouth.

The development of other adverse reactions depends to a large extent on the dose and may include anorexia, nausea, vomiting, abdominal discomfort, paralytic ileus, toxic megacolon (especially in patients with acute ulcerative colitis), dizziness, headache, malaise, restlessness, euphoria, numbness of the extremities, respiratory depression, pruritus, angioedema, gum swelling, and urticaria. Atropine-related side-effects (more common in children) include flushing, tachycardia, blurred vision, urinary retention, hyperthermia, reduced secretions, and dry skin and mucous membranes.

Diphenoxylate can prolong or aggravate diarrhea due to organisms such as Salmonella, Shigella sp. and toxigenic E. coli that penetrate the intestinal mucosa, or diarrhea that is the result of antibiotic-induced pseudomembranous enterocolitis.

CONTRAINDICATIONS AND PRECAUTIONS

Diphenoxylate with atropine sulfate is contraindicated in patients with obstructive jaundice or antibiotic-induced pseudomembranous colitis and in children under age 2. Cautious use is required in the presence of dehydration, cirrhosis, hepatic or renal disease, ulcerative colitis, or glaucoma, and in persons with a history of drug abuse, children, pregnant women, or nursing mothers.

Although the presence of atropine discourages use of high doses, overdosage has occurred and can lead to lethargy, hypotonic reflexes, nystagmus, respiratory depression, and coma. Treatment includes gastric lavage, maintenance of an open airway, and administration of the opiate-antagonist naloxone for respiratory depression (see Chap. 22).

INTERACTIONS

(See also Chap. 14 and Chap. 22.)
1. Diphenoxylate may potentiate the depressant effects of barbiturates, alcohol, narcotics, and other tranquilizers, and sedatives.
2. Concurrent use with MAO inhibitors may precipitate a hypertensive crisis.

NURSING CONSIDERATIONS

See general Nursing Process.

Diphenoxylate may produce anticholinergic side-effects such as dry mouth, dizziness, and sedation. The patient taking them should be told to use caution in driving or engaging in any hazardous activity, including climbing stairs, until response to the drug is known. In addition, to decrease the chance of dehydration, the patient should avoid sitting in the sun until symptoms pass.

This drug can lead to physical dependence with long-term use although the anticholinergic side-effects tend to discourage deliberate abuse.

Loperamide

(Imodium)

A structural analogue of meperidine with a reduced risk of dependence at recommended doses, loperamide is similar to diphenoxylate in action, but it does not contain atropine; therefore, anticholinergic side-effects are reduced. It is claimed to have slightly less abuse potential than diphenoxylate for chronic therapy, but caution is required during prolonged use, especially in patients with a history of drug abuse.

MECHANISM AND ACTIONS

Loperamide binds to opiate receptors and decreases intestinal motility, and reduces peristalsis by a direct effect on circular and longitudinal smooth muscle. Tolerance to the antidiarrheal action is minimal, and CNS action is slight. Opiate-like effects are not observed at recommended doses.

USES
1. Control of acute nonspecific diarrhea and chronic diarrhea associated with inflammatory bowel disease
2. Reduction of volume of discharge from ileostomies

ADMINISTRATION AND DOSAGE

Loperamide is available as capsules (2 mg) and liquid (1 mg/5 ml). In treating acute diarrhea, the initial adult dosage is 4 mg, followed by 2 mg after each loose stool to a maximum of 16 mg/day. Children are given the following initial doses:

Age (yr)	Weight (kg)	Dose
2–5	13–20	1 mg tid
5–8	20–30	2 mg bid
8–12	above 30	2 mg tid

Subsequent total daily dosage should not exceed the first day recommended doses.

For managing chronic diarrhea in adults, an average daily dose of 4 mg to 8 mg in divided doses has been established.

Treatment for 10 days at a dose of 16 mg/day without apparent benefit suggests that diarrhea cannot be controlled by the drug.

FATE
Loperamide is *not* well absorbed orally and does not penetrate well into the brain. Peak plasma levels occur in about 4 hours with capsule administration and within 3 hours with liquid usage. The elimination half-life is 10 hours to 12 hours. A large proportion of the dose is excreted in the feces.

SIDE-EFFECTS/ADVERSE REACTIONS
The most common side-effect with loperamide is abdominal cramping. Other adverse effects, noted especially during chronic therapy, are abdominal distention, constipation, dry mouth, nausea, vomiting, drowsiness, dizziness, and allergic reactions, such as skin rash. Overdosage is infrequent; doses up to 60 mg have resulted in no apparent harm. In the event of CNS depression with very large amounts, naloxone may be given as an antidote (see Chap. 22).

CONTRAINDICATIONS AND PRECAUTIONS
Loperamide should not be used in patients in whom constipation should be avoided, such as those with severe cardiac disease or intestinal obstruction, nor in cases of acute diarrhea associated with organisms that penetrate the intestinal mucosa (*e.g.*, *Salmonella*, *Shigella*, toxigenic *E. coli*). It should not be given to persons with antibiotic-induced pseudomembranous colitis. A *cautious* approach to therapy is warranted in the presence of acute ulcerative colitis because toxic megacolon

can result. The drug is not recommended for use in children under age 2 and must be given cautiously to pregnant women or nursing mothers. Physical dependence has not been observed with loperamide.

INTERACTIONS
1. Loperamide may enhance the sedative effects of other CNS depressants (*e.g.*, barbiturates, alcohol, narcotics, hypnotics).

NURSING CONSIDERATIONS
See general Nursing Process.

Camphorated Opium Tincture
(Paregoric)

Camphorated opium tincture contains 2 mg of morphine equivalent per 5 ml together with 45% alcohol. Its antidiarrheal action is due to its morphine content. *Camphorated* opium tincture should not be confused with *deodorized* opium tincture, a liquid containing 25 times the morphine equivalency (*i.e.*, 10 mg/ml). Paregoric reduces GI motility and peristalsis, suppresses secretion and slows the passage of intestinal contents. It is used for the control of acute diarrhea. Adult dosage is 5 ml to 10 ml one to four times a day after loose bowel movements. Children may be given 0.25 ml/kg to 0.5 ml/kg up to four times a day.

Side-effects are relatively infrequent but may include drowsiness, lightheadedness, constipation, sweating, allergic reactions, and habituation. Large doses or prolonged administration can lead to symptoms of narcotic overdosage (see Chap. 22). Because paregoric can depress the CNS in large amounts, it may enhance the CNS depressive effects of alcohol, tranquilizers, and other narcotics. Paregoric is a Schedule III controlled drug, and is also available in combination with other antidiarrheal medications, which are listed in Table 45-1.

Locally Acting Antidiarrheals

A large number of compounds exhibiting diverse pharmacologic effects have been employed in the treatment of diarrhea. Other than those drugs previously discussed in this chapter, most other frequently used antidiarrheal agents are locally acting drugs; that is, they are primarily nonabsorbable chemicals that act within the lumen of the GI tract by a variety of mechanisms. The most commonly employed classes of locally acting antidiarrheal drugs are the adsorbents, antiseptics, and bacterial cultures, although astringents, antacids, bulk laxatives, digestive enzymes, and electrolytes have all been tried in the treatment of diarrhea. These locally acting agents, while essentially safe in recommended doses, have not been conclusively demonstrated to be clinically effective. Nevertheless, they are widely available over-the-counter, usually as combination products containing several different locally acting ingredients, and frequently including small doses of paregoric or other opium equivalents. Because they are readily available and relatively safe, they are most often the initial agents tried in cases of occasional, uncomplicated diarrhea, and in many instances they provide sufficient relief. The warning that appears on every product should be heeded, however, and these agents should not be used for longer than 2 days to 3 days, or when a high fever is present. Further, children under 3 years should be given these drugs only by prescription from a physician.

A general review of the pharmacology of the most frequently used locally acting antidiarrheals is presented here, followed by a listing of the ingredients of the commonly employed combination products in Table 45-1.

Adsorbents

The adsorbents are the antidiarrheal products most frequently used for the treatment of mild diarrhea. Commercial products usually contain two or more adsorbents, frequently combined with small amounts of opium derivatives or anticholinergics, or both. The extent to which the adsorbents contribute to the overall antidiarrheal efficacy of such mixtures is a subject of controversy, however. These compounds have the ability to bind to their particle surface toxins, bacteria, and other irritants that may be present in the GI tract; in addition, some adsorbents (e.g., pectin) may also exert a soothing demulcent action on the mucosal surface of the irritated bowel. The adsorptive activity of these compounds is not selective for irritants or toxins, however, and they may also adsorb other drugs found in the intestinal tract at the same time. Thus, adsorbents can potentially interfere with the normal GI absorption of many drugs, and this possibility should be noted whenever an adsorbent substance is given to a patient receiving medications for other conditions.

The most frequently encountered adsorbents in commercial preparations are kaolin, pectin, activated attapulgite, and certain bismuth salts (e.g., subgallate, subsalicylate). Cholestyramine, an anion-exchange resin discussed in Chapter 37, has also been employed in some cases of severe diarrhea. It is thought to complex with bacterial toxins in the GI tract. Anion-exchange resins are not approved as antidiarrheal drugs, and their use in this matter is strictly experimental.

Antiseptics/Astringents

Drugs such as zinc phenolsulfonate, phenyl salicylate, and zinc sulfocarbolate are included in several proprietary antidiarrheal mixtures based on their astringent and reputed antiseptic action. It is doubtful whether inclusion of these substances significantly improves the antidiarrheal activity of the mixture.

Bacterial Cultures

Cultures of viable strains of *Lactobacillus acidophilus* and *Lactobacillus bulgaricus* have been used in the treatment of diarrhea resulting from a disruption of normal intestinal microorganism balance. Seeding the bowel with bacterial cultures is believed to reestablish the normal intestinal flora and suppress the growth of undesired microorganisms, thus improving those GI disturbances, including diarrhea, resulting from an altered intestinal flora. While possibly effective in those cases of diarrhea induced by treatment with antibiotics that can upset the normal bacterial population of

Table 45-1
Antidiarrheal Combination Products

Trade Name	Dosage Form	Opiate Derivative	Adsorbents/ Astringents	Anticholinergics	Other Ingredients
Amogel PG	Suspension	Powdered opium	Kaolin, pectin	Hyoscyamine, atropine, scopolamine	
Bacid	Capsules				*Lactobacillus acidophilus*, sodium carboxymethylcellulose
Banatol	Liquid	Opium	Pectin, bismuth subsalicylate, zinc phenolsulfonate		Extract Irish moss
BPP Lemmon	Tablets	Powdered opium	Kaolin, pectin, bismuth subgallate, zinc phenolsulfonate		
Corrective Mixture with Paregoric	Suspension	Paregoric	Bismuth subsalicylate, zinc sulfocarbolate, phenyl salicylate		Pepsin
Devrom	Chewable tablets		Bismuth subgallate		
Diabismul	Tablets	Powdered opium	Bismuth subcarbonate, calcium carbonate		
Diabismul	Suspension	Opium	Kaolin, pectin		
Dia-Eze	Suspension		Kaolin, bismuth subgallate		
Dia-Quel	Suspension	Opium tincture	Pectin	Homatropine	
Diar Aid	Tablets		Activated attapulgite, pectin		
Diasorb	Tablets Liquid		Activated attapulgite		
Donnagel	Suspension		Kaolin, pectin	Hyoscyamine, atropine, scopolamine	
Donnagel-PG	Suspension	Powdered opium	Kaolin, pectin	Hyoscyamine, atropine, scopolamine	
Infantol Pink	Liquid	Opium	Pectin, bismuth subsalicylate, zinc phenosulfonate		Extract Irish moss
Kaodene with Codeine	Suspension	Codeine phosphate	Kaolin, pectin, bismuth subsalicylate, sodium carboxymethylcellulose		
Kaodene with Paregoric	Suspension	Anhydrous morphine	Kaolin, pectin, bismuth subsalicylate, so-		

(continued)

Table 45-1 (continued)
Antidiarrheal Combination Products

Trade Name	Dosage Form	Opiate Derivative	Adsorbents/ Astringents	Anticholinergics	Other Ingredients
Kaodene with Paregoric (continued)			dium carboxy-methylcellu-lose		
Kaodene Non-narcotic	Suspension		Kaolin, pectin, bismuth subsa-licylate, so-dium carboxy-methylcellu-lose		
Kaodonna PG	Suspension	Powdered opium	Kaolin, pectin	Hyoscyamine, atropine, sco-polamine	
Kaopectate	Suspension Tablets		Kaolin, pectin Attapulgite		
Kao-tin	Suspension		Kaolin, pectin		
Kapectolin	Suspension		Kaolin, pectin		
Kapectolin Gel with Bella-donna	Suspension		Kaolin, pectin	Hyoscyamine, atropine, sco-polamine	
Kapectolin with Paregoric	Liquid	Paregoric	Kaolin, pectin		
Kapectolin PG	Suspension	Powdered opium	Kaolin, pectin	Hyoscyamine, atropine, sco-polamine	
KBP/O	Capsules	Powdered opium	Kaolin, pectin, bismuth sub-carbonate		
K-C	Suspension		Kaolin, pectin, bismuth sub-carbonate		
K-P	Suspension		Kaolin, pectin		
K-Pek	Suspension		Kaolin, pectin		
Lactinex	Granules Tablets				*Lactobacillus bulgaricus* *Lactobacillus acidophilus*
Mitrolan	Chewable tablets				Calcium polycar-bophil
Parepectolin	Suspension	Opium	Kaolin, pectin		
PectoKay	Liquid		Kaolin, pectin		
Pepto-Bismol	Suspension Chewable tablets		Bismuth subsali-cylate		
Polymagma Plain	Tablets		Activated atta-pulgite, pectin		
Quiagel	Suspension		Kaolin, pectin	Hyoscyamine, atropine, sco-polamine	
Quiagel PG	Suspension	Powdered opium	Kaolin, pectin	Hyoscyamine, atropine, sco-polamine	
Rheaban	Tablets		Colloidal acti-vated attapul-gite		

the GI tract, *Lactobacillus* preparations are not recommended for most episodes of diarrhea, inasmuch as they are somewhat more costly than other locally acting drugs, and there is no conclusive evidence that modification of intestinal flora has a beneficial effect in acute diarrhea.

Other

Among the other types of locally acting products that have been used in the treatment of diarrhea are the bulk-producing laxatives or hydrophilic colloids (*e.g.*, carboxymethylcellulose, polycarbophil, psyllium seed). The rationale behind this apparently paradoxical action is that these substances have the ability to absorb excess fecal fluid as they swell in the intestinal tract, thus aiding in the production of formed stools. Their suitability for most forms of diarrhea, however, remains speculative.

An important facet of the adjunctive treatment of persistent or severe, acute diarrhea is replenishment of fluid and electrolyte loss, especially in infants and young children. Various oral and parenteral fluids and electrolyte solutions are available for this purpose (see Chap. 78).

CASE STUDY

Sandy Carroll, age 42, was getting ready for a party when she had an attack of diarrhea. She had a prescription for diphenoxylate (Lomotil) left over from a trip to the Far East and decided to take a dose of the drug to control her symptoms so she wouldn't miss the event. She took 5 mg and about 20 minutes later had another bowel movement. She took another 5 mg, began to feel cramping after about 15 minutes, and took 10 mg more. In about an hour she developed severe abdominal pain, cramping, and nausea, and her husband brought her to the Emergency Room when she passed out from the pain.

The examining physician found her to be in acute pain, the abdominal wall was rigid and tender in all four quadrants, and Sandy was very nauseated. A nasogastric (NG) tube was inserted, an IV of 5D/NSS was started, and Sandy was admitted for observation with a diagnosis of "rule out intestinal obstruction." She was given Demerol, 100 mg IM, for pain.

Within 36 hours the pain abated, and the NG tube was removed. Once out of bed, Sandy began to pass some flatus, and plans were made for discharge.

Discussion Questions

1. How did Sandy's use of Lomotil cause the symptoms that brought her to the Emergency Room? What advice did Sandy neglect to follow regarding the use of antidiarrheal agents in general and systemic agents in particular?
2. Outline a basic teaching plan for this patient on use of antidiarrheal agents.

REVIEW QUESTIONS

1. What is the major danger of severe, acute diarrhea?
2. List the most widely used types of antidiarrheal drugs.
3. Which agents may be used to prevent "travellers' diarrhea"? What dietary precautions should the individual take to prevent the problem?
4. How do diphenoxylate and loperamide differ from other narcotic drugs?

5. Why is atropine combined with diphenoxylate?
6. In what conditions must diphenoxylate and loperamide be used with caution?
7. How does *camphorated* opium tincture differ from *deodorized* opium tincture?
8. List several different kinds of drugs found in over-the-counter antidiarrheal medications.
9. Should all episodes of diarrhea be treated with antidiarrheal medications? Explain. What other measures should be employed to treat diarrhea?

BIBLIOGRAPHY

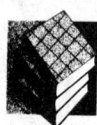

Anderson BJ: Tubefeeding: Is diarrhea inevitable? Am J Nursing 86:710F, 1986

Awouters CJ, Niemegeers E, Janssen PAJ: Pharmacology of antidiarrheal drugs. Annu Rev Pharmacol Toxicol 23:279, 1983

Black RE: The prophylaxis and therapy of secretory diarrhea. Med Clin North Am 66(3):621, 1982

Feldman M: Travelers' diarrhea. Am J Med Sci 288(3):136, 1984

Heel RC, Brogden RN, Speight TM, Avery GS: Loperamide: A review of its pharmacological properties and therapeutic efficacy in diarrhea. Drugs 15:33, 1978

Netchvolodoff CV, Hargrove MD: Recent advances in the treatment of diarrhea. Arch Intern Med 139:813, 1979

Satterwhite TK, DuPont HL: Infectious diarrhea in office practice. Med Clin North Am 67(1):203, 1983

Weiss BD: Travelers' diarrhea: Update 1983. Am Fam Physician 27:193, 1983

Emetics and Antiemetics

46

895

Drugs having the ability to enhance the vomiting reflex, either through a peripheral (*i.e.*, local gastric mucosal irritation) or central (*i.e.*, stimulation of the medullary chemoreceptor trigger zone) action are termed emetics. They are used primarily to induce vomiting in cases of drug overdosage or poisoning with other types of chemicals or toxins.

Antiemetics are those agents that reduce the hyperreactive vomiting reflex, largely by a central action, either at the level of the vomiting center or chemoreceptor trigger zone (CTZ), or on the vestibular apparatus in the inner ear. The various mechanisms that may be involved in eliciting the vomiting reflex are reviewed below.

Chemoreceptor Trigger Zone (CTZ)

Located in the floor of the fourth ventricle of the brain near the vomiting center, the CTZ may be stimulated by the following:

1. Drugs, chemicals, and toxins (*e.g.*, cardiac glycosides and apomorphine)
2. Pathologic states (*e.g.*, uremia and diabetic ketoacidosis)
3. Variations in gonadotropin and progesterone levels (*e.g.*, pregnancy)
4. Radiation
5. Altered metabolic states

The CTZ exerts a tonic influence on the vomiting center, maintaining a state of excitability to other incoming vestibular impulses (see below).

Drug-, chemical-, or toxin-induced neuronal excitation of the CTZ is probably mediated by the release of *dopamine* from surrounding cells (*e.g.*, astrocytes) that form synaptic connections with the neurons of the CTZ.

Cortical Stimulation

Emesis may follow cortical stimulation induced by psychic factors, such as unpleasant scenes or disagreeable odors, or increased intracranial pressure, for example, hydrocephalus, brain tumors, or inflammation. Other cortically mediated causes of vomiting include pain, vascular changes, and emotional disturbances.

Disturbances of the Inner Ear (Labyrinth)

Motion (through mechanical stimulation of receptors in the labyrinth of the ear) and disorders affecting the vestibular apparatus may produce emesis. Impulses are carried by the vestibulocochlear (VIII) nerve and are transmitted through the cerebellum and CTZ to the vomiting center. *Acetylcholine* is thought to be the neurotransmitter involved with impulse transmission along the labyrinthine pathway to the vomiting center.

Visceral Stimulation

Afferent impulses from the abdominal viscera may be generated by visceral distention or visceral irritation, and these impulses can directly stimulate the vomiting center. Destruction of the CTZ abolishes vomiting of labyrinthine origin (suggesting a modulatory role for the CTZ in vestibular activation of the vomiting center) but does not alter the emetic effect of visceral stimulation. Other conditions that may result in vomiting include appendicitis, pancreatitis, myocardial infarction, and congestive heart failure.

Nodose Ganglion

Certain drugs may produce vomiting by stimulating the nodose ganglion of the vagus (X cranial) nerve.

Following stimulation of the vomiting center, the esophagus, gastroesophageal sphincter, and the body of the stomach relax, while the pyloric antrum and duodenum contract. Forced inspiration follows, and sudden, powerful contraction of the diaphragm and abdominal muscles generates increased intragastric pressure that propels the gastric contents through the esophagus and pharynx into the mouth. Reflex elevation of the soft palate prevents the vomitus from entering the nasopharynx, and closure of the glottis prevents pulmonary aspiration.

Emesis is often preceded by nausea and profuse salivary secretion. Severe nausea may be accompanied by sweating, pallor of the skin, and dizziness.

A schematic representation of vomiting reflex mechanisms is presented in Figure 46-1.

Emetics

Vomiting is an efficient means of removing unabsorbed drugs or toxins from the stomach; thus, emetics are frequently used in instances of drug overdosage or accidental ingestion of toxic chemi-

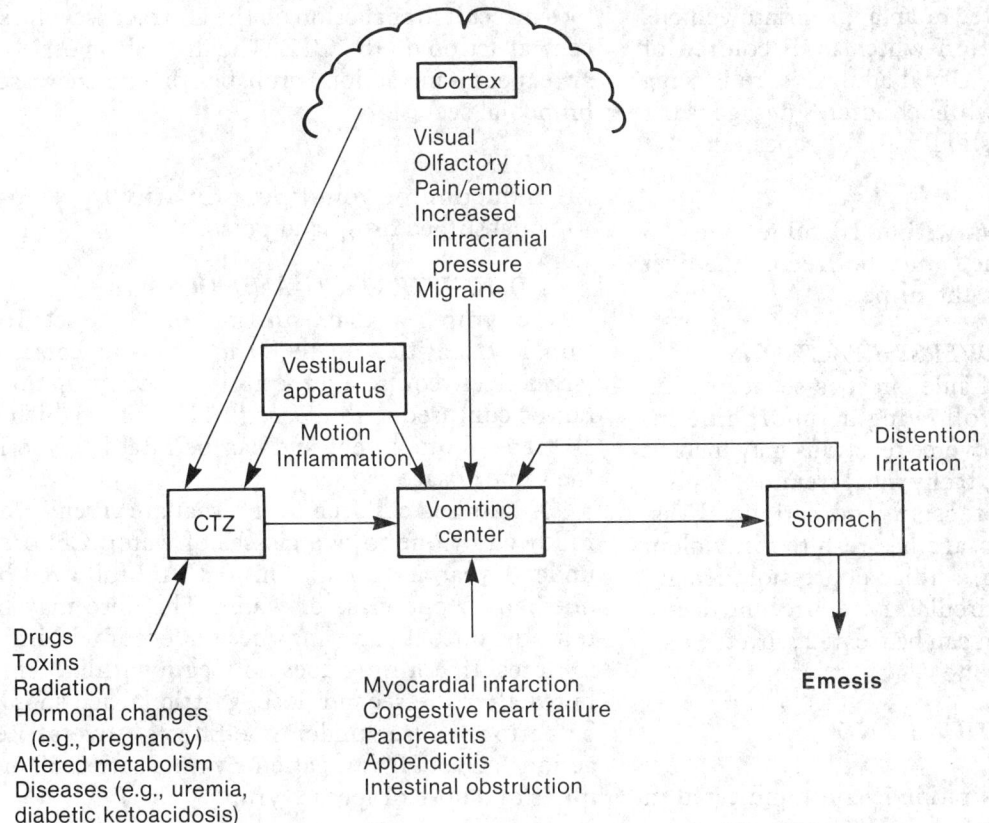

Figure 46-1. *Mechanisms involved in the vomiting reflex.*

cals or other substances. Prompt administration is essential in order to remove as much of the toxin as possible before significant amounts are absorbed into the system. Emetics generally should not be used, however, in certain types of poisoning, for example, with corrosive or caustic agents or petroleum products, because the expulsion of these substances by vomiting can severely irritate or damage the epithelium of the upper digestive tract. Likewise, patients who are comatose or semiconscious or who demonstrate hyperactive or convulsive activity should not receive emetics. Whenever possible, adjunctive drugs and *other* measures (e.g., materials for gastric lavage or suction, adsorbents such as activated charcoal, oxygen, or specific antidotes to the common poisons) should be available and employed when necessary. Drug overdosage or chemical poisoning is a potentially serious problem, and everyone, especially parents, should have ready access to a poisoning chart giving explicit instructions for handling poisoning emergencies. The phone number of the closest poison prevention center should be on hand, because speed of recognition and treatment is very often a critical factor for successful recovery. A listing of common poisons is found in the appendix.

Apomorphine

MECHANISM AND ACTIONS

Apomorphine is a synthetic derivative of morphine with potent dopamine agonistic activity. It stimulates the CTZ, thus activating the medullary vomiting center, resulting in emesis. Vomiting occurs within 10 minutes to 15 minutes after injection, and the drug is virtually 100% effective. Apomorphine can depress several areas of the CNS, including the respiratory and vasomotor centers, and the degree of CNS depression is dose-dependent. Its analgesic effects, however, are greatly diminished compared to that of most other opiates. Because it exhibits dopamine receptor-stimulating action, it may reduce secretion of prolactin and alter central motor regulatory function (e.g., reduce akinesia or rigidity).

USES

1. Production of emesis by a central action at the level of the CTZ

ADMINISTRATION AND DOSAGE

Apomorphine is available as *soluble tablets* (6 mg), but it is administered as a SC injection following dissolution of the tablet in an appropriate vehicle. Do not use any solution which is discolored or contains a precipitate. Usual adult dosage is 5 mg (range 2 mg–10 mg), while children's dosage is 0.1 mg/kg. The injection should *not* be repeated.

FATE
The onset of action is within 10 minutes to 15 minutes. Apomorphine is metabolized by the liver and excreted chiefly in the urine.

SIDE-EFFECTS/ADVERSE REACTIONS
The most often noted side-effect is sedation, and most patients sleep following apomorphine-induced emesis. Other adverse reactions may include euphoria, restlessness, tachypnea, tremors, depression, orthostatic hypotension, and peripheral vascular collapse. Overdosage has resulted in violent retching and vomiting, cardiac depression, irregular respiration, acute circulatory failure, and death. Severe CNS depression can be treated with the narcotic antagonist naloxone.

CONTRAINDICATIONS AND PRECAUTIONS
Apomorphine administration is contraindicated in impending shock, poisoning with corrosives or petroleum products, or overdosage with opiates, barbiturates, alcohol, or other CNS depressants. It must be used with *caution* in patients with cardiac decompensation, in children, and in elderly or debilitated persons. If vomiting does not result from the first dose, do *not* give additional amounts.

INTERACTIONS
1. Apomorphine may enhance the effects of levodopa or bromocriptine, as they are also dopamine agonists.

NURSING CONSIDERATIONS
The patient should have ready access to bathroom or emesis basin because stimulation of vomiting by this drug will be rapid and forceful. The nurse should provide support and privacy and try to keep the patient comfortable. Drowsiness will occur soon after the vomiting stops, so this patient should not be left alone. Respiratory depression may occur several hours after injection; therefore, vital signs should be performed at least every 2 hours for the first 6 hours after injection.

Ipecac Syrup

MECHANISM AND ACTIONS
An alkaloidal mixture containing principally emetine and cephaline, ipecac exerts its emetic effect by a direct irritant action on the GI tract as well as a central action on the CTZ. The drug also possesses an expectorant action, probably due to increased bronchial secretions.

USES
1. Induction of vomiting, primarily to remove unabsorbed drugs and poisons

ADMINISTRATION AND DOSAGE
Ipecac syrup is available in 1.5% or 2% concentration in quantities up to 30 ml over-the-counter; larger sizes require a prescription. The syrup must not be confused with *ipecac fluid extract*, which is 14 times more potent and can be fatal if given in the same dosage as the syrup.

Adults and children over 1 year are given 15 ml followed by one to two glasses of water. Children under 1 year are given 5 ml to 10 ml followed by one-half to one glass of water. The dose may be repeated once if vomiting does not occur within 20 minutes. If vomiting does not begin within 30 minutes after the second dose, gastric lavage should be performed (see under Side-Effects/Adverse Reactions). Over 90% of patients vomit within 30 minutes of a dose of ipecac syrup.

SIDE-EFFECTS/ADVERSE REACTIONS
Diarrhea and mild CNS depression are common with ipecac syrup. GI upset may persist for several hours. Large doses can result in cardiac conduction disturbances, fibrillation, or myocarditis, probably due to significant systemic absorption of the alkaloid emetine. Ipecac is cardiotoxic if absorbed, and serious cardiac disturbances can occur in cases of overdosage. Gastric lavage with activated charcoal is recommended along with appropriate cardiovascular support when necessary.

CONTRAINDICATIONS AND PRECAUTIONS
Ipecac syrup should *not* be given to unconscious, semiconscious, or convulsing patients, to pregnant or lactating women, or if corrosives, strong acids or alkalis, or strychnine has been ingested. Patients should be cautioned to contact an emergency room, physician, or Poison Control Center if vomiting does not occur within 20 minutes after a second dose.

INTERACTIONS
1. Activated charcoal may absorb ipecac syrup, nullifying its emetic effect.
2. Simultaneous administration of milk or carbonated beverages may interfere with the action of ipecac.

NURSING CONSIDERATIONS

Although parents of young children frequently receive a recommendation to keep this drug on hand in case of accidental poisoning they should receive other instructions as well. Syrup of ipecac should not be administered if the substance ingested is unknown. If the parent knows the substance but is unsure if it is corrosive, he or she should call the Poison Control Center *before* administering the drug. Last, the parent should never give a child more than two doses of the drug without medical help.

Parents should be warned to discard any unused portion of the drug once it is opened because efficacy will diminish. Expiration dates should be checked periodically, and old drug should be discarded as appropriate.

Antiemetics

The mechanisms involved in the vomiting reflex can involve several pathways and are outlined in detail in Figure 46-1 and reviewed at the beginning of the chapter.

A variety of drugs have been successfully employed for the prophylaxis and treatment of vomiting of diverse etiology. Although vomiting may have many causes, for example, drug or chemical poisoning, motion sickness, radiation exposure, bacterial or viral infection, pregnancy, endocrine disorders, neurologic or psychic disturbances, most successful antiemetic drugs act primarily by inhibition of the CTZ in the medulla or depression of vestibular apparatus sensitivity in the inner ear. The major groups of drugs used to control nausea and vomiting are the phenothiazines, anticholinergics, antihistamines, and sedatives, along with a group of miscellaneous drugs, most of which also exhibit a central mechanism of action. These agents are listed in the box entitled Antiemetic Drugs, with brief descriptions of their pharmacologic effects. In addition, a variety of other drugs, predominately local acting, have been used in the treatment of nausea and vomiting, and include antacids, adsorbents, antiflatulents, demulcents, and local anesthetics. The efficacy of most of these regionally acting antiemetic drugs is subject to considerable debate; nevertheless, the placebo effect of such medications cannot always be discounted, and their occasional use to settle an "upset stomach" is probably not harmful in the otherwise healthy patient.

The majority of clinically useful antiemetic drugs are considered elsewhere in the text. Thus, the phenothiazines, which are potent dopamine blocking agents and therefore very effective against drug-induced emesis at the level of the CTZ, are discussed in Chapter 27. Antihistamines, which are primarily useful in preventing the nausea and vomiting of motion sickness because they apparently reduce vestibular activation of the vomiting center, are reviewed in Chapter 18. Scopolamine, a highly effective antinauseant for motion

---

Antiemetic Drugs

I. Phenothiazines (*e.g.*, chlorpromazine, perphenazine, prochlorperazine, promethazine, thiethylperazine, triflupromazine)
Potent antiemetic drugs acting by inhibition of CTZ by a dopaminergic blocking action; primarily effective for drug-induced emesis and nausea and vomiting associated with surgery, anesthesia, radiation, carcinoma, and severe infections; little usefulness in motion sickness because drugs do not affect the vestibular apparatus; possibility of numerous side-effects (some serious); thus recommended for short-term use only; most drugs are also useful in managing psychotic behavior and are discussed in Chapter 27, *except* thiethylperazine, which is used exclusively as an antiemetic and is reviewed in this chapter.

II. Antihistamines (*e.g.*, buclizine, cyclizine, dimenhydrinate, diphenhydramine, meclizine)
Act by decreasing sensitivity of vestibular apparatus of inner ear; thus most effective in treating nausea and vomiting of motion sickness, Meniere's disease, or labyrinthitis; all elicit varying degrees of drowsiness and may have significant anticholinergic activity (see Chap. 18)

III. Anticholinergics (*e.g.*, scopolamine)
Depress the vestibular apparatus and inhibit cholinergic activation of the vomiting center; very effective in preventing motion sickness; high incidence of side-effects limits oral usefulness, but scopolamine is also available as Transderm-Scop in the form of a circular, flat disk that adheres to the skin behind the ear and provides for a continuous steady rate of drug release (0.5 mg over 3 days) with minimal side-effects (see Chap. 14).

IV. Sedatives (*e.g.*, barbiturates, hydroxyzine)
Decrease anxiety and possibly reduce excess stimulation of the vomiting center; largely ineffective and associated with a high incidence of drowsiness (see Chaps. 24 and 28).

V. Miscellaneous (*e.g.*, benzquinamide, diphenidol, dronabinol, nabilone, thiethylperazine, trimethobenzamide)
Predominantly centrally acting antiemetics possessing various mechanisms of action; individual drugs are discussed in this chapter.

sickness, is now frequently used as a transdermal patch, which provides a prolonged action (i.e., 3 days) and greatly reduces the side-effects previously associated with oral administration of the drug. Scopolamine is considered in Chapter 14. A number of other drugs exhibiting an antiemetic action do not fall into one of the above categories and therefore are reviewed individually in this chapter, including metoclopramide, a drug with several GI indications, including antineoplastic drug-induced nausea and vomiting. In addition, dronabinol (the psychoactive principal in marijuana) and nabilone (a synthetic cannabinoid) have been demonstrated to be effective in controlling refractive cases of nausea and vomiting resulting from cancer chemotherapy, and are presented here.

■ Nursing Process

□ ASSESSMENT
For many patients vomiting represents a humiliating loss of control, and some fear that once it starts it will never stop. Therefore, the person who seeks antiemetic medication, whether for motion sickness or to control the side-effects of chemotherapy, will be motivated to follow a successful plan.

Antiemetics should only be given if the cause of nausea is known. Therefore a thorough history should be taken and a relationship established between the symptom, the disease, and the treatment.

The nurse needs to find out when the individual gets nauseated. For the person on chemotherapy the sequence may be very clear-cut, but for others, external stimulation may be a factor. For example, a person may experience motion sickness only when he loses a view of the horizon (i.e., goes inside a ship cabin); a pregnant woman may experience nausea only when arising in the morning. Others may report nausea when specific movement, noise, or odors occur. Helping the patient become aware of environmental stimuli may also help him to begin to discover ways to control it.

The nurse should explore the patient's use of home remedies as well. Some patients report eating dry crackers, taking flat cola or ginger ale, or drinking Coca-Cola syrup over ice to be effective. These remedies may be used in addition to prescribed medication, and strategies can be developed to include them.

□ NURSING DIAGNOSES
Knowledge deficit related to action, dose, exacerbating stimuli, and drug side-effects.

Potential for injury, trauma, related to drowsiness, a drug side-effect.

□ PLAN
The nursing care goal is to help the patient develop a routine to eliminate or manage nausea and vomiting until the causative stimuli can be eliminated.

□ INTERVENTION
The main intervention is to help the patient establish strategies for taking antiemetics effectively. Most of the drugs act best if taken on an empty stomach and in advance of any activity which causes vomiting. Therefore, an antiemetic should be given before chemotherapy, but the whole regimen should be given several hours after a meal for best results.

Once vomiting has begun, the antiemetics are less effective but may still be given. Other useful strategies are to try to eliminate bothersome stimuli such as noise and odors, keep the environment clean, and remove vomitus as quickly as possible. If the patient can tolerate some food, offer small amounts of whatever he desires. This is a time when a home remedy might be requested and might be useful from a physical as well as a psychologic standpoint.

Most antiemetics cause drowsiness, and many cause dry mouth. The nurse should teach the patient to frequently rinse his mouth, take sips of fluids, and suck on candy if it helps. Drowsiness may lessen over time, but in the interim the patient should avoid activities where mental alertness is important such as driving or operating any machinery.

□ EVALUATION
The best outcome criterion against which to measure success is elimination of vomiting. However, this is not always possible. Other useful criteria include increased patient comfort, ability to eat, and ability to maintain fluid and electrolyte balance.

Benzquinamide
(Emete-Con)

MECHANISM AND ACTIONS
Benzquinamide possesses antiemetic, antihistaminic, anticholinergic, and sedative effects. Although its exact mechanism of action in relieving nausea and vomiting is unknown, it is believed to depress CTZ activation.

USES
1. Prevention and treatment of nausea and vomiting related to general anesthesia or surgery

ADMINISTRATION AND DOSAGE
The drug is available as powder for IM or IV injection, containing 50 mg/vial. The powder is reconstituted with 2.2 ml sterile water for injection. This yields 2 ml of a solution containing 25 mg drug/ml which is stable for 14 days at room temperature. For IM use, 50 mg is given initially, repeated in 1 hour, then every 3 hours to 4 hours as necessary. To prevent nausea and vomiting, it should be given at least 15 minutes prior to emergence from anesthesia.

IV administration is more hazardous and should *not* be used in patients with cardiovascular disease. The initial IV dose is 25 mg at a rate of 1 ml/min; subsequent doses should be given IM.

FATE
Benzquinamide is rapidly absorbed from IM sites, and effects occur within 15 minutes. Approximately 50% to 60% of the drug in the plasma is protein bound. Metabolism occurs in the liver, and the drug is excreted largely as metabolites in the urine. The elimination half-life is approximately 45 minutes.

SIDE-EFFECTS/ADVERSE REACTIONS
Benzquinamide injection frequently results in drowsiness and dry mouth. A number of other untoward reactions have occurred during use and are listed below:

Autonomic—Flushing, shivering, sweating, salivation, increased temperature, blurred vision, hiccups

Cardiovascular—Hypotension, dizziness, atrial fibrillation, premature ventricular contractions (Sudden hypertension may follow IV injection.)

CNS—Restlessness, headache, excitement, fatigue, insomnia, weakness, tremors

GI—Anorexia, nausea

Other—Allergic reactions (rash, chills, fever, urticaria)

CONTRAINDICATIONS AND PRECAUTIONS
There are no absolute contraindications to use of benzquinamide. IV injection must be undertaken with *caution* because sudden increases in blood pressure and arrhythmias have been reported. Benzquinamide should also be used cautiously in elderly or debilitated patients, and during pregnancy.

INTERACTIONS
1. Markedly increased blood pressure may result from use of benzquinamide with other pressor agents.
2. Benzquinamide may enhance the effects of other CNS depressants.

NURSING CONSIDERATIONS
(See general Nursing Process.)

Diphenidol
(Vontrol)

MECHANISM AND ACTIONS
Diphenidol depresses the excitability of the vestibular apparatus and inhibits the CTZ. In addition, the drug exhibits relatively weak antihistaminic, anticholinergic, and CNS depressant activity.

USES
1. Control of nausea and vomiting due to surgery, vestibular disturbances, infectious diseases, neoplasms, and radiation therapy
2. Treatment of vertigo due to Meniere's disease, labyrinthitis, or middle or inner ear surgery

ADMINISTRATION AND DOSAGE
Diphenidol is administered orally as 25-mg tablets. Usual adult dosage is 25 mg to 50 mg every 4 hours. Children should receive 0.4 mg/lb (0.88 mg/kg) every 4 hours, to a maximum of 2.5 mg/lb/day.

FATE
Diphenidol is well absorbed orally, and the onset of action is within 30 minutes to 60 minutes. It is metabolized by the liver and excreted by the kidney.

SIDE-EFFECTS/ADVERSE REACTIONS
A principal concern with diphenidol is the potential of the drug to cause auditory or visual hallucinations, disorientation, and confusion. The incidence is approximately one in 350 patients, and the reaction usually occurs within 3 days. Symptoms subside within several days after discontinuation of the drug. Other adverse effects associated with diphenidol are drowsiness, depression, dizziness, insomnia, headache, blurred vision, dry mouth, transient hypotension, skin rash, and mild jaundice.

CONTRAINDICATIONS AND PRECAUTIONS

Diphenidol is contraindicated in patients with anuria due to the danger of cumulation, and for controlling the nausea and vomiting of pregnancy. It must be given with *caution* to patients with glaucoma, obstructive GI or urinary lesions, or prostatic hypertrophy, because the drug has mild anticholinergic activity. *Cautious use* is also necessary in nursing mothers and in very young children; it is not recommended for children less than 50 lb.

INTERACTIONS

1. Additive CNS-depressant effects can occur with diphenidol in combination with other sedative or hypnotic drugs.

NURSING CONSIDERATIONS

(See general Nursing Process.)

Phosphorated Carbohydrate Solution

(Calm-X Liquid, Eazol, Emetrol, Especol, Nausetrol)

MECHANISM AND ACTIONS

Phosphorated carbohydrate solution is a hyperosmolar solution of carbohydrates (*e.g.,* fructose, dextrose) and orthophosphoric acid that relieves nausea and vomiting by a local action in the GI tract to reduce smooth muscle contraction and delay gastric emptying.

USES

1. Symptomatic relief of nausea and vomiting. (Effectiveness has *not* been conclusively demonstrated.)

ADMINISTRATION AND DOSAGE

These solutions are administered undiluted orally, and no other fluids should be taken for 15 minutes before or after ingestion. The recommended doses are:

Acute vomiting: Adults—15 ml to 30 ml;
  Children—5 ml to 10 ml (may be taken at
  15-minute intervals until vomiting ceases)
Regurgitation in infants: 5 ml to 10 ml, 10
  minutes to 15 minutes before each feeding
Morning sickness: 15 ml to 30 ml on arising
  and every 3 hours as needed
Motion sickness: 15 ml as needed (5 ml for
  very young children)

SIDE-EFFECTS/ADVERSE REACTIONS

Large doses have resulted in diarrhea and abdominal pain.

CONTRAINDICATIONS AND PRECAUTIONS

These products should not be used by diabetics due to the significant content of carbohydrates, nor by patients with hereditary fructose intolerance.

NURSING CONSIDERATIONS

(See general Nursing Process.)

Thiethylperazine

(Torecan)

MECHANISM AND ACTIONS

Thiethylperazine is a phenothiazine derivative used *exclusively* as an antiemetic agent. The mechanism of action is unknown, but the drug may exert a depressant effect on the CTZ by its dopamine blocking activity and directly depress the vomiting center as well.

USES

1. Symptomatic control of nausea and vomiting

ADMINISTRATION AND DOSAGE

Thiethylperazine is available as tablets (10 mg), suppositories (10 mg), and for IM injection (5 mg/ml). Adult dosage is 10 mg to 30 mg daily in divided doses by either the oral, rectal, or deep IM route. The drug should not be injected IV because it may cause severe hypotension. Children's dosage has not been established, and the drug is not recommended in children under age 12.

FATE

The onset of action is 30 minutes to 60 minutes with oral or rectal administration and 15 minutes to 30 minutes following IM injection. The drug is metabolized in the liver and excreted both in the urine and feces.

SIDE-EFFECTS/ADVERSE REACTIONS

Drowsiness frequently occurs following thiethylperazine administration. Other adverse reactions include headache, dizziness, blurred vision, restlessness, fever, altered taste perception, orthostatic hypotension, and cholestatic jaundice.

Because the drug is a phenothiazine, the potential to elicit other adverse effects characteristic of the phenothiazines exists; refer to Chapter 27 for a complete discussion of phenothiazines.

CONTRAINDICATIONS AND PRECAUTIONS

Thiethylperazine is contraindicated in pregnancy, children under 12 years of age, comatose states, and severe CNS depression. It should *not* be administered IV. *Cautious use* is warranted in patients with hepatic or renal disease, in nursing mothers, and following intracranial or intracardiac surgery. Patients should be kept recumbent following injection to minimize orthostatic hypotension.

NURSING CONSIDERATIONS
The main nursing responsibilities with this drug are managing the side-effects and teaching the patient to watch for their development.

The most worrisome side-effect is the potential for development of extrapyramidal movements. Teach the patient to watch for unusual eye movements, changes in speech, gait, or extremity control. All of these indicate potential drug toxicity and must be reported to the physician immediately. The patient on thiethylperazine for any length of time should be periodically evaluated using the AIMS scale in Chapter 27.

This drug may occasionally result in severe hypotension which warrants immediate treatment. Remember the drug of choice in such a crisis is norepinephrine or phenylephrine. Epinephrine is contraindicated because it may cause further hypotension.

Trimethobenzamide
(Tigan, and various other manufacturers)

MECHANISM AND ACTIONS
The precise mechanism of action of trimethobenzamide is not established. It may directly depress the CTZ and also interfere with vestibular activation of the CTZ or the vomiting center. It does not appear to block *direct* activation of the vomiting center.

USES
1. Symptomatic control of nausea and vomiting (combined with other antiemetics if vomiting is severe)

ADMINISTRATION AND DOSAGE
Trimethobenzamide is used as capsules (100 mg, 250 mg), suppositories (100 mg, 200 mg) or by injection (100 mg/ml). The usual dosage ranges are:
Oral: Adults—250 mg three or four times a day; Children—100 mg to 200 mg three or four times a day
Rectal: Adults—200 mg three or four times a day; Children—100 mg to 200 mg three or four times a day
IM: Adults only—200 mg three or four times a day. Inject deep IM in outer gluteal region, and rotate injection sites with each dose. Solution is very irritating to tissue.

FATE
The onset of action following oral or rectal administration is 15 minutes to 45 minutes, with a duration of 3 hours to 4 hours. Following IM injection, onset is 15 minutes and duration is 2 hours to 3 hours. Trimethobenzamide is metabolized in the liver and excreted primarily in the urine.

SIDE-EFFECTS/ADVERSE REACTIONS
Adverse reactions to trimethobenzamide include hypersensitivity reactions, hypotension (especially with IM use), blurred vision, depression, diarrhea, dizziness, drowsiness, jaundice, muscle cramping, and blood dyscrasias.

In addition, especially in the presence of acute fever, gastroenteritis, dehydration, or electrolyte imbalance, the drug has produced CNS reactions such as opisthotonos (tetanic spasm of back muscles), convulsions, extrapyramidal symptoms (rigidity, akathisia, tremor), and coma.

Following IM injection, redness, irritation, stinging, swelling, or burning at injection site has been reported.

CONTRAINDICATIONS AND PRECAUTIONS
Trimethobenzamide should not be given parenterally to children nor rectally to premature infants or neonates. The drug is contraindicated in persons hypersensitive to benzocaine or other local anesthetics, because it is a structural analogue. *Cautious use* is required in elderly or debilitated patients (increased likelihood of CNS reactions) and in pregnant women or nursing mothers. Extreme caution must be observed when giving trimethobenzamide to patients receiving other centrally acting drugs, such as phenothiazines, barbiturates, and anticholinergics (see under *Interactions*).

Patients, especially children, should be observed for abrupt onset of vomiting, confusion, lethargy, or irrational behavior, *possible* signs of Reye's syndrome, a potentially fatal condition terminating in convulsions, liver degeneration, encephalopathy, coma, and death. Although trimethobenzamide and other antiemetic drugs have not been definitely linked to Reye's syndrome, it has been associated with their use during acute febrile periods. Immediate medical attention is imperative if the above symptoms occur. See Chapter 23 for additional discussion of Reye's syndrome associated with use of aspirin in children with viral infections.

INTERACTIONS

1. Additive depressant effects can occur when trimethobenzamide is used with other CNS depressant drugs (e.g., narcotics, alcohol, barbiturates).
2. Extrapyramidal reactions, convulsions, and other CNS disturbances may be enhanced if trimethobenzamide is given together with phenothiazines or barbiturates.

NURSING CONSIDERATIONS

Trimethobenzamide is frequently ordered to be administered by IM route when nausea is already present. However, the solution is extremely irritating to tissue so careful monitoring of injection sites is imperative. A flow sheet or body diagram may be a useful tool if multiple doses are anticipated. If tissue begins to appear reddened or swollen, it may be necessary to switch to a rectal route of administration. Absorption of the drug will diminish if the tissue site is damaged, and abscess formation may occur.

The patient who is on prolonged therapy and the nurse who frequently administers this drug need to know what side-effects to watch for. Hypersensitivity reaction may occur early on. Encourage the patient to report any rash, fever, or itching. Central nervous system toxicity will manifest itself through disorientation, lethargy, or tremors, and occasionally, extrapyramidal movements may develop (altered gait, tremors, changes in speech). All of these must be reported immediately and the drug must be discontinued.

Metoclopramide

(Clopra, Maxolon, Octamide, Reclomide, Reglan)

MECHANISM AND ACTIONS

Metoclopramide is a smooth muscle stimulant that acts largely on the upper GI tract to increase the tone and amplitude of gastric contractions and facilitate peristaltic movements in the duodenum and jejunum. Its exact mechanism of action is unclear, but the drug probably blocks dopamine receptors, sensitizing the tissues to the action of acetylcholine. The action of metoclopramide is *not* dependent on intact vagal nerve innervation, but its effects on motility can be abolished by anticholinergic drugs. In addition to its effects on motility, metoclopramide relaxes the pyloric sphincter and duodenal bulb, and the net effect of the drug's action is to accelerate gastric emptying and increase upper intestinal transit time. The drug has little effect on colonic or gallbladder motility or intestinal, biliary, or pancreatic secretions. There is a dose-related increase in lower esophageal sphincter pressure. Other actions of metoclopramide include sedation, increased prolactin release, and elevated circulating aldosterone levels.

USES

1. Symptomatic treatment of acute or chronic diabetic gastroparesis (gastric stasis). Symptoms of delayed gastric emptying, such as nausea, vomiting, anorexia, and abdominal fullness are progressively relieved over several weeks.
2. Treatment of gastroesophageal reflux (short-term, *i.e.*, 4 weeks to 12 weeks, course of therapy in patients who do not respond to conventional therapy)
3. Prevention of nausea and vomiting associated with cancer chemotherapy
4. Facilitation of small bowel intubation in patients in whom the tube does not pass the pylorus by conventional measures
5. Stimulation of gastric emptying and intestinal transit of barium where delayed emptying interferes with radiologic examination
6. Investigational uses include facilitation of lactation and symptomatic treatment of gastric ulcers, anorexia nervosa, and nausea and vomiting due to pregnancy or a variety of other causes.

ADMINISTRATION AND DOSAGE

Metoclopramide is available as tablets (5 mg, 10 mg), syrup (5 mg/5 ml), and injection (5 mg/ml). The following dosage ranges are recommended:

Diabetic gastroparesis: 10 mg orally 30 minutes before each meal and at bedtime for 2 weeks to 8 weeks. Severe symptoms may necessitate IM or IV administration.

Gastroesophageal reflux: 10 mg to 15 mg orally up to four times/day 30 minutes before meals and at bedtime. Alternately 20 mg as a single dose prior to the provoking situation.

Chemotherapy-induced emesis: Initially, 1 mg/kg to 2 mg/kg by slow infusion at least 30 minutes before beginning cancer chemotherapy. Dose may be repeated every 2 hours for two doses, then every 3 hours for three doses. The higher dose should be used when highly emetogenic antineoplastic drugs such as cisplatin or dacarbazine are used.

Small bowel intubation:

Adults—10 mg by slow IV injection (1 minute–2 minutes)

Children (6 years–14 years)—2.5 mg to 5 mg as above

Children (under 6 years)—0.1 mg/kg as above

Injectable solutions should not be mixed with solutions of cephalothin, chloramphenicol, or sodium bicarbonate, because they are incompatible.

FATE

Onset of action is 1 minute to 2 minutes IV, 10 minutes to 15 minutes IM, and 30 minutes to 60 minutes orally. Effects persist for 1 hour to 2 hours. Protein binding is minimal. The drug is primarily excreted in the urine (80% in 24 hours) as both unchanged drug and metabolites. Elimination half-life is 3 hours to 6 hours.

SIDE-EFFECTS/ADVERSE REACTIONS

Side-effects noted with greatest frequency, especially at higher parenteral doses, are drowsiness, restlessness, fatigue, nausea, and diarrhea. Less frequently occurring adverse reactions are extrapyramidal (parkinsonian-like) reactions, akathisia, dizziness, dystonias, insomnia, headache, anxiety, myoclonus, transient hypertension, and, rarely, depression and persistent dyskinesia.

Extrapyramidal symptoms are more common in children and young adults and at higher doses. Manifestations include involuntary limb movements, facial grimacing, torticollis, oculogyric crisis, rhythmic tongue protrusion, and dystonic reactions resembling tetanus. Symptoms may be controlled by 50 mg of diphenhydramine IM.

CONTRAINDICATIONS AND PRECAUTIONS

Metoclopramide is contraindicated in persons with GI obstruction, perforation or hemorrhage, pheochromocytoma, and epilepsy. The drug should be given cautiously in the presence of diabetes, depression, galactorrhea, or gynecomastia and to pregnant women or nursing mothers.

INTERACTIONS

1. The action of metoclopramide can be antagonized by anticholinergics and narcotic analgesics.
2. Metoclopramide may impair absorption of drugs from the stomach (*e.g.*, digitalis glycosides, cimetidine) but can *increase* absorption of drugs from the small intestine (*e.g.*, acetaminophen, ethanol, tetracyclines, levodopa).
3. Increased sedation may be observed when metoclopramide is given with alcohol, barbiturates, narcotics, or other sedatives and hypnotics.

4. Metoclopramide may alter insulin requirements by influencing the timing of food delivery to the intestines.

NURSING CONSIDERATIONS

Initial assessment of the patient receiving metoclopramide should include weight, vital signs, especially heart rate and blood pressure, and evidence of dehydration through review of mucous membranes, skin turgor, and urinary output. The diabetic should have a baseline blood glucose level drawn as well.

If the patient receives the drug intravenously the solution should be covered to protect it from light, and the rate of flow should be monitored with an infusion pump. Side-effects and adverse reactions are more likely to occur with intravenous administration, especially intravenous injection.

The most common side-effect is drowsiness. The outpatient should be cautioned against driving or engaging in any activity requiring alertness while taking this drug until its effects are known. Usually drowsiness is transient.

Diarrhea and an increase in nausea are other side-effects. Fluid intake should be monitored and the use of antidiarrheal agents considered if the drug is preventing vomiting or facilitating gastric emptying.

Extrapyramidal side-effects, described above, are rare but may occur with intravenous administration and in children. Routine assessment using a guide such as the AIMS scale in Chapter 27 may facilitate early diagnosis of the problem. If symptoms are noted, the physician should be notified, the drug discontinued, and treatment started with anticholinergic or antiparkinsonism drugs as ordered.

Cannabinoids

Dronabinol
(Marinol)

Nabilone
(Cesamet)

MECHANISM AND ACTIONS

Dronabinol is delta-9-tetrahydrocannabinol (THC), the principal psychoactive substance found in *Cannabis sativa* or marijuana. Nabilone is a synthetic cannabinoid. They are effective antiemetics, especially in controlling vomiting due to cancer chemotherapy, but their use should be reserved for those patients not responding to conventional anti-emetic therapy, as they are capable of causing profound CNS effects. Cannabinoid administration has been associated with extreme mood changes (euphoria, anxiety, depression, panic, paranoia), altered states of reality, impaired memory, distorted perception, and hallucinations. In addition, tachycardia is noted frequently, and orthostatic hypotension and fainting have been reported. These drugs are highly addicting and are Schedule II controlled substances (see Chap. 7).

USES

1. Treatment of nausea and vomiting due to cancer chemotherapy in patients who have not responded to more conventional antiemetic therapy.

ADMINISTRATION AND DOSAGE

Dronabinol is available as liquid-filled capsules containing 2.5 mg, 5 mg, or 10 mg. The initial dose is 5 mg/m^2 body surface 1 hour to 3 hours prior to chemotherapy, then every 2 hours to 4 hours thereafter to a total of four to six doses/day. Dosage may be increased by 2.5-mg/m^2 increments, if necessary, to a maximum of 15 mg/m^2 per dose. The incidence of psychiatric side-effects increases significantly with increasing dosage.

Nabilone is available as 1-mg capsules. The recommended dose is 1 mg to 2 mg twice daily; the initial dose should be given 1 hour to 3 hours before an antineoplastic agent is administered. Nabilone may be given two to three times a day up to a maximum dose of 6 mg/day during the course of chemotherapy.

FATE

Oral absorption is adequate, although there is extensive first-pass hepatic metabolism, especially with dronabinol. Peak plasma concentrations occur within 2 hours to 3 hours. Within 72 hours, approximately one-half of an oral dose is recovered in the feces, biliary excretion being the major route of elimination. Smaller amounts are excreted in the urine. Chronic use may result in drug accumulation to toxic amounts.

SIDE-EFFECTS/ADVERSE REACTIONS

Many untoward reactions are possible with use of cannabinoids, the most common being drowsiness, elation and giddiness, dizziness, anxiety, impaired thinking ability, altered perception, decreased coordination, irritability, depression, weakness,

headache, memory impairment, and ataxia. In addition, vertigo and dry mouth are very common occurrences with nabilone. Other untoward reactions associated with cannabinoids are paresthesias, visual distortions, confusion, disorientation, paranoia, tinnitus, nightmares, speech difficulty, flushing, sweating, tachycardia, hypotension, fainting, diarrhea, and muscle pain.

CONTRAINDICATIONS AND PRECAUTIONS

Cannabinoids are not intended for treating nausea and vomiting due to causes other than cancer chemotherapy. Due to their profound effects on mental status, they should be used only under close patient supervision. Cannabinoids must be given *cautiously* to depressive, schizophrenic, or manic patients, to patients with heart disease or hypertension, and to patients receiving other psychoactive drugs. Their use should be avoided in pregnant women or nursing mothers. Dependence can occur, and a withdrawal syndrome (*e.g.*, irritability, insomnia, restlessness) has occurred within 12 hours after abrupt withdrawal of dronabinol. The likelihood of physical dependence with nabilone has not been adequately determined, but is probably similar to that of dronabinol.

INTERACTIONS

1. Enhanced CNS effects may occur with combined use of cannabinoids and alcohol, sedatives, hypnotics, or other psychotomimetic substances.

NURSING CONSIDERATIONS

The patient who considers street drug use a taboo may have difficulty using cannabinoids when he realizes their relationship to marijuana. The psychologic side-effects of giddiness and elation may rapidly progress to more disturbing effects, such as paranoia, and act as a deterrent for future use. It is necessary to discuss with the patient his feelings about the use of such drugs before subjecting him to it.

Clinical trials have found cannabinoids moderately effective but less useful for nausea and vomiting caused by cisplatin and doxorubicin than with other antineoplastic drugs. Evidence varies among tests, and some researchers believe the drugs may work better among patients who have had previous experience with marijuana, suggesting the importance of psychologic effect in the usefulness of cannabinoids.

REVIEW QUESTIONS

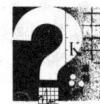

1. In what ways can the medullary vomiting center be stimulated?
2. What are the principal indications for the use of emetic drugs?
3. How does apomorphine cause emesis?
4. What is the difference between ipecac syrup and ipecac fluid extract?
5. Absorption of large amounts of ipecac can result in what type of toxicity?
6. List several classes of drugs that can function as antiemetics.
7. What environmental cues may trigger vomiting? How can the nurse help the patient to manipulate these factors?
8. What part do "home remedies" play in control of vomiting? How can the nurse use them to help the patient?
9. For what type of nausea and vomiting is scopolamine most effective?
10. What adverse reactions are most dangerous with large doses of diphenidol?
11. Briefly state how phosphorated carbohydrate solution relieves nausea and vomiting.
12. In what dosage forms is trimethobenzamide useful as an antiemetic?
13. What is the major danger in IM administration of trimethobenzamide? What actions can the nurse take to minimize its development?
14. Describe the major pharmacologic actions of metoclopramide.
15. List the principal indications of metoclopramide. In what conditions is its use contraindicated?
16. What type of drugs are dronabinol and nabilone? In which patients may they be most useful?
17. List the principal adverse reactions associated with use of dronabinol and nabilone.

BIBLIOGRAPHY

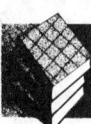

Albibi R, McCallom PW: Metoclopramide: Pharmacology and clinical application. Ann Intern Med 98:86, 1983

Barbezat GO: The vomiting patient: The rational approach. Drugs 22:246, 1981

DiGregorio GJ, Froncillo RJ: Antiemetics. Am Fam Physician 26(1):200, 1982

Fiori JJ, Gralla RJ: Pharmacologic treatment of chemotherapy-induced nausea and vomiting. Cancer Invest 2(5):351, 1984

Frytak S, Moertel CG: Management of nausea and vomiting in the cancer patient. JAMA 245:393, 1981

Hanson SJ, McCallum RW: The diagnosis and treatment of nausea and vomiting. Prac Gastroenterol 9(3):22, 1985

Schulze-Delrieu R: Drug therapy: Metoclopramide. N Engl J Med 305:28, 1981

Wood CD: Antimotion sickness and antiemetic drugs. Drugs 17:471, 1979

Wyman JB: The vomiting patient. Am Fam Physician 21:139, 1980

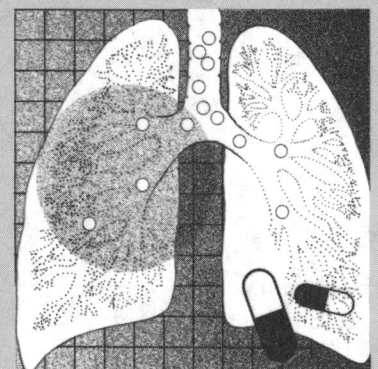

Drugs Affecting Respiratory Function

VII

Antitussives and Expectorants

Antitussives

Narcotic Antitussives
    Codeine
    Hydrocodone

Non-Narcotic Antitussives
    Benzonatate
    Dextromethorphan
    Diphenhydramine

Expectorants
    Ammonium Chloride
    Guaifenesin

Iodine Products
    Hydrogen Iodide
    Iodinated Glycerol
    Potassium Iodide
    Potassium Iodide/
      Niacinamide

Terpin Hydrate

Combination Cough Mixtures

47

Coughing is a protective mechanism initiated by chemical or mechanical stimulation of the tracheobronchial tree by which the body attempts to remove foreign particles or accumulated secretions from the respiratory tract. The cough reflex may be initiated by a number of factors, such as local inflammation of the bronchioles (e.g., smoking), mechanical or physical obstruction (e.g., foreign bodies, emboli), local or systemic disease states (e.g., pulmonary edema, bronchogenic carcinoma, or congestive heart failure), and emotional stress. To the extent that the cough is annoying or debilitating, proper drug therapy should be undertaken to eliminate the condition. Not all coughing is undesirable, however, and the productive type of cough that aids in removing excessive bronchiolar mucus in the form of sputum generally should not be suppressed. Of course, if the cough is secondary to some other disease, every effort should be made to identify and eliminate the underlying pathologic condition, such as pneumonia, bronchitis, or tuberculosis.

The most frequently employed drugs for the control of coughing may be divided into the *antitussives* and the *expectorants*. Antitussives are cough suppressants that may act centrally at the level of the "cough center" in the brain stem or peripherally at various sites along the tracheobronchial tree. Antitussives are primarily indicated in the treatment of annoying, dry, unproductive coughing, especially where it interferes with other functions (e.g., talking, sleeping) or leads to excessive weakness or progressive irritation.

Expectorants, on the other hand, increase and liquefy bronchial secretions. These drugs act either on the secretory glands of the respiratory tract or by irritation of the gastric mucosa, which reflexly increases respiratory secretions. They find their major clinical application in the treatment of obstructive pulmonary diseases associated with the accumulation of excessive tenacious mucus, where they may reduce the viscosity of bronchial secretions, thus facilitating elimination. They are also frequently employed in treating common respiratory disorders such as the common cold, as they are claimed to produce secretions which soothe inflamed mucosa and reduce dry, irritative coughing. There is doubt, however, as to the efficacy of the usual amounts of expectorants found in over-the-counter cough formulations in reducing bronchial irritation or lessening the severity of nonproductive coughing. Exposure to humidified air and especially adequate fluid intake have proven as effective as most expectorants in relieving nonpro-

ductive coughing, liquefying thick, tenacious mucus, and facilitating removal of respiratory secretions.

■ Nursing Process for Antitussives and Expectorants

□ ASSESSMENT

□ Subjective Data
Most of the products discussed below are available over the counter and with few exceptions are used to treat common cold symptoms. However, the nurse may have an opportunity to interact with an individual through an office visit or phone call and should make use of such time to facilitate careful drug taking by the patient.

Establish the cause of the cough. If it is related to cold or allergy symptoms, it may be self-limiting and the use of any of the OTC remedies may bring relief. Ask how long the cough has lasted. A history of cough for over 1 week may indicate a more serious problem, such as an infection and should be evaluated. Ask the individual to describe the cough. Is it wet and productive or dry and hacking? Either may be present with a cold, but the dry, hacking type is more common and irritating. Determine if there has been fever, associated pain (throat, head, chest), or other symptoms of infection or complicating illness.

A drug history is also important. Ask the patient what remedies he has already tried. Some home concoctions, frequently containing alcohol, are contraindicated with the use of narcotic antitussives, but other remedies may be useful to soothe irritated mucous membranes. Ask about the use of any drugs which might adversely interact with an antitussive (see under Interactions for specific drugs). Also ask about current use of street drugs. While the addiction potential to narcotic antitussives is fairly low, some patients do seek prescriptions from multiple physicians in order to obtain narcotics.

□ Objective Data
Assessment should include visual inspection of the nose and throat, palpation of head and neck lymph nodes, and a temperature. Lungs should be auscultated. In most cases there will be no evidence of crackling or rhonchi, and any moisture heard will be located in the upper respiratory tree. If rales are heard or there is an absence of sounds, the condition may be more serious.

□ *NURSING DIAGNOSES*

Actual nursing diagnoses may include:

Knowledge deficit related to drug action, dose, and side-effects

Alteration in respiratory function related to cough

Potential nursing diagnoses are generally related to side-effects which vary with each drug. Some examples may include:

Potential for injury: trauma related to drowsiness or dizziness

Sleep pattern disturbance if the drug is ineffective

Alteration in thought processes: excitation, a paradoxical drug effect

□ *PLAN*

The nursing care goals are to attempt to provide relief from coughing and to minimize side-effects from drug therapy.

□ *INTERVENTION*

Whatever remedy used, the nurse should encourage the patient to take only the recommended dosage because the incidence of side-effects increases if the doses are increased too much. With some of these drugs the side-effects are benign, but others may be dangerous. Patients who are not getting relief from a product may tend to overuse it to try to relieve the cough. Instead, suggest they try an-

other product or contact the physician for another prescription or further evaluation of the problem.

Many of the drugs cause drowsiness or dizziness, and patients should be warned to limit their activities until the effect of the drug is known. Children and elderly patients may have the opposite response of paradoxical excitation. They must also be observed closely, and dosages must be reduced as necessary.

The patient may enhance the effect of the drugs by drinking plenty of fluids, especially water, and increasing the humidity of his dwelling. This can be accomplished by a sophisticated ultrasonic nebulizer, a cool-mist vaporizer, or by placing pans of water close to heat sources. He may also find sucking on throat lozenges or hard candy helps. This action works by increasing saliva production which coats irritated mucous membranes. It may also work because the patient is more likely to keep his mouth closed while sucking which will reduce mucosal irritation and dryness caused by talking.

□ *EVALUATION*

The outcomes sought by the patient who takes an antitussive or expectorant are relief from coughing. In cases where this interferes with sleep or talking, reports of relief may also be a measure of success. Nursing Care Plan 47-1 contains a summary of the nursing process for the child receiving antitussives and expectorants. Care for the adult is similar.

Antitussives

The antitussive drugs are used to reduce the frequency of dry, unproductive coughing, and most act to depress the cough reflex by a direct inhibition of the cough center in the medulla. Drugs possessing antitussive activity can be divided into two groups, the narcotic and the non-narcotic cough suppressants. Although many narcotic drugs exhibit an antitussive action, most are unsuitable for use in controlling simple coughing as they are potent drugs with many adverse reactions and a significant danger of habituation. Of the many narcotic drugs available (see Chap. 22), only codeine and hydrocodone are routinely used for the relief of coughing, usually as a component of a combination product.

The non-narcotic antitussives are a structurally diverse group of pharmacologic agents that possess

a variety of both central and peripheral mechanisms of action. In most cases, they are nearly as effective as codeine, with a somewhat lower incidence of disturbing side-effects and a reduced likelihood of dependence. Because they have various mechanisms of action as well as different patterns of side-effects, they are discussed individually.

Narcotic Antitussives

Codeine is the most commonly used narcotic antitussive because it is very effective in reducing the frequency of coughing, but is much less likely to depress respiration or result in habituation than other narcotic agents. Although it is available in tablet form, it is most frequently administered as a component of liquid cough preparations, in which it may be combined with antihistamines, decongestants, expectorants, or analgesics.

Hydrocodone (dihydrocodeinone) is comparable to codeine in efficacy but is somewhat more habituating. It is not available for use *alone* but is found in a number of cough preparations in combination with expectorants, antihistamines, and decongestants. It is considered briefly in this chapter; however, the general information presented for codeine below applies to hydrocodone as well.

Codeine

MECHANISM AND ACTIONS
Codeine suppresses the cough reflex by exerting a depressant effect on the cough center in the medulla. Respiratory depressant effects are minimal at recommended doses.

USES
1. Suppression of nonproductive cough
2. Relief of mild to moderate pain (see Chap. 22)

ADMINISTRATION AND DOSAGE
Codeine is available as tablets (15 mg, 30 mg, 60 mg) of either the sulfate or phosphate salt, although for relief of coughing, it is most often used as a liquid preparation in combination with one or more ingredients. A list of representative codeine-containing cough preparations is presented in Table 47-1. Adults should receive 10 mg to 20 mg every 4 hours to 6 hours to a maximum of 120 mg/day. Children 6 years to 17 years are given 5 mg to 10 mg every 4 hours to 6 hours to a maximum of 60 mg/day, while younger children (2 years–6 years) may be given 2.5 mg to 5 mg every 4 hours to 6 hours, with a maximum of 30 mg/day.

FATE
Codeine is well absorbed orally, and effects are noted within 15 minutes to 30 minutes. The duration of action is approximately 3 hours to 4 hours. Codeine is metabolized in the liver and excreted primarily in the urine within 24 hours as metabolites. The plasma half-life of codeine is approximately 3 hours.

SIDE-EFFECTS/ADVERSE REACTIONS
The most frequently noted side-effects are lightheadedness, dizziness, sedation, sweating, nausea, and vomiting, and these occur with greater frequency at higher doses. Because codeine is a narcotic, a wide range of other adverse reactions can

occur during usage, especially in large amounts and over prolonged periods of time; these are listed below:

GI—Dry mouth, anorexia, constipation, biliary spasm

CNS—Euphoria, weakness, insomnia, headache, anxiety, fear, mood changes, disorientation, agitation, tremors, impaired physical performance, psychologic dependence, delirium, hallucinations, coma, miosis, visual disturbances, respiratory and cardiovascular depression (especially with large doses)

CV—Flushing, tachycardia, palpitations, hypotension

Other—Allergic reactions (rash, urticaria, pruritus, edema), urinary retention, decreased libido or potency, faintness, syncope, ureteral spasm

Serious overdosage is characterized by extreme miosis, cold and clammy skin, cyanosis, respiratory depression, somnolence, muscle flaccidity, stupor, and coma. Treatment is generally accomplished with naloxone (see Chap. 22).

CONTRAINDICATIONS AND PRECAUTIONS
Codeine should not be given to patients with known narcotic addiction, although the abuse potential of codeine is quite low compared to most other opiates. *Cautious use* of codeine is necessary in persons with asthma or other chronic obstructive pulmonary diseases, cardiac disease (including arrhythmias), convulsive disorders, renal or hepatic impairment, prostatic hypertrophy, severe CNS depression, acute abdominal conditions, toxic psychoses, head injuries, intracranial lesions, hypothyroidism, Addison's disease, and in alcoholics, pregnant women, and in elderly or debilitated patients.

INTERACTIONS
1. Increased CNS depression (*e.g.*, sedation, hypotension, respiratory depression) may occur if codeine is used in combination with alcohol, barbiturates, other narcotics, phenothiazines, and other drugs having a CNS depressant action. (See also Chap. 22 for other potential interactions of narcotic drugs.)

Hydrocodone

Hydrocodone (dihydrocodeinone) is a relatively weak analgesic and a strong antitussive found in combination with other agents, such as expecto-

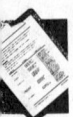

Assessment

Subjective Data	1. Medication history
	  a. See Interactions section to formulate pertinent questions
	  b. Remember to ask about specific remedies already tried. Because many are OTC drugs, they may be overlooked.
	  c. Sedative effect of codeine formulations is increased by simultaneous administration of CNS depressants, including alcohol.
	2. Medical history
	  a. Progression of cough symptoms
	  b. Age of child (these medications are not usually recommended for children under 2 years)
	  c. Pre-existing conditions that may contraindicate drug use or that warrant cautious use, such as respiratory disease, cardiovascular disease, renal disease, convulsive disorders, hepatic disease
	  d. Current pregnancy or lactation
	3. Personal history/compliance: Parent's past experience in getting child to take medication; use of folk remedies that may contain alcohol

Objective Data	1. Physical assessment: may not be obtained if OTC drugs are used. If completed, focus on
	  a. Vital signs, especially temperature
	  b. Respiratory examination
	  c. Head, neck, nose, and throat examination
	2. Laboratory data: not usually obtained. Guaifenesin may interfere with some lab values (see text).

Nursing Diagnosis	*Expected Client Outcome*	*Intervention*
Knowledge deficit: related to drug action, correct administration, and potential side-effects	Will verbalize knowledge of expected action, correct administration, and potential side-effects.	Explain that drug action of an antitussive will reduce cough but may not eliminate it. Expectorants will facilitate secretion removal. Encourage an increase in fluid intake to liquefy secretions and hydrate mucous membranes. Encourage patient/family to seek medical care if drug is ineffective or if cough persists over 1 week. Recommend drugs be used for short periods (1 week) and that dose *not* be increased if the drug is ineffective. Instead, seek physician recommendations and follow-up to avoid habituation and tolerance. Encourage patient/family to monitor temperature and report any elevation of 101°F or greater, which may indicate onset of more serious infection.
Potential for injury: trauma related to drowsiness from drug	Safety precautions will be maintained.	Teach family to monitor drowsiness within 1 hour of administration. Limit child's climbing and activity; attempt to interest child in sedentary play.

(continued)

Nursing Diagnosis	Expected Client Outcome	Intervention
Potential for injury: trauma related to drowsiness from drug (continued)		Notify physician if child seems excessively drowsy or is difficult to arouse from sleep. Dose may need adjustment.
Potential alteration in thought processes: related to paradoxical excitation from drug	Hyperactivity will be minimized.	Teach family to monitor irritability, crying, decreased attention span, and aggressive play and to contact physician if changes from norm occur. Dose may need to be reduced or drug may need to be discontinued.

rants and antihistamines in many cough formulations. It exhibits a relatively low degree of respiratory depression and physical dependence, although the likelihood of habituation appears to be greater than that of codeine. Commercial preparations containing hydrocodone include:

Entuss (with guaifenesin)
Hycodan (with homatropine)
Hycomine (with phenylpropanolamine)
Tussionex (with phenyltoloxamine)
Tussend (with pseudoephedrine and guaifenesin)

The recommended dosage for hydrocodone in these preparations is 5 mg up to four times a day. Refer to the preceding discussion of codeine for additional information regarding side-effects, precautions, and interactions.

NURSING CONSIDERATIONS FOR CODEINE AND HYDROCODONE

Although the danger of habituation with codeine or hydrocodone-containing cough syrups is relatively low, it can occur. Laws vary from state to state, but in most a patient who is 21 years old can sign for a codeine cough mixture which contains 60 mg of drug in 30 ml of fluid. The pharmacist can dispense only one bottle per patient in 48 hours and will usually ask the patient to seek medical attention at the time of a second request.

An individual can seek prescriptions from multiple care givers and have them filled at different pharmacies. In this manner, a patient who started out seeking cough relief may wind up habituated. Early signs for the patient and family to watch for include evidence that the cough mixture does not

Table 47-1
Codeine-Containing Cough Preparations

Trade Names	Other Ingredients
Actifed with Codeine	pseudoephedrine, triprolidine
Ambenyl	bromodiphenhydramine
Cheracol	guaifenesin
Dimetane-DC	brompheniramine, phenylpropanolamine
Isoclor Expectorant	guaifenesin, pseudoephedrine
Naldecon-CX	guaifenesin, phenylpropanolamine
Novahistine Expectorant	guaifenesin, pseudoephedrine
Nucofed	pseudoephedrine
Phenergan with Codeine	promethazine
Phenergan VC with Codeine	promethazine, phenylephrine
Robitussin A-C	guaifenesin
Terpin Hydrate with Codeine	terpin hydrate
Tussar-2	guaifenesin, chlorpheniramine, carbetapentane
Tussi-Organidin	iodinated glycerol

provide relief for the expected time period, and restlessness and agitation on the part of the individual. If possible, this is when the patient should seek help to avert more serious side-effects.

If the drug is given in tablet form, the patient should be encouraged to drink fluids to facilitate liquefication of secretions. If, however, the medication is given in liquid form, no fluids should be taken for at least a half hour after taking the drug.

One bothersome side-effect of codeine use is constipation. Encourage increased fluid intake, bulk and fiber foods, and use of a stool softener or bulk laxative if needed.

Non-Narcotic Antitussives

Benzonatate
(Tessalon Perles)

MECHANISM AND ACTIONS
Benzonatate is structurally related to tetracaine and exerts a local anesthetic action on stretch receptors in the respiratory passages, lungs, and pleural cavity. As a result, the activity of these receptors is suppressed and the cough reflex is dampened. The drug does not appear to alter the function of the respiratory center at recommended doses.

USES
1. Symptomatic relief of nonproductive cough

ADMINISTRATION AND DOSAGE
Benzonatate is used as capsules containing 100 mg. The recommended dosage is 100 mg three times a day to a maximum of 600 mg/day.

FATE
The onset of action following oral administration is within 15 minutes to 20 minutes, and the cough suppressive effects persist for 3 hours to 6 hours.

SIDE-EFFECTS/ADVERSE REACTIONS
Adverse reactions can include sedation, dizziness, nasal congestion, constipation, nausea, GI upset, pruritus, skin eruptions, burning in the eyes, a "chilly" sensation, and numbness in the chest. Large doses can lead to CNS stimulation (restlessness, tremor, convulsions).

CONTRAINDICATIONS AND PRECAUTIONS
Benzonatate is contraindicated in persons who are allergic to tetracaine or related local anesthetics.

The drug should be used *cautiously* in pregnant women or nursing mothers. Capsules should be swallowed whole and not chewed because release of the drug in the mouth can anesthetize the oral mucosa.

NURSING CONSIDERATIONS
See Nursing Process for Antitussives and Expectorants.

Dextromethorphan
(Benylin DM, Congespirin Liquid, Cremacoat 1, Delsym, DM Cough, Hold, Mediquell, Pediacare 1, Pertussin, St. Joseph Cough, Sucrets Cough Control)

Dextromethorphan is a widely used non-narcotic antitussive with minimal CNS depressant action and no analgesic effect. Its administration is unlikely to produce constipation or result in tolerance. It is commonly found in over-the-counter cough formulations, frequently combined with antihistamines, decongestants, and expectorants. A 30-mg dose of dextromethorphan is approximately equivalent to 15 mg of codeine in relieving coughing.

MECHANISM AND ACTIONS
The precise mechanism of action of dextromethorphan is unknown. The drug appears to exert a depressant effect on the medullary cough center.

USES
1. Control of nonproductive cough

ADMINISTRATION AND DOSAGE
Dextromethorphan is available as lozenges (5 mg), chewy squares (15 mg), syrup (5 mg/5 ml, 7.5 mg/5 ml, 10 mg/5 ml, 15 mg/5 ml), and a controlled-release suspension (i.e., Delsym; 30 mg/5 ml). Dextromethorphan is also available in combination with benzocaine in various dosages as throat lozenges (Formula 44 Cough Control Discs, Spec-T, Vicks Cough Silencers). The dosage schedules for the various preparations are as follows:
Lozenges/Syrup
    Adults: 10 mg to 30 mg every 4 hours to 8 hours; maximum 120 mg/24 hours
    Children (6 years–12 years): 5 mg to 10 mg every 4 hours or 15 mg every 6 hours to 8 hours; maximum 60 mg/24 hours
    Children (2 years–6 years): 2.5 mg to 5 mg every 4 hours or 7.5 mg every 6 hours to 8 hours; maximum 30 mg/24 hours

Controlled-Release Liquid (Delsym)
    Adults: 60 mg twice a day
    Children (6 years–12 years): 30 mg twice a day
    Children (2 years–6 years): 15 mg twice a day

FATE

The onset of action is within 15 minutes to 30 minutes, and the antitussive effects persist 3 hours to 6 hours depending on the dose (up to 12 hours with controlled release liquid).

SIDE-EFFECTS/ADVERSE REACTIONS

Side-effects are minimal with dextromethorphan; occasionally, use of the drug can result in gastric distress, drowsiness, or dizziness.

CONTRAINDICATIONS AND PRECAUTIONS

Dextromethorphan should not be given to persons with a chronic, persistent cough or with a cough associated with excessive secretions. It should not be used in combination with MAO inhibitors because hyperpyrexia, muscular rigidity, and hypotension can occur. *Cautious use* of dextromethorphan should be undertaken in persons with chronic obstructive pulmonary disease, high fever, persistent headache, or vomiting; these symptoms may indicate underlying conditions that require proper diagnosis and treatment.

Diphenhydramine
(Benylin and various other manufacturers)

Diphenhydramine is an antihistamine (see Chap. 18) that is used as a syrup to control coughing due to colds or allergies. It is available as a syrup containing 12.5 mg/5 ml or 13.3 mg/5 ml. Oral dosage is 25 mg every 4 hours for adults, and 6.25 mg to 12.5 mg every 4 hours for children. The major side-effect with diphenhydramine is drowsiness. The drug is also found in 25-mg and 50-mg strengths as the principal ingredient in over-the-counter sleep aids such as Nytol, Sleep-Eze 3, Sominex 2, Compoz, and Twilite.

Expectorants

Expectorants are claimed to facilitate removal of viscous mucus from the respiratory tree and provide a soothing, demulcent action on the respiratory mucosa by stimulating secretion of a lubricating fluid. While large doses of certain prescription-only expectorants (such as potassium iodide) may decrease the tenacity of mucus associated with chronic obstructive pulmonary diseases, the efficacy of most other nonprescription expectorants is subject to considerable debate. They are probably no more effective in providing relief of bronchial irritation or facilitating mucus liquefaction than high fluid intake, that is, 6 to 10 glasses/day, and humidification of the environment. There is little support for the claim that expectorants relieve dry, irritative coughing by increasing production of a soothing fluid any more than would be produced by use of a cough drop or throat lozenge. Therefore, their inclusion in cough/cold formulations containing antitussives, antihistamines, and decongestants among other medications is probably an example of therapeutic overkill.

On the other hand, adverse reactions are rare at usual therapeutic doses, the most frequent complaint being GI distress. Thus, the drugs are quite safe when taken as directed, and if patients believe the compounds are effective, it may be difficult to convince them otherwise.

Ammonium Chloride

Ammonium chloride is primarily used as a systemic and urinary acidifier to treat metabolic alkalosis, to correct chloride depletion, and to assist in the urinary excretion of certain basic drugs. These indications are considered in Chapter 78. The drug has also been used as an expectorant and is found in a number of over-the-counter cough preparations, although its efficacy is subject to considerable doubt and its use in this manner should be discouraged.

The action of ammonium chloride is apparently mediated by an irritating action on the GI mucosa, which elicits a reflex stimulation of respiratory secretions. Average adult dosage when used as a component of proprietary combination products is 100 mg to 200 mg several times a day.

GI upset is common with oral administration of ammonium chloride. Too large doses can result in metabolic acidosis, which is characterized by vomiting, thirst, weakness, lethargy, confusion, and hyperventilation.

The excretion of basic drugs (*e.g.*, amphetamines, antidepressants, antihistamines, anti-anxiety agents, catecholamines, narcotic analgesics, quinidine, theophylline) may be enhanced by ammonium chloride, whereas the systemic actions of acidic drugs (*e.g.*, barbiturates, clofibrate, mercurial diuretics, pyrazolones, salicylates, oral antidiabetics, thyroid hormones) may be potentiated by ammonium chloride, because their renal excretion may be retarded.

Guaifenesin
(Breonesin, Cremacoat 2, Robitussin, and various other manufacturers)

MECHANISM AND ACTIONS
Guaifenesin, formerly known as glyceryl guaicolate, is the most commonly used over-the-counter expectorant. The drug is believed to increase output of respiratory tract fluid by reducing its adhesiveness and surface tension, thus facilitating removal of mucus. The increased fluid flow is also claimed to soothe dry, irritated membranes, thereby relieving dry, hacking cough. Large doses may have a gastric stimulant action. There is *no* evidence that the drug is effective.

USES
1. Symptomatic relief of dry, unproductive coughing associated with common respiratory disorders, such as colds, bronchitis, bronchial asthma (efficacy not conclusively established)

ADMINISTRATION AND DOSAGE
Guaifenesin is used as tablets (100 mg, 200 mg), capsules (200 mg), sustained-release tablets (600 mg), and most frequently as a syrup containing either 67 mg/5 ml or 100 mg/5 ml. Dosage recommendations are as follows:
   Adults: 100 mg to 400 mg every 3 hours to 6
      hours; maximum 1.2 g/day
   Children (6 years–12 years): 100 mg to 200
      mg every 4 hours; maximum 600 mg/day
   Children (2 years–6 years): 50 mg to 100 mg
      every 4 hours; maximum 300 mg/day

SIDE-EFFECTS/ADVERSE REACTIONS
Side-effects are generally rare with ordinary doses of guaifenesin. There have been occasional reports of nausea, GI distress, drowsiness, and vomiting. Decreased platelet aggregation may occur during guaifenesin treatment, but it is rarely of clinical significance.

CONTRAINDICATIONS AND PRECAUTIONS
Guaifenesin should not be given for prolonged periods of time, especially if cough persists or recurs frequently or if it is accompanied by high fever, rash, or headache. Guaifenesin may cause color interference with laboratory determinations of 5-hydroxyindoleacetic acid (a serotonin metabolite) and vanillylmandelic acid (a catecholamine metabolite). The drug should be discontinued several days before these laboratory tests are performed.

NURSING CONSIDERATIONS
(See Nursing Process for Antitussive and Expectorants.)

Iodine Products

Hydrogen Iodide
(Hydriodic Acid)

Iodinated Glycerol
(Iophen, Organidin, R-Gen Elixir)

Potassium Iodide
(Pima and other manufacturers)

Potassium Iodide/Niacinamide
(Iodo-Niacin)

Several iodine-containing preparations are used as expectorants, although their clinical efficacy is subject to doubt. In addition, they have the potential to cause a number of adverse reactions, and many persons display allergic reactions to iodine-containing drugs. Iodinated glycerol is claimed to be less irritating to the GI tract than other iodides, but is probably less effective as well.

MECHANISM AND ACTIONS
Iodides enhance the secretion of respiratory fluid and may decrease the viscosity and tenacity of mucus. They may also facilitate breakdown of fibrous material at inflammatory sites and stimulate digestion of mucoprotein.

USES
1. Adjunctive treatment of respiratory conditions associated with increased mucus, such as bron-

chitis, asthma, emphysema, and cystic fibrosis, and following surgery to help prevent atelectasis (efficacy not conclusively established)

ADMINISTRATION AND DOSAGE

Potassium iodide is available as enteric-coated tablets (300 mg), liquid (500 mg/15 ml), syrup (325 mg/5 ml), and as a saturated solution (1 g/ml). It is also available in combination with niacinamide (135 mg/25 mg) as tablets. Hydrogen iodide is used as a syrup (70 mg/5 ml), while iodinated glycerol is available as tablets (30 mg), elixir (60 mg/5 ml), and sugar-free solution (50 mg/ml). Iodinated glycerol is also used in combination products such as Theo-Organidin (with theophylline), Tussi-Organidin (with codeine), or Tussi-Organidin DM (with dextromethorphan).

Recommended doses are as follows:

Potassium Iodide

Adults—300 mg to 600 mg every 4 hours to 6 hours

Children—150 mg to 300 mg every 4 hours to 6 hours

Hydrogen Iodide

Adults—70 mg three to four times a day

Iodinated Glycerol

Adults—60 mg four times a day

Children—Up to one half adult dosage based on weight

Potassium Iodide/Niacinamide

Adults—2 tablets three times a day

Dilute liquid formulations in plenty of water or juice and encourage increased fluid intake with all formulations. Measure children's doses carefully in drops.

FATE

Iodides are absorbed in conjunction with amino acids. They accumulate in the thyroid gland and attain higher levels in gastric and salivary secretions than in extracellular fluids. Iodides are excreted chiefly by the kidney.

SIDE-EFFECTS/ADVERSE REACTIONS

Side-effects seen with iodides include GI distress, nausea, epigastric pain, diarrhea, sore throat, metallic taste, mucosal ulceration, sneezing, coryza, and increased salivation. Hypersensitivity to iodides may be manifested as fever, arthralgia, angioedema, cutaneous and mucosal bleeding, lymph node enlargement, and eosinophilia. Large doses can lead to thyroid adenoma, goiter, and myxedema.

CONTRAINDICATIONS AND PRECAUTIONS

Iodides are contraindicated in the presence of hyperthyroidism, hyperkalemia, and acute bronchitis, and in persons hypersensitive to iodides. Iodide administration should be undertaken *cautiously* in persons with goiter, high fever, persistent cough, inflammatory bowel lesions, cystic fibrosis, tuberculosis, acne, dermatoses, and in pregnant women or nursing mothers. Enteric-coated preparations have resulted in small bowel lesions leading to hemorrhage, obstruction, and perforation. Iodide preparations may interfere with laboratory determinations of protein-bound iodine.

INTERACTIONS

1. The hypothyroid and goitrogenic effects of potassium iodide may be potentiated by lithium or other antithyroid drugs.
2. Iodide-induced hyperkalemia can be intensified by potassium supplements or potassium-sparing diuretics (see Chap. 41).

Terpin Hydrate

Terpin hydrate is used in liquid form to stimulate respiratory secretions, presumably by a direct action on respiratory tract secretory glands. The drug is occasionally used alone (85 mg every 3 hours–4 hours) for minor bronchial irritations but is most frequently employed in combination with codeine (85 mg/10 mg per 5 ml) as terpin hydrate and codeine elixir for control of minor coughing. This preparation contains approximately 40% alcohol and may cause drowsiness. Gastric upset can occur, especially if it is given on an empty stomach. A glass of water should be taken after each dose to facilitate loosening of mucus.

Combination Cough Mixtures

Although this chapter has dealt with individual antitussive and expectorant drugs, the most frequent use of these products, as indicated, is in combination cough mixtures. Such formulations may contain several other types of drugs, in addition to an antitussive and an expectorant. The most commonly used of these other agents are listed below, along with the rationale for their inclusion.

1. Analgesics
   For example, aspirin, acetaminophen, sodium salicylate; used to provide relief of headache, fever, and muscle aches often accompanying an upper respiratory condition (see Chap. 23)
2. Anticholinergics
   For example, atropine, belladonna alkaloids, methscopolamine; employed for their drying action on mucous membranes; thus are only beneficial in conditions characterized by excessive secretions (e.g., rhinorrhea); should be avoided in chronic obstructive pulmonary diseases (see Chap. 23)
3. Antihistamines
   For example, chlorpheniramine, pyrilamine; provide symptomatic relief of running nose, sneezing, itching, watery eyes; may be effective in relieving chronic cough resulting from postnasal drip (e.g., allergic rhinitis, chronic sinusitis); exhibit an anticholinergic (drying) action, therefore should not be used in respiratory conditions characterized by excessive congestion; most have a sedative effect (see Chap. 18)
4. Bronchodilators
   For example, ephedrine, theophylline; relax bronchiolar smooth muscle, thus are of great-

est benefit in conditions characterized by excessive bronchiolar muscle tone (e.g., asthma) rather than mucus accumulation (see Chap. 48)
5. Decongestants
   For example, phenylephrine, phenylpropanolamine, pseudoephedrine; used to reduce mucosal congestion by activating alpha-adrenergic receptor sites, thus eliciting vasoconstriction; probably not significantly effective and can lead to systemic side-effects (e.g., hypertension) (see Chap. 15)

The principal disadvantage of combination products is that the fixed dosage ratio of the ingredients precludes individualization of the dosage of each drug according to the needs of the patient. Moreover, the "shotgun" approach to drug therapy—inclusion of several different kinds of drugs in one preparation—is usually unnecessary from a therapeutic standpoint and most often simply increases the likelihood of untoward reactions without significantly improving the desired therapeutic effect. Finally, the cost of combination formulas is frequently in excess of the cost of the necessary individual ingredients used separately. Nevertheless, antitussive and expectorant combinations remain the most widely used over-the-counter preparations for the relief of cough, and it is essential that users of such medications be advised of the potential hazards inherent in the indiscriminate consumption of these readily available cough mixtures.

REVIEW QUESTIONS

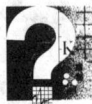

1. How do antitussives differ from expectorants in their pharmacologic actions?
2. What other measures can a patient take to reduce cough symptoms in conjunction with drug therapy?
3. What steps should a patient take if relief is not obtained from the cough mixture currently being used?
4. What is the most frequently used narcotic antitussive? What are its advantages over other narcotic drugs in relieving cough?
5. List several side-effects associated with use of codeine.
6. Mention several other kinds of drugs found in combination with codeine in commercially available cough preparations.

7. Briefly describe the mechanism of action of benzonatate in suppressing cough.
8. What is the most widely used non-narcotic cough suppressant? In what dosage forms is it available?
9. How do expectorants act to remove excess mucus secretions?
10. List several expectorants in clinical use. Which is the most commonly used expectorant in combination cough/cold preparations?
11. What are the dangers associated with use of iodides as expectorants?

BIBLIOGRAPHY

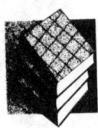

Eigen H: The clinical evaluation of chronic cough. Ped Clin North Am 29:67, 1982

Kuhn JJ, Hendley JO, Adams KF, Clark JW, Gwaltney JM: Antitussive effect of guaifenesin in young adults with natural colds: Objective and subjective assessment. Chest 82:713, 1982

Mullan PA: Cough/cold preparations. Am Pharmacy 21:42, 1981

Zanjanian MH: Expectorants and antitussive agents: Are they helpful? Ann Allergy 44:290, 1980

Bronchodilators

48

Drugs capable of relaxing bronchiolar smooth muscle (*i.e.*, dilating the bronchioles) have their principal clinical application in three common respiratory disorders: bronchial asthma, chronic bronchitis, and emphysema. Although these three diseases differ in etiology and overall pathology, they share one important common characteristic, namely, a reduced respiratory flow due to obstructed airways.

In order to better understand the action of drugs affecting bronchiolar function, a brief review of respiratory physiology will be presented.

Respiratory Physiology

Anatomy–Histology

The respiratory system has two major functional divisions: the conducting division and the respiratory division.

CONDUCTING DIVISION

The components of the conducting division serve primarily as air conduits to the gas-exchanging areas of the lungs. During its passage through the upper segments of the conducting division, the air is filtered, warmed, and humidified. Components of the conducting division are the nose, pharynx, larynx, trachea, bronchi, bronchioles, and terminal bronchioles.

RESPIRATORY DIVISION

The respiratory bronchioles, alveolar ducts, alveolar sacs, and alveoli form the respiratory division of the lungs wherein the oxygen-rich, water-saturated air is exposed to the blood for gaseous exchange.

THE RESPIRATORY TREE

During inspiration the air passes through the nose (or mouth), pharynx, and larynx before entering the trachea. The trachea is structurally characterized by the presence of 16 to 20 C-shaped rings of hyaline cartilage (completed posteriorly by smooth muscle and connective tissue), which support the trachea and keep it patent. The tissue lining the trachea is pseudostratified ciliated epithelium with goblet cells. The trachea terminates in the thorax by dividing into two primary bronchi that pass to the roots of the lungs. The right bronchus is shorter, wider, and more vertical than the left.

Within the lungs, the primary bronchi undergo successive branching to form a tree-like arrangement of smaller bronchi and bronchioles, often called the *bronchial tree.* The successive branching within the bronchial tree results in the formation of successively narrower tubes that collectively offer a greater total cross-sectional area of the lumina than the parent tubes.

The following histologic modifications occur with progressive branching:

1. The rings of cartilage are replaced by irregular plates of cartilage that gradually become smaller and finally disappear in the bronchioles.
2. As the amount of cartilage decreases, the amount of smooth muscle progressively increases. The smooth muscle layer plays a major role in determining the airway resistance because it governs the caliber of the bronchioles (which no longer have cartilage rings to maintain tubular patency).
3. The pseudostratified ciliated epithelium loses its goblet cells and then the cilia and is eventually replaced by simple cuboidal epithelium in the terminal bronchioles.

Arising from the terminal bronchioles are the first components of the respiratory division—the respiratory bronchioles—whose free terminations open into alveolar ducts. The alveolar ducts communicate with spaces called *alveolar sacs*, which in turn open into a number of pocket-like expansions, the alveoli.

Histologically, the smooth muscle prominent in the latter segments of the conducting division is replaced by elastic connective tissue within the respiratory division.

The respiratory epithelium loses its cilia and thins out to a single squamous configuration, thus allowing gaseous exchange to occur. Increasing vascularity and a greater cross-sectional surface area further promote efficient exchange of gases. It has been estimated that human lungs contain approximately 300 million alveoli and provide a total surface area of 70 m^2 for gaseous exchange.

THE LUNGS

All the components of the respiratory tract beyond the primary bronchi are contained within the lungs. The lungs are cone-shaped, paired structures located in the thoracic cavity, surrounded by a cage-like framework composed of the sternum, costal cartilage, ribs, and vertebrae. The muscular, dome-shaped diaphragm serves as the floor of the thoracic cage.

Blood vessels, lymphatics, nerves, and the bronchi enter the lungs at the hilus and form the root of the lung. The parietal pleura, which lines the thoracic cavity, and the visceral pleura, which

923

covers the lung surface, are continuous serous membranes that reflect upon each other at the root of each lung. The potential space between these two membranes (the pleural cavity) contains a thin film of lubricating fluid that minimizes friction during respiratory movements.

The right lung contains three lobes and the left lung contains two lobes, each of which is supplied by a secondary (or lobar) bronchus. Each lung is further subdivided into bronchopulmonary segments supplied by tertiary (or segmental) bronchi.

Each bronchopulmonary segment contains smaller anatomical units called *lobules*, supplied by a terminal bronchiole, arteriole, venule, and lymphatic vessel.

BLOOD SUPPLY

The pulmonary artery and its branches carry blood from the right ventricle of the heart to the respiratory tissue of the lung for oxygenation and removal of CO_2. Venules, arising from the vast network of pulmonary capillaries that surround the alveoli, collect oxygenated blood, which is then returned to the left atrium of the heart by the pulmonary veins.

Oxygenated blood reaches the visceral pleura and other portions of the lung through the bronchial arteries and their branches. Some bronchial veins empty into the superior vena cava through the azygos system, while others drain into the pulmonary veins.

In contrast to the systemic circulation, the pulmonary circulation is a low-pressure, low-resistance circuit.

NERVE SUPPLY

The bronchial tree is innervated by fibers from both divisions of the autonomic nervous system. Activation of parasympathetic (vagal) nerve fibers causes contraction of respiratory smooth muscle, whereas sympathetic stimulation brings about relaxation.

Autonomic nerves also supply pulmonary and bronchial blood vessels.

Respiratory Defense Mechanisms

Large particulate matter inhaled through the nares (nostrils) is filtered by the coarse hairs lining the nasal vestibule. A blanket of mucus (secreted by goblet cells and mucous glands in the upper respiratory tract) traps dust and fine particulate matter. The mucus and entrapped materials are swept toward the mouth by ciliary movements. The cough reflex provides a more forceful mechanism for the expulsion of secretions and particulate matter from the respiratory tract.

Alveolar macrophages ("dust cells") provide a major defense against bacterial invasion of the lungs. These unique phagocytic cells migrate freely over the alveolar surface, engulfing and lysing bacteria and other particulate matter.

Pulmonary Ventilation

Pulmonary ventilation operates on the principle that the pressure and volume of a closed cavity are inversely related. Therefore, if the volume of a closed cavity increases, the pressure within it will fall.

The lungs lie in separate air-tight cavities within the thorax, surrounded by the pleura. The elastic recoil of the lungs tends to pull them away from the thoracic wall, creating a partial vacuum within the pleural cavity. The flow of air through the respiratory tract follows pressure gradients between the atmosphere and the lungs. Just before inspiration, the pressure inside the lungs (the intrapulmonary pressure) is equal to atmospheric pressure, whereas the pressure within the pleural cavity (the intrapleural pressure) is always below atmospheric.

Inspiration is an active process resulting from the expansion of the thorax. It is initiated by nervous activity leading to the contraction of respiratory muscles. During normal quiet inspiration the contraction and descent of the diaphragm increase the vertical dimensions of the thoracic cavity, while contraction of the external intercostal muscles widens the thorax by elevating the ribs and sternum. The lungs expand as they follow the movements of the thoracic wall because the surface tension generated by the serous fluid in the pleural cavity causes the visceral and parietal pleura to adhere closely, much as two moist plates of glass resist separation.

As the lungs expand and the pulmonary volume increases, the intrapulmonary pressure falls below atmospheric, creating a pressure gradient that causes air to flow from the atmosphere through the conducting passageways into the lungs. As the lungs expand, elastic components of the lung stretch and develop tension.

Quiet expiration occurs passively through relaxation of the inspiratory muscles. As the diaphragm ascends and the ribs and sternum return to their resting positions, the size of the thoracic cavity decreases. As the thorax assumes its original size, the potential energy stored in the elastic elements of the lung is converted into kinetic energy. These events cause the intrapulmonary pressure temporarily to exceed the atmospheric pressure, thus reversing the flow of air.

Accessory muscles of respiration include the scalene and pectoralis minor, which contract during forceful inspiration to further expand the thorax. During active, forceful expiration, coughing, or vomiting, the internal intercostal muscles contract to pull the ribs downward and inward, while the abdominal muscles contract to push the diaphragm upward.

RESPIRATORY COMPLIANCE

Respiratory compliance, which may be defined as the lung volume change per unit of pressure, is a term often used to describe the ease with which the lungs may be inflated. Two major factors that affect respiratory compliance are surface tension and resistance to airflow.

Surface Tension

Surface tension is a phenomenon resulting from the forces of attraction between molecules on a fluid surface at a liquid–gas interface. The inner surface of the alveoli is coated with a thin film of fluid that exerts a surface tension tending to impair expansion of alveoli on inspiration (and favor collapse on expiration).

The surface tension and tendency for collapse are particularly great in the smaller alveoli. Normally, the alveolar septal (type II) cells secrete a lipoprotein surfactant that reduces the surface tension and lowers the resistance of the alveoli to expansion on inspiration. Pulmonary surfactant therefore increases respiratory compliance and reduces the work required for breathing.

A deficiency of pulmonary surfactant characterizes respiratory distress syndrome (also known as *hyaline membrane disease*), a condition often afflicting premature infants.

Resistance to Airflow

Any obstruction or resistance to the flow of air would increase the force required to bring air into the alveoli. Airway resistance is encountered chiefly in the bronchi and bronchioles. It can be increased by the contraction of respiratory smooth muscle (bronchoconstriction) or by swelling of the respiratory mucosa (mucosal edema).

Reflex bronchoconstriction may follow mechanical or chemical stimulation of airway receptors. Parasympathetic stimulation, acetylcholine, histamine, prostaglandins F and D, and leukotrienes can cause bronchoconstriction. Sympathetic stimulation, cyclic adenosine monophosphate (AMP), and prostaglandins E and I_2 are effective bronchorelaxants.

EXCHANGE AND TRANSPORT OF RESPIRATORY GASES

In a mixture of gases (such as the atmosphere), the portion of the total pressure contributed by a particular gas in the mixture is termed the *partial pressure* or *tension*. The partial pressure exerted by each individual gas varies directly with its concentration in the mixture. For example, O_2, which makes up approximately 21% of atmospheric air, exerts a partial pressure (PO_2) of 160 mm Hg under standard total atmospheric pressure of 760 mm Hg, that is, $0.21 \times 760 = 160$.

Atmospheric (inspired) air is composed primarily of nitrogen and O_2 with very small amounts of CO_2, water vapor, and inert gases. Alveolar air differs from atmospheric air in composition because the inspired air becomes saturated with water vapor and mixed with old anatomical deadspace air during its passage through the conducting components of the respiratory tract. Alveolar PO_2 is 100 mm Hg in contrast with the atmospheric PO_2 of 160 mm Hg.

The exchange of gases within the body occurs through diffusion, with each gas diffusing according to its partial pressure gradient. As shown in Figure 48-1, pressure gradients cause O_2 to diffuse from the alveoli into the blood, and from the blood into the tissues. The pressure gradients are reversed for CO_2, causing it to diffuse from the tissues into the blood and subsequently into the alveoli.

Within the alveoli, large volumes of water-saturated air are exposed to a vast volume of blood to effect efficient exchange of gases. Pulmonary venous blood is not maximally oxygenated because alveolar ventilation and perfusion are not uniform throughout the lung. During normal ventilation (in an upright person at rest) the lower (basal) segments of the lungs receive a relatively greater blood flow than the upper (apical) portions due to gravitational forces. Most respiratory disorders are characterized by even greater ventilation–perfusion inequalities. Possible pathologic causes of uneven ventilation include obstruction of airways (as in asthma), altered elasticity of airways (as in advanced emphysema), and reduced pulmonary expansion (as in atelectasis). Uneven capillary perfu-

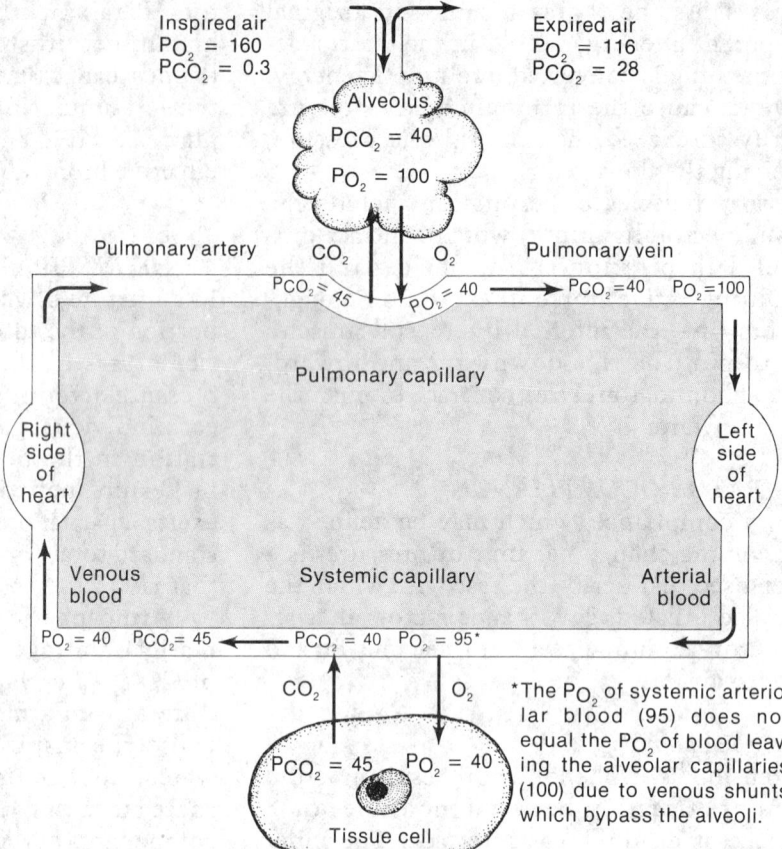

Figure 48-1. Gaseous exchange according to partial pressure gradients.

sion may result from shunts, embolization, and compression of pulmonary blood vessels.

During pulmonary exchange of gases, O_2 and CO_2 must diffuse across a functional respiratory membrane composed of the following: (1) alveolar membrane, (2) interstitial fluid, (3) capillary endothelium and basement membrane, (4) plasma, and (5) erythrocyte (red blood cell) membrane.

The rate at which O_2 diffuses from the alveoli into the blood depends on (1) the partial pressure gradient for oxygen, (2) the total functional surface area of the alveolar and capillary membranes, (3) the thickness of the respiratory membrane, and (4) the ventilation–perfusion ratio.

The diffusion of a gas into a liquid medium, such as plasma, depends on the partial pressure gradient and the solubility of the gas in that fluid. Immediately on entering the blood, the respiratory gases dissolve in the fluid portion of blood—the plasma (CO_2 is about 20 times more soluble in plasma than is O_2).

Erythrocytes play an essential role in the transport of both O_2 and CO_2 because mere physical solution of these gases in blood plasma would not be adequate to meet even minimal body needs. The gas-carrying capacity of blood is greatly increased by rapidly reversible chemical reactions that remove O_2 and CO_2 from solution, thus steepening their gradients for diffusion.

Oxygen Transport

The amount of O_2 in the blood is essentially determined by three factors: (1) the amount of O_2 dissolved in the plasma, (2) the amount of hemoglobin (Hb) in the blood, and (3) the affinity of Hb for O_2.

Normally, the amount of O_2 physically dissolved in plasma is very small because of its low solubility in this fluid. Most (approximately 98%) of the O_2 in the blood is transported in combination with Hb, a conjugated protein present in erythrocytes. Hb contains four iron atoms, each of which can reversibly bind one molecule of oxygen. While the oxygenation of Hb occurs in a stepwise fashion, the overall process is generally represented by the simple equation

$$Hb + O_2 \rightarrow HbO_2$$
$$\text{(hemoglobin)} \quad \text{(oxygen)} \quad \text{(oxyhemoglobin)}$$

When fully saturated with the gas, each gram of Hb can hold 1.34 ml of O_2. At an average Hb concentration of 15 g per 100 ml of blood, the O_2-carrying capacity of Hb is 20.1 volumes percent (15 × 1.34).

In arterial blood, Hb is 97% saturated with O_2, whereas in venous blood the degree of saturation falls to 75%. The color of Hb reflects the degree of its saturation with O_2. HbO_2 is bright crimson, explaining the bright red color of arterial blood, whereas reduced Hb is dark purple, imparting a port-wine color to venous blood.

The affinity of Hb for O_2 is greatly affected by the P_{O_2}. When the P_{O_2} is high, as it is in the lungs, Hb binds large amounts of O_2 and becomes nearly saturated with it. In the tissue capillaries, where P_{O_2} is substantially lower, the affinity of Hb for O_2 is reduced, and O_2 is released for diffusion into the tissues.

The amount of O_2 in combination with Hb also depends on the P_{CO_2}, pH, and temperature of the blood. Under conditions of increased P_{CO_2}, low pH (acidity), or elevated temperature of the blood, the amount of O_2 that binds to hemoglobin at any given P_{O_2} is diminished.

The reduced affinity of Hb for O_2 that occurs when blood pH falls is termed the *Bohr effect*. The pH of the blood falls as its CO_2 content increases because CO_2 combines with water to form carbonic acid (H_2CO_3), which rapidly dissociates into hydrogen (H^+) and bicarbonate ions (HCO_3^-), as shown below:

$$CO_2 + H_2O \leftrightharpoons H_2CO_3 \leftrightharpoons H^+ + HCO_3^-$$

Another metabolic factor that favors the dissociation of O_2 from Hb is 2,3-diphosphoglycerate (2,3-DPG), an organic phosphate present in erythrocytes that binds to Hb and decreases its affinity for O_2. Erythrocyte 2,3-DPG concentration increases during prolonged exercise, anemia, and in various diseases marked by chronic hypoxia.

As the O_2 dissociates from Hb, it becomes available for diffusion into tissue cells. Metabolically active tissues tend to accumulate CO_2 and acidic metabolites and undergo temperature elevation—conditions that favor O_2 dissociation from Hb and increase availability of O_2 to the tissue cells.

Carbon Dioxide Transport

CO_2, a principal end product of cellular metabolism, diffuses from the tissues into the blood for transport to the lungs (for elimination). It is transported by the blood in three forms as follows:

1. Dissolved in the plasma
2. As carbamino compounds
3. As bicarbonate ions

CO_2 is highly soluble in plasma and nearly 10% of the total CO_2 in the blood is carried in physical solution within the plasma.

Approximately 20% of blood CO_2 combines with amino groups of various blood proteins (principally Hb) to form carbamino compounds. Some of the CO_2 that diffuses from the plasma into the erythrocytes combines with Hb to form the compound carbaminohemoglobin. However, most of the CO_2 in the erythrocytes is readily hydrated in the presence of carbonic anhydrase enzyme, forming H_2CO_3. H_2CO_3 rapidly dissociates into H^+ and HCO_3^- ions. The H^+ ions are buffered, principally by Hb, while the HCO_3^- ions diffuse into the plasma. Electrochemical neutrality is maintained by the rapid diffusion of chloride (Cl^-) ions into the erythrocytes (the so-called chloride shift). Approximately 70% of the CO_2 in the blood is transported in the form of HCO_3^- ions.

Disorders of respiratory function are a major cause of morbidity and mortality among the population, and chronic obstructive pulmonary diseases (COPDs) afflict millions of Americans. Two such diseases, chronic bronchitis and emphysema, are discussed in the accompanying Disease Briefs. The third, and most common, bronchial asthma, is reviewed in detail below.

Bronchial Asthma: Pathophysiology

Bronchial asthma is a bronchospastic disease characterized by increased airway resistance frequently manifested as coughing, wheezing, shortness of breath, and dyspnea.

Major factors contributing to the heightened airway resistance are respiratory muscle spasm, thickening of the respiratory mucosa due to edema, and excessive secretion of viscous mucus. Bronchospasm associated with asthma is frequently due to increased responsiveness of bronchiolar smooth muscle to various external stimuli, such as dust and pollen, which trigger, by way of an antigen–antibody reaction, release of endogenous allergenic mediators (*e.g.*, histamine, leukotrienes, eosinophil chemotactic factor) from mast cells (Fig. 48-2). These substances then interact with bronchiolar smooth muscle cells to cause contraction. Asthma of this type is often termed *extrinsic asthma* or

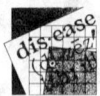

DISEASE BRIEF

■ Chronic Bronchitis

Chronic bronchitis is a prolonged inflammation of the bronchi that often is associated with emphysema and occasionally with bronchial asthma. It is characterized by a chronic cough, frequently with production of excessive sputum due to mucous gland hyperplasia and increased numbers of goblet cells in the bronchioles. The sputum may become purulent, either intermittently or chronically, and airflow obstruction may develop. Many factors may be responsible for causing this condition, most prominently smoking, air pollution, and infection. Treatment is multidimensional, and includes suppression of nonproductive coughing with codeine preparations, relief of bronchial spasm with theophylline or beta-2 agonists, and amelioration of bronchial inflammation with prednisone. If the sputum is purulent, use of penicillin, ampicillin, or tetracycline is also indicated. Of course, cessation of smoking is imperative.

atopic asthma. It is commonly noted in younger persons and usually becomes progressively more severe. A second important mechanism contributing to bronchospasm is activation of parasympathetic reflex pathways, which appear to become hypersensitive in many asthmatics. This reflex parasympathetic response results in release of acetylcholine (ACh) from vagal nerve endings, and may be elicited by the allergens extruded from the mast cells, although many other nonimmunologic factors, such as cold, stress, infection, or exercise, can also trigger an attack. ACh constricts bronchiolar smooth muscle cells, resulting in narrowing of the airways. This form of asthma has been termed "intrinsic" and most attacks of this type can *not* be related to exposure to antigens. Because the increased airway resistance is muscular in origin, it frequently responds to systemic or local bronchodilators, and these drugs, in fact, represent the mainstay in the treatment of bronchial asthma.

Distinction must be made between the therapeutic aims in treating acute versus chronic bronchospastic conditions. Sudden bronchial constriction, as seen during acute attacks of asthma, requires immediate and vigorous therapy, and may be treated with epinephrine subcutaneously (SC) or intramuscularly (IM), or, in less acute situations, with one of the inhaled beta-adrenergic bronchodilators. Aminophylline administered intravenously (IV) may also be effective in terminating acute bronchospastic attacks. Maintenance therapy of the COPDs, on the other hand, is directed toward decreasing the overall tone and responsiveness of bronchiolar smooth muscle, which are usually considerably higher in the asthmatic than in the non-asthmatic, even in the "resting" state. In addition, therapy is also intended to keep the respiratory

passages free of obstruction, thus reducing the incidence and severity of acute bronchospastic attacks. To accomplish these aims, a variety of pharmacologic agents are often employed, including oral or inhaled bronchodilators (*e.g.*, aminophylline, beta-adrenergic agonists), expectorants, mucolytics, corticosteroids, and cromolyn, an agent that has a prophylactic effect in certain asthmatic patients. In addition, persons with bronchospastic disorders should employ adjunctive measures such as adequate hydration, cessation of smoking, and avoidance of precipitating factors such as irritants, cold, and allergens to minimize the disturbing symptoms associated with diseases and to avoid potentially dangerous complications.

Many of the drugs used in the management of COPDs have been reviewed in other chapters and are not considered here. Thus, *adrenergic bronchodilators* are discussed in Chapter 15; *corticosteroids*, in Chapter 55 (although mention is made later in this chapter of the inhaled steroids useful in severe asthma); *expectorants*, in Chapter 47; and *mucolytics*, in Chapter 49. Xanthine derivatives, of which the most widely used is theophylline, are discussed in detail in this chapter, and cromolyn, an agent used to *prevent* asthmatic attacks, is also reviewed in this chapter.

Xanthine Derivatives

Aminophylline, Dyphylline, Oxtriphylline, Theophylline

The methylated xanthine derivatives (methylxanthines) include theophylline, its soluble salts (*e.g.*,

DISEASE BRIEF

■ *Emphysema*

Emphysema is characterized by loss of elasticity in the terminal pulmonary passages, alveolar distention, breakdown of intra-alveolar partitions, and reduced pulmonary function, leading to impaired ventilation and hypoxia. Clinical findings include chronic productive cough (most frequent), intermittent wheezing, prolonged expiratory phase, exertional dyspnea, weakness, and weight loss, the latter two symptoms probably being due to the increased muscular demand required for breathing. Typically, the chest is "barrel-shaped," the neck appears shortened, and the lips and nails frequently become cyanotic. Respiratory infections can be quite serious in the patient with emphysema. The condition can occur in the absence of chronic lung disease or secondary to bronchial obstructive disorders such as bronchitis or asthma. Smoking appears to be a major causative or exacerbating factor. Genetic predisposition has been noted. Treatment is symptomatic, and includes bronchodilators, mucolytics, expectorants, corticosteroids, and appropriate anti-infectives as necessary.

aminophylline, oxtriphylline), and a chemically related derivative, dyphylline. These products are available in a number of different dosage forms. Theophylline itself has been used as an effective bronchodilator for over a quarter of a century, and many of the problems associated with its early use —gastrointestinal (GI) upset, poor or erratic absorption—have been largely overcome by the synthesis of various theophylline salts as well as by the incorporation of theophylline into different dosage vehicles. Currently, theophylline and its derivatives are available in tablets, capsules, coated tablets, sustained-release tablets and capsules, aqueous solutions and suspensions, hydroalcoholic elixirs, suppositories, rectal solutions, and IV and IM injections. This multiplicity of available preparations may create confusion among clinicians concerning the appropriate dose and dosage form of theophylline to be employed for a particular clinical situation. Proper prescribing of methylxanthines, therefore, requires recognition of the many factors that may contribute to the often marked therapeutic variation observed in different patients using these products.

Clinical efficacy is a direct function of theophylline blood levels, the desired therapeutic range being 10 mcg to 20 mcg per milliliter of serum. Principal causes of difficulty in determining the appropriate dose of theophylline are (1) variations in anhydrous theophylline content among different preparations; (2) varying rates of absorption, metabolism, and elimination; (3) altered availability of theophylline from different dosage forms; and (4) age and health status of the patient. A closer look at some of these factors may aid in selecting the proper dose of theophylline for each patient.

Because of differences in anhydrous theophylline base content, the various available salt preparations are not therapeutically equal on a weight basis, and equivalent doses of the different theophylline products can vary by as much as 100%. Table 48-1 lists the percent of theophylline base and approximate equivalent doses for each clinically available preparation. These differences become important if patients are transferred from one theophylline product to another, because the plasma concentration, and thus clinical efficacy, varies directly with the intake of theophylline base.

Oral absorption of theophylline appears to be related primarily to the dosage form. Although it was formerly believed to be poorly or erratically absorbed from the GI tract, most data indicate that theophylline is inherently well absorbed, tablet disintegration being the major rate-limiting step. Thus, oral liquids are the most rapidly absorbed form of theophylline, followed very closely by uncoated tablets, especially if they are chewed. Enteric-coated or sustained-release forms of the drug, on the other hand, may be erratically or incompletely absorbed, and can yield variable plasma levels. However, newer continuous-release formulations have provided more consistent serum drug levels for 8 hours to 12 hours and represent a major advance in the chronic treatment of asthma. However, experience with preparations that claim to provide 24-hour steady-state plasma levels with single daily dosing has been less than successful. Food generally has little effect on theophylline

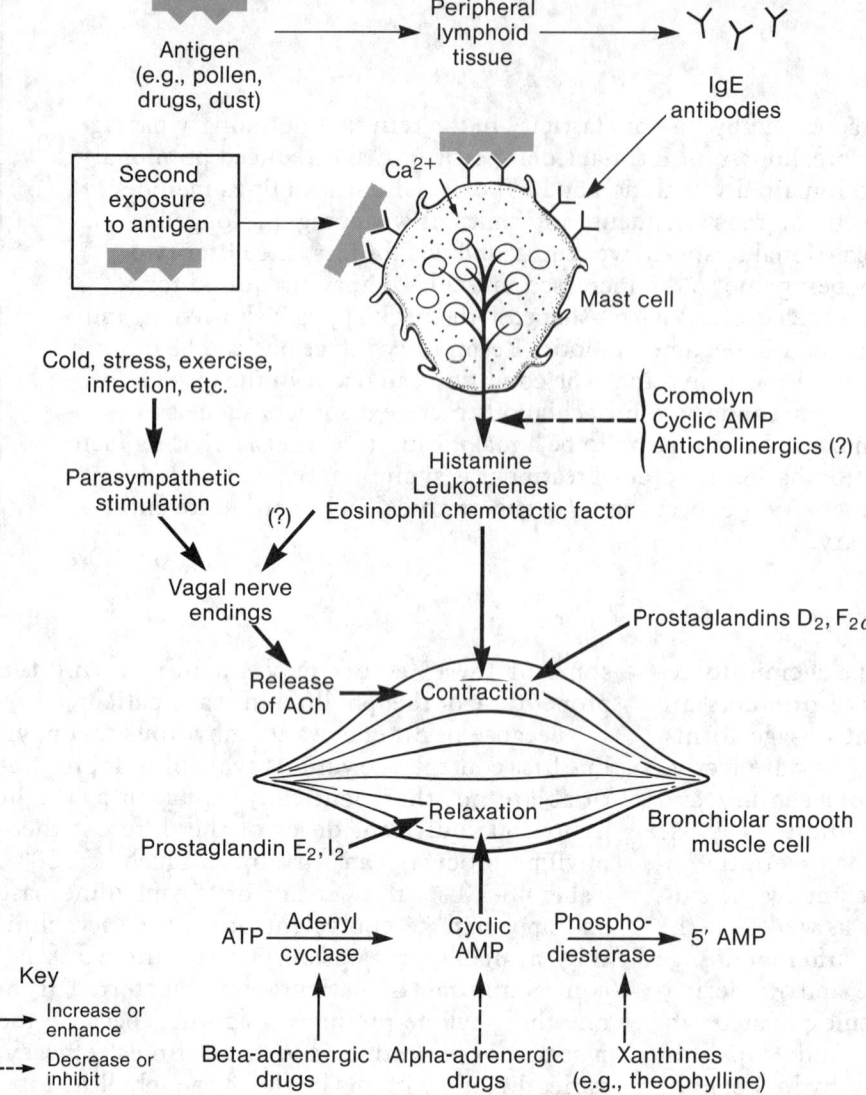

Figure 48-2. Factors regulating bronchiolar smooth muscle contraction and relaxation. On exposure to an antigen, lymphoid tissue forms IgE antibodies, which then attach to the surface of mast cells. Reexposure to antigen triggers an antigen–antibody reaction on the mast cell surface (termed IgE bridging), resulting in release of endogenous allergens from the mast cell, probably by way of increased calcium influx. The allergens elicit contraction of bronchiolar smooth muscle cells either by a direct action on the cells or by activating parasympathetic pathways.

availability, although oral absorption of theophylline from sustained-release formulations may be somewhat slower when food is present than from an empty stomach. Rectal absorption in adults is generally considered to be slow and unreliable with suppositories but nearly equivalent to oral absorption when concentrated rectal solutions are used. IM administration yields effective serum levels about equal to that of oral dosing, although not quite as rapid as with use of oral liquids.

Rates of metabolism and excretion of theophylline also vary widely. Hepatic metabolism is extensive (80%–90%), and the major metabolite is 3-methylxanthine, which exhibits approximately one-third to one-half the bronchodilator activity of theophylline itself. The plasma elimination half-life can range from 3 hours to 12 hours in adults and 1½ hours to 9 hours in children (see Fate, below). Decreased clearance is noted in patients with heart failure, liver dysfunction, and pulmo-

Table 48-1
Theophylline Content of Xanthine Derivatives

Preparation	Percent Theophylline Base	Equivalent Dosage
theophylline, anhydrous	100%	100 mg
aminophylline, anhydrous	86%	115 mg
aminophylline dihydrate	79%	127 mg
dyphylline	*	*
oxtriphylline	64%	156 mg
theophylline sodium glycinate	49%	204 mg

* A derivative of theophylline that is not metabolized to theophylline *in vivo*; it is approximately one-tenth as potent as theophylline.

nary edema, whereas smoking enhances plasma clearance. Table 48-2 lists several factors that can alter theophylline clearance. Children over 9 years of age generally respond to theophylline in a manner similar to adults, and should be given comparable doses. Younger children, however, require higher infusion rates and larger oral doses of theophylline than adults to maintain effective plasma concentrations (see Administration and Dosage, below). However, some children are unusually sensitive to the central nervous system (CNS)-stimulating effects of theophylline, and caution is recommended when administering this drug to pediatric patients.

Dosage must, of course, be individualized and carefully titrated, and serum levels maintained in the range of 10 mcg to 20 mcg/ml for optimal therapeutic effect. To achieve a rapid effect, an initial loading dose can be given, although many clinicians prefer to start at lower doses and gradually increase the dosage based on the response. Dosage adjustments are usually made on the basis of clinical signs and careful monitoring of toxicity. Once the plasma levels have stabilized, they tend to remain reasonably constant as long as the dose and dosage form are kept consistent. Dosage intervals with immediate-release products are usually maintained at 6 hours in children and nonsmoking adults to provide stable blood levels, whereas sustained-release formulations may be given to nonsmokers every 12 hours. Smokers, however, may require sustained-release dosage forms every 8 hours due to the increased rate of theophylline clearance. IV administration of aminophylline is usually accomplished by giving an initial loading dose over a 20-minute to 30-minute period, followed by a continuous maintenance infusion (see Dosage, below).

Owing to the difficulties in individualizing theophylline dosage, the use of fixed-combination bronchodilator products (e.g., theophylline, ephedrine, sedatives, or expectorants) should be strongly discouraged. Although frequently employed, such combination formulations do not allow the dosage flexibility necessary in bronchodilator therapy, and may increase the overall incidence of untoward reactions. Moreover, inclusion of barbiturates in

Table 48-2
Factors Capable of Altering Clearance of Theophylline

Factors That Increase Clearance (Decrease Half-Life)

Age under 12 years
Cigarette/marijuana smoking
High-protein/low-carbohydrate diet
Phenobarbital
Phenytoin
Aminoglutethimide

Factors That Decrease Clearance (Increase Half-Life)

Congestive heart failure
Liver disease
Age over 50 years
Chronic obstructive pulmonary disease
Pulmonary edema
Respiratory infections
Alcoholism
Prolonged fever
Obesity
High-carbohydrate/low-protein diet
Cimetidine
Erythromycin/troleandomycin
Influenza virus vaccine
Oral contraceptives

these preparations may enhance the hepatic metabolism of theophylline, necessitating use of large doses to maintain steady-state blood levels. Ephedrine, another frequent inclusion in such formulations, may potentiate the CNS-excitatory action of the methylxanthines.

MECHANISM AND ACTIONS
Xanthines exert a competitive inhibitory effect on the enzyme phosphodiesterase, thus preventing the breakdown of cyclic AMP (see Fig. 48-2). Increased levels of cyclic AMP relax bronchiolar smooth muscle (in part through release of epinephrine) and may inhibit release of endogenous allergens such as histamine and leukotrienes from sensitized mast cells. Xanthines also antagonize prostaglandin-mediated bronchoconstriction and block receptors for adenosine, a naturally occurring purine nucleoside bronchoconstrictor. Adenosine antagonism may represent the major mechanism of action of theophylline.

Other pharmacologic actions of the xanthines include myocardial stimulation, mild diuresis, decreased uterine contractions, CNS excitation, increased respiration and gastric acid secretion, glycogenolysis, lipolysis, and weak inotropic and chronotropic effects.

USES
1. Symptomatic relief or prevention of bronchial asthma, bronchospasm associated with chronic bronchitis, emphysema, and other obstructive pulmonary diseases
2. Treatment of bradycardia and apnea in premature infants (investigational use only)

ADMINISTRATION AND DOSAGE
Dosage is highly individualized and is adjusted to provide theophylline serum levels of 10 mcg/ml to 20 mcg/ml. The initial loading dose (see below) is determined by the volume of distribution and is based on *lean* body weight, since theophylline does *not* distribute into fatty tissue. It varies little from patient to patient. Conversely, the maintenance dose is determined largely by the rate of clearance of theophylline from the plasma and varies considerably from patient to patient (see Table 48-2).

The following dosage recommendations are for *anhydrous theophylline*. Refer to Table 48-1 for conversion factors for other salts of theophylline and to Table 48-3 for dosage schedules for individual theophylline preparations.

Acute Symptoms Requiring Rapid Oral Dosing

Patients Not Receiving Theophylline
Adults: 6 mg/kg as a loading dose, then 3 mg/kg every 6 hours for 2 doses, then 3 mg/kg every 8 hours
Older adults: 6 mg/kg as a loading dose, then 2 mg/kg every 6 hours for 2 doses, then 2 mg/kg every 8 hours
Adults with congestive heart failure: 6 mg/kg as a loading dose, then 2 mg/kg every 8 hours for 2 doses, then 1 mg to 2 mg/kg every 12 hours
Children (9 yr–16 yr) and adult smokers: 6 mg/kg as a loading dose, then 3 mg/kg every 4 hours for three doses, then 3 mg/kg every 6 hours
Children (under 9 yr): 6 mg/kg as a loading dose, then 4 mg/kg every 4 hours for three doses, then 4 mg/kg every 6 hours
Note: The *loading dose* is equivalent in all patient populations.

All Patients Currently Receiving Theophylline
Initially 2.5 mg/kg; subsequent doses are based on serum theophylline levels; each 0.5 mg/kg of theophylline will raise the serum theophylline concentration approximately 1.0 mcg/ml

Chronic Oral Therapy
Initially 16 mg/kg/day or 400 mg/day (whichever is less) of anhydrous theophylline in divided doses every 6 hours to 8 hours; increase in approximately 25% increments at 2-day to 3-day intervals, if tolerated, until optimal response or maximum dose is attained; maximum doses are the following:
Adults: 13 mg/kg/day, or 900 mg
Children (12 yr–16 yr): 18 mg/kg/day
Children (9 yr–12 yr): 20 mg/kg/day
Children (under 9 yr): 24 mg/kg/day

FATE
Theophylline is generally well absorbed orally, except for some enteric-coated and sustained-release formulations, which may be erratically absorbed. Food may alter the rate of absorption of some sustained-release preparations. Rectal absorption from suppositories is slow and unreliable, while concentrated rectal solutions yield good absorption. Peak effects differ among the various preparations and dosage forms, ranging from 1 hour with most liquids to 10 hours with some sustained-release tablets and capsules. The plasma elimination half-life of theophylline averages 7 hours to 9 hours in adult nonsmokers, 4 hours to 5 hours in adult

Table 48-3
Xanthine Bronchodilators

Drug	Preparations	Usual Dosage Range	Clinical Considerations
aminophylline (Amoline, Phyllocontin, Somophyllin, Truphylline)	Tablets—100 mg, 200 mg Timed-release tablets—225 mg Liquid (alcohol-free)—315 mg/15 ml Suppositories—250 mg, 500 mg Rectal solution—300 mg/5 ml Injection (IV)—250 mg/10 ml, 500 mg/20 ml Injection (IM)—500 mg/2 ml Injection (with 0.45% sodium chloride)—100 mg/100 ml, 200 mg/100 ml	*Oral* Adults—500 mg initially, then 200 mg–300 mg every 6 h–8 h Children—7.5 mg/kg initially, then 5 mg/kg–6 mg/kg every 6 h–8 h Timed-release tablets—1 to 2 tablets every 8 h–12 h before meals and at bedtime (not recommended in children under 12) *Rectal solutions* Adults—300 mg 1 to 3 times a day or 450 mg twice a day Children—5 mg/kg every 6 h–8 h *Suppositories* Adults—500 mg 1 to 2 times a day Children—7 mg/kg *IM* Adults—500 mg *IV* Initially 6 mg/kg loading dose by IV injection at a rate not exceeding 25 mg/minute For continuous infusion, the rates (mg/kg/h) are as follows:	Ethylenediamine salt of theophylline with similar pharmacologic properties; contains 79% theophylline; only xanthine derivative used IV for acute attacks of bronchial asthma; sensitivity reactions and dermatitis have occurred, especially with parenteral use; suppositories may produce rectal irritation; IM injections are very painful and should be avoided if possible; use only diluted solutions (25 mg/ml) for IV injection and warm to room temperature; 5% dextrose injection or normal saline solution preferred diluents; inject very slowly (maximum 25 mg/min) to avoid cardiovascular disturbances, and closely monitor vital signs during infusion. Drug is incompatible in IV fluids with many drugs (see Appendix).

	0–12 h	After 12 h
Nonsmoking adults	0.7	0.5
Smoking adults and children 9 yr–16 yr	1.0	0.8
Children 6 mo–9 yr	1.2	1.0
Older patients	0.6	0.3
Patients with congestive heart failure	0.5	0.1–0.2

Drug	Preparations	Usual Dosage Range	Clinical Considerations
dyphylline (Dilor, Dyflex, Lufyllin, Neothylline)	Tablets—200 mg, 400 mg Elixir—100 mg/15 ml, 160 mg/15 ml Injection (IM)—250 mg/ml	*Oral* Adults—up to 15 mg/kg every 6 h depending on response *IM* Adults—250 mg–500 mg (maximum 15 mg/kg every 6 h)	A chemically related derivative of theophylline that is not metabolized to theophylline *in vivo*; equivalent to approximately 70% theophylline by molecular weight ratio; claimed to produce *(continued)*

Table 48-3 (continued)
Xanthine Bronchodilators

Drug	Preparations	Usual Dosage Range	Clinical Considerations
dyphylline (Dilor, Dyflex, Lufyllin, Neothylline) (*continued*)		Children—4.4 mg–6.6 mg/kg/day in divided doses	less GI upset and fewer overall side-effects, but blood levels and activity are somewhat lower than theophylline; peak plasma levels ocur in 1 hour; short half-life (2 h) requires frequent dosing to maintain effective blood levels; inject drug slowly IM and aspirate to avoid inadvertent IV injection; excreted essentially unchanged in the urine; specific dyphylline blood levels must be used to monitor therapy; serum *theophylline* levels are *not* indicative of dyphylline levels.
oxtriphylline (Choledyl)	Tablets—100 mg, 200 mg Sustained-release tablets— 400 mg, 600 mg Elixir—100 mg/5 ml Syrup—50 mg/5 ml (pediatric)	Adults—200 mg 4 times a day *or* 400-mg–600-mg sustained-release tablets every 12 h Children—3.6 mg/kg 4 times a day (100 mg/60 lb)	Choline salt of theophylline containing 64% theophylline; claimed to be more uniformly absorbed and more stable than theophylline, and to produce less GI distress and tolerance; regular tablets are *partially* enteric coated, which delays onset but not completeness of absorption.
theophylline (Aerolate, Bronkodyl, Elixophyllin, Slo-Phyllin, Somophyllin, Theo-Dur, Theolair, and various other manufacturers)	Tablets—100 mg, 125 mg, 200 mg, 225 mg, 250 mg, 300 mg Timed-release tablets—100 mg, 200 mg, 250 mg, 300 mg, 400 mg, 450 mg, 500 mg	*Oral* Adults—100 mg–250 mg every 6 h or 1 to 2 timed-release preparations every 8 h–12 h Children—4 mg–6 mg/kg every 6 h (see Dosage	Standard xanthine derivative widely used as a bronchodilator; available in various forms, allowing flexibility in dosing; sustained-release preparations provide for gradual *(continued)*

smokers, and 3 hours to 5 hours in children. Decreased plasma clearance occurs in patients with congestive heart failure, liver dysfunction, pulmonary edema, cor pulmonale, respiratory infections, and in alcoholics (see Table 48-2). The xanthines are metabolized in the liver and excreted by the kidneys. Less than 15% of the drug is excreted unchanged.

SIDE-EFFECTS/ADVERSE REACTIONS

Adverse effects are generally minimal at plasma levels below 20 mcg/ml. The most frequently occurring side-effects with theophylline preparations are nausea, nervousness, and urinary frequency.

Other common side-effects noted at plasma levels between 20 mcg/ml and 25 mcg/ml are diarrhea, vomiting, headache, irritability, and insomnia. Higher plasma levels can result in arrhythmias, hypotension, tachycardia, hyperglycemia, and seizures. A variety of other untoward reactions have occurred during theophylline therapy, the incidence and frequency of which are generally related to high plasma levels, and these are listed by organ system below.

    GI—Anorexia, hematemesis, intestinal bleeding, activation of ulcer pain
    CNS—Restlessness, dizziness, muscle twitching, reflex hyperexcitability,

Table 48-3 (continued)
Xanthine Bronchodilators

Drug	Preparations	Usual Dosage Range	Clinical Considerations
theophylline (Aerolate, Bronkodyl, Elixophyllin, Slo-Phyllin, Somophyllin, Theo-Dur, Theolair, and various other manufacturers) (continued)	Capsules—100 mg, 200 mg, 250 mg Timed-release capsules—50 mg, 60 mg, 65 mg, 100 mg, 125 mg, 130 mg, 200 mg, 250 mg, 260 mg, 300 mg Encapsulated powder (Theo-Dur Sprinkle)—50 mg, 75 mg, 125 mg, 200 mg Elixir—80 mg/15 ml, 150 mg/15 ml Liquid (alcohol-free)—80 mg/15 ml, 150 mg/15 ml, 160 mg/15 ml Syrup—80 mg/15 ml, 150 mg/15 ml Suspension—100 mg/5 ml	under general discussion of xanthines)	release of active drug so that they may be given every 8 h–12 h depending on formulation; a 24-h timed-release preparation is available (Theo-24), but plasma levels may not remain constant for the entire time; liquid formulations may be hydroalcoholic elixirs or alcohol-free syrups or suspensions; aqueous solutions provide similar serum levels as alcoholic elixirs, but lack CNS-depressant effects and are better tasting; some timed-release products may exhibit unpredictable absorption; found in many combination products with ephedrine, sedatives, or expectorants; fixed-combination preparations do not allow individual dosage adjustments that are often necessary to obtain optimal action.
theophylline sodium glycinate (Synophylate)	Elixir—330 mg/15 ml	Adults—330 mg–660 mg every 6 h–8 h Children (6 yr–12 yr)—220 mg–330 mg every 6 h–8 h Children (under 6 yr)—55 mg–165 mg every 6 h–8 h	Mixture of sodium theophylline and glycine containing 47% theophylline; claimed to elicit fewer adverse GI effects than theophylline itself; it is an infrequently used preparation.

depression, speech difficulties, tonic or clonic convulsions
Cardiovascular—Palpitations, flushing, extrasystoles, circulatory failure
Renal—Diuresis, dehydration, proteinuria
Other—Tachypnea, respiratory arrest, fever, rash, rectal irritation and strictures with use of suppositories

Rapid IV injection or infusion can result in flushing, palpitations, dizziness, hyperventilation, hypotension, and angina-like pain.

Overdosage is marked by vomiting, nervousness, agitation, tachycardia, tachypnea, tonic/clonic convulsions, and arrhythmias (which may be the initial sign of toxicity). Children are particularly likely to show hyperactivity, which may proceed to convulsions. Treatment is symptomatic and may include induction of vomiting, gastric lavage, anticonvulsants (if seizures occur), antiarrhythmics if necessary, and, in severe overdosage, charcoal hemoperfusion.

CONTRAINDICATIONS AND PRECAUTIONS

Xanthine bronchodilators are contraindicated in the presence of active gastritis and in patients in whom myocardial stimulation might prove dangerous. Rectal suppositories are also contraindicated in the presence of rectal or lower colonic irritation or infection. These drugs must be given with *caution* to persons with acute cardiac disease, renal or hepatic disease, severe hypoxemia, hypertension, myocardial damage, cor pulmonale, congestive heart failure, glaucoma, hyperthyroidism, peptic ulcer, diabetes, or prostatic hypertrophy. Cautious use is also warranted during pregnancy or lactation, and in children and alcoholics.

INTERACTIONS

1. Xanthines may increase the CNS stimulation seen with amphetamines, ephedrine, and other sympathomimetic drugs.
2. Increased theophylline plasma levels (decreased clearance) may occur with use of cimetidine, oral contraceptives, allopurinol, influenza virus vaccine, erythromycin, clindamycin, lincomycin, and troleandomycin (see Table 48-2).
3. The effects of theophylline may be decreased by nicotine, marijuana, phenobarbital and aminoglutethimide by way of increased hepatic metabolism (see Table 48-2).
4. Xanthines can increase the excretion of lithium and phenytoin, and decrease their effectiveness.
5. Xanthines and beta-adrenergic blocking agents (e.g., propranolol, metoprolol, nadolol) may be mutually antagonistic.
6. Xanthines can enhance the diuretic action of other types of diuretics.
7. The toxicity of digitalis glycosides may be increased by xanthines.
8. Tachycardia can result when xanthines are given together with reserpine.
9. Concurrent use of theophylline and tetracyclines may result in an increased incidence of GI side-effects.
10. Dosage requirements for nondepolarizing muscle relaxants (e.g., pancuronium) may be increased by concurrent use of theophylline.
11. Antacids can retard the rate of absorption of orally administered theophylline, but *not* the overall extent.
12. An increased likelihood of cardiac arrhythmias can result from concurrent use of theophylline and halothane.

■ Nursing Process

□ ASSESSMENT

□ Subjective Data

The patient with a chronic respiratory problem has been treated with a variety of drugs and may have actually been on a theophylline derivative at one time or another. Therefore, a complete drug history is essential before therapy is initiated. The nurse needs to ask about use of over-the-counter drugs and inhalers, which the patient may forget to report, and, if possible, ask to see the drugs themselves since many have multiple formulations of varying effectiveness. The patient should describe how he takes his current drugs since pattern times and concurrent food intake may affect blood levels.

A smoking history is also important since theophylline levels will be affected by nicotine. In addition, a history of cardiovascular illness and respiratory problems should be highlighted.

An exploration of the patient's and family's perception of the illness will help improve the treatment plan. Reactions to chronic respiratory illness range from anxiety over the inability to breathe to depression about the hopelessness of the condition. Parents of children with chronic respiratory problems may feel the disease is their fault and may become overprotective. The patient who smokes may express anger or guilt over his smoking and its relationship to the disease process or he may deny the extent of the problem. Exploring these feelings will help the nurse to determine the patient's attitude and what problems may develop in ensuring compliance to the proposed drug regimen. In addition, such a discussion provides an opportunity to determine what the patient and family understand about the illness; if understanding is incomplete, the patient may be unnecessarily limiting activities or, conversely, he may be doing things that may make the condition worse.

□ Objective Data

Physical examination will be extensive, especially of the cardiopulmonary system. Lung auscultation should focus on the ratio of the length of inspiration to the length of expiration and the presence of adventitious sounds, especially wheezing. Observation of breathing patterns, use of accessory muscles, shape of chest, and ease of breathing is essential. Incentive spirometry may be ordered to determine inspiratory, expiratory, and tidal volume. These parameters can serve as a baseline against which to measure the effectiveness of the medication.

Laboratory evaluation should include electrolyte studies, arterial blood gases, and a theophylline level, especially if it is suspected that the patient may already be taking one of the drug forms. The presence of theophylline in the plasma will influence the dosing of the current and future prescription. The patient should be asked about recent ingestion of coffee, tea, chocolate, acetaminophen, or cephalosporins since these may falsely increase the laboratory report of theophylline level.

□ *NURSING DIAGNOSES*

Actual nursing diagnoses may include
    Knowledge deficit related to drug action, administration, and side-effects
Potential nursing diagnoses may include
    Alteration in comfort: pain from injection site, nausea or headache, drug side-effects
    Alteration in cardiac output: decreased, related to arrhythmias, a drug side-effect usually signaling toxicity
    Alteration in respiratory function: worsening of condition, a symptom of drug toxicity
    Alteration in bowel elimination: diarrhea
    Noncompliance with the prescribed drug regimen, especially if side-effects are uncomfortable or if symptoms disappear
    Sleep pattern disturbance: insomnia
    Alteration in thought processes: confusion, restlessness, and irritability, an early sign of toxicity especially in the elderly
    Alteration in patterns of urinary elimination: increased frequency

□ *PLAN*

Nursing care goals may include
1. Administering the drug safely and correctly during the time the patient is acutely ill
2. Monitoring side-effects during the acute treatment phase
3. Teaching the patient
   a. To take the medication correctly in order to control and prevent respiratory symptoms
   b. The major side-effects of the drug and what to do if they occur
   c. The relationship between drug therapy and other activity such as exercise and relaxation techniques in management of symptoms (especially important for parents who may limit the activities of an asthmatic child)
   d. The importance of follow-up clinic visits to measure drug levels, breathing changes, and drug effectiveness

□ *INTERVENTION*

Xanthine drugs may be given by various routes, including IV, oral, rectal, and IM. The intramuscular route is rarely used and should be avoided if at all possible. Xanthines are extremely irritating to tissue, can cause severe pain, and may result in abscess formation.

Absorption following rectal administration by suppository is slow in adults and highly erratic in children. If the rectal route must be used in a child, a retention enema using aminophylline solution is the preferred method since the drug is much more efficiently absorbed. If a suppository is used it should be inserted before meals, with the individual in the recumbent position where he should remain for 15 to 20 minutes or until the defecation reflex subsides.

Aminophylline is the only xanthine administered by intravenous route and is usually reserved for acute bronchial emergencies such as status asthmaticus. The administration schedules given in Table 48-3 should be closely followed. The drug is best given by IV infusion. IV injection should be used only in extreme emergencies and the rate of administration should never exceed 25 mg/minute regardless of method. Serious drug toxicity can occur rapidly during intravenous administration characterized by tachyarrhythmias, hypotension, and seizures. The patient should be placed on a cardiac monitor and lidocaine and a defibrillator should be immediately available if needed. Frequent blood pressures (every 5 minutes for at least the first 15 minutes then every 10 minutes for 1 hour, then as condition warrants) must be taken and the rate of infusion slowed if significant changes occur. Seizure precautions should be observed. An infusion pump should be used to monitor rate and will be helpful when the dose is titrated down to be discontinued. While the patient is on IV aminophylline, frequent arterial blood gases should be drawn to help determine drug effectiveness, and serum drug levels must be closely monitored to avoid overdosage.

Oral xanthine derivatives are available in multiple formulations, and this large array of products can create confusion for the nurse when administering the drug or teaching the patient and family self-administration at home. Medication formulations should not be interchanged (*i.e.*, liquid for time-released capsules) since strength and absorption vary widely. If a formulation must be changed the theophylline level must be closely monitored to be sure it stays within the desired therapeutic range. Consequently, the tablets should not be crushed nor time-released capsules opened unless a liquid formulation cannot be substituted.

The patient needs to be reminded that the medication must be taken even when he is feeling well, not just when he is short of breath. It is also critical that the doses be evenly spaced throughout the day so the plasma levels remain consistent.

If the patient has been using prescription or over-the-counter sympathomimetic bronchodilators before the theophylline drug was prescribed he needs to discontinue their use until the effects of theophylline on his condition are known. The combination of xanthine and sympathomimetic drugs can cause CNS excitation, hyperactivity, and arrhythmias. The most common side-effect, GI distress, which may include nausea, vomiting, or diarrhea, may be averted by taking the drug with milk or food. There has been some controversy about dumping of the time-released formulas when taken with food because of the increased gastric acidity associated with digestion. While responses will be individual, the patient should be aware that all but a few of the 24-hour release capsules can be taken with food; if one formula produces GI distress another may not and changes may be made. If a patient begins to take the drug with milk or food he should continue to do so with each dose so that the release of drug is uniform with each dose. His subsequent dosage will then be based on serum theophylline levels. If symptoms persist the physician should be notified.

Another common side-effect, urinary frequency, is somewhat difficult to manage if the patient is on a every-6-hours regimen around the clock. If a sustained-action dosage form can be prescribed, the patient may opt to take the drug early in the morning and early in the evening to minimize the inconvenience of frequent bathroom use during the day and during sleep.

In general, the elderly have a more variable response to xanthine derivatives because of the drug's narrow therapeutic index and the older person's lessened ability to clear the drug. Clearance may take as long as 24 hours; such variation must be calculated in the dose or the elderly patient will be likely to develop toxicity. Symptoms of early toxicity in the older person are vomiting, dizziness, restlessness, insomnia, and irritability and should be reported at once. Cardiovascular changes may occur late or early depending on the patient's pretreatment cardiovascular status but should be closely monitored because life-threatening arrhythmias can occur. Children may exhibit marked hyperactivity and quickly develop generalized convulsions when toxic drug levels are reached. See Side-Effects/Adverse Reactions, above, for a complete list of signs and symptoms as well as treatment. The best method to prevent drug toxicity is frequent evaluation of serum theophylline levels, especially during initial therapy, when a drug formulation or dose is changed, or when the patient experiences other problems (see Table 48-2). The patient and family must understand the importance of these laboratory tests and become aware of body changes that provide an early signal of drug toxicity. In all age groups, irritability and hyperactivity are the two most common parameters. Occasionally, patients report worsening respiratory symptoms as an early sign of toxicity.

The patient needs encouragement to learn adjunctive measures to facilitate drug therapy such as pursed-lip or abdominal–diaphragmatic breathing techniques and body relaxation strategies to reduce anxiety about dyspnea and to improve air exchange. If possible, he can participate in a gradually increased exercise program, which is especially important for children whose parents tend to be overprotective and restrict activity. It may be useful to teach the family postural drainage and chest percussion techniques to help the patient expectorate thick mucous secretions, which will facilitate bronchodilation with the drug therapy. All of these measures require follow-up and assistance since the disease is a continuing process.

The nurse also needs to help the patient understand that the drug therapy is only part of a therapeutic regimen for a chronic incurable disease. Clinic follow-up is essential for measuring drug effectiveness and providing support and encouragement to improve compliance. The patient will need strong family and health-team supports. He will occasionally lapse from the treatment routine if he becomes depressed or tired of spending so much energy on a therapy that cannot cure him. Self-help groups, health-facility–sponsored groups, and family groups may help the patient cope and actually improve therapeutic outcomes.

□ *EVALUATION*

Outcome criteria that may indicate successful drug therapy in the acute phase of treatment include improved blood gas readings, decreased respiratory rate, improved breath sounds, decreased wheezing, and decreased respiratory effort measured by incentive spirometer. Long-term outcomes might be improved activity tolerance, decrease in frequency or severity of symptoms, minimal development of side-effects, and improved patient self-perception. Nursing Care Plan 48-1 provides a summary of the nursing process for the patient taking xanthine drugs.

(*Text continues on p. 941.*)

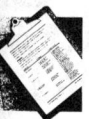

Nursing Care Plan 48-1
The Patient Receiving Oral Xanthine Drugs

Assessment

Subjective Data

1. Medication history: see Interactions section to formulate pertinent questions.
   a. Ask about current use of xanthines, use of OTC bronchial aids
   b. Use of street drugs, alcohol, smoking history
   c. Allergies/hypersensitivity to xanthines
2. Medical history
   a. Description of symptoms, duration of problem, previous treatment that helped/failed
   b. Pre-existing conditions that may contraindicate use, *e.g.*, gastritis
   c. Pre-existing conditions that warrant cautious use, such as hypertension, congestive heart failure, cor pulmonale, renal or hepatic disease, glaucoma, hyperthyroidism, diabetes mellitus, peptic ulcer, prostatic hypertrophy
3. Personal history/compliance issues
   a. Perception of illness: may be colored by progression, duration, effect on life activity
   b. Evidence of anger, guilt, denial
   c. Ability to self-medicate, follow a regimen, seek follow-up care
   d. Personal, financial resources; supportive network to maintain compliance

Objective Data

1. Physical assessment
   a. Cardiovascular status: pulse, blood pressure, evidence of murmurs, arrhythmias
   b. Respiratory status: inspiration/expiration ratio, rate, effort, lung sounds, use of accessory muscles, chest shape
   c. Neurologic status: memory, mental acuity, psychomotor function, sensation
2. Laboratory/diagnostic data
   a. Incentive spirometry: inspiratory, expiratory, and tidal volume
   b. Blood gases (arterial)
   c. Serum electrolytes
   d. Serum theophylline level—ask about recent ingestion of coffee, tea, chocolate, or drugs, which may cause false increase in lab report.

Nursing Diagnosis	Expected Client Outcome	Intervention
Knowledge deficit: related to drug action and effect on disease process, correct administration, potential side-effects	Will verbalize understanding of the drug action, effect, administration, and side-effects.	Explain the relationship between chronic respiratory problems, drug therapy, exercise, and other factors that affect drug level (see Table 48-2). Teach patient to monitor common side-effects as described below and follow preventive and reactive strategies given.
	Will maintain a therapeutic theophylline level between 10 mcg/ml and 20 mcg/ml.	Emphasize need for correct drug taking to maintain therapeutic drug levels. Drug should be taken at the same time every day. If multiple doses are ordered, drug must be taken around the clock at evenly spaced intervals to maintain level. Drug should be taken even when the patient is feeling well.

(continued)

Nursing Diagnosis	Expected Client Outcome	Intervention
Knowledge deficit: related to drug action and effect on disease process, correct administration, potential side-effects (continued)		Teach the patient that formulations of theophylline are not interchangeable. If a different formulation is needed, close monitoring must be completed.
		Teach the patient to avoid all other drugs and alcohol unless approved by physician first.
		Stress the importance of early reporting of any illness that might alter theophylline clearance (see Table 48-2).
Potential noncompliance: related to chronic nature of disease and length of drug therapy	Will keep appointments for follow-up. Will build a trust relationship with the health team.	Attempt to build a trust relationship. Provide support, a ready resource to answer questions and concerns.
		Initiate follow-up to monitor progress, express concern for client.
		Set realistic goals for exercise, smoking cessation, increasing daily activities as necessary.
		Encourage clinical follow-up to measure goal achievements.
		Teach patient parameters used to measure drug effectiveness: therapeutic drug levels with minimal side-effects, improvement in lung sounds and incentive spirometry.
		Use clinical follow-up to provide support and encouragement, and to allow time for discussion about regimen, perceptions, and effects on daily life.
	Will contact health team before abruptly withdrawing from drug.	Encourage patient to contact health team before abruptly discontinuing drug. Discuss patient's reasons for wanting to withdraw. Acknowledge that patient will make the ultimate decision.
Potential alteration in respiratory function: decreased related to disease process or ineffective drug levels	Respiratory volumes as measured on incentive spirometry improve.	Teach breathing techniques, relaxation exercises, postural drainage, and chest percussion as appropriate to enhance breathing and facilitate expectoration of secretions.
		Encourage adequate fluid intake.
		Encourage early reporting of dyspnea or illness that affects respiratory function (cold, sinus infection) because theophylline dose may need adjustment.
Potential alteration in cardiac output: decreased related to drug-induced arrhythmias	Will maintain a normal sinus rhythm.	Provide continuous ECG monitoring when theophylline toxicity is suspected or when dosage adjustment is difficult.

(continued)

Nursing Diagnosis	Expected Client Outcome	Intervention
Potential alteration in cardiac output: decreased related to drug-induced arrhythmias (*continued*)		Obtain periodic ECG as prescribed during follow-up.
		Teach the patient to report immediately any palpitations, sensation of a rapid heart rate, weakness, or dizziness.
Potential alteration in thought processes: related to drug-induced confusion, irritability, or hyperactivity	Symptoms of drug toxicity will be reported early.	Be aware that confusion and irritability are early signs of toxicity in the elderly; hyperactivity is an early sign in children.
		Teach patient/family to seek immediate medical attention if symptoms appear and to hold all doses until physician can be contacted. Serum drug level should be drawn.
Potential sleep pattern disturbance: insomnia related to drug toxicity	Normal sleep pattern will be maintained.	Teach patient to report early any changes in sleep cycle.
Potential alteration in comfort: GI distress related to drug effect	GI side-effects will be minimized.	Teach patient to take drug with food if discomfort starts. If drug is taken with food, each dose must be taken the same way to maintain consistent drug release.
		Encourage early reporting of persistent symptoms. Dose or formula may need to be changed.
Potential alteration in patterns of urinary elimination: increased frequency related to drug effect	Will minimize disruption of daily activities.	Teach patient to arrange dosage to minimize sleep disruption as much as possible while keeping a schedule that maintains drug level.
		Encourage physician to use sustained-release capsules whenever possible for appropriate patients.

Cromolyn Sodium

(Intal, Nasalcrom, Opticrom)

Cromolyn is a prophylactic agent that is used as an adjunctive drug in the management of severe bronchial asthma. Cromolyn may decrease the severity of the clinical symptoms of asthma or reduce the requirements for concomitant drug therapy, or both. It is strictly a prophylactic drug and possesses no intrinsic bronchodilator, antihistaminic, or anti-inflammatory activity and thus is of no value in the treatment of acute asthmatic attacks. The drug is available for *oral* inhalation as powder-containing capsules, a solution for nebulization, or an aerosol, and *no* significant difference in effectiveness between these dosage forms has been demonstrated. Cromolyn is also marketed as a nasal spray (Nasalcrom) for treatment of chronic allergic rhinitis and as ophthalmic drops (Opticrom) for treatment of allergic ocular disorders such as allergic keratoconjunctivitis or vernal keratitis. These latter two dosage forms are considered briefly following the discussion of the orally inhaled form of cromolyn.

MECHANISM AND ACTIONS

By stabilizing the mast cell membrane, cromolyn inhibits the release of endogenous allergens such as histamine and leukotrienes from mast cells, which normally occurs following exposure to specific antigens.

USES

1. Prophylactic management of severe, perennial bronchial asthma (reduces severity of symp-

toms or bronchodilator drug dosage requirements). Improvement is usually noted within 4 weeks.

2. Prevention of exercise-induced bronchospasm
3. Symptomatic control of chronic allergic rhinitis (Nasalcrom) or ocular allergies (Opticrom) —see below
4. Investigational uses include treatment of food allergies, systemic mastocytosis, eczema, dermatitis, urticaria pigmentosa, chronic urticaria, hay fever, and postexercise bronchospasm.

ADMINISTRATION AND DOSAGE

Cromolyn is available for oral inhalation as powder-containing capsules (20 mg), a solution (20 mg/2 ml) for use with a power-assisted nebulizer, and an aerosol that delivers approximately 800 mcg per activation. A nasal spray (40 mg/ml) and ophthalmic solution (4%) are also available (see below). Recommended dosage for asthma prophylaxis is 20 mg four times a day. The capsules are placed into a special inhaler device (Spinhaler turbo-inhaler), and the powder is inhaled according to the instructions provided with the package. The nebulizer solution is administered using a power-operated nebulizer having an adequate flow rate and equipped with a suitable face mask. Hand-operated nebulizers are *not* suitable. Cromolyn should not be given until an acute bronchospastic episode has been controlled and the patient is capable of inhaling satisfactorily. An inhaled bronchodilator may be administered prior to cromolyn to facilitate its penetration into the lungs.

The recommended dose using the oral aerosol spray is 2 sprays 4 times a day. For prevention of exercise-induced bronchospasm, 10 mg is inhaled 30 minutes to 60 minutes prior to the exercise. A repeat inhalation may be given as required for protection during prolonged exercise.

FATE

Approximately 8% to 10% of the dose is absorbed by the lungs following inhalation, then rapidly excreted unchanged in the bile and urine. The remainder of the dose is either exhaled or swallowed and then excreted in the feces (GI absorption is poor). The elimination half-life is 80 minutes to 90 minutes.

SIDE-EFFECTS/ADVERSE REACTIONS

Coughing and nasal congestion can occur with oral inhalation of cromolyn. The drug is only absorbed to a limited degree and adverse reactions are generally infrequent but can include lacrimation, nausea, dizziness, headache, swollen parotid glands, dysuria, urinary frequency, rash, urticaria, joint swelling and pain, wheezing, sneezing, nose bleed, and abdominal pain.

Other untoward reactions noted in patients receiving orally inhaled cromolyn (although a direct causal relationship is not established) are hoarseness, myalgia, vertigo, photosensitivity, peripheral neuritis, nephrosis, anemia, exfoliative dermatitis, vasculitis, pericarditis, eosinophilia, and anaphylactic reactions.

CONTRAINDICATIONS AND PRECAUTIONS

Cromolyn should not be used to abort an acute attack of bronchospasm. The safety and efficacy of cromolyn powder in children under 6 years (under 2 years for the nebulizer solution) have not been established. Cromolyn should be employed *cautiously* in persons with impaired renal or hepatic function, and in pregnant or nursing mothers.

NURSING CONSIDERATIONS

The primary nursing responsibility is to teach the patient the correct use of the inhaling device prescribed, either the Spinhaler or the power nebulizer. Many nurses do not know the correct method of using either device. Refer to Tables 48-4 and 48-5 for information on teaching the patient self-administration and refer to the package inserts for further information. Use the pharmacist or respiratory therapist as a resource if necessary.

Patients must understand that cromolyn is a preventative drug and should not be taken if an asthmatic attack begins. Use of the drug at such a time may actually worsen the symptoms.

Cromolyn Intranasal

(Nasalcrom)

Cromolyn is also available as a nasal spray for the management of symptoms of allergic rhinitis. Repeated inhalation of the drug is believed to decrease the occurrence and severity of attacks of allergic rhinitis. One spray is administered into each nostril three to six times a day using the inhaler supplied with the drug cartridge. Side-effects are rare, and the drug is well tolerated, although there are occasional reports of sneezing and nasal stinging or burning. Headaches, bad taste in the mouth,

Table 48-4
Teaching Self-Administration of Cromolyn Sodium by Turbo-inhaler (Spinhaler)

It is extremely important for the patient to learn the correct use of this administration tool. If the turbo-inhaler is used incorrectly the patient will not derive full benefit from the drug. When teaching the technique, allow the patient plenty of time for supervised practice (refer to the product insert) and emphasize the following points:

1. Clear mucus from lungs prior to procedure to enhance the effectiveness of the drug.
2. Put the cromolyn capsule in the propellor cup, put the top on and push the sleeve down to pierce the capsule.
3. Pull the sleeve up, but not off.
4. Place inhaler in mouth.
5. Exhale through nose, close lips around mouthpiece and inhale deeply through mouth. Repeat this process until all the powder is inhaled. (*Note:* A small amount of powder may be left at the end and repeated inhalations will not dislodge it. This sometimes occurs if too much moisture reaches the powder. To avoid this the patient should avoid breathing into the inhaler.)
6. If an asthma attack begins do not use cromolyn, because it may worsen symptoms.
7. The drug should be effective within 4 weeks if it is going to help. If no change is noted contact the physician.
8. Wash the turbo-inhaler at least once a week in warm water.

If the patient cannot coordinate the technique of the turbo-inhaler, cromolyn sodium can be given in a power nebulizer using a liquid form of the drug. See Table 48-5.

Table 48-5
Teaching Self-Administration of Bronchodilators by Power Nebulizer

Although this tool requires less coordinated effort to operate, the patient must still perform the technique correctly to get the full benefit of the drug. When teaching the technique, allow the patient plenty of time for supervised practice, refer to the product insert, and emphasize the following points:

1. Place the prescribed amount of solution in the nebulizer.
2. Plug the compressor into an appropriate wall outlet. Test to make sure it is grounded (will not blow a fuse at that location).
3. Open mouth; hold nebulizer horizontal about 2 inches away from mouth.
4. Exhale, then inhale through mouth. At the same time close the nebulizer valve with finger to release the mist of medication. Hold your breath for several seconds and release finger valve. Repeat this process until the medication is gone.
5. Wash the nebulizer, finger valve, and tubing daily, because the liquid medium from the medication is an excellent reservoir for bacteria. Use a mild detergent such as Ivory to clean the units, then soak in a solution of 2 parts white vinegar and 3 parts water for 20 minutes. Rinse and thoroughly dry the units on a clean towel. Store in a dust-free area.

and epistaxis occur rarely. Nasal passages should be cleared by blowing prior to inhalation. Effects should become apparent within several weeks; however, antihistamines or decongestants will probably be required during this initial period, but the need for these drugs should diminish with continued use of intranasal cromolyn.

Cromolyn Ophthalmic

(Opticrom 4%)

Cromolyn is also used as a 4% solution in the eye for the treatment of allergic ocular disorders. Decreased itching, redness, tearing, or discharge usually occurs within several days but treatment is often continued for up to 6 weeks. Dosage is 1 to 2 drops in each eye four to six times a day at regular intervals. Most frequent side-effects are a transient stinging or burning on instillation. Other infrequent reactions are ocular irritation; dryness; watery, puffy eyes; and styes. Soft contact lenses should not be worn during treatment, but may be reinserted within a few hours after discontinuation of the drug. Corticosteroids may be used concomitantly.

Inhaled Corticosteroids

Beclomethasone, Dexamethasone, Flunisolide, Triamcinolone

Several corticosteroids are available for inhalation in the treatment of steroid-dependent bronchial asthma. These agents are synthetic steroids with glucocorticoid activity, and the basic pharmacology of glucocorticoids is reviewed in detail in Chapter 55. This discussion is limited to their application in treating bronchial asthma, and a listing of the four drugs, with recommended doses and pertinent remarks, is given in Table 48-6.

Although the precise mechanism of action of the inhaled corticosteroids is unknown, several actions probably contribute to their effectiveness. They are believed to reduce the number and activity of inflammatory cells, retard bronchoconstrictor mechanisms, facilitate the action of beta-adrenergic drugs to elevate cyclic AMP levels, and possibly exert a direct smooth muscle-relaxing effect.

Inhaled corticosteroids are indicated for the control of bronchial asthma in patients who are either presently receiving such therapy systemically or who are inadequately controlled with a nonsteroid regimen, which may include beta-agonists, theophylline, or cromolyn sodium. These drugs are generally not necessary for relief of bronchial asthma, which can be adequately managed by bronchodilators, or in patients who only require corticosteroid therapy on an infrequent basis. Moreover, they are not suitable for control of acute bronchospastic episodes. The advantage of inhaled corticosteroid therapy versus systemic therapy is a reduced incidence of adverse effects, since the amount of inhaled drug that is absorbed is less than with systemic administration. Most common side-effects with these drugs are throat irritation, coughing, dry mouth, and hoarseness. Oral and pharyngeal fungal infections have occurred but respond promptly to discontinuation of medication and appropriate antifungal medication. An inhaled bronchodilator should be administered several minutes prior to the inhaled steroid to enhance its penetration into the lungs. Following inhalation, the mouth should be rinsed with water or mouthwash to reduce the likelihood of dry mouth or hoarseness.

Asthmatic patients transferred from systemic to inhaled corticosteroids are at risk for adrenal insufficiency and deaths have occurred. Chronic systemic steroid therapy results in suppression of hypothalamic–pituitary–adrenal (HPA) function through a negative feedback mechanism as illustrated in Figure 55-2, in Chapter 55. However, systemic steroid levels remain high due to the presence of the exogenously administered steroid. Following withdrawal of systemic steroids, many months are often required for HPA function to return to normal, and the inhaled steroid can no longer supply the high plasma concentrations of exogenous steroid. During this period (i.e., while patients are being transferred from systemic steroid to inhaled steroid and for several months thereafter), symptoms of adrenal insufficiency can occur if a sudden demand is made on adrenal function, such as with trauma, stress, severe infection, or surgery. Thus, during periods of stress or in the event of an acute asthmatic attack, patients receiving only inhaled corticosteroids should immediately resume systemic steroid treatment and contact their physician for further instructions. Although the inhaled steroid is usually sufficient to control asthmatic symptoms during these periods, it can not provide the systemic steroid necessary in these emergencies. Transfer from systemic to inhaled steroid must be accomplished gradually.

Table 48-6
Inhaled Corticosteroids

Drug	Preparations	Usual Dosage Range	Clinical Considerations
dexamethasone (Decadron)	Aerosol—each activation releases 84 mcg dexamethasone	Adults—3 inhalations 3 to 4 times a day (maximum 3/dose and 12/day) Children—2 inhalations 3 to 4 times a day (maximum 2/dose and 8/day)	Dose is gradually reduced when a favorable response is noted. Aerolized particles dissolve rapidly in bronchial secretions. Systemic absorption is about 50% (higher with larger doses or more frequent inhalation).
beclomethasone (Beclovent, Vanceril)	Aerosol—each activation delivers approximately 42 mcg	Adults—2 inhalations 3 to 4 times a day up to 20 inhalations/day in severe asthma Children—1 to 2 inhalations 3 to 4 times a day up to 10 inhalations a day	Systemic absorption is rapid, and drug and metabolites are eliminated primarily in the feces. Improvement in symptoms is generally noted in 1 week to 4 weeks. Not recommended in children under 6 years.
flunisolide (AeroBid)	Aerosol—each activation delivers approximately 250 mcg	Adults—2 inhalations twice a day (maximum 4 inhalations twice a day) Children (6 yr–15 yr)—2 inhalations twice a day	Systemic absorption is approximately 40%. Rapidly and extensively metabolized during first pass through the liver. Half-life is about 2 h. Not recommended in children under 6 years.
triamcinolone (Azmacort)	Aerosol—each activation delivers approximately 100 mcg	Adults—2 inhalations 3 to 4 times a day (maximum 16 inhalations/day) Children (6 yr–15 yr)—1 to 2 inhalations 3 to 4 times a day (maximum 12 inhalations/day)	Drug disappears rapidly from the lungs. Blood levels are maximum in 1 h–2 h. The major route of elimination is the feces. Not recommended in children under 6 years. Improvement is usually noted within 1 week to 2 weeks.

The aerosol should be initiated while the patient is still receiving normal maintenance doses of systemic steroids. After 1 week, the systemic steroid dosage should be reduced gradually at 1-week to 2-week intervals while observing the patient for signs of adrenal insufficiency. A slow rate of withdrawal cannot be overemphasized.

NURSING CONSIDERATIONS

See Nursing Considerations under Bronchodilators, Chapter 15, for information on teaching patients how to administer medication correctly through a metered-dose inhaler. Correct technique is very important for ensuring adequate intake of the drug. Always read the package insert before commencing to teach any patient the use of a particular inhaler and always ask the patient for a return demonstration.

After the patient inhales the drug he should rinse his mouth and gargle. This will reduce symptoms of dry mouth and hoarseness that often accompany drug use but will also decrease the incidence of fungal infections of the mouth. Teach the patient to look for redness on gums and mucosa and white patches on his tongue and to report such symptoms immediately. Treatment with antifungal medications is usually very effective.

Teach the patient not to use the drug during an acute asthmatic attack because it will not be effective and may actually worsen the condition.

Anticholinergics

Anticholinergic agents are effective bronchodilators, and the naturally occurring belladonna alkaloids (*e.g.*, atropine) have been used for hundreds of years in treating bronchial asthma. Unfortunately, the wide range of side-effects associated with systemic anticholinergic drugs greatly limits their usefulness in the routine management of bronchoconstrictive disorders. However, there has been a resurgence of interest in cholinergic antagonists as potential therapeutic agents for treating bronchial asthma with the clarification of the role played by the parasympathetic nervous system in intrinsic (*i.e.*, nonallergic) forms of asthma (see Fig. 48-2).

Anticholinergic, or more properly antimuscarinic, drugs can block the contraction of bronchiolar smooth muscle and the increase in mucus secretion resulting from increased vagal (*i.e.*, parasympathetic) activity. In addition, these drugs can inhibit acetylcholine-induced release of allergenic mediators from the mast cells. There appears to be substantial interpatient variation in the bronchial response to anticholinergic drugs, perhaps because these agents primarily interfere with parasympathetic activity, which plays a highly variable role in regulating bronchial function.

Ipratropium
(Atrovent)

MECHANISM AND ACTIONS
Ipratropium is a quaternary ammonium compound that exerts an anticholinergic action in the bronchioles to prevent the increase in cyclic GMP resulting from parasympathetic nerve activation. Thus, bronchial smooth muscle is relaxed and airway flow is improved. Since the drug is a quaternary salt, little systemic absorption occurs following inhalation and side-effects are minimal compared with systemic use of anticholinergics.

USES
1. Treatment of bronchospasm associated with chronic obstructive lung diseases, such as asthma, chronic bronchitis, or emphysema.

ADMINISTRATION AND DOSAGE
Ipratropium is used as an orally administered aerosol, which delivers 18 mcg of drug with each activation. The usual dose is 2 inhalations 4 times a day, although more frequent administration may be used in severe episodes, up to a maximum of 12 inhalations within 24 hours.

FATE
Much of an inhaled dose is swallowed, and is eliminated in the feces. Systemic absorption is minimal due to the quaternary configuration of the drug, which lowers its lipid solubility. The elimination half-life is about 2 hours following inhalation.

SIDE-EFFECTS/ADVERSE REACTIONS
Most frequently encountered side-effects with ipratropium are coughing, dryness of the oropharynx, nervousness, and gastric distress (especially if significant amounts are swallowed). Other reported adverse reactions include headache, dizziness, palpitations, skin rash, blurred vision, and drying of mucosal secretions. Rarely, tachycardia, drowsiness, coordination difficulties, itching, constipation, tremor, paresthesias, and mucosal ulceration have occurred.

CONTRAINDICATIONS AND PRECAUTIONS
Ipratropium should not be used to treat acute bronchospastic episodes where a rapid response is needed. The drug must be given *cautiously* to patients with narrow-angle glaucoma, prostatic hypertrophy, or bladder neck obstruction. The usual cautions should be observed in pregnant women, nursing mothers, and young children.

NURSING CONSIDERATIONS
See Nursing Considerations under Bronchodilators, Chapter 15 for information on teaching patients how to administer medication correctly through a metered-dose inhaler. Always read the instructions in the package to determine the proper method for activating the inhaler. Advise patients that use of the inhaler may result in drying of the mouth and pharynx. Suggest frequent rinsings to minimize this problem.

In addition to ipratropium, an inhaled dosage form of atropine sulfate may also be useful in preventing bronchial spasm, although systemic side-effects are more likely with atropine due to its greater systemic absorption. Dey-Dose Atropine Sulfate is administered by a nebulizer three to four times a day. 0.025 mg/kg of atropine sulfate diluted with 3 ml to 5 ml of saline provides bronchodilation without significant changes in heart rate or salivation. Bronchodilator activity varies inversely with the degree of preexisting airway obstruction and appears to be more marked on large airways compared to smaller airways. The effects of atropine are largely additive to those of inhaled beta-agonists. Systemic absorption of atropine can occur, and doses greater than 2.5 mg are likely to result in increased side-effects with little improvement in clinical efficacy. Adverse reactions include dry mouth, flushing, blurred vision, headache, tachycardia, slurred speech, and confusion.

CASE STUDY

Patricia Small, aged 30, had her first asthma attack at 14 years of age. She is allergic to many plants, animals, and molds. Although her treatment regimen has varied over the years she has most recently been controlled on theophylline time-release capsules, 300 mg every 12 hours, and cromolyn sodium, 20-mg capsules by spinhaler four times a day.

Over the last month Mrs. Small started a new job as an office manager in a small town where she recently moved with her husband. The couple bought an older home with an acre of property and are looking forward to fixing it up.

Mrs. Small awakened one night short of breath and heard herself wheezing. Although frightened, she got a metered-inhaler of metaproterenol and managed 3 inhalations. When she got no relief within 5 minutes she took another 300-mg tablet of theophylline. In the meantime, Mr. Small awakened, heard her breathing, and insisted they go to the local hospital emergency room. Mrs. Small was seen by the emergency room physician who decided to admit her with a diagnosis of acute asthma. An IV was started and an aminophylline drip begun. O_2 was administered by nasal cannula and theophylline level was drawn. Within 20 minutes Mrs. Small began to feel relief.

Discussion Questions

1. Why is it essential to obtain a theophylline level on Mrs. Small early in treatment?
2. An infusion of 250 mg aminophylline in 500 ml 5% dextrose in water was started on Mrs. Small and the physician ordered that she receive 16 mg per hour. How many milliliters per hour should be infused?
3. What factors may have precipitated Mrs. Small's asthma attack? How can the nurse incorporate these factors into a teaching plan for the patient?
4. Mrs. Small took metaproterenol, a drug she was not currently taking, when the attack began. Why did she do so? (See Chap. 15 for more information on this drug.) Should she have done so? Why did she take an additional theophylline tablet? Was this appropriate? How can the nurse use Mrs. Small's actions to develop a teaching plan for home care once Mrs. Small is discharged?

REVIEW QUESTIONS

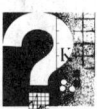

1. Briefly describe the anatomy of the respiratory system.
2. List several factors that can cause (1) bronchoconstriction and (2) bronchodilation.
3. Distinguish between "extrinsic" and "intrinsic" asthma.
4. Give the various treatments that can be used in managing an *acute* asthmatic attack.

5. Describe the mechanism of the bronchodilating action of (1) beta-adrenergic agonists and (2) xanthines (*e.g.*, theophylline).
6. List several factors that can (1) increase and (2) decrease the half-life of theophylline.
7. How do theophylline doses in children compare with those in adults? Explain.
8. What other pharmacologic actions in addition to bronchodilation are noted with theophylline?
9. How do differences in dosage forms for theophylline and its salts affect oral absorption?
10. What are the most frequently encountered side-effects with theophylline?
11. List several other types of drugs that may be found in fixed combination with theophylline? What are the disadvantages of these fixed-combination products?
12. What information does the nurse need to establish an adequate data base for the patient about to receive one of the theophylline drugs?
13. Outline the techniques to be taught to a patient who will take theophylline at home.
14. How can a patient manage the gastrointestinal distress sometimes associated with theophylline drugs?
15. What adjunctive measures may help the patient manage the activity associated with dyspnea and may also contribute to success of drug therapy?
16. What is the mechanism of action of cromolyn sodium? In what dosage forms is it available?
17. Give the major indications for cromolyn sodium.
18. In what types of patients are the inhaled corticosteroids indicated?
19. What are the principal adverse effects of inhaled corticosteroids?
20. What is the major danger associated with transferring patients from systemic to inhaled corticosteroids? Explain briefly.
21. What is the role of anticholinergics in treating bronchial asthma? What are their limitations?

BIBLIOGRAPHY

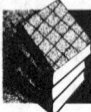

Au WY, Dutt AK, DeSoyza N: Theophylline kinetics in chronic obstructive airway disease in the elderly, Clin Pharmacol Ther 37:472, 1985

Bukowskyj M: Theophylline: An overview. Rational Drug Therapy 22(1):1, 1988

Burton AJ: Asthma inhalation devices: What do we know? Br Med J 288:1650, June 2, 1984

Cherniak RM: Current Therapy of Respiratory Disease, 1984–1985. Philadelphia, BC Decker, 1984

Corticosteroid aerosols for asthma. Med Lett Drugs Ther 27:5, 1985

Dwyer JM: A pharmacological approach to the management of asthma. Rational Drug Therapy 18(10):1, 1984

Flenley DC: New drugs in respiratory disorders. Br Med J 266:995, 1983

Fredholm BB, Persson CG: Xanthine derivatives as adenosine receptor antagonists. Eur J Pharmacol 81:673, 1982

Gillilland JL: Asthma Rx: Which drug for which patient? Modern Medicine 54(3):106, 1986

Henney HR et al: Knowledge of nurses and respiratory therapists about using cannister nebulizers. Am J Hosp Pharm 41:2402, Nov 1984

Kirilloff LH, Tibbals SC: Drugs for asthma—A complete guide. Am J Nurs 83(1):55, 1983

Lynch JP: Bronchoconstriction: Drugs that help patients breathe easier. Modern Medicine 53(1):104, 1985

McDonald G: A home program for patients with chronic lung disease. Nurs Clin North Am 16(2):259, 1981

Morris H: Pharmacology of corticosteroids in asthma. In Middleton E, Reed C, Ellis E (eds): Allergy—Principles and Practice. St Louis, CV Mosby, 1983

Petty TL: Drug strategies for airflow obstruction. Am J Nurs 87:180, 1987

Rall TW: Evolution of the mechanism of action of methylxanthines: From calcium mobilizers to antagonists of adenosine receptors. Pharmacologist 24:277, 1982

Shapiro GG, Konic P: Cromolyn sodium: A review. Pharmacotherapy 5:156, 1985

Sustained-release theophylline. Med Lett Drugs Ther 26:1, 1984

Todd B: Precautions in using bronchodilators. Geriatric Nursing 328, Sept/Oct 1984

Wang VA, Dworetzky M: How to manage the asthmatic patient. Drug Ther 13(9):79, 1983

Weissman G: The Eicosanoids of asthma. N Engl J Med 308:454, 1983

Wickland S (ed): 24-Hour theophylline—who can use it? Nurse's Drug Alert. Am J Nurs 85(4):428, 1985

Mucolytics

Acetylcysteine

49

Mucolytic agents have the ability to liquefy mucus and thus facilitate its removal from the respiratory passages by normal physiologic processes such as ciliary action, bronchiolar peristalsis, coughing, or through suction. Although various proteolytic enzymes and detergents have been tried previously as mucolytic agents, most exhibited undesirable side-effects and were unsuitable for clinical use. The only currently available mucolytic drug is acetylcysteine, an amino acid derivative that disrupts the molecular structure of mucus. It is a relatively nontoxic compound when used by inhalation for adjunctive therapy of a number of broncho-obstructive conditions resulting from excessive or highly viscous mucus.

Acetylcysteine may be administered by nebulization, using a face mask or mouthpiece, or if large volumes are required, by use of a tent or croupette. The drug may also be instilled directly into the bronchial tree by a tracheostomy tube or intratracheal cannula. However, when administered by an ordinary aerosol nebulizer, its effectiveness is compromised by its inability to penetrate deeply enough into the obstructed bronchiolar passages. Acetylcysteine is not indicated for routine use in bronchial asthmatic patients with mucus accumulation, inasmuch as it is frequently irritating and may elicit reflex bronchospasm, further impairing the patients' respiratory function.

Prompt removal of the liquefied secretions is necessary following use of a mucolytic agent. When coughing is unsuccessful in eliminating the liquefied mucus, or in the case of elderly or debilitated patients who are unable to encourage productive coughing, the airway must be kept clear by mechanical suction.

Acetylcysteine has also been employed to prevent or to minimize hepatotoxicity associated with acetaminophen overdosage by blocking the formation of a toxic metabolite. The drug is given orally for this indication, and the dosage is outlined below.

Acetylcysteine

(Mucomyst, Mucosol)

MECHANISM AND ACTIONS

Acetylcysteine contains a sulfhydryl group which acts to split disulfide linkages in the mucoprotein structures of mucus, thus reducing its viscosity. The mucolytic action of acetylcysteine is unaffected by the presence of DNA and increases with increasing *p*H, becoming optimal between *p*H 7 and 9.

Acetylcysteine also reduces the extent of liver damage following acetaminophen overdosage. Mechanisms of action include restoration (or maintenance) of glutathione levels and detoxification of the hepatotoxic metabolite of acetaminophen by serving as an alternative substrate for conjugation of the metabolite.

USES

1. Adjunctive therapy for the relief of abnormal, viscous mucus accumulation associated with a variety of chronic respiratory conditions, such as emphysema, asthmatic bronchitis, bronchiectasis, tuberculosis, or amyloidosis of the lung
2. Minimization of bronchiolar obstructive complications associated with tracheostomy, cystic fibrosis, atelectasis, surgery, anesthesia, or trauma
3. Facilitation of diagnostic bronchial studies (*e.g.*, bronchogram, bronchospirometry)
4. Prevention of hepatotoxicity due to acetaminophen overdosage (treatment must be initiated within 24 hours of ingestion)
5. Investigational uses include ophthalmic administration for treatment of keratoconjunctivitis sicca (dry eye) and as an enema for treating bowel obstruction due to meconium ileus.

ADMINISTRATION AND DOSAGE

Acetylcysteine sodium is available as a 10% or 20% solution. It is administered in several ways depending on the indication and condition of the patient. The various means of administration and recommended doses are listed below. In preparing the solutions, the 20% concentration is diluted with either normal saline or water for injection, while the 10% concentration may be given undiluted. Solutions should be used within 96 hours after opening.

Nebulization (face mask, mouthpiece, tracheostomy): 1 ml to 10 ml (20% solution) or 2 ml to 20 ml (10% solution) every 2 hours to 6 hours; usual dose is 6 ml to 10 ml of 10% solution three to four times a day

Nebulization (tent, croupette): volume of 10% to 20% solution sufficient to maintain a heavy mist in the area for the desired time period

Direct instillation: 1 ml to 2 ml of 10% to 20% solution every 1 hour to 4 hours by a tracheostomy tube or tracheal cannula

Diagnostic bronchograms: 1 ml to 2 ml (20% solution) or 2 ml to 4 ml (10% solution) by nebulization or direct instillation for two or three administrations before diagnostic procedure

Antidote to acetaminophen overdosage: (oral use—20% is diluted with soft drinks to a final concentration of 5%; dilutions should be used within 1 hour; undiluted solutions may be kept refrigerated up to 96 hours.) Initially, 140 mg/kg is given as a loading dose followed by 70 mg/kg every 4 hours thereafter for a total of 17 doses, *unless* an acetaminophen assay reveals a nontoxic plasma level.

If the patient vomits within 1 hour of any dose, repeat that dose. Refer to the package instructions for further diluting and dosing instructions.

SIDE-EFFECTS/ADVERSE REACTIONS
Large doses of oral acetylcysteine are likely to result in nausea, vomiting, and other GI symptoms. In addition, the drug has caused stomatitis, rhinorrhea, fever, rash, urticaria, tracheal and bronchial irritation, bronchospasm, and other allergic reactions.

CONTRAINDICATIONS AND PRECAUTIONS
There are no absolute contraindications to use of acetylcysteine. The drug should be given *cautiously* to patients with bronchial asthma (danger of bronchospasm) or a history of allergies and to elderly or debilitated patients or patients unable to elicit a productive cough to remove the accumulated mucus breakdown products (mechanical suction may be necessary in such instances).

Use of hand-held nebulizers provides insufficient output to deliver enough drug and should be avoided.

INTERACTIONS
1. Acetylcysteine is incompatible in solution with many antibiotics (*e.g.*, tetracyclines, amphotericin B, sodium ampicillin, erythromycin) and should not be mixed in the same solution. The drug is also incompatible in solution with trypsin, chymotrypsin, and hydrogen peroxide.

■ *Nursing Process*

See Chapter 23 for discussion of acetylcysteine in acetaminophen overdose.

□ ASSESSMENT
Prior to any inhalation treatment with acetylcysteine a baseline assessment of lungs should be performed. Look at respiratory rate and effort, and auscultate for diminished breath sounds, rhonchi, and so forth. If bronchospasm is suspected as manifested by wheezing, dyspnea, increased effort, increased pulse, and anxiety, notify the physician. Acetylcysteine should not be given until bronchospasm is relieved.

□ NURSING DIAGNOSES
Actual nursing diagnoses for the patient receiving acetylcysteine may include:

Knowledge deficit related to drug action, method of administration, effective expectoration after treatment, and potential side-effects

Potential nursing diagnoses may include:

Ineffective airway clearance after treatment related to weakness

Alteration in comfort related to nausea from the odor of the drug

Alteration in oral mucous membranes related to drug irritation

□ PLAN
The patient care goal is to facilitate removal or expectoration of mucus in order to clear the airway and enhance breathing.

□ INTERVENTION
Inhalation therapy with acetylcysteine is frequently ordered for patients who have difficulty expelling mucus. In addition to patients with respiratory diseases, candidates may include other patients with bronchial congestion such as the elderly bedridden patient, the postoperative patient especially after abdominal or chest surgery, the patient with a chest tube, and the immobilized patient. The nurse needs to encourage such patients to include adjunctive measures to facilitate mucus removal in addition to inhalation therapy. Coughing and deep breathing, forcing fluids, and changing positions or walking frequently are very important and will assist acetylcysteine therapy.

If the nurse is responsible for administering inhalation treatment, it is important to be aware of several factors which affect administration of the drug. The drug may develop a light purplish cast once opened. As long as acetylcysteine is used within 96 hours of opening, a color change will not impair its effectiveness. Prolonged nebulization with acetylcysteine will result in drug concentration and may impair delivery. In order to avoid this, monitor the drug reservoir chamber closely. Once the chamber has approximately one-fourth of the total drug left, add an equal amount of sterile water to dilute the solution.

Many patients find the odor of acetylcysteine very disagreeable and compare it to the odor of rotten eggs. Over time, the odor may become less apparent and more tolerable, but in some patients it may produce nausea and vomiting. Monitor the patient closely, be prepared to disconnect the inhalation device quickly, and keep an emesis basin close at hand.

Once liquefaction of mucus begins, be sure the patient has the strength to expectorate. Provide pillows to splint a wound if necessary, and have suction apparatus ready for use for the patient who is too weak to cough productively or for the patient with a tracheostomy or endotracheal tube.

Once the treatment is completed wash the patient's face and the apparatus mask and container to remove the sticky coating acetylcysteine produces. Encourage the patient to rinse his mouth after each treatment because acetylcysteine is irritating to mucous membranes.

Continue to monitor for signs and symptoms of bronchospasm.

□ *EVALUATION*

Outcome criteria against which to measure success of drug therapy include improved lung sounds, increased mucus production and expectoration, patient perception of improved breathing and ease of respiration.

REVIEW QUESTIONS

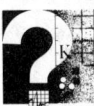

1. By what various means may acetylcysteine be administered?
2. What are the mechanisms of the (a) mucolytic and (b) hepatic-protective actions of acetylcysteine?
3. With what solutions are acetylcysteine solutions incompatible?
4. What baseline data are needed before administering acetylcysteine?
5. What adjunctive measures should the nurse advocate to improve expectoration of mucus?

BIBLIOGRAPHY

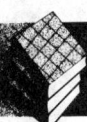

Bailey BO: Acetaminophen hepatotoxicity and overdose. Am Fam Physician 22:83, 1980
Prescott LF, Critchley J: The treatment of acetaminophen poisoning. Annu Rev Pharmacol Toxicol 23:87, 1983

Respiratory Stimulants

50

Drugs having the ability to enhance depressed respiratory function are termed respiratory stimulants or *analeptics.* Such agents act both at the level of the respiratory center in the brain stem and on the peripheral carotid chemoreceptors to increase the depth and, frequently, the rate of respiration also.

A brief review of respiratory control mechanisms will aid in understanding the action of the respiratory stimulant drugs.

Neural Control of Respiration

The rhythmic pattern of normal respiration is maintained by the cyclic discharge of neurons located in the brain stem. Three bilateral interconnected respiratory "centers" (located in the medulla and pons) are generally recognized: the medullary center, the apneustic center, and the pneumotaxic center.

Medullary Respiratory Center

The medullary respiratory center consists of two anatomically intermingled but functionally distinct and reciprocally active aggregates of neurons: inspiratory neurons and expiratory neurons. The inspiratory neurons exhibit spontaneous bursts of activity during which the expiratory neurons are inhibited due to the operation of oscillating negative feedback circuits.

Simultaneously, impulses originating in the inspiratory neurons travel along the phrenic and intercoastal nerves to the diaphragm and external intercoastal muscles, respectively, causing their contraction and the subsequent enlargement of the thorax, leading to inspiration. The medullary respiratory center receives afferent (sensory) input from central chemoreceptors, various peripherally located receptors, and from higher brain centers (including the apneustic and pneumotaxic centers of the pons). The afferent input can modify the basic rhythmic discharge of the medullary respiratory neurons. For example, impulses originating in the cerebral cortex allow voluntary interruption of the normal breathing cycle for activities such as speaking, laughing, and breath holding.

Apneustic Center

The apneustic center, located in the reticular formation of the lower pons, provides tonic solution to the medullary inspiratory neurons, thereby facilitating and prolonging inspiration. The apneustic center is not necessary for the maintenance of a basic respiratory rhythm, and its level of activity can be modified (inhibited) by afferent input from the pneumotaxic center and from pulmonary stretch receptors.

Pneumotaxic Center

The pneumotaxic center (located in the superior pons) periodically inhibits inspiration and facilitates expiration by inhibiting the apneustic center and possibly by inhibiting the medullary inspiratory neurons directly. The pneumotaxic center does not possess an inherent rhythmicity but is activated by a feedback mechanism during discharge of medullary inspiration neurons. Inhibition of the inspiratory neurons deprives the pneumotaxic center of its stimulation, causing it to become inactive.

Chemical Control of Respiration

The CO_2, O_2, and H^+-ion levels of the blood (and other body fluids) are of major importance in the control of respiration. CO_2 is the most potent physiologic stimulant of respiration, exerting its effects chiefly through central chemoreceptors. It must be noted, however, that very high concentrations of CO_2 (in excess of 30% in inspired air) produce central nervous system (and respiratory) depression and may be lethal.

Central Chemoreceptors

The ventral surface of the medulla contains chemosensitive cells that respond to elevations of CO_2 and H^+ ions in arterial blood and cerebrospinal fluid by stimulating the medullary respiratory center.

CO_2 readily diffuses from the blood plasma into the cerebrospinal fluid, where it combines with water to form H_2CO_3, which then dissociates into H^+ and HCO_3^- ions.

Because cerebrospinal fluid is not as well buffered as the blood, the H^+-ion concentration rises quickly, effectively stimulating the central chemoreceptors and thereby increasing pulmonary ventilation.

Peripheral Chemoreceptors

Located peripherally in the carotid and aortic bodies are chemoreceptors neurally connected to the medullary respiratory center by afferent glossopharyngeal and vagal nerve fibers.

These peripheral chemoreceptors are primarily sensitive to arterial O_2 levels, responding to lowered arterial P_{O_2} (hypoxemia) by stimulating respiration. They serve as an important emergency mechanism of respiratory stimulation in states of low O_2 intake.

Carotid and aortic chemoreceptors also respond to elevations in arterial P_{CO_2} and H^+-ion concentrations, mechanisms of importance in acidosis.

Reflex Regulation of Respiration

In addition to chemoreceptors, there are a number of peripheral receptors whose stimulation initiates reflex changes in respiration.

Sensory modalities such as pain, temperature, and touch affect respiration, with pain exerting a strong excitatory effect on the medullary respiratory center.

Movements of joints, whether active or passive, stimulate respiration by way of afferent pathways originating in the proprioceptors of muscles, tendons, and joints. These pathways, which converge on the respiratory center, augment pulmonary ventilation during exercise.

Sneezing and coughing are reflex, modified respiratory responses to irritants of the respiratory mucosa.

Inflation of the lungs stimulates pulmonary stretch receptors that lead to vagally mediated inhibition of inspiration. This "inflation reflex" (also termed the vagal or Hering-Breuer reflex) does not appear to be of great importance during normal respiration in humans.

Respiratory Stimulant Drugs

The various central nervous system respiratory centers are sensitive to the depressant effects of a variety of drugs, including sedative-hypnotics, narcotics, anesthetics, and alcohol.

Respiratory stimulants are primarily indicated as adjuncts to overcome respiratory depression due to drug overdosage with these various classes of CNS depressants or to manage postanesthesia respiratory depression resulting from general anesthetic drugs. Their clinical effectiveness in many cases of drug-induced respiratory depression has been questioned, however, and their potential for eliciting untoward reactions is rather high. Thus, they should be used with caution and only by those individuals skilled in their administration.

Foremost among the disadvantages of these drugs is that doses needed to elicit sufficient respiratory stimulation in cases of marked respiratory depression often stimulate other CNS areas as well (e.g., vasomotor center, vomiting center, brain stem reticular formation), resulting in a variety of undesirable effects ranging from mild cardiovascular stimulation to marked central activation leading to vomiting, hyperreflexia, and convulsions. Because respiratory stimulants have a rather narrow safety margin, they must be administered cautiously by trained personnel and only in conjunction with appropriate resuscitative measures (e.g., oxygen, suction, anticonvulsants, muscle relaxants) as necessary.

Analeptics are merely physiologic antagonists of respiratory depressants and do not specifically block the effects of narcotics, barbiturates, muscle relaxants, or other drugs. In fact, analeptics alone are often insufficient in arousing a severely depressed individual and should be used only in conjunction with adequate adjunctive measures, such as mechanical assistance, narcotic antagonists, or cholinergic drugs, depending on the particular drug involved. Obviously, maintenance of an open airway is essential with use of respiratory stimulants.

Although these drugs are not routinely employed to overcome postanesthetic respiratory depression and to shorten recovery time, some clinicians advocate a single IV injection or a slow IV infusion of doxapram, the preferred analeptic, together with oxygen following surgery to encourage "deep breathing" and prevent development of postoperative atelectasis, especially in patients with compromised respiratory function. A danger in such a procedure is that the analeptic can mask the residual effects of a muscle relaxant if one was administered during surgery.

In addition to doxapram, a specific analeptic drug, caffeine and sodium benzoate injection has also been employed as a respiratory stimulant under certain conditions, and this combination is considered in Chapter 32 with other CNS stimulants.

Doxapram
(Dopram)

MECHANISM AND ACTIONS
Doxapram enhances the depth and to a lesser degree the rate of respiration by activating the peripheral carotid chemoreceptors and, in large doses, by directly stimulating the medullary respiratory centers. Tidal volume is increased, and respiratory rate may also be slightly elevated. Increasing doses stimulate other areas of the brain, although there is little direct action on the cortex. Convulsions can occur with large doses. Blood pressure may be elevated, largely due to increased cardiac output as a result of stimulation of the medullary vasomotor center. Increased catecholamine release can occur.

USES
1. Reversal of postanesthetic respiratory depression or apnea (*except* due to muscle relaxants) and facilitation of emergence from anesthesia (May also be given with O_2 to stimulate deep breathing in the postoperative patient)
2. Adjunctive treatment of drug-induced CNS and respiratory depression, to hasten arousal and facilitate return of laryngopharyngeal reflexes (*Note*: Respiratory depression due to CNS-depressant overdosage is best managed by mechanical ventilation.)
3. Prevention of elevated arterial carbon dioxide tension during oxygen administration in patients with chronic obstructive pulmonary disease with acute respiratory insufficiency (*not* to be used in conjunction with mechanical ventilation)

ADMINISTRATION AND DOSAGE
Doxapram is available as an injection solution in a concentration of 20 mg/ml. Recommended dosages for the various indications are as follows:
Postanesthesia: 0.5 mg to 1 mg/kg IV injection (maximum 2 mg/kg when given as multiple injections at 5-minute intervals) *or* 5 mg/minute by IV infusion until a satisfactory response is obtained, then 1 mg to 3 mg/minute to maintain respiration (maximum dose is 300 mg).
Drug-induced respiratory depression: 2 mg/kg IV injection; repeat in 5 minutes, than at 1-hour to 2-hour intervals until arousal is sustained (total maximum dose is 3 g); *alternately*, 1 mg to 3 mg/minute by IV infusion following initial priming dose of 2 mg/kg by IV injection. Discontinue at end of 2 hours or if patient awakens (total maximum dose is 3 g).
Chronic obstructive pulmonary disease: 1 mg to 3 mg/minute by IV infusion (2 mg/ml solution) for a maximum of 2 hours.
Note: Admixture of doxapram solution with alkaline solutions (*e.g.*, aminophylline, bicarbonate) will result in precipitation.

FATE
Following IV injection, respiratory stimulation occurs within 20 seconds to 40 seconds with the peak effect at 1 minute to 2 minutes. Duration of action ranges from 6 minutes to 12 minutes. The drug is rapidly and completely metabolized and excreted in the urine. Plasma half-life ranges from 2 hours to 4 hours.

SIDE-EFFECTS/ADVERSE REACTIONS
A slight pressor response frequently occurs during doxapram administration but is seldom of clinical consequence except in hypertensive patients. A variety of other adverse effects have been noted during doxapram administration, most of which are the result of its increased central stimulatory action in larger doses, and these are listed by organ system below.
CNS/autonomic—Flushing, sweating, feeling of warmth, pruritus, paresthesias, headache, dizziness, disorientation, mydriasis, tremors, involuntary movements, muscle spasticity, hyperactivity, convulsions, increased deep tendon reflexes, clonus
Respiratory—Cough, dyspnea, bronchospasm, laryngospasm, hiccups, rebound hypoventilation
Cardiovascular—Chest pain and tightness, phlebitis, depressed T waves, arrhythmias
GI—Nausea, vomiting, diarrhea, urge to defecate
Other—Urinary retention, incontinence, proteinuria, decreased hemoglobin, hematocrit, or red blood cell count
Overdosage can result in an excessive pressor effect, tachycardia, skeletal muscle spasticity, and convulsive seizures. Seizures are unlikely at recommended doses, however.

CONTRAINDICATIONS AND PRECAUTIONS
Doxapram administration is contraindicated in patients with epilepsy or other convulsive states, airway obstruction, incompetence of the ventilatory

mechanism, pneumothorax, extreme dyspnea, acute bronchial asthma, suspected or confirmed pulmonary embolism, respiratory failure due to neuromuscular disorders, pulmonary fibrosis, severe hypertension, acute cerebrovascular accident, head injury, coronary artery disease, and uncompensated heart failure.

The drug must be given with extreme *caution* and under close supervision to patients with cerebral edema, severe tachycardia, arrhythmias, cardiac disease, pheochromocytoma, history of bronchial asthma, hyperthyroidism, peptic ulcer, acute agitation, to pregnant women or to children under 12 years.

Extravasation of the infusion solution should be avoided because thrombophlebitis and localized skin irritation can occur. Too rapid infusion may result in hemolysis. Doxapram is not a specific narcotic antagonist nor an antagonist to muscle relaxant drugs. In patients who have received muscle relaxants, doxapram may temporarily mask the effects of muscle-relaxing drugs.

Intravenous short-acting barbiturates or diazepam, along with oxygen and resuscitative equipment, should be readily available to manage overdosage marked by excessive CNS stimulation.

INTERACTIONS
1. Additive pressor effects may occur if doxapram is combined with sympathomimetics or MAO inhibitors.
2. Doxapram releases epinephrine, and thus may increase the incidence of arrhythmias with those general anesthetics that sensitize the myocardium (*e.g.*, halothane, enflurane, cyclopropane). Doxapram administration should be delayed for at least 10 minutes to 15 minutes following discontinuation of the general anesthetic to minimize the danger of this interaction.

■ Nursing Process

□ ASSESSMENT
Doxapram should be used only in an environment where a patient can be continuously observed and where cardiovascular and hemodynamic monitoring can be performed. The nurse must make sure resuscitative equipment, oxygen and emergency drugs are immediately available and should strongly urge the physician in charge to remain in attendance or close at hand while the drug is infus-

ing. Follow institution policy regarding IV injection of this drug, but in most cases it should be given by a physician.

Prior to drug administration baseline data should be collected. Assess the rate and depth of respiration and note effort. Obtain arterial blood gases, and, if possible, ensure the correct insertion of an arterial line to facilitate continuous monitoring. Cardiac rate and rhythm should also be noted, and the patient should be placed on a cardiac monitor. Muscle contractility, strength, and depth of deep tendon reflexes need to be tested and recorded for later comparison.

□ PLAN
The goal of this drug therapy is to stimulate respiration to facilitate adequate air exchange.

□ NURSING DIAGNOSES
Potential nursing diagnoses are based on the drug side-effects and may include:

Alteration in cardiac output: decreased related to hypertension and arrhythmias

Alteration in respiratory function: hyperventilation

Alteration in comfort: vomiting related to the drug's effect on the central nervous system

Alteration in thought processes: seizures related to the drug's effect on the central nervous system

Urinary retention: related to the drug's effect on the central nervous system

Alteration in tissue perfusion: thrombophlebitis at IV site

□ INTERVENTION
The nurse may not actually administer doxapram but may be responsible for preparing the injection or infusion and monitoring the rate of administration. The drug should be given very slowly; if possible, an infusion pump should be used if the drug is given by continuous or intermittent infusion. Doxapram will precipitate with alkaline IV solutions, such as sodium bicarbonate and thiopental. The drug can be mixed with normal saline, 5% or 10% dextrose and water, or a combination of these two. The drug should not be administered through a line with other drugs. Watch the infusion site closely; extravasation can cause tissue damage, and thrombophlebitis may occur. If pain, redness, or swelling develop, the IV should be discontinued and a new site found.

The nurse's main responsibility is close patient monitoring to observe for improved respiratory function, and to prevent or detect side-effects of the drug early so overdosage can be avoided.

A flow sheet may be useful for documentation because monitoring will be frequent and overdosage may first be seen through subtle changes. Blood pressure must be taken every 2 minutes to 5 minutes early in the infusion because the hypertension secondary to doxapram can be severe. The frequency of blood pressure monitoring can be decreased as the infusion progresses but should be done at least every half hour. If there is a significant fall in blood pressure or dyspnea, the drug should be discontinued. The cardiac monitor should be watched for signs of arrhythmias, and heart rate should be taken regularly. Arterial blood gases should be drawn every half hour paying particular attention to any increase in PCO_2 or decrease in PO_2. Respiratory rate, volume of air exchange, and effort should also be watched closely. A respirometer may be used to test volume. An excessive increase in respiratory rate, hyperventilation, can result from overdosage and lead to respiratory alkalosis and, ultimately, apnea. Should respiratory arrest occur, resuscitation and mechanical ventilation should be initiated and doxapram immediately discontinued. Deep tendon reflexes and muscular contractility should be tested regularly throughout the infusion; an increase in reflexes or muscle twitching may be the first signs of overdose.

Doxapram may stimulate the central nervous system resulting in vomiting, seizures, or urinary retention. Position the patient to prevent aspiration if vomiting should occur because the response may be projectile and without warning. Have suction equipment ready. Have intravenous anticoagulants on hand and protect the patient in bed to reduce the chance of injury should a seizure occur. Palpate the bladder, and record urine output hourly during initial drug infusion and every 2 hours throughout the course of therapy.

Doxapram can mask the respiratory depressant effect of anesthetics and depressants so the drug should be withdrawn slowly and the patient continuously monitored for about 1 hour to 2 hours afterward to ensure respiratory depression does not recur. Voluntary respiration should be effortless, and all reflexes should return to normal.

□ EVALUATION

The outcomes by which to measure successful therapy are improved minute volume indicating adequate air exchange, improved rate and depth of respiration, improved arterial blood gas picture with a lowering of PCO_2 and responsiveness of the patient.

REVIEW QUESTIONS

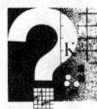

1. What is an analeptic?
2. What are the principal disadvantages associated with the use of analeptics?
3. Describe the mechanism of action of doxapram.
4. What are the major symptoms of doxapram overdosage?
5. Why should doxapram *not* be given concurrently with halogenated general anesthetics such as halothane?
6. What baseline data should be collected before administering an analeptic?
7. What are the nurse's main responsibilities during doxapram administration?
8. What outcome criteria can be used to judge the effectiveness of doxapram therapy?

BIBLIOGRAPHY

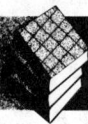

Calverly PMA, Robson RH, Wraith PK, Prescott LF, Flenley DC: The ventilatory effects of doxapram in normal man. Clin Sci 65:65, 1983

Hirsh K, Wang SC: Selective respiratory stimulating action of doxapram compared to pentylenetetrazol. J Pharmacol Exp Ther 189:1, 1974

Wang SC, Ward JW: Analeptics. Pharmacol Ther 3:123, 1977

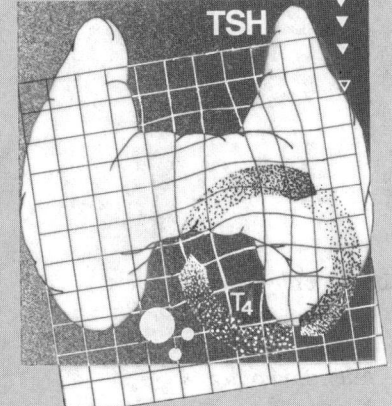

Hormones and Drugs Affecting Hormonal Function

Hypophyseal Hormones

51

The hypophysis, or pituitary gland, is composed of two major divisions, the adenohypophysis (anterior lobe), which secretes at least six hormones, and the neurohypophysis (posterior lobe), which releases two hormones. Virtually no bodily function is exempt from the influence of at least one of the hypophyseal hormones, which collectively serve to regulate and integrate the physiologic and metabolic processes necessary for the maintenance of homeostasis. Before beginning a discussion of the clinically useful hypophyseal hormones, however, a review of the anatomy and physiology of the hypophysis is presented.

Pituitary Gland (Hypophysis)

The pituitary gland, previously called the "master gland," secretes several polypeptide hormones that directly or indirectly regulate a wide variety of metabolic and physiologic processes essential to normal growth and development, as well as to the maintenance of homeostasis. Many of the hormones secreted by the pituitary gland are critical to the activity of peripheral target glands, including the thyroid, adrenals, and gonads.

Anatomy

The pituitary gland (hypophysis cerebri) is located at the base of the brain, resting within the sella turcica of the sphenoid bone. The pituitary gland maintains elaborate neural and vascular connections with the hypothalamus of the brain, which plays a central role in the integration of neuroendocrine activity (Fig. 51-1).

The pituitary gland has two major components: the neurohypophysis and the adenohypophysis.

NEUROHYPOPHYSIS
The neurohypophysis, which is connected directly to the hypothalamus by the infundibular (pituitary) stalk, is rich in nerve fibers of hypothalamic origin (the hypothalamicohypophyseal tract).

Neurosecretory cells in the supraoptic and paraventricular nuclei of the hypothalamus produce two hormones: antidiuretic hormone (ADH, or vasopressin) and oxytocin. These hormones are then transported along the axons of the hypothalamicohypophyseal tract to the pars nervosa (posterior lobe) of the pituitary gland for storage and ultimate release.

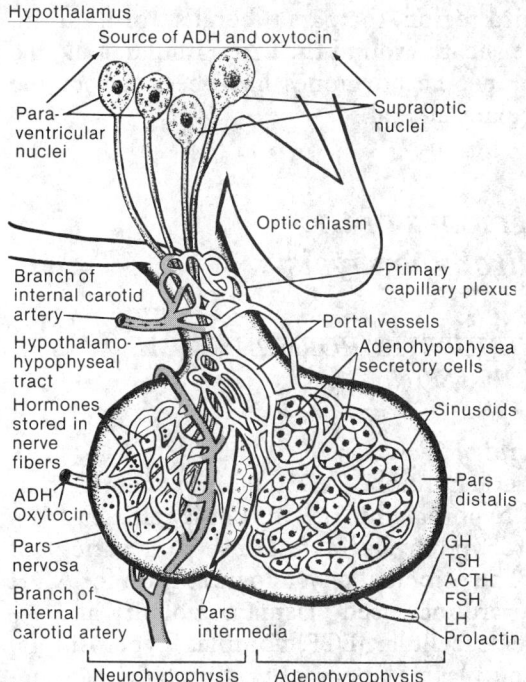

Figure 51-1. *The pituitary gland (hypophysis) and its relationship with the hypothalamus.*

ADENOHYPOPHYSIS
The adenohypophysis is served by an elaborate vascular system, including the hypothalamicohypophyseal portal system, which transports hypothalamic regulating hormones (factors) to the glandular cells of the adenohypophysis.

The largest portion of the adenohypophysis is the pars distalis (anterior lobe). Its secretory chromophilic cells include the following:

1. Acidophils (alpha cells), which constitute 40% of the cellular population, and which secrete growth hormone (GH; somatotropin; STH) and prolactin (luteotropic hormone; LTH)
2. Basophils (beta cells), which represent 10% of the glandular cells, and which secrete four hormones: thyroid-stimulating hormone (TSH; thyrotropin); adrenocorticotropic hormone (ACTH; corticotropin); follicle-stimulating hormone (FSH); and luteinizing hormone (LH)

The remaining 50% of the cells in the adenohypophysis are chromophobes. Chromophobe tumors have been associated with excessive secretion of ACTH and GH.

The pars intermedia (intermediate lobe) of the adenohypophysis contains basophilic (beta) cells, which secrete melanocyte-stimulating hormone (MSH, or intermedin).

A third region, the pars tuberalis, forms an incomplete sheath around the infundibular stalk. To date, no specific hormones have been associated with the pars tuberalis.

Hormones of the Neurohypophysis

ANTIDIURETIC HORMONE (ADH; VASOPRESSIN)

Control of Secretion

Antidiuretic hormone (ADH) is a nonapeptide hormone of hypothalamic origin that is released from the neurohypophysis in response to a variety of stimuli. The principal physiologic stimuli for ADH secretion are increased plasma osmolality and decreased extracellular (ECF) volume. Hyperosmolality of the plasma apparently stimulates osmoreceptors in the anterior hypothalamus, producing a reflex secretion of ADH. Decreased circulating blood volume is a potent stimulus for ADH release, operating by way of volume receptors (low-pressure baroreceptors) located in the left atrium, the great veins, the aortic arch, and the carotid sinus.

Other stimuli for ADH release include pain, hypoxia, and such pharmacologic agents as morphine, nicotine, and barbiturates.

ADH secretion is inhibited by decreased plasma osmolality, increased ECF volume, alcohol, and phenytoin.

Actions

The principal physiologic role of ADH is to regulate ECF volume and osmolality by controlling the final volume and concentration of urine.

ADH, acting through the second messenger cyclic AMP, increases the permeability of the collecting tubules to water. The enhanced reabsorption of water from the renal tubules results in the production of a concentrated urine that is reduced in volume.

Pharmacologic amounts of ADH produce a pressor (hypertensive) effect that results from a direct constrictor action of the hormone on vascular smooth muscle.

The early observations that posterior pituitary extracts produce a marked elevation of arterial blood pressure led to the initial naming of this hormone as *vasopressin*.

Clinical States

Diabetes Insipidus

Inadequate ADH secretion results in the excretion of large volumes of dilute urine (polyuria). Intense thirst and consumption of large amounts of liquid (polydipsia) are also characteristic of diabetes insipidus.

This disorder may be idiopathic or it may follow trauma or cranial injury, central nervous system (CNS) disease, infection, or emotional shock. The deficit may be related to the supraoptic nuclei, the hypothalamicohypophyseal tract, or the neurohypophysis.

A rare ADH-resistant or nephrogenic diabetes also exists. In this inherited disorder, ADH secretion is normal; however, the renal tubules are unresponsive to the hormone. Treatment of diabetes insipidus is discussed later in this chapter under the uses for vasopressin.

Inappropriate ADH Syndrome

The inappropriate ADH syndrome, a clinical state characterized by hypersecretion of ADH, may result from generalized infection, mediastinal tumors, metastatic tumors to the brain, pathologic CNS changes, or intracranial surgery.

Abnormal fluid retention leads to dilution of plasma sodium (dilutional hyponatremia), and urine becomes inappropriately concentrated. Fluid intake must be stringently restricted to minimize water intoxication.

OXYTOCIN

Control of Secretion and Actions

The two major physiologic actions of oxytocin are exerted on female reproductive structures.

Galactokinetic Action

The ejection of milk from a primed, lactating mammary gland follows a neuroendocrine reflex in which oxytocin serves as the efferent limb. The reflex is normally initiated by suckling, which stimulates cutaneous receptors in the areola of the breast. Afferent nerve impulses travel to the paraventricular nuclei of the hypothalamus to effect the release of oxytocin from the neurohypophysis. Oxytocin is carried by the blood to the mammary gland, where it causes contraction of myoepithelial cells surrounding the alveoli and lactiferous ducts to bring about the ejection of milk (milk let-down).

In lactating women, tactile stimulation of the

breast areola, emotional stimuli, and genital stimulation may also lead to oxytocin release.

Oxytocic Action

Oxytocin acts directly on uterine smooth muscle to elicit strong, rhythmic contractions of the myometrium. Uterine sensitivity to oxytocin varies with its physiologic state and with hormonal balance. The gravid (pregnant) uterus is highly sensitive to oxytocin, particularly in the late stages of gestation. Uterine sensitivity to oxytocin is greatly enhanced by estrogen and inhibited by progesterone.

Oxytocin release appears to follow a neuroendocrine reflex initiated by genital stimulation.

There is some evidence that oxytocin may affect sperm transport through the female genital tract.

Hormones of the Adenohypophysis

The secretion of hormones by the adenohypophysis (pars distalis and pars intermedia) is controlled by hypothalamic regulatory hormones (factors) that are transported to the pituitary gland by the hypothalamohypophyseal portal system, illustrated in Figure 51-1.

There appear to be several regulatory (hypophysiotropic) hormones produced by the hypothalamus:

1. Thyrotropin-releasing hormone (TRH)
2. Corticotropin-releasing hormone (CRH)
3. Growth hormone-releasing hormone (GHRH)
4. Growth hormone release-inhibiting hormone (GHRIH), or *somatostatin*
5. Gonadotropin-releasing hormone (GnRH)
6. Prolactin release-inhibiting hormone (PRIH)
7. Prolactin-releasing hormone (PRH)
8. Melanotropin-releasing hormone (MRH)
9. Melanotropin-inhibiting hormone (MIH)

The secretion of hypothalamic regulatory hormones is controlled by neurotransmitters, many of which have been specifically identified.

GROWTH HORMONE (GH; SOMATOTROPIN; STH)

Control of Secretion

Growth hormone secretion is largely controlled by two hypothalamic hypophysiotropic hormones. These and other factors affecting GH secretion are listed below.

Factors Promoting GH Secretion
GHRH
Hypoglycemia and fasting
Elevated plasma levels of amino acids (*e.g.*, arginine)
Stress
Exercise
Levodopa (or other dopamine agonists)
GH secretion in response to hypoglycemia, fasting, and exercise appears to be reduced by obesity.

Factors Inhibiting GH Secretion
GHRIH (somatostatin)
Hyperglycemia
Elevated plasma levels of free fatty acids
Cortisol (glucocorticoids)
Alpha-adrenergic blocking agents
GH (negative feedback mechanism)

Actions

Effects on Growth
GH accelerates overall body growth by increasing the mass of both skeletal and soft body tissues through hyperplasia (increased cell number) and hypertrophy (increased cell size).

The effects of GH are particularly evident in hard tissues where chondrogenesis (cartilage formation) and osteogenesis (bone formation) are enhanced, leading to an increase in linear growth and stature before epiphyseal closure and in bone thickness following closure of the epiphyses.

GH stimulates certain tissues, notably the liver and kidneys, to produce somatomedins (formerly termed *sulfation factor*). Somatomedins are polypeptides that mediate certain effects of GH, including the stimulation of collagen synthesis, chondrogenesis, and incorporation of sulfate into cartilage. Somatomedins exhibit some insulin-like effects, including increased glucose and amino acid transport into certain cells.

Metabolic Effects
1. Protein metabolism—GH increases protein synthesis and nitrogen retention by enhancing the incorporation of amino acids into protein. The protein anabolic action results from (1) accelerated entry of amino acids into cells and (2) increased ribonucleic acid (RNA) synthesis.
2. Lipid metabolism—GH stimulates the mobilization and utilization of fats, enabling the body to use stored fats as an energy source. The ele-

vation of plasma levels of free fatty acids resulting from the hydrolysis of triglycerides (stored neutral fats) is potentially ketogenic.

3. Carbohydrate metabolism—GH causes hyperglycemia by increasing the hepatic output of glucose and impairing glucose transport into muscle ("anti-insulin" action on muscle).

Excessive secretion of GH may precipitate or increase the severity of clinical diabetes mellitus ("diabetogenic" effect).

PROLACTIN (MAMMOTROPIN; LACTOGENIC HORMONE)

Control of Secretion
Prolactin secretion is controlled by the hypothalamus, with PRIH normally dominating. Tactile stimulation of the breast may initiate neuronal activity leading to the release of prolactin-releasing hormone (PRH) from the hypothalamus, thus promoting prolactin secretion from the alpha cells of the adenohypophysis. Activation of dopamine receptors can inhibit prolactin secretion by liberating PRIH from the hypothalamus.

Actions
Prolactin initiates and maintains milk secretion from breasts primed for lactation by other hormones such as estrogens, progesterone, insulin, corticosteroids, and thyroid hormones.

Prolactin also appears to act synergistically with estrogen to stimulate growth of the mammary glands.

Prolactin and GH are very closely related structurally and may, therefore, exert some overlapping functions.

FOLLICLE-STIMULATING HORMONE

Control of Secretion
FSH secretion is controlled by the hypothalamus by way of gonadotropin-releasing hormone (GnRH). Circulating levels of androgens (testosterone) and estrogens participate in this control by inhibiting GnRH secretion by the hypothalamus. Shortly before ovulation, estrogen exerts a positive feedback on gonadotropin secretion, causing a burst of FSH secretion. The pineal gland has also been implicated in the control of gonadotropin secretion.

Actions
FSH stimulates the germinal epithelium of testicular seminiferous tubules, thereby promoting spermatogenesis in the male. In the female, FSH stimulates follicular growth and development within the ovaries. FSH is the dominant gonadotropin during the follicular or preovulatory phase of the ovarian cycle.

LUTEINIZING HORMONE (LH; INTERSTITIAL CELL-STIMULATING HORMONE; ICSH)

Control of Secretion
LH secretion is controlled by the hypothalamus through GnRH.

The release of LH is inhibited by testosterone and by estrogens, except for a brief priming effect exerted by estrogen to allow a surge of LH needed to effect ovulation.

Actions
In the male, this hormone stimulates testosterone production by testicular interstitial cells (of Leydig); hence the name interstitial cell-stimulating hormone.

In the female, LH stimulates ripening of the ovarian follicles, controls ovulation, and promotes the formation and maintenance of the corpus luteum.

In many animals, LH elicits the behavioral manifestations of estrus (heat).

THYROTROPIN (THYROID-STIMULATING HORMONE; TSH)

Control of Secretion
TRH and cold promote secretion of TSH by the beta cells of the adenohypophysis. Elevated plasma levels of free thyroid hormones inhibit thyrotropin secretion.

Actions
TSH stimulates growth (hypertrophy) of the thyroid gland and promotes the synthesis and release of thyroid hormones thyroxine and triiodothyronine. The actions of TSH on the thyroid gland are mediated by cyclic AMP, and they are detailed later in this chapter in the section on the thyroid gland.

TSH may also act directly on the ocular orbital tissue to cause exophthalmos (protrusion of the eyeballs).

CORTICOTROPIN (ADRENOCORTICOTROPIC HORMONE; ACTH)

Control of Secretion
ACTH secretion is regulated by neural factors and by a hormonal negative feedback mechanism.

ACTH is secreted in response to CRH and to various forms of stress, including fear, pain, cold, trauma, and hypoglycemia.

Elevated plasma glucocorticoid (cortisol) levels inhibit CRH and ACTH secretion.

Actions

ACTH exerts its tropic effects on the adrenal glands, promoting growth and steroidogenesis in the adrenal cortex. The stimulation of corticosteroid production (steroidogenesis) in response to ACTH is mediated by the second messenger, cyclic AMP.

MELANOTROPIN (MELANOCYTE-STIMULATING HORMONE; MSH; INTERMEDIN)

Control of Secretion

MSH secretion by the pars intermedia is controlled by hypothalamic inhibiting and releasing hormones.

Actions

MSH acts on the skin of fish, reptiles, and amphibians to disperse melanophore granules, leading to changes in skin coloration.

Mammals, including humans, do not possess melanophores, but rather melanin-containing cells called *melanocytes*. Thus, there appears to be no major physiologic role for MSH in humans. Some neurotropic effects of MSH have been observed; however, the physiologic significance of these remains unclear.

Abnormally large amounts of MSH (such as with functional pituitary tumors) may produce hyperpigmentation of skin in humans.

ACTH and alpha-MSH are structurally similar, so that hyperpigmentation associated with certain pathologic states may result from ACTH or alpha-MSH hypersecretion.

Disorders of the Adenohypophysis

HYPOFUNCTIONAL STATES

Hypopituitarism (Pituitary Insufficiency)

In the adult, hypopituitarism may be manifested in a variety of forms, such as panhypopituitarism, Simmonds' disease (pituitary cachexia), or Sheehan's syndrome.

Pituitary insufficiency may result from hypothalamic lesions, cysts or tumors affecting the pituitary, surgical hypophysectomy, infiltrative granulomatous disease, vascular collapse, or thrombosis.

The deficiency in the production of tropic hormones leads to functional deficiency and atrophy of target glands such as the adrenal cortex, thyroid, and gonads. Symptoms of pituitary insufficiency may include weakness; decreased resistance to stress, cold, and infection; sexual dysfunction (*e.g.,* infertility, amenorrhea, decreased secondary sex characteristics); sallow, dry, wrinkled skin; and hypotension.

Pituitary Dwarfism

The hallmark of hypopituitarism in children is growth retardation or dwarfism. Despite the small stature, the pituitary dwarf has normal body proportions. Hypoglycemia, hypogonadism, and hypothyroidism may also occur.

HYPERFUNCTIONAL STATES

Gigantism and Acromegaly

Excessive secretion of GH is usually caused by acidophilic adenomas. Hypersecretion of GH occurring before closure of the epiphyses leads to proportional but immense growth. An individual may grow to 7 or 8 feet in height; hence the term *gigantism.*

Excessive secretion of GH following epiphyseal closure results in acromegaly. Because the bones can no longer increase in length, overall height (stature) is not affected. However, the bones thicken considerably, an effect particularly noticeable in the face, hands, and feet. Overgrowth of the mandible results in prognathism (jaw protrusion) and separation of the lower teeth. The skeletal changes predispose to joint disorders such as osteoarthritis.

Increased sweating, thickening of the skin, and increased body hair (in women) are common. Hyperglycemia and glucose intolerance may be noted. Headaches and visual disturbances may result from pressure by the tumor.

Clinical Uses of Hypophyseal Hormones
Neurohypophysis

The neurohypophysis or posterior lobe of the pituitary contains two hormones, oxytocin and vasopressin, both of which are available for clinical use. In addition, a posterior pituitary preparation, an extract of pituitary glands possessing the activity of both oxytocin and vasopressin, is used both by injection and by inhalation for certain therapeutic indications.

Vasopressin is also referred to as the antidiuretic hormone (ADH), because it promotes reabsorption of water from the distal tubules and collecting ducts of the kidney. Its other pharmacologic effects include contraction of vascular smooth muscle, especially of the portal and splanchnic (visceral) vessels, and a direct spasmogenic effect on gastrointestinal (GI) smooth muscle. Available preparations of vasopressin include a synthetic derivative of the naturally occurring hormone possessing marked pressor and antidiuretic activity and two structural analogs, desmopressin and lypressin, which exhibit relatively selective antidiuretic activity with minimal pressor effects. These drugs are reviewed individually in this chapter.

Oxytocin exerts two principal actions in the body: contraction of uterine smooth muscle (oxytocic effect) and contraction of the myoepithelial cells surrounding the ducts of the mammary gland, resulting in ejection of milk (galactokinetic effect). The sensitivity of the uterus to the effects of oxytocin is dependent both on the stage of gestation (maximal at term and immediately postpartum) as well as on the existing balance of female sex hormones (increased in the presence of estrogen and reduced in the presence of progesterone). Natural oxytocin is no longer available for clinical use and has been replaced by a synthetic derivative. It is most frequently employed to enhance uterine contractions during labor. Although not derived from pituitary sources, two other drugs used for their oxytocic effects, ergonovine and methylergonovine, are also considered in this chapter.

Posterior Pituitary Injection

(Pituitrin-S)

MECHANISM AND ACTIONS
Posterior pituitary injection is a sterile aqueous extract from pituitary glands of domesticated animals used for food by humans. It contains the equivalent of 20 USP (United States Pharmacopeia) U/ml. Posterior pituitary injection possesses oxytocic, vasopressor, smooth muscle spasmogenic, and antidiuretic activity.

USES
1. Control of postoperative ileus and to facilitate expulsion of gas before pyelography

2. Aid to achieving hemostasis in surgical procedures and in treating esophageal varices
3. Treatment of enuresis of diabetes insipidus

ADMINISTRATION AND DOSAGE
Posterior pituitary injection (20 U/ml) may be administered either subcutaneously (SC) or preferably intramuscularly (IM). The usual dosage is 10 U, although a range of 5 U to 20 U may be given.

SIDE-EFFECTS/ADVERSE REACTIONS
Most common side-effects with posterior pituitary injection are increased GI activity (e.g., nausea, cramping, flatus, abdominal discomfort), facial pallor, and uterine cramps. In addition, tinnitus, mydriasis, visual disturbances, anxiety, diarrhea, proteinuria, eclampsia, and loss of consciousness have occurred with injection of the drug.

CONTRAINDICATIONS AND PRECAUTIONS
Injection of posterior pituitary extract is contraindicated in patients with cardiac disease, hypertension, epilepsy, advanced arteriosclerosis, or toxemia of pregnancy. In addition, the drug is not to be used as an oxytocic or in the treatment of surgical shock, since the drug can produce vasoconstriction and increased peripheral resistance, which may result in decreased coronary blood flow and cardiac output, further aggravating the conditions that may have led to shock. Cautious use is warranted in patients with arrhythmias or coronary insufficiency (see Interactions) or in patients receiving barbiturates.

INTERACTIONS
1. An increased incidence of cardiac arrhythmias and coronary insufficiency can occur if Pituitrin-S is combined with barbiturates or general anesthetics, especially cyclopropane.
2. The antidiuretic effects can be potentiated by chlorpropamide, clofibrate, and carbamazepine.

NURSING CONSIDERATIONS
The actions of this drug are intense and relatively short-lived. As such, the patient who receives it should be closely monitored. Vital signs should be taken frequently immediately following injection, watching for signs of vasoconstriction as evidenced by increases in blood pressure and pulse rate and intense abdominal pain. Any changes should be reported immediately to the physician.

Since posterior pituitary extract is derived from

animals (primarily from pigs and cows), it is important to ask about allergies to beef or pork before administering the drug. In addition, the patient whose religion prohibits the use of animal protein may object to administration of this drug, which will pose ethical problems since few alternatives are available.

Posterior Pituitary, Intranasal (Posterior Pituitary)

An intranasal dosage form of posterior pituitary extract is available for the control of symptoms of diabetes insipidus (*e.g.*, polyuria, polydipsia) due to an endogenous deficiency of ADH. The drug is supplied as capsules containing 40 mg of posterior pituitary powder, which is administered 3 to 4 times a day using an Armour Powder Inhalator. Dosage is individualized according to response, and the technique for using the inhalator should be demonstrated to the patient. Nasal irritation, rhinorrhea, and nasal mucosal ulceration have occurred, and inadvertent inhalation deep into the bronchioles has resulted in dyspnea and coughing. Intranasal posterior pituitary extract should be used cautiously in patients with coronary artery disease, because vasoconstriction can occur if appreciable amounts are absorbed systemically. Use of the product in pregnant women may induce abortion, due to the drug's oxytocic activity. Since the product is derived from animal pituitary glands, allergic reactions can occur in hypersensitive individuals.

Vasopressin

(Pitressin Synthetic)

Vasopressin Tannate

(Pitressin Tannate in Oil)

Vasopressin is a synthetic compound structurally identical to naturally occurring vasopressin, possessing vasopressor and antidiuretic activity. Its principal indication is the treatment of diabetes insipidus (see above). Vasopressin provides replacement therapy to correct the symptoms of polyuria and polydipsia. Occasionally, however, the problem is unresponsiveness of the renal tubules to the action of vasopressin. In these cases, vasopressin is *ineffective* in treating the condition. Successful therapy of this latter type of diabetes insipidus is difficult, but clinical benefit has been reported

with use of thiazide diuretics and chlorpropamide. Vasopressin is also used to reduce excessive bleeding based on its ability to contract vascular smooth muscle strongly. The drug is being used increasingly to control variceal bleeding, when infused either intravenously or occasionally intra-arterially, although the latter route is significantly more hazardous.

MECHANISM AND ACTIONS
Vasopressin increases the reabsorption of water by increasing the permeability of the tubular epithelium *via* activation of cyclic AMP in cells of the renal collecting ducts. The drug also enhances contraction of vascular and nonvascular smooth muscle, resulting in decreased peripheral blood flow and GI, urinary, and uterine smooth muscle spasm. Vasopressin-induced constriction of coronary arteries may precipitate or worsen existing angina. Vasoconstriction is most marked in the portal and splanchnic vessels and somewhat less intense in peripheral, cerebral, and pulmonary vessels.

USES
1. Treatment of diabetes insipidus of central (hypophyseal) origin
2. Prevention and treatment of postoperative abdominal distention
3. Dispersion of gas shadows to aid abdominal roentgenography
4. Control of bleeding esophageal varices and hemorrhage due to abdominal surgery

ADMINISTRATION AND DOSAGE
Vasopressin is available for injection as an aqueous solution containing 20 pressor U/ml. Vasopressin *tannate* injection is a water-insoluble tannate salt of vasopressin suspended in peanut oil, containing 5 pressor units/ml and having a prolonged (24 hours–72 hours) duration of action. Vasopressin injection is usually given either IM or SC, although it has been used IV or intra-arterially for esophageal varices. The tannate salt is *only* given IM and injection may be painful. Recommended dosages are as follows:

Vasopressin Injection
Diabetes insipidus—5 U to 10 U 2 to 3 times a day IM, SC, or intranasally on cotton pledgets
Abdominal distention—5 U IM initially; increase to 10 U every 3 hours to 4 hours as necessary
Abdominal roentgenography—10 U IM 2 hours and ½ hour before films are exposed

Bleeding episodes—20 U by IV infusion or
 occasionally intra-arterially over 5 minutes
 to 10 minutes

Vasopressin Tannate in Oil
 0.3 ml to 1 ml (1.5 U–5 U) IM; repeat as
 needed every 24 hours to 96 hours

FATE

The duration of action with the aqueous injection
is 2 hours to 8 hours; effects of tannate injection
persist 24 hours to 96 hours, primarily due to slow,
cumulative absorption from the IM injection site.
The drug is rapidly removed from the plasma
(half-life 15 minutes) and inactivated by the liver
and kidneys. Vasopressin is excreted in the urine as
metabolites and unchanged drug.

SIDE-EFFECTS/ADVERSE REACTIONS

Side-effects with vasopressin occur most frequently with higher doses and may include facial
pallor, nausea, skin blanching, and abdominal or
uterine cramping. Other reported adverse reactions
are vertigo, sweating, headache, vomiting, tremor,
urticaria, bronchoconstriction, hypersensitivity reactions, anaphylactic reaction, and anginal pain.

Following nasal insufflation (see Lypressin,
below), congestion, irritation, rhinorrhea, headache, conjunctivitis, and mucosal ulceration have
occurred.

Vasopressin can produce water intoxication, of
which the early signs are drowsiness, listlessness,
and headache; convulsions and coma have occurred
in severe cases.

CONTRAINDICATIONS AND PRECAUTIONS

Vasopressin is contraindicated in patients with severe coronary artery disease, chronic nephritis, or
advanced arteriosclerosis. Extreme *caution* is necessary when administering vasopressin to patients
with epilepsy, asthma, cardiovascular disease, migraine, renal disease, goiter, or any state in which
an increase in extracellular fluid volume would be
hazardous.

INTERACTIONS

1. The action of vasopressin may be potentiated
 by antidiabetics, acetaminophen, fludrocortisone, ganglionic blocking agents, neostigmine,
 and general anesthetics.
2. The antidiuretic activity of vasopressin can be
 increased by chlorpropamide, clofibrate, or
 carbamazepine.
3. The antidiuretic action of vasopressin may be

reduced by alcohol, epinephrine, cyclophosphamide, heparin, and lithium.

■ *Nursing Process*

□ ASSESSMENT

□ *Subjective Data*

History taking includes information about current
medications, especially use of antidiabetic agents
or acetaminophen that can potentiate vasopressin
and alcohol use, which may interfere with the
drug's antidiuretic effect. The patient is also asked
about a history of cardiovascular disease, renal disease, seizures, and migraine, all of which warrant
cautious use of vasopressin.

□ *Objective Data*

Physical assessment varies depending on the rationale for treatment. On all patients a baseline blood
pressure, body weight, and intake-to-output ratio
are obtained, because these parameters will be used
throughout therapy to determine drug effectiveness and to detect the onset of side-effects such as
water intoxication. Laboratory values for serum
electrolytes and urine specific gravity are essential.

When vasopressin is used to treat diabetes insipidus a hormone challenge test is performed to
determine baseline hormone levels. To test hormone suppression, the patient is deprived of fluids;
to test hormone stimulation, a saline infusion is
administered. Blood samples are then collected to
determine circulating hormone levels, and urine
samples are evaluated for hormone metabolite
levels.

When vasopressin is used in the treatment of
abdominal distention, baseline information includes abdominal girth measurement, palpation of
the abdomen for evidence of pain, percussion for
evidence of gas pockets, and auscultation for bowel
sounds. These parameters are used to measure drug
effectiveness throughout therapy.

□ NURSING DIAGNOSIS

Actual nursing diagnoses may include
 Knowledge deficit related to the drug's action,
  administration, and side-effects.
 Anxiety related to multiple injections
  throughout therapy
Potential nursing diagnoses may include
 Alteration in fluid volume: excess related to
  water intoxication
 Fluid volume deficit related to hypovolemia

Impaired tissue integrity related to multiple injections

□ *PLAN*

Nursing care goals focus on

1. Administering the drug safely and correctly
2. Monitoring drug side-effects, especially water intoxication and hypovolemia
3. Teaching the patient and family correct injection techniques, early symptoms of problems, how to manage changes, and when to seek assistance

□ *INTERVENTION*

The patient with diabetes insipidus may require long-term treatment with vasopressin. If tannate injections are used the patient or significant other must learn correct injection technique in order to avoid lipodystrophy. The solution is warmed to body temperature and vigorously shaken to ensure uniform dispersion. The injection is given deep IM in a muscular site such as the gluteus muscle or the thigh. Sites are rotated on each injection using a body map (see Chap. 8) to avoid random rotation. The injection site is massaged after drug administration to facilitate absorption of the tannate oil. The patient should be encouraged to drink at least 2 glasses of water after each dose to reduce vasospastic side-effects such as cramping, skin blanching, and nausea. In spite of good technique, tannate injections are painful and may cause abscesses. If site rotation does not prevent such problems nasal insufflation or subcutaneous administration using another form of vasopressin may be appropriate. However, it is essential to teach the patient that the only appropriate administration route for vasopressin tannate is intramuscular injection.

The patient must also learn to monitor the drug's effectiveness. In doing so he will also be able to catch early warning signs of problems. The patient needs to weigh himself daily and to report any sudden changes. He must also learn to monitor his intake and output and to keep an accurate record. Intake/output (I/O) ratios vary widely, but for the patient receiving appropriate drug therapy they should be approximately equal. If intake rapidly exceeds output or the reverse occurs, the patient must contact the physician immediately since hypovolemia or water intoxication may occur. In addition to monitoring I/O ratio, the patient may be taught to take urine specific gravity levels on a daily basis and to replace fluids based on that value. Regardless of method the patient must learn to monitor himself closely and to report any changes.

The major side-effects the patient learns to watch for are water intoxication and hypovolemia. Early signs of water intoxication are nausea, vomiting, confusion, drowsiness, and headaches. Signs of hypovolemia include weight loss, decreased skin turgor, and decrease in blood pressure, giving the patient a sense of lightheadedness and dizziness. To avoid these problems the patient is generally seen by the health team on a regular basis to monitor sodium levels, urine specific gravity, and fluid I/O ratios.

□ *EVALUATION*

Outcome criteria will vary depending on the rationale for drug treatment. If vasopressin is given to reduce abdominal distention the parameters used to judge the drug's effectiveness may include decreased abdominal girth, increased peristalsis, return of bowel function, and patient reports of decreased pain and discomfort.

If the drug is given for diabetes insipidus the outcome criteria to judge success may include urine specific gravity of at least 1.015, appropriate I/O ratio, and normal serum sodium levels. In addition, the patient or a significant other will be able to demonstrate correct administration of the drug and can verbalize the major side-effects to watch for and what to do if they occur.

Desmopressin Acetate
(DDAVP, Stimate)

MECHANISM AND ACTIONS

Desmopressin acetate is a synthetic analog of arginine vasopressin that elicits a prompt antidiuretic action that is more specific and more prolonged than that of vasopressin. Urine volume is reduced, and urine osmolality is increased. At normal therapeutic doses, there is very little vasopressor or oxytocic activity. It is administered either by IV or SC injection or intranasally. The injection form possesses approximately 10 times the antidiuretic effect of an equivalent intranasal dose. Desmopressin also elicits a dose-related increase in Factor VIII levels and may be useful in maintaining hemostasis in certain Factor VIII deficiency states (see Uses, below).

USES

1. Treatment of diabetes insipidus of central (hypophyseal) origin (intranasal or parenteral)
2. Treatment of polyuria and polydipsia associated with trauma or surgery of the pituitary gland

3. Treatment of hemophilia A and certain forms of von Willebrand's disease where Factor VIII levels are greater than 5% (parenteral form is approved; intranasal form is still investigational)

ADMINISTRATION AND DOSAGE

Desmopressin is available for injection (4 mcg/ml) and for intranasal use as a nasal solution (0.1 mg/ml; equivalent to 400 IU/ml). For treating polyuria associated with diabetes insipidus or pituitary surgery, the drug may be administered either intranasally or parenterally.

Intranasal

The drug is supplied with a flexible calibrated plastic tube (rhinyle). The desired quantity of solution is drawn into the tube, one end of the tube is inserted into the nostril, and the patient blows on the other end of the tube to deposit the drug deep into the nasal cavity. Infants and young children may require the assistance of an air-filled syringe attached to the plastic tube.

> Adults: 0.1 ml to 0.4 ml/day, either as a single dose or in 2 or 3 divided doses
> Children (under age 12): 0.05 ml to 0.3 ml/day in a single or 2 divided doses

Parenteral

The drug is given either SC or by direct IV injection.

> Adults: 0.5 ml to 1 ml daily in 2 divided doses
> For the adjunctive treatment of hemophilia A or von Willebrand's disease (type 1): 0.3 mcg/kg of desmopressin diluted in sterile saline is infused over 15 minutes to 30 minutes. The necessity for repeat administration is assessed by laboratory response and the patient's clinical condition. In adults, 50 ml of diluent is used; children weighing less than 10 kg are given only 10 ml of diluent.

FATE

A single dose of desmopressin produces an antidiuretic effect that persists for 8 hours to 20 hours. Increases in Factor VIII levels are evident within 30 minutes after injection and are maximal within 90 minutes to 120 minutes. The drug is metabolized by the liver and kidney and excreted in the urine.

SIDE-EFFECTS/ADVERSE REACTIONS

Adverse reactions are generally infrequent. High doses have produced headache, nausea, abdominal cramping, vulval pain, mild elevation of blood pressure, and flushing. Local erythema, swelling, or burning pain has occurred at the site of injection. Intranasal administration can elicit nasal irritation, sneezing, and congestion. Excessive water retention may result in drowsiness or listlessness.

CONTRAINDICATIONS AND PRECAUTIONS

Desmopressin should not be used to treat hemophilia B or type IIB von Willebrand's disease, since platelet aggregation can be increased. *Cautious* use is necessary in patients with coronary artery disease or hypertension, in pregnant or nursing mothers, and in very young or elderly persons, since the risk of water intoxication is increased.

INTERACTIONS

See Vasopressin.

NURSING CONSIDERATIONS

See Nursing Process for vasopressin.

Lypressin

(Diapid)

Lypressin is a synthetic lysine vasopressin analog with minimal vasopressor oxytocic action. It is administered as a *nasal spray* (50 U/ml) for the control or prevention of the symptoms (polyuria, polydipsia) of neurogenic diabetes insipidus. One to two sprays (1 spray = 2 U) are administered in one or both nostrils four times a day, with an additional bedtime dose given to reduce nocturia not controlled by the daily dosage regimen. More than 3 sprays into the nostril at one time is generally wasted, since the unabsorbed excess is swallowed and inactivated. Instruct the patient to clear nasal passages before taking the drug, to hold the bottle upright while spraying, and to keep head in an upright position to ensure that a fine mist is evenly dispersed over the nasal mucosa rather than placed in one small area. This may help reduce vasospasm and skin breakdown.

The maximal antidiuretic effect occurs within 30 minutes to 60 minutes and effects usually persist for 4 hours to 6 hours. Side-effects are mild and infrequent; nasal irritation, congestion, pruritus, and rhinorrhea have been reported. Systemic adverse effects are minimal; however, large or frequent doses may eventually result in headache, heartburn, abdominal cramping, drowsiness, and dyspnea. Cautious use is necessary in patients with coronary artery disease. The effectiveness of intranasal lypressin may be impaired in the presence of nasal congestion, allergic rhinitis, or upper respiratory infections, since absorption may be reduced; larger doses may be required. The patient should be instructed to contact the physician for advice in these situations.

NURSING CONSIDERATIONS
See Nursing Process for vasopressin.

Oxytocin, Parenteral
(Pitocin, Syntocinon)

Oxytocin, Nasal
(Syntocinon)

MECHANISM AND ACTIONS
Oxytocin is a synthetic peptide possessing the pharmacologic effects of the endogenous hormone. It exerts a direct spasmogenic effect on uterine smooth muscle, presumably by increasing the permeability of the cell membranes of myofibrils to sodium ions, thereby augmenting contractile activity. Oxytocin also contracts myoepithelial cells surrounding the ducts and alveoli of the mammary gland, facilitating ejection of milk from the properly primed gland. The sensitivity of the uterus to oxytocin gradually increases during gestation and becomes maximal immediately before parturition. Estrogens increase and progestins decrease the sensitivity of uterine smooth muscle to oxytocin. The drug has a weak antidiuretic effect and also exhibits a transient relaxing effect on vascular smooth muscle.

USES
1. Initiation or augmentation of uterine contractions to assist in delivery of the fetus *for valid fetal or maternal reasons only*, such as the following:
   a. Maternal diabetes
   b. Rh problems
   c. Uterine inertia
   d. Premature rupture of membranes
   e. Preeclampsia or eclampsia
2. Facilitation of uterine contractions during the third stage of labor
3. Control of postpartum hemorrhage
4. Management of inevitable, incomplete, or missed abortion, usually during the second trimester

5. Aid in milk let-down during breast-feeding or relief of postpartum breast engorgement (*only* indication for the nasal spray)

ADMINISTRATION AND DOSAGE
Oxytocin is available as an injection for IM or IV use containing 10 U/ml, and as a nasal spray containing 40 U/ml. Never give undiluted solution IV, nor give oxytocin by more than one route at any one time.

Recommended doses are as follows.

Injection
Induction or enhancement of labor—0.001 U to 0.002 U/minute (0.1 ml–0.2 ml/min of a 1:1000 dilution; see below) by IV infusion; increase gradually in 0.001-U to 0.002-U/minute increments at 15-minute to 30-minute intervals until a desirable contraction pattern has been established; adjust rate according to uterine response. Dose should rarely exceed 0.020 U/minute.
Dilution—1-ml ampule (10 U) added to 1000 ml of 0.9% aqueous sodium chloride or other suitable IV fluid; mix well by rotating the bottle or agitating the bag gently; use constant infusion pump to control dose accurately.
Postpartum urine bleeding
   IV—10 U to 40 U/1000 ml diluent infused at a rate to control bleeding (usually 0.001 U to 0.002 U/min)
   IM—10 U after delivery of the placenta
Incomplete abortion—10 U/500 ml diluent infused IV at a rate of 0.020 U to 0.040 U/minute

Nasal Spray
One spray into one nostril or both nostrils 2 minutes to 3 minutes before nursing or pumping of breasts. Hold container upright and maintain an upright position while taking the drug to decrease surface contact with nasal mucosa.

FATE
The onset of effect is within 1 minute with IV infusion, 3 minutes to 7 minutes with IM injection, and 5 minutes to 10 minutes with nasal spray. Nasal absorption is erratic. Oxytocin has a short plasma half-life (several minutes) and is rapidly cleared from the plasma by the liver, kidney, and mammary gland. The drug is primarily excreted as metabolites by the kidney, with small amounts as active drug.

SIDE-EFFECTS/ADVERSE REACTIONS

Adverse reactions to oxytocin include nausea, vomiting, premature ventricular contractions, arrhythmias, uterine hypertonicity or spasm, pelvic hematoma, afibrinogenemia, postpartum hemorrhage, anaphylactic reaction, and hypertension. In addition, fetal bradycardia and neonatal jaundice have occurred. Excessive doses can result in uterine rupture due to severe tetanic contraction. Water intoxication has occurred during slow IV infusion over 24 hours, with convulsions and coma.

CONTRAINDICATIONS AND PRECAUTIONS

Oxytocin is contraindicated in the following situations: unfavorable fetal position, significant cephalopelvic disproportion, fetal distress where delivery is not imminent, hypertonic uterine patterns, undilated cervix, prolonged use in uterine inertia, or severe toxemia, conditions in which vaginal delivery is contraindicated (e.g., prolapsed cord, total placenta previa, vasa praevia), invasive cervical carcinoma, dead fetus, and abruptio placentae. Nasal administration of oxytocin is also contraindicated during pregnancy.

Except in unusual circumstances, oxytocin should not be used in the following conditions: prematurity, partial placenta previa, borderline cephalopelvic disproportion, previous surgery on the cervix or uterus, overdistention of the uterus, grand multiparity, or history of uterine sepsis.

During prolonged infusion, signs of developing water intoxication should be noted, such as confusion, headache, or drowsiness. Edema or anuria should be recognized immediately.

INTERACTIONS

1. Severe persistent hypertension can occur if oxytocin is given in the presence of other vasopressor drugs (e.g., epinephrine, ephedrine, methoxamine, metaraminol).
2. Estrogens may augment and progestins may decrease the uterine spasmogenic action of oxytocin.
3. Oxytocin can be potentiated by cyclophosphamide.

■ Nursing Process

□ ASSESSMENT

□ Subjective Data

Information about obstetric history is obtained especially of complications such as cephalopelvic

disproportion, grand multiparity, prematurity, partial placenta previa, or previous uterine surgery. A history of hypertension warrants extreme caution.

If the mother is to receive nasal oxytocin to facilitate milk let-down it is important to help her find a quiet, relaxing atmosphere, which will enhance the process. A discussion of stressors may help her identify factors that are prohibiting adequate relaxation; breathing and focusing techniques may be used to facilitate relaxation. The nurse can also assist by helping the mother to recognize the tingling, pulling sensation that signals the milk let-down response.

□ Objective Data

Physical assessment when the patient receives oxytocin to enhance contractions includes maternal heart rate, blood pressure, and fetal heart rate. A fetal monitor will be hooked up to facilitate measurements of contractions and heart rate during drug administration. A complete blood count with differential is drawn to rule out hemorrhage and electrolytes are evaluated to determine the presence of water intoxication.

□ NURSING DIAGNOSIS

Actual nursing diagnoses may include
   Knowledge deficit related to the drug's action and effects and the management of subsequent contractions
   Anxiety related to the anticipated increase in strength of contractions
Potential nursing diagnosis may include
   Alteration in fluid volume: excess related to water intoxication

□ PLAN

Nursing goals focus on
1. Safe and correct drug administration
2. Monitoring of side-effects such as hypertension and water intoxication
3. Safe delivery of a child without injury to mother or child
4. Effective breast-feeding or pumping (when used to stimulate milk let-down response)

□ INTERVENTION

When oxytocin is administered intravenously the infusion rate must be closely monitored since small quantities exert significant effects. Infusion should be adequately diluted (see Dosage, above) and administered via infusion pump whenever possible.

Flow rate should be regulated to achieve effective uterine contractions, which will help labor progress without causing fetal distress or maternal hypertension. Consequently, fetal heart rate, uterine contractions, and maternal blood pressure and pulse must be monitored frequently. Significant changes should be reported immediately. Most institution protocols recommend that oxytocin be stopped or infusion rate decreased if contractions occur more frequently than every 2 minutes, last longer than 60 seconds, or are greater than 50 mm Hg. The nurse needs to check hospital policy before administering this drug. In addition, because it is a dangerous drug, many facilities permit oxytocin to be given only by a physician or an IV certified nurse in constant attendance. The mother should never be left alone during drug titration and should be coached to help her breathe through the contractions.

Though rarely used, oxytocin may be given intramuscularly usually after delivery of the placenta. Absorption by this route is less controlled and the danger of uterine spasm exists. Before administering the drug by either the IM or IV route, magnesium sulfate must be on hand to facilitate myometrium relaxation if necessary.

The most significant adverse effect of oxytocin is water intoxication. Early signs are confusion, headache, and drowsiness. Intake/output ratio should be closely monitored throughout drug infusion and the patient observed for signs of edema and anuria. Blood pressure should be monitored every 15 minutes to 30 minutes during titration. Any changes must be reported promptly.

The patient should be carefully monitored (heart rate, blood pressure, and intake/output) following delivery, because drug complications can occur after administration has ceased.

□ EVALUATION
The outcome criteria against which to measure the success of drug therapy might include increase in effectiveness and progression of labor to successful delivery, reduction in postpartum bleeding, successful facilitation of the milk let-down reflex, and absence of any side-effects such as fetal distress, maternal injury, maternal hypertension, or water intoxication.

Non-hypophyseal Oxytocics

In addition to oxytocin, other compounds also possess a uterine spasmogenic action and are used for some of the same indications as oxytocin, particularly to control postpartum atony and hemorrhage. *Ergonovine*, an alkaloid obtained from ergot, a fungus that grows on the rye plant, and *methylergonovine*, a semisynthetic derivative of ergonovine, exert a somewhat more prolonged oxytocic action than oxytocin itself and appear to be more selective spasmogens for uterine smooth muscle.

Ergonovine
(Ergotrate)

Methylergonovine
(Methergine)

MECHANISM AND ACTIONS
Ergonovine and methylergonovine exert a direct stimulating effect on smooth muscle of the uterus. In small doses, they increase the force and frequency of uterine contractions, but a normal relaxant phase follows. Larger doses produce *sustained*, forceful contractions, with markedly elevated resting tone. Cerebral vasoconstriction is moderate, and less than that observed with ergotamine, a related alkaloid used in migraine (see Chap. 18).

USES
1. Management of postpartum atony, hemorrhage, or subinvolution of the uterus following delivery of the placenta
2. Facilitation of labor (given in the second stage following delivery of the anterior shoulder)—methylergonovine *only*
3. Investigational uses include alternate therapy of migraine (especially when use of ergotamine causes paresthesias) and diagnosis of Prinzmetal's variant angina during coronary arteriography (see Administration and Dosage, below)

ADMINISTRATION AND DOSAGE

Ergonovine
Ergonovine is available as tablets (0.2 mg) and for injection (0.2 mg/ml). It is used *orally* to minimize late postpartum bleeding in a dose of 0.2 mg to 0.4 mg every 6 hours to 12 hours, generally for 48 hours. Tablets may be given sublingually and cramping is an indication of effectiveness but if severe may necessitate a dosage reduction.

Parenterally, the preferred route of administration is IM, although the drug may be given IV in emergency situations. The usual IM or IV dose is

0.2 mg, which may be repeated in 2 hours to 4 hours if necessary to control severe bleeding. IV administration is associated with a greater risk of side-effects.

For *investigational use to diagnose Prinzmetal's variant angina:* 0.05 mg to 0.2 mg IV during coronary arteriography will provoke coronary arterial spasms, which are reversible with nitroglycerin.

Methylergonovine

Methylergonovine is also available as tablets (0.2 mg) and for injection (0.2 mg/ml). Oral dosage is 0.2 mg three to four times a day for a maximum of 7 days. The drug may also be given IM in a dose of 0.2 mg after delivery of the placenta and repeated if necessary at 2-hour to 4-hour intervals. Methylergonovine can also be administered IV in a dose of 0.2 mg infused slowly over 60 seconds, but the danger of a sudden hypertensive reaction is greater with IV use.

FATE

The drugs are well absorbed orally, sublingually, and parenterally. The onset of action is 30 seconds to 60 seconds IV, 3 minutes to 7 minutes IM, and 8 minutes to 10 minutes orally. Uterine contractions may continue for up to 3 hours to 4 hours.

SIDE-EFFECTS/ADVERSE REACTIONS

Side-effects are generally infrequent at normal doses; nausea, diarrhea, vomiting, increased blood pressure, headache, tinnitus, dyspnea, and chest pain have been reported. Other adverse reactions occasionally noted are allergic reactions, paresthesias, sweating, palpitations, dizziness, confusion, abdominal cramping, and muscle weakness.

Overdosage can lead to diarrhea, numbness or coldness of the extremities, weak pulse, dyspnea, chest pain, hypercoagulability, gangrene of the fingers or toes, confusion, delirium, convulsions, and coma. Treatment is symptomatic and can include anticonvulsants, heparin, nitroglycerin for coronary vasospasm, and nitroprusside for peripheral vasospasm. Blood pressure elevations may be controlled with IV chlorpromazine.

CONTRAINDICATIONS AND PRECAUTIONS

Ergonovine and methylergonovine are contraindicated for induction of labor, in cases of threatened spontaneous abortion, in severe hypertension, and in toxemia of pregnancy. *Caution* must be exercised in using these drugs in patients with sepsis, obliterative vascular disease, hepatic or renal dysfunction, heart disease, or mitral valve stenosis. These drugs should be given IV only in emergencies (*e.g.*, uterine hemorrhage), and careful monitoring of blood pressure must be carried out. Pulse and uterine contractions should be closely monitored. Prolonged use is not advisable, as decreased circulatory function can occur.

INTERACTIONS

1. The pressor effects of ergonovine and methylergonovine may be intensified by other pressor agents.

NURSING CONSIDERATIONS

See Chapter 18 for a discussion of nursing considerations for drugs used in the treatment of migraine. The ergot alkaloids are given primarily by the oral, sublingual, and intramuscular route. Intravenous administration is reserved for emergencies and is far more hazardous than the other routes because of the number of significant side-effects.

Response to the ergot alkaloids depends on adequate calcium in the muscle cells to facilitate contractility. If a patient does not respond to the drug, she may be hypocalcemic. Consequently, serum calcium levels should be obtained before drug therapy begins. If calcium levels are low, calcium gluconate may be needed as a replacement.

Ergot alkaloids can cause significant side-effects that require close monitoring. Blood pressure should be taken at regular intervals; elevations should be reported promptly. The patient who takes the drug at home should have the blood pressure monitored regularly and be told to report any blinding headaches, dizziness, or extremity weakness at once.

Ergot poisoning can occur and is evidenced by pale, cold, or numb extremities; seizures; nausea; vomiting; diarrhea; headache; and muscle pain. Examination of extremities must be performed on a regular basis and the patient should report any change in color or temperature. Ergot poisoning can cause severe vasoconstriction leading to gangrene of the fingers and toes. Seizure precautions should be maintained.

Uterine hypotonicity is another possible side-effect and is characterized by increased bleeding and a decrease in uterine firmness. The size and firmness of the uterine fundus and volume and color of vaginal discharge must be monitored every

15 minutes to 30 minutes and then hourly until vaginal discharge decreases or color darkens.

Uterine hypertonicity may also occur. Cramps are considered a sign that the drug is working but excessive pain is an indication for medical intervention and the physician should be notified.

Adenohypophysis

Of the six principal hormones of the adenohypophysis, only growth hormone (GH), adrenocorticotropic hormone (ACTH), and thyroid-stimulating hormone (TSH) are available for clinical use. Growth hormone is a purified polypeptide of recombinant DNA origin containing the identical sequence of the 191 amino acids constituting endogenous growth hormone. Adrenocorticotropic hormone is a 39 amino acid polypeptide extracted from pituitary glands of animals. Thyroid-stimulating hormone is a purified extract of the hormone from bovine pituitary glands. Since these three hormones are peptides, they must be given parenterally, because they would be quickly destroyed in gastric juice if taken by mouth. Further, since ACTH and TSH are naturally derived products, their use is associated with the possibility of allergic reactions. GH, on the other hand, is now prepared synthetically and is virtually devoid of hypersensitivity problems. ACTH and GH are reviewed individually below; TSH is used strictly in a diagnostic capacity, and is considered in Chapter 80.

The two adenohypophyseal gonadotropins, follicle-stimulating hormone (FSH) and luteinizing hormone (LH), are extracted from the urine of pregnant and postmenopausal women. The commercial preparation, human menopausal gonadotropin (HMG), is used in the treatment of infertility and cryptorchidism (undescended testes) and is discussed in Chapter 57. The remaining adenohypophyseal hormone, prolactin (luteotropic hormone, LTH), is unavailable for therapeutic use.

All adenohypophyseal hormones except GH exert their effects on selective target organs, such as the adrenal cortex, thyroid gland, or gonads. Replacement therapy in cases of hormonal deficiency states is usually best accomplished by supplying the individual target gland hormones (thyroxine, hydrocortisone, estrogen, progesterone) instead of the pituitary hormones for many of the reasons mentioned above. In the case of the gonadal hormones, moreover, the individual purified hypophyseal hormones are not clinically available.

Adrenocorticotropic Hormone

Corticotropin Injection
(Acthar, ACTH)

Repository Corticotropin Injection
(ACTH Gel, Cortigel, Cortrophin Gel, Cotropic-Gel, H.P. Acthar Gel)

Corticotropin Zinc
(Cortrophin-Zinc)

Adrenocorticotropic hormone (ACTH) is a polypeptide containing 39 amino acids and it is extracted from the pituitary glands of various animals. ACTH is commercially available either as a stable aqueous solution for injection, an aqueous solution containing gelatin to delay absorption and prolong the action (repository form), or a zinc hydroxide complex to prevent tissue destruction, which also prolongs the effect. A synthetic subunit (*i.e.*, 24 amino acids) of ACTH that is identical in action to natural ACTH is available as cosyntropin, and is used to test for adrenocortical insufficiency. Cosyntropin is reviewed in Chapter 80. A second diagnostic agent, metyrapone, can also be employed to ascertain whether pituitary secretion of ACTH is adequate, and is likewise considered in Chapter 80.

MECHANISM AND ACTIONS
ACTH (corticotropin) stimulates the adrenal cortex to synthesize and secrete its various hormones, such as glucocorticoids (*e.g.*, hydrocortisone), mineralocorticoids (*e.g.*, aldosterone), and adrenogenital corticoids (*e.g.*, testosterone). This action is mediated by activation of adenyl cyclase in adrenal cell membranes, leading to increased production of cyclic AMP. Adequate adrenal function, therefore, is necessary for the action of ACTH. Increased plasma levels of adrenal corticoids suppress endogenous ACTH secretion by way of a negative feedback mechanism (Fig. 51-2). Thus, chronic administration of exogenous corticosteroids will gradually lower ACTH secretion and can lead to adrenal hypofunction and atrophy.

USES
Note: Corticotropin has a rather limited therapeutic application. Although it can theoretically be

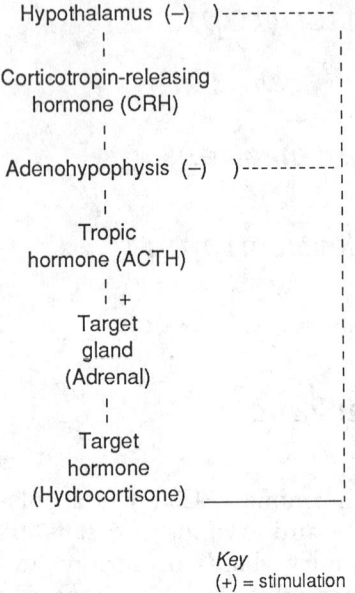

Key
(+) = stimulation
(−) = inhibition

Figure 51-2. *Negative feedback mechanism regulating endocrine hormone secretion. Increased plasma levels of the target hormone (e.g., hydrocortisone) reduce the secretion of the tropic hormone (e.g., ACTH) by a negative feedback either at the level of the adenohypophysis or at the level of the hypothalamus (by decreasing release of a corticotropin-releasing hormone).*

used in most conditions responsive to corticosteroid therapy, specific treatment of these conditions with *individual* corticosteroids is generally preferred to reduce the likelihood of allergic reactions to the naturally derived corticotropin. In addition, many synthetic corticosteroids are given orally (see Chap. 55), whereas corticotropin must be administered parenterally. The various conditions for which corticotropin injection may be useful are

1. Management of severe myasthenia gravis and acute exacerbations of multiple sclerosis
2. Treatment of nonsuppurative thyroiditis, tuberculous meningitis (with appropriate antibacterial therapy), trichinosis with neurologic or myocardial involvement, and hypercalcemia associated with cancer
3. Treatment of rheumatic, collagen, respiratory, allergic, hematologic, GI, edematous, and neoplastic disorders, and as an *alternative* to more specific glucocorticoid therapy
4. Diagnostic testing of adrenocortical function (see Chap. 80; cosyntropin is the preferred agent).

ADMINISTRATION AND DOSAGE

Corticotropin is available for IM, SC, or IV injection as an aqueous solution containing 25 U/vial or 40 U/vial; for IM or SC injection as a gelatinized solution providing delayed absorption and prolonged action (repository injection) containing 40 U/ml or 80 U/ml; and for IM injection *only* as a solution of ACTH adsorbed onto zinc hydroxide (which also delays absorption) containing 40 U ACTH and 2 mg zinc per milliliter of suspension.

Corticotropin should not be administered until adrenal responsiveness has been verified with the route of administration selected. An increase in urinary and plasma corticosteroid levels is direct evidence of adequate adrenal function. After adrenal responsiveness has been verified, dosage should be individualized. The *usual* SC or IM dose is 20 U four times a day initially, with gradual reduction as response permits. Recommended doses for specific indications are as follows:

Diagnosis—10 U to 25 U/500 ml 5% dextrose by IV infusion over 8 hours
Myasthenia—100 U/day to total of 2000 U
Multiple sclerosis—80 U to 120 U/day IM for 2 weeks to 3 weeks

The average dose of the *repository* injection is 40 U to 80 U IM or SC every 1 to 3 days.

FATE

Corticotropin injection (IM, SC, IV) has a rapid onset and effects may persist 2 hours to 4 hours. The repository and zinc injections provide for a slower onset but more prolonged effects (24 hours–72 hours). The drug can bind to plasma proteins. Excretion is largely in the urine.

SIDE-EFFECTS/ADVERSE REACTIONS

During therapy with corticotropin, a wide variety of untoward reactions can occur; these are listed by organ system below:

GI—Peptic ulcer, abdominal distention, pancreatitis, ulcerative esophagitis
Musculoskeletal—Weakness, osteoporosis, steroid myopathy, loss of muscle mass, vertebral compression fractures, fracture of long bones
Dermatologic—Erythema, petechiae, ecchymoses, delayed wound healing, sweating, hyperpigmentation, acneiform reactions, thinning skin
CNS—Convulsions, vertigo, headache, insomnia, depression, mood swings, euphoria, personality alterations, seizures

Endocrine—Menstrual irregularities, hirsutism, diabetes, decreased carbohydrate tolerance, growth suppression

Electrolyte—Hypernatremia, hypokalemia, hypocalcemia, weight gain, fluid retention

Cardiovascular—Hypertension, necrotizing angiitis

Other—Subcapsular cataracts, increased intraocular pressure, exophthalmos, negative nitrogen balance, allergic reactions, decreased resistance to infections

Prolonged use of corticotropin can result in reduced adrenal stimulatory effects, presumably due to antibody production. In addition, chronic treatment with exogenous corticotropin may suppress signs of chronic disease without altering the natural course of the disease.

CONTRAINDICATIONS AND PRECAUTIONS

Contraindications to use of corticotropin include osteoporosis, scleroderma, systemic fungal infections, ocular herpes simplex, recent surgery, peptic ulcer, congestive heart failure, hypertension, IV use (*except* diagnostic testing), alone in active tuberculosis, and sensitivity to proteins of porcine origin.

Corticotropin must be used with *caution* in the presence of diabetes, hypothyroidism, cirrhosis, pyogenic infections, diverticulitis, renal insufficiency, myasthenia gravis, in pregnant and lactating women, and in emotionally unstable individuals.

Patients should be observed for signs of electrolyte imbalances (*e.g.*, thirst, weakness, muscle cramping), sodium or water retention, or psychic changes (*e.g.*, mood swings, insomnia, depression, euphoria).

Immunization procedures should be undertaken with extreme caution during ACTH therapy, because lack of antibody response and neurologic complications have been reported. Do *not* vaccinate against smallpox during treatment with ACTH, and avoid immunization with *live* vaccines during corticotropin therapy.

INTERACTIONS

1. Increased requirements for antidiabetic drugs may occur with use of ACTH, because of the hyperglycemic action of corticosteroids.
2. ACTH may enhance the hypoprothrombinemic action of aspirin.
3. Marked hypokalemia may result if ACTH is given with diuretics that cause potassium loss.
4. ACTH may antagonize oral anticoagulants.
5. The adverse effects of vaccines may be enhanced if given during ACTH therapy.

NURSING CONSIDERATIONS

See Chapter 55 for a complete discussion of nursing considerations for steroid drugs. Baseline data required before administration of ACTH include skin sensitivity testing if porcine allergy is suspected, plasma and urine corticosteroid levels (to determine adrenal responsiveness), electrolyte levels, complete blood count, weight, and intake/output ratio.

Nursing care centers around monitoring side-effects that are typical of steroid drugs: electrolyte disturbances, weight gain and water retention, mood swings and possible depression, and increased susceptibility to infection due to the immunosuppressive effect of the drug. Chapter 55 contains specific strategies for dealing with these problems.

Dosage adjustment and withdrawal must be done gradually and under close supervision since drug therapy effectively suppresses the body's own feedback system for production of the hormone. If this drug has been given in large doses over a prolonged period and is to be withdrawn it must be tapered off very gradually and the patient observed for signs of adrenal insufficiency such as water retention, hypoglycemia, and lethargy or depression.

Synthetic Growth Hormone

Somatrem

(Humatrope, Protropin)

Somatrem is a synthetic polypeptide hormone obtained by a recombinant DNA technique containing the identical sequence of 191 amino acids comprising endogenous growth hormone plus an additional amino acid, methionine. It is useful in treating growth retardation in children lacking endogenous growth hormone. Previously, the growth hormone used clinically was obtained from cadavers, but this product was discontinued following several reports of deaths due to a degenerative neurologic disorder in young men who had received the drug. This disorder resembled Creutzfeldt-Jakob disease (CJD) and was believed to be due to a "slow" virus that apparently was present in at least one of the many cadavers from which a pituitary extract was obtained and then subsequently transmitted to the recipient of the pooled human growth hormone product. Since each patient may have received extracts from over 100,000 cadavers during a 3- to 4-year course of therapy, it is believed that at least one of the cadavers was the probable source of the viral pathogen responsible for the neurologic changes. Since the virus is resistant to most chemical and physical methods for decontamination, the procedures utilized in extracting and purifying human growth hormone from cadaver pituitary glands may not have removed the pathogen. The new synthetic growth hormone is apparently not associated with a similar danger.

MECHANISM AND ACTIONS

The principal action of somatrem is stimulation of linear growth, in a manner therapeutically equivalent to that of endogenous human growth hormone. Skeletal growth is enhanced and the length of long bones is increased at the epiphyses. The number and size of skeletal muscle cells are increased, as is red cell mass. Somatrem enhances cellular protein synthesis and nitrogen retention and decreases blood urea nitrogen. There is increased synthesis of chondroitin sulfate and collagen, and serum levels of phosphate are increased. Urinary calcium excretion is facilitated, but GI absorption of calcium is enhanced; thus, serum calcium levels are relatively unchanged. Potassium and sodium retention can also occur. Large doses may increase blood glucose levels, decrease glucose tolerance, and lower sensitivity to exogenous insulin, leading to a diabetogenic state. The anabolic effects of growth hormone are apparently mediated by a group of substances termed *somatomedins*, which are peptides whose hepatic synthesis is stimulated by growth hormone. Somatomedins promote uptake of sulfate into cartilage and appear to be the mediators of cellular processes involved with bone growth.

USES

1. Treatment of growth failure resulting from a deficiency of endogenous growth hormone

ADMINISTRATION AND DOSAGE

Somatrem is available as a lyophilized powder for injection containing 5 mg (approximately 10 IU per vial). The powder is reconstituted with 1 ml to 5 ml of bacteriostatic water for injection (benzyl alcohol preserved). Dosage is individualized; up to 0.1 mg/kg (0.2 IU/kg) is given IM three times a week

for 6 months to 36 months. Larger doses should not be used, since the potential for adverse reactions is increased.

SIDE-EFFECTS/ADVERSE REACTIONS

Myalgia, pain, and swelling have occurred at the injection site. Other adverse reactions noted are hypothyroidism, hyperglycemia, and ketosis. Approximately one third of all patients develop persistent antibodies to growth hormone but these seldom interfere with the growth response to somatrem.

CONTRAINDICATIONS AND PRECAUTIONS

Somatrem is contraindicated in patients with closed epiphyses, when there is evidence of progression of an underlying intracranial lesion, and in persons with sensitivity to benzyl alcohol. *Cautious* use is necessary in patients with diabetes or hypothyroidism.

INTERACTIONS

1. Accelerated epiphyseal closure (fusion of ends of long bones) can occur if somatrem is combined with androgens or thyroid hormones.
2. Hydrocortisone and other anti-inflammatory steroids may inhibit the response of somatrem.
3. Somatrem may decrease responsiveness to insulin or to oral antidiabetic drugs by increasing blood glucose levels.

■ Nursing Process

□ ASSESSMENT

□ Subjective Data

Lack of growth hormone resulting in growth failure is devastating to both children and their parents. Height and stature are an integral part of a positive body image and provide the visual cues for believing a child is passing from childhood to adulthood. Therefore, throughout therapy the nurse must allow the family and the child opportunities to verbalize their concerns about this problem. They must be constantly aware of the success or limits of the therapy and be assisted in learning to deal with everyday problems that may occur.

□ Objective Data

Extensive diagnostic information is collected before a decision is made to administer growth hormone. Immunoassay of growth hormone level will be obtained at baseline and in response to a challenge test. In individuals who are producing adequate growth hormone, insulin-induced hypoglycemia, intravenous administration of arginine hydrochloride, oral administration of levodopa, or intramuscular administration of glucagon will result in increases in growth hormone level. Failure of growth hormone levels to rise above 5 mg to 7 mg/ml in response to at least two of these stimuli indicates the need for therapy.

A bone age assessment (x-ray) must also be completed to determine whether epiphyseal closure has occurred. Therapy will be ineffective if the epiphysis is already closed. Height and weight should be compared to standard pediatric growth charts.

Thyroid function and pancreatic function must also be tested since somatrem can produce hypothyroidism and hypoglycemia. These can be treated during drug therapy if necessary.

□ *NURSING DIAGNOSES*
Actual nursing diagnoses may include
> Knowledge deficit related to the drug's action and effects, correct injection technique, and side-effects to monitor
> Anxiety related to multiple injections

Potential nursing diagnoses may include
> Altered growth and development
> Impaired tissue integrity related to changes at injection sites

□ *PLAN*
Nursing care goals focus on
1. Safe and correct administration of the drug
2. Monitoring side-effects such as alterations in insulin/glucose balance, thyroid function, and electrolytes, and minimizing pain at injection sites
3. Teaching the patient and family correct injection techniques, safe drug administration, and how to monitor for side-effects

□ *INTERVENTION*
Responsible family members can be taught correct injection techniques and site rotation in order to limit pain at the injection site. A site rotation chart may be useful to help them remember where the last injection was administered. In addition, the family should be taught to examine tissue for lumps, sponginess, pain, swelling, and redness before administering each injection. Such changes should be reported immediately and the injection administered in a different location.

Family and health professionals need to establish a relationship that will facilitate communication and encourage clinical follow-up. The patient must be seen regularly to evaluate growth, thyroid and pancreatic function, and status of the epiphyses. Once-a-month evaluations may be recommended. Bone x-ray studies may be done yearly, or more frequently as the child reaches the end of his bone growth period. But the child and family may need continuing support to deal with body image and school and peer relationships.

The two major side-effects to watch for are hypothyroidism and hypoglycemia. Parents may have difficulty distinguishing the early warning signs from behavior typical of preadolescence: tiredness, thirst, lack of energy. They must be encouraged to report sudden changes in behavior or anything they think may be a change. Blood work can easily confirm or deny suspicions but early intervention is better than delayed follow-up.

□ *EVALUATION*
The main outcome criterion for judging treatment success is increased growth (height and weight) prior to epiphyseal closure. Other outcomes the nurse may seek include successful management of body image concerns by the patient or family, early reporting of side-effects, and clean, pain-free injection sites with no evidence of swelling or abscess.

REVIEW QUESTIONS

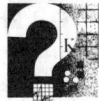

1. Distinguish between the neurohypophysis and adenohypophysis with respect to the hormones secreted from each structure.
2. What are the two types of secretory cells found in the adenohypophysis and what hormones does each secrete?
3. What are the major stimuli responsible for secretion of antidiuretic hormone?
4. List the principal regulatory hormones (peptides) of the hypothalamus.
5. Give the major pharmacologic effects of vasopressin.
6. How does posterior pituitary injection differ from vasopressin injection?

7. Briefly describe the symptoms of diabetes insipidus. What are the two types of diabetes insipidus and how do they differ?
8. In what conditions is use of vasopressin injection contraindicated?
9. What data must be collected before initiating vasopressin therapy?
10. What strategies must be taught to the patient and family to ensure correct administration of vasopressin?
11. How must the patient monitor himself to ensure drug effectiveness while on vasopressin therapy? Outline a brief teaching plan for such monitoring.
12. What advantages does desmopressin have over vasopressin?
13. What are the pharmacologic effects of oxytocin?
14. List the principal indications for oxytocin.
15. What are the major dangers associated with oxytocin use?
16. What is the major difference between administering oxytocin by nasal spray and using other nasal sprays?
17. What baseline data are needed before administering oxytocin?
18. What are the principal advantages of ergonovine over oxytocin?
19. For what indications is ergonovine recommended?
20. What are the major dangers associated with ergonovine overdosage?
21. What three adenohypophyseal hormones are available for clinical use?
22. How is the secretion of ACTH from adenohypophysis influenced by administration of corticotropin injection?
23. List the major indications for corticotropin injection.
24. To what major side-effects of ACTH must the nurse be ready to respond?
25. How is the clinically available growth hormone prepared?
26. Why was the human (i.e., cadaver)-derived human growth hormone preparation discontinued?
27. Briefly describe the major actions of growth hormone.
28. What are the contraindications to use of growth hormone?
29. How can the nurse help the patient taking growth hormone deal with his body image in relation to others his age?

BIBLIOGRAPHY

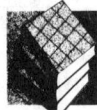

Altura BM, Altura BT: Actions of vasopressin, oxytocin and synthetic analogs on vascular smooth muscle. Fed Proc 43:80, 1984
Brownstein MJ: Biosynthesis of vasopressin and oxytocin. Annu Rev Physiol 45:129, 1983
Chrousos GP, et al: Clinical applications of corticotropin releasing factor. Ann Intern Med 102:344, 1985
Gash DM, Thomas GJ: What is the importance of vasopressin in memory processes. Trends in Neuroscience 6:197, 1983
Hays RM: Alteration of luminal membrane structure by antidiuretic hormone. Am J Physiol 245:1289, 1983
Hintz RL: The somatomedins. Adv Pediatr 28:293, 1981

Hintz RL, Rosenfeld RG: Clinical uses of synthetic growth hormone. Hosp Pract 18:115, 1983

Horowitz L: Nursing implications of selected pediatric endocrine problems. Nurs Clin North Am 15(3):525, 1980

McCann SM: Control of anterior pituitary hormone release by brain peptides. Neuroendocrinology 31:355, 1980

Meisenberg G, Simmons WH: Centrally-mediated effects of neurohypophyseal hormones. Neurosci Biobehav Rev 7:263, 1983

Muthe N: Endocrinology: A Nursing Approach. Boston, Little, Brown & Co., 1981

Reichlin S: Somatostatin. N Engl J Med 309:1495 and 1556, 1983

Share L, Crofton JT: The role of vasopressin in hypertension. Fed Proc 43:103, 1984

Sklar AH, Schrier RW: Central nervous system mediators of vasopressin release. Physiol Rev 63:1243, 1983

Solomon B: The hypothalamus and the pituitary gland. Nurs Clin North Am 15(3):435, 1980

VanVliet G, Styne DM, Kaplan SL, Grumbach MM: Growth hormone treatment for short stature. N Engl J Med 309:1016, 1983

Zimmerman EA, Nilaver G, Hou-Yu A, Silverman AJ: Vasopressinergic and oxytocinergic pathways in the central nervous system. Fed Proc 43:91, 1984

Thyroid Hormones and Antithyroid Drugs

52

The hormones of the thyroid gland exert a wide spectrum of metabolic and physiologic actions that affect virtually every tissue in the body. Before considering the clinical applications of thyroid drugs, however, a brief review of thyroid anatomy and physiology will be presented.

The Thyroid Gland

Anatomy

The thyroid gland is a bilobed organ overlying the trachea anteriorly. The gland is composed of numerous closely packed spheres or follicles. Each follicle consists of a simple cuboidal epithelium (follicular cells) enclosing a lumen or cavity containing a viscous hyaline substance termed *colloid*. The chief constituent of the colloid is the iodinated glycoprotein thyroglobulin. Interspersed among the follicles are small clusters of parafollicular (C) cells, which secrete calcitonin (thyrocalcitonin), a hormone affecting calcium metabolism.

Thyroid Hormones

The follicular cells of the thyroid gland secrete two hormones, thyroxine (tetraiodothyronine or T_4) and triiodothyronine (T_3). The plasma levels of these hormones are regulated by the hypothalamo-pituitary axis, as outlined in Figure 52-1. Intrinsic (intrathyroidal) mechanisms, as well as bioavailability of iodine, influence thyroid hormone production.

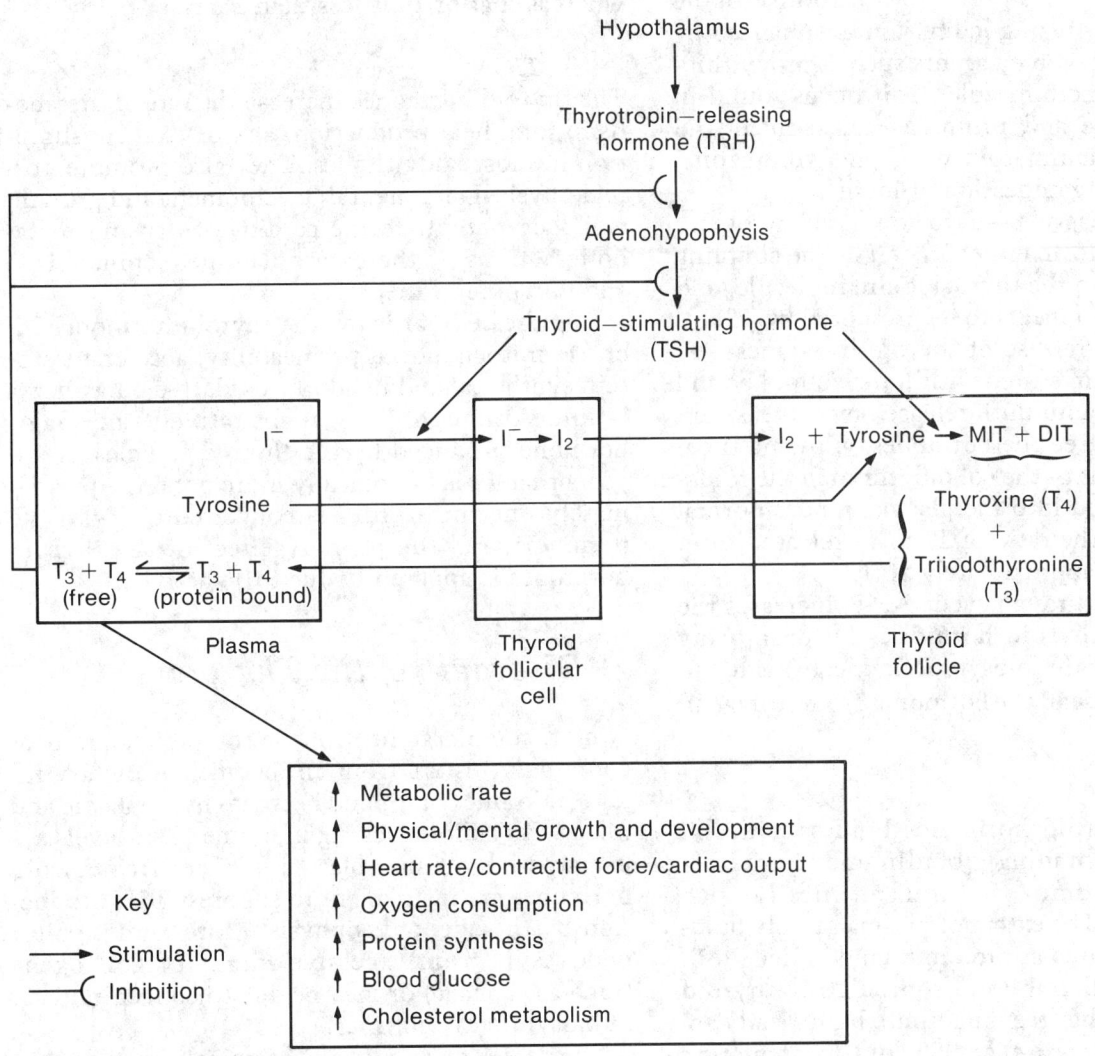

Figure 52-1. *Synthesis, storage, release, and actions of thyroid hormones.*

985

BIOSYNTHESIS

1. Iodide uptake—Ingested iodine is readily absorbed from the gastrointestinal (GI) tract in the reduced iodide state. Iodide ions are actively transported from the blood into the thyroid follicles by an energy-requiring "trapping" mechanism, often termed the *iodide pump*. The normal thyroid/serum ratio of iodide is 25:1. The uptake of iodide is enhanced by thyroid-stimulating hormone (TSH) and may be blocked by anions such as perchlorate and thiocyanate.
2. Oxidation to iodine—On entering the colloid, iodide is rapidly oxidized to iodine in the presence of peroxidase enzymes. Thiouracil appears to inhibit peroxidase activity.
3. Iodination of tyrosine—Free molecular iodine spontaneously combines with tyrosine residues on the thyroglobulin to form 3-monoiodotyrosine (MIT) and 3,5-diiodotyrosine (DIT). This organic iodination is enhanced by TSH and blocked by agents such as propylthiouracil and methimazole. Goitrogens found in cabbage, kale, and turnips, as well as cobalt and the anti-inflammatory drug phenylbutazone, also block organification of iodine.
4. Coupling reaction—Two iodinated tyrosines combine to form either T_3 or T_4. The coupling occurs within the thyroglobulin molecule, and the reaction appears to be promoted by TSH.
5. Storage and release of thyroid hormones—T_4 and T_3 remain stored within the colloid bound to thyroglobulin until released by protease enzymes that free the hormones, allowing them to diffuse out of the colloid, through the follicular cells, and into the plasma. Under normal conditions, the ratio of T_4 to T_3 released from the gland is approximately 20:1.

TSH, acting through cyclic AMP, increases the production of thyroid hormones by promoting various steps in the biosynthetic mechanism, including the release of the hormones from storage in thyroglobulin.

TRANSPORT

Circulating thyroid hormones bind specifically with thyroxine-binding globulin and thyroxine-binding pre-albumin, and nonspecifically with serum albumin. The extent of plasma protein binding can be measured as protein-bound iodine (PBI).

Only a small fraction of circulating thyroid hormones is in the free (unbound), biologically active form, since more than 99% of the circulating stores of thyroid hormones are bound to serum proteins.

Several drugs, including phenytoin and salicylates, compete for plasma protein binding sites, thus lowering the PBI and increasing the percentage of free, active hormones. High levels of estrogen, such as those occurring in pregnancy or during oral contraceptive therapy, elevate plasma protein levels, thereby increasing PBI levels.

FATE

Thyroid hormones are inactivated by deiodination, deamination, decarboxylation, or conjugation with glucuronic acid or sulfate. Much of the iodine released during biodegradation is recycled and reutilized for synthesis of new hormones. The remainder is excreted in the urine. Metabolism occurs chiefly in the liver, and excretion is mainly through the kidneys. The conjugated hormones are excreted through the bile and eliminated in the feces. The plasma half-life of T_4 is 6 to 7 days, whereas that of T_3 is less than 2 days.

ACTIONS

The thyroid hormones increase the rate of metabolism, total heat production, and oxygen consumption in most body tissues. They also promote normal physical and mental development and growth, and they potentiate the cardiovascular and metabolic actions of the catecholamines (epinephrine and norepinephrine).

At the cellular level, the thyroid hormones increase mitochondrial permeability, accelerate protein synthesis, and uncouple oxidative phosphorylation. Although T_4 is quantitatively the major hormone produced by the thyroid follicles, it appears that T_3 is biologically more potent. Approximately one third of T_4 is converted to T_3 in the periphery and the primary effect of the thyroid hormones is apparently due to T_3 activity.

Disorders of the Thyroid

Goiter, an enlargement of the thyroid gland, most commonly results from an insufficient dietary intake of iodine. The gland becomes hyperplastic and filled with colloid lacking in iodine. TSH levels are usually high because plasma levels of free thyroid hormones are insufficient to suppress TSH production by the adenohypophysis. More rarely, goiter may result from excessive intake of goitrogens (such as cabbage) or may be due to congenital lack of biosynthetic enzymes.

Transient simple goiter may occur during pregnancy or at the onset of puberty, when the demand for the hormones increases.

HYPOTHYROIDISM

Hypothyroidism may result from primary disease of the thyroid gland itself, or it may be secondary to a deficiency of pituitary TSH or hypothalamic thyrotropin-releasing hormone (TRH).

Because thyroid hormones affect a wide range of physiologic and metabolic processes, including growth and development, the time of onset of a deficiency state is most important.

Cretinism (Congenital or Neonatal Hypothyroidism)

Cretinism results from fetal or neonatal thyroid hormone deficiency, which may be due to anatomical dysgenesis of the thyroid, iodine deficiency, or inborn errors of iodine metabolism.

Cretinism is characterized by mental retardation and dwarfism due to delayed skeletal maturation. Other signs of this disorder include the presence of thick, dry skin, large protruding tongue, and umbilical hernia. The child appears apathetic or lethargic and has a low body temperature. TSH and serum cholesterol levels are elevated.

Myxedema (Adult Hypothyroidism)

Primary myxedema may follow thyroidectomy, eradication of the thyroid by radioactive iodine, excessive ingestion of goitrogens, or chronic thyroiditis. Idiopathic atrophy, possibly involving autoimmune mechanisms, may also lead to hypothyroidism.

Early symptoms of myxedema include cold intolerance, weakness, fatigue, dryness of the skin, thinning hair, and thin brittle nails. Among later signs are weight gain, pallor, dyspnea, peripheral edema, anginal pain, bradycardia, and slow speech. Cardiac enlargement may result from pericardial effusion, and macrocytic anemia may occur.

The low turnover of protein leads to the accumulation of a protein-rich fluid under the skin, lending a puffiness and thickness to the skin.

Manifestations of personality changes and organic psychoses ("myxedema madness") may also occur.

It is noteworthy that myxedematous patients are unusually sensitive to opiates, and may die from average doses of these agents.

HYPERTHYROIDISM (THYROTOXICOSIS)

Hyperthyroid states are characterized by some degree of glandular hyperplasia and excessive thyroid hormone production, the most common cause of which is overstimulation of the gland by circulating immunoglobulins, synthesized by B-lymphocytes. One such antibody is thyroid-stimulating immunoglobulin (TSI), sometimes referred to as long-acting thyroid stimulator (LATS), which interacts with receptor sites on the thyroid cell to stimulate hormonal output.

Nervousness, excessive sweating, heat intolerance, warm moist skin, weight loss despite increased appetite, restlessness, and tremor are common signs of hyperthyroidism. Tachycardia, wide pulse pressure, and systolic hypertension frequently occur.

When associated with toxic diffuse goiter, elevated metabolic rate, and exophthalmos, hyperthyroidism is termed *Graves' disease.* Thyroid-stimulating immunoglobulin has been isolated from the serum of patients with Graves' disease, and can bind to TSH binding sites, resulting in stimulation of thyroid function.

Therapy of hyperthyroidism can include surgical removal of a part of the gland (subtotal thyroidectomy), use of radioactive iodide (^{131}I) to destroy thyroid tissue, or administration of antithyroid drugs that interfere with synthesis and release of thyroid hormones. The relative usefulness of these three approaches is compared in Table 52-1. The antithyroid drugs methimazole and propylthiouracil are reviewed in this chapter and a discussion of ^{131}I is also presented.

Certain types of thyroid disorders can also be effectively treated with elemental iodine preparations, and these products are considered at the end of the chapter. Two other thyroid-related drugs are protirelin, a synthetic thyrotropin-releasing hormone, and thyrotropin, a highly purified form of thyroid-stimulating hormone of bovine origin. These two agents are used for diagnosis of thyroid dysfunction and are reviewed in Chapter 80 along with various other diagnostic drugs.

Determination of Thyroid Functioning

Effective treatment of thyroid disorders depends on accurate assessment of the thyroid state. Several laboratory parameters used to ascertain thyroid functioning are listed in Table 52-2, with average (normal) values given beside each test.

Because of the possibility of false increases or decreases in the readings of any one of the thyroid function tests as a result of other medications taken by the patient (see Interactions under Thyroid Hormones), or the presence of certain disease states (*e.g.,* hepatitis, nephrosis), *several* tests should be performed before a final diagnosis is made, and the results should be used only in combination with a thorough clinical assessment of the patient.

Table 52-1
Approaches to the Treatment of Hyperthyroidism

Treatment	Advantages	Disadvantages
antithyroid drugs (propylthiouracil, methimazole)	No thyroid tissue damage Effects are reversible Rapid control of symptoms Dose is adjustable Can be given to pregnant women and to children	Relapse is common. Prolonged therapy is required. Blood dyscrasias can occur. Many side-effects are possible.
radioactive iodide (^{131}I)	Limited tissue damage Relapse is rare Multiple dosing usually not required	Dosage determination is not precise. Myxedema is common, requiring thyroid supplementation. Contraindicated in pregnancy
thyroidectomy (subtotal)	Provides rapid benefit Suspicious lesions can be removed Very effective if gland is greatly enlarged	Requires surgical skill Loss of thyroid function is irreversible. Discomfort and pain Complications can involve parathyroid glands and vocal cords.

Thyroid Hormones

Levothyroxine, Liothyronine, Liotrix, Thyroglobulin, Thyroid Desiccated

Several types of thyroid hormone preparations are available, both natural extracts of animal thyroid glands and synthetic derivatives. The natural animal extracts (*e.g.*, desiccated thyroid, thyroglobulin) exhibit more variation in potency than the synthetic derivatives and are much less frequently employed today than the synthetic derivatives.

The available thyroid preparations are the following:

1. Desiccated thyroid—Powdered, dried thyroid glands of domesticated animals, standardized on the basis of iodine content
2. Thyroglobulin—Purified extract of porcine thyroid gland, standardized by iodine content and bioassayed for metabolic activity
3. Levothyroxine sodium—Sodium salt of the synthetic L-isomer of T_4

Table 52-2
Laboratory Parameters Used to Ascertain Thyroid Gland Function

Commonly Used

1. Free thyroxine index (FT_4I): 1.4 ng/100 ml–4.2 ng/100 ml
2. Resin uptake of radioactive T_3 *in vitro* (RT_3U): 27%–37% uptake of T_3
3. TSH levels: up to 10 μU/ml
4. Radioimmunoassays for T_3 and T_4:
   T_3 (RIA)—80 ng/100 ml–180 ng/100 ml (adults)
   T_4 (RIA)—5 mcg/100 ml–12 mcg/100 ml (adults)

Infrequently Used

1. Basal metabolic rate (BMR): ±10%
2. Protein-bound iodine (PBI): 4 mcg/100 ml–8 mcg/100 ml serum
3. Radioactive iodine uptake: 5%–10% at 2 hours; 10%–20% at 6 hours; 20%–40% at 24 hours
4. Thyroxine-binding globulin levels: 10 mcg/100 ml–26 mcg/100 ml
5. Free T_3 index (FT_3I): 20 ng/100 ml–60 ng/100 ml (confirm diagnosis of hyperthyroidism only)

4. Liothyronine sodium—Sodium salt of the synthetic L-isomer of T_3

5. Liotrix—Combination of levothyroxine sodium (T_4) and liothyronine sodium (T_3) in a 4:1 ratio, on a weight basis

MECHANISM AND ACTIONS

The precise mechanism of action of the thyroid hormones is incompletely understood. High-affinity binding sites for these substances have been found in the nucleus, mitochondria, and plasma membrane of cells, suggesting multiple sites of action. Thyroid hormones probably bind to receptors on cellular surfaces, increasing uptake of glucose and amino acids. They may also diffuse into cells and interact with receptors on mitochondria and chromatin material, resulting in increased synthesis of RNA, which leads to accelerated protein synthesis and enhanced enzymatic and cellular activity. Thyroid hormones appear to stimulate sodium–potassium–ATPase directly, thus facilitating membrane transport of sodium and potassium and increasing cellular utilization of oxygen.

Thyroid hormones are necessary for the optimal growth, development, and functioning of virtually all body tissues and are especially vital for early development of the central nervous system (CNS). Effects of these hormones include increases in body temperature, respiratory rate, heart rate, cardiac output, blood volume, carbohydrate, fat and protein metabolism, and enzymatic activity. Conversely, serum cholesterol levels may be reduced.

USES

1. Replacement or substitution therapy of primary hypothyroidism (*e.g.*, cretinism, myxedema, nontoxic goiter, hypothyroid state of childhood) or hypothyroidism resulting from surgery, radiation, drugs, pregnancy, or aging

2. Adjuncts to thyroid-inhibiting agents when they are used to reduce release of thyrotropic hormones in the treatment of thyrotoxicosis (thyroid drugs prevent development of goiter and hypothyroidism)

3. Prevention or treatment of various euthyroid goiters, such as thyroid nodules, multinodular goiter, or chronic, lymphocytic thyroiditis

4. Differentiation of hyperthyroidism from euthyroidism (T_3 *only* in the T_3 suppression test)

5. Adjunctive therapy of follicular and papillary carcinoma of the thyroid, in conjunction with radioactive iodine

ADMINISTRATION AND DOSAGE

See Table 52-3.

FATE

Oral absorption is variable, T_3 being absorbed to a greater extent (95% within 4 hours) than T_4 (50%–75%). The onset of action is within 6 hours to 8 hours for T_3, but much slower with T_4 (2 to 3 days). Peak effects generally require up to 8 to 10 days to develop, although full therapeutic effects may not be evident for several weeks. Plasma half-lives are 1 to 2 days for T_3 and 6 to 7 days for T_4. Both hormones are highly bound (99%–100%) to plasma proteins (thyroxine-binding globulin, thyroxine-binding pre-albumin, and albumin), although T_4 has a higher affinity for both globulin and pre-albumin than does T_3, which contributes to its higher serum levels and longer half-life. Approximately 35% of T_4 is deiodinated in the periphery to T_3. The thyroid hormones are metabolized at a number of sites and excreted in the urine (70%–80%) or bile (20%–30%) both as free drugs and conjugated metabolites.

SIDE-EFFECTS/ADVERSE REACTIONS

Adverse reactions to the thyroid hormones are almost always the result of excessive dosage or too-rapid increases in dosage. Most often, palpitations, sweating, nervousness, and heat intolerance are noted, although other reported adverse effects include fever, headaches, diarrhea, weight loss, arrhythmias, anginal pain, tremors, insomnia, menstrual irregularities, allergic skin reactions, congestive heart failure, and shock.

A partial loss of hair can occur in children during the first few months of therapy, but is usually transient and recovery is complete.

Chronic excessive dosage will produce symptoms of hyperthyroidism such as nervousness, tachycardia, increased bowel motility, and menstrual irregularities. Angina or congestive heart failure may be aggravated or induced and shock and cardiac failure can develop. Dosage should be reduced or temporarily discontinued and gradually reinstituted at a lower dose.

CONTRAINDICATIONS AND PRECAUTIONS

Thyroid hormones are contraindicated in patients with thyrotoxicosis, nephrosis, acute myocardial infarction, and untreated hypoadrenalism. In addition, thyroid hormones should not be used to treat obesity, infertility, or depression, conditions for which these drugs have been used previously but for which there exists no evidence for their effectiveness.

Thyroid hormone preparations should be given with *caution* to patients with cardiovascular dis-

(*Text continues on p. 992.*)

Table 52-3
Thyroid Hormones

Drug	Preparations	Usual Dosage Range	Clinical Considerations
thyroid, desiccated (Armour Thyroid, S-P-T, Thyrar, Thyro-Teric)	Tablets—16 mg, 32 mg, 65 mg, 98 mg, 130 mg, 195 mg, 260 mg, 325 mg Coated tablets—32 mg, 65 mg, 130 mg, 195 mg Capsules (timed-release)—65 mg, 130 mg, 195 mg, 325 mg	*Adults* Myxedema—16 mg/day for 2 weeks; 32 mg/day for 2 weeks; then 65 mg/day; increase daily dosage at monthly or greater intervals based on laboratory tests (usual range 65 mg–195 mg/day) Hypothyroidism without myxedema—65 mg/day increased by 65 mg every 30 days until desired response *Children* Dosage regimen same as adults, with increments made at 2-week intervals; maintenance doses may be higher in growing child than in adult.	Desiccated animal thyroid glands containing active thyroid hormones (T_3 and T_4) in their natural state and ratio; potency can vary significantly from lot to lot; clinical effects develop slowly and are very prolonged; caution in transferring patient from thyroid to T_3 alone; discontinue thyroid, begin T_3 at very low doses, and gradually increase dosage levels; drug should be stored in dark, moisture-free bottles.
thyroglobulin (Proloid)	Tablets—32 mg, 65 mg, 100 mg, 130 mg, 200 mg	Initially 32 mg/day; increase at 2-week to 3-week intervals until optimal response is attained; usual maintenance doses are 65 mg–200 mg and may be higher in growing child than in adult	Purified extract of hog thyroid containing T_4 and T_3 in an approximate 2.5:1 ratio; biologically assayed and standardized in animals; action is similar to that of desiccated thyroid with comparable onset and duration.
levothyroxine sodium—T_4 (Levothroid, Levoxine, Synthroid, Synthrox, Syroxine)	Tablets—0.025 mg, 0.05 mg, 0.075 mg, 0.1 mg, 0.125 mg, 0.15 mg, 0.175 mg, 0.2 mg, 0.3 mg Injection—200 mcg/vial, 500 mcg/vial	*Oral* Adults—0.1 mg/day initially; increased by 0.05-mg–0.1-mg increments every 1 week to 3 weeks until desired response is obtained; in elderly, myxedematous, or cardiovascular patients, initial dose 0.025 mg with 0.025-mg–0.05-mg increments as needed; usual range 0.1 mg–0.2 mg/day *Children* 0.025 mg–0.05 mg initially, with increments of 0.05 mg–0.1 mg/day at 1-week to 3-week intervals until desired response is obtained; usual range 0.2 mg–0.4 mg/day *Parenteral* Myxedematous coma—0.2 mg–0.5 mg by IV injection (0.1 mg/ml) on the first day; 0.1 mg–0.3 mg	Synthetic monosodium salt of the naturally occurring l-isomer of thyroxine; 0.1 mg is equivalent to 65 mg of desiccated thyroid; used orally for hypothyroid replacement therapy and IV for treatment of myxedema coma or stupor demanding immediate replacement; may be given IM when oral route is not feasible; slower onset and longer duration than synthetic T_3; discontinue T_4 before switching to T_3; conversely, begin T_4 several days before stopping T_3; parenteral solution is prepared with sodium chloride injection (without bacteriostatic agent) and shaken until clear, use immediately; do *not* add to IV fluids; administer IV very cautiously to patients

(continued)

Table 52-3 (continued)
Thyroid Hormones

Drug	Preparations	Usual Dosage Range	Clinical Considerations
levothyroxine sodium— T₄ (Levothroid, Levoxine, Synthroid, Synthrox, Syroxine) (*continued*)		second day if necessary; daily injections maintained until patient can accept a daily oral dose	with heart disease; inject slowly in small doses, and carefully observe patient.
liothyronine sodium— T₃ (Cytomel, Cyronine)	Tablets—5 mcg, 25 mcg, 50 mcg	*Adults and children over 3 years* Mild hypothyroidism—25 mcg/day initially, increase by 12.5 mcg/day–25 mcg/day every 1 week to 2 weeks; usual maintenance is 25 mcg–75 mcg/day in divided doses Myxedema—5 mcg/day initially; increased by 5 mcg–10 mcg/day every 1 week to 2 weeks; usual maintenance is 50 mcg–100 mcg/day Simple nontoxic goiter—see Myxedema (above) T₃ suppression test—75 mcg–100 mcg/day for 7 days; then repeat ¹³¹I uptake test; in hyperthyroid patient, uptake is not affected; in normal patient, uptake will fall to less than 20%. *Children under 3 years* Cretinism—initially 5 mcg/day; increase by 5 mcg every 3 to 4 days until desired response is achieved; infants a few months old require about 20 mcg/day; at 1 year, 50 mcg/day is required; above 3 years full adult dose may be necessary.	Synthetic form of the naturally occurring l-triiodothyronine (T₃): 25 mcg is equivalent to 65 mg of desiccated thyroid; possesses similar actions and uses of other thyroid hormones, but has a more rapid onset of maximal effect and shorter duration (half-life 1–2 days), allowing quicker dosage adjustments; serum TSH levels are most reliable laboratory index for monitoring T₃ replacement; also used in T₃ suppression test to differentiate borderline hyperthyroid from euthyroid (normal); useful in patients allergic to naturally extracted derivatives; be alert for possible additive effects due to residual action of longer-acting thyroid drugs when T₃ is substituted for them; potential for cardiotoxicity is high; use extreme caution when administering to patients with cardiac disease

liotrix (Euthroid, Thyrolar)

Tablets containing T₄ and T₃ in a fixed 4:1 ratio

T₄ (mcg)	T₃ (mcg)	Thyroid Equivalent (mg)
12.5	3.1	15
25	6.25	30
30	7.5	30
50	12.5	60
60	15	60
100	25	120
120	30	120
150	37.5	180
180	45	180

Usual Dosage Range: Dosage given in thyroid equivalents Initially 15 mg–30 mg/day; increased gradually every 1 to 2 weeks until desired response is obtained Replacement therapy for other thyroid products is based on the equivalency: 60 mg liotrix = 65 mg desiccated thyroid or thyroglobulin = 0.1 mg T₄ = 25 mcg T₃

Clinical Considerations: A constant mixture of synthetic T₄ and T₃ in a fixed 4:1 ratio by weight; although the product is claimed to more closely approximate the endogenous ratio of T₄:T₃, when differences in potency, absorption, binding, peripheral conversion of T₄ to T₃, and metabolism are considered, the fixed ratio offers no apparent advantage over other thyroid hormones used at optimal doses (except in those few intolerant persons); tablets have a shelf life of 2 years; it is given as a single daily dose before breakfast.

orders (especially angina or arrhythmias), and dosage must be reduced if chest pain, dyspnea, or rhythm disturbances occur. Cautious use is also necessary in patients with concomitant diabetes mellitus or adrenal insufficiency, since symptoms may be exacerbated by thyroid hormone therapy.

Prolonged hypothyroidism frequently results in decreased adrenocortical function. Initiation of thyroid replacement therapy does not concomitantly increase adrenocortical activity, and a state of adrenocortical insufficiency can develop. Therefore, supplemental adrenocorticosteroid therapy may be necessary.

INTERACTIONS

1. The cardiovascular effects of catecholamines may be potentiated by thyroid hormones, possibly resulting in coronary insufficiency or arrhythmias.
2. Highly protein-bound drugs (e.g., anti-inflammatory drugs) may compete with thyroid hormones for plasma protein binding sites, resulting in increased plasma levels of thyroid hormones.
3. Thyroid hormones can potentiate the effects of oral anticoagulants by increasing catabolism of vitamin-K–dependent clotting factors.
4. Thyroid hormones may increase blood sugar levels, thus increasing requirements for insulin and oral hypoglycemic drugs.
5. Estrogens may decrease plasma levels of free T_4 by increasing levels of thyroid-binding globulin.
6. Cholestyramine binds T_3 and T_4 in the intestine, thus impairing their absorption.
7. Thyroid hormone therapy may decrease the effectiveness and increase the likelihood of toxicity of the digitalis glycosides.
8. The activity of tricyclic antidepressants can be enhanced by thyroid hormones, possibly resulting in cardiac arrhythmias.
9. Tachycardia and hypertension may occur with ketamine in patients receiving thyroid hormones.

■ Nursing Process

□ ASSESSMENT

□ Subjective Data
Accurate diagnosis of a hypothyroid state is essential before drug therapy is initiated since administration of thyroid hormone when the body is al-ready producing a sufficient quantity will disrupt hormonal balance on multiple levels. Laboratory tests will confirm suspicions but data collection begins with an accurate history of symptoms.

Although the common symptoms of hypothyroidism in the adult include weakness, sluggishness, dry skin, edema, facial puffiness, constipation, and sensation of being cold, these may be absent in the elderly individual and in the infant or child. The older adult may exhibit slowness in thinking and fatigue and isolate himself from social activities, behaviors that are sometimes perceived as normal for this age group. The nurse must be acutely aware of behavioral changes that may signal hormonal imbalance rather than "old age." Likewise, the infant may exhibit respiratory distress, lethargy, poor feeding patterns, slow passage of meconium (in the neonate), and temperature fluctuations below 95° F, all symptoms of hypothyroidism. Laboratory testing is always in order when the disorder is suspected in the newborn and is routinely done in some nurseries to ensure any problems are discovered early.

A complete drug history is essential before thyroid medication is given since the drug may enhance the effect of many drugs, creating the potential for toxicity. Examples of such drugs include tricyclic antidepressants, oral anticoagulants, and catecholamines. See Interactions, above, for ideas on how to frame appropriate drug history questions. In addition, a history of other endocrine disorders should be identified since in most cases treatment and response will be closely related. The patient with cardiovascular problems must be given thyroid hormone with caution.

□ Objective Data
A complete physical examination will be necessary before drug therapy begins. Cardiovascular assessment is essential, including resting heart rate and auscultation to detect any arrhythmias. An electrocardiogram will be performed, and is especially important in the elderly who are prone to arrhythmias while taking thyroid hormones.

Children need a complete growth and development assessment. An evaluation of the risks versus the benefits is crucial since thyroid hormone can accelerate growth processes including premature epiphyseal closure.

The laboratory tests used to evaluate thyroid function are listed in Table 52-2. Several drugs that may alter the values of these tests are listed in Table 52-4. The nurse needs to review these items with the patient before specimens are drawn to de-

Table 52-4
Effects of Drugs on Thyroid Function Tests

Test	Drugs That Increase Values	Drugs That Decrease Values
Serum T_4	estrogens insulin methadone phenothiazines topical betadine	androgens barbiturates diazepam heparin nitroprusside phenytoin salicylates antidiabetics sulfonylureas
Serum T_3	estrogens methadone thiazide diuretics	corticosteroids phenytoin propranolol
T_3 uptake	anabolic steroids corticosteroids danazol phenylbutazone salicylates	estrogens fluorouracil methadone
Free thyroxine index	heparin propranolol	aminosalicyclic acid barbiturates lithium phenylbutazone phenothiazines

termine the accuracy of the tests. Other laboratory data will include cardiac enzymes, serum glucose level, and renal function studies.

□ *NURSING DIAGNOSES*
Actual nursing diagnoses may include
Knowledge deficit related to the action and effect of the hormone, administration, duration of therapy, and side-effects to monitor
Potential nursing diagnoses are related to hypothyroidism, indicating insufficient drug, or hyperthyroidism, indicating excessive drug. Examples of some nursing diagnoses that may occur include
Alteration in cardiac output: decreased related to tachycardia, arrhythmias (hyperthyroid response)
Sleep pattern disturbance: insomnia related to hyperthyroid response; increased length of sleep time, tiredness related to hypothyroid response

Alteration in bowel elimination: constipation related to hypothyroid response

□ *PLAN*
Nursing care goals may include:
1. Helping the patient and his family to incorporate correct drug taking into daily activities since, in most cases, thyroid hormone must be taken for life; and
2. Teaching the patient
   a. The importance of follow-up blood studies,
   b. How to manage dosage adjustment periods,
   c. Symptoms of overdosage and underdosage, and
   d. Major drug side-effects and what to do if they occur.

□ *INTERVENTION*
The most important point the patient must learn about taking thyroid medication is that the regimen must usually continue for life. Since the drug remains in the body for several weeks after being discontinued, it is easy for the patient to believe he no longer needs it since symptoms will return very slowly; but symptoms will return. Consequently, the patient needs to establish a pattern to the drug taking so he won't forget it. Many patients tie the therapy in with breakfast or morning hygiene routines. This is effective since these routines are completed on a daily basis and ensure the drug is less likely to interfere with sleeping patterns. However, if a dose is missed one day, no attempt should be made to take an extra dose the next day.

Patients need to learn first the signs of an adequate therapeutic response by which to judge the drug's effectiveness. The adult may experience a sense of well-being, increase in energy, weight loss, mild diuresis, increased appetite, decreased facial edema, and an increase in heart rate and basal temperature. In the infant and child, mental alertness improves, as does appetite and growth; heart rate, and basal temperature increase and the child sleeps on a more normal curve for his age group. Such symptoms will enable the patient to recognize when a dosage adjustment is needed and will encourage early medical follow-up.

A patient may go through a dosage-adjustment period during initial therapy or after years on the medication. Introduction of a new medication may alter the need for thyroid hormone. Life factors that may instigate the need for dosage adjustments include an increase in stress, menopause, pregnancy and the postpartum period, and changes in activity level. Patients need to learn about these factors early in treatment so they can seek medical advice. Some patients claim they require an adjustment about every 7 years regardless of other factors. The change may produce symptoms of hypothyroidism or hyperthyroidism. The patient may already be aware of *hypothyroid* symptoms that signal the need for more medication since these may have been the symptoms that caused him to seek help in the first place. However, the nurse should provide a list as a reminder. These are mentioned under Assessment, above, and in the discussion of hypothyroidism earlier in this chapter. Early symptoms of hyperthyroidism or of therapeutic overdosage are nervousness, sweating, tachycardia, heat intolerance, palpitations, and sleep disturbances. In either case, as the dose is adjusted the patient must monitor closely for symptoms and have regular blood work completed. He should be encouraged to learn to take his pulse and know symptoms of cardiotoxicity (chest pain, dyspnea, and palpitations) since cardiovascular changes may be early indicators of drug effect.

The pregnant patient on thyroid hormones needs regular laboratory work and close monitoring. Dosage requirements will usually vary in each trimester. The newborn should also be monitored for thyroid function especially if the mother breast-feeds since the hormone is excreted in breast milk.

Children taking thyroid hormones need special attention. The child may actually start out on a higher dose than an adult, resulting in a more dramatic initial response. Symptoms of hypothyroid or hyperthyroid states may be more exaggerated, and therapeutic effects may occur quickly. The child's activity level may increase dramatically and may even be viewed as aggressive or hyperactive. However, these behaviors will generally become more moderate as the child becomes accustomed to the new hormone level. It is important that parents be cautioned about such behavior so they can deal with it more easily if it occurs. Partial loss of hair can occur in early stages of drug therapy in children. The child needs to be monitored more frequently than the adult. Blood levels, growth and development assessment, and bone age assessments should be done throughout therapy to ensure that the dosage of the hormone does not impair growth and development.

□ *EVALUATION*

Outcome criteria that can be used to judge drug effectiveness may include adequate serum values of T_3, T_4, and PBI; timely renewal of medications, which ensures the patient has taken the hormone as prescribed; absence of hypothyroid or hyperthyroid symptoms; early reporting of symptomatology indicating changes; and returns to clinic/office for follow-up therapy but especially during dosage-adjustment periods.

Antithyroid Drugs

Methimazole, Propylthiouracil

The antithyroid drugs impair the synthesis of the thyroid hormones T_3 and T_4 in the thyroid gland, and are used in the treatment of hyperthyroid states. Unlike other means of hyperthyroid therapy, such as subtotal thyroidectomy or ^{131}I, antithyroid drugs do not damage thyroid tissue beyond repair and thus are usually the initial treatment of choice. Long-term therapy may produce remission of the disease in some cases, but relapse is not uncommon. Patients who fail to respond fully to drug therapy or who show evidence of relapse should be considered as candidates for either surgery or radioisotope therapy (see Table 52-1).

Because the antithyroid drugs do not interfere with the release or activity of previously formed thyroid hormones, their clinical effects are delayed for several weeks, until body stores of preformed T_3 and T_4 are exhausted. Likewise, the action of exogenously administered thyroid hormones is unimpaired by antithyroid drugs.

Several kinds of compounds are capable of exerting an antithyroid effect. Large amounts of the iodide ion (6 mg–10 mg/day) can quickly suppress release of thyroid hormones from the gland, and are thus occasionally used for treating some forms of acute hyperthyroidism such as thyroid storm and for reducing the size and vascularity of the gland before thyroidectomy. Certain monovalent inorganic anions (*e.g.*, perchlorate, thiocyanate, periodate) block uptake of iodide by the gland and can exert an antithyroid action. They are rarely used clinically, however, because of the availability of more effective and less toxic drugs. The principal antithyroid agents are the thioamide derivatives methimazole and propylthiouracil; they are discussed below, and summarized in Table 52-5.

MECHANISM AND ACTIONS

The antithyroid drugs inhibit the synthesis of T_3 and T_4 by interfering with the action of the peroxidase enzyme, thus preventing oxidation of iodide to the reactive iodine compound in the thyroid

Table 52-5
Antithyroid Drugs

Drug	Preparations	Usual Dosage Range	Clinical Considerations
methimazole (Tapazole)	Tablets—5 mg, 10 mg	Adults—15 mg–60 mg initially depending on degree of hyperthyroidism in 3 daily doses at 8-h intervals; maintenance is 5 mg–15 mg/day Children—0.4 mg/kg initially in 3 divided doses at 8-h intervals; maintenance is 1/2 initial dose	More potent than propylthiouracil, longer duration of action, and somewhat more toxic; skin rash is an indication for discontinuing drug.
propylthiouracil	Tablets—50 mg	Adults—initially 100 mg 3 times/day, every 8 h; maintenance is 100 mg–150 mg/day Children (over 10 yr)—50 mg–100 mg 3 times/day every 8 h Children (6 yr–10 yr)—50 mg–150 mg/day in divided doses	Least toxic antithyroid drug; administer with meals to reduce GI distress; monitor prothrombin time regularly during therapy because drug can cause hypoprothrombinemia.

gland. These drugs may also block the oxidative coupling of monoiodotyrosine (MIT) and diiodotyrosine (DIT) to form T_3 and T_4. Evidence has also accrued that the peripheral deiodination of T_4 to T_3 is retarded by propylthiouracil. These agents do *not* inactivate existing T_3 and T_4, nor interfere with the action of exogenous thyroid hormones; thus, their effects are slow in developing.

Antithyroid drug-induced depression of thyroid hormone synthesis leads to a gradual reduction in plasma levels of T_3 and T_4, which results in a compensatory increase in TSH secretion from the adenohypophysis. Excess TSH stimulates the thyroid gland and can lead to an increase in its size and vascularity, a condition referred to as *goiter*.

USES
1. Treatment of hyperthyroidism (most effective in milder cases in which thyroid gland is not excessively enlarged)
2. Preparation for subtotal thyroidectomy or radioactive iodine therapy (to reduce hyperthyroidism and to lessen surgical risks)

ADMINISTRATION AND DOSAGE
See Table 52-5.

FATE
The antithyroid drugs are well absorbed orally and oral bioavailability is high. Peak serum levels occur within 1 hour. Plasma half-lives are relatively short (1–2 hours for propylthiouracil and 3–5 hours for methimazole) but do *not* reflect the duration of the antithyroid effect, which is due to an action within the thyroid gland. Dosing frequency is usually every 6 hours to 8 hours. Most of a dose of propylthiouracil is excreted by the kidney within 24 hours as inactive metabolites. Excretion of methimazole is slower, approximately 75% of a dose being recovered in the urine within 48 hours.

SIDE-EFFECTS/ADVERSE REACTIONS
The most frequently encountered side-effects with antithyroid drugs are skin rash, itching, and epigastric distress. The most serious adverse reaction is agranulocytosis, which occurs in approximately 0.5% of patients receiving antithyroid drugs. Large doses appear to increase the risk of agranulocytosis, which is usually rapidly reversible on drug discontinuation. A variety of other untoward reactions have occurred during antithyroid drug therapy and include

> CNS—Headache, vertigo, drowsiness, paresthesias, stimulation, neuropathies
> GI—Nausea, vomiting, loss of taste, sialadenopathy
> Hepatic/renal—Jaundice, hepatitis, nephritis
> Hematologic—Granulocytopenia, thrombocytopenia, hypoprothrombinemia, vasculitis, periarteritis

Dermatologic—Urticaria, pigmentation of skin, lupus-like syndrome, exfoliative dermatitis (rare)

Other—Myalgia, arthralgia, edema, lymphadenopathy, fever

Goiter can also occur (see Mechanism and Actions, above) and is manifested as periorbital edema, fatigue, paresthesias, muscle cramping, cold sensitivity, and bradycardia.

CONTRAINDICATIONS AND PRECAUTIONS

Antithyroid drugs should not be used in nursing mothers. A *cautious* approach to therapy is required in persons with bleeding tendencies or liver dysfunction, and in pregnant women (because the drugs can induce goiter in the fetus).

INTERACTIONS

1. Antithyroid drugs can magnify the effects of oral anticoagulants by causing hypoprothrombinemia.
2. Antithyroid drugs should be used cautiously in the presence of other drugs known to cause agranulocytosis (*e.g.*, carbamazepine, clofibrate, indomethacin, methyldopa, meprobamate, phenylbutazone, procainamide, quinidine, and tolbutamide).

■ Nursing Process

□ ASSESSMENT

□ Subjective Data

A history of the patient's symptoms usually identifies hyperthyroidism clearly but data must be accurately collected before drug treatment is selected. Common signs of hyperthyroidism include some gland enlargement, warm moist skin, weight loss in spite of increased appetite, tachycardia, systolic hypertension, and some degree of insomnia. The patient may also complain of being jittery, nervous, or anxious. Clinical signs are usually confirmed by laboratory findings. A drug history is also essential since antithyroid drugs may enhance the effects of oral anticoagulants and result in increased risk of agranulocytosis when combined with a variety of agents (see Interactions, above).

□ Objective Data

Laboratory data should be collected before therapy with antithyroid drugs begins. Thyroid function studies such as T_3 and T_4 levels are completed for diagnosis although overwhelming symptoms of hyperthyroidism or thyroid storm are the key indicators of the disease. Baseline levels of T_3 and T_4 can be used for later comparison to measure the effectiveness of drug therapy. In addition, a complete blood count, coagulation studies, and a pregnancy test should be obtained.

□ NURSING DIAGNOSES
Actual nursing diagnoses may include
Knowledge deficit related to the drug action, correct administration, and side-effects
Potential nursing diagnoses may include
Alteration in cardiac output: decreased, related to drug-induced hypothyroidism
Alteration in fluid volume: excess, related to drug-induced hypothyroidism
Alteration in thought processes: depression, related to drug-induced hypothyroidism
Impaired skin integrity, bruising, rashes related to drug-induced agranulocytosis
Potential for infection related to drug-induced agranulocytosis
Alteration in tissue perfusion related to drug-induced hypoprothrombinemia

□ PLAN
The nursing care goals focus on
1. Helping the patient learn to take the drug correctly
2. Teaching the patient to monitor for side-effects such as hypothyroidism, the development of blood dyscrasias, or coagulation problems

□ INTERVENTION
Patients with hyperthyroidism may have a sufficiently enlarged thyroid gland to produce difficulty in swallowing. Antithyroid tablets may be crushed to make swallowing easier.

Antithyroid medications require a period of dosage adjustment while existing thyroid hormone is excreted. Consequently the patient must be willing to take the prescribed dose consistently, have periodic thyroid function tests, and monitor himself for drug effectiveness. Signs of inadequate dose response include increased pulse rate, anxiety, weight loss, and tremor, and an increase in medication is indicated. Teach the patient to take his pulse, if possible, since cardiovascular effects may be early indicators of inappropriate dose. If the dose is too high the patient will develop signs and symptoms of *hypothyroidism* such as depression, fluid retention, cold intolerance, and bradycardia, and should report the onset of these to the physician.

Once an appropriate dose has been established, periodic thyroid function studies must be done to ensure the patient's need for the drug has not changed. It is important that the patient be willing and able to continue follow-up. One life change that must be reported is pregnancy. Since antithyroid drugs readily cross the placental barrier, they may produce hypothyroidism and possibly cretinism in the developing fetus. During pregnancy doses of antithyroid drugs may be reduced and may be given concurrently with thyroid hormones to decrease the risk to the fetus. Since the mother's metabolism changes drastically during pregnancy, thyroid hormones may actually be indicated to prevent her from developing hypothyroidism. Breast-feeding should be avoided if the mother continues to take antithyroid medications. It is important that this discussion be initiated before delivery to prepare the mother and help her make some decisions about drug therapy.

Patients taking antithyroid medications should learn to read the labels of over-the-counter medications carefully. Preparations containing iodide such as cough syrups and asthma preparations may interfere with the effectiveness of antithyroid drugs. The patient should be provided with a list of medications to avoid.

Antithyroid drug therapy usually lasts 1 to 2 years whereupon remission is attained in about 50% of patients. When the drug is withdrawn, the patient must continue to monitor himself for increased pulse rate or weight loss and report any significant changes since these can be early indicators of returning hyperthyroidism.

Aside from hyperthyroid or hypothyroid symptoms two serious side-effects, agranulocytosis and hypoprothrombinemia, may occur during treatment with antithyroid drugs. Periodic complete blood count and coagulation studies can detect problems early but the patient needs to know what symptoms to report immediately as well. Early symptoms of agranulocytosis include bruising, sore throat, rash, fever, headache, and malaise. Symptoms of coagulation problems include petechiae, frequent bruising or unexplainable nosebleeds, gum bleeding, rectal bleeding, or hematuria.

□ *EVALUATION*

Outcome criteria that may be used to measure the success of drug therapy include return to a euthyroid state as indicated by absence of symptoms and a T_3 or T_4 level within normal range, attendance at follow-up appointments, timely renewal of prescription, absence of serious side-effects such as hypoprothrombinemia or blood dyscrasia, and early reporting of any symptoms of side-effects.

Iodine/Iodide Products

Strong Iodine Solution, Sodium Iodide, Potassium Iodide, Saturated Solution of Potassium Iodide

At one time, iodine and iodide were commonly used as treatment for hyperthyroidism. In spite of their rapid beneficial action, effects were short-lived, and within a few weeks symptoms usually returned and in many instances were intensified. Largely for this reason, these drugs have only a limited therapeutic application today, and are primarily used to suppress hyperthyroidism and reduce the size and vascularity of the thyroid gland before thyroidectomy. They also can provide a thyroid blocking action in a radiation emergency. The available compounds include strong iodine solution (5% iodine and 10% potassium iodide), sodium iodide injection, saturated solution of potassium iodide (SSKI), and tablets or solution containing potassium iodide. The pharmacology of these agents is discussed in general terms and individual drugs are then listed in Table 52-6. In addition, certain iodide-containing products useful as expectorants are detailed in Chapter 47.

MECHANISM AND ACTIONS

The precise mechanism of action of the iodides is not completely known. These substances may suppress release of thyroid hormones from thyroglobulin, and interfere with the synthesis of thyroid hormones. Improvement in symptoms is rapid; hence, these drugs may be of value in treating thyroid storm. Iodides reduce the size and vascularity of the thyroid gland and increase the quantity of bound iodine within the gland.

USES

1. Preparation for thyroidectomy in hyperthyroid patients, in conjunction with an antithyroid drug (reduce size and vascularity of gland)
2. Acute treatment of thyrotoxic crisis (thyroid storm) or neonatal thyrotoxicosis

Table 52-6
Iodine/Iodide Compounds

Drug	Preparations	Usual Dosage Range	Clinical Considerations
potassium iodide (Iosat,* PIMA, Thyro-Block*)	Liquid—500 mg/15 ml Syrup—325 mg/5 ml Enteric-coated tablets—300 mg Solution—21 mg/drop* Tablets—130 mg*	Expectorant—325 mg–650 mg every 4 h–6 h Radiation emergency Adults: 130 mg daily Children (under age 1): 65 mg daily	Useful for hyperthyroidism, thyrotoxic crisis (with antithyroid drugs), preoperatively for thyroidectomy, and to facilitate bronchial drainage and cough in chronic pulmonary diseases; also used in radiation emergencies to block uptake of radioactive iodine by the thyroid gland; discontinue if skin rash appears; see also Chapter 47.
saturated solution potassium iodide (SSKI)	Solution—1 g/ml	0.3 ml–0.6 ml 3 to 4 times/day diluted in water, juice, or milk (maximum 12 times/day)	Used presurgically for reducing size and fragility of thyroid gland; do not allow to stand uncovered for prolonged periods of time because solution may evaporate; slight discoloration of solution does not affect potency.
sodium iodide (various manufacturers)	Injection—10%	Thyroid crisis—2 g/day by IV infusion	Primarily used for acute treatment of thyroid crisis; be alert for development of acute iodism (e.g., metallic taste, stomatitis, sneezing, vomiting, swollen salivary glands) and pulmonary edema.
strong iodine solution (Lugol's solution)	Solution—5% iodine and 10% potassium iodide	0.1 ml–0.3 ml (approximately 2–6 drops) 3 times/day (usually for 10 days–14 days before thyroidectomy)	Principally used to prepare thyroid gland for surgery; also used with an antithyroid drug for treating thyrotoxic crisis; discontinue if signs of iodism appear (see above); administer solution diluted in juice, milk, or water, preferably after meals.

* Available only to state and federal agencies for radiation emergencies. See Uses.

3. Provide a thyroid blocking action in a radiation emergency

ADMINISTRATION AND DOSAGE
See Table 52-6.

FATE
Iodides and iodine-containing products are generally well absorbed orally, effects are usually noted within 24 hours to 48 hours, and maximal effects occur within 2 weeks. The drugs are rapidly cleared from the plasma, primarily by thyroid uptake. Elimination is by way of either the urine or the feces.

SIDE-EFFECTS/ADVERSE REACTIONS
Side-effects observed with oral iodides include an unpleasant metallic taste, gum soreness, mucosal ulceration, salivary gland enlargement, excessive salivation, rhinitis, fever, joint pain, dyspnea, edema, skin rash, vomiting, headache, and goiter (enlarged thyroid gland).

IV administration can result in acute iodide poisoning, characterized by edema (bronchial, laryngeal); mucosal hemorrhaging; serum sickness; acneiform, maculopapular, vesicular, or bullous eruptions; and generalized inflammation.

Chronic use of iodides may result in "iodism," which is characterized by skin eruptions, bronchial irritation, generalized swelling, conjunctivitis, coryza, erythema, purpura, fever, and restlessness.

CONTRAINDICATIONS AND PRECAUTIONS

These preparations are contraindicated in persons sensitive to iodides. Sodium iodide is also contraindicated in patients with pulmonary edema or tuberculosis and potassium iodide is contraindicated in patients with hyperkalemia. Iodide preparations should be used cautiously in pregnant or nursing women. The parenteral form of sodium iodide should not be given to children.

INTERACTIONS

1. Lithium may enhance the hypothyroid action of iodide preparations.
2. Estrogens can increase the amount of protein-bound iodine.

NURSING CONSIDERATIONS

Since iodine preparations are now considered adjunctive to antithyroid medication therapy, the reader is referred to the Nursing Process in the section on antithyroid drugs. Care of the pregnant patient, use of over-the-counter preparations containing iodine, and concerns about developing symptoms of hypothyroidism or hyperthyroidism are the same.

In addition, the principal nursing concerns are to ensure appropriate administration and the detection of adverse reactions. Iodine preparations must be taken as prescribed before thyroidectomy to avoid the possibility of gland enlargement and revascularization. This task may be difficult to accomplish since the preparations have a very unpleasant, salty taste. In addition to clear explanations about the importance of taking the medication, the nurse may achieve more success in compliance by diluting the medication in a well-chilled glass of water, juice, or milk and offering it after meals to decrease GI upset. Iodine solutions should be taken through a straw since the preparations can stain teeth.

The patient must also be taught to watch for symptoms of "iodism," which are listed under Side-Effects/Adverse Reactions, and told to report them immediately, for the drug may be discontinued. To prevent development of iodism, the patient also needs to limit foods high in iodine such as seafood, iodized salt, and many processed foods including some cereals, soups, and canned vegetables that contain iodized salt. Teach the patient to read labels carefully and mutually agree on a daily intake goal of sodium to limit iodine intake.

Severe adverse reactions such as laryngeal or bronchial edema may occur following intravenous administration of iodine. Emergency equipment must be available including endotracheal and tracheostomy equipment, mechanical ventilation, oxygen, and emergency drugs such as epinephrine and corticosteroids to decrease edema.

Radioactive Iodide

Of the several different radioactive isotopes of iodine that can be prepared, ^{131}I is the preferred agent for clinical use, since it has favorable emission characteristics and a rather short physical half-life.

Radioactive Sodium Iodide:[131]I

(Iodotope)

MECHANISM AND ACTIONS

Radioactive sodium iodide is trapped (i.e., taken up) by the thyroid gland in the same efficient manner as ordinary iodide and is rapidly converted to protein-bound iodine and stored within the follicles of the gland. [131]I decays by both beta and gamma emissions (approximately 90% beta and 10% gamma). Beta radiation has a short wavelength and penetrates only a few millimeters of thyroid tissue, thus destroying very small amounts of tissue. Low amounts of long wavelength gamma radiation are also emitted, which can be detected and measured by external monitoring. Destruction of thyroid tissue results in a gradual reduction in thyroid hormone secretion and amelioration of the symptoms of hyperthyroidism. The amount of radioactive iodine administered is carefully controlled to minimize the danger of destroying too much tissue, leading to a hypothyroid state. However, some degree of hypothyroidism almost always occurs following use of radioactive iodine.

USES

1. Treatment of hyperthyroidism, especially in patients over 30 years of age who do not respond to other antithyroid medications
2. Treatment of selected types of thyroid carcinoma (papillary or follicular) and metastases

(effectiveness is questionable in other forms because some thyroid neoplasms, *e.g.*, giant cell, spindle cell, and amyloid solid carcinomas, do not concentrate sufficient iodide ion)

ADMINISTRATION AND DOSAGE

Radioactive sodium iodide is available as capsules or solution for oral use containing variable amounts of radioactivity, measured in millicuries (mCi). The amount of radioactivity contained in each dose is measured by a radioactivity calibration procedure just prior to administration. Specific calibration and dosing instructions are provided with the product literature. Solution may darken on standing but this does not affect potency.

The average recommended doses are as follows:

Hyperthyroidism: 4 mCi to 10 mCi as a single dose. Toxic nodular goiter and severe hyperthyroidism may require larger amounts. If a second treatment is necessary, it is generally given 6 months to 12 months later, after the patient's thyroid function has been completely assessed.

Thyroid carcinoma: 50 mCi to 150 mCi depending on extent of thyroid involvement

FATE

Sodium iodide ^{131}I is rapidly absorbed orally and quickly and efficiently concentrated by the thyroid gland as well as by the stomach and salivary glands. Radioactivity can be detected in the thyroid within minutes. The half-life of ^{131}I is 8 days. Thyroid function begins to decrease within 2 weeks, and maximum effects are observed in 8 weeks to 12 weeks. The isotope is excreted mainly by the kidneys.

SIDE-EFFECTS/ADVERSE REACTIONS

Tenderness and soreness in the neck area, pain on swallowing, and cough can occur within a few days of treatment but usually disappear spontaneously. The principal adverse reactions resulting from radioiodide administration occur with larger amounts (as in treating thyroid carcinoma) and include nausea, vomiting, sialoadenitis, thinning of the hair, acute thyroid crisis, chromosomal abnormalities, bone marrow depression, leukemia, anemia, leukopenia, and thrombocytopenia. Destruction of excessive thyroid tissue can result in symptoms of hypothyroidism such as weakness, fatigue, cold intolerance, peripheral edema, bradycardia, dyspnea, puffiness of the skin, and angina-like pain.

CONTRAINDICATIONS AND PRECAUTIONS

Radioactive iodide should not be given to pregnant or nursing mothers, very young children, in the presence of preexisting nausea and vomiting, or following a recent myocardial infarction.

Prior to giving radioactive iodide, antithyroid drugs should be discontinued for 3 to 4 days. Use *caution* in women of childbearing age who may become pregnant during therapy. If necessary, the drug should be administered within 10 days following the onset of menses.

Thyroid hormone therapy may be necessary following radioactive iodide to minimize the incidence and severity of hypothyroidism. Hypothyroidism is often insidious in development but probably occurs in almost everyone receiving radioiodide treatment, although it may take years to become manifest. Continual replacement therapy with thyroid hormones should be employed for as long as necessary should hypothyroidism develop.

INTERACTIONS

1. The uptake of ^{131}I by the thyroid gland can be impaired by the recent intake of iodine in any form (*e.g.*, x-ray contrast media) or by use of thyroid or antithyroid drugs. Thyrotropin, however, can stimulate radioiodide uptake by the thyroid gland.

NURSING CONSIDERATIONS

Nursing care for the patient receiving ^{131}I should focus on appropriate administration, teaching the patient how to monitor the development of hypothyroidism, and following hospital/clinic policies on handling the patient receiving a radioactive isotope.

The patient must understand the need to discontinue any antithyroid medication 3 to 4 days before the isotope is given and to fast starting at midnight on the evening before drug administration. Food in the GI tract delays absorption of ^{131}I.

The patient receiving ^{131}I may be asked to sign a consent since there is a low incidence of destruction of reproductive organs following administration of the drug. This information should be shared with the patient before arrangements are made to give the drug and the patient should be given time to think about the possible consequences. To minimize the incidence of reproductive problems, women of childbearing age should be given ^{131}I during or within 10 days after the onset of menstruation. Information on hazards to the fetus must be provided to encourage birth control.

^{131}I is radioactive and specific guidelines

should be followed when handling patients receiving it. Check the institution's policy before commencing care and if no policy exists contact the radiation department for written guidelines. The nurse must seek to protect herself as well as minimize danger to her patient when dealing with radiation.

In general, the patient who receives a dose of 30 mCi of ^{131}I or less will be allowed to go home. This patient should receive the following instructions:

1. Minimize contact with small children on the first day and sleep alone for 2 nights.
2. To dilute the concentration of ^{131}I in the urine and feces, increase fluid intake to at least 2000 ml/day for about 1 week. Flush the toilet at least twice after use.
3. Attempt to minimize coughing or expectoration for 24 hours, if possible.

Be sure the patient understands that the risk to others is very minimal, if at all, when these steps are followed and allow time for him to ask questions and work through strategies for implementing the guidelines at home.

If a patient must receive a dose of ^{131}I greater than 30 mCi, hospitalization is recommended. In addition to the guidelines recommended for the patient at home, hospital personnel must take other precautions. The extent of these will be determined by the dose and radiation regulations in the facility. A sign indicating use of radioactive substance should be above the patient's bed and on the door. Only nonpregnant personnel should care for the patient and contact should be limited to 30 minutes per person on the first day and 1 hour per person on the second day. Urine, feces, and linen should be considered contaminated and gloves should be worn by anyone handling them. Special procedures may be needed for disposal since use of the regular sewage system may be prohibited. Visiting is usually limited on the first day.

Such stringent guidelines may be frightening to the patient and to personnel. Planning and information can diminish this anxiety. Staff should have an opportunity to be briefed on the expected procedures before caring for the patient and given time to ask questions. Regular interactions with radiation specialists in the facility and easily accessible information will also help. The patient needs to understand the need for limited contact and plans should be made to help him occupy his time while alone on the first day. A staff rotation schedule should be devised on each shift to facilitate care but also to assign someone just to visit with the patient on an hourly basis to decrease his sense of isolation.

CASE STUDY

Donna Donahue, age 30, is married and has two children. Mrs. Donahue developed symptoms of hypothyroidism about 10 years ago and was started on levothyroxine sodium (Synthroid), 0.2 mg daily. She had been asymptomatic until 6 weeks ago, when she began to have difficulty sleeping, noticed her heart rate seemed very fast at times, and developed a sense of anxiety. At first she thought the symptoms were related to increased stress at work and to a problem that had developed with her son at school. The symptoms persisted for about 2 weeks and Mrs. Donahue decided to see her physician.

On questioning, the physician found that Mrs. Donahue was experiencing dry skin, itching, increased thirst, and a localized skin infection around her breasts along her bra line. He ordered a serum thyroxine test (T_4), which showed an elevated level of 16.7 mg/dl. Synthroid was reduced to 0.15 mg daily and arrangements were made to have repeat laboratory work completed on a weekly basis.

After 2 weeks Mrs. Donahue's T_4 level was 13.8 mg/dl but increased heart rate and anxiety persisted. Synthroid was reduced to 0.1 mg daily. After 2 weeks the T_4 level was 8.4 mg/dl and Mrs. Donahue's symptoms were gone except for the dry skin and skin rash, which was responding to medication.

Discussion Questions

1. Mrs. Donahue missed the early symptoms of hyperthyroidism caused by excessive dosage of

replacement hormone. What other symptoms would the
nurse or physician want to explore with her? How could
she plan for the next incident should it occur?

2. Why might a patient suddenly need less hormone after
years of stability? During dosage adjustment how might
the nurse help Mrs. Donahue monitor the need further?

3. Outline a review teaching plan for Mrs. Donahue to
ensure her knowledge of the medication, its side-effects,
and how to respond to an episode of hypothyroidism or
hyperthyroidism.

REVIEW QUESTIONS

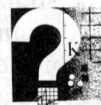

1. Briefly describe the steps in the biosynthesis of thyroid
hormones.
2. List the major pharmacologic actions of the thyroid
hormones.
3. What are the principal differences between T_3 and T_4?
4. What is goiter? What are the principal causes of goiter?
5. Distinguish between cretinism and myxedema.
6. Which tests are most often performed to assess the state
of thyroid function?
7. What are the three major approaches to the treatment of
hyperthyroidism?
8. List the available thyroid hormone preparations.
9. Briefly describe the mechanism of action of the thyroid
hormones.
10. Describe the most commonly encountered side-effects
during thyroid hormone therapy.
11. Why may supplemental adrenocorticoid therapy be
required during thyroid hormone treatment of
hypothyroidism?
12. List several drugs that may alter the results of thyroid
function tests.
13. What symptoms may the elderly patient with
hypothyroidism exhibit that may delay diagnosis? What
are typical symptoms in the infant?
14. How can the nurse facilitate incorporation of drug taking
into the patient's daily routine when thyroid hormones are
prescribed?
15. How should dosage-adjustment periods be handled?
16. What are some of the differences seen in children taking
thyroid hormones? How can the nurse help parents handle
these responses?
17. How do antithyroid drugs work on the treatment of
hypothyroidism?
18. Why is goiter a complication of antithyroid drug therapy?
19. What laboratory data should be collected before and
during antithyroid drug therapy?
20. How should the pregnant patient on antithyroid drugs be
handled?
21. What are the major indications for iodide products such as
sodium iodide or potassium iodide?

22. Which isotope of iodine is most often used clinically? What are its emission characteristics?
23. For what indications is radioactive iodine approved?
24. What are the major disadvantages of radioactive iodine versus antithyroid drugs in controlling hyperthyroidism?
25. What guidelines should the nurse follow when caring for a patient receiving radioactive iodine?

BIBLIOGRAPHY

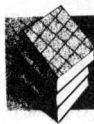

Cooper DS: Antithyroid drugs. N Engl J Med 311:1353, 1984

Dunn JT: Choice of therapy in young adults with hyperthyroidism of Graves' disease: A brief case-directed poll of 54 thyroidologists. Ann Intern Med 100:891, 1984

Evangelisti J, Thorpe C: Thyroid storm—A nursing crisis. Heart Lung 12:184, 1983

Horita A, Carino MA, Lai H: Pharmacology of thyrotropin releasing hormone. Annu Rev Pharmacol Toxicol 26:311, 1986

Jackson I: Thyrotropin-releasing hormone. N Engl J Med 306:145, 1982

Larsen PR: Thyroid pituitary interaction: Feedback regulation of thyrotropin secretion by thyroid hormones. N Engl J Med 306:23, 1982

Larsen PR: Tests of thyroid function. Med Clin North Am 59:1063, 1975

McKenzie JM, Zakarija M: LATS in Graves' disease. Recent Prog Horm Res 33:29, 1977

Morkin E, Flink IL, Goldman S: Biochemical and physiological effects of thyroid hormones on cardiac performance. Prog Cardiovasc Dis 25:435, 1983

Murphy D: Iodide—An Rx for radiation accident. Am J Nurs 82:96, 1982

Nunez J, Pommier J: Formation of thyroid hormones. Vitam Horm 39:175, 1982

Oppenheimer JH: Thyroid hormone action at the nuclear level. Ann Intern Med 102:374, 1985

Refetoff S: Thyroid hormone therapy. Med Clin North Am 59:1147, 1975

Slingerland DW, Burrows BA: Long-term antithyroid treatment in hyperthyroidism. JAMA 242:2408, 1979

Sterling K: Thyroid hormone action at the cell level. N Engl J Med 300:117, 1979

Volpe R: The pathogenesis of Graves' disease: An overview. Clin Endocrinol Metab I:3, 1978

Wake MM, Brensinger JF: The nurse's role in hypothyroidism. Nurs Clin North Am 15:453, 1980

Parathyroid Drugs, Calcitonin, and Calcium

53

Calcium, the most abundant cation in the body, plays an important role in many vital physiologic processes, such as bone formation, blood coagulation, muscle contraction, nerve conduction, hormone secretion, and enzyme activity. The level of free calcium and phosphate in the blood is dependent on a complex series of interactions among several substances, most important of which are parathyroid hormone and vitamin D.

Regulation of Plasma Calcium

Parathyroid hormone is a polypeptide synthesized by the parathyroid glands, small oval bodies (usually four or five in number) embedded in the dorsal surface of the thyroid gland. Two types of epithelial cells comprise the bulk of the gland, the *chief (principal)* cells, which produce and secrete parathyroid hormone, and the *oxyphil* cells, whose precise function is uncertain. Parathyroid hormone (PTH) is released in response to hypocalcemia (low serum calcium) and is capable of regulating serum calcium by primarily affecting three target tissues:

1. Bone—PTH stimulates bone resorption by activating the bone-destroying osteoclasts. The demineralization of bone elevates serum calcium and phosphate levels.
2. Kidneys—PTH promotes renal tubular reabsorption of calcium and increases renal excretion of phosphate by blocking its reabsorption.
3. Gastrointestinal (GI) tract—PTH enhances calcium and phosphate absorption from the small intestine in the presence of adequate amounts of vitamin D.

Vitamin D is the term commonly applied to two biologically similar substances, ergocalciferol (D_2) and cholecalciferol (D_3). Its major actions on calcium metabolism are essentially identical to those of PTH, namely increased calcium resorption from bone and enhanced gastrointestinal (GI) absorption of calcium.

A third endogenous substance, calcitonin, can also influence calcium and phosphate metabolism. Calcitonin (thyrocalcitonin) is a polypeptide hormone secreted by the parafollicular cells of the *thyroid* gland in response to hypercalcemia (elevated blood calcium). Calcitonin lowers serum calcium primarily by inhibiting the rate of calcium release from bone. In addition, calcitonin appears to accelerate bone formation and mineral deposition. Calcitonin may also inhibit the renal calcium reabsorptive action of parathyroid hormone.

In addition to the parafollicular cells of the thyroid, calcitonin-secreting cells have been found in the parathyroid and thymus glands. Because calcitonin is not the principal calcium-regulating hormone, there are no clinical syndromes associated with abnormal rates of calcitonin secretion.

Serum levels of calcium are normally maintained within a narrow range (10 ± 1 mg/100 ml), and deviation from this level results in the appearance of symptoms of either hypercalcemia or hypocalcemia. Hypercalcemia may result from hyperparathyroidism, excessive vitamin D intake, malignant tumors, or hyperthyroidism. It is characterized by vomiting, constipation, muscle weakness, electrocardiographic abnormalities, and deposition of calcium in soft tissues such as the kidney. Significant elevations in serum calcium can lead to progressive clouding of the sensorium and eventually coma.

Principal causes of hypocalcemia are hypoparathyroidism, inadequate vitamin D levels, and dietary calcium deficiency. Symptoms include muscle twitching, tetanic spasms, and convulsions. In addition, sedation and coma can occur.

Drugs discussed in this chapter are used to regulate body calcium stores, to provide replacement for inadequate calcium, and to treat Paget's disease, a decalcification of bone leading to skeletal deformities, joint impairment, and development of vascular fibrous tissue in marrow spaces (see Disease Brief).

Although once used clinically, bovine extracts of parathyroid hormone are no longer available, because tolerance usually developed quickly and allergic reactions were noted in a number of patients. Synthetic calcitonin and a nonhormonal substance, etidronate, two drugs used in moderate to severe forms of Paget's disease, are reviewed individually below. Mention is also made of plicamycin, an antibiotic used to treat hypercalcemia and hypercalciuria in patients not responsive to conventional treatment. Plicamycin is also used to treat testicular tumors, and that aspect of its pharmacology is reviewed in Chapter 75. Oral calcium salts, employed as dietary supplements for calcium-deficiency states, are also considered in this chapter.

Calcitonin

Calcitonin, Salmon
(Calcimar, Miacalcin)

Calcitonin, Human
(Cibacalcin)

The calcitonin products available for clinical use are synthetic compounds that resemble the poly-

DISEASE BRIEF

■ Hypoparathyroidism

Hypoparathyroidism is not common. When it occurs, usually following accidental removal of or damage to the parathyroid glands during thyroidectomy, signs of hypocalcemia ensue. Among these are neuromuscular hyperexcitability related in severity to the degree of hypocalcemia, tetany, and mental disturbance. Respiratory difficulties mimicking asthma may occur. Treatment may include calcium supplements, vitamin D, and high-calcium diet.

peptide hormones of salmon calcitonin and human calcitonin.

The salmon calcitonin, while essentially similar in action to mammalian calcitonin, is considerably more potent in humans than is human calcitonin, and it is also longer acting, perhaps because it is cleared from the circulatory system more slowly. However, circulating antibodies can form to salmon calcitonin and its efficacy may decline with continued use. The risk of reduced effectiveness due to antibody formation appears to be less with synthetic human calcitonin, and this product may be effective in patients who have developed resistance to nonhuman calcitonin.

MECHANISM AND ACTIONS

Calcitonin lowers serum calcium and phosphate by acting primarily on bone and kidney function. The drug inhibits osteoclastic bone resorption, although this inhibitory effect decreases over time, perhaps due to accumulation of neutralizing antibodies. Bone formation is largely unaffected initially, but is reduced with prolonged administration. The rate of bone turnover is slowed, with a corresponding fall in serum alkaline phosphatase and urinary hydroxyproline. The renal excretion of calcium and phosphorus is increased, due to impaired renal absorption. There is a transient decrease in the volume and acidity of gastric juice and pancreatic secretions.

USES

1. Treatment of moderate to severe Paget's disease (osteitis deformans), characterized by polyostotic involvement, and elevated serum alkaline phosphatase and urinary hydroxyproline excretion
2. Treatment of hypercalcemia, especially hypercalcemic emergencies (salmon calcitonin)
3. Adjunctive treatment of postmenopausal osteoporosis, in conjunction with adequate in-

take of calcium and vitamin D (salmon calcitonin)

ADMINISTRATION AND DOSAGE

Salmon Calcitonin

Salmon calcitonin is available for injection as a solution containing 100 U/ml or 200 U/ml. The drug may be given subcutaneously (SC) or intramuscularly (IM). The following doses are recommended:

Paget's disease: Initially, 100 U/day, preferably SC. Effects are assessed by evaluation of clinical symptoms and measurement of serum alkaline phosphatase. Biochemical abnormalities and bone pain should improve within several months; neurologic lesions may respond more slowly. Maintenance dosage is 50 U to 100 U every day or every other day to maintain improvement.

Hypercalcemia: Initially, 4 U/kg every 12 hours SC or IM; may be increased to 8 U/kg every 12 hours after 1 day to 2 days, then to a maximum of 8 U/kg every 6 hours if response is still unsatisfactory. If injection volume exceeds 2 ml, *IM* injection is preferred and multiple sites should be utilized.

Postmenopausal osteoporosis: 100 U/day SC or IM in conjunction with supplemental calcium and an adequate vitamin D intake

Skin testing for allergy: 0.1 ml of a 10-U/ml dilution intracutaneously on the forearm; appearance of more than mild erythema or wheal indicates a positive allergic response.

Human Calcitonin

Human calcitonin is used as a powder for injection containing 0.5 mg/vial. In treating Paget's disease, the starting dose is 0.5 mg/day SC. Dosage is adjusted based on clinical response and serum alka-

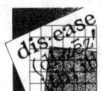 DISEASE BRIEF

■ *Pseudohypoparathyroidism*

Pseudohypoparathyroidism, also rare, is an inherited metabolic disorder resulting in increased production of parathyroid hormone, but lack of tissue response results in low serum calcium and high phosphorus levels. Children exhibit short stature, round facies, short fingers, tetanic seizures, and mental retardation.

line phosphatase. Some patients improve with 0.5 mg two to three times a week, while others may require 0.25 mg daily up to 0.5 mg twice daily. Treatment should be continued for 6 months and may be discontinued if symptoms have been relieved. Reconstituted solution should be used within 6 hours.

FATE
The calcium-lowering effect occurs within 2 hours after injection and persists for 6 hours to 8 hours. When given every 12 hours, the calcium-lowering effect lasts for up to 8 days. Calcitonin is rapidly converted to smaller fragments in the kidney, blood, and other organs, and these fragments are excreted in the urine.

SIDE-EFFECTS/ADVERSE REACTIONS
Nausea (with or without vomiting) is the most frequently reported side-effect with calcitonin administration. This reaction (twice as common with human versus salmon calcitonin) usually disappears with continued administration. Anorexia, diarrhea, salty taste, abdominal pain, and gastric discomfort may also occur and facial flushing and paresthesias have been noted. Inflammatory reactions at the injection site have developed with salmon calcitonin. Other adverse reactions that have occurred during calcitonin treatment are urticaria, skin rash, chills, dyspnea, metallic taste, dizziness, and diuresis. Hypocalcemic tetany is theoretically possible. Since calcitonin is a protein, systemic allergic reactions can occur and are more common with salmon calcitonin. In addition, antibodies may form to calcitonin with repeated use, reducing its efficacy. This latter effect is seen more frequently with salmon calcitonin as well.

CONTRAINDICATIONS AND PRECAUTIONS
Calcitonin is not recommended for use in pregnant or nursing mothers or in children unless a definite need exists. The drug should be given with *caution*

to persons with osteoporosis in the absence of adequate calcium and vitamin D supplementation, and in the presence of renal impairment or pernicious anemia.

INTERACTIONS
1. Calcitonin may antagonize the hypercalcemic action of PTH, dihydrotachysterol, and vitamin D.
2. The effects of calcitonin can be augmented by androgens.

■ *Nursing Process*

□ ASSESSMENT

□ *Subjective Data*
A history of the symptoms is useful in determining the rationale for drug use and will determine the type of diagnostic tests to be performed before the drug is administered. For example, the patient with Paget's disease may complain of frequent headaches, changes in gait, and deep bone pain. A history of renal dysfunction or pernicious anemia, asthma, or multiple allergies warrants cautious use.

A drug history should be obtained and any potential adverse interactions noted. The patient will also be asked to give a 24-hour diet recall to determine if calcium and vitamin D intake is adequate or excessive. Modifications may be necessary to ensure drug absorption but prevent further hypercalcemia.

Treatment with calcitonin is long term and requires commitment on the part of the patient and his support system to administer injections regularly and seek follow-up care. The nurse must explore with the patient and his family their willingness and ability to learn self-injection techniques and their perceptions of the long-term nature of the illness. The patient who is highly motivated and has support is more likely to be compliant.

DISEASE BRIEF

■ Hyperparathyroidism

Primary hyperparathyroidism may result from adenoma, carcinoma, or primary hyperplasia of the parathyroid glands. It may also be associated with ectopic production of PTH by carcinomas elsewhere in the body.

Signs and symptoms characteristic of hyperparathyroidism include hypercalcemia, anorexia, thirst, polyuria, and renal calculi (kidney stones). Skeletal manifestations may range from simple joint or back pain to pathologic fractures and cystic bone lesions throughout the skeleton (osteitis fibrosa cystica). The skeletal abnormalities result from the excessive demineralization of bone, while the occurrence of kidney stones is related to excessive renal excretion of minerals (calcium and phosphate). Treatment may include calcitonin or plicamycin; furosemide may also be effective.

□ Objective Data

If a patient suffers from multiple food or drug allergies or has a history of asthma, a skin test is performed prior to drug administration. A 0.1-ml (1 MRC unit) of calcitonin diluted to a solution of 10 MRC/ml is given by intracutaneous injection. Presence of more than mild erythema or slight wheal formation within 15 minutes of injection is a positive sign of hypersensitivity. In such cases, human calcitonin may be tested and given since it is associated with a reduced incidence of hypersensitivity.

Other laboratory data collected will include serum calcium, serum phosphorus, and alkaline phosphatase; elevations in these are indications for the drug. A 24-hour urine for hydroxyproline will be obtained if Paget's disease is suspected. Such diagnosis will be further confirmed by bone scans and other bone x-ray studies.

□ NURSING DIAGNOSIS

Actual nursing diagnoses may include
Knowledge deficit related to drug action and administration, symptoms of antibody resistance, and side-effects
Anxiety related to multiple injections
Potential nursing diagnoses are based on the three major side-effects hypersensitivity, hypocalcemia from excessive dosage, or hypercalcemia from the development of antibody resistance to the drug. Nursing diagnoses may include
Alteration in respiratory function related to dyspnea from hypersensitivity reaction
Hyperthermia from hypersensitivity
Alteration in cardiac output: decreased related to tachycardia from hypersensitivity

Alteration in mobility related to tetanic spasms from hypocalcemia
Alteration in thought processes related to sedation, seizures, or coma from hypocalcemia
Alteration in comfort: nausea and vomiting from hypercalcemia
Alteration in bowel elimination: constipation related to hypercalcemia
Alteration in cardiac output: decreased, bradycardia related to hypercalcemia
Alteration in thought processes: confusion, lethargy related to central nervous system effects of hypercalcemia

□ PLAN

Nursing care goals focus on
1. Correct and safe drug administration
2. Careful monitoring of drug effectiveness and emergence of side-effects such as hypersensitivity, hypocalcemia, or antibody resistance emerging as hypercalcemia
3. Teaching the patient and family how to administer the drug correctly and the side-effects to monitor and report

□ INTERVENTION

Initial therapy with calcitonin will be closely observed. Symptoms of hypersensitivity may occur quickly or be delayed in spite of a negative reaction to the drug on testing. Symptoms may include urticaria, rash, difficulty breathing, itching, fever, or tachycardia and may vary in degree of intensity. Mild symptoms may be treated with antipyretics and antihistamines and a switch to human calcitonin will be made. Severe symptoms require

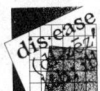

DISEASE BRIEF

■ Paget's Disease

Paget's disease (osteitis deformans) is a bone disorder characterized by excessive osteoclastic bone resorption and successive repair. However, the repair occurs in an unorganized manner, and bone deformities are created. The early stages are usually asymptomatic and deep bone pain is frequently the initial sign. Bones become softened, frequently the skull is involved, and headaches are common. The gait may be unsteady, kyphosis is noted, neurologic function may be impaired, and frequent fractures often occur on slight trauma. Serum alkaline phosphatase is elevated, as is urinary hydroxyproline; however, serum calcium and phosphate are usually within normal limits. Radiologic findings and bone scans are helpful in diagnosis. Treatment is directed toward reducing bone pain and slowing or preventing progressive deformity. Drugs that reduce bone resorption may be useful in treating Paget's disease, and include calcitonin and etidronate. Plicamycin may also be used for more resistant forms. Preparations with vitamin D-like activity (calcifediol, calcitriol, dihydrotachysterol) can be used to control hypocalcemic states resulting from a number of conditions, and these agents are discussed with the other fat-soluble vitamins in Chapter 77.

emergency measures including equipment to maintain respiration such as airways, mechanical ventilation and oxygen, cardiac monitoring, and emergency drugs such as lidocaine, corticosteroids, and epinephrine. In severe reactions the drug must be discontinued.

Effective drug therapy will result in gradual cessation of symptoms. The patient with Paget's disease will experience a reduction in bone pain; the patient with hypercalcemia will experience increasing muscle strength, clearing of senses, and improved GI function; and the patient with postmenopausal osteoporosis will show a slowing of bone degeneration on bone scan. However, throughout treatment serum calcium and alkaline phosphatase levels and 24-hour urine hydroxyproline levels must be monitored to ensure that the patient does not develop hypocalcemia, which results when the drug reduces serum calcium below normal levels. Symptoms of hypocalcemia that the nurse must observe for during initial treatment and teach the patient and family to observe for throughout therapy include muscle twitching; numbness, tingling, and tetanic spasms of the hands, wrists, ankles, and feet (also called *carpopedal spasm*); and facial muscle twitching when the facial nerve is tapped in front of the ear (Chvostek's sign). If untreated, hypocalcemia will lead to sedation, seizures, and coma. In infants and small children, early symptoms may include abdominal distention and hypotonia, which will progress to laryngeal stridor and tetany. A parenteral form of calcium, as prescribed by the physician, should be on hand for emergencies.

Sometimes a patient will initially have a positive response to calcitonin but will experience a return of the symptoms of hypercalcemia over time. If this happens the formation of antibodies against the drug must be suspected since it is a protein substance foreign to the body. To test antibody presence the patient is asked to fast overnight. In the morning, a serum calcium level is drawn and a dose of 100 MRC units of calcitonin is administered. Blood samples are drawn 3 hours and 6 hours after injection. A *decrease* in serum calcium of 0.3 mg/100 ml or *less* suggests antibody presence and the drug should be discontinued because it is ineffective.

Patients should also be aware of the early symptoms of returning hypercalcemia, which may include anorexia, nausea, vomiting, constipation, lethargy, and confusion, and report them immediately. Cardiovascular changes may also occur, resulting in bradycardia. Symptoms of hypercalcemia, hypocalcemia, and hypersensitivity should be listed for the patient on an easy-to-read card along with instructions on what to do if problems occur.

Chapter 8 contains an extensive discussion of self-injection techniques for the patient or family member who will give the medication. A home nursing consultation may be helpful to facilitate learning and help overcome fears about managing the procedure. Calcitonin may be given SC or IM but must be given by the latter route if the dose volume is greater than 2 ml. Initially, one route of administration should be taught to minimize confusion.

□ **EVALUATION**
Outcome criteria that may demonstrate drug effectiveness include a decrease in serum calcium and alkaline phosphatase levels, decrease in urinary hydroxyproline excretion, a reduction in bone pain and neurologic problems, appropriate return demonstration of injection technique, timely reporting of changes in symptoms, and return for clinical follow-up as required.

Etidronate
(Didronel)

MECHANISM AND ACTIONS
Etidronate is a nonhormonal substance that reduces the rate of bone turnover. It adsorbs onto the surfaces of hydroxyapatite crystals, disrupting the formation, growth, and dissolution of these crystals. Inhibition of crystal resorption occurs at lower doses than those required to retard crystal growth. Accelerated bone turnover in Paget's disease is slowed, and bone pain and the incidence of fractures are often reduced. The elevated cardiac output associated with Paget's disease and the increased vascularity of pagetic bone may also be reduced. Etidronate can prevent or retard heterotopic ossification of bone following total hip replacement or that resulting from spinal cord injury. The drug does not appear to affect *mature* heterotopic bone. Fracture healing or spinal stabilization following spinal cord injury is not impaired.

Etidronate does not adversely affect serum levels of parathyroid hormone or calcium, but decreases serum alkaline phosphatase levels and urinary hydroxyproline excretion. Increased tubular reabsorption of phosphate by the kidney can occur, possibly resulting in hyperphosphatemia, which is readily reversible on termination of therapy. Advantages of etidronate over calcitonin are its lack of antigenicity, lower cost, and oral effectiveness.

USES
1. Treatment of moderate to severe Paget's disease (osteitis deformans); symptomatic improvement occurs in approximately three out of five patients.
2. Reduction of heterotopic bone ossification due to spinal cord injury or that complicating total hip replacement
3. Treatment of hypercalcemia of malignancy, by

IV infusion, usually following rehydration and use of high-ceiling diuretics to restore urine output

ADMINISTRATION AND DOSAGE
Etidronate is administered orally as 200-mg or 400-mg tablets or as an injection solution (300 mg/6 ml), which is diluted for IV infusion. It is generally given orally as a single daily dose 2 hours before a meal; however, if gastric discomfort occurs, the dose may be divided.

Recommended doses for the approved oral indications of etidronate are
  Paget's disease: Initially 5 to 10 mg/kg/day for up to 6 months or 11 mg to 20 mg/kg/day for up to 3 months (maximum dose 20 mg/kg/day); retreatment at the same doses may be initiated after at least a 3-month drug-free period if reactivation of the disease has occurred.
  Heterotopic ossification due to spinal cord injury: 20 mg/day for 2 weeks, followed by 10 mg/kg/day for 10 weeks, instituted as soon as possible following the injury
  Heterotopic ossification complicating total hip replacement: 20 mg/kg/day for 1 month preoperatively; then 20 mg/kg/day for 3 months postoperatively
  For IV infusion in treating hypercalcemia of malignancy: The recommended dose is 7.5 mg/kg/day for 3 successive days, given over at least 2 hours. The daily dose must be diluted in *at least* 250 ml of sterile normal saline. Retreatment may be undertaken if appropriate after at least a 7-day rest interval. Oral tablets may be started on the day after the last infusion in a dose of 20 mg/kg/day for up to 30 days.

FATE
Only a small fraction of the oral dose is absorbed (1% at 5 mg/kg to 6% at 20 mg/kg). Absorption is usually complete within 2 hours, but may be retarded by the presence of food or substances containing divalent cations (e.g., Ca^{2+}, Mg^{2+}, Fe^{2+}). Most of the absorbed drug is cleared from the blood within 6 hours. Etidronate is not metabolized and one half of the absorbed dose is excreted in the urine within 24 hours. The remainder is absorbed onto bone and slowly eliminated. The half-life of etidronate on bone is 3 to 6 months. Unabsorbed drug is excreted intact into the feces. A large fraction of the infused dose is eliminated unchanged in the urine. Plasma half-life is 5 to 7 hours. The fraction of drug taken up by bone is slowly eliminated

from the body over several months through bone turnover.

SIDE-EFFECTS/ADVERSE REACTIONS

The most frequently encountered side-effects during oral etidronate therapy are loose stools and nausea, especially with elevated doses. Increased bone pain or pain at previously asymptomatic sites has occurred during treatment of Paget's disease with etidronate. Pain may decrease with continued therapy in some patients, but may persist in others. Osteomalacia has also been reported. Mineralization of osteoid laid down during bone accretion may be suppressed by etidronate and fracture healing may be retarded. Elevated BUN or serum creatinine have occurred with IV infusion of etidronate, and reports of a metallic taste or altered taste sensation have also been received.

CONTRAINDICATIONS AND PRECAUTIONS

Etidronate is contraindicated in patients with class Dc or higher renal functional impairment (serum creatinine greater than 5 mg/dl). *Cautious* use is warranted in patients with less severe renal impairment, enterocolitis, long bone fractures (see above), and in pregnant or nursing women and in children. Adequate intake of calcium and vitamin D should be maintained during etidronate therapy. If a fracture occurs during treatment, the drug should be discontinued until the fracture has healed.

NURSING CONSIDERATIONS

Nursing care goals should focus on helping the patient learn how to take the drug to maximize effectiveness and minimize side-effects and how to incorporate adequate calcium and vitamin D in the patient's diet.

Etidronate should be taken on an empty stomach with water or juice to maximize drug absorption. However, many people cannot follow this guideline realistically since rapid absorption may increase GI distress and diarrhea. The patient who has problems can be encouraged to split the dose and take it twice a day instead of once or take it with a meal without calcium-containing foods. If problems continue to persist the dose may need to be reduced.

The nurse needs to teach the patient to include adequate sources of calcium and vitamin D in the daily diet. Milk, yogurt, and hard cheese are ideal sources of calcium but may be poorly tolerated by some people who are lactose intolerant. Other sources include shellfish, oily fish, rhubarb, nuts, beans, broccoli, greens, and some bottled mineral waters. Vitamin D is added to milk but is rarely found in quantity in any other foods. Encourage the patient to get at least 30 minutes of exposure to sunshine daily and to take a supplement as necessary.

The patient with Paget's disease should be warned that there can be an increase in bone pain in existing pathologic sites, and appearance of pain in new sites as well.

Outcome criteria that may indicate drug effectiveness include a decrease in serum alkaline phosphatase, a decrease in urinary hydroxyproline levels, a decrease in bone pain and fractures, and evidence of inclusion of foods rich in calcium in the diet.

Plicamycin
(Mithracin)

Plicamycin (also known as mithramycin) is an antibiotic produced by *Streptomyces plicatus*. It is administered by intravenous infusion to treat hypercalcemia and hypercalciuria in patients not responsive to conventional therapy, such as those with advanced neoplasms. Due to its potential to elicit serious toxicity (thrombocytopenia, hemorrhage, liver or kidney dysfunction), however, the potential benefit from the drug must be carefully weighed against the risk. Plicamycin is contraindicated in patients with thrombocytopenia, coagulation disorders, increased susceptibility to bleeding, and bone marrow depression. Platelet counts, prothrombin time, and bleeding time must be determined frequently during therapy and for several days following the last dose. Epistaxis or hematemesis may be an early indication of a developing hemorrhagic syndrome and should be reported immediately. GI symptoms (nausea, diarrhea, anorexia, stomatitis) represent the most frequent side-effects. The recommended dose is 25 mcg/kg/day by IV infusion over 4 hours to 6 hours for 3 or 4 days. If the desired degree of reversal of hypercalcemia is not attained, the dosage may be repeated at intervals of one week or longer. Normal calcium balance can often be maintained with single weekly doses or two to three doses per week. Rapid IV injections should be avoided, because the incidence of GI disturbances is much greater with this method. Extravasation of the solution should be avoided, because local irritation, cellulitis, and possibly thrombophlebitis can occur. Moderate heat applied to the site of extravasation may help disperse the compound and minimize discomfort.

Plicamycin is also employed in the treatment of testicular neoplasms, and that application is considered in detail in Chapter 75.

Oral Calcium Salts

Calcium Carbonate, Calcium Glubionate, Calcium Gluconate, Calcium Lactate, Dibasic Calcium Phosphate, Tricalcium Phosphate

Adequate intake of calcium is essential for normal homeostasis, and is particularly critical during periods of active bone growth, for example, during childhood, adolescence, pregnancy, or lactation. In addition, sufficient calcium intake is necessary for the prevention and treatment of disease-induced calcium-deficiency states such as hypoparathyroidism, postmenopausal osteoporosis, and tetany of the newborn. The use of oral calcium supplements, particularly as they apply to the adjunctive treatment of calcium-deficiency states resulting from hypoparathyroidism, is discussed here. Parenteral therapy with calcium, on the other hand, is indicated for treatment of hypocalcemic states requiring a prompt elevation in plasma calcium, for example, neonatal tetany, severe vitamin D deficiency, systemic alkalosis, and cardiac resuscitation following open-heart surgery. Parenteral calcium therapy is reviewed along with other parenteral electrolytes in Chapter 79. The pharmacology of the oral calcium preparations is detailed for the group, and individual drugs are listed in Table 53-1.

MECHANISM AND ACTIONS
Oral calcium salts provide replacement for deficient calcium stores in the body. The presence of sufficient calcium is essential for bone development, blood coagulation, muscle contraction, cardiac functioning, and many other physiologic processes.

USES
1. Prevention or treatment of calcium-deficiency states, such as those associated with hypoparathyroidism, osteoporosis, rickets, and osteomalacia
2. Dietary supplement where calcium intake is inadequate, such as in childhood, pregnancy, lactation, and postmenopause

ADMINISTRATION AND DOSAGE
See Table 53-1.

FATE
Absorption is good when taken orally in the presence of adequate levels of vitamin D and PTH. The metabolism of calcium is likewise controlled by vitamin D and PTH and the ion is excreted largely in urine.

SIDE-EFFECTS/ADVERSE REACTIONS
Side-effects are rare with normal doses; occasional GI distress is noted. Excessive amounts can lead to hypercalcemia, symptoms of which include nausea, anorexia, vomiting, abdominal pain, constipation, dry mouth, polyuria, fatigue, bradycardia, and arrhythmias.

CONTRAINDICATIONS AND PRECAUTIONS
Supplemental calcium is contraindicated in persons with hypercalcemia or renal calculi. Oral calcium should be administered *cautiously* to patients with a history of renal stones or cardiac arrhythmias, to patients receiving digitalis glycosides and to persons with renal insufficiency.

INTERACTIONS
1. The GI absorption of calcium is enhanced by vitamin D and may be impaired by corticosteroids, phosphorus (*e.g.*, milk, dairy products), oxalic acid (*e.g.*, spinach, rhubarb), and phytic acid (*e.g.*, bran cereals).
2. Calcium may reduce the muscle-relaxing effects of neuromuscular-blocking agents.
3. Elevated serum calcium levels may increase digitalis toxicity.
4. Oral calcium products can retard the oral absorption of tetracyclines.
5. Calcium may antagonize the action of calcium channel blocking drugs (see Chap. 36).

■ Nursing Process

Recent media emphasis on the ability of calcium to reduce the risk of osteoporosis has resulted in a tremendous increase in the sale of calcium supplements, including those found in antacids. However, there are serious questions about the ability of this drug to avert osteoporosis, especially in postmenopausal women whose estrogen levels are diminished. Consequently, the nurse needs to counsel the patient who will take calcium supplements to ensure maximum benefit.

Table 53-1
Oral Calcium Salts

Drug	Preparations	Usual Dosage Range	Clinical Considerations
calcium carbonate (BioCal, Caltrate, Os-Cal 500, and various other manufacturers)	Tablets—650 mg, 667 mg, 750 mg, 1.25 g, 1.5 g Chewable tablets—350 mg, 420 mg, 500 mg, 625 mg, 750 mg, 850 mg, 1.25 g, 1.5 g Capsules—1.5 g Oral suspension—1.25 g/5 ml	1 g–1.5 g 3 times/day (maximum 8 g/day)	Contains 40% calcium; very potent antacid (see Chap. 42); high incidence of constipation; tablet may be chewed before swallowing or dissolved in mouth and followed by water.
calcium glubionate (Neo-Calglucon)	Syrup—1.8 g/5 ml	Adults—15 ml 3 times/day Pregnancy—15 ml 4 times/day Children—10 ml 3 times/day Infants—5 ml 3 times/day	Contains 6.5% calcium; GI disturbances are rare; administer before meals to enhance absorption.
calcium gluconate	Tablets—500 mg, 650 mg, 975 mg, 1 g Injection—10%	1 g–2 g orally 3 to 4 times/day Children—500 mg/kg/day in divided doses	Contains 9% calcium; can be given IV (see Chap. 79); GI irritation is minimal, but may be constipating.
calcium lactate	Tablets—325 mg, 650 mg	325 mg–1.3 g 3 times/day	Contains 13% calcium; tablets may be dissolved in hot water, then cool water added to taste; absorption may be enhanced by lactose; administer with meals.
dibasic calcium phosphate dihydrate (dicalcium phosphate)	Tablets—486 mg	1–3 tablets 2 to 3 times/day	Contains 23% calcium; administer with meals.
tricalcium phosphate (Posture)	Tablets—300 mg, 600 mg	1–2 tablets 2 to 4 times/day	Contains 39% calcium

□ *ASSESSMENT*

□ *Subjective Data*

A drug history is important to determine if the patient is taking corticosteroids, which may impair calcium absorption. Supplements must be given with caution to patients on digitalis drugs since digitalis toxicity may occur as calcium levels increase.

A diet history is also essential. If the patient consumes excessive amounts of foods high in phosphorus, oxalic acid, or phytic acid (see Interactions, above), calcium absorption may be impaired. The patient's calcium intake must also be determined. A diet that provides adequate calcium intake in foods, which is usually readily absorbed by the body, may require little or no supplementation. Overabundant intake of calcium may actually impair absorption. A patient who is fearful of osteoporosis may have a familial predisposition to the disease. Osteoporosis tends to run in families and may be related to a genetic inability to absorb adequate calcium. Smoking and coffee or alcohol ingestion all increase the risk. Other risk factors include small bone structure, lack of exercise, early menarche or early menopause, and long-term steroid or anticonvulsant therapy.

□ *Objective Data*

Musculoskeletal assessment of bone formation and muscle strength is important to rule out potential hypercalcemia. Laboratory evaluation of serum calcium and phosphorus levels will help confirm diagnosis.

A bone scan may be ordered on a woman considered at high risk for osteoporosis but is not necessary for most patients receiving calcium supplements.

☐ *NURSING DIAGNOSES*

Actual nursing diagnoses may include

Knowledge deficit related to the relationship between supplement effectiveness and diet, exercise, and sunshine, and drug administration and side-effects

Potential nursing diagnoses may include

Alteration in bowel function: constipation related to drug effect

Alteration in nutrition: less than body requirements for calcium and other minerals related to inappropriate supplementation

Alteration in patterns of urinary elimination related to calciuria

☐ *PLAN*

Nursing care goals focus on helping the patient

1. Develop a realistic view of the benefits of calcium therapy
2. Manage and prevent side-effects
3. Incorporate calcium in the diet

☐ *INTERVENTION*

Any patient receiving calcium supplement must understand that adequate absorption depends on many factors. The patient should eat vitamin D-fortified foods and get a minimum of 30 minutes of sunshine per day. If necessary, a vitamin D supplement can be taken. This is especially important for the elderly patient who naturally produces 30% to 50% less vitamin D than the adolescent. Reduction or elimination of caffeine-containing beverages, alcohol, and tobacco is beneficial since these interfere with calcium absorption. Weight-bearing exercise is also a boost to calcium utilization and should be suggested. Walking is extremely helpful and available to almost everyone.

Side-effects with calcium supplements are usually minimal. Some patients suffer from constipation or gastrointestinal distress usually from calcium carbonate. If this occurs the patient can switch to the lactate or gluconate form. The disadvantage of these formulations is that the patient may have to increase the number of pills taken to achieve the same dose. Constipation can be relieved by increasing fluids and bulk-containing foods and occasional use of a mild laxative.

Calciuria occurs infrequently but may develop in a predisposed patient. Any individual with a family history of kidney stones should consult with his physician before beginning a supplement. Increases in fluid intake will decrease the risk of calciuria.

Calcium supplements may interfere with the absorption of zinc, copper, magnesium, and iron as well as of calcium itself. In addition, foods containing oxalic acid, phosphorus, or phytic acid (see Interactions, above) may interfere with calcium absorption. To minimize this problem, encourage the patient to take several smaller doses throughout the day, preferably 1 hour before or 2 hours after meals.

The patient should also learn to include calcium-rich foods in the diet since these are well absorbed. Foods rich in calcium include milk, yogurt, cheese, shellfish, oily fish such as salmon and sardines, rhubarb, nuts, beans, broccoli, greens, and some bottled mineral waters.

☐ *EVALUATION*

Outcome criteria that may measure drug effectiveness include improved serum calcium levels, a decrease in or elimination of deficiency symptoms, incorporation of calcium into the daily diet, inclusion of exercise in a daily routine, and ability to avoid or manage common side-effects.

CASE STUDY

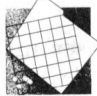

Ruth Francis, age 54, has been menopausal for 5 years. After reading several articles in lay magazines she decides to start taking a calcium supplement. She purchases calcium carbonate, 500-mg tablets, from the supermarket and begins taking one tablet twice a day at lunch and dinner.

During a routine history and physical examination about two weeks later, Mrs. Francis reports taking the supplement but complains about recent constipation and upset stomach and wonders if the calcium is to blame. When asked why she started taking the supplement she replies "Because my mother was told she has brittle bones and I don't want the same thing to happen to me."

Discussion Questions

1. What information is needed to determine if Mrs. Francis is at risk for osteoporosis?
2. How might Mrs. Francis' menopausal state affect calcium absorption?
3. What guidelines can the nurse provide Mrs. Francis to improve her absorption of calcium?
4. How can the gastrointestinal problems caused by the calcium carbonate be handled?

REVIEW QUESTIONS

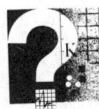

1. List the major actions of the parathyroid hormone.
2. What are the principal causes of (1) hypercalcemia and (2) hypocalcemia?
3. What is Paget's disease? Describe the symptoms.
4. Why might salmon calcitonin be preferred over human calcitonin? What advantages might human calcitonin have over salmon calcitonin?
5. Give the principal effects of calcitonin on the body.
6. Describe 2 methods to test hypersensitivity to calcitonin.
7. What outcome criteria can be used to measure the effectiveness of a drug treatment plan with calcitonin?
8. Briefly describe the mechanism of action of etidronate.
9. What are the approved indications for etidronate?
10. In what conditions should etidronate be used with caution?
11. What information should a patient be given to enable him to derive full benefit from etidronate therapy?
12. Give the indications for plicamycin.
13. Which salts of calcium are employed as oral supplements?
14. What substances can interfere with the oral absorption of calcium?
15. How can the nurse help a patient learn to use calcium supplements safely and effectively?

BIBLIOGRAPHY

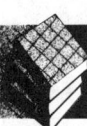

Anghileri LJ, Tuffer-Anghileri AM (eds): The Role of Calcium in Biological Systems. Boca Raton, Fla, CRC Press, 1982

Austin LA, Heath H: Calcitonin: Physiology and pathophysiology. N Engl J Med 304:269, 1981

Broadus AE, Rasmussen H: Clinical evaluation of parathyroid function. Am J Med 70:475, 1981

Deftos LJ, First BP: Calcitonin as a drug. Ann Intern Med 95:192, 1981

Elliott GI, KcKenzie MW: Treatment of hypercalcemia. Drug Intell Clin Pharm 17(1):12, 1981

Krane SM: Etidronate disodium in the treatment of Paget's disease of bone. Ann Intern Med 96(5):619, 1982

Neimark J: Beyond calcium: Why milk is just a start. American Health 5(8):53, 1986

Rosen JF, Chesney RW: Circulating calcitriol concentrations in health and disease. J Pediatr 103:1, 1983

Stewart AF: Therapy of malignancy-associated hypercalcemia. Am J Med 74:475, 1983

Synthetic calcitonin for postmenopausal osteoporosis. Med Lett Drugs Ther 27:53, June, 1985

VanDop C, Bourne HR: Pseudohypoparathyroidism. Ann Rev Med 34:259, 1983

Antidiabetic and Hyperglycemic Agents

54

Alterations in blood glucose levels can occur in a variety of diseases as well as in response to use of a number of different drugs. Increased blood glucose, or *hyperglycemia*, is primarily the result of diabetes mellitus, a chronic metabolic disorder characterized by a deficiency of *functional* insulin, a polypeptide secreted by the beta cells of the pancreas. Decreased blood glucose, or *hypoglycemia*, may result from several disease states, such as pancreatic carcinoma or liver dysfunction, or may occur as a consequence of overdosage with antidiabetic drugs used to control diabetes mellitus.

Because endogenous regulation of blood glucose levels is primarily a function of hormones secreted by the pancreas, a brief review of pancreatic function is presented prior to consideration of the drugs used to control blood glucose.

Pancreas

The pancreas is a flat organ consisting of a head, body, and tail located behind and slightly below the stomach (Fig. 54-1). The endocrine functions of the pancreas are performed by the islets of Langerhans, which are small, highly vascularized masses of cells scattered throughout the pancreas and representing only 1% to 3% of the entire organ.

The islets of Langerhans contain at least four types of secretory cells:

1. Alpha (A) cells, which secrete glucagon
2. Beta (B) cells, which secrete insulin
3. Delta (D) cells, which secrete somatostatin
4. *PP* (F) cells, which secrete pancreatic polypeptide

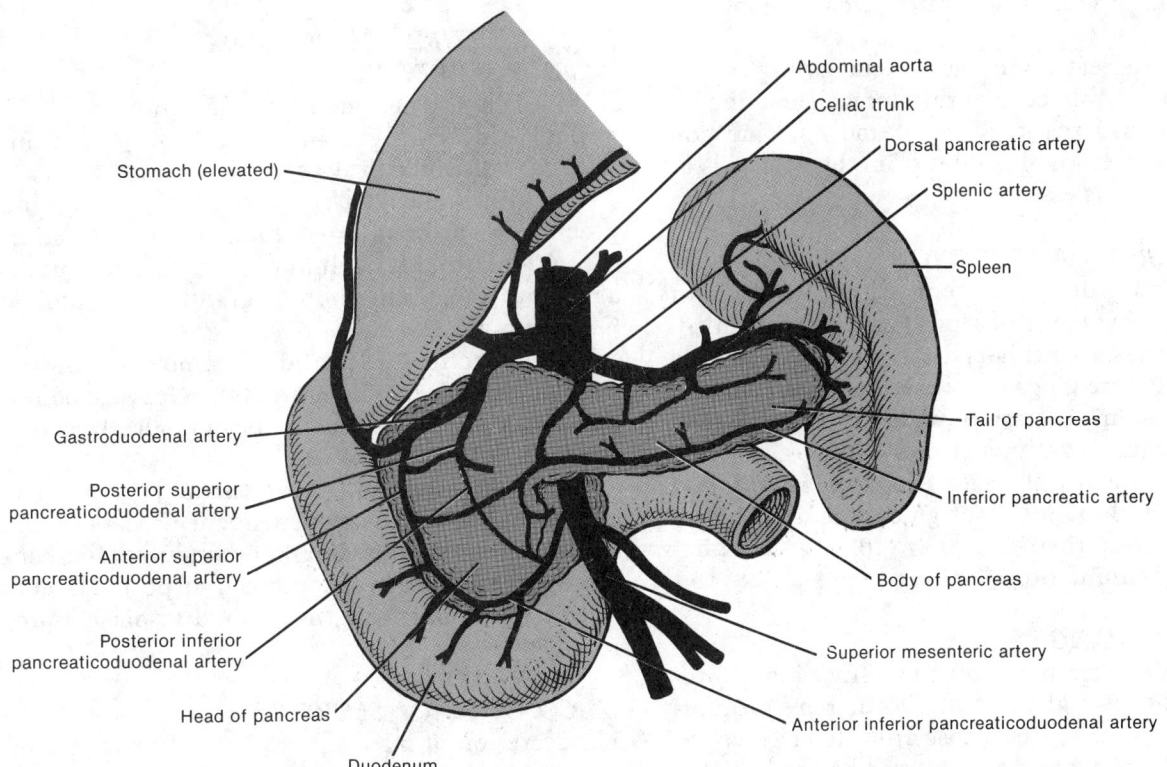

Figure 54-1. Location of the pancreas. (Tortora GJ, Anagnostakos NP: Principles of Anatomy and Physiology, 5th ed, p 425. New York, Harper & Row, 1987)

Insulin-secreting beta cells are the most numerous, making up 70% to 80% of the islet cell population. The A cells containing glucagon comprise approximately 20% of islet cell mass, whereas the somatostatin-containing D cells account for 3% to 5% of pancreatic islet cells. The F cells make up less than 2% of islet cells and contain a polypeptide that is believed to assist in digestion in a yet undetermined manner.

The physiologic roles of glucagon and insulin in the regulation of intermediary metabolism are well established; however, the exact physiologic role of pancreatic somatostatin remains unclear. Because somatostatin inhibits the release of both glucagon and insulin from the pancreatic islets, it may function, at least in part, as a *hormone-regulating* pancreatic secretion.

Glucagon

Glucagon is a 29 amino-acid polypeptide hormone secreted by the alpha cells of the pancreatic islets primarily in response to hypoglycemia. Glucagon is essentially a catabolic hormone that decreases carbohydrate and lipid energy stores and increases the amount of glucose and fatty acids available for oxidation.

Extrapancreatic glucagon ("gut glucagon") is secreted by certain cells of the stomach and duodenum. Both pancreatic glucagon and gut glucagon stimulate secretion of insulin from the beta cells of the pancreatic islets.

CONTROL OF SECRETION
The plasma glucose concentration is the major physiologic regulator of glucagon secretion. In addition to hypoglycemia and fasting, the following factors promote glucagon secretion: ingestion of a high-protein meal (amino acids), exercise, stress, gastrin, pancreozymin, and beta-adrenergic stimulation. The rate of glucagon secretion is inhibited by elevated blood levels of glucose and free fatty acids, by somatostatin, phenytoin, and alpha-adrenergic stimulation.

MAJOR ACTIONS
1. Carbohydrate metabolism—Glucagon stimulates hepatic glycogenolysis, thereby promoting the release of glucose from liver glycogen stores. This action is mediated by cyclic AMP, which stimulates protein kinase activity leading to the activation of phosphorylase, the glycogenolytic enzyme. In addition to stimulating

hepatic glycogenolysis, glucagon inhibits glycogenesis and increases the rate of hepatic gluconeogenesis. The net effect is an elevation of blood glucose (hyperglycemia).
2. Lipid metabolism—Glucagon stimulates lipolysis, thereby increasing the release of free fatty acids and glycerol from adipose tissue. Glucagon also promotes the uptake and oxidation of fatty acids by liver and muscle.
3. Protein metabolism—Glucagon exerts a catabolic action on proteins and inhibits the incorporation of amino acids into hepatic protein.
4. Cardiac effects—Large amounts of exogenous glucagon produce a positive inotropic effect on the heart by increasing myocardial levels of cyclic AMP. A direct chronotropic effect has also been reported. The net effect is an increased force of myocardial contraction and increased heart rate.

All the major actions of glucagon—hepatic glycogenolysis, lipolysis, stimulation of insulin release, and the inotropic effect on the heart—are mediated by cyclic AMP.

Insulin

STRUCTURE, BIOSYNTHESIS, AND SECRETION
Insulin is a polypeptide hormone composed of 51 amino acids arranged in two chains (A and B), linked by disulfide bridges.

Insulin is derived from a large, polypeptide precursor—proinsulin—which is synthesized in the endoplasmic reticulum of beta cells and packaged into membrane-bound granules within the Golgi complex.

A connecting (C) peptide is removed from the proinsulin molecule by proteolytic cleavage before the secretion of insulin in its biologically active form.

Insulin secretion occurs through exocytosis (emiocytosis), a calcium-dependent process that is enhanced by cyclic AMP and potassium. Upon entering the circulation, insulin is transported largely in free molecular form, not bound to plasma proteins.

CONTROL OF SECRETION
The secretion of insulin is controlled primarily by the blood glucose level, with an elevation of blood glucose (hyperglycemia) increasing both production and release of insulin. Ingested glucose effects a far greater secretion of insulin than an equivalent

amount of intravenously administered glucose because several gastrointestinal hormones, including gastrin, secretin, pancreozymin, and glucagon, stimulate insulin secretion.

Insulin secretion is also increased by mannose, fructose, certain amino acids, vagal stimulation (acetylcholine), cyclic AMP, potassium, and oral hypoglycemic drugs such as tolbutamide. Hyperglycemia, somatostatin, alpha-adrenergic stimulation, thiazide diuretics, phenytoin, and diazoxide inhibit insulin secretion.

MAJOR ACTIONS

1. Cellular membrane permeability—Insulin facilitates the transport of glucose across selected cell membranes, thereby accelerating the entry of glucose into muscle, adipose tissue, fibroblasts, leukocytes, mammary glands, and the anterior pituitary. The transport of glucose into the liver, brain, renal tubules, intestinal mucosa, and erythrocytes is independent of insulin. Exercise and hypoxia mimic the effect of insulin on cellular permeability to glucose in skeletal muscle. The insulin requirements of diabetics engaging in strenuous exercise may be reduced substantially, and therefore must be monitored carefully to avoid hypoglycemia. Insulin also increases cellular permeability to amino acids, fatty acids, and potassium, particularly in muscle and adipose tissue.
2. Carbohydrate metabolism—Insulin effectively lowers the level of blood glucose by enhancing the transport and peripheral utilization of glucose. Insulin increases muscle and liver glycogen stores by activating enzymes involved in glycogenesis, while inhibiting those that produce glycogenolysis. Glycolytic enzymes are also activated by insulin, while several enzymes involved in gluconeogenesis are inhibited.
3. Protein metabolism—Insulin is strongly anabolic, increasing protein synthesis and inhibiting protein catabolism. Insulin increases the incorporation of amino acids into protein by accelerating the entry of amino acids into the cell and possibly by increasing RNA synthesis.
4. Lipid metabolism—Insulin stimulates forma-

tion of triglycerides (lipogenesis) and inhibits their breakdown (lipolysis). Insulin accelerates fatty acid and glycerol phosphate synthesis and enhances cellular permeability to fatty acids, leading to increased deposition of triglycerides in adipose tissue.

Somatostatin (Growth Hormone Release Inhibiting Hormone)

Somatostatin is a tetradecapeptide that has been isolated from the hypothalamus, the pancreas, and the upper gastrointestinal tract. Within the pancreatic islets, the somatostatin-secreting delta (D) cells are located between the glucagon-secreting alpha (A) cells and the central mass of insulin-secreting beta (B) cells. Such an arrangement could permit the product of the D cells—somatostatin—to directly influence the secretion of glucagon and insulin by the A and B cells, respectively.

ACTION

Although the precise role or roles of somatostatin remain unclear, several endocrine and nonendocrine activities have been attributed to this hormone. These biologic actions include the following:

Endocrine
Inhibition of secretion of:
  GH (growth hormone)
  TSH (thyroid-stimulating hormone)
  Glucagon
  Insulin
  Gastrin
  Secretin
  Renin
Nonendocrine
Inhibition of:
  Gastric acid secretion and gastric emptying
  Pancreatic bicarbonate and enzyme release
  Gallbladder contraction
  Xylose absorption
  Splanchnic blood flow
  Platelet aggregation
  Electrical activity of CNS neurons
  Acetylcholine release from peripheral nerves

Disorders of Glucose Metabolism

Hypoglycemia

Hypoglycemic states are characterized by the presence of an abnormally low blood glucose level. This represents a threat to the brain, which depends on glucose as its source of energy.

Normally, when the blood glucose falls below a critical level, insulin secretion is inhibited and release of glucagon, epinephrine, GH, and glucocorticoids is increased. Only the release of the catecholamine epinephrine leads to observable symptoms, such as sweating, palpitation, anxiety, and weakness.

Impairment of brain function, confusion, amnesia, bizarre behavior, or blurred vision may occur if the blood glucose falls below a level of 40 mg/100 ml. Severe hypoglycemia may ultimately lead to hypothermia, convulsions, and coma. Hypoglycemic disorders may be divided into two types: fasting (food-deprived) and postprandial (food-stimulated or reactive).

Possible causes of fasting hypoglycemia are listed below:

1. Hyperinsulinism—Insulinomas (insulin-secreting tumors of the pancreas), overdosage with exogenous insulin or sulfonylurea drugs (oral hypoglycemic agents)
2. Endocrine disorders—Addison's disease (adrenocortical insufficiency), hypopituitarism (e.g., Simmonds' disease), myxedema
3. Liver disease—Hepatic necrosis, malignancy, or advanced cirrhosis, which may lead to impairment of glycogenesis and gluconeogenesis, thereby reducing liver glycogen stores and hepatic output of glucose
4. Acute alcoholism
5. Extrapancreatic tumors

The possible causes of postprandial (reactive) hypoglycemia include early or alimentary hypoglycemia, which may follow gastric intestinal surgery or result from increased vagal tone, and late hypoglycemia (early or occult diabetes mellitus).

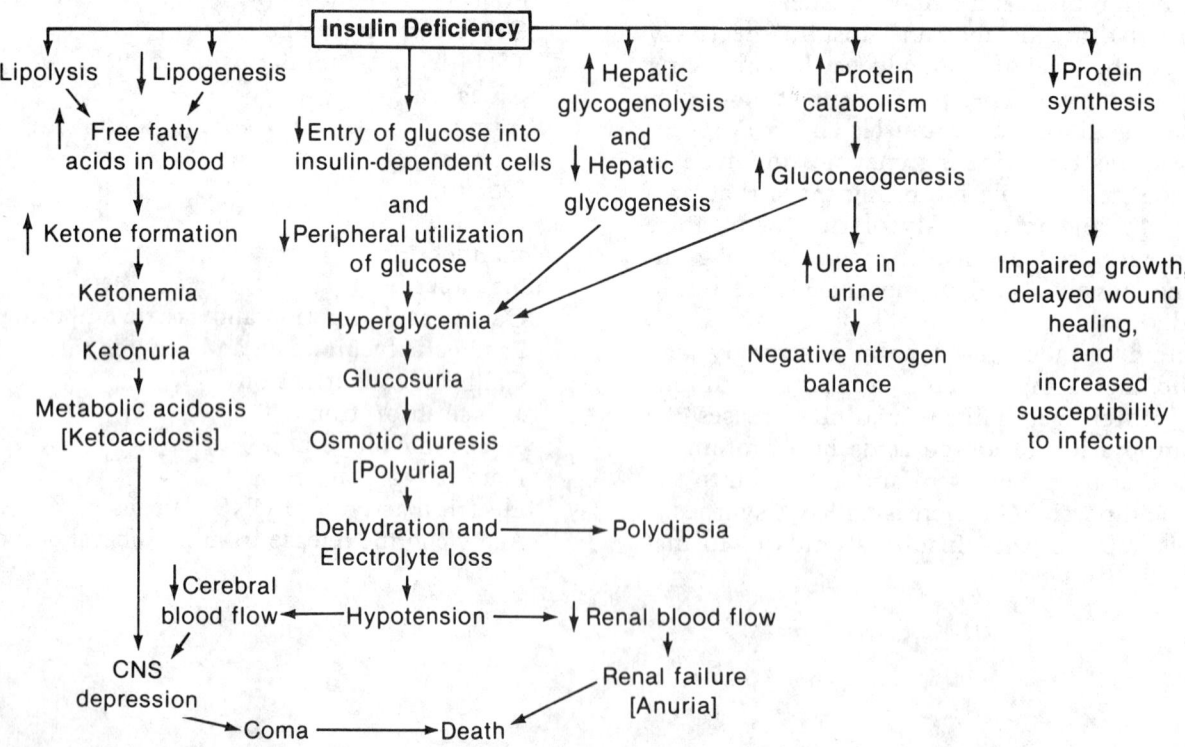

Figure 54-2. Metabolic consequences of severe insulin deficiency.

Diabetes Mellitus

Diabetes mellitus is a chronic disorder of metabolism characterized by carbohydrate intolerance and inappropriate hyperglycemia resulting from a deficiency of insulin secretion or a reduction in its biologic efficacy ("relative" insulin deficiency).

The insulin deficiency, be it absolute or relative, triggers a series of biochemical changes in the metabolism of carbohydrates, lipids, and proteins, as outlined in Figure 54-2. These metabolic abnormalities lead to the classic symptoms of diabetes mellitus—polyuria (frequent urination), polydipsia (excessive thirst), polyphagia (hunger), and fatigue.

Long-term, serious complications of diabetes mellitus include gangrene, visual impairment resulting from proliferative retinopathy, myocardial infarction, polyneuropathy, and uremia. Pathologic changes in the blood vessels, particularly in the microcirculation (microangiopathy), appear to underlie the majority of these complications.

Diabetes mellitus is a disorder of heterogenous etiology. Predisposition to diabetes is inherited, although the genetic factors are complex. There are two generally recognized types of diabetes mellitus: (1) insulin dependent (type I or juvenile onset) and (2) noninsulin dependent (type II or maturity onset). Major characteristics of each type of diabetes are presented in Table 54-1.

Insulin-Dependent (Type I) Diabetes

Insulin-dependent diabetes generally occurs in nonobese persons before the age of 30, most commonly in adolescence. Circulating insulin is virtually absent, and the beta pancreatic cells fail to respond to all normal stimuli for insulin secretion. The islet beta cell reserve is markedly reduced or totally absent, and ketosis usually develops in the course of the disease. Patients respond to exogenous insulin, which is required to reverse the hyperglycemia and the general catabolic state and to prevent ketosis.

Immunopathologic mechanisms have been strongly implicated in this type of diabetes. Specific histocompatibility (HLA) antigens have been linked to this disorder, and circulating antibodies to islet cells have been detected in some patients early in the course of the disease.

Viruses such as mumps, coxsackie B4 virus, and rubella have been associated epidemiologically with the onset of juvenile-onset diabetes. It is possible that an underlying genetic defect of the im-

Table 54-1
Types of Diabetes Mellitus and Major Characteristics

	Type I (Insulin dependent)	Type II (Noninsulin dependent)
Onset	Sudden, usually during adolescence	Gradual, usually after age 30–35
Major symptoms	Polydipsia, polyuria, polyphagia	Often none (patients frequently obese)
Stability of blood glucose levels	Very unstable; wide fluctuations are common	Fairly stable; fluctuations are minimal
Presence of ketones	Usually present	Rare
Presence of insulin	None	Usually present, occasionally *in excess*; but is ineffective
Effective treatment	Insulin is required; oral hypoglycemics are seldom used	Oral hypoglycemics are frequently effective alone; insulin may be necessary in some patients
Diet	Balanced diet is necessary but cannot control symptoms alone	Balanced diet and weight loss may be effective without drug therapy in some patients

mune system may predispose an individual to beta cell destruction following these viral infections.

Noninsulin-Dependent (Type II) Diabetes

Noninsulin-dependent diabetes usually has its onset after the age of 40, although it may occur at any age. Obesity is a major risk factor to the development of this disease, beta cell mass may be only moderately reduced, and autoimmunity is not demonstrable. There is no correlation with HLA antigens; however, there is a strong genetic component. Ketosis rarely occurs.

In at least some cases of noninsulin-dependent diabetes, a defect in insulin binding to cellular receptors is likely. Insulin apparently exerts a nega-

tive feedback control over its own receptors. In the presence of obesity, certain tissues (such as muscle and adipose tissue) display insensitivity to insulin. Perhaps the hyperinsulinism that results from chronic excessive caloric intake and sustained beta cell stimulation actually reduces the number of available insulin receptors and leads to glucose intolerance.

In addition to obesity and excessive carbohydrate intake, diabetes mellitus may be precipitated by pancreatitis, pregnancy, and endocrine disorders associated with overproduction of GH, glucocorticoids, or catecholamines.

Almost all forms of clinical and experimental diabetes mellitus are associated with increased secretion of glucagon, a potent hyperglycemic hormone whose glycogenolytic, gluconeogenic, lipolytic, and ketogenic actions are intensified by insulin deficiency.

Antidiabetic Drugs

Antidiabetic drugs are used to control the symptoms of diabetes mellitus. Drug therapy of diabetes mellitus may be undertaken by providing replacement insulin obtained from either bovine or porcine sources or synthesized in vitro or by oral administration of synthetic, sulfonamide-related hypoglycemic drugs (sulfonylureas), which increase release of endogenous insulin and increase the number and affinity of insulin receptors on body cells.

The antidiabetic drugs considered in this chapter include the various kinds of insulin preparations that are primarily indicated in absolute insulin-deficient forms of diabetes (type I, insulin-dependent diabetes or juvenile-onset diabetes) and the oral hypoglycemic drugs, which are used primarily in milder diabetes, frequently associated with obesity, in which insulin levels are near normal but the hormone is relatively ineffective (type II, noninsulin-dependent diabetes or maturity-onset diabetes).

Successful treatment of diabetes mellitus, however, requires more than mere drug therapy. Among the many adjunctive measures that should be considered in properly managing the diabetic state are (1) weight reduction, (2) regulation of the diet, (3) proper amounts of exercise, (4) maintenance of good hygiene, and (5) education of the

patient about proper monitoring procedures to avoid untoward effects. In fact, milder forms of noninsulin-dependent diabetes can be adequately controlled in many instances without resorting to drugs, simply by weight loss and careful regulation of the diet. Drug treatment of diabetes mellitus, when necessary, is a highly individualized matter and requires accurate diagnosis, continual monitoring of the patient, and proper drug dosage modifications as necessitated by changes in patient status.

Insulins

Insulin Injection; Insulin Zinc Suspension (Lente); Insulin Zinc Suspension, Extended (Ultralente); Insulin Zinc Suspension, Prompt (Semilente); Isophane Insulin Suspension (NPH); Protamine Zinc Insulin Suspension (PZI)

Endogenous insulin is a 51 amino-acid polypeptide hormone secreted by the beta (B) cells of the islets of Langerhans of the pancreas. The clinically available insulin preparations include purified extracts from beef or pork pancreas which possess biologic effects qualitatively identical to those of human insulin, differing from human insulin by only three amino acids (beef) or one (pork) amino acid in the sequence. In addition, human insulin (*i.e.*, exact amino acid sequence of endogenous insulin) is also available and is derived by either recombinant DNA techniques utilizing strains of *Escherichia coli* or chemical modification of animal-extracted pork insulin to replace the lone amino acid that is different from that of human insulin.

All commercially available insulins extracted from animal sources contain certain quantities of proinsulin and other proteins or substances resulting from incomplete conversion of the prohormone. These "contaminants" may contribute to the various immunogenic reactions that some insulin users experience, such as lipodystrophy and other local and systemic allergic reactions. Generally, beef-derived insulins are somewhat more immunologic than pork-derived products. All commercially available insulins in the United States contain less than 25 parts per million (ppm) of proinsulin and are termed *single-peak* insulins because their purification by gel chromatography yields a single spectrographic peak.

Over the years, the various purification techniques used to remove allergenic contaminants (*e.g.*, proinsulin) have been refined to the point that a new class of further purified single-peak insulins is available. These products, indicated by the term "purified insulin" on the label, contain less than 10 ppm of proinsulin and may elicit even fewer allergic reactions in hypersensitive patients than conventional single-peak insulins.

The newer "human" insulins are prepared by recombinant DNA techniques, and several different human insulin preparations are available. They appear to be as safe and effective as the conventional insulins and may be less immunogenic than the beef or pork insulins in certain patients because

Table 54-2
Characteristics of Insulin Preparations

Drug	Synonym	Composition	Onset	Peak Action	Duration
Rapid Acting					
Insulin injection	regular insulin	Precipitate of insulin with zinc chloride	½ h–1 h	2 h–4 h	6 h–8 h
insulin zinc suspension, prompt	semilente insulin	Precipitate of amorphous (noncrystalline) insulin with zinc	½ h–1 h	4 h–8 h	12 h–16 h
Intermediate Acting					
insulin zinc suspension	lente insulin	Stable mixture of 70% extended insulin zinc suspension and 30% insulin zinc suspension, prompt	1 h–2 h	8 h–14 h	18 h–24 h
isophane insulin suspension	NPH insulin	Crystalline complex of insulin, zinc, and protamine	1 h–1½ h	6 h–12 h	18 h–24 h
Long Acting					
insulin zinc suspension, extended	ultralente insulin	Large insulin crystals suspended with high zinc content without protein	4 h–8 h	12 h–24 h	30 h–36 h
protamine zinc insulin suspension	protamine zinc insulin (PZI)	Insulin and zinc in a protein complex	4 h–8 h	14 h–20 h	30 h–36 h

Table 54-3
Insulin Preparations

Drug	Preparations and Sources	Remarks
Rapid Acting		
insulin injection (Regular Insulin, Regular Iletin I) purified (Regular Purified Pork, Regular Iletin II, Velosulin) human (Novolin R, Humulin R, Velosulin Human)	Injection—40 U/ml, 100 U/ml (pork, beef and pork) Purified injection—100 U/ml (beef, pork) Human—100 U/ml	Short acting; solution is clear; may be administered SC 15 min–30 min before meals for control of diabetes, or IV (only insulin suitable for IV use) for severe ketoacidosis or diabetic coma; give 1 g dextrose/U insulin when administered IV, and monitor blood sugar, blood pressure, and intake/output ratio every hour until stable; be alert for development of rapid hypoglycemia and insulin shock.
insulin injection, concentrated (Regular Concentrated Iletin II)	Purified injection—500 U/ml (pork)	Indicated for control of diabetes in patients with marked insulin resistance; may be administered SC or IM: concentrated from pork pancreas, solution is clear and colorless; accuracy in dosage is essential due to potency; marked hypoglycemia can occur
insulin zinc suspension, prompt (Semilente Iletin I, Semilente insulin) purified (Semilente Purified Pork)	Injection—40 U/ml, 100 U/ml (beef, beef and pork) Purified injection—100 U/ml (pork)	Suspension of small particles of insulin and zinc chloride; solution is cloudy; administered SC 30 min before meals, usually breakfast; may only be mixed with other lente insulins; mix thoroughly by rolling vial and inverting end to end; do not shake; if suspension is granular or clumped, discard vial
Intermediate Acting		
insulin zinc suspension (Lente Iletin I, Lente insulin) purified (Lente Iletin II, Lente Purified Pork) human (Humulin L, Novolin L)	Injection—40 U/ml, 100 U/ml (beef, beef and pork) Purified injection—100 U/ml (beef, pork) Human—100 U/ml	Cloudy suspension containing a mixture of 30% prompt zinc suspension and 70% extended zinc suspension; contains no proteins, thus allergic reactions are rare; administered SC 30 min–60 min (continued)

they contain neither proinsulin nor any other contaminants found in animal-derived insulins.

Most diabetes can be managed equally well on conventional single-peak insulin or purified insulin. Generally, candidates for the purified insulins are those patients who exhibit local or systemic allergic reactions or severe lipodystrophy with conventional insulin preparations. A few patients may require dosage adjustments when switched from conventional to highly purified insulins, because the highly purified preparations are less bound by insulin antibodies and therefore may be slightly more potent. All stabilized diabetics being switched to a purified insulin preparation should be monitored closely to determine if a dosage modification is required. The possible advantages of human insulin over purified porcine insulin remain to be definitely established, and the number of patients who *absolutely* require human insulin remains quite small. Should the methods for synthesizing human insulins become more cost-effective than animal-extraction procedures over time, however, the use of human insulin products will greatly increase.

Several different types of insulin preparations are available. In addition to regular insulin, modified forms of insulin have been formulated which display important differences in onset, peak, and

Table 54-3 (continued)
Insulin Preparations

Drug	Preparations and Sources	Remarks
Intermediate Acting (continued)		
insulin zinc suspension (Lente Iletin I, Lente insulin) purified (Lente Iletin II, Lente Purified Pork) human (Humulin L, Novolin L) (continued)		before breakfast; action closely approximates that of NPH insulin, although duration of action may be slightly longer; see insulin zinc suspension, prompt for mixing instructions and compatabilities
isophane insulin suspension (NPH Insulin, NPH Iletin I) purified (Insulatard NPH, NPH Iletin II, NPH Purified Pork) human (Humulin N, Novolin N)	Injection—40 U/ml, 100 U/ml (beef, beef and pork) Purified injection—100 U/ml (beef, pork) Human—100 U/ml	Suspension of protamine zinc insulin crystals; administered SC 30 min before breakfast; a second injection in the evening may be required; see insulin zinc suspension, prompt for mixing instructions; it may be mixed with regular insulin injection, but not lente forms; available in fixed combination (70% NPH with 30% Regular Insulin Injection as Mixtard and Novolin 70/30)
Long Acting		
insulin zinc suspension, extended (Ultralente Iletin I, Ultralente insulin) purified (Ultralente Purified Beef)	Injection—40 U/ml, 100 U/ml (beef, beef and pork) Purified injection—100 U/ml (beef)	Cloudy suspension of large particles of zinc insulin, which delay absorption and prolong effects; no protein and low incidence of allergic reactions; administered SC 30 min–90 min before breakfast; may be mixed with other lente preparations
protamine zinc insulin suspension (Protamine, Zinc and Iletin I) purified (Protamine, Zinc and Iletin II)	Injection—40 U/ml, 100 U/ml (beef, beef and pork) Purified injection—100 U/ml (beef)	Cloudy suspension of fine particles of protamine zinc insulin; administered 30 min–60 min before breakfast; duration of action may exceed 36 h; balanced diet and regular meals are essential; may be mixed with regular insulin only; clinical effects may be delayed several days, supplemental doses of regular insulin may be needed during that time; hypoglycemia may be gradual in onset and often unnoticed.

duration of action, thereby allowing the physician to control the response carefully in each patient. The time course of action of the different insulins is largely dependent on the physical properties of the various preparations, such as the presence of conjugating metals or proteins (such as zinc or protamine), types of buffers, and the pH of the medium. Thus, insulin preparations can conveniently be divided into three groups based on their onset and duration of action. This classification is outlined in Table 54-2, where several characteristics of the different insulins are listed. All available insulin preparations are presented in Table 54-3 where specific indications and other pertinent information are given for each individual drug.

Insulin preparations are standardized on the base of their hypoglycemic action in fasted rabbits, and doses are measured in units. One insulin unit possesses the activity of $1/24$ mg of zinc insulin crystals reference standard. Insulin is marked in 10-ml vials containing 40 U/ml or 100 U/ml as well as a 20-ml concentrated solution containing 500 U/ml. The U100 insulins have virtually replaced the older U40 insulins today, because they allow for greater ease in measuring the correct dosage. Regular insulin preparations are close to a neutral pH and are therefore quite stable at room temperature, unlike the older preparations which had to be refrigerated. In addition, the mixing of certain types of insulins in the same syringe can now be accomplished without incompatibility problems (see under Administration and Dosage).

MECHANISM AND ACTIONS
Insulin facilitates uptake of glucose by cells of striated muscle and adipose tissue, probably by activating a carrier system for transport of glucose across the cell membrane. It also stimulates glycogen synthesis in muscle and liver by increasing enzyme activity, and suppresses gluconeogenesis. Insulin enhances formation of triglycerides, retards release of free fatty acids from adipose tissue, and facilitates incorporation of amino acids into muscle protein-promoting protein synthesis. Restoration of efficient glucose utilization decreases hyperglycemia, reduces glucosuria, and prevents diabetic acidosis and coma.

USES
1. Treatment of diabetes mellitus, especially the insulin-dependent type and complicated forms of noninsulin-dependent (i.e., maturity-onset) diabetes not adequately controlled by diet and weight loss
2. Emergency treatment of severe ketoacidosis or diabetic coma (regular insulin IV or IM)
3. Induction of hypoglycemic shock for therapy of certain psychiatric states (essentially obsolete)

ADMINISTRATION AND DOSAGE
Insulin dosage is tailored to each individual's needs and is based on blood and urinary glucose and ketone levels. The frequency and size of daily insulin doses must be carefully determined and closely monitored. Many factors can alter insulin requirements, and patient education is of vital importance in ensuring proper drug therapy. The various insulin preparations are listed in Table 54-3, along with their source and pertinent remarks. The drug is given SC, and sites of administration are rotated to minimize the occurrence of lipodystrophy (i.e., localized hollowing of the skin at the injection site, presumably due to alterations in lipid metabolism).

Preparations available as suspensions should be rolled gently between the hands before administration to facilitate uniform dispersion; vigorous shaking should be avoided, because frothing may result in withdrawal of improper amounts of drug for injection.

Insulin preparations are stable if stored at room temperature away from direct heat and sunlight. Refrigeration can be provided, but it is not necessary.

Insulin Admixtures
Some types of insulin may be mixed in the same syringe. If regular insulin is used, always draw it into the syringe first. Regular insulin may be mixed with protamine-zinc insulin in any proportion. Mixtures of regular insulin with NPH or lente insulins may not be stable beyond 5 minutes to 10 minutes and should be injected immediately. Semilente, lente, and ultralente insulins may be combined in any proportion.

Insulin can absorb onto plastic IV infusion sets; the extent of absorption is approximately 20% to 30% and is inversely proportional to the concentration of insulin. If administered in this manner, the response should be closely monitored.

FATE
Insulin is not active when taken orally. Following the injection, it is absorbed at varying rates depending on the composition of the preparation. Insulin circulates largely as the free hormone, and the plasma half-life is less than 10 minutes. Insulin is inactivated during its first passage through the liver as well as by the kidney.

SIDE-EFFECTS/ADVERSE REACTIONS
Mild hypoglycemic reactions are frequently encountered during the initial period of dosage adjustments if dosage is excessive. Symptoms may include fatigue, headache, drowsiness, nausea, and mild tremor. Local allergic reactions at the site of injection may be marked by itching, swelling, and erythema.

More severe hypoglycemic episodes can result in the appearance of tremor, sweating, hunger, weakness, nervousness, palpitations, paresthesias, blurred vision, irritability, confusion, delirium, convulsions, and unconsciousness.

Other adverse reactions resulting from insulin usage are lipodystrophy of the injection sites, characterized by disappearance of subcutaneous fat and a "pitted" appearance to the skin, visual disturbances, and systemic allergic reactions, such as urticaria, angioedema, and anaphylactic shock.

In some patients, especially obese diabetics on intermittent insulin therapy, a high level of circulating anti-insulin antibodies develops, necessitating very large doses of insulin. Often, this is a transient condition and clears spontaneously. In addition, switching from beef to the less antigenic pork or human insulin can overcome this resistance.

CONTRAINDICATIONS AND PRECAUTIONS

Insulins of animal origin should not be used in persons hypersensitive to the specific animal proteins. Because insulin requirements in diabetes can change quickly, for example due to fever, vomiting, dehydration, stress, infection, altered eating habits, and so forth, patients should be cautioned to be alert for early signs of hypoglycemia, such as fatigue, nervousness, tachycardia, nausea, and sweating. Persons using insulin should wear some sort of identification in the event an insulin reaction occurs in an unfamiliar setting. Pregnancy may make diabetic management more difficult; however, insulin is the drug of choice during pregnancy.

If signs of hypoglycemia occur, patients should be instructed to immediately take sugar (2 tsp) or a sugar-sweetened product, which usually will correct the imbalance and prevent further symptoms. If the reaction is more severe, a 40% glucose gel and chewable glucose tablet are available for oral use. Alternately, glucagon may be given SC, IM, or IV, or dextrose may be administered IV (see below).

INTERACTIONS

1. The hypoglycemic effects of insulin may be enhanced by acetaminophen, alcohol, anabolic steroids, fenfluramine, beta-blockers, monoamine oxidase inhibitors, phenylbutazone, salicylates, tetracyclines, and theophylline.
2. Insulin needs may be increased by concomitant use of corticosteroids, dobutamine, epinephrine, levodopa, nicotine, oral contraceptives, phenytoin, thiazide diuretics, and thyroid hormones.
3. Insulin may increase the likelihood of toxicity with digitalis drugs by altering serum potassium levels.

■ *Nursing Process*

□ ASSESSMENT

□ *Subjective Data*

Accurate diagnosis of diabetes is essential before starting a patient on insulin. The classic symptoms of polyuria, polydipsia, and polyphasia will generally be evident in adults and children. Children and young adults may also exhibit rapid weight loss. Blood glucose levels will be elevated. In adults, a fasting blood glucose of 140 mg/dl or higher is cause for concern. In children, a level of 200 mg/dl or higher indicates the need for intervention. Usually blood studies will be done at different times of day to allow for error, metabolic changes, or other variables before a definitive diagnosis is made.

Once the patient is labeled diabetic, the nurse must begin an extensive assessment of the patient's psychomotor skills, cognitive skills, and support systems to help him cope with the disease and to learn to manage the required regimen. The first step may be to learn his perceptions of the illness and what it means in his life. The patient should personalize the disease early on so he can begin incorporating it into his daily routine. Diabetes, unlike most chronic illnesses, affects everything from sleep and eating to daily hygiene and exercise. Therefore, the earlier the patient recognizes this and accepts the challenge to learn the care plan, the more successful he will be at maintaining the regimen. (See Chap. 6 for a discussion on assessing and facilitating learner readiness.) Children may need a different approach to assessing learner readiness. Through doll play, needle play, and drawing pictures, they may better vent their frustrations and fears.

The nurse must also assess the patient's ability to read. Much diabetes literature is commercially available and is typically given as a packet. It is of little use to the nonreader or to the person with limited reading abilities. Other formats using pictures, audiotapes, and movies or videotapes are available. A patient who cannot read can become very competent in self-care if the appropriate tools are used to guide him.

The patient's support system must also be reviewed. Regardless of willingness and capability, the patient who has diabetes needs to have the support of someone who will motivate him and who can check on him at least daily. If hypoglycemia or illness should occur, the patient may be unable even to telephone for help. In addition, a supportive friend or relative would know what to do if either incident occurred and could prevent a major problem by taking quick action on the patient's behalf. If a support person can be identified early in the nursing care, both individuals can learn the regimen together, which provides added impetus for learning.

Necessary supports also include the physical environment. Does the patient have a telephone, which is essential for getting help quickly? Is refrigeration available if insulin needs to be stored for an extended period? Does the patient have running water or access to water to maintain some asepsis and skin care? What facilities are available in the home for storage of needles, insulin, and other equipment? What is the patient's financial situation? How will he purchase syringes and other needed equipment? These may seem like basics, but not everyone has them. By knowing this information in advance, however, the nurse can plan a regimen to include variations.

Other subjective data may include a drug history. The effect of insulin is enhanced by many drugs (see under Interactions), including acetaminophen, alcohol, aspirin, and others. Conversely, some drugs increase the need for insulin, including corticosteroids, thiazide diuretics, and thyroid hormones. How these drugs will interact in a specific patient and how they will affect his insulin requirement will vary, but such information must be considered. In addition, the patient should be asked about allergies to animals or animal products because many of the insulins are derived from pork or beef. It is also prudent to ask if the patient's religious beliefs preclude use of certain animal products. Appropriate substitutions can then be made at the onset of treatment.

☐ *Objective Data*

Once learner readiness, acceptance, and patient resources are assessed, psychomotor skills can be reviewed. Self-administration of insulin, self-blood-glucose monitoring (SBGM), and urine testing require a certain degree of manual skill, vision, and memory. The patient must be able to see clearly, to manipulate the tools, and to remember correctly a sequence of steps in order to perform the task safely and accurately. Children under 8 years old may lack the motor skills to administer insulin safely, but they should be evaluated. Because diabetes may affect peripheral circulation of the hands, finger dexterity may be limited. In addition, vision may be impaired by diabetic retinopathy, age-related ocular changes, or transient blurring of vision which may occur during hyperglycemic episodes. Although patients with such limitations have successfully learned insulin injection techniques, it is important to be aware of these problems before teaching begins.

☐ *NURSING DIAGNOSES*

Actual nursing diagnoses for the patient taking insulin may include:

Knowledge deficit related to the drug's action, administration, and side-effects; the relationship between diet, exercise, and insulin; symptoms and appropriate management of hyper- and hypoglycemia

Anxiety related to self-injection, the impact of a chronic illness, and the ability to cope with a complex regimen

Potential nursing diagnoses for the patient taking insulin include:

Potential for infection at the injection sites

Impaired tissue integrity related to lipodystrophy or atrophy of tissue from chronic insulin injection

☐ *PLAN*

The nursing care goals for the newly diagnosed diabetic must be realistic. Hospital policies are such that a patient may be discharged within a few days of learning his diagnosis; in other cases he may not be hospitalized at all. Consequently, the nurse must establish short-term, intermediate, and long-term goals with the patient and plan to involve multiple health-care providers in order to accomplish these goals (see suggested outcomes under Evaluation). Attempting to overload the patient with all of the information he'll need within a few days, when he is still reacting emotionally to the news of his diagnoses, may prevent him from remembering even the simplest task. Consequently, for some patients the only goal in the hospital may be to help the patient begin to accept the diagnoses, especially if the hospital stay is short. Then most teaching will begin at home. Early goals should focus on the strategies the patient needs to survive with his illness. These may include basic self-injection techniques, proper drug storage, how to test blood or urine, how to recognize hypoglycemia, and what to do if it occurs. Intermediate goals may expand on these techniques and include injection site rotation schedules, skin assessment, utilization of a sugar source when hypoglycemia occurs, and institution of a sick-day regimen. Long-term goals should focus on helping the patient to understand how stress, illness, meals, and exercise affect insulin utilization, how to use the blood glucose measurement to make appropriate changes in insulin dose, and to develop a degree of confidence in his ability to manage his illness. Each patient is different; consider these flexible guidelines. Some information may be more important to one patient than to another. In diabetes, more than most illnesses, the plan must be extremely individualized and well-coordinated with all those involved, understanding that up to 1 year may be required to complete the teaching plan.

□ INTERVENTION

Teaching self-administration of insulin is frequently seen as the first step in a diabetic teaching plan. However, a more logical approach is to begin teaching with information about what diabetes is and what symptoms the patient has which indicate he is a diabetic. It is extremely important that the patient recognize how diabetes affects him and what he can do to manage it. Several excellent programs exist to help the nurse make this introduction, including the "Getting Started" program by Becton Dickinson Pharmaceutical Company.*

The patient must grasp the process of insulin–blood glucose regulation. If there is no insulin, blood glucose increases. Insulin decreases blood glucose (by helping the body to utilize glucose); therefore, too much insulin decreases glucose to dangerous levels. Both diet and exercise influence the need for insulin and glucose utilization, a further component to understanding the process of insulin–blood glucose regulation.

Once the patient understands that diabetes control is a three-part process influenced by diet, exercise, and drug therapy, he may be more open to learning about self-injection. Most people fear injections, and self-injection is frequently perceived as self-mutilating, especially if blood glucose-monitoring finger sticks are also required. The nurse must explore these fears regardless of the patient's age. Most nurses recognize the need for needle play with children before teaching self-injection, but it is equally important with adults. All patients need an opportunity to manipulate the equipment and practice on other objects such as a piece of styrofoam or an orange. They need time to become comfortable with the whole idea of injection management. Although time may be limited, it is important to plan to allow some space between practice on other objects and the actual first self-stick.

In addition to helping the patient cope with the concept of self-injection, the nurse must determine whether the patient will be able to draw up accurately the prescribed dose of insulin. The patient must be able to see and read the calibrations and identify the type of syringe he has been given. Most patients will use the U100 system, but the patient should be able to identify the markings of a U100 syringe and a U100 bottle of insulin. To determine

* Becton Dickinson Consumer Products, Rochelle Park, NJ 07662.

the patient's ability to read the calibrations, he should be asked to identify the marking on the syringe scale that identifies his dose and be able to line up the syringe plunger end with the marking after a demonstration. If the patient cannot safely measure the insulin dose, arrangements must be made for a support person to learn the technique and provide the patient with premeasured insulin doses.

The first stick will be traumatic, at least in thought. One patient told of a dream about needles and syringes dancing around her bed the night before she gave her first insulin injection. If fear is high, it may be better to allow the patient to give a self-injection of sterile saline first so the procedure is not tied to a specific time. Once the first injection is given, most patients agree that it hurts very little. The needle is extremely sharp and the lumen very narrow, usually at least 25 gauge. If the insulin is at room temperature, the angle of the needle correct, insertion deep enough, and the thrust of the needle gentle but firm, the pain is usually minimal. The nurse can help the patient control these factors by teaching correct technique and guiding early injections to correct any problems.

Teaching correct technique will be difficult if the nurse is wedded to only one method. Although drawing up insulin is universally standard (see under Insulin Admixtures), actual injection will depend on the patient's size, weight, and motor skills. The angle of insertion can vary from 45 degrees to 90 degrees, the steeper angle being used by patients with a larger mass and in body sites with higher fat content such as the abdomen and thigh. Literature also varies on whether or not to pinch a roll of skin, a factor which can also vary depending on fat content. The goal is to inject insulin in subcutaneous tissue. If that can be accomplished without pinching a roll of skin, there is no need to do it, and elimination of this step may be easier for some patients to manage. Another source of disagreement is whether to pull back on the plunger before injection to test for blood. If the patient can manage this action, some clinicians prefer it because the chance for injecting insulin into the bloodstream is eliminated. The patient should be taught to watch for any tinge of blood. If blood is observed, the patient should pull back the needle slightly and then inject. However, if the patient correctly inserts the needle into subcutaneous tissue, chances of hitting a blood vessel are extremely low. Therefore, if he cannot manage the pull-back technique, it is usually safe to eliminate it providing his site selection technique is good.

A last source of disagreement centers around

whether a patient can safely reuse a needle and syringe. The patient may do this without seeking approval as a cost-saving measure, especially if he must take several injections a day. Because syringes cost 17 cents to 20 cents each, the cost may be high to a patient with limited resources. Research indicates that the incidence of site infection from needle reuse is relatively low, about 9%, approximately the same as the rate for patients who use needles only once. If a patient indicates he reuses syringes, he should be encouraged to use a new needle and syringe daily or at least every 2 days, and after each injection, to flush the needle with air, wipe it with alcohol, and replace the cap until the next dose. (See the box entitled Teaching Self-Administration of Insulin.)

Site selection is another component of the injection teaching plan. Early in therapy the patient may prefer to use the thighs or abdomen because these are the easiest sites to inject. Over time he needs to learn to use auxiliary sites and to get a

support person to learn to inject him in the back sites so all areas can be utilized. One of the side-effects of insulin injection is lipodystrophy or atrophy, which occurs when a site is overutilized. Once the site atrophies it cannot be used, so the best approach is prevention by routine site rotation and skin assessment. Teach the patient to palpate the skin regularly and to report any bumps or crevices at once. Figure 54-3 shows an example of a site rotation plan.

An alternate administration technique is the insulin pump, also called the continuous subcutaneous insulin infusion system. The system delivers a continuous flow of insulin to the body at a rate that more closely resembles the normal physiologic process. The pump also allows for administration of a premeal bolus of insulin. However, use of the pump is limited to people who are highly motivated to comply with a strict blood glucose-testing schedule, who have a clear understanding of the relationship between insulin, diet, and exercise, and are willing to observe strict aseptic technique in the care of the needle. The pump delivers insulin through a subcutaneous needle site, which must be rotated every 48 hours to 72 hours. The patient must be taught how to antiseptically prepare the skin, insert the needle, and secure with sterile tape. Adherence to a strict regimen reduces the risk of site infection, a major side-effect of insulin infusion devices. However, the pump is extremely valuable in regulating patients who cannot achieve therapeutically acceptable blood glucose levels through injections. Included in this group are type I diabetics at various stages of their illness and pregnant women who must take insulin.

The patient must also be taught proper storage of insulin. Today's insulin products do not need to be refrigerated although refrigeration is recommended if the solution is not currently in use. Teach the patient to watch for precipitation and to be aware of product expiration dates so that the insulin he uses is at full strength.

In addition to learning correct administration techniques and all its components, the patient must learn when his body needs more or less insulin and how his insulin dose is affected by diet and exercise. To do this effectively, he must learn to do self-blood-glucose monitoring (SBGM) a technique by which he takes a blood sample by a small finger stick and tests it on a commercial reagent strip. He may also need to learn urine testing to determine the existence of ketones in the urine. Learning these techniques will help him know when to seek medical advice. Early in therapy the goal of teaching SBGM or urine testing may be only to use the

---

Teaching Self-Administration of Insulin

1. Teach the patient to read the insulin bottle labels. He must know the difference between the types of insulin he is using. Most patients use NPH and regular insulin or another variation and regular insulin. Most also use U100 strength, although occasionally a patient will continue to use U40. If the patient must take two insulins at the same time, to avoid extra injections he may wish to learn an admixture routine (see under Insulin Admixtures). Successful teaching depends on the patient's eyesight and motor skills. Syringe magnifiers are available and may help some patients. Others may have to rely on a support person to mix the insulins. Premixing longer than 15 minutes before injection should be discouraged because potency changes quickly even when the mixture is refrigerated.
2. Plan several sessions of needle play. Encourage practice in all steps of the process.
3. Have the person self-inject sterile saline first, especially if he is nervous.
4. Follow this injection format.
   a. Wash your hands.
   b. Map out the selected injection site.
   c. Clean the site with alcohol.
   d. Pinch a roll of skin or stretch skin slightly depending on weight, site location, availability of skin folds, patient's manual skill.
   e. Insert needle using a firm downward stroke at predetermined angle (45 degrees–90 degrees).
   f. Pull back plunger to check for blood (may be optional).
   g. Inject, pushing the plunger quickly.
   h. Remove needle, releasing skin at the same time.
   i. Massage skin site to facilitate absorption.

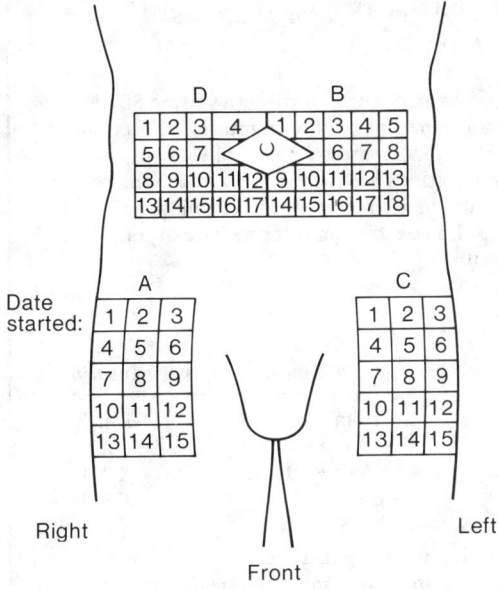

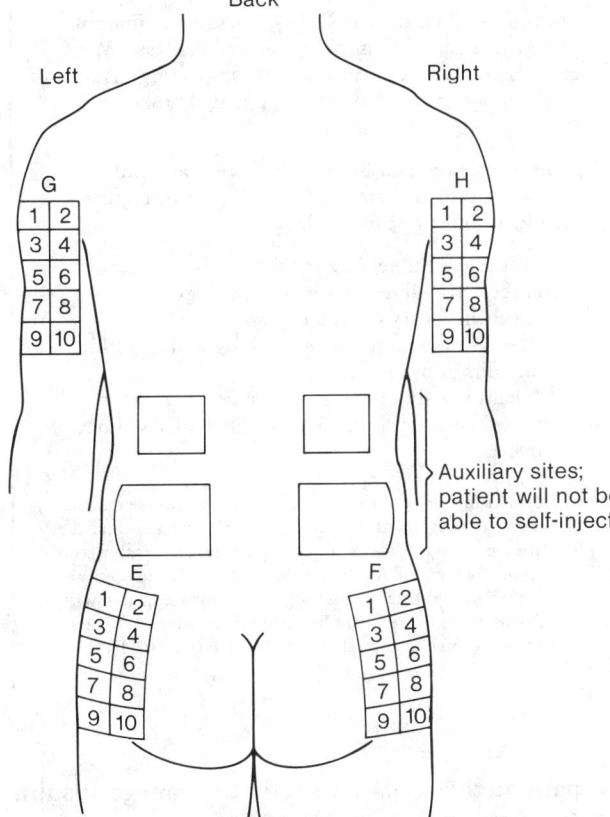

Figure 54-3. Sample injection site rotation schedule.

1. *Start injections at Section A (right thigh).*
2. *After each injection site is used, cross out the numbered box that indicates its location.*
3. *Use the schedule sheet for reference before each injection.*
4. *Rotate to the next numbered site, about 1½ inches (or one knuckle width) from the last needle mark.*

technique to alert the patient about developing hypo- or hyperglycemia. But in the patient who seeks more independence and flexibility in controlling his diabetes, SBGM can be used to help him make changes in insulin, diet, or exercise. If the patient is so motivated and has been effective in managing his care, he may be taught an algorithm for managing his diabetes. An algorithm is a step-by-step procedure for regulating blood glucose levels with insulin. These may be simple or complex and may vary according to the physician. (See boxes entitled A Conservative Algorithm for Diabetes Management and A "Tight" Algorithm for Diabetes Management.)

Another component of monitoring is recognizing when periods of hypoglycemia occur and knowing what actions to take. The patient may need to learn what sugar sources are appropriate, such as orange juice or sugar solution, or may be encouraged to carry and take glucagon when symptoms occur. The key is for the patient to learn how to avert a crisis situation and what to do if one occurs. Symptoms of early hypoglycemia in addition to low blood glucose level include sweating, hunger, nervousness, and weakness, but these can rapidly deteriorate into convulsions and coma if action is not taken.

A third component of monitoring is knowing how to handle sick days. Some patients assume that if they are ill or not eating regular meals they do not need insulin. The danger in this thinking is the rapid development of hyperglycemia because the body's metabolic needs actually increase during illness and infection. See the box entitled Guidelines for Sick Days for Diabetics for an example of a sick-day regimen.

If the patient has not learned other management techniques or is a new diabetic, he should be encouraged to seek attention immediately to avert problems. The patient should be told what sick days are; a cold, sore throat, vomiting, and diarrhea can all be serious to a diabetic and need some supervision, although the long-term goal is to teach

5. *Use each numbered site only once, rotate to a new site for each injection. For example, if you self-inject four times a day you will use four numbered sites.*
6. *Cross out the lettered body site as you complete it and move to the next one.*

This chart is designed to indicate body sites the patient can use for self-injection; auxiliary sites are indicated if the patient has a significant other who will also give him injections.

The rotation schedule is designed to give a body site a minimum of 5 weeks' rest before it is reused.

A Conservative Algorithm for Diabetes Management

Guidelines for a conservative algorithm for diabetics on two injections/day:

Document blood glucose (BG) values in log book two to four times each day.

Look for patterns (3 or more days) of high or low BG values.

Example A (four times/day SMBG)

	7 AM	11 AM	4 PM	10 PM
Day 1	64 mg/dl	90 mg/dl	350 mg/dl	200 mg/dl
Day 2	102	128	275	230
Day 3	220	102	290	140
Day 4	130	110	302	165
Day 5	80	89	285	189

Example B (two times/day SMBG)

	7 AM	11 AM	4 PM	10 PM
Day 1	240 mg/dl		200 mg/dl	
Day 2		178 mg/dl		64 mg/dl
Day 3	163		100	
Day 4		140		70
Day 5	145		122	

Guidelines for adjusting insulin:

· Decide which insulin is peaking (or working hardest) at the time of the need for change. In Example A, BGs are all high. For a person on split/mixed NPH/regular insulins, morning NPH probably is affecting the 4 PM values. In Example B, low 10 PM values are most likely affected by presupper regular insulin.

· Change the appropriate insulin by 1 to 2 units.

· Avoid changing more than one insulin at a time.

· Monitor and document the results of the insulin change over the next 3 days.

· If BG values have improved satisfactorily, no further change is necessary.

· If BG values worsen or cause other than expected changes with the insulin adjustment, call the physician or designated health professional for help.

· If BG values improve with the changes, but are still too low or too high, adjust appropriate insulin by another 1 to 2 units and observe for next 3 days.

Note: The above insulin adjustments should not be guided by urine glucose values.

(Adapted from handout by Dr. Neil White for course entitled "Intensive Management of Diabetes" for physicians and the health-care team, Diabetes Education Center, Washington University School of Medicine, St. Louis, MO. Copyright 1986, American Journal of Nursing Company. Reprinted with permission from Haire-Joshu D, Flavin K, Santiago JV: Intensive conventional insulin therapy. Am J Nurs 86(11):1253, 1986.

A "Tight" Algorithm for Diabetes Management

Example of an algorithm for diabetics using SBGM four or more times per day with multiple injections of regular insulin preprescribed by physician. (Multiple injections are two or more injections per day of regular insulin by injection or pump, or regular insulin added to an intermediate or long-acting insulin.)

Sample Algorithm Glucose	Time (before meal)	Dose of Regular Insulin
under 70	−15 min	X-1 or X-2
70–150	−30 min	X
150–200	−45 to −60 min	X + 1
over 200	−60 min	X + 2

Guidelines for adjusting insulin:
• Monitor BG an hour before each mealtime.
• Guided by premeal BGs, select appropriate dose and time for regular insulin.

Example A: Prebreakfast BG = 120. Give X amount of regular insulin 30 minutes before breakfast. May give regular with intermediate or long-acting insulin if within an hour of the time you usually take intermediate or long-acting.

Example B: Prelunch BG = 280. Give X amount of regular insulin plus two additional units of regular insulin 1 hour prior to lunch.

• Never select the regular insulin dosage by the way you feel. BG value must be used as a guide.
• If mealtimes vary considerably:
Always take intermediate or long-acting within an hour of usual time.
Mealtimes should be at least 4 hours apart so that the action of regular insulin peaks will not overlap.

(Adapted from handout by Dr. Neil White for course entitled "Intensive Management of Diabetes" for physicians and the health-care team, Diabetes Education Center, Washington University School of Medicine, St. Louis, MO. Copyright 1986, American Journal of Nursing Company. Reprinted with permission from Haire-Joshu D, Flavin K, Santiago JV: Intensive conventional insulin therapy. Am J Nurs 86(11):1253, 1986.

the patient the tools he needs to manage insulin therapy during illness.

In addition to hypoglycemic reactions, insulin has two side-effects that the nurse must monitor. The first, allergic reaction, usually occurs early in therapy and may be local or systemic. An allergic reaction can be suspected if stinging, itching, or redness occurs at the injection site soon after drug administration. An antihistamine may be used to

Guidelines for Sick Days for Diabetics

1. Take your regular dose of insulin. If additional insulin is needed, based on blood glucose readings, use *regular* insulin.
2. Increase the number of times you test your blood glucose and/or urine to at least four times a day. In some cases, testing may have to be done every 4 hours to 6 hours.
3. Drink fluids every hour. If you are unable to eat solids, try to take in foods that have some carbohydrates such as soups, ginger ale, sherbet.
4. Keep warm and rest. Avoid strenuous activity and exercise.
5. Have someone available to help you because hyperglycemia can occur rapidly during illness.
6. Contact your physician or health resource especially if you have vomiting or diarrhea. Do not attempt to treat yourself without supervision. If you can reach no one, go to the emergency department of your local hospital.

relieve discomfort, and switching to purified insulin may avert further problems. Systemic reactions are rare but must be suspected in any patient allergic to animal proteins. In such a case, the best strategy may be to use purified or human insulin from the start.

Another side-effect, insulin resistance, occurs more frequently in patients who are overweight, have other hormonal imbalances, or in type I diabetics who have a period of remission during which they discontinue insulin therapy. The patient responds less and less to insulin. While this problem is extremely complex, the nurse must suspect it if the patient has frequent episodes of hyperglycemia in spite of faithful adherence to the prescribed diet and drug regimen.

The pregnant woman who is diabetic must be closely monitored throughout pregnancy. Insulin requirements will decrease in the first trimester, then increase in the second and third trimesters, making SBGM and infusion pump injections vital to accurate maintenance. The pregnant diabetic needs to be followed on a weekly basis to prevent complications to the mother and child and to ensure that the mother follows closely the guidelines provided.

□ *EVALUATION*

The outcome criteria for judging drug effectiveness are tied to criteria for diabetes management through exercise, diet, and hygiene. In addition, proof of success must also be judged along a continuum to allow the patient sufficient time to learn the regimen and incorporate the disease into his life.

Therefore, outcome criteria fall into several categories, and examples of each are given below:

Blood studies: Blood glucose levels remain between 60 mg and 120 mg/dl depending on the degree of control sought and the incidence of patient hypoglycemia episodes; measurements of glycosylated hemoglobin (HgA) show adequate glucose attachment to the hemoglobin molecule over the 60-day to 120-day lifespan of a red blood cell. This test, more than SBGM, gives the patient positive feedback on his long-term ability to use glucose effectively.

Short-term outcomes: The patient or family understands and verbalizes the need for insulin and the need for regular eating habits, can prepare and self-inject insulin, tests blood and urine accurately, knows proper storage of insulin, knows the symptoms of hypo- and hyperglycemia, and knows what to do if they occur.

Intermediate outcomes (several weeks after diagnosis): In addition to the above, the patient knows how to rotate injection sites, knows how to check for fatty tissue changes, carries and correctly uses a sugar source for hypoglycemic episodes, plans a sick-day regimen and verbalizes how to implement it, expresses a beginning understanding of the relationship between diet, exercise, stress, illness, and insulin requirements.

Long-term outcomes (several months after diagnosis): The patient uses blood glucose measurements to make changes in insulin requirements, changes insulin dose when meals, exercise, and wellness vary, independently initiates a sick-day regimen, and calls health resources as needed. Nursing Care Plan 54-1 summarizes the nursing process for the patient receiving insulin. The care plan is based on childhood needs but is adaptable to many adults.

Oral Antidiabetic Drugs

Acetohexamide, Chlorpropamide, Glipizide, Glyburide, Tolazamide, Tolbutamide

The orally effective hypoglycemic agents are sulfonamide derivatives classified as sulfonylureas. The clinically useful oral antidiabetics have similar mechanisms of action, that is, release of endoge-

(Text continues on p. 1036.)

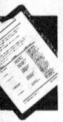

Assessment

Subjective Data	1. Medication history
	  a. Refer to Interactions section to formulate pertinent questions.
	  b. Include a history of allergies to animal products.
	2. Medical history
	  a. Parent's/child's description of symptoms, progress of the disease, knowledge about regimen. Focus on presence of polyuria, polydipsia, polyphagia, weight loss, skin changes, visual changes.
	  b. Determine presence of renal or cardiovascular disease.
	  c. Determine presence of family history of diabetes.
	3. Personal history/compliance issues
	  a. Parent's/child's ability to manage a complex therapeutic regimen
	  b. Age and development of child
	  c. Financial, personal resources; support systems
	  d. Parent's perception of illness: explore anger, guilt, denial

Objective Data	1. Physical assessment: complete, highlighting
	  a. Vital signs, peripheral pulses
	  b. Height and weight
	  c. Neurologic status: vision, peripheral sensation, reflexes, mental acuity, psychomotor function
	  d. Renal: urinary output
	2. Laboratory data
	  a. CBC with differential
	  b. Fasting blood sugar, glucose tolerance test
	  c. Serum electrolytes
	  d. Renal function studies

Nursing Diagnosis	Expected Client Outcome	Intervention
Knowledge deficit related to drug's action, administration, side-effects; the relationship between diet, exercise and insulin; symptoms and management of hypoglycemia and hyperglycemia, need for follow-up care	Will verbalize knowledge of the disease and the relationship of drug therapy, diet, and exercise	Teach the family/teacher/child the basic components of diabetes, how insulin works to control it, and what role diet, exercise, and growth play in the process.
	Blood glucose levels will remain within normal limits (or prescribed goal)	Instruct the family in correct drug-taking, including: • Following the prescribed time of administration; • The importance of maintaining regularly scheduled meals and snacks; • How to measure, mix, and inject insulin; and • Systematic site rotation and recording.
	Will verbalize knowledge of the causes and symptoms of hypo- and hyperglycemia and appropriate actions to take	Teach the family/teacher/child the symptoms of hyper- and hypoglycemia and appropriate actions to take if symptoms develop. Put information on an easy-to-read card. Teach the family causes for hypo- and hyperglycemia and strategies to prevent development. Teach the family an appropriate sick-day regimen and how to enact it to *(continued)*

Nursing Care Plan 54-1 (continued)
The Child Receiving Insulin

Nursing Diagnosis	Expected Client Outcome	Intervention
Knowledge deficit related to drug's action, administration, side-effects; the relationship between diet, exercise and insulin; symptoms and management of hypoglycemia and hyperglycemia, need for follow-up care *(continued)*	Will demonstrate correct testing technique Will return to health care provider for frequent monitoring Will wear a Medic-alert device at all times	minimize the development of problems (see box, Guidelines for Sick Days for Diabetics). Teach the correct use of SBGM or urine glucose/ketone testing to monitor body glucose levels. Emphasize the need for follow-up care to measure growth, obtain laboratory data, monitor vascular changes, provide support, and answer questions about the regimen. Teach family to inform all caregivers that child is a diabetic. Inform family of the importance of the child wearing some identification in the case of an emergency.
Anxiety related to self-injection, the impact of a chronic illness, and attempting to cope with a complex regimen	Will learn self-injection if age is appropriate	Plan practice sessions for parent and child so that gradually, self-medication and disease management are attained. Many children from age 8 years onward can learn to administer their own insulin. Attempt to provide a supportive network for child and family through support groups, meeting with other patients in the practice, family counseling.
Potential for infection at injection sites related to poor aseptic technique	Infection is prevented.	Teach proper aseptic technique including cleansing of injection site, use of syringe and vials. Alert parents and child to watch for signs of local infection, which include pain, redness, swelling, and increased temperature, all of which should be reported immediately. Monitor injection technique periodically on follow-up visits.
Potential for impaired tissue integrity related to lipodystrophy or tissue atrophy from poor site selection	Tissue will remain intact	Teach proper site selection and rotation. Teach patient/family to assess site *before* injection for redness, bogginess, soft, spongy feeling, or induration. Sites that are not smooth and firm should be avoided, and physician should be notified.
Potential alteration in tissue perfusion related to microcirculatory changes	Will have no changes in vision, kidney, periphery as a result of vascular changes	Encourage family to return for frequent follow-up visits to monitor vision, renal function, peripheral vascular function. Keep a close check on blood glucose and effectiveness of drug dose in maintaining normal glucose levels. Monitor the hospitalized child closely to avoid wide swings in glucose levels.

nous insulin from functional beta cells in the pancreas and enhanced sensitivity of insulin receptor sites on cellular membranes. However, they display significant differences in the duration of their hypoglycemic action. These differences are detailed in Table 54-4, which lists the available drugs, dosages, and other pertinent characteristics.

The principal indication for the oral hypoglycemic agents is management of mild, stable, noninsulin-dependent, maturity-onset diabetes that cannot be adequately controlled by diet alone. They arc of no value in diabetes complicated by acidosis or coma, and there is no justification for and significant hazard in their use in labile, insulin-dependent forms of diabetes.

Considerable support exists for the view that initial control of most if not all noninsulin-dependent diabetes should be attempted by diet and weight reduction alone, especially in the obese diabetic. Oral antidiabetic drugs are primarily used in those patients not stabilized by diet and weight loss who display fasting serum glucose less than 200 mg/dl, and absence of ketoacidosis. This cautious approach to oral antidiabetic drug therapy has evolved from earlier reports of increased cardiovascular mortality in patients receiving oral antidiabetic drugs compared to patients being controlled with diet or diet plus insulin. Although the conclusions of this study conducted in a number of American clinics some years ago have been challenged, largely based on faulty experimental design, the status of oral hypoglycemic drugs is still somewhat uncertain and their use remains largely a matter of clinician preference and experience.

MECHANISM AND ACTIONS
Oral hypoglycemic drugs act to stimulate release of preformed endogenous insulin from functional beta cells in the pancreas. They also appear to increase the number and sensitivity of insulin receptor sites on tissues, thus increasing the utilization of available insulin. The drugs may inhibit hepatic glucose production and reduce serum glucagon concentrations.

USES
1. Treatment of stable, nonketotic, or nonacidotic type II (noninsulin-dependent) diabetes mellitus not adequately controlled by diet and weight reduction
2. Adjunct to insulin in certain types of insulin-dependent diabetes (allows reduced insulin dosage)
3. Diagnosis of pancreatic insulinoma (tolbutamide)

4. Adjunctive treatment of nephrogenic diabetes insipidus (chlorpropamide only)

ADMINISTRATION AND DOSAGE
See Table 54-4.

FATE
The oral hypoglycemic drugs are well absorbed orally, tolazamide being the most slowly absorbed and having the slowest onset of action (4 hours–6 hours) compared to the other drugs (1 hour–2 hours). All of the drugs are highly bound to plasma proteins. They are metabolized in the liver to both active and inactive metabolites which are excreted primarily in the urine, except for glyburide, whose metabolites are eliminated in both the bile and urine. Tolbutamide is the shortest acting oral hypoglycemic drug (6 hours–12 hours) and is given two to three times a day. The duration of action of chlorpropamide is up to 60 hours, whereas the remaining drugs exhibit durations of action ranging from 12 hours to 24 hours.

SIDE-EFFECTS/ADVERSE REACTIONS
The most commonly encountered side-effects with oral hypoglycemic drugs are dose-related and include GI distress (nausea, heartburn, fullness), headache, anorexia, weakness, and paresthesias.

Other adverse reactions to these drugs include:
Dermatologic—Urticaria, pruritus, photosensitivity, morbilliform or maculopapular rash, erythema multiforme, exfoliative dermatitis
Hepatic—Cholestatic jaundice, altered liver function tests, hepatic porphyria
Hematologic (rare)—Thrombocytopenia, leukopenia, mild anemia, eosinophilia, agranulocytosis

Overdosage with these agents results in the appearance of symptoms of hypoglycemia, which usually occur in approximately the following sequence: tingling of the lips and tongue, hunger, nausea, yawning, lethargy, nervousness, tachycardia, sweating, confusion, tremor, agitation, irritability, delirium, convulsions, stupor, and, ultimately, coma.

Mild hypoglycemic episodes can be treated with oral glucose (*i.e.*, glucose gel) or adjustment in drug dosage or eating schedules. Severe hypoglycemia is infrequent but is a medical emergency and is usually managed by IV dextrose (see below).

Although the association of oral hypoglycemic drug usage and cardiovascular toxicity is tenuous, as discussed in the introduction, long-term use of these drugs in patients with known or suspected cardiac disease should be undertaken with caution.

CONTRAINDICATIONS AND PRECAUTIONS

Oral hypoglycemic drugs are contraindicated in persons with insulin-dependent diabetes; hepatic or renal dysfunction; diabetes complicated by uremia, ketosis, acidosis, coma; stress, fever, infection, or trauma; and pregnancy.

Cautious use of oral hypoglycemic drugs should be undertaken in persons with cardiac impairment, adrenal or thyroid dysfunction, in women of childbearing age, in elderly or debilitated patients, and in alcoholics. Safety and efficacy for use in children have not been established. Persons taking beta-blockers concurrently may not evidence early symptoms of hypoglycemia, such as tachycardia, sweating, or tremor.

INTERACTIONS

1. The effects of oral hypoglycemic drugs may be prolonged or enhanced by oral anticoagulants, alcohol, allopurinol, anti-inflammatory drugs, chloramphenicol, insulin, MAO inhibitors, probenecid, phenytoin, salicylates, sulfonamides, and other highly protein-bound drugs.
2. Diazoxide and beta-blocking agents can reduce the response to oral antidiabetic drugs.
3. Alcohol may elicit a "disulfiram-like" reaction especially in patients taking chlorpropamide (see Chap. 26) and may also produce photosensitivity reactions.
4. Chlorpropamide and possibly other sulfonylureas may prolong the effects of barbiturates.
5. Oral hypoglycemics may increase the metabolism of digitoxin.
6. Oral hypoglycemic requirements can be increased by drugs that produce hyperglycemia, such as calcium channel blockers, corticosteroids, estrogens, isoniazid, nicotinic acid, phenothiazines, phenytoin, sympathomimetics, thiazide diuretics, and thyroid drugs.
7. Rifampin may stimulate the hepatic metabolism of tolbutamide and chlorpropamide, reducing their effectiveness.

■ Nursing Process

Many similarities exist between nursing care for the diabetic taking oral hypoglycemics and one taking insulin. Thorough assessment of cognitive and psychomotor skills is essential because the patient must learn about diabetes and the relationship between diet, exercise, stress, or illness and drug therapy. The patient may need to learn SBGM and urine testing to monitor the effect of the oral hypoglycemic on blood sugar and urine. Assessment of support systems is also essential because episodes of hypoglycemia may occur. A sick-day regimen must be learned because changed metabolic needs from infection may change drug needs. (See box entitled Guidelines for Sick Days for Diabetics.) The reader is referred to the section on insulin for a detailed discussion of these topics.

□ ASSESSMENT

□ Subjective Data

A newly diagnosed type II diabetic may tend to deny the permanent nature of his illness because symptoms are not severe and therapy may, initially, be aimed at diet therapy. The patient may perceive the addition of an oral hypoglycemic either as a sign of failure on his part or as a crutch which will free him from having to worry about what he eats. Therefore, the nurse needs to explore these perceptions to determine whether the patient truly understands the disease and his role in managing it. Only when some degree of acceptance has been established is the patient ready to learn a diabetic regimen. Support systems can be very influential in establishing an accepting environment, but the patient must take responsibility for his care.

A thorough drug history should also be obtained. It must be determined if the patient is taking any other drugs that could interact with oral hypoglycemic agents (OHA) (see under Interactions). The patient should be asked about alcohol use, which may produce a severe disulfiram reaction in combination with OHA; demonstrated allergies to sulfa drugs may react to oral hypoglycemics.

□ Objective Data

Laboratory data will be collected before an oral hypoglycemic is started. Fasting blood sugar will be obtained, usually in a series to determine the severity of the disease. Hepatic and renal function studies will be performed because evidence of kidney or liver dysfunction may contraindicate drug use.

□ NURSING DIAGNOSES

The *actual* nursing diagnosis is:

Knowledge deficit related to the drug's action, administration, and side-effects; the relationship between drug, diet, and exercise; symptoms of hyper- and

(Text continues on p. 1040.)

Table 54-4
Oral Antidiabetic Drugs

Drug	Preparations	Usual Dosage Range	Clinical Considerations
acetohexamide (Dymelor)	Tablets–250 mg, 500 mg	250 mg to 1500 mg/day in a single dose of two divided doses if over 1000 mg/day	Intermediate acting drug (duration 12 h–24 h); possesses significant uricosuric activity at therapeutic doses; metabolized to active intermediate by the liver (two and one-half times as potent as parent compound); use with caution in renal insufficiency because action of metabolite may be significantly prolonged
chlorpropamide (Diabinese)	Tablets—100 mg, 250 mg	Initially 250 mg/day (100 mg to 125 mg/day in older patients); maintenance 100 mg to 500 mg/day (usual 250 mg/day) depending on condition	Longest acting oral antidiabetic drug (duration up to 60 h); more potent and generally more toxic than other oral drugs; also indicated for treatment of polyuria of diabetes insipidus; may enhance effects of antidiuretic hormone (ADH); give as a single morning dose, with food, to minimize GI upset; if hypoglycemia occurs, give frequent feedings or glucose for at least 3 days to 5 days, because drug is very long acting, and observe patient closely during this time
glipizide (Glucotrol)	Tablets—5 mg, 10 mg	Initially, 5 mg before breakfast; increase in 2.5-mg to 5-mg increments every 7 days until optimal response; maximum daily dose is 40 mg	Peak plasma concentrations occur in 1 h–3 h; serum half-life is 2 h–4 h but blood sugar control persists for up to 24 h; liver metabolism is rapid and extensive; daily doses greater than 15 mg should be divided and given before meals; reduce dosage in elderly, debilitated, or malnourished persons, and in the presence of impaired *(continued)*

Table 54-4 (continued)
Oral Antidiabetic Drugs

Drug	Preparations	Usual Dosage Range	Clinical Considerations
glipizide (Glucotrol) (continued)			renal or hepatic function; may elicit a mild diuresis.
glyburide (DiaBeta, Micronase)	Tablets—1.25 mg, 2.5 mg 5 mg	Initially 2.5 mg to 5 mg before breakfast; usual maintenance dose ranges from 1.25 mg to 20 mg daily in a single dose or two divided doses; maximum daily dose is 20 mg	Peak plasma levels are attained within 4 h, and effects persist for at least 24 h. Serum half-life is approximately 10 h. Excreted in the bile and urine, 50% by each route; thus, can be used in patients with renal impairment with greater safety than other oral antidiabetics; use is associated with a higher incidence of hypoglycemia than most other sulfonylureas due to its long half-life.
tolazamide (Ronase, Tolamide, Tolinase)	Tablets—100 mg, 250 mg, 500 mg	Initially 100 mg to 250 mg/ day in a single dose depending on fasting blood sugar; maintenance 100 mg to 500 mg/day	Intermediate-acting drug (duration 10 h–14 h); may be effective in patients who do not respond to other sulfonylureas or in some patients with a history of ketoacidosis or coma; converted to several weakly active metabolites by the liver
tolbutamide (Orinase, Oramide)	Tablets—250 mg, 500 mg Vials (Sodium Salt)—1 g with diluent	Initially 1 g to 2 g/day orally; Maintenance 0.25 g to 2 g/day, usually in divided doses IV—1 g given over 2 min–3 min	Short-acting drug (duration 6 h–12 h); mildly goitrogenic at high doses and may reduce radioactive iodide uptake after prolonged administration without producing clinical hypothyroidism; rapidly metabolized to inactive metabolites; useful in patients with kidney disease; Orinase IV is used to diagnose islet cell adenoma (see Chap. 80); in presence of tumor, there is a rapid, marked drop in blood glucose which persists for up to 3 h; IV injection may produce local irritation or thrombophlebitis

hypoglycemia and appropriate management; urine or SBGM testing; and sick-day regimens

Potential nursing diagnoses may include:

Alteration in comfort related to nausea, heartburn, or headache, drug side-effects

Impaired skin integrity related to photosensitivity or hypersensitivity reactions

☐ PLAN

Nursing care goals must be very realistic. The patient receiving oral hypoglycemics may be diagnosed and treated completely as an outpatient. Therefore, patient teaching will take place over an extended period of time and include multiple care givers. The patient may be referred to a diabetic teaching program through a local hospital or community health center. He may be followed by an office nurse, a community health nurse, or an industrial nurse in addition to his physician. These people need to coordinate a teaching plan to decrease confusion and repetition. Immediate, intermediate, and long-range goals may be established as discussed in the section Insulins. The main goals should focus on helping the patient learn to administer the drug correctly; how drug taking, diet, and exercise are related; common side-effects to watch for; how to recognize hypoglycemia and what to do if it occurs, and how and when to seek medical attention.

☐ INTERVENTION

The most important point to emphasize when teaching a patient how to take an oral hypoglycemic is the need to eat on a regular schedule. In fact, before the decision is made on whether to treat a patient with a long-acting or a short-acting agent, a 24-hour diet recall should be collected. If a patient eats regularly scheduled, balanced meals he may do well with a long-acting drug. If he eats more sporadically, tends to eat small portions, or skips meals, he may do better with a short-acting drug several times a day. The outcome sought is to achieve some measure of control without having the patient develop a hypoglycemic reaction. Focus attention on helping the patient establish a realistic routine and show him how it can be safely altered. Use of nutritious snacks when a full meal is not possible and incorporation of exercise in the daily regimen can help the patient have more control.

Oral hypoglycemics can occasionally produce side-effects. The ones to mention when teaching the patient about the drug are gastrointestinal upset, photosensitivity, hypersensitivity, lack of adequate control, and, most important, hypoglycemia.

The patient can avoid GI upset by taking the drug with meals or with a glass of milk. Photosensitivity varies among patients. The patient should be encouraged to extend time in the sun very gradually and to avoid direct sun if rash, heat sensitivity, or eye irritation occurs. Hypersensitivity reactions are very rare but should be reported immediately. Symptoms include itching, rash, fever, sore throat, diarrhea, and vomiting. Due to the long-acting nature of many of the drugs, hypersensitivity may not manifest itself until several days after the drug has been started. Therefore, the patient using a new compound should be closely monitored for at least a week, and dosage adjustments should be made slowly.

Hypoglycemia and lack of adequate control are at opposite poles on the spectrum of reactions to the drug, but are essential to watch for. The long-acting nature of the drugs means that when hypoglycemia occurs it may last for days. Teach the patient to recognize the common symptoms (see under Side-Effects/Adverse Reactions) and to carry some form of soluble glucose such as candy, sweetened juice, or glucagon. If symptoms do not subside 30 minutes after ingestion of the glucose source, the patient should seek medical attention immediately because drug dose may have been too high. Treatment of a hypoglycemic reaction may take several days of extra carbohydrates and simple sugars and a change in drug therapy. It is best accomplished under direct supervision with the health team.

The patient should be taught to be alert also for lack of control with oral hypoglycemia, which will be manifested by signs of hyperglycemia. Symptoms include consistent elevation of blood glucose levels, thirst, polyuria, flushing, fatigue, weight loss, fruity odor on breath, and urine ketones. The patient should contact his health resources immediately if these symptoms develop.

☐ EVALUATION

Many of the outcome criteria listed in the insulin section also apply here. Patient outcomes sought include euglycemia, evidenced by blood glucose levels between 60 mg and 120 mg/dl; ability to verbalize and appropriately demonstrate knowledge of the relation between drug therapy, diet, exercise and stress; ability to verbalize knowledge of and to manage side-effects, including gastrointestinal distress, photosensitivity, hypersensitivity, and hypoglycemia; ability to recognize and report any evidence of lack of control from drug therapy; ability to perform SBGM and urine testing when appropriate and to know and be able to initiate an appropriate sick-day regimen. Nursing Care Plan 54-2 summarizes the nursing process for the patient receiving an oral hypoglycemic agent.

Hyperglycemic Agents

Although the most rapid and effective means of elevating the blood glucose level in cases of marked hypoglycemia is direct IV injection of glucose, this method is not always available or feasible. Alternatives include the oral administration of *glucose* as a gel or chewable tablet, or diazoxide, a thiazide-like drug which inhibits release of insulin from the pancreas and is used in the management of hypoglycemia due to hyperinsulinism. In addition, parenteral use of glucagon, a polypeptide produced by pancreatic alpha cells, can increase conversion of glycogen to glucose in the liver and stimulate hepatic gluconeogenesis, thus increasing blood glucose levels.

Most drug-induced hypoglycemic episodes are mild and, if detected in the early stages, generally can be reversed by oral ingestion of some form of glucose (such as candy, soda, sweetened orange juice). However, in those instances in which the hypoglycemic response is severe (*e.g.*, insulin shock), is prolonged (when symptoms persist longer than 30 minutes), or fails to respond to oral consumption of glucose, the use of IV glucose or glucagon is indicated.

Glucose

(B-D Glucose, Glutose, Insta-Glucose, Monoject)

Symptoms of mild hypoglycemic reactions can often be controlled by the oral use of glucose as either chewable tablets or a 40% liquid gel-like solution. Glucose is rapidly absorbed from the GI tract, and a rapid increase (*i.e.*, 5 minutes–10 minutes) in blood glucose concentration occurs following oral administration. The recommended dose is 10 g to 20 g, which may be repeated in 10 minutes if consciousness is not regained.

Glucose is *not* absorbed from the buccal cavity and must be swallowed to be effective. Thus, whenever possible, other drugs should be employed to treat hypoglycemia in the *unconscious* patient, because the swallowing reflex does not always occur, and the absence of the normal gag reflex can lead to aspiration. Occasional reports of nausea have appeared, but the drug is virtually nontoxic when taken as directed. It is not recommended in children under 2 years of age.

Glucagon

(Glucagon)

Glucagon is a polypeptide hormone secreted by the alpha cells of the islets of Langerhans. Purified glucagon may be administered SC or IM to counteract severe hypoglycemic episodes when the IV administration of glucose is not feasible. For example, members of a diabetic's family may be taught to give a dose of glucagon IM or SC while awaiting emergency assistance for a hypoglycemic episode, whereas IV administration in such a situation is hazardous. Glucagon is of benefit in treating hypoglycemia providing liver glycogen is available; it is of little value in states of starvation, *chronic* hypoglycemia, or adrenal insufficiency. The response to glucagon in *juvenile* diabetes is generally less dramatic, and supplementary carbohydrates are usually required.

MECHANISM AND ACTIONS
Glucagon accelerates synthesis of cyclic AMP, thus increasing phosphorylase activity resulting in glycogenolysis and increased blood glucose levels. It also inhibits glycogen synthetase, promotes uptake of amino acids into liver, and stimulates hepatic gluconeogenesis. Hepatic and adipose tissue lipolysis is enhanced, supplying free fatty acids and glycerol, which further stimulates gluconeogenesis and ketogenesis. Glucagon also relaxes GI smooth muscle and increases the rate and force of contraction of the heart.

USES
1. Treatment of severe drug-induced hypoglycemic reactions in diabetic patients or persons undergoing insulin shock therapy (minimal effectiveness in states of starvation, adrenal insufficiency, or chronic hypoglycemia)
2. Production of GI hypotonia as an aid for diagnostic radiologic examination of stomach, duodenum, small intestine, or colon
3. Investigational uses include treatment of beta-blocker overdosage and GI spasm.

ADMINISTRATION AND DOSAGE
Glucagon is available as powder for injection containing 1 mg (1 unit) or 10 mg (10 units) per vial. Recommended doses are:

(Text continues on p. 1044.)

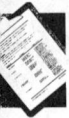

Nursing Care Plan 54-2
The Patient Receiving Oral Hypoglycemic Agents (OHAs)

Assessment

Subjective Data

1. Medication history: see Interactions section to formulate appropriate questions.
   a. Ask about use of alcohol and street drugs.
   b. If patient uses oral contraceptives encourage an alternate method of contraception.
   c. Ask about allergies/hypersensitivity to sulfa drugs.
2. Medical history
   a. Progression of symptoms leading to need for OHA. Type II diabetes mellitus may first be treated with diet and excrcise.
   b. Pre-existing conditions that may alter the drug dosage requirement or require cautious use such as hepatic or renal dysfunction, cardiac disease, adrenal or thyroid disorders
   c. Presence of fever, infection, trauma, or increased stress
   d. Pregnancy or lactation
3. Personal history/compliance issues
   a. Cognitive understanding of disease process and drug effect, ability to manage self-care.
   b. Personal, financial resources; supportive network

Objective Data

1. Physical assessment
   a. Neurologic status: memory, mental acuity, psychomotor function, vision
   b. Cardiovascular status: heart rate, blood pressure, peripheral pulses, presence of edema
   c. Renal function: urine output, weight
   d. Hepatic: liver size
2. Laboratory data
   a. Serial fasting blood glucose levels
   b. Hepatic and renal function studies

Nursing Diagnosis	Expected Client Outcome	Intervention
Knowledge deficit related to the relationship between the disease, drug, diet, and exercise; correct drug taking; symptoms of and appropriate responses to hypo- and hyperglycemia; use of a sick-day regimen; testing of urine glucose or SBGM, potentially dangerous drug interactions	Will verbalize an understanding of the relationship between drug therapy, diet, and exercise in managing diabetes	Teach the patient the importance of correct drug taking, diet, and exercise in managing diabetes, what the drug can and cannot do, and the importance of consistent monitoring of potential side-effects and follow-up care.
	Blood glucose levels will remain within normal limits (or prescribed goal)	Emphasize correct drug-taking techniques. OHAs should be taken at the same time every day. Meals must be eaten on a regular schedule, but snacks, if nutritious, can be used when a meal must be missed.
	Will verbalize causes, symptoms, and actions to take for hypo- and hyperglycemia	Teach the symptoms of hypo- and hyperglycemia, relating them to symptoms the patient has already had.
		Be aware that long-acting OHAs may cause hypoglycemia for days; therefore, the patient must seek care.
		Encourage patient to carry a rapid-acting glucose source at all times.
	Will enact a sick-day routine when appropriate and seek help as necessary	Teach the patient the importance of establishing a sick-day routine (see box entitled Guidelines for Sick Days for Diabetics).

(continued)

Nursing Diagnosis	Expected Client Outcome	Intervention
Knowledge deficit related to the relationship between the disease, drug, diet, and exercise; correct drug taking; symptoms of and appropriate responses to hypo- and hyperglycemia; use of a sick-day regimen; testing of urine glucose or SBGM, potentially dangerous drug interactions (continued)		Identify what constitutes a sick day for a diabetic, what actions to take, and when to seek help.
		Teach self-injection of insulin, if appropriate, for use during times of illness or other increased stress.
	Will demonstrate urine glucose or SBGM testing	Teach patient to monitor blood or urine glucose regularly as prescribed to identify early any changes in glucose utilization by the body.
	Verbalizes knowledge of dangerous drug interactions	Emphasize the adverse effects that can occur if the patient ingests alcohol.
		Make a list of drugs to avoid. Encourage the patient not to take any new drug without seeking the advice of the primary health care provider.
	Will wear a Medic-alert appliance	Stress the importance of telling any health-care provider that the patient is diabetic and takes OHAs.
		Encourage patient to obtain and wear a Medic-alert device in case of emergency.
	Will keep appointments for follow-up care and report symptoms of side-effects early	Encourage patient to make follow-up appointments to monitor blood glucose levels, hepatic function, and progress in managing the regimen.
		Encourage patient to report immediately jaundice, fever, dark urine, bleeding, or light-colored stools—symptoms of hepatic problems.
		Teach patient to report and manage common side-effects as described below.
Potential alteration in comfort: headache, nausea, heart burn, related to drug side-effects	Will learn management of minor side-effects and when to report problems	Encourage patient to take drug with milk if GI distress occurs.
		Teach patient to use mild analgesics for headache.
		Encourage early reporting of persistent symptoms.
Potential alteration in skin integrity related to photosensitivity or hypersensitivity reactions	Will maintain intact skin surface	Encourage patient to obtain sun exposure very gradually if at all, to avoid sun in midday, and to use sunscreens and protective clothing as much as possible. If rash occurs, patient should avoid exposure.
		If a patient is beginning OHAs for the first time or if a new compound is being tried, close monitoring is essential for hypersensitivity to the drug.
		Teach the patient to report immediately any itching, rash, fever, sore throat, diarrhea, or vomiting—early symptoms of hypersensitivity.

Hypoglycemia: 0.5 mg to 1 mg SC, IM, or IV; repeat once or twice at 10-minute to 20-minute intervals if no response has occurred. If patient still fails to respond, give glucose IV to prevent cerebral hypoglycemia. Once patient has responded, supplemental carbohydrate is administered to restore liver glycogen and prevent secondary hypoglycemia.

Insulin shock therapy: 0.5 mg to 1 mg SC, IM, or IV, after 1 hour of coma; if no response within 15 minutes to 25 minutes, repeat. In very deep coma, IV glucose can be given concurrently.

Diagnostic aid: 0.25 mg to 2 mg IV or IM, depending on the onset and duration of action desired. Onset is within 1 minute IV and 5 minutes to 10 minutes IM. Duration of effect is largely dose-dependent.

Glucagon added to IV drug tubing is incompatible with solutions of sodium, potassium, or calcium chloride; it is compatible, however, with dextrose solutions.

FATE
Consciousness is restored within 5 minutes to 20 minutes after injection of glucagon. The plasma half-life is 3 minutes to 6 minutes. The drug is degraded by the liver and kidney, as well as in the plasma and at tissue receptor sites.

SIDE-EFFECTS/ADVERSE REACTIONS
Adverse effects with glucagon are rare. Occasional nausea and vomiting have occurred, but these effects are also seen with hypoglycemia. Hypokalemia can occur in large doses.

CONTRAINDICATIONS AND PRECAUTIONS
There are no absolute contraindications to glucagon. The drug must be given with *caution* to patients with a history of insulinoma (may result in *hypo*glycemia due to insulin release) or pheochromocytoma (may stimulate catecholamine release leading to increased blood pressure). Cautious use is also necessary in pregnant women or nursing mothers.

INTERACTIONS
1. Glucagon may potentiate the action of oral anticoagulants.

NURSING CONSIDERATIONS FOR GLUCOSE AND GLUCAGON
Nursing care is aimed at two levels with these drugs. The first is patient/family teaching of appropriate home use and the second is safe intravenous management during emergency situations.

The patient and his support system must know the symptoms of hypoglycemia and how and when to take action. At the first sign of hypoglycemia, the patient should try to take an oral glucose source. If that does not work within 15 minutes, if the patient vomits, or if symptoms worsen, then the support person should know how to give an IM or SC injection of glucagon and seek emergency assistance. The most glucagon the support person should give is two doses. Hopefully, emergency help will reach them before this so an intravenous line can be inserted.

Glucagon and glucose are given intravenously once oral ingestion is ineffective or no longer safe. The nurse should maintain seizure precautions, obtain blood glucose levels, and monitor vital signs and respiration. The swallow reflex is lost when the patient becomes unconscious so aspiration is possible and tracheal suctioning equipment should be available.

If the patient does not respond to glucose or glucagon within 20 minutes of infusion, there may be cause for loss of consciousness other than hypoglycemia, and a thorough work-up should be completed. It is not appropriate to continue giving the drug when no evidence of response occurs either through blood glucose changes or changes in level of consciousness.

Diazoxide, Oral
(Proglycem)

Diazoxide is a structural analogue of the thiazide diuretics which is available orally for the management of persistent hypoglycemia due to hyperinsulinism. It is also available for IV injection as Hyperstat for treating hypertensive emergencies (see Chap. 35).

MECHANISM AND ACTIONS
Diazoxide produces a prompt increase in blood glucose by inhibiting release of insulin from the pancreas and possibly by increasing glycogen synthesis. The hyperglycemic effects are potentiated by hypokalemia. Other actions of diazoxide are decreased sodium, chloride, and water excretion, increased serum uric acid, and increased serum free fatty acids. Blood pressure is relatively unchanged with oral diazoxide in recommended doses; conversely, IV diazoxide elicits a rapid, marked drop in blood pressure due to a direct relaxant effect on vascular smooth muscle.

USES

1. Management of hypoglycemia due to hyperinsulinism (*e.g.*, islet cell proliferation, hyperplasia, or carcinoma; extrapancreatic malignancy; leucine sensitivity) where other medical or surgical treatment is ineffective or inappropriate

ADMINISTRATION AND DOSAGE

Orally, diazoxide is used as either capsules (50 mg) or an oral suspension (50 mg/ml). It is also available for IV injection as a solution containing 300 mg/20 ml. (See Chap. 35.) The initial oral dose in adults and children is 3 mg to 8 mg/kg/day in two or three divided doses every 8 hours to 12 hours. The starting dose in an average adult is approximately 200 mg/day. Infants and newborns should receive 8 mg to 15 mg/kg/day in two to three divided doses every 8 hours to 12 hours.

FATE

The hyperglycemic effect of oral diazoxide begins in approximately 1 hour and persists from 6 hours to 8 hours. The drug is extensively bound to plasma proteins (90%), and the plasma half-life in adults is 24 hours to 36 hours (shorter in younger children). Half-life is prolonged in patients with impaired renal function because diazoxide is excreted by the kidneys.

SIDE-EFFECTS/ADVERSE REACTIONS

The most common side-effects with oral diazoxide are sodium and fluid retention (which may precipitate congestive heart failure in patients with decreased cardiac reserve), GI distress (nausea, diarrhea, abdominal pain, vomiting, ileus), tachycardia, palpitations, loss of taste, increased serum uric acid, headache, weakness, skin rash, hirsutism, and thrombocytopenia (may require discontinuation of the drug).

Other untoward reactions noted during diazoxide therapy include:

Cardiovascular—Hypotension, chest pain
CNS—Anxiety, dizziness, insomnia, extrapyramidal symptoms
Hematologic—Thrombocytopenia, neutropenia, eosinophilia, excessive bleeding, decreased hemoglobin
Ocular—Transient cataracts, subconjunctival bleeding, blurred vision, scotoma, lacrimation
Hepatic/renal—Azotemia, hematuria, proteinuria, decreased urinary output, nephrotic syndrome, increased alkaline phosphatase and SGOT
Other—Fever, lymphadenopathy, pancreatitis, galactorrhea, gout, dermatitis, pruritus, herpes, loss of scalp hair, paresthesias, hyperglycemia, glycosuria, ketoacidosis

Overdosage is characterized by marked hyperglycemia which may be associated with ketoacidosis. Treatment includes prompt administration of insulin and restoration of fluid and electrolyte balance.

CONTRAINDICATIONS AND PRECAUTIONS

Diazoxide, oral, is contraindicated in the presence of functional hypoglycemia and in persons sensitive to thiazide or sulfonamide drugs. The drug should be used *cautiously* in pregnant women and in patients with diabetes, impaired cardiac or cerebral circulation, compromised cardiac reserve, gout, renal dysfunction, and hypertension.

INTERACTIONS

1. The hypotensive effects of diazoxide may be intensified by antihypertensives and diuretics.
2. Thiazides may potentiate the hyperglycemic and hyperuricemic action of diazoxide.
3. The effects of diazoxide may be enhanced by other protein-bound drugs (*e.g.*, anti-inflammatory agents, anticoagulants, barbiturates, phenytoin, sulfonamides).
4. Chlorpromazine can strongly potentiate the hyperglycemic effect of diazoxide.
5. The inhibition of insulin release by diazoxide is antagonized by alpha-adrenergic blocking agents.
6. Concurrent use of diazoxide and sulfonylurea antidiabetic drugs may result in reduced effects of both drugs.
7. Diazoxide may decrease the effects of phenytoin by increasing its hepatic metabolism.

NURSING CONSIDERATIONS

Oral use of this drug for unusual cases of hypoglycemia requires careful history taking and close monitoring and supervision. A medication history is essential because diazoxide interacts with many drugs, most notably, diuretics (see under Interactions) which could lead to multiple problems. Medical history taking should determine whether the patient has congestive heart failure or gout, both of which warrant cautious use of the drug.

Diazoxide is most frequently used preoperatively to restore euglycemia before the source of the problem, usually a tumor, is removed. Therefore, the nurse should establish a flow sheet and obtain frequent blood glucose and urine ketone levels. These should be recorded with the drug dose. Dosage may have to be altered if hyperglycemia or urine ketones occur. Serum electrolyte levels should also be obtained regularly to monitor renal function and intake/output ratios should be closely watched. If evidence of fluid retention occurs diuretic therapy may be necessary.

Patients at risk for the onset of congestive heart failure should be monitored for increasing weight, shortness of breath, and peripheral edema. Sodium and fluid retention are most common in young infants.

Side-effects from diazoxide are unpleasant, but most GI effects such as anorexia, nausea, vomiting, and diarrhea disappear when the drug is withdrawn. Transient cataracts have been reported; therefore, the patient should report any changes in vision. Hematologic, hepatic, and renal changes can be monitored by frequent blood studies of CBC with differential, liver enzymes, bilirubin, serum creatinine, BUN, and uric acid. Hirsutism, which occurs more frequently in women and children, will subside when the drug is withdrawn.

If the patient will take the drug at home, he must receive instruction on urine testing of glucose and ketones to monitor drug effectiveness. Daily weights may also be advised if fluid retention is a potential problem.

Some individuals show higher diazoxide blood levels with the liquid than with the capsule formulation of the drug. Caution should be used when changing formulations because the incidence of side-effects may increase. If diazoxide does not adequately reduce serum glucose after 2 weeks to 3 weeks, therapy should be discontinued.

CASE STUDY

Diabetes Mellitus

Marjory Williams, a 65-year-old woman, was brought to a clinic by her grandson with an open lesion of the left foot. She said she had been nursing it at home for several weeks. Upon examination, the physician found three toes affected with gangrene and a wound that was draining and foul smelling. Mrs. Williams said she knew it was serious when her toes changed color. She also complained of recent weight loss, nausea, thirst, and dizziness which she thought was related to her infected foot.

Mrs. Williams was admitted with suspected diabetic gangrene of the left foot. Fasting blood glucose level was 240 mg/dl. She was started on NPH insulin 20 U before breakfast and regular insulin 8 U at 4 PM. daily. Plans were made for surgery.

Surgery was done 3 days later with a partial amputation of the left foot. In the postoperative period, Mrs. Williams learned crutch walking and began to learn about diabetes and her care.

Mrs. Williams lived in an urban community, was widowed, and had been raising her five grandchildren for 6 years since their mother was killed in an auto accident. The children ranged in age from 10 years to 18 years old. In addition to daily visits by these children, others also came frequently. Mrs. Williams had apparently been a foster parent to ten other children over the past 20 years, all of whom kept in touch with her. Her only financial resources were her Social Security and the benefits her grandchildren received. She was also eligible for Medicare. But her people resources were great. In addition to her grandchildren, she had the support of many neighbors and friends from church.

As the nurse began planning a teaching program for Mrs. Williams, she discovered the woman had never been taught to read. In addition, the patient complained of needing glasses and admitted to occasional blurred vision. Eye examination revealed some diabetic changes in the retina.

Discussion Questions

1. Given the known variables from this study, list the strengths and weaknesses for this patient in terms of learning insulin administration and diabetic care.
2. What other factors should the nurse try to find out about this patient?
3. Outline a basic teaching plan for teaching Mrs. Williams self-injection of insulin.

REVIEW QUESTIONS

1. Name the four types of pancreatic secretory cells and their respective products.
2. What are the major actions of (a) glucagon and (b) insulin in the body?
3. What is the role of somatostatin in the secretion of pancreatic hormones?
4. List several causes of fasting hypoglycemia.
5. Distinguish between type I and type II diabetes mellitus.
6. Discuss the various measures that may be employed in treating noninsulin-dependent diabetes.
7. How does "human" insulin differ from "pork" insulin in structure and mode of preparation?
8. What are the advantages of newer "purified" insulins over older insulins?
9. How are insulin preparations modified to alter their duration of action?
10. List the different types of insulins and their synonyms.
11. How is assessment of cognitive and psychomotor skills and support systems used to teach the diabetic about insulin therapy?
12. What factors must be considered before teaching a patient self-injection of insulin?
13. Why does a diabetic on insulin need a readily available support system?
14. What are some realistic nursing goals for the newly diagnosed insulin-dependent diabetic?
15. Outline a self-injection teaching program for a child with diabetes.
16. How should the health team determine whether a patient is a good candidate for an insulin pump?
17. Outline the steps a patient should take to determine insulin dosage adjustments.
18. What symptoms of hypoglycemia should the patient be taught? What actions should he take? What should the support person know?
19. What is a sick-day regimen for diabetes?
20. List some outcome criteria to evaluate the effectiveness of insulin on a patient who has been taking the drug for 6 weeks.

21. How do the oral antidiabetic drugs act?
22. What are the principal contraindications to use of oral antidiabetic drugs?
23. How are the perceptions of a noninsulin-dependent diabetic different from those of the patient who takes insulin?
24. What side-effects of oral hypoglycemics must the patient learn when he takes them?
25. List the various drugs that can be used to elevate blood glucose levels.
26. Why shouldn't oral glucose be given to an unconscious patient?
27. Outline a brief teaching plan for a patient and his support person on using glucagon to control hypoglycemia.
28. What information should be recorded on a flow sheet for monitoring diazoxide therapy?

BIBLIOGRAPHY

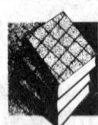

Baker DE, Campbell RK: The second generation sulfonylureas: Glipizide and glyburide. Diabetes Educator 11(3):29, 1985

Dillon R: Improved serum profiles in diabetic individuals who massage their insulin injection sites. Diabetes Care 6:399, 1983

Donohue-Porter P: Insulin dependent diabetes mellitus. Nurs Clin North Am 20:191, 1985

Dupre J: Insulin therapy: Progress and prospects. Hosp Pract 18:171, 1983

Eisenbarth GS: Type I diabetes mellitus: A chronic autoimmune disease. N Engl J Med 314:1360, 1986

Essig M: Oral antidiabetic drugs. Nursing 83 13:59, 1983

Flavin K, Haire-Joshu D: Drugs for diabetes: The pharmacologic repertoire. Am J Nurs 86:1244, 1986

Flier JS: Insulin receptors and insulin resistance. Ann Rev Med 34:145, 1983

Guthrie D, Guthrie R: Nursing Management of Diabetes Mellitus, 2nd ed. St. Louis, CV Mosby, 1982

Haire-Joshu D, Flavin K, Santiago JV: Intensive conventional insulin therapy. Am J Nurs 86:1251, 1986

Home PD, Alberti KG: Human insulin. Clin Endocrinol Metab 11:453, 1982

Jacobs S, Cuatrecasas P: Insulin receptors. Ann Rev Pharmacol Toxicol 23:461, 1983

McCall AL: How drugs work: The new human insulins. Mod Medicine 53(9):112, 1985

Peden N, Newton RW, Feely J: Oral hypoglycemic agents. Br Med J 286:1564, 1983

Price MJ: Insulin and oral hypoglycemic agents. Nurs Clin North Am 18:687, 1983

Salans LB: Diabetes mellitus: A disease that is coming into focus. JAMA 247:590, 1982

Seltzer HS: Efficacy and safety of oral hypoglycemic agents. Am Rev Med 31:261, 1980

Turner JG, Lancaster J: Multiple use of disposable syringe units by insulin-dependent diabetes. Diabetes Educator 10(3):38, 1984

Adrenocortical Steroids

55

The adrenal gland plays a critical role in bodily functions. Its secretory products, primarily in the form of their synthetic derivatives, are also used clinically in a variety of disorders. In order to understand the action of the adrenal hormones better, a discussion of the adrenal gland and adrenal gland disorders will be presented.

Adrenal Glands

The adrenal (suprarenal) glands are paired, yellowish masses of tissue situated at the superior pole of each kidney (Fig. 55-1). Each gland consists of two distinct entities—an outer adrenal cortex and an inner adrenal medulla—that differ in embryologic origin, character, and function.

Adrenal Medulla

The adrenal medulla develops from the embryonic ectoderm. It remains functionally associated with the sympathetic nervous system, being essentially a modified sympathetic ganglion whose postganglionic neurons have lost their axons and become secretory.

Histologically, the adrenal medulla contains large, ovoid cells arranged in clumps or irregular cords around numerous blood vessels. The medullary cells, often termed *chromaffin cells* because their granules possess affinity for chromium salts, secrete the catecholamine hormones epinephrine (adrenalin) and norepinephrine (noradrenalin). The *principal* secretory product is epinephrine, with norepinephrine normally accounting for only 20% of the total secretion.

Adrenal medullary secretion of the catecholamines is physiologically controlled by the posterior hypothalamus. The hormones are stored in cellular granules, bound to adenosine triphosphate (ATP) and protein, and are released in response to the following stimuli: sympathetic nervous system activation, hypoglycemia, pain, hypoxia, hypotension, cold, emotional stress, acetylcholine, histamine, and nicotine.

Epinephrine and norepinephrine are rapidly metabolized to inactive products, principally by the liver and kidneys. Major products of biodegradation include metanephrine, normetanephrine, and vanillylmandelic acid (VMA). These appear in the urine and may be assayed during the course of clinical diagnosis.

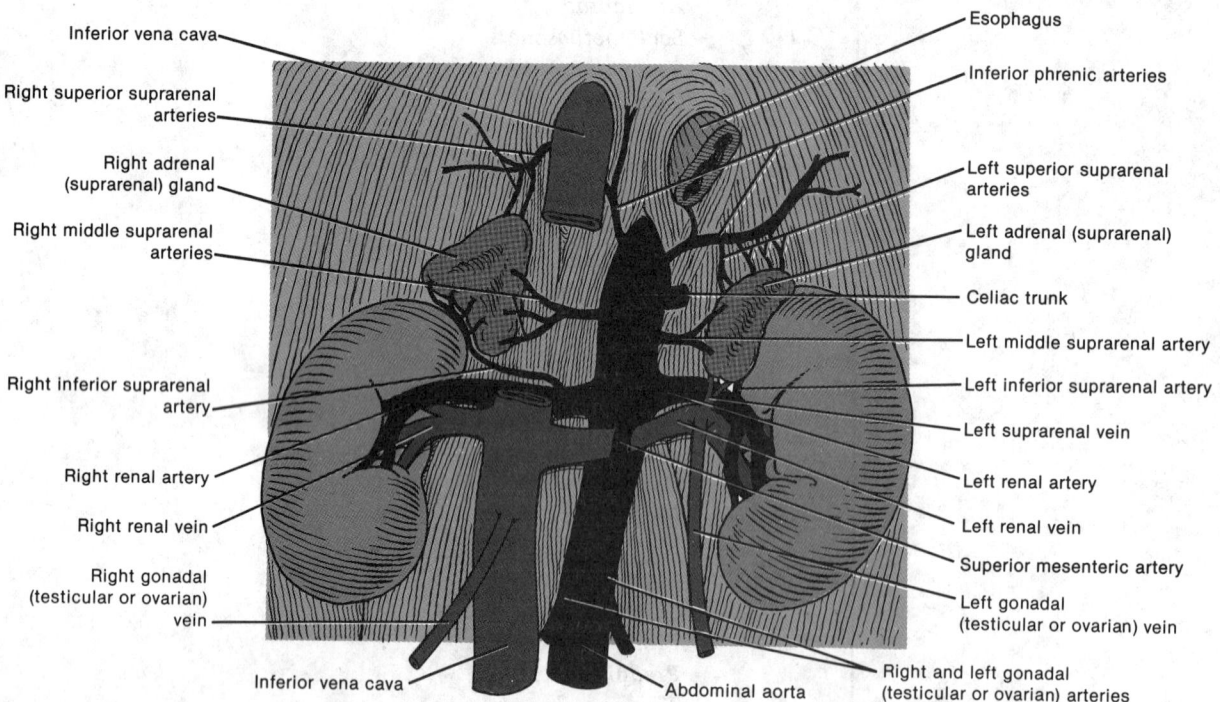

Figure 55-1. *Location of the adrenal glands. (Tortora GJ, Anagnostakos NP: Principles of Anatomy and Physiology, 5th ed, p 419. New York, Harper & Row, 1987)*

ACTIONS OF ADRENAL MEDULLARY HORMONES

Epinephrine and norepinephrine mimic the effects of sympathetic nerve discharge, producing the following effects:

1. Direct increase in cardiac rate and myocardial force of contraction
2. Elevation of blood pressure
3. Dilation of coronary and skeletal muscle blood vessels
4. Constriction of the cutaneous and visceral vasculature
5. Relaxation of respiratory smooth muscle
6. Inhibition of gastrointestinal (GI) motility
7. Pupillary dilation (mydriasis)
8. Glycogenolysis in liver and muscle
9. Lipolysis

The cardiac excitatory effects and the metabolic actions of lipolysis and glycogenolysis are mediated by cyclic AMP, the latter involving the activation of phosphorylase enzyme by protein kinase.

The catecholamines also elevate the metabolic rate (calorigenic action), stimulate the central nervous system, increase alertness, and stimulate respiration. The pharmacologic application of epinephrine and norepinephrine is presented in Chapter 15.

CLINICAL DISORDERS

Adrenal medullary function is not essential to life; therefore, *hypo*secretion of adrenal medullary hormones does not constitute a recognized clinical entity.

Pheochromocytoma

Pheochromocytoma is a chromaffin-cell tumor of the sympathoadrenal system, most commonly involving one of the adrenal glands or both (see Disease Brief in Chapter 16). It is characterized by hypersecretion of the catecholamines epinephrine and norepinephrine, the latter usually dominating. Clinical manifestations of pheochromocytoma include paroxysmal or persistent hypertension, severe headaches, tachycardia, profuse sweating, epigastric pain, nausea, irritability, and dyspnea. Metabolic signs of this disorder include fasting hyperglycemia, increased basal metabolic rate, weight loss, and elevated levels of urinary catecholamines or their metabolites. Treatment of pheochromocytoma may be accomplished with alpha-adrenergic blocking agents (Chap. 16) or metyrosine (Chap. 35), although the condition frequently requires surgery.

Adrenal Cortex

The adrenal cortex develops from the mesoderm during embryonic life. The cells of the adrenal cortex, which are arranged in continuous cords separated by capillaries, are characterized by an abundance of mitochondria, endoplasmic reticulum, and accumulation of lipid.

Adrenal cortical tissue is structurally arranged into three concentric regions or zones: a thin outer *zona glomerulosa*, a thick middle *zona fasciculata*, and an inner *zona reticularis* bordering on the adrenal medulla.

Chemically, the steroid hormones of the adrenal cortex, the adrenocorticoids, are all derivatives of cholesterol. The adrenocorticoid hormones are usually divided into three functional groups: the mineralocorticoids, such as aldosterone, which regulate electrolyte and water balance; the glucocorticoids, such as cortisol (hydrocortisone), which affect carbohydrate, protein, and fat metabolism; and the adrenogenital steroids, or sex hormones.

The adrenogenital steroids are of three types: androgens (such as dehydroepiandrosterone), estrogens (such as estradiol), and progestins (such as progesterone).

Under normal physiologic conditions the adrenogenital steroids are secreted (under the control of adrenocorticotropic hormone, ACTH) in minute amounts and, therefore, they exert minimal effects on reproductive functions. Excessive secretion of adrenal androgens results in precocious pseudopuberty in boys, and causes masculinization of females (adrenogenital syndrome). The pharmacologic properties of these hormones are discussed in Chapters 56 to 58.

MINERALOCORTICOIDS

Control of Secretion and Actions

Aldosterone is the principal physiologic mineralocorticoid secreted by the zona glomerulosa. Its secretion is regulated primarily by the renin–angiotensin mechanism described in Figure 35-1, Chapter 35. The plasma concentrations of sodium and potassium are central factors in the control of aldosterone secretion, since low sodium or elevated potassium levels stimulate the zona glomerulosa both directly and indirectly (by way of the renin–angiotensin system). Other factors contributing to the control of aldosterone secretion include blood volume and level of ACTH, the latter exerting a limited, nonselective stimulatory effect.

Aldosterone plays a major physiologic role in the maintenance of electrolyte and fluid balance by promoting the renal tubular reabsorption of sodium and the secretion of potassium and hydrogen. Aldosterone binds to nuclear receptors and stimulates DNA-directed RNA synthesis, leading to increased formation of specific proteins involved in sodium transport.

A similar sodium-retaining, potassium-excreting action is exerted on other target tissues, including salivary glands and sweat glands.

GLUCOCORTICOIDS

Control of Secretion and Actions

Glucocorticoid secretion, which occurs primarily in the zona fasciculata, is controlled by ACTH. A variety of stressful stimuli, including anxiety, fear, hypoglycemia, hypotension, and hemorrhage, increase secretion of corticotrophin-releasing hormone (CRH) from the hypothalamus. CRH promotes ACTH release from the adenohypophysis, and ACTH stimulates adrenal cortical secretory activity, thereby elevating blood levels of cortisol (the principal physiologic glucocorticoid). Elevated blood levels of free cortisol normally exert a negative feedback control over further secretion of CRH and ACTH (Fig. 55-2). Constant adrenal stimulation by prolonged ACTH secretion can result in hypertrophy and hyperplasia of the adrenal cortex and excessive secretion of all adrenocorticoid hormones. In addition, use of exogenous corticosteroids can also increase the degree of negative feedback on CRH and ACTH release.

The metabolic and physiologic actions of the glucocorticoids are summarized below and their pharmacologic actions and clinical uses are considered later in the chapter.

1. *Carbohydrate metabolism*—Glucocorticoids stimulate hepatic gluconeogenesis and inhibit peripheral uptake and utilization of glucose, thereby promoting hyperglycemia. Hepatic glycogenesis is also enhanced.
2. *Protein metabolism*—Glucocorticoids exert protein catabolic and antianabolic actions, promoting the breakdown of existing proteins while inhibiting the incorporation of amino acids into new proteins, except in the liver, where protein synthesis is stimulated.
3. *Lipid metabolism*—Glucocorticoids inhibit lipogenesis and favor mobilization of fats from adipose tissues. When present in large amounts, these hormones favor redistribution of adipose stores by promoting loss of fat from the extremities and accumulation of fat depots in central body regions (*e.g.*, "moon face" and "buffalo hump" formation).
4. *Blood and immunologic effects*—Glucocorticoids inhibit the immune response, cause involution of lymphoid tissue, and reduce blood levels of lymphocytes, eosinophils, and basophils. These hormones also stimulate erythropoiesis and elevate circulating levels of platelets and neutrophils.
5. *GI tract effects*—Glucocorticoid hormones stimulate gastric acid and pepsin secretion and inhibit the production of protective mucus, thereby favoring development of gastric ulcers.

DISORDERS OF THE ADRENAL CORTEX

Addison's Disease

Addison's disease (chronic adrenocortical insufficiency) may result from idiopathic adrenocortical atrophy, adrenocortical destruction by disease (*e.g.*, tuberculosis or cancer), or deficiency of ACTH or CRH secretion.

Weakness and fatigability are early signs of the disease, and weight loss, dehydration, and hypotension are characteristic. Emotional changes and GI disturbances (such as anorexia, nausea, vomiting, diarrhea) frequently occur. Hyperpigmentation is a major characteristic of primary adrenocortical insufficiency, with increased pigmentation being prominent on skin folds, pressure points (bony prominences), extensor surfaces, nipples, perineum, tongue, and buccal mucosa.

In Addison's disease, aldosterone (mineralocorticoid) deficiency results in increased excretion of sodium and retention of potassium. The salt and

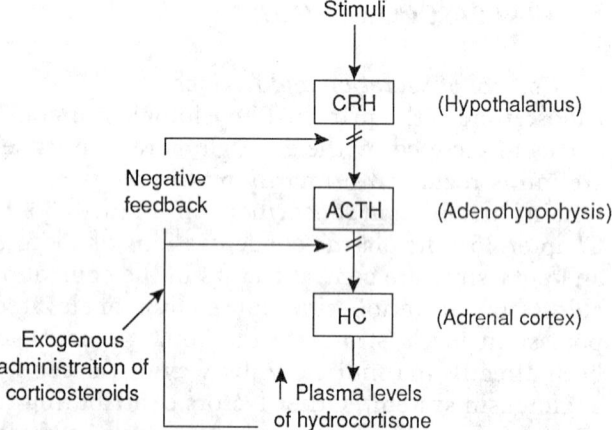

Figure 55-2. Control of secretion of adrenocorticoids and regulation by negative feedback mechanism.

water depletion causes severe dehydration and reduces circulatory volume, leading to hypotension and eventual circulatory collapse.

Glucocorticoid (cortisol) deficiency leads to reduced gluconeogenesis, hypoglycemia, diminished hepatic glycogen, and extreme insulin sensitivity. The inability to withstand stress (such as infection, trauma, surgery) may result in acute adrenal insufficiency (adrenal crisis).

Cushing's Syndrome

Cushing's syndrome is a clinical state characterized by glucocorticoid excess resulting from adrenocortical tumors, hypersecretion of ACTH, or from the administration of large amounts of exogenous corticosteroids or ACTH.

Clinical manifestations of this syndrome include truncal obesity, moon face, and buffalo hump, resulting from the characteristic redistribution of fat from the extremities to central body regions (abdomen, face, and upper back). The increased central subcutaneous fat depots stretch the skin, rupturing the subdermal tissue and causing formation of purple striae.

Excessive protein catabolism results in protein depletion and causes thin skin, muscular wasting, easy bruising, and poor wound healing. Osteoporosis develops, predisposing the patient to fractures and skeletal deformities.

Increased gluconeogenesis and decreased peripheral utilization of glucose result in hyperglycemia and glucose intolerance, and frank diabetes mellitus may develop in genetically predisposed individuals.

Hypertension and renal calculi frequently occur, and psychiatric disturbances are common.

Primary Hyperaldosteronism (Conn's Syndrome)

Conn's syndrome, a clinical state resulting from excessive production of the mineralocorticoid aldosterone, is usually due to an aldosterone-secreting adenoma. Occasionally, however, it may be the result of bilateral hyperplasia of the adrenal cortex. The condition is generally characterized by potassium depletion, sodium retention, hypertension, polyuria, fatigue, and muscular weakness. Hypokalemic alkalosis and tetany may also be observed.

Adrenocorticosteroids

As indicated above, the adrenal cortex secretes a large number of steroidal compounds possessing a variety of physiologic actions. These substances are termed *adrenocorticoids*, or simply *corticoids*. According to their predominant action in the body, they may be divided into one of the three following categories:

1. Mineralocorticoids (*e.g.*, aldosterone)
2. Glucocorticoids (*e.g.*, hydrocortisone)
3. Adrenogenital corticoids (*e.g.*, dehydroepiandrosterone)

To review briefly, mineralocorticoids, of which aldosterone is the major endogenous representative, exert their principal action on electrolyte and water metabolism, especially in the kidney; there they facilitate the reabsorption of sodium and water from the urine by the ionic exchange mechanisms in the distal segments of the tubule. Aldosterone itself is not available for therapeutic use, and those mineralocorticoids employed clinically are the synthetic derivatives desoxycorticosterone and fludrocortisone.

The glucocorticoids are those compounds that primarily influence carbohydrate, fat, and protein metabolism and thus can elicit varied effects in the body and alter the body's immune response to diverse stimuli. Hydrocortisone and cortisone are the major endogenous glucocorticoids. Metabolic actions of the glucocorticoids include gluconeogenesis, hyperglycemia, increased protein catabolism, decreased utilization of amino acids, impaired lipogenesis, and increased lipolysis. In addition, they can suppress the inflammatory process, and this action is responsible for their major clinical application, the control of symptoms of inflammation. Both naturally occurring glucocorticoids (such as cortisone, hydrocortisone) as well as a plethora of synthetic glucocorticoids (*e.g.*, betamethasone, prednisone) are available for therapeutic use, and they differ in potency and degree of side-effects.

The adrenogenital corticoids are male and female sex hormones (such as estrogen, progesterone, and testosterone) found in very small amounts in the adrenal cortex. Other than dehyroepiandrosterone, a precursor of both testosterone and the estrogens, the adrenogenital corticoids are present in the adrenal cortex in amounts too small to be of clinical significance. The sex hormones are discussed in Chapters 56 to 58.

Although the classification of the major adrenocorticoids into mineralocorticoids and glucocorticoids is convenient for discussion purposes, it represents an oversimplification from a functional standpoint. With the exception of a few potent synthetic glucocorticoids, complete separation of mineralocorticoid activity from glucocorticoid activity has not been achieved and considerable overlapping of activity exists with most compounds, especially when employed in large doses. This overlapping is responsible for many of the side-effects associated with adrenocorticosteroid therapy, although in some cases it may represent a desirable extension of the clinical activity of a particular drug. For example, in the treatment of primary adrenal cortical hypofunction (Addison's disease), the mineralocorticoid action (salt and water retention) of glucocorticoid compounds such as hydrocortisone is desirable from a therapeutic point of view. In fact, mineralocorticoid supplementation is often provided with glucocorticoid therapy in the treatment of Addison's disease. On the other hand, a mineralocorticoid action might prove undesirable in the cardiac patient, because salt and water retention may aggravate the already compromised cardiac function.

Synthesis of adrenocorticoids is controlled primarily by ACTH (corticotropin) released from the adenohypophysis as described above. ACTH itself is used in certain clinical situations and is discussed in Chapter 51; the remaining adrenal cortical drugs are reviewed in this chapter. In addition, aminoglutethimide and trilostane, drugs used in the treatment of adrenal cortical hyperfunction (Cushing's syndrome) will be considered at the end of the chapter.

Mineralocorticoids

Desoxycorticosterone Acetate
(Doca Acetate, Percorten Acetate)

Desoxycorticosterone Pivalate
(Percorten Pivalate)

Fludrocortisone Acetate
(Florinef Acetate)

MECHANISM AND ACTIONS
Both desoxycorticosterone (DOCA) and fludrocortisone exhibit potent salt- and water-retaining activity. The drugs act on the renal distal tubules to promote reabsorption of sodium (and water) and excretion of potassium and hydrogen. Sodium retention is also facilitated in sweat glands, salivary glands, and gastric mucosal cells. A rise in blood pressure can occur especially with the more potent fludrocortisone. DOCA is virtually devoid of glu-

cocorticoid activity, whereas fludrocortisone exhibits marked (i.e., 15 times that of hydrocortisone) glucocorticoid activity. In large doses, fludrocortisone inhibits endogenous adrenal cortical secretion and promotes deposition of liver glycogen. Unless protein intake remains adequate, a negative nitrogen balance can ensue.

USES
1. Partial replacement therapy for primary and secondary adrenocortical insufficiency (in combination with glucocorticoids, fluids, electrolytes, and other adjunctive measures)
2. Treatment of salt-losing adrenogenital syndrome (with adequate glucocorticoid therapy)
3. Management of severe orthostatic hypotension (fludrocortisone only)

ADMINISTRATION AND DOSAGE
Desoxycorticosterone is a synthetic form of the naturally occurring 11-desoxycorticosterone available as a short-acting injection (acetate) containing 5 mg/ml; a repository (long-acting) injection (pivalate) containing 25 mg/ml; and long-acting implantable pellets (acetate), which contain 125 mg each. Fludrocorticose is used as oral tablets containing 0.1 mg. Therapy with these agents is usually accompanied by a glucocorticoid (e.g., 10 mg to 30 mg hydrocortisone or 10 mg to 37.5 mg cortisone per day). Dosage recommendations for the various dosage forms are as follows:

Desoxycorticosterone
Injection (acetate): 2 mg to 5 mg/day IM (gluteal site is preferred—avoid deltoid)
Repository injection (pivalate): 25 mg to 100 mg once every 4 weeks depending on daily requirement of regular injection (25 mg pivalate for 1 mg acetate). Pivalate is very viscous; therefore, give injection with a 20-gauge needle in a large muscle mass such as the outer quadrant of the buttock.
Pellets: 1 pellet for each 0.5 mg of DOCA acetate required daily; pellet is implanted SC every 8 months to 12 months. Implantation is usually in the infrascapular region.

Fludrocortisone
Addison's disease: 0.1 mg 3 times/week orally to 0.2 mg/day (usually 0.1 mg/day)
Dose should be reduced to 0.05 mg/day if hypertension develops

Salt-losing adrenogenital syndrome: 0.1 mg/
day to 0.2 mg/day

Orthostatic hypotension: 0.1 mg to 0.5 mg/
day; dosage is titrated by clinical response
or development of ankle edema.

FATE

Desoxycorticosterone is destroyed in the GI tract.
The duration of action is approximately 24 hours
to 48 hours with regular injection, 4 weeks with
repository injection, and 8 months to 12 months
with pellets.

Fludrocortisone is readily absorbed orally; peak
plasma levels occur in 1.5 hours to 2 hours. Effects
persist for up to 24 hours to 36 hours.

Both drugs are excreted in the urine as both
metabolites and some unchanged drug.

SIDE-EFFECTS/ADVERSE REACTIONS

Muscle weakness or cramping, paresthesias, arrhythmias, and fatigue can occur if potassium loss
is excessive. Edema, hypertension, and congestive
heart failure may result from marked fluid retention. Other adverse reactions noted during mineralocorticoid therapy are frontal or occipital
headaches, arrhythmias, pulmonary congestion,
arthralgia, and hypersensitivity reactions. Pain and
irritation at the injection site have been reported
with DOCA.

In addition, since fludrocortisone possesses significant glucocorticoid activity, refer to the side-
effects/adverse reactions listed under glucocorticoids later in this chapter for additional possible
untoward reactions.

CONTRAINDICATIONS AND PRECAUTIONS

The mineralocorticoids are contraindicated in patients with severe hypertension, congestive heart
failure, or other severe cardiac disease. Safety for
use in children has not been established. A *cautious*
approach to therapy is necessary during times of
stress, trauma, or severe illness when using fludrocortisone; additional glucocorticoid therapy may
be required to prevent symptoms of adrenal insufficiency. Cautious use is also necessary in nursing
mothers (since the drugs enter breast milk) and
during pregnancy (since adrenocortical insufficiency can be precipitated in the newborn infant).

INTERACTIONS

See glucocorticoid discussion for potential interactions, especially involving fludrocortisone.

NURSING CONSIDERATIONS

See Glucocorticoids, below.

Table 55-1
Comparative Activities of Systemic Glucocorticoids

Drug	Equivalent Oral Doses (mg)	Relative Anti-Inflammatory Activity	Relative Mineralocorticoid Potency
Short-Acting			
cortisone	25	0.8	++
hydrocortisone	20	1	++
Intermediate-Acting			
prednisone	5	3–4	+
prednisolone	5	3	+
methylprednisolone	4	5	0
triamcinolone	4	5	0
Long-Acting			
paramethasone	2	10	0
dexamethasone	0.75	25–30	0
betamethasone	0.6	25–30	0

Key: ++, high mineralocorticoid activity; +, low mineralocorticoid activity; 0, no mineralocorticoid activity

Table 55-2
Relative Potencies of Topically Applied Corticosteroids*

Generic Name	Trade Name	Dosage Form/ Strength	
Group I			
amcinonide	Cyclocort	Ointment	0.1%
		Cream	0.1%
		Lotion	0.1%
betamethasone dipropionate	Alphatrex, Diprolene, Diprosone, Maxivate	Ointment	0.05%
		Cream	0.05%
		Lotion	0.05%
clobetasol propionate	Temovate	Cream	0.05%
		Ointment	0.05%
desoximetasone	Topicort	Cream	0.25%
		Ointment	0.25%
diflorasone diacetate	Florone, Maxiflor, Psorcon	Ointment	0.05%
		Cream	0.05%
fluocinolone acetonide	Synalar HP	Cream	0.2%
fluocinonide	Lidex, Lidex-E	Cream	0.05%
		Ointment	0.05%
		Solution	0.05%
		Gel	0.05%
halcinonide	Halog, Halog-E	Cream	0.1%
		Ointment	0.1%
		Solution	0.1%
mometasone	Elocon	Cream	0.1%
		Ointment	0.1%
Group II			
betamethasone benzoate	Benisone, Uticort	Cream	0.025%
		Ointment	0.025%
		Lotion	0.025%
betamethasone valerate	Betatrex, Beta-Val, Valisone	Ointment	0.1%
		Cream	0.1%
		Lotion	0.1%
desoximetasone	Topicort	Cream	0.05%
		Gel	0.05%
triamcinolone acetonide	Aristocort, Kenalog	Cream	0.5%
		Ointment	0.5%

(continued)

Glucocorticoids

*Alclometasone, Amcinonide,
Beclomethasone, Betamethasone,
Clobetasol, Clocortolone,
Cortisone, Desonide,
Desoximetasone, Dexamethasone,
Diflorasone, Flunisolide,
Fluocinolone, Fluocinonide,
Fluorometholone,*

*Flurandrenolide, Halcinonide,
Hydrocortisone, Medrysone,
Methylprednisolone,
Mometasone, Paramethasone,
Prednisolone, Prednisone,
Triamcinolone*

The glucocorticoids encompass a large number of naturally occurring and synthetic steroids, possessing similar pharmacologic actions but differing widely in potency and the type and severity of

Table 55-2 (continued)
*Relative Potencies of Topically Applied Corticosteroids**

Generic Name	Trade Name	Dosage Form/Strength	
Group III			
fluocinolone acetonide	Synalar, Synemol	Ointment	0.025%
		Cream	0.025%
flurandrenolide	Cordran	Ointment	0.05%
		Cream	0.05%
		Lotion	0.05%
halcinonide	Halog	Cream	0.025%
triamcinolone acetonide	Aristocort, Kenalog	Ointment	0.1%
		Cream	0.1%
		Lotion	0.1%
Group IV			
betamethasone valerate	Betatrex, Valisone	Cream	0.01%
clocortolone pivalate	Cloderm	Cream	0.1%
fluocinolone acetonide	Synalar, Synemol	Cream	0.01%
		Solution	0.01%
flurandrenolide	Cordran	Cream	0.025%
		Ointment	0.025%
hydrocortisone valerate	Westcort	Ointment	0.2%
		Cream	0.2%
triamcinolone acetonide	Aristocort, Kenalog	Cream	0.025%
		Lotion	0.025%
		Ointment	0.025%
Group V			
alclometasone dipropionate	Aclovate	Cream	0.05%
		Ointment	0.05%
desonide	DesOwen, Tridesilon	Cream	0.05%
dexamethasone	Hexadrol	Cream	0.05%
hydrocortisone	Alphaderm, Hytone	Cream	1.0%
	Cortril	Ointment	1.0%
	Cort-Dome	Lotion	1.0%
methylprednisolone acetate	Medrol	Ointment	1.0%

* Group I drugs are the most potent; group V drugs are the least potent. Drugs in each list are listed alphabetically; there is no significant difference among agents in each group.

side-effects. The principal naturally occurring adrenocorticosteroids are cortisone and hydrocortisone (cortisol), and they exhibit both mineralocorticoid (salt-retaining) as well as glucocorticoid (anti-inflammatory) effects. As such, they are primarily used as replacement therapy for adrenocortical deficiency states.

Synthetic glucocorticoids are characterized by their greater glucocorticoid potency compared to natural adrenocorticosteroids and by their reduced (and in some cases complete absence of) mineralocorticoid action. The synthetic drugs are used principally for their potent anti-inflammatory ac-

tion and are available in many different dosage forms. The relative potencies of the various systemically employed glucocorticoids are listed in Table 55-1, which compares their oral effectiveness, anti-inflammatory activity, and mineralocorticoid potency.

It is important to recognize that the majority of adverse reactions associated with glucocorticoid use occur following the systemic use of these compounds. When a local effect is desired, the drug may be applied topically in various dosage forms (*e.g.*, ointment, cream, lotion, aerosol, nasal spray, ophthalmic drops) or administered by an intralesional or intra-articular injection. A number of different corticosteroids are used topically, and the relative potency of topical steroids is dependent on several factors, including the concentration of drug applied, the basic characteristics of the drug molecule, and the type of vehicle used. For example, fluorinated derivatives (e.g., betamethasone, fluocinonide, halcinonide) are more potent than non-fluorinated agents (e.g., hydrocortisone, desonide) and are less likely to cause sodium retention but may have a higher incidence of local adverse effects. A relative potency ranking of the various topical steroid preparations is presented in Table 55-2.

This discussion of glucocorticoids focuses mainly on their systemic pharmacology. Following is a general review of glucocorticoids; individual drugs, both systemic and local, are listed in Table 55-3, where the available dosage forms are given along with recommended dose levels for each dosage form, and specific remarks pertaining to each drug are presented.

MECHANISM AND ACTIONS

Glucocorticoids exert a variety of metabolic effects and alter the body's immune responses to various stimuli. They possess significant anti-inflammatory activity, which may be due to a number of specific actions, namely (1) stabilization of lysosomal membranes, reducing release of tissue-destructive enzymes; (2) inhibition of capillary dilation and permeability; (3) interference with the biosynthesis, storage, or release of allergic substances (e.g., bradykinin, histamine); (4) suppression of leukocyte migration and phagocytosis; (5) inhibition of fibroblast formation and collagen deposition; and (6) reduction of antibody formation by lymphocytes and plasma cells.

When applied topically, cortisteroids exhibit anti-inflammatory, antipruritic, and tissue antiproliferative actions. The clinical effectiveness of topical corticosteroids depends in large part on the degree of percutaneous absorption, which is influenced by a number of factors, such as vehicle, concentration of drug, site of application, and use of occlusive dressings.

Systemic glucocorticoids may also enhance the responsiveness of the cardiovascular system to circulating catecholamines, thus increasing cardiac output as well as local perfusion pressure. Those derivatives possessing mineralocorticoid activity as well, such as hydrocortisone and prednisone, exert effects on fluid and electrolyte balance as detailed in the discussion of mineralocorticoids earlier in the chapter.

USES

1. Replacement therapy in primary or secondary adrenal cortical insufficiency (hydrocortisone is drug of choice; synthetic analogs may be used *with* mineralocorticoid supplementation)
2. Treatment of congenital adrenal hyperplasia
3. Symptomatic treatment of various inflammatory, allergic, or immunoreactive disorders, including the following:
   a. Rheumatic—Rheumatoid arthritis, bursitis, osteoarthritis, acute gouty arthritis, tenosynovitis, synovitis, ankylosing spondylitis
   b. Collagen—Acute rheumatic carditis, systemic lupus erythematosus, polymyositis
   c. Allergic — Allergic rhinitis, bronchial asthma, status asthmaticus, dermatitis, serum sickness, drug hypersensitivity, laryngeal edema
   d. Dermatologic—Erythema multiforme (Stevens-Johnson syndrome), exfoliative dermatitis, severe psoriasis, angioedema, urticaria, chronic eczema
   e. Ophthalmic—Conjunctivitis, keratitis, iritis, uveitis, acute optic neuritis, chorioretinitis, allergic corneal marginal ulcers, corneal injury resulting from chemical, radiation, or thermal burns, or foreign body infiltration
   f. Gastrointestinal—Ulcerative colitis, regional enteritis, intractable sprue
   g. Hematologic/neoplastic—Thrombocytopenic purpura, hemolytic anemia (autoimmune), erythroblastopenia, leukemias, Hodgkin's disease, multiple myeloma
   h. Other—Nephrotic syndrome, gout, hypercalcemia associated with cancer, acute exacerbations of multiple sclerosis, acute myasthenic episodes, anaphylactic shock, tuberculous meningitis, nonsuppurative thyroiditis, trichinosis with neurologic or myocardial involvement
4. Testing of adrenal cortical hyperfunction or relief of cerebral edema due to metastatic brain tumors, head injury, or craniotomy (dexamethasone *only*)
5. Treatment of pulmonary emphysema with bronchospasm and edema and diffuse interstitial pulmonary fibrosis (triamcinolone)
6. Investigational uses include prevention of cisplatin-induced vomiting (dexamethasone), prevention of respiratory distress syndrome in premature neonates (usually betamethasone), treatment of septic shock (methylprednisolone

(Text continues on p. 1064.)

Table 55-3
Glucocorticoids

Drug	Preparations	Usual Dosage Range	Clinical Considerations
alclometasone (Aclovate)	Ointment—0.05% Cream—0.05%	Apply to affected area 2 to 3 times/day	Synthetic corticosteroid used for treatment of inflammatory and pruritic manifestations of steroid-responsive dermatoses. Side-effects include localized itching, burning, erythema, dryness, irritation, and rash.
amcinonide (Cyclocort)	Cream—0.1% Ointment—0.1%	Apply 2 to 3 times/day	Effective against steroid-responsive dermatoses; cream is formulated in nonsensitizing hydrophilic base.
beclomethasone (Beclovent, Beconase, Vancenase, Vanceril)	Aerosol for oral inhalation —42 mcg/dose Aerosol for intranasal inhalation—42 mcg/dose	*Oral inhalation* Adults—2 inhalations 3 to 4 times/day (maximum 20/day) Children—1 or 2 inhalations 3 to 4 times/day (maximum 10/day) *Nasal inhalation* 1 inhalation 2 to 4 times/day	Synthetic corticosteroid related to prednisolone; used by oral inhalation for chronic management of bronchial asthma not controlled by bronchodilators and other nonsteroidal drugs; dry mouth, hoarseness, and localized fungal infections of mouth and pharynx can occur; danger of adrenal insufficiency if patients are transferred from oral to inhaled steroids too quickly or during periods of stress; oral steroids should be available at all times; not indicated for relief of acute asthmatic attack; intranasal solution is used for relief of symptoms of seasonal or perennial rhinitis; minimal systemic effects; do not use in children under 12; nasal irritation and dryness are most common side-effects; effects are evident only with several days' use; patients with blocked nasal passages should use a decongestant (see Chap. 15) prior to administration; do not use longer than 3 weeks if no effect.
betamethasone (Celestone)	Tablets—0.6 mg Syrup—0.6 mg/5 ml	Oral—0.6 mg–7.2 mg/day IM, IV (phosphate only) —up to 9 mg/day	Long-acting agent with no mineralocorticoid activity; phosphate salt has a *(continued)*

Table 55-3 (continued)
Glucocorticoids

Drug	Preparations	Usual Dosage Range	Clinical Considerations
betamethasone phosphate (Betameth, Celestone Phosphate, Selestoject)	Injection—4 mg/ml Repository injection—3 mg acetate and 3 mg phosphate/ml Cream—0.01%, 0.025%, 0.05%, 0.1%	IM (repository)—0.5 mg to 9.0 mg/day Intra-articular—2 mg–8 mg (0.25 ml–2 ml) depending on joint size and disease Topical—apply 1 to 3 times/day	prompt onset of action and is given IV or IM; phosphate salt is available in combination with acetate salt as Celestone Soluspan for repository IM injections, given once a day into joints, lesions, or bursae; up to 2 ml may be injected into very large joints; not used in Addison's disease, as salt- and water-retaining action is minimal; used topically for dermatoses, pruritus, and psoriatic lesions; use aerosol cautiously, because systemic absorption may be substantial, resulting in increased adverse effects. Dipropionate salt is available in a specially formulated waxy vehicle that enhances drug absorption (Diprolene).
betamethasone benzoate (Benisone, Uticort)	Ointment—0.025% Cream—0.025% Lotion—0.025% Gel—0.025%		
betamethasone dipropionate (Alphatrex, Diprolene, Diprosone, Maxivate)	Ointment—0.05% Cream—0.05% Lotion—0.05% Aerosol—0.1%		
betamethasone valerate (Betatrex, Beta-Val, Valisone, Valnac)	Ointment—0.1% Cream—0.01%, 0.1% Lotion—0.1%		
clobetasol (Temovate)	Cream—0.05% Ointment—0.05%	Apply twice a day	Very potent topical corticosteroid; limit treatment to 14 days; adrenal suppression has occurred with doses as low as 2 g/day; use very sparingly and do not cover with occlusive dressings.
clocortolone (Cloderm)	Cream—0.1%	Apply 1 to 3 times/day	Indicated for relief of inflammatory manifestations of corticosteroid-responsive dermatoses
cortisone (Cortone)	Tablets—5 mg, 10 mg, 25 mg Injection—25 mg/ml, 50 mg/ml	Oral, IM—20 mg–300 mg/day; reduce to lowest effective dosage	Short-acting glucocorticoid with prominent mineralocorticoid activity; injection has a relatively slow onset but long duration of action; drug is largely converted to hydrocortisone, which is responsible for most of its pharmacologic action.
desonide (DesOwen, Tridesilon)	Cream—0.05% Ointment—0.05%	Apply 2 to 3 times/day	Possesses anti-inflammatory, antipruritic, and vasoconstrictive activity; discontinue if irritation develops; less potent than most other topical steroids
desoximetasone (Topicort)	Cream—0.05%, 0.25% Gel—0.05% Ointment—0.25%	Apply 1 to 2 times/day	Higher-strength (0.25%) cream is very potent; weaker-strength cream *(continued)*

Table 55-3 (continued)
Glucocorticoids

Drug	Preparations	Usual Dosage Range	Clinical Considerations
desoximetasone (Topicort) (continued)			(Topicort LP) and gel are of moderate potency.
dexamethasone (Decadron, Hexadrol, various other manufacturers)	Tablets—0.25 mg, 0.5 mg, 0.75 mg, 1.0 mg, 1.5 mg, 2 mg, 4 mg, 6 mg Oral solution—0.5 mg/5 ml Drops—0.5 mg/0.5 ml Elixir—0.5 mg/5 ml Injection—4 mg/ml, 10 mg/ml, 20 mg/ml, 24 mg/ml Repository injection (acetate salt)—8 mg/ml, 16 mg/ml Ophthalmic solution—0.1% Ophthalmic suspension—0.1% Ophthalmic ointment—0.05%, 0.1% Cream—0.1% Gel—0.1% Aerosol—0.01%, 0.04% Aerosol (Respihaler)—12.6 g (84 mcg/dose) Aerosol (Turbinaire)—12.6 g (84 mcg/dose)	Oral—0.75–9 mg/day Children—0.2 mg/kg/day Parenteral—$\frac{1}{3}$ to $\frac{1}{2}$ oral dose every 12 h (usual range 0.5 mg–5 mg/day) Repository injection—8 mg–16 mg IM every 1 week to 3 weeks Intra-articular, intralesion, or soft-tissue injection—0.4 mg–6 mg depending on area Ophthalmic—1 to 2 drops or thin film of ointment 3 to 4 times/day Topical—2 to 4 times/day as needed Respihaler—2 to 3 inhalations 3 to 4 times/day Turbinaire—2 sprays in nostril 2 to 3 times/day	Widely used, potent corticosteroid; long-acting, and not recommended for alternate-day dosing; phosphate salt is freely soluble and is given IM or IV; prompt onset of action; acetate salt is largely insoluble and has a prolonged effect when given IM; aerosol therapy may result in nasal or bronchial irritation, drying of mucosa, rebound congestion, asthmatic-like reaction, and other systemic effects; Turbinaire aerosol is used for nasal inflammation, whereas Respihaler aerosol is indicated for bronchial asthma; available with lidocaine for soft-tissue injection (e.g., bursitis, tenosynovitis); systemic adverse effects may follow long-term or high-dose topical, intralesional, or inhalation therapy; protect eyes from topical spray in the face area; discontinue ophthalmic use if eye irritation develops; may cause hiccoughs at high doses, which are not easily controlled until the drug is stopped.
diflorasone (Florone, Maxiflor, Psorcon)	Ointment—0.05% Cream—0.05%	Apply 2 to 3 times/day	Used in steroid-responsive dermatoses; cream is in an emulsified hydrophilic base.
flunisolide (AeroBid, Nasalide)	Aerosol—7 g (250 mcg/dose) Nasal spray—25 mcg/dose	*Oral inhalation* Adults—2 inhalations twice/day (maximum 2 mg/day) Children (age 6–15)—1 to 2 inhalations twice/day (maximum 1 mg/day) *Nasal inhalation* Adults—2 sprays each nostril 2 to 3 times/day Children (age 6–14)—1 spray 3 times/day or 2 sprays twice/day	Oral inhalation used to control steroid-dependent bronchial asthma (*not* for relief of acute attacks); transfer from oral steroids should be done *gradually*; during periods of stress or severe asthma attacks, oral steroids should be reinstituted; side-effects include cough, dry mouth, hoarseness, and local fungal infections. Nasal spray is used to relieve symptoms *(continued)*

Table 55-3 (continued)
Glucocorticoids

Drug	Preparations	Usual Dosage Range	Clinical Considerations
flunisolide (AeroBid, Nasalide) (continued)			of rhinitis; not recommended in children under age of 6; discontinue after 3 weeks if no improvement is noted; after clinical effect is observed reduce dose to lowest effective maintenance dose.
fluocinolone (Fluocet, Fluonid, Flurosyn, Synalar, Synemol)	Ointment—0.025% Cream—0.01%, 0.025% 0.2% Solution—0.01%	Apply sparingly 2 to 4 times/day in a thin layer	Possesses moderate anti-inflammatory and antipruritic activity; high-potency cream (0.2%) should be used for short periods of time only; it can be used as an otic solution for excessive cerumen; also available with neomycin (Neo-Synalar).
fluocinonide (Lidex, Lidex-E)	Ointment—0.05% Cream—0.05% Gel—0.05% Solution—0.05%	Apply 3 to 4 times/day	Used for anti-inflammatory action in steroid-responsive dermatoses; one of the more potent topical corticosteroids; it is available in several different vehicles.
fluorometholone (Fluor-Op, FML Liquifilm)	Ophthalmic suspension—0.1% Ophthalmic ointment—0.1%	Ophthalmic—1 to 2 drops or small ribbon of ointment 3 to 4 times/day	Be alert for ocular irritation and discontinue drug; transient burning can occur when first applied but disappears within minutes.
flurandrenolide (Cordran)	Ointment—0.025%, 0.05% Cream—0.025%, 0.05% Lotion—0.05% Tape—4 mcg/cm²	Apply 2 to 3 times/day Tape—cut tape to size of area; apply to clean dry skin and replace every 12 h	Good anti-inflammatory, antipruritic, and vasoconstrictive activity; ointment is slightly more effective than cream; both preparations are available with neomycin (Cordran-N) for use in dermatoses complicated by bacterial infections; tape is usually removed every 12 h but may be left in place for 24 h if well tolerated; if irritation or infection develops, remove tape and advise physician.
halcinonide (Halog, Halog-E)	Ointment—0.1% Cream—0.025%, 0.1% Solution—0.1%	Apply 2 to 3 times/day in a thin film	Similar to most other topical corticosteroids; ointment is formulated in a polyethylene and mineral oil gel base; cream (0.1%) is available in a vanishing base (Halog-E).

(continued)

Table 55-3 (*continued*)
Glucocorticoids

Drug	Preparations	Usual Dosage Range	Clinical Considerations
hydrocortisone (Cort-Dome, Cortef, and various other manufacturers)	Tablets—5 mg, 10 mg, 20 mg Oral suspension—10 mg/5 ml Injection—25 mg/ml, 50 mg/ml; 100 mg/vial, 250 mg/vial, 500 mg/vial, 1,000 mg/vial Repository injection (acetate)—25 mg/ml, 50 mg/ml Enema—100 mg/60 ml Rectal foam aerosol—90 mg/application Ointment—0.1%, 0.2%, 0.5%, 1%, 2.5% Cream—0.1%, 0.2%, 0.25%, 0.5%, 1%, 2.5% Lotion—0.25%, 0.5%, 1%, 2%, 2.5% Gel—1% Aerosol spray—0.5%	Oral—20 mg–240 mg/day in divided doses Parenteral—⅓ to ½ oral dose IM every 12 h *Acute adrenal insufficiency* Adults—100 mg IV, followed by 100 mg every 8 h in IV fluids Children—1 mg–2 mg/kg IV bolus, then 150 mg–250 mg per day IV in divided doses Enema—100 mg/night for 21 days Intralesional, intra-articular, or soft-tissue injection—10 mg–50 mg depending on area Ophthalmic—a thin film of ointment 3 to 4 times/day Topical—a thin film or spray onto area 2 to 4 times/day	Short-acting corticosteroid possessing mineralocorticoid activity; similar in action but less potent than many other synthetic derivatives; local injection as acetate provides long-lasting effect due to low solubility; phosphate and succinate salts are water soluble and may be given IV; topical hydrocortisone preparations of 0.5% or weaker are available over the counter; also available with neomycin as both cream and ointment (Neo-Cort-Dome, Neo-Cortef).
medrysone (HMS Liquifilm)	Ophthalmic suspension—1%	1 to 2 drops 2 to 4 times/day as needed	Used for steroid-responsive inflammatory conditions of the eye; discontinue if irritation develops; prolonged use has resulted in cataract formation; shake suspension well before using
methylprednisolone (Medrol, and various other manufacturers)	Tablets—2 mg, 4 mg, 8 mg, 16 mg, 24 mg, 32 mg Injection—40 mg/vial, 125 mg/vial, 500 mg/vial, 1000 mg/vial Repository injection (acetate)—20 mg/ml, 40 mg/ml, 80 mg/ml Powder for injection—2000 mg/vial Enema—40 mg Ointment—0.25%, 1%	Oral—4 mg–48 mg/day in divided doses Repository injection—40 mg–120 mg IM every 1 week to 4 weeks depending on condition Intra-articular—4 mg–80 mg depending on joint size Injection—10 mg–40 mg IV over several minutes; subsequent doses may be given IM or IV Children—not less than 0.5 mg/kg/day Topical—2 to 3 times/day	Available as base (tablets), sodium succinate (rapid-acting injection), or acetate (repository injection, topical ointment); use alternate-day regimen when administered orally over extended periods of time; used as a dosepak (*i.e.*, 21 tablets) for short-term (6-day) therapy; acetate salt is *not* given IV.
mometasone (Elocon)	Cream—0.1% Ointment—0.1%	Apply thin film once daily	Potent topical corticosteroid used for steroid-responsive dermatoses. Do *not* use occlusive dressings.
paramethasone (Haldrone)	Tablets—1 mg, 2 mg	2 mg–24 mg/day in divided doses depending on severity of condition	Approximately 10 times more potent than hydrocortisone, with minimal mineralocorticoid activity; hypocalcemia is common with prolonged high doses.

(*continued*)

Table 55-3 (continued)
Glucocorticoids

Drug	Preparations	Usual Dosage Range	Clinical Considerations

prednisolone (various manufacturers)	Tablets—5 mg
	Syrup—15 mg/5 ml
	Oral liquid—5 mg/5 ml
	Injection
	  Sodium phosphate—20 mg/ml
	  Acetate—25 mg/ml, 50 mg/ml, 100 mg/ml
	  Tebutate—20 mg/ml
	Ophthalmic drops—0.12% 0.125%, 0.5%, 1%
		Oral—5 mg–60 mg/day (up to 200 mg/day for acute exacerbation of multiple sclerosis)
		Injection (IM, IV)—4 mg–60 mg/day
		Intralesional, intra-articular, or soft-tissue injection—4 mg–30 mg (tebutate) or 5 mg–100 mg (acetate)
		Ophthalmic—1 to 2 drops into conjunctival sac every 4 h
			Synthetic derivative of hydrocortisone, approximately 5 times more potent; administer orally with meals to minimize GI irritation; sodium and water retention is minimal with normal doses; alternate-day therapy is advisable with prolonged use to reduce incidence of adverse effects; ophthalmic use may increase intraocular pressure; frequent examinations are advisable during extended therapy; injections are available as phosphate (rapid onset; short duration), acetate (prolonged action), tebutate (prolonged action), and a combination of acetate and phosphate (prompt onset and prolonged effect).

prednisone (various manufacturers)	Tablets—1 mg, 2.5 mg, 5 mg, 10 mg, 20 mg, 25 mg, 50 mg Syrup—5 mg/5 ml Oral concentrate—5 mg/ml	5 mg–60 mg/day in divided doses Children—0.1 mg–0.15 mg/kg/day divided every 12 h	Synthetic derivative of hydrocortisone; therapeutic action is due to metabolism to prednisolone; use with caution in patients *(continued)*

IV), and diagnosis of depression (dexamethasone).

ADMINISTRATION AND DOSAGE
See Table 55-3.

Endogenous adrenal cortical activity is maximum between 2 AM and 8 AM and minimal between 4 PM and midnight. Therefore, exogenous corticosteroids should be given before 9 AM, since suppression of adrenocortical activity by exogenous drugs is *least* when the activity of the gland is maximal and the danger of adrenal suppression is minimized.

FATE
Most drugs are well absorbed from the GI tract and circulate in the blood partially bound to plasma proteins. The duration of action varies among the derivatives. Most drugs are metabolized in the liver and excreted largely by the kidney in conjugated

form; induction of hepatic enzymes will increase the metabolic clearance of glucocorticoids. The renal clearance is accelerated when plasma levels are increased. (See Table 55-3 for specific data for individual drugs.)

SIDE-EFFECTS/ADVERSE REACTIONS
The most frequently encountered side-effects with systemic glucocorticoids are GI distress with oral administration, salt and water retention, and increased appetite. Most significant adverse reactions occur with prolonged use and can involve a variety of organ systems:

GI—Vomiting, peptic ulcer, pancreatitis, abdominal distention, ulcerative esophagitis

Cardiovascular—Hypertension, arrhythmias (especially with rapid IV injection), congestive heart failure, shock, thrombophlebitis, fat embolism, necrotizing angiitis

Table 55-3 (*continued*)
Glucocorticoids

Drug	Preparations	Usual Dosage Range	Clinical Considerations
prednisone (various manufacturers) (*continued*)			with liver disease; may produce sodium and water retention and potassium loss, especially at high doses; administer on alternate days during prolonged therapy; frequently combined with antineoplastic drugs in certain forms of carcinoma (see Chap. 75); it is a very inexpensive and widely used drug.
triamcinolone (Aristocort, Azmacort, Kenalog, and various other manufacturers)	Tablets—1 mg, 2 mg, 4 mg, 8 mg Syrup—2 mg/5 ml, 4 mg/5 ml Injection—25 mg/ml, 40 mg/ml Repository injection—5 mg/ml, 10 mg/ml, 20 mg/ml, 40 mg/ml Ointment—0.025%, 0.1% 0.5% Cream—0.025%, 0.1%, 0.5% Lotion—0.025%, 0.1% Topical spray—delivers approximately 0.2 mg/spray Oral inhaler—approximately 100 mcg delivered with each activation.	Oral—4 mg–60 mg/day depending on condition Repository injection (IM)—40 mg once a week Intralesional, intra-articular injection Diacetate—5 mg–40 mg Acetonide—2.5 mg–15 mg Hexacetonide—2 mg–20 mg Topical—apply 2 to 4 times/day as needed Inhalation—2 inhalations 3 to 4 times/day	Synthetic corticosteroid approximately 5 times more potent than hydrocortisone; no significant mineralocorticoid activity at normal doses; diacetate has an intermediate onset and moderate duration of action; acetonide and hexacetonide derivatives possess a slow onset and prolonged duration of action; do not use in children; injections should be made IM; do not administer IV; oral inhalation (Azmacort) is used in steroid-responsive bronchial asthma (see Chap. 48).

Dermatologic—Petechiae, ecchymoses, purpura, hirsutism, acne, thinning of skin, striae, fatty redistribution in subcutaneous layers, impaired wound healing, abnormal pigmentation

Musculoskeletal—Osteoporosis, muscle weakness, tendon rupture, vertebral compression fractures, spontaneous fractures, steroid myopathy (loss of muscle mass)

Neurologic—Vertigo, headache, syncope, personality changes, irritability, insomnia, convulsions, catatonia, steroid-induced psychosis

Fluid/electrolyte—Hypokalemia, hypocalcemia, alkalosis

Endocrine—Menstrual irregularities, growth retardation, decreased carbohydrate tolerance, steroid diabetes, hyperglycemia, glycosuria

Ophthalmic—Posterior subcapsular cataracts, glaucoma, exophthalmos, secondary viral or fungal infections

Other—Increased susceptibility to or masking of infections, reactivation of tuberculosis, fatty embolism, negative nitrogen balance, growth suppression in children, hypersensitivity and anaphylactic reactions, renal stones, leukocytosis

Intra-articular injection has resulted in erythema, tendon rupture, local infection, skin atrophy, and osteonecrosis. Intraspinal administration can lead to meningitis.

With prolonged use, adrenal insufficiency can occur if dosage levels are not maintained. Corticosteroid therapy longer than 5 days may lead to suppression of the hypothalamic–pituitary–adrenal axis through a negative feedback mechanism (see Fig. 55-2). The degree of adrenal suppression varies with the dosage and duration of therapy. Since recovery of adrenal function is slow in developing, abrupt discontinuation of therapy will remove the *exogenous* source of corticosteroids; however, the endogenous source (*i.e.*, adrenal gland) is unable to supply sufficient corticosteroids, since its function has been suppressed, and a state of adrenal insufficiency occurs. Signs of adrenal insufficiency include nausea, fatigue, anorexia, diarrhea, weakness, weight loss, dizziness, and hypoglycemia. Abrupt withdrawal of therapy should be avoided, and rapid-acting steroids should be available during and following any period of stress or trauma that might increase steroid requirements.

CONTRAINDICATIONS AND PRECAUTIONS

Glucocorticoids given by any route of administration are contraindicated in the presence of systemic fungal infections. Systemically administered drugs are contraindicated in combination with any live virus vaccine and in patients receiving immunosuppressive doses of corticosteroids. IM steroids are also contraindicated in idiopathic thrombocytopenic purpura. Ocular and topical administration of corticosteroids is not recommended in the presence of herpes simplex infections, or other viral or tubercular infections of the cornea or skin.

Glucocorticoids given by any route should be used *cautiously* in patients with hypothyroidism, ulcerative colitis, fresh intestinal anastomoses, diverticulitis, cirrhosis, active or latent peptic ulcer, diabetes mellitus, chronic nephritis, hypertension, congestive heart failure, osteoporosis, renal insufficiency, thrombophlebitis, glaucoma, myasthenia gravis, convulsive disorders, metastatic carcinoma, pyogenic infections, Cushing's syndrome, vaccinia or varicella infections, and in pregnant or nursing women.

Steroids should not be injected into a joint suspected of being unstable, since permanent damage to the joint can occur.

Corticosteroids may mask signs of infection, encourage their spread, and decrease the patient's resistance. Signs of slow wound healing, prolonged inflammation, or persistent fever or sore throat should be reported immediately.

INTERACTIONS

1. The pharmacologic effects of corticosteroids may be reduced by barbiturates, phenytoin, ephedrine, and rifampin, drugs that enhance the metabolic clearance of steroids.
2. Corticosteroids may increase the dosage requirements for insulin and oral antidiabetic agents, isoniazid, salicylates, and oral anticoagulants.
3. Increased intraocular pressure can result from combinations of corticosteroids and anticholinergics, tricyclic antidepressants, or adrenergics.
4. Excessive hypokalemia has resulted from concomitant use of corticosteroids and potassium-depleting diuretics or amphotericin.
5. Corticosteroids can increase digitalis toxicity as a result of increased potassium loss.
6. The action of corticosteroids may be enhanced by estrogens by way of reduced hepatic clearance.
7. GI absorption of corticosteroids can be impaired by cholestyramine and colestipol.
8. Corticosteroids may increase the pharmacologic effects of theophylline.
9. Concurrent use of corticosteroids and salicylates may result in reduced salicylate levels and an increased likelihood for gastric ulceration.

■ Nursing Process

Corticosteroids are given by many routes. Topical applications, otic drops, nasal drops or sprays, and ophthalmic ointment or drops are used with great success for inflammatory conditions. Systemic absorption via these routes is generally negligible. Consequently, most of the following discussion does not usually apply to the above administration routes but systemic effects may occur if therapy is prolonged or there is increased permeability in the injured tissue being treated.

□ ASSESSMENT

□ Subjective Data

A complete drug history is essential since corticosteroids adversely interact with many drugs (see Interactions, above). Patients taking insulin, oral antidiabetic agents, or oral anticoagulants may need dosage increases during therapy. Patients on digitalis may need careful monitoring of potassium and serum drug levels to avoid digitalis toxicity. Patients on theophylline may require similar monitoring to avoid a toxic drug reaction. Use of over-the-counter drugs including aspirin and cold or allergy remedies must be explored. Aspirin can increase the anti-inflammatory action of these drugs; cold and allergy remedies may contain anticholinergics or adrenergics, which can dangerously increase intraocular pressure.

Few drugs affect as many body systems as corticosteroids. Consequently, whenever possible, the patient should have a complete history and physical examination before therapy begins. However, these drugs are frequently started in emergency situations. In such cases, it is necessary to determine whether the patient has an active infection, such as a fungus or tuberculosis, or has recently received any type of vaccination that would contraindicate use. In addition, a history of cardiovascular disease, gastrointestinal dysfunction, renal problems, hematologic disorders, endocrine problems such as hypothyroidism or diabetes mellitus, glaucoma, or neurologic disorders should be identified. Corticosteroids must be used with caution and the nurse must be aware of how certain disorders may influence the patient's reaction to the drug. For example, the patient with coronary artery disease may be likely to develop congestive heart failure while on the drug.

For the patient starting long-term treatment, the nurse also assesses attitude about drug therapy, willingness to comply with the regimen, and understanding of the drug effects on the body as well as its benefits. Body function may change dramatically while the drug provides great benefits in a disease process. The patient needs an explanation of the risks and benefits of treatment to make a decision. While there are usually few other alternatives when corticosteroid therapy is chosen, the patient who has a clear understanding of the drug and who feels honest explanations about its effects have been given is more likely to follow the prescribed therapy. The patient's support systems can be extremely helpful with decision-making and in assisting the patient to cope with changes in body image.

□ *Objective Data*

Physical examination of the cardiovascular, respiratory, renal, gastrointestinal, and neurologic systems is essential before treatment begins. Blood pressure, pulse, respiration, weight, current fluid intake to urinary output ratio, mental status, and reflexes should be highlighted since these form the basic parameters that may change during drug treatment. In children, height measurements must also be recorded. They will be closely monitored throughout therapy since corticosteroids may interfere with normal growth.

Laboratory data may include a complete urinalysis, electrolytes, complete blood count with differential, serum and urine glucose, renal function studies, and plasma cortisol level, all of which will be monitored regularly during treatment. A chest x-ray study may be ordered to rule out respiratory infection.

□ *NURSING DIAGNOSES*

For the patient starting on steroid therapy an *actual* nursing diagnosis may be

> Knowledge deficit related to the administration and side-effects of steroid therapy

Other diagnoses may develop as therapy progresses. The following are *potential* problems and are related to the side-effects of the drug. This is not an exclusive list.

> Alterations in cardiac output: decreased
> Alteration in comfort related to gastrointestinal pain
> Excess fluid volume
> Altered growth and development (in children)
> Potential for infection related to delayed healing
> Self-concept: disturbance in body image
> Potential for injury: trauma
> Sensory–perceptual alteration: visual changes
> Alteration in thought processes related to drug effect or perception of drug effect
> Alteration in tissue integrity
> Alteration in nutrition: potential for less than body requirements of potassium and protein
> Alteration in nutrition: potential for more than body requirements of sodium and calcium

□ *PLAN*

Nursing care goals focus on

1. Safe and correct drug administration during the acute treatment phase
2. Monitoring for side-effects, which are numerous, but especially adrenal insufficiency and Cushing's syndrome
3. Teaching the patient how to take the drug correctly, how to monitor side-effects and when to report problems, how to withdraw from the drug when necessary, and what dietary restrictions may be necessary

□ *INTERVENTION*

Corticosteroids are most frequently administered by the oral or intravenous route. Rectal or intramuscular routes are used occasionally. Rectal administration is usually through retention enema for treatment of colitis and must be given with caution to avoid perforation since the rectal wall is very fragile in this condition. The patient is usually mildly sedated and given antidiarrheal medication to increase comfort and aid enema retention. Systemic absorption is usually minimal but may occur if tissue permeability is increased. The patient should be told to report any pain or burning immediately.

Intramuscular injections of the respiratory corticosteroid drug form must be given deep in a large muscle mass and sites must be rotated using a body map to avoid random rotation (see Chap. 8 for an example). Sterile abscesses and tissue atrophy can occur; consequently, sites should be palpated for pain, swelling, or fissures before each injection.

Corticosteroids can be administered intravenously by injection, intermittent infusion, or continuous drip. Injection should be at a rate no greater than 100 mg per minute since too rapid injection can cause perineal burning or tingling, nystagmus, and vertigo. Intermittent and continuous infusions should be monitored by an infusion pump. Corticosteroids come in multiple formulations but only a few are appropriate for intravenous use and such information should be clearly stated on the container label. Nurses should clarify any orders that seem ambiguous since certain forms used for intramuscular injections are inappropriate for IV use (see Table 55-3). Corticosteroids are physically incompatible with many other drugs (see Appendix). Therefore, a separate IV line should be used for drug administration. If the patient's condition makes finding a separate line impossible, the timing of corticosteroid administration should be 1 to 2 hours away from administration of other drugs and the IV line must be completely flushed before the next drug is given.

Regardless of the route of drug administration, there are several guidelines to follow when administering corticosteroids or teaching the patient about taking them at home. The goal of therapy is to use the minimum effective dose to achieve the desired response in order to minimize the occurrence of side-effects, some of which can be fatal. The dose should never be withheld due to vomiting, illness, or problems in swallowing. The physician should be notified and an alternate route chosen. Allowing cortisol levels to drop may increase the risk of side-effects.

Except in emergencies, dosing of steroids should be timed so the normal diurnal pattern of cortisol secretion is disrupted as little as possible. If the dose is once per day the medication should be taken before 9 AM; if twice a day, the second dose should be taken before 4 PM. During early therapy plasma cortisol levels will be monitored to indicate the effectiveness of the drug, how it is influencing the diurnal cortisol pattern, and what adjustments in dosage are needed. Once a therapeutic dose is established the patient may be placed on an alternate-day pattern of therapy. He will be advised to take a dose of the steroid large enough to work for 48 hours and will take the drug every other day. Such a pattern has been found to be least disruptive to the diurnal cortisol level, to lessen the chance of the development of cushingoid symptoms, and, in children, to minimize the growth retardation that frequently occurs with steroid therapy. Some manufacturers supply oral preparations in calendar boxes to assist the patient in taking every-other-day doses accurately. A calendar marked with the dosage days may also be helpful.

Once a patient has been taking a steroid the equivalent of 20 mg of hydrocortisone daily for 2 weeks, he is considered on long-term therapy and must be gradually withdrawn from the drug when therapy is discontinued. Withdrawal must be done under supervision and the patient closely monitored for the development of adrenal insufficiency. Generally, a protocol is initiated whereby the patient reduces the dose of steroid approximately 5 mg every 3 to 7 days. If no side-effects occur within that period the drug dose is further reduced until it is completely eliminated. Even after a steroid is safely withdrawn several months may pass before the adrenal glands consistently maintain a normal cortisol level. Consequently, the patient must be aware of the symptoms of insufficiency for at least 6 months after treatment cessation. If the patient faces a major stress such as a family death, injury, surgery, or disease in that period, the adrenal gland may not respond sufficiently and steroid therapy may need to be reinitiated. All patients on long-term corticosteroid therapy should be encouraged to wear a Medic-Alert appliance to identify their drug therapy readily in case of emergency.

The patient on steroid therapy must know specific sets of symptoms to watch for in order to avert or manage side-effects. Failure to catch changes early can lead to serious injury or death.

Of the common side-effects, GI irritability is usually preventable. The patient should be taught to take steroid medication with milk or food and never on an empty stomach and should try to avoid gastric irritants such as caffeine, alcohol, and smoking because they can increase the risk of ulcer development. Early symptoms of ulceration include a gnawing sensation in the epigastric region, dark stools, nausea, bloating, and hematemesis. If any symptoms occur the health team should be notified immediately. Some patients are given anti-ulcer therapy to prevent ulceration, such as antacids or histamine antagonists. The most dangerous side-effect occurs when the patient is either not getting a sufficient quantity of corticosteroid or the body is not responding to the dose. If this occurs, adrenal insufficiency will develop. Early symptoms include fatigue, loss of appetite, nausea, vomiting, and diarrhea. The patient may fail to relate these symptoms to steroid therapy, thinking instead that he has the flu. But symptoms left untreated can rapidly progress to weakness, coma, hypoglycemia, and vascular collapse as a result of rapid alterations in potassium and sodium. Acute adrenal insufficiency can be fatal. Therefore, the patient needs to learn the early symptoms and set up a "sick-day routine." If symptoms worsen within several hours, he should call the physician. If they do not worsen but do not improve, he should still call the physician. Sometimes a patient will be given instructions to automatically increase the steroid dose when symptoms occur and if symptoms do not subside the patient must contact the health team. These same rules may be applied if a patient on steroids develops a cold, sore throat, or flu symptoms.

At the other end of the spectrum of side-effects from steroids is the development of cushingoid symptoms. The patient may develop drug-induced Cushing's syndrome (see Introduction) or exhibit only a few of the symptoms. Early symptoms may include amenorrhea and fat pads on the chest and abdomen as well as facial puffiness. Cushingoid symptoms may indicate steroid overdose and will disappear as the drug dosage is reduced or drug is withdrawn. Sometimes the dose cannot be lowered to maintain the therapeutic response and the patient must choose between the symptoms of the disease being treated and the changed body image from the drug. This is difficult to cope with and is a frequent cause of noncompliance. The nurse needs to allow the patient opportunities to discuss this problem in order to try to maintain the therapy. Sometimes the patient will refuse to continue therapy. In such a case it is safer to help the patient *gradually* withdraw from the steroid than to abandon him, since he will surely stop on his own.

Delayed healing and masked infection are other side-effects of steroid therapy and can be extremely dangerous. The patient needs to make any dentist or surgeon he sees aware of the drug regimen since even a tooth filling can be complicated in the steroid-dependent individual. If the patient suffers any cut that doesn't heal within a few days

he should report it to the health team. Since corticosteroid therapy reduces the body's response to infection, even a minor injury may need treatment. Patients need to be taught to report any slight temperature elevation; a sore, scratchy, or reddened throat; cough; or redness, swelling, or drainage at an infection site. The patient should limit contact with anyone who has an infection, even a cold, but especially with children during the season for chickenpox. In the hospital all visitors should be screened for symptoms of infection. Delayed healing may result in wound separation in the postsurgical patient or can result in serious wound infection of even a small cut or abrasion the patient gets at home.

Skin integrity becomes more fragile during long-term corticosteroid therapy and is a factor in the development of decubitus ulcers in patients with limited mobility. Frequent position changes, careful turning to avoid skin abrasion, and use of padding or special pressure-reducing devices in chairs and beds can decrease the development of ulcers. But skin assessment must be routinely completed. Such nursing intervention can also decrease the incidence of pathologic fractures, another side-effect of long-term corticosteroid therapy.

An increase in intraocular pressure may occur, especially in susceptible patients. Measurements of ocular pressure should be periodically performed on any patient receiving long-term therapy but all patients should be told to report immediately any eye pain, blurred vision, or scleral redness.

Mental status changes are not infrequent, especially in long-term therapy. Women report premenstrual mood swings and many patients report mild depression. The elderly are very prone to confusion, especially if the dose is too high. Patients with a history of psychoses may have a recurrence of previously controlled symptoms. Any change in mental status should be reported. Changes may be situational, especially if the drug is beginning to cause changes in appearance or body function, or may signal the need to reduce the dose.

Electrolytes and serum protein should be monitored throughout therapy. Electrolyte changes may occur as a function of drug action or as a precursor to adrenal crisis. Potassium may decrease, requiring supplements. Calcium and sodium levels may increase and may require dietary restrictions. Serum protein levels may drop, requiring an increase in protein intake.

An increase in serum sodium may be an early sign of fluid retention, which frequently occurs during corticosteroid therapy, especially in patients with preexisting cardiac problems. Patients should have their weight taken daily; vital signs monitored regularly for potential tachycardia, dyspnea, and hypertension; routine lung auscultation done for signs of rales; and extremities and sacrum examined for signs of peripheral edema. Any changes should be reported.

All patients are prone to the hypoglycemic effects of corticosteroids; therefore, serum and urine glucose levels should be monitored every six hours for patients on high doses of the drug, those who are known diabetics, and those who show increases in serum glucose. All patients on long-term therapy should do urine glucose testing daily and have periodic serum glucose levels drawn. Patients should report early signs of hypoglycemia such as thirst, dizziness or weakness, and hunger. Insulin may be needed during treatment of nondiabetics; known diabetics may require increases in dose.

The pregnant patient must be monitored even more closely when steroids are given since pregnancy increases the risk of side-effects to the mother and the fetus. After birth, the newborn must be closely monitored for signs of hypoadrenalism, which include vomiting, lethargy, poor feeding, hypotension, rapid weight loss, and low serum glucose. Breast-feeding must be avoided if the mother must continue taking the drug since corticosteroids readily enter the breast milk and pose a continuing threat to the newborn.

The patient on long-term therapy may want to keep a flow sheet at home to monitor himself for the development of other side-effects. He should watch his weight and for signs of edema since changes in these can occur suddenly. He may need to take his pulse or at least learn to be aware of its regularity and he may be taught to test urine glucose. All of these parameters can help him detect changes in his body that may warrant care. To treat the side-effects of steroid therapy successfully one must catch subtle changes early.

☐ **EVALUATION**
The outcome criteria the nurse may use to judge the success of steroid therapy include normal blood pressure, blood glucose, and plasma or urine cortisol levels; cortisol levels that remain higher in the morning than in the evening (indicating the maintenance of the diurnal pattern); absence of cushingoid symptoms or symptoms of insufficiency or other side-effects; and early reporting of problems and evidence of patient compliance with the regimen and follow-up visits. Nursing Care Plan 55-1

contains a summary of the nursing process for the patient on long-term therapy with oral adrenocortical steroids.

Adrenal Steroid Inhibitors

Two drugs are available for suppressing adrenal cortical hyperfunctioning in patients with Cushing's syndrome (see Disorders of the Adrenal Cortex, above). They are reviewed below.

Aminoglutethimide
(Cytadren)

MECHANISM AND ACTIONS
Aminoglutethimide reduces the synthesis of adrenal corticoids by binding to the hemoprotein cytochrome P450, thus limiting the conversion of cholesterol to delta-5-pregnenolone, a necessary step in the biosynthetic pathway of adrenal steroid production. Plasma hydrocortisone levels were reduced to at least 50% of baseline values in at least one third of patients studied.

USES
1. Suppression of adrenal function in selected patients with adrenocortical hyperfunction (Cushing's syndrome); usually given until more definitive therapy (*i.e.*, surgery) can be undertaken
2. Investigational uses include treatment of advanced mammary carcinoma in postmenopausal women and metastatic prostatic carcinoma.

ADMINISTRATION AND DOSAGE
Aminoglutethimide is available as tablets containing 250 mg. The initial dose is 250 mg four times a day at 6-hour intervals. If hydrocortisone suppression is inadequate, increase by 250 mg daily at 1-week to 2-week intervals to a total daily dose of 2 g.

Mineralocorticoid replacement may be necessary and may be accomplished with concurrent use of fludrocortisone.

If adverse reactions occur (*e.g.*, skin rash, extreme drowsiness), dosage reduction may be required. Persistent skin rash (*e.g.*, longer than 7 days) is an indication for discontinuing the drug.

FATE
Oral absorption is good and the plasma half-life is 12 hours to 16 hours initially but decreases to 5

(Text continues on p. 1074.)

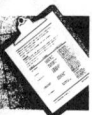

Assessment

Subjective Data

1. Medication history: see Interactions section to formulate appropriate questions.
   a. Focus on use of alcohol or street drugs, OTC cold or allergy remedies, digitalis, antidiabetic agents, xanthine drugs, oral anticoagulants.
   b. Allergies
2. Medical history
   a. Description of symptoms and progression of problem to present
   b. Complete medical history because all body systems can be affected by steroid therapy
   c. History of any recent vaccination
   d. Presence of any active infection especially fungus, eye infection, tuberculosis, herpes
3. Personal history/compliance issues
   a. Knowledge of proposed regimen, ability to manage long-term therapy
   b. Perception of self; acknowledgment of the risks versus benefits of treatment
   c. Personal resources; family supports

Objective Data

1. Physical assessment
   a. Cardiovascular: heart rate, rhythm, blood pressure, peripheral edema
   b. Gastrointestinal: motility, bowel sounds, presence of any epigastric pain
   c. Neurologic: mental acuity, reality orientation, memory, psychomotor function
   d. Growth and development: height, weight, and cognitive and motor skills for age (for children)
2. Laboratory data
   a. Blood, urine glucose levels
   b. Serum electrolytes
   c. Renal and hepatic function studies
   d. Plasma cortisol
   e. CBC with differential

Nursing Diagnosis	Expected Client Outcome	Intervention
Knowledge deficit: related to drug action, correct self-administration, potential side-effects, the need for supervised withdrawal, and the importance of informing all caregivers that steroids are taken	Will verbalize understanding of drug action and administration.	During dosage adjustment monitor response to drug closely to ensure use of the minimum effective dose. Goal is to provide effective drug action, but to maintain a normal cortisol level that is higher in the AM than in PM.
		Encourage patient on long-term therapy to follow prescribed regimen closely, usually every other day dosing.
	Will seek assistance when unable to take drug or when withdrawal is desired/necessary.	Teach patient never to withhold a dose but to seek medical advice if unable to take the drug for any reason.
		Inform the patient that the drug must be gradually withdrawn under supervision, even when side-effects occur, to prevent adrenal insufficiency.

(continued)

Nursing Diagnosis	Expected Client Outcome	Intervention
Knowledge deficit: related to drug action, correct self-administration, potential side-effects, the need for supervised withdrawal, and the importance of informing all caregivers that steroids are taken (*continued*)	Will seek follow-up care during and after treatment as appropriate.	Teach the patient to contact physician during any period of stress or illness while on the medication and for 6 months after medication is discontinued.
		Encourage frequent follow-up care to monitor changes in laboratory levels and to detect any symptoms of side-effects.
	Will obtain and wear a Medic-Alert device.	Encourage the patient to wear a Medic-Alert device to inform any caregiver of drug and dose in case of emergency.
	Will monitor, manage, and report side-effects as appropriate.	Teach the patient to monitor urine glucose or SBGM during therapy to ensure glucose remains within normal limits. Teach the patient symptoms of hypoglycemia, which should be reported immediately to the physician.
		Be aware that diabetic or pregnant patients are at greater risk of developing hypoglycemia and other drug-induced side-effects.
		Teach the patient to monitor other drug side-effects as described below and follow preventive/reactive strategies given.
Potential alteration in comfort: GI distress related to drug effect	Drug-induced ulcer will be prevented.	Emphasize the importance of taking the drug with food or milk, never on an empty stomach.
		Encourage use of anti-ulcer medications as prescribed, *i.e.*, antacids, histamine₂ antagonists.
		Teach patient to report nausea, hematemesis, gnawing epigastric pain immediately.
Potential alteration in cardiac output: decreased, related to vascular changes from adrenal insufficiency	Normal sinus rhythm is maintained.	Encourage patient to keep laboratory appointments for routine plasma cortisol and serum electrolyte levels, which may facilitate early detection.
		Establish a sick day routine by identifying what a sick day is for a patient on steroids, when to contact the physician, and what drug dose to take, as prescribed.
		Teach the patient to report immediately any fatigue, anorexia, nausea, vomiting, or diarrhea.

(continued)

Nursing Diagnosis	Expected Client Outcome	Intervention
Potential disturbance in body image: related to cushingoid symptoms from drug (adults and children)	Will verbalize concerns about change in body.	Teach the patient to report amenorrhea, fat pads, facial puffiness. Drug dose may need to be reduced.
		Discuss changes in body image that may have to be accepted for length of needed drug therapy.
Potential alteration in growth and development: related to cushingoid symptoms (children)	Growth will remain normal for age.	Monitor child's growth (height) at least monthly, especially during times of expected growth spurts. Radiographic exam of long bones may be ordered if stunted growth is suspected.
Potential for infection: related to delayed healing and suppressed immune response	Will use preventive measures to reduce risk of infection.	Teach the patient to limit contact with anyone who has any type of infection.
		Encourage safety measures to decrease risk of cuts and scrapes. Tell the patient to report any wound that does not heal within 7 days or if color and drainage of wound change.
		Teach patient to report any sore throat, temperature elevation, flu-like symptoms immediately.
Potential for impaired tissue integrity: related to tissue fragility	Pressure ulcers will be prevented.	Set up a routine turning and position change schedule for any debilitated or elderly bedridden.
		Use padding or bed devices to reduce pressure on bony prominences.
		Prevent shearing against skin during turning to decrease skin abrasions from bed linen.
Potential for injury: trauma related to brittle bones	Pathologic fractures will be prevented.	Be aware that elderly, debilitated patients or those with pre-existing osteoporosis are most susceptible to this problem.
		Use caution in turning and positioning to decrease pressure and stress on bones.
		Encourage ambulation as much as possible when a patient is able to do so. Encourage safety devices and assistance to decrease the risk of falls.
Potential sensory–perceptual alterations in vision: related to increased intraocular pressure	Will report any change in vision immediately.	Ensure that patient has periodic tonometric examinations throughout therapy.
		Teach the patient to report immediately any blurred vision, scleral redness, eye pain.

(continued)

1073

Nursing Diagnosis	Expected Client Outcome	Intervention
Potential alteration in thought processes: related to drug effect	Changes in mental status will be reported promptly.	Be aware that drug-induced depression and psychoses are more likely to occur in the elderly, in children, and in the patient with a psychiatric history of such problems.
		Teach family to report any change in patient's level of alertness, sociability, reality orientation. Drug will be gradually withdrawn.
Potential alteration in nutrition: related to drug effect · less than body requirements of protein and potassium · more than body requirements of sodium and calcium	Serum protein and electrolytes will remain within normal limits.	Encourage patient to increase protein intake during therapy to reduce risk of protein depletion.
		Encourage patient to keep laboratory appointments for periodic monitoring of electrolytes.
		If sodium levels increase, sodium restriction is warranted.
		If potassium levels fall, supplements and foods rich in potassium must be added. Patients on digitalis must be monitored closely for the development of cardiac arrhythmias.
		If calcium levels increase, the patient must restrict calcium, increase fluid intake, and monitor for development of renal calculi.
Potential alteration in fluid volume: excess	Weight gain will be minimal during therapy.	Be aware that fluid retention is usually related to an increase in sodium.
		Teach the patient to report immediately any rapid weight gain, dyspnea, or palpitations.
		Monitor patient for peripheral edema, elevated heart rate, elevated blood pressure.
		Teach patient to keep input and output record. Monitor any shift in input/output ratio where input > output. Report to physician.

hours to 8 hours after 1 week to 2 weeks of therapy. Approximately one half of a dose is excreted unchanged in the urine, and the remainder as metabolites. Protein binding is minimal.

SIDE-EFFECTS/ADVERSE REACTIONS
The most frequently encountered side-effects with aminoglutethimide are drowsiness, skin rash, anorexia, nausea, and dizziness. Other adverse reactions can include the following:

Hematologic—Neutropenia, transient leukopenia, pancytopenia, thrombocytopenia
Cardiovascular—Orthostatic hypotension, tachycardia
GI—Vomiting
Dermatologic—Pruritus, urticaria

Other—Adrenal insufficiency, hypothyroidism, hirsutism, fever, myalgia, altered liver function tests, cholestatic jaundice

CONTRAINDICATIONS AND PRECAUTIONS

The drug should be given with *caution* to persons with hypothyroidism, hepatic disease (drug can elevate serum glutamic-oxaloacetic transaminase, alkaline phosphatase, and bilirubin), acute illness (increased likelihood of adrenal cortical *hypo*function), and to pregnant or nursing mothers. The safety for use in children has not been established.

INTERACTIONS

1. Aminoglutethimide can accelerate the metabolism of dexamethasone. If glucocorticoid supplementation is necessary, hydrocortisone is preferred.

NURSING CONSIDERATIONS

See Nursing Considerations for trilostane, below.

Trilostane

(Modastrane)

MECHANISM AND ACTIONS

Trilostane lowers circulating glucocorticoid levels by inhibiting enzyme systems essential for their production. There is a corresponding increase in urinary 17-ketosteroid levels. The above effects become apparent within the first few days of treatment. Trilostane exhibits *no* intrinsic hormonal activity.

USES

1. Temporary treatment of adrenal cortical hyperfunction (Cushing's syndrome) until more definitive measures (*e.g.*, surgery) can be undertaken.

ADMINISTRATION AND DOSAGE

Trilostane is available as 30-mg and 60-mg capsules. The initial dose is 30 mg four times a day, which may be increased gradually at 3-day to 4-day intervals. Most persons respond to doses less than 360 mg/day. Failure to respond within 2 weeks is reason for discontinuing therapy. Careful monitoring of plasma or urinary hormones and electrolytes is essential during therapy.

SIDE-EFFECTS/ADVERSE REACTIONS

The most common side-effects with trilostane are diarrhea, abdominal discomfort and cramping, burning sensations of the oral or nasal membranes, flushing, and headache. Other adverse reactions noted include bloating, belching, nasal stuffiness, lacrimation, muscle or joint pain, erythema, skin rash, numbness or tingling of extremities, fever, and fatigue.

CONTRAINDICATIONS AND PRECAUTIONS

Trilostane is contraindicated in persons with adrenal insufficiency or severe renal or hepatic disease and in pregnant women. The drug should be given *cautiously* to patients receiving other drugs that suppress adrenal function, to patients with an acute illness, and to nursing mothers. The safety for use of trilostane in children has not been established.

INTERACTIONS

1. Concurrent use of trilostane and aminoglutethimide or mitotane can cause severe adrenal cortical hypofunction.

NURSING CONSIDERATIONS

The nurse must coordinate close monitoring of the patient receiving an adrenal steroid inhibitor since multiple laboratory studies must be performed and the patient must watch closely for side-effects. Initially, a complete blood count, thyroid function studies, liver function studies, serum electrolytes, and cortisol levels should be obtained since all of these can be altered during therapy and changes will signal the development of toxic side-effects. This patient will benefit from having a carefully maintained laboratory flow sheet, so comparisons can be made quickly.

Cortisol levels are expected to decrease on steroid suppression therapy but a balance must be maintained. The drug may become too effective or the patient may suffer increased stress, both of which may produce symptoms of adrenal insufficiency. Early symptoms such as fatigue, nausea, vomiting, loss of appetite, and diarrhea should be reported. However, nausea and loss of appetite may be transient early in therapy so cortisol levels are a more accurate indicator of the development of insufficiency.

Teach the patient that orthostatic hypotension may occur throughout therapy. The patient needs to get in the habit of rising slowly and sitting down as soon as dizziness or lightheadedness occurs. Caution the patient to limit driving, heavy lifting, and quick changes in position until he knows how this symptom affects him.

Hypothyroidism may develop as a result of adrenal suppression. Teach the patient to watch for early side-effects, such as fatigue, weakness, or a sense of heaviness, and to report them immediately. Thyroid supplement therapy may be necessary.

CASE STUDY

Ellen Casey, age 32, has been an asthmatic for 20 years. Mrs. Casey was brought to the emergency room by her husband after suffering for several days with increasing symptoms. At the time she was admitted, she had difficulty breathing, was wheezing, had an irregular heart rate of 160, and was diaphoretic. She was started on hydrocortisone, 50 mg by intravenous piggyback every 12 hours for the first 24 hours, after Mrs. Casey reported that she had been unresponsive to all theophylline preparations prescribed for her. Initial diagnosis was status asthmaticus but after blood work showed an elevated theophylline level the diagnosis was changed to theophylline toxicity.

As Mrs. Casey's breathing improved she was switched to prednisone, 60 mg in two divided doses. She continued to improve rapidly and was discharged on prednisone, 30 mg daily.

Over the next few weeks the physician attempted to gradually wean Mrs. Casey from steroids. After 2 weeks at 30 mg daily, he reduced the dose to prednisone, 20 mg daily for 1 week, then prednisone, 10 mg daily for 1 week. At this point Mrs. Casey developed a tooth infection and the prednisone had to be increased to 30 mg daily until the infection resolved 2 weeks later.

The weaning process began again but by this time Mrs. Casey had begun to develop steroid side-effects. In the 2½ months Mrs. Casey had taken steroids she had gained 25 lb and developed extra facial hair, moderate moon facies, some gastrointestinal discomfort, dry skin, and amenorrhea. She was anxious to get off the drug but understood the necessity for gradual withdrawal. The withdrawal dosage schedule was as follows: prednisone, 20 mg daily for 1 week, then 10 mg daily for 1 week, then 5 mg daily for 1 week, then 5 mg daily every other day, then 2.5 mg daily for 1 week, then 1 mg daily for 5 days, and then the drug was discontinued.

Mrs. Casey remained symptom-free with no signs of adrenal insufficiency until she developed flu symptoms 3 months later. Cortisol levels dropped and she complained of nausea, vomiting, and diarrhea. The physician ordered prednisone, 20 mg PO daily. On interview, the patient told the nurse she did not want to take steroids again because she was "very afraid of getting hooked again."

Discussion Questions

1. Why would the physician want to use steroids again on Mrs. Casey after 3 months off the drug?
2. Why does Ellen Casey perceive steroid therapy as "getting hooked again"?

3. Outline a strategy for encouraging Mrs. Casey to agree to the therapy.
4. What administration strategies should the nurse recommend to decrease the amount of disruption to Mrs. Casey's normal diurnal cortisol pattern?
5. What side-effects should this patient be taught to watch for?

REVIEW QUESTIONS

1. What are the principal secretory products of the (1) adrenal medulla and (2) adrenal cortex?
2. Briefly describe the major actions of the glucocorticoids.
3. What are the three types of adrenocorticosteroids?
4. How does fludrocortisone differ from desoxycorticosterone in action?
5. What are the principal side-effects associated with mineralocorticoids used clinically?
6. Describe the actions of glucocorticoids that may contribute to their anti-inflammatory activity.
7. Why is the timing of daily glucocorticoid dosing so important?
8. What are the dangers associated with prolonged use of glucocorticoids?
9. For what indicators are inhaled corticosteroids used?
10. What cautions must be observed when transferring patients from oral to inhaled corticosteroids?
11. What assessment parameters are essential to watch when monitoring a patient for side-effects from steroid drugs?
12. What two factors should the nurse remember when administering or teaching about steroid therapy?
13. Describe the purpose of an alternate-day dosing schedule for the patient taking a steroid.
14. What are the early symptoms of adrenal insufficiency? What actions should be taken if they occur?
15. Why does a patient develop cushingoid symptoms from steroids? What actions may be taken if such symptoms develop?
16. Describe the mechanism of action of adrenal steroid inhibitors.
17. What laboratory data must be closely monitored in the patient taking adrenal steroid inhibitors?

BIBLIOGRAPHY

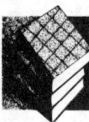

Adams CE: Pulling your patient through an adrenal crisis. RN 46(10):36, October, 1983

Baxter JD, Rosseau GG (eds): Glucocorticoid Hormone Action. New York, Springer-Verlag, 1979

Baylink DJ: Glucocorticoid-induced osteoporosis. N Engl J Med 309:306, 1983

Cornell RC, Stoughton RB: The use of topical steroids in psoriasis. Dermatol Clin 2:397, 1984

Corticotropin-releasing factor (symposium). Fed Proc 44:145, 1985

Cupps TR, Fauci AS: Corticosteroid-mediated immunoregulation in man. Immunol Rev 65:133, 1982

Donham J: The weakness of steroids. Am J Nurs 86:917, 1986

Gotch PM: Teaching patients about adrenal corticosteroids. Am J Nurs 81:78, 1981

Larson CA: The critical path of adrenocortical insufficiency. Nursing '84 14:66, 1984

Messer J, Reitman D, Sacks HS et al: Association of adrenocorticosteroid therapy and peptic ulcer disease. N Engl J Med 309:21, 1983

Miller JA, Munro DD: Topical corticosteroids: Clinical pharmacology and therapeutic use. Drugs 19:119, 1980

Schleimer RP: The mechanisms of anti-inflammatory steroid action in allergic diseases. Ann Rev Pharmacol Toxicol 25:381, 1985

Streeten DH: Corticosteroid Therapy. 1. Pharmacologic properties and principles of corticosteroid use. JAMA 232:944, 1975

Swatz SL, Dluhy RG: Corticosteroids: Clinical pharmacology and therapeutic use. Drugs 16:238, 1978

Young C: Drugs: Actions and reactions—topical corticosteroids. J Enterost Therapy 11:245, Nov-Dec, 1984

Estrogens and Progestins

56

The female hormones may be categorized into two types—estrogens and progestins. Both groups are composed of steroidal compounds secreted by the ovaries beginning around the time of puberty, by the placenta during pregnancy, and in much lesser amounts by the adrenal cortex throughout life. The female sex hormones play a major role in the development and maintenance of the reproductive system and also affect the functioning of many other physiologic systems.

Secretion of female hormones is cyclical in nature and a brief review of this process is presented below.

The Menstrual Cycle

The menstrual cycle is characterized by a series of alterations in the uterine lining of a nonpregnant woman that result from changes in circulatory levels of estrogens and progestins. Figure 56-1 is a graphic representation of the hormonal and anatomical changes occurring during a single menstrual cycle.

The release of gonadotropins from the anterior pituitary gland is controlled by a peptide termed gonadotropin-releasing hormone (GnRH), which is secreted by the hypothalamus into the portal circulation that perfuses the anterior pituitary. GnRH stimulates the release of follicle-stimulating hormone (FSH) and luteinizing hormone (LH) from the pituitary, and these hormones in turn facilitate the development of the follicles in the ovary and the release of the ovum from the mature follicle, respectively. Specifically, FSH encourages the initial maturation of several follicles within the ovary, one of which eventually becomes dominant while the others eventually regress. Under the influence of both FSH *and* LH, the follicles continue to grow and produce estrogens. These in turn act on the uterine lining to increase its vascularity and facilitate its thickening in preparation for implantation of a fertilized egg. This phase of the cycle is termed the *proliferative phase*. The rapidly rising estrogen levels stimulate further release of GnRH and spur the LH-releasing mechanism so that on approximately day 10 or 11 of the cycle there occurs a sudden sharp increase in LH secretion, the so-called LH surge. The high level of LH triggers the rupture of the mature, dominant follicle, and ovulation occurs. Following ovulation, the follicle is transformed into a corpus luteum, which secretes considerable amounts of progesterone in addition to estrogens, and under the influence of both of these hormones, the endometrial glands continue to grow, the arteries become enlarged and spiraled, and the endometrium is now prepared to accept a fertilized egg. In addition, the elevated levels of estrogen and progesterone together exert a *negative* feedback on further release of GnRH from the hypothalamus and on the subsequent release of FSH and LH from the anterior pituitary. Coupled with the degeneration of the corpus luteum, in the absence of fertilization, estrogen and progesterone levels begin to decline rapidly and the endometrial tissue degenerates and is sloughed off, resulting in the appearance of menses. As the levels of estrogen and progesterone continue to fall, the negative feedback inhibition on GnRH release is removed and a new cycle begins with the secretion of FSH and LH from the anterior pituitary.

If fertilization occurs, the corpus luteum remains and continues to secrete estrogen and progesterone during the early weeks of pregnancy. The other important source of hormones during pregnancy is the placenta, and by the end of the second month of pregnancy the placenta becomes the major source of estrogen and progesterone for the duration of the pregnancy.

Therapeutic Uses of Estrogens

The estrogens are a group of both naturally occurring and synthetic derivatives that exhibit similar pharmacologic and toxicologic effects, differing primarily in their suitability for a particular route of administration, their potency, and their therapeutic indications. One useful classification of the estrogens divides them into the following categories:

1. Natural (endogenous) estrogens (*e.g.*, estradiol, estriol, estrone)
2. Esters and conjugates of natural estrogens (*e.g.*, estradiol valerate, estropipate, polyestradiol phosphate, conjugated estrogens)
3. Semisynthetic and synthetic estrogens (*e.g.*, ethinyl estradiol, chlorotrianisene, dienestrol, diethylstilbestrol)

The endogenous estrogens are composed of several related substances, the principal one being estradiol, which is the most potent. Estradiol is rapidly converted to estrone, which is approximately one half as potent. Estrone in turn is metabolized in estriol, the weakest in action of the three. These endogenous estrogens promote the growth and de-

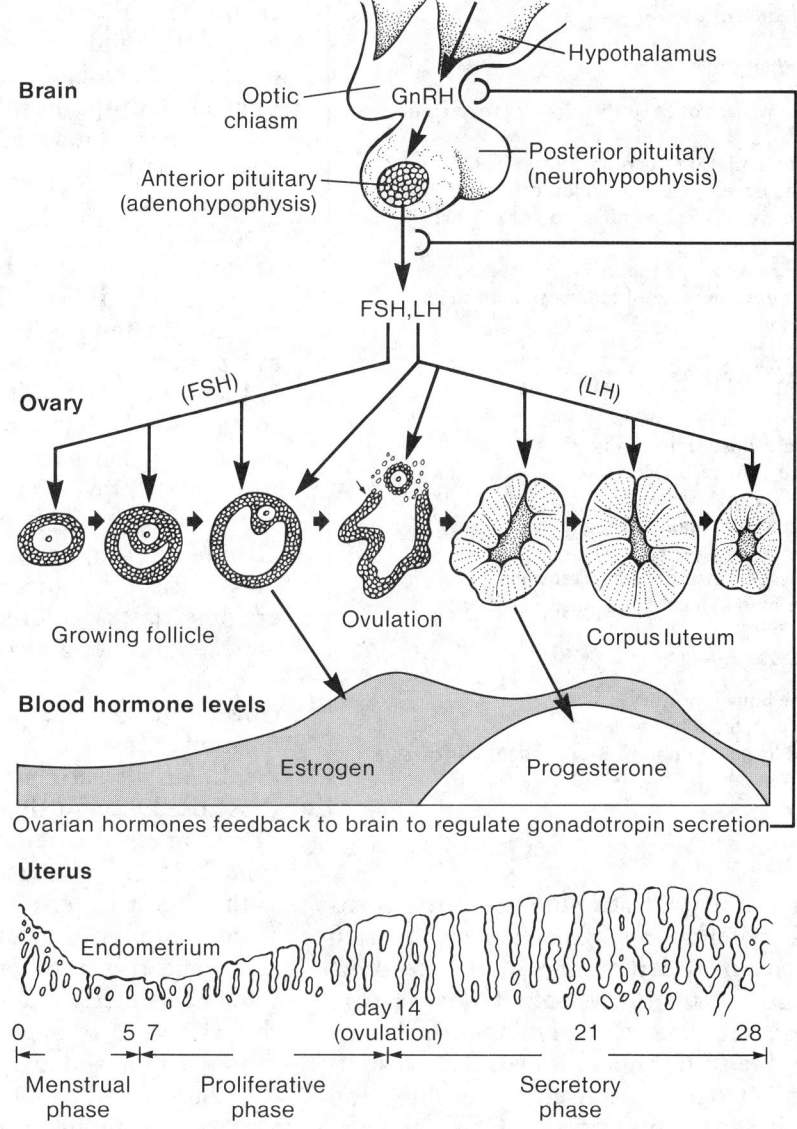

Brain

Hypothalamus

Optic chiasm — GnRH

Anterior pituitary (adenohypophysis)

Posterior pituitary (neurohypophysis)

FSH,LH

Ovary   (FSH)   (LH)

Growing follicle   Ovulation   Corpus luteum

Blood hormone levels

Estrogen   Progesterone

Ovarian hormones feedback to brain to regulate gonadotropin secretion

Uterus

Endometrium

0   5 7   day 14   21   28
                              (ovulation)

Menstrual phase   Proliferative phase   Secretory phase

Figure 56-1. The menstrual (endometrial) cycle.

Key: ➝ stimulation; ─⟅ inhibition; GnRH, gonadotropin-releasing hormone; FSH, follicle-stimulating hormone; LH, luteinizing hormone.

velopment of the endometrium and exert a wide range of effects on other body structures (see Effects of Estrogens).

Naturally occurring estrogens are poorly absorbed when administered orally, are rapidly inactivated, and are quickly eliminated; thus, they are largely unsuited for oral therapy. Estradiol is available for injection as either the cypionate or valerate salt in an oily vehicle (long acting), whereas estrone is available as an aqueous suspension (short acting). Crystalline estrone sulfate stabilized with piperazine (estropipate) can be used as a vaginal cream, as

can dienestrol, a synthetic estrogen. Orally effective estrogens include micronized estradiol, estropipate, conjugated and esterified estrogenic substances, and a number of semisynthetic and synthetic derivatives. Estradiol is also available as a transdermal patch. Two very potent orally effective semisynthetic estrogens, ethinyl estradiol and mestranol, are the estrogens found in the combination oral contraceptive formulations; these products are reviewed in Chapter 57.

Principal indications for use of estrogens include relief of the symptoms of menopause, symp-

Effects of Estrogens

Reproductive Effects

1. Decrease release of FSH (through negative feedback)
2. Facilitate ovulation (increase release of LH)
3. Stimulate development of endometrium
4. Promote growth and cornification of vaginal epithelium
5. Increase sensitivity of uterus to oxytocin
6. Promote development of duct system in mammary glands

Metabolic Effects

1. Increase protein synthesis
2. Accelerate closure of epiphyses
3. Decrease bone resorption rate
4. Increase serum triglycerides
5. Decrease serum cholesterol and low-density lipoproteins
6. Enhance sodium and water retention
7. Increase blood glucose (anti-insulin action)

Miscellaneous Effects

1. Decrease bowel motility
2. Reduce platelet adhesiveness
3. Increase levels of vitamin-K-dependent clotting factors

tomatic management of atrophic vaginitis, treatment of primary female hypogonadism and ovarian failure, palliation of certain types of carcinoma, suppression of lactation, relief of postpartum breast engorgement, and control of abnormal uterine bleeding due to hormonal imbalance. In addition, certain estrogens are used in combination with progestins for contraception. Of these uses, the treatment of menopause has been the most controversial application for estrogens, and division of opinion still exists on the safety and efficacy of oral estrogen replacement therapy for menopausal symptomatology.

Uses of Estrogens in Menopause

Between the approximate ages of 45 and 55, a woman's menstrual cycle begins to show increasing variability and a reduced frequency of ovulation. The ovaries become less responsive to the action of gonadotropic hormones, the number of primary follicles is eventually depleted, menses are irregular and eventually cease, and degenerative changes gradually appear in many organs. The endome-

trium becomes atrophic, vaginal epithelium becomes thin and dry as glycogen production is reduced, and atrophic changes may also occur in the ovaries, fallopian tubes, and breasts. Clinical symptoms of menopause include vasomotor reactions (hot flashes, extreme sweating), headache, muscular aches, gradual loss of bone structure, and emotional instability.

Since menopause is related to a decreased production of estrogen, replacement therapy with estrogen has long been employed for treating the symptoms of menopause. Although this procedure is theoretically sound, the potential for estrogens to cause a variety of untoward reactions, some quite serious, has tempered the enthusiasm for this form of therapy. The principal hazards associated with estrogen replacement therapy are thromboembolic complications, gallbladder disease, and, most critically, endometrial carcinoma. The risk of endometrial carcinoma has been estimated to be between 5 times and 14 times greater than in nonusers, and is closely dependent on the dose of estrogens being used and the duration of therapy. Currently, the doses of estrogens being used in menopausal treatment are significantly lower than those used previously, and it is hoped that the risk of endometrial carcinoma will be reduced. Additionally, estrogens are now being given cyclically with progestins (i.e., 3 weeks estrogen followed by 1 week progestin or estrogen–progestin combination), and this regimen has also been reported to reduce the likelihood of endometrial carcinoma (although cyclic withdrawal bleeding is more common with the added progestin).

There is little doubt that low-dose oral estrogen therapy can reduce the incidence and severity of vasomotor symptoms associated with the menopause (such as sweating, flushing, "hot flashes") or that topical application is effective in retarding the atrophic changes in the vaginal epithelium (as in senile vaginitis). Conversely, there is no substantial evidence to support the use of estrogenic substances for the control of the mental and emotional changes that often accompany the onset of menopause. The use of estrogens to retard the progression of osteoporosis in menopausal women has been the subject of some debate; however, the current consensus of opinion seems to favor use of low doses of estrogen together with supplemental calcium as a safe and effective means of retarding bone loss and reducing the incidence of spontaneous fractures. The estrogen is usually given for 25 days each month and a progestin is added for the last 10 days for the reasons outlined above. Many clinicians prescribe supplemental calcium as well and it appears that the doses necessary to maintain a positive calcium balance in perimenopausal and postmenopausal women are 1.0 g to 1.5 g of calcium per day. Concurrent use of vitamin D is also recognized as safe and effective, but doses should be restricted to 400 U/day or less. Large doses of vitamin D have actually been demonstrated to *increase* bone resorption. Use of other therapeutic agents, such as calcitonin or sodium fluoride, is much less generally accepted.

The use of estrogens in menopausal women must be undertaken cautiously, minimal effective doses must be used, and cyclic administration should be employed. Therapy should be reevaluated at 3-month to 6-month intervals. Appropriate tests and physical examinations should be performed frequently because of the possibility of significant adverse effects.

The discussion of the estrogens considers the agents together as a group. Individual drugs and dosages are listed in Table 56-1 along with comments pertaining to each individual drug. Several estrogenic substances (diethylstilbestrol diphosphate, estramustine phosphate, polyestradiol phosphate) as well as an antiestrogen (tamoxifen) are used in treating various forms of carcinoma and are considered in detail in Chapter 75.

Estrogens

Chlorotrianisene, Conjugated Estrogens, Dienestrol, Diethylstilbestrol, Esterified Estrogens, Estradiol, Estrone, Estropipate, Ethinyl Estradiol, Polyestradiol Phosphate, Quinestrol

MECHANISM AND ACTIONS

The principal actions of the estrogens are listed above under Effects of Estrogens. They are essential for the development and maintenance of the female reproductive system and the secondary sex characteristics.

The biochemical actions of estrogens are apparently due to their interaction with receptor proteins on estrogen-responsive tissues (*e.g.*, breasts,

genitalia). As a result, there is increased synthesis of DNA, RNA, and various proteins that alter the function of these tissues. These receptor effects are blocked by inhibitors of RNA or protein synthesis.

The effects of estrogens to decrease resorption of bone are probably due to an antagonism of the action of parathyroid hormone on bone; however, estrogens do not appear to stimulate bone formation.

USES
See Table 56-1 for specific indications for each drug.
1. Relief of vasomotor, atrophic, and osteoporotic symptoms of the menopause
2. Treatment of atrophic vaginitis and kraurosis vulvae (dryness and pruritus of genitalia)
3. Replacement therapy in female hypogonadism, female castration, and primary ovarian failure
4. Palliative treatment of advanced prostatic carcinoma and mammary carcinoma in women who are at least 5 years postmenopausal (See Chap. 75)
5. Relief of postpartum breast engorgement (benefit versus risk must be critically weighed; use is largely obsolete)
6. Control of abnormal uterine bleeding due to lack of estrogen secretion (parenteral conjugated estrogens)
7. Relief of severe acne resistant to more conventional therapy (investigational use in female patients only)
8. Postcoital contraception (investigational use for diethylstilbestrol, 25 mg twice daily for 5 days; emergency *only*)

ADMINISTRATION AND DOSAGE
See Table 56-1 for specific dosing recommendations for each drug.

Most indications for estrogens require cyclical therapy (*i.e.*, 3 weeks on and 1 week off). A progestin may be given during the final week to mimic the normal physiological cycle more closely and reduce the likelihood of endometrial carcinoma. Likewise, during chronic estrogen therapy (*e.g.*, cancer), use of a progestin is recommended during the last 10 dosing days each month.

FATE
Estradiol is metabolized to estrone and further to estriol, which is then conjugated and excreted in the urine. Natural estrogens are rapidly inactivated in the gastrointestinal (GI) tract. Esterification of

(*Text continues on p. 1088.*)

**Table 56-1
Estrogens**

Drug	Preparations	Usual Dosage Range	Clinical Considerations
chlorotrianisene (Tace)	Capsules—12 mg, 25 mg, 72 mg	Menopause—12 mg–25 mg/day cyclically for 30 days Breast engorgement—12 mg 4 times/day for 7 days or 50 mg every 6 h for 6 doses or 72 mg twice a day for 2 days Female hypogonadism—12 mg–25 mg/day cyclically for 21 days, followed by 100 mg progesterone IM Prostatic carcinoma—12 mg–25 mg/day	Synthetic estrogen with delayed onset and prolonged duration of action; stored in adipose tissue; 72-mg capsule is used *only* for postpartum breast engorgement in non-nursing mothers; first dose should be given within 8 h of delivery; drug is not recommended for mammary carcinoma, because it induces uterine bleeding and endometrial hyperplasia (see Chap. 75).
conjugated estrogens (Estrocon, Premarin, Progens)	Tablets—0.3 mg, 0.625 mg, 0.9 mg, 1.25 mg, 2.5 mg Injection—25 mg/vial with 5 ml diluent Vaginal cream—0.625 mg/g	Menopause—0.3 mg–0.9 mg/day cyclically Hypogonadism, ovarian failure—2.5 mg–7.5 mg/day in divided doses for 20 days; oral progestin during last 5 days Prostatic carcinoma—1.25 mg–2.5 mg 3 times/day for several weeks (maintenance ½ initial dose) Breast cancer—10 mg 3 times/day for 2 months–5 months as needed to obtain desired response Vaginitis, kraurosis vulvae—insert vaginal cream 1 to 2 times/day Abnormal uterine bleeding—25 mg IV or IM; repeat in 6 h if necessary	Water-soluble mixture of conjugated estrogens (sodium estrone sulfate, 50%–65%, and sodium equilin sulfate, 20%–35%) obtained from the urine of pregnant mares; commonly used orally for treating menopausal symptoms; recommended doses are 0.3 mg–0.625 mg daily, usually in combination with calcium and vitamin D. Vaginal cream is employed for atrophic vaginitis and pruritus vulvae and injection can be used to control abnormal uterine bleeding due to hormonal imbalance; perform IV injection slowly to minimize flushing; do not use if solution is darkened or a precipitate is noted; solution is incompatible with other solutions having an acid *p*H; it is also available in combination with meprobamate (Milprem and PMB) for menopause.
dienestrol (DV, Estraguard, Ortho Dienestrol)	Vaginal cream—0.01%	Atrophic vaginitis, kraurosis vulvae—1 to 2 applicators of cream daily for 1 week to 2 weeks, then 1 applicatorful every other day	Synthetic estrogen employed vaginally for treating atrophic vaginitis; systemic absorption may be significant during prolonged use.

(continued)

Table 56-1 (continued)
Estrogens

Drug	Preparations	Usual Dosage Range	Clinical Considerations
diethylstilbestrol (DES)	Tablets—1 mg, 5 mg Enteric-coated tablets—0.1 mg, 0.25 mg, 0.5 mg, 1 mg, 5 mg	Menopause—0.2 mg–0.5 mg/day cyclically Female hypogonadism—0.2 mg–0.5 mg/day cyclically Breast cancer—15 mg/day Prostatic carcinoma—1 mg–3 mg/day Postcoital contraception—25 mg twice a day for 5 days (emergency *only*)	Potent synthetic estrogen, usually given orally; frequently produces nausea, vomiting, and headache; should be administered cyclically when given for prolonged periods; contraindicated during pregnancy, because drug has been implicated in causing vaginal and cervical cancer in offspring of women receiving the drug during first trimester; when used as a postcoital contraceptive, drug is most effective if given within 24 h of coitus but no later than 72 h.
diethylstilbestrol diphosphate (Stilphostrol)	Tablets—50 mg Injection—0.25 g/5 ml	Advanced prostatic carcinoma—50–200 mg orally 3 times/day or 0.5 g IV infusion first day, then 1 g/day on subsequent 5 days; maintenance 0.25 g–0.5 g 1 to 2 times/week	High-dose diethylstilbestrol used for treatment of prostatic carcinoma unresponsive to other estrogens; be alert for early signs of thrombotic complications; for IV administration, dissolve 0.5 g–1 g of drug in 300 ml saline or 5% dextrose and infuse slowly (20 drops–30 drops/min) during first 10 minutes–15 minutes; adjust rate thereafter so that entire amount is given over 1 hour (see Chap. 75).
esterified estrogens (Estratab, Menest)	Tablets—0.3 mg, 0.625 mg, 1.25 mg, 2.5 mg	Menopause—0.3 mg–1.25 mg/day Hypogonadism, ovarian failure—2.5 mg–7.5 mg/day in divided doses for 20 days, stop for 10 days, then repeat if necessary Breast cancer—10 mg 3 times/day for 3 months Prostatic carcinoma—1.25 mg–2.5 mg 3 times/day	Mixture of sodium estrone sulfate (75%–85%) and sodium equilin sulfate (6%–15%); action is similar to conjugated estrogens; also available in combination with chlordiazepoxide as Menrium.
estradiol, oral (Estrace)	Tablets—1 mg, 2 mg	Menopause—1 mg–2 mg/day orally for 3 weeks; then 1 week off Prostatic carcinoma—1 mg–2 mg 3 times/day Breast cancer—10 mg 3 times/day for 3 months	Estrogenic hormone derived from estrone, but more potent; readily absorbed orally; it is available in salt form for injection (see below) providing slow onset and more prolonged duration of action. *(continued)*

Table 56-1 (continued)
Estrogens

Drug	Preparations	Usual Dosage Range	Clinical Considerations
estradiol cypionate (Depo-Estradiol and various other manufacturers)	Injection—1 mg/ml, 5 mg/ml	Menopause—1 mg–5 mg IM every 3 weeks to 4 weeks Hypogonadism—1.5 mg–2 mg IM once a month	Salt of estradiol in cotton-seed oil providing a depot effect; duration of action 3 weeks–6 weeks; it is administered IM only (see Chap. 75).
estradiol valerate (Delestrogen and various other manufacturers)	Injection—10 mg/ml, 20 mg/ml, 40 mg/ml	Menopause, hypogonadism, ovarian failure—10 mg–20 mg IM every 4 weeks Prostatic carcinoma—30 mg IM every 1 week–2 weeks	Salt of estradiol in sesame or castor oil provides 2 weeks–3 weeks of estrogenic activity following a single IM dose (see Chap. 75).
estradiol transdermal system (Estraderm)	Transdermal patch—releasing either 0.05 mg/24 h or 0.1 mg/24 h	Apply patch to skin twice weekly; usually given on a cyclic schedule (i.e., 3 weeks on, 1 week off)	Transdermal patch used to control vasomotor symptoms of the menopause, atrophic vaginitis, kraurosis vulvae, and symptoms of primary ovarian failure and female hypogonadism; system is placed on a clean, dry area of skin, preferably the abdomen; do not apply to breasts; rotate application sites; apply patch immediately after opening pouch and ensure good contact between patch and skin.
estrone (Theelin Aqueous and various other manufacturers)	Injection—aqueous suspension containing 2 mg/ml, 5 mg/ml	Menopause—0.1 mg–0.5 mg IM 2 to 3 times/week Hypogonadism, ovarian failure—0.1 mg–2 mg/week IM in single or divided doses Prostatic carcinoma—2 mg–4 mg IM 2 to 3 times/week	Estrogenic hormone derived from both natural and synthetic sources; response to therapy for prostatic carcinoma should become apparent within 3 months; if response occurs, continue drug until disease again becomes progressive (see Chap. 75).
estropipate (Ogen)	Tablets—0.625 mg, 1.25 mg, 2.5 mg, 5 mg (equivalent to 0.75 mg, 1.5 mg, 3 mg, and 6 mg estropipate, respectively) Vaginal cream—1.5 mg/g	Menopause—0.625 mg–5 mg/day, cyclically each month Hypogonadism, ovarian failure—1.25 mg–7.5 mg/day for 3 weeks, followed by 8-day–10-day	Crystalline form of estrone solubilized as sulfate and stabilized with piperazine, making preparation orally effective; tablets contain 83% sodium estrone sulfate equivalent; *(continued)*

***Table* 56-1** (continued)
Estrogens

Drug	Preparations	Usual Dosage Range	Clinical Considerations
estropipate (Ogen) (continued)		rest period repeated as needed Atrophic vaginitis—1 g–2 g vaginal cream only	formerly known as piperazine estrone sulfate.
ethinyl estradiol (Estinyl, Feminone)	Tablets—0.02 mg, 0.05 mg, 0.5 mg	Menopause—0.02 mg–0.05 mg/day for 21 days cyclically each month Hypogonadism—0.05 mg 1 to 3 times/day for 2 weeks, followed by an oral progestin for 2 weeks; continue for 3 months–6 months Breast cancer—1 mg 3 times/day Prostatic carcinoma—0.15 mg–2 mg/day	Potent, orally effective synthetic estrogen is found in many oral contraceptives (see Chap. 57); also used for menopausal symptoms, female hypogonadism, and certain carcinomas (see Chap. 75).
polyestradiol phosphate (Estradurin)	Injection—40 mg/vial with 2 ml diluent	Advanced prostatic carcinoma—40 mg IM every 2 weeks to 4 weeks up to 80 mg	Provides a stable level of active estrogen over a prolonged period; quickly cleared from blood (24 h) and passively stored in reticuloendothelial system; estradiol levels are maintained constant by continuous replacement from storage sites; increasing the dose prolongs the duration of action but does not significantly enhance the response; may produce temporary burning at IM injection site; clinical response should be evident within 3 months; continue drug until disease becomes progressive (see Chap. 75).
quinestrol (Estrovis)	Tablets—100 mcg	Menopause, hypogonadism, ovarian failure, kraurosis vulvae, atrophic vaginitis—100 mcg once daily for 7 days, then 100 mcg–200 mcg once a week thereafter	A derivative of ethinyl estradiol that is stored in body fat and slowly released, thus providing a prolonged duration of action; once-weekly administration is as effective as cyclic therapy with shorter-acting estrogens, and may improve patient compliance.

natural estrogens delays metabolism and prolongs action. Aqueous solutions of estrogens provide rapid onset and relatively short duration of action. Suspensions or solutions in oil allow slower absorption from intramuscular (IM) injection sites, delayed onset, and prolonged duration of action. Oral absorption of synthetic estrogens is good, and the synthetic estrogens are less rapidly inactivated than are the natural derivatives. They circulate in both free and conjugated forms. Metabolism of estrogens occurs primarily in the liver; less active conjugated products are produced. Estrogens are excreted largely in the urine, although some excretion occurs by way of the bile.

SIDE-EFFECTS/ADVERSE REACTIONS

■ WARNING

Use of estrogens is associated with an increased risk of endometrial carcinoma. The risk is dose and duration dependent, and is estimated to be between 5 times and 15 times that of non-users. There appears to be no difference in risk between "natural" versus synthetic estrogens. Close supervision is essential, use of the lowest effective dose is mandatory, and discontinuation of therapy as early as possible is recommended.

Use of estrogens during early pregnancy may damage the fetus. Female offspring exposed in utero to diethylstilbestrol display an increased incidence of cervical or vaginal adenocarcinoma. Congenital anomalies have also been reported in male offspring whose mothers ingested the drug while pregnant. Patients using estrogens must be apprised of the risks of becoming pregnant while taking the drugs.

Many adverse effects have occurred during therapy with estrogens, often when used as oral contraceptives in combination with a progestin (See Chap. 57). In general, the incidence of adverse effects is dependent on the dose of estrogen and on the length of treatment. The most frequently encountered side-effects are nausea, fluid retention, breakthrough (mid-cycle) bleeding, changes in menstrual flow, and breast fullness or tenderness. Other adverse reactions include the following:

GI—Vomiting, abdominal cramps, bloating, diarrhea, anorexia, cholestatic jaundice, colitis

Dermatologic—Skin rash, pruritus, hirsutism, chloasma, photosensitivity, melasma, erythema multiforme, erythema nodosum, alopecia, acne

Central nervous system—Irritability, depression, headache, migraine attacks, dizziness, insomnia, paresthesias

Genitourinary—Dysmenorrhea, amenorrhea, vaginal candidiasis, increased cervical secretions, cystitis-like reaction, endometrial hyperplasia, increase in size of uterine fibromyomata; in males, feminization of genitalia, testicular atrophy, impotence

Other—Endometrial carcinoma, gallbladder disease (2- to 3-fold increase), thromboembolic complications, hepatic adenoma, hypertension, hypercalcemia, decreased carbohydrate tolerance, aggravation of porphyria, changes in libido, pain at injection site, sterile abscess, fetal damage (see Warning)

CONTRAINDICATIONS AND PRECAUTIONS

Estrogens are contraindicated in the presence of pregnancy, known or suspected breast cancer in premenopausal women, estrogen-dependent neoplasia, undiagnosed genital bleeding, or a history of or active thromboembolic disease.

Estrogens must be used cautiously in persons with cerebrovascular or coronary artery disease, severe hypertension, epilepsy, asthma, migraine headaches, renal or hepatic dysfunction, diabetes mellitus, depression or other emotional disturbances, gallbladder disease, metabolic bone disease associated with hypercalcemia, thyroid dysfunction, endometriosis, and in patients with a history of jaundice or a family history of breast or genital cancer. Judicious use is also warranted in young patients with incomplete bone growth, since premature epiphyseal closure can occur.

INTERACTIONS

See also the discussion of oral contraceptives in Chapter 57.

1. Estrogens may reduce the effectiveness of oral anticoagulants, chenodiol, and insulin, resulting in increased dosage requirements.
2. The incidence of adverse effects with tricyclic antidepressants may be increased by estrogens.
3. The effects of estrogens may be attenuated by phenobarbital, phenytoin, carbamazepine, pri-

midone, rifampin, and other drugs that can induce hepatic microsomal enzymes, thus accelerating the metabolism of estrogens.

4. Estrogens increase the effects of oxytocin on the uterus.
5. Estrogens can alter many laboratory values; for example, they may increase prothrombin, thyroid-binding globulin, serum triglycerides, phospholipids, sulfobromophthalein retention, and norepinephrine-induced platelet aggregability, and they may decrease serum folate, glucose tolerance, pregnanediol excretion, antithrombin III levels, and triiodothyronine (T_3) uptake; in addition, estrogens may cause an impaired response to the metyrapone test.

■ *Nursing Process*

□ ASSESSMENT

□ *Subjective Data*

A thorough history of other endocrine problems and genitourinary problems must be obtained, and a thorough menstrual history is important for the patient being treated for PMS. A family history of breast cancer, coronary artery disease, thromboembolic disease, or diabetes, or known use of DES by the mother during pregnancy with this patient may contraindicate estrogen therapy or at least indicate the need for cautious use. A medication history is also important since estrogens interfere with oral anticoagulants, chenodiol, and insulin, resulting in the need for increased doses of these drugs to maintain effectiveness. Certain anticonvulsants, phenobarbital, and rifampin decrease estrogen effectiveness by accelerating its metabolism, and changes may be necessary before therapy begins. A smoking history is also essential since nicotine increases the risk of cardiovascular side-effects from estrogen.

The nurse also needs to discuss the risks of estrogen therapy as well as the benefits. The patient who is experiencing hot flashes may initially feel she cannot live without estrogen. When the risks are explained, however, she may decide to manage her symptoms rather than risk the development of cancer or another side-effect. Discussions prior to therapy allow the patient to make a conscious decision about following the regimen and taking responsibility for the decision to initiate therapy. On the other hand, if the patient is to take estrogen for cancer therapy the risk versus benefit discussion

may present the potential side-effects in light of the benefit of the drug in treating the malignancy. Evaluate the patient's perception of the malignancy. Some men may accept the temporary feminization of body parts caused by estrogen therapy if told how the drug will benefit them in the long run.

□ *Objective Data*

Physical assessment of the genitourinary tract and breasts is essential prior to treatment. A baseline measurement of weight, peripheral edema and intake-to-output ratios will be helpful in monitoring fluid retention later in therapy.

Laboratory data must also be obtained. A pregnancy test should be done since pregnancy contraindicates estrogen use. Blood lipids, liver enzymes, fasting blood sugar, complete blood count, and Pap smear must also be completed. Patients being treated for malignancy should also have serum calcium tested. Estrogen blood level may be done and occasionally an endometrial biopsy or progesterone challenge test will be performed to determine appropriateness of therapy.

□ NURSING DIAGNOSES

Nursing diagnoses for the patient taking estrogens include

Knowledge deficit related to the administration, action, and side-effects of this drug

Other nursing diagnoses are *potential* problems related to the side-effects of estrogen therapy:

Alteration in bowel elimination: diarrhea
Ineffective individual coping
Alteration in fluid volume: excess
Altered growth and development (in children)
Sexual dysfunction
Altered peripheral tissue perfusion related to thromboembolic complications

□ PLAN

Nursing care goals focus on

1. Safe, correct drug administration
2. Monitoring of significant side-effects such as fluid retention, increased blood pressure, vaginal candidiasis, thromboembolism, jaundice, or depression
3. Teaching the patient
   a. Correct drug-taking techniques to minimize gastrointestinal distress
   b. Techniques that may reduce discomfort and improve sexual relations, when appropriate

    c. How to monitor and manage significant side-effects

    d. How to incorporate other activities that will decrease or eliminate the need for estrogen (postmenopausal patient)

□ *INTERVENTION*

Estrogens are used to treat hypogonadism but should be used with caution in adolescent females since premature epiphyseal closure can occur. Bone age assessments through bone scans and x-ray films must be done periodically and height measurements should be taken at regular intervals to prevent growth and development problems.

Use of estrogens to treat carcinoma and mammary carcinoma is discussed in more detail in Chapter 75. Male patients may suffer gynecomastia as a result of therapy, which will disappear once therapy is completed. Both sexes may suffer significant nausea and vomiting, which should be managed with antiemetics as needed. Hypercalcemia may also occur. Consequently, serum calcium levels should be obtained periodically and the patient should be told to report early symptoms, which include constipation, lethargy, and confusion. Nausea and vomiting may occur but may not be recognized as symptoms of calcium changes if the patient has suffered problems during treatment. All patients are subject to the side-effects mentioned below and should be encouraged to report any problems immediately.

The diabetic patient receiving estrogen must have frequent blood glucose monitoring until the effect of the drug on glucose is known. Most patients will need an increase in the dose of insulin or oral antidiabetic drug during treatment.

Estrogen used for treatment of menopause or hypogonadism usually follows a cyclical pattern of 3 weeks on medication, 1 week off, at as low a dose as possible to eliminate symptoms. The menopausal patient is also encouraged to increase her diversional activity level to involve herself in an effort to minimize the effects of symptoms, to exercise, and, occasionally, to increase intake of vitamins B and E.

The patient may experience some transient side-effects, which can usually be managed. Nausea, which may occur in the first few weeks of therapy, will usually disappear. The patient can eat smaller, more frequent meals and take medication with meals. Diarrhea may also occur and can be managed with mild antidiarrheal drugs. Persistent problems should be reported. Some patients may experience vaginal dryness, which can interfere with sexual pleasure. Encourage the patient to use a lubricant such as K-Y jelly and explain the importance of the arousal phase during intercourse as well as performance of Kegel exercises to enhance muscle tone. Sexual discussions of this type are delicate and may not be broached by the patient unless the nurse allows opportunity and provides an atmosphere of privacy and trust. A woman may also experience withdrawal bleeding soon after the cycle of estrogen has been completed. The nurse needs to provide reassurance that this is a normal side-effect and is not a return of menses and fertility, but that the patient should report any prolonged bleeding.

The patient taking estrogen is prone to other more disturbing side-effects of the drug and should be taught symptoms to watch for.

Fluid retention, weight gain, and increased blood pressure can occur. Patients should weigh themselves every few days and be aware of tight-fitting rings, shoes, and waistbands. Patients with a history of congestive heart failure should also watch for increased shortness of breath and ankle edema. If more than a few pounds are gained or if swelling or dizziness is noted the physician should be contacted immediately.

The patient taking estrogen is also more susceptible to the development of vaginal candidiasis. She should be told to report any thick, white vaginal secretion accompanied by local itching or inflammation because such conditions require treatment and usually respond to appropriate antifungal agents.

Thromboembolic complications can occur particularly when high doses are used, as in the treatment of carcinoma. The patient should be taught to report immediately any symptoms of severe headache, numbness, weakness of one side of the body, dizziness, dyspnea, calf pain, leg swelling, or visual disturbances. If thromboembolism is suspected, estrogen should be discontinued immediately.

Jaundice is another serious symptom that should be reported immediately and indicates the drug should be discontinued since hepatic function may be compromised. Symptoms include yellow skin or sclera, itching, dark urine, and light-colored stools. Patients receiving high doses for treatment of carcinoma are at greater risk for hepatic toxicity than are patients treated for menopause.

Depression may occur during estrogen therapy but seems to be more likely in patients with previous mental problems. The patient and family need to be aware of symptoms such as lack of appetite, lack of motivation, and withdrawal from family and social activities. Estrogen therapy can exacerbate these symptoms. The patient should notify the physician if these symptoms occur and the drug should be discontinued.

☐ *EVALUATION*

Outcome criteria the nurse may use to judge the success of estrogen therapy vary with the reason for therapy. In the menopausal patient absence or control of menopausal symptoms may indicate drug effectiveness. In all patients, the absence of significant side-effects is also an important measurement of treatment success.

Progestins

Hydroxyprogesterone, Medroxyprogesterone, Megestrol, Norethindrone, Norgestrel, Progesterone

The term *progestins* refers to a group of naturally occurring and synthetic steroids having the physiologic effects of progesterone, the principal endogenous progestational hormone. Progesterone is normally secreted by the corpus luteum and also by the placenta during pregnancy, and elicits a variety of actions in the body, which are listed below under Effects of Progestins. Due to its rapid inactivation following oral ingestion, progesterone is administered intramuscularly only, either in an aqueous or oily vehicle. A group of synthetic progestational steroids are also available, which exhibit effects qualitatively similar to progesterone itself, but which differ from the endogenous progestin in that they possess greater potency, longer duration of action, and, in some cases, oral or sublingual effectiveness.

Primary indications for the various progestins are amenorrhea, abnormal uterine bleeding, endometriosis, and endometrial carcinoma. In addition, several of the orally effective synthetic derivatives are used either alone or in fixed combinations with estrogen for the prevention of conception. A discussion of the oral contraceptive agents is presented in Chapter 57.

Progestins were previously used during the first trimester of pregnancy in an attempt to prevent habitual abortion or to treat threatened abortion. However, this use of progestational drugs is no longer considered valid. There is no conclusive evidence that such treatment is effective, since the usual cause of abortion is a defective ovum, on which progestins have minimal influence. Moreover, several reports have suggested that fetal damage (*i.e.*, congenital heart or limb reduction defects) and delayed spontaneous abortion of defective ova due to a uterine-relaxant effect can result from use of progestational agents during early pregnancy. If exposed to progestins during the initial stages of pregnancy, patients should be apprised of the potential risks to the fetus.

This discussion of the progestational drugs treats them as a group, inasmuch as their pharmacology is similar. Individual drugs are listed in Table 56-2.

(*Text continues on p. 1094.*)

Effects of Progestins

Reproductive Effects

1. Inhibit ovulation (decrease release of LH)
2. Induce biochemical changes in endometrium in preparation for implantation of fertilized egg
3. Stimulate cervical mucus secretion
4. Decrease sensitivity of uterus to oxytocin
5. Facilitate development of secretory apparatus in mammary glands

Metabolic Effects

1. Increase body temperature
2. Elevate basal insulin levels and potentiate response to glucose
3. Promote hepatic glycogen storage and ketogenesis
4. Decrease plasma levels of amino acids

Miscellaneous Effects

1. Decrease renal sodium reabsorption (? aldosterone antagonist)
2. Increase ventilatory response to CO_2
3. Decrease T-cell activity

Table 56-2
Progestins

Drug	Preparations	Usual Dosage Range	Clinical Considerations
hydroxyprogesterone caproate (Duralutin, Gesterol L.A., Hy-Gestrone, Hylutin, Hyprogest 250, Hyproval-P.A., Hyroxon, Pro-Depo)	Injection—125 mg/ml, 250 mg/ml	Amenorrhea, uterine bleeding—375 mg IM; if no bleeding after 21 days, begin cyclic therapy (20 mg estradiol on day 1, followed by 250 mg hydroxyprogesterone + 5 mg estradiol on day 15) and repeat every 4 weeks for 4 cycles. Uterine adenocarcinoma—1 g or more IM initially; repeat 1 or more times each week (maximum 7 g/week); stop when relapse occurs or after 12 weeks with no response. Test for endogenous estrogen production—250 mg IM; repeat in 4 weeks; bleeding 7 days–14 days after injection indicates endogenous estrogen is present	Long-acting synthetic progestin, available in either sesame oil or castor oil; duration of action is approximately 10 days–17 days; devoid of estrogenic activity and does not prevent conception; may produce dyspnea, coughing, constriction of the chest, and allergic-like reactions, especially at high doses; solution should be protected from light and stored at room temperature (see also Chap. 75).
medroxyprogesterone acetate (Amen, Curretab, Depo-Provera, Provera)	Tablets—2.5 mg, 5 mg, 10 mg. Injection (Depo-Provera)—100 mg/ml, 400 mg/ml	Amenorrhea—5 mg–10 mg/day orally for 5 days–10 days (withdrawal bleeding usually occurs 3 days–7 days after therapy is terminated). Uterine bleeding—5 mg–10 mg/day for 5 days–10 days beginning on 16th or 21st day of cycle. Endometrial or renal carcinoma—400 mg–1000 mg/week IM; maintenance therapy following improvement 400 mg a month	Synthetic progestin used orally for inducing secretory changes in the estrogen-primed endometrium and IM in a depot injectable form for adjunctive therapy of inoperable, recurrent, or metastatic endometrial or renal carcinoma; also has been used orally to stimulate respiration in the obesity–hypoventilation syndrome; has produced malignant mammary nodules in dogs; the human significance of this finding is not established (see Chap. 75).
megestrol acetate (Megace, Pallace)	Tablets—20 mg, 40 mg	Breast or endometrial carcinoma—40 mg–80 mg 4 times/day for at least 2 months	Orally effective synthetic progestin indicated for palliative treatment of advanced breast or endo-

(continued)

Table 56-2 (continued)
Progestins

Drug	Preparations	Usual Dosage Range	Clinical Considerations
megestrol acetate (Megace, Pallace) (continued)			metrial carcinoma; may cause back pain, nausea, vomiting, and breast tenderness; no serious side-effects in humans in doses as high as 800 mg a day (see also Chap. 75).
norethindrone (Micronor, Norlutin, Nor-Q.D.)	Tablets—0.35 mg, 5 mg	Amenorrhea, uterine bleeding—5 mg–20 mg/day from days 5 to 25 of cycle Endometriosis—10 mg/day for 2 weeks, then increase by 5 mg/day every 2 weeks to 30 mg/day Contraception—0.35 mg daily	Synthetic progestin possessing androgenic, anabolic, and antiestrogenic properties, especially in high doses; component of several oral contraceptive products and used alone (0.35 mg) as well as a progestin-only contraceptive (see Chap. 57).
norethindrone acetate (Aygestin, Norlutate)	Tablets—5 mg	Amenorrhea, uterine bleeding—2.5 mg–10 mg/day from days 5 to 25 of cycle Endometriosis—5 mg/day for 2 weeks; then increase by 2.5 mg/day every 2 weeks to 15 mg/day	Potent synthetic progestin possessing androgenic, anabolic, and antiestrogenic activity; component of several oral contraceptive drugs (see Chap. 57).
norgestrel (Ovrette)	Tablets—0.075 mg	Contraception—0.075 mg/day	Potent progestational hormone used as a progestin-only oral contraceptive ("mini-pill") (see Chap. 57).
Progesterone (Bay Progest, Femotrone, Gesterol-50, Progestaject)	Injection Aqueous—25 mg/ml, 50 mg/ml Oil—25 mg/ml, 50 mg/ml, 100 mg/ml	Amenorrhea—5 mg–10 mg IM for 6 to 8 consecutive days (withdrawal bleeding occurs within 48 h–72 h) Uterine bleeding—5 mg–10 mg/day IM for 6 days (bleeding should cease within 6 days)	Endogenous progestin possessing antiestrogenic activity; large doses may have a catabolic action and produce loss of sodium and chloride; warm solution before injecting to ensure dissolution of all particles; should not be used for diagnosis of pregnancy; progesterone suppositories have been used for treatment of premenstrual syndrome (PMS) but are not approved for this indication.

MECHANISM AND ACTIONS

The principal actions of the progestins are outlined under Effects of Progestins on p. 1091. These agents transform a proliferative endometrium into a secretory endometrium, and prevent follicular maturation and ovulation. Progestins also exhibit some estrogenic, androgenic, and anabolic activity. Although the precise biochemical mechanism of action of progesterone is not completely delineated, the drug has been shown to bind to cellular receptors, thereby increasing the synthesis of proteins and nucleic acids.

USES

See Table 56-2 for specific indications for each drug.

1. Treatment of primary and secondary amenorrhea and dysmenorrhea
2. Control of abnormal uterine bleeding due to hormonal imbalance, in the absence of organic pathology
3. Treatment of endometriosis
4. Palliative and adjunctive treatment of advanced, inoperable, or metastatic breast or endometrial carcinoma (see Chap. 75)
5. Prevention of conception (alone or combined with estrogens; see Chap. 57)
6. *Investigational uses* include use of medroxyprogesterone acetate for relief of menopausal symptoms and to stimulate respiration in obstructive sleep apnea, and use of progesterone suppositories or tablets for treatment of premenstrual syndrome (see Disease Brief)

ADMINISTRATION AND DOSAGE

See Table 56-2 for specific dosing recommendations for each drug.

FATE

Progesterone is quickly inactivated orally; other derivatives are rapidly absorbed following oral administration or aqueous IM injection. Progestins are quickly metabolized by the liver and excreted both in the urine and the feces.

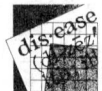

DISEASE BRIEF

■ Premenstrual Syndrome

During the later stages of the menstrual cycle, when levels of both estrogen and progesterone are high but prior to the onset of menses, a number of symptoms occur in many women and have been termed the *premenstrual syndrome* (PMS). Typically, these symptoms include swollen or tender breasts, fluid retention (bloating, weight gain), muscle or joint aching, irritability, restlessness, headaches, increased appetite, binge eating, cravings for sweet or salty foods, and, occasionally, depression. In addition, cramping and abdominal pain are often noted shortly before the onset of or during menses. Symptoms may be similar to those of dysmenorrhea but begin earlier in the menstrual cycle and are abruptly relieved at the onset of menses, whereas symptoms of dysmenorrhea begin later and are not relieved until the second or third day of menstruation. Cramping and abdominal pain are believed to be due to increased synthesis of prostaglandins in the uterus (see Chap. 82). Other theories about the cause of the syndrome include estrogen/progesterone imbalance, vitamin deficiency, and hypoglycemia, although none has been proven as yet.

Assessment frequently includes a complete physical examination, nutritional history, and a history of symptoms recorded over a period of time (usually 2 to 3 months). Psychological screening is also performed at some centers. If a cycle of symptoms consistently occurs over the last half of each menstrual cycle (the luteal phase) the patient is considered to have PMS.

Treatment may include changes in diet such as small, frequent meals with increased protein and complex carbohydrates, stress-reduction therapy, behavior therapy, exercise, and possible vitamin supplementation with B complex and E. Diuretics may be used if fluid retention is found to be excessive. If symptoms do not remit with diet, exercise, and life-style changes, some clinicians treat the patient with progesterone suppositories during the luteal phase of the menstrual cycle. Such treatment is still controversial and studies vary on the drug's effectiveness. However, for patients with severe symptoms, progesterone has provided some relief.

SIDE-EFFECTS/ADVERSE REACTIONS

Note: Progestins are most frequently used in combination with estrogens as oral contraceptives. Refer to Chapter 57 for a complete review of adverse effects associated with these products.

When used alone, the most commonly encountered side-effects are changes in menstrual flow and breakthrough bleeding. *Other adverse* effects noted during therapy with progestins, especially with large doses, are amenorrhea, changes in cervical secretion, altered libido, masculinization of the female fetus, fluid retention (edema, weight gain), breast tenderness, hirsutism, alopecia, rash, melasma, chloasma, decreased glucose tolerance, photosensitivity, cholestatic jaundice, pruritus, diarrhea, depression, nervousness, migraine, coughing, dyspnea, allergic reactions, and retinal vascular lesions. In addition, medroxyprogesterone has been associated with thromboembolic episodes, including pulmonary embolism.

CONTRAINDICATIONS AND PRECAUTIONS

Progestins are contraindicated in the presence of thromboembolic disorders, markedly impaired liver function, known or suspected genital or breast malignancy, undiagnosed vaginal bleeding, missed abortion, and cerebral hemorrhage. They are also not recommended to prevent abortion (see above) or as a diagnostic test for pregnancy. *Cautious* use is necessary in patients with diabetes (may decrease glucose tolerance), migraine, epilepsy, cardiac or renal disease, hypertension, asthma, and depression (because there may be exacerbation of these conditions with progestins), and in nursing mothers. Patients should be cautioned to note the occurrence of any visual changes or other unusual ocular manifestations and to report such incidents immediately. If ophthalmic examination reveals papilledema or retinal vascular lesions, the drug should be discontinued.

INTERACTIONS

1. Progestins can impair the action of sympathomimetic drugs by enhancing their metabolism and can reduce the effectiveness of antidiabetic drugs by decreasing glucose tolerance.
2. The effects of progestins may be reduced by phenylbutazone, phenytoin, phenobarbital, and other hepatic enzyme inducers.

NURSING CONSIDERATIONS

See Nursing Process for estrogens, earlier in this chapter, especially on responsibilities for significant side-effects. See also Chapter 57, for a discussion of oral contraceptives. Progesterone is used alone to treat symptoms of PMS (see Disease Brief). For this patient or for any other being treated for dysmenorrhea it is extremely important to emphasize the need to use an effective method of contraception during therapy since progesterone can be extremely damaging to the fetus. Teach the patient the difference between normal withdrawal bleeding, which occurs about 3 to 4 days after discontinuation of the drug, and breakthrough bleeding or spotting, which occurs during therapy. The latter should be reported because dosage adjustment may be necessary.

The patient should be told to report any visual changes, eye pain, or loss of vision immediately since retinal damage can occur.

Photosensitivity can also occur. The patient needs to avoid prolonged exposure to sunlight and to use sunscreens and protective clothing as much as possible when in the sun.

CASE STUDY

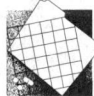

Ellen Fry, age 51, goes to her gynecologist, accompanied by her husband, at the urging of her family who are worried about the change in her behavior. Mrs. Fry has been menopausal for approximately 1 year and has been experiencing progressively more frequent hot flashes during the last 3 months. She reports that the hot flashes leave her completely drenched and she must change all her clothing after each episode. The episodes occur randomly but at least once every 2 days and sometimes she has several in one day. She has started to refuse to go out for fear of being embarassed by one of these episodes. Mr. Fry tells the doctor that his wife has always been well dressed and sociable; now he often comes home from work to find that she has not gotten dressed, has not left the house, and is frequently quiet and withdrawn. Mrs. Fry agrees that she feels isolated and that she cries frequently.

After a thorough history, physical examination, and laboratory evaluation the physician prescribes conjugated estrogens (Premarin), 0.625 mg PO daily, cyclically, to control hot flashes and other symptoms of menopause.

Discussion Questions

1. What information should Mrs. Fry be given about taking estrogen on a cyclical basis?
2. Outline a list of discussion topics to tell Mrs. Fry about the risks versus the benefits of treatment.
3. Develop a teaching plan that includes significant side-effects for the Fry family to monitor while Mrs. Fry is taking estrogen.
4. The physician feels Mrs. Fry's depression is related to her feelings of powerlessness over control of hot flashes and decides to postpone any other treatment until the effect of the estrogen is known. What should the family be told to watch for and immediately report about Mrs. Fry's emotional status?

REVIEW QUESTIONS

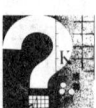

1. Briefly describe the major hormonal events during the menstrual cycle.
2. What are the principal indications for use of the estrogens?
3. List the major reproductive and metabolic effects of estrogens.
4. For what symptoms of the menopause are estrogens most effective? Least effective?
5. What are the major risks associated with chronic use of estrogens?
6. Discuss the rationale behind *cyclical* therapy with estrogens that includes a progestin for a portion of the treatment duration.
7. In what conditions are estrogens contraindicated?
8. What baseline laboratory data should be obtained before estrogens are administered?
9. What other aspects of therapy should the menopausal woman pursue to enhance estrogen therapy and prepare for gradual drug reduction and discontinuation?
10. Give the major actions of progestins.
11. List the principal indications for use of progestins.
12. What are the most important adverse reactions associated with progestin use?

BIBLIOGRAPHY

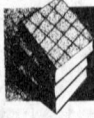

Aloia JF et al: Risk factors for postmenopausal osteoporosis. Am J Med 78:95, 1985

Frank EP: What are nurses doing to help PMS patients? Am J Nurs 86:137, 1986

Gambrell RD: Menopause: Benefits and risks of estrogen-progestogen replacement therapy. Fertil Steril 37:457, 1982

Gambrell RD, Maier RC, Sanders BI: Decreased incidence of breast cancer in postmenopausal estrogen-progestogen users. Obstet Gynecol 62:435, 1983

Hammond MG: Managing menopausal signs and symptoms. Drug Ther 14(12):35, 1984

Horsman A, Jones M, Francis R, Nordin C: The effect of estrogen dose on postmenopausal bone loss. N Engl J Med 309:1405, 1983

Judd HL, Meldrum DR, Deftos LJ, Henderson BE: Estrogen replacement therapy: Indications and complications. Ann Intern Med 98:195, 1983

Kalkhoff RK: Metabolic effects of progesterone. Am J Obstet Gynecol 142:735, 1982

Kase NG: Progestin therapy for perimenopausal women. J Reprod Med 27:522, 1982

Ladewig PA: Protocol for estrogen replacement therapy in menopausal women. Nurse Pract 10(10):44, 1985

Maltrasian GD: Exogenous estrogens: A continuing controversy. Geriatrics 37(3):79, 1982

Mann JI: Progestogens in cardiovascular disease: An introduction to the epidemiologic data. Am J Obstet Gynecol 142:752, 1982

Meade TW: Effects of progestogens on the cardiovascular system. Am J Obstet Gynecol 142:776, 1982

O'Brien PM: The premenstrual syndrome: A review of the present status of therapy. Drugs 24:140, 1982

Quigley MM: Postmenopausal hormone R_x: Time for a fresh clinical look. Mod Med 54(8):34, 1986

Raisz LG, Smith JA: Prevention and therapy of osteoporosis. Ration Drug Ther 19(8):1, 1985

Ryan KJ: Postmenopausal estrogen use. Annu Rev Med 33:171, 1982

Stampfer MJ et al: A prospective study of postmenopausal estrogen therapy and coronary heart disease. N Engl J Med 313:1044, 1985

Utian WH: Menopause in Modern Perspective. New York, Appleton-Century-Crofts, 1980

Wentz AC: Assessment of estrogen and progestin therapy in gynecology and obstetrics. Clin Obstet Gynecol 20:461, 1977

Drugs Used in Fertility Control

57

Several different kinds of pharmacologic agents are employed to control female fertility. They may be grouped according to their action as follows:

1. Steroid contraceptives (*e.g.*, estrogen–progestin combinations)
2. Ovulation stimulants (*e.g.*, clomiphene, menotropins, urofollitropin)
3. Abortifacients (*e.g.*, prostaglandins, sodium chloride 20%)
4. Tocolytics (*e.g.*, ritodrine, ethyl alcohol)

Steroid contraceptives are the most effective drug-based means of preventing conception and are widely used today. They are discussed in detail below. Ovulation stimulants are drugs capable of inducing ovulation in infertile women, provided ovarian responsiveness is adequate. These agents are likewise considered in detail in this chapter. Drugs used to abort a fetus include several prostaglandin derivatives, which are discussed in Chapter 82, and hypertonic sodium chloride solution, which is briefly considered in this chapter. Tocolytic drugs relax uterine smooth muscle and are used in controlling premature labor. Several different agents have been used for this purpose, such as ethyl alcohol (see Chap. 26), isoxsuprine (see Chap. 15), and the drug of choice, ritodrine, which is also discussed in Chapter 15.

Steroid Contraceptives

The widest application for estrogens and progestins is in the prevention of pregnancy. Combinations of estrogens and progestins, commonly referred to as oral contraceptives or "the pill," are the most frequently employed and most effective means for preventing pregnancy in fertile women. The many fixed-combination products differ both in the amount and potency of the two components and in the relative estrogen–progestin activity ratio.

There are three basic types of combination oral contraceptives currently available:

Monophasic: A fixed dose of estrogen and progestin in every tablet; the majority of oral contraceptives are of this type.

Biphasic (*e.g.*, Ortho-Novum 10/11): A fixed amount of estrogen in every tablet; the amount of progestin in the first 10 tablets is one-half the amount in the remaining 11 tablets.

Triphasic (*e.g.*, Ortho-Novum 7/7/7, Tri-Levlen, Tri-Norinyl, Triphasil): Amounts of estrogen *and* progestin vary throughout the tablets.

The latter two types, biphasic and triphasic, are formulated to deliver the hormones in a manner that more closely resembles their physiologic secretion than is possible with the monophasic preparations. However, contraceptive efficacy is *equivalent* for all three types of products and the potential advantages of phasic delivery of the hormones remains to be established.

The two estrogens that are found in all of the oral contraceptives, either ethinyl estradiol or mestranol, are essentially equivalent in their activity. They are present in varying amounts in the different products, as indicated in Table 57-1. The most popular products are those that contain relatively low amounts of estrogens (*i.e.*, 35 mcg or less), because they are associated with a lower incidence of estrogen-related side-effects than combinations containing 50 mcg to 100 mcg of estrogen.

The progestin component of these preparations may be comprised of one of five different compounds (see Table 57-1). These vary not only in potency, but also in degree of estrogenic or antiestrogenic and androgenic activity. Although contraceptive efficacy varies little among the currently available oral contraceptive combinations, frequency and severity of side-effects are often related to the relative strength of the estrogen or progestin component. Achieving the proper hormonal balance of estrogen–progestin activity in each individual can often significantly reduce the degree of untoward effects and thus maximize patient compliance. Table 57-2 presents the important side-effects resulting from either estrogen or progestin excess and provides a listing of currently available oral contraceptives grouped according to their relative estrogen-to-progestin ratio.

While the estrogen–progestin combination products are generally recognized as being the most effective nonsurgical means of contraception, other types of steroidal and nonsteroidal products are used to prevent conception. Progestin-only oral contraceptives (the "mini-pill") are claimed to elicit fewer adverse effects than the combination products, but are also somewhat less effective, having approximately a threefold higher incidence of pregnancy than the estrogen–progestin combinations.

Another steroidal preparation is the intrauterine progesterone contraceptive system, a T-shaped device containing a reservoir of progesterone that is continuously released in small amounts into the uterine cavity following implantation. The unit is effective for up to 1 year and contraceptive efficacy is equivalent to that of progestin-only drugs. This preparation is discussed below.

Table 57-1
Oral Contraceptives

Drug	Estrogen	Progestin
Estrogen Dominant		
Enovid-E	mestranol 100 mcg	norethynodrel 2.5 mg
Norinyl 2 mg	mestranol 100 mcg	norethindrone 2 mg
Ortho-Novum 2 mg	mestranol 100 mcg	norethindrone 2 mg
Ovulen	mestranol 100 mcg	ethynodiol diacetate 1 mg
Intermediate Estrogen–Low Progestin		
Norinyl 1 + 80	mestranol 80 mcg	norethindrone 1 mg
Norlestrin 1/50	ethinyl estradiol 50 mcg	norethindrone 1 mg
Ortho-Novum 1/80	mestranol 80 mcg	norethindrone 1 mg
Ovcon-50	ethinyl estradiol 50 mcg	norethindrone 1 mg
Intermediate Estrogen–Intermediate Progestin		
Demulen 1/50	ethinyl estradiol 50 mcg	ethynodiol diacetate 1 mg
Enovid 5 mg	mestranol 75 mcg	norethynodrel 5 mg
Norlestrin 2.5/50	ethinyl estradiol 50 mcg	norethindrone 2.5 mg
Ovral	ethinyl estradiol 50 mcg	norethindrone 0.5 mg
Low Estrogen–Low Progestin		
Brevicon	ethinyl estradiol 35 mcg	norethindrone 0.5 mg
Genora 1/35	ethinyl estradiol 35 mcg	norethindrone 1 mg
Genora 1/50	mestranol 50 mcg	norethindrone 1 mg
Gynex 0.5/35E	ethinyl estradiol 35 mcg	norethindrone 0.5 mg
Gynex 1/35E	ethinyl estradiol 35 mcg	norethindrone 1.0 mg
Loestrin 1/20	ethinyl estradiol 20 mcg	norethindrone 1 mg
Modicon	ethinyl estradiol 35 mcg	norethindrone 0.5 mg
Norinyl 1 + 50	mestranol 50 mcg	norethindrone 1 mg
Norinyl 1 + 35	ethinyl estradiol 35 mcg	norethindrone 1 mg
Ortho-Novum 1/50	mestranol 50 mcg	norethindrone 1 mg
Ortho-Novum 1/35	ethinyl estradiol 35 mcg	norethindrone 1 mg
Ortho-Novum 10/11	ethinyl estradiol 35 mcg	norethindrone (10 tablets 0.5 mg; 11 tablets 1.0 mg)
Ortho-Novum 7/7/7	ethinyl estradiol 35 mcg	norethindrone (7 tablets 0.5 mg; 7 tablets 0.75 mg; 7 tablets 1.0 mg)
Ovcon-35	ethinyl estradiol 35 mcg	norethindrone 0.4 mg
Tri-Levlen, Triphasil	ethinyl estradiol (6 tablets 30 mcg; 5 tablets 40 mcg; 10 tablets 30 mcg)	levonorgestrel (6 tablets 0.05 mg; 5 tablets 0.75 mg; 10 tablets 0.125 mg)
Tri-Norinyl	ethinyl estradiol 35 mcg	norethindrone (7 tablets 0.5 mg; 9 tablets 1.0 mg; 5 tablets 0.5 mg)
Low Estrogen—Intermediate Progestin		
Levlen	ethinyl estradiol 30 mcg	levonorgestrel 0.15 mg
Lo/Ovral	ethinyl estradiol 30 mcg	norgestrel 0.3 mg
Nordette	ethinyl estradiol 30 mcg	levonorgestrel 0.15 mg
Progestin Dominant		
Demulen 1/35	ethinyl estradiol 35 mcg	ethynodiol deacetate 1 mg
Loestrin 1.5/30	ethinyl estradiol 30 mcg	norethindrone 1.5 mg
Progestin Only		
Micronor		norethindrone 0.35 mg
Nor-Q.D.		norethindrone 0.35 mg
Ovrette		norgestrel 0.075 mg

Table 57-2
Hormonal Balance of Oral Contraceptive Products and Relation to Adverse Effects

Hormone Balance

Estrogen dominant: Enovid-E, Norinyl 2 mg, Ortho-Novum 2 mg, Ovulen

Intermediate estrogen–low progestin: Norinyl 1 + 80, Norlestrin 1/50, Ortho Novum 1/80, Ovcon-50

Intermediate estrogen–intermediate progestin: Demulen 1/50, Enovid 5 mg, Norlestrin 2.5/50, Ovral

Low estrogen–low progestin: Brevicon, Genora 1/35 and 1/50, Gynex 0.5/35E, 1.0/35E, Loestrin 1/20, Modicon, Norinyl 1 + 35 and 1 + 50, Ortho-Novum 1/35, 1/50, 10/11 and 7/7/7, Ovcon-35, Tri-Levlen, Triphasil, Tri-Norinyl

Low estrogen–intermediate progestin: Levlen, Lo/Ovral, Nordette

Progestin dominant: Demulen 1/35, Loestrin 1.5/30

Adverse Effects

Estrogen excess: Cervical mucorrhea, edema, nausea, bloating, breast tenderness, migraine, hypertension, chloasma

Estrogen deficiency: Early or mid-cycle breakthrough bleeding, spotting, nervousness, hypomenorrhea

Progestin excess: Acne, depression, hirsutism, fatigue, increased appetite, weight gain, monilial vaginitis, oily skin, pruritus, hypomenorrhea

Progestin deficiency: Late-cycle bleeding, dysmenorrhea, delayed withdrawal bleeding

Diethylstilbestrol (DES), a synthetic estrogen reviewed in Chapter 56, has been used as a postcoital contraceptive in large doses (25 mg twice a day for 5 days), provided the drug is given within 72 hours after intercourse. At these doses, DES apparently blocks implantation of the fertilized ovum. Because of the hazards of such large doses of DES, this method of contraception is not recommended for routine use, but should be restricted to emergency situations, such as rape or incest.

Many other chemical (spermicidal foams, gels, and creams) and mechanical (diaphragm, intrauterine device, condom) methods of contraception are available, and although usually somewhat less reliable than steroidal drugs, do not present as great a risk of potentially serious untoward reactions as does the use of steroid drugs. Choice of a contraceptive method is a highly personal one, and the advantages and disadvantages of the available methods should be clearly understood by both prescriber and user before a decision is reached.

Oral Contraceptives

The oral contraceptives are discussed as a group, inasmuch as they are essentially alike in their pharmacologic action. A complete list of available products is given in Table 57-1, along with their respective estrogen and progestin content. A review of the intrauterine progestin system is also presented.

MECHANISM AND ACTIONS

Oral contraceptive combination products interfere with follicular maturation (estrogen decreases release of follicle-stimulating hormone [FSH]) and inhibit ovulation (progestin suppresses release of luteinizing hormone [LH]) (see Fig. 56-1); these products also induce structural and biochemical changes in the endometrium, making it unfavorable for implantation of the fertilized ovum. Progestins reduce the amount and increase the viscosity of cervical mucus, thus interfering with motility of sperm cells. Oral contraceptives may also impair the ciliary and peristaltic activity of the fallopian tubes, impeding movement of the ova.

USES
1. Prevention of pregnancy (Products containing more than 50 mcg of estrogen are *not* recommended, since the risk of thromboembolic complications and other adverse effects increases significantly at higher doses.)

ADMINISTRATION AND DOSAGE

Combination products are available as either a 21-day or a 28-day supply. The 21-day products contain active ingredients in every tablet. The 28-day products contain active ingredients in the first 21 tablets, the last 7 tablets being inert, and permit continuous daily dosage throughout the cycle.

Dosages are as follows:

21-day regimen—1 tablet daily beginning on day 5 of cycle. No tablets are taken for 7 days at end of cycle whether bleeding has stopped or not.

28-day regimen—1 tablet daily during the entire 28-day cycle

Although the likelihood of ovulation is minimal if one tablet is missed, it increases with each succeeding day that a dose is missed. If *one* tablet is missed, it may be taken later that day or 2 tablets may be taken the following day. If tablets are missed for 2 consecutive days, 2 tablets should be taken daily for the next 2 days before resuming the regular schedule. If 3 consecutive days of therapy are missed, a new package of tablets should be started 7 days after the last tablet was taken and alternate means of birth control should be used during this interval.

FATE

Estrogens

Ethinyl estradiol is rapidly absorbed and undergoes significant first-pass hepatic metabolism. Mestranol is converted to ethinyl estradiol, which is highly bound to plasma proteins (97%–98%). Plasma half-life ranges from 6 hours to 18 hours. The drugs are excreted in both the bile and the urine.

Progestins

Progestins are well absorbed orally. Norethynodrel and ethynodiol diacetate are converted to norethindrone. Peak plasma levels occur in 0.5 hour to 3 hours. Progestins are bound to plasma proteins and are primarily metabolized in the liver.

SIDE-EFFECTS/ADVERSE REACTIONS

■ WARNING

Use of oral contraceptives has been associated with increased risk of thromboembolic episodes, hemorrhagic stroke, hypertension, myocardial infarction, hepatic tumors, visual disturbances, gallbladder disease, and fetal abnormalities. In addition, cigarette smoking *significantly* increases the risk of cardiovascular side-effects.

Many side-effects noted with oral contraceptives are related to the ratio of estrogen to progestin in the product. Table 57-2 outlines the common side-effects that may occur as a consequence of either an excess or a deficiency of estrogen or progestin. Many commonly occurring side-effects can be minimized or eliminated by choice of a product having an optimal estrogen-to-progestin ratio relative to the side-effects being reported.

The most frequently encountered side-effects during the initial weeks of therapy with oral contraceptives are nausea, vomiting, headache, fluid retention, bloating, breast tenderness, and spotting and breakthrough bleeding.

The most serious adverse effects related to oral contraceptive use are the following:

1. *Thromboembolic episodes*—Users have a two to eleven times greater risk than non-users; risk *increases* with smoking, larger estrogen doses, and age; the risk of hemorrhagic stroke is two times greater than in nonusers and risk of thrombotic stroke in oral contraceptive users is four to ten times greater than in non-users.

2. *Myocardial infarction*—Risk is doubled in nonsmokers who use oral contraceptives versus non-users; risk increases dramatically with smoking (5- to 12-fold), age, hypertension, hypercholesterolemia, and obesity; risk may persist for years after discontinuation of therapy.

3. *Hepatic adenomas*—Risk increases with age and with increasing doses of estrogen and progestin.

4. *Gallbladder disease*—Risk increases with duration of therapy.

5. *Hypertension*—Risk increases with duration of use and age; incidence is higher in women with a history of fluid retention or weight gain during the menstrual cycle.

6. *Ocular lesions* (*e.g.*, retinal thrombosis, optic neuritis)

7. *Fetal abnormalities*—Use of female sex hormones during early pregnancy may seriously damage the fetus; pregnancy must be ruled out before initiating or continuing oral contraceptive use.

Many other adverse effects have been reported in oral contraceptive users and these are listed below by organ system. *Not all* of these effects, however, have been definitely related to the presence of the drugs.

Gastrointestinal/hepatic—Abdominal cramping, diarrhea, cholelithiasis, and cholestatic jaundice

Genitourinary—Dysmenorrhea, amenorrhea, infertility after discontinuation, change in cervical secretions, increased urinary tract and vaginal infections

Ophthalmic—Papilledema, change in corneal curvature, intolerance to contact lenses

Central nervous system—Migraine, depression, menstrual tension, fatigue

Other—Rash, melasma, photosensitivity, reduced lactation, impaired carbohydrate tolerance, altered laboratory values (*e.g.*, liver function, thyroid function, serum triglycerides, blood glucose)

There appears to be *no* statistically documented increased risk of breast or endometrial cancer in oral contraceptive users. In fact, the drugs appear to have a protective effect on development of ovarian and endometrial carcinoma. In addition, a reduced incidence of benign breast tumors in oral contraceptive users has been documented. However, close observation is necessary in all women receiving these drugs, especially those women with a family history of breast cancer or with breast nodules, fibrocystic breast disease, abnormal mammogram findings, or cervical dysplasia. Recurrent or undiagnosed vaginal bleeding during therapy must be evaluated immediately to rule out malignancy.

CONTRAINDICATIONS AND PRECAUTIONS

Oral contraceptives are contraindicated in women with thromboembolic disorders, coronary artery or cerebrovascular disease, myocardial infarction, or previous history of these disorders; known or suspected breast or other estrogen-dependent carcinoma; undiagnosed vaginal bleeding; known or suspected pregnancy; severe liver disease or liver tumors; and in nursing mothers since the drugs decrease lactation.

A *cautious* approach to therapy must be undertaken in the presence of diabetes, hypertension, obesity, migraine, amenorrhea, depression, anemia, or porphyria.

INTERACTIONS

See also Chapter 56.

1. Reduced contraceptive efficacy and an increased incidence of breakthrough bleeding may occur with concurrent use of barbiturates, penicillin, ampicillin, chloramphenicol, sulfonamides, primidone, phenytoin, meprobamate, carbamazepine, rifampin, isoniazid, phenylbutazone, nitrofurantoin, griseofulvin, analgesics, antimigraine drugs, and antihistamines.

2. Oral contraceptives may impair the effectiveness of anticonvulsants, anticoagulants, antihypertensives, tricyclic antidepressants, antidiabetics, insulin, and certain vitamins such as folic acid and B_6.

3. Oral contraceptives may impair the metabolism of caffeine, chlordiazepoxide, corticosteroids, diazepam, metoprolol, imipramine, phenytoin, and phenylbutazone.

4. The metabolism of acetaminophen, lorazepam, and oxazepam may be accelerated by oral contraceptives.

5. Use of aminocaproic acid with oral contraceptives may increase clotting factors, leading to a hypercoagulable state.

6. Concurrent use of troleandomycin and oral contraceptives may result in jaundice.

■ *Nursing Process*

See also Chapter 56 on estrogens and progestins.

□ ASSESSMENT

□ *Subjective Data*

A complete history should be taken on any woman about to start taking oral contraceptives. A thorough drug history should also be obtained (see Interactions, above). In addition to asking about diseases (listed above under Contraindications and Precautions), the nurse should determine whether the patient is obese, anticipates surgery in the near future, or has limited mobility for any reason since such factors may increase the risk of developing thromboembolic side-effects from the drug. Also ask about smoking. The women who are most at risk of developing complications from oral contraceptives are those who are smokers and over 35 years of age and all women over age 45. The best candidate is the healthy young woman under 35 years of age, a nonsmoker, who is able to use a low-dose oral contraceptive and whose menses began at least 2 years prior to contraceptive use. A thorough menstrual history is essential.

Candidates should be thoroughly screened and made aware of the risks of oral contraceptives. However, the low-risk candidate described above should also be told the benefits of using oral contraceptives over other means of birth control. For many patients, the risks are minimal and if screening is done carefully the concerns expressed by the patient can be allayed. Oral contraceptives have recently been the subject of negative publicity, much of which stems from indiscriminate prescription of the drug. This should be avoided.

□ *Objective Data*

A thorough physical examination should be completed, including pelvic examination, blood pressure, apical rate, and peripheral pulses.

Laboratory evaluations should also be completed before beginning oral contraceptive use. A complete blood count with platelets should be performed, as well as liver function studies, blood glucose, serum triglycerides, and thyroid function studies. A pregnancy test should also be performed and a Pap smear completed. This baseline data can help determine potential risks for the patient as well as serve as a basis for comparison in the early detection of problems.

□ *NURSING DIAGNOSES*

The main nursing diagnosis for the patient taking oral contraceptives is

Knowledge deficit related to safe drug taking and monitoring side-effects

Potential nursing diagnoses related to possible side-effects of oral contraceptive use include

Alteration in comfort: pain

Alteration in fluid volume: excess

Alteration in nutrition: less than body requirements

Sensory–perceptual alteration: vision

Alteration in tissue perfusion: cardiopulmonary, cerebral, or peripheral

□ *PLAN*

Nursing care goals focus on teaching the patient

1. How to take the drug correctly
2. What bodily changes may occur
3. What side-effects to watch for and what to do if side-effects develop

□ *INTERVENTION*

Safe, effective drug taking of oral contraceptives depends on the woman's memory. She must remember to take them every day and should be encouraged to develop a habit of taking them at the same time every day as part of an already established routine such as morning hygiene or sleep preparation. The prescription of a 28-day supply or a 21-day supply is strictly a matter of patient preference. Some patients establish the habit of drug taking more easily when there is no interruption. Others may resent the implication that they are not responsible enough to resume the contraceptive on the seventh day of the cycle. A discussion of the alternatives is appropriate before a course is prescribed.

The woman should be advised to use another form of contraception during the initial first week of pill taking. She should be alerted that transient nausea may occur but will generally subside after the first cycle. If it persists the physician should be notified since the dose may need to be adjusted. A reduction in menstrual flow may also occur as a normal consequence of the drug. The health team should be notified if withdrawal bleeding does not occur following a course of therapy. The absence of bleeding or any other sign of pregnancy may indicate pregnancy and the woman should not resume therapy until a pregnancy test is completed since oral contraceptives can cause fetal damage. Conversely, if the patient desires to become pregnant, she should discontinue the oral contraceptives and use an alternative form of birth control for 2 to 3 months to minimize the risk of congenital abnormalities from residual effects of the steroidal hormones.

The patient needs to learn to watch for any patterns of side-effects and report them since dosages may need to be changed. For example, early or mid-cycle breakthrough bleeding may indicate estrogen deficiency and the dose of the estrogen component of the oral contraceptive may need to be increased. See Table 57-1 for other side-effects that indicate hormonal imbalance. Teach the patient to do routine breast self-examination to detect early any breast changes resulting from oral contraceptive use.

The most serious and most publicized side-effects of oral contraceptive use are cardiovascular complications ranging from thrombophlebitis to stroke, myocardial infarction, or embolism. If the patient has been adequately screened, her risk of developing these side-effects should be minimal. However, the patient should learn to report immediately any of the following symptoms: persistent headaches, dizziness, unilateral weakness, blurred vision, chest pain, shortness of breath, or leg or calf pain, tenderness, or redness. Advise patients of other side-effects based on their potential susceptibility. For example, the patient who wears contact lenses should know that corneal curvature may change leading to incorrect fit or contact lens intolerance, and this symptom should be reported.

There is also recent evidence that oral contraceptive use may increase the body's need for vitamins C, B_6, B_{12}, and folacin. Although most studies focus on deficiencies in adolescents and young adults whose eating habits are frequently irregular and imbalanced, the nurse should do a brief diet history to determine the patient's eating habits. Symptoms of vitamin C deficiency may be recurring infections and nosebleeds; lack of B_6 may result in depression and lack of confidence; lack of

B$_{12}$ may manifest as anemia, as will lack of folacin. The patient should be advised to increase her intake of foods high in these vitamins or to add vitamin supplements while taking oral contraceptives. Foods high in vitamin C include citrus fruits, broccoli, tomatoes, and cabbage; those high in B$_6$ are red meats, liver, whole grains, and eggs; foods high in B$_{12}$ include eggs, milk, cheese, liver, and red meat; and foods high in folacin include citrus fruits, yogurt, bananas, and dark green leafy vegetables.

The postpartum patient who chooses to breast-feed should be told not to resume oral contraceptive use because the hormones will pass through breast milk and adversely affect the baby. An alternative form of birth control must be used.

The patient should be encouraged to have a yearly gynecological examination and breast examination as well as a Pap smear to detect any changes early. Health-care providers should limit prescription refills to encourage clinical follow-up.

If the patient is having planned surgery, oral contraceptives should be discontinued 4 weeks before the procedure to reduce the risk of vascular problems that may occur. If the patient is placed on antibiotics (see Interactions, above) an alternative form of contraception must be used for the duration of treatment. The patient should be told to report oral contraceptive use to any health-care provider.

The diabetic patient taking oral contraceptives should closely monitor blood glucose since levels may rise requiring an increase in insulin or oral antidiabetic agents for the duration of drug use.

□ *EVALUATION*
The outcome criteria the nurse may use to judge drug effectiveness include
  1. The patient does not become pregnant while taking the drug.
  2. Drug dose is adjusted so that no patterned side-effects occur.
  3. No major cardiovascular side-effects develop.
  4. The patient complies with the advised nutrition supplements and shows no symptoms of deficiency.

Intrauterine Progesterone Contraceptive System

(Progestasert)

The intrauterine progesterone contraceptive system is a T-shaped intrauterine device (IUD) containing 38 mg of progesterone dispersed in silicone oil. Following insertion of the unit into the uterine cavity, progesterone is continuously released at an average rate of 65 mcg/day. The contraceptive effectiveness approximates that of oral progestin-only tablets and is retained for a period of 1 year, after which the system must be replaced. The system apparently acts to suppress proliferation of endometrial tissue, creating an environment unfavorable for implantation. It also may decrease sperm survival time, possibly by altering cervical mucus, but does *not* appear to prevent ovulation.

The intrauterine progesterone system is contraindicated in the presence of pregnancy or suspicion of pregnancy, previous ectopic pregnancy, pelvic inflammatory disease, venereal disease, previous pelvic surgery, uterine abnormalities, uterine or cervical malignancy, vaginal bleeding of undetermined origin, and acute cervicitis.

Adverse reactions associated with the system include dysmenorrhea, amenorrhea, cervical erosion, pelvic infection, vaginitis, endometritis, spotting, prolonged menstrual flow, delayed menses, dyspareunia, septicemia, septic abortion, cervical or uterine perforation, ectopic pregnancy, and pain, bleeding, bradycardia, or syncope upon insertion.

The device should be inserted during or immediately following menstruation to ensure that pregnancy has not occurred. An increased risk of pelvic inflammatory disease (PID) is associated with the use of intrauterine devices. Users should be apprised of the usual symptoms of PID (fever, nausea, vomiting, abdominal pain, malaise, purulent vaginal discharge) and if present, should report to their physician.

Ovulation Stimulants

Anovulation is an infrequent cause of infertility. When it occurs, however, it has responded to the use of ovulation-stimulating drugs, which have made conception possible in previously anovulatory women. Because therapy with these agents is expensive, often tedious, and potentially hazardous, selection of patients with a reasonable expectation for success is important. Thus, women with primary ovarian failure, uterine abnormalities, fallopian tube obstruction, or endometrial carcinoma should be excluded as potential candidates. Likewise, impaired or absent sperm production in the partner should be ruled out. When careful patient selection is observed, 25% to 50% of those persons completing a course of therapy can be expected to conceive. However, treatment with ovulation-inducing drugs is not without its hazards, such as ovarian enlargement, often accompanied by pain and ascites. The incidence of early abortion is increased with use of these drugs, and the occurrence of multiple pregnancies even with recommended dosage schedules has been estimated to be as high as 20%.

Ovulation-inducing agents include clomiphene, a drug capable of increasing release of FSH and LH from the adenohypophysis, and human menopausal gonadotropins (HMG, menotropins) and urofollitropin, two preparations that are purified extracts of FSH and LH. Clomiphene is used alone, while HMG therapy and urofollitropin therapy are followed by an injection of human chorionic gonadotropin (HCG) to induce ovulation. These drugs are reviewed individually below, following the Nursing Process related to use of ovulation-inducing drugs.

■ Nursing Process

□ ASSESSMENT

□ Subjective Data
Drug therapy is a major part of the treatment of infertility secondary to failure of ovulation, and couples tend to put a lot of faith in the ability of the drug to help them conceive a child. By the time drug treatment is started the couple may have been trying to conceive for several years, subjected themselves to multiple tests or operations, seen various physicians, and sought adoption alternatives. Their relationship may be strained and their patience exhausted. The nurse needs to get a thorough history of what they have done already and what they are willing to continue to do to conceive a child. She needs to build a supportive and trusting environment for the couple and give them a realistic view of the potential for success before therapy begins.

A sexual history also needs to be obtained. The couple may feel that intercourse has only one objective now, procreation, and its failure to do that makes the act abhorrent. Such couples need to have an opportunity to discuss past romantic moments and given some feedback and encouragement in helping to make intercourse enjoyable again. Since the timing of sexual intercourse during drug therapy is critical the couple may see it as another mechanical intrusion and need to learn techniques to focus on the pleasure of the act rather than on the

expected outcome. This is not easy to accomplish and may work as a deterrent to successful drug therapy. Couples experiencing difficulties may need to take a break from the infertility work-up, seek therapy, or get involved in a support group such as RESOLVE, a group specific for infertile couples.

□ Objective Data
An infertility work-up can be completed in various stages depending on the initial review of the woman's basal body temperature. The woman should take her temperature orally each morning at the same time before arising and record it on a graph (Fig. 57-1). This should be done for 2 to 3 months. The record indicates when ovulation occurs and gives a rough idea of whether luteinizing hormone and progesterone are secreted. At the same time, the woman's thyroid function, liver function, and progesterone levels during the luteal phase of the menstrual cycle should be tested. The man's sperm count and sperm motility should also be evaluated.

The woman should also have a complete pelvic examination, including an evaluation of ovarian cysts since ovarian enlargement can occur with ovulation stimulants. A routine pregnancy test should also be performed since ovulation stimulants will cause fetal damage.

□ NURSING DIAGNOSES
Actual nursing diagnoses for the patient taking ovulation stimulants will generally include
>   Anxiety related to inability to conceive
>   Alteration in comfort related to ovarian
>   stimulation by the drug
>   Knowledge deficit: about administration of
>   the drug in the correct sequence, timing of
>   sexual intercourse during drug therapy, and
>   monitoring for side-effects

Potential nursing diagnoses are related to the drug's side-effects and include
>   Ineffective family coping: compromised by
>   the drug therapy course (particularly if it
>   becomes extended)
>   Sexual dysfunction related to the
>   requirements for sexual intercourse during
>   therapy

□ INTERVENTION
Drugs must be taken exactly as prescribed (see Administration and Dosage for each drug, below). The usual protocol is to try gradually increased doses of clomiphene, and if that is unsuccessful to attempt

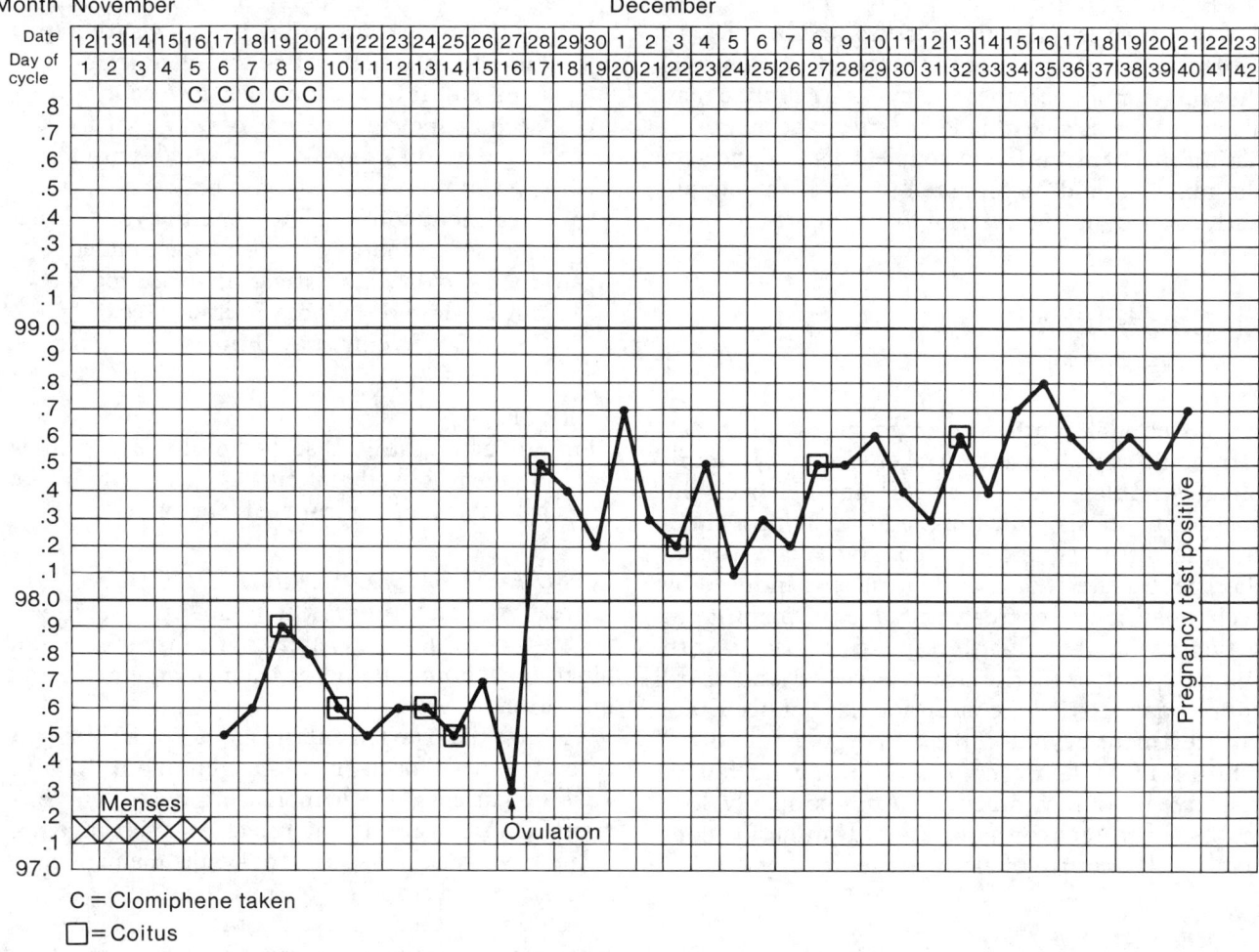

Figure 57-1. *Basal body temperature chart showing conception on Clomiphene.*

fertilization using HMG and HCG or urofollitropin and HCG. Since fertilization can only occur for a few days during each cycle and is optimal only for a 24-hour period the woman must continue to take basal body temperature readings and the couple should learn at least one method of determining whether ovulation is occurring. A drop in the basal body temperature at the expected time of ovulation (around the 14th day of the menstrual cycle) is the easiest sign to learn. The patient may also learn to test cervical mucus for the spinnbarkeit effect. Cervical mucus becomes extremely elastic at ovulation and can be stretched as much as 3 to 4 inches between the thumb and index finger. Some patients may also be able to perceive the wink sign, a momentary contraction of the cervical os during penetration. Intercourse should take place during the time that ovulation is most likely to occur.

Side-effects are listed with each drug but the most dangerous among them is ovarian hyperstimulation, which can lead to multiple pregnancy. All ovarian stimulants cause some ovarian pain and enlargement. Pain can generally be relieved by rest, limited activity, and a warm bath. If the pain persists 7 days after ovulation, the physician should be notified and the couple should refrain from intercourse. Rupture of the ovary can occur so the patient should be evaluated at once.

The couple should also understand the risk of multiple births associated with the use of ovarian stimulants. The rates vary with the individual drugs and are more likely to produce twins than other multiples. However, the couple should be prepared for the possibility. Sonograms are sometimes used to determine if multiple follicles have formed so that fertilization can be avoided.

□ EVALUATION

The outcome criteria most patients and health-care professionals use to determine drug effectiveness is that the woman becomes pregnant. The nurse may also use the absence of side-effects as another evaluation mechanism. If the couple fails to conceive, the nurse should be prepared to assist the couple with counseling and referral to a support group.

Clomiphene

(Clomid, Serophene)

A nonsteroidal, synthetic estrogen possessing weak estrogenic as well as antiestrogenic activity, clomiphene stimulates release of FSH and LH from the adenohypophysis, and thus requires both a functioning pituitary and a responsive ovary for its therapeutic effect. Ovulation is usually induced by each 5-day course of treatment, and the majority of patients who are going to respond will do so with the first course of therapy. A second and third course may be tried if conception has not occurred, but treatment beyond three courses in patients exhibiting no evidence of ovulation or who fail to conceive is not recommended. Approximately 30% to 40% of women with ovulatory dysfunction conceive with a course of clomiphene therapy.

MECHANISM AND ACTIONS

Clomiphene binds to estrogenic receptors in the cytoplasm, thus decreasing the number of available estrogenic receptor sites (antiestrogenic action). This action is interpreted by the hypothalamus and pituitary that estrogen levels are low, and the secretion of FSH and LH is increased in response to the removal of the negative feedback. The increased release of FSH and LH stimulates maturation of the follicle, ovulation, and development of the corpus luteum.

USES

1. Treatment of ovulatory failure in properly selected patients desiring pregnancy, whose partners are fertile (therapy is ineffective in persons with primary pituitary or ovarian failure)
2. Treatment of male infertility (investigational use)

ADMINISTRATION AND DOSAGE

Clomiphene is available as 50-mg tablets. Dosage is as follows:

Female infertility: Beginning on the fifth day of the cycle, 50 mg/day for 5 days (therapy may be started anytime in amenorrheic women); if ovulation does not occur, a second and third course of therapy (at 100 mg/day for 5 days) may be tried, with a minimum 30-day interval between treatment courses. Treatment beyond three courses of therapy is *not* recommended.

Male infertility (investigational): 25 mg/day for 25 days or 100 mg 3 times/week (Monday, Wednesday, Friday)

FATE

Clomiphene is readily absorbed orally. The drug is partially metabolized and appears primarily in the feces by way of an enterohepatic circulation.

SIDE-EFFECTS/ADVERSE REACTIONS

At recommended doses the common side-effects are vasomotor flushing, abdominal discomfort and bloating, abdominal and ovarian enlargement, and breast tenderness.

Abnormal ovarian enlargement is infrequent at recommended doses and occurs in about 10% to 15% of patients. With increasing doses, enlargement is more common and luteal cysts can develop. Patients with polycystic ovary syndrome may have an exaggerated response to the drug.

Other adverse reactions observed in patients receiving clomiphene are nausea, vomiting, diarrhea, visual disturbances (*e.g.*, blurring, photophobia, diplopia, scotomata), headache, nervousness, lightheadedness, dizziness, vertigo, insomnia, depression, abnormal uterine bleeding, ovarian hemorrhage, urinary frequency, rash, allergic dermatitis, reversible hair loss, fluid retention, weight gain; increased incidence of early abortion, and multiple births. The incidence of multiple births with clomiphene is approximately 7% and less than 1% results in triplets or greater. It appears there is a direct correlation between dosage and the likelihood of multiple births. The incidence of birth defects does *not* appear to exceed that of the general population.

CONTRAINDICATIONS AND PRECAUTIONS

Use of clomiphene is contraindicated in pregnant women and in women with liver dysfunction or a history of liver disease, ovarian cysts, thrombophlebitis, or abnormal uterine or vaginal bleeding. Therapy is ineffective in patients with primary pituitary or ovarian failure.

INTERACTIONS

1. Clomiphene can elevate levels of serum thyroxine and thyroxine-binding globulin.

NURSING CONSIDERATIONS

See also Nursing Process, above.

The timing of intercourse is important during clomiphene therapy. Couples are usually advised to watch for the signs of ovulation and, if unsure, have sexual intercourse on the day of the temperature drop and for 2 days after that.

The woman should also be aware that clomiphene can cause dizziness and lightheadedness. She should use caution in driving or engaging in other hazardous activities during the 5 days of treatment. Any visual disturbances should be reported and the drug stopped.

Menotropins—Human Menopausal Gonadotropins

(Pergonal)

Menotropins or human menopausal gonadotropins (HMG) is a purified preparation of gonadotropins extracted from the urine of postmenopausal women. Menotropins is biologically standardized for FSH and LH activity, and provides an exogenous source of pituitary gonadotropins. Unlike clomiphene, it does not require the presence of functional hypophyseal gonadotropins for its activity. Treatment with menotropins usually results *only* in follicular growth and maturation; subsequent ovulation is effected by subsequent administration of HCG (see Human Chorionic Gonadotropin, below) when sufficient follicular maturation has occurred.

MECHANISM AND ACTIONS

Menotropins provides a source of FSH and LH, thus promoting growth of ovarian follicles in women who do *not* have primary ovarian failure. The drug does not usually elicit ovulation, which must be induced by injection of HCG, a polypeptide possessing significant LH activity (see below).

In males, menotropins given concurrently with HCG for at least 3 months induces spermatogenesis in men with primary or secondary pituitary hypofunction.

USES

1. Treatment of infertility in women with primary or secondary amenorrhea (with or without galactorrhea), polycystic ovary syndrome, anovulatory cycles, or irregular menses (not effective in primary ovarian failure)

2. Stimulation of spermatogenesis in men who have primary or secondary hypogonadotropic hypogonadism (in combination with HCG)

ADMINISTRATION AND DOSAGE

Menotropins is used as a powder for injection containing either 75 U FSH activity and 75 U LH activity per 2-ml ampule, or 150 U FSH activity and 150 U LH activity per 2-ml ampule.

The contents of 1 ampule is dissolved in 1 ml to 2 ml of sterile saline and administered IM. Unused portions should be discarded.

Dosage recommendations are as follows:

Women (must be individualized): usually 1 ampule/day of 75 U each of FSH and LH IM for 9 days to 12 days, followed by HCG, 10,000 U IM 1 day after the last dose of menotropins. If ovulation occurs without pregnancy, repeat course of therapy twice with same dosage levels at monthly intervals. If ovulation does not occur, repeat treatment with 1 ampule/day of 150 U each of FSH and LH for 9 days to 12 days, followed by 10,000 U HCG IM. Do not exceed this latter dose.

Men (to increase spermatogenesis): HCG alone (5000 IU three times/week for 4 months to 6 months) to achieve normal serum testosterone levels; then, 1 ampule of 75 U each IM 3 times/week plus HCG, 2000 IU, twice a week for 4 months

SIDE-EFFECTS/ADVERSE REACTIONS

The principal adverse effect with a recommended dosage of menotropins is ovarian enlargement, with or without abdominal pain, which occurs in approximately 20% of patients and usually regresses without treatment within 2 weeks to 3 weeks. Other adverse effects, most often noted with large doses, are ovarian hyperstimulation syndrome (*e.g.*, abdominal pain, ascites, pleural effusion, sudden ovarian enlargement), fever, nausea, vomiting, diarrhea, hemoperitoneum, arterial thromboembolism (rare), and ovarian cysts.

Multiple births have occurred with HMG–HCG treatment; approximately 15% of pregnancies resulted in twins, of which over 90% were viable, and 5% have resulted in 3 or more fetuses, of which less than one fourth were viable.

In men receiving HMG–HCG, gynecomastia has occurred.

CONTRAINDICATIONS AND PRECAUTIONS

Contraindications to use of menotropins in women include primary ovarian failure, pregnancy, ovarian cysts or enlargement not due to polycystic ovary syndrome, thyroid or adrenal dysfunction, intracranial lesion, abnormal bleeding of unknown origin, and infertility due to factors other than anovulation.

In men, primary testicular failure and infertility not due to hypogonadotropic hypogonadism are contraindications to HMG.

Urofollitropin

(Metrodin)

MECHANISM AND ACTIONS
Urofollitropin is a purified preparation of gonadotropin extracted from the urine of postmenopausal women. The drug stimulates ovarian follicular growth in women who do not have primary ovarian failure. Treatment results in follicular growth and maturation only; ovulation is effected by subsequent administration of HCG (see below) where laboratory assessment indicates that sufficient follicular maturation has occurred.

USES
1. Induction of ovulation in patients with polycystic ovarian disease who display elevated LH/FSH ratio and who have failed to respond to clomiphene therapy. Treatment with urofollitropin must be followed by administration of HCG to induce ovulation from the mature follicle.

ADMINISTRATION AND DOSAGE
Urofollitropin is available as powder for injection containing 0.83 mg (75 U FSH activity) per ampule with diluent. The recommended initial dose is 75 U/day IM for 7 days to 12 days followed by 5,000 U to 10,000 U of HCG 1 day after the last urofollitropin dose.

If there is evidence of ovulation but no pregnancy, repeat the above course of therapy at least two more times at monthly intervals before increasing the dose of urofollitropin to 150 U/day for 3 additional monthly treatments. Do not increase the dose further.

SIDE-EFFECTS/ADVERSE REACTIONS
Approximately 10% of patients experience ovarian hyperstimulation, characterized by abdominal pain and distention, ovarian enlargement, and rash, pain, swelling, or irritation at the injection site.

Less frequently reported side-effects with urofollitropin are nausea, vomiting, diarrhea, abdominal cramping, bloating, headache, breast tenderness, fever, muscle aching, chills, malaise, fatigue, dry skin, hair loss, and ectopic pregnancy. Thromboembolic episodes have occurred with the similar-acting drug menotropins and must be considered a possibility with urofollitropin as well.

Multiple births have occurred with a frequency estimated to be in the range of 15% to 20%.

Sudden ovarian enlargement, occasionally accompanied by ascites and pleural effusion, has been reported in approximately 5% of treated patients.

CONTRAINDICATIONS AND PRECAUTIONS
Urofollitropin is contraindicated in the presence of high levels of LH and FSH, indicating primary ovarian failure, overt thyroid or adrenal dysfunction, intracranial lesions, abnormal bleeding of undetermined origin, or ovarian cysts *not* due to polycystic ovary syndrome. Urofollitropin is also contraindicated in pregnancy. The drug should be used cautiously in persons with thromboembolic disorders, and in nursing mothers.

NURSING CONSIDERATIONS
(See Nursing Process for ovulation stimulants and the following discussion of human chorionic gonadotropin.)

Human Chorionic Gonadotropin

(A.P.L., Chorex, Chorigon, Choron-10, Corgonject-5, Follutein, Glukor, Gonic, Pregnyl, Profasi HP)

MECHANISM AND ACTIONS
A purified polypeptide hormone, HCG is produced by the human placenta and extracted from the urine of women during the first trimester of pregnancy. The effect of HCG is due primarily to its LH-like activity, although it exhibits a slight degree of FSH-like activity as well. HCG stimulates the corpus luteum to produce progesterone, and triggers ovulation from FSH-primed follicles. In males, it stimulates the interstitial cells of the testes to produce androgens, thus promoting development of secondary sex characteristics and descent of the testicles.

USES
1. Induction of ovulation in the anovulatory female who has been properly pretreated with HMG or urofollitropin
2. Treatment of cryptorchidism (undescended testes) in instances not due to anatomical ob-

struction; therapy is usually instituted between ages 4 years and 9 years.

3. Treatment of male hypogonadism secondary to a pituitary deficiency

ADMINISTRATION AND DOSAGE

HCG is available as powder for injection containing, after reconstitution, 200 U/ml, 500 U/ml, 1000 U/ml, and 2000 U/ml. The drug is given IM *only* and dosage is highly individualized. Representative doses for the various indications are as follows:

Induction of ovulation
5000 U to 10,000 U 1 day following last dose of HMG or urofollitropin

Cryptorchidism
1. 4000 U three times a week for 3 weeks
2. 5000 U every other day for four injections
3. 15 injections of 500 U to 1000 U over 6 weeks
4. 500 U three times a week for 4 weeks to 6 weeks; if unsuccessful, repeat after one month with 1000 U per injection

Hypogonadism
1. 500 U to 1000 U three times a week for 3 weeks, then twice a week for 3 weeks
2. 1000 U to 2000 U three times a week
3. 4000 U three times a week for 6 months to 9 months, then 2000 U three times a week for 3 months

SIDE-EFFECTS/ADVERSE REACTIONS

The major adverse effects associated with HCG administration are ovarian hyperstimulation, rupture of ovarian cysts with resultant hemoperitoneum, multiple births, and arterial thromboembolism. Other adverse reactions include headache, irritability, restlessness, fatigue, depression, fluid retention and edema, gynecomastia in males, precocious puberty, and pain at the site of injection.

CONTRAINDICATIONS AND PRECAUTIONS

HCG is contraindicated in persons with prostatic carcinoma or other androgen-dependent neoplasms and in the presence of precocious puberty. The drug must be used with caution in persons with asthma, cardiac or renal disease, epilepsy, or migraine, since fluid retention may aggravate these conditions. Excessive treatment with HCG may damage a mechanically obstructed, undescended

testis. Cryptorchidism failing to respond to HCG within a reasonable period of time (6 weeks to 12 weeks) usually requires surgical intervention.

Although HCG has been used in the treatment of obesity, there is no substantial evidence that the drug alters fat mobilization or distribution, retards appetite, or reduces hunger associated with low-calorie diets. Its use as an anti-obesity drug should be avoided.

NURSING CONSIDERATIONS

See also Nursing Process, above. (*Note:* The following applies to use of both urofollitropin and HCG.)

Before initiating HMG–HCG or urofollitropin–HCG therapy the woman should undergo a 24-hour urine testing to determine total estrogen secretion and a total plasma estradiol level. Another test should be done at the end of therapy. Pregnancy is most likely to occur if the 24-hour estrogen level is between 100 mcg and 200 mcg per 24 hours. If the level exceeds 200 mcg per 24 hours ovarian hyperstimulation may occur. The urinary levels are used to determine the best time to give HMG or urofollitropin.

The patient should be closely monitored during the course of therapy and for 2 weeks after therapy since this is the time period during which ovarian hyperstimulation is most likely to occur. (See Side-Effects/Adverse Reactions, above.) The condition can be life threatening if rupture occurs and hospitalization may be necessary.

Timing of intercourse is also critical during therapy. The couple is usually advised to have intercourse on the day that HCG is given and for 2 days following drug administration. They should be aware of the signs of ovulation, as described earlier.

The child who receives HCG for cryptorchidism must have good support systems since the development of secondary sex characteristics may be somewhat exaggerated and development of gynecomastia during a period of identity crisis is disturbing. The child should have an opportunity to share his feelings about being "different" and parents should be given some strategies to help him get through this period. In addition, since the child is subjected to multiple painful injections the nurse and family may expect periods of rebellion, anger, and withdrawal. Contracting with the child for something he would like, limit setting on rebellious behaviors, with verbalization about understanding the frustration of treatment, and clear explanations about the treatment and its effects may be useful in getting the child to participate.

Abortifacients

Termination of pregnancy can be accomplished by both mechanical and pharmacologic methods. During the early weeks of pregnancy, there is no safe and reliable method for pharmacologically inducing fetal expulsion, and suction curettage is the commonly performed procedure. Beginning at about the start of the second trimester, however, pharmacologic methods are usually employed; these consist of injections of either hypertonic (i.e., 20%) saline solution or prostaglandin $F_{2\alpha}$ into the amniotic sac, IM administration of a prostaglandin salt, or use of a prostaglandin (E_2) vaginal suppository. Certain prostaglandins (PGE_2, PGF_2) have been detected in amniotic fluid during labor or spontaneous abortion and appear to play a role in fetal expulsion by facilitating myometrial contractions. These observations have led to the development of several prostaglandin preparations indicated for the induction of second-trimester elective abortion. These agents are preferable to intra-amniotic injection of hypertonic sodium chloride (see below) because they have a more rapid onset of action, although their use may be associated with a greater frequency of systemic adverse reactions such as nausea, vomiting, diarrhea, and fever. The prostaglandins used as abortifacients are reviewed in Chapter 82, where the pharmacology and clinical applications of all of the prostaglandins are considered.

Sodium Chloride 20%

Intra-amniotic injection of hypertonic sodium chloride can be used for second-trimester abortion (i.e., 16 weeks' to 22 weeks' gestation), but has been largely replaced by the prostaglandins (see Chap. 82), which have a much faster rate of induction and may be given by more convenient, less technically difficult routes of administration (e.g., IM, intravaginally). The principal indication for sodium chloride injection is in the patient desiring abortion who has not responded successfully or completely to one of the prostaglandins. When prostaglandin-induced abortion is incomplete, however, injection of hypertonic saline should be delayed until the uterus is no longer contracting. The volume of solution instilled should not exceed the volume of amniotic fluid removed. Injection should be performed at a relatively slow rate and fluid samples taken at regular intervals to ensure

that the needle remains in the amniotic cavity. The maximum dose is considered to be 250 ml. Inadvertent intravascular injection should be avoided, because sudden, severe hypernatremia may result, possibly leading to cardiovascular shock, extensive hemolysis, and renal necrosis. The drug should be administered only in a medical unit with intensive care facilities readily available. If labor has not begun within 48 hours after instillation, reevaluation of the patient status is indicated.

Tocolytics

Tocolytic drugs reduce uterine contractions and are used in the management of premature labor. The most widely used tocolytic is ritodrine, a beta-adrenergic agonist that is administered IV to arrest the acute stage of labor and also orally to avert a relapse until the proper stage of gestation. Ritodrine is considered in detail in Chapter 15. Another beta-agonist, terbutaline, is also used as a tocolytic, and is also reviewed in Chapter 15. Isoxsuprine, another drug exhibiting a degree of uterine-relaxant activity, has been employed to manage premature labor, although this is neither an approved nor a recommended indication. Maternal and fetal tachycardia has occurred, pulmonary edema has been reported in mothers given the drug for this purpose, and hypotension, hypoglycemia, and ileus have been reported in infants whose mothers have received isoxsuprine.

IV infusion of a 10% solution of ethyl alcohol at a rate of 7.5 ml/kg/hour for 2 hours, followed by 1.5 ml/kg/hour for up to 10 hours has been used for many years to reduce uterine activity during premature labor. The drug apparently acts by inhibiting release of oxytocin from the posterior pituitary. This procedure is largely obsolete today with the availability of ritodrine, since infusion of alcohol can result in maternal intoxication and a depression of fetal and neonatal function.

Recent evidence suggests that calcium channel blockers such as nifedipine can relax the myometrium and may be effective in delaying parturition. The potential clinical usefulness of these agents remains to be established.

High doses of magnesium sulfate can inhibit uterine contractions and this agent may be a useful alternative when beta-agonists such as ritodrine are contraindicated. However, large doses of magnesium can impair cardiac conduction, neuromuscular transmission, and respiratory function and can prove quite hazardous.

CASE STUDY

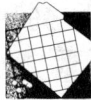

Gwen Simon and her husband, Rob, were evaluated by an infertility specialist after trying unsuccessfully to conceive for 2 years. A review of Gwen's basal body temperature records for 3 months revealed anovulation. Examination of Rob's sperm showed slightly decreased quantity and normal motility. Gwen's thyroid function was within normal limits and progesterone levels during the luteal phase of her cycle were at normal levels. The decision was made to start Gwen on clomiphene, 50 mg for days 5 to 9 of her next menstrual cycle.

On day 28 Gwen's menses began. Her basal body temperature reading had dropped during the period of ovulation but cervical mucus did not achieve desired elasticity. The physician increased her dose of clomiphene to 100 mg for 5 days. On day 11 Gwen began to notice ovarian tenderness and had pain walking to her car from her office. She drove home and called the physician, who advised her to come to the office.

Discussion Questions

1. What parameters will the physician assess to determine the cause of Gwen's pain?
2. Gwen is upset that she may not be able to have intercourse due to the pain. What actions should the nurse take to allay her fears?
3. Gwen's pain diminishes the following day and she calls the office to ask if it is safe for her to have intercourse. What symptoms should she continue to watch for?

REVIEW QUESTIONS

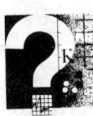

1. Describe the three basic types of oral contraceptive combination products.
2. Briefly list the mechanisms by which oral contraceptives prevent pregnancy.
3. How does the ratio of estrogen to progestin in the product influence the choice of the particular drug for a patient?
4. What are the principal symptoms of (1) estrogen excess and (2) progestin excess in these products?
5. Describe the major adverse effects associated with the use of oral contraceptives.
6. What other factors increase the risk of myocardial infarction in oral contraceptive uses?
7. List the principal contraindications to oral contraceptive use.
8. What information should a woman be given about taking oral contraceptives? What effects of the drug should she be told to expect?
9. What nutritional information should a woman receive about the effects of oral contraceptives?
10. How is the intrauterine progesterone contraceptive system used?
11. List the database needed for any couple who are being considered for ovulation-stimulant drug therapy.

12. What parameters can a couple use to determine whether ovulation is occurring?
13. What are the symptoms of ovarian hyperstimulation?
14. What are the risks of multiple births with ovarian stimulants?
15. Briefly discuss the mechanism of action of clomiphene.
16. Give several dangers associated with clomiphene use.
17. How does menotropins facilitate ovulation? Is it used alone or with another agent?
18. From what source is human chorionic gonadotropin obtained? What is its principal action?
19. What types of drugs may be used as second-trimester abortifacients?
20. What type of drug is a tocolytic? List several different classes of drugs that can be used as tocolytics.

BIBLIOGRAPHY

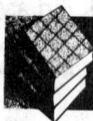

Alexander NB, Cotanct PH: The endrocrine basis of infertility in women. Nurs Clin North Am 15:511, 1980

Brenner PF: The pharmacology of progestogens. J Reproduc Med 27(suppl):490, 1982

Bronson RA: Oral contraception: Mechanism of action. Clin Obstet Gynecol 24:869, 1981

Dickerson J: The pill, a closer look. Am J Nurs 83(10):1392, 1983

Durand JL, Bressler R: Clinical pharmacology of the steroidal oral contraceptives. Adv Intern Med 24:97, 1979

Frederiksen MC: Tocolytic therapy with beta-adrenergic agonists. Ration Drug Ther 17(6):1, 1983

Friedman BM: Infertility work up. Am J Nurs 81:2041, 1981

Goldzieher JW (ed): Advances in oral contraception: An international review of levonorgestrel and ethinyl estradiol. J Reprod Med 28:53, 1983

Jordan VC: Biochemical pharmacology of antiestrogen action. Pharmacol Rev 36:245, 1984

Kanell RG: Oral contraceptives: the risks in perspective. Nurse Pract 9(9):25, 1984

Meade TW: Oral contraceptives, clotting factors and thrombosis. Am J Obstet Gynecol 142:758, 1982

Oral contraceptives and the risk of cardiovascular disease. Med Lett Drugs Ther 25:69, 1983

Price MC, Henderson BE, Krailo MD, et al: Breast cancer in young women and use of oral contraceptives: possible modifying effect of formulation and age at use. Lancet 2:920, 1983

Sands CD, Robinson JD, Orlando JB: The oral contraceptive PPI: Its effect on patient knowledge, feelings, and behavior. Drug Intell Clin Pharm 18:730, 1984

Speroff L: Formulation of oral contraceptives: Does the amount of estrogen make any clinical difference. Johns Hopkins Med J 150:170, 1982

Stedel BV: Oral contraceptives and cardiovascular disease. N Engl J Med 305:612, 672, 1981

Weiss NS, Sayvetz TA: Incidence of endometrial cancer in relation to the use of oral contraceptives. N Engl J Med 302:551, 1980

Wynn V: Cardiovascular effects and progestins in oral contraceptives. Am J Obstet Gynecol 142:718, 1982

Veninga KS: Effects of oral contraceptives on vitamins B_6, B_{12}, C, and folacin. Journal of Nurse-Midwifery 29(6):386, 1984

Androgens and Anabolic Steroids

58

The term androgen refers to a number of naturally occurring or synthetic steroidal compounds exhibiting the masculinizing and tissue-building (anabolic) actions of testosterone, the principal endogenous physiologic androgenic hormone. Testosterone is produced in and secreted by the interstitial (Leydig's) cells of the testes under the stimulus of interstitial cell-stimulating hormone (ICSH), which is identical to luteinizing hormone (LH) of the female.

At the time of puberty, the pituitary begins to secrete increased amounts of FSH and ICSH. These hormones together are responsible for controlling testicular growth, formation of sperm cells (spermatogenesis), and synthesis of testosterone and other gonadal hormones (steroidogenesis). Specifically, ICSH increases the formation of cyclic AMP in the interstitial cells of the testes, resulting in the synthesis of androgens from cholesterol and acetate. The major effect of FSH, on the other hand, is believed to be on the formation of sperm cells in the seminiferous tubules.

Androgens are also normally secreted by the adrenal cortex and by the ovaries. Approximately 7 mg to 8 mg of testosterone are produced daily in the adult male, 95% of which is derived from the interstitial cells of the testes. Much smaller amounts of other androgens are also produced by the testes, including dihydrotestosterone, androstenedione, and dehydroepiandrosterone.

Physiologic Effects of Androgens

The principal androgen, testosterone, is responsible for the development and support of the male sex organs and the appearance of the secondary sex characteristics (e.g., deep voice, body hair) at the time of puberty. In addition, testosterone exerts a protein anabolic action (thus stimulating growth of skeletal muscle tissue), reduces excretion of sodium, potassium, chloride, nitrogen, and phosphorus, and enhances growth of long bones in prepubertal males. However, it also accelerates the ossification (hardening) process of the ends of long bones, eventually resulting in a conversion of cartilage into bone in the active growth areas (epiphyses) and cessation of further bone growth. For this reason, use of large amounts of androgens in young boys may actually result in a reduction of full potential growth due to a premature closing of the epiphyses after an initial spurt in growth. Like-

wise, androgenic therapy in young males can result in precocious puberty, that is, premature development of the male sex organs and secondary sex characteristics, with possible attendant psychologic trauma.

Other physiologic actions of testosterone include increased sebaceous gland activity, thickening of the vocal cords, darkening of the skin, loss of subcutaneous fat, and increased skin vascularization. In addition, psychologic and behavioral changes occur as production of testosterone is increased.

Anabolic Action

As noted above, testosterone exhibits a protein anabolic action, in addition to its effects on the gonads. In addition to testosterone, a group of synthetic steroids structurally related to testosterone have been developed that display some separation of anabolic from androgenic activity, although the degree of separation is incomplete and variable. These compounds are termed anabolic steroids and have been used for a variety of conditions in which an anabolic activity is desired, such as retarded growth and development in children; senile, postmenopausal, or corticosteroid-induced osteoporosis; debilitation resulting from trauma, surgery, or illness; and certain types of anemia (e.g., aplastic). Of course, sufficient caloric and protein intake must be maintained during drug therapy to achieve and maintain a positive nitrogen balance. While these compounds exhibit a higher anabolic-to-androgenic ratio (e.g., 3:1 or 4:1) than testosterone or methyltestosterone, which demonstrate equal degrees of anabolic and androgenic activity, excessive dosage or prolonged administration is associated with most of the same untoward effects as seen with testosterone itself. Moreover, anabolic steroids have not been proven to enhance athletic prowess to the extent that their routine administration justifies the potential health hazards that can result from their use. Thus, anabolic steroid administration, especially in women and children, should be closely supervised and restricted to the valid indications listed below.

Other steroids that bear structural resemblance to testosterone but exhibit reduced androgenic activity are used in the treatment of advanced or metastatic breast cancer in postmenopausal women. These drugs, dromostanolone and testolactone, are reviewed in Chapter 75.

Therapeutic Use of Androgens

Testosterone itself, although adequately absorbed from the GI tract, is not administered orally because it is rapidly inactivated by the liver, and very large oral doses (*e.g.*, 400 mg/day) would be necessary to provide clinically effective blood levels. Testosterone may be given by IM injection (aqueous suspension); again, it is relatively short acting when administered by this route, due to rapid metabolism. Several esters of testosterone (propionate, cypionate, enanthate) exhibit greater stability and slower metabolism and, when injected IM in an oily vehicle, display a prolonged duration of action. Other structural modifications of testosterone (*e.g.*, methyltestosterone, fluoxymesterone) can increase potency and, in addition, can confer resistance to hepatic metabolism, thus permitting use by the oral or buccal route.

In addition to the androgens mentioned above, several other structural analogues of testosterone are used primarily for their anabolic action. Because the androgenic and anabolic steroids are similar in their pharmacology, they are discussed as a group and then are listed in Table 58-1 along with their specific indications and recommended doses. Danazol, a synthetic androgen possessing antigonadotropic and androgenic activity, is used in the treatment of endometriosis and is also reviewed at the end of this chapter.

Androgens and Anabolic Steroids

Ethylestrenol, Fluoxymesterone, Methandrostenolone, Methyltestosterone, Nandrolone, Oxandrolone, Oxymetholone, Stanozolol, Testosterone

MECHANISM AND ACTIONS
Androgens appear to bind to a cytoplasmic protein receptor, and this interaction results in increased synthesis of protein and RNA. At some sites, testosterone must first be converted to dihydrotestosterone in order to interact with the receptors, while at other sites, testosterone itself is active. Other derivatives appear to stimulate protein synthesis directly.

Androgens increase growth of muscle, bone, skin, and hair and accelerate closure of epiphyses at ends of long bones. They also increase production of red blood cells and may decrease renal excretion of nitrogen, phosphorus, sodium, and probably calcium and potassium as well. Androgens can temporarily arrest progression of estrogen-dependent carcinomas. Large doses can suppress pituitary gonadotropin secretion, and decrease spermatogenesis through feedback inhibition of FSH.

USES
(See Table 58-1 for specific indications.)
1. Replacement therapy in androgen deficiency states, such as testicular hypofunction, pituitary dysfunction, eunuchism (complete testicular failure), eunuchoidism, (partial testicular failure), cryptorchidism, castration, or male climacteric
2. Treatment of low sperm count or impotence due to androgen deficiency (low doses only)
3. Palliative therapy of androgen-responsive inoperable breast cancer in 1-year to 5-year postmenopausal women
4. Production of a positive nitrogen balance in those conditions in which an anabolic action is desired (*e.g.*, retarded growth and physical development in children, osteoporosis, anemia, corticosteroid-induced nitrogen loss, and debilitation resulting from injury, trauma, illness, and other causes)

■ *NOTE*
Use of anabolic steroids will *not* significantly enhance athletic ability. These are dangerous drugs that can cause serious adverse effects, and their use has resulted in death. There is *no* conclusive evidence that anabolic steroids can significantly increase muscle mass, muscle strength, or athletic performance level in *males*. In fact, much of the increased body weight noted with use of these drugs is probably the result of increased sodium and fluid retention. In addition, any increased muscle mass is *not* accompanied by increased tendon strength, and ruptured tendons are common if the muscle mass becomes too great for the tendon to support under increased physical demand.

While nitrogen retention and increased body mass can occur with *females* taking anabolic steroids, the inevitable virilizing side-effects must be recognized and seem a high price to pay for possible improvement in athletic performance. Moreover, use of other drugs with anabolic steroids, such as diuretics to reduce fluid retention, can further increase the likelihood of toxicity, and resultant electrolyte imbalances may have serious adverse consequences. Use of anabolic steroids for improving athletic prowess should be strongly discouraged.

5. Relief of postpartum breast pain and engorgement (rarely used)

ADMINISTRATION AND DOSAGE
See Table 58-1.

FATE
Testosterone is adequately absorbed when given orally, but as much as 50% of a dose undergoes first-pass hepatic metabolism and very high doses are necessary to achieve effective plasma levels. Synthetic androgens are less extensively metabolized and exhibit longer half-lives. Esterification of testosterone increases its stability, and when administered in an oily vehicle it possesses a long duration of action (2 weeks–4 weeks). Testosterone is highly (98%) bound to plasma proteins, especially testosterone-estradiol-binding globulin. Androgens are metabolized in the liver, and conjugated metabolites are excreted largely in the urine.

SIDE-EFFECTS/ADVERSE REACTIONS

■ *WARNING*
Use of androgens or anabolic steroids can result in development of peliosis hepatis, a condition in which the liver and spleen may become engorged with blood-filled cysts. Liver failure has resulted, and intra-abdominal hemorrhage has also occurred. Liver cell tumors have been reported, and while usually benign, fatal malignant tumors can occur. Adverse serum lipid changes, such as decreased high-density lipoproteins and elevated low-density lipoproteins, have also been noted with androgen therapy. Cholestatic hepatitis and jaundice can occur with fluoxymesterone and methyltestosterone at relatively low doses; the drug-induced jaundice is reversible when the medication is discontinued.

The most common side-effects of androgens in females are amenorrhea, menstrual irregularities, and virilization, characterized by hirsutism, voice deepening, and clitoral enlargement. In males, gynecomastia is a frequent occurrence. Nausea occurs commonly with use of the oral preparations, and flushing and changes in libido are also noted with frequency.

Other adverse effects reported in males include phallic enlargement, increased erections, testicular atrophy, bladder irritability, decreased sperm count, epididymitis, chronic priapism, and oligospermia with high doses. Impotence can occur following withdrawal, due to inhibition of endogenous testosterone production.

In females, male pattern baldness, hypercalcemia, and suppression of ovulation and lactation have occurred with androgen use.

Many other adverse reactions have been noted in both sexes and include acne; oily skin; excitation; insomnia; anxiety; depression; headache; paresthesia; chills; leukopenia; polycythemia; rash, dermatitis, muscle cramping, pain; swelling, urticaria, and irritation at injection sites; sodium and water retention; increased serum cholesterol; and alterations in many other clinical laboratory tests.

CONTRAINDICATIONS AND PRECAUTIONS
Androgen use is contraindicated in pregnant women and in the presence of breast or prostatic carcinoma in males. In addition, anabolic steroids are also contraindicated in patients with pituitary insufficiency, a history of myocardial infarction, prostatic hypertrophy, hepatic dysfunction, nephrosis, hypercalcemia, and in infants and young children.

These agents must be given with *caution* to persons with hypertension, coronary artery disease, gynecomastia, renal disease, hypercholesterolemia, and to prepubertal males because early closure of the epiphyses can occur and stunted growth may result. Geriatric patients given androgens may be at increased risk for developing prostatic hypertrophy and prostatic carcinoma.

INTERACTIONS
1. Androgens may decrease oral anticoagulant requirements.
2. Barbiturates and other hypnotics, phenytoin, and phenylbutazone may decrease the action of androgens by accelerating their hepatic metabolic breakdown.

(Text continues on p. 1122.)

Table 58-1
Androgens and Anabolic Steroids

Drug	Preparations	Usual Dosage Range	Clinical Considerations
Androgens			
fluoxymesterone (Android-F, Halotestin, Ora-Testryl)	Tablets—2 mg, 5 mg, 10 mg	Hypogonadism, impotence—5 mg to 20 mg a day Delayed puberty—2 mg a day initially; increase gradually as necessary, up to 20 mg a day Breast cancer—10 mg to 40 mg a day in divided doses Postpartum breast engorgement—2.5 mg shortly after delivery; thereafter, 5 mg to 10 mg in divided doses for 4 days to 5 days	Potent, orally effective, short-acting derivative of testosterone, approximately five times more active than testosterone itself; minimal sodium and water retention, but frequent GI distress (administer drug with food); be alert for symptoms suggestive of peptic ulcer; confirmatory tests should be performed (see also Chap. 75)
methyltestosterone (Android, Metandren, Oreton, Testred, Virilon)	Tablets: Oral—10 mg, 25 mg Buccal—5 mg, 10 mg Capsules—10 mg	Male hypogonadism, impotence, male climacteric—10 mg to 40 mg a day (oral) or 5 mg to 20 mg a day (buccal) Cryptorchidism—30 mg a day (oral) or 15 mg a day (buccal) Postpartum breast pain and engorgement—80 mg a day (oral) or 40 mg a day (buccal) for 3 days to 5 days Breast cancer—200 mg a day (oral) or 100 mg a day (buccal)	Orally effective, short-acting androgen, somewhat less effective than testosterone esters; does not produce full sexual maturation in prepubertal testicular failure unless patient has been pretreated with testosterone; creatinuria is a common finding, although its significance is not known; buccal tablets should be placed between cheek and gum and allowed to dissolve; do not chew or swallow, and avoid eating, drinking, or smoking for at least 1 hour after ingestion; advise patient to report any inflammation or pain in oral cavity following drug usage; good oral hygiene should be stressed to reduce infection or irritation (see also Chap. 75)
testosterone, aqueous (Andro 100, Andronaq-50, Histerone, Testamone 100, Testaqua, Testoject)	Injection (aqueous suspension)—25 mg/ml, 50 mg/ml, 100 mg/ml	Male hypogonadism, impotence, male climacteric—25 mg to 50 mg IM two to three times a week Postpartum breast engorgement—25 mg to 50 mg a day for 3 days to 4 days Breast carcinoma—50 mg to 100 mg three times a week	Male sex hormone used as replacement therapy in deficiency states, for relief of breast engorgement and treatment of mammary carcinoma in women; inject IM only, deep into gluteal muscle; if crystals are present in the vial, warming and shaking will disperse them; absorption is slow and effects persist for several days; do not administer more frequently than recommended; regression of mammary
testosterone propionate (Testex)	Injection (in oil)—25 mg/ml, 50 mg/ml, 100 mg/ml		

(continued)

Table 58-1 (continued)
Androgens and Anabolic Steroids

Drug	Preparations	Usual Dosage Range	Clinical Considerations
Androgens *(continued)*			
testosterone propionate (Testex) *(continued)*			tumors should be apparent within 3 months; occasionally, acceleration of tumor growth is encountered, in which case discontinue immediately; in some of these cases, estrogens will then cause regression (see also Chap. 75). Testosterone propionate is formulated in an oily vehicle; absorption may be somewhat slower than testosterone aqueous, but duration of action is comparable.
testosterone cypionate (Andro-Cyp, Andronate, Andronaq LA, dep Andro, Depotest, Depo-Testosterone, Duratest, Testa-C, Testadiate-Depo, Testoject LA) testosterone enanthate (Andro L.A., Andropository, Andryl, Delatest, Delatestryl, Durathate, Everone, Testone L.A., Testrin-P.A.)	Injection (in oil)—50 mg/ml, 100 mg/ml, 200 mg/ml	Hypogonadism, male climacteric—50 mg to 400 mg IM every 2 wk to 4 wk Oligospermia—100 mg to 200 mg every 4 wk to 6 wk Delayed puberty—50 mg to 200 mg every 2 wk to 4 wk Inoperable mammary cancer—200 mg to 400 mg every 2 wk to 4 wk	Long-acting esters of testosterone providing a therapeutic effect for approximately 4 wk with a single injection; not recommended for use in treating *metastatic* breast carcinoma; inject deep into gluteal muscle; shaking and warming of vial will redissolve any crystals that have formed; use of a wet needle or syringe may cloud solution but potency is unaffected.
Anabolic Steroids			
ethylestrenol (Maxibolin)	Tablets—2 mg Elixir—2 mg/5 ml	Weight gain, osteoporosis, anemias: Adults—4 mg to 8 mg a day initially if needed Children—2 mg a day (range 1 mg–3 mg a day)	Anabolic steroid given for a 6-wk period, then stopped for 4 wk; if indication for its use is still evident, it may be resumed for additional 6-wk period; in children, x-rays should be taken before reinstating therapy to determine stage of bone maturation
methandrostenolone (Methandrostenolone)	Tablets—2.5 mg, 5 mg	Adults—5 mg initially; usual maintenance dose 2.5 mg to 5 mg daily	Used as adjunctive therapy in senile and postmenopausal osteoporosis; intermittent therapy is recommended for long-term use
nadrolone decanoate (Anabolin LA, Androlone-D, Deca-Durabolin, Decolone, Hybolin, Nandrobolic L.A., Neo-Durabolic)	Injection (in oil)—50 mg/ml, 100 mg/ml, 200 mg/ml	Anemia of renal disease: Men—100 mg to 200 mg per week Women—50 mg to 100 mg per week Children—25 mg to 50 mg every 3 wk to 4 wk	Long-acting ester of nandrolone (duration 3 wk–4 wk) used for management of anemia of renal insufficiency; rated *possibly* effective for adjunctive therapy of senile or postmeno-*(continued)*

Table 58-1 (continued)
Androgens and Anabolic Steroids

Drug	Preparations	Usual Dosage Range	Clinical Considerations
Anabolic Steroids (continued)			
nandrolone decanoate (Anabolin LA, Androlone-D, Deca-Durabolin, Decolone, Hybolin, Nandrobolic L.A., Neo-Durabolic) (continued)		Osteoporosis, tissue building (investigational): Adults—50 mg to 100 mg IM every 3 wk to 4 wk Children—25 mg to 50 mg every 3 wk to 4 wk Metastatic breast cancer: 100 mg to 200 mg a week	pausal osteoporosis, for increasing tissue-building activity postsurgically, for control of metastatic breast carcinoma, and in certain types of refractory anemia
nandrolone phenpropionate (Anabolin-IM, Androlone, Durabolin, Hybolin Improved, Nandrobolic)	Injection (in oil)—25 mg/ml, 50 mg/ml	Metastatic breast cancer: 25 mg to 100 mg/week IM Osteoporosis, anemia, tissue building (investigational): Adults—50 mg to 100 mg a week Children—12.5 mg to 25 mg every 2 wk to 4 wk	Synthetic androgen approved for use in metastatic breast cancer; also used for tissue-building action and for adjunctive therapy of osteoporosis and anemia. Possesses a high anabolic–androgenic ratio; effects persist 1 wk to 3 wk; injection should be made deeply into gluteal muscle in adults; intermittent therapy is recommended, with 4-wk to 8-wk rest periods every 4 mo (see Chap. 75)
oxandrolone (Anavar)	Tablets—2.5 mg	Osteoporosis, tissue building: Adults—2.5 mg two to four times a day (up to 20 mg a day) for 2 wk to 4 wk; repeat after a rest period if desired Children—0.25 mg/kg a day	Synthetic anabolic steroid with low androgenic activity; used to help promote weight gain following trauma, severe illness, major surgery, or prolonged corticosteroid administration; do not administer longer than 3 mo
oxymetholone (Anadrol-50)	Tablets—50 mg	Anemias—(adults and children) 1 mg to 2 mg/kg/day to a maximum of 5 mg/kg/day (highly individualized)	Synthetic anabolic steroid used primarily for anemias due to deficient red cell production, congenital or acquired aplastic anemia, and anemias resulting from administration of myelotoxic drugs; a minimum of 3 mo to 6 mo should be allowed because response is often slow; following remission, some patients may be able to stop drug, while others may require a minimum daily dosage
stanozolol (Winstrol)	Tablets—2 mg	Hereditary angioedema: Adults—initially 2 mg three times a day. Decrease gradually to maintenance dosage of 2 mg/day.	Primarily used to decrease frequency and severity of attacks of hereditary angioedema; exhibits minimal androgenic effects at normal doses; administer with meals to decrease GI distress

3. Androgens can antagonize the action of calcitonin and parathyroid hormone.
4. Corticosteroids may increase the severity of androgen-induced edema.
5. Anabolic steroids may decrease blood glucose in diabetics, reducing insulin or oral hypoglycemic drug requirements.
6. Androgens can alter the results of laboratory tests for glucose tolerance, thyroid function, blood coagulation, liver function, creatinine clearance, and 17-ketosteroid excretion.

■ Nursing Process

□ ASSESSMENT

□ Subjective Data
To do a thorough assessment, the nurse must first determine why anabolic steroids have been prescribed (see under Uses). By seeking a history of the present illness and the symptoms the patient is experiencing, the nurse will be able to determine the patient's needs and plan his care. The patient who receives an androgen for treatment of metastatic breast cancer may want information about the drug's ability to slow the disease process and ease pain. The adolescent male suffering testicular hypofunction needs to discuss his self-image and his hopes that the drug will bring his appearance more in line with that of his peers. The adult male being treated for low sperm count may have concerns about his virility and may question the drug's ability to help him reproduce. Each of these patients has very different needs, will require different information about the drug prescribed, and will be looking for different outcomes. Compliance with the prescribed regimen will also depend on the patient's perception of the drug's value to him.

A complete systems history should also be obtained with particular focus on cardiovascular, hepatic, or renal problems, or presence of a prostate condition or of diabetes mellitus. A thorough drug history should also be obtained because interactions occur frequently.

□ Objective Data
Although a complete physical is essential, the nurse may want to highlight a few parameters in the assessment to use for later comparison. These include weight, blood pressure, and a complete genital examination. In the prepubescent male, height and the presence of any secondary sex characteristics should also be noted.

Laboratory data may include liver studies, cholesterol level, serum calcium, and a complete blood count because the red blood cell count may increase during therapy leading to polycythemia. A sperm count will be performed in the male treated for infertility. The adolescent with testicular hypofunction may have other tests performed such as an immunoassay for gonadotropin, testosterone level, and a 24-hour urine for 17-ketosteroids. Serum protein level may be obtained in any patient for whom the anabolic action of the drug will be important.

□ Nursing Diagnoses
Every patient who receives androgens/anabolic steroids will have the following diagnosis:
> Knowledge deficit related to the action, administration, and side-effects of the drug

Other nursing diagnoses may emerge during assessment or throughout therapy depending on the patient's diagnosis and/or side-effects which may develop.

The following are *potential* nursing diagnoses for the patient taking these drugs:
> Anxiety
> Altered cardiac output: decreased
> Altered growth and development
> Alteration in oral mucous membrane
> Disturbance in self-concept: body image, personal identity
> Sexual dysfunction
> Sleep pattern disturbance
> Alteration in thought processes: depression
> Urinary retention related to prostatic enlargement

□ PLAN
The nursing care goals should focus on (1) safe administration of the drug and (2) teaching the patient and family correct drug administration and how to monitor closely for side-effects.

□ INTERVENTION
If intramuscular injection is the route of administration the injection site should be a deep one into a substantial muscle mass such as the gluteus. Most of the steroids and androgens are viscous; therefore, a large 18- to 20-gauge needle about 1½ inches long should be used. Sites should be rotated with each dose regardless of the time span between them because drug absorption is slow, and injection sites should be examined regularly for signs of inflammation or abscess.

Buccal tablets should be placed under the tongue or in the space between cheek and gum. Teach the patient to rotate between the four possible locations in the mouth to reduce the chance of ulceration. Encourage the patient not to eat, drink, or smoke until the tablet is completely dissolved because these activities will alter absorption and may also cause ulcer formation. Oral tablets should be taken with food to minimize gastrointestinal distress.

The patient taking androgens/anabolic steroids is subject to a number of unpleasant and possibly damaging side-effects. Consequently, it is important to teach the patient steps to minimize the occurrence of problems and how to detect early signs which should be reported. In general, a patient should not be treated with these drugs for more than 90 days without careful reassessment and comparison of the risks versus the benefits of continued therapy.

Hypercalcemia may develop, most frequently in the bedridden, immobilized patient or in the patient with metastatic breast cancer. This effect can be minimized if the patient can perform some regular exercise even as simple as flexion/extension exercises of the extremities. Early symptoms of hypercalcemia such as vomiting, constipation, lethargy, polyuria, and muscle weakness should be reported immediately. A serum calcium level will be drawn, the drug will be discontinued, and fluids will be encouraged in large quantities to prevent development of renal calculi.

Jaundice may occur if liver function is diminished by drug therapy. Early signs such as yellow skin or sclera, abdominal pain, and itching should be reported immediately.

The adolescent receiving these drugs may have an initial growth surge but should be closely monitored for signs of premature epiphyseal closure. Radiologic examination of the long bones should be done at regular intervals.

Gonadal symptoms such as priapism, reduced ejaculatory volume, or impotence in males should also be reported. Symptoms may be controlled by dosage reduction, or the physician may opt to temporarily discontinue therapy until symptoms subside.

The patient needs to weigh himself daily and watch closely for signs of fluid retention. A rapid increase in weight of more than 2 lb or 3 lb or a feeling of tightness in waist or extremities should be reported.

The nurse who sees young athletes in his or her practice may deal with anabolic steroids from a different perspective. The nurse may see a patient suffering from overdose of these drugs, also called "sports doping." Athletes sometimes abuse these drugs in an effort to increase their muscle mass, strength, speed, and mental toughness. Some are encouraged by coaches, trainers, and peers to use steroids this way. The athlete is unlikely to readily report the drugs as the cause of symptoms because such use is illegal in sports. Therefore, the nurse must ask questions carefully to determine a problem. The athlete who has abused steroids may complain of headaches, gastrointestinal distress, muscle aches, dizziness, and sleeping problems. He or she may feel these are flu symptoms. Physical exam will reveal bruises, scratch marks from itchy skin, needle marks, evidence of increased bleeding either in nosebleeds, body petechiae, or bleeding gums, and reddened conjunctiva. Males will probably have an enlarged spleen, liver, and prostate, decreased testicular size and extremity edema. Females may also exhibit increased facial hair, menstrual irregularities, and enlarged clitoris. Laboratory values may show increases in testosterone, red blood cells, liver function, and cholesterol.

The nurse who suspects steroid abuse should seek physician referral immediately because the patient is likely to suffer irreversible liver damage if drug use continues. The athlete who agrees to go through withdrawal from these drugs also faces a hard road. He or she is likely to lose weight and strength, the very effects the athlete sought to increase. Withdrawal also produces a variety of mood swings, ranging from violent rage to depression. Some patients have attempted suicide. Withdrawal should be controlled and closely monitored. The effect on athletic ability may be very demoralizing to the young person whose life revolves around the sport.

☐ EVALUATION
Outcome criteria depend on the reason treatment was initiated. For all patients, hopefully, the drug will be taken safely and correctly and the patient will learn to watch for side-effects. For the adolescent with androgen deficiency outcome criteria may include development of appropriate secondary sex characteristics, increased testosterone level, and continued ability to grow based on siting of open epiphysis on radiologic examination. For the woman with metastatic breast cancer the outcomes sought are evidence that tumor growth has slowed down or stopped and decrease in pain. In the male with low sperm count the outcome sought would be an increase in sperm production.

Danazol
(Danocrine)

MECHANISM AND ACTIONS

Danazol is a synthetic derivative of 17-alpha-ethinyl testosterone that inhibits the release of gonadotropins from the pituitary gland and exhibits a weak androgenic effect. No estrogenic or progestational activity has been demonstrated. Danazol suppresses release of FSH and LH and also acts by inhibiting enzymes involved in the biosynthesis of gonadal hormones. The drug may also competitively interfere with binding of sex steroids to the cytoplasmic receptors in body tissues.

In endometriosis, danazol alters the tissue so that it becomes atrophic, and complete resolution of endometrial lesions occurs in the majority of cases.

The drug also corrects the principal biochemical abnormality associated with hereditary angioedema (see Disease Brief: Angioedema).

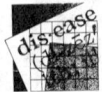

DISEASE BRIEF

■ Angioedema

Angioedema or angioneurotic edema is characterized by localized swelling of subcutaneous tissue throughout the body. The swelling results from dilatation of small vessels and capillary leakage. Angioedema occurs in two forms, a relatively rare hereditary form and a more common nonhereditary or sporadic form. The hereditary form is apparently due to a lack of specific enzyme inhibitors of the first component of complement as well as of serum globulin permeability factor and plasma kallikrein. Thus, there is unopposed activation of permeability factors, and development of localized edema, especially involving respiratory and gastrointestinal systems as well as subcutaneous tissue. The nonhereditary type is usually the result of food or drug allergy, infection, or emotional change and often occurs with urticaria. This latter type is frequently seen in persons with a history of allergic disorders.

The lesion usually consists of a rounded swelling, several centimeters in diameter. There is no pain or itching, and the principal sensation is distention. Areas involved include the face, hands, legs, tongue, genitalia, and feet. In the hereditary form, GI involvement is common and is manifested by abdominal pain and vomiting. Laryngeal edema is a possible cause of death. Drug therapy includes epinephrine, antihistamines, corticosteroids, and orally effective androgens.

USES

1. Treatment of endometriosis in those patients who cannot tolerate or who fail to respond to other means of therapy (not indicated in cases in which surgery is the treatment of choice)
2. Symptomatic treatment of severe fibrocystic breast disease
3. Prevention of attacks of hereditary angioedema (*e.g.*, cutaneous, laryngeal, abdominal)
4. Treatment of gynecomastia, infertility, and menorrhagia (investigational use only)

ADMINISTRATION AND DOSAGE

Danazol is used as 50-mg, 100-mg, or 200-mg capsules. Treatment with danazol should be initiated during menstruation or where pregnancy has been absolutely ruled out. Doses for the various indications are:

Endometriosis—200 mg to 400 mg twice a day uninterrupted for 3 months to 9 months; titrate dosage downward to a dose sufficient to maintain amenorrhea if possible; may reinstitute therapy if symptoms recur after terminating therapy.

Fibrocystic breast disease—100 mg to 400 mg/day in two divided doses for 3 months to 6 months. Breast pain is usually relieved within 2 months to 3 months, but resolution of nodules may require 4 months to 6 months of uninterrupted therapy. Amenorrhea or irregular menses may occur in up to one-third of patients. If symptoms recur after therapy is terminated, treatment may be reinstituted.

Hereditary angioedema—Initially, 200 mg two to three times a day; reduce dosage at

1-month to 3-month intervals if clinical response is favorable. If an attack occurs, dosage may be temporarily increased up to 200 mg/day.

SIDE-EFFECTS/ADVERSE REACTIONS

Common side-effects occurring with use of danazol include flushing, sweating, and vaginitis. Androgenic effects, such as edema, hirsutism, acne, oily skin, weight gain, voice deepening, decreased breast size, and clitoral hypertrophy, have also been noted during therapy with danazol. Other adverse effects are vaginal bleeding, nervousness, emotional lability, and hepatic dysfunction. A variety of adverse effects occurring in patients taking danazol for which a direct causal relationship has not been established are loss of hair, changes in libido, pelvic pain, muscle cramps, back, neck, or leg pain, skin rash, nasal congestion, nausea, vomiting, gastroenteritis, dizziness, headache, tremor, paresthesias, and visual disturbances.

CONTRAINDICATIONS AND PRECAUTIONS

Danazol is contraindicated in persons with undiagnosed abnormal vaginal bleeding, impaired cardiac, renal, or hepatic function, and in pregnant women or lactating mothers. Prior to initiating treatment for fibrocystic breast disease, carcinoma of the breast should be excluded. *Cautious use* of danazol is necessary in persons with migraine, epilepsy, cardiac disease, hypertension, and renal dysfunction because the drug can cause fluid retention. The androgenic effects of the drug may *not* be reversible following long-term use; patients must be closely observed for signs of virilization, and the dose must be reduced or the drug discontinued if possible.

INTERACTIONS

1. Danazol may result in prolongation of prothrombin time in patients stabilized on warfarin.
2. Therapy with danazol may increase insulin requirements and result in abnormal glucose tolerance tests.

NURSING CONSIDERATIONS

The main nursing goal is to help the patient to minimize and to tolerate some of the drug's side-effects long enough for it to be effective. Most of the androgenic effects listed under Side-Effects/Adverse Reactions are reversible once the drug is withdrawn, however, some may remain. The patient needs to be told of this possibility before therapy begins.

The patient treated with danazol who hopes to get pregnant after therapy may be concerned if amenorrhea and anovulation develop. Reassure her that these are reversible symptoms which will return within 60 days to 90 days after termination of therapy.

REVIEW QUESTIONS

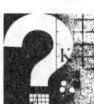

1. Briefly outline the actions of FSH and ICSH in the male.
2. List the various sources of androgens in the body.
3. Describe the physiologic effects of the androgens.
4. What are anabolic steroids?
5. Give several approved uses for androgens.
6. What are the common side-effects associated with use of androgens in (a) males and (b) females?
7. Under what circumstances is use of androgens contraindicated?
8. What are the principal damages associated with use of anabolic steroids?
9. Briefly describe the various clinically available preparations of testosterone. What are the principal differences among them?
10. What types of carcinomas are androgens most often used in treating?
11. What data must be collected before placing a patient on androgen therapy?
12. How can pain from intramuscular injection of androgens be minimized?

13. What side-effects of androgens should the adolescent watch for?
14. What are the symptoms of anabolic steroid abuse? Outline a strategy the nurse might use to help an athlete come to terms with his drug problem.
15. What is the mechanism of action of danazol?
16. List the principal indications for danazol.
17. Give the most frequently encountered adverse reactions with danazol.

BIBLIOGRAPHY

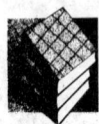

Barbieri RL, Ryan KJ: Danazol: Endocrine pharmacology and therapeutic applications. Am J Obstet Gynecol 141:453, 1981
Burger H, DeKretzer D (eds): The Testis. New York, Raven Press, 1981
Danazol and other androgens for hereditary angioedema. Med Lett Drugs Ther 23:83, 1981
Duncan DJ, Shaw EB: Anabolic steroids: Implications for the nurse practitioner. Nurse Pract 10(12):8, 1985
Griffin JE, Leshin M, Wilson JD: Androgen resistance syndromes. Am J Physiol 243:81, 1982
Lipsett MB: Physiology and pathology of the Leydig cell. N Engl J Med 303:682, 1980
Mandanes AE, Farber M: Danazol Ann Intern Med 96:625, 1982
Neumann F: Pharmacology and clinical use of antiandrogens. Ir J Med Sci 15:61, 1982
Pardridge WM, Gorski RA, Lippe BM, Green R: Androgens and sexual behavior. Ann Intern Med 96:488, 1982
Perlmutter G, Lowenthal DT: Use of anabolic steroids by athletes. Am Fam Physician 32:203, 1985
Ryan AJ: Anabolic steroids are fool's gold. Fed Proc 40:2682, 1982
Wilson JD, Griffin JE: The use and misuse of androgens. Metabolism 29:1278, 1980

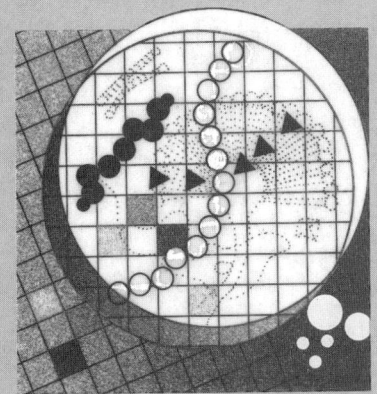

Anti-infective and
Antineoplastic Agents

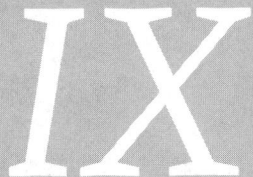

Anti-infective Therapy: General Considerations

59

Drugs used for the treatment of infectious diseases may be termed antibiotics, anti-infectives, antimicrobials, or chemotherapeutic agents. While these terms are often used interchangeably, antibiotics, anti-infectives, and antimicrobials are properly used to describe those drugs commonly employed for the treatment of infections. The designation chemotherapeutic agent has come to be more closely associated with those drugs used in the treatment of cancer.

Antibiotics are strictly defined as natural substances produced by various microorganisms and capable of inhibiting the growth of other microorganisms. Little distinction is made, however, between those substances having a natural origin and those with a synthetic origin. In fact, the term semisynthetic is often applied to the product of a chemical alteration of a naturally derived anti-infective compound.

Although the use of substances extracted from soil, plants, or living organisms to kill other organisms has been described for centuries, the modern age of antibacterial chemotherapy had its origin in the late 1930s and early 1940s with the introduction of sulfonamides and penicillins, respectively. Since that time a variety of antimicrobial agents that differ in spectrum of action, mechanism, and side-effects have become available, and the overall morbidity and mortality due to infectious diseases has steadily diminished. Nevertheless, the search for newer anti-infective drugs continues unabated, because some infectious diseases still have not been completely eradicated, while other previously unknown or unrecognized diseases are just beginning to appear. In addition, the treatment of some previously susceptible microorganisms by currently available antimicrobial drugs is becoming more difficult with the emergence of increasing numbers of resistant strains due to the previously widespread use of certain anti-infectives. While many different antibiotics are now available to the clinician, enabling treatment of a wide range of bacterial infections, no single agent yet represents the "ideal" antimicrobial drug in terms of spectrum of action, efficacy, safety, and cost.

Classification

There are several different characteristics that may be used to classify the currently available antimicrobial drugs. However, no single classification is sufficient to completely categorize a particular

drug; rather, complete description of any agent requires reference to a number of these characteristics. The most commonly used classifying characteristics are outlined below.

Spectrum of Activity

A broad classification of antibiotics divides them according to the range of their antimicrobial activity into broad spectrum and narrow spectrum. Broad-spectrum antibiotics exert their effects against a number of different types of bacteria and other microorganisms. Tetracyclines are, for example, active against a wide range of both gram-positive and gram-negative bacteria, as well as several other categories of microorganisms, such as *Rickettsia*, *Chlamydia*, and *Mycoplasma* species. Generally, if an agent is effective against both gram-positive and gram-negative organisms, it is referred to as broad spectrum, although some broad-spectrum antibiotics are active against a much wider range of organisms than others.

Antibacterial drugs that primarily affect only one group of microorganisms are termed narrow-spectrum antibiotics. For example, penicillin G affects only gram-positive bacteria and *Neisseria* at normal therapeutic doses and therefore is considered narrow spectrum. It is worth noting here, however, that spectrum of activity does not necessarily correlate with antimicrobial effectiveness. In fact, because of excessive use and subsequent emergence of resistant strains, many broad-spectrum antibiotics are much less active against many microorganisms than the more selective narrow-spectrum drugs.

Antimicrobial Activity

Antimicrobial agents may also be categorized on the basis of their antibacterial activity as either *bacteriostatic* or *bactericidal*. Bacteriostatic drugs (e.g., tetracyclines, sulfonamides) suppress the growth of microorganisms without actually killing existing microbes. The invading microorganisms are removed by the host defense mechanisms. Bactericidal drugs (such as penicillins), on the other hand, are capable of directly destroying organisms, especially those in an active state of replication. Theoretically, bactericidal drugs are more desirable from a therapeutic standpoint, but it is important to recognize that their lethal action on microorganisms is dependent on their being present in sufficient concentrations. In subtherapeutic doses, bactericidal drugs may be merely bacteriostatic, and conversely, at very high doses some bacteriostatic drugs may exert a bactericidal action. Nevertheless, even the most potent bactericidal drug is usually incapable of totally eliminating an infection without intervention of the patient's own natural defense mechanisms, such as antibody production, phagocytosis, and leukocyte proliferation. Impaired defense mechanisms can result from disease states (neoplasms, diabetes, hematologic disorders) or drugs (e.g., antineoplastics, corticosteroids) and can severely compromise the action of antimicrobial drugs.

Mechanism of Action

Antimicrobial agents exhibit several different mechanisms of action and may also be categorized on this basis. Most antibiotics exert their effects on microorganisms in one of five ways:

1. *Inhibition of bacterial cell wall synthesis* (e.g., penicillins, cephalosporins, bacitracin). Unlike animal cells, bacteria possess a rigid cell wall composed of macromolecules cross-linked by peptide chains. This arrangement serves to maintain the shape of the cell and to prevent cell rupture, because most bacteria, especially gram-positive microorganisms, have a high internal osmotic pressure. Thus, the viability of these bacterial cells depends on the integrity of the cell wall. Drugs acting by inhibiting cell wall synthesis do so by interfering with various steps in the assembly of the peptide chains that impart rigidity to the wall. The weakened cell wall can then no longer support the internal pressure, and the cells undergo lysis and disintegrate. Drugs acting in this manner are bactericidal.

2. *Alteration in cell membrane function* (e.g., amphotericin, nystatin, polymyxins). The semipermeable bacterial cell membrane (located between the cell wall and cytoplasm) helps control the internal environment of the cell by functioning as a selective barrier to penetration of cell constituents and nutrients. Disruption of this membrane by antibiotics alters its permeability, allowing escape of proteins, nucleotides, sugars, amino acids, and other cell constituents, resulting in damage to the cell and ultimately cellular death. Drugs acting in this manner may be either bacteriostatic or bactericidal depending on the drug, dose, and organism.

3. *Inhibition of protein synthesis* (e.g., aminoglycosides, erythromycin, tetracyclines). Certain antibiotics can interfere with ribosomal-mediated protein synthesis in bacterial cells without affecting protein synthesis in normal mammalian cells. It is believed that this occurs because the composition of the ribosomes in bacterial cells is different (i.e., bacteria have 70S ribosomes whereas mammalian cells have 80S ribosomes). Antibiotics may disrupt bacterial protein synthesis at several stages; for example, by binding to the ribosomes, blocking attachment of transfer RNA, causing a misreading of the genetic code, interfering with attachment of amino acids to the developing peptide chain, or tying up essential cofactors such as calcium, magnesium, or iron. Drugs inhibiting protein synthesis may be either bactericidal or bacteriostatic.

4. *Inhibition of nucleic acid metabolism* (e.g., nalidixic acid, rifampin, trimethoprim). Although most agents interfering with nucleic acid metabolism are used as antineoplastic drugs, a few antibacterial compounds act in this manner as well. Nalidixic acid inhibits DNA synthesis, rifampin interferes with DNA-dependent RNA synthesis, and trimethoprim can inhibit dihydrofolate reductase, an enzyme essential for production of tetrahydrofolic acid, an intermediate in the formation of DNA. These drugs are bacteriostatic.

5. *Interference with intermediate cell metabolism* (e.g., sulfonamides). All bacteria require dihydrofolic acid for production of nucleic acids; however, certain bacteria cannot assimilate preformed dihydrofolic acid but must synthesize it themselves from precursors within the cell. An essential precursor is para-aminobenzoic acid (PABA), and because sulfonamides are close structural analogues of PABA, they compete with it for active sites within bacterial cells, impairing synthesis of dihydrofolic acid and thus cell replication. Sulfonamides are bacteriostatic at normal dose levels.

Selection of Appropriate Drug

The aim of anti-infective drug therapy is to choose an agent that is most likely active against the offending pathogen and has the least potential to cause adverse reactions. Several important considerations go into the choice of a suitable antimicrobial drug for use in a particular patient. The most important of these factors are examined below:

1. *Necessity of therapy.* Even before a decision is made as to which antibiotic should be prescribed, the necessity for antibiotic therapy at all must be determined. Many infectious conditions do not require systemic antimicrobial therapy, and the clinician should make a careful assessment of the patient's status and the location and severity of the infection before undertaking antibiotic therapy. Unfortunately, overprescribing of antibiotics, especially in children with "colds" or "flu," occurs to a significant extent and is responsible for an undue number of untoward reactions as well as increased development of resistant strains of microorganisms. Likewise, indiscriminate medication of children by parents with "refillable" antibiotics has contributed to the reduced effectiveness of these drugs in many infectious conditions. While occupying a deservedly important place in pharmacotherapy, antibiotics are indeed frequently misused, usually to the detriment of the patient.

2. *Diagnosis of the pathogen.* Accurate determination of the infecting organism or organisms is the cornerstone of safe and effective antimicrobial therapy. Appropriate anti-infective therapy is best accomplished by bacteriologic culture of the infected material (sputum, pus, urine), subsequent isolation and identification of the pathogen, and selection of an antibiotic known to be effective against the offending organism. While it is always desirable to have the results of bacterial culturing before initiating antimicrobial treatment, this is not always practical or feasible. For example, in acute, life-threatening infections (such as septicemia, peritonitis, pneumonia), a delay in initiating treatment of 24 hours to 48 hours while awaiting results of culture testing can prove fatal and cannot be justified. In these situations, as well as others requiring administration of an antibiotic without bacteriologic identification, the initial choice of an antibiotic should be made on the basis of patient history, physical examination, clinical symptoms, and, most especially, an awareness on the part of the clinician as to what microorganisms are *likely to be present* based on the site of infection and the circumstances under which it developed. In some cases the probable organism can be determined by the attending physician by performing a simple Gram's stain on smears of exudate from the infected area. However, proper bacteriologic culturing is essential for accurate diagnosis of the infecting pathogen, and should be ordered as soon as possible. Once the microbiologic information has been obtained, definitive antimicrobial therapy can be initiated. The physician will either continue with the antibiotic prescribed initially if appropriate or switch to one that is more active or more selective against the bacterial species shown to be present.

3. *Sensitivity testing.* Because many common microorganisms exhibit varying degrees of antibacterial resistance, once a pathogen has been identified by bacteriologic culturing, the sensitivity of the infecting organism to different antimicrobial drugs is often determined. Sensitivity testing, however, is not always necessary, because some microorganisms are uniformly susceptible to certain antibiotics. For example, *Pneumococcus*, group A beta-hemolytic *Streptococcus*, *Clostridia*, and *Treponema pallidum* respond predictably to penicillin G. Conversely, *Staphylococcus aureus*, *Streptococcus viridans*, and several gram-negative bacilli (such as *Escherichia coli*, *Pseudomonas aeruginosa*, *Klebsiella pneumoniae*, *Salmonella*, *Shigella*, *Hemophilus influenzae*) exhibit varying degrees of resistance to different antibiotics and should be tested for susceptibility *in vitro*.

The most widely used procedure for sensitivity testing is the Kirby-Bauer or disk diffusion method, in which paper disks containing known amounts of various antibiotics are placed on an agar surface that has been swabbed with bacteria isolated from the patient. After an 18-hour incubation, the size of the clear zone of inhibition around each disk is a measure of the activity of each antibiotic to inhibit the growth of the particular microorganism. While useful as an index of microbial susceptibility to various antibiotics, the disk method of sensitivity testing measures only growth inhibition, and thus is an indication of bacteriostatic activity only. In addition, there are several false-positive reactions to cephalosporins with this method, including enterococci, *Shigella*, and methicillin-resistant *Staphylococcus*.

Where a bactericidal action is essential (as

for bacterial endocarditis), demonstration of sensitivity by the disk method is meaningless. In these situations, more reliable tube dilution sensitivity testing may be employed to determine both the minimum inhibitory concentration (*i.e.*, lowest concentration of drug that prevents visible growth after 24 hours) and the minimum bactericidal concentration (*i.e.*, lowest concentration that sterilizes the medium) of an antibiotic against a particular organism. There is frequently a discrepancy between *in vitro* results and clinical response, due to a number of factors such as *p*H, temperature, and the ability of the drug to reach the site of infection. Demonstration of *in vitro* bacterial susceptibility does not guarantee clinical success but merely provides another parameter on which to base selection of an antimicrobial agent.

4. *Location of the infection.* Generally, once the offending pathogen has been identified and its susceptibility ascertained, a selective choice of an antimicrobial agent can be made. However, consideration must also be given to the location of the infection when choosing an appropriate antibiotic. The distribution of an antibacterial drug in the body is an important determinant of its ultimate efficacy. Although the concentration of an antimicrobial agent in the body is usually defined in terms of blood or plasma levels, the *critical* concentration is that which is achieved in the infected tissues themselves. Plasma levels often do not accurately reflect tissue levels, and in spite of high plasma concentrations, some drugs may never attain sufficient tissue concentrations at the desired site of action. It is difficult to generalize about the distribution of antibiotics because the attainment of adequate infected tissue levels is dependent on a multitude of factors such as dose and route of administration, protein binding, lipid solubility, presence of tissue fluid or abscesses, *p*H, site of infection, and causative organism. For example, drugs used in meningitis must be able to readily penetrate the CNS (meninges), while drugs excreted largely unchanged in the urine are quite effective in urinary tract infections (provided they are active at a *p*H of 5 to 6) in spite of the fact that they may exhibit very low plasma levels.

There are, of course, other factors that can influence the choice of an antibiotic; these include severity of the infection, a previous hypersensitivity or serious adverse reaction to a particular drug, patient acceptance of parenteral administration, and cost of the drug. While proper selection of antimicrobial agents can result in quick eradication of most infections with minimal adverse effects or complications, injudicious use of antibiotics may ultimately prove harmful to the patient. The decision to initiate antibacterial therapy must be based on careful assessment of the patient and the choice of drugs must be determined by accurate bacteriologic and sensitivity testing whenever possible. Antibiotic therapy in the absence of proper culturing should be undertaken only with those drugs most likely to be effective against the suspected pathogen, and should be modified if necessary as soon as the culture and sensitivity test results are known. Further, adequate dosage and duration of therapy are essential to ensure complete drug efficacy. These factors are considered next.

Dosage and Duration of Therapy

Anti-infective drug dosage should always be high enough and duration of treatment long enough to provide effective drug concentrations in infected tissues in order to render the culture from the infected site sterile. As indicated earlier, blood levels of the antibiotic do not always reflect tissue concentrations at the infection site; nonetheless, they are frequently used as a guide to determine if proper dosage is being administered. Despite the importance of maintaining treatment long enough to completely eradicate the microorganism, antibiotics are sometimes discontinued too early. The result of this may be either reinfection with the same organism or emergence of mutant strains resistant to the drug being used.

Although different infections require variable treatment durations, oral antimicrobial therapy of most common respiratory and urinary infections should be continued for a minimum of 7 days to 10 days. Patients may decide to discontinue antimicrobial drugs as soon as the overt symptoms (*e.g.*, fever, sore throat, painful urination) of their disease subside. For this reason, they should be carefully instructed to continue the drugs for at least 48 hours to 72 hours after symptoms disappear to ensure that the pathogen is completely eliminated. Follow-up cultures are also desirable to confirm the effectiveness of therapy.

More severe infections, such as endocarditis and staphylococcal pneumonia, generally require parenteral administration of higher doses of antibiotics and for longer periods than the more common infections, which can be treated orally. Large doses of antimicrobial drugs may also be necessary in debilitated patients or in patients with disease- or drug-impaired defense mechanisms.

Adjunctive Treatment of Infections

In infections characterized by the presence of purulent exudates or large abscesses, drainage of these areas is often necessary; antibiotics frequently are unable to penetrate these infected lesions sufficiently to eradicate the large quantity of pathogens at these sites. Similarly, patients with urinary infections associated with the presence of renal stones will continue to suffer recurrent infections despite the use of antibiotics unless the stones are removed. It is important to recognize that no antibiotic alone can be expected to completely control every infection, and appropriate adjunctive measures are frequently necessary to treat certain types of infections.

Antipyretic drugs (*e.g.*, aspirin, acetaminophen) may be useful in keeping body temperature below dangerous levels and making patients with infections more comfortable. These drugs should be given on a regular basis during the febrile period (*i.e.*, every 4 hours), and their usage will seldom "mask" the presence of an infection.

Other supportive measures that may be undertaken to facilitate recovery from severe infections include correction of electrolyte or acid–base disturbances, support of respiration, and maintenance of an adequate nutritional status.

Prophylactic Use of Antibiotics

The use of antimicrobial drugs to prevent rather than treat infections is a very controversial area of chemotherapy. While doubtless effective in certain situations, anti-infective prophylaxis is without proven value in many conditions and may, in fact, be detrimental in certain instances. There is general agreement that successful chemoprophylaxis is most often attained when a single drug known to be effective against a specific pathogen is used to prevent invasion of that pathogen before it has a chance to become established. Some generally ac-

cepted indications for antimicrobial prophylaxis are as follows:

1. Penicillin G—for prophylaxis of Group A streptococcal infection in patients with rheumatic heart disease, recurrent cellulitis in lymphedema, and subacute bacterial endocarditis
2. Rifampin or minocycline—prophylaxis of meningococcal meningitis
3. Isoniazid—prophylaxis of tuberculosis
4. Doxycycline—prevention of "traveler's diarrhea"
5. Chloroquine—prevention of malaria
6. Amantadine—prevention of influenza A
7. Trimethoprim + sulfamethoxazole—prophylaxis of recurrent urinary tract infections and *Pneumocystis carinii* pneumonia

In addition, there is evidence that prophylactic use of first generation cephalosporins such as cefazolin during certain abdominal, cardiac, and gynecologic surgical procedures in which the incidence of wound infection is high can prevent development of secondary infections and reduce morbidity. Treatment should be initiated not more than 6 hours prior to surgery and continued for not more than 12 hours to 24 hours following surgery. Prophylactic antimicrobial usage has also been advocated for reducing postoperative infections following surgery for head or neck cancer.

On the other hand, conclusive evidence is lacking concerning the effectiveness of antibiotics used prophylactically in patients with chronic obstructive pulmonary disease, in patients undergoing urologic, dental, or neurologic surgical procedures, and in patients with acute pancreatitis. Finally, chemoprophylaxis is considered to be ineffective in preventing (1) secondary bacterial infection in "common colds," influenza, or other viral diseases; (2) urinary infections in the presence of stones, obstruction, or indwelling urinary catheters; (3) recurring herpes simplex ulcers of the mouth; (4) secondary infections in burn patients; and (5) infections associated with prolonged use of corticosteroids, immunosuppressants, or antineoplastic drugs.

A major danger of chemoprophylaxis is the development of superinfections with drug-resistant strains, the incidence of which is closely related to the duration of exposure to the antibiotic. Therefore, short-term prophylaxis is preferred whenever possible; there is no conclusive evidence to indicate the incidence of wound infections is lower if anti-infectives are given beyond the day of surgery. Conversely, antibiotic-resistant strains are much more likely to develop if the drugs are given for longer than 24 hours.

Situations necessitating prolonged use of prophylactic antibiotics, such as rheumatic fever, endocarditis, or chronic bronchitis, must be continually monitored and patients must be closely observed for signs of a developing superinfection (diarrhea, glossitis, perianal or vaginal itching).

Other disadvantages to antimicrobial chemoprophylaxis include an increased incidence of allergic reactions and diarrhea, and frequently a substantially higher cost to the patient.

Combined Antimicrobial Therapy

Although most infections can be adequately treated with a single anti-infective agent, simultaneous administration of two or more antimicrobial agents is justifiable under certain circumstances. When combination antimicrobial therapy is indicated, it should be accomplished by administration of two or more individual drugs whose doses can be titrated independently to provide an optimal effect. The once widespread use of "fixed-dose" antibiotic combinations has essentially been eliminated by the removal of most of these combinations from the market, on the grounds that many contained subtherapeutic amounts of antibiotic drugs, were often ineffective, and favored emergence of resistant bacterial populations.

Use of two or more antibacterial drugs concurrently increases the risk of drug interactions, which may either be beneficial or harmful to the patient. An awareness of potential drug interaction problems among the different anti-infective drugs can minimize the likelihood of an adverse drug interaction and increase the beneficial effects of the selected drug combination. A general discussion of drug interactions is presented in Chapter 5, and specific interaction problems with each class of anti-infective drugs are addressed in the respective chapters which follow.

The primary indications for combination anti-infective therapy are the following:

1. *Treatment of mixed bacterial infections.* Some infections (*e.g.*, intra-abdominal, urinary, genital, inner ear) may be complicated by the presence of two, or possibly more, microorganisms possessing different antimicrobial susceptibility. Although broad-spectrum antibiotics are occasionally successful when used alone in such infections, combination therapy is frequently necessary to ensure complete eradication of all pathogens present in mixed infections. Sensitivity testing is essential in such cases.

2. *Initial treatment of severe infections where the causative agent is unknown.* Before the results of bacteriologic culturing in an unknown infection are obtained, combination therapy is often undertaken to ensure that the widest range of possible organisms is covered. Such treatment, of course, should be modified if necessary as soon as culture and sensitivity data are available; prolonged use of several broad-spectrum anti-infective drugs is not only expensive, but may result in serious toxicity as well.

3. *Postponement of the emergence of resistant strains.* Development of resistance to antibiotic agents is often delayed (but not necessarily prevented) when a sensitive pathogen is exposed to two drugs simultaneously. This is particularly apparent with the combined use of two or more antitubercular drugs (*e.g.*, isoniazid, rifampin) or combinations of carbenicillin and gentamicin or tobramycin for severe pseudomonal infections.

4. *Enhancement of antibacterial activity.* Increased antibacterial activity is frequently observed with simultaneous use of two antibiotics, compared to that observed with each drug alone. This synergistic effect is noted, for example, with an extended spectrum penicillin and an aminoglycoside for pseudomonal infections, with isoniazid and ethambutol in treating tuberculosis, with tetracycline and streptomycin in treating brucellosis or glanders, and with amphotericin B and flucytosine in treating certain systemic fungal infections.

A relatively new combination is the use of a penicillin such as ampicillin or ticarcillin with clavulanic acid, an inhibitor of beta-lactamase enzyme (see below under Resistance). Clavulanic acid prevents the destruction of the penicillin by the beta-lactamase enzymes secreted by certain microorganisms (*e.g.*, staphylococci, *H. influenzae*), thus allowing successful eradication of the microbe by the penicillin drug. Preventing enzymatic destruction can expand the usefulness of certain antibiotics previously ineffective against beta-lactamase-producing organisms.

5. *Reduction of toxicity.* In certain instances, combined use of anti-infective drugs may

allow a reduced dosage of one or both drugs, with a possible corresponding reduction in toxicity. On the other hand, the addition of a second drug to the regimen, especially at full dosage, can *increase* the likelihood of adverse effects compared to that seen with a single drug. Again, a knowledge of the potential toxicities of the various anti-infective drugs is essential in order to maximize the therapeutic effects while minimizing the potential for untoward reactions.

As indicated, combination anti-infective drug therapy can result in undesirable effects, reduced clinical effectiveness, and superinfections. For example, combined use of two or more aminoglycosides can increase the incidence of ototoxicity and nephrotoxicity above that observed with each drug alone. Therefore, other than those circumstances outlined above in which combination antimicrobial therapy has proven beneficial, use of more than one carefully selected anti-infective drug to treat a particular infectious condition should be avoided.

Adverse Effects of Antimicrobial Drugs

A wide range of adverse reactions have been reported with the various classes of drugs used in the treatment of infections, and these are reviewed in detail in the individual chapters dealing with each group of drugs. The most frequently encountered untoward reactions with antibiotics are considered briefly at this time.

1. *Hypersensitivity reactions.* Both acute and delayed allergic responses have occurred with a number of antimicrobial drugs, most frequently with the penicillins and sulfonamides. These may range from mild dermatologic manifestations, such as skin rash, itching, and urticaria, to severe anaphylactic reactions, which have proved fatal in a number of instances. The importance of obtaining a careful patient history before administration of an antimicrobial agent known to be associated with hypersensitivity reactions cannot be overemphasized.
2. *Organ toxicity.* Various classes of antibiotics are known to exert selective toxic effects on certain structures or organs of the body. For example, aminoglycosides and vancomycin cause both renal and eighth cranial nerve damage. Amphotericin B and polymyxins, among others, impair kidney function while lincomy-

cin and clindamycin often induce severe diarrhea and colitis. Tetracyclines may damage teeth, nails, or bones, and rifampin and the estolate salt of erythromycin can be hepatotoxic.
3. *Superinfection.* Development of secondary infections is a potentially serious problem connected with antibiotic usage. It occurs most often as a result of prolonged anti-infective therapy, insufficient drug dosage, impaired host defense mechanisms, concurrent therapy with immunosuppressive drugs, or a combination of these factors. Pathogens frequently responsible for secondary infections include *Pseudomonas*, *Proteus*, *Candida*, and drug-resistant staphylococci and fungi. These organisms may be especially difficult to eradicate because they often represent strains resistant to conventional antimicrobial agents. Although superinfection can theoretically occur anywhere in the body, it is found most commonly in the GI tract and may be manifested by diarrhea, glossitis, stomatitis, "furry" tongue, and perineal irritation. Prompt recognition of a secondary infection is critical to its effective management. Therapy is best accomplished by discontinuing the initial antibiotic, culturing the infected area, and administering an antimicrobial drug shown by sensitivity testing to be effective against the new organism.
4. *Resistance.* Bacteria are susceptible to elimination by some anti-infective drugs but not others. The phenomenon whereby certain organisms are unaffected by a particular antimicrobial agent is called resistance. Bacterial resistance may be broadly categorized into either *natural* or *acquired* resistance. *Natural* resistance is genetically determined and may be characteristic of either an entire species or only certain strains within a species. It is not a significant therapeutic problem, inasmuch as the resistance is usually to a particular mechanism of antimicrobial action, and there are other antibiotics with different mechanisms of action to which the organism will be susceptible. *Acquired* resistance, on the other hand, can develop in previously susceptible pathogens for a number of reasons and is a major clinical problem with many anti-infective drugs. Development of bacterial resistance has severely limited the usefulness of many antibiotics in certain infections.

Unfortunately, the more an antimicrobial agent is employed in clinical practice, the greater the likelihood that resistant strains of once susceptible bacteria will develop. This further underscores the importance of sensitivity testing whenever there is doubt as to the susceptibility of an infecting microorganism to a chosen antibiotic. Complicating the picture is the problem of cross-resistance, that is, not only the resistance of a certain bacteria to all members of a particular antibiotic group (e.g., penicillins, tetracyclines, sulfonamides) but resistance to other chemically related drugs (e.g., penicillins and cephalosporins) or in some cases chemically unrelated drugs (e.g., erythromycin and lincomycin).

Microbial resistance has presented a serious dilemma in many hospitals where a variety of anti-infective agents must be used to control the many types of infections frequently encountered in this setting. As a result, secondary infections occur to a significant extent, and these are often caused, as indicated above, by strains or mutants of pathogens resistant to conventional therapy. Control of many of these hospital-acquired infections is therefore often difficult.

Microorganisms can develop resistance to anti-infective drugs in a number of ways, the most important of which are listed below:

· Elaboration of enzymes (e.g., beta-lactamases such as penicillinases or cephalosporins) that destroy the drug
· Decreased permeability of the microbial cell membrane to certain antibiotics (e.g., tetracyclines, aminoglycosides, chloramphenicol) that depend on penetration into the bacteria for their effectiveness
· Development of altered binding sites (e.g., loss of specific ribosomal proteins) within the bacterial cell for certain antibiotic drugs (e.g., aminoglycosides, erythromycins) that normally interrupt ribosomal function by chemically binding to ribosomal proteins
· Development of altered enzymatic or metabolic pathways that either entirely bypass the reaction inhibited by the antimicrobial drug or that become less susceptible to interruption by antibiotic drugs such as sulfonamides
· Production by bacteria of a direct antibiotic drug antagonist (e.g., PABA vs sulfonamides)

In many cases, the emergence of resistant bacterial strains has necessitated the use of less effective and more toxic antimicrobial agents to treat an infection formerly controlled by a more desirable drug. Moreover, the increasing

numbers of anti-infective drugs proving ineffective against certain infectious organisms (e.g., staphylococci, gram-negative bacilli) have raised the specter of some diseases eventually becoming largely uncontrollable by the currently available antibiotic drugs. To minimize this possibility, it is essential that antimicrobial drugs be used sensibly and that only those drugs necessary to eliminate the organisms known to be present should be prescribed.

Antibiotics in Renal Failure

Kidney function is a major determinant of the response to many antimicrobial drugs. Drugs eliminated principally by the kidney are potentially more hazardous when employed in the patient with renal impairment because serum levels are more elevated for longer periods of time due to the slowed elimination. Therefore, clinicians should be aware of the mode of excretion of any anti-infective agent they administer. Further, renal function should be determined not only before administration of an anti-infective agent that is cleared by the kidney, but throughout the course of therapy as well, particularly if the course of treatment is prolonged. Antibiotics eliminated largely by the kidneys include the penicillins, cephalosporins, aminoglycosides, polymyxins, vancomycin, trimethoprim-sulfamethoxazole, and most tetracyclines. The penicillins and cephalosporins are relatively nontoxic even at high plasma levels and therefore can be used safely in the presence of limited renal dysfunction. The tetracyclines are cleared by the kidney at varying rates, and those derivatives with extended half-lives (except doxycycline) should not be used when renal function is impaired. The aminoglycosides, polymyxins, and vancomycin will accumulate rapidly when kidney function is reduced; thus, the dosage or frequency of administration of these drugs must be reduced in the patient with renal impairment. Moreover, these latter drugs are themselves nephrotoxic, and thus can elicit or aggravate renal failure, further reducing their own excretion. It is unfortunate that patients with renal failure are often subject to precisely those infections (e.g., gram-negative bacilli) that are usually most responsive to nephrotoxic antibacterial drugs such as aminoglycosides, thus setting up a potentially vicious cycle. Nevertheless, there are a number of effective antimicrobial agents that may be employed with reasonable safety in patients with kidney impairment provided that the appropriate dosage adjustments are undertaken. The excretion patterns and related cautions to be observed with the use of each class of antibiotic drug are noted in the individual drug monographs in succeeding chapters.

Drugs of Choice for Various Infections

The selection of an individual antimicrobial agent as a drug of choice for a particular infection is sometimes subject to debate, and opinions often change as new drugs become available or resistant strains of previously susceptible organisms emerge. Nevertheless, some agreement does exist on the first-line drugs for a number of common infections, providing sensitivity tests have confirmed pathogen susceptibility. While by no means definitive, Table 59-1 outlines recommended drugs of choice as well as alternative drugs for the treatment of infections resulting from a number of microorganisms, and also lists the type of organism and the most common illnesses associated with it. The recommendations made in Table 59-1 represent a distillate of several sources and are presented only as a guide to aid the clinician in choosing an appropriate antibiotic. They are not intended as a substitute for careful sensitivity testing, and the drug ultimately used to treat a specific infectious state should be chosen on the basis of as much laboratory and clinical data as can be obtained.

■ Nursing Process

While the drugs used in anti-infective therapy are very diverse, nursing considerations common to all of them are outlined below. The reader is referred to specific drug chapters for more detailed information.

□ ASSESSMENT

□ Subjective Data
The nurse needs to obtain a detailed medication history to ensure safe antibiotic therapy. Most antibiotics interact with many other drugs, sometimes resulting in severe or fatal consequences. Adverse effects can range from a reduction or inhibition of expected drug action to electrolyte or coagulation abnormalities, changes in glucose metabolism or

nephrotoxicity. Be aware of the drugs listed under Interactions in each of the following chapters and plan the questions about medications with those drugs in mind. The nurse should also ask about previous treatment with antibiotics and a history of allergic response to any drugs. Any drug allergies should be highlighted on the patient's chart.

Ask the patient why he sought treatment and what symptoms he now has. Try to find out what his expectation is of the prescribed antibiotic. Such information will help the nurse determine what information the patient has and how realistic his view is on therapy and may give clues about whether he will complete the proposed regimen.

Systemic history should focus on the presence of any liver, kidney, or gastrointestinal disorders because many antibiotics tax these systems. The patient with a positive history needs careful screening before a drug is prescribed. The pregnant woman and nursing mother should also be identified because many antibiotics are toxic to the fetus and young infant.

□ Objective Data
The nurse should locate and examine the site of infection if possible and try to obtain a direct culture before therapy begins unless circumstances are life-threatening. Other data should be collected including temperature, a description of the infectious site (i.e., appearance of a wound, lung sounds of a patient with pneumonia) including the presence of pain, warmth, sensation, and pulses above and below the site. A flow sheet may be useful to record such information and to provide a guideline for future assessments throughout care.

Laboratory studies will vary with the drug prescribed. A complete blood count should include a white cell count which will probably be elevated and red blood cell count because thrombocytopenia is a side-effect of long-term antibiotic therapy. Liver and renal function studies should be done whenever a major infection is suspected, when the patient is elderly, or when a young child has been unresponsive to therapy for a common problem such as otitis media.

□ NURSING DIAGNOSES
For most patients receiving antibiotics the first *actual* nursing diagnosis will be:

Knowledge deficit regarding the actions of the drug, how to take it safely, and what side-effects to watch for

Other nursing diagnoses will be determined by the responses the patient has to the specific drug and any side-effects that develop.

□ *PLAN*

Nursing care goals focus on:
1. Correct, safe administration in the acute care setting
2. Monitoring for side-effects
3. Teaching the patient
   a. How to take the drug safely and correctly at home
   b. How to manage intravenous therapy techniques at home when necessary
   c. What foods to avoid while on medication
   d. Common side-effects, how to manage them, and what drug effects to report immediately

□ *INTERVENTION*

Antibiotics may be administered by a variety of routes; intravenous, oral, oral liquid, and intramuscular are the most common. In acute care, the nurse will administer these drugs most frequently by the intravenous route and, consequently, needs to follow certain guidelines to ensure safe administration.

Antibiotics are irritating to veins, so sites should be carefully monitored and rotated frequently; lines should be removed at the first sign of pain or swelling. Therapeutic plasma levels and cell action are rapidly achieved when intravenous antibiotics are administered; therefore, anaphylactic or allergic reactions and serious side-effects can also occur quickly. This is especially true in the pediatric and geriatric patient.

With the advent of the intravenous heparin lock, subcutaneous venous access ports, and use of central lines such as the Hickman, Broviac, or Groshong catheter, a patient may not need to have a continuous intravenous infusion in order to receive IV antibiotics. In fact, he may be discharged on antibiotic therapy using a protocol whereby he is carefully supervised, returns to the health-care facility every other day, and is taught how to self-administer the drug at home according to specific guidelines. The infusion may be given by a small bag of medication or by a syringe infusion pump (see Chap. 8 for more information). The nurse working with such a patient must determine the patient's ability and willingness to learn such an exact regimen and help the patient plan home man-

agement and resumption of life activities while on the drug. The nurse must also be comfortable with the use of different types of infusion lines and must know the various supply companies and support services available to this patient. The teaching plan for such a patient is complex and usually must be completed in a short period of time. Consequently, the patient must have ready access to the discharging health-care facility or receive coordinated care from the home-care program.

Intramuscular injection of antibiotics occurs less frequently now than in the past because of the availability of multiple intravenous access devices. However, a patient may occasionally receive single or multiple injections of antibiotics. Most antibiotics are irritating to tissue and may cause abscess formation and tissue damage. If multiple injections are ordered, administration using a body map rotation tool (such as the one shown in Chap. 8) will decrease risk of the pain, swelling, and tissue necrosis at the injection site.

Oral administration of antibiotics is the other common route. While taking a pill may seem simple, the nurse needs to focus attention on spacing medications throughout the day and what to do if a dose is missed. A patient may not understand the need to waken through the night in order to space doses evenly. With many antibiotics, exact time spacing is not essential; a close approximation will suffice. Therefore, if a drug is ordered every 6 hours, the patient will probably derive therapeutic benefit from the drug is he takes the medicine at 7 AM, 1 PM, 6 PM, and 12 midnight. If a dose is missed and the patient remembers several hours later, he should take it then. If he forgets until the next dose, he should continue taking the regular dose rather than doubling the dose which may increase irritating side-effects. He needs to be taught to complete the prescription, adding missed doses at the end by extending the number of days of therapy if necessary.

Liquid administration of antibiotics, frequently used for children, may produce special problems. Many of the liquids have an unpleasant aftertaste which the child will dislike. Young children, especially those under age 4, will have little understanding of the benefit of such drugs and may refuse to take them. The nurse who spends time with the parents of such a child teaching about restraint techniques, various administration devices, how to gain the child's trust, and how to correctly measure the dose will do a lot to improve compliance with the regimen and completion of the pre-

(Text continues on p. 1146.)

Table 59-1
Antimicrobial Drugs of Choice for Common Infections

Organism	Classification	Representative Clinical Illnesses	Drugs of First Choice	Alternate Drugs
Acinetobacter (Mima, Herellea) species	Gram (−) bacilli	Bacteremia, endocarditis, meningitis, urethritis	gentamicin, tobramycin	amikacin, imipenem, netilmicin, doxycycline, minocycline, carbenicillin, ticarcillin, mezlocillin, piperacillin, azlocillin, ceftizoxime, ceftriaxone, ceftazidime
Actinomyces israelli	Actinomycetes	Actinomycosis	penicillin G	tetracycline, erythromycin, cephalosporin
Alcaligenes faecalis	Gram (−) bacilli	Urinary infections, wound infections	chloramphenicol, tetracycline	colistimethate, polymyxin B, gentamicin, kanamycin
Aspergillus	Fungi	Systemic fungal infections, (*e.g.*, skin, lung, bone)	amphotericin B	flucytosine
Bacillus anthracis	Gram (+) bacilli	Anthrax, pneumonia, meningitis	penicillin G	erythromycin, tetracycline, cephalosporins (first generation), chloramphenicol
Bacteroides (various strains)	Gram (−) bacilli	Bacteremia, brain and lung abscesses, genital infections, pulmonary infections, endocarditis	penicillin G (oropharyngeal strains) clindamycin, metronidazole, (GI strains, endocarditis)	tetracycline, piperacillin, mezlocillin, azlocillin, chloramphenicol, cefoxitin, third generation cephalosporins, imipenem, erythromycin
Blastomyces dermatitidis	Fungi	Blastomycosis	amphotericin B	hydroxystilbamidine, ketoconazole
Bordetella pertussis	Gram (−) bacilli	Whooping cough	erythromycin	Ampicillin, tetracycline, trimethoprim-sulfamethoxazole
Borrelia recurrentis	Spirochetes	Relapsing fever	tetracycline	penicillin G
Branhamella catarrhalis	Gram (−) bacilli	Respiratory infections, sinusitus, otitis media	amoxicillin-clavulanic acid	cefuroxime
Brucella	Gram (−) bacilli	Brucellosis	tetracycline with or without streptomycin	chloramphenicol (with or without streptomycin), trimethoprim-sulfamethoxazole
Calymmato-bacterium granulomatis	Gram (−) bacilli	Granuloma inguinale	tetracycline	streptomycin, ampicillin
Candida (various species)	Fungi	Local and systemic fungal infections	Systemic—amphotericin B (with or without flucytosine)	Systemic—flucytosine *alone*

(continued)

Table 59-1 (continued)
Antimicrobial Drugs of Choice for Common Infections

Organism	Classification	Representative Clinical Illnesses	Drugs of First Choice	Alternate Drugs
Candida (various species) *(continued)*			Gastrointestinal—oral nystatin Local—miconazole, clotrimazole, nystatin	
Chlamydia psittaci	Chlamydiae	Psittacosis, ornithosis	tetracycline	chloramphenicol
Chlamydia trachomatis	Chlamydiae	Inclusion conjunctivitis	erythromycin	tetracycline, sulfonamide
		Pneumonia	erythromycin	sulfonamide
		Trachoma	tetracycline	sulfonamide
		Urethritis	tetracycline	erythromycin
		Lymphogranuloma venereum	tetracycline	erythromycin, sulfonamide
Clostridium difficile	Gram (+) bacilli	Pseudomembranous colitis (antibiotic associated)	vancomycin	metronidazole
Clostridium perfringens	Gram (+) bacilli	Gas gangrene	penicillin G	chloramphenicol, cephalosporins, clindamycin, tetracycline, metronidazole
Clostridium tetani	Gram (+) bacilli	Tetanus	penicillin G	tetracycline, cephalosporins, erythromycin
Coccidioides immitis	Fungi	Systemic fungal infections	amphotericin B	miconazole, ketoconazole
Corynebacterium diphtheriae	Gram (+) bacilli	Laryngitis, pharyngitis, pneumonia, tracheitis	erythromycin, penicillin G	cephalosporin (first generation), rifampin
Cryptococcus neoformans	Fungi	Systemic fungal infections	amphotericin B, (with or without flucytosine)	ketoconazole, miconazole
Dermatophytes (tinea)	Fungi	Infections of the skin, hair, and nails	clotrimazole, miconazole	Oral—griseofulvin Topical—tolnaftate, haloprogin
Enterobacteriaceae (*Aerobacter aerogenes*)	Gram (−) bacilli	Urinary infections, bacteremia, wound infections	gentamicin, tobramycin, mezlocillin, piperacillin, azlocillin, third generation cephalosporins	amikacin, aztreonam, netilmicin, imipenem, carbenicillin, ciprofloxacin, ticarcillin, amdinocillin, tetracycline, cefonicid
Escherichia coli	Gram (−) bacilli	Urinary infections, bacteremia, meningitis, gastroenteritis	gentamicin, tobramycin, mezlocillin, piperacillin, azlocillin, cephalosporin (third generation)	ampicillin, aztreonam, carbenicillin, amdinocillin, norfloxacin, ticarcillin, netilmicin, amikacin, kanamycin, imipenem, trimethoprim-sulfamethozazole, ciprofloxacin

(continued)

Table 59-1 (continued)
Antimicrobial Drugs of Choice for Common Infections

Organism	Classification	Representative Clinical Illnesses	Drugs of First Choice	Alternate Drugs
Francisella tularensis	Gram (−) bacilli	Tularemia	streptomycin	tetracycline, chloramphenicol
Hemophilus ducreyi	Gram (−) bacilli	Chancroid	trimethoprim-sulfamethoxazole	tetracycline, erythromycin, streptomycin, cephalothin
Hemophilus influenzae	Gram (−) bacilli	Pharyngitis, pneumonia, meningitis, otitis media, tracheobronchitis, epiglottiditis	Life-threatening—chloramphenicol plus ampicillin Other infections—ampicillin, amoxicillin	aztreonam, moxalactam, trimethoprim-sulfamethoxazole, imipenem tetracycline, sulfonamide, cefonicid, cefaclor, third generation cephalosporins, trimethoprim-sulfamethoxazole, ciprofloxacin
Hemophilus vaginalis	Gram (−) bacilli	Vaginal infections	metronidazole	
Herpes simplex	Virus	Keratitis Encephalitis	Topical—acyclovir, trifluridine vidarabine	Topical—idoxuridine, vidarabine acyclovir
Histoplasma capsulatum	Fungi	Pneumonia, meningitis, skin, lung, and bone lesions	amphotericin B	ketoconazole
Influenza A	Virus	Influenza	amantadine (prophylaxis)	
Klebsiella pneumoniae	Gram (−) bacilli	Pneumonia, urinary and biliary infections, osteomyelitis	gentamicin, tobramycin, cephalosporin	aztreonam, imipenem, mezlocillin, piperacillin, azlocillin, amikacin, netilmicin, tetracycline, amdinocillin, trimethoprim-sulfamethoxazole, chloramphenicol, ciprofloxacin
Legionella pneumophila	Gram (−) bacilli	Legionnaires' disease	erythromycin (with or without rifampin)	tetracycline
Leptospira	Spirochetes	Meningitis, Weil's disease	penicillin G	tetracycline
Leptotrichia buccalis	Gram (−) bacilli	Vincent's infection	penicillin G	tetracycline, erythromycin
Listeria monocytogenes	Gram (+) bacilli	Bacteremia, meningitis, endocarditis, recurrent abortion	ampicillin or penicillin G (with or without gentamicin or streptomycin)	tetracycline, erythromycin, chloramphenicol
Mucor	Fungi	Systemic fungal infections	amphotericin B	
Mycobacterium (atypical)	Acid-fast bacilli	Lymphadenitis, pulmonary lesions	isoniazid with rifampin (with or without ethambutol)	erthromycin, cycloserine, ethionamide
Mycobacterium leprae	Acid-fast bacilli	Leprosy	dapsone with rifampin	ethionamide

(continued)

Table 59-1 (continued)
Antimicrobial Drugs of Choice for Common Infections

Organism	Classification	Representative Clinical Illnesses	Drugs of First Choice	Alternate Drugs
Mycobacterium tuberculosis	Acid-fast bacilli	Pulmonary, renal, meningeal, or other tuberculosis infections	isoniazid with rifampin	streptomycin, pyrazinamide, ethambutol, cycloserine, ethionamide, kanamycin
Mycoplasma hominis	Mycoplasmas	Nonspecific urethritis, septicemia	clindamycin, tetracycline	erthromycin, chloramphenicol, gentamicin
Mycoplasma pneumoniae	Mycoplasmas	Atypical viral pneumonia	erythromycin, tetracycline	
Neisseria gonorrhoeae	Gram (−) cocci	Gonorrhea, meningitis, urethritis, vaginitis, endocarditis, arthritis	penicillin G, amoxicillin, tetracycline, spectinomycin	ampicillin, cefotaxime, cefoxitin, trimethoprim-sulfamethoxazole
Neisseria meningitidis	Gram (−) cocci	Meningitis, bacteremia	penicillin G, rifampin (carrier state)	chloramphenicol, moxalactam, cefotaxime
Nocardia	Actinomycetes	Pulmonary lesions, brain abscess	trisulfapyrimidines (with or without minocycline or ampicillin)	trimethoprim-sulfamethoxazole, cycloserine, ampicillin plus erythomycin
Pasteurella multocida	Gram (−) bacilli	Bacteremia, meningitis	penicillin G	tetracycline, cephalosporin
Pneumocystis carinii	Protozoan	Pneumonia in immunologically compromised patients	trimethoprim-sulfamethoxazole	pentamidine
Proteus mirabilis	Gram (−) bacilli	Urinary and other infections	ampicillin, gentamicin, tobramycin	aztreonam, carbenicillin, ticarcillin, amikacin, mezlocillin, azlocillin, piperacillin, norfloxacin, ciprofloxacin, cephalosporin
Proteus (other species)	Gram (−) bacilli	Urinary and other infections	gentamicin, tobramycin, amikacin, third generation cephalosporins	carbenicillin, ticarcillin, mezlocillin, azlocillin, piperacillin, norfloxacin, ciprofloxacin, tetracycline, imipenem, chloramphenicol, cefonicid, cefoxitin
Providencia (*Proteus inconstans*)	Gram (−) bacilli	Urinary and other infections	amikacin, third generation cephalosporins	gentamicin, tobramycin, carbenicillin, ticarcillin, mezlocillin, azlocillin, chloramphenicol, cefonicid
Pseudomonas aeruginosa	Gram (−) bacilli	Urinary and other infections (*e.g.*, respiratory, skin)	Antipseudomonal penicillins (*e.g.*, mezlocillin, azlocillin, piperacillin) with an aminoglycoside (such as gen-	Aminoglycoside (*e.g.*, amikacin, gentamicin, tobramycin, netilmicin) with a third generation cephalosporin (*e.g.*, (continued)

Table 59-1 (continued)
Antimicrobial Drugs of Choice for Common Infections

Organism	Classification	Representative Clinical Illnesses	Drugs of First Choice	Alternate Drugs
Pseudomonas aeruginosa (continued)			tamicin, amikacin, or tobramycin)	cefoperazone, cefotaxime, ceftizoxime, moxalactam), aztreonam, norfloxacin, ciprofloxacin, imipenem
Pseudomonas mallei	Gram (−) bacilli	Glanders	streptomycin with tetracycline	streptomycin with chloramphenicol
Pseudomonas pseudomallei	Gram (−) bacilli	Melioidosis	trimethoprim-sulfamethoxazole	sulfonamide, tetracycline (with or without chloramphenicol, kanamycin)
Rickettsia (various species)	Rickettsiae	Rocky Mountain spotted fever, typhus, Q fever, tick-bite fever	tetracycline	chloramphenicol
Salmonella typhosa	Gram (−) bacilli	Typhoid fever	chloramphenicol	ampicillin, amoxicillin, cefoperazone, trimethoprim-sulfamethoxazole
Salmonella (other species)	Gram (−) bacilli	Paratyphoid fever, gastroenteritis, bacteremia	ampicillin, amoxicillin	chloramphenicol, trimethoprim-sulfamethoxazole
Serratia	Gram (−) bacilli	Various systemic infections (usually secondary to immunosuppressive therapy)	gentamicin, amikacin, netilmicin, third generation cephalosporins	aztreonam, imipenem, trimethoprim-sulfamethoxazole, carbenicillin, ticarcillin, mezlocillin, azlocillin, piperacillin
Shigella	Gram (−) bacilli	Acute gastroenteritis	trimethoprim-sulfamethoxazole	chloramphenicol, ampicillin, tetracycline
Spirillum minus	Gram (−) bacilli	Rat-bite fever	penicillin G	tetracycline, streptomycin
Sporothrix schenckii	Fungi	Sporotrichosis	amphotericin B	potassium iodide (for cutaneous form only)
Staphylococcus aureus	Gram (+) cocci	Pneumonia, meningitis, endocarditis, bacteremia, abscesses, osteomyelitis	Nonpenicillinase-producing—penicillin G or V Penicillinase-producing—penicillinase-resistant penicillin, ciprofloxacin, imipenem	cephalosporin, clindamycin, vancomycin, amoxicillin plus clavulanic acid

(continued)

Table 59-1 (continued)
Antimicrobial Drugs of Choice for Common Infections

Organism	Classification	Representative Clinical Illnesses	Drugs of First Choice	Alternate Drugs
Streptobacillus moniliformis	Gram (−) bacilli	Rat-bite fever, Haverhill fever, bacteremia	penicillin G	tetracycline, streptomycin
Streptococcus (anaerobic species)	Gram (+) cocci	Bacteremia, endocarditis, peritonitis, brain abscess	penicillin G	clindamycin, tetracycline, erythromycin, chloramphenicol, cephalosporins
Streptococcus bovis	Gram (+) cocci	Urinary infections, endocarditis, bacteremia, meningitis	penicillin G (with or without gentamicin)	cephalosporin, vancomycin
Streptococcus faecalis (enterococcus group)	Gram (+) cocci	Endocarditis, septicemia, meningitis, severe systemic infection Urinary infections	ampicillin or penicillin G with gentamicin or tobramycin ampicillin, amoxicillin	vancomycin with gentamicin or streptomycin, imipenem nitrofurantoin, tetracycline
Streptococcus (Diplococcus) pneumoniae	Gram (+) cocci	Pneumonia, meningitis, endocarditis, arthritis	penicillin G or V	erythromycin, cephalosporin, (first generation), clindamycin, chloramphenicol, ciprofloxacin
Streptococcus pyogenes (Groups A, C, G)	Gram (+) cocci	Various infections	penicillin G or V	Erythromycin, cephalosporin, vancomycin (bacteremia), ciprofloxacin
Streptococcus pyogenes (Group B)	Gram (+) cocci	Various infections	penicillin G, ampicillin	chloramphenicol, erythromycin, imipenem, cephalosporins, clindamycin
Streptococcus (viridans group)	Gram (+) cocci	Urinary infections, dental infections, endocarditis, meningitis, bacteremia	penicillin G (with or without streptomycin or gentamicin)	cephalosporin, vancomycin, norfloxacin, clindamycin
Treponema pallidum	Spirochetes	Syphilis	penicillin G	tetracycline, erythromycin
Treponema pertenue	Spirochetes	Yaws	penicillin G	tetracycline
Vibrio cholerae	Gram (−) bacilli	Cholera	tetracycline	trimethoprim-sulfamethoxazole, chloramphenicol, erythromycin
Yersinia (Pasteurella) pestis	Gram (−) bacilli	Plague	streptomycin (with or without tetracycline)	tetracycline, chloramphenicol

scription. Refer to Chapter 9 for some specific techniques.

The nurse may occasionally participate in administering a single dose of antibiotic to a patient. Single dose therapy is sometimes used in treating congenital syphilis, uncomplicated gonorrhea, group A beta-hemolytic streptococcus, and, occasionally, urinary tract infection. Physician preference and patient selection may vary, but there is clinical evidence that these infections will respond to a single sufficient dose of antibiotic.

The nurse also needs to discuss scheduling drug taking around meals. Many antibiotics are adversely affected by food, leading to a decrease in the therapeutic benefit of the drug. Table 59-2 is a partial listing of drug–food interactions and their potential outcomes. The best vehicle to use for drug taking is water. Refer to Chapter 5 and to specific drug chapters for more information.

Side-effects from antibiotics are common, but most are self-limiting and can be easily managed either by altering the dose or changing the drug. The most common reactions are skin rash which may spontaneously abate, diarrhea, and gastrointestinal distress. Other side-effects are discussed under specific drugs, especially those which may manifest during long-term therapy. If signs of an allergic reaction occur, the drug should be discontinued immediately and the physician should be notified.

Compliance is another issue the nurse deals with when teaching the patient about antibiotics. Because symptoms usually abate within 48 hours of drug therapy the patient may think he no longer needs the drug. Such thinking, coupled with the appearance of side-effects, and in children, the dif-

ficulty the parent experiences in giving the drug, may lead to premature discontinuation. The patient, or parent, will make the ultimate decision, but the nurse can minimize this problem by explaining the need to continue drug therapy to eliminate the infecting organism and helping the patient or family plan how to deal with problems that may arise.

Drug cost may also be a factor in determining whether the patient takes it. Many antibiotics are expensive, especially when therapy is prolonged. The nurse can offset this problem by inquiring about the patient's resources and knowing which antibiotics will be most financially draining. The nurse may be able to find resources or facilitate application for funds through insurance or public programs.

☐ *EVALUATION*
The outcome criteria the nurse may use to judge the success of anti-infective therapy include resolution of the infection and accompanying symptoms, a decrease in fever and in white cell count, and absence of side-effects. In outpatient care, criteria may also include completion of the prescription within the time frame proposed, follow-up visit if the problem is not resolved within the expected time (usually 7 days to 10 days). In the patient receiving intravenous antibiotics, additional criteria may include absence of infiltration or inflammation at the IV site and evidence that the patient knows and follows the protocol taught if he is at home on IV therapy.

Nursing Care Plan 59-1 summarizes the nursing process for the patient taking an anti-infective drug.

(Text continues on p. 1149.)

Table 59-2
Examples of Antibiotic Drug–Food Interactions

Drug	Food(s)	Potential Outcome
erythromycin stearate	Acidic fruit, fruit juice, carbonated beverages	Premature drug decomposition
griseofulvin	Insufficient fat intake	Incomplete drug absorption
lincomycin	Any food or beverage	Decreased absorption
tetracycline	Any food, especially dairy products	Incomplete absorption
rifampin	Any food	Delayed absorption

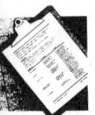

Nursing Care Plan 59-1
The Patient Receiving Anti-infective Drugs

Assessment

Subjective Data

1. Medication history: see Interactions section for each drug to formulate appropriate questions.
   a. Previous experience with antibiotic regimens
   b. Multiple food or drug allergies: increase the risk of hypersensitivity to antibiotics
2. Medical history
   a. Patient's description of symptoms for which drug is to be prescribed, knowledge of the rationale for a proposed regimen
   b. Presence of pre-existing conditions that may contraindicate or complicate anti-infective drug therapy such as hepatic, renal, or gastrointestinal disorders; pregnancy or breast-feeding
3. Personal history/compliance issues
   a. Knowledge of the regimen, ability to manage drug therapy
   b. Personal, financial resources; many anti-infectives are extremely expensive
   c. Past compliance with anti-infective treatment related to completing the course of therapy
   d. Parent's past experiences with attempting to convince a child to swallow a drug

Objective Data

1. Physical assessment
   a. Temperature, pulse respiration
   b. Examination of the site of infection, if possible
2. Laboratory data
   a. CBC with differential, noting WBC count
   b. Renal and hepatic function studies in patients receiving long-term therapy or compromised patients
   c. Culture and sensitivity testing of the site of infection, if possible

Nursing Diagnosis	Expected Client Outcome	Intervention
Knowledge deficit: related to drug action, correct administration and potential side-effects	Will verbalize understanding of drug action, correct dose and administration, and common side-effects.	Teach patient/family to space drug administration evenly throughout the day to maximize therapeutic levels. For some drugs this is essential, whereas for others more leeway is permitted. Explain how this facilitates drug action.
		Encourage the patient to take the drug with water and to avoid foods that may alter absorption (see specific drugs).
		Teach parents how to measure a correct dose using appropriate tools when giving antibiotics to a child, how to gain the child's trust, and how to use restraint if necessary. Provide parent with support.
		Plan detailed instructions for the patient who will be discharged on intravenous anti-infectives and make arrangements for 24-hour emergency care.

(continued)

Nursing Diagnosis	Expected Client Outcome	Intervention
Knowledge deficit: related to drug action, correct administration and potential side-effects (*continued*)		Teach patient to monitor common side-effects and serious adverse reactions as described in each chapter and follow preventive/reactive strategies given.
Potential noncompliance with drug regimen: related to cost, lack of symptoms	Will complete the course of drug therapy as prescribed.	Encourage the patient to complete the entire drug course as prescribed even though most symptoms will abate within 48 hours.
		Identify financial problems early to decrease the chance that the patient will stop taking the drug before the infection is completely cleared.
Potential for infection: related to inadequate or inappropriate drug therapy or drug-induced phlebitis at the IV site	Physical signs of infection will resolve, *i.e.*, reduction in temperature, decreased WBC counts, and reduced pain, swelling, redness at the infected site.	Review response to anti-infective treatment every 7–10 days or sooner if symptoms do not subside.
		In acute infection maintain a flow sheet to monitor vital signs, culture and sensitivity test results, WBC counts, RBC count, and, in long-term therapy or in susceptible patients such as the elderly and young children, renal and hepatic function studies to determine drug appropriateness.
	Phlebitis will be prevented.	Monitor IV sites closely, rotate peripheral lines every 48 hours, and discontinue IV at the first sign of pain, swelling, or redness at the IV site.
Potential alteration in skin integrity: related to drug hypersensitivity reaction	Drug reactions will be avoided or reported early.	Closely monitor a patient who is receiving an anti-infective agent for the first time or who has a history of multiple food or drug allergies.
		Teach the patient to report immediately any itching, rash, redness, facial angioedema, or difficulty breathing. The drug must be discontinued.
		Have on hand antihistamines, corticosteroids, epinephrine, and resuscitative equipment to manage drug anaphylaxis if it should occur.

REVIEW QUESTIONS

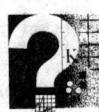

1. List several different ways in which anti-infective drugs may be classified.
2. Distinguish between (a) broad-spectrum and narrow-spectrum drugs and (b) bacteriostatic and bactericidal drugs.
3. Briefly describe several mechanisms by which anti-infective drugs act.
4. What methods may be utilized to test for sensitivity of an organism for a particular antimicrobial drug?
5. What factors can influence the choice of an appropriate anti-infective drug?
6. Briefly discuss the importance of administering anti-infective drugs for a sufficient duration of time.
7. List several examples of anti-infective drugs that may be used prophylactically.
8. What are the principal dangers associated with prophylactic use of antibiotics?
9. Describe several situations in which combined antimicrobial drug therapy might be indicated.
10. List the principal types of adverse drug reactions associated with antimicrobial drug use.
11. Briefly describe several ways in which microorganisms can develop resistance to antimicrobial drugs.

BIBLIOGRAPHY

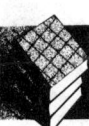

Antimicrobial prophylaxis for surgery. Med Lett Drugs Ther 25:113, 1983

Burnakis TG: Surgical antimicrobial prophylaxis: Principles and guidelines. Pharmacotherapy 4:248, 1984

Calderwood SB, Moellering RC: Principles of anti-infective therapy, In Stein JH (ed): Internal Medicine. p. 1139. Boston, Little, Brown & Co, 1983

Coleman DL, Horwitz RI, Andriole VT: Association between serum inhibitory and bactericidal concentrations and therapeutic outcome in bacterial endocarditis. Am J Med 73:260, 1982

Conte JE, Barriere SL: Manual of Antibiotics and Infectious Diseases, 4th ed. Philadelphia, Lea & Febiger, 1981

Cunha BA, Ristuccia AM: Adverse effects of antibiotics. Heart Lung 13:465, 1984

Gleckman RA, Gants NM (eds): Infections in the Elderly. Boston, Little, Brown & Co, 1983

Johnston JB, Davidson MR: Use of a mini-infuser syringe pump for the self-administration of IV antibiotics in the home. NITA 7:381, 1984

Kogan BM (ed): Antimicrobial Therapy, 3rd ed. Philadelphia, WB Saunders, 1980

Mandell GL, Douglas RG, Bennett JE (eds): Principles and Practice of Infectious Diseases, 2nd ed. New York, John Wiley & Sons, 1985

Neuman M (ed): Useful and harmful interactions of antibiotics. Boca Raton, CRC Press, 1985

Prevention of bacterial endocarditis. Med Lett Drugs Ther 26:3, 1984

Ristuccia AM, Cunha BA (eds): Antimicrobial Therapy. New York, Raven Press, 1984

Root RK, Sande MA (eds): New Dimensions in Antimicrobial Therapy. New York, Churchill Livingstone, 1984

Sanford JP: Guide to Antimicrobial Therapy. Bethesda, MD, Sanford, 1983

Snavely SR, Hodges GR: The neurotoxicity of antibacterial agents. Ann Intern Med 101:92, 1984

Tipper DJ: Mode of action of beta-lactam antibiotics. Rev Infect Dis 1:39, 1979

Toby LE, Covington TR: Antimicrobial drug interactions. Am J Nurs 75:1470, 1975

Washington AE: Update on treatment recommendations for gonococcal infections. Rev Infect Dis 4(Suppl):5758, 1982

Yoos L: Factors influencing maternal compliance to antibiotic regimens. Pediatric Nursing 10:141, 1984

Sulfonamides

Sulfonamides were the first group of systemic antimicrobial agents to be effective when used clinically and were the mainstay of anti-infective therapy before the introduction of the penicillins in the 1940s. Sulfonamides are widely distributed in the body and are bacteriostatic against a broad spectrum of both gram-positive and gram-negative organisms. Their use, however, has declined from that of the early years with the introduction of more potent and, in some cases, more selective antibacterial drugs. Resistance of many organisms to the action of sulfonamides has also contributed to their relatively limited clinical usefulness. Nonetheless, they remain valuable therapeutic agents in certain infectious conditions, most notably acute urinary tract infections, because the high solubility in urine of certain derivatives allows them to reach effective concentrations without danger of kidney damage.

A major deterrent to the continuing effective use of sulfonamides has been the emergence of resistant strains of microorganisms that were once sensitive to the action of these drugs (e.g., gonococci, beta-hemolytic streptococci, meningococci, coliform organisms). Development of sulfonamide resistance in these organisms has been greatly abetted by the previous widespread prophylactic use of the drugs in subtherapeutic doses for the attempted control of gonorrhea, upper respiratory infections, and urinary infections. Among the major causes of increased sulfonamide resistance among microorganisms are production of excessive amounts of para-aminobenzoic acid (PABA) by the bacteria (PABA is an essential component of folic acid synthesis necessary for cell growth and is competitively antagonized by sulfonamides—see under Mechanisms and Actions); enhanced destruction of the sulfonamide molecule by the microorganism; or development of alternate metabolic pathways for handling essential amino acids. Acquired bacterial resistance plays a major role in therapeutic failures with sulfonamides, and the clinical usefulness of these agents, in spite of their relatively low cost, is therefore limited. Cross-resistance between sulfonamides is very common as well.

Significant differences exist among the various sulfonamide drugs in their rates of absorption, metabolism, and excretion, and these differences are important with regard to the indications, efficacy, and toxicity of the various compounds. Based upon such differences, the sulfonamides may be categorized into several groups; such a classification is presented in the box entitled Sulfonamides. Among

Sulfonamides

I. Systemic
   A. Short Acting
      sulfacytine
      sulfadiazine
      sulfamerazine
      sulfamethazine
      sulfamethizole
      sulfisoxazole
   B. Intermediate Acting
      sulfamethoxazole
      sulfapyridine
II. Local
   A. Intestinal
      sulfasalazine
   B. Ophthalmic
      sulfacetamide
      sulfisoxazole
   C. Vaginal
      sulfabenzamide
      sulfacetamide
      sulfathiazole
      sulfisoxazole
   D. Topical
      mafenide
      silver sulfadiazine

the systemic agents, the short-acting compounds are rapidly absorbed and quickly eliminated by the kidney. Sulfamethoxazole, an intermediate-acting sulfonamide, is somewhat more slowly absorbed and excreted than the short-acting drugs, and thus may be used twice a day rather than four to six times a day, possibly improving dosing compliance.

While most systemic sulfonamide use is by oral ingestion, sulfisoxazole is available for injection. Parenteral use of sulfonamides should be undertaken only where oral administration is impractical (as in a comatose patient) and is best accomplished by slow IV injection. The solutions are highly alkaline and can be quite irritating, and the drug may precipitate out of solution.

Locally acting sulfonamides may be employed in several ways. Sulfasalazine is administered orally for the treatment of ulcerative colitis. The compound is split by the action of intestinal microflora into sulfapyridine and 5-aminosalicylate, the latter agent accumulating in significant amounts in the colon, where it may exert an anti-inflammatory action. 5-aminosalicylic acid is also available alone as mesalamine (Rowasa) in the form of a suspension enema for treating ulcerative colitis or proctitis.

Other indications for use of locally acting sulfonamides are eye and vaginal infections (sulfacetamide, sulfathiazole, sulfisoxazole) and prevention and treatment of sepsis in second- and third-degree burns (mafenide, silver sulfadiazine). Topical application of sulfonamides occasionally elicits allergic hypersensitivity reactions and local ocular irritation.

Sulfonamides have little likelihood of causing serious toxicity and are relatively inexpensive drugs. Thus they can be very valuable anti-infective agents in treating those infections where the causative pathogen has been demonstrated to be sensitive to the sulfonamide. Because their basic pharmacology is similar, the sulfonamide drugs are reviewed as a group. Individual drugs are then presented in Table 60-1 where specific indications and characteristics are mentioned. Mafenide and silver sulfadiazine are then discussed individually, as is trimethoprim-sulfamethoxazole, a synergistic combination of two antibacterial agents (one a sulfonamide) that is used in both acute and chronic urinary tract infections as well as for several other indications. The sulfonamide discussion focuses principally on the systemic effects of the drugs, with mention being made of specific points pertaining to their local application wherever necessary.

Sulfonamides

Sulfacetamide, Sulfabenzamide, Sulfacytine, Sulfadiazine, Sulfamethizole, Sulfamethoxazole, Sulfapyridine, Sulfasalazine, Sulfathiazole, Sulfisoxazole, Multiple Sulfonamides

MECHANISMS AND ACTIONS
Sulfonamides are structural analogues of para-aminobenzoic acid (PABA), which is an essential component for formation of folic acid by bacterial cells, a step leading ultimately to synthesis of purines and nucleic acids (see Fig. 60-1). The sulfonamide drugs are bacteriostatic, as they compete with PABA for the enzyme necessary to form folic acid. The result is reduced production of folic acid and impaired bacterial cell replication. Some microorganisms do not synthesize folic acid internally but obtain it from exogenous sources and are not susceptible to the action of sulfonamides. Like-

wise, bacterial cells that produce large quantities of PABA can overcome the competitive blocking action of sulfonamides on folic acid synthesis and are also largely resistant to these drugs.

Microorganisms that have remained largely susceptible to sulfonamides include *Escherichia coli, Hemophilus influenzae, Nocardia asteroides, Chlamydia trachomatis,* and *Proteus mirabilis.* In addition, some strains of *Enterobacter, Klebsiella,* staphylococci, meningococci and streptococci may respond to the sulfonamides. The various indications for the different sulfonamide drugs are listed below.

USES
(See also Table 60-1 for specific indications for each drug.)
1. Acute, recurrent, or chronic urinary tract infections in the absence of obstruction. Acute infections generally respond to a single sulfonamide drug, usually sulfisoxazole or sulfamethoxazole; recurrent infections or infections complicated by obstruction or bacteremia are less effectively controlled by a sulfonamide alone, and usually require adjunctive therapy.
2. Chancroid
3. Trachoma
4. Nocardiosis

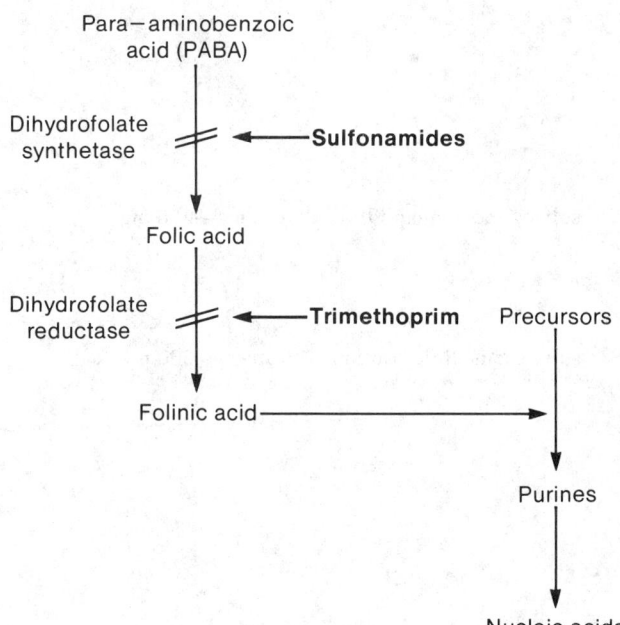

Figure 60-1 *Mechanism of action of sulfonamides and trimethoprim. Sulfonamides block conversion of PABA to folic acid and trimethoprim impairs the reduction of folic acid to folinic acid.*

(Text continues on p. 1156.)

Table 60-1
Sulfonamides

Drug	Preparations	Usual Dosage Range	Clinical Considerations
sulfacetamide (Ak-Sulf, Bleph 10, Cetamide, Isopto Cetamide, Ophthacet, Sebizon Lotion, Sodium Sulamyd, Sulf-10, Sulfair-15, Sulten-10)	Ophthalmic drops—10%, 15%, 30% Ophthalmic ointment—10% Lotion—10%	Drops—1 drop to 2 drops every 1 h–4 h as condition dictates Ointment—small amount in conjunctival sac two to four times a day Lotion—apply two to four times a day for bacterial infections or at bedtime for seborrheic dermatitis	Ophthalmic drops or ointment is indicated for treatment of conjunctivitis, corneal ulcers, superficial ocular infections, and as adjunctive therapy with systemic sulfonamides for trachoma; lotion is used for seborrheic dermatitis and cutaneous bacterial infections with susceptible organisms; solutions are incompatible with silver preparations; nonsusceptible organisms may proliferate with use of sulfacetamide; drug may be inactivated by PABA produced by purulent exudates; ophthalmic ointment may impair corneal healing; 30% drops may be irritating upon application; do not use if ophthalmic solution is dark brown; discontinue drug if signs of hypersensitivity develop; apply topical lotion cautiously to abraded or denuded skin areas; available with phenylephrine as ophthalmic solution (Vasosulf) and combined with sulfathiazole and sulfabenzamide as vaginal cream and vaginal tablets (Sultrin, Triple Sulfa, Sulfa-Gyn, Trysul)
sulfacytine (Renoquid)	Tablets—250 mg	Adults—500 mg initially; then 250 mg four times a day for 10 days	Short-acting sulfonamide not recommended in children under 14 years of age; *only* used for treatment of urinary tract infections
sulfadiazine (Microsulfon)	Tablets—500 mg	Adults—2 g to 4 g initially, then 2 g to 4 g/day in three to six divided doses Children—75 mg/kg initially, followed by 150 mg/kg/day in four to six divided doses (maximum 6 g/day) Rheumatic fever prophylaxis —0.5 g to 1 g once daily	Short-acting sulfonamide indicated for most sulfonamide-susceptible infections but rather infrequently used because drug is poorly soluble in acid urine and danger of nephrotoxicity exists; high urine volume must be maintained to prevent crystalluria; component of triple sulfa formulations with sulfamerazine and sulfamethazine; combination claimed to reduce

(continued)

Table 60-1 (continued)
Sulfonamides

Drug	Preparations	Usual Dosage Range	Clinical Considerations
sulfadiazine (Microsulfon) (*continued*)			chance of crystalluria; alkalinization of urine is recommended
sulfamethizole (Proklar, Thiosulfil-Forte)	Tablets—500 mg	Adults—0.5 g to 1 g three to four times a day Children—30 mg to 45 mg/kg day in four divided doses	Short-acting sulfonamide used for acute and chronic urinary infections; highly bound to plasma proteins; use with caution with other protein-bound drugs; rapidly excreted in urine, mostly in active form; drug may impart an orange-yellow color to urine or skin; available in combination with phenazopyridine (Thiosulfil-A) and oxytetracycline (Urobiotic)
sulfamethoxazole (Gamazole, Gantanol, Urobak)	Tablets—500 mg, 1000 mg Suspension—500 mg/5 ml	Adults—2 g initially, followed by 1 g two to three times a day Children—50 mg to 60 mg/kg initially, then 25 mg to 30 mg/kg morning and night (maximum 75 mg/kg/day) Lymphogranuloma venereum—1 g twice a day for at least 2 wk	Intermediate-acting sulfonamide similar to sulfisoxazole but with somewhat slower oral absorption and urinary excretion; used twice a day in most cases to prevent accumulation; available in combination with trimethoprim (Bactrim, Septra; see separate discussion) and phenazopyridine (Azo Gantanol), the latter drug serving as a urinary analgesic for relief of dysuria associated with urinary tract infection
sulfapyridine	Tablets—500 mg	Adults—500 mg four times a day until improvement is noted, then reduce by 500 mg/day at 3-day intervals to effective maintenance level	Intermediate-acting agent used in the treatment of dermatitis herpetiformis (recurrent, inflammatory skin disease, herpetic in nature, characterized by erythema, vesicles, and pustules); slowly absorbed from GI tract (peak levels in 6 h–8 h); excreted both as intact drug and conjugated metabolites, largely within 3 days to 4 days; administer with sufficient fluids to prevent crystalluria
sulfasalazine (Azaline, Azulfidine, S.A.S.-500)	Tablets—500 mg Enteric-coated tablets (EN-Tabs)—500 mg Suspension—250 mg/5 ml	Adults—1 g to 4 g/day initially in evenly divided doses; maintenance dose is 500 mg four times/day (maximum 8 g/day) Children—40 mg to 60 mg/kg/day in three to six	Locally-acting sulfonamide used orally in the treatment of mild to moderate ulcerative colitis; hydrolyzed in intestinal tract to sulfapyridine (antibacterial) and 5-aminosalicylic *(continued)*

Table 60-1 (continued)
Sulfonamides

Drug	Preparations	Usual Dosage Range	Clinical Considerations
sulfasalazine (Azaline, Azulfidine, S.A.S.-500) (continued)		divided doses initially followed by 30 mg/kg/day in four divided doses	acid (anti-inflammatory); systemic absorption of parent drug and hydrolysis products are variable (increased in the presence of severe ulceration); frequently produces GI intolerance; if noted early in therapy, space daily dosage more evenly or use enteric-coated tablets; enteric-coated tablets have passed through GI tract without disintegrating; if this is noted, discontinue therapy; if GI distress is observed after several days of therapy, reduce dosage or stop drug for 5 days to 7 days, then resume at a lower dose; doses above 4 g/day are associated with increased incidence of adverse effects; drug is often continued at reduced levels even when clinical symptoms, including diarrhea, are controlled; dosage and duration of therapy are primarily governed by endoscopic evaluation; if diarrhea recurs, increase dosage to previously effective level; infertility has been reported in men; withdrawal of drug reverses this effect; advise patient that drug may impart an orange-yellow color to skin and to alkaline urine; sulfasalazine may impair absorption of folic acid

(continued)

5. Toxoplasmosis (with pyrimethamine)
6. Acute otitis media due to *Hemophilus influenzae* (with penicillin or erythromycin); also, prophylaxis of recurrent otitis media (sulfisoxazole)
7. Adjunctive therapy of malaria (chloroquine-resistant strains of *Plasmodium falciparum*)
8. Prophylaxis and treatment of sulfonamide-sensitive group A strains of meningococcal meningitis or hemophilus meningitis (with streptomycin)
9. Prophylaxis of recurrent rheumatic fever (sulfadiazine *only*)
10. Conjunctivitis and superficial eye infections (sulfacetamide, sulfisoxazole)
11. *Hemophilus vaginalis* vaginitis (sulfabenzamide, sulfacetamide, sulfathiazole, sulfisoxazole)

Table 60-1 (continued)
Sulfonamides

Drug	Preparations	Usual Dosage Range	Clinical Considerations
sulfisoxazole (Gantrisin, Gulfasin, Lipo Gantrisin)	Tablets—500 mg Syrup—500 mg/5 ml (chocolate) Pediatric suspension—500 mg/5 ml (raspberry) Emulsion (Lipo Gantrisin)—1 g/5 ml in homogenized vegetable oil (long-acting) Ophthalmic drops—4% Ophthalmic ointment—4%	Oral (except emulsion, see Clinical Considerations): Adults—2 g to 4 g initially, then 4 g to 8 g/day in four to six divided doses Children—150 mg/kg/day in four to six divided doses (initial dose is one-half the 24-h dose) Ophthalmic: 1 drop to 2 drops every 1 h to 4 h as condition warrants or small amount of ointment three to four times a day	Short-acting sulfonamide used orally and locally (eye) for a number of bacterial infections; peak blood levels occur within 3 h–4 h following oral administration; highly protein bound but rapidly excreted in the urine (95% within 24 h); emulsion (Lipo Gantrisin) is long acting and is administered every 12 h (adults 4 g–5 g; children 60 mg–75 mg/kg); see under sulfacetamide for remarks concerning ophthalmic and vaginal application; available in combination with phenazopyridine (*e.g.*, Azo Gantrisin), which provides an analgesic effect for relief of dysuria associated with urinary infections, or with erythromycin (Pediazole) which is used for acute otitis media in children caused by resistant *Hemophilus influenzae*
Multiple sulfonamides (Neotrizine, Sul-Trio MM, Terfonyl, Triple Sulfa)	Tablets—162 mg or 167 mg each of sulfadiazine, sulfamerazine, and sulfamethazine Suspension—167 mg each of sulfadiazine, sulfamerazine, and sulfamethazine per 5 ml	Adults—2 g to 4 g initially, then 2 g to 4 g/day in four to six divided doses Children—75 mg/kg initially then 150 mg/kg/day in four to six divided doses	A combination of three short-acting sulfonamides that provides the therapeutic effect of the total sulfonamide content, but reduces the risk of precipitation in the kidneys, because the solubility of each sulfonamide is independent of the others; infrequently used preparation, because other equally effective and more soluble sulfonamides are available (*e.g.*, sulfisoxazole)

12. Ulcerative colitis (sulfasalazine)
13. Dermatitis herpetiformis (sulfapyridine *only*)

ADMINISTRATION AND DOSAGE
See Table 60-1.

FATE
Orally administered sulfonamides, except for those designed for their local effects in the bowel, are readily absorbed from the GI tract. Absorption from other sites, such as the skin or vagina, is considerably more variable and unreliable. The drugs distribute widely in the body and may be found in cerebrospinal fluid as well as pleural, peritoneal, synovial, ocular, placental, and other body fluids. Protein binding is variable (20%–90%) but can be significant. Interpatient variations in serum levels may be considerable. The duration of action is largely dependent on the rate of metabolism and

renal excretion. The drugs are metabolized in the liver by several pathways, one of which, acetylation, can occur at varying rates. "Slow acetylators" have an increased risk of drug accumulation and subsequent toxicity. Sulfonamides are eliminated in the urine as both unchanged drug and metabolic products, glomerular filtration playing the major role in excretion. Tubular reabsorption occurs to a different extent with each drug, and, as indicated above, variations in the rate of excretion influence the duration of action. Urinary solubility of sulfonamides is pH dependent; alkalinization of the urine favors excretion (increases ionization of molecule and solubility of drug) and reduces danger of crystallization in the urinary fluid.

Some derivatives (e.g., sulfacytine, sulfadiazine, sulfisoxazole) are readily absorbed and quickly excreted and must be given up to six times a day to maintain adequate plasma concentrations. Sulfamethoxazole is somewhat more slowly absorbed and excreted and is given less frequently (two to three times a day). "Long-lasting" sulfonamides (i.e., drugs slowly absorbed and excreted) are no longer used because the incidence of crystalluria was higher with these drugs and toxic reactions were more difficult to manage. Sulfasalazine is an orally administered drug which is only very slightly absorbed and is excreted largely in the feces; it is used for its local effects in the bowel.

SIDE-EFFECTS/ADVERSE REACTIONS

Although the overall incidence of adverse effects with sulfonamides is relatively low, the drugs can elicit a wide variety of untoward reactions. Most commonly noted with oral administration of these drugs are GI symptoms such as abdominal discomfort, nausea, and diarrhea. Drug fever occurs in approximately 3% of patients, may be sudden in onset, and frequently represents an allergic manifestation. It may be accompanied by chills, malaise, pruritus, and headache. Patients evidencing drug fever must be closely observed for signs of more serious toxicity, such as blood dyscrasias or serum sickness, which also present initially as fever among their symptoms.

The incidence of hypersensitivity reactions to sulfonamides is variable. Among the effects reported are urticaria, generalized skin eruptions, photosensitivity, arthralgia, periorbital edema, erythema multiforme, exfoliative dermatitis, serum sickness, anaphylactic reactions, and myocarditis.

Pneumonia characterized by eosinophilic infiltrates may occur. Toxic nephrosis and hepatitis can also result from an allergic reaction to sulfonamides.

Serum sickness has appeared after several days of sulfonamide use and may be heralded by fever, joint pain, conjuctivitis, bronchospasm, dermal eruptions, and leukopenia.

Many other untoward effects have occurred during sulfonamide therapy although the incidence may vary widely among the different drugs. These are outlined below by organ system involved.

GI—Vomiting, diarrhea, anorexia, stomatitis, pancreatitis, jaundice, hepatitis, impaired folic acid absorption

CNS—Headache, drowsiness, dizziness, insomnia, vertigo, tinnitus, ataxia, depression, convulsions, hallucinations, peripheral neuritis, hearing loss, psychosis

Renal—Proteinuria, albuminuria, hematuria, oliguria, anuria, crystalluria, nephrotic syndrome

Hematologic—Petechiae, hemolytic or macrocytic anemia, blood dyscrasias, hypoprothrombinemia, methemoglobinemia, purpura

Other—Alopecia, cyanosis, goiter, hypothyroidism, diuresis, hypoglycemia, reduction in sperm count, infertility, periarteritis nodosum, lupus-like syndrome

Sulfonamides given to pregnant women near term or to neonates may cause a serious disorder known as kernicterus (see Disease Brief: Kernicterus).

Sulfasalazine may produce an orange-yellow color in the urine and occasionally in the skin.

Severe overdosage with a sulfonamide is marked by vomiting, dizziness, fever, acidosis, acute hemolytic anemia, maculopapular dermatitis, toxic neuritis, jaundice, agranulocytosis, anuria, and occasionally death.

Treatment is directed toward removal of unabsorbed drug, forced excretion, and symptomatic management as necessary.

CONTRAINDICATIONS AND PRECAUTIONS

Use of sulfonamides is contraindicated in persons with hypersensitivity to sulfonylurea antidiabetics or thiazide diuretics, persons with porphyria, or advanced kidney disease, near term of pregnancy or during the early nursing period, and in infants under 2 months of age (except for treating congenital toxoplasmosis).

In addition, sulfasalazine is contraindicated in intestinal or urinary obstruction, in children under 2 years of age, and in patients with salicylate allergy.

Sulfonamides should be used with caution in persons with liver or kidney dysfunction, blood

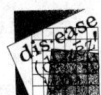

DISEASE BRIEF

■ *Kernicterus*

Neonates have a temporary deficiency of the hepatic enzyme glucuronyl transferase, which is not fully developed at birth. This results in decreased conjugation of bilirubin. The resultant increased serum levels of unconjugated bilirubin are normally bound to serum albumin, preventing diffusion into the central nervous system. Sulfonamides however, can displace bilirubin from its serum protein binding sites. Higher levels of unbound bilirubin in plasma can lead to increased brain levels of unconjugated bilirubin because the pigment readily crosses the immature blood–brain barrier.

Kernicterus, or bilirubin encephalopathy, results from abnormal pigmentation of the gray matter due to the increased levels of bilirubin in the brain. Clinically, the neonate displays spasticity, head retraction, opisthotonos, muscle twitching, and convulsions. Death occurs frequently, and survivors commonly display mental retardation and spastic paraplegia. Exchange transfusion can lower serum bilirubin levels and phenobarbital may be useful to increase the rate of bilirubin degradation and elimination. Metabolic acidosis must be treated vigorously. Sulfonamides, which can displace bilirubin from its serum binding sites, must be avoided during the latter stages of pregnancy and in nursing mothers.

dyscrasias, a history of allergic reactions, bronchial asthma, or a glucose-6-phosphate dehydrogenase deficiency (hemolytic anemia can occur). Cautious use is also warranted in persons receiving anticoagulant or antiplatelet drugs because increased bleeding tendency has occurred. Sulfonamides should not be used to treat group A beta-hemolytic streptococcal infections because they will not eradicate the organism nor prevent sequelae such as glomerulonephritis or rheumatic fever. Sulfasalazine must be administered carefully to patients with extensive intestinal ulceration because increased systemic absorption can occur, leading to increased toxicity.

INTERACTIONS

1. Due to competition for protein-binding sites, sulfonamides may potentiate or be potentiated by other protein-bound drugs (*e.g.*, oral anticoagulants, oral antidiabetics, methotrexate, phenytoin, salicylates, anti-inflammatory agents, sulfinpyrazone, probenecid, and barbiturates).
2. The effects of sulfonamides on localized infections may be impaired by infiltration of local anesthetics that are metabolized to PABA (*e.g.*, chloroprocaine, procaine, and tetracaine).
3. Concurrent use of sulfonamides may reduce oral contraceptive efficacy and increase the incidence of breakthrough bleeding.
4. Tolbutamide and methotrexate may increase sulfonamide plasma levels by competing for renal tubular excretory mechanisms.
5. The effects of tolbutamide, chlorpropamide, and phenytoin may be potentiated by sulfonamides through inhibition of their hepatic metabolism.
6. The incidence of crystalluria with sulfonamides can be increased by paraldehyde, methenamine, or urinary acidifiers (*e.g.*, ammonium chloride).
7. Sulfasalazine can reduce the bioavailability of digoxin and can retard absorption of folic acid.
8. Antacids and possibly mineral oil may decrease the effects of sulfonamides by impairing absorption.

Mafenide

(Sulfamylon)

Mafenide in a topical sulfonamide that is bacteriostatic against a variety of gram-positive and gram-negative organisms, including *Pseudomonas aeruginosa* and certain strains of anaerobes. It is active even in the presence of pus and serum, and its activity is not altered by changes in *p*H.

Mafenide retards bacterial invasion of avascular burn sites, facilitating spontaneous healing of partial thickness burns. It is indicated as adjunctive therapy in second- and third-degree burns.

The drug is used as a cream (85 mg/g) and is applied aseptically twice a day over the burned surface to a depth of 1 mm to 2 mm. Mafenide should be reapplied whenever necessary to maintain continuous covering of area. Application should be continued until healing is well along or skin is ready for grafting. The drug diffuses through devascularized areas and is quickly absorbed from the burn surface, with peak plasma concentrations in 2 hours to 4 hours. It is rapidly metabolized and eliminated by the kidney.

Mafenide and its metabolite inhibit the enzyme carbonic anhydrase which can lead to development of metabolic acidosis. Impaired renal function may exaggerate this response. Close monitoring of acid–base balance is necessary, especially where the burn area is extensive.

The most frequently encountered side-effects with mafenide are pain, burning, and stinging upon application. Allergic reactions, such as rash, itching, facial edema, swelling, hives, erythema and eosinophilia have also been noted during therapy with mafenide. Other adverse reactions reported on occasion include hyperventilation (with resultant respiratory alkalosis), hyperchloremia, fungal colonization in the wound area, and excoriation and bleeding of skin.

Patients should be bathed daily to aid in debridement. Dressings are usually not necessary, but a *thin* covering may be used if desired. Mafenide must be used with caution in patients with acute renal failure, pulmonary infection, or impaired pulmonary function and in pregnant women.

Silver Sulfadiazine

(Silvadene, Thermazine)

A condensation product of silver nitrate with sulfadiazine, silver sulfadiazine possesses broad antimicrobial activity. In contrast to mafenide, it is *bactericidal* against a number of both gram-positive and gram-negative bacteria as well as yeasts and is used topically to prevent invasion as well as to eradicate sensitive microorganisms from burns. In addition, the drug, unlike mafenide, does not affect electrolyte or acid–base balance, and application is less painful.

Silver is slowly released from the preparation in concentrations that are *selectively* toxic to bacteria. Although less than 1% of the silver content is absorbed, as much as 10% of the sulfadiazine may reach the systemic circulation depending on the extent of the burn area of application.

Silver sulfadiazine is used to prevent *or* treat sepsis in second- or third-degree burns. It is used as a cream (10 mg/g) and applied aseptically one or two times a day to a thickness of 1 mm to 2 mm.

Reapplication is done as often as necessary to maintain continuous covering. Treatment is continued, as with mafenide, until healing has occurred or the site is ready for grafting.

Burning at the application site is the most commonly reported side-effect; other adverse reactions include rash, itching, fungal overgrowth, and, rarely, leukopenia and interstitial nephritis. Because sulfadiazine may be absorbed in substantial amounts in some patients, the adverse reactions listed under the discussion of sulfonamides earlier in the chapter must be considered as possibilities.

The drug should not be used in pregnant women near term, premature infants, or in neonates under 2 months of age, because the danger of kernicterus exists (see Disease Brief: Kernicterus). *Cautious use* of silver sulfadiazine is warranted in patients with a history of sulfonamide hypersensitivity, impaired renal or hepatic function, or glucose-6-phosphate dehydrogenase deficiency (danger of hemolysis), and during pregnancy.

Trimethoprim-Sulfamethoxazole

(Bactrim, Septra, and various other manufacturers)

Trimethoprim-sulfamethoxazole (co-trimoxazole, TMP-SMZ) is a synergistic combination of antimicrobial drugs that interfere with two sequential steps in an essential enzymatic reaction necessary for bacterial multiplication (see Fig. 60-1). Consequently, clinical efficacy is enhanced, and development of resistance is significantly reduced when compared to the use of either agent alone. Its antibacterial spectrum includes common urinary pathogens (except *Pseudomonas aeruginosa*) and middle ear pathogens (e.g., *Hemophilus*) as well as several organisms associated with respiratory conditions such as acute bronchitis and pneumonitis. A severe form of pneumonitis due to *Pneumocystis carinii* can occur in immunocompromised persons such as those receiving cancer chemotherapy, other immunosuppressant drugs, or those afflicted with AIDS. This opportunistic infection is difficult to eradicate, and trimethoprim-sulfamethoxazole has now become a favored drug in treating this serious disease.

MECHANISM AND ACTIONS

Sulfamethoxazole inhibits synthesis of dihydrofolic acid (folic acid) by competitive antagonism of PABA; trimethoprim inhibits the dihydrofolate reductase enzyme, thus blocking production of tetrahydrofolic acid (folinic acid). Thus, two consecutive steps in the synthesis of essential proteins and nucleic acids in many bacteria are impaired.

USES
1. Recurrent or chronic urinary tract infections due to susceptible organisms (i.e., *Escherichia coli, Klebsiella-Enterobacter, Proteus mirabilis, Proteus vulgaris, Proteus morgani*)

   Note: Initial episodes of uncomplicated acute urinary tract infections should be treated with a single agent rather than this combination.
2. Acute otitis media in children over 2 years of age due to susceptible strains of *Hemophilus influenzae* (including ampicillin- and amoxicillin-resistant strains) or *Streptococcus pneumoniae*
3. Acute exacerbations of chronic bronchitis in adults due to susceptible strains of *H. influenzae* or *S. pneumoniae*
4. Enteritis due to susceptible strains of *Shigella*
5. *Pneumocystis carinii* pneumonitis in children and adults immunosuppressed by cancer chemotherapy or other immunosuppressive therapy or suffering from AIDS.
6. Treatment of *Nocardia asteroides* infections (usually for 6 months to 12 months)
7. Investigational uses include treatment of cholera, salmonella type infections, melioidosis, brucellosis, chancroid, penicillinase-producing *Neisseria gonorrhoeae*, and prophylaxis of traveler's diarrhea.

In addition, once daily or thrice weekly administration of low doses (see under Administration and Dosage) has been used to prevent recurrent urinary tract infections in women.

ADMINISTRATION AND DOSAGE
Trimethoprim-sulfamethoxazole is available as regular strength (80 mg TMP/400 mg SMZ) and double strength (160 mg TMP/800 mg SMZ) tablets, oral suspension (40 mg TMP/200 mg SMZ per 5 ml), and a solution for IV infusion (80 mg TMP/400 mg SMZ per 5 ml).

The following are recommended doses for the various indications, with dosage ratios given as the amount of trimethoprim/sulfamethoxazole in the preparation:

Urinary infections, bronchitis, shigellosis, otitis media:

Adults: 160 mg TMP/800 mg SMZ every 12 hours for 10 days to 14 days (7 days in shigellosis)

Children: 8 mg TMP/kg/day and 40 mg SMZ/kg/day in two divided doses every 12 hours for 10 days (5 days in shigellosis) (Children weighing 40 kg or more should receive an adult dose.)

Severe urinary infections or shigellosis:

8 to 10 mg/kg/day (trimethoprim equivalent) by IV infusion in two to four divided doses for up to 14 days in urinary infections and 5 days in shigellosis.

Prevention of recurrent urinary infections in females:

40 mg TMP/200 mg SMZ daily at bedtime or 80 mg/400 mg two to three times a week

Prostatitis:

Acute—160 mg TMP/800 mg SMZ twice daily until patient is afebrile 48 hours.

Chronic—160 mg TMP/800 mg SMZ twice daily for 4 weeks to 12 weeks

Pneumocystis carinii pneumonitis:

Adults and children: 20 mg/kg/day TMP and 100 mg/kg/day SMZ orally or by IV infusion in equally divided doses every 6 hours for 14 days

Chancroid:

160 mg TMP/800 mg SMZ orally twice daily for a minimum of 7 days

Penicillinase-producing Neisseria gonorrhoeae:

Pharyngeal infection—9 tablets (80 mg TMP/400 mg SMZ) in a single dose daily for 5 days

When administering IV, give slowly over 60 minutes to 90 minutes. Do *not* give IM. Infusion solution (5-ml ampule) is diluted with 125 ml of 5% dextrose in water, and the dilution should not be mixed with other drugs or solutions.

FATE
The drug combination is rapidly absorbed when taken orally. Peak serum levels occur in 1 hour to 4 hours with oral use and 1 hour to 1.5 hours following IV administration. Half-lives for both drugs are 10 hours with oral administration and 11 hours to 13 hours with IV infusion. The ratio for trimethoprim to sulfamethoxazole in the blood is approximately 1:20 which is optimum for synergistic antibacterial activity. Roughly 45% of trimethoprim and 70% of sulfamethoxazole are protein-bound. The drugs are widely distributed in the body, including the cerebrospinal fluid. Both agents are metabolized, although trimethoprim only to a limited extent, and are excreted primarily by kidneys.

Urine concentrations are significantly higher than serum concentrations.

SIDE-EFFECTS/ADVERSE REACTIONS
The most commonly encountered side-effects are nausea, vomiting, rash, and mild thrombocytopenia. A variety of other adverse reactions have been noted during therapy with trimethoprim-sulfamethoxazole and, as expected, closely resemble those reported with use of the two component drugs on an individual basis. In addition to the effects listed below, reference should be made to the sections on side-effects/adverse reactions under sulfonamides in this chapter and trimethoprim in Chapter 67 for additional information on potential untoward reactions with this drug combination.

GI—Abdominal pain, glossitis, stomatitis, pseudomembranous colitis, jaundice, hepatitis, pancreatitis

CNS—Headache, tinnitus, vertigo, fatigue, insomnia, muscle weakness, ataxia, convulsions, peripheral neuritis, depression, hallucinations

Allergic—Pruritus, urticaria, periorbital edema, generalized skin eruptions, photosensitivity, arthralgia, myocarditis, anaphylactic reactions, serum sickness, erythema multiforme, Stevens-Johnson syndrome, epidermal necrolysis

Hematologic—Blood dyscrasias, purpura, hemolytic anemia, hypoprothrombinemia, methemoglobinemia

Other—Chills, fever, oliguria, anuria, lupus-like syndrome, goiter, diuresis, hypoglycemia, periarteritis nodosa

Patients with AIDS frequently react adversely when trimethoprim-sulfamethoxazole is administered to treat pneumocystis pneumonia. Fever, rash, malaise, and pancytopenia are common occurrences.

IV use at high doses or for prolonged periods may result in bone marrow depression.

CONTRAINDICATIONS AND PRECAUTIONS
Use of trimethoprim-sulfamethoxazole is contraindicated in persons with megaloblastic anemia due to folate deficiency, in pregnant women near term, nursing mothers, and infants less than 2 months of age. A cautious approach to therapy must be undertaken in patients with reduced hepatic function, folate deficiency, bronchial asthma, severe allergy, or glucose-6-phosphate dehydroge-

nase deficiency. The drug should not be used to treat streptococcal pharyngitis because it will not eradicate the organism nor prevent complications.

INTERACTIONS
Refer to the interactions listed under sulfonamides in this chapter and under trimethoprim in Chapter 67 for potential interactions with the combination of trimethoprim and sulfamethoxazole.

■ Nursing Process

(See also Chap. 59, Nursing Process for anti-infective drugs.)

The extent of the assessment performed will be determined by the rationale for treatment. Sulfonamides are commonly used in the treatment of otitis media and urinary tract infections and as such are generally given for a short course of about 10 days. When used for other problems listed under Uses, the course of therapy is of longer duration and the consequences of therapy are greater. Therefore, initial assessment must also be more detailed.

□ ASSESSMENT

□ Subjective Data
A complete history is needed on any patient receiving a sulfonamide drug. Renal, hematologic, and hepatic disease should be ruled out, as should pregnancy. A woman should also be asked if she is nursing because sulfonamides pass through breast milk and can be damaging to the young infant. A history of diabetes should be noted, and the patient should be asked about insulin or oral hypoglycemic drug use. Sulfonamides can alter blood glucose level; therefore, antidiabetic drug doses may need to be altered during therapy. In addition, the patient should be asked to describe the course of the present symptoms to determine the appropriateness of the prescribed therapy. A medication history is also essential because sulfonamides adversely interact with a wide variety of drugs. Refer to the section on interactions earlier in this chapter to formulate questions in this area. Ask about drug allergies and previous experience with antibiotics. Many patients are allergic to sulfa drugs but may have never taken them before. If a patient reports allergies to salicylates or thiazide drugs he may be allergic to sulfonamides. Any patient with multiple

drug allergies should be treated with caution and carefully observed during initial doses.

□ *Objective Data*

If the patient is a burn victim, the burn site must be carefully assessed to provide a baseline against which to measure the effectiveness of the topical agent as well as the development of infection resistant to the drug. The size of the wound, location of eschar, presence of edema, and evidence of drainage, pus, redness, or other signs of infection are carefully recorded. A flow sheet and schematic diagram are useful for this purpose and can be referred to throughout therapy.

The extent of laboratory data collection will again be determined by the length of the therapy. Renal and hepatic function studies and hematologic evaluations should be done initially if an extended course of therapy is expected, in the elderly patient whose function may be diminished, or in anyone suspected of having problems. All patients should have a culture and sensitivity study of the infected site, in wound or urine. Urine acidity should also be tested because acidic urine may make long-acting sulfonamides insoluble.

□ *NURSING DIAGNOSES*

For many patients receiving sulfonamides the *actual* nursing diagnosis will be:

Knowledge deficit: about administration of the drug, actions of the drug, and side-effects to watch for.

Other nursing diagnoses may develop based on side-effects which can occur.

Potential nursing diagnoses for the patient taking a sulfonamide may include:

Alteration in bowel elimination: diarrhea

Alteration in breathing pattern: wheezing, if an allergic reaction occurs

Potential for infection if there is a lack of response to the drug

Noncompliance related to completion of the course of therapy; especially in an extended treatment time

Sexual dysfunction: infertility or decreased sperm count (more likely with an extended course or on sulfasalazine; usually reversible on discontinuation of therapy)

Alteration in patterns of urinary elimination related to development of crystalluria

□ *PLAN*

Nursing care goals center around assisting the patient to learn how to:

1. Take the drug correctly, noting effectiveness of therapy
2. Prevent or manage common side-effects and know which ones to report immediately.

□ *INTERVENTION*

Sulfonamides are administered by many routes (see box entitled Sulfonamides), but the most common are the oral and topical route. Orally, the drug should be taken on an empty stomach and with lots of fluids to decrease the chance of crystalluria. Some patients complain of nausea and diarrhea with sulfonamides, especially with sulfasalazine. This drug may be taken with food to decrease symptoms because absorption is not impaired. Patients on other types of sulfonamides may be able to manage gastrointestinal symptoms by switching to a long-acting formulation or by taking the drug, having something to eat within an hour of ingestion, and incorporating binding foods such as rice, bananas, and other starches into their diets to minimize diarrhea.

Topical administration of sulfonamides, specifically mafenide and silver sulfadiazine, is used for burn treatment. The drug works best if the wound is clean because its action may be slowed by pus or cell breakdown products, and it must be applied to all parts of the wound using sterile technique. Wound care of the burn victim is usually tedious and painful but is essential for tissue growth. The sulfonamide should be applied after the wound has been thoroughly cleaned. The drug may be applied by applicator, which can be messy, and may not spread evenly across the surface. It may also be applied, using sterile technique, to gauze pads or rolled gauze and then applied to the wound surface. This technique allows the nurse to prepare the gauze in advance and store it in a sterile container, minimize the amount of contact with the wound, and maximize the application of the drug to the burn site. The patient or family can also be taught this technique when wound care will be done at home.

Many patients are allergic to sulfonamide drugs so each should know signs to watch for. The nurse should also be aware that a patient receiving a parenteral sulfonamide is more likely to develop a rapid and dangerous allergic reaction. All signs of allergic reaction should be reported immediately. The patient using a topical drug may notice burning or itching at the site. The burn patient may only notice this if the drug touched undamaged skin, so a small patch of skin should be tested. Early symptoms of severe erythema multiforme, an acute sensitivity reaction, are severe headache, rash, rhinitis, and urticaria and should be reported immediately because this syndrome can be fatal.

Evidence of another serious side-effect of sulfonamides, hematologic toxicity, should also be reported immediately. Symptoms include sore throat, fever, malaise, mucosal ulceration, and jaundice, as well as bleeding tendencies. Hematologic and hepatic function studies should be done periodically on any patient receiving sulfonamides for more than 4 weeks to detect any changes early before symptoms occur.

Many patients will exhibit increased photosensitivity while on sulfonamides. The patient should be cautioned against sunbathing, because severe burns and rash can occur, and encouraged to wear protective clothing and sunglasses whenever in direct sun during therapy.

A minor side-effect of sulfonamides is a color change of urine to orange. While this is not dangerous, it may be frightening to a patient who doesn't expect it. The patient should be warned of the possibility but assured it is harmless and will disappear when the drug is discontinued.

Many organisms have become resistant to sulfonamide drugs. An organism which initially responds may become resistant during the course of therapy, or a new organism resistant to sulfonamides may emerge. This is a particular problem for the burn victim and should be closely monitored. Early signs of infection in a burn site include tissue discoloration and rapid development of edema in burn tissue and in surrounding tissue where none was evident before. Such changes should be reported immediately. In addition, wound cultures with sensitivity tests should be done periodically to ensure the drug is still effective.

□ EVALUATION

Physical outcome criteria the nurse can use to judge drug effectiveness include culture of site showing no growth; absence of side-effects; and decrease in white blood cell count, pain, fever, or other physical symptoms. Evidence of patient compliance can be seen if the patient returns for follow-up, if appropriate; if he completes the prescription; and if he reports early any side-effects of the drug.

CASE STUDY

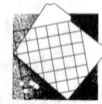

Ronnie Howell, age 2, is brought to the pediatrician by his mother. He has had cold symptoms: runny nose, congestion, and fever of around 101°F for 3 days. Today he began pulling on his ears, and he had difficulty sleeping last night. On examination the physician finds bilateral bulging of the tympanic membranes and cerumen accumulation. He diagnoses Ronnie as having bilateral otitis media and prescribes amoxicillin liquid, 125 mg PO, every 8 hours. (Ronnie weighs 35 lb.)

Two days later Mrs. Howell brings Ronnie back to the office. His fever is down, but he continues to pull on his ears and awaken in his sleep. The physician notes there is little change in the tympanic membrane bulging and decides to switch Ronnie's prescription to co-trimoxazole oral suspension (40 mg TMP/200 mg SMZ per 5 ml) 5 ml every 12 hours. Mrs. Howell expresses concern about this medication working because the other one didn't.

Discussion Question

Develop a teaching plan that incorporates strategies to deal with:
  a. Mrs. Howell's fears about the effectiveness of the drug and compliance issues
  b. The need to increase Ronnie's fluid intake
  c. Getting Ronnie to take the medication (see Chap. 8 for information on giving medicine to 2-year-old children)
  d. Side-effects of the drug

REVIEW QUESTIONS

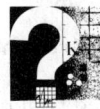

1. What are the major limitations to the use of sulfonamides in many infections?
2. How may the various sulfonamide antibiotics be categorized?
3. Briefly discuss the mechanism of action of sulfonamides.
4. What microorganisms are generally highly susceptible to the action of sulfonamides?
5. Give the principal indications for the sulfonamides.
6. What information is needed when assessing a patient about to receive a sulfonamide drug?
7. How may the likelihood of crystalluria with sulfonamides be minimized?
8. What are the most frequently encountered side-effects during sulfonamide therapy? What strategies can the nurse offer the patient to deal with them?
9. What are early signs that a burn wound is getting infected? What action is needed if the patient is already receiving mafenide topically?
10. What are the early symptoms of erythema multiforme? Why must action be taken immediately when sensitivity to sulfonamide results in such a reaction?
11. What is kernicterus? Why may use of sulfonamides in infancy lead to this condition?
12. Which sulfonamide is used orally for its local action in the colon? How does this drug act in treating symptoms of ulcerative colitis?
13. Name two sulfonamides that are applied topically in burn patients. What is the rationale for their use in this situation?
14. List the major indications for the combination of trimethoprim-sulfamethoxazole.
15. What are the advantages of such a combination over use of either drug alone?
16. In what conditions is use of trimethoprim-sulfamethoxazole contraindicated?

BIBLIOGRAPHY

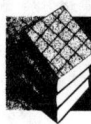

Abshagen D: Topical agents and emergency care for minor burn injuries. J Emerg Nurs 10:325, 1984

Harrison HN: Pharmacology of sulfadiazine silver. Arch Surg 114:281, 1979

Hughes WT: Trimethoprim-sulfamethoxazole. Ped Clin N Am 30:27, 1983

Keys TF: Urinary tract infection: New perspectives on diagnosis and treatment. Mod Medicine 54(6):34, 1986

Lang PG: Sulfones and sulfonamides in dermatology today. J Am Acad Dermatol 1:479, 1979

Patel RB, Welling PG: Clinical pharmacokinetics of co-trimoxazole (trimethoprim-sulphamethoxazole). Clin Pharmacokin 5:405, 1980

Robertson KE, et al: Burn care: The first crucial days. Am J Nurs 85:30, 1985

Robin RH, Swartz MN: Trimethoprim-sulfamethoxazole. N Engl J Med 303:426, 1980

Sattler FR, Remington JR: Intravenous trimethoprim-
    sulfamethoxazole therapy for *Pneumocystis carinii* pneumonia.
    Arch Intern Med 143:1709, 1983
Stamm WE: Prevention of urinary tract infections. Am J Med 76:146,
    1984
Wharton M, et al: Prospective randomized trial of trimethoprim-
    sulfamethoxazole versus pentamidine for *Pneumocystis carinii*
    pneumonia in the acquired immunodeficiency syndrome. Am Rev
    Respir Dis 129:1, 1984
Wormser GP, Keusch GT, Rennie CH: Cotrimoxazole (trimethoprim-
    sulfamethoxazole): An updated review of its antibacterial activity
    and clinical efficacy. Drugs 24:459, 1982

Penicillins, Carbapenems, and Monobactams

Penicillins
*Amdinocillin, Amoxicillin,
Ampicillin,
Azlocillin,
Bacampicillin,
Carbenicillin,
Cloxacillin,
Cyclacillin,
Dicloxacillin,
Methicillin,
Mezlocillin,
Nafcillin, Oxacillin,
Penicillin G,
Penicillin V,
Piperacillin,
Ticarcillin*

Carbapenems
Imipenem-Cilastatin

Monobactams
Aztreonam

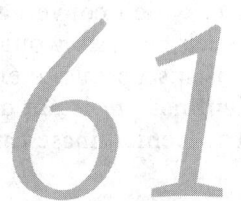

The penicillin group of antibiotics includes natural extracts from several strains of the *Penicillium* mold and a number of semisynthetic derivatives. Of the many natural fermentation products first developed in the early 1940s, penicillin G (benzylpenicillin) proved to be the most active and is still frequently used. Penicillin G, however, possesses several undesirable characteristics, such as instability in gastric acid, susceptibility to inactivation by penicillinase enzyme, rapid renal excretion, and a relatively narrow antimicrobial spectrum of action. Some of these problems have been at least partially eliminated in many of the newer semisynthetic penicillin derivatives, which represent structural modifications of the basic 6-amino-penicillanic acid nucleus. Because this nucleus contains a four-member beta-lactam ring, these drugs, together with the structurally similar cephalosporins and carbapenems are sometimes referred to as beta-lactam antibiotics. The cephalosporins are reviewed in Chapter 62, while the carbapenems are considered following the penicillins in this chapter. Another structurally unique beta-lactam related group of anti-infectives are the monobactams, which possess a very wide spectrum of activity against gram-negative organisms. These agents are also considered in this chapter.

The semisynthetic penicillins have been prepared by incorporating specific precursors into the mold cultures (*e.g.,* penicillin V) or, more commonly, by chemically replacing a side chain on the 6-aminopenicillanic nucleus, as in ampicillin. Although these chemically modified derivatives of penicillin G each possess distinct advantages in certain aspects, it must be recognized that none of these agents represents the "ideal" penicillin in terms of activity and toxicity. In fact, penicillin G, by virtue of its good antibacterial activity, minimal toxicity, and low cost is still the preferred drug for a number of infections due to susceptible organisms, especially the more common gram-positive cocci such as streptococci, gonococci, and meningococci.

Many different penicillin derivatives are currently available, differing principally in stability in gastric acid, resistance to inactivation by penicillinase (a beta-lactamase enzyme produced by many bacteria that disrupts the beta-lactam ring in the penicillin molecule, rendering the drug inactive), degree of protein binding, and spectrum of antimicrobial activity. The important characteristics of the various penicillins are outlined in Table 61-1. The usefulness of these derivatives in treating specific bacterial infections may be ascertained by ref-

erence to Chapter 59, Table 59-1, a list the preferred antimicrobial drugs for treating a number of microorganisms.

Penicillins exert their antibacterial effects by blocking biosynthesis of cell wall mucopeptide, rendering the bacteria osmotically unstable and thus unable to survive. Penicillins, in adequate concentrations, are bactericidal and are most effective when active bacterial cell multiplication is occurring. Moreover, the penicillins are virtually nontoxic toward human cells, inasmuch as these cells do not have rigid walls like those of bacteria but merely a limiting cytoplasmic membrane. The greater activity of most penicillins against gram-positive organisms opposed to gram-negative organisms is due to the higher proportion of mucopeptide in the cell walls of gram-positive bacteria and their higher internal osmotic pressure. Unlike some other antibiotics, such as sulfonamides, the activity of the penicillins is not inhibited by blood, pus, or other tissue breakdown products.

The major untoward reaction associated with use of the penicillins is hypersensitivity. This can range from mild skin rash and contact dermatitis to severe allergic reactions, including exfoliative dermatitis, serum sickness, and anaphylaxis. The incidence of allergic reactions to penicillin is higher in patients with previously demonstrated hypersensitivity to multiple allergens or a history of hay fever or asthma, and the drugs should be used with extreme caution in such persons. No one penicillin derivative is safer in this respect than any other. Penicillin-sensitive patients can also exhibit cross-sensitivity to certain other antibacterial agents, notably cephalosporins, and caution must be exercised in using cephalosporins in penicillin-sensitive patients and vice versa.

Bacterial resistance to the penicillins is variable. In spite of extensive clinical use of penicillin for over 25 years, some species of bacteria have remained uniformly susceptible (*e.g., Diplococcus pneumoniae, Neisseria meningitidis*), whereas other species have developed progressively increasing resistance. This variability in development of resistance may be explained in part by the fact that there are several mechanisms responsible for resistance to penicillins. Most commonly, resistance occurs because some bacteria (such as staphylococci) can synthesize beta-lactamase enzymes, notably penicillinase, which convert the drugs to inactive products. Such bacteria would display resistance to penicillins susceptible to enzyme activity, but not to penicillinase-resistant derivatives.

Drugs resistant to penicillinase can be synthesized either by a modification of the basic structure or by combination with a second agent which binds to the beta-lactamase enzymes and inactivates them. An example of such an enzyme-inactivating agent is clavulanic acid; this agent is now available in combination with several different penicillins ordinarily destroyed by beta-lactamases (see Table 62-2). Addition of clavulanic acid to the penicillin extends the spectrum of action of these antibiotics by protecting them against breakdown in the presence of penicillinase-secreting organisms.

Conversely, bacteria may become resistant to the action of penicillins because they lack specific receptor sites for the drugs, because their cell surfaces have become impermeable to the drugs, or because they have developed alternate metabolic pathways that avoid steps sensitive to the action of the drugs. Finally, microorganisms that lack cell walls, such as certain strains of mycoplasma, are resistant to penicillins inasmuch as the drugs act to interfere with bacterial cell wall formation, and are thus ineffective against microbes without cell walls.

The various penicillin drugs may be categorized into several classes based on their respective characteristics, such as spectrum of activity, resistance to penicillinase, and source. The major groups of penicillin drugs are briefly described below.

NATURAL PRODUCTS

1. Penicillin G—First penicillin in extensive clinical use; still considered a first-line drug against most gram-positive bacteria (except penicillinase-producing staphylococci) when given by IM injection; virtually nontoxic to human cells, thus can be given safely in large amounts; widely distributed in the body, especially following IM injections and rapidly bactericidal; very low cost; major disadvantages are irregular oral absorption, destruction by gastric acid, inactivation by penicillinase enzyme, and rather narrow antimicrobial spectrum of action. Effects may be prolonged by parenteral (IM) use of benzathine or procaine salts of penicillin G, repository forms of the drug producing lower serum blood levels but longer duration of action.

SEMISYNTHETIC DERIVATIVES

1. Penicillin V—Semisynthetic analogue of penicillin G with similar spectrum of activity; More completely absorbed orally than penicillin G and not destroyed by gastric acid, thus yielding three to five times higher blood levels; preferred over penicillin G for oral therapy of *mild* infections of the throat, upper respiratory tract, or soft tissues caused by non-penicillinase-producing staphylococci and other gram-positive cocci, but not recommended for seriously ill patients; ineffective for gonorrhea; only used orally, therefore not indicated during acute stages of serious infections with susceptible organisms, because these usually require parenteral penicillin G; potassium salt is the preferred form, because it is better absorbed than plain penicillin V.

2. Penicillinase-resistant penicillins (cloxacillin, dicloxacillin, methicillin, nafcillin, oxacillin)—Resistant to inactivation by penicillinase and are used in the treatment of infections due to penicillinase-producing *Staphylococcus aureus*; cloxacillin or dicloxacillin are indicated for oral use, because they are acid stable and well absorbed, although their GI absorption is reduced by food; parenteral methicillin, nafcillin, or oxacillin is usually employed in serious infections; all of these agents are less effective than penicillin G against non-penicillinase-producing staphylococci and other gram-positive organisms and are inactive against gram-negative organisms.

3. Broad-spectrum penicillins (amoxicillin, ampicillin, bacampicillin, cyclacillin)—Effective against a range of both gram-positive and gram-negative organisms; no real advantage over the less costly penicillin G or V in treating most gram-positive infections, but are significantly more active against many gram-negative organisms, especially *Hemophilus influenzae*, *Escherichia coli*, *Proteus mirabilis*, *Salmonella*, and *Shigella*; not effective against *Pseudomonas*, *Klebsiella*, *Enterobacter*, *Serratia*, and anaerobic organisms; frequently employed empirically as *initial* drugs where the identity of the microorganism has not been conclusively determined, for example, urinary infections, respiratory infections such as sinusitis or bronchitis, and otitis media; drugs are not resistant to penicillinase enzyme, but are all acid stable.

4. Extended-spectrum penicillins—antipseudomonal penicillins—(azlocillin, carbenicillin, mezlocillin, piperacillin, ticarcillin)—Wide antimicrobial spectrum, including *Pseudomonas* and many other gram-negative bacilli resistant to the broad-spectrum penicillins; in addition to the organisms listed under broad-

Table 61-1
Penicillins—General Characteristics

Drug	Routes of Administration	Oral Absorption	Protein Binding	Acid Stable	Penicillinase Resistant	Remarks
amdinocillin	IV, IM		5%–10%		Yes	Structurally unique penicillinase-resistant drug active against *E. coli, Klebsiella* sp., *Enterobacter* sp.; not effective vs gram (+) organisms; synergistic with other beta-lactam drugs, because mechanism is different
amoxicillin	Oral	Excellent	20%–25%	Yes	No	Similar to ampicillin but better absorbed, thus giving more rapid and higher serum levels
ampicillin	Oral, IV, IM	Good	20%–25%	Yes	No	Broad spectrum; effective against many gram (−) organisms, but no real advantage over penicillin G for most gram (+) infections
azlocillin	IV		20%–40%		No	Broad spectrum; good effectiveness against *Pseudomonas* and most other gram (−) bacilli
bacampicillin	Oral	Excellent	20%–25%	Yes	No	Rapidly hydrolyzed to ampicillin during GI absorption; peak ampicillin blood levels three times those obtained with ampicillin itself
carbenicillin	Oral, IV, IM	Good	50%	Yes	No	Broad spectrum, with high activity against most strains of *Pseudomonas*; less active than ampicillin against gram (+) bacteria
cloxacillin	Oral	Good	95%	Yes	Yes	Effective against penicillinase-producing staphylococci as well as most other gram (+) organisms

(continued)

spectrum penicillins, above, carbenicillin and ticarcillin are also effective against *Pseudomonas*, several *Proteus* species, *Citrobacter*, *Enterobacter*, *Bacteroides*, *Peptococcus*, and *Serratia*; azlocillin, mezlocillin, and piperacillin have the broadest *in vitro* spectrum of all penicillins, including *Klebsiella, Acinetobacter, Shigella* and contain less than one-half the sodium content of carbenicillin and ticarcillin. Their activity is nearly comparable to that of the aminoglycosides, but they are considerably less toxic; extended-spectrum penicillins are not penicillinase-resistant.

5. Amidinopenicillin (amdinocillin)—Possesses good activity against *E. coli, Klebsiella, Enterobacter, Serratia, Salmonella,* and *Shigella. Not* active against gram-positive organisms or anaerobes; binds to different proteins than other penicillins and thus has a synergistic effect with other beta-lactam drugs; action is primarily bacteriostatic, although drug attains high levels in urinary tract, which provide a bactericidal action.

The discussion of the penicillins focuses on these agents as a group, inasmuch as the basic pharmacology and toxicology of all derivatives are identical.

Table 61-1 (continued)
Penicillins—General Characteristics

Drug	Routes of Administration	Oral Absorption	Protein Binding	Acid Stable	Penicillinase Resistant	Remarks
cyclacillin	Oral	Excellent	20%	Yes	No	Broad spectrum but somewhat less active than ampicillin in spite of higher peak blood levels
dicloxacillin	Oral	Good	95%–98%	Yes	Yes	Similar to but slightly more active than cloxacillin or oxacillin
methicillin	IV, IM		40%–50%	Yes		Parenteral antibiotic active against penicillinase-producing staphylococci but less effective than penicillin G against most other gram (+) infections
mezlocillin	IV, IM		20%–40%	No		Broad spectrum; highly active against *Enterobacter*; good activity versus most other gram (−) organisms
nafcillin	Oral, IV, IM	Fair	90%	Yes	Yes	Highly resistant to penicillinase but erratically absorbed orally; good activity against gram (+) organisms
oxacillin	Oral, IV, IM	Good	90%–95%	Yes	Yes	Similar to cloxacillin; most effective when given parenterally
penicillin G	Oral, IV, IM	Poor	50%–60%	No	No	Highly active against gram (+) bacteria; much less active against gram (−) organisms
penicillin V	Oral	Good	80%–90%	Yes	No	Similar to penicillin G; much more reliably absorbed but less potent
piperacillin	IV, IM		20%–40%	No		Broad spectrum; very effective against *Pseudomonas* and *Enterobacter*; uniformly active against gram (−) bacilli
ticarcillin	IV, IM		45%–50%	No		Broad spectrum, including *Pseudomonas, Serratia, Citrobacter*; only effective parenterally

Drugs are listed in Table 61-2, where appropriate dosages and individual characteristics are given.

Penicillins

Amdinocillin, Amoxicillin, Ampicillin, Azlocillin, Bacampicillin, Carbenicillin, Cloxacillin, Cyclacillin,

Dicloxacillin, Methicillin, Mezlocillin, Nafcillin, Oxacillin, Penicillin G, Penicillin V, Piperacillin, Ticarcillin

MECHANISM AND ACTIONS

Penicillins inhibit the synthesis of bacterial cell wall mucopeptide, thus rendering the cells osmotically unstable. The high internal osmotic pressure then causes the cells to swell and burst. Cellular lysis is also facilitated by inactivation of inhibitors of autolytic enzymes in the bacterial cell wall. The

(Text continues on p. 1184.)

Table 61-2
Penicillins

Drug	Preparations	Usual Dosage Range	Clinical Considerations
penicillin G, potassium or sodium (Pentids, Pfizerpen, and various other manufacturers)	Tablets—200,000 U, 250,000 U, 400,000 U, 500,000 U, 800,000 U Powder for oral solution—200,000 U/5 ml, 400,000 U/5 ml. Powder for injection—200,000 U/vial, 500,000 U/vial; 1-, 5-, 10-, 20-million U/vial *Note:* 400,000 U = 250 mg	Adults: Oral—200,000 U to 500,000 U every 6 h–8 h for at least 10 days IM, IV—300,000 U to 8 million U daily (some severe infections [*e.g.*, meningococcal meningitis, gram (−) bacteremia, clostridial infections] may require up to 20 million to 30 million U/day) Children under age 12: Oral—25,000 U to 90,000 U/kg/day in three to six divided doses IM, IV—300,000 U to 1.2 million U/day in divided doses (up to 10 million U/day may be required)	Natural penicillin preparation derived from the *Penicillium* mold; considered drug of choice for treating infections due to susceptible organisms such as staphylococci; also effective against *Bacillus anthracis, Listeria monocytogenes, Neisseria gonorrhoeae, Treponema pallidum,* and several other microorganisms (see Table 59-1); rapid-acting, inexpensive, and very effective against many organisms, but destroyed by gastric acid and penicillinase; administer orally on an empty stomach; refrigerate reconstituted oral solution and discard within 14 days; do not use oral penicillin G as prophylaxis for genitourinary instrumentation or surgery, sigmoidoscopy, or childbirth; IM is the preferred parenteral route; keep injection volume small and inject deeply into a large muscle mass; maximal plasma concentrations are attained within 30 minutes to 60 minutes; doses exceeding 10 million U/day must be given by IV infusion only; administer large doses slowly, because electrolyte overload may occur depending on which salt is used; use extreme caution in renal insufficiency; half-life (normally 30 min) increases to 10 h in patients with anuria; perform periodic serum electrolyte determinations during high-dose therapy and be alert for symptoms of hyperkalemia (hyperreflexia, convulsions, arrhythmias) when using potassium salts

(continued)

Table 61-2 (continued)
Penicillins

Drug	Preparations	Usual Dosage Range	Clinical Considerations
pencillin G, benzathine (Bicillin L.A., Permapen)	Tablets—200,000 U Injection—300,000 U/ml, 600,000 U/ml, 1,200,000 U/dose, 2,400,000 U/dose	Adults: Oral—400,000 U to 600,000 U every 4 h–6 h IM—1,200,000 U as a single injection Children under age 12: Oral—25,000 U to 90,000 U/kg/day in three to six divided doses IM—600,000 U to 1,200,000 U depending on weight Syphilis (early): 2.4 million units IM as a single dose Syphilis (of more than 1 year's duration: 2.4 million U IM/wk for three successive weeks Prophylaxis of rheumatic fever: 200,000 U orally twice a day, 1.2 million U IM once a month, or 600,000 U IM every 2 wk	Benzathine salt of penicillin G providing a slowly absorbed and hence long-acting dosage form; oral preparations are less effective than IM forms due to unpredictable GI absorption; use a large-gauge needle for administration, inject deeply into a large muscle, and do not massage injection site; not for IV or SC use; when high sustained serum levels of penicillin are desired, use aqueous penicillin G, because benzathine salt provides fairly low serum concentrations; in small children, divide dose between two injection sites if necessary
penicillin G, procaine (Crysticillin A.S., Duracillin A.S., Pfizerpen-AS, Wycillin)	Injection—300,000 U/ml, 500,000 U/ml Injection—300,000 U; 600,000 U; 1.2-, 2.4-million U per unit dose	600,000 U to 1.2 million U every 1 day to 3 days Gonorrheal infections: 1 g probenecid followed by 4.8 million U divided into two doses and injected at different sites	Long-acting form of penicillin G, similar to benzathine penicillin G in most respects; indicated in moderately severe infections due to organisms (*e.g.*, pneumococci, streptococci) sensitive to persistent low serum levels of penicillin G; may also be effective in treating syphilis, acute pelvic inflammatory disease, diphtheria, anthrax, Vincent's gingivitis, and for perioperative prophylaxis against bacterial endocarditis; only given IM; contains procaine, which provides for slow release and absorption of penicillin; may be allergenic; procaine may impart a local anesthetic effect, making injections less painful than benzathine preparation; single-dose therapy for gonorrhea has elicited anxiety, confusion, depression, hallucinations, seizures, and ex- *(continued)*

Table 61-2 (continued)
Penicillins

Drug	Preparations	Usual Dosage Range	Clinical Considerations
penicillin G, procaine (Crysticillin A.S., Duracillin A.S., Pfizerpen-AS, Wycillin) *(continued)*			treme weakness; also available in a combination package with probenecid tablets, which delay the excretion of penicillin G
penicillin G, benzathine and procaine combined (Bicillin C-R)	Injection—150,000 U–150,000 U; 300,000 U–300,000 U; 600,000 U–600,000 U; 900,000 U–300,000 U; per ml each, respectively, benzathine and procaine penicillin G	Streptococcal infections: Adults—2.4 million U IM Children (30 to 60 lb)—900,000 to 1.2 million U IM Children (under 30 lb)—600,000 U IM Pneumococcal infections: 600,000 U in children or 1.2 million U in adults every 2 days to 3 days until patient is afebrile for 48 hours	Combination of long-acting forms of penicillin G, used to treat moderate to severe streptococcal and pneumococcal infections sensitive to the serum levels attainable with this drug formulation, *eg,* upper respiratory tract, skin and soft tissues, erysipelas; only administered IM; not effective against streptococcal group D; do not use in venereal diseases; see benzathine penicillin G and procaine penicillin G
penicillin V; penicillin V, potassium (Pen-Vee-K, V-Cillin-K, and various other manufacturers)	Tablets—125 mg, 250 mg, 500 mg Powder for oral suspension —125 mg/5 ml, 250 mg/5 ml Powder for oral solution (potassium salt)—125 mg/5 ml, 250 mg/5ml	Adults—125 mg to 500 mg every 6 h–8 h depending on severity of infection Children—25 mg to 50 mg/kg/day in three to six divided doses *Prevention of bacterial endocarditis:* Adults—2 g, 30 min–60 min prior to procedure, then 1 g every 6 h for eight doses Children—1 g, 30 min–60 min prior to procedure, then 500 mg every 6 h for eight doses	Phenoxymethyl derivative of penicillin G, with identical range of activity but more resistant to inactivation by gastric acid, hence better absorbed, yielding two to five times higher blood levels; potassium salt is preferred due to better overall GI absorption; only used orally for mild infections of the throat, respiratory tract, or soft tissue due to streptococci, pneumococci, and susceptible staphylococci; also useful to prevent bacterial endocarditis in patients with rheumatic or acquired valvular heart disease about to undergo surgery or dental procedures; not indicated as initial therapy when parenteral penicillins are necessary (*e.g.,* in severe infections); highly bound to plasma proteins; rapidly excreted in the urine; effective when given with food, but blood levels are higher if administered on an empty stomach

(continued)

Table 61-2 (continued)
Penicillins

Drug	Preparations	Usual Dosage Range	Clinical Considerations
Penicillinase-Resistant Penicillins			
cloxacillin (Cloxapen, Tegopen)	Capsules—250 mg, 500 mg Powder for oral solution—125 mg/5 ml	Adults—250 mg to 1 g every 6 h Children—50 mg to 100 mg/kg/day in divided doses every 6 h	Primarily used to treat infections caused by penicillinase-producing staphylococci; may also be used to initiate therapy in patients in whom a staphylococcal infection is suspected; somewhat less effective than penicillin G against most other gram (+) cocci; best absorbed from an empty stomach; highly protein-bound
dicloxacillin (Dicloxacil, Dycill, Dynapen, Pathocil)	Capsules—125 mg, 250 mg, 500 mg Powder for oral suspension—62.5 mg/5 ml	Adults—125 mg to 250 mg every 6 h (maximum 4 g/day) Children under 40 kg—12.5 mg to 25 mg/kg/day in divided doses every 6 h	Similar to cloxacillin and oxacillin, but producing slightly higher plasma levels than equivalent doses of these other related penicillins; do not use in neonates; see under cloxacillin for indications
methicillin (Staphcillin)	Powder for injection—1-g, 4-g, 6-g, 10-g vials	Adults: IM/IV infusion—4 g to 12 g/day in divided doses every 4 h–6 h Children: 100 to 300 mg/kg/day in divided doses every 4 h–6 h Infants: 50 to 150 mg/kg/day in divided doses every 6 h–12 hr	Indications are similar to those for cloxacillin but used by injection only; considerably less active than penicillin G against streptococci and pneumococci; acid labile and therefore used by injection only; well tolerated by deep IM injection, slow IV injection, or continuous IV infusion; observe injection sites for signs of irritation, inflammation, or hypersensitivity; be alert for development of drug-induced febrile reactions with IV administration; drug has produced interstitial nephritis within 2 wk–4 wk of start of therapy; observe for early indications (*e.g.*, cloudy urine, oliguria, spiking fever) and discontinue drug; achieves high levels in the CSF; methicillin is incompatible in solution with a wide range of drugs; do not mix with other drugs, including antibiotics but administer

(continued)

Table 61-2 (continued)
Penicillins

Drug	Preparations	Usual Dosage Range	Clinical Considerations
Penicillinase-Resistant Penicillins (continued)			
methicillin (Staphcillin) (continued)			separately; carefully follow instructions on container when diluting powder for injection; higher concentrations (10 mg–30 mg/ml) are stable for 8 h at room temperature, but weaker dilutions (2 mg/ml) are only stable for 4 h
nafcillin (Nafcil, Nallpen, Unipen)	Capsules—250 mg Tablets—500 mg Powder for oral solution— 250 mg/5 ml Powder for injection—500-mg, 1-g, 2-g, 4-g, 10-g vials	Adults: Oral—250 mg to 1 g every 4 h–6 h depending on severity of infection IM—500 mg every 4 h–6 h IV—500 mg to 1 g every 4 h Children: Oral—50 mg/kg/day in four divided doses Scarlet fever/pneumonia: 25 mg/kg/day in four divided doses Neonates: IM—10 mg/kg twice a day	Penicillinase-resistant penicillin with same indications as cloxacillin; oral absorption is inferior to that of other similar penicillins; major route of elimination is by way of the bile; parenteral therapy is indicated initially in severe infections; change to oral therapy should be made as condition warrants; not as active as penicillin G against nonpenicillinase-producing organisms; for IV use, dilute powder in 15 ml to 30 ml sterile water for injection or sodium chloride injection and inject over 5 min–10 min; avoid extravasation because tissue necrosis can occur; IV injection may result in thrombophlebitis; limit therapy to 48 h; reconstitute solution for IM injection with sterile or bacteriostatic water for injection; administer immediately by deep intragluteal injection; solution may be kept refrigerated for up to 48 h
oxacillin (Bactocill, Prostaphlin)	Capsules—250 mg, 500 mg Powder for oral solution— 250 mg/5 ml Powder for injection—250-mg, 500-mg, 1-g, 2-g, 4-g, 10-g vials	Adults: Oral—500 mg to 1 g every 4 h–6 h for a minimum of 7 days depending on severity of infection IM, IV—250 mg to 1 g every 4 h–6 h depending on severity of infection Children under 40 kg:	Penicillinase-resistant drug, similar in most respects to cloxacillin and dicloxacillin, but slightly less potent orally, highly protein bound; in serious infections parenteral therapy is indicated, because oral absorption may be unreli- *(continued)*

Table 61-2 (continued)
Penicillins

Drug	Preparations	Usual Dosage Range	Clinical Considerations
Penicillinase-Resistant Penicillins (continued)			
oxacillin (Bactocill, Prostaphlin) *(continued)*		Oral—50 mg to 100 mg/kg/day in divided doses IM, IV—50 mg to 100 mg/kg/day in divided doses	able; following initial control of infection, oral therapy may then be substituted; drug should be taken on an empty stomach; solutions for IM or IV use should be prepared by diluting powder with sterile water for injection or sodium chloride injection; discard unused IM injection after 3 days at room temperature or 7 days with refrigeration; consult package for suitable diluents for IV infusion solutions; at concentrations of 0.5 mg to 40 mg/ml, dilutions are stable for approximately 6 h–8 h at room temperature; adjust rate of infusion to deliver intended drug dose within this time; transient elevations in serum enzymes (SGOT, SGPT, LDH) may occur with oxacillin; high doses have resulted in transient hematuria, proteinuria, and azotemia in infants
Broad-Spectrum Penicillins			
amoxicillin (Amoxil, Larotid, Polymox, Trimox, Utimox, Wymox)	Capsules—250 mg, 500 mg Chewable tablets—125 mg, 250 mg Powder for oral suspension—125 mg/5 ml, 250 mg/5 ml Drops—50 mg/ml	Adults and children over 20 kg—250 mg to 500 mg every 8 h Chilren under 20 kg—20 to 40 mg/kg/day in divided doses every 8 h Uncomplicated gonorrhea (Adults): 3 g with 1 g oral probenecid as a single dose Disseminated gonococcal infection: As above, followed by 500 mg oral amoxicillin four times a day for 7 days to 10 days Pelvic inflammatory disease: As above, followed by 100 mg oral doxycycline twice daily for 10 to 14 days	Broad-spectrum, acid-stable penicillin rapidly and completely absorbed from the GI tract; absorption is not significantly affected by food; activity similar to ampicillin but less effective against *Shigella*; widely used in acute otitis media due to *Hemophilus*, although resistant strains are emerging; also effective against *E. coli, Proteus, Neisseria gonorrhoeae*, streptococci, pneumococci, and non-penicillinase-producing staphylococci; less likely to disturb GI flora than ampicillin; often used as initial therapy before culture and sensitiv- *(continued)*

Table 61-2 (continued)
Penicillins

Drug	Preparations	Usual Dosage Range	Clinical Considerations
Broad-Spectrum Penicillins (continued)			
amoxicillin (Amoxil, Laro-tid, Polymox, Trimox, Utimox, Wymox) (continued)			ity tests because of broad spectrum of action; no more effective than penicillin G or V against susceptible gram (+) organisms; available in combination with potassium clavulanate (see below)
amoxicillin and potassium clavulanate (Augmentin)	Tablets—250 mg, 500 mg with 125 mg clavulanic acid (as potassium salt) Chewable tablets—125 mg, 250 mg with 31.25 mg and 62.5 mg clavulanic acid (as potassium salt) respectively Powder for suspension—125 mg/5 ml (with 31.25 mg clavulanic acid) and 250 mg/5 ml (with 62.5 mg clavulanic acid)	(Dose is given as amoxicillin equivalent) Adults—250 mg to 500 mg every 8 h Children—20 mg/kg/day to 40 mg/kg/day in divided doses every 8 h Pelvic inflammatory disease —500 mg three times a day for 10 days with doxycycline, 100 mg twice a day	Contains the potassium salt of clavulanic acid, a beta-lactam that inactivates beta-lactamase enzymes which destroy amoxicillin; combination serves to protect amoxicillin from degradation by beta-lactamase enzymes produced by certain bacteria thereby extending the spectrum of action of amoxicillin to include organisms normally resistant to the drug (*e.g.*, *Klebsiella*, beta-lactamase-producing strains of *Hemophilus, E. coli, Branhamella catarrhalis,* and staphylococci). Both 250-mg and 500-mg oral tablets contain the same amount of clavulanic acid; thus two 250-mg tablets are *not* equivalent to one 500-mg tablet
ampicillin (Amcill, Omnipen, Polycillin, Principen, Totacillin, and various other manufacturers)	Capsules—250 mg, 500 mg Capsules with probenecid —389 mg/111 mg Powder for oral suspension —125 mg/5 ml, 250 mg/5 ml, 500 mg/5 ml Drops—100 mg/ml Oral suspension with probenecid—3.5 g/1 g per bottle Powder for injection (sodium salt)—125-mg, 250-mg, 500-mg, 1-g, 2-g, 10-g vials	Respiratory and soft tissue infections: *Adults* Oral—250 mg every 6 h IM, IV—250 mg to 500 mg every 6 h *Children under 40 kg* Oral—50 mg/kg/day in divided doses IM, IV—25 mg to 50 mg/kg/day in divided does GI and urinary infections: *Adults* Oral, IM, IV—500 mg every 6 h *Children under 40 kg* Oral—100 mg/kg/day in divided doses IM, IV—50 mg/kg/day in divided doses	Broad-spectrum penicillin widely used in respiratory, GI, urinary, and soft tissue infections primarily due to susceptible strains of *E. coli, Hemophilus influenzae, Proteus mirabilis, Neisseria gonorrhoeae, Shigella, Salmonella,* and enterococci; skin rash can occur, especially in patients with mononucleosis or hyperuricemia; parenteral form should be used only for severe infections or in patients unable to take oral medications; treatment should be continued 48 h–72 h after symptoms have dis-

(continued)

Table 61-2 (continued)
Penicillins

Drug	Preparations	Usual Dosage Range	Clinical Considerations
Broad-Spectrum Penicillins (continued)			
ampicillin (Amcill, Omnipen, Polycillin, Principen, Totacillin, and various other manufacturers) (continued)		Bacterial meningitis and septicemia: *Adults and children*—150 mg to 200 mg/kg/day in divided doses every 3 h–4 h; begin with IV administration, then continue with IM. Gonorrheal urethritis: 3.5 g with 1 g probenecid orally or 500 mg IM every 8 h–12 h. Gonorrhea: 3.5 g with 1 g probenecid orally as single dose. Disseminated gonococcal infection: As above, followed by 500 mg oral ampicillin four times a day for 7 days. Pelvic inflammatory disease: As above, followed by 100 mg oral doxycycline twice a day for 14 days. Prevention of bacterial endocarditis: 1 g IM or IV plus gentamicin 1.5 mg/kg; give initial doses 30 min–60 min prior to procedure and then two additional doses every 8 h thereafter	appeared; administer on an empty stomach to enhance GI absorption; during extended therapy (*e.g.*, chronic urinary infections), frequent bacteriologic tests should be performed and sufficient doses must be given; clinical and bacteriologic follow-up should be maintained for several months after cessation of therapy; use only freshly prepared solutions for parenteral administration, dilute according to package directions with suitable diluent, and use within 1 h after preparation; powder for injection contains 3 mEq sodium/g
ampicillin and sulbactam sodium (Unasyn)	Powder for injection—1 g ampicillin/0.5 g sulbactam; 2 g ampicillin/1 g sulbactam	(Dosage given in ampicillin equivalents) 1 g–2 g ampicillin IV or IM every 6 h (maximum 4 g/day). Reduce frequency of dosing in patients with renal impairment.	Sulbactam inhibits a wide range of beta-lactamases found in many microorganisms, thereby extending the spectrum of action of ampicillin to include many bacteria normally resistant to it (*e.g.*, beta-lactamase-producing strains of *E. coli, Klebsiella, Enterobacter, Proteus, Bacteroides*, and *Staph. aureus*). Pain at injection site occurs frequently; both drugs are eliminated largely unchanged in the urine—caution in kidney impairment.
bacampicillin (Spectrobid)	Tablets—400 mg Powder for oral suspension —125 mg/5 ml	Upper respiratory, urinary and skin infections: *Adults*—400 mg to 800 mg every 12 h	Rapidly hydrolyzed to ampicillin during GI absorption; each tablet equivalent to 280 mg ampicil-*(continued)*

Table 61-2 (continued)
Penicillins

Drug	Preparations	Usual Dosage Range	Clinical Considerations
Broad-Spectrum Penicillins (continued)			
bacampicillin (Spectrobid) (continued)		Lower respiratory infections: 800 mg every 12 h. Gonorrhea: 1.6 g with 1 g probenecid as a single dose. Children—25 mg to 50 mg/kg/day in two equally divided does	lin; more completely absorbed than ampicillin, yielding effective serum levels for up to 12 h; much more costly than ampicillin; see under ampicillin for additional remarks; do not administer with disulfiram; may be given without regard to meals
cyclacillin (Cyclapen-W)	Tablets—250 mg, 500 mg. Powder for oral suspension—125 mg/5 ml, 250 mg/5 ml	Adults—250 mg to 500 mg four times a day in equally spaced doses. Children—125 mg to 250 mg three to four times a day in equally spaced doses	Broad-spectrum agent, rapidly and completely absorbed when taken orally; peak serum levels within 30 min; rapidly excreted in the urine; dosage frequency must be reduced in renal impairment; spectrum of action is virtually identical to ampicillin; indicated for treatment of bronchitis, pneumonia, upper respiratory infections, urinary infection, and otitis media due to susceptible organisms; not used in children under 2 months; somewhat lower incidence of skin rash and diarrhea than with ampicillin or amoxicillin; should *not* be used for infections caused by *Escherichia coli* or *Proteus mirabilis* other than urinary tract infections
Extended-Spectrum Penicillins			
azlocillin (Azlin)	Powder for injection—2-g, 3-g, 4-g vials	Urinary infections: IV only—100 mg to 200 mg/kg/day (2 g–3 g every 6 h). Serious systemic infections: 200 mg to 300 mg/kg/day in four to six divided doses (3 g every 4 h). Life-threatening infections: Up to 350 mg/kg/day (4 g every 4 h)	Extended-spectrum antipseudomonal penicillin used either by slow IV injection (over 5 min–10 min) or by IV infusion (30 min); very effective *in vitro* against *Pseudomonas, Proteus, Salmonella,* and *Acinetobacter*; rapid IV administration has elicited transient chest discomfort; contains 2.17 mEq/g of sodium, less than one-half the amount in carbenicil- *(continued)*

Table 61-2 (continued)
Penicillins

Drug	Preparations	Usual Dosage Range	Clinical Considerations
Extended-Spectrum Penicillins *(continued)*			
azlocillin (Azlin) *(continued)*			lin or ticarcillin; dosage should be reduced in patients with significant renal impairment; synergistic with aminoglycosides against pseudomonal infections but must be administered in a separate syringe; solutions are stable at room temperature for 24 h; to minimize venous irritation, do not use solutions more concentrated than 10%; bile levels of drug are 10 to 15 times greater than serum levels— danger in biliary obstruction; drug may depress serum uric acid level; in immunosuppressed patients, azlocillin is combined with a cephalosporin or aminoglycoside
carbenicillin disodium (Geopen)	Powder for injection—1-g, 2-g, 5-g vials; 2-g, 5-g, 10-g piggyback units; 10 g, 20-g, 30-g bulk packages	Urinary infections: Adults—200 mg/kg/day IV drip or 1 g to 2 g IM or IV every 6 h Children—50 mg to 200 mg/kg/day IM or IV in divided doses Soft tissue or respiratory infections, septicemia: Adults—15 g to 40 g daily IV in divided doses or by continuous drip Children—250 mg to 500 mg/kg/day IM or IV in divided doses (maximum dose 40 g/day) Gonorrhea: 1 g probenecid orally followed in 1 h by 4 g carbenicillin IM Presence of renal insufficiency: (creatinine clearance less than 5 ml/min)—2 g IV every 8 h–12 h	Extended-spectrum penicillin especially effective against many gram (−) organisms such as *Pseudomonas, Proteus, Acinetobacter, Escherichia, Salmonella,* and *Enterobacter;* attains very high levels in urine when given IM or IV; most *Klebsiella* and some *Pseudomonas* species are resistant; clinical efficacy is enhanced by combination with gentamicin or tobramycin, especially against *Pseudomonas* and *Providencia;* may elicit increased bleeding tendencies associated with abnormal coagulation tests; be alert for signs of hemorrhage (bruising, petechiae); fairly high in sodium content; monitor serum electrolytes during extended administration; use very cautiously in patients with impaired renal function; IV therapy is recommended for

(continued)

Table 61-2 (continued)
Penicillins

Drug	Preparations	Usual Dosage Range	Clinical Considerations
Extended-Spectrum Penicillins (continued)			
carbenicillin disodium (Geopen) (continued)			serious urinary or systemic infections; IM injections should not exceed 2 g/dose and are given well into the body of a large muscle (*e.g.*, gluteus or mid-lateral thigh); reconstitute solutions according to package directions and discard unused solutions after 24 h at room temperature (72 h in refrigerator); do not mix carbenicillin and gentamicin together in the same IV fluid; administer separately
carbenicillin indanyl sodium (Geocillin)	Tablets—382 mg	382 mg to 764 mg four times a day	Indanyl ester of carbenicillin, suitable for oral use; primarily indicated for acute and chronic upper and lower urinary tract infections and prostatitis, due to *Escherichia coli*, *Proteus*, *Pseudomonas*, *Enterobacter*, and *Enterococcus*; readily absorbed orally and hydrolyzed to carbenicillin, which is rapidly excreted in the urine, attaining high levels
mezlocillin (Mezlin)	Powder for injection—1-g, 2-g, 3-g, 4-g vials or infusion bottles	Adults: IV—1.5 g to 4 g every 4 h–6 h depending on the severity of infection (life-threatening infections—4 g every 4 h) IM—1.5 g to 2 g every 6 h Acute gonococcal urethritis: 1 g to 2 g, as a single IV or IM injection, together with 1 g probenecid orally Prevention of postoperative infection in contaminated surgery—4 g IV 1 h before surgery, and again 6 h and 12 h after surgery Children: IV, IM—75 mg/kg every 6 h–8 h (neonates—75 mg/kg every 12 h)	Similar in activity to piperacillin, but somewhat less effective against *Pseudomonas*; may be used with an aminoglycoside or cephalosporin in severe infections in cases in which the causative agent is unknown; do not inject more than 2 g IM, and give slowly (15 sec) well into the body of a large muscle mass; inject IV over a period of 3 min–5 min (concentration of drug in solution should not exceed 10% to minimize venous irritation); IV infusion should be given over 30 min; follow package directions for mixing and diluting, for dosage reductions in pa- *(continued)*

Table 61-2 (continued)
Penicillins

Drug	Preparations	Usual Dosage Range	Clinical Considerations
Extended-Spectrum Penicillins (continued)			
mezlocillin (Mezlin) (continued)			tients with impaired renal function (based on creatinine clearance), and for compatibility and stability data; low sodium content (1.85 mEq/g)
piperacillin (Pipracil)	Powder for injection—2-g, 3-g, 4-g vials or infusion bottles; 40 g per bulk vial	**Adults:** 3 g to 4 g every 4 h–6 h over 20 min–30 min (maximum 24 g/day) **Uncomplicated gonorrheal infection:** 2 g IM in a single dose with 1 g probenecid ½ h before injection **Prophylaxis during surgery:** 2 g IV just prior to surgery, 2 g during or immediately following surgery and 2 g 6 h—12 h following surgery	Extended-spectrum penicillin, used IM or IV for treatment of a variety of gram (+) and gram (−) infections; similar to mezlocillin in spectrum of activity and efficacy; synergistic with aminoglycosides against *Pseudomonas aeruginosa*, but do not mix in the same bottle because aminoglycoside will be inactivated; sodium content (1.88 mEq/g) is lower than that of carbenicillin or ticarcillin; reduce dose in patients with renal impairment according to creatinine clearance values; not recommended for use in children under age 12; maximum adult daily dosage is 24 g; do not inject more than 2 g at any one IM injection site; refer to package insert for mixing diluting, and storage instructions; solutions are stable for 24 h at room temperature, and up to 1 wk refrigerated
ticarcillin (Ticar)	Powder for injection—1-g, 3-g, 6-g vials; 20-g, 30-g bulk vials	**Adults:** IV infusion—150 mg to 300 mg/kg/day in divided doses every 3 h–6 h IV, IM injection—1 g every 6 h **Children:** IV infusion—150 mg to 300 mg/kg/day in divided doses every 4 h–6 h IV, IM injection—50 mg to 100 mg/kg/day in divided doses every 6 h–8 h **Neonates:** Under 7 days:	Extended-spectrum penicillin, not absorbed when taken orally; similar in activity to carbenicillin, but more active against most strains of *Pseudomonas*; synergistic with gentamicin and tobramycin against *Pseudomonas* organisms; high in sodium content, therefore monitor serum electrolytes during prolonged therapy and use with caution in sodium-restricted

(continued)

Table 61-2 (continued)
Penicillins

Drug	Preparations	Usual Dosage Range	Clinical Considerations
Extended-Spectrum Penicillins (continued)			
ticarcillin (Ticar) *(continued)*		150 to 225 mg/kg/day in divided doses every 8 h–12 h by IM injection or IV infusion Over 7 days: 225 to 300 mg/kg/day in divided doses every 8 h by IM injection or IV infusion	patients; IM injections should not exceed 2 g/dose; children weighing more than 40 kg should receive the adult dose; administer IM deeply into large muscle mass; discard IM solutions after 24 h at room temperature or 72 h if refrigerated; inject slowly IV to avoid vein irritation; reduce dosage according to package instructions in patients with renal insufficiency based on creatinine clearance; do not mix ticarcillin and gentamicin or tobramycin in same solution, because latter drugs may be inactivated; available with potassium clavulanate (see below)
ticarcillin and potassium clavulanate (Timentin)	Powder for injection—3 g ticarcillin and 0.1 g clavulanic acid (as potassium salt) per vial	Adults—3.1 g ticarcillin/ 0.1 g clavulanic acid every 4 h–6 h by IV infusion Children (over 12)—200 mg/kg/day to 300 mg/kg/day (ticarcillin content) in divided doses every 4 h–6 h	Combination of ticarcillin and potassium salt of clavulanic acid which protects ticarcillin from destruction by beta-lactamase enzymes produced by certain bacteria, thereby extending its spectrum of action. Use in children under age 12 has not been established; dose must be reduced in *(continued)*

activated enzymes then destroy the integrity of the cell.

The initial step in the penicillin reaction appears to be binding of the drugs to cellular receptor proteins which are several in number. Receptor affinity differs for different penicillins; thus, while most derivatives bind to proteins 1B and 3, amdinocillin appears to preferentially bind to protein 2, and may therefore exert an additive effect with other penicillins. Upon binding to cellular proteins, penicillins inhibit the action of enzymes necessary for the formation of cell wall peptidoglycans, substances that provide rigidity to the cellular wall by virtue of their latticework-like arrangement.

In adequate concentrations, penicillins are bactericidal and are most effective during stages of active multiplication when peptidoglycan synthesis is occurring. Less than optimal concentrations of these drugs may exert only a bacteriostatic action.

Gram-positive microorganisms possess much larger amounts of peptidoglycan in their cell walls than gram-negative organisms, and these walls are up to fifty times thicker. The greater susceptibility of some gram-positive organisms to penicillins

Table 61-2 (continued)
Penicillins

Drug	Preparations	Usual Dosage Range	Clinical Considerations
Extended-Spectrum Penicillins (continued)			
ticarcillin and potassium clavulanate (Timentin) (continued)			presence of renal impairment; solutions are stable up to 6 h at room temperature and up to 72 h if refrigerated; drug is reconstituted for infusion with either sterile water for injection or sodium chloride injection
Amidinopenicillins			
amdinocillin (Coactin)	Powder for injection—500-mg, 1-g vials	Adults—60 mg/kg/day in divided doses by IM injection or IV infusion over 15 min–30 min. In combination with other beta-lactam antibiotics or in patients with renal impairment, reduce dose to 40 mg/kg/day in divided doses	Chemically unique penicillin primarily used in serious urinary tract infections caused by susceptible strains of *E. coli*, *Klebsiella* sp. and *Enterobacter* sp. Synergistic with other beta-lactam antibiotics due to different mechanisms of action (see general discussion under Mechanism and Actions). Penicillinase resistant and minimally protein bound; no demonstrated activity against gram (+) organisms or anaerobes; when used in combination with another anti-infective drug, administer by separate means; may be given IM into a large muscle mass; safety and efficacy in children under 12 have not been established

compared to gram-negative organisms is the result of several factors, including the relative amounts of cell wall peptidoglycans, increased affinity of cellular receptors for the drugs, and higher internal osmotic pressure, which causes rupture of the cells as the cell wall is weakened.

USES

The various penicillins are used against a wide range of microorganisms depending on their microbial spectrum of action and on the susceptibility of the organism to the drug.

The principal clinical indications for the individual penicillins are given in Table 61-2 under Clinical Considerations. In addition, Table 59-1 lists the drugs of choice for most infections, and many of the penicillins are recognized as either first or second choice agents for a number of infectious states.

ADMINISTRATION AND DOSAGE
See Table 61-2.

FATE
The oral absorption of penicillins ranges from excellent (amoxicillin, bacampicillin, cyclacillin) to fair or poor (penicillin G, nafcillin); the other oral

drugs are reasonably well absorbed by the oral route although absorption is usually retarded in the presence of food (except for amoxicillin, bacampicillin, and penicillin V).

Following IM injection, most drugs yield rapid and high serum levels, except for the procaine and benzathine salts of penicillin G, which provide lower blood levels but more prolonged effects. Peak serum levels following oral absorption generally occur within 1 hour to 2 hours.

The drugs diffuse readily into most body tissues. Tissue levels equal serum levels at most sites except the CNS and the eye, where significant penetration occurs only when the meninges are inflamed. The penicillins are protein-bound to varying extent, ranging from 5% with amdinocillin to 98% with dicloxacillin. Penicillin V and oxacillin are the only derivatives metabolized to any extent; the others are rapidly excreted, largely in an unchanged form in the urine. Elimination half-life is less than 1 hour for most of these drugs, although it is slightly longer for ampicillin and amoxicillin. Most of the penicillins are secreted into the bile, but this is only a minor route of elimination for most. Nafcillin and oxacillin differ in that they are excreted in more significant amounts in the bile.

SIDE-EFFECTS/ADVERSE REACTIONS

The most frequently noted side-effects during penicillin treatment are hypersensitivity reactions. These can occur in up to 10% of patients, especially those with a history of allergy, hay fever, or asthma. The incidence of allergic reactions is somewhat higher with parenteral administration, although serious, and sometimes fatal anaphylactic reactions have occurred with oral administration. A variety of allergic symptoms have been reported, ranging from skin rash, pruritus, urticaria, and sneezing, to more serious manifestations such as angioedema, wheezing, laryngeal edema, serum sickness, exfoliative dermatitis, erythema multiforme, arthralgia, hypotension, prostration, anaphylaxis, and vascular collapse. In addition, a maculopapular rash which is not a true allergic response has been reported with ampicillin.

Many other adverse reactions have been associated with penicillin administration, although the overall incidence is rather infrequent and their occurrence is often dose dependent. A listing of adverse reactions possible with penicillin usage is as follows:

GI—Nausea, vomiting, epigastric distress, glossitis, stomatitis, dry mouth, abnormal taste, "hairy" tongue, diarrhea, flatulence, enterocolitis (due to secondary microbial overgrowth), abdominal pain, GI bleeding

Electrolyte—Hypokalemia (especially extended-spectrum penicillins), hypernatremia (especially carbenicillin, ticarcillin)

Renal—Hepatic-interstitial nephritis (most frequently with methicillin), glomerulonephritis, cholestatic hepatitis, elevated SGOT, SGPT, LDH, and alkaline phosphatase (especially oxacillin)

CNS—Neurotoxicity (irritability, lethargy, hallucinations, seizures), anxiety, confusion, agitation, depression

Hematologic—Blood dyscrasias, bone marrow depression, hemolytic anemia, hemorrhagic manifestations associated with abnormalities of coagulation tests (especially extended-spectrum penicillins)

Other—Pain and irritation at injection site, phlebitis, oral and rectal candidiasis, overgrowth of nonsusceptible organisms, vaginitis, neuropathy, sciatic neuritis

CONTRAINDICATIONS AND PRECAUTIONS

The only absolute contraindication to use of penicillins is in patients who have demonstrated a previous hypersensitivity to the drugs. However, these agents must be used with *caution* in persons with asthma, hay fever, or a history of other allergies. Cautious use is also necessary in patients with impaired renal function, and in nursing mothers because excretion of the drugs in breast milk may cause diarrhea or fungal overgrowth in the nursing infant.

During parenteral administration, care must be taken to avoid inadvertent intravascular injection because severe neurovascular damage has occurred, including necrosis and sloughing at the injection site, and gangrene. Repeated IM injections into the anterolateral thigh have resulted in development of fibrosis and localized tissue atrophy. IV injection can result in thrombophlebitis, neuromuscular excitability, and convulsions.

Penicillin preparations containing a sodium salt may alter the electrolyte balance, especially if given in large amounts. The sodium content of the different penicillin preparations is variable and the amount of sodium received per day depends on the sodium content of the preparation and the daily dose. The approximate sodium load per 24 hours resulting from maximum daily doses of representative penicillins is as follows:

Drug	Approximate Daily Sodium Load (mEq)
ampicillin	25
azlocillin	50
carbenicillin	200
methicillin	10
mezlocillin	45
nafcillin	10
oxacillin	20
piperacillin	45
ticarcillin	120

Likewise, potassium levels can be altered by penicillin preparations. Increased serum potassium may occur if large amounts of potassium penicillin G or V are administered. Conversely *hypokalemia* has been reported in some patients receiving carbenicillin, mezlocillin, piperacillin, or ticarcillin. Careful monitoring of serum electrolytes is necessary during high-dose or prolonged therapy with any of the above drugs.

INTERACTIONS

1. Concurrent use of bacteriostatic antibiotics (*e.g.,* tetracyclines, erythromycin) may diminish the effectiveness of penicillins by slowing the rate of bacterial growth, because penicillins are most effective during phases of rapid bacterial multiplication.
2. Probenecid prolongs blood levels of penicillins by blocking their elimination by renal tubular secretion.
3. Highly protein-bound penicillins (*e.g.,* cloxacillin, dicloxacillin, nafcillin, and oxacillin) can be potentiated by other highly protein-bound drugs (*e.g.,* salicylates, oral anticoagulants, anti-inflammatory agents) as a result of displacement from protein binding sites.
4. Antacids, other alkalinizing agents, cholestyramine, colestipol and oral neomycin, can inhibit the action of oral penicillins by impairing absorption.
5. Increased incidence of skin rash can occur with combined use of ampicillin and allopurinol.
6. The effectiveness of oral contraceptives may be reduced and the incidence of breakthrough bleeding increased by ampicillin or penicillin V.
7. Penicillins mixed in solution with an aminoglycoside may inactivate the aminoglycoside.
8. High doses of IV penicillins (especially carbenicillin) may increase the risk of bleeding in patients receiving heparin or oral anticoagulants.
9. Use of penicillin and chloramphenicol together may reduce the effectiveness of penicillin and slow the elimination of chloramphenicol.
10. Extended-spectrum penicillins may be synergistic with aminoglycosides against certain gram-negative organisms, such as *Pseudomonas, Providencia,* and enterococci.

■ Nursing Process for Penicillins

See also Chapter 59, under Nursing Process.

□ ASSESSMENT

□ Subjective Data

A drug history is essential and should begin with questions about allergy to penicillin drugs. Demonstrated allergy (hives, temperature, rash, or the more serious respiratory or vascular symptoms) contraindicates drug use. Other drugs which may cause problems are antacids which will decrease drug absorption and oral contraceptives. Penicillin drugs decrease the effectiveness of oral contraceptives thus reducing protection against pregnancy. The woman on a penicillin drug who takes oral contraceptives should be advised to use an alternate method of birth control throughout the entire cycle during which the penicillin was taken.

Medical history should focus on the symptoms for which the drug is to be prescribed as well as a history of renal, hepatic, or hematologic disorders. Penicillins are not contraindicated in any disorder, but the patient with renal disease or hepatic dysfunction may need dosage adjustments to accommodate alterations in metabolism and excretion. The patient with hematologic problems may require more frequent monitoring of blood studies especially platelets and clotting times. A history of allergy, asthma, hay fever, or first time use of penicillin also warrants caution because such patients may be more susceptible to hypersensitivity reactions.

□ Objective Data

Physical assessment focuses on the site of infection as well as the GI tract. Auscultation of bowel sounds will detect hypermotility, which may be aggravated by oral doses of the penicillin drugs.

Laboratory data should include hepatic, renal, and hematologic function studies. Electrolytes should be drawn on patients who are suspected of having an electrolyte imbalance, who receive high dose intravenous therapy, or who must restrict sodium intake.

□ NURSING DIAGNOSES
Actual nursing diagnoses may include:
Knowledge deficit related to action, administration, and side-effects of the drug
Potential nursing diagnoses may include:
Alteration in bowel elimination: diarrhea
Potential for infection related to super infection from resistant bacteria
Sensory-perceptual alterations: gustatory (taste)
Impaired tissue integrity related to intravenous extravasation or long-term intramuscular injections
Alteration in body temperature related to hypersensitivity reaction
Alteration in cardiac output: decreased related to neurovascular changes and hypotension in hypersensitivity reaction
Alteration in respiratory function related to hypersensitivity reaction

□ PLAN
Nursing care goals should focus on:
1. Administering the drug correctly and safely according to the prescribed route
2. Monitoring for side-effects, especially hypersensitivity and gastrointestinal distress
3. Teaching the patient correct drug-taking techniques, side-effects, and what to do if problems develop

□ INTERVENTION
The penicillin drugs are administered by oral, intramuscular, and intravenous routes and should be given around the clock to ensure adequate serum level and therapeutic effectiveness. In general, the intravenous route provides the most consistent serum levels and as such should always be used in acute infections. Penicillins are extremely irritating to tissue and should be well diluted prior to parenteral administration. Most are best mixed with sodium chloride to alkalinize the solution (see Table 61-2 for specific dilution recommendations for each drug). Therefore, penicillins should never be given by intravenous injection. Accidental injections have caused neurovascular damage, gangrene, and paralysis. The drug should be given by slow intravenous infusion, usually ranging from 30 minutes to 1 hour, depending on the dose. Site should be carefully monitored for signs of thrombophlebitis, warmth, pain, red streaking, or swelling; if any of these signs develop, the IV should be

immediately removed. IV sites should be rotated every 48 hours to decrease venous irritability. In long-term therapy, a central line may be used to decrease the risk of problems.

Intramuscular administration also irritates muscle tissue. A large muscle such as the gluteus in adults or the vastus lateralis in children under age 3 years is the most appropriate site, and sites should be rotated with each injection. If multiple injections are to be given, a body map (see Chap. 8 for example) will help ensure systematic rotation. Muscle atrophy and abscess formation have occurred with intramuscular injection of penicillins. Site location and aspiration prior to injection also is important because accidental drug injection into a vein or nerve can cause permanent damage.

Each dose of the oral forms of the drug should be given with at least a full glass of water, including the liquid form for children. Penicillins should not be given with acidic fruit juices because premature decomposition of the drug may occur. This information should be shared with parents who may be tempted to combine the drug with juice in order to get a small child to take it. Most penicillins are best taken on an empty stomach either 1 hour before or 2 hours to 3 hours after a meal. Penicillin V, bacampicillin, and amoxicillin are exceptions to this rule because their absorption is not diminished by food. All liquid penicillins should be refrigerated throughout the therapy and discarded upon completion of the course, usually 10 days to 14 days, because drug potency gradually decreases on exposure to air and heat.

Several forms of penicillin may alter laboratory values during therapy. Table 61-3 lists the drugs, tests, and reactions that may develop. Patients on these drugs should be appropriately monitored and should be given alternate tests whenever possible.

Potential side-effects of the penicillins include hypersensitivity, gastrointestinal distress, superinfection, electrolyte disturbances, and central nervous system disturbances. Of all of these, hypersensitivity is the most common and, potentially, the most serious. A hypersensitivity reaction may occur immediately or take several days to develop. Serious anaphylactic reactions usually occur soon after the drug is started especially when the intravenous route is used. At the start of penicillin therapy, especially IV, the nurse should plan to stay with the patient for the first 5 minutes to 15 minutes, take baseline vital signs, and monitor for early symptoms such as hives, nasal congestion, dyspnea, wheezing, facial swelling, or local reactions. In all acute care settings where penicillins are given, emergency equipment should be available to

Table 61-3
Changes in Laboratory Values Resulting From Penicillin Drugs

Drug	Test	Reaction
ampicillin	Clinitest urine glucose	False positive
	Plasma estrogen	Decreased
azlocillin	Serum uric acid	Decreased
carbenicillin (IV)	Coombs' test	Positive
mezlocillin	Serum proteins	False positive
piperacillin	Coombs' test	Positive

deal with hypersensitivity reactions which can lead to anaphylactic shock and respiratory or cardiac arrest. Epinephrine, antihistamines, corticosteroids, calcium preparations, vasopressors, antiarrhythmics such as lidocaine, and respiratory equipment such as oxygen, ambu-bag, tracheostomy set, and endotracheal tubes form the core of equipment essential to treat a hypersensitivity emergency. The patient going home on a penicillin should be taught the early warning signs and seek emergency care immediately should any develop. Delayed reactions may consist of fever, rash, and some edema and may be treated by antipyretics and antihistamines. In most cases, the drug will be immediately discontinued.

Superinfections may develop during the course of drug therapy either as a result of the penicillin being ineffective against an organism at the infection site or because the penicillin disrupts the normal bacterial flora in the mouth, gastrointestinal tract, or perineum. General signs of increasing infection include fever, malaise, cough, and redness, inflammation or discharge from the infected site. Signs of disruption of normal bacterial flora include white patches in the mouth and gums (thrush), foul-smelling watery diarrhea, or white, cheesy vaginal discharge and itching (monilia). Treatment may be symptomatic to decrease diarrhea, topical to treat thrush or vaginal monilia, or the penicillin may be discontinued.

Other gastrointestinal side-effects may include gastrointestinal upset and changes in taste, which frequently occur with carbenicillin. Taste loss will return when the drug is discontinued. If gastrointestinal upset prevents drug taking, the formulation may be changed to a comparable drug that can be taken with food.

Electrolyte disturbances can occur if the patient is sodium sensitive (hypernatremia) or if high doses of intravenous penicillin V or G, which contain potassium, are given (hyperkalemia). Serum electrolyte studies can be done to determine early electrolyte changes. The nurse should monitor the patient for signs of hypernatremia, which also signal the development of congestive heart failure. These include weight gain, edema, increased heart rate and respiration, and the presence of rales. Symptoms of hyperkalemia include numbness or tingling in the extremities, listlessness, muscle weakness, and hypotension. This can lead to cardiac arrhythmias, especially bradycardia. The healthcare team should be immediately notified if any of these occur.

Several adverse toxic reactions have been reported immediately following intramuscular administration of aqueous procaine penicillin G which is frequently used in high single doses for several sexually transmitted diseases. Symptoms range from hallucinations, agitation, paranoia, and severe anxiety to appearance of a generalized seizure. The episode usually passes quickly, but nurses in outpatient facilities where the drug is given should closely monitor the patient for about 15 minutes after administration and conduct a mental status check before discharge. Intravenous diazepam (for seizures) and oxygen need to be among the emergency equipment available in the facility to deal with such a toxic reaction.

Children receiving penicillin antibiotics, especially in high intravenous doses, should have fluid, electrolytes, and central nervous system status monitored closely. The young child is more susceptible to diarrhea and subsequent dehydration, electrolyte imbalance, and CNS irritability than adults receiving the same drugs.

Patients with renal impairment also warrant close monitoring using periodic evaluations of BUN and creatinine clearance. If renal function diminishes as a result of penicillin, creatinine clearance levels will decrease and the patient will develop a decrease in platelet aggregation leading to thrombocytopenia and bleeding. Early symptoms may include petechiae, hematomas, and bleeding gums after toothbrushing, but may progress to rectal or vaginal bleeding and hemoptysis. Any signs of bleeding should be immediately reported. Either the drug dose will be lowered, or the drug will be discontinued. Similar symptoms may develop in any patient receiving nafcillin. Consequently, coagulation studies and platelet counts should be done on any patient receiving extended therapy.

□   EVALUATION

The outcome criterion usually used to measure treatment success with any antibiotic is resolution of infection through a decrease or disappearance of symptoms. With penicillins, other criteria may include *absence* of side-effects such as hypersensitivity, superinfection, thrombophlebitis (intravenous administration), gastrointestinal distress, and electrolyte disturbances.

Carbapenems

Imipenem-Cilastatin

(Primaxin)

Imipenem, a thienamycin antibiotic, is a beta-lactam that is structurally unique from the penicillins and cephalosporins but which possesses a similar mechanism of action. It is effective against a wide range of gram-positive, gram-negative, and anaerobic microorganisms and is useful in treating serious infections due to a variety of bacteria resistant to many other antimicrobial drugs. It may be useful as a *single agent* in infections that would ordinarily require multiple anti-infective drug therapy. Imipenem is rapidly hydrolyzed by an enzyme in the proximal tubule of the kidney, resulting in very low levels of the drug in the urine, which are probably inadequate for an antibacterial action. This problem has been overcome by the addition of cilastatin to the formulation, which is an inhibitor of the renal enzyme that destroys imipenem.

MECHANISM AND ACTIONS

Imipenem readily penetrates gram-positive and gram-negative bacterial cells and binds avidly to penicillin-binding proteins 1B and 2, thus interfering with synthesis of peptidoglycan and subsequent cell wall formation. The drug is highly resistant to destruction by beta-lactamase enzymes. Imipenem appears to inhibit over 90% of the clinically important pathogens, the notable exceptions being *Pseudomonas maltophilia*, *Streptococcus faecium*, groups A, C, and G streptococci, and

methicillin-resistant staphylococci. The combination of imipenem and cilastatin is as effective as aminoglycosides or third generation cephalosporins for severe gram-negative infections.

USES

1. Treatment of serious infections due to most common pathogens, except those mentioned under Mechanism and Actions above.

> *Note:* Many infections resistant to antibiotics such as penicillins, cephalosporins, or aminoglycosides have responded to treatment with imipenem-cilastatin.

ADMINISTRATION AND DOSAGE

Imipenem-cilastatin is available as powder for injection containing either 250 mg or 500 mg *each* of imipenem and cilastatin. Dosages are given in terms of imipenem equivalent. The drug is administered by IV infusion over 20 minutes to 30 minutes as a dilution in one of several compatible diluents (see package instructions). Recommended doses range from 250 mg every 6 hours for milder infections to 1 g every 6 hours to 8 hours for severe, life-threatening infections. The maximum daily dose is 4 g/day. Reduced doses are necessary in persons with impaired renal function. Reconstituted solutions vary from colorless to yellow; this variation does not affect potency. The drug should not be mixed with other anti-infective drug solutions but should be infused separately.

FATE

Following IV infusion, the plasma half-life of each component is approximately 1 hour. Plasma levels decline to 1 mcg/ml or less within 4 hours to 6 hours. Imipenem is approximately 20% protein bound. If administered alone, imipenem is rapidly metabolized in the kidneys by a dihydropeptidase enzyme; this metabolism is markedly slowed by cilastatin. Approximately 75% of a dose of imipenem and cilastatin appears in the urine within 10 hours after administration.

SIDE-EFFECTS/ADVERSE REACTIONS

The most frequently reported side-effects with imipenem-cilastatin are nausea, diarrhea, and thrombophlebitis (approximately 3%). Other adverse reactions associated with administration of the drug include vomiting, fever, dizziness, seizures, hypotension, rash, urticaria, pruritus, pain and erythema at injection site, fatigue, confusion, headache, paresthesia, tachycardia, palpitations, and vein induration. Rarely encountered adverse effects include chest discomfort, dyspnea, hyperventilation, transient hearing loss, weakness, oliguria, anuria, polyarthralgia, facial edema, cyanosis, candidal infection, glossitis, salivation, gastroenteritis, pseudomembranous colitis, myoclonus, and encephalopathy.

CONTRAINDICATIONS AND PRECAUTIONS
Other than known hypersensitivity to either component, there are no absolute contraindications to use of imipenem-cilastatin. *Cautious use* of this product is warranted in patients with a history of seizure disorders, thrombophlebitis, renal impairment, or allergic reactions. Care must also be exercised in using imipenem-cilastatin in pregnant women or nursing mothers. The safety and efficacy of the drug have not been conclusively established in children under 12 years of age. Prolonged use of this drug can result in overgrowth of nonsusceptible organisms and possibly development of pseudomembranous colitis.

INTERACTIONS
There are no specific interactions reported with imipenem-cilastatin. Because the drug is a beta-lactam antibiotic, the interactions listed for both the penicillins and cephalosporins are possible with this drug. Refer to the list of interactions for penicillins earlier in this chapter and those for the cephalosporins in Chapter 62.

NURSING CONSIDERATIONS
See also Nursing Process for Penicillins earlier in this chapter and Nursing Process for anti-infective therapy in Chapter 59.

Imipenem-cilastatin should be reconstituted with normal saline which increases the diluted drug's stability both at room temperature and under refrigeration. While the drug can be reconstituted with dextrose and water it must be used within 4 hours at room temperature and 24 hours under refrigeration. If mixed with normal saline it will remain stable for 10 hours at room temperature and 48 hours under refrigeration.

The drug must be mixed with a sufficient quantity of diluent to avoid the formation of a milky white suspension with particulate matter. Recommendations are to use 100 ml of solution for a 500-mg dose and 250 ml of solution for a 1-g dose.

Although the drug is thought to be extremely effective, the nurse must watch for signs of superinfection especially if the organism being treated is *Pseudomonas aeruginosa*, which may develop drug resistance. Most side-effects are similar to the other penicillins, except transient hearing loss which should be reported.

Monobactams

Aztreonam

(Azactam)

The monobactam group of anti-infective agents are a relatively new class of drugs that are structurally different from other beta-lactams. Aztreonam is the first of the clinically available monobactams. It possesses a wide spectrum of action against gram-negative aerobic pathogens.

MECHANISM AND ACTIONS
Aztreonam is bactericidal towards gram-negative aerobic pathogens, including *Pseudomonas, E. coli, Enterobacter, Klebsiella, Serratia, Proteus,* and *Hemophilus* among many others. Its action is the result of inhibition of bacterial cell wall synthesis due to a high affinity of aztreonam for penicillin-binding protein 3. The drug exhibits a high degree of beta-lactamase resistance and its antibacterial activity is maintained over a range of pH from 6 to 8. Aztreonam and aminoglycosides are synergistic against *Pseudomonas*, many strains of Enterobacteriaceae, and other gram-negative aerobic bacilli.

USES
1. Treatment of infections resulting from susceptible strains of the above-named organisms; responsive infections include urinary tract, lower respiratory tract, intra-abdominal, gynecologic, skin and soft tissue, and septicemia.
   Note: Aztreonam is usually given initially with another antimicrobial agent in seriously ill patients, because it is largely ineffective against gram-positive organisms and anaerobic organisms.

ADMINISTRATION AND DOSAGE
Aztreonam is available as powder for injection containing 500 mg, 1 g, or 2 g per vial or infusion bottle. The drug is given IM or IV, with the IV route being preferred when the dose exceeds 1 g or if the patient is seriously ill. Recommended doses are 500 mg to 1 g every 8 hours to 12 hours for urinary infections and 1 g to 2 g every 6 hours to 12 hours for other systemic infections depending upon the severity of the infection. Dosage should

be reduced by one half in patients with impaired renal function (*i.e.*, creatinine clearance between 10 ml and 30 ml per minute after an initial loading dose of 1 g to 2 g). Treatment should be continued for at least 48 hours after the patient becomes asymptomatic or bacterial eradication has been confirmed.

FATE
Following IM injection, peak serum levels occur within 1 hour. The serum half-life is 1.5 hour to 2 hours in patients with normal renal function. Approximately 70% of an IV or IM dose is recovered in the urine within 8 hours; smaller amounts are found in the feces. Serum protein binding is approximately 50% and single doses given every 8 hours do not appear to result in cumulation of drug in the body.

SIDE-EFFECTS/ADVERSE REACTIONS
Swelling and pain at the injection site can occur following IM administration, and phlebitis has been noted upon IV administration. Other systemic reactions noted in some patients are nausea, diarrhea, vomiting, and skin rash. A variety of adverse reactions have occurred in the occasional patient, and include confusion, headache, weakness, paresthesia, insomnia, abdominal cramping, hypotension, tinnitus, altered taste, nasal congestion, urticaria, petechiae, muscular aching, fever, malaise, breast tenderness, blood dyscrasias, jaundice, and hepatitis. Alterations in liver function enzymes, prothrombin and partial thromboplastin times, serum creatinine, and a positive direct Coombs' test have also been reported during aztreonam treatment.

CONTRAINDICATIONS AND PRECAUTIONS
Aztreonam has no absolute contraindications. A *cautious* approach to therapy should be observed in patients with liver or kidney dysfunction, in patients with previous hypersensitivity reactions to other beta-lactam antibiotics (*e.g.*, penicillins, cephalosporins) and in pregnant women or nursing mothers. Superinfection can occur with nonsusceptible organisms such as gram-positive cocci or fungi and appropriate measures should be taken to minimize this danger.

INTERACTIONS
1. Beta-lactamase inducing antibiotics (*e.g.*, cefoxitin, imipenem) should not be used concurrently with aztreonam, because they may reduce its effectiveness against beta-lactamase secreting gram-negative aerobes.
2. Aztreonam is incompatible in solution with nafcillin, cephradine, and metronidazole.

NURSING CONSIDERATIONS
See also Nursing Process for Penicillins earlier in this chapter, and Nursing Process for anti-infective therapy in Chapter 59.

IM injections should be made well into a large muscle mass. When giving the drug IV, a bolus injection may be used to initiate therapy and is given over 3 minutes to 5 minutes directly into a vein or into the tubing of an administration set. Powder for injection should be reconstituted with Sterile Water for Injection. Subsequent dilution for infusion may be made into one of several IV infusion solutions (refer to package directions for appropriate solutions). Reconstituted solutions are stable at room temperature for 48 hours and for up to 7 days if refrigerated.

The nurse must observe for signs of superinfection, because the drug is only effective against gram-negative aerobes. Renal function should also be monitored, especially if aztreonam is given together with an aminoglycoside, because the potential for nephrotoxicity is enhanced.

CASE STUDY

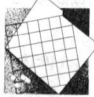

During the flu season, Jane Harris, age 34, a fifth-grade school teacher, is diagnosed with a sore throat which cultures as *Streptococcus pyogenes*. The physician prescribes rest, increased fluids, and penicillin V (Pen-Vee-K) 250 mg every 6 hours for 14 days.

Discussion Questions

1. What information should the nurse give Jane about taking this drug?
2. What side-effects should she watch for?

3. Five days into therapy Jane calls the office complaining of vaginal itching and a milky discharge which is diagnosed as candida. What caused this problem? How is it likely to be treated (refer to Table 59-1)? What should Jane know about this treatment (see Chap. 73)?

REVIEW QUESTIONS

1. List the major classes of penicillins.
2. What are the principal differences between (a) penicillin V and penicillin G, and (b) broad-spectrum and extended-spectrum penicillins?
3. Which penicillins are penicillinase resistant? What is the advantage of this property?
4. Give several ways in which bacteria may become resistant to penicillins.
5. Briefly describe the mechanism of action of the penicillins.
6. Why are gram-positive organisms more susceptible to the action of penicillins than gram-negative organisms?
7. Why may electrolyte levels be altered during penicillin administration?
8. How is penicillin G modified to confer a longer duration of action to the drug?
9. Name the extended spectrum penicillins.
10. What is the rationale for combining clavulanic acid with penicillins?
11. With what class of drugs are the extended-spectrum penicillins synergistic?
12. Against what organisms is amdinocillin most effective?
13. Why should a drug history be taken on a patient receiving penicillins? What information should a patient be given if she takes antacids or birth control pills?
14. Describe the range of symptoms that can develop in a hypersensitivity reaction to penicillin. What preventive measures should the nurse take for a patient receiving penicillin for the first time?
15. What are some of the potential sites of superinfection from penicillin? How might they be treated?
16. Which electrolyte disturbances may occur during penicillin therapy? Describe the symptoms and appropriate nursing actions.
17. To which side-effects of penicillin are children more susceptible? How should they be monitored?
18. Why is cilastatin combined with imipenem?
19. What is the spectrum of activity of aztreonam?
20. Why should aztreonam be given with another anti-infective in seriously ill patients?

BIBLIOGRAPHY

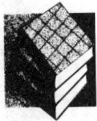

Bauk NV, Kammer RB: Hematologic complications associated with beta-lactam antibiotics. Rev Infect Dis 5(Suppl 7):5380, 1983
Brooks GF, Barriere SL: Clinical use of the new beta-lactam antimicrobial drugs. Ann Intern Med 98:530, 1983
Cleeland R, Squires E: Enhanced activity of beta-lactam antibiotics with amdinocillin. Am J Med 75(Suppl):21, 1983

Eliopoulos GM, Moellering RC: Azlocillin, mezlocillin and piperacillin: New broad-spectrum penicillins. Ann Intern Med 79:755, 1982

Erffmeyer JE: Adverse reactions to penicillin. Ann Allergy 47:288, 1981

Geddes AM, Stille W (eds): Imipenem: The first thienamycin antibiotic. Rev Infect Dis 7(Suppl 3):353, 1985

Landis BJ, Dunn L: Adverse toxic reaction to aqueous procaine penicillin G. Nurs Pract 9(11):36, November 1984

McCloskey WW, Jeffrey LP: Drug stop: Newer beta-lactam antimicrobials. J Neurosurg Nursing 17:210, 1985

Mills J: A guide to using the newer penicillins and beta-lactam antibiotics. Mod Med 55:46, 1987

Neu HC: The *in vitro* activity human pharmacology and clinical effectiveness of new beta-lactam antibiotics. Annu Rev Pharmacol Toxicol 22:599, 1982

Neu HC: Structure-activity relations of new β-lactam compounds and *in-vitro* activity against common bacteria. Rev Infect Dis 5(Suppl 2):5319, 1983

Neu HC: Penicillins. In Mandell GL, Douglas RG, Bennett JE (eds): Principles and Practice of Infectious Diseases, 2nd ed, p 166. New York, John Wiley & Sons, 1985

Neu HC (ed): Proceedings of a Symposium. Aztreonam: A monocyclic beta-lactam antibiotic. Am J Med 78:1, 1985

Neu HC, Reeves DS, Leigh DA: Azlocillin—An antipseudomonas penicillin. J Antimicrob Chemotherap 11(Suppl B):1, 1983

Parry MF, Pancoast SJ: Antipseudomonal penicillins. In Ristuccia AM, Cunha BA (eds): Antimicrobial Therapy, p 197. New York, Raven Press, 1984

Root RK, Sande MA (eds): Contemporary Issues in Infectious Diseases. Vol. I, New Dimensions in Antimicrobial Therapy. New York, Churchill Livingstone, 1984

Salvio K, Apuzzio JJ: New antibiotics in the treatment of pelvic infections. JOGN Nurs 13:308, 1984

Scheife RT, Neu HC: Bacampicillin hydrochloride: chemistry, pharmacology and clinical use. Pharmacotherap 2:313, 1982

Scherer P: New drugs of 1985 in theory and in practice. Am J Nursing 86:407, 1986

Stein GE, Gurwith MJ: Amoxicillin-potassium clavulanate: A beta-lactamase-resistant antibiotic combination. Clin Pharmacol 3:591, 1984

Symposium. An international review of amdinocillin: A new beta lactam antibiotic. Am J Med 75:1, 1983

Symposium. Carbapenem (imipenem). Am J Med 78(Suppl 6A):1, 1985

Wright AJ, Wilkowski CJ: The penicillins. Mayo Clin Proc 58:21, 1983

Cephalosporins

Cephalosporins
Cefaclor, Cefadroxil,
Cefamandole,
Cefazolin, Cefonicid,
Cefoperazone,
Ceforanide,
Cefotaxime,
Cefotetan, Cefoxitin,
Ceftazidime,
Ceftizoxime,
Ceftriaxone,
Cefuroxime,
Cephalexin,
Cephalothin,
Cephapirin,
Cephradine,
Moxalactam

62

The cephalosporins are an extensive group of semisynthetic, broad-spectrum antibiotics mostly derived from cephalosporin C, a natural product of the fungus *Cephalosporium acremonium.* In addition to the various cephalosporin C derivatives, cefoxitin and cefotetan, derivatives of the structurally related cephamycin C, and moxalactam, a beta-lactam derivative are also viewed as cephalosporins due to their structural and pharmacologic similarities to other derivatives.

Cephalosporins are divided into first-, second-, and third-generation drugs. Table 62-1 presents some of the principal differences among the three groups of cephalosporins, although it must be recognized that some exceptions exist to the information indicated in the table. In general, activity against gram-negative bacilli increases from first- to third-generation drugs, as does efficacy against resistant organisms as well as drug cost. Conversely, efficacy against gram-positive organisms is greatest with the first-generation drugs and progressively decreases through the second- and third-generation compounds.

Another major difference among the various cephalosporins is in their spectrum of action. The principal microorganisms susceptible to each of the three groups of cephalosporins are indicated in Table 62-2. Within each group of drugs, the individual agents differ primarily in their efficacy, half-lives, protein binding, and principal routes of excretion. Some of these differences are also presented in Table 62-2.

Cephalosporin antibiotics are usually bactericidal against most gram-positive cocci (except enterococci, which are unaffected by all drugs except possibly cefoperazone) and many gram-negative bacilli. In general, the older, first-generation drugs are the most effective against staphylococci and streptococci, whereas the second- and third-generation drugs display increased activity against gram-negative enterobacteria. However, although widely prescribed, cephalosporins are recognized as drugs of choice for only a few infections, primarily due to the availability of more specific, more effective, or less costly alternatives.

Cephalosporins are indicated for surgical prophylaxis when extended gram-negative activity is desired, for treating *Klebsiella* infections, and for treatment of gram-positive infections (except enterococci) in patients allergic to penicillin. However, cross-allergenicity exists between the penicillins and the cephalosporins (estimated incidence is 5%–15%), so caution is indicated when cephalosporins must be given to patients with a history of penicillin allergy. Second- and third-generation drugs should not be routinely used for gram-positive infections, because they are less effective than first-generation agents and significantly more expensive as well. More active, and less costly alternatives (*e.g.,* penicillins, erythromycins) are readily available.

Because many gram-negative bacilli are susceptible to the second- and third-generation cephalosporins (see Table 62-2), these drugs are frequently used in respiratory, genitourinary, skin, and soft-tissue infections due to a variety of gram-negative microorganisms. In addition, the third-generation drugs display varying degrees of activity against *Pseudomonas, Serratia,* and possibly *Salmonella* and *Acinetobacter* and are often employed as alternatives to the more toxic (however more effective) aminoglycosides. Cefoxitin, as well as the third-generation drugs are also active against *Bacteroides fragilis,* but this activity is not as great or as predictable as with other non-cephalosporin drugs. Moreover, many gram-negative bacilli have developed resistance to the cephalosporins, greatly restricting their usefulness in many infections. Specific indications for the individual cephalosporins are given in Table 62-3.

Most first-generation drugs are susceptible to inactivation by beta-lactamase (*i.e.,* cephalosporinase) enzymes. Conversely, second-generation drugs (except cefamandole) and all third-generation drugs display greater resistance to enzymatic inactivation, including the cephalosporinases produced by

(Text continues on p. 1208.)

Table 62-1
General Characteristics of Cephalosporins

	First-Generation Drugs	Second-Generation Drugs	Third-Generation Drugs
Activity vs gram (+) organisms	+++	++	+
Activity vs gram (−) organisms	+	++	+++
Resistance to beta-lactamase enzymes	0(+)	+ to ++	++ to +++
Cost	Moderate	High	Very high

Key: 0(+), very weakly active; +, weakly active; ++, moderately active; +++, very active.

Table 62-2
Cephalosporins: Pharmacokinetics and Bacterial Spectrum of Action

Drug	Routes of Administration	% Protein Binding	Plasma Half-Life (min)	Urinary Excretion (% Unchanged)	Sodium Content (mEq/g)	Susceptible Microorganisms*
First Generation						
cefaclor	Oral	25	40–50	60–80		Staphylococci
cefadroxil	Oral	20	70–80	90–95		Streptococci (including
cephalexin	Oral	10–15	30–50	80–100		beta-hemolytic),
cephradine	Oral, IM, IV	10–15	45–60	80–90	6	*Escherichia coli,*
cephapirin	IM, IV	40–50	20–40	50–75	2.4	*Hemophilus*
cephalothin	IM, IV	65–75	30–60	50–75	2.8	*influenzae* (except
cefazolin	IM, IV	75–85	90–120	75–100	2	cefadroxil), *Klebsiella,*
						Proteus mirabilis
Second Generation						
cefamandole	IM, IV	65–75	30–60	60–80	3.3	All the above, plus:
cefonicid	IM, IV	90–95	240–300	99	2.7	*Neisseria gonorrhoeae*
cefoxitin	IM, IV	65–75	30–60	90–100	2.3	(except cefamandole),
cefuroxime	Oral, IM, IV	40–50	60–120	70–95	2.4	*Proteus morganii,*
ceforanide	IM, IV	80	150–180	80–95	0	*Proteus vulgaris,*
						Providencia (except
						cefonicid,
						cefamandole),
						Enterobacter (except
						cefoxitin,
						cefamandole),
						Neisseria
						meningitidis
						(cefuroxime only),
						Clostridium,
						Peptococcus,
						Peptostreptococcus,
						Bacteroides fragilis
						(cefoxitin only),
						Fusobacterium
						(except cefoxitin),
						Salmonella
						(cefuroxime only),
						Shigella (cefuroxime
						only).
Third Generation						
cefotaxime	IM, IV	30–50	60–70	50–60	2.2	All the above, plus:
ceftizoxime	IM, IV	30	100–120	75–80	2.6	*Pseudomonas*
cefoperazone	IM, IV	80–90	100–150	20–25	1.5	*aeruginosa* (except
moxalactam	IM, IV	45–55	120–210	70–90	3.8	cefotetan), *Serratia,*
ceftriaxone	IM, IV	85–95	350–500	30–60	3.6	*Acinetobacter*
cefotetan	IM, IV	80–90	180–270	50–80	3.5	(ceftizoxime,
ceftazidime	IM, IV	5–15	100–120	80–90	2.3	ceftriaxone,
						cefoperazone,
						ceftazidime only),
						Eubacterium
						(cefoperazone,
						moxalactam,
						ceftizoxime, only),
						Clostridium difficile
						(cefoperazone,
						cefotetan only).

* Susceptibility may vary with individual members of the group, and in some cases has only been demonstrated *in vitro.*

Table 62-3
Cephalosporins

Drug	Preparations	Usual Dosage Range	Clinical Considerations
First Generation			
cefaclor (Ceclor)	Capsules—250 mg, 500 mg Oral suspension—125 mg/5 ml, 250 mg/5 ml	Adults—250 mg to 500 mg every 8 h (maximum 4 g/day) Children—20 mg to 40 mg/kg/day in divided doses every 8 h (maximum 1 g/day)	Orally effective, short-acting cephalosporin used in respiratory, urinary, skin, and soft-tissue infections and otitis media; a single 2-g dose has been used in acute, uncomplicated urinary tract infections; skin rash, fever, polyarthritis and erythema multiforme can occur within 1 wk–2 wk; corticosteroids and antihistamines may be used to treat symptoms, which usually resolve within several days after drug is stopped
cefadroxil (Duricef, Ultracef)	Capsules—500 mg Tablets—1 g Oral suspension—125 mg/5 ml, 250 mg/5 ml, 500 mg/5 ml	Adults—1 g to 2 g/day in a single or two divided doses Children—30 mg/kg/day in divided doses every 12 h	Orally effective drug used principally to treat infections due to *Escherichia coli*, *Proteus mirabilis*, or *Klebsiella*; also used in staphylococcal and streptococcal infections of skin, pharynx, and tonsils; not metabolized to any extent and excreted essentially intact in the urine; oral absorption is not signficantly affected by food; adjust dosage according to package instuctions in patients with renal impairment
cefazolin (Ancef, Kefzol)	Injection—250 mg, 500 mg, 1 g, 5 g, 10 g per vial	Adults—250 mg to 1.5 g IV or IM every 6 h–8 h depending on severity of infection (maximum 12 g/day) Children—25 mg to 100 mg/kg/day divided into three or four doses depending on severity of infection *Acute uncomplicated urinary tract infections*—1 g every 12 h *Perioperative prophylaxis:* 1 g ½ h to 1 h before surgery, 0.5 g to 1 g during surgery of 2 h or longer, then 0.5 g to 1 g every 6 h–8 h for 24 h following surgery	Parenteral cephalosporin similar to cephalothin but claimed to be less irritating and less nephrotoxic; used in treatment of respiratory, urinary, and biliary tract infections, skin and soft-tissue infections, septicemia, bone and joint infections, and endocarditis; also indicated perioperatively to reduce risk of infection following certain surgical procedures; highly protein bound; do not use in children under 1 month; follow manufacturer's recommendations for dosing in renal impairment; hemiparesis and confusion have occurred *(continued)*

Table 62-3 (continued)
Cephalosporins

Drug	Preparations	Usual Dosage Range	Clinical Considerations
First Generation (continued)			
cefazolin (Ancef, Kefzol) (continued)			following large doses in patients with renal failure; pain on injection is infrequent; diluted solutions are stable for 24 h at room temperature and 96 h under refrigeration
cephalexin (Keflex, Keflet, Keftab)	Capsules—250 mg, 500 mg Tablets—250 mg, 500 mg, 1 g Oral suspension—125 mg/5 ml, 250 mg/5 ml Pediatric drops—100 mg/ml	Adults—250 mg to 500 mg every 6 h (maximum dose is 4 g/day) Children—25 mg to 100 mg/kg/day in four divided doses depending on severity of infection	Orally effective cephalosporin indicated for streptococcal respiratory infections, bone infections caused by staphylococci or *Proteus mirabilis*, skin and soft tissue infections caused by staphylococci or streptococci, urinary infections due to *E. coli*, *Proteus mirabilis*, or *Klebsiella* and otitis media in penicillin-allergic patients; some staphylococci are resistant; stable in gastric acid, well absorbed, and only slightly protein-bound; if doses greater than 4 g/day are necessary, parenteral cephalosporins should be used; refrigerate oral suspension, and discard unused portion in 14 days
cephalothin (Keflin, Seffin)	Powder for injection—500 mg, 1 g, 2 g, 4 g, 20 g/vial Injection—1 g, 2 g, 10 g per vial or infusion packs	Adults—500 mg to 1000 mg IM or IV injection every 4 h–6 h (up to 2 g every 4 h IV in life-threatening infections) Children—80 mg to 160 mg/kg/day in divided doses Perioperative prophylaxis: Adults—1 g to 2 g IM or IV ½ h–1 h before surgery, during surgery as needed, and every 6 h following surgery for 24 h Children—20 mg/kg to 30 mg/kg following the above schedule	Prototype first-generation parenteral cephalosporin used to treat respiratory, GI, urinary, skin, bone, joint, and soft-tissue infections as well as septicemia and meningitis due to staphylococci, streptococci, *E. coli*, *Proteus mirabilis*, *Hemophilus*, and *Klebsiella*; not effective against *Pseudomonas*, *Serratia*, indole-positive *Proteus* or *Enterococcus*; may be employed perioperatively to reduce incidence of certain infections in high-risk situations (*e.g.*, vaginal hysterectomy, intestinal or colorectal surgery, open heart surgery, cholecystectomy, prosthetic athroplasty); IM in- (continued)

Table 62-3 (continued)
Cephalosporins

Drug	Preparations	Usual Dosage Range	Clinical Considerations
First Generation (continued)			
cephalothin (Keflin, Seffin) (continued)			jection often elicits pain, induration, and sloughing; IV administration may lead to phlebitis or other inflammatory reactions; may be added to peritoneal dialysis fluid in concentrations up to 6 mg/100 ml and instilled throughout the dialysis procedure; due to short half-life (30 min–45 min), initial perioperative dose should be given just before start of surgery and readministered at appropriate intervals throughout procedure to maintain sufficient blood levels; prophylactic use should be discontinued within 24 h following surgery; maintenance dose must be reduced in patients with impaired renal function based on creatinine clearance; solutions are stable for 12 h–24 h at room temperature and 96 h under refrigeration; slight darkening does not affect potency
cephapirin (Cefadyl)	Powder for injection—500 mg, 1 g, 2 g, 4 g, 20 g per vial	Adults—500 mg to 1000 mg IM or IV every 4 h–6 h (up to 12 g/day IV in serious infections) Children—40 mg to 80 mg/kg/day IM in divided doses Perioperative prophylaxis: 1 g to 2 g IM or IV ½ h–1 h before surgery, during surgery if needed, and every 6 h after surgery for 24 h	Parenteral cephalosporin similar to cephalothin in action but causing less tissue irritation; clinical evidence of renal damage is lacking but jaundice has been reported; do not use in children under 3 mo of age; dilutions are stable for 24 h at room temperature and up to 10 days with refrigeration; check package instructions for compatibility with various infusion solutions
cephradine (Anspor, Velosef)	Capsules—250 mg, 500 mg Oral suspension—125 mg/5 ml, 250 mg/5 ml Powder for injection—250 mg, 500 mg; 1 g, 2 g, 4 g per vial or infusion bottle	Oral: Adults—250 mg to 500 mg every 6 h or 1 g every 12 h Children (over 9 mo)—25 mg to 100 mg/kg/day in divided doses every 6	Only cephalosporin available in both oral and parenteral dosage forms; oral preparations are primarily used as follow-up therapy to parenteral *(continued)*

Table 62-3 (continued)
Cephalosporins

Drug	Preparations	Usual Dosage Range	Clinical Considerations
First Generation (continued)			
cephradine (Anspor, Velosef) (continued)		h—12 h maximum 4 g/day) IV, IM: Adults—500 mg to 1000 mg four times a day (maximum 8 g/day) Children (over 12 mo)—50 mg to 100 mg/kg/day in four divided doses Perioperative prophylaxis: 1 g IV or IM 30 min–40 min before surgery, then 1 g every 4 h—6 h thereafter up to 24 h Cesarean section: 1 g IV when cord is clamped, then again at 6 h and 12 h	treatment; may be given without regard to meals, because drug is acid-stable; excreted largely unchanged in urine, mostly within 6 h, thus is effective in urinary infections due to susceptible organisms; very slightly protein-bound following reconstitution; IM or direct IV solutions should be used within 2 h at room temperature; continuous IV solutions retain potency for 10 h at room temperature; infusion solution should be replaced at that time; do not combine cephradine solutions with those of other antibiotics; doses smaller than those indicated should not be used; persistent infections may require several weeks therapy
Second Generation			
cefamandole (Mandol)	Injection—500 mg, 1 g, 2 g, 10 g per vial	Adults—500 mg to 1000 mg IM or IV every 4 h–8 h (up to 2 g/4 h in severe infections) Children—50 mg to 100 mg/kg/day in divided doses every 4 h–8 h *Perioperative prophylaxis:* Adults—1 g to 2 g IM or IV ½ h to 1 h prior to incision, then 1 g to 2 g every 6 h for 24 h—48 h Children—50 mg to 100 mg/kg/day in equally divided doses according to above schedule	Parenteral cephalosporin indicated for infections of the respiratory or urinary tracts and skin, for surgical prophylaxis, and for septicemia and peritonitis caused by susceptible organisms; effective against anaerobic organisms (*Clostridium, Peptococcus*), indole-positive *Proteus* and some strains of *Bacteroides fragilis*; also used in combination with an aminoglycoside for gram-positive or gram-negative sepsis (danger of nephrotoxicity, see under Interactions); reduce dose as indicated in package insert in patients with renal impairment; may cause acute tubular necrosis; bleeding episodes have occurred—monitor

(continued)

Table 62-3 (continued)
Cephalosporins

Drug	Preparations	Usual Dosage Range	Clinical Considerations
Second Generation (continued)			
cefamandole (Mandol) (continued)			prothrombin time and platelet count; jaundice has been noted in some patients; do not mix with aminoglycoside in same container; dilute drug solution as instructed with appropriate diluent; reconstituted cefamandole is stable for 24 h at room temperature and 96 h under refrigeration; IV dosage can be up to 12 g/day depending on severity of infection (e.g., bacterial septicemia), possible false-positive readings for urine glucose and proteinuria
cefonicid (Monocid)	Powder for injection—500 mg, 1 g, 10 g per vial	Adults—0.5 g to 1 g IM or slow IV injection once every 24 h (maximum dose is 2 g once daily) Perioperative prophylaxis: Adults—1 g given 1 h prior to incision; intraoperative administration is unnecessary; may be given once a day for 2 days following surgery	Long-acting cephalosporin given once daily for respiratory, urinary, skin, bone, and joint infections, and septicemia; not active against *Pseudomonas, Serratia, Enterococcus, Acinetobacter,* and most strains of *Bacteroides fragilis;* may cause pain on injection; doses larger than 1 g should be divided and given at two different IM sites; reduce dosage in patients with impaired renal function according to package directions; dilutions are stable for 24 h at room temperature and 72 h if refrigerated; very highly protein bound
ceforanide (Precef)	Powder for injection—500 mg, 1 g, 10 g per vial	Adults—0.5 g to 1 g IM or IV every 12 h Children—20 to 40 mg/kg/day in equally divided doses every 12 h *Perioperative prophylaxis:* 0.5 g to 1 g IM or IV 1 h prior to start of surgery; intraoperative administration is not necessary	Long-acting parenteral cephalosporin given twice a day for respiratory, urinary, and skin and soft-tissue infections due to staphylococci, streptococci, *Klebsiella, Hemophilus, E. coli, Proteus mirabilis,* also effective in bone and joint infections and endocarditis caused by staphylococci, septicemia due to staphylococci, streptococci or *E. coli,* and for perioperative *(continued)*

Table 62-3 (continued)
Cephalosporins

Drug	Preparations	Usual Dosage Range	Clinical Considerations
Second Generation (continued)			
ceforanide (Precef) (continued)			tive prophylaxis, active against *Enterobacter, Citrobacter,* and *Providencia.* Reduce dosage in renal impairment; elevated creatinine phosphokinase has occurred following IM injection. Contains *no* sodium
cefoxitin (Mefoxin)	Injection—1 g, 2 g, 10 g per vial and infusion bottles	Adults—1 g to 2 g every 6 h–8 h IV or IM (maximum is 12 g/day) *Gonorrhea (see remarks):* 2 g IM with 1 g oral probenecid *Disseminated gonorrhea:* 1 g IV four times a day for at least 7 days *Acute pelvic inflammatory disease:* 2 g IV four times a day with 100 mg doxycycline IV twice a day for at least 4 days; continue 100 mg doxycycline oral twice a day for an additional 10 days to 14 days *Perioperative prophylaxis:* 2 g IV or IM ½ h–1 h before surgery and every 6 h thereafter for up to 24 h Children—80 to 160 mg/kg/day in four to six divided doses (maximum 12 g/day).	Effective against a variety of organisms susceptible to first-generation cephalosporins as well as anaerobic organisms, indolepositive *Proteus, Bacteroides fragilis,* and some gram-negative bacteria resistant to other cephalosporins and broad-spectrum penicillins; may reduce incidence of postoperative infections in patients undergoing surgical procedures that are classified as potentialy contaminated (*e.g.,* GI surgery, vaginal hysterectomy); also indicated for penicillinase-producing *Neisseria gonorrhoeae* resistant to spectinomycin and for acute pelvic inflammatory disease; highly resistant to beta-lactamase; reconstituted solutions maintain potency for 24 h at room temperature, 1 wk under refrigeration, and up to 26 wk frozen; dry material may darken with time but potency is not affected; frequently painful upon IM injection; follow package directions for dosing patients with renal impairment; may cause false-positive urine glucose
cefuroxime (Kefurox, Zinacef) cefuroxime axetil (Ceftin)	Powder for injection—750 mg, 1.5 g, 7.5 g per vial Tablets—125 mg, 250 mg, 500 mg	Oral: Adults—125 mg to 500 mg every 12 h depending on severity of infection Children (under 12)—125 mg every 12 h	Cephalosporin which, unlike other first- and second-generation drugs, attains significant concentrations in the cerebrospinal fluid, espe- *(continued)*

Table 62-3 (continued)
Cephalosporins

Drug	Preparations	Usual Dosage Range	Clinical Considerations
Second Generation (continued)			
cefuroxime (Kefurox, Zinacef) cefuroxime axetil (Ceftin) (continued)		Parenteral: Adults—2.25 g to 6 g/day IM or IV in divided doses every 6 h–8 h (maximum dose is 9 g/day in bacterial meningitis) *Uncomplicated gonorrhea:* 1.5 g IM as a single dose with 1 g oral probenecid *Perioperative prophylaxis:* 1.5 g IV just prior to surgery, then 750 mg IV or IM every 8 h for 24 h Children (over 3 mo)—50 mg to 100 mg/kg/day in divided doses every 6 h–8 h *Bacterial meningitis (children's dosage only):* 200 mg to 240 mg/kg/day IV in divided doses every 6 h–8 h; reduce to 100 mg/kg/day IV upon improvement	cially if the meninges are inflamed; effective against many gram (−) bacilli, including *Enterobacter* and *Citrobacter* (some strains, however, are resistant); administer single 1.5-g IM dose for gonorrhea at two different sites; dosage is reduced according to package instructions in patients with renal dysfunction; inject slowly (3 min–5 min) IV or infuse either intermittently or continuously; do not mix with aminoglycosides; powder and solutions may darken with time, but potency of solution is unaffected for 24 h at room temperature and 48 h refrigerated
Third Generation			
cefotaxime (Claforan)	Injection—1 g, 2 g, 10 g per vial	Adults—1 g to 2 g every 6 h–12 h IV or IM (maximum dose 12 g/day) Children—50 mg to 180 mg/kg/day in four to six divided doses *Perioperative prophylaxis:* 1 g IV or IM 30 min–90 min before surgery, *Gonorrhea:* 1 g IM as a single injection *Disseminated gonorrhea:* 500 mg IV four times/day for at least 7 days	Parenteral cephalosporin used in the treatment of serious infections of the abdomen, lower respiratory tract, urinary tract, skin, and genital tract; also indicated as a surgical prophylactic agent and for pencillinase-producing *Neisseria gonorrhoeae* infections resistant to spectinomycin; many strains of *Pseudomonas* and enterococci are resistant; most common adverse reactions are pain, tenderness, and inflammation at injection site; reduce dose according to package instructions in patients with renal impairment; does not appear to be nephrotoxic, may be used concurrently with an aminoglycoside, but do not mix in same syringe; durg and metabolite attain high concentrations in the bile *(continued)*

Table 62-3 (continued)
Cephalosporins

Drug	Preparations	Usual Dosage Range	Clinical Considerations
Third Generation (continued)			
cefoperazone (Cefobid)	Powder for injection—1 g, 2 g per vial	Adults—2 g to 4 g/day IM or IV in equally divided doses every 12 h; up to 16 g/day have been given by constant infusion in severe infections	Cephalosporin with an extensive spectrum of action; used in respiratory, intra-abdominal, and urogenital infections, bacterial septicemia, and infections of the skin and associated structures; highly protein-bound; extensively excreted in the bile—do not exceed 4 g/day in patients with hepatic disease or biliary obstruction; no dosage adjustment is required in the presence of renal failure; long half-life requires only twice-a-day dosing, although more frequent administration can be used in severe infections; highly resistant to beta-lactamase enzymes produced by most gram (−) pathogens; pseudomembranous colitis has occurred, be alert for development of diarrhea; symptoms of hepatitis have been reported; may interfere with hemostasis resulting in bleeding
cefotetan (Cefotan)	Powder for injection—1 g, 2 g per vial	Adults—1 g to 2 g IV or IM every 12 h for 5 days to 10 days (maximum 3 g every 12 h in life-threatening infections) *Perioperative prophylaxis:* 1 g to 2 g IV 30 min–60 min before surgery	Long-acting parenteral cephamycin effective against most common organisms *except Pseudomonas* and *Acinetobacter*; highly resistant to beta-lactamases; use cautiously in persons with bleeding tendencies because drug may interfere with hemostasis; may produce acute alcohol intolerance; reconstituted solutions retain potency for 24 h at room temperature, 96 h refrigerated, and at least 1 wk frozen; do not refreeze; dose is reduced in patients with renal failure based on creatinine clearance
ceftazidime (Fortaz, Tazicef, Tazidime)	Powder for injection—500 mg, 1 g, 2 g, 6 g per vial or infusion pack	Adults—usually 1g to 2 g IV or IM every 8 h–12 h *Urinary infections:*	Very broad-spectrum cephalosporin used for a variety of infections (respira-*(continued)*

Table 62-3 (continued)
Cephalosporins

Drug	Preparations	Usual Dosage Range	Clinical Considerations
Third Generation (continued)			
ceftazidime (Fortaz, Tazicef, Tazidime) (*continued*)		250 mg to 500 mg every 8 h–12 h *Pseudomonal lung infection in cystic fibrosis patients:* 30 mg to 50 mg/kg IV every 8 h to a maximum of 6 g/day Children—30 mg to 50 mg/kg IV every 8 h (neonates every 12 h) *Dialysis*—1-g loading dose followed by 1 g after each hemodialysis period	tory, urinary, bone, skin, gynecologic, intra-abdominal, CNS, septicemia); good activity against *Pseudomonas* but poorly active vs *Bacteroides fragilis*; protein binding is minimal; very stable in the presence of beta-lactamases; administer separately from aminoglycosides
ceftizoxime (Cefizox)	Powder for injection—1 g, 2 g per vial Injection—1 g/50 ml, 2 g/50 ml	Adults—1 g to 2 g IM or IV every 8 h–12 h (maximum dose is 12 g/day) *Uncomplicated gonorrhea:* 1 g IM as a single dose Children—50 mg/kg every 6 h–8 h	Broad-spectrum drug used in a variety of infections due to both gram (+) and gram (−) organisms; given as twice-daily dosing in less severe infections, but serious infections require administration every 8 h; stable against beta-lactamase enzymes and only slightly (30%) protein-bound; may be active against some microorganisms that have developed resistance to other cephalosporins; dosage must be reduced in patients with impaired renal function; may be injected directly IV (3 min–5 min) or given by intermittent or continuous infusion; use in children has been associated with elevated levels of SGOT, SGPT, CPK, and eosinophils; reconstitute powder in sterile water for injection; stable for 8 h at room temperature and 48 h if refrigerated
ceftriaxone (Rocephin)	Powder for injection—250 mg, 500 mg, 1 g, 2 g, 10 g per vial	Adults—1 g to 2 g daily in a single or two divided doses IM or IV (maximum 4 g/day) Children—50 to 75 mg/kg/day in divided doses every 12 h (maximum 2 g/day)	Very long-acting cephalosporin usually given once daily (except for meningitis); very stable against beta-lactamase enzymes; highly protein-bound; excreted in both the urine and the bile; may alter (continued)

Table 62-3 (continued)
Cephalosporins

Drug	Preparations	Usual Dosage Range	Clinical Considerations
Third Generation (continued)			
ceftriaxone (Rocephin) (continued)		*Meningitis*—100 mg/kg/ day in divided doses IV every 12 h following a loading dose of 75 mg/kg *Uncomplicated gonorrhea:* 250 mg as a single IM dose *Surgical prophylaxis:* 1 g IM or IV ½ h–2 h before surgery	prothrombin time; casts in urine have occurred during therapy; dosage adjustment is seldom necessary in patients with renal or hepatic impairment; solutions should not be mixed with other antimicrobial drugs due to incompatability
moxalactam (Moxam)	Powder for injection—1 g, 2 g, 10 g per vial	Adults—500 mg to 2 g IV or IM every 8 h–12 h for most mild to moderate infections; serious or life-threatening infections— up to 4 g every 8 h Children—50 mg/kg every 6 h–8 h Infants—50 mg/kg every 6 h Neonates—50 mg/kg every 8 h–12 h	Long-acting cephalosporin, highly resistant to inactivation of beta-lactamases; indicated in lower respiratory, urinary, intra-abdominal, CNS (penetrates blood–brain barrier), skin, bone, and joint infections due to susceptible organisms; effective against many strains of *Pseudomonas* but high doses are necessary and other therapy (e.g., aminoglycosides) should be instituted if a clinical response does not occur promptly; may be given concomitantly with an aminoglycoside; probenecid does not alter the elimination of moxalactam; hypoprothombinemia and increased bleeding tendency have been reported; monitor bleeding time (especially if dose exceeds 4 g/day) and observe for signs of bleeding; discontinue drug or provide supplemental vitamin K (10 mg/wk); IV administration of moxalactam is preferred for more serious infections (i.e., slow injection [3 min–5 min] or infusion); reconstituted solution is stable for 90 h if stored under refrigeration; can cause a disulfiram-like reaction in patients who drink alcohol

many gram-negative pathogens, such as *Pseudomonas*, *Hemophilus*, *Acinetobacter*, *Neisseria*, and some strains of *Bacteroides*.

Compared to many other antibacterial drugs, cephalosporins are relatively nontoxic. The most commonly occurring adverse reactions are allergic in nature, and include rash, urticaria, fever, angioedema, and occasionally serum sickness, eosinophilia, and anaphylaxis (for additional untoward reactions, refer to general discussion of cephalosporins which follows).

A major factor in the selection of cephalosporins is their cost. Parenterally administered cephalosporins are among the most expensive antibiotics in use today, and their cost increases substantially with broadened spectrum. Thus, second-generation drugs are approximately twice as expensive as first-generation drugs, while third-generation drugs can exceed the cost of first-generation drugs by a factor of four or five. It becomes cost imperative, then, to use the least expensive cephalosporin that is effective against the microorganisms shown to be present. Empiric therapy with third-generation cephalosporins is a frightfully expensive undertaking, and considerable justification should be established for this procedure, such as the presence of severe ototoxicity or nephrotoxicity that would contradict the use of aminoglycosides.

The cephalosporins are considered here as a group. Individual drugs are then listed in Table 62-3, together with specific information pertaining to each drug. In addition, reference should be made to Table 59-1 for the recommended indications for the cephalosporins.

Cephalosporins

Cefaclor, Cefadroxil, Cefamandole, Cefazolin, Cefonicid, Cefoperazone, Ceforanide, Cefotaxime, Cefotetan, Cefoxitin, Ceftazidime, Ceftizoxime, Ceftriaxone, Cefuroxime, Cephalexin, Cephalothin, Cephapirin, Cephradine, Moxalactam

MECHANISM AND ACTIONS
Cephalosporins inhibit mucopeptide synthesis in the bacterial cell wall, resulting in a defective, osmotically unstable wall. They are usually bactericidal, depending on dose, tissue concentrations of drug, organism susceptibility, and rate of bacterial replication. The drugs are most effective against rapidly growing organisms.

USES
1. Alternates to penicillins for treatment of infections of the respiratory tract, skin and soft tissues, genitourinary tract, middle ear, and bloodstream caused by susceptible organisms (see Table 59-1 and Table 62-2 for susceptible microorganisms)
2. Surgical (*i.e.*, perioperative) prophylaxis when expanded gram-negative activity is desired, in procedures where there is a significant risk of contamination (*e.g.*, GI surgery, cholecystectomy, vaginal hysterectomy) (Usually first-generation drugs)
3. Treatment of serious *Klebsiella* infections, frequently in conjunction with an aminoglycoside
4. Treatment of meningitis caused by gram-negative enteric bacteria
5. Adjunctive treatment (with an aminoglycoside) of bacteremia of unknown origin in debilitated or immunosuppressed patients
6. Adjunctive therapy in septicemia, acute endocarditis, and bone and joint infections

ADMINISTRATION AND DOSAGE
See Table 62-3.

FATE
Oral drugs are well absorbed from GI tract, but absorption may be delayed by food. Absorption from IM sites is good. Peak blood levels are attained rapidly (usually 30 minutes–60 minutes). Half-lives are given in Table 62-2. Cephalosporins are distributed extensively, but only cefuroxime and the third-generation drugs diffuse into the cerebrospinal fluid in significant amounts, and especially when the meninges are inflamed. Penetration into bone is variable. The drugs readily cross the placental barrier and are also secreted into the milk of nursing mothers. Most derivatives (except cefotaxime, cephalothin, ceftriaxone, and cephapirin) are not appreciably metabolized and are excreted largely unchanged in the urine. Cefoperazone, however, is eliminated predominantly in the bile, and half-life and serum levels are unaltered in the presence of renal impairment, but may be increased in hepatic dysfunction or biliary stasis. Ceftriaxone and cefotaxime are also found in appreciable amounts in the bile.

First-generation drugs are usually inactivated by beta-lactamase-producing organisms. Of the second-generation agents, most are relatively stable in the presence of beta-lactamases except for cefamandole. Most third-generation cephalosporins display a high degree of stability in the presence of both cephalosporinases and penicillinases.

SIDE-EFFECTS/ADVERSE REACTIONS

The most commonly encountered side-effects with oral administration of cephalosporins are GI reactions, which include nausea, diarrhea, and vomiting and occur in up to one-third of patients receiving the drugs. The other group of frequently occurring side-effects are hypersensitivity reactions, especially in patients with a history of allergies, hay fever, or bronchial asthma. Hypersensitivity reactions may range from mild (pruritus, urticaria, drug fever, joint pain, erythema, edema) to extremely serious (erythema multiforme, serum sickness, anaphylactic reactions). Skin rash, accompanied by fever and polyarthritis are fairly common with cefaclor and may develop from 3 days to 21 days after initiation of therapy. These reactions resolve within a few days of discontinuation of therapy.

Many other adverse reactions have occurred in persons receiving cephalosporins and are listed below. Untoward reactions that may be associated with individual cephalosporins are indicated in Table 62-3 for the specific drugs involved.

GI—Anorexia, abdominal pain, dyspepsia, heartburn, severe diarrhea, oral candidiasis, glossitis, GI bleeding, enterocolitis

Allergic—Urticaria, pruritus, skin rash, fever, chills, serum sickness, eosinophilia, angioedema, exfoliative dermatitis, anaphylactic reactions

Hematologic—Neutropenia, leukopenia, thrombocytopenia, agranulocytosis, hemolytic anemia, bleeding due to hypoprothrombinemia (see below), positive direct Coombs' test

Genitourinary—Dysuria, elevated BUN, proteinuria, hematuria, vaginal discharge, candidal vaginitis, genitoanal pruritus, genital candidiasis

Hepatic—Elevated SGOT, SGPT, bilirubin, alkaline phosphatase, and LDH levels; hepatitis (rare)

Other—Headache, weakness, dizziness, dyspnea, paresthesia, candidal overgrowth, hepatomegaly; IM administration, especially of cephalothin and cefoxitin, may cause pain, induration, tenderness, fever,

and tissue sloughing; IV injection has produced thrombophlebitis

Coagulation abnormalities associated with bleeding episodes, some of a severe nature, have occurred with use of several cephalosporins, including cefamandole, cefoperazone, and especially moxalactam. These drugs can interfere with hemostasis in several ways: (a) they may destroy vitamin K-producing intestinal bacteria, resulting in hypoprothrombinemia; (b) they may inhibit platelet function; and (c) they may induce an allergic thrombocytopenia. Predisposing factors to cephalosporin-induced bleeding include hepatic or renal dysfunction, thrombocytopenia, and concomitant use of anticoagulants or other drugs that adversely affect hemostasis. Elderly or debilitated persons are more likely to have bleeding episodes with cephalosporins than younger, healthier patients.

The inhibition of platelet function is generally dose-dependent and can be minimized by reducing the dose of the drugs. Bleeding resulting from hypoprothrombinemia can be prevented by administration of vitamin K (e.g., 10 mg K$_1$/week) prophylactically.

Bleeding during cephalosporin therapy may not necessarily be due to the drugs but may result from complications of an underlying disease state, such as malignancy, sepsis, or hepatic or renal disease. Accurate diagnosis is essential.

Pseudomembranous colitis has developed with use of cephalosporins (as well as other broad-spectrum antibiotics). Diarrhea is usually the initial symptom. Mild cases are relieved by discontinuation of the drug. More severe cases may require fluid and electrolyte supplementation, and, if due to overgrowth of *Clostridium difficile*, oral vancomycin or metronidazole infusion may be effective.

CONTRAINDICATIONS AND PRECAUTIONS

Other than hypersensitivity to cephalosporins, there are no absolute contraindications to use of these drugs. A *cautious* approach to therapy, however, is warranted in patients with a history of GI disease, allergies, asthma, hay fever, penicillin sensitivity (see introductory comments), impaired renal function during pregnancy, and in small children and nursing mothers.

In addition, cefoperazone, ceftriaxone, and cefotaxime should be given cautiously to persons with impaired liver function, as they are excreted in the bile.

Inflammatory reactions with parenteral cephalosporin administration are relatively common. The drugs should be given deep into a large muscle mass. Sterile abscesses have occurred following inadvertent SC injection.

INTERACTIONS

1. Use of bacteriostatic antibiotics (e.g., tetracyclines, erythromycins) may reduce the effectiveness of the bactericidal cephalosporins, especially in acute infections where the organisms are proliferating rapidly.
2. The nephrotoxic effects of cephalosporins may be augmented by aminoglycosides, colistin, vancomycin, polymyxin B, ethacrynic acid, furosemide, bumetanide, probenecid, and sulfinpyrazone.
3. Cephalosporins are incompatible in parenteral mixtures with tetracyclines, erythromycins, calcium chloride, and magnesium salts.
4. Probenecid may increase and prolong cephalosporin plasma levels (except moxalactam) by inhibiting renal tubular secretion of the drugs.
5. Alcohol may elicit a disulfiram-like reaction (see Chap. 26) with cefamandole, cefoperazone, cefotetan, or moxalactam.

■ Nursing Process

(See also Nursing Process for anti-infective therapy in Chapter 59.)

□ ASSESSMENT

□ Subjective Data

A drug history should be obtained focusing on antibiotic use. Concurrent use of a bacteriostatic antibiotics such as erythromycin may reduce cephalosporin effectiveness and may increase the risk of superinfection. Concurrent use of any nephrotoxic drugs (see under Interactions) may increase the nephrotoxic effects of cephalosporins. The patient should also be asked about alcohol use. Certain cephalosporins when combined with alcohol will cause a disulfiram-like reaction described below. This information is especially important if the patient is a chronic abuser being treated for an acute illness. The patient should also be asked about drug allergies, especially to penicillin because cross-hypersensitivity between these drugs is likely to occur.

General history should focus on the symptoms of infection for which the antibiotic is being prescribed as well as presence of renal or gastrointestinal disease, pregnancy, or lactation all of which warrant use only when the benefits outweigh the therapeutic risks. Cephalosporins should be used cautiously in patients with known allergies, asthma, and hay fever because drug hypersensitivity is more likely to occur.

Except in emergencies where no other drug is appropriate, the patient should be asked about ability to pay for the drug. Cephalosporins are among the most expensive antibiotics marketed and may be prohibitively expensive to the outpatient not covered by insurance. The cost may result in noncompliance; financial resources should be explored before treatment begins.

□ Objective Data

Physical assessment of the site of infection is appropriate. Bowel sounds should be auscultated to detect hypermotility which may be aggravated by drug therapy. Urinary output should be measured, and extremities examined for evidence of edema. The nurse should also obtain a heart rate and listen to breath sounds. All of these latter are measures of cardiac function and will be used as a baseline should the patient develop fluid retention and congestive heart failure.

Laboratory data should include a complete blood count with differential, renal function studies, liver enzymes, coagulation studies, and a direct Coombs' test on any patient with compromised renal function (especially the elderly) or young children or any patient receiving high dose or intravenous drug therapy.

□ NURSING DIAGNOSES

Actual nursing diagnoses may include:
    Knowledge deficit related to action, administration, and side-effects of the drug
Potential nursing diagnoses may include:
    Alteration in bowel elimination: diarrhea, a drug side-effect
    Alteration in comfort: pain from IM injection or phlebitis, a drug side-effect of intravenous administration
    Alteration in fluid volume: excess; may be related to sodium retention or to development of nephrotoxicity
    Other nursing diagnoses may be appropriate if the patient develops hypersensitivity (see Chap. 61) or a disulfiram-like reaction (see Chap. 26).

□ PLAN

Nursing care goals should focus on:
1. Administering the drug correctly and safely according to the prescribed route
2. Monitoring for side-effects, especially gastrointestinal problems, hypersensitivity, hematologic changes, and nephrotoxicity
3. Teaching the patient correct drug-taking tech-

niques, side-effects, especially use of alcohol during treatment, and what to do if problems occur

☐ *INTERVENTION*

Oral doses of cephalosporin drugs are best absorbed on an empty stomach but can be given with food if gastrointestinal upset develops. Food may delay drug absorption but will not decrease therapeutic effectiveness.

Intramuscular injections should be given deep in a large muscle mass such as the gluteus in adults or the vastus lateralis in small children. Sites should be carefully rotated using a body map (see Chap. 8) to decrease the pain and inflammation which can develop from the drug. Sites should be palpated for pain and lumps before injection to ensure tissue is not further damaged. Needle length must be sufficient to ensure intramuscular placement; short needles can produce a subcutaneous injection which has resulted in sterile abscesses in some cases.

Some cephalosporin drugs can be given by intravenous injection although infusion is preferred. The manufacturer's instructions for dilution and time period for injection should be strictly followed. If directions are not specific, a general guideline is that each 500 mg of drug should be mixed in 10 ml of diluent and total injection time should be at least 3 minutes to 5 minutes. The pharmacist or the manufacturer should be consulted if exact guideline cannot be determined from the product literature. Most cephalosporins are very irritating to veins; therefore, intermittent infusion of the drug dose in a larger volume of solution (50 ml–100 ml) over a 30-minute period is preferred. Large veins should be used as infusion sites and the IV should be changed every 48 hours to decrease the chance of phlebitis. Sites should be routinely checked for pain, swelling, and redness; if such signs are noted the IV must be removed immediately. Intravenous lines should be completely flushed if other parenteral antibiotics or other drugs are being given. Cephalosporins are physically incompatible with many other drugs (see Appendix).

Many of the side-effects seen with cephalosporins are similar to those with the penicillins. See Nursing Process for Penicillins in Chapter 61 for a discussion of the symptoms and nursing actions for hypersensitivity reactions, electrolyte imbalances (hypernatremia occurs with cephalosporins), and superinfections. The patient on cephalosporins is most likely to develop perineal monilia or gastrointestinal diarrhea from disruption of bacterial flora.

Although the incidence of diarrhea is low in adults and children, it must be monitored closely and any severe or prolonged bouts (over 24 hours) should be reported immediately. Pseudomembranous colitis can develop allowing proliferation of *Clostridium difficile*, a dangerous bacteria which elaborates a toxin and must be treated immediately.

Laboratory values can be altered by cephalosporins. A false-positive reading for urine glucose will be obtained with Clinitest tablets. Tes-Tape or Clinistix should be used during drug therapy. A positive direct Coombs' test (the measure of the development of red blood cell antibodies) may occur without any clinical evidence of RBC breakdown or anemia. However, the patient who develops a positive Coomb's test should be monitored for signs of anemia.

Cephalosporins, especially moxalactam, cefamandole, and cefoperazone, can interfere with hemostasis by decreasing the availability of vitamin K and interfering with normal platelet function. Bleeding tendencies are most common in elderly patients receiving these drugs. Platelet levels and prothrombin times should be drawn throughout therapy to monitor changes. Vitamin K can be given weekly, as necessary, if prothrombin times rise above normal. Other hematologic changes can occur (see under Side-Effects/Adverse Reactions), therefore, a CBC with differential should be taken periodically.

Moxalactam, cefamandole, and cefaperazone can also induce a disulfiram-like reaction when mixed with alcohol. Symptoms include nausea, vomiting, throbbing headache, weakness, and vertigo when small quantities are ingested but may lead to congestive heart failure, arrhythmias, respiratory depression, and death if larger quantities have been taken. Blood alcohol levels diminish slowly; therefore a patient should always be asked about the quantity and timing of recent alcohol ingestion because the reaction can occur even several days after the last drink if a large quantity was ingested or if the individual is a chronic abuser. All patients should be told to avoid alcohol completely during the course of treatment. Treatment of a disulfiram-like reaction includes fluids, rest, and drug therapy for treatment of symptoms. The cephalosporin should be discontinued.

The patient with impaired renal function should receive reduced doses of a cephalosporin to decrease the chance of toxicity. However, nephrotoxicity is a possibility with any patient, especially the young child and the elderly patient; therefore urinary output, urine protein, BUN, and serum creatinine should be closely monitored throughout treatment and the cephalosporin discontinued if enzymes become elevated or symptoms of jaundice, fever, lethargy occur.

☐ *EVALUATION*

Outcome criteria used to measure treatment success may include resolution of infection, evidence that the nurse or patient uses correct administration techniques, and the absence of side-effects such as hypersensitivity, superinfection, hypernatremia, phlebitis (IV route), diarrhea or colitis, hematologic changes or bleeding tendencies, disulfiram-like reaction (from alcohol ingestion), nephrotoxicity, or hepatic toxicity.

CASE STUDY

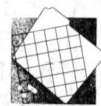

Alexander Morgan, aged 58, was diagnosed with colorectal carcinoma, and a decision was made to perform exploratory surgery for removal of the tumor and possible temporary colostomy. In addition to the other preoperative orders written, the physician prescribes cephalothin (Keflin) 1 g IV piggyback in 50 ml of normal saline to infuse in 30 minutes; dose to be given ½ hour before surgery. He also requests 2 g cephalothin to accompany the patient to the OR. Two doses of cephalothin are given during the operative procedure. Postoperatively, Mr. Morgan returns to his room. A colostomy has been performed.

Discussion Questions

1. Why was cephalothin ordered pre- and perioperatively for this patient?
2. What postoperative drug orders should the nurse expect to see regarding antibiotic drug therapy?
3. Outline a flow sheet for monitoring Mr. Morgan while he is receiving cephalothin.

REVIEW QUESTIONS

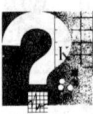

1. In what way are the cephalosporins usually classified?
2. How do third-generation cephalosporins differ from first-generation cephalosporins with respect to (a) activity against gram-positive organisms, (b) resistance to beta-lactamase enzymes, and (c) cost?
3. Against which microorganisms are first-generation drugs most effective?
4. List the recognized indications for the cephalosporin drugs.
5. What are the only cephalosporins used orally?
6. Give the most commonly encountered side-effects with cephalosporins. How are they treated? What should the patient be told to monitor?
7. With what cephalosporins is the risk of bleeding complications increased? What mechanisms may be involved in these bleeding abnormalities?
8. What is the usual dosing procedure when cephalosporins are used for *perioperative prophylaxis*?
9. Name the only injectable cephalosporin that does not contain sodium.
10. Which cephalosporin is eliminated predominantly in the bile?
11. Which cephalosporin has the longest half-life?
12. Name the two cephalosporins which are derivatives of cephamycin C.

13. What should a patient be asked in a drug history before cephalosporins are administered?
14. What preliminary laboratory samples should be collected before drug administration? Why?
15. Outline the nursing actions for a patient receiving an intravenous cephalosporin.

BIBLIOGRAPHY

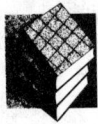

Bank NV, Kammer RB: Hematologic complications associated with beta-lactam antibiotics. Rev Infect Dis 5(suppl 2):380, 1983

Baumgartner J, Glauser MP: Single daily dose treatment of severe refractory infections with ceftriaxone. Arch Intern Med 143:1868, 1983

Bertino JS, Speck WT: The cephalosporin antibiotics. Pediatr Clin North Am 30:17, 1983

Bodey G, Fainstein V, Hinkle A: Comparative *in vitro* study of new cephalosporins. J Antimicrob Agents 20:226, 1981

Byrd HJ, Fischer RG: Cephalosporins: A brief overview of three generations. Ped Nursing 9:330, 1983

Ceftriaxone sodium (Rocephin). Med Lett Drugs Ther 27:37, 1985

Garzone P, Lyon J, Yu VL: Third-generation and investigational cephalosporins, Parts I and II. Drug Intell Clin Pharm 17:507, 615, 1983

Klein JO, Neu HC: Empiric therapy for bacterial infections: Evaluation of cefoperazone. Rev Infect Dis 5:S1, 1983

Mandell GL: Cephalosporins. In Mandell GL, Douglas RG, Bennett JE (eds): Principles and Practice of Infectious Diseases, 2nd ed, p 180. New York, John Wiley & Sons, 1985

McCloskey WW, Jeffrey LP: Drug stop: New beta-lactam antimicrobials. J Neurosurg Nursing 17:210, 1985

Mullaney DT, John JF: Cefotaxime therapy. Arch Intern Med 143:1705, 1983

Murray BE, Moellering RC: Cephalosporins. Annu Rev Med 32:559, 1981

Neu HC: New beta-lactamase-stable cephalosporins. Ann Intern Med 97:408, 1982

Neu HC: Clinical uses of cephalosporins. Lancet 1:252, 1982

Phillips I, Wise R, Leigh DA: Cefotetan: A new cephamycin. J Antimicrob Chemother 11(Suppl B):1, 1983

Polk R: Moxalactam (Moxam). Drug Intell Clin Pharm 16:104, 1982

Quintiliana R, et al: Cephalosporins: An overview. In Ristuccia AM, Cunha BA (eds): Anti-microbial Therapy, p 289. New York, Raven Press, 1984

Schumacher GE: Pharmacokinetic and microbiologic evaluation of dosage regimens for newer cephalosporins and penicillins. Clin Pharm 2:448, 1983

Smith BR, LeFrock JL: Cefuroxime: Antimicrobial activity, pharmacology and clinical efficacy. Ther Drug Monit 5:149, 1983

Sykes RB, Bush K: Interaction of new cephalosporins with beta lactamases and beta-lactamase-producing gram negative bacilli. Rev Infect Dis 5:S356, 1983

Thompson RL, Wright AJ: Cephalosporin antibiotics. Mayo Clin Proc 58:79, 1983

Weinstein AJ: The cephalosporins: Activity and clinical use. Drugs 19:137, 1980

Weitekamp MR, Aber RC: Prolonged bleeding times and bleeding diathesis associated with moxalactam administration. JAMA 249:69, 1983

Tetracyclines

Tetracyclines
> *Chlortetracycline,*
>> *Demeclocycline,*
>> *Doxycycline,*
>> *Meclocycline,*
>> *Methacycline,*
>> *Minocycline,*
>> *Oxytetracycline,*
>> *Tetracycline*

63

The tetracycline group of antibiotics is composed of a number of naturally derived and semisynthetic compounds possessing similar pharmacologic properties. These bacteriostatic anti-infective agents exhibit a broad spectrum of activity which overlaps that of some other antibacterial drugs, but because of their extensive and often indiscriminate use in the past, their current clinical usefulness has been restricted by the emergence of a number of resistant bacterial strains. Many previously sensitive staphylococcal, streptococcal, pneumococcal, and other gram-positive organisms are now largely resistant to the tetracyclines, and in vitro laboratory susceptibility tests are necessary to determine the usefulness of a given tetracycline in a particular patient.

While essentially alike in their antimicrobial activity, the various tetracyclines differ in some of their pharmacokinetic properties, and these differences are indicated in Table 63-1. Oral absorption is variable and erratic and, except for doxycycline and minocycline, may be reduced by elevated gastric pH and the presence of food or polyvalent cations such as iron, calcium, magnesium, and aluminum. Plasma protein binding varies throughout a wide range. Tetracyclines diffuse readily into most body tissues, attaining highest concentrations in the lungs, liver, kidney, spleen, bone marrow, and lymph. Penetration of the drugs into the CNS is largely determined by the respective lipid solubility, minocycline and doxycycline being the most lipophilic derivatives and thus best able to enter the CNS while oxytetracycline is the least lipo-

philic. In addition, minocycline attains high levels in saliva, making it useful in eliminating meningococci from the nasopharynx of carriers (see under Uses).

The drugs cross the placental barrier, and concentrations in the fetal circulation may reach as high as 70% of the maternal circulation. Due to the high affinity of tetracyclines for calcium, any fetal tissue undergoing active calcification (e.g., bone, teeth) may have its development impaired by the presence of tetracyclines. Likewise, prolonged use of tetracyclines during the entire period of tooth development (fourth fetal month through the eighth year of life) may cause inadequate calcium deposition and discoloration of both deciduous and permanent teeth. Therefore, these drugs should be avoided during pregnancy and lactation (because they are secreted in breast milk), and in young children up to the age of 8 years.

With the exception of minocycline, the other tetracyclines are not metabolized to an appreciable extent. Except for minocycline and doxycycline, they are excreted largely in the urine. Doxycycline is secreted into the intestinal lumen where it forms insoluble complexes with intestinal solids and is eliminated predominately in the feces. Minocycline and its metabolites are recoverable in both the feces and urine, but renal clearance is low (see below). Renal clearance of all tetracyclines is by glomerular filtration and varies widely among the different derivatives. Drugs having a high renal clearance (e.g., oxytetracycline, tetracycline) are more effective in treating urinary tract infections

Table 63-1
Characteristics of Tetracyclines

Drug	Routes of Administration	Approximate Percentage Oral Absorption (%)	Protein Binding (%)	Plasma Half-Life (h)	Major Route of Elimination	Urinary Excretion (% Unchanged Drug)
chlortetracycline	Opthalmic Topical					
demeclocycline	Oral	60–70	50–80	10–16	Kidney	40–50
doxycycline*	Oral, IV	90–95	60–90	12–24	Feces	30–40
meclocycline	Topical					
methacycline	Oral	30–60	75–90	12–16	Kidney	40–50
minocycline*	Oral, IV	95–100	60–75	12–20	Kidney/feces (metabolites)	5–10
oxytetracycline	Oral, IV, IM	50–60	20–30	6–10	Kidney	50–70
tetracycline	Oral, IV, IM Ophthalmic Topical	70–80	20–60	6–10	Kidney	60–70

* Absorption is not significantly decreased by the presence of food, dairy products, or antacids.

than drugs with low renal clearances, but they may be more dangerous in the presence of renal impairment because of accumulation of drug in the body.

The systemic tetracyclines can be divided arbitrarily into two broad groups based on their serum half-lives. Tetracycline and oxytetracycline are considered short-acting drugs, having half-lives of 6 hours to 10 hours. The remaining derivatives possess half-lives of approximately 10 hours to 20 hours and thus exhibit a longer duration of action. There is no convincing evidence, however, that one derivative is significantly more effective than any other for treating most susceptible infections. The more completely absorbed, longer acting drugs (i.e., doxycycline, minocycline) require less frequent administration (twice a day vs three or four times a day) than the other derivatives, and thus may improve patient compliance; however, they are considerably more expensive, and minocycline is associated with a high incidence of vestibular disturbances (e.g., dizziness, ataxia, lightheadedness). Because doxycycline and minocycline are not appreciably excreted by the kidney, they are preferred tetracyclines for use in patients with renal impairment.

As noted previously, the emergence of resistant strains has severely limited the clinical application of the tetracyclines. Currently they are considered first-choice drugs for only the following infections: cholera, brucellosis, granuloma inguinale, meloidosis, chlamydial infections (ornithosis, psittacosis, trachoma, urethritis, cervicitis, lymphogranuloma venereum), Mycoplasma pneumoniae infections, rickettsial infections (Rocky Mountain spotted fever, tick-bite fever, typhus, Q fever), relapsing fever, and gonorrhea and syphilis in penicillin-allergic patients. Tetracyclines are also indicated as alternate drugs for a number of gram-positive and gram-negative infections (see Table 59-1), although sensitivity tests are necessary to confirm susceptibility. Although active in vitro against many gram-positive cocci, tetracyclines should not be used to treat staphylococcal, group A beta-hemolytic streptococcal or Streptococcus pneumoniae infections, because of the occurrence of many resistant strains. Oral tetracyclines have been used as adjunctive therapy for severe acne because they reduce the amount of free fatty acids in acne lesions as well as decrease the population of Propionibacterium acnes in sebaceous glands. Topical application of tetracycline solution or meclocycline cream is also effective in treatment of acne vulgaris lesions, although the mechanism is not well established. Both oral and topical tetracy-

clines may be employed for treatment of inclusion conjunctivitis. Finally, doxycycline appears to be useful in preventing "travelers' diarrhea" caused by Escherichia coli, and minocycline can be used to treat asymptomatic carriers of Neisseria meningitidis.

Tetracyclines

Chlortetracycline, Demeclocycline, Doxycycline, Meclocycline, Methacycline, Minocycline, Oxytetracycline, Tetracycline

The following discussion considers the tetracyclines as a group. Individual members of the class are then listed in Table 63-2.

MECHANISM AND ACTIONS
Tetracyclines are bacteriostatic against a wide range of gram-positive and gram-negative microorganisms. Their site of action is the bacterial ribosome, to which the drugs gain access by one of two processes: either passive diffusion through pores in the bacterial cell membrane or by an active transport system in the inner cytoplasmic membrane. Once inside the bacterial cells, tetracyclines bind specifically to 30S ribosomes. They appear to prevent binding of transfer RNA to the acceptor site on the messenger RNA–ribosome complex, thus inhibiting protein synthesis. High doses of tetracyclines may also interfere with replication of DNA on the cell membrane. Although high doses can interfere with protein synthesis in mammalian cells as well, these cells lack the active transport system for uptake of the tetracycline drugs.

USES
1. Treatment of the following infections: Rickettsiae (i.e., Rocky Mountain spotted fever, typhus, Q fever, rickettsial pox, tick fever); Mycoplasma pneumoniae, chlamydial infections, brucellosis, granuloma inguinale, cholera, relapsing fever, and chancroid
2. Treatment of susceptible strains of Escherichia coli, Enterobacter, Shigella, Acinetobacter, Hemophilus influenzae, Klebsiella, streptococci, and Diplococcus pneumoniae
(Note: Many strains of streptococci and most of the other above-named organisms are resistant.

Tetracyclines are not drugs of choice in staphylococcal infections.)

3. Adjunctive therapy for severe acne or inclusion conjunctivitis (oral or combined oral/topical administration)
4. Adjunctive therapy (with amebicides) in the treatment of acute intestinal amebiasis
5. Treatment of uncomplicated urethral, endocervical, or rectal infections in adults caused by *Chlamydia trachomatis*
6. Alternate therapy for gonorrhea or syphilis in penicillin-sensitive patients
7. Elimination of meningococci from the nasopharynx of asymptomatic carriers of *Neisseria meningitidis* (oral minocycline only). *Not* for treatment of meningococcal infections
8. Investigational uses include:
   a. Prevention of travelers' diarrhea due to enterotoxic *Escherichia coli* (doxycycline)
   b. Management of chronic inappropriate antidiuretic hormone secretion (demeclocycline)
   c. Alternative to sulfonamides in treatment of nocardiosis (minocycline)
   d. Sclerosing agent (by chest tube) in malignant pleural effusion (tetracycline)

ADMINISTRATION AND DOSAGE
See Table 63-2.

FATE
Oral absorption of the tetracyclines is variable and incomplete; the percentage of the oral dose absorbed ranges from as low as 30% (methacycline) to nearly 100% (minocycline) but rises as the dose is increased. Absorption is greater in the fasting state, except for doxycycline and minocycline which should be taken with food. Oral absorption of tetracyclines is reduced in the presence of milk or dairy products, calcium, magnesium, aluminum, and iron probably due to chelation (see under Interactions). Distribution of tetracyclines is variable; most derivatives are widely distributed in the body, except for the CNS, where only highly lipophilic derivatives (*e.g.*, doxycycline, minocycline) attain appreciable levels. Minocycline is also highly concentrated in saliva and tears. Plasma half-lives vary from 6 hours to 24 hours (see Table 63-1), and extent of protein binding differs considerably among the different drugs. Other than minocycline, the drugs are not metabolized to a significant extent. Doxycycline and minocycline and its metabolites are excreted largely in the feces whereas other derivatives are eliminated primarily by the kidneys, a considerable amount as unchanged drug. Thus, dosage reduction in patients with renal impairment may be necessary.

SIDE-EFFECTS/ADVERSE REACTIONS
The most often encountered side-effects with tetracycline usage are gastrointestinal irritation, nausea, diarrhea, anorexia, and photosensitivity reactions (most frequent with demeclocycline, less frequent with doxycycline, and relatively infrequent with the other derivatives). In addition, minocycline frequently elicits vestibular disturbances characterized by lightheadedness, dizziness, and vertigo. Oncholysis (*i.e.*, loosening of nails) has been noted in approximately one-fourth of patients exhibiting a photosensitivity reaction.

Other reported adverse reactions during therapy with tetracyclines include:

GI—Stomatitis, glossitis, sore throat, dysphagia, vomiting, enterocolitis, steatorrhea, inflammation in the anogenital region, esophageal ulceration

Dermatologic—Macropapular and erythematous rash, exfoliative dermatitis

Hypersensitivity—Fever, urticaria, angioedema, headache, impaired vision, papilledema, pericarditis, anaphylaxis, exacerbation of systemic lupus erythematosus

Hematologic—Hemolytic anemia, eosinophilia, neutropenia, thrombocytopenia, leukopenia, leukocytosis

Other—Increased BUN, permanent discoloration of teeth (see under Contraindications and Precautions), enamel hypoplasia, impaired calcification of bony structures, increased intracranial pressure and bulging fontanels in young infants, nephrogenic diabetes insipidus (demeclocycline only), irritation at IM injection sites, thrombophlebitis with IV administration, overgrowth of nonsusceptible organisms

Outdated tetracycline products are potentially nephrotoxic and have resulted in development of the Fanconi syndrome, characterized by nausea, vomiting, polyuria, polydipsia, proteinuria, glycosuria, and acidosis. Symptoms disappear within several weeks after cessation of therapy.

Doses in excess of 2 g/day have resulted in hepatic toxicity, and pregnant women appear to be particularly susceptible to hepatic damage. Symptoms include fatty deposition, azotemia, acidosis, and jaundice.

(*Text continues on p. 1222.*)

Table 63-2
Tetracyclines

Drug	Preparations	Usual Dosage Range	Clinical Considerations
chlortetracycline (Aureomycin)	Ophthalmic ointment—1% Topical ointment—3%	Ophthalmic—place small amount of ointment into lower conjunctival sac every 3 h as needed Topical—apply small amount every 3 h–6 h as needed	Tetracycline derivative not given systemically and infrequently used topically due to risk of sensitization; be alert for appearance of allergic reactions and discontinue drug; ophthalmic ointment may retard corneal healing; topical use should be supplemented by appropriate systemic antibiotics
demeclocycline (Declomycin)	Tablets—150 mg, 300 mg Capsules—150 mg	Adults—150 mg four times a day or 300 mg twice a day Children—3 mg to 6 mg/lb (6.6 mg–13.2 mg/kg) divided into two to four doses Gonorrhea in penicillin-sensitive patients—600 mg initially, followed by 300 mg every 12 h for 5 days Uncomplicated chlamydial infections—300 mg four times a day for at least 7 days	Orally effective tetracycline that is slowly excreted in part because of enterohepatic circulation; among tetracyclines, produces highest incidence of photosensitivity reactions; may result in diabetes insipidus-like syndrome (polyuria, polydipsia, weakness) on prolonged therapy; syndrome is caused by interference with action of vasopressin (ADH) on the kidneys, is dose-dependent, and is reversible upon discontinuation of drug; intake-to-output ratio should be monitored routinely; drug has been used investigationally in managing the chronic form of syndrome of inappropriate anti-diuretic hormone secretion (SIADH)
doxycycline (AK-Ramycin, Doryx, Doxy-Caps, Doxychel, Doxy-Tabs, Vibramycin, Vibra Tabs, Vivox)	Tablets—50 mg, 100 mg Capsules—50 mg, 100 mg Slow-release capsules (coated pellets)—100 mg Powder for oral suspension —25 mg/5 ml Syrup—50 mg/5 ml Powder for injection—100 mg/vial, 200 mg/vial	Oral: Adults:200 mg in two divided doses initially followed by 100 mg/day in single or two divided doses; severe infections require 100 mg every 12 h Children—2 mg/lb (4.4 mg/kg) in divided doses the first day; then 1 mg to 2 mg/lb (2.2 mg–4.4 mg/kg) as a single dose or two divided doses each day IV infusion: Adults—200 mg the first day; then 100 mg to 200	Semisynthetic tetracycline that is well absorbed orally, exhibits a prolonged duration of action, and is slowly excreted, primarily in the feces; may be used safely in patients with renal impairment; IV infusion is not recommended in children under 8 years of age; oral absorption is not significantly affected by food; drug has low affinity for calcium binding; infrequent incidence of photosensitivity; duration of *(continued)*

***Table 63-2** (continued)*
Tetracyclines

Drug	Preparations	Usual Dosage Range	Clinical Considerations
doxycycline (AK-Ramycin, Doryx, Doxy-Caps, Doxychel, Doxy-Tabs, Vibramycin, Vibra Tabs, Vivox) *(continued)*		mg/day in one to two infusions Children—2 mg/lb (4.4 mg/kg) first day in one to two infusions; then 1 mg to 2 mg/lb (2.2 mg to 4.4 mg/kg) in one to two infusions each day Gonococcal infections: 100 mg twice a day for 7 days following a single dose of penicillin or cephalosporin. Patients allergic to penicillin and cephalosporins—100 mg twice a day for 7 days Acute pelvic inflammatory disease: 100 mg twice a day for 10 days to 14 days following a single dose of amoxicillin, cefoxitin, or ceftriaxone Syphilis: 300 mg/day orally or IV for at least 10 days Uncomplicated chlamydial infections: 100 mg twice day for at least 7 days Prevention of "travelers' diarrhea"—100 mg/day as a single dose	IV infusion varies with the dose, and ranges from 1 h–4 h; minimum infusion time for 100 mg of a 0.5 mg/ml solution is 1 h; therapy should be continued for at least 24 h–48 h after symptoms have subsided; follow package instructions for preparation and storage of IV infusion solution; do not inject solutions IM or SC and avoid extravasation, because solutions are irritating; drug is used experimentally to prevent "travelers' diarrhea" (see under Usual Dosage Range)
meclocycline (Meclan)	Cream—1%	Apply twice a day in generous amounts until skin is thoroughly wet	Locally acting tetracycline that is not absorbed to a significant extent; used in treatment of mild to moderate acne vulgaris; avoid contact with eyes, nose, or mouth; may produce skin irritation and transient stinging and burning; slight yellowing of the skin can occur but may be removed by washing; cosmetics may be applied in the usual manner during treatment; caution in patients allergic to formaldehyde, as it is a component of the vehicle
methacycline (Rondomycin)	Capsules—150 mg, 300 mg	Adults—600 mg/day in two to four divided doses Children—3 mg to 6 mg/lb/day (6.6 mg–13.2 mg/kg/day) in two to four divided doses Gonorrhea—900 mg initially, then 300 mg four	Semisynthetic, orally effective tetracycline; incompletely absorbed orally; highly bound to plasma protein; excreted largely in urine; use with caution in presence of renal impairment; similar to tet- *(continued)*

Table 63-2 (continued)
Tetracyclines

Drug	Preparations	Usual Dosage Range	Clinical Considerations
methacycline (Rondomycin) (*continued*)		times/day to a total of 5.4 g Syphilis—18 g to 24 g in equally divided doses over 10 days to 15 days	racycline in most other respects, and significantly more expensive
minocycline (Minocin)	Capsules—50 mg, 100 mg Tablets—50 mg, 100 mg Syrup—50 mg/5 ml Powder for injection—100 mg/vial	Adults—200 mg initially, then 100 mg every 12 h or 50 mg four times a day Children (over 8 yr)—4 mg/kg initially; then 2 mg/kg every 12 h Gonorrhea—200 mg initially then 100 mg every 12 h for a minimum of 5 days Syphilis—100 mg every 12 h for 10 days to 15 days Meningococcal carrier state—100 mg every 12 h for 5 days Chlamydial infections—100 mg twice a day for at least 7 days IV infusion: Adults—200 mg initially then 100 mg every 12 h (maximum 400 mg/day) Children—4 mg/kg initially, then 2 mg/kg every 12 h	Semisynthetic tetracycline that is almost completely absorbed orally; very lipid soluble and possesses a long half-life (up to 20 h): low renal clearance; oral absorption is not appreciably altered by food; only tetracycline drug metabolized to any extent; photosensitivity occurs rarely; vestibular side-effects are very common (lightheadedness, dizziness, vertigo), therefore, urge caution in driving or operating machinery; indicated in treatment of asymptomatic carriers of *Neisseria meningitidis* to eliminate organism from nasopharynx because drug attains high levels in saliva; *not* recommended for treatment of meningococcal infection; also used in treatment of nocardiosis; may result in blue-gray pigmentation of the skin and mucous membrane; IV solutions are stable at room temperature for 24 h
oxytetracycline (E. P. Mycin, Terramycin, Uri-Tet)	Capsules—250 mg IM injection—50 mg/ml, 125 mg/ml (with 2% lidocaine) Powder for IV infusion—250 mg/vial, 500 mg/vial	Oral: Adults—1 g to 2 g/day in two to four equally divided doses Children—10 mg to 20 mg/lb/day (22 mg–44 mg/kg/day) in two to four equal doses IM: Adults—250 mg/day in a single dose or 300 mg/day in divided doses every 8 h–12 h Children—15 mg to 25 mg/kg/day in divided doses every 8 h–12 h (maximum 250 mg/day)	Naturally derived tetracycline with actions similar to tetracycline itself; oral absorption is incomplete, half-life is 6 h–10 h, and protein binding is minimal; renal clearance is highest of all tetracyclines, thus drug may be more effective than other derivatives in urinary infections; use with caution in presence of renal impairment, because drug may accumulate rapidly; IM solution contains 2% lidocaine; do not inject (*continued*)

Table 63-2 (continued)
Tetracyclines

Drug	Preparations	Usual Dosage Range	Clinical Considerations
oxytetracycline (E. P. Mycin, Terramycin, Uri-Tet) (continued)		IV infusion: Adults—250 mg to 500 mg every 12 h (maximum 2 g/day) Children—12 mg/kg/day in two divided doses (range 10 mg–20 mg/kg/day)	IV; use only injection marked "IV" for IV administration; reconstituted solutions for injection are stable for 48 h with refrigeration
tetracycline (Achromycin, Panmycin, Sumycin, and various other manufacturers)	Capsules—100 mg, 250 mg, 500 mg Tablets—250 mg, 500 mg Syrup—125 mg/5 ml Powder for IM injection—100 mg/vial, 250 mg/vial with 2% procaine Powder for IV injection—250 mg/vial, 500 mg/vial Ophthalmic drops—1% Ophthalmic ointment—1% Topical ointment—3% Topical solution—2.2 mg/ml	Oral: Adults—1 g to 2 g/day in two to four equal doses Children—25 mg to 50 mg/kg/day in two to four equal doses Gonorrhea—1.5 g initially; then 0.5 g every 6 h for 5 days to 7 days Syphilis—30 g to 40 g in equally divided doses over 10 days to 15 days Brucellosis—500 mg four times a day for 3 wk, with 1 g streptomycin IM twice a day for the first week, then once daily the second week Chlamydial infections—500 mg four times a day for at least 7 days Acne—1 g/day initially; reduce to 125 mg to 500 mg daily for chronic therapy IM: Adults—250 mg/day in a dose or 300 mg/day in divided doses every 8 h–12 h (maximum 800 mg/day) Children—15 mg to 25 mg/kg/day in divided doses every 8 h–12 h IV: Adults—250 mg to 500 mg every 12 hours (maximum 2 g/day) Children—10 mg to 20 mg/kg/day in two divided doses Ophthalmic: 1 drop to 2 drops or small amount of ointment in affected eye two to four times a day Topical: Apply two to four times a day	Semisynthetic tetracycline produced from chlortetracycline or obtained naturally; widely used and least expensive of the tetracyclines; used orally, parenterally, or locally; available in combination with amphotericin B (Mysteclin-F); combination is claimed to reduce the incidence of Candida superinfections; topical application may result in hypersensitivity reactions; discontinue drug at first sign of allergic response; ophthalmic use may retard corneal healing; IM injections contain procaine and are not suitable for IV administration; injection of IM solution into subcutaneous layer may cause pain and induration; do not dilute injectable solutions with calcium-containing diluents, because precipitate can form especially in an alkaline medium; reconstituted solutions are stable for 12 h at room temperature

CONTRAINDICATIONS AND PRECAUTIONS

Tetracyclines should not be used in pregnant women or nursing mothers, young children, or in patients with severe renal damage (*except* possibly doxycycline or minocycline).

These agents must be given with extreme *caution* to children under 8 years of age because they may cause permanent discoloration of teeth and inadequate calcification due to their ability to complex with calcium and deposit in the teeth. Tetracyclines can also form stable calcium complexes in developing bone and may retard normal bone growth if given over extended periods of time, especially in very young children.

Because most tetracycline derivatives are excreted largely by the kidney (except for doxycycline and minocycline), they may accumulate in the body in persons with impaired renal function. Dosage reduction may be necessary to avoid development of adverse effects.

INTERACTIONS

1. Oral absorption of tetracyclines (*except* doxycycline and minocycline) may be impaired by the presence of food. In addition, dairy products, antacids, iron, or other polyvalent cations (*e.g.*, calcium, magnesium, aluminum), and alkali (*e.g.*, sodium bicarbonate) can also retard GI absorption of tetracyclines.
2. Because they are bacteriostatic, tetracyclines can reduce the effectiveness of penicillins and other bactericidal antibiotics.
3. The action of doxycycline may be shortened by barbiturates, other sedative-hypnotics, phenytoin, and carbamazepine, because of hepatic enzyme induction.
4. BUN elevation can occur with combined tetracycline–diuretic use.
5. Tetracycline may enhance the effects of oral anticoagulants by interfering with synthesis of vitamin K by intestinal microorganisms.
6. Plasma levels of digoxin and lithium can be increased by tetracyclines.
7. Tetracyclines may enhance methoxyflurane-induced nephrotoxicity.
8. The effects of oral contraceptives may be reduced by tetracyclines, possibly resulting in breakthrough bleeding or pregnancy.
9. Theophylline and tetracyclines can result in increased GI side-effects.
10. Tetracyclines may increase serum levels of creatinine, urea nitrogen, bilirubin, alkaline phosphatase, SGPT, SGOT, and urinary levels of catecholamines and protein, and may decrease hemoglobin and platelet values. They may also yield a false-negative result with Clinistix or Tes-Tape and a false-positive urinary glucose test with Clinitest.

■ Nursing Process

See Nursing Process for anti-infective therapy in Chapter 59.

□ ASSESSMENT

□ Subjective Data

A thorough history is essential. The nurse should ask questions about oral contraceptive use because tetracyclines decrease oral contraceptive effectiveness; an alternate method of birth control should be used during the entire menstrual cycle that tetracycline is taken. Tetracycline may also interfere with the effectiveness of other antibiotics and may enhance the effects of digoxin, lithium, and oral anticoagulants. Patients taking theophylline-based drugs may suffer more gastrointestinal side-effects, and patients taking diuretics may suffer renal impairment when those drugs are combined with tetracycline. Patients taking these drugs need to be identified early to avoid serious drug reactions. A history of drug allergy or allergy to "caine" drugs such as lidocaine should also be reported because several tetracyclines contain lidocaine.

A history of symptoms for which the antibiotic is prescribed should be noted as well as any renal or hepatic problems, pregnancy, or lactation. If pregnancy is suspected, a confirming pregnancy test should be done to ensure that fetal damage is avoided. Tetracycline should not be used in children under age 8 except where the therapeutic benefits clearly outweigh the risks of potential problems with tooth calcification and bone growth.

□ Objective Data

Physical assessment focuses on the site of infection, the gastrointestinal tract, and liver and kidney function. Bowel sounds should be auscultated for hypermotility, the liver should be palpated, and urinary output should be measured.

Laboratory data should include hepatic and renal function studies in anyone starting on high dose or long-term therapy or in whom hepatic or renal dysfunction is suspected.

□ NURSING DIAGNOSES

Actual nursing diagnosis may include:

Knowledge deficit related to the action, dose, and side-effects of the drug

Potential nursing diagnoses may include:

Alteration in bowel elimination: diarrhea

Potential for injury: trauma, related to drug-induced dizziness

Alteration in oral mucous membranes due to superinfection

Impairment of skin integrity related to photosensitivity

□ PLAN

The nursing care goals focus on

1. Administering the drug safely and correctly according to the prescribed route
2. Monitoring for side-effects, especially gastrointestinal irritation, photosensitivity, dizziness, superinfection, and renal or hepatic impairment
3. Teaching the patient correct drug-taking techniques, dietary restrictions, side-effects, and what to do if problems occur

□ INTERVENTION

Most oral tetracyclines should be taken on an empty stomach, except doxycycline and minocycline which are not affected by food. If gastrointestinal problems or nausea develop the drug can be taken with water and a small quantity of food such as crackers or other bread products, but calcium-containing products should be avoided. The drug should not be taken with any calcium-containing food (such as dark green vegetables or dairy products) or drugs such as antacids or antidiarrheals because impaired absorption and possible drug inactivation will occur. Any tetracycline products left at the end of a treatment course should be discarded because the drugs readily decompose, frequently to toxic products, with age or exposure to light, heat, or humidity. Fanconi syndrome, described above, and nephrotoxicity can develop if outdated products are used.

Parenteral administration of tetracyclines includes the intramuscular and intravenous routes. Intramuscular injections should be given deep in a large muscle mass such as the gluteus in adults and the vastus lateralis in young children, and sites should be rotated using a body map (see Chap. 8) if multiple injections are given. Intravenous administration is usually by slow infusion over 30 minutes to 60 minutes and should be used with caution; the incidence of hepatotoxicity is higher with this route than with others. The IV site should be rotated every 48 hours and carefully observed for signs of redness, pain, or swelling because thrombophlebitis can occur. Development of any signs of thrombophlebitis warrants immediate removal of the IV.

The most common side-effects seen with tetracycline drugs are gastrointestinal irritation, photosensitivity, and dizziness (primarily with minocycline). Gastrointestinal irritation may be alleviated, as described above, with food or by changing the formulation to one which can be well tolerated with food. Photosensitization, including a severe rash and swelling, can occur with all tetracyclines but especially with demeclocycline. The patient should be advised to minimize direct sun exposure and to use sunscreens and protective clothing and sunglasses for the duration of therapy. Dizziness and lightheadedness may be transient or persist throughout the treatment course. The patient should be warned to avoid driving and any potentially hazardous activity (including climbing stairs) until reaction to the drug is known. One method to reduce dizziness is to take the drug with food to slow absorption; another is to rise slowly from a sitting or standing position.

Superinfection of the mouth and perineum are possible with tetracycline therapy. Symptoms may include black or "furry" tongue, sore mouth, and rectal, vaginal, or perineal itching. Diarrhea may also develop secondary to disruption of intestinal flora. Appropriate anti-infective drugs and comfort measures are employed to treat symptoms.

The patient with renal impairment usually requires a dosage reduction or an increase in dosage intervals to prevent excessive drug accumulation (except doxycycline and minocycline). However, BUN and creatinine clearance should be closely monitored throughout therapy and the physician should be notified immediately if vomiting, azotemia, weight loss, dehydration, or changes in mental affect (signs of acidosis) develop.

During long-term therapy, the potential for hepatic toxicity and hematologic dysfunction increases. Consequently hepatic function and hematologic blood studies (CBC with differential) should be performed at regular intervals.

□ EVALUATION

Outcome criteria used to measure drug effectiveness include evidence that the infection has subsided, evidence that the patient avoids ingesting

calcium-containing drugs and food with the tetracycline, and absence of such side-effects as
thrombophlebitis (IV administration), gastrointestinal irritation, photosensitivity, dizziness, superinfection, and renal, hepatic, or hematologic
toxicity.

CASE STUDY

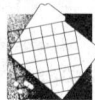

Mary Mueller, age 33, was preparing for a vacation to Mexico
with her husband. Prior to leaving she contacted her physician
for advice because she had a history of diverticulitis and was
worried about getting travelers' diarrhea on the trip. The
physician gave Mrs. Mueller a prescription for doxycycline and
advised her to obtain Pepto-Bismol to take on the trip. He also
advised her to eat only peeled fruit, to drink bottled water, and
to avoid ice or vegetables or fruits that may have been washed
in local water.

On the third day of her vacation, Mrs. Mueller became
nauseated and developed watery diarrhea. She started
doxycycline, 100 mg PO in the morning, and took 100 mg in
the evening that day. She also took three doses of Pepto-Bismol
(two chewable tablets) spaced evenly through the day but not at
the same time as the doxycycline. On the second day she took
doxycycline, 100 mg in the morning, and continued to take the
drug each morning for the rest of the vacation. She also
continued taking Pepto-Bismol, tid, for the duration of the
trip. The diarrhea subsided within 4 days, and the nausea
passed with 24 hours.

Three days after Mrs. Mueller began doxycycline she was
lying in the sun after applying sunscreen and noticed a red,
flat, itchy rash on her right hand, arm, and both feet. She
immediately moved to the shade, and the intensity of the rash
decreased within minutes.

Discussion Questions

1. What side-effect of doxycycline did Mrs. Mueller
   experience? Why may it have occurred only on the sites
   mentioned?
2. What advice should Mrs. Mueller have been given about
   treatment of diarrhea, in addition to drug taking? (See
   Chap. 45 for further information.)

REVIEW QUESTIONS

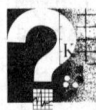

1. List the tetracyclines that can be given both orally and
   parenterally.
2. Name the tetracycline drugs that are only used topically.
3. What substances can retard the oral absorption of
   tetracyclines?
4. Why are tetracyclines contraindicated in very young
   children?
5. Which tetracycline derivatives are safest?
6. Briefly describe the mechanism of action of tetracyclines.
7. List the principal approved indications for the tetracyclines.
8. Why is minocycline effective in eliminating meningococci
   from the nasopharynx of carriers of *Neisseria meningitidis*?

9. What are the most frequently encountered side-effects with tetracyclines? How can patients be taught to manage these symptoms?
10. What is the danger in using outdated tetracycline products?
11. Why is doxycycline preferred over monocycline in most instances?
12. Which tetracycline is associated with the highest incidence of photosensitivity reactions?
13. For what indication is meclocycline used? What are its principal side-effects?
14. Why is amphotericin B combined with tetracycline in an oral dosage form?
15. Which drugs and drug allergies should a patient be asked about in a drug history prior to treatment with a tetracycline?
16. What dietary restrictions must the patient follow during tetracycline use? Are these absolute or related to time of drug taking?

BIBLIOGRAPHY

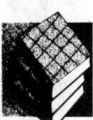

Banza M, Schiefe RJ: Antimicrobial spectrum, pharmacology and therapeutic use of antibiotics. 1. Tetracyclines. Am J Hosp Pharm 34:49, 1977

Baptista RJ, Harvie RJ, Guen R: The tetracyclines: An overview. US Pharmacist 4:33, Aug. 1979

Chopra I, Howe TG: Bacterial resistance to the tetracyclines. Microbiol Rev 42:707, 1978

Elmore MF, Rogge JD: Tetracycline-induced pancreatitis. Gastroenterology 81:1134, 1981

Neu HC: A symposium on tetracyclines: A major appraisal. Bull NY Acad Med 54:111, 1978

Ory EM: The tetracyclines. In Kagan BM (ed): Antimicrobial Therapy, 3rd ed, p 117. Philadelphia, WB Saunders, 1980

Siegel D: Tetracyclines: New look at old antibiotic. NY State J Med 78:950, 1978

Standiford HC: The tetracyclines and chloramphenicol. In Mandell GL, Douglas RG, Bennett JE (eds): Principles and Practice of Infectious Diseases, 2nd ed, p 206. New York, John Wiley & Sons, 1985

Wilson WB, Cockerill FR: Tetracyclines, chloramphenicol, erythromycin, clindamycin. Mayo Clin Proc 58:92, 1983

Winckler K: Tetracycline ulcers of the oesophagus: Endoscopy, histology and roentgenology in two cases and a review of the literature. Endoscopy 13:225, 1981

Erythromycins

64

The erythromycins are members of the macrolide group of antibiotics, so named because the chemical structure of the compounds consists of a large lactone ring to which one or more sugars are attached. Erythromycin itself as a base is an orally effective antibiotic originally isolated from a strain of *Streptomyces erythreus.* Although erythromycin base is a biologically active form, it is unstable in gastric acid and thus must be formulated in an enteric-coated preparation for oral administration. Absorption of enteric-coated products is occasionally less than adequate, however, and blood levels may not reach sufficient concentrations. Therefore, to avoid destruction of the drug by gastric juices and to facilitate absorption, erythromycin has also been formulated in several salt forms (estolate, ethylsuccinate, stearate), all of which are largely acid-stable and yield biologically effective plasma levels of free erythromycin base. The strength of erythromycin products is expressed in terms of base equivalents. Thus, 400 mg of the ethylsuccinate salt provides serum levels of free erythromycin equivalent to those resulting from administration of 250 mg of erythromycin base or the stearate or estolate salts. Two other soluble salts of erythromycin (gluceptate, lactobionate) are available for IV use and are indicated mainly in severe infections where high serum levels of the drug are required immediately. The other clinically available macrolide antibiotic is troleandomycin, an agent resembling erythromycin in both structure and pharmacologic activity, but somewhat less effective and more toxic, and hence infrequently used today. It is discussed briefly at the end of this chapter.

Erythromycins inhibit protein synthesis and are usually bacteriostatic at normal therapeutic doses. However, they may be bactericidal against certain organisms at high concentrations. This bactericidal activity is greatest if the organisms are rapidly dividing and increases significantly as the pH is elevated. Their antibacterial spectrum of action is similar to that of the penicillins, being most effective against certain gram-positive cocci, such as staphylococci, streptococci, enterococci, and pneumococci. Erythromycin has been demonstrated to be synergistic with sulfonamides against *Hemophilus influenzae.* Although used principally as alternatives to penicillin in treating susceptible organisms, the erythromycins may be considered first-line drugs against the following organisms: *Bordetella pertussis* (whooping cough), *Corynebacterium diphtheriae, Legionella pneumophila* (legionnaires' disease), *Mycoplasma pneumoniae*

(atypical viral pneumonia), and strains of *Chlamydia trachomatis* causing pneumonia and inclusion conjunctivitis (refer to Table 59-1 for a listing of the organisms for which erythromycin is considered an alternate drug).

Microbial resistance has become a problem with use of the erythromycins and is especially frequent in staphylococci. Prolonged use of erythromycin in staphylococcal infections is almost invariably associated with the emergence of resistance, and alternative drugs should be used in treating severe staphylococcal infections. Erythromycin-resistant streptococci and pneumococci are likewise developing with increasing frequency. Although cross-resistance is not a significant problem between erythromycin and most other antibiotics, it has been reported with lincomycin and clindamycin, and is virtually complete among all the members of the macrolides. Gram-negative organisms are largely impermeable to erythromycin and are usually resistant to the drug unless their cell walls are altered.

As noted earlier, erythromycin is used as the free base as well as several salts, and the various preparations are available for oral, IV, topical, and ophthalmic administration. Absorption of the base and the stearate preparations are impaired by the presence of food, and these drugs should be administered on an empty stomach, if possible. Conversely, absorption of the estolate and ethylsuccinate salts are either unaffected or enhanced by the presence of food. However, the estolate salt has been associated with cholestatic hepatitis, especially in adults, and its use in this group cannot be justified. Erythromycins in general, however, are among the safest antibiotics, and their administration is accompanied by relatively few and predominately minor adverse effects. For this reason, these agents are commonly prescribed in children, although as previously mentioned, they should not be considered first-line drugs except in those few infections listed above.

Following a general discussion of erythromycin, the various salts, their doses and dosage forms, and pertinent comments are presented in Table 64-1. The other macrolide antibiotic, troleandomycin, is then reviewed at the end of the chapter.

Erythromycins

Erythromycin Base, Erythromycin Estolate, Erythromycin

(*Text continues on p. 1230.*)

Table 64-1
Erythromycins

Drug	Preparations	Usual Dosage Range	Clinical Considerations
erythromycin base (Ak-mycin, E-Mycin, Ery-Tab, Eryc, Ilotycin, PCE, Robimycin)	Enteric-coated tablets—250 mg, 333 mg, 500 mg Film-coated tablets—250 mg, 500 mg Capsules (enteric-coated pellets)—125 mg, 250 mg Ointment—2% Opthalmic ointment—0.5%	Oral: Adults—250 mg to 500 mg every 6 h–12 h up to 4 g/day for severe infections Children—30 mg/kg to 50 mg/day in three to four divided doses up to 100 mg/kg/day Syphilis—30 g to 40 g in divided doses over 10 days to 15 days Legionnaires' disease—1 g to 4 g daily in divided doses Pertussis—40 mg to 50 mg/kg/day in divided doses for 5 days to 15 days Sexually-transmitted diseases (syphilis, gonorrhea, nongonococcal urethritis, chanchroid, lymphogranuloma)—500 mg four times a day for at least 7 days to 10 days (up to 30 days for syphilis) Topical—apply to skin two to four times a day as necessary Ophthalmic: Prevention of neonatal conjunctivitis due to *Neisseria* or *Chlamydia*—apply to eye two to three times a day	Free-base form of erythromycin, which is acid-labile and thus administered orally in enteric-coated form; absorption is variable depending on product used; should be administered on an empty stomach if possible; do not break or crush enteric-coated tablets; opthalmic ointment may retard corneal healing; be alert for hypersensitivity reactions with topical application; see below for discussion of topical solution used in acne
erythromycin base topical solution (Akene-mycin, A/T/S, C-Solve-2, E-Solve-2, ETS-2%, Erycette, Eryderm, Erymax, Staticin, T-Stat)	Topical solution—1.5%, 2%	Apply morning and evening to areas usually affected by acne	Alcohol solution of erythromycin base used in the treatment of acne vulgaris; avoid contact with eyes, nose, mouth, or other mucous membranes; use cautiously with other topical acne treatment, because severe irritation can occur; most common side-effect is excessive drying of treated area; erythema, pruritus, burning, and desquamation have also been reported; wash, rinse, and dry area to be treated before application
erythromycin estolate (Ilosone)	Tablets—500 mg Chewable tablets—125 mg, 250 mg Capsules—125 mg, 250 mg Drops—100 mg/ml	Adults—250 mg every 6 h (or 500 mg every 12 h) up to 4 g/day Children—30 mg/kg to 50 mg/kg/day orally in di-	Ester salt of erythromycin that is acid-stable, well absorbed in the presence of food, and yields higher and more sustained blood *(continued)*

Table 64-1 (*continued*)
Erythromycins

Drug	Preparations	Usual Dosage Range	Clinical Considerations
erythromycin estolate (Ilosone) (*continued*)	Suspension—125 mg/5 ml, 250 mg/5 ml	vided doses, up to 100 mg/kg/day Syphilis—20 g over 10 days	levels than other derivatives; may produce hepatotoxicity; thus be alert for early signs of liver dysfunction (vomiting, malaise, cramping, right upper-quadrant pain, fever, jaundice), and discontinue drug; symptoms usually occur with 1 wk–2 wk of continuous therapy and are reversible upon discontinuation of medication; not indicated for prolonged administration (*e.g.*, acne, prophylaxis of rheumatic fever) or for treatment of syphilitic infections in pregnant women; regular tablets (500 mg) should be swallowed whole; liquid should be kept refrigerated and unused portion discarded after 14 days
erythromycin ethylsuccinate (E.E.S., E-Mycin E, EryPed, Pediamycin, Wyamycin-E)	Film-coated tablets—400 mg Chewable tablets—200 mg Drops—100 mg/2.5 ml Suspension—200 mg/5 ml, 400 mg/5 ml Powder for suspension—200 mg/5 ml, 400 mg/5 ml	Adults—400 mg every 6 h up to 4 g/day for severe infections Children—30 mg/kg to 50 mg/kg/day up to 100 mg/kg/day Syphilis—48 g to 64 g over 10 days in divided doses	Acid-stable salt of erythromycin that is reliably absorbed from the GI tract; requires a higher dose (*i.e.*, 400 mg vs 250 mg) than other oral salts to yield comparable blood levels of erythromycin base; oral liquids are stable for 14 days with refrigeration; reconstituted powder is stable for 10 days
erythromycin gluceptate (Ilotycin Gluceptate)	Powder for injection—250 mg, 500 mg, 1 g in 30 ml vials	Adults and children—15 mg/kg to 20 mg/kg/day by continuous (preferred) or intermittent infusion; up to 4 g/day can be used in severe infections Acute pelvic inflammatory disease due to *Neisseria gonorrhoeae*—500 mg every 6 h for 3 days, followed by 250 mg oral erythromycin every 6 h for 7 days	Soluble salt of erythromycin indicated in severe infections requiring immediate, high serum levels, or when oral administration is not possible or feasible; may produce pain, irritation, and possibly phlebitis upon administration; solution is prepared initially by adding sterile water for injection to the vial according to package directions and shaking until dissolved; no preservatives should be used; reconstituted solution is stored refrigerated and used within 7

(*continued*)

Table 64-1 (continued)
Erythromycins

Drug	Preparations	Usual Dosage Range	Clinical Considerations
erythromycin gluceptate (Ilotycin Gluceptate) (continued)			days; intermittent infusion is performed by administering 250 mg to 500 mg in 100 ml to 250 ml of sodium chloride injection or 5% dextrose over 30 min–60 min four times a day; initial solution may be added to sodium chloride injection or 5% dextrose in water to give 1 g/L for slow IV infusion; pH of diluted solution should be kept between 6 and 8; do *not* give by IV push because irritation is common; high doses have resulted in alterations in liver function; periodic hepatic function tests are required during prolonged therapy
erythromycin lactobionate (Erythrocin Lactobionate-IV)	Powder for injection—500 mg/vial, 1 g/vial Piggyback single dose vial—500 mg powder/vial when reconstituted	Adults and children—15 mg/kg to 20 mg/kg/day by continuous (preferred) or intermittent infusion; up to 4 g/day may be given in severe infections	Soluble salt of erythromycin used in a similar manner as the gluceptate salt; see Gluceptate for mixing and diluting intructions; IV infusion of 4 g/day or (continued)

Ethylsuccinate, Erythromycin Gluceptate, Erythromycin Lactobionate, Erythromycin Stearate

MECHANISM AND ACTIONS

Erythromycin inhibits bacterial protein synthesis by attaching to 50S ribosomal subunits of sensitive microorganisms, thereby interfering with the binding of t-RNA to the donor site. These drugs do *not* alter the bacterial cell wall. Gram-positive bacteria concentrate approximately 100 times more erythromycin than gram-negative bacteria. Because the nonionized form of the drug penetrates the cells most efficiently, the antimicrobial activity of erythromycin is increased in an alkaline pH, as the drug exists predominantly in the unionized form in such an environment.

USES

1. Treatment of respiratory infections caused by susceptible organisms, such as the following: *Mycoplasma pneumoniae* (drug of choice), *Legionella pneumophila*, (drug of choice), *Streptococcus pneumoniae*, group A beta-hemolytic streptococcus (in penicillin-sensitive patients), and *Bordetella pertussis* (eliminates organism from the nasopharynx)
2. Treatment of acute skin and soft-tissue infections due to *Staphylococcus aureus* (resistant organisms usually emerge during extended therapy)
3. Prophylaxis of subacute bacterial endocarditis and recurrence of acute rheumatic fever in penicillin-sensitive patients
4. Treatment of *Neisseria gonorrhoeae* and *Treponema pallidum* infections in penicillin- and tetracycline-sensitive patients
5. Treatment of chlamydial infections (*e.g.*, uncomplicated adult urethritis, endocervicitis, or rectal infections; conjunctivitis or pneumonia in infants) in tetracycline-sensitive patients
6. Treatment of *Campylobacter jejuni* gastroenteritis (especially if begun within several days of onset of symptoms)

Table 64-1 (continued)
Erythromycins

Drug	Preparations	Usual Dosage Range	Clinical Considerations
erythromycin lactobionate (Erythrocin Lactobionate-IV) (continued)		Acute pelvic inflammatory disease—see gluceptate above	more has caused reversible hearing loss; do not exceed this dose; intermittent IV administration is accomplished by giving one-fourth the daily dose over 30 min–60 min every 6 h by slow injection of 250 mg to 500 mg in 100 ml to 250 ml of sodium chloride or 5% dextrose; IV therapy should be replaced by oral therapy as soon as is feasible
erythromycin stearate (Eramycin, Erypar, Erythrocin, Ethril, Wyamycin-S)	Film-coated tablets—250 mg, 500 mg	Adults—250 mg every 6 h (or 500 mg every 12 h) up to four grams a day in divided doses Children—30 mg/kg to 50 mg/kg/day in divided doses four times a day, up to 100 mg/kg/day Syphilis—30 g to 40 g in divided doses over 10 days to 15 days	Acid-stable salt of erythromycin claimed to be the most completely and reliably absorbed of all the derivatives when taken on an empty stomach; may be associated with a slightly higher incidence of allergic reactions than other forms of erythromycin

7. Treatment of upper respiratory and middle ear infections due to *Hemophilus influenzae* (in combination with sulfonamides)
8. Adjunctive treatment of *Corynebacterium* infections (with antitoxin)
9. Topical control of mild to moderate acne vulgaris
10. Treatment of intestinal amebiasis due to *Entamoeba histolytica*
11. Reduction of wound complications when given with neomycin prior to colorectal surgery

ADMINISTRATION AND DOSAGE
See Table 64-1.

FATE
Erythromycin base is destroyed by gastric acid and must be formulated in enteric-coated products for oral administration. The various salts are acid stable and are well absorbed; absorption of the ethylsuccinate and estolate salt is unaffected (or possibly enhanced) by the presence of food. Erythromycin base and stearate should be given on an empty stomach. Erythromycin diffuses into most body fluids, and antimicrobial activity is apparent in all tissues except the brain and cerebrospinal fluid. Passage of the drug across the blood–brain barrier is increased if the meninges are inflamed. It is one of the few antibiotics to enter prostatic fluid, where concentrations up to 40% of those in the plasma can be attained. The drug crosses the placental barrier and is found in breast milk. Protein binding is approximately 70% to 75%. Erythromycin is concentrated in the liver and excreted in the bile. Less than 5% of orally administered and 15% of IV-administered drug is eliminated in the urine. The plasma half-life is 1 hour to 2 hours, but is prolonged to 6 hours in severe renal dysfunction.

SIDE-EFFECTS/ADVERSE REACTIONS
The overall incidence of adverse effects with erythromycin is among the lowest of any antibiotic drug. Gastrointestinal symptoms such as cramping and abdominal discomfort are most often noted following oral administration; nausea, vomiting, and diarrhea occur much less frequently. Other

untoward reactions which have been reported during erythromycin therapy include allergic reactions (rash, pruritus, urticaria, eczema, fever, anaphylaxis), reversible hearing loss at high doses, and cholestatic hepatitis (most often with the estolate salt but occasionally with the ethylsuccinate and stearate salts as well. Symptoms of liver toxicity include severe abdominal pain, fever, jaundice, and vomiting. The symptoms usually disappear quickly when the drug is discontinued, and permanent liver damage is rare.

A few instances of psychiatric reactions have been recorded during erythromycin treatment, and symptoms have included uncontrollable crying, abnormal thought processes, hysteria, fear, confusion and feeling of impending loss of consciousness.

IV administration of erythromycin can result in pain, venous irritation, and trauma to the vessel on rare occasions.

As with use of most other antibiotics, superinfection (*i.e.,* bacterial or fungal overgrowth) may occur following repeated administration of erythromycin.

CONTRAINDICATIONS AND PRECAUTIONS
The estolate salt of erythromycin should not be given to persons with pre-existing liver disease. The remaining erythromycin preparations must be used with *caution* in such individuals. Cautious use of all erythromycins is necessary in pregnant women or nursing mothers.

INTERACTIONS
1. The activity of erythromycins may be enhanced by urinary alkalinizers (*e.g.,* sodium bicarbonate, acetazolamide) and decreased by urinary *acidifiers* (*e.g.,* ammonium chloride, citric acid beverages).
2. The effects of lincomycin and clindamycin may be antagonized by erythromycin, which competes for ribosomal binding sites.
3. Tetracyclines and cephalothin are incompatible with erythromycin in parenteral mixtures.
4. Erythromycin can elevate serum digoxin levels in a small percentage of patients who metabolize digoxin in the GI tract by slowing its metabolism in the gut.
5. Erythromycins can increase serum levels of theophylline, methylprednisolone and carbamazepine by reducing their hepatic clearance.
6. Erythromycin, being primarily bacteriostatic, may impair the antimicrobial activity of penicillins or other bactericidal antibiotics.

7. The effects of oral anticoagulants may be increased by erythromycins.
8. Erythromycin may increase the pharmacologic effects of cyclosporin by reducing its clearance.

■ Nursing Process

See also Nursing Process for anti-infective therapy in Chapter 59.

☐ ASSESSMENT

☐ Subjective Data
A drug history is useful prior to administration of erythromycins and should include questions about digoxin, theophylline, or oral anticoagulant use. The effect of all these drugs may be enhanced when given with erythromycins; therefore, dosage adjustments may be necessary to avoid toxic drug reactions. The patient should also be asked about the current use of other antibiotics whose effect may be antagonized by erythromycin. Information about drug allergies is also essential; hypersensitivity to any "mycin" may preclude further therapy with these drugs. In addition, patients with multiple drug allergies may be more susceptible to reactions from erythromycins than other patients.

Further history taking focuses on the symptoms of infection for which the erythromycin will be prescribed as well as evidence of hepatic disease, pregnancy, or lactation, all of which may contraindicate erythromycin use. The drugs should also be used cautiously when first administered to any patient with a history of allergies or hay fever.

☐ Objective Data
Physical assessment of the site of infection is important. Auscultation of bowel sounds will detect hypermotility which may be aggravated by the drug; palpation of the liver will detect any enlargement which should be further evaluated. Skin should also be assessed for evidence of pre-existing rash or break in integrity because some hypersensitivity reactions from erythromycins are local in nature. Temperature should also be noted.

Laboratory data might include hepatic or renal function studies if dysfunction is suspected or if the patient will be on long-term therapy.

☐ NURSING DIAGNOSES
Actual nursing diagnoses may include:
   Knowledge deficit related to the action, dose, and side-effects of the drug

Potential nursing diagnoses may include:

Alteration in comfort: pain at IM injection site or at IV site at the onset of phlebitis, a side-effect of the drug

Impaired tissue integrity related to rash from hypersensitivity reaction or superinfection

Alteration in bowel elimination: diarrhea related to disruption of normal intestinal flora

Alteration in oral mucous membranes related to superinfections

□ PLAN

The nursing care goals focus on:

1. Administering the drug safely and correctly according to the prescribed route
2. Monitoring for side-effects, especially local hypersensitivity, gastrointestinal cramping, and superinfection
3. Teaching the patient correct drug-taking techniques, dietary restrictions, side-effects, and what to do if problems occur

□ INTERVENTION

Erythromycins are given by multiple routes and in general are very safe, but each has some specific concerns for the nurse. Intermittent intravenous doses should be well diluted in a minimum of 100 ml of 5% dextrose and water or normal saline and should be infused slowly over a 20-minute to 60-minute period (see Table 64-1). The drug may also be administered in a continuous infusion usually at a ratio of 1 g to 1000 ml. Continuous infusions may need to have buffering compounds added to maintain a *p*H between 6 and 8 and ensure drug efficacy. The manufacturer's instructions and pharmacist's advice should be sought before the infusion begins. Although erythromycins are less irritating than many antibiotics, the IV site should be rotated every 48 hours and closely observed throughout therapy for signs of phlebitis: redness, pain, or swelling. If any of these develop, the IV should be immediately removed.

Oral doses of erythromycin may be taken with food to decrease gastrointestinal irritability except for oral forms of erythromycin base (see Table 64-1), which must be taken on an empty stomach. However, the drug should be taken with water, not acidic liquids such as fruit juice or carbonated beverages because these will prematurely decompose the drug. All oral erythromycin drugs are formulated in enteric-coated tablets; therefore, none can be crushed or chewed. One advantage of the drug is that it can be taken every 12 hours instead of every 6 hours and still maintain therapeutic serum levels.

This may be helpful to the patient who forgets to take medicine or who may not be able to take a drug frequently throughout the day.

Intramuscular injections of erythromycin should be given in a large muscle mass such as the gluteus in adults or the vastus lateralis in young children to decrease pain. Sites should be rotated using a body map (see Chap. 8), and palpation for lumps, or hardness or pain should be done before the injection is given.

Topical ointments or solutions should be applied to a cleansed skin surface unless the physician directs otherwise. The person applying the drug should be careful to avoid contact with eyes, nose, mouth, or other mucous membranes until hands are thoroughly washed. Erythromycin can cause local hypersensitivity reactions in these areas and can be systemically absorbed.

Erythromycin ophthalmic ointment should be applied in small ribbon along the inside of the lower lid but not touching the lid. After application, the lid should be closed and the eye should be massaged to ensure even distribution.

Common side-effects which the nurse may manage include gastrointestinal cramping, allergic reactions, and possible superinfection. Liver toxicity, while quite rare, must also be monitored.

Gastrointestinal cramping is usually alleviated by drug administration with food or meals as long as concurrent ingestion of acidic beverages is avoided. Symptoms rarely become severe, but persistent problems should be reported.

Most hypersensitivity reactions are local in nature (as described under Side-Effects/Adverse Reactions). Patients should be told to report any development of skin rash or itching especially at a site being treated with a topical formulation. Systemic hypersensitivity, while rare, is also possible. Refer to Chapter 59 for a discussion on precautions and treatment.

Superinfection by nonsusceptible organisms is possible with erythromycin therapy. Common sites include the mouth, characterized by the development of black, "furry" tongue, and the vaginal area, characterized by vaginal discharge and perianal itching or irritation. Diarrhea may indicate a disruption of the normal intestinal flora; fever may be present with any of the above. Treatment depends on the organisms cultured and will resolve completely when the erythromycin is discontinued.

Liver toxicity may develop and will manifest itself by the symptoms listed under Side-Effects/Adverse Reactions. All patients should be taught to immediately report the development of such symptoms. In addition, periodic hepatic function studies should be performed on anyone receiving high dose or extended therapy. Elevations may occur in SGOT, SGPT, and alkaline phosphatase.

Erythromycin therapy may cause changes in other laboratory values which may or may not be clinically significant. These include a decrease in serum glucose and cholesterol levels and false elevations in urinary catecholamines and 17-keto steroids.

□ **EVALUATION**

The outcome criteria which may be used to measure drug effectiveness include resolution of infection, decrease in temperature, evidence that the patient takes the drug with water, and the absence of such effects as phlebitis (IV administration) site pain (IM administration), allergic reactions at topical or ophthalmic sites, gastrointestinal cramping, superinfection, and liver toxicity.

Troleandomycin

(Tao)

Troleandomycin, a semisynthetic derivative of oleandomycin, is a macrolide antibiotic obtained from *Streptomyces antibioticus*. It is similar to erythromycin in activity but somewhat less effective and more toxic, hence its clinical usefulness is limited. Troleandomycin is generally effective in eradicating streptococci from the nasopharynx.

Its mechanism of action resembles that of erythromycin, and the drug is capable of inhibiting protein synthesis in susceptible bacteria. Principal indications for troleandomycin are treatment of pneumococcal pneumonia in susceptible strains and group A beta-hemolytic streptococcal infections of the upper respiratory tract. Although it is effective in eradicating streptococci from the nasopharynx, there is inconclusive evidence that it is useful for long-term prophylaxis of rheumatic fever.

The drug is given orally as capsules (250 mg). The adult dose is 250 mg to 500 mg four times a day, while children are given 125 mg to 250 mg every 6 hours.

The most frequently encountered side-effects are abdominal cramping and discomfort. Allergic reactions are occasionally associated with its usage, and the drug has been associated with development of an allergic cholestatic hepatitis marked by nausea, vomiting, fever, upper right quadrant pain, eosinophila, and leukocytosis. Liver function should be monitored during troleandomycin therapy, and caution must be observed when administering the drug to persons with impaired liver function, as it is principally eliminated in the liver.

Concurrent use of troleandomycin and oral contraceptives has resulted in marked cholestatic jaundice, while its use in conjunction with ergotamine-like drugs can lead to ischemic reactions. Troleandomycin can also impair the hepatic metabolism of theophylline, corticosteroids, and carbamazepine.

Troleandomycin represents an alternative to the erythromycins but is infrequently used today. Nursing considerations are the same as for other erythromycins.

REVIEW QUESTIONS	
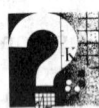	1. List the different forms of erythromycin that are available.

1. List the different forms of erythromycin that are available.
2. Why must erythromycin base be formulated in enteric-coated preparations for oral use?
3. What factors enhance the bactericidal activity of erythromycin against certain organisms?
4. Why are many gram-negative organisms resistant to erythromycin?
5. Which salts of erythromycin may be taken with food? Which salts are best taken on an empty stomach?
6. Name the two erythromycin salts used parenterally. What actions should be taken to ensure safe administration by this route?
7. Briefly describe the mechanism of action of erythromycin.
8. In what infections may erythromycin be considered a drug of choice?
9. What is the major disadvantage of treating staphylococcal infections with erythromycin for extended periods of time?

10. What are the most often encountered side-effects with erythromycin? What actions can be taken to counteract them?
11. With what salt of erythromycin is cholestatic hepatitis most frequently associated? What are the symptoms of this disorder?
12. Why may use of erythromycin together with penicillin reduce the effectiveness of penicillin in treating certain infections?
13. What is the principal indication for topical application of erythromycin?
14. Give the major indications for troleandomycin. What disadvantages does it possess compared to erythromycin?
15. What information should be collected on a drug history prior to administration of any erythromycin?

BIBLIOGRAPHY

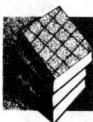

Anders BJ, Laver BA, Paisley JW, Reller LB: Double-blind placebo controlled trial of erythromycin for treatment of campylobacter enteritis. Lancet 1:131, 1982

Balows A, Fraser D (eds): International symposium on legionnaires' disease. Ann Intern Med 90:489, 1976

Bernstein G, Davis J, Katcher M: Prophylaxis of neonatal conjunctivitis. Clin Pediatr 21:545, 1982

Derrick CW, Reilly KM: Erythromycin, lincomycin, and clindamycin. Pediatr Clin North Am 30:63, 1983

Istre GR, Welch DF, Marks MI, Moyer N: Susceptibility of group A beta-hemolytic *Streptococcus* isolates to penicillin and erythromycin. Antimicrob Agents Chemother 20:244, 1981

Karmody CS, Weinstein L: Reversible sensorineural hearing loss with intravenous erythromycin lactobionate. Ann Otol Rhinol Laryngol 86:9, 1977

May DC, Jarboe CH, Ellenburg DT, Roe EJ, Karibo J: The effects of erythromycin on theophylline elimination in normal males. J Clin Pharmacol 22:125, 1982

Meade RH: Antimicrobial spectrum, pharmacology and therapeutic use of erythromycin and its derivatives. Am J Hosp Pharm 36:1185, 1979

Omura S: Macrolide Antibiotics. New York, Academic Press, 1984

Sasso SC: Erythromycin for eye prophylaxis. Matern Child Nurs 9:417, 1984

Steigbigel NH: Erythromycin, lincomycin and clindamycin. In Mandell GL, Douglas RG, Bennett JE (eds): Principles and Practice of Infectious Diseases, 2nd ed, p 224. New York, John Wiley & Sons, 1985

Aminoglycosides

Aminoglycosides
Amikacin, Gentamicin,
Kanamycin,
Neomycin,
Netilmicin,
Streptomycin,
Tobramycin

65

The aminoglycosides are a group of broad-spectrum bactericidal antibiotics that exhibit similar pharmacologic, antimicrobial, and toxicologic properties. Despite their extended spectrum of action, however, their use is generally restricted to treatment of serious systemic gram-negative enteric infections caused by *Pseudomonas, Proteus, Klebsiella, Enterobacter, Serratia,* and *Escherichia* species. Aminoglycoside treatment of infections due to other organisms, both gram-negative and gram-positive, is generally reserved for those instances where less toxic agents have failed. The major limitation to the routine use of aminoglycoside antibiotics is their potential for eliciting serious untoward reactions, most notably ototoxicity (both auditory and vestibular) and nephrotoxicity. Toxicity with aminoglycosides can develop even with conventional therapeutic doses, especially in patients with impaired renal function, although it is much more common at higher doses. *Persistent* exposure to the drugs rather than brief exposure to high doses is most closely associated with toxicity. Adverse effects are considered in more detail below.

Due to the narrow margin between the therapeutic and toxic serum levels with aminoglycosides, serum concentrations should be monitored frequently in critically ill patients and in persons with renal impairment. Peak serum concentrations are determined 30 minutes after completion of IV infusion or 1 hour after IM injection. Minimum (*i.e.,* trough) levels are taken immediately prior to the next dose. Therapeutic serum levels (mcg/ml) are maintained between these two extremes as indicated in Table 65-1. Peak and trough levels are determined several times a week (more often if renal function is impaired or declining) to ensure both the adequacy of antibacterial drug activity (*i.e.,* peak levels) as well as to protect against drug cumulation (*i.e.,* trough levels).

Absorption of aminoglycosides from the GI tract is negligible, and the drugs must be administered parenterally for treatment of systemic infections. Several aminoglycosides may also be given orally for localized intraintestinal infections or as adjunctive therapy in the treatment of hepatic coma. Some drugs are also applied topically to the eye, skin, or mucous membranes for treatment of superficial infections due to susceptible organisms. Thus, despite similar chemical and pharmacologic properties, the aminoglycosides do not share similar modes of administration or clinical indications.

Table 65-2 lists the various routes of administration for each of the aminoglycosides, as well as

Table 65-1
Therapeutic and Toxic Serum Levels for Aminoglycosides

	Therapeutic Serum Levels (mcg/ml)	Minimum Toxic Serum Levels (mcg/ml)	
		Peak*	Trough†
amikacin	8–16	35	5
gentamicin	4–10	12	2
kanamycin	8–16	30	5
neomycin	5–10	‡	‡
netilmicin	1–10	16	4
streptomycin	25–28	50	5
tobramycin	4–8	12	2

* Obtained 1 h after IM administration.
† Obtained immediately prior to next dose.
‡ Systemic use is not recommended.

Example: Physician's order for: Gentamicin, 80 mg IV piggyback, to run 30 min every 8 h with peak and trough levels daily.
If administration schedule was 6 AM, 2 PM, 10 PM, *peak level* would be drawn 7:30 AM (1 h after IV dose is completed) and *trough levels* would be drawn between 1:45 and 2:00 PM (immediately before the next dose).

their major antimicrobial spectrum of action. The aminoglycosides, while active against a variety of gram-positive organisms are rarely used clinically against these organisms due to the availability of more effective and less toxic antibacterial agents. As indicated above, their principal application is in treating severe systemic infections caused by a number of gram-negative aerobic bacilli. Of the various available aminoglycosides, gentamicin, tobramycin, amikacin, and netilmicin are the most often use derivatives and are virtually interchangeable in the treatment of most infections due to *Acinetobacter, Enterobacter, Escherichia coli, Klebsiella pneumoniae, Proteus* species, *Pseudomonas aeruginosa, Providencia,* and *Serratia.* In many instances a synergistic action is obtained against these organisms when an extended-spectrum penicillin (such as carbenicillin or ticarcillin) or a third-generation cephalosporin (such as cefoperazone or ceftizoxime) is combined with one of these aminoglycosides.

Streptomycin is the agent of choice for treating infections due to *Francisella tularensis* (tularemia), *Pseudomonas mallei* (melioidosis), and *Yersinia pestis* (plague), and may also be useful in treating tuberculosis (see Chap. 69). Parenteral neomycin is usually reserved for serious infections unrespon-

Table 65-2
Administration and Antimicrobial Spectrum of Aminoglycosides

Drug	Routes of Administration	Plasma Half-Life (h)	Principal Antimicrobial Spectrum of Action*†
amikacin	IM, IV	2–3	1, 2, 3, 7, 10, 11, 12, 15
gentamicin	IM, IV, intrathecal, ophthalmic, topical	1–4	2, 3, 7, 10, 12, 13, 14, 15
kanamycin	IM, IV, intraperitoneal, aerosol, oral	2–4	1, 3, 6, 7, 9, 10, 13, 14, 15
neomycin	IM, ophthalmic, topical, oral	2–3	3, 7, 10, 12
netilmicin	IM, IV	2–3	1, 2, 3, 7, 10, 12, 13, 14, 15
streptomycin	IM	2–3	3, 4, 5, 6, 7, 8, 10, 16, 17
tobramycin	IM, IV, ophthalmic	2–3	2, 3, 7, 10, 11, 12, 15

* *Organisms*
† Does not necessarily indicate drug of choice (see Table 59-1).

1. *Acinetobacter* species
2. *Citrobacter freundii*
3. *Escherichia coli*
4. *Francisella tularensis*
5. *Hemophilus ducreyi*
6. *Hemophilus influenzae*
7. *Klebsiella-Enterobacter-Serratia* species
8. *Mycobacterium tuberculosis*
9. *Neisseria gonorrhoeae*

10. *Proteus* species
11. *Providencia* species
12. *Pseudomonas aeruginosa*
13. *Salmonella* species
14. *Shigella* species
15. *Staphylococcus* species
16. *Streptococcus* (group D)
17. *Yersinia pestis*

sive to other aminoglycosides, because it is the most toxic of the group. Orally administered neomycin has been used for preoperative bowel sterilization, relief of *E. coli*-induced diarrhea, and as adjunctive therapy for hepatic coma. Kanamycin has a somewhat more limited spectrum of action than other aminoglycosides, and its use has declined in recent years.

Resistance to aminoglycosides is becoming more prevalent as their use increases. Resistant strains of *Enterobacter, Klebsiella, Proteus, Pseudomonas,* and *Serratia* have appeared in many hospitals where the aminoglycosides are widely used. This resistance can occur in a number of ways, the most common being decreased penetration of the drug into the bacterial cell, a deficiency of the ribosomal receptor (see under Mechanism and Action), or increased enzymatic destruction of the drug. The newer derivatives (amikacin, netilmicin) may still be effective, however, against certain organisms that have become resistant to the action of the older agents such as kanamycin, tobramycin, and gentamicin. In addition, amikacin is not degraded by most aminoglycoside-inactivating enzymes that affect other derivatives, and thus may be useful against enzyme-producing organisms resistant to the other systemic aminoglycosides. Nevertheless, culture and sensitivity tests should be performed to determine the susceptibility of an infecting organism to a particular aminoglycoside.

The possibility of serious adverse reactions is a major limitation to the routine use of the aminoglycosides, and all derivatives exhibit essentially the same range of toxic effects, although some effects occur less frequently with some of the newer agents. In general, the likelihood of toxicity with aminoglycosides increases with increased dosage, increased duration of therapy, and increased degree of kidney dysfunction.

Foremost among the untoward reactions seen with aminoglycoside use is ototoxicity, which can involve both the auditory and vestibular functions of the eighth cranial nerve. The risk is greatest in patients with renal impairment or preexisting hearing loss, and the incidence of ototoxicity is generally related to the dose and especially to the duration of treatment. Patients should be observed closely for early signs of impending toxicity (tinnitus, vertigo, high-frequency deafness), and the dosage should be lowered or the drug discontinued to prevent irreversible deafness. Vestibular toxicity is more common with gentamicin and streptomycin, whereas auditory toxicity is more prevalent with kanamycin, neomycin, amikacin, and netilmicin. The *relative* ototoxicity of aminoglycosides is neomycin > streptomycin = kanamycin > amikacin = gentamicin = tobramycin > netilmicin.

Because aminoglycosides are eliminated almost entirely by the kidneys, they may accumulate in patients with compromised renal function. Moreover, the drug's own toxic effects may further reduce the organ's ability to excrete nitrogenous wastes. The result is increased nitrogen retention (*i.e.*, elevated BUN or serum creatinine), frequently accompanied by oliguria, proteinuria, azotemia, and the presence of red and white cell casts in the urine. Because renal tubular damage is usually reversible if detected early enough, careful monitoring of renal function and serum creatinine levels is essential during prolonged aminoglycoside therapy, especially in the patient with preexisting renal dysfunction. Decreased creatinine clearance necessitates a reduction in drug dosage or an increase in dosing intervals, or both; the presence of casts in the urine suggests that hydration of the patient should be increased; the appearance of symptomatic azotemia or a progressive decrease in urine output is usually an indication to discontinue the drug. It should be noted, however, that when patients are well hydrated and kidney function is normal the risk of nephrotoxicity with aminoglycosides is comparatively low, provided dosage limits are not exceeded. The relative nephrotoxicity of these agents is approximately neomycin > amikacin = gentamicin = kanamycin = netilmicin > tobramycin > streptomycin.

Interference with neuromuscular transmission, possibly leading to respiratory depression or paralysis, has occurred with aminoglycosides, especially when given either simultaneously with or shortly after general anesthetics or muscle relaxants. Reversal of aminoglycoside-induced neuromuscular blockade (characterized by apnea and muscle paralysis) may be accomplished with either neostigmine or calcium salts.

Inasmuch as the different aminoglycosides share the same properties, they are considered as a group. Characteristics of individual drugs are then presented in Table 65-3. The discussion focuses primarily on the parenteral use of the drugs, with references to their oral and topical application where appropriate.

Aminoglycosides

Amikacin, Gentamicin, Kanamycin, Neomycin, Netilmicin, Streptomycin, Tobramycin

MECHANISM AND ACTIONS
Aminoglycosides are bactericidal to a wide range of microorganisms. Their principal site of action is the 30S ribosomal subunit, to which they bind and subsequently interfere with the first step in protein synthesis. The presence of the drugs also results in a misreading of the genetic code of the m-RNA template, leading to incorporation of incorrect amino acids into growing polypeptide chains. The drugs are more active in an alkaline medium; thus, their efficacy against urinary pathogens can be increased by alkalinization of the urine.

USES
(See Tables 59-1 and 65-2 for susceptible organisms.)
1. Treatment of severe gram-negative infections of the GI, respiratory or urinary tracts, CNS, bone, and soft tissues due to susceptible organisms (parenteral use only)
2. Preoperative suppression of intestinal bacterial (kanamycin or neomycin orally)
3. Treatment of acute or chronic intestinal amebiasis (paromomycin orally, see Chap. 72)
4. Adjunctive therapy of hepatic coma to reduce concentration of ammonia-forming bacteria in the GI tract (oral administration of kanamycin, neomycin, or paromomycin—see Chap. 72).
5. Treatment of superficial infections of the eye, skin, or mucous membranes, due to susceptible organisms (gentamicin or neomycin)
6. Treatment of severe diarrhea due to *Escherichia coli* (neomycin orally)

ADMINISTRATION AND DOSAGE
See Table 65-3.

FATE
Aminoglycosides are not absorbed to an appreciable extent from the GI tract; absorption from IM sites is usually rapid, with peak blood levels occurring within 1 hour. The drugs are widely distributed in the extracellular fluids but do not attain significant levels in cerebrospinal fluid unless the meninges are inflamed. Plasma protein binding is negligible, and plasma half-lives generally range from 1 hour to 3 hours with normal kidney function. The half-life may be prolonged in young infants and elderly persons and markedly lengthened in the presence of renal impairment (up to 80 hours–100 hours). Serum levels in febrile patients may be lower than those of afebrile patients, and the half-life of the drugs may be shortened. A decreased half-life is also noted in severely burned patients. Aminoglycosides are not metabolized to any extent but are eliminated by the kidney largely as the unchanged drug (up to 98% of a single IV dose within 24 hours). Accumulation of drug does not occur in patients with normal renal function,

(*Text continues on p. 1246.*)

Table 65-3
Aminoglycosides

Drug	Preparations	Usual Dosage Range	Clinical Considerations
amikacin (Amikin)	Injection—100 mg/2 ml; 500 mg/2 ml; 1 g/4 ml	IM, IV: Adults and older children—15 mg/kg/day in two to three divided doses (maximum 1.5 g/day) Urinary tract infections: 250 mg IM twice a day Neonatal sepsis: Initially 10 mg/kg, followed by 7.5 mg/kg every 12 h	Semisynthetic aminoglycoside derived from kanamycin, exhibiting a similar spectrum of action; not degraded by most aminoglycoside-inactivating enzymes, therefore may be effective against organisms resistant to other derivatives; amikacin resistance is emerging, however, as its use increases; duration of treatment should be 7 days to 10 days; longer therapy necessitates daily monitoring of renal and auditory function; if a clinical response does not occur within 5 days, stop drug and reevaluate; may be used in uncomplicated urinary tract infections (dose: 250 mg IM twice a day) due to organisms not susceptible to other, less toxic agents; urine should be examined during treatment for the presence of protein, blood cells, or casts; maintain high degree of hydration to minimize renal irritation; solution for IV use is prepared by adding contents of 500 mg vial to 200 ml of appropriate diluent (see package instructions) and administered over a 30-min to 60-min period (1 h–2 h for neonates); do not premix with other drugs; stable for extended period of time at room temperature; dosage interval must be lengthened or dose reduced in patients with renal impairment according to package instructions
gentamicin (Garamycin, Genoptic, Gentacidin, Gentafair, Gentak, Jenamicin)	Injection—10 mg/ml, 40 mg/ml Piggyback injection or disposable syringe—60 mg/dose, 80 mg/dose, 100 mg/dose Intrathecal injection—2 mg/ml	IM, IV: Adults—3 mg/kg/day to 5 mg/kg/day in three to four divided doses Children—6 mg/kg to 7.5 mg/kg/day in three divided doses Infants and neonates—7.5	Broad-spectrum aminoglycoside obtained from an *Actinomyces* organism; drug of choice against several gram-negative organisms (see Table 59-1), synergistic with extended-spectrum penicil- *(continued)*

Table 65-3 (continued)
Aminoglycosides

Drug	Preparations	Usual Dosage Range	Clinical Considerations
gentamicin (Garamycin, Genoptic, Gentacidin, Gentafair, Gentak, Jenamicin) (continued)	Ophthalmic drops—0.3% Ophthalmic ointment—0.3% Topical ointment—0.1% Topical cream—0.1%	mg/kg/day in three divided doses Premature infants and neonates (less than 1 wk)—5 mg/kg/day in two equal doses Intrathecal: Adults—4 mg to 8 mg/day in a single dose Children and infants (over 3 mo)—1 mg to 2 mg once a day Ophthalmic: 1 drop to 2 drops or small amount of ophthalmic ointment two to four times/day Topical: Apply sparingly to affected area three to four times/day	lins against *Pseudomonas* infections; may be used in combination with a penicillin or cephalosporin in treating serious unknown infections before sensitivity testing; but must also be administered separately; also used with antistaphylococcal penicillins for treatment of staphylococcal endocarditis; generally given IM, but may be used IV in patients with septicemia, shock, congestive heart failure, severe burns, or hematologic disorders; do not mix with other drugs before injection; intrathecal administration is used as an adjunct to systemic administration in serious CNS infection (*e.g.*, meningitis, ventriculitis) due to *Pseudomonas* species; injections are continued as long as sensitive microorganisms are demonstrable in the CSF; may also be given into subdural space or into a ventricle by an implanted cannula; topical application is used to treat superficial infections of the skin and mucous membranes due to susceptible organisms; photosensitivity reactions have occurred following topical use; systemic toxicity can result from application to large abraded areas of skin; use cautiously on burns or large wounds; reduce dose or increase dosage interval in patients with impaired renal function
kanamycin (Kantrex, Klebcil)	Injection—500 mg/2 ml; 1 g/3 ml Pediatric injection—75 mg/2 ml Capsules—500 mg	IM: Adults and children—7.5 mg/kg every 12 h (maximum 1.5 g/day) IV: Up to 15 mg/kg/day in two to three divided doses in-	Aminoglycoside derived from a species of *Streptomyces*; similar in activity to neomycin but not as toxic; effective against many common gram (−) organisms (except *Pseu-* (continued)

Table 65-3 (continued)
Aminoglycosides

Drug	Preparations	Usual Dosage Range	Clinical Considerations
kanamycin (Kantrex, Klebcil) (continued)		fused over a 30-min to 60-min period Intraperitoneal: 500 mg/20 ml sterile distilled water instilled into peritoneal cavity through a wound catheter Aerosol: 250 mg (1 ml) diluted with 3 ml saline two to four times a day, using a nebulizer Oral: Suppression of intestinal bacteria—1 g every hour for 4 h, then 1 g every 6 h for 36 h to 72 h Hepatic coma—8 g to 12 g/day in divided doses	domonas) but not considered drug of choice for any infection; primarily used as alternate to gentamycin or tobramycin; occasionally used as adjunctive therapy of *Mycobacterium tuberculosis*; inject deeply IM and rotate sites; extend dosing interval according to package directions in patients with reduced kidney function; discontinue drug if a clinical response does not occur within 5 days; prepare IV solutions by adding 500 mg to 200 ml, or 1 g to 400 ml, of sterile diluent, and infuse over 30 min to 60 min two to three times a day; do not mix dilution with other drug solutions; solution in vials may darken on shelf with no loss of potency; intraperitoneal instillation for established peritonitis or fecal spill during surgery should be postponed until patient has recovered from effects of anesthesia and muscle relaxants (danger of respiratory depression and muscle paralysis); may be used as an irrigating solution (0.25%) in abscess cavities, peritoneal, ventricular, or pleural spaces; when used orally, be alert for malabsorption syndrome (*e.g.,* increased fecal fat) or secondary bacterial or fungal infections (*e.g.,* diarrhea, stomatitis); used with caution orally in patients with GI ulceration, because enhanced systemic absorption can occur; oral use may increase effects of oral anticoagulants by impairing absorption of vitamin K; nausea, vomiting, and diarrhea are common with oral ingestion

(continued)

Table 65-3 (continued)
Aminoglycosides

Drug	Preparations	Usual Dosage Range	Clinical Considerations
neomycin (Mycifradin, Myciguent)	Tablets—500 mg Oral solution—125 mg/5 ml Topical ointment—0.5% Topical cream—0.5%	Oral: Preoperative bowel preparation—on day prior to surgery, give 2 oral doses of neomycin (1 g each) with 1 g erythromycin base 1 h apart, then give a third dose at bedtime Hepatic coma— Adults—4 g to 12 g/day in divided doses Children—50 mg to 100 mg/kg/day in divided doses Infectious diarrhea—50 mg/kg/day in divided doses for 2 days to 3 days Topical: Apply two to four times/day	Broad-spectrum antibiotic obtained from a species of *Streptomyces*; similar in action to kanamycin, but is the most potent neuromuscular blocker and reportedly the *most toxic* of all aminoglycosides; many organisms exhibit moderate to marked resistance against neomycin; principal indications for oral neomycin are severe diarrhea due to *Escherichia coli* and preoperative bowel sterilization in conjunction with a low-residue diet; a saline cathartic is administered before first dose of neomycin; may interfere with absorption of other drugs (*e.g.*, digitalis glycosides, methotrexate, penicillins; see under Interactions); nausea and diarrhea are fairly common with oral administration; widest application is topically, either alone or more commonly with bacitracin and/or polymyxin (*e.g.*, Neosporin, Mycitracin, Neo-Polycin) for superficial infections of eye, skin, and mucous membranes; hypersensitivity reactions are common with topical application; discontinue drug if irritation, redness, or itching occurs; do not use over large body surface areas, or if skin is broken or abraded, because increased systemic absorption and toxicity can occur
netilmicin (Netromycin)	Injections—100 mg/ml	IM, IV: Adults—3 mg to 6.5 mg/kg/day in divided doses every 8 h–12 h Children—5.5 mg to 8 mg/kg/day in divided doses every 8 h–12 h Neonates—4 mg to 6 mg/kg/day in divided doses every 12 h	Semisynthetic derivative similar to gentamicin in activity but somewhat less effective against *Pseudomonas*; may be slightly less nephrotoxic and ototoxic than other aminoglycosides; used in serious staphylococcal infections where penicillins *(continued)*

Table 65-3 (continued)
Aminoglycosides

Drug	Preparations	Usual Dosage Range	Clinical Considerations
netilmicin (Netromycin) (continued)			are contraindicated, and in suspected or confirmed gram (−) infections; usual duration of treatment is 7 days to 14 days; for longer therapy, carefully monitor renal, auditory, and vestibular functions; follow package instructions for dosage adjustment in the presence of impaired renal function
streptomycin (Streptomycin)	Powder for injection—1 g/vial, 5 g/vial, Injection—400 mg/ml	IM use only: Tuberculosis—1 g/day, together with other antitubercular drugs (e.g., isoniazid, ethambutol, rifampin); may reduce to 1 g two to three times a week as condition improves Tularemia—1 g to 2 g/day in divided doses for 7 days to 10 days Plague—2 g to 4 g/day in divided doses Bacterial endocarditis—0.5 g to 1 g twice a day for 2 wk in combination with pencillin Prophylaxis of bacterial endocarditis in patients undergoing intestinal or urinary surgery—1 g IM ½–1 h before surgery in combination with 2 million U penicillin G or 1 g ampicillin, IM or IV Other infections—1 g to 4 g/day in divided doses depending on severity of infection Children—20 mg to 40 mg/kg/day in divided doses every 6 h–12 h	Aminoglycoside isolated from a species of Streptomyces; fairly high toxicity and rapid development of resistance limits its usefulness to those infections not controlled by other less toxic drugs, except in tularemia, plague, and melioidosis, where it is the drug of choice, and tuberculosis, where it is commonly used in combination with several other tuberculostatic agents; (See Chap. 69); total treatment period for tuberculosis is a minimum of 1 year; also indicated for prophylaxis of bacterial endocarditis in high-risk patients undergoing respiratory, dental, gastrointestinal, or genitourinary surgery or instrumentation, in combination with penicillin G or ampicillin; most frequent adverse effect is vestibular toxicity; observe for headache, vomiting, dizziness, difficulty in reading, or ataxia, and consult physician; incidence of nephrotoxicity is lowest of all aminoglycosides, but use with caution in renal impairment and perform frequent determinations of serum drug concentration; adequate hydration is important, especially during prolonged therapy (e.g., for tuberculosis); com-(continued)

Table 65-3 (continued)
Aminoglycosides

Drug	Preparations	Usual Dosage Range	Clinical Considerations
streptomycin (Streptomycin) *(continued)*			mercially available IM solutions contain a preservative and should not be injected IV or SC; solution may darken during storage, but potency is not affected
tobramycin (Nebcin, Tobrex)	Injection—40 mg/ml, 60 mg/1.5 ml Pediatric injection—20 mg/2 ml Powder for injection—30 mg/ml, 40 mg/ml when reconstituted Ophthalmic solution—0.3% Ophthalmic ointment—3 mg/g	IM, IV: Adults and children—3 mg to 5 mg/kg/day in three to four equally divided doses depending on severity of infection Children—6 mg to 7.5 mg/kg/day in three or four equally divided doses Neonates (1 wk or less)—up to 4 mg/kg/day in two equal doses every 12 h Ophthalmic: 1 drop to 2 drops or ½-inch ribbon of ointment every 4 h; in severe infections 2 drops every hour until improvement is noted	Aminoglycoside antibiotic with pharmacologic properties, indications, and overall toxicity similar to gentamicin; somewhat lower incidence of vestibular toxicity has been reported; do not exceed 5 mg/kg/day unless serum levels are monitored; prolonged serum concentrations above 12 mcg/ml should be avoided; urine should be observed for presence of protein, cells, and casts; follow package directions for dosage reduction in patients with renal impairment; reduced doses may be calculated based on creatinine clearance or serum creatinine; IV dose should be diluted to 50 ml to 100 ml for adults (and proportionately less for children) with sodium chloride or 5% dextrose injection and infused over 20 min–60 min; do not premix with other drugs but administer separately; usual duration of treatment is 7 days to 10 days; in severe or complicated infections, a longer course of therapy may be necessary; auditory, vestibular, and renal function should be monitored frequently during prolonged therapy; conjunctival erythema, itching and swelling of the eyelids, and local allergic reactions have occurred with use of eye drops or ointment; safe use of eye drops or ointment in pregnant women or nursing mothers has not been established.

but significant accumulation and subsequent toxicity can occur rapidly if renal function is impaired. The drugs exhibit a narrow margin between the therapeutic and toxic serum levels, and serum levels should be closely monitored. Aminoglycosides administered orally (i.e., kanamycin, neomycin) are eliminated largely as unabsorbed drug in the feces.

SIDE-EFFECTS/ADVERSE REACTIONS

The principal adverse reactions associated with aminoglycoside use are ototoxicity and nephrotoxicity. (See introduction for relative incidence among the various derivatives.) The ototoxicity can manifest itself as either *auditory* dysfunction (cochlear damage), which is usually heralded by high-pitched tinnitus and high frequency deafness which usually progresses through the lower sound ranges with continued drug use, or *vestibular* dysfunction, which is usually evident by the appearance of vertigo and ataxia. The half-lives of the aminoglycosides are several times longer in the otic fluids than in the plasma, and persistently elevated levels of the drugs result in progressive destruction of vestibular and cochlear cells, leading eventually to irreversible deafness. Because the initial symptoms are reversible, however, careful monitoring of patients receiving these drugs is essential. Therapy should be discontinued as soon as possible, because the incidence of ototoxicity is directly proportional to the duration of therapy and the amount of drug administered.

Aminoglycosides are concentrated by proximal tubular cells in the renal cortex, and, depending on the levels attained at these sites, varying degrees of renal toxicity can occur. Early signs of renal toxicity include mild proteinuria, appearance of cells or casts in the urine, decreased creatinine clearance and urine specific gravity, and increased BUN and nonprotein nitrogen. Glomerular filtration rate may be reduced with continued drug exposure. Acute tubular necrosis has occurred but is an infrequent complication. The impaired renal function is usually reversible because proximal tubular cells have a regenerative capacity. However, the renal tubular damage may result in impaired excretion of the aminoglycoside, increasing the risk of ototoxicity and other untoward reactions. Neomycin is highly concentrated by the renal tubular cells and is the most nephrotoxic aminoglycoside; it should not be given systemically. Streptomycin, on the other hand, is not nephrotoxic because it does not concentrate in the tubular cells.

Aminoglycosides possess a curare-like action at the neuromuscular junction and can elicit skeletal muscle weakness, especially when given in conjunction with or immediately following administration of neuromuscular blocking agents or general anesthetics. Patients with myasthenia gravis are particularly susceptible to this action. The effect is most pronounced with neomycin and streptomycin but has occurred with the other derivatives as well. Respiratory paralysis has occurred with these drugs, especially when administered at high doses. Intravenous calcium is the preferred means of treatment, although cholinesterase inhibitors have been used successfully as well.

In general, allergic reactions to aminoglycosides are rare. Their administration has been associated with a range of adverse reactions, most of which are observed more frequently with prolonged high dose therapy; these adverse effects are listed below by organ system.

CNS—Confusion, disorientation, lethargy, depression, visual disturbances, amblyopia, nystagmus, optic neuritis, numbness and paresthesias, muscle twitching, tremor, convulsions

Allergic (infrequent)—Rash, pruritus, urticaria, alopecia, laryngeal edema, fever, exfoliative dermatitis, anaphylaxis

Hematologic—Agranulocytosis, leukopenia, thrombocytopenia, eosinophilia, pancytopenia, anemia

Hepatic—Increased serum transaminase and bilirubin, hepatomegaly, hepatic necrosis

Other—Palpitations, myocarditis, splenomegaly, arthralgia, hypotension, pulmonary fibrosis, superinfections, muscle weakness, respiratory depression, pain and irritation with IM injection

Oral administration of aminoglycosides has resulted in development of the "malabsorption syndrome" (i.e., decreased absorption of vitamins, minerals, electrolytes, fats) as well as steatorrhea, anorexia, stomatitis, and salivation. Burning, itching, urticaria, erythema, photosensitivity, and macropapular dermatitis have occurred following topical application of these agents.

CONTRAINDICATIONS AND PRECAUTIONS

Aminoglycosides should not be used for extended periods of time in patients with impaired renal function or in conjunction with other drugs that may be ototoxic or nephrotoxic (see under Interactions). Neomycin should not be given to infants or small children.

Aminoglycosides must be used *cautiously* in patients with neuromuscular disorders, such as myasthenia gravis or parkinsonism or in conjunction with skeletal muscle relaxants, because increased muscle weakness can develop. Cautious use is also necessary in children, elderly persons, and in pregnant or nursing mothers. Because aminoglycosides reach high levels in the kidney, patients must be kept well hydrated to minimize the degree of irritation and damage to the renal tubules.

INTERACTIONS

1. Concurrent use of aminoglycosides and amphotericin, bacitracin, cephalothin, colistimethate, polymyxin, or vancomycin can increase the incidence of nephrotoxicity.
2. The ototoxic effects of the aminoglycosides can be enhanced by potent diuretics such as ethacrynic acid, bumetanide, furosemide, and mannitol.
3. Dimenhydrinate, meclizine, cyclizine, and other antivertigo drugs may mask the early symptoms of the ototoxic effects of aminoglycosides.
4. Aminoglycosides can enhance the muscle-relaxing effects of neuromuscular blocking agents and general anesthetics, possibly leading to respiratory depression.
5. Aminoglycosides exert a synergistic effect with antipseudomonal penicillins (*e.g.,* carbenicillin, ticarcillin, piperacillin, mezlocillin, azlocillin) against *Pseudomonas* infections at normal concentrations; however, at high concentrations the penicillins may inhibit the antibacterial activity of aminoglycosides. In addition, penicillins and cephalosporins may inactivate aminoglycosides when admixed or coadministered (see under Nursing Process).
6. Oral administration of neomycin may impair the absorption of penicillin VK, digitalis drugs, vitamin K, and methotrexate.

■ Nursing Process

See also Nursing Process for anti-infectives in Chapter 59.

□ ASSESSMENT

□ Subjective Data

A thorough drug history is essential because drug interactions that occur with aminoglycosides can be devastating. (See under Interactions.) Use of other nephrotoxic antibiotics should be listed; when used with aminoglycosides the risk of nephrotoxicity increases. Likewise, drugs with the potential for ototoxicity such as diuretics and antivertigo drugs must be identified because they can lead to an increased incidence of that side-effect. Any oral drug can be affected if oral or rectal use of an aminoglycoside is planned because these formulations will decrease or eliminate absorption of almost any drug. Alternative administration methods of essential drugs such as digitalis may be needed. Penicillins may act synergistically with aminoglycosides, so their use must also be identified. However, at high doses these same drugs may impair the bactericidal activity of aminoglycosides, so their concurrent use is not without hazards. Drug allergies, especially to aminoglycosides, should also be identified.

A history of the symptoms of infection for which the aminoglycoside is prescribed is necessary. A medical history should also be obtained; the presence of neuromuscular disease such as myasthenia gravis or parkinsonism, hearing loss, renal dysfunction, pregnancy, or lactation warrants extremely cautious drug use.

□ Objective Data

Physical assessment may focus on evaluation of the infected site, neuromuscular function, hearing, especially high-pitched sounds, and gastrointestinal motility. A weight and urine output should be obtained as baseline data to monitor renal function throughout therapy.

Diagnostic data may include a baseline audiogram if long-term therapy is expected. Laboratory studies of hematologic, hepatic (bilirubin and enzymes), and renal (BUN and creatinine) function are appropriate. A culture and sensitivity of infected site and urinalysis are also important.

□ NURSING DIAGNOSIS

Actual nursing diagnoses may include:
  Knowledge deficit related to dose, effect on body, and side-effects of the drug
Potential nursing diagnoses may include:
  Alteration in respiratory function related to neuromuscular blockade, a drug side-effect, or a sign of superinfection
  Alteration in bowel elimination: diarrhea related to the bowel-cleansing effect of oral drug forms or a sign of superinfection
  Alteration in fluid volume: excess related to nephrotoxicity

Potential for injury: trauma related to
dizziness, an ototoxic drug effect
Alteration in nutrition: less than body
requirements related to malabsorption
during oral or rectal drug administration
Sensory-perceptual alteration related to
auditory changes and ototoxicity
Impaired thought processes: related to central
nervous system changes, a drug side-effect
(rare)
Impaired tissue integrity related to
photosensitivity from topical drug
application or superinfection

□ *PLAN*
Nursing care goals focus on:
1. Safe and correct administration of the drug by
the route prescribed
2. Close monitoring of side-effects, especially
nephrotoxicity, ototoxicity, superinfection,
and photosensitivity (topical use)
3. Teaching the patient, as necessary, correct
drug-taking techniques, side-effects, and what
to do if problems occur

□ *INTERVENTION*
The main routes of aminoglycoside administration
are intravenous and intramuscular. Topical administration is used occasionally, and oral administration is used rarely, in specific situations.

Intravenous administration must be closely
monitored to reduce the incidence of untoward effects. The drugs should be reconstituted immediately before use, according to current manufacturers' instructions, because solutions are
relatively unstable. Refer to Table 65-2 for dilution
instructions on each drug. Rate of infusion should
be closely monitored by an infusion pump or other
rate-control device to avoid too rapid administration which can increase the risk of ototoxicity and
neuromuscular blockade. The nurse must be aware
that while aminoglycosides and certain penicillins
may be given concurrently in a treatment regimen,
many drugs are physically incompatible; if possible, separate IV lines should be used for each drug;
if not possible, lines should be completely flushed
after each administration, and doses should be separated from each other by at least 1 hour. For example, if both drugs are ordered q 6 hours, the aminoglycoside might be given at 6 AM, 12 noon, 6 PM,
and 12 midnight, and penicillin might be given at 8
AM, 2 PM, 8 PM, and 2 AM to avoid problems.

Intramuscular injections should be given in a
large muscle mass such as the gluteus in adults or
the vastus lateralis in young children, and sites
should be rotated using a body map (see Chap. 8) to
decrease the chance of tissue damage. Injections are
painful.

Oral aminoglycosides are rarely given, except
for bowel cleansing prior to gastrointestinal surgery or in treatment of severe diarrhea, and are
administered rectally to reduce ammonia-forming
bacteria in hepatic coma. Both of these administration routes can be extremely hazardous to any patient with a lesion of the GI tract because systemic
absorption is then more likely and can rapidly lead
to nephrotoxicity. A GI series or barium enema
may be appropriate before therapy begins, and the
nurse should watch closely for signs of hematemesis, gastric pain, rectal bleeding, or blackened
stools throughout therapy, all symptoms of gastrointestinal lesions. If any symptoms develop, the
drug should be held and the physician notified at
once.

Topical formulations of neomycin and gentamicin are different for the eyes, ears, and skin and
cannot be interchanged. Tubes should be clearly
marked to avoid confusion and potentially toxic
systemic absorption. Sites should be checked for
ulceration, burns, or other breaks, and drugs
should be used with caution in these instances because the risk of systemic absorption is increased.
Local allergic reaction may occur with topical use.
The patient should be told to immediately report
the development of rash, pruritis, urticaria, or
angioedema (localized swelling). The drug will generally be discontinued.

Aminoglycoside administration can result in
serious ototoxicity and nephrotoxicity even in normal therapeutic doses. In an attempt to avoid irreversible damage, the physician may order peak and
trough serum drug levels checked on a routine
basis to catch early any developing toxicity. (See
Table 65-1.) The nurse is usually responsible to ensure the blood levels are drawn at the appropriate
times and that results are checked before the next
dose is given. Frequently, the serum levels will be
listed on a flow sheet or on the medication administration record (MAR) so the drug will not be inadvertently continued if the serum level approaches the toxic range.

A list of therapeutic and toxic ranges such as
the one shown in Table 65-1 should be posted as a
ready reference for all clinicians.

However, blood studies are only part of the
dose monitoring needed during aminoglycoside administration. To check for developing ototoxicity,
frequent tests for the ability to hear high-pitched
sounds can be performed at the bedside. Loss of

this ability may be the first sign of auditory damage. A periodic audiogram should also be performed. Other early symptoms include fullness and vertigo (signs of vestibular dysfunction) or tinnitus (a sign of cochlear damage). Any sign should be reported immediately, and the drug should be discontinued. Hearing loss may be reversible if caught early, but monitoring should be continued for 3 weeks to 4 weeks after the drug is stopped to determine the full extent of the impairment.

Nephrotoxicity is an equally important side-effect to monitor because it may occur first, speeding the development of ototoxicity. Preventive care includes close monitoring of BUN, creatinine, and fluid intake and urinary output. Dosages should be reduced if renal function becomes impaired. Renal irritation, often a precursor to renal dysfunction, is manifested by the development of red or white blood cells, albumin, or casts in the urine detectable on urinalysis. If this occurs, fluids should be increased to 2000 ml to 3000 ml per day, and other parameters should be monitored more closely. If BUN rises, serum creatinine falls, oliguria develops, or intake is greater than output, nephrotoxicity is developing and the drug should be discontinued.

Superinfection is another side-effect of aminoglycoside therapy most frequently manifesting as an upper respiratory infection. The patient should have frequent vital signs, monitoring temperature and respiratory rate specifically, and lungs should be routinely auscultated. Other signs of bacterial or fungal overgrowth which may occur include diarrhea (with parenteral therapy), "furry" tongue, stomatitis, glossitis, or perianal itching or irritation. Treatment with an appropriate anti-infective is usually effective.

Photosensitivity may occur with topical drug administration. Patients should be warned to avoid direct sunlight, wear protective clothing, sunglasses, and sun screens as necessary.

Most of the other side-effects of aminoglycosides develop when high doses are used or therapy is prolonged. Hematologic and hepatic dysfunction can be monitored by periodic blood studies. However, if central nervous system symptoms (see under Side-Effects/Adverse Reactions) develop, respiratory depression, hypotension, and cardiac palpitations are likely to occur. Appropriate emergency equipment should be on hand to treat a possible respiratory arrest.

□ *EVALUATION*

The outcome criteria used to measure drug effectiveness may include resolution of infection seen by fever reduction and absence of growth in cultures as well as evidence of appropriate administration techniques and routine peak and trough level results documented as ordered. Other criteria may include the absence or early treatment of such side-effects as ototoxicity, nephrotoxicity, superinfection, or central nervous system problems.

CASE STUDY

Lester Jones, age 21, was shot in the abdomen by the owner of the liquor store he was attempting to rob. Mr. Jones was rushed, unconscious, to the emergency room of a local hospital and taken immediately for exploratory surgery. The bullet, which had perforated the bowel, was removed, and a wound excision and temporary colostomy were performed.

A wound culture and sensitivity were obtained during surgery, but gentamicin, 80 mg by IV piggyback every 6 hours, was ordered postoperatively until lab results were known. The wound culture showed multiple gram-negative bacilli including *Pseudomonas* and *Enterobacter* strains. The physician decided to continue gentamicin and to add azlocillin, 2 g by IV piggyback every 6 hours. (Refer to Chap. 61 for information on azlocillin).

Discussion Questions

1. Mr. Jones was taken quickly to surgery because of his injury, and basic assessment data were not evaluated before the early postoperative period. In light of the drugs prescribed, which laboratory studies should be checked?

What physical assessment should also be highlighted? What historic information should be obtained?

2. How should administration of these drugs be timed? In what should each of them be diluted? How fast can each be infused?

3. Design a flow sheet of the basic information which should be periodically monitored to detect early any side-effects from these drugs.

4. At what point might the physician order peak and trough levels for gentamicin? Based on the answer developed in Question 2, when should each level be drawn?

REVIEW QUESTIONS

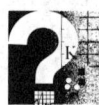

1. List the clinically available aminoglycosides.
2. Against which organisms are aminoglycosides most often employed?
3. By what routes of administration are systemically acting aminoglycosides given?
4. Why is it necessary to determine plasma levels of aminoglycosides frequently during therapy? Describe peak and trough levels and how they are used clinically. What is the nurse's responsibility?
5. How can microorganisms develop resistance to the aminoglycosides?
6. What are the major types of toxicity associated with aminoglycoside usage? What actions will facilitate early detection of these problems?
7. What factors increase the likelihood of these toxic reactions with aminoglycosides?
8. How are aminoglycosides excreted?
9. Briefly describe the mechanism of action of these agents.
10. What are the two principal forms of ototoxicity? What are the initial symptoms of each?
11. How do aminoglycosides interfere with renal function?
12. What is the action of aminoglycosides on skeletal muscle? How may this effect be reversed?
13. What are the principal side-effects of oral neomycin?
14. What other drugs can increase the incidence of nephrotoxicity with aminoglycosides?
15. Which aminoglycoside is (a) most nephrotoxic and (b) least nephrotoxic?
16. What baseline physical assessments should be performed before aminoglycosides are administered?

BIBLIOGRAPHY

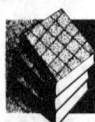

Aminoglycosides. Nursing 83 13(2):64A, 1983

Betts RF et al: Five year surveillance of aminoglycoside usage in a university hospital. Ann Intern Med 100:219, 1984

Blumer JL, Reed MD: Clinical pharmacology of aminoglycoside antibiotics in pediatrics. Pediatr Clin North Am 30:195, 1983

Brummett RE: Drug-induced ototoxicity. Drugs 19:412, 1980

Bryan LE: Mechanisms of action of aminoglycoside antibiotics. In Root RK, Sande MA (eds): Contemporary Issues in Infectious

Diseases, Vol. 1: New Dimensions in Antimicrobial Therapy, p 1. New York, Churchill Livingstone, 1984

Edson RS, Keys TF: The aminoglycosides. Mayo Clin Proc 58:99, 1983

Gever LN: Parenteral aminoglycosides: Administering them safely. Nursing 84 14(3):90, 1984

Langslet J, Habel ML: The aminoglycoside antibiotics. Am J Nurs 81:1144, 1981

Lerner AM et al: Randomized controlled trial of the comparative efficacy, auditory toxicity and nephrotoxicity of tobramycin and netilmicin. Lancet 1:1123, 1983

Lietman PS: Aminoglycosides and spectinomycin: Aminocyclitols. In Mandell GL, Douglas RG, Bennett JE (eds): Principles and Practice of Infectious Diseases, 2nd ed, p 192. New York, John Wiley & Sons, 1985

Lietman PS, Smith CR: Aminoglycoside nephrotoxicity in humans. J Infect Dis 5(suppl 2):284, 1983

Moore RD, Smith CR et al: Risk factors for nephrotoxicity in patients treated with aminoglycosides. Ann Intern Med 100:352, 1984

Moore RD, Smith CR, Lietman PS: Risk factors for the development of auditory toxicity in patients receiving aminoglycosides. J Infect Dis 149:23, 1984

Shannon K, Phillips I: Mechanisms of resistance to aminoglycosides in clinical isolates. J Antimicrob Chemother 9:91, 1982

Silverblatt FJ: Unraveling the mechanisms of aminoglycoside toxicity. Drug Therapy 9(8):55, 1979

Silverblatt FJ: Pathogenesis of nephrotoxicity of cephalosporins and aminoglycosides: A review of current concepts. Rev Infect Dis 4(suppl):360, 1982

Smith CR, Lietman PS: Effect of furosemide on aminoglycoside-induced nephrotoxicity and auditory toxicity in humans. Antimicrob Agents Chemother 23:133, 1983

Whelton A, Neu HC (eds): The Aminoglycosides: Microbiology, Clinical Use and Toxicity. New York, Marcel Dekker, 1982

Polypeptides

Bacitracin
Colistimethate

Colistin Sulfate
Polymyxin B Sulfate

66

The polypeptide group of antibiotics comprises polymyxin B, colistin (polymyxin E), the methane-sulfonate salt of colistin (colistimethate), and bacitracin. The first three of these drugs are commonly termed the polymyxins, and while certain similarities exist between these agents and bacitracin, significant differences are noted as well.

The polymyxins are a group of strongly basic polypeptides obtained from *Bacillus polymyxa* and variants and are designated as polymyxins A, B, C, D, and E. Of these only polymyxins B and E (colistin) are employed clinically, because the remaining derivatives are too toxic for human use.

The polymyxins are bactericidal, primarily against gram-negative bacilli such as *Pseudomonas*, *Escherichia coli*, *Klebsiella*, *Enterobacter*, *Salmonella*, and *Shigella*. However, most strains of *Proteus* and *Neisseria* and virtually all gram-positive organisms are unaffected by the polymyxins. They exert their antibacterial action by disrupting the bacterial cell membrane, thus allowing cell constituents to escape. The drugs are not absorbed orally, and, following parenteral administration, they do not reach the CNS (unless given intrathecally), the joints, or the eye in appreciable amounts. Excretion is by way of the kidney (except oral colistin), thus cumulation toxicity can occur in the presence of renal impairment. The polymyxins are used systemically for severe infections only, especially those of the urinary tract, caused by susceptible gram-negative organisms not sensitive to other less toxic antimicrobial drugs. The drugs find their widest application for topical treatment of skin and mucous membrane infections (including the eye and ear), especially if *Pseudomonas* is the offending pathogen. Principal adverse effects are of two major types, neurotoxicity and nephrotoxicity, and the incidence and severity of these untoward reactions severely limit the systemic usefulness of the polymyxins to all but very severe infections.

Polymyxin B is available as an injection, a powder for preparing ophthalmic drops, and in several combination products (*e.g.*, with neomycin, bacitracin, gramicidin, and corticosteroids) as drops or ointment for ophthalmic or otic use. Colistin sulfate (polymyxin E) can be used either as an oral suspension for control of diarrhea and gastroenteritis or in combination with hydrocortisone and neomycin as ear drops (Coly-Mycin S Otic). Colistimethate, as a powder for injection, may be administered either IV or IM for serious systemic or urinary infections, particularly when caused by *Pseudomonas*. Because there are many differences among these three polymyxin preparations, they are considered individually in this chapter.

Bacitracin is a mixture of several polypeptides isolated from a strain of *Bacillus subtilis*, the major constituent being bacitracin A. This antibiotic appears to inhibit bacterial cell wall formation and is bactericidal against a variety of gram-positive bacteria as well as a few gram-negative organisms. The drug is available for IM injection, and as a topical and ophthalmic ointment. Because of its potential for serious toxicity, however, it is used parenterally only for treatment of staphylococcal pneumonia or empyema in infants. Bacitracin is most often used topically, alone or in combination with neomycin and polymyxin, for treatment of cutaneous or ocular infections, because it is highly effective against susceptible organisms and rarely causes hypersensitivity reactions. Kidney damage is a major danger with parenteral use of bacitracin, and renal function must be closely monitored during therapy.

Bacitracin
(AK-Tracin, Baciguent)

MECHANISM AND ACTIONS
Bacitracin appears to inhibit bacterial cell wall synthesis and may alter cell membrane permeability. Most gram-positive organisms are susceptible as well as *Neisseria*, *Hemophilus influenzae*, *Treponema pallidum*, *Actinomyces*, and *Fusobacterium*. Systemic use of the drug is virtually obsolete because parenteral administration is highly nephrotoxic. Bacitracin has been employed previously in infants with staphylococcal pneumonia and empyema demonstrated to be sensitive to the drug. It is commonly used topically (see below).

USES
1. Treatment of superficial infections of the skin, mucous membrane, and eye due to susceptible organisms (topical use *only*)
2. Treatment of antibiotic-induced pseudomembranous colitis caused by *Clostridium difficile* (investigational use for *oral* bacitracin)

ADMINISTRATION AND DOSAGE
Bacitracin is available for IM injection in vials containing 10,000 units and 50,000 units. It is also used as an ophthalmic ointment and a topical ointment, each containing 500 units/g. When administered IM in infants, the recommended dosage is 900 units/kg/day for children under 2.5 kg and

1000 units/kg/day for heavier children, given in two or three divided doses. The diluent solution should be sodium chloride injection containing 2% procaine, and the concentration of bacitracin should be between 5,000 units and 10,000 units per ml. The ointments may be applied several times a day as necessary.

FATE
Absorption of bacitracin following IM injection is rapid and virtually complete. The drug is widely distributed throughout the body and is slowly excreted by glomerular filtration. Absorption from topical sites is minimal.

SIDE-EFFECTS/ADVERSE REACTIONS
The most serious adverse effect with parenteral bacitracin is nephrotoxicity, which may result in renal failure due to glomerular and tubular necrosis. Renal function must be closely monitored before and during parenteral therapy, and fluid intake and urinary output must be maintained at adequate levels. Other symptoms of renal toxicity include proteinuria, azotemia, hematuria, increased BUN, and uremia. Other adverse reactions noted with parenteral bacitracin are pain and irritation at the injection site, nausea, diarrhea, vomiting, tinnitus, altered taste sensations, skeletal muscle weakness, and hypersensitivity reactions (e.g., rash, urticaria). Topical use of bacitracin has resulted in contact dermatitis. Ophthalmic application can produce irritation, burning, itching, and stinging in the eyes.

CONTRAINDICATIONS AND PRECAUTIONS
Systemic bacitracin is contraindicated in persons with severe renal impairment. Intraocular bacitracin should not be used in patients with viral, fungal, or mycobacterial infections of the eye. *Cautious use* of bacitracin is necessary in persons with a history of allergic reactions or myasthenia gravis.

INTERACTIONS
1. The nephrotoxic effects of bacitracin may be additive to those of other antibiotics having similar toxicity (e.g., aminoglycosides, polymyxins, vancomycin).
2. Bacitracin can enhance or prolong the muscle-relaxing effects of neuromuscular blocking agents and anesthetics, or other drugs with neuromuscular blocking actions such as aminoglycosides, procainamide, or succinylcholine.

NURSING CONSIDERATIONS
See also Nursing Process for anti-infective therapy in Chapter 59.

Although rarely used, intramuscular bacitracin may still be administered occasionally. Injection solution is mixed with 2% procaine hydrochloride to decrease pain. Solutions are unstable at room temperature but can be kept up to 1 week if refrigerated. The patient should be asked about a history of allergy to "caine" drugs or to bacitracin before administration. The injection should be given in a large muscle mass such as the gluteus in adults or the vastus lateralis in young children, and sites should be rotated using a body map (see Chap. 8) to decrease tissue damage.

The main side-effect of parenteral bacitracin is nephrotoxicity. Baseline evaluation of urinary output, intake-to-output ratio, BUN, serum creatinine, and protein in urine should be obtained before therapy begins and should be done periodically throughout treatment. Changes in any of these values indicate renal dysfunction, and the drug should be immediately discontinued and the physician should be notified.

Topical use of bacitracin is widespread, especially in combination with neomycin and polymyxin. Ophthalmic use is also frequent. Topical and ophthalmic ointments are not interchangeable and should be clearly marked to avoid confusion. Prior to use, the patient should be asked about any known allergies to the drug. The most common side-effect is local hypersensitivity characterized by rash, pruritis, and urticaria. The patient should be told to report such symptoms immediately.

Superinfection, especially by *Candida albicans*, is possible with long-term bacitracin use and depends on the extent of systemic absorption. Potential sites are the mouth (characterized by white patches) and perianal area (characterized by white, cheesy vaginal discharge and itching or irritation).

Colistimethate
(Coly-Mycin M)

MECHANISM AND ACTIONS
Colistimethate penetrates into and subsequently disrupts the integrity of bacterial cell membranes, allowing escape of cell constituents. The drug is bactericidal against *Enterobacter, Escherichia coli, Klebsiella pneumoniae,* and *Pseudomonas aeruginosa.*

USES

1. Treatment of acute or chronic infections due to sensitive strains of the above-named organisms

ADMINISTRATION AND DOSAGE

Colistimethate is available as powder for injection containing 150 mg colistin (as colistimethate sodium) per vial. It may be administered either IM or IV. Adults and children receive 2.5 mg/kg/day to 5 mg/kg/day in two to four divided doses (maximum dose in persons with normal renal function is 5 mg/kg/day.

IV administration may be by direct injection (one-half daily dose over 3 minutes–5 minutes every 12 hours) or by infusion (one-half dose over 3 minutes–5 minutes, then 5 mg–6 mg/h starting 1 hour–2 hours after initial injection).

FATE

IM absorption is good, and maximum blood levels are attained within 1 hour to 2 hours. The serum half-life is 2 hours to 3 hours. Colistimethate does not enter the CNS in appreciable amounts but readily crosses the placental barrier. The drug is excreted primarily in the urine.

SIDE-EFFECTS/ADVERSE REACTIONS

Renal toxicity can occur, especially with large doses or prolonged therapy, and may be marked initially by decreased urinary output, increased BUN or serum creatinine, proteinuria, and azotemia. Renal failure has occurred. Other adverse effects include paresthesia, itching, urticaria, fever, dermatoses, numbness in the extremities, GI upset, vertigo, and slurred speech. Neuromuscular blockade possibly resulting in muscle weakness or respiratory depression has been reported, especially in patients with reduced renal function.

CONTRAINDICATIONS AND PRECAUTIONS

Colistimethate should not be used in persons with severe renal impairment. A *cautious* approach to therapy is warranted in persons with myasthenia gravis, persons receiving skeletal muscle relaxants, persons with a neurologic deficit, pregnant women, or nursing mothers.

INTERACTIONS

1. Additive nephrotoxic effects can result from concurrent use of colistimethate and other drugs which impair renal function (*e.g.*, aminoglycosides, vancomycin).
2. Extreme muscle weakness and muscle paralysis can occur if colistimethate is administered with several anesthetics, neuromuscular blocking agents, aminoglycosides, or other drugs having a neuromuscular blocking action.

■ Nursing Process

See also Nursing Process for anti-infective therapy in Chapter 59.

□ ASSESSMENT

□ Subjective Data

A drug history regarding use of skeletal muscle relaxants or any nephrotoxic drugs is essential to avoid toxic drug reactions. A history of renal disease contraindicates drug use, and a history of any neurologic or neuromuscular disorder, pregnancy, or lactation warrants cautious use.

□ Objective Data

Physical assessment of neuromuscular function is essential. Urinary output and weight should be measured as a baseline to evaluate later renal function. Laboratory data include a baseline urinalysis, BUN, and serum creatinine.

□ NURSING DIAGNOSIS

Actual nursing diagnoses may include:
　Knowledge deficit related to drug effects and potential side-effects
Potential nursing diagnoses may include:
　Alteration in respiratory function related to neuromuscular blockade
　Alteration in fluid volume: excess related to nephrotoxicity
　Potential for injury: trauma, related to dizziness or paresthesias
　Sensory-perceptual alteration related to auditory or visual changes, signs of neurotoxicity

□ PLAN

The nursing care goals include:
1. Safe, correct drug administration
2. Close monitoring for renal and neurologic side-effects

□ INTERVENTION

Colistimethate is administered intravenously by injection, intermittent infusion, or by continuous infusion. The reconstituted drug should be further diluted with 20 ml of sterile water for injection and should be injected slowly over 3 minutes to 5 minutes or according to institution policy. When the drug is administered by intermittent infusion (piggyback), it should be diluted in 100 ml of normal saline or 5% dextrose and water and infused over 30 minutes to 60 minutes. The drug can also be administered by continuous infusion in a variety of dextrose and water or dextrose and saline solutions if the dosage must be reduced because of renal impairment. A continuous infusion should be attached to an infusion pump to ensure accurate dosing, and the solution should be changed every 24 hours to ensure drug stability and maintain efficacy.

Intramuscular injection is painful and should be administered in a large muscle mass such as the gluteus in adults or the vastus lateralis in children. Sites should be rotated using a body map (see Chap. 8) to decrease the chance to tissue damage.

The main side-effects of colistimethate are nephrotoxicity, neurotoxicity, and superinfection. Throughout therapy, BUN, creatinine, urinalysis intake-to-output ratio, and serum drug levels should be closely monitored. Output should remain at least 30 ml/h in adults; if it falls below that the physician should be notified. Routine urinalysis will show protein or casts, early signs of renal dysfunction, and elevation of BUN or fall in serum creatinine. All are signs of nephrotoxicity. They should be immediately reported to the physician, and the drug should be discontinued.

Neurotoxicity may begin as changes in vision, hearing, or speech, drowsiness, dizziness, or paresthesia. Routine neurologic assessments and arterial blood gases should be done on every patient receiving colistimethate to ensure early detection of problems. Toxicity can progress to neuromuscular blockade leading to dyspnea, chest pain, labored breathing, and respiratory arrest secondary to chest muscle paralysis. Emergency resuscitative equipment should be available to support respiration until the drug is eliminated. Calcium chloride may be used to attempt to reverse respiratory depression.

Superinfection with drug-resistant bacterial strains may occur. The patient should be closely monitored for fever, diarrhea, and perianal irritation. Appropriate anti-infective therapy should alleviate symptoms.

☐ EVALUATION

Outcome criteria which may be used to determine drug effectiveness include resolution of infection and absence or early treatment of side-effects such as nephrotoxicity, neurotoxicity, and superinfection.

Colistin Sulfate
(Coly-Mycin S)

MECHANISM AND ACTIONS
Colistin, like the other polymyxins, disrupts the bacterial cell membrane. It is bactericidal against most gram-negative enteric microorganisms, especially Escherichia coli, and Shigella. Proteus species appear to bc resistant. It is used as an oral suspension for treating GI infections and as an ear drop in combination with hydrocortisone and neomycin for treating superficial bacterial infections of the external auditory canal.

USES
1. Control of diarrhea in infants and children due to susceptible strains of enteropathogenic Escherichia coli (oral suspension)
2. Treatment of gastroenteritis due to Shigella organisms (oral suspension)
3. Treatment of superficial infections of the ear canal (combination with neomycin and hydrocortisone as Coly-Mycin S Otic)

ADMINISTRATION AND DOSAGE
Colistin is used either as an oral suspension containing 25 mg per 5 ml when reconstituted or as an otic suspension (3 mg/ml) in combination with hydrocortisone (1%) and neomycin (3.3 mg/ml). The recommended oral dose of colistin is 5 mg to 15 mg/kg/day in three divided doses. Higher doses may be required in severe infections. The otic suspension (3 drops to 4 drops) is administered three to four times a day into the external ear canal.

FATE
When administered orally, colistin is not absorbed to a significant extent from the GI tract and is excreted primarily in the feces.

SIDE-EFFECTS/ADVERSE REACTIONS
Adverse reactions are rare with recommended doses. Intestinal superinfection with nonsusceptible organisms can occur with oral use of colistin.

CONTRAINDICATIONS AND PRECAUTIONS
Colistin should not be used in the ear if a viral or fungal infection is present. If systemic absorption is significant (e.g., with prolonged administration),

renal toxicity can occur. The drug should be given with *caution* to patients with pre-existing kidney damage.

NURSING CONSIDERATIONS
See also Nursing Process for anti-infective therapy in Chapter 59.

If diarrhea remits during therapy and then returns before treatment is completed, superinfection by disruption of normal bacterial flora may have occurred and must also be treated. It will usually remit when colistin is discontinued. The drug is very safe; however, the otic solution contains neomycin and should therefore be used cautiously when the eardrum is perforated or if chronic otitis media exists, because neomycin is ototoxic.

Polymyxin B Sulfate
(Aerosporin)

MECHANISM AND ACTIONS
Polymyxin B increases the permeability of bacterial cell membranes, resulting in leakage of cellular constituents and ultimately cell death. The drug possesses a bactericidal action against most gram-negative bacilli, except *Proteus* species. Gram-positive bacteria, gram-negative cocci, *Neisseria*, and fungi are resistant.

USES
1. Treatment of acute infections due to susceptible strains of *Pseudomonas aeruginosa* (IM, IV)
2. Alternate treatment of severe infections of the blood, meninges, or urinary tract due to *Escherichia coli*, *Klebsiella pneumoniae*, *Enterobacter aerogenes*, or *Hemophilus influenzae*, when less toxic drugs are ineffective (IM, IV)
   (*Note*: In meningeal infections, polymyxin B is given by the intrathecal route and is a treatment of choice for pseudomonal meningitis)
3. Treatment of superficial infections of the eye, ear, mucous membranes, or skin due to susceptible organisms (topical combination products containing polymyxin B)

ADMINISTRATION AND DOSAGE
Polymyxin B is used as an injectable solution containing 500,000 units/vial or as a powder for ophthalmic solution containing 500,000 units for reconstitution with 20 ml to 50 ml of diluent. Polymyxin B is also available as either a solution or ointment for ophthalmic use with neomycin (Statrol), bacitracin (Polysporin), oxytetracycline (Terramycin), neomycin plus bacitracin (Neosporin Ophthalmic, Ak-Spore), and neomycin plus a corticosteroid (Cortisporin, Dexacidin, Maxitrol). It is also available as an otic solution or suspension with hydrocortisone (Pyocidin-Otic, Otobiotic), and hydrocortisone plus neomycin (Cortisporin Otic, Ak-Spore H.C.) for treatment of superficial ear infections.

In addition, polymyxin B is available in combination with neomycin as a bladder irrigant solution (Neosporin G.U. Irrigant), containing 200,000 units polymyxin and 40 mg neomycin per ml (see below for dosage).

For topical application, the drug is found in combination with other antibiotics, such as neomycin, gramicidin, bacitracin, and oxytetracycline in various ointments and solutions.

The recommended dosages for the various routes of administration of polymyxin are as follows:

IV infusion:
   Adults and children—15,000 U/kg to 25,000 U/kg/day; infusions may be given every 12 hours
   Infants—Up to 40,000 U/kg/day
IM: (May cause severe pain at injection site)
   Adults and children—25,000 U/kg to 30,000 U/kg/day, divided and given at 4-hour to 6-hour intervals
   Infants—up to 40,000 U/kg/day
Intrathecal (*e.g.*, in pseudomonal meningitis):
   Adults and children (over 2 years)—50,000 U once daily for 3 days to 4 days; then 50,000 U every other day for at least 2 weeks after cultures of the cerebrospinal fluid are negative and glucose content has returned to normal
   Children (under 2 years)—20,000 U once daily for 3 days to 4 days; then 25,000 U every other day for at least 2 weeks (as above)
Bladder irrigation (Neosporin G.U. Irrigant):
   Add 1 ml irrigant to 1 L isotonic saline solution. Infuse by catheter at a rate of 1 L/24 h *continuously*. If urine output exceeds 2 L/day, increase flow rate to 2 L/24 h.
Ophthalmic:
   One or two drops in affected eye several times a day, as necessary

FATE

Polymyxin B is not significantly absorbed from the GI tract or mucous membranes. Peak plasma concentrations are reached within 2 hours after IM injection. Plasma half-life is 4 hours to 6 hours. Active blood levels are low, because the drug loses up to one-half its activity in the serum; blood levels are higher in infants and children than in adults. Diffusion into many tissues is poor, and the drug does not enter the CNS unless it is given intrathecally. Polymyxin is slowly excreted by the kidneys, largely in unchanged form.

SIDE-EFFECTS/ADVERSE REACTIONS

The principal toxic reactions with systemic use of polymyxin B are nephrotoxicity and neurotoxicity. Nephrotoxicity is manifested as proteinuria, azotemia, cellular casts, decreased urine output, and rising BUN levels. Because the drug is excreted in the urine, cumulation can occur if renal function is impaired.

Neurotoxic reactions may be manifested by irritability, weakness, ataxia, drowsiness, blurred vision, perioral paresthesia, and numbness in the extremities. Respiratory depression and apnea can occur, especially if the drug is given in association with or immediately following anesthetics or neuromuscular blocking agents.

Intrathecal administration can lead to meningeal irritation, characterized by fever, headache, stiff neck, and increased cells and proteins in the cerebrospinal fluid. Other reported adverse reactions with polymyxin B include rash, urticaria, severe pain at IM injection sites, and thrombophlebitis at IV injection sites. Ophthalmic administration can result in burning, stinging, itching, and temporary swelling in the eyes. Prolonged systemic use of the drug can result in overgrowth of nonsusceptible organisms (superinfection).

CONTRAINDICATIONS AND PRECAUTIONS

Polymyxin B should not be used in persons with serious renal impairment or in conjunction with other nephrotoxic or neurotoxic drugs (see under Interactions). The drug should be used in a hospital setting, where constant supervision of the patient is possible. Safety for use during pregnancy has not

been established. A *cautious* approach to therapy is necessary in persons with neurologic disorders.

INTERACTIONS

1. Concurrent use of polymyxin and other nephrotoxic drugs (*e.g.,* aminoglycosides, vancomycin, bacitracin, colistimethate) may increase the danger of kidney damage
2. Use of polymyxin with neuromuscular blocking agents, general anesthetics, or aminoglycosides can lead to extreme muscle weakness and respiratory paralysis.

NURSING CONSIDERATIONS

See Nursing Process for anti-infective therapy in Chapter 59. See also Nursing Process for colistimethate—Assessment, Nursing Diagnoses, Plan, and Evaluation are the same.

Polymyxin B sulfate alone or in combination with other drugs is administered by multiple routes. Intramuscular injection is very painful, however, especially in children and infants, and should be avoided if at all possible.

Intrathecal administration, essential in pseudomonal meningitis because the drug will not pass the blood–brain barrier when given intravenously, must be done under sterile technique and is usually performed by the physician unless an intrathecal reservoir has been inserted and the nurse is allowed to administer the drug according to institutional policy. The drug should be mixed with sterile physiologic saline.

Intravenous administration is usually by continuous infusion with a new solution hung every 12 hours. The drug should be mixed in 5% dextrose and water or normal saline.

Major side-effects of the drug are neurotoxicity, nephrotoxicity, and superinfection.

See Nursing Process for colistimethate for appropriate nursing actions and precautions. Fluid intake should be sufficient to maintain a urinary output of at least 1500 ml/day in adults to reduce the risk of nephrotoxicity.

Note that many of the symptoms of meningitis and neurotoxicity are the same (irritability, dizziness, paresthesias). Frequent neurologic assessment with careful notation of changes in status or recurrence of previously remitting symptoms may facilitate early detection of neurotoxic side-effects.

REVIEW QUESTIONS

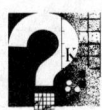

1. Name the anti-infective drugs classified as polypeptides.
2. What is the principal mechanism of action of the polymyxins?
3. Against what microorganisms are they most effective?
4. What are the most important adverse reactions associated with their use?
5. How does bacitracin differ from the polymyxins?
6. By what routes of administration may bacitracin be given? How is it most often used?
7. What are the symptoms of the principal toxic effect of bacitracin? How can the nurse monitor its development?
8. What other types of drugs can increase the likelihood of adverse effects with colistimethate?
9. In what dosage forms is colistin administered?
10. What are the indications for colistin?
11. For what type of infection may polymyxin B be considered the drug of choice? How must it be administered in this situation?
12. What are the principal adverse reactions with polymyxin B? What are the appropriate nursing actions for dealing with them?
13. What data should be collected before colistimethate or polymyxin B are administered?
14. How can the nurse distinguish between the symptoms of meningitis and neurotoxicity from polymyxin B?

BIBLIOGRAPHY

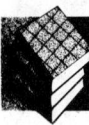

Brown MR, Wood SM: Relation between cation and lipid content of cell walls of *Pseudomonas aeruginosa*, *Proteus vulgaris*, and *Klebsiella aerogenes* and their sensitivity to polymyxin B and other antibacterial agents. J Pharm Pharmacol 24:215, 1972
Petersdorf RG: Colistin—A reappraisal. JAMA 183:123, 1963
Pratt WB: Chemotherapy of Infection. p 128. New York, Oxford University Press, 1977

Urinary Anti-infectives

Urinary Anti-infectives
 Cinoxacin
 Methenamine Hippurate
 Methenamine Mandelate
 Methylene Blue
 Nalidixic Acid
 Nitrofurantoin
 Nitrofurantoin
  Macrocrystals
 Norfloxacin
 Trimethoprim

Urinary Analgesic
 Phenazopyridine

Urease Inhibitor
 Acetohydroxamic Acid

67

Although the term urinary anti-infective refers theoretically to any drug capable of eradicating pathogens present in the urinary tract, it is generally applied only to those agents used specifically for urinary infections and which do not achieve effective plasma concentrations with recommended doses. Thus, while other antimicrobial drugs, such as broad-spectrum penicillins, cephalosporins, tetracyclines, sulfonamides, aminoglycosides, and polypeptides, have all been employed successfully in the treatment of urinary tract infections, they are not considered *specific* urinary anti-infectives because *they* attain significant plasma levels throughout the body and can therefore be used to treat a number of systemic infections as well. The drugs considered to be selective urinary anti-infectives include cinoxacin, methenamine, nalidixic acid, nitrofurantoin, norfloxacin, and trimethoprim. Although specific for urinary infections by virtue of their rapid elimination in the urine and concentration in the renal tubules and their lack of significant systemic antimicrobial activity, these agents are usually *not* considered drugs of choice for acute, uncomplicated urinary tract infections, inasmuch as they are not as effective against many common urinary pathogens as are the sulfonamides, broad-spectrum penicillins, or cephalosporins. The urinary anti-infectives are most often reserved for those persons who are either intolerant of or unresponsive to one of the first-line drugs. Urinary anti-infectives are also of value for the control of chronic urinary infections due to organisms that have developed resistance to commonly used antibiotics. For example, low doses of nitrofurantoin, administered once a day at bedtime, have been used successfully for long-term prophylaxis in chronic urinary infections. Likewise, trimethoprim-sulfamethoxazole (see Chap. 60) and methenamine have also been employed for chemoprophylaxis of chronic urinary infections.

The fact that urinary anti-infectives generally do not attain effective antibacterial blood levels does not mean that they are free of systemic toxic effects. On the contrary, with the exception of methenamine, the other agents in this group all have the potential to elicit serious untoward reactions, and their use should be accorded the same respect as any other antimicrobial drug.

A urine culture and sensitivity test should be completed when therapy begins, although a medication will be started before the results are available. Patients should be encouraged to force fluids (about 1500 ml per day) throughout the treatment course.

Patients receiving a urinary anti-infective drug should be advised to continue taking the prescribed dose for the recommended period of time (usually 10 days–14 days) even though the symptoms of the infection, such as low back pain, burning on urination, or fever, may have disappeared within 48 hours. Complete eradication of the infecting organism, not simply symptomatic relief, is the goal of urinary chemotherapy, because relapses and reinfection are major problems in the treatment of urinary infections. A relapse, the result of failure to eliminate completely the original pathogen from the urinary system with the initial course of therapy, is most often due to insufficient dose or duration of therapy, or both. Recurring infections are frequently noted some time after successful recovery from an initial attack, and are often caused by microorganisms different from those responsible for the initial infection. These may include resistant forms that have emerged during the first course of therapy.

Perhaps the most troublesome situation is the chronic urinary infection that often complicates an anatomical or physiologic abnormality such as urinary stones, urethral strictures, or prostate enlargement. Treatment of these conditions requires prolonged therapy with a urinary anti-infective capable of interfering with bacterial growth without favoring emergence of resistant organisms. The most commonly employed drugs for chronic urinary conditions are trimethoprim-sulfamethoxazole (see Chap. 60), nitrofurantoin, and methenamine. Of course, surgical intervention is often necessary when a blockage or some other anatomical lesion is present.

In addition to the urinary anti-infectives mentioned above, several other drugs may be employed in urinary infections. *Methylene blue*, a dye, is a weak germicide and is occasionally used orally as a mild urinary antiseptic. *Phenazopyridine*, another dye, is excreted in the urine following oral ingestion and exerts a mild analgesic effect. It is used to relieve irritation and pain in conjunction with an appropriate anti-infective. *Acetohydroxamic acid* (AHA) inhibits the urease-mediated hydrolysis of urea and the subsequent production of ammonia in urine infected with urea-splitting organisms. It is indicated as adjunctive therapy in chronic urea-splitting urinary infections. The above drugs are considered in this chapter along with the other urinary anti-infectives.

Urinary Anti-infectives

Cinoxacin

(Cinobac)

MECHANISM AND ACTIONS
Cinoxacin is an organic acid structurally related to nalidixic acid. The drug inhibits DNA replication in susceptible bacteria within the range of urinary pH. It is bactericidal at normal dose levels and is active against most strains of *Escherichia coli*, *Klebsiella* species, *Enterobacter* species, and *Proteus* species. It is *not* effective, however, against *Pseudomonas*, staphylococci, or enterococci.

There is cross-resistance between cinoxacin and nalidixic acid, but bacterial resistance to cinoxacin occurs in less than 5% of patients given recommended doses.

USES
1. Treatment of initial and recurrent urinary tract infections resulting from susceptible organisms (see above)

ADMINISTRATION AND DOSAGE
Cinoxacin is used as capsules containing either 250 mg or 500 mg. The usual adult dose is 1 g/day, in two to four divided doses for 7 days to 14 days. Dosage should be reduced in patients with impaired renal function based on creatinine clearance or serum creatinine according to package instructions.

FATE
Cinoxacin is rapidly absorbed from the GI tract. Peak serum concentrations occur within 1 hour to 2 hours, and detectable levels persist for 10 hours to 12 hours. Food decreases peak serum levels by about one-fourth but does not alter the total amount absorbed. The drug is excreted almost entirely in the urine, 60% as unaltered drug and the remainder as metabolites. Peak urine levels are noted within 2 hours to 4 hours. Approximately 97% of an oral dose is excreted in the urine within 24 hours. The drug is 60% to 80% protein bound. Serum half-life is 1 hour to 2 hours with normal renal function but increases markedly in the presence of impaired renal function.

SIDE-EFFECTS/ADVERSE REACTIONS
Side-effects observed with greatest frequency during cinoxacin therapy are nausea and abdominal cramping. Other untoward reactions include diarrhea, vomiting, anorexia, perineal burning, headaches, dizziness, nervousness, insomnia, confusion, photophobia, blurred vision, tinnitus, rash, pruritus, urticaria, edema, and increased BUN, SGOT, SGPT, serum creatinine, and alkaline phosphatase.

CONTRAINDICATIONS AND PRECAUTIONS
Cinoxacin is contraindicated in patients with anuria, and also in pregnant women and in prepubertal children because the drug has caused cartilage erosion in weight-bearing joints in immature animals of various species. Cinoxacin must be used *cautiously* in persons with reduced renal or hepatic function and in nursing mothers.

INTERACTIONS
1. Probenecid blocks tubular secretion of cinoxacin, reducing its elimination rate in the urine and increasing its half-life and serum concentration.
2. The rate of cinoxacin excretion may be slowed by acidification and enhanced by alkalinzation of the urine.

NURSING CONSIDERATIONS
Pregnancy should be ruled out in women of childbearing age before cinoxacin is prescribed because the potential for fetal damage is great. If the patient has a history of renal or hepatic problems, BUN, serum creatinine, liver enzymes, and alkaline phosphatase should be obtained before treatment and evaluated again at the end of the therapy. Urinary output should also be closely monitored if renal disease exists. If input exceeds output, the physician should be notified at once. The patient at home can be taught to measure urine output so changes can be reported early.

The main side-effect of cinoxacin is gastrointestinal distress which can usually be alleviated by taking the drug with food.

Methenamine Hippurate, Methenamine Mandelate

Methenamine is a urinary antibacterial agent whose action depends on its hydrolysis to ammonia and formaldehyde in an acidic urine. Formaldehyde is bactericidal against a variety of gram-positive and gram-negative organisms (see under Mechanism and Actions). Methenamine is used in the form of an acid salt (hippurate, mandelate), which helps maintain a low urinary pH. Characteristics of the different methenamine salts are presented in Table 67-1.

MECHANISM AND ACTIONS
In an acid urine (pH 5.5 or lower), methenamine is hydrolyzed to form ammonia and formaldehyde, the latter being bactericidal. The acid liberated from the salt (i.e., mandelic or hippuric) may also exert a weak antibacterial action, although it is probably of little clinical significance. Susceptible organisms include *Escherichia coli*, staphylococci, and enterococci. *Enterobacter aerogenes* is resistant, as are *Pseudomonas* and *Proteus* species, the latter two being urea-splitting organisms that can raise urinary pH above the effective level.

Most bacteria are sensitive to free formaldehyde at concentrations above 25 mcg/ml. A dose of 2 g/day of methenamine yields a formaldehyde concentration of 18 mcg to 60 mcg/ml when urinary pH is below 6 and daily urine volume is 1000 ml to 1500 ml. Bacteria do *not* appear to develop resistance to formaldehyde, thus, methenamine is well suited for *chronic* therapy.

USES
1. Treatment of chronic bacteriuria associated with cystitis, pyelonephritis, or other chronic urinary conditions
2. Treatment of infected residual urine (e.g., accompanying certain neurologic diseases)
3. Adjunctive treatment of patients with anatomical abnormalities of the urinary tract

ADMINISTRATION AND DOSAGE
See Table 67-1.

FATE
Methenamine salts are readily absorbed orally; absorption is decreased 30% by enteric coating. The generation of formaldehyde is dependent on urinary pH (peak levels are seen at a pH of 5.5 or less), the dose of methenamine, and the length of time the urine is retained in the bladder. A urinary concentration of 25 mcg/ml is necessary for antibacterial activity. Peak formaldehyde levels are attained within 2 hours after a dose of the hippurate salt, and within 3 hours to 6 hours after the mandelate salt. Steady state urinary formaldehyde levels are reached in 2 days to 3 days with regular dosing. Methenamine excretion occurs by way of glomerular filtration and tubular secretion, and up to 90% of a dose is eliminated within 24 hours.

SIDE-EFFECTS/ADVERSE REACTIONS
The most likely side-effect with methenamine is gastric upset, especially with large doses. Other adverse reactions include abdominal pain, cramping,

Table 67-1
Methenamine Derivatives

Drug	Preparations	Usual Dosage Range	Clinical Considerations
methenamine hippurate (Hiprex, Urex)	Tablets—1 g	Adults—1 g twice a day Children (6 yr–12 yr)—0.5 g to 1 g twice a day	Effective in lower daily doses than mandelate salt; safe use in early pregnancy has not been established; may transiently elevate serum transaminase levels; periodic liver function tests are indicated
methenamine mandelate (Mandameth, Mandelamine)	Tablets—0.5 g, 1 g Enteric-coated tablets—0.5 g, 1 g Oral suspension—0.25 g/5 ml Suspension forte—0.5 g/5 ml Granules—1 g/packet	Adults—1 g four times a day Children (6 yr–12 yr)—0.5 g four times a day Children (under 6 yr)—0.25 g/30 lb four times a day	Most commonly used methenamine salt; enteric-coated tablets are claimed to lower incidence of GI upset; oral suspensions have a vegetable oil base; use cautiously in elderly or debilitated patients due to danger of aspiration (lipid) pneumonia; granules are orange flavored

vomiting, diarrhea, stomatitis, anorexia, urinary frequency or urgency, hypersensitivity reactions (rash, pruritus), and in large doses, bladder irritation, dysuria, proteinuria, and hematuria.

CONTRAINDICATIONS AND PRECAUTIONS

Contraindications to use of methenamine are renal insufficiency, severe dehydration, and severe hepatic disease (drug liberates ammonia). The drug must be administered *cautiously* to patients with gout, because methenamine salts may cause precipitation of urate crystals in the urine. Oral suspensions of methenamine have a vegetable oil base and must be used carefully in elderly or debilitated patients due to the danger of aspiration lipid pneumonia. Safe use of methenamine in pregnant women or nursing mothers has not been established. The drug is not intended to be used alone for acute infections with renal parenchymal involvement associated with systemic symptoms. Adequate fluids should be taken during therapy, but excessive hydration can reduce the concentration of free formaldehyde in the urine.

INTERACTIONS

1. Sulfonamides can form insoluble precipitates with formaldehyde in the urine.
2. The effectiveness of methenamine can be reduced by drugs or foods that raise urinary pH (*e.g.*, sodium bicarbonate, acetazolamide, thiazide diuretics, milk products).
3. Methenamine may interfere with laboratory urine determinations of 17-hydroxycorticosteroids and catecholamines (false increases) as well as 5-hydroxyindoleacetic acid (false decrease).

NURSING CONSIDERATIONS

If the patient has a history of renal or hepatic disease, renal function studies and hepatic enzymes should be performed before treatment with methenamine begins. Periodic renal and hepatic laboratory studies should be performed on all patients who receive long-term therapy, especially those on prophylactic treatment.

The patient must be aware of the importance of maintaining urinary pH at 5.5 or lower. To monitor pH urine can be tested with Nitrazine paper (see Chap. 80). If pH exceeds 5.5, ascorbic acid 4 g to 12 g/day in divided doses may be prescribed. The patient should be advised to limit intake of milk and citrus fruits and juices which have an alkalinizing effect on urine. Some think cranberry juice may facilitate acidification, but conflicting information exists on its worth in this regard.

The adult patient taking methenamine should increase fluid intake to maintain a daily urine output of about 1500 ml/day. Most patients can achieve this by drinking about eight glasses of water per day in addition to their regular fluids unless normal intake is high. The patient should be cautioned against excessive intake which will decrease the amount of free formaldehyde in the urine and decrease drug effectiveness. Likewise, if the patient is unable to take sufficient fluids because of illness, the physician should be notified. Methenamine can become toxic if an individual is dehydrated, and the drug may have to be discontinued.

Methenamine is suitable for long-term prophylaxis in chronic urinary infections because bacteria and fungi do not develop resistance to formaldehyde. However, treatment success depends on free formaldehyde remaining in the bladder long enough to be effective. Therefore, methenamine is not suitable for prevention of urinary infections in patients with indwelling catheters because the bladder is continuously emptied.

The most common side-effects from methenamine are gastrointestinal distress and dysuria. To minimize gastric upset, the drug can be taken with any food except as noted above. Dysuria is more likely to occur with high doses or if urine is inadequately acidic and will remit with dosage adjustment and appropriate acidification.

Oral suspensions of methenamine have a vegetable oil base and should be cautiously administered to children, elderly patients, and debilitated patients. The patient's ability to swallow and level of alertness should be tested before administering the drug to decrease the risk of lipid aspiration pneumonia.

Methylene Blue

(Urolene Blue)

MECHANISM AND ACTIONS

Methylene blue is a dye possessing a weak germicidal action. When given orally, it exerts a bacteriostatic action and is used as a genitourinary antiseptic. In high concentrations, methylene blue converts the *ferrous* iron of reduced hemoglobin to *ferric* iron, resulting in production of methemoglobin. This latter action is the basis for its use IV as an antidote in cyanide poisoning, because methemoglobin competes with cytochrome oxidase, a vital enzyme, for the cyanide ion, resulting in formation of cyanmethemoglobin and the resulting preservation of cytochrome oxidase.

USES
1. Symptomatic treatment of cystitis and urethritis (infrequent use)
2. Treatment of idiopathic and drug-induced methemoglobinemia and as an antidote for cyanide poisoning (IV)
3. Investigational uses include management of patients with oxalate urinary tract calculi and diagnostic confirmation of rupture of amniotic membranes

ADMINISTRATION AND DOSAGE
Methylene blue is available as tablets (55 mg, 65 mg) and an injection containing 10 mg/ml. Orally, the recommended dosage for urinary antisepsis is 55 mg to 130 mg three times a day. Parenterally, the drug is injected slowly IV in a dose of 1 mg to 2 mg/kg for treating cyanide poisoning and drug-induced methemoglobinemia.

SIDE-EFFECTS/ADVERSE REACTIONS
Oral administration of methylene blue may color the urine and possibly the stool blue-green. Other adverse effects attributed to oral administration include nausea, vomiting, diarrhea, fever, and bladder irritation. Large doses may result in abdominal or precordial pain, dizziness, headache, sweating, or confusion. Prolonged administration has resulted in anemia and hemolysis. Cyanosis has occurred during treatment with methylene blue.

CONTRAINDICATIONS AND PRECAUTIONS
Methylene blue is contraindicated in persons with renal insufficiency. The drug should not be administered by intraspinal injection. *Cautious* administration of the drug is necessary in patients with anemia, glucose-6-phosphate dehydrogenase deficiency, and decreased hemoglobin levels. IV administration must be undertaken carefully in patients with cardiovascular disease because cyanosis and cardiovascular abnormalities have occurred.

NURSING CONSIDERATIONS
When used orally the drug should be administered with a full glass of water after meals. The patient should be told that urine and stool may take on a blue-green color for the duration of therapy.

Intravenous drug administration is usually in an emergency situation because cyanide poisoning leads rapidly to hypoxia, respiratory failure, and death, depending on the amount ingested. Emergency equipment to support respiration should be available, and the patient should be placed on a cardiac monitor. Methylene blue, especially in intravenous doses, can cause cardiac arrhythmias.

Nalidixic Acid
(NegGram)

MECHANISM AND ACTIONS
Nalidixic acid is bactericidal over the entire urinary pH range against most gram-negative bacteria causing urinary infections. The drug probably acts by inhibiting DNA polymerization and may impair RNA synthesis as well. It exhibits good activity against *Proteus* species, *Escherichia coli*, *Enterobacter*, and *Klebsiella*, but is ineffective against *Pseudomonas*. Resistance has developed in some cases.

USES
1. Treatment of urinary tract infections caused by susceptible organisms (see under Mechanism and Actions)

ADMINISTRATION AND DOSAGE
Nalidixic acid may be administered as tablets (250 mg, 500 mg, 1 g) or an oral suspension (250 mg/5 ml). Adults are given an initial dose of 1 g four times a day for 2 weeks. For prolonged therapy, the dose is reduced to 2 g daily thereafter. Children under age 12 may be administered 55 mg/kg/day in four equally divided doses for 1 week to 2 weeks; for prolonged therapy, the dose is reduced to 33 mg/kg/day.

Note: Initial dosage should be as recommended (and not lower) to minimize the emergence of resistant strains.

FATE
Oral absorption is nearly complete and peak serum levels are attained within 1 hour to 2 hours after an oral dose of 1 g. The drug concentrates largely in renal tissue and seminal fluid but does not appear to enter prostatic tissue. Nalidixic acid is approximately 90% to 95% protein bound. The drug is metabolized to hydroxynalidixic acid (which is many times more active than the parent drug) and inactive conjugates, and the metabolites are rapidly excreted by the kidneys. The plasma half-life is 1 hour to 3 hours in persons with normal renal function, and the half-life in the urine is 6 hours. A

small amount of nalidixic acid is eliminated in the feces.

SIDE-EFFECTS/ADVERSE REACTIONS

Gastrointestinal upset, abdominal pain, nausea, and diarrhea may occur following administration of nalidixic acid. Photosensitivity reactions, characterized by erythema, pruritus, and painful bullae on exposed skin surfaces, have occurred with as little as 15 minutes of exposure but usually resolve completely within several weeks after discontinuation of therapy. Other adverse effects linked to nalidixic acid are listed below.

CNS—Drowsiness, dizziness, weakness, headache, vertigo, visual disturbances (e.g., difficulty in focusing, overbrightness of lights, decreased visual acuity, double vision, altered color perception).
Convulsions and toxic psychosis have been reported with large doses.
Infants and children may experience increased intracranial pressure, papilledema, severe headache, and bulging anterior fontanel.
Allergic—Rash, pruritus, urticaria, angioedema, eosinophilia, arthralgia, anaphylactic reaction (rare)
Other—(Rare) GI bleeding, cholestasis, paresthesias, metabolic acidosis, blood dyscrasias, hemolysis in patients with glucose-6-phosphate dehydrogenase deficiency.

CONTRAINDICATIONS AND PRECAUTIONS

Nalidixic acid should not be given to patients with a history of convulsive disorders nor should it be used during early pregnancy or in infants less than 3 months of age. The drug should be administered with *caution* to elderly or debilitated persons, to patients with liver disease, epilepsy, cerebral arteriosclerosis, severe renal failure, and to young children, because cartilage erosion can occur in weight-bearing joints.

INTERACTIONS

1. Nalidixic acid may potentiate the action of other strongly protein-bound drugs (e.g., oral anticoagulants, phenytoin, oral hypoglycemics, anti-inflammatory agents).
2. Nitrofurantoin may inhibit the antibacterial activity of nalidixic acid.
3. Urinary acidifiers can potentiate the antibacterial activity of nalidixic acid by reducing its urinary excretion rate.
4. Antacids may impair GI absorption of nalidixic acid, reducing its activity.
5. Cross-resistance has occurred between nalidixic acid and cinoxacin.
6. Nalidixic acid may falsely elevate urinary 17-ketosteroids, and the drug's urinary metabolites may produce false-positive urinary glucose results with Clinitest tablets or Benedict's or Fehling's reagent (Tes-Tape and Clinistix can be used).

NURSING CONSIDERATIONS

A thorough drug history is essential. Doses of oral anticoagulants, oral hypoglycemics and anti-inflammatory drugs may need to be reduced during therapy. The patient who frequently takes antacids should be told to discontinue use during therapy or space doses at least 2 hours after the dose of nalidixic acid is taken.

Pregnancy should be ruled out in women of child-bearing age because fetal damage may occur. Patients with a history of renal or hepatic disease should have baseline and periodic monitoring of BUN, creatinine, and liver enzymes, as well as urinary output, weight, and intake-to-output ratio.

The most common side-effect of nalidixic acid is gastrointestinal upset, which can be relieved by taking the drug with food. Dairy products should not be taken at the same time to decrease the risk of impaired absorption. Patients should also be cautioned against exposure to direct sun during treatment because serious photosensitivity reactions can occur even with minimum exposure. The patient should avoid being outside in midday sun, especially in the summer, and should always wear sunscreen, protective clothing, and sunglasses.

Parents of young children and care givers of elderly debilitated patients taking this drug should be told which signs to monitor for development of CNS side-effects. Infants and young children (under 18 months) may experience irritability, crying, vomiting, and a bulging anterior fontanelle. The older patient may complain of dizziness, headache, and vision changes (see under Side-Effects/Adverse Reactions). All symptoms should be immediately reported, and the drug should be discontinued. Transient dizziness may occur at the beginning of therapy. The patient should be cautioned to avoid driving or engaging in any hazardous activity until the effect of the drug is known.

Nitrofurantoin
(Furadantin, Furalan, Furan, Furanite, Nitrofan)

Nitrofurantoin Macrocrystals
(Macrodantin)

Nitrofurantoin is a synthetic nitrofuran effective against most gram-negative bacilli and gram-positive cocci associated with urinary infections. Nitrofurantoin macrocrystals is a preparation containing larger crystal-size particles than the regular nitrofurantoin preparation and that produces less gastric upset (see under Side-Effects/Adverse Reactions below).

MECHANISM AND ACTIONS
Nitrofurantoin is bacteriostatic in low concentrations and bactericidal in higher concentrations. Its probable mechanism of action is interference with carbohydrate metabolism by inhibition of acetyl coenzyme A. The drug may also impair bacterial cell wall formation. Nitrofurantoin is most effective against *Escherichia coli, Klebsiella, Enterobacter,* and *Citrobacter* species, group B streptococci, enterococci, and staphylococci. Some strains of *Enterobacter* and *Klebsiella* are resistant, as are most strains of *Proteus, Serratia,* and *Acinetobacter. Pseudomonas* is highly resistant. Organisms that are sensitive to nitrofurantoin show little acquired clinical resistance, even with prolonged treatment.

USES
1. Treatment of urinary tract infections due to susceptible strains of the above named organisms
2. Prophylaxis against recurrent bacteriuria (small doses of Macrodantin)

ADMINISTRATION AND DOSAGE
Nitrofurantoin is available as tablets (50 mg, 100 mg), regular capsules (50 mg, 100 mg), and oral suspension (25 mg/5 ml). The drug is also used as a macrocrystalline form in capsules containing 25 mg, 50 mg, or 100 mg. The oral drug is generally administered with food or milk to minimize gastric upset. Therapy should be continued for at least 10 days to 14 days and at least 3 days after a sterile urine is obtained. Recommended doses are as follows:

>Adults—50 mg to 100 mg four times a day for 10 days to 14 days; for long-term suppressive therapy, 50 mg to 100 mg is given once daily at bedtime
>Children (over 1 month)—5 mg to 7 mg/kg/day in four divided doses; for long-term suppressive therapy, 1 mg/kg/day may be used in a single or two divided doses.
>Prophylaxis of recurrent infections (Macrodantin)—50 mg daily at bedtime for at least 6 months

FATE
Nitrofurantoin is well absorbed orally; the macrocrystalline form is absorbed more slowly than other oral forms but causes less GI distress. Absorption is enhanced by ingestion of food; therapeutic serum and tissue levels are *not* attained following the usual oral doses *except* in the urinary tract. The plasma half-life is 20 minutes to 30 minutes in persons with normal renal function. Plasma protein binding is approximately 60% to 75%. One-half to two-thirds of a dose is rapidly inactivated by body tissues and excreted in the urine and bile. Up to one-half of a dose may be eliminated unchanged in the urine. Renal clearance is reduced (*i.e.*, tubular reabsorption is increased) in an acidic urine, and antibacterial activity is enhanced.

SIDE-EFFECTS/ADVERSE REACTIONS
The most frequent side-effects noted with nitrofurantoin administration are nausea, anorexia, and vomiting. A sudden onset of dyspnea, chest pain, cough, chills, and fever may occur within hours of initiating therapy or up to 3 weeks following therapy. Chest x-rays have revealed alveolar infiltrates and effusions; eosinophilia and elevated sedimentation rate have also occurred. These abnormalities generally disappear within 24 hours to 48 hours after discontinuing therapy. A more insidious condition may develop with prolonged therapy and is marked by dyspnea, nonproductive cough, and malaise. Interstitial pneumonitis often develops as well. Although symptoms generally regress over several weeks to months with discontinuation of therapy, pulmonary function can be permanently impaired, and respiratory failure and death have occurred.

Peripheral neuropathy can occur and may become severe and irreversible. Predisposing factors include anemia, renal impairment, diabetes, vitamin B deficiency, and electrolyte imbalance.

A variety of other untoward reactions have been associated with nitrofurantoin use and are listed below.

GI—Diarrhea, abdominal pain, pancreatitis, parotitis

Pulmonary—Chills, cough, chest pain, dyspnea, pulmonary infiltration with consolidation or pleural effusion, diffuse interstitial pneumonitis or fibrosis (with prolonged therapy)

Dermatologic—Rash, pruritus, urticaria, angioedema, alopecia; rarely, exfoliative dermatitis, erythema multiforme

Hematologic—Hemolytic anemia (due to glucose-6-phosphate dehydrogenase deficiency), megaloblastic anemia, leukopenia, granulocytopenia, eosinophilia, thrombocytopenia, agranulocytosis

Allergic—Drug fever, asthmatic attack, arthralgia, anaphylaxis

Hepatic—Chronic active hepatitis, cholestatic hepatitis, and cholestatic jaundice (*not* dose-related)

Neurologic—Dizziness, paresthesias, headache, drowsiness, nystagmus, peripheral neuropathy

Other—Hypotension, myalgia, superinfections, tooth staining from oral suspension

CONTRAINDICATIONS AND PRECAUTIONS

Use of nitrofurantoin is contraindicated in persons with anuria, oliguria, or significant renal impairment (creatinine clearance less than 40 ml/min). It is also contraindicated in pregnant women at term and in infants under 3 months (possibility of hemolytic anemia due to immature enzyme systems).

A *cautious* approach to therapy is warranted in patients with anemia, diabetes, vitamin B deficiency, chronic lung disease, electrolyte imbalance, or other debilitating diseases, because these conditions may predispose to development of peripheral neuropathy. Cautious use is also indicated in pregnant women or nursing mothers, and in persons with glucose-6-phosphate dehydrogenase deficiency or hepatic disease.

INTERACTIONS

1. Nitrofurantoin can antagonize the action of nalidixic acid.
2. Urinary acidifying agents (*e.g.,* ammonium chloride, ascorbic acid) may potentiate nitrofurantoin by slowing its excretion, whereas urinary alkalinizing agents (*e.g.,* acetazolamide, sodium bicarbonate) can reduce its effectiveness by accelerating its elimination.

3. Probenecid reduces the renal clearance of nitrofurantoin and may increase its toxicity.
4. Antacids can reduce the effectiveness of nitrofurantoin by impairing its GI absorption.
5. Anticholinergics, other GI antispasmodic drugs, and the presence of food may increase GI absorption of nitrofurantoin by prolonging gastric emptying time.
6. Nitrofurantoin may cause false-positive tests for serum glucose, bilirubin, alkaline phosphatase, and BUN levels.

NURSING CONSIDERATIONS

Nitrofurantoin should be used cautiously because it has the potential to produce a variety of serious irreversible side-effects. Therefore, the patient should be thoroughly evaluated before treatment commences, and the benefits of therapy must be carefully weighed against the risks. General history taking should determine the presence of renal dysfunction, hepatic disease, anemia, diabetes, dehydration or other electrolyte imbalances, and pregnancy or lactation. Laboratory data should include a CBC with differential to rule out anemia, a pregnancy test in women of child-bearing age, and renal and hepatic function studies in any patient with suspected problems. Baseline vital signs and weight are also important.

Oral drug forms should be taken with food to enhance absorption and decrease gastrointestinal distress. If GI upset persists, the macrocrystalline dosage form may further minimize the problem. The patient should be advised to space the doses evenly over a 24-hour period to maintain serum levels. Oral drug forms should be stored in amber bottles away from strong light which can cause a loss of potency.

Patients taking oral suspensions should rinse the mouth thoroughly after use to prevent staining of teeth. Parents of toddlers should also rinse the child's mouth using a cup and a swab or small toothbrush. Offering the child liquids through a bottle will not rinse the teeth.

One of the harmless side-effects of nitrofurantoin is brown discoloration of urine, which will subside when the drug is stopped. However, patients should be informed of the color change to avoid concern that they might be bleeding.

The other major side-effects of nitrofurantoin require close monitoring and rapid action to avoid irreversible damage. Patients may develop an immediate or latent pulmonary sensitivity to the drug which can begin with a variety of symptoms (see under Side-Effects/Adverse Reactions). Early symptoms include cough, fever, dyspnea, and eosinophilia. Consequently, the patient should take a temperature daily throughout therapy, have a CBC performed every 2 weeks, and report immediately any symptoms of cold, flu, or pulmonary congestion. Even after the initial 3-week period has passed, insidious pulmonary problems can occur characterized by the same symptoms. Patients on long-term therapy should also have periodic chest x-rays. Early recognition of the problem and prompt drug discontinuation are the only methods of avoiding permanent lung damage.

Peripheral neuropathy is another serious and potentially irreversible side-effect of nitrofurantoin and is more likely to occur in the patient with diabetes, anemia, dehydration, or vitamin B deficiency. If possible, dehydration and electrolyte or vitamin deficiencies should be corrected before beginning therapy. Patients should be told to watch closely for signs of numbness, tingling, or weakness, especially in hands or feet, and to report such changes immediately. The only way to prevent irreversible neuropathy is to identify it early and discontinue the drug.

Renal, hepatic, and hematologic dysfunction can occur at any time during therapy and should be closely monitored by periodic laboratory evaluations of BUN, creatinine, liver enzymes, bilirubin, CBC, and direct Coomb's test. Patients should be told to monitor intake and output, weight, and edema at home and report if output decreases, weight increases, or if swelling of hands or feet occurs, all early signs of renal problems. Hepatitis may develop, characterized by flank pain, weakness, fever, and jaundice, which must also be reported. Anemia may only be characterized by weakness. With all of these problems the patient should be encouraged to report any illness or change in his symptoms so they can be properly evaluated.

Urinary tract superinfections may occur during nitrofurantoin therapy, characterized by fever, dysuria, and foul-smelling urine. Most are *Pseudomonas*, but the urine should be sent for culture and sensitivity testing so treatment can be initiated with an appropriate antibiotic.

Norfloxacin

(Noroxin)

MECHANISM AND ACTIONS
Norfloxacin is a synthetic fluoroquinolone anti-infective possessing *in-vitro* activity against a broad spectrum of gram-positive and gram-negative organisms. The drug is bactericidal against many organisms, including gram-negative aerobic bacteria and *Pseudomonas aeruginosa*. Norfloxacin inhibits bacterial DNA synthesis. Resistance to norfloxacin is rare. Its action is generally limited to the urinary tract, bile, and gut.

USES
1. Treatment of uncomplicated or complicated urinary tract infections caused by susceptible strains of *E. coli*, *Klebsiella pneumoniae*, *Proteus* species, *Enterobacter*, *Pseudomonas aeruginosa*, *Citrobacter freundii*, *Staphylococcus aureus*, and group D streptococci

ADMINISTRATION AND DOSAGE
Norfloxacin is available as 400-mg film-coated tablets. For uncomplicated urinary infections, the recommended dose is 400 mg twice a day for 7 days to 10 days. Complicated infections may require 400 mg twice a day for up to 21 days. Dosage may have to be reduced to 400 mg once daily in patients with impaired renal function.

FATE
Oral absorption is incomplete (30%–40%) but generally rapid following single doses. Peak plasma levels occur in approximately 1 hour. The plasma half-life is 3 hours to 4 hours, and steady-state plasma levels are attained within 2 days. Serum protein binding is minimal (10%–15%). Norfloxacin is eliminated both as unchanged drug and metabolites in both the urine and feces.

SIDE-EFFECTS/ADVERSE REACTIONS
The most commonly encountered side-effects during norfloxacin therapy are nausea, headache, and dizziness. Eosinophilia and elevated SGPT, SGOT, and alkaline phosphatase have also been reported during therapy. Other potential adverse reactions include rash, fatigue, depression, insomnia, abdominal pain, constipation, flatulence, heartburn, dry mouth, fever, visual disturbances, vomiting, and increased BUN, serum creatinine, and LDH. Large doses may result in crystalluria; the recommended dosage should not be exceeded, and fluid intake should be adequate during therapy.

CONTRAINDICATIONS AND PRECAUTIONS
Norfloxacin should *not* be given to pregnant women or young children because the drug has been shown to produce cartilage lesions in imma-

ture animals, resulting in lameness and arthropathy. The drug must be used *cautiously* in patients with impaired renal function (dosage reduction is required), a predisposition to seizures and in nursing mothers.

INTERACTIONS
1. Probenecid can reduce the urinary excretion of norfloxacin during concomitant administration.
2. Concurrent use of nitrofurantoin can impair the antibacterial activity of norfloxacin.
3. Antacids may reduce the oral absorption of norfloxacin.

NURSING CONSIDERATIONS
A drug history is useful, especially if the patient has been treated with other urinary anti-infectives, such as nitrofurantoin which may impair norfloxacin's antibacterial activity. Antacid use should also be documented because they can interfere with norflaxin absorption. A history of drug allergies should also be obtained. A patient who is hypersensitive to other quinolone drugs (nalidixic acid and cinoxacin) will probably be hypersensitive to norfloxacin.

A history of seizures contraindicates drug use as does pregnancy. Women of child-bearing age who are not using contraceptives should have a pregnancy test done before the drug is prescribed because norfloxacin can cause fetal damage. Patients with renal disease or liver disease also need to be identified because such conditions warrant cautious use and may require dosage reduction.

Initial laboratory evaluations on any patient with renal or hepatic problems or who will be on extended therapy should include: CBC with differential, BUN, serum creatinine, liver enzymes, and alkaline phosphatase. These should be repeated periodically as abnormalities can occur.

To maximize absorption the drug should be taken either 1 hour before or 2 hours after meals with a full glass of water. If the patient complains of nausea or other gastrointestinal discomfort, the drug may be taken with a small amount of food such as toast or crackers but should never be taken with dairy products which might impair absorption.

The patient should be encouraged to increase fluid intake to 1500 ml to 2000 ml per day for the duration of therapy to minimize the risk of crystalluria, a rare but dangerous side-effect. Urine output should increase to respond to fluid intake; if no change is noted or swelling of hands or feet are noted, the physician should be notified.

Aside from nausea, the most common side-effects are headache and dizziness, both of which may be transient. Headaches can be treated with mild analgesics as necessary. Dizziness can be eased by taking the drug with food and encouraging the patient to rise slowly from a sitting or standing position if position-related and to sit down immediately if an episode occurs. The patient should be warned to exercise caution in driving or performing any tasks requiring mental alertness until response to the drug is known. Persistent symptoms should be immediately reported. Hematologic abnormalities can occur. The patient should be told to immediately report any fever, rash, sore throat, or fatigue.

Trimethoprim
(Proloprim, Trimpex)

MECHANISM AND ACTIONS
Trimethoprim is a synthetic antibacterial agent with a spectrum of action encompassing common urinary tract pathogens, *except Pseudomonas*. The drug blocks production of tetrahydrofolic acid from dihydrofolic acid by reversible inhibition of dihydrofolate reductase, thus interfering with synthesis of proteins and nucleic acids in susceptible bacteria. Trimethoprim demonstrates good activity against *Escherichia coli*, *Proteus mirabilis*, *Klebsiella pneumoniae*, *Enterobacter* species, and *Staphylococcus* species (coagulase-negative).

Trimethoprim acts synergistically with sulfonamides by blocking sequential steps in the synthesis of folic acid and is also available in fixed combination with sulfamethoxazole (as Bactrim, Septra). This combination is reviewed in Chapter 60.

USES
1. Initial treatment of uncomplicated urinary tract infections due to susceptible strains of the organisms listed above

ADMINISTRATION AND DOSAGE
Available preparations of trimethoprim are 100-mg and 200-mg tablets. The recommended dose for adults and children over age 12 is 100 mg every 12 hours or 200 mg once daily for 10 days. If creatinine clearance is 15 ml to 30 ml/min, dosage should be reduced to 50 mg every 12 hours. The

drug should not be used if creatinine clearance is less than 15 ml/min.

FATE
Trimethoprim is rapidly and completely absorbed, and peak serum levels occur within 1 hour to 4 hours. Urine levels are considerably higher than blood levels. Less than 50% is protein bound in the plasma. Less than 20% of trimethoprim is metabolized, and excretion is primarily by way of the kidneys. The elimination half-life is 8 hours to 16 hours, and up to 60% of a single dose is excreted in the urine within 24 hours.

SIDE-EFFECTS/ADVERSE REACTIONS
Most common side-effects observed during therapy with trimethoprim are rash, epigastric distress, nausea, vomiting, and glossitis. High doses may result in the frequent occurrence of maculopapular, morbilliform, and pruritic rashes. Other adverse effects reported with trimethoprim include fever; elevated levels of BUN, serum creatinine, bilirubin and serum transaminase; thrombocytopenia; leukopenia; neutropenia; megaloblastic anemia; and methemoglobinemia.

CONTRAINDICATIONS AND PRECAUTIONS
Trimethoprim is contraindicated in patients with megaloblastic anemia due to folate deficiency and severe renal dysfunction (i.e., creatinine clearance below 15 ml/min). The drug should be administered cautiously to patients with liver impairment, reduced renal function, folate deficiency, and to pregnant women or nursing mothers. Safety for use in infants under 2 months of age has not been established.

INTERACTIONS
1. Trimethoprim may potentiate the action of oral anticoagulants and possibly phenytoin due to impairment of hepatic metabolism.

NURSING CONSIDERATIONS
See also Nursing Process for sulfonamides in Chapter 60.

Baseline and periodic data should include a complete blood count with differential, liver enzymes, bilirubin, serum creatinine clearance, and BUN, especially if long-term therapy is anticipated, because changes in these laboratory values may be early signs of dysfunction. A urine culture and sensitivity should also be performed, but treatment will usually be initiated before results are available.

Symptoms of blood dyscrasias (such as thrombocytopenia, leukopenia, and neutropenia) may include sore throat, fever, bruising, mucosal ulceration, pallor, and weakness. The physician should be informed immediately, and the drug will be discontinued and a CBC with differential will be ordered. If the laboratory results show signs of bone marrow depression (i.e., thrombocytopenia, leukopenia, megaloblastic anemia), the physician may order leucovorin (see Chap. 38) to restore hematopoiesis.

A more common side-effect, skin rash, may appear 7 days to 14 days after initiation of therapy. Symptoms should be reported and will usually disappear after the drug is discontinued.

Urinary Analgesic

Phenazopyridine
(Pyridium and various other manufacturers)

MECHANISM AND ACTIONS
Phenazopyridine is an azo dye that is excreted in the urine, where it exerts a topical analgesic action on the urinary tract mucosa. Its mechanism of action is unknown. Phenazopyridine is most often used together with a urinary anti-infective such as sulfamethizole (Thiosulfil-A), sulfamethoxazole (Azo Gantanol), or sulfisoxazole (Azo Gantrisin, Suldiazo) to help control pain and discomfort before the infection is controlled.

USES
1. Symptomatic relief of pain, burning, irritation, and urinary urgency or frequency resulting from a lower urinary tract infection, trauma, surgery, catheterization, or endoscopic procedures

ADMINISTRATION AND DOSAGE
Phenazopyridine is used orally as tablets containing 100 mg or 200 mg. It may also be found in combination with hyoscyamine and butabarbital (Pyridium Plus) or atropine, scopolamine, and hyoscyamine (Urogesic) as well as several sulfonamides (see Chap. 60).

Adult dosage is 200 mg three times a day after meals. Children (6 years–12 years) are given 100 mg three times a day. Therapy should not exceed 2 days when used concurrently with a urinary anti-bacterial agent because there is no evidence that combined phenazopyridine–antibacterial drug administration is of greater benefit than use of the antibacterial drug itself after 2 days.

FATE

Oral absorption is good, and the drug is rapidly excreted into the urine, approximately 65% in unchanged form.

SIDE-EFFECTS/ADVERSE REACTIONS

Phenazopyridine may cause some gastric upset and may discolor the urine a reddish-orange. Adverse reactions are rare with recommended doses. An occasional report of headache or rash has appeared. Very large doses may result in methemoglobinemia, hemolytic anemia, and renal or hepatic damage on rare occasions.

Overdosage may be treated with ascorbic acid (100 mg–200 mg, orally), which should result in prompt reduction of methemoglobinemia and cyanosis. Severe overdosage may require IV methylene blue (1 mg–2 mg/kg). (See discussion earlier in this chapter.)

CONTRAINDICATIONS AND PRECAUTIONS

Phenazopyridine is contraindicated in patients with renal insufficiency, uremia, or chronic glomerulonephritis. The drug should be used with caution in pregnant women or nursing mothers, and in patients with chronic, recurrent urinary infections.

NURSING CONSIDERATIONS

Patients who have taken this drug before know it reduces the pain and burning on urination associated with urinary tract infections almost immediately. Therefore, they may be tempted to save a few doses "for the next time" and may delay reporting a future infection. The patient must be made aware that phenazopyridine does not treat the cause of the symptoms and may complicate the therapy if anti-infective treatment is not initiated early.

The azo dye which causes the urine to turn reddish-orange is oily and will stain clothing. The patient may wish to use light padding during therapy to prevent fabric damage.

Patients may develop a yellowish tinge to sclera or skin, a possible indication of reduced renal excretion and accumulation toxicity. The physician should be immediately notified if this happens, and the drug should be discontinued.

Urease Inhibitor

Acetohydroxamic Acid
(Lithostat)

MECHANISM AND ACTION

Acetohydroxamic acid is a reversible inhibitor of the bacterial enzyme urease and, therefore, retards the hydrolysis of urea and the production of ammonia in urine infected with urea-splitting organisms. The decreased ammonia levels and reduced pH resulting from the action of acetohydroxamic acid enhance the effectiveness of antimicrobial agents and can increase the cure rate. Acetohydroxamic acid does not possess antibacterial activity itself, nor does it directly acidify the urine.

USES

1. *Adjunctive* treatment of urinary infections due to urea-splitting organisms.
   Note: Acetohydroxamic acid should *not* be used in place of appropriate antimicrobial therapy or surgery where indicated (*e.g.*, patients with stones).

ADMINISTRATION AND DOSAGE

Acetohydroxamic acid is administered orally as 250-mg tablets. In adults, the initial dose is 250 mg three to four times a day to a total of 12 mg/kg/day. Dosage may be increased to a maximum of 1.5 g/day. The drug should be given on an empty stomach. The recommended dose in children is 10 mg/kg/day in two or three divided doses.

Patients with a serum creatinine in excess of 1.8 mg/dl should *not* receive more than 1 g/day in two divided doses every 12 hours. The drug should not be given if the serum creatinine is above 2.5 mg/dl.

FATE

Acetohydroxamic acid is well absorbed orally, and peak blood levels occur within 1 hour. The plasma half-life is approximately 5 hours to 10 hours in patients with normal renal function and is prolonged in persons with impaired renal function. From one-third to two-thirds of a dose is excreted unchanged in the urine and constitutes the active fraction of the drug.

SIDE-EFFECTS/ADVERSE REACTIONS

Approximately 30% of patients receiving acetohydroxamic acid experience adverse effects. The incidence of adverse effects appears to be higher in patients with advanced renal disease or thrombophlebitis. The most often encountered side-effects with the drug are headache, nausea, vomiting, anorexia, malaise, nervousness, tremor, anxiety, and depression. Laboratory evidence of a Coombs' negative hemolytic anemia has occurred in approximately 15% of patients. A mild reticulocytosis occurs even more frequently. A small number of these patients develop a hemolytic anemia severe enough to require discontinuation of therapy. Other adverse reactions associated with acetohydroxamic acid include superficial phlebitis, nonpruritic skin rash on the upper extremities and face, and alopecia.

In experimental animals, large doses of acetohydroxamic acid have caused bone marrow depression and hepatocellular carcinoma, but these effects have not been reported in humans.

CONTRAINDICATIONS AND PRECAUTIONS

Use of acetohydroxamic acid is contraindicated in persons with impaired renal function (i.e., serum creatinine greater than 2.5 mg/dl) or urinary infections due to non-urease-producing organisms. It is also contraindicated in pregnant women or females of child-bearing age not using contraceptive measures because the drug is teratogenic in rats at high doses. The drug should be administered with caution to persons with anemia, blood dyscrasias, bone marrow depression, thrombophlebitis, skin rash, depression, and in nursing mothers.

INTERACTIONS
1. Alcohol has produced a rash in the presence of acetohydroxamic acid.

2. Acetohydroxamic acid can reduce oral absorption of iron and possibly other metal ions by forming a chelate with the metal.

NURSING CONSIDERATIONS
Baseline laboratory data should include a pregnancy test in women of child-bearing age who are not using contraceptives, a complete blood count with differential and renal functions studies if the patient is suspected having renal problems, anemia, or blood dyscrasias.

The drug should be taken 1 hour before meals or 2 hours after meals, not on a full stomach. The patient needs to know that ingestion of any alcohol may result in a macular skin rash ranging from mild and transient to severe. Alcohol should be avoided. If the patient takes iron supplement, absorption may be impaired by acetohydroxamic acid. A parenteral form may be given as a substitute, if necessary.

A complete blood count with differential should be obtained 2 weeks after initial therapy begins and every 3 months thereafter until therapy is completed. A mild elevation of the reticulocyte count is expected, but an elevation of greater than 6% usually requires a dosage reduction, and the physician should be notified. If the reticulocyte count continues to rise the patient may develop hemolytic anemia characterized by nausea, vomiting, anorexia, and malaise. Drug therapy must be discontinued. A very common side-effect, headache, occurs within the first 48 hours to 72 hours of treatment and will usually disappear spontaneously. Mild analgesics will usually help control pain, if necessary.

REVIEW QUESTIONS

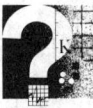

1. What distinguishes *urinary anti-infective* drugs from other drugs also having an effect on urinary pathogens?
2. Why must urinary anti-infectives usually be administered for at least 10 days to 14 days?
3. Against what organisms is cinoxacin usually effective?
4. What are the contraindications to use of cinoxacin?
5. What is the mechanism of action of methenamine?
6. Why is the drug more effective when given as the mandelate or hippurate salt?
7. List the principal uses for mandelamine.
8. What strategies can the nurse give the patient to help maintain adequate fluid intake and appropriate urine acidification with methenamine therapy?
9. Why is methenamine ineffective in prophylaxis of urinary tract infection for patients with indwelling catheters?
10. Describe the effect of methylene blue responsible for its action to antidote cyanide poisoning.

11. What are the other indications for methylene blue?
12. What is the mechanism of action of nalidixic acid? What other urinary anti-infective does it closely resemble in action?
13. What laboratory studies should be obtained before therapy with nalidixic acid begins?
14. List the major adverse reactions associated with use of nalidixic acid.
15. Briefly describe the mechanism of action of nitrofurantoin. What types of microorganisms are generally susceptible to nitrofurantoin?
16. What is the advantage of the macrocrystalline dosage form of nitrofurantoin over the regular oral tablets or capsules?
17. What are the early signs of pulmonary sensitivity from nitrofurantoin? What steps should be taken to attempt to prevent permanent damage?
18. What are the major indications for norfloxacin? How does it differ from other urinary anti-infectives in its spectrum of action?
19. What are the major adverse effects of nitrofurantoin?
20. What factors may predispose a patient to peripheral neuropathy while taking nitrofurantoin?
21. How does trimethoprim exert its antibacterial activity? With what other anti-infective drugs is it synergistic and why?
22. What are the most commonly observed side-effects with trimethoprim?
23. Give the principal indications for phenazopyridine.
24. What is the danger with overdosage with phenazopyridine, and what drugs may be given to treat overdosage?
25. Describe the action and uses of acetohydroxamic acid.
26. List the major adverse effects with acetohydroxamic acid.

BIBLIOGRAPHY

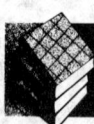

Andriole VT: Urinary tract agents: Nalidixic acid, oxolinic acid, cinoxacin, nitrofurantoin and methenamine. In Mandell GL, Douglas RG, Bennett JE (eds): Principles and Practice of Infectious Diseases, 2nd ed, p 244. New York, John Wiley & Sons, 1985

Black M, Robin L, Schatz N: Nitrofurantoin-induced chronic active hepatitis. Ann Intern Med 92:62, 1980

Bushby SR, Hitchings GH: Trimethoprim, a sulfonamide potentiator. Br J Pharmacol Chemother 33:72, 1968

Gleckman R, Alvarez S, Jouvert DW, Matthews SJ: Drug therapy reviews: Methenamine mandelate and methenamine hippurate. Am J Hosp Pharm 36:1509, 1979

Hamilton-Miller JM, Brumfitt W: Methenamine and its salts as urinary antiseptics. Invest Urol 14:287, 1977

Holmberg L, Boman G, Bottiger LE, Eriksson BA, Spross R, Wessling A: Adverse reactions to nitrofurantoin. Am J Med 69:733, 1980

Muytjens HL, vanderRos-vandeRepe J, vanVeldhuizen G: Comparative activities of ciprofloxacin, norfloxacin, pipemidic acid and nalidixic acid. Antimicrob Agents Chemother 24:302, 1983

Norrby SR, Jonsson M: Antibacterial activity of norfloxacin. Antimicrob Agents Chemother 23:15, 1982

Scavone JM, Gleckman RA, Fraser DG: Cinoxacin: Mechanisms of action, spectrum of activity, pharmacokinetics, adverse reactions and therapeutic indications. Pharmacotherap 2:266, 1982

Spielberg SP, Gordon GB: Nitrofurantoin cytotoxicity. J Clin Invest 67:37, 1981

Stamey TA, Bragonjie J: Resistance to nalidixic acid: A misconception due to underdosage. JAMA 236:1857, 1976

Vainrub B, Musher DM: Lack of effect of methenamine on suppression of, or prophylaxis against chronic urinary infection. Antimicrob Agents Chemother 12:625, 1977

Miscellaneous Antibiotics

Chloramphenicol
Ciprofloxacin
Clindamycin
Lincomycin
Clofazimine
Dapsone
Furazolidone
Hydroxystilbamidine

Nitrofurazone
Novobiocin
Pentamidine
Spectinomycin
Vancomycin

68

A number of antimicrobial drugs in clinical use today cannot be precisely categorized based on their chemical structure or biologic activity. These drugs are most conveniently grouped under a miscellaneous heading and are reviewed here individually.

Chloramphenicol

(AK-Chlor, Chloracol, Chlorofair, Chloromycetin, Chloroptic, Ophthochlor)

Chloramphenicol is a synthetic, broad-spectrum, bacteriostatic antibiotic effective against a wide range of gram-positive and gram-negative bacteria, rickettsiae, and chlamydiae. Its potential for eliciting serious toxicity, however, largely restricts its systemic use to severe infections in which other, less toxic drugs are ineffective or contraindicated. The drug is also employed locally in the eye for treating superficial ocular infections and in the ear for infections of the external auditory canal. Currently, it is considered to be the drug of choice for acute *Salmonella typhi* infections (typhoid fever), but should not be used for routine treatment of the typhoid "carrier state." Other organisms against which it is quite active are *Hemophilus influenzae*, *Bacteroides fragilis*, other *Salmonella* species, rickettsiae, lymphogranuloma-psittacosis group, and various gram-negative bacteria causing bacteremia or meningitis. The major danger associated with chloramphenicol is bone marrow depression, and fatal blood dyscrasias have occurred following both its short-term and long-term use. Frequent blood studies are therefore essential during its administration. Other untoward reactions noted with chloramphenicol are neurotoxicity and the "gray syndrome" in newborns (see under Side-Effects/ Adverse Reactions). While it is a valuable anti-infective for certain severe infections, chloramphenicol should *never* be used for trivial infections (*e.g.*, colds, flu, throat infections) or as a prophylactic agent.

MECHANISM AND ACTIONS
Chloramphenicol binds to the 50S ribosomal subunits of bacteria, and, by preventing binding of t-RNA to the ribosome, it inhibits bacterial protein synthesis by cellular ribosomes. It is bacteriostatic at normal concentrations. The drug can also inhibit mitochondrial protein synthesis in mammalian cells, because mitochondrial ribosomes resemble bacterial ribosomes.

USES
1. Treatment of acute infections caused by *Salmonella typhi* (drug of choice)
2. Alternative treatment of severe infections due to susceptible organisms for which less toxic drugs are ineffective or contraindicated (see Table 59-1). Principal indications include *Hemophilus influenzae* meningitis, pneumococcal or meningococcal meningitis in penicillin-sensitive patients, *Bacteroides fragilis* infections, and rickettsial infections in tetracycline-sensitive patients.
3. Adjunctive therapy in cystic fibrosis regimens
4. Superficial infections of the skin, eye, and external auditory canal due to susceptible microorganisms (topical application only)

ADMINISTRATION AND DOSAGE
Chloramphenicol is available in the following dosage forms: capsules (250 mg, 500 mg), oral suspension (150 mg/5 ml), powder for injection (100 mg/ml as sodium succinate), ophthalmic solution (5 mg/ml), powder for ophthalmic solution (25 mg/vial), ophthalmic ointment (10 mg/g), otic solution (0.5%), and topical cream (1%).
Recommended doses are as follows:
Oral, IV:
　　Adults and children—50 mg/kg/day in divided doses every 6 hours (maximum 100 mg/kg/day in very severe infections)
　　Newborns and infants with immature metabolic processes—25 mg/kg/day in four equally divided doses every 6 hours
Topical:
　　Apply several times a day to affected area
Ophthalmic:
　　One drop or two drops or small amount of ointment to infected eye two to four times a day
Otic:
　　Two to three drops three times a day
The parenteral solution is only intended for IV injection as a 10% solution injected over at least 1 minute. Chloramphenicol is ineffective when given IM. When administered IV, oral dosage should be substituted as soon as possible.

FATE
Chloramphenicol is rapidly absorbed orally, and peak serum levels occur in 1 hour to 2 hours. Its total body distribution is variable with highest concentrations occurring in the liver and kidney, while lowest amounts are found in the brain and

cerebrospinal fluid (about one half the levels in the blood). The drug is approximately 50% to 60% protein-bound. The elimination half-life is 3 hours to 4 hours. Chloramphenicol is metabolized by the liver and excreted in the urine, largely as the glucuronic acid conjugate, with small amounts (8%–12%) of unchanged drug; minor quantities of active drug are found in the bile and feces. The drug readily crosses the placental barrier and appears in breast milk.

SIDE-EFFECTS/ADVERSE REACTIONS

The most serious toxicities associated with chloramphenicol use are bone marrow depression and blood dyscrasias (especially aplastic anemia).

Serious and potentially fatal blood dyscrasias (e.g., agranulocytosis, aplastic anemia, thrombocytopenia) have occurred with both short-term and prolonged use of chloramphenicol. Although more likely with systemic administration, the hematologic abnormalities can occur with topical or local application of chloramphenicol. Thus, it should be employed only in severe infections unresponsive to other, less hazardous antibiotics, and careful blood studies should be performed at least every 2 days during therapy. A dose-related reversible type of bone marrow depression may occur during treatment and is characterized by a decrease in red cell iron uptake, saturation of iron-binding globulin, reduced reticulocyte count, and leukopenia. It is readily detectable by blood studies and responds promptly to discontinuation of the drug. An irreversible type of bone marrow depression leading to aplastic anemia with a high mortality rate has also been reported (estimated incidence 1:25,000–40,000) but does not appear to be dose-related. It may occur weeks or even months following therapy and is characterized by bone marrow aplasia or hypoplasia and pancytopenia. Most importantly, it is not readily predictable by routine blood studies performed during treatment. Follow-up blood tests and close observation of the patient are necessary.

Another serious toxic reaction, termed the gray syndrome, has occurred with chloramphenicol when given systemically to premature or newborn infants within the first 48 hours of life. Symptoms appear after 3 days to 4 days of treatment, especially with high doses and usually occur in the following order: abdominal distention, emesis, pallid cyanosis, vasomotor collapse, irregular respiration, and hypothermia. Death may occur within a few hours after onset of symptoms; however, discontinuation of therapy upon appearance of the initial symptoms frequently leads to complete recovery.

Other adverse reactions reported during chloramphenicol treatment are:

Hematologic—Blood dyscrasias (leukopenia, reduction in erythrocytes, granulocytopenia, hypoplastic anemia, thrombocytopenia, aplastic anemia)

Neurologic—Headache, confusion, depression, delirium, optic and peripheral neuritis

Hypersensitivity—Fever, rash, urticaria, angioedema, anaphylaxis; itching or burning with topical application

GI—Vomiting, glossitis, stomatitis, diarrhea, enterocolitis (rare)

Other—Jaundice, superinfections

CONTRAINDICATIONS AND PRECAUTIONS

Chloramphenicol should not be used to treat trivial infections, such as influenza, colds, or throat infections, nor should it be used as a prophylactic agent against bacterial infections. Concurrent therapy with other bone marrow-depressing drugs should also be avoided. Chloramphenicol must be used with extreme caution and careful monitoring in pregnant women, nursing mothers, infants, and patients with impaired renal or hepatic function, acute intermittent porphyria, diabetes, seizure disorders, or glucose-6-phosphate-dehydrogenase deficiency. Repeat courses of therapy should be avoided, and treatment should not be continued longer than is necessary to effect a cure. Patients must be advised to report the appearance of sore throat, fever, unusual bruising or bleeding, excessive fatigue, or mucosal ulceration, because these are frequently early indicators of a developing blood dyscrasia.

INTERACTIONS

1. Chloramphenicol can inhibit the metabolism of oral anticoagulants, oral antidiabetic drugs, cyclophosphamide, barbiturates, and phenytoin, thus potentiating their effects.
2. Chloramphenicol may inhibit the hematinic activity of vitamin B_{12}, folic acid, and iron.
3. The bactericidal action of other antibiotics (e.g., penicillins) may be reduced by chloramphenicol.
4. Chloramphenicol can interfere with the immune response to diphtheria and tetanus toxoids.
5. Concomitant administration of acetaminophen may elevate serum levels of chloramphenicol.

6. A disulfiram-like reaction to alcohol may occur with use of chloramphenicol (see Chap. 26).

■ *Nursing Process*

□ *ASSESSMENT*

□ *Subjective Data*

A thorough drug history is essential. The patient should be asked about the use of oral anticoagulants, oral antidiabetics, barbiturates, or phenytoin because the effectiveness of these drugs may be enhanced in the presence of chloramphenicol. Dosage adjustments may be needed. The use of acetaminophen (Tylenol) and alcohol must be determined because both of these must be completely avoided during therapy. If the patient has received a recent DPT shot or tetanus shot, the effects of these vaccines may be negated by chloramphenicol, and such a history should be reported before therapy begins. The patient should also be asked about allergy to chloramphenicol, a contraindication to further use, and about current use of other antibiotics because chloramphenicol may reduce the bactericidal action of other drugs.

Medical history should determine the presence of hepatic, renal, or hematologic problems such as acute intermittent porphyria, pregnancy, lactation, or diagnoses of glucose-6-phosphate-dehydrogenase deficiency. The benefits of therapy must clearly outweigh the risks when the drug is used on patients with any of these conditions.

□ *Objective Data*

Physical assessment of the nervous system is especially important in the newborn receiving this drug to quickly detect changes if gray syndrome occurs. Vital signs should be recorded, and breath sounds auscultated. Pretreatment urinary output and weight are essential. The infected site should be thoroughly examined. Laboratory data should include a complete blood count with differential, liver enzymes, BUN, serum creatinine, and urinalysis.

□ *NURSING DIAGNOSES*

Actual nursing diagnoses may include:

Knowledge deficit related to the drug action, administration, and side-effects

Anxiety related to drug side-effects, which can be very serious

Potential nursing diagnoses may include:

Alteration in respiratory function related to drug toxicity

Alteration in comfort: headache (a drug side-effect)

Potential for hypothermia related to drug toxicity (gray syndrome)

Potential for infection related to blood dyscrasias, or superinfection

Potential for injury: trauma related to mental confusion

Alteration in oral mucous membranes: related to drug side-effects

Sensory-perceptual alteration in vision related to optic neuropathy

Sensory-perceptual alteration in tactile sense related to peripheral neuropathy

Impaired skin integrity related to local hypersensitivity reaction

Alteration in tissue perfusion related to blood dyscrasias

□ *PLAN*

The nursing care goals focus on

1. Safe, correct drug administration techniques
2. Close monitoring of side-effects, including blood dyscrasias, gray syndrome, oral lesions, neuropathies, gastrointestinal side-effects, headache, superinfection, hypersensitivity
3. Careful monitoring of patients with special needs such as the diabetic or the patient on oral anticoagulants
4. Teaching the patient correct drug-taking techniques, about side-effects, and what to do if problems occur

□ *INTERVENTION*

Treatment with chloramphenicol should not extend longer than required to resolve the infection with minimal risk of relapse (*i.e.*, a normal temperature for 48 hours). Repeated courses of therapy should be avoided regardless of the route used. The patient taking this drug should know about the *extremely* serious adverse reactions possible with chloramphenicol.

Oral doses should be administered on an empty stomach but may be given with small amounts of food if gastrointestinal distress occurs. Doses should be spaced evenly over a 24-hour period to ensure therapeutic serum levels.

Topical doses should be administered with the same care as other routes because systemic toxicity can occur. Prolonged administration to the eye, ear, or skin should be avoided. Local hypersensitivity reactions are not uncommon. The patient should be told to report immediately any itching, burning, or angioedema because anaphylaxis can occur.

Intravenous chloramphenicol is physically incompatible with many antibiotics including most penicillins, polymyxin B and tetracyclines, and phenothiazines and must be administered in a separate IV line or 1 hour to 2 hours after an incompatible drug has been given and the line has been completely flushed.

Chloramphenicol can be given by direct IV injection if the drug is diluted to 100 mg/ml of diluent and infused over 1 minute, but it is most often given by intermittent infusion. The dose is mixed in 50 ml to 100 ml of 5% dextrose in water and infused over a 15-minute to 30-minute period. It can also be administered by continuous infusion if necessary. A fresh solution must be given every 24 hours.

The side-effects of chloramphenicol make the drug extremely dangerous because toxicity is not dose related and is therefore difficult to prevent.

To monitor the development of blood dyscrasias, a CBC with differential should be performed every 48 hours during therapy and at monthly intervals for 4 months to 6 months after therapy is ended. Special attention must be paid to platelets, white blood cells, and reticulocytes. Any significant changes warrant drug discontinuation. If platelets fall below 100,000/mm^3, the patient should be monitored for signs of bleeding from any orifice and all secretions. If WBC count falls below 2000, the patient should be placed on protective (reverse) isolation until immune response returns. Superinfection at multiple sites is likely if WBC count is low. If reticulocyte count changes, anemia or bone marrow depression may be developing. Patients should be advised to report immediately any fever, sore throat, fatigue, bruising, or bleeding so the drug can be discontinued.

Gray syndrome (see under Side-Effects/Adverse Reactions) in infants can quickly lead to respiratory arrest and death. Close monitoring of the neonate using a flow sheet to record abdominal tenderness, vomitus, skin color and capillary refill, respiration, heart rate, and temperature is essential to identify the syndrome early. Emergency resuscitative equipment including drugs for vascular collapse and respiratory depression and equipment to support ventilation must be on hand at all times.

Headache and mental confusion are not uncommon with administration of chloramphenicol. Headache may be relieved with a mild analgesic such as aspirin, but the patient should not take any product containing acetaminophen. The patient should avoid driving or tasks requiring concentration until drug effects are known.

Peripheral and optic neuropathies can occur with chloramphenicol use and can be irreversible if not identified early. Symptoms of peripheral neuropathy include pain, tingling, numbness, or weakness, especially in hands, fingers, feet, and toes. Optic neuropathy is characterized by a change in visual acuity, appearance of scotoma, and eye pain or tenderness. Symptoms should be reported immediately, and the drug should be discontinued.

Gastrointestinal side-effects may be transient, but persistent vomiting or diarrhea should be reported. Glossitis and stomatitis are treated by frequent mouth rinses and by avoiding irritating food and fluids. Symptoms will subside when the drug is discontinued.

Superinfection may occur with chloramphenicol use even if WBC count remains normal. Likely sites are the primary infected site, upper respiratory tract, perineum (*Monilia*), and the GI tract (diarrhea from overgrowth). Treatment with appropriate anti-infectives will usually resolve the problem.

□ *EVALUATION*
Outcome criteria by which to judge drug effectiveness include resolution of infection (absence of fever, improved symptoms) and a treatment duration for a short period to achieve resolution, absence or early detection and adequate treatment of side-effects such as blood dyscrasias, gray syndrome, headache, mental confusion, neuropathy gastrointestinal upset, and superinfection.

Ciprofloxacin
(Cipro)

Ciprofloxacin is a synthetic fluoroquinolone anti-infective agent that exerts a bactericidal action against a wide range of gram-positive and gram-negative organisms. Unlike its structurally related analog, norfloxacin (see Chap. 67), it is useful not only in treating urinary infections but also in managing respiratory, skin, soft tissue, bone, and joint infections due to susceptible organisms.

MECHANISM AND ACTIONS
Ciprofloxacin interferes with the enzyme DNA gyrase, which is necessary for the synthesis of bacterial DNA. The drug is effective against most of the common gram-positive and gram-negative organisms, with the exception of *Streptococcus fecalis*, *Mycobacterium tuberculosis*, and *Chlamydia trachomatis*. Ciprofloxacin has additive antibac-

terial effects when combined with beta-lactams, aminoglycosides, clindamycin, or metronidazole.

USES
1. Treatment of infections caused by most strains of gram-positive and gram-negative organisms except those listed above

ADMINISTRATION AND DOSAGE
Ciprofloxacin is available as tablets containing 250 mg, 500 mg, or 750 mg. Recommended dosage ranges are 250 mg to 750 mg every 12 hours, depending on the severity of the infection. The usual duration of therapy is 7 to 14 days but may be more prolonged in bone or joint infections. Doses are reduced in patients with impaired renal function.

FATE
Oral absorption is rapid and complete. First pass metabolism is minimal. Food delays the rate of absorption but not the total amount absorbed. Peak serum levels are attained within 1 hour to 2 hours after dosing. Serum protein binding is minimal (20%–30%). Approximately one half of an oral dose is excreted in the urine as unchanged drug. Up to one third of an oral dose is recovered in the feces within 5 days. The plasma half-life of ciprofloxacin in patients with normal renal function is about 4 hours. The urinary excretion is virtually complete within 24 hours.

SIDE-EFFECTS/ADVERSE REACTIONS
The most frequently noted side-effects during ciprofloxacin therapy are nausea, diarrhea, vomiting, abdominal discomfort, headache, and skin rash. Other adverse effects are listed below by organ system:

CNS: dizziness, restlessness, insomnia, nightmares, irritability, tremors, weakness, convulsions, depression
GI: dysphagia, oral candidiasis, intestinal bleeding
Cardiovascular: palpitations, ventricular ectopy, hypertension, angina
Respiratory: epistaxis, laryngeal edema, hiccoughs, dyspnea, bronchospasm
Dermatologic: pruritus, urticaria, photosensitivity, flushing, angioedema, hyperpigmentation
Other: blurred vision, diplopia, tinnitus, altered taste perception, joint or back pain, polyuria, urinary retention, vaginitis, nephritis

Altered laboratory values observed during ciprofloxacin therapy include elevations in SGPT, SGOT, LDH, alkaline phosphatase, and serum bilirubin.

CONTRAINDICATIONS AND PRECAUTIONS
There are no absolute contraindications to the use of ciprofloxacin. The drug should be given *cautiously* to patients with CNS disorders, such as epilepsy, and to pregnant or nursing mothers. Ciprofloxacin should not be used in children, because it has caused arthropathy in immature animals.

INTERACTIONS
1. Antacids may decrease the oral absorption of ciprofloxacin.
2. Increased serum levels of ciprofloxacin may occur if probenecid is administered concurrently.
3. Plasma concentrations of theophylline may be elevated if given together with ciprofloxacin.

Clindamycin
(Cleocin)

Lincomycin
(Lincocin)

Clindamycin and lincomycin are two chemically related antibiotics frequently termed lincosamides. They exhibit antibacterial activity similar to but not identical to that of the erythromycins. Lincomycin and its chlorine-substituted derivative, clindamycin, are effective against most of the common gram-positive pathogens, particularly *Staphylococcus, Pneumococcus, Streptococcus, Corynebacterium*, and *Nocardia*, as well as many anaerobic organisms, such as *Bacteroides, Actinomyces, Peptococcus, Eubacterium*, and most strains of *Clostridium* (except *Clostridium difficile*). Most gram-negative organisms, on the other hand, are resistant. Because of their toxic potential, however, lincomycin and clindamycin are usually recommended only for treatment of serious anaerobic infections for which penicillin or erythromycin is ineffective or inappropriate (*e.g.*, when penicillin hypersensitivity is present). The major dangers associated with use of clindamycin and lincomycin are related to the GI tract, and include persistent profuse diarrhea, severe abdominal cramping, and pseudomembranous colitis. These effects, although most frequent with systemic use, have oc-

Table 68-1
Clindamycin and Lincomycin

Drug	Preparations	Usual Dosage Range	Clinical Considerations
clindamycin (Cleocin)	Capsules—75 mg, 150 mg Granules for suspension—75 mg/5 ml Injection—300 mg/2 ml, 600 mg/4 ml, 900 mg/6 ml Topical solution—10 mg/ml (Cleocin-T)	Oral: Adults—150 mg to 450 mg every 6 h depending on severity of infection Children—8 mg to 12 mg/kg/day in three to four divided doses (up to 25 mg/kg/day) in severe infections IM, IV: Adults—600 mg to 2700 mg/day in two to four equally divided doses depending on severity of infection Children—15 mg to 40 mg/kg/day in three to four equal doses depending on severity of infection or 350 mg to 450 mg/M²/day *Acute pelvic inflammatory disease:* 600 mg IV every 6 h plus gentamicin or tobramycin (2 mg/kg initially, followed by 1.5 mg/kg 3 times/day for 4 days). Continue clindamycin orally (450 mg 4 times/day for at least 7–10 days). Topical: Apply thin film to affected area twice a day	Do not use in children under 1 month; minimum recommended oral dose in children weighing 10 kg or less is 37.5 mg three times a day; do not refrigerate reconstituted granules because it may thicken and become difficult to pour; oral solution is stable for 2 weeks at room temperature; use parenteral therapy initially in children to treat anaerobic infections; follow with oral administration when appropriate; in severe infections children should receive no less than 300 mg a day parenterally, regardless of body weight; adults may be given up to 4.8 g a day IV in life-threatening infections; single IM injections of more than 600 mg are not recommended; do not give more than 1200 mg an hour by IV infusion; physically incompatible with ampicillin, phenytoin, aminophylline, barbiturates, calcium gluconate, and magnesium sulfate; applied topically to (continued)

curred with topical application of clindamycin as well. Clindamycin is generally regarded as the preferred drug of the two for systemic use, because it is better absorbed orally, has a somewhat broader spectrum of action, including *Bacteroides fragilis*, and is reported to elicit fewer GI side-effects. Although the two drugs are alike enough in their pharmacologic properties to be discussed together, some important differences do exist, and these are noted whenever appropriate in the following discussion as well as in Table 68-1.

MECHANISM AND ACTIONS
These agents interfere with protein synthesis in susceptible organisms by binding to the 50S subunits of bacterial ribosomes. Resistance develops slowly, possibly due to chromosomal alterations.

Both drugs possess neuromuscular blocking activity and are active against most common gram-positive pathogens. Clindamycin demonstrates a slightly wider range of action against anaerobic gram-positive organisms (e.g., *Actinomyces, Peptococcus, Clostridium*, microaerophilic streptococci) and anaerobic gram-negative bacilli (e.g., *Bacteroides, Fusobacterium*).

USES
1. Alternate therapy for serious streptococcal, pneumococcal, or staphylococcal infections in patients in whom penicillins and erythromycins are ineffective or inappropriate
2. Alternate treatment of serious infections due to anaerobic organisms, such as *Bacteroides, Fusobacterium, Peptococcus*, or *Actinomyces*

Table 68-1 (continued)
Clindamycin and Lincomycin

Drug	Preparations	Usual Dosage Range	Clinical Considerations
clindamycin (Cleocin) *(continued)*			acne vulgaris lesions; alcohol base may be irritating to sensitive surfaces (eye, mucous membranes, wounds)
lincomycin (Lincocin)	Capsules—250 mg, 500 mg Injection—300 mg/ml	Oral: Adults—500 mg three to four times a day Children—30 mg to 60 mg/kg/day in three to four divided doses depending on severity of infection IM: Adults—600 mg every 12 h–24 h Children—10 mg/kg every 12 h–24 h IV infusion: Adults—600 mg to 1 g every 8 h–12 h Children—10 mg to 20 mg/kg/day in divided doses Subconjunctival injection: 0.25 ml (75 mg)	Do not use in children under 1 month; administer orally on an empty stomach; IM injections should be made deeply and slowly to minimize pain; severe cardiopulmonary reactions have occurred when drug has been given IV at higher than recommended doses or rates; in life-threatening situations, daily IV doses of up to 8 g have been used; dilute 1 g lincomycin in 100 ml of a compatible infusion solution (see package insert) and infuse over a period of not less than 1 h; repeat as often as needed to a maximum of 8 g a day; subconjunctival injection results in effective ocular fluid levels of antibiotics for 5 h; drug is incompatible with novobiocin and kanamycin as well as phenytoin sodium and protein hydrolysates

species, in penicillin-sensitive patients (clindamycin is most effective)

3. Treatment of acute pelvic inflammatory disease (endometritis, pelvic cellulitis, nongonococcal tubo-ovarian abscess). See Table 68-1.
4. Treatment of acne (topical application of clindamycin solution)

ADMINISTRATION AND DOSAGE
See Table 68-1.

FATE
Oral absorption is rapid and virtually complete (90%) for clindamycin, whereas only about 20% to 30% of an oral dose of lincomycin is absorbed. Food markedly impairs absorption of lincomycin but not clindamycin. Peak plasma levels occur within 45 minutes with oral clindamycin and 2 hours to 4 hours with oral lincomycin. IM injection yields peak serum levels within 30 minutes with lincomycin and 1 hour to 3 hours with clindamycin. Plasma half-lives are 2 hours to 3 hours for clindamycin and 4 hours to 6 hours for lincomycin. Both drugs are widely distributed in the body and are approximately 70% protein-bound. Penetration into the cerebrospinal fluid is minimal unless the meninges are inflamed. Effective antibacterial blood levels are maintained for 6 hours to 8 hours after oral administration, and up to 12 hours following IM injection or IV infusion. Most of a dose of clindamycin is metabolized in the liver and excreted in the urine and bile. Less than 15% is eliminated unchanged by the kidneys. Lincomycin is partially metabolized in the liver and excreted both

in the urine and the feces. A dosage reduction is necessary for lincomycin in patients with impaired renal function.

SIDE-EFFECTS/ADVERSE REACTIONS

The most common side-effects seen with clindamycin and lincomycin are nausea, vomiting, diarrhea, and skin rash. Diarrhea may be persistent and severe and indicate the presence of colitis, which develops in up to 10% of patients receiving the drugs orally. Toxins produced by resistant strains of clostridia are a primary cause of the colitis, which is also characterized by severe abdominal cramps and passage of blood and mucus. This reaction can prove fatal, and the development of severe diarrhea, abdominal pain, or bloody stools warrants immediate discontinuation of the drug. Diarrhea and colitis can begin up to several weeks following cessation of therapy. Mild cases of diarrhea and colitis usually respond to discontinuation of therapy. Other measures that may become necessary depending on severity of the condition are fluid and electrolyte replacement, protein supplementation, and either systemic or rectal corticosteroids to relieve the colitis. Antidiarrheal drugs, such as diphenoxylate, loperamide, or opiates, should be avoided because they may prolong or aggravate the condition. Pseudomembranous colitis resulting from toxins produced by *Clostridium difficile* may respond to oral vancomycin, and this agent is discussed later in this chapter.

Many other adverse reactions have occurred during therapy with these agents, and, while some are more closely associated with one or the other of these drugs, all of the following untoward reactions must be considered a possible consequence of usage of *either* drug:

GI—Abdominal pain, glossitis, esophagitis, stomatitis, pruritus ani, jaundice, abnormal liver function tests, acute enterocolitis, or pseudomembranous colitis (occasionally fatal)

Hypersensitivity—Maculopapular or morbilliform rashes, urticaria, angioedema, serum sickness, erythema multiforme (rare), Stevens-Johnson syndrome (rare), exfoliative dermatitis (rare)

Hematologic—Eosinophilia, infrequent blood dyscrasias (neutropenia, leukopenia, thrombocytopenia, agranulocytosis, aplastic anemia)

Cardiovascular—Hypotension and possible cardiopulmonary arrest following too rapid IV injection

Other—Vaginitis, polyarthritis, tinnitus, vertigo, pain or induration on IM injection

Topical application of clindamycin can result in contact dermatitis, skin dryness, oily skin, facial swelling, stinging sensation and gram-negative folliculitis.

CONTRAINDICATIONS AND PRECAUTIONS

Clindamycin and lincomycin should *not* be used to treat trivial bacterial or viral infections. In addition, clindamycin is not indicated in treating meningitis because it does not diffuse into the CNS in adequate amounts and lincomycin is not recommended in newborns, nursing mothers, or in patients with severe liver disease.

Both drugs must be given with *caution* to patients with renal or hepatic disease, myasthenia gravis, a history of bronchial asthma or other allergic diseases, GI disease, to pregnant women, and to elderly or debilitated patients.

INTERACTIONS

1. The activity of clindamycin and lincomycin may be reduced by concurrent use of erythromycin or chloramphenicol because they bind to the same ribosomal site.
2. Clindamycin and lincomycin can enhance the action of neuromuscular blocking drugs.
3. Use of antiperistaltic drugs such as opiates, loperamide, and diphenoxylate may prolong or aggravate the diarrhea observed with clindamycin and lincomycin.
4. The oral absorption of clindamycin and lincomycin can be impaired by kaolin, pectin, other antidiarrheal medications, and cyclamates.
5. Clindamycin and lincomycin can increase serum levels of SGOT, SGPT and alkaline phosphatase.

NURSING CONSIDERATIONS

A drug history, focusing on previous drug allergies, is important because hypersensitivity to both drugs is more likely in individuals with multiple allergies, asthma, and hay fever. Prior to treatment, laboratory data, including liver enzymes, renal function studies and a CBC with differential, should be complete, especially if the patient has a history of liver, kidney, or hematologic problems.

See Table 68-1 for specific information on administration. Intravenous administration can cause thrombophlebitis. Intravenous sites should be rotated every 48 hours and closely observed for signs of pain, redness, and swelling, at which point the IV should be removed.

The most serious side-effect of these drugs is the development of bloody diarrhea and colitis, which can occur at any time during therapy and up to 1 month after discontinuation. The patient should be told to report immediately any abdominal cramping, nausea, vomiting, or bloody stool. See under Side-Effects/Adverse Reactions for treatment guidelines. Hydration and electrolyte balance must be closely monitored with replacements provided as necessary to correct any problems. Diarrhea can cause rapid hypokalemia, characterized by muscle cramping and weakness, and must be treated with a parenteral potassium replacement.

Treatment with clindamycin or lincomycin may result in superinfection by nonsusceptible organisms. Sites most likely to be affected include the original site of infection, upper respiratory tract, and gastrointestinal tract (diarrhea). Diarrhea must be distinguished from that resulting from drug-induced colitis in order to determine effective treatment.

Clofazimine
(Lamprene)

MECHANISM AND ACTIONS

Clofazimine is a bactericidal and anti-inflammatory leprostatic drug that is slowly bactericidal toward *Mycobacterium leprae* or Hansen's bacillus. The drug binds preferentially to mycobacterial DNA and can inhibit growth of the organism. Its anti-inflammatory effects are useful for controlling erythema nodosum leprosum reactions.

Clofazimine is a reddish-brown powder that is deposited in tissues upon systemic absorption. As a result, pigmentation (pink to brownish-black) usually occurs on the skin conjuctivae, on other tissues, and in urine. Clearing of the discoloration occurs gradually on drug withdrawal.

USES

1. Treatment of leprosy including dapsone-resistant leprosy and lepromatous leprosy complicated by erythema nodosum leprosum. (Drug is generally administered in combination with one or more other antileprosy drugs, such as dapsone or rifampin.) See under Administration and Dosage.

ADMINISTRATION AND DOSAGE

Clofazimine is administered as capsules containing 50 mg or 100 mg. The recommended dosage is 100 mg daily in combination with one (or more) other antileprosy drugs for 3 years, followed by monotherapy with 100 mg clofazimine daily thereafter. Clinical improvement is usually evident within 3 months to 6 months.

When corticosteroids are necessary to treat symptoms of erythema nodosum leprosum, daily doses of 100 mg to 200 mg clofazimine for up to 3 months can reduce or possibly eliminate corticosteroid requirements.

FATE

Absorption is variable and can range from approximately 45% to 65% of an oral dose. Clofazimine is highly lipophilic and is deposited primarily in fatty tissue and in the reticuloendothelial system. The drug is retained by the body for long periods of time; the half-life with repeated dosage is at least 60 days to 70 days. Some drug is recoverable in the feces, probably by biliary excretion.

SIDE-EFFECTS/ADVERSE REACTIONS

Side-effects occurring most frequently with clofazimine are discoloration of the skin, urine, feces, sweat, tears, conjunctiva and cornea, dryness of the skin, and GI intolerance (nausea, diarrhea, vomiting, abdominal or epigastric pain).

Other adverse effects occur rather infrequently (generally less than 1% incidence) and include:

GI—Bleeding, constipation, weight loss, bowel obstruction, hepatitis, jaundice, enteritis, enlarged liver

CNS—Dizziness, drowsiness, fatigue, depression, neuralgia, taste alteration

Skin—Rash, pruritus, phototoxicity, acneiform eruptions, monilial cheilosis

Ocular—Dryness, itching, or burning of the eyes

Other—Cystitis, anemia, edema, fever, bone pain, lymphadenopathy, reduced vision, splenic infarction, thromboembolism, vascular pain, elevated serum albumin, bilirubin and SGOT, eosinophilia, hypokalemia

CONTRAINDICATIONS AND PRECAUTIONS

There are no known absolute contraindications to clofazimine. The drug should be given with *caution* to patients with GI problems, and to pregnant or nursing women. The drug crosses the placenta and can cause pigmentation of neonatal skin. Doses above 100 mg a day should be given for as short a period of time as possible, as the incidence of adverse reactions increases significantly at higher doses.

NURSING CONSIDERATIONS

The patient should be informed about skin discoloration from the drug because the change occurs in 75% to 100% of all patients taking it. Because the patient must already cope with a disfiguring disease it is important to inform him of any further visible change that can be expected. Likewise he should be aware of potential changes in the color of urine, tears, and feces to reduce anxiety that another problem may be developing.

Gastrointestinal distress may be alleviated by taking the drug with food. Constipation can be managed by encouraging the patient to increase fluids and fiber in the daily diet. However, persistent epigastric or gastrointestinal pain, abdominal tenderness or bloating, and prolonged constipation should be reported because bowel obstruction and GI bleeding have occurred.

Clofazimine causes skin dryness, which can usually be treated by a mild lubricant. Eye drops can be used if eye dryness is a problem. (See also Dapsone.)

Dapsone

Sulfones, of which the sole clinically available representative is dapsone, are chemical analogues of the sulfonamides that are used in the treatment of all forms of leprosy (Hansen's disease). Although clinical benefit is often noted within a few months, the more severe skin lesions characteristic of the disease may require several years for complete resolution. Because of its high potential for toxicity, dapsone is usually used only for the treatment of leprosy, although it has been shown to be effective in the treatment of dermatitis herpetiformis, for the management of relapsing polychondritis, and in the prophylaxis of malaria.

MECHANISM AND ACTIONS

The action of dapsone is probably similar to the sulfonamides, that is, interference with essential components of bacterial nutrition. The drug also possesses immunosuppressant action and may inhibit certain bacterial enzymes. Dapsone is bacteriostatic and probably also bactericidal for *Mycobacterium leprae*, the causative agent in leprosy; however, the organism may become resistant to the drug during the course of therapy, which is usually quite lengthy (see under Administration and Dosage).

USES

1. Treatment of all forms of leprosy
2. Treatment of dermatitis herpetiformis
3. Management of relapsing polychondritis (investigational use only)
4. Prophylaxis of malaria (investigational use only)

ADMINISTRATION AND DOSAGE

Dapsone is used as tablets containing either 25 mg or 100 mg. In treating leprosy, the recommended adult dosage is 50 mg to 100 mg per day; children's doses are generally one-quarter to one-half the adult dose. Therapy is continued for at least several years. The World Health Organization recommends continuing drug therapy for *at least* 10 years after the patient has become bacteriologically negative.

In treating dermatitis herpetiformis, the initial dosage is 50 mg/day for adults, which is increased gradually until an optimal effect is noted. The usual dosage range is 50 mg to 300 mg daily. Dosage should be reduced to a minimum maintenance level as soon as possible following clearance of skin lesions and reduction of pruritus.

FATE

Dapsone is slowly and completely absorbed orally; peak plasma concentrations occur in 4 hours to 8 hours. The drug is 70% to 90% protein-bound, and undergoes enterohepatic circulation. It is metabolized in the liver by acetylation and excreted slowly in the urine (70%–85%) as both unchanged drug and metabolites. The plasma half-life averages 25 hours to 30 hours (range 10 hours–50 hours).

SIDE-EFFECTS/ADVERSE REACTIONS

The most common side-effect with dapsone is hemolysis, which may occur to varying degrees. Hemolysis develops in almost every patient given 200 mg to 300 mg a day; however, lower doses (50 mg–100 mg) generally do not cause hemolysis. Methemoglobinemia is also common at higher doses, and most patients show an increased reticulocyte count and a shortened red cell life span. Hemolytic anemia, however, is unusual. Hemolysis may be exaggerated or may occur at lower doses in patients with glucose-6-phosphate-dehydrogenase deficiency.

Other adverse reactions to dapsone include:
Dermatologic—Dermatitis, pruritus, phototoxicity, drug-induced lupus erythematosus
Hematologic—Leukopenia, granulocytopenia, agranulocytosis

GI—Nausea, vomiting, anorexia, abdominal pain

CNS—Headache, paresthesias, tinnitus, insomnia, vertigo, psychotic reactions (rare)

Other—Muscle weakness, back or leg pain, drug fever, blurred vision, toxic hepatitis, cholestatic jaundice, hyperbilirubinemia, hematuria, albuminuria, nephrotic syndrome, renal papillary necrosis, motor neuropathy, infertility, infectious mononucleosis-like syndrome

A lepromatous lepra reaction, sometimes termed the "sulfone syndrome," can occur in up to 50% of patients during the first year of therapy and is thought to be due to elevated circulating immune complexes. The symptoms include fever, malaise, neuritis, orchitis, joint swelling, epistaxis, proteinuria, depression, and tender erythematous skin nodules. Dapsone therapy is usually continued, and the reaction can be ameliorated with analgesics, corticosteroids, or clofazimine.

CONTRAINDICATIONS AND PRECAUTIONS

Dapsone must be administered *cautiously* to patients with liver or kidney disease, anemia, glucose-6-phosphate-dehydrogenase deficiency, diabetes and to pregnant women or nursing mothers. Frequent blood counts must be done (weekly for first month, then monthly), and, if a significant change is noted, the drug should be discontinued. Cutaneous allergic reactions can occur and may be serious. If toxic dermatologic reactions occur, dapsone therapy should be discontinued.

Distinction must be made, however, between these reactions and the cutaneous manifestations of the lepromatous lepra reaction described above, because the latter reaction does not require discontinuation of therapy.

INTERACTIONS

1. Probenecid inhibits the renal tubular secretion of dapsone, thus elevating its plasma level.
2. Rifampin and phenobarbital can reduce the effects of dapsone by increasing hepatic microsomal enzyme activity.
3. The leprostatic effects of dapsone can be antagonized by para-aminobenzoic acid (PABA).
4. The GI absorption and enterohepatic recirculation of dapsone may be impaired by activated charcoal.

NURSING CONSIDERATIONS

Patients receiving dapsone should have baseline and periodic blood studies of hematologic and hepatic function to monitor the development of problems. Patients should also be asked about previous drug hypersensitivity before therapy begins.

The most common side-effect, hemolysis, is characterized by fatigue and hemoglobinuria. The symptom will usually remit if the drug dose is lowered; however, reticulocyte count should be monitored periodically to ensure anemia is not developing.

Other blood dyscrasias characterized by fever, sore throat, bruising, and malaise will be difficult to distinguish from "sulfone syndrome" (see under Side-Effects/Adverse Reactions). A complete blood count with differential can be done; if abnormalities have developed, the drug must be discontinued.

Hepatic dysfunction can occur and can also be monitored by periodic evaluation of liver enzymes and bilirubin. Symptoms of hepatotoxicity, such as anorexia, vomiting, abdominal pain, and light-colored stools, necessitate drug withdrawal.

Cutaneous hypersensitivity reactions to the drug can be severe. A baseline skin assessment should be performed at the beginning of therapy. Any cutaneous changes must be immediately reported because they can rapidly progress. The drug must be discontinued.

Dapsone therapy is very long term and may be taken for life in complex cases of leprosy. The patient needs tremendous support to maintain compliance and to cope with the severe disfigurement caused by the disease. Treatment can be paid for by the federal government through admission to Carville Hospital, Baton Rouge, Louisiana.

Furazolidone

(Furoxone)

Furazolidone is a synthetic nitrofuran with both antibacterial and antiprotozoal activity. It is effective against many common GI pathogens, such as *Escherichia coli*, *Salmonella*, *Shigella*, *Enterobacter aerogenes*, *Proteus*, *Vibrio cholerae*, staphylococci, as well as the protozoan *Giardia lamblia*. Furazolidone is poorly absorbed orally, and its action is largely restricted to the GI tract.

MECHANISM AND ACTIONS

Furazolidone is bactericidal by virtue of its ability to interfere with several bacterial enzyme systems. The drug does not alter normal bowel flora nor lead to fungal overgrowth. The development of resistant organisms is minimal. Furazolidone may exert an MAO-inhibitory action if used for more that 4 days to 5 days, which is probably due in part to accumulation of a metabolite, 2-hydroxyethylhydrazine.

USES
1. Symptomatic treatment of bacterial or protozoal diarrhea and enteritis due to susceptible organisms

ADMINISTRATION AND DOSAGE
Furazolidone is available as tablets (100 mg) or liquid (50 mg/15 ml). Recommended doses are as follows:

  Adults: 100 mg four times a day
  Children (over 5 years): 25 mg to 50 mg four times a day
  Children (1 year to 4 years): 17 mg to 25 mg four times a day
  Children (under 1 year): 8 mg to 17 mg four times a day

The maximal daily dose is 8.8 mg/kg; higher doses are associated with a significant degree of nausea and vomiting. If a satisfactory response is not obtained within 7 days, the drug should be discontinued.

FATE
Oral absorption is minimal. The drug is metabolized in the intestine and excreted largely in the feces. Approximately 5% is eliminated in the urine, along with colored metabolites, which may color the urine brown.

SIDE-EFFECTS/ADVERSE REACTIONS
Untoward reactions with furazolidone include nausea, vomiting, anal pruritus, proctitis, colitis, staphylococcal enteritis, headache, malaise, allergic reactions (fever, urticaria, morbilliform rash, arthralgia, hypotension), reversible intravascular hemolysis and disulfiram-like reaction to alcohol (see Chap. 26), characterized by flushing, dyspnea, chest tightness, and fever. Symptoms disappear generally within 24 hours with no lasting ill effects. Alcohol should be avoided during and for 4 days following termination of furazolidone therapy.

CONTRAINDICATIONS AND PRECAUTIONS
Furazolidone should not be given to infants under 1 month of age because hemolytic anemia can occur due to immature enzyme systems. Concurrent use of alcohol should be avoided (see under Side-Effects/Adverse Reactions). During extended therapy (i.e., longer than 5 days), the intake of tyramine-containing foods (see Chap. 29) or concurrent use of sympathomimetic amines should be avoided to minimize the danger of a hypertensive reaction, because furazolidone inhibits the enzyme monoamine oxidase which normally metabolizes pressor amines such as tyramine. Cautious use of furazolidone must be undertaken in persons with diabetes (may potentiate hypoglycemia), glucose-6-phosphate-dehydrogenase deficiency, and in pregnant women or nursing mothers.

INTERACTIONS
1. Alcohol may elicit a mild disulfiram-like reaction (flushing, hyperthermia, sweating, dyspnea, tachycardia, palpitations) in the presence of furazolidone.
2. Hypertension can result from concurrent use of furazolidone with other MAO inhibitors, sympathomimetic amines, or tyramine-containing foods.
3. The actions of sedatives, narcotics, and other CNS depressants can be enhanced by furazolidone, resulting in hypotension and excessive drowsiness.
4. A toxic psychosis can result from concurrent use of furazolidone and tricyclic antidepressant.
5. The antihypertensive effectiveness of guanethidine may be reduced by furazolidone.
6. Furazolidone may potentiate the hypoglycemic effect of insulin and sulfonylurea antidiabetics.
7. Concurrent use of furazolidone and meperidine may result in sudden development of hypertension, restlessness, agitation, seizures, and coma.

NURSING CONSIDERATIONS
A complete drug history should be obtained (see under Interactions) prior to therapy to avoid toxic drug reactions from combination with a variety of drugs. The patient should be told to avoid all alcohol, over-the-counter cold and allergy medications which may contain vasopressor agents, and all foods high in tyramine (unpasteurized cheeses, beer, wine, broad beans, yeasts, and fermented products) for the duration of therapy and for about 5 days after therapy is completed.

Diarrhea can rapidly lead to dehydration and electrolyte imbalances, especially in children and debilitated patients. Symptoms of muscle cramping, weakness, hypotension, "sunken eyes," irregular pulse, weak cry (in children), and poor skin

Although novobiocin is better absorbed on an empty stomach, it can be given with a small amount of food if nausea occurs. If GI symptoms persist or worsen, the drug may have to be discontinued.

A CBC with differential should be performed periodically throughout therapy to monitor the development of blood dyscrasias. If laboratory values change (see under Side-Effects/Adverse Reactions) or the patient develops fever, sore throat, bruising, or bleeding the drug should be withheld and the physician informed.

Hepatic function studies will indicate early development of liver disease. Other symptoms such as yellowing of skin or sclera, abdominal pain, light-colored stools indicate the need to immediately discontinue the drug and inform the physician.

Pentamidine
(Pentam 300)

MECHANISM AND ACTIONS
Pentamidine is a diamidine antiprotozoal agent that is effective against several protozoa and fungi. The exact mechanism of action has not been established, but there is some indication that the drug may interfere with nuclear metabolism and inhibit the synthesis of DNA, RNA, proteins, and phospholipids. Pentamidine was previously recognized as the primary agent for treating pneumocystis pneumonia (due to *Pneumocystis carinii*), a serious, opportunistic respiratory infection occurring frequently in immunocompromised patients, such as patients with acquired immune deficiency syndrome (AIDS). However, trimethoprim-sulfamethoxazole (see Chap. 60) is now viewed as the drug of choice for pneumocystis pneumonia because it is less toxic than pentamidine and equally effective.

USES
1. Alternative treatment of *Pneumocystis carinii* pneumonia
2. Treatment of trypanosomiasis and visceral leishmaniasis (investigational uses)

ADMINISTRATION AND DOSAGE
Pentamidine is available as a powder for injection containing 300 mg/single dose vial. It is administered either by IV infusion or deep IM injection. The recommended dosage is 4 mg/kg once daily for 14 days. Dosage should be reduced in persons with renal failure. IV solutions are stable at room temperature for up to 24 hours.

FATE
Pentamidine is well absorbed from IM injection sites but exists in the bloodstream only temporarily, because it is extensively bound to tissues. Approximately one-half to two-thirds of a dose is excreted unchanged by the kidneys within 6 hours. The remainder is very slowly eliminated over several weeks. The drug does not enter the CNS in appreciable amounts.

SIDE-EFFECTS/ADVERSE REACTIONS
Side-effects noted most frequently with pentamidine administration are elevated serum creatinine, sterile abscess or pain at IM injection site, elevated liver function tests, leukopenia, nausea, anorexia, fever, hypotension, rash, and hypoglycemia. Too rapid IV administration often leads to tachycardia, dizziness, headache, vomiting, and fainting, probably due to excessive hypotension.

Other untoward reactions reported with pentamidine include confusion, hallucinations, anemia, neuralgia, hyperkalemia, phlebitis, thrombocytopenia, acute renal failure, hypocalcemia, ventricular tachycardia, arrhythmias, and Stevens-Johnson syndrome. The incidence of adverse reaction is significantly higher in patients with AIDS receiving pentamidine than in patients with other conditions.

CONTRAINDICATIONS AND PRECAUTIONS
There are no absolute contraindications to the use of pentamidine in treating pneumocystis pneumonia. The drug should be given *cautiously* to patients with hypertension, hypotension, hypoglycemia, hypocalcemia, leukopenia, thrombocytopenia, anemia, renal or hepatic disease, and arrhythmias. Severe hypotension can occur after a single dose, and fatalities due to severe hypoglycemia or cardiac arrhythmias have occurred following both IM and IV administration. Safety for use in pregnancy has not been established, and the drug should be given to pregnant women only when absolutely needed.

NURSING CONSIDERATIONS
Although pentamidine can be administered both IM and IV, intermittent infusion IV is preferred. IM injections are painful, and sterile abscesses may form. To decrease the chance of tissue injury, the drug should be injected into a large muscle mass with warm compresses applied after injection and sites rotated using a body map (see Chap. 8). However, most patients with pneumocystis pneumonia

are debilitated and have substantial loss of muscle, making IM injections extremely painful.

IV administration may cause phlebitis. IV sites should be routinely rotated and evaluated for pain, redness, and swelling.

Prior to intravenous administration, the patient should lie down and blood pressure should be taken. As the drug is administered, blood pressure should be monitored every 15 minutes. If significant hypotension develops, emergency resuscitative equipment should be available as well as vasopressors. However, hypotension may respond to an increase in IV fluids. Blood pressure should be monitored after infusion until stable and the patient no longer feels dizzy. The patient should rise slowly and limit activity until dizziness passes.

Hypoglycemia may occur during therapy and can be monitored by finger stick blood glucose levels. The patient may be able to manage hypoglycemia by increasing food intake, attempting to eat five or six small meals per day.

Acute renal failure may occur with drug therapy. Periodic BUN and serum creatinine levels should be monitored. Fluid retention and decreased urinary output must be immediately reported. The drug may have to be discontinued.

Patients with pneumocystis pneumonia secondary to AIDS may be reluctant to report drug side-effects because there are few alternatives for treatment. These patients need close monitoring and support to help them manage the devastating effects of the disease but need to be reminded that the drug side-effects can also be fatal.

Pentamidine can alter taste sensation.

Spectinomycin
(Trobicin)

MECHANISM AND ACTIONS
Spectinomycin selectively inhibits protein synthesis in gram-negative bacteria by binding to the 30S ribosomal subunit. The drug is active against most strains of Neisseria gonorrhoeae, and there appears to be little bacterial resistance or cross resistance between spectinomycin and penicillin. Reinfection is the most common cause of treatment failure.

USES
1. Treatment of acute gonorrheal urethritis, proctitis, and cervicitis due to susceptible strains of Neisseria gonorrhoeae (usually in patients sensitive to penicillins, cephalosporins, or tetracyclines, or when organisms are resistant to these drugs)

ADMINISTRATION AND DOSAGE
Spectinomycin is available as powder for injection containing 400 mg/ml when reconstituted with diluent (bacteriostatic water for injection). The drug is administered IM only. Individuals known to have had recent exposure to gonorrhea should be treated the same as those proven to have gonorrhea by culture. Dosage recommendations are:

Adults and children over 45 kg: usually 2 g (5 ml) IM in a single dose; in areas where antibiotic resistance is known to be present, 4 g (10 ml) divided into two equal parts and injected at different sites; inject in large muscle mass such as gluteus and use a large (20) gauge needle.

Children under 45 kg (safety has not been established): 40 mg/kg IM

Injections may be followed by a course of therapy with oral erythromycin or a tetracycline.

FATE
Absorption from IM injection sites is rapid. Serum levels peak in 1 hour to 2 hours, and effective levels are still present at 8 hours. The drug is not significantly protein-bound and is excreted by the kidneys in a biologically active form.

SIDE-EFFECTS/ADVERSE REACTIONS
Single doses produce few side-effects. Occasionally, chills, fever, urticaria, dizziness, nausea, insomnia, and pain at the injection site have occurred. Repeated administration has infrequently resulted in decreased hemoglobin, hematocrit, and creatinine clearance and increased alkaline phosphatase, BUN, and SGPT. Reduced urine output has occurred on occasion.

CONTRAINDICATIONS AND PRECAUTIONS
Use of spectinomycin must be undertaken with caution in infants and young children, pregnant women and nursing mothers and in persons with a history of allergies. The drug is not indicated for the treatment of pharyngeal infections due to Neisseria gonorrhoeae, nor is it effective in treating syphilis. Use of spectinomycin may delay or mask the symptoms of incubating syphilis.

Vancomycin
(Lyphocin, Vancocin, Vancoled)

Vancomycin is a bactericidal glycopeptide antibiotic selectively active against gram-positive bacteria, such as streptococci, staphylococci (including penicillinase-producing), Clostridium difficile, Corynebacterium, and *Listeria.* In addition, it is bacteriostatic against enterococci. The potential for serious toxicity, however, limits its parenteral usefulness to treatment of life-threatening infections in patients allergic or unresponsive to less toxic antibacterial drugs. It may also be administered orally for treatment of staphylococcal enterocolitis and antibiotic-induced pseudomembranous colitis (for which it is generally considered to be the drug of choice), because it is poorly absorbed from the GI tract.

MECHANISM AND ACTIONS

Vancomycin inhibits bacterial cell wall synthesis by binding to precursors of the cell wall, such as the D-alanyl-D-alanine portion of the precursor units. The drug may also inhibit bacterial RNA synthesis and damage bacterial cytoplasmic membranes. There appears to be no cross-resistance between vancomycin and any other antibiotic.

USES

1. Treatment of serious staphylococcal infections (*e.g.*, endocarditis, septicemia, pneumonia, osteomyelitis) in patients who cannot tolerate or who do not respond to penicillins, cephalosporins, or other less toxic antibiotics (may be used alone or in conjunction with an aminoglycoside or rifampin)
2. Treatment of staphylococcal enterocolitis (oral use only)
3. Treatment of antibiotic-induced (*e.g.*, clindamycin, lincomycin) pseudomembranous colitis caused by *Clostridium difficile* (drug of choice)

ADMINISTRATION AND DOSAGE

Vancomycin is available as capsules (125 mg, 250 mg), powder for oral solution (1 g, 10 g) and powder for injection (500 mg/vial). The various dosage recommendations for the different indications are given below:

Oral
    Adults—500 mg every 6 hours or 1 g every 12 hours
    Children—40 mg/kg/day in divided doses, not to exceed 2 g/day
    Neonates—10 mg/kg/day in divided doses
IV
    Adults—500 mg every 6 hours or 1 g every 12 hours by slow IV infusion over at least 60 minutes
    Children—40 mg/kg/day in divided doses, added to fluids
    Infants/neonates—15 mg/kg initially, followed by 10 mg/kg every 12 hours

during the first week of life up to age 1 month
Prevention of bacterial endocarditis in penicillin-allergic patients undergoing dental procedures or upper respiratory tract surgery:
    Adults—1 g IV infused over 30 minutes to 60 minutes, ½ hour to 1 hour before surgery; then oral erythromycin 500 mg every 6 hours for eight doses
    Children—20 mg/kg IV infused over 30 minutes to 60 minutes as above; then 10 mg/kg oral erythromycin every 6 hours for eight doses
Prevention of bacterial endocarditis in penicillin-allergic patients undergoing GI or genitourinary surgery:
    Adults—1 g IV infused over 60 minutes *plus* 1.5 mg/kg gentamicin IM or IV concurrently 1 hour prior to procedure
    Children (less than 27 kg)—20 mg/kg IV slowly over 1 hour and 2 mg/kg gentamicin IM or IV concurrently 1 hour prior to procedure
Pseudomembranous colitis:
    Adults—500 mg to 2 g a day *orally* in divided doses every 6 hours to 8 hours for 7 days to 10 days

Dosage of vancomycin must be reduced in patients with renal impairment depending on the creatinine clearance or serum creatinine according to the package literature.

Oral and parenteral solutions are stable for 14 days if refrigerated following reconstitution. Refer to product information for a list of compatible diluents.

FATE

Vancomycin is poorly absorbed orally, although significant plasma levels have been noted following oral administration in patients with colitis. IV administration yields rapid attainment of effective serum levels. The elimination half-life is 4 hours to 8 hours in adults and 2 hours to 3 hours in children but increases in renal failure. The drug is widely distributed in the body, does not readily cross the blood–brain barrier, but penetrates into pleural, pericardial, ascitic, and synovial fluid in the presence of inflammation. Approximately 80% of the injected drug is excreted by the kidneys.

SIDE-EFFECTS/ADVERSE REACTIONS

Vancomycin is both nephrotoxic and ototoxic, and the risk of these toxicities is increased appreciably by large doses or prolonged therapy. Tinnitus and high-frequency hearing loss may be early indicators of ototoxicity. Deafness may progress despite cessation of treatment.

Too rapid IV administration may result in development of the "red-neck syndrome," characterized by a sudden, profound drop in blood pressure, often accompanied by fever, chills, and a maculopapular rash over the face, neck, upper chest, and extremities. Antihistamine fluids or corticosteroids may be useful in controlling the symptoms, which usually resolve within several hours.

IV administration of vancomycin has also resulted in dyspnea, wheezing, pruritus, hypotension, phlebitis, increased serum creatinine or BUN, and thrombocytopenia. Other adverse reactions attributed to vancomycin include nausea, urticaria, macular rashes, eosinophilia, reversible neutropenia, drug fever, and anaphylactic reactions. IM injection is not recommended, because tissue irritation and necrosis can occur. Fungal or bacterial overgrowth may occur, leading to secondary infections.

CONTRAINDICATIONS AND PRECAUTIONS

Vancomycin should not be used in combination with other nephrotoxic or ototoxic antibiotics (see under Interactions). A *cautious* approach to therapy is necessary in patients with renal impairment or hearing disturbances, in neonates, in pregnant women, in nursing mothers, and in elderly patients.

INTERACTIONS

1. Increased ototoxicity and nephrotoxicity can result from concurrent use of vancomycin with aminoglycosides, polymyxin B, colistin, amphotericin B, cisplatin, furosemide, and ethacrynic acid.
2. The action of vancomycin may be reduced by concurrent use of bacteriostatic antibiotics, for example, tetracyclines, erythromycins.
3. Antivertigo and antinausea drugs (*e.g.*, meclizine, dimenhydrinate, promethazine) may mask the ototoxic effects of vancomycin.

NURSING CONSIDERATIONS

A drug history, focusing on recent or concurrent use of nephrotoxic or otoxic antibiotics is essential. Use of antivertigo or antinausea drugs should be discontinued (see under Interactions). Baseline tests should include audiogram if hearing loss is suspected and testing of the eighth cranial nerve by tuning fork. Initial and periodic laboratory evaluation of renal and hepatic function, CBC with differential, and urinalysis should be done on all patients receiving the drug. Changes in laboratory values may be the first indication of hepatic dysfunction, nephrotoxicity, or blood dyscrasias.

If renal function is compromised, drug dose should be lowered and laboratory and clinical signs watched closely. Nephrotoxicity increases the risk of ototoxicity. Early signs of renal failure include proteinuria and casts in urine on urinalysis, elevated BUN, elevated serum creatinine levels, oliguria, weight gain, and evidence of flura retention. The physician should be notified at once if any of these symptoms occur, and the drug must be discontinued to prevent further damage.

Ototoxicity is characterized by tinnitus, roaring in the ears, and loss of high-pitch hearing which can be tested using a tuning fork. Periodic tests of hearing should be performed throughout therapy. The patient should be told to report any perceived change immediately, because even after the drug is discontinued hearing loss may progress.

Vancomycin is administered primarily by intermittent intravenous infusion but may be given by continuous infusion if necessary. Infusion rate should be carefully monitored by an infusion pump or other rate-control device to decrease the risk of "red-neck syndrome" (see under Side-Effects/Adverse Reactions). The IV site should be closely monitored for signs of phlebitis or extravasation characterized by pain, swelling, or redness, and the IV should be removed promptly should symptoms develop. Extravasation of the drug into the tissue may cause irritation and necrosis. Warm compresses should be applied continuously if infiltration occurs.

REVIEW QUESTIONS

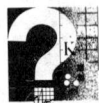

1. Against which organisms is chloramphenicol most effective? In what infection is it the drug of choice?
2. List the principal types of toxicity associated with chloramphenicol use. What routine monitoring techniques can be used to detect symptoms of toxicity early?
3. Why is a drug history essential before treatment with chloramphenicol commences? How will certain drugs affect therapy?

4. What type of organisms respond best to clindamycin?
5. Why is clindamycin generally preferred over lincomycin?
6. What are the major dangers associated with clindamycin and lincomycin?
7. How is clindamycin used topically?
8. What is the mechanism of action of clofazimine? Give its principal indications.
9. What are the principal indications for dapsone?
10. Describe the most common side-effect of dapsone. What is the "sulfone syndrome" observed with dapsone?
11. What laboratory data can help in early detection of side-effects from dapsone?
12. What is the principal use for furazolidone?
13. Why should alcohol be avoided during furazolidone therapy? Why should tyramine-containing foods be avoided as well?
14. Give the indications for hydroxystilbamidine.
15. Against what types of organisms is nitrofurazone most effective? How is the drug administered?
16. What is the mechanism of action of novobiocin? What organisms are most susceptible to novobiocin?
17. List the major adverse reactions with novobiocin.
18. What is the principal use for pentamidine? What other agent is also effective for this particular indication?
19. What is the danger of too rapid IV administration of pentamidine? How can the nurse plan close monitoring to catch this side-effect early?
20. Which organism is highly responsive to spectinomycin? What is the mechanism of action of this drug?
21. How does vancomycin exert its antibacterial action?
22. For what condition is vancomycin considered the drug of choice? List the other indications for vancomycin.
23. Briefly describe the major adverse effects associated with vancomycin.

BIBLIOGRAPHY

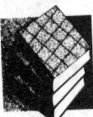

Bullock WE: *Mycobacterium leprae* (leprosy). In Mandell GL, Douglas RG, Bennett JE (eds): Principles and Practice of Infectious Disease, 2nd ed, p 1406. New York, John Wiley & Sons, 1985

Cook FV, Farrar WE: Vancomycin revisited. Ann Inter Med 88:813, 1978

Cunha BA, Ristuccia AM: Clinical usefulness of vancomycin. Clin Pharm 2:417, 1983

Dhawan VK, Thadepalli H: Clindamycin: A review of fifteen years of experience. Rev Infect Dis 4:1133, 1982

Farber BF, Moellering RC: Retrospective study of the toxicity of preparations of vancomycin from 1974 to 1981. Antimicrob Agents Chemother 23:138, 1983

Feder HM, Osler C, Maderazo FG: Chloramphenicol: A review of its use in clinical practice. Rev Infect Dis 3:479, 1981

Fekety R: Vancomycin. Med Clin North Am 66:175, 1982

Jacobson RR: The treatment of leprosy (Hansen's disease). Hosp Formulary 17:1076, 1982

Kucers A: Good antimicrobial prescribing: Chloramphenicol, erythromycin, vancomycin, tetracyclines. Lancet 2:425, 1982

Morer NA: New drugs: Hands-on experience. Am J Nurs 85:252, 1985

Perkins HR: Vancomycin and related antibiotics. Pharmacol Ther 16:181, 1982

Powell DA, Nahata MC: Chloramphenicol: A new perspective on an old drug. Drug Intell Clin Pharm 16:295, 1982

Scherer P: New drugs: Hands-on experience, Part 1. Am J Nurs 87:448, 1987

Schietinger H: A home care plan for AIDS. Am J Nurs 86:1021, 1986

Sharpe SM: Pentamidine and hypoglycenia. Ann Intern Med 99:128, 1983

Smith AL, Weber A: Pharmacology of chloramphenicol. Pediatr Clin North Am 30:209, 1983

Steigbigel NH: Erythromycin, lincomycin and clindamycin. In Mandell GL, Douglas RG, Bennett JE (eds): Principles and Practice of Infectious Diseases, 2nd ed, p 224. New York, John Wiley & Sons, 1985

Waters MF: New approaches to chemotherapy for leprosy. Drugs 26:465, 1983

World Health Organization (WHO) Study Group: Chemotherapy of leprosy for control programs. WHO Technical Report, Series No. 675, WHO, Geneva, 1982, p 7

Antitubercular Drugs

69

Tuberculosis, an infection caused by *Mycobacterium tuberculosis*, is characterized by severe inflammation, tissue necrosis, and frequently by the development of open cavities in the lungs, all of which can impair pulmonary function. In some cases, the offending pathogen gains access to the blood or lymph, and the infection may spread to other body tissues as well. Transmission of the disease is usually by inhalation of droplets of cough from infected persons.

Mycobacteria are strict aerobes and therefore must have an oxygen-rich environment to survive. Because of this, infections most commonly occur in the lungs, but may also occur in other tissues with high oxygen tension, such as the kidneys, CNS, and the ends of long bones. The disease progresses through several stages. The initial infection occurs in the lungs as a consequence of inhaling droplets of cough containing live organisms from persons with active tuberculosis. In the alveoli, the organisms are phagocytized and begin to multiply. These organisms may either remain in the lungs or be carried to other sites in the body by the lymphatic system and the bloodstream. An inflammatory reaction develops in response to the presence of the bacilli, and local necrosis can occur as cellular immunity reactions attempt to isolate the infection. *Severe* necrosis may result in the development of large cavities in the lungs, which can greatly compromise respiratory function.

A person is considered infected with the tubercle bacilli upon its entrance into the body. If the body's immune system successfully checks the invasion, there are usually no symptoms and the person appears healthy. The clinical disease becomes apparent with the onset of symptoms such as cough, malaise, weight loss, and night sweats and is usually diagnosed by chest x-ray and confirmed by the presence of the organism in the sputum.

Current chemotherapy for tuberculosis is very effective, provided strict patient compliance can be ensured, but it may be complex, difficult, and prolonged. Infections tend to be chronic, and the microorganisms can exhibit extended periods of inactivity, making complete eradication difficult. The pathogen rapidly develops resistance to single-drug antitubercular therapy and, perhaps even more serious, increasing numbers of bacterial strains are proving resistant to some multiple-drug regimens. To minimize the emergence of resistant strains, therefore, antitubercular agents are almost always administered as combinations of two or three drugs. Moreover, combination therapy allows use of lower doses of each individual drug than would be required if each were used alone, thereby reducing the likelihood of adverse effects.

Antitubercular drugs vary markedly, both in efficacy and toxicity, and based on the differences, may be divided into first-line drugs and second-line drugs. The first-line drugs are almost always used to initiate treatment of a newly diagnosed infection, inasmuch as they are the most dependable and least toxic agents when employed in low to moderate dose combination therapy. Second-line drugs, on the other hand, are often less effective and usually more toxic than the first-line drugs, and thus are reserved for treatment of resistant infections. Classification of the available antitubercular drugs is as follows:

First-line drugs
· ethambutol
· isoniazid (INH)
· rifampin
· streptomycin

Second-line drugs
· aminosalicylic acid and salts
· capreomycin
· cycloserine
· ethionamide
· pyrazinamide

Note: Some references group the antitubercular agents into three categories, that is, primary (isoniazid, rifampin), secondary (ethambutol, pyrazinamide, streptomycin), and tertiary (aminosalicylic acid, capreomycin, cycloserine, ethionamide).

Treatment of an active case of tuberculosis is almost always initiated with isoniazid (INH), the most active antitubercular drug, usually in combination with rifampin, both given in single daily doses. These agents are bactericidal and are capable of sterilizing the tuberculous lesions. Clinical effectiveness (*i.e.*, cessation of *Mycobacterium tuberculosis* growth in culture of sputum) is usually demonstrated within 1 month with this regimen. However, approximately one fourth of these patients show laboratory evidence of impaired liver function, and about 5% of these persons develop symptoms (nausea, anorexia, vomiting, jaundice). Although liver function usually returns to normal with continued therapy, the drug regimen should be discontinued if the above symptoms persist.

Other treatment regimens used successfully are (1) INH–rifampin for 20 weeks followed by INH–ethambutol for 12 months following sputum conversion; (2) INH–streptomycin–ethambutol initially, followed by INH–ethambutol for 18 months to 24 months; and (3) INH–ethambutol–rifampin for 2 months to 3 months, then INH–ethambutol for 18 months to 24 months.

Although para-aminosalicylic acid (PAS) was formerly widely used with INH, it is poorly tolerated by many patients, and the GI distress resulting from the large doses that are required reduced patient compliance. PAS is still a valuable adjunctive drug, but, as indicated above, it has been replaced in many INH drug regimens by ethambutol or rifampin. Streptomycin is likewise an effective antitubercular drug, but it must be given only in combination with other drugs such as INH, PAS, ethambutol, and rifampin, because resistance develops rapidly. It is used primarily for extensive pulmonary or disseminated tuberculosis. The second-line drugs, because of their toxicity, are indicated only where treatment with the first-line drugs has failed. In addition, pyrazinamide is only effective for approximately 2 months and should not be continued for longer periods of time.

Resistance to antitubercular drugs is variable. Nearly 5% of patients do not respond to INH, and nearly 10% of patients do not show adequate response to one or more of the other drugs. However, less than 0.5% of patients do not respond to rifampin.

A *short-course regimen* consisting of a 9-month course of therapy with INH (15 mg/kg) plus rifampin (600 mg) has been recommended as an alternative in adults with previously untreated, uncomplicated pulmonary tuberculosis. Patients with extrapulmonary tuberculosis or who have received previous therapy for tuberculosis are not considered candidates for the short-course regimen.

Prophylaxis of Tuberculosis

Administration of INH for 1 year at a daily dose of 300 mg (10 mg/kg for children) can prevent active tuberculosis and reduce morbidity in treated persons. Not only is the risk of active disease reduced, but the spread of the disease to uninfected persons is diminished. Persons with fibrotic chest lesions taking INH for 6 months to 12 months showed a 65% to 95% reduction in the development of active tuberculosis. However, *generalized* prophylaxis of tuberculosis is subject to controversy, inasmuch as INH is potentially hepatotoxic. Candidates for chemoprophylaxis of tuberculosis with INH fall into one of the following categories:

1. Household members and close associates of those with recently diagnosed tuberculosis or those in high-risk groups, such as immigrants from Southeast Asia
2. Tuberculin reactors with radiographic evidence of nonprogressive, healed, or quiescent lesions without positive bacteriologic findings
3. Persons whose tuberculin reaction has become positive within the last 2 years
4. Tuberculin reactors at increased risk, such as persons with diabetes, leukemia, Hodgkin's disease, postgastrectomy, and persons receiving immunosuppressive or prolonged glucocorticoid therapy
5. Positive tuberculin reactors under 35 years of age

■ Nursing Process for Patients Receiving Antitubercular Drugs

□ ASSESSMENT

□ Subjective Data
A complete drug history is essential because many of the antitubercular drugs adversely interact with other drugs which may pose potential problems given the projected length of therapy. Refer to the Interaction sections of each drug for specific guidelines. Most of the drugs adversely interact with alcohol; consequently, the extent of alcohol use needs to be explored. Chronic alcohol abuse is a statistical factor of noncompliance with antitubercular therapy. The patient identified as a potential chronic abuser may need close monitoring and frequent clinical follow-up.

Nurses need to be aware of populations which appear at risk for development of tuberculosis. In addition to alcoholics, these include frail elderly patients in nursing homes, residents of single-room hotels or boarding houses in inner cities, and recent immigrants from Southeast Asia.

The patient's perception of the disease will affect treatment success and should be discussed. Many people think of tuberculosis as a disease of poor, unclean people, and it carries great stigma. Perceptions of illness may reflect compliance patterns; the patient may choose to ignore the disease and the required drug therapy, may accept both and begin incorporating the change into his life, or become depressed by the prospect of long-term care and respond by acting in a dependent or passive manner. Thorough discussion of the disease process, the drug therapy, and the potential outcome of successful therapy may help the patient gain perspective, control, and a willingness to participate.

Alcohol use and perception of illness are only two factors that will influence compliance. Any long-term therapy that relies on consistent drug taking has the potential for failure simply because patients may, at times, forget to take the drugs. Memory may be faulty or a workday so busy that the drug is forgotten. By asking several nonjudgmental questions such as "Lots of people sometimes forget to take their medicine. How often does this happen to you?" the nurse may uncover a patient who may have such difficulty.

Exposure of family members or significant others to the disease should be assessed. All others in close contact or in the same household with the patient need to be tested and will probably need chemoprophylaxis for tuberculosis. If such is the case, resources also need to be explored to determine how such long-term drug therapy will be financed and what community resources can be utilized for follow-up.

□ Objective Data
Regardless of the drug used, physical assessment should be completed on the respiratory system noting lung sounds in all lobes. Baseline assessment of renal and hepatic function is also important because these sites may become compromised in long-term therapy.

Laboratory and diagnostic data for all patients undergoing antitubercular drug therapy should include liver enzymes, bilirubin, BUN, serum creatinine, urinalysis, sputum culture and sensitivity, and chest x-rays. A tuberculin skin test using purified protein derivative (PPD) may also be completed if the chest x-ray and cultures are not definitive. However, a PPD is contraindicated if active tuberculosis is strongly suspected because the local reaction to the test may be severe enough to cause tissue necrosis.

□ NURSING DIAGNOSIS
Actual nursing diagnoses for the patient receiving antitubercular drugs may include:
   Knowledge deficit related to the actions, administration, and side-effects of the drug
   Alteration in respiratory function related to disease process although symptoms may vary
   Potential for infection of family members or

close contacts related to the mode of disease transmission (airborne droplets)
Potential nursing diagnoses may include:
   Noncompliance with a prolonged drug regimen
   Disturbance in self-concept: body image, related to the "stigma" of the disease

□ PLAN
Nursing care goals focus on:
1. Safe, correct administration while the patient is hospitalized (usually brief or not at all except in severe cases)
2. Teaching the patient:
   a. Safe drug-taking techniques including mcmory joggers to establish the habit
   b. How to monitor and manage side-effects and which ones to report
   c. The importance of follow-up visits
   d. Inclusion of nutritious diet to facilitate healing process

□ INTERVENTION
Patients need to know the sequence of drug taking (daily or several times a week) and must incorporate it as part of a daily routine. The primary cause of treatment failure with antitubercular drugs is that the drugs were not taken, and the primary cause of the development of resistant strains is insufficient dose. Memory joggers may be used, such as a calendar or drug box, or drug taking can be attached to a morning routine, such as brushing teeth. However, some patients will not remember to take the drug because of impaired memory, alcohol abuse, or mental status changes. These patients may require a daily home health visit or may have to be taken to a clinic on a daily or twice weekly basis to ensure the drug is taken. The cost of such follow-up is substantially less than the cost of treating the individual for diffuse tuberculosis. Statistically, the patient who is most likely to be noncompliant with antitubercular therapy is the single, unemployed, inner city, male alcoholic.

The nurse needs to follow even patients who seem willing to comply because most individuals will occasionally forget to take any drug. The patient on antitubercular therapy needs the support of a consistent care giver and needs to have a regular resource available to respond to questions and deal with potential drug side-effects (see individual drug monographs).

All patients should follow a nutritious, well-balanced diet with adequate calorie intake. Any infectious process increases metabolism and the body's need for food. The drug therapy will only be successful if the body can successfully fight the infection, and, because the course of tuberculosis is slow, optimum nutritional status must be maintained. Vitamin supplements may be necessary; dieting during the course of drug therapy should be discouraged.

Family members and close contacts who have been identified as candidates for chemoprophylaxis also need follow-up and close monitoring. Compliance in this group may be even more difficult because few are likely to show any symptoms of the disease at the onset of treatment. Chest x-ray and PPD screening may be completed periodically to determine the development of symptoms, and are sometimes the first indication that the individual has not continued with drug therapy.

□ *EVALUATION*
The outcome criteria used to judge successful antitubercular drug therapy include evidence of infection resolution on chest x-ray and in sputum cultures. Other criteria may include evidence that the patient understands the rationale for drug therapy, the reason for a prolonged course of treatment, and the consequences of early drug discontinuation. Further criteria of treatment success include timely renewal of prescriptions for the duration of therapy and attendance at appointed clinic follow-up visits.

First-Line Drugs

Isoniazid

(Laniazid, Nydrazid, Teebaconin)

A first-line drug of choice for most cases of active tuberculosis, isoniazid (INH) is usually prescribed in combination with ethambutol or rifampin, or both, to delay the emergence of resistant strains. It is also indicated for prophylactic use in high-risk patients, as outlined above. A major danger associated with INH is severe and sometimes fatal hepatitis. The risk of developing hepatitis increases with advancing age (see under Side-Effects/Adverse Reactions), which is why *prophylaxis* with INH is not recommended in those over 35 years of age.

MECHANISM AND ACTIONS
INH is bactericidal against actively multiplying organisms and probably interferes with lipid and nucleic acid synthesis in the growing organisms. The drug also can produce a vitamin B_6 (pyridoxine)

deficiency, presumably by competing for an enzyme necessary for its production. Primary resistance of the *Mycobacterium tuberculosis* organism to INH occurs in up to 5% of patients but may be much higher in certain populations, such as Asians and Hispanics.

USES
1. Treatment of all forms of active tuberculosis due to susceptible organisms, usually in combination with other tuberculostatic drugs
2. Prophylaxis in high-risk patients, such as those groups outlined in the introduction to this chapter

ADMINISTRATION AND DOSAGE
INH is usually administered orally as tablets (50 mg, 100 mg, 300 mg) but is also available for IM injection (100 mg/ml). For treating active tuberculosis, the recommended adult dose is 5 mg/kg/day in a single dose to a maximum of 300 mg/day. Children are given 10 mg to 20 mg/kg/day in a single daily dose to a maximum of 500 mg/day. Preventive therapy is undertaken with a single daily dose of 300 mg in adults and 10 mg/kg/day in children.

The drug is preferably taken on an empty stomach but may be administered with food to decrease GI upset. Pyridoxine (Vitamin B_6), 15 mg to 50 mg daily, is generally given concurrently to minimize the danger of peripheral neuropathy (see below), especially in malnourished, alcoholic, or uremic patients. Fixed combinations of INH and pyridoxine in various doses are available (Teebaconin and Vitamin B_6, P-I-N Forte) and INH and rifampin as Rifamate or Rimactane/INH Dual Pack are also available.

FATE
INH is rapidly and completely absorbed from the GI tract, but absorption is reduced by food. Peak blood levels occur within 1 hour to 2 hours but decline to 50% or less within 6 hours. The drug is widely distributed in the body, including cerebrospinal, pleural, and ascitic fluids as well as other tissues and organs. Less than one half of a dose is excreted unchanged in the urine; most of the remainder is acetylated or hydrolyzed by the liver, and metabolites are removed by the kidney. The rate of acetylation is genetically determined and may be slow (in approximately 50% of blacks and whites) or rapid (rest of blacks and whites as well as most Orientals and Eskimos). However, the rate of acetylation does not alter the clinical efficacy of

INH, but it may influence its toxicity (*i.e.*, slow acetylators are more prone to elevated blood levels and increased toxic reactions, including peripheral neuropathies; rapid acetylators are more likely to develop hepatitis). Liver disease can prolong clearance of INH.

SIDE-EFFECTS/ADVERSE REACTIONS
The most frequently encountered adverse effects with INH are numbness and tingling in the extremities, the incidence of which is dose-dependent and which occurs to a greater extent in malnourished, diabetic, alcoholic, or elderly patients. Transient elevations in serum transaminase levels (SGOT, SGPT) occur in up to 25% of patients within the first 4 months to 6 months of therapy but generally return to normal with continued treatment. Occasionally, progressive liver damage occurs, especially in older patients.

Severe and occasionally fatal hepatitis has developed, usually with prolonged therapy. The risk is greatest in patients between ages 50 and 65 and is increased with daily consumption of alcohol. Early symptoms include fatigue, malaise, weakness, anorexia, or vomiting.

Other adverse reactions occurring less frequently with INH include:
- CNS—Optic neuritis, toxic encephalopathy, memory impairment, toxic psychosis, convulsions
- GI—Nausea, vomiting, epigastric distress
- Hepatic—Bilirubinemia, bilirubinuria, jaundice
- Hematologic—Hemolytic or aplastic anemia, agranulocytosis, eosinophilia, thrombocytopenia
- Allergic—Fever, skin rashes (morbilliform, maculopapular, purpuric, exfoliative), vasculitis, lymphadenopathy
- Other—Vitamin B$_6$ deficiency, hyperglycemia, metabolic acidosis, gynecomastia, pellagra, rheumatoid or systemic lupus-like symptoms, irritation at IM injection site

CONTRAINDICATIONS AND PRECAUTIONS
Patients with acute liver disease should not be given INH, nor should persons who have demonstrated severe adverse reactions to a previous course of therapy with INH. The drug must be used with *caution* in patients with chronic liver disease, renal dysfunction, diabetes, a history of allergic reactions, convulsive disorders, psychoses,

in alcoholics and in pregnant women or nursing mothers.

Overdosage is characterized initially by nausea, vomiting, dizziness, slurred speech, blurred vision, and visual hallucinations. Marked overdosage may be associated with CNS and respiratory depression, stupor, severe seizures, metabolic acidosis, hyperglycemia, and coma. Fatalities have occurred. Treatment includes gastric lavage (within the first 2 hours to 3 hours), anticonvulsants (*e.g.*, diazepam IV) followed by IV pyridoxine, control of metabolic acidosis (*e.g.*, sodium bicarbonate IV), and forced osmotic diuresis. Hemodialysis may be indicated in very severe cases.

INTERACTIONS
1. INH can increase serum levels of phenytoin by reducing its metabolism.
2. The efficacy of INH may be reduced when given concurrently with corticosteroids.
3. Alcohol increases the risk of INH-induced hepatitis.
4. INH can potentiate the pharmacologic and toxicologic effects of carbamazepine and benzodiazepine antianxiety agents, possibly by inhibiting their hepatic metabolism.
5. Antacids reduce GI absorption of INH if they are given together.
6. Disulfiram and INH can impair coordination and produce behavioral changes.
7. Concurrent use of INH and rifampin may increase the likelihood of hepatotoxicity, while combined use of INH and cycloserine can increase CNS toxicity.
8. INH may exhibit MAO inhibitory activity and can potentiate sympathomimetic amines, leading to increased blood pressure (see Chap. 29).
9. INH has been reported to potentiate anesthetics, anticoagulants, anticonvulsants, antidiabetics, antihypertensives, antiparkinsonian agents, anticholinergics, antidepressants, narcotics, and sedatives, although the clinical importance of these potential interactions has not been definitely established.

NURSING CONSIDERATIONS
(See also Nursing Process for Patients Receiving Antitubercular Drugs.)

A drug history is important because INH potentiates the action of many drugs such as anticoagulants, anticonvulsants, antidiabetics, antihypertensives, and antiparkinsonian drugs among others. Consequently, patients taking these drugs while on INH need closer monitoring and may need dosage adjustments. For example, the diabetic patient may need a dosage adjustment in antidiabetic medication because INH can elevate serum blood sugar as well as potentiate the action of the antidiabetic drug taken.

Throughout therapy the patient should have periodic neurologic examinations testing for vision changes and peripheral neuropathy. Vision changes are characterized by scotoma, blurring, and eye pain. Peripheral neuropathies are characterized by numbness, tingling, weakness or pain in hands, fingers, feet, or toes. Sensation must be tested to determine gradual changes. Neurotoxicity may be prevented by administering vitamin B_6 to all patients receiving INH and by closely monitoring patients who are diabetic, malnourished, or "slow" acetylators of INH (see under Fate) because they are more likely to develop neurotoxicity.

Monthly liver function studies are also essential because hepatic dysfunction and hepatitis may occur. Although some transient elevations of liver enzymes may be expected, patients should be told to report immediately any symptoms such as anorexia, malaise, nausea, vomiting, darkening of the urine, paresthesias, or jaundice. The drug must be discontinued and alternative therapy employed. Patients on INH who are at higher risk for the development of liver dysfunction and hepatitis are the elderly, the alcoholic, and individuals who are known to be "rapid" acetylators of INH. If the patient develops liver dysfunction, drug toxicity may occur. (See symptoms and treatment of overdosage under Contraindications and Precautions.)

Oral INH should be taken on an empty stomach with water to facilitate absorption. Food can be taken if gastrointestinal problems develop during drug therapy, but absorption will be slowed. Milk and antacids should not be taken simultaneously with the drug because they may reduce absorption. Intramuscular administration of INH should be avoided if possible. Injections are irritating and painful. Sites must be rotated using a body map to ensure planned rotation, but because the drug must be given in a large muscle mass, rotation sites are limited and an alternative drug route may be needed.

Rifampin

(Rifadin, Rimactane)

A derivative of the antibiotic rifamycin B, rifampin is a first-line bacteriostatic antitubercular drug. It is most often used in combination with INH and ethambutol, because resistance can develop rapidly if it is given alone. The drug should be taken on an uninterrupted schedule, because intermittent therapy has resulted in the more frequent occurrence of adverse effects, especially a "flu-like" syndrome (see below).

MECHANISMS AND ACTIONS

Rifampin inhibits DNA-dependent RNA polymerase activity in mycobacterial cells, blocking nucleic acid chain formation. The drug can inhibit the growth of most gram-positive bacteria as well as many gram-negative microorganisms. There appears to be no cross-resistance with other antitubercular drugs.

USES

1. Treatment of pulmonary tuberculosis in conjunction with at least one other tuberculostatic drug (*e.g.*, INH or ethambutol)
2. Treatment of asymptomatic carriers of *Neisseria meningitidis* to eliminate meningococci from the nasopharynx (*not* indicated for meningococcal infections)
3. Investigational uses include treatment of staphylococcal infections, legionnaire's disease not responsive to erythromycin, gram-negative bacteremia in infancy, leprosy (with dapsone), and prophylaxis of *Hemophilus* meningitis.

ADMINISTRATION AND DOSAGE

Rifampin is used orally as capsules (150 mg, 300 mg). In treating pulmonary tuberculosis, adults should receive 600 mg once daily, while children may be given 10 mg to 20 mg/kg not to exceed 600 mg a day.

For treating meningococcal carriers, the above doses are given daily for four consecutive days. The drug is not indicated in children under age 5. For patients unable to swallow capsules, an oral suspension may be prepared from the capsules, using simple syrup according to package directions. The suspension is stable for up to 6 weeks if refrigerated.

FATE

Rifampin is almost completely absorbed orally and achieves peak plasma levels within 1 hour to 4 hours. Absorption is slowed by the presence of food. The drug is widely distributed throughout the body and is approximately 75% protein bound. Rifampin is metabolized in the liver to an active metabolite and is excreted both as the metabolite in the bile (40%) and urine (30%–60%) as well as the intact drug. Dosage adjustment is necessary in patients with hepatic dysfunction but not in patients with renal impairment. The half-life varies from 1.5 hours to 5 hours but is progressively shortened during the initial weeks of therapy due to microsomal enzyme induction which accelerates the drugs metabolism.

SIDE-EFFECTS/ADVERSE REACTIONS
The most often encountered side-effects with rifampin are elevation of liver enzymes, rash, and mild GI distress. Use of larger doses on an intermittent schedule (*i.e.*, less than twice weekly) is frequently associated with development of a "flu-like" syndrome marked by fever, chills, and myalgia, but which may also lead to eosinophilia, thrombocytopenia, hemolytic anemia, and shock. Intermittent therapy may also result in hemoglobinuria, hematuria, renal insufficiency, and acute renal failure. A number of other adverse reactions have occurred during rifampin therapy and are listed below:

GI—Anorexia, vomiting, diarrhea, cramping, flatulence, sore mouth, pancreatitis, pseudomembranous colitis

CNS—Headache, drowsiness, fatigue, dizziness, ataxia, confusion, visual disturbances, muscle weakness, generalized numbness, hearing disturbances

Allergic—Pruritus, urticaria, flushing, acneiform lesions, fever

Hepatic/renal—Hepatitis, proteinuria

Hematologic—"flu-like" syndrome (described above), transient leukopenia, thrombocytopenia, decreased hemoglobin, hemolytic anemia, eosinophilia

Other—Conjunctivitis, elevated serum uric acid, menstrual irregularities, osteomalacia, myopathy

Rifampin may impart an orange-red color to urine, feces, sputum, saliva, and tears; this reaction is not harmful.

Overdosage is characterized by nausea, vomiting, lethargy, liver enlargement, jaundice, and loss of consciousness. Antiemetics may control the nausea and vomiting, and gastric lavage can remove unabsorbed drug. Forced diuresis will promote excretion, but bile drainage may be indicated in the presence of serious liver impairment.

CONTRAINDICATIONS AND PRECAUTIONS
Rifampin is *not* recommended for intermittent therapy, and interruption of the daily dosage regimen should be avoided. The use of rifampin should be undertaken *cautiously* in the presence of hepatic or renal disease, in alcoholics, in pregnant women, and in nursing mothers. Because the effectiveness of oral contraceptives may be reduced by rifampin (see under Interactions), the drug should be given cautiously to women of childbearing potential taking contraceptive drugs. As indicated above, the importance of taking rifampin on a continual basis must be stressed to minimize the likelihood of adverse effects.

INTERACTIONS
1. Rifampin induces microsomal enzymes and thus may decrease the effects of other drugs metabolized by these liver enzymes, for example, oral anticoagulants, oral contraceptives, estrogens, progestins, metoprolol, propranolol, quinidine, clofibrate, corticosteroids, oral antidiabetics, and methadone.
2. PAS administered concurrently can impair GI absorption of rifampin and can reduce rifampin serum levels.
3. The action of rifampin can be potentiated by probenecid or isoniazid which compete for hepatic uptake.
4. Concomitant use of rifampin and alcohol may increase the incidence of hepatotoxicity.
5. Rifampin may interfere with standard assays for serum folate and vitamin B_{12}.

NURSING CONSIDERATIONS
(See also Nursing Process for Patients Receiving Antitubercular Drugs.)

Oral administration of rifampin to children or adults exposed to meningococcal or *Hemophilus influenzae* meningitis may be preceded by a nasopharyngeal or throat culture. However, if exposure is verified by history, the drug will be given before cultures return. Oral doses to young children may be given in a syrup as described under Dosage and Administration. If syrup is not available, the capsule can be opened and the drug can be given in applesauce or ice chips. It is unstable in juice or water.

In general, for treatment of tuberculosis, the drug should be taken on an empty stomach because food may delay absorption. However, small amounts of food can be used if gastrointestinal distress occurs during therapy.

A drug history should be obtained before treatment begins because rifampin can decrease the effects of oral anticoagulants, oral antidiabetics, propranolol, and steroids among others, necessitating close monitoring and possible dosage adjustments during the course of therapy. Rifampin also decreases the effectiveness of estrogen and progestin drugs, including oral contraceptives. Consequently, the woman who uses them as a birth control method needs to use an alternative during the course of drug therapy.

The most serious side-effect of rifampin is liver dysfunction, which may take several forms. Monthly liver function studies should be completed throughout therapy to monitor the development of elevations, and patients should be told to immediately report symptoms of jaundice, pruritus, darkened urine, or light-colored stools. Alcoholics are at great risk of hepatotoxicity from rifampin. Liver dysfunction may also occur if the patient takes the drug intermittently rather than on the regular schedule as prescribed. Intermittent dosing may result in the flu-like syndrome described under Side-Effects/Adverse Reactions, but is a signal of impending hepatic dysfunction.

Allergic rash is a common side-effect of rifampin. Patients should be told to report pruritus, urticaria, fever, or rash because drug hypersensitivity may develop, necessitating drug withdrawal.

Hematologic function must also be tested periodically to detect blood dyscrasias. The patient should also be taught to report immediately fever, sore throat, weakness, or unusual bleeding or bruising—all possible indications of blood dyscrasias.

Patients should also be told that urine, feces, saliva, sputum, sweat, and tears may take on a harmless red-orange color that will disappear when the drug therapy is complete.

Ethambutol

(Myambutol)

A synthetic, orally administered tuberculostatic drug effective against actively dividing mycobacteria, ethambutol is a first-line drug for treatment of pulmonary tuberculosis. It is most often used in combination with INH, with or without rifampin or streptomycin, depending on the severity of the condition because it is somewhat less active alone than other first-line drugs. Previously unexposed microorganisms are uniformly sensitive to ethambutol, but resistance does develop in a stepwise manner. Ethambutol may have adverse effects on visual acuity, thus, monthly eye examinations are recommended during therapy.

MECHANISM AND ACTIONS
Ethambutol enters actively growing mycobacterial cells and may inhibit the synthesis of one or more metabolites, thus arresting multiplication, impairing cell metabolism, and causing cell death. There is no apparent cross-resistance with other antitubercular agents. Bacterial resistance is unpredictable and appears to develop slowly.

USES
1. Treatment of pulmonary tuberculosis, in combination with at least one other antituberculosis drug

ADMINISTRATION AND DOSAGE
Available preparations of ethambutol are 100-mg and 400-mg tablets. In patients who have not received previous antituberculosis therapy, the recommended dose is 15 mg/kg as a single oral dose every 24 hours in conjunction with a single daily dose of isoniazid.

In patients who have received previous antimycobacterial drug therapy, retreatment is accomplished with 25 mg/kg as a single daily dose in combination with another antitubercular drug. After 60 days, the dose may be reduced to 15 mg/kg/day.

FATE
Ethambutol is adequately absorbed orally, and absorption is unaffected by the presence of food. Peak serum levels occur in 2 hours to 4 hours and fall to minimal levels within 24 hours. The serum half-life is approximately 3 hours to 4 hours. During the 24 hour period, approximately 20% of a dose is metabolized by the liver. Nearly one-half of the unchanged drug is excreted in the urine, 20% to 25% is eliminated unchanged in the feces, and 10% to 15% is excreted as metabolites by the kidney.

SIDE-EFFECTS/ADVERSE REACTIONS
Untoward reactions with daily doses of 15 mg/kg are infrequent. Diminished visual acuity may occur, but the incidence and severity are related to the dose and duration of therapy. These changes, presumably due to optic neuritis, may be unilateral or bilateral, and changes in color perception are usually the first sign of toxicity. The effects are generally reversible upon drug discontinuation, but complete reversal may require months. Other adverse effects are:

CNS—Fever, malaise, headache, dizziness, confusion, disorientation, paresthesias, hallucinations

GI—Abdominal pain, GI upset, vomiting, anorexia

Allergic—Pruritus, dermatitis, joint pain, anaphylactic reactions

Other—Elevated serum uric acid, acute gout, transient impairment of liver function, epidermal necrolysis, thrombocytopenia

CONTRAINDICATIONS AND PRECAUTIONS
Use of ethambutol is not recommended in patients with optic neuritis or in children under age 12. The drug should be used with *caution* in patients with hepatic or renal dysfunction, hyperuricemia, or acute gout, and in pregnant women. Periodic eye examinations should be performed during therapy with ethambutol.

INTERACTIONS
1. Ethambutol may reduce the effectiveness of uricosuric drugs such as probenecid and sulfinpyrazone.
2. Aluminum-containing antacids may impair oral absorption of ethambutol.

NURSING CONSIDERATIONS
(See also Nursing Process for Patients Receiving Antitubercular Drugs.)

Baseline liver enzymes and uric acid level should be performed before therapy begins and monitored periodically. Although transient elevation of liver enzymes may occur, ethambutol can cause liver dysfunction in susceptible patients such as the elderly and the alcoholic.

The main side-effect of the drug is a change in vision. A baseline ophthalmic examination, including testing of color vision, is important. Periodic checks of visual acuity, color vision, and field of vision will help detect problems early. In addition to changes in color vision, other early symptoms may include scotoma, eye pain, and blurring.

Because the drug absorption is not affected by food, ethambutol can be taken with a meal to decrease gastrointestinal distress.

Streptomycin

An aminoglycoside antibiotic effective against *Mycobacterium tuberculosis*, streptomycin is considered a primary drug. It is most often used in combination with INH, rifampin, or ethambutol for control of more severe infections. Resistance develops rapidly; hence, combination therapy is necessary to maintain effectiveness. It is administered IM only, thus, patient compliance during prolonged therapy may be poor. The principal danger associated with use of streptomycin is ototoxicity,

both vestibular and auditory, and patients receiving the drug must be observed carefully. Streptomycin has been discussed in detail in Chapter 65, and only those aspects of its use in treating tuberculosis are discussed here.

The action of streptomycin is to suppress, not eradicate, the tubercle bacillus, presumably because the drug does not readily enter living cells. When used alone, up to 80% of patients demonstrate some degree of resistance to streptomycin, and the longer therapy is continued, the greater the incidence of resistance.

Streptomycin is given by IM injection. The usual regimen is 1 g streptomycin together with an appropriate dose of additional antitubercular drugs, such as INH, ethambutol, or rifampin. The dose of streptomycin should be reduced to 1 g two or three times a week as symptoms improve. Smaller doses should be used in elderly patients or in patients with impaired renal function. (Refer to Chap. 65 for a complete discussion of streptomycin.)

Second-Line Drugs

Aminosalicylate Sodium
(P.A.S. Sodium, Teebacin)

Aminosalicylate sodium is the sodium salt of para-aminosalicylic acid (PAS) and contains 73% aminosalicylic acid equivalent and 10.9% sodium. It is used in combination with isoniazid, rifampin, or streptomycin to delay the emergence of bacterial resistance to these first-line antitubercular drugs. PAS should never be used as the sole therapeutic agent in treating tuberculosis.

MECHANISM AND ACTION
Aminosalicylate sodium is bacteriostatic against *Mycobacterium tuberculosis*. The drug is a structural analogue of para-aminobenzoic acid, and its mechanism of action is similar to that of the sulfonamides; that is, it appears to inhibit mycobacterial folic acid synthesis by competing with enzyme systems for incorporation of para-aminobenzoic acid. Resistant strains do emerge during aminosalicylic acid therapy, but much more slowly than with streptomycin.

USES
1. Adjunctive treatment of tuberculosis, in combination with other antitubercular drugs (PAS is a second-line drug that is occasionally

used as a part of the regimen, possibly to delay the onset of resistance to first-line drugs.)

ADMINISTRATION AND DOSAGE
Aminosalicylate sodium is used as tablets containing either 0.5 g or 1 g. A powder is also available. Adult dosage is 14 g to 16 g a day in two or three divided doses. Children are given 275 mg to 420 mg/kg/day in three or four divided doses. If solutions are used, they must be protected from heat and moisture because they are very unstable and should be used within 24 hours of mixing.

FATE
The drug is readily absorbed from the GI tract and widely distributed in the body, concentrating in pleural tissue. The half-life is approximately 1 hour. Aminosalicylate sodium is metabolized in the liver, primarily by acetylation, and excreted through the kidneys as both metabolites and free acid.

SIDE-EFFECTS/ADVERSE REACTIONS
The most common side-effects encountered with aminosalicylate sodium are nausea, diarrhea, abdominal pain, and vomiting. Other adverse reactions include fever, skin rash, malaise, joint pain, infectious mononucleosis-like syndrome, jaundice, hepatitis, pancreatitis, blood dyscrasias (leukopenia, agranulocytosis, thrombocytopenia), hemolytic anemia, goiter, encephalopathy, vasculitis, and Löffler's syndrome. Crystalluria can occur at high doses.

Aminosalicylate sodium deteriorates rapidly in the presence of heat, light, or water. A brownish or purplish color indicates deterioration, and such products should not be used.

CONTRAINDICATIONS AND PRECAUTIONS
Aminosalicylate sodium should not be used in persons with a known salicylate hypersensitivity and must be given with *caution* to persons with impaired renal or hepatic function, gastric ulcers, congestive heart failure, and other situations requiring sodium restriction.

INTERACTIONS
1. PAS plasma levels may be increased by probenecid, salicylates, or sulfinpyrazone.
2. PAS may decrease absorption of rifampin, folic acid, and vitamin B_{12}.
3. PAS may increase INH plasma levels by reducing its rate of metabolism.
4. Urinary acidifiers (*e.g.*, ammonium chloride, ascorbic acid) increase the possibility of PAS crystalluria.
5. PAS may potentiate the action of oral anticoagulants.
6. PAS may interfere with certain laboratory tests such as urinary protein, urobilinogen, and VMA and urinary glucose determination with Clinitest tablets.

NURSING CONSIDERATIONS
(See also Nursing Process for Patients Receiving Antitubercular Drugs.)

A drug history is essential to identify use of aspirin or other salicylates or allergies to any of these drugs before therapy begins. A history of ulcers or bleeding tendencies must also be identified; cautious use is warranted in such patients.

The drug should be taken with food to minimize significant GI upset and to decrease the chance of ulcers. The patient should be told to report any increase in gastrointestinal pain, tarry or bloody stools, or hematemesis. The drug may produce a sour or bitter taste in the mouth, which can be alleviated by chewing gum or sucking on hard candy. Fluid intake should be increased to about 2000 ml/day, and urine should be kept alkaline to prevent crystalluria. Urine *p*H should be periodically checked using Nitrazine paper; if *p*H drops too low, the physician may prescribe sodium bicarbonate or antacids to increase alkalinity. The patient should be told to avoid foods that acidify urine such as ascorbic acid and cranberry juice.

PAS is very high in sodium, which may cause problems for patients with heart disease or those who retain fluids. The patient should be told to report any sudden weight gain, shortness of breath, or swelling of hands, feet, or legs, which may indicate early symptoms of heart failure or renal dysfunction.

Hypersensitivity to PAS may occur early in therapy and is characterized by fever, malaise, joint pain, pruritus, and skin rash. Symptoms should be immediately reported, and the drug will be discontinued although it may be resumed at a lower dose once symptoms subside. If the physician opts for drug resumption the patient must be closely monitored for further signs of hypersensitivity as well as signs of hepatic dysfunction.

Blood dyscrasias can develop during PAS therapy; therefore a periodic CBC with differential should be completed. Patients should be told to report immediately any fever, sore throat, unusual bleeding, or bruising.

Capreomycin

(Capastat)

Capreomycin is a polypeptide antibiotic used in combination with other appropriate drugs as an alternate antitubercular agent when the first-line drugs are ineffective. Capreomycin is both ototoxic and nephrotoxic and must be administered cautiously.

MECHANISM AND ACTIONS

The mechanism of action of capreomycin is not completely established. The drug is bacteriostatic against human strains of *Mycobacterium tuberculosis*. No cross-resistance has been observed between capreomycin and other antitubercular drugs.

USES

1. Alternate therapy of pulmonary tuberculosis in patients intolerant of or resistant to first-line drug regimens, such as INH, ethambutol, rifampin, and streptomycin (used concomitantly with other antitubercular drugs)

ADMINISTRATION AND DOSAGE

Capreomycin is available as powder for injection containing 1 g per 5 ml vial. The drug is administered by deep IM injection into a large muscle mass. The usual dose is 1 g daily for 60 days to 120 days, followed by 1 g two to three times weekly. The maximum daily dose is restricted to 20 mg/kg.

Prepare solution by dissolving powder in 2 ml of sodium chloride injection or sterile water for injection. Complete dissolution may take 2 minutes to 3 minutes of mixing. Store at room temperature for 48 hours; store for 14 days if refrigerated.

FATE

Capreomycin is not absorbed in significant amounts when given orally and is only administered IM. Peak serum concentrations are attained in 1 hour to 2 hours. The drug is excreted essentially unchanged in the urine, over half of a dose within 12 hours.

SIDE-EFFECTS/ADVERSE REACTIONS

The principal adverse reactions with capreomycin are ototoxicity and nephrotoxicity. In many patients, there is elevation of BUN above 20 mg/100 ml and of nonprotein nitrogen (NPN) above 35 mg/100 ml, and the appearance of casts, red cells, and white cells in the urine has occurred in a high percentage of these cases. The clinical significance of these slight changes has not been established;

however, elevation of BUN above 30 mg/100 ml or other evidence of decreasing renal function requires dosage reduction or drug withdrawal.

Subclinical auditory loss (*i.e.*, 5 decibel to 10 decibel loss) occurs in over 10% of patients, and clinically apparent hearing loss may occur in 2% to 4% of patients. Tinnitus and vertigo have also been reported. Most patients receiving capreomycin evidence eosinophilia exceeding 5% with daily injections, but this reaction subsides when doses are reduced to 2 g to 3 g weekly.

Other untoward reactions reported during capreomycin therapy are hematuria, proteinuria, renal tubular necrosis, anorexia, leukocytosis, leukopenia, abnormal liver function tests, pain and induration at IM injection site, urticaria, maculopapular skin rash, and hypokalemia.

CONTRAINDICATIONS AND PRECAUTIONS

Capreomycin should be administered with *caution* to patients with renal or hepatic dysfunction, auditory impairment, a history of allergies, myasthenia gravis; to pregnant women; and to children. The drug should also be used cautiously in combination with other nephrotoxic or ototoxic drugs (see under Interactions).

INTERACTIONS

1. Capreomycin may enhance the muscle-relaxing action of neuromuscular blocking agents, polypeptide antibiotics, aminoglycosides, and general anesthetics.
2. The potential for nephrotoxicity is increased by combined use of capreomycin with aminoglycosides, cephalothin, ethacrynic acid, furosemide, polymyxins, and vancomycin.
3. The ototoxic effects of capreomycin may be potentiated by aminoglycosides, ethacrynic acid, furosemide, and vancomycin.

NURSING CONSIDERATIONS

(See also Nursing Process for Patients Receiving Antitubercular Drugs.)

A thorough drug history is essential, focusing especially on other drugs the patient takes that are also potentially ototoxic or nephrotoxic (see under Interactions), because the danger of adverse reactions increases and may actually contraindicate drug use unless adjustments can be made.

Capreomycin must be given by intramuscular injection—not a pleasant prospect for the patient facing a course of therapy of 18 months' to 24 months' duration. A body map (see Chap. 8) should be used to rotate injection sites in a systematic fashion. All muscles with substantial mass, including the deltoid, if possible, should be used in order to decrease pain and swelling. Sites should be palpated for swelling, hardness, induration, or presence of soft pockets, all evidence of underlying tissue damage. If such changes are noted an alternate site should be used. Efforts should be made to change to oral therapy as soon as possible during the treatment course, especially if tissue damage develops or if the patient begins to oppose injections, because noncompliance with the regimen is likely.

Ototoxicity is a dangerous drug side-effect necessitating immediate drug discontinuation to avoid permanent damage. Baseline and periodic audiograms should be done to evaluate hearing. Between audiograms, high-pitch hearing can be tested using a tuning fork. Any changes in ability to respond to these tests or reports by the patient of dizziness or tinnitus are cause to discontinue the drug.

Ototoxicity is more likely if the patient develops nephrotoxicity. Regular renal function tests should be performed, monitoring BUN carefully. The patient should also be taught to monitor his intake and urinary output. If output is less than intake over 24 hours or if hematuria occurs, the physician should be notified, and the drug should be discontinued to prevent permanent damage.

Serum potassium levels should also be periodically monitored to detect early signs of hypokalemia. Signs of deficiency which should be reported include paresthesias, muscle cramping, weakness, and palpitations.

Cycloserine

(Seromycin)

A broad-spectrum antibiotic, cycloserine is effective against a variety of gram-positive and gram-negative bacteria as well as *Mycobacterium tuberculosis*. A second-line drug in the treatment of tuberculosis, it can also be used for acute urinary tract infections unresponsive to commonly employed drugs. Its major untoward reactions are CNS toxicity (*e.g.*, convulsions, psychosis, depression) and allergic reactions.

MECHANISM AND ACTIONS

Cycloserine is a structural analogue of D-alanine and antagonizes its role in bacterial cell wall synthesis. Thus, the formation of cell walls in susceptible strains of gram-positive and gram-negative bacteria as well as *Mycobacterium tuberculosis* is

inhibited. The drug is bactericidal at usual therapeutic doses.

USES
1. Alternate treatment of active tuberculosis in conjunction with other tuberculostatic drugs when first-line therapy has failed
2. Alternate treatment of acute urinary tract infections, especially those due to *Enterobacter* and *Escherichia coli* (only where other antimicrobial agents are ineffective and the infecting organism has demonstrated sensitivity to cycloserine)

ADMINISTRATION AND DOSAGE
Cycloserine is administered orally as 250-mg capsules. The initial dosage is 250 mg twice a day for 2 weeks. The maintenance dosage is 500 mg to 1 g daily in divided doses, not to exceed 1 g daily.

FATE
Cycloserine is rapidly absorbed orally and reaches peak plasma levels in 3 hours to 4 hours. It is widely distributed throughout the body, and cerebrospinal levels are equivalent to those of the plasma. Approximately one-third of the drug is metabolized, and both metabolites and unchanged drug are excreted in the urine. Cumulation may occur in patients with renal insufficiency.

SIDE-EFFECTS/ADVERSE REACTIONS
The most common untoward reactions to cycloserine involve the CNS and are largely dose related, occurring with increased frequency at doses greater than 500 mg/day. The central effects of cycloserine include paresthesias, drowsiness, vertigo, confusion, headache, tremor, dysarthria, nervousness, irritability, hyperreflexia, convulsions, clonic seizures, loss of memory, psychoses (possibly with suicidal tendencies), and coma.

Other adverse reactions may include skin rash, allergic dermatitis, photosensitivity, vitamin B_{12} or folic acid deficiency, megaloblastic anemia, and elevated serum transaminase levels.

Overdosage may be marked by depression, dizziness, confusion, hyperreflexia, and convulsions. Treatment is symptomatic and includes anticonvulsants, vitamin B_6, oxygen, IV fluids, and supportive therapy.

CONTRAINDICATIONS AND PRECAUTIONS
Contraindications to use of cycloserine include epilepsy, depression, severe anxiety or psychosis, renal insufficiency, and excessive use of alcohol

(see below). Safety for use during pregnancy and in young children has not been established. Toxicity is closely related to blood levels, which should be maintained below 30 mcg/ml. Periodic hematologic renal and liver function studies should be performed, and weekly blood levels should be determined in patients with reduced renal function.

INTERACTIONS

1. Cycloserine can potentiate the effects of MAO inhibitors and phenytoin.
2. Ethionamide, isoniazid, and alcohol can enhance the neurotoxic effects of cycloserine.
3. Cycloserine can increase the excretion of the B-complex vitamins.

NURSING CONSIDERATIONS

(See also Nursing Process for Patients Receiving Antitubercular Drugs.)

Central nervous system side-effects range from mild to severe and are related to higher doses, alcohol ingestion, and impaired renal function leading to slowed drug clearance. The patient should be urged to use caution when driving or performing any hazardous task (including household chores) until the effects of the drug are known. Drowsiness, dizziness, and confusion may be transient, but if symptoms persist, the physician should be notified. Patients should avoid alcohol consumption, which increases CNS side-effects and may result in toxicity and convulsions.

The patient suffering CNS toxicity from cycloserine should be hospitalized. Emergency equipment, including oxygen, mechanical ventilators, vasopressors, anticonvulsants, and intravenous fluids, should be readily available.

Allergic dermatitis may also develop during cycloserine therapy. The patient should immediately report any pruritus, urticaria, or angioedema and seek treatment. The drug will be discontinued, and antihistamines may be used. Allergic dermatitis can proceed to anaphylaxis.

The patient taking cycloserine is likely to experience photosensitivity. He should be told to wear protective clothing and sunglasses and to avoid direct sun, especially during the summer, throughout the course of therapy.

Anemia may develop while the patient is taking cycloserine. A periodic CBC with differential as well as serum folate and vitamin B_{12} levels will facilitate identification. Vitamin replacement may resolve symptoms, but if not, the drug must be discontinued.

Ethionamide

(Trecator-SC)

MECHANISM AND ACTIONS

Ethionamide is a second-line antitubercular drug that is bacteriostatic against *Mycobacterium tuberculosis*. Its mechanism of action is not known. Resistance develops rapidly *in vitro*.

USES

1. Alternate therapy of active tuberculosis in combination with other effective antitubercular drugs, when treatment with first-line drugs (INH, ethambutol, rifampin, streptomycin) has failed

ADMINISTRATION AND DOSAGE

Ethionamide is used orally as 250-mg tablets. The average adult dose is 0.5 g to 1 g daily in divided doses, with at least one other antitubercular drug. Concomitant administration of pyridoxine (50 mg/day) is recommended. The drug should be taken with food to minimize gastric upset.

FATE

Ethionamide is well absorbed orally and widely distributed throughout the body including the CNS. Peak serum concentrations are attained within 3 hours. The drug is metabolized in the liver and excreted in the urine, almost entirely as metabolites.

SIDE-EFFECTS/ADVERSE REACTIONS

The most common adverse reactions to ethionamide are anorexia, nausea, and vomiting, and up to one-half of patients cannot tolerate doses above 500 mg a day. Other frequently encountered side-effects are diarrhea, metallic taste, stomatitis, drowsiness, depression, and asthenia. Hepatitis has occurred in approximately 5% of patients; however, the signs of hepatotoxicity resolve when the drug is discontinued. Among the other untoward reactions reported with use of ethionamide are blurred vision, diplopia, dizziness, headache, restlessness, tremors, peripheral neuropathy, olfactory disturbances, convulsions, psychotic behavior, jaundice, postural hypotension, skin rash, acne, alopecia, gynecomastia, impotence, menorrhagia, pellagra-like syndrome, and thrombocytopenia.

CONTRAINDICATIONS AND PRECAUTIONS

Ethionamide must be given *cautiously* to persons with hepatic or renal dysfunction, diabetes (control of diabetic symptoms by antidiabetic drugs is more difficult during ethionamide therapy), and to pregnant women and children.

INTERACTIONS

1. Ethionamide can enhance the neurotoxicity of cycloserine and may intensify the adverse effects of other tuberculostatic agents.
2. Ethionamide may increase the neurotoxic effects of alcohol.
3. Ethionamide may potentiate the hypotensive effects (especially orthostatic) of antihypertensive drugs.
4. Ethionamide may interfere with the management of diabetes by antidiabetic drugs.

NURSING CONSIDERATIONS

(See also Nursing Process for Patients Receiving Antitubercular Drugs.)

A thorough drug history is essential because ethionamide potentiates the action of antihypertensive and antidiabetic drugs necessitating close monitoring and periodic dosage adjustments. The hypertensive patient may have an increase in hypotensive episodes unless blood pressure is evaluated regularly and drug dose changed. The diabetic may have periodic changes in blood glucose even after a dosage adjustment is made in the oral antidiabetic drug. Consequently, blood glucose monitoring must be frequent during the entire course of treatment with ethionamide.

Gastrointestinal distress from ethionamide may be decreased if the drug is taken with a meal. If symptoms persist and oral intake is inadequate due to nausea and vomiting, the drug may have to be discontinued.

Liver enzymes should be evaluated every 2 weeks to 4 weeks during therapy to detect early liver dysfunction. The patient should be told to report immediately evidence of hepatitis such as fever, malaise, darkening urine, light-colored stools, or jaundice. The drug must be discontinued.

Pyrazinamide

Pyrazinamide is a second-line tuberculostatic agent, used only in combination with primary drugs (INH, ethambutol, rifampin, streptomycin) in resistant patients, or for short-term therapy before pulmonary surgery to minimize further spread of infection in advanced cases. Principal adverse effects are hepatotoxicity (the incidence of which ranges from 2%–20% and is dependent on the dosage) and hyperuricemia.

MECHANISMS AND ACTIONS

Pyrazinamide is a structural analogue of nicotinamide and is bacteriostatic against *Mycobacterium tuberculosis.* Its mechanism of action is unknown. If used alone, resistance develops rapidly.

USES

1. Adjunctive therapy of tuberculosis in combination with other first-line drugs in patients in whom these primary agents are ineffective

ADMINISTRATION AND DOSAGE

Pyrazinamide is available as 500 mg-tablets. The average adult dose is 20 mg to 35 mg/kg/day in three or four divided doses. The maximum recommended dose is 3 g/day.

FATE

Oral absorption is rapid, and peak serum levels are noted within 2 hrs. The drug distributes widely throughout the body including the CNS. Metabolism occurs primarily in the liver, and the metabolites are excreted, together with a small fraction of unchanged drug, by the kidney.

SIDE-EFFECTS/ADVERSE REACTIONS

The principal adverse effect with pyrazinamide is hepatic injury, the incidence of which ranges from 2% to 20% depending on dosage. The reaction can vary from alterations in liver function tests without clinical symptoms through a mild syndrome characterized by fever, malaise, anorexia, liver tenderness, hepatomegaly, and splenomegaly to a more serious situation leading to jaundice, acute yellow atrophy, and occasionally death.

Other adverse reactions noted during pyrazinamide therapy are hyperuricemia, acute gout, nausea, diarrhea, vomiting, skin rash, photosensitivity, arthralgia, dysuria, urinary retention, and anemia.

CONTRAINDICATIONS AND PRECAUTIONS

Pyrazinamide is contraindicated in the presence of severe liver damage. It should not be used in children unless absolutely necessary and should be discontinued immediately if signs of hepatocellular damage or hyperuricemia accompanied by acute gouty arthritis occur. *Cautious use* of pyrazinamide is necessary in patients with a history of or active gout, diabetes mellitus, acute intermittent porphyria, or impaired renal function and in chronic alcoholics.

INTERACTIONS
1. Pyrazinamide can interfere with the uricosuric action of probenecid and sulfinpyrazone.
2. Pyrazinamide may alter the dosage requirements for insulin or oral hypoglycemic drugs in diabetics.

NURSING CONSIDERATIONS
(See also Nursing Process for Patients Receiving Antitubercular Drugs.)

Liver function studies should be performed every 2 weeks to 4 weeks throughout therapy to monitor changes. Although minor elevations in enzymes without clinical symptoms require no dosage change, any persistent elevations accompanied by any of the symptoms listed under Side-Effects/Adverse Reactions warrant discontinuation of the drug. The patient should be taught early symptoms to report, such as fever, malaise, and abdominal tenderness.

Serum uric acid levels should be obtained at the beginning of therapy and monthly throughout treatment to monitor the development of hyperuricemia. Patients should be told to report any joint pain especially in ankles, heels, or toes.

The diabetic taking pyrazinamide needs frequent blood glucose monitoring because the drug may alter insulin or oral antidiabetic drug effects. Finger sticks for blood glucose may be needed daily until control is reestablished.

The patient taking pyrazinamide may experience photosensitivity and should be told to wear protective clothing, sunglasses, and sunscreens and to avoid midday sun, especially in the summer.

REVIEW QUESTIONS

1. Briefly describe the development of tuberculosis following infection by *Mycobacterium tuberculosis*. What are the principal symptoms?
2. How may the various antitubercular drugs be classified?
3. What are the principal reasons for using combination drug therapy in treating tuberculosis?
4. List three popular antitubercular drug regimens.
5. In what situation is *prophylaxis* of tuberculosis recommended?
6. What subjective data should be collected before a patient begins therapy with antitubercular drugs? How will perception of illness influence the success of treatment?
7. What population is, statistically, the most at risk for being noncompliant with antitubercular drug therapy? How can care givers improve compliance in all patients treated for tuberculosis?
8. What outcome criteria can be used to judge the success of drug therapy for tuberculosis?
9. Describe the mechanism of action of isoniazid.
10. What is the major danger associated with use of isoniazid? What are the most common side-effects?
11. What information should be asked in a drug history for a patient initiating treatment with isoniazid?
12. What are the principal indications for rifampin?
13. Why should rifampin be taken on an uninterrupted schedule rather than intermittently?
14. Why is the half-life of rifampin shortened with chronic therapy?
15. List the most frequently encountered side-effects with rifampin.
16. Why may oral contraceptives be ineffective during treatment with rifampin? What other drugs may be affected by rifampin?
17. How does ethambutol act in treating tuberculosis?
18. Describe the most often noted side-effects with ethambutol.

19. What are the major disadvantages to use of streptomycin in treating tuberculosis?
20. Briefly describe the mechanism of action of aminosalicylic acid in treating tuberculosis.
21. List the most common side-effects with aminosalicylic acid.
22. How is capreomycin used in tuberculosis?
23. Describe the major adverse reactions with capreomycin?
24. How can information obtained in a drug history decrease the risk of adverse reactions with capreomycin?
25. Outline a plan for IM administration of capreomycin.
26. What is the mechanism of action of cycloserine?
27. List the indications for cycloserine.
28. In what situation is the use of cycloserine contraindicated?
29. Under what conditions must ethionamide be used cautiously?
30. What is the principal danger associated with pyrazinamide administration?

BIBLIOGRAPHY

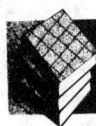

Addington WW: Treatment of pulmonary tuberculosis: Current options. Arch Intern Med 139:1391, 1979

Banner AS: Tuberculosis: Clinical aspects and diagnosis. Arch Intern Med 139:1387, 1979

Bullock WE: Rifampin in the treatment of leprosy. Rev Infect Dis 5(Suppl 3):606, 1983

Centers for Disease Control: Primary resistance to antituberculosis drugs. Ann Intern Med 32:521, 1983

Coleman DA: TB: The disease that's not dead yet. RN 47(9):48, 1984

DesPrez RM, Goodwin RA: *Mycobacterium tuberculosis.* In (Mandell GL, Douglas RG, Bennett JR (eds): Principles and Practice of Infectious Diseases, 2nd ed, p 1383. New York, John Wiley & Sons, 1985

Drugs for tuberculosis. Med Lett Drugs Therap 24:17, 1982

Dutt AR, Stead WW: Present chemotherapy for tuberculosis. J Infect Dis 146:698, 1982

Farr B, Mandell GL: Rifampin. Med Clin North Am 66:157, 1982

Glassroth J, Robins AG, Snider DE: Tuberculosis in the 1980's. N Engl J Med 302(26):1441, 1980

Grosset J, Leventis S: Adverse effects of rifampin. Rev Infect Dis 5(suppl 3):S440, 1983

Hauser M, Baier H: Interactions of isoniazid with foods. Drug Intell Clin Pharm 16:617, 1982

Lester TW: Drug-resistant and atypical mycobacterial disease: Bacteriology and treatment. Arch Intern Med 139:1399, 1979

Mangione RA, Souse RB: Antimicrobial management of pulmonary tuberculosis. Pharmacy Times 50:74, 1984

Pilhev JA, DeSalvo MD, Koch O: Liver alterations in antituberculosis regimens containing pyrazinamide. Chest 80:720, 1981

Reed MD, Blumer JL: Clinical pharmacology of antitubercular drugs. Pediatr Clin North Am 30:177, 1983

Snider DE et al: Standard therapy for tuberculosis 1985. Chest 87(suppl):1175, 1985

Stead WW, Dutt AK: Chemotherapy for tuberculosis today. Am Rev Respir Dis 125(3):94, 1982

Van Scoy RE, Wilkowske CJ: Antituberculous agents. Mayo Clin Proc 58:233, 1983

Wehrli W: Rifampin: Mechanisms of action and resistance. Rev Infect Dis 5(suppl 3):S407, 1983

Antimalarial Drugs

70

Malaria is a parasitic disease which is still prevalent in many areas of the world, especially Southeast Asia, Africa, and Central and South America. Estimates place the number of people afflicted with malaria at over 200 million, and well over 1 million deaths a year can be attributed to the disease.

Although malaria has been virtually eradicated in the United States, travel to and from regions in which the disease is present is responsible for many Americans contracting malaria. Increased numbers of immigrants from malaria-infected countries have also become a risk factor for United States residents.

Four species of the protozoan *Plasmodium* can cause malaria in humans, and these are described briefly below.

1. *Plasmodium falciparum*—Cause of malignant tertian (MT) malaria; a severe, often fulminating infection that may progress to a fatal outcome if not treated quickly and vigorously; prompt therapy is usually highly successful, however, and relapses generally do not occur; inadequate treatment, however, can lead to periodic outbreaks due to multiplication of parasites persisting in the blood.
2. *Plasmodium vivax*—Cause of benign tertian (BT) malaria; a less severe disease than that produced by the *Plasmodium falciparum* strain, having a low mortality rate but characterized by periodic relapses which may continue for years if untreated.
3. *Plasmodium malariae*—Cause of quartan malaria; so named because the attacks of chills and high fever recur every 4 days rather than every 3 days as in the tertian form of the disease; outbreaks tend to appear in localized regions of the tropics; clinical signs may remain dormant for many years, and relapses do occur, but less frequently than with the *Plasmodium vivax* organism.
4. *Plasmodium ovale*—Cause of ovale tertian malaria, a rare form of relapsing malaria similar to but milder and more readily cured than the vivax infection.

Etiology of Malaria

Although malaria can be transmitted by transfusion of infected blood, it is usually transmitted to humans by the bite of the female *Anopheles* mosquito, which deposits the infective sporozoites, formed in the blood of the mosquito by the union of male and female gametocytes, into the human.

The sporozoites localize in the liver, where they multiply to form primary tissue schizonts. These then grow and multiply further into merozoites. This is called the preerythrocytic, exoerythrocytic, or symptom-free stage of the infection. When mature, the merozoites are released from the liver by rupture of the tissue schizonts, and enter the circulation where they invade the erythrocytes (red blood cells) to begin the blood-cycle (or *erythrocytic*) phase of the infection. Young parasites in the red blood cell are termed trophozoites, and they grow and divide into mature schizonts, also known as blood merozoites. Periodically, the blood merozoites burst from the ruptured red cells and invade a new group of erythrocytes, beginning the process anew. This periodic (every 2 days–4 days) rupturing of infected erythrocytes occurs repeatedly until death of the host or termination of the cycle by drug therapy and is responsible for the characteristic fever and chills that accompany acute attacks of malaria.

Once human plasmodial cells enter the erythrocytic cycle, they generally do *not* reinvade other tissues. Thus, tissue infection does not occur in those forms of malaria induced by blood transfusion. However, another phase of the plasmodial life cycle occurs in infections caused by *P. vivax*, *P. ovale*, and possibly *P. malariae*, and is termed the exoerythrocytic cycle. Following the release of most of the mature merozoites from the liver, some parasites in the merozoite stage of the above three forms of *Plasmodium* remain in the liver and continue to multiply in liver cells for extended periods of time. Relapses occurring months or even years following the initial infection can then result as new merozoites are released from the liver cells to reinvade erythrocytes.

Thus, acute malarial attacks can occur for several years unless these exoerythrocytic forms are eradicated during the primary treatment phase. This process does not occur with *P. falciparum*, because no forms of the parasite remain in the liver following the initial infection.

Finally, some of the merozoites that invade erythrocytes do not undergo the above described process of asexual reproduction, but instead differentiate into male and female gametocytes. Upon ingestion into a female mosquito (i.e., when the mosquito draws blood from an infected human by a bite), sexual fertilization of the female gametocyte by the male gametocyte occurs in the gut of the mosquito, giving rise to new infective sporozoites.

Drug therapy of malaria may be directed either toward prevention of infection, suppression of clinical symptoms, treatment of acute attacks, or prevention of relapses. These methods are reviewed below:

1. Prevention of infection—Drugs that kill the malarial organisms during their preerythrocytic (exoerythrocytic) stages are termed *causal prophylactics*; however, no drug is currently available that can selectively destroy sporozoites at therapeutic levels that are considered safe. Prophylaxis of malaria is best accomplished by mosquito control.

2. Suppression of clinical symptoms—Inhibition of the erythrocytic stage of the cycle can prevent development of clinical symptoms in an infected individual. Several antimalarial drugs (*i.e.*, chloroquine, hydroxychloroquine, pyrimethamine) act in this manner, but acute attacks can occur when therapy is discontinued if exoerythrocytic forms of the organism are still present.

3. Treatment of acute attacks—Interruption of erythrocytic parasite multiplication can terminate the symptoms of an acute malarial attack, and drugs acting in this way are termed *schizonticides*. The 4-amino-quinolines are generally considered drugs of choice in this case, but they do not completely eliminate the parasite from the body; hence the possibility of relapse exists, especially with the vivax strains.

4. Prevention of relapse—Drugs that eradicate the exoerythrocytic parasite (secondary tissue forms) can prevent relapse infections, and such treatment is sometimes referred to as a radical cure. The only currently available drug producing a radical cure in vivax malaria is primaquine, and it is usually given in combination with a drug (*e.g.*, chloroquine) that suppresses the erythrocyte cycle as well.

Combination suppressive therapy and radical cure (*e.g.*, with chloroquine and primaquine) is widely employed in travelers to areas in which malaria is endemic. Therapy is begun before arrival and repeated at weekly intervals during the stay and for at least 2 months after returning from the malarial region to ensure that, in the event infection occurs, clinical symptoms are suppressed and any secondary tissue forms are eradicated.

Prophylaxis may also be accomplished by use of the combination product sulfadoxine and pyrimethamine (Fansidar) beginning 1 day to 2 days before exposure to an endemic area, continuing during the stay, and then for 4 weeks to 6 weeks following departure.

Resistance to Antimalarial Drugs

An increasingly prevalent problem in treating malaria is the extent of acquired resistance that has developed to many antimalarial drugs. The most serious problem with resistance appears to be with *P. falciparum*, because this species is responsible for the large majority of cases of malaria and most of the human mortality associated with the disease. Resistance of *P. falciparum* to chloroquine, a mainstay in the treatment of malaria for many years, is increasing dramatically throughout the world, and there is increasing resistance to pyrimethamine-sulfadoxine, a combination considered to be the preferred alternative to chloroquine for prophylaxis of falciparum malaria. This increasing resistance to conventional antimalarial therapy illustrates the necessity of developing newer, improved, and perhaps unique antimalarial drugs that may act by different mechanisms, to treat effectively those forms of malaria presently unaffected by current modes of treatment.

4-Aminoquinolines

Chloroquine, Hydroxychloroquine

MECHANISM AND ACTIONS

The 4-aminoquinolines are synthetic drugs which are particularly active against the erythrocytic forms of *Plasmodium vivax* and *Plasmodium malariae* and against most strains of *Plasmodium falciparum*. The action of the drugs is to fix protozoal DNA in its double-stranded form so that it is unable to replicate or be transcribed by RNA. The synthesis of protozoal protein and nucleic acid is blocked. Chloroquine also possesses an amebicidal and anti-inflammatory action. Because they are ineffective against the exoerythrocytic forms, they do not prevent relapses in infected persons. Their principal indications are as suppressive agents in vivax or malariae malaria and for terminating acute attacks of all types of malaria. In falciparum malaria, they abolish the acute attack and cure the infection, unless due to a resistant strain. The two drugs are reviewed together, inasmuch as their pharmacology is identical, then listed individually in Table 70-1.

USES

1. Suppression and treatment of acute attacks of malaria due to *Plasmodium vivax*, *Plasmodium malariae*, *Plasmodium ovale*, and susceptible strains of *Plasmodium falciparum*
2. Treatment of extraintestinal amebiasis (chloroquine, see Chap. 72)
3. Treatment of systemic lupus erythematosus and rheumatoid arthritis (investigational use)

ADMINISTRATION AND DOSAGE
See Table 70-1.

FATE
The drugs are readily absorbed from the GI tract, and peak plasma levels occur in 1 hour to 2 hours. Plasma protein binding is approximately 50%. The drugs are widely distributed and concentrate in the liver, spleen, kidney, heart, and brain and in melanin-containing cells such as in the eyes and skin, where they are highly bound to melanin. Elimination occurs very slowly by the kidney, as both unchanged drugs and metabolites, and is enhanced by acidification of the urine. Tissue levels may be detectable for months and occasionally years, especially after termination of prolonged therapy.

SIDE-EFFECTS/ADVERSE REACTIONS
Use of chloroquine and hydroxychloroquine for treating acute malarial attacks is frequently accompanied by GI upset, pruritus, transient headache, and visual disturbances such as blurred vision or difficulty in focusing. These symptoms readily disappear upon discontinuation of therapy. Prolonged therapy is generally well tolerated, especially at low doses. Higher doses increase the likelihood of adverse effects such as hypotension, ECG changes (*e.g.*, widening of QRS complex, T-wave inversion), skin eruptions, alopecia, skin pigmentary changes, anorexia, and muscle weakness.

Ophthalmologic changes have occurred, especially during long-term high-dose therapy. Reported disturbances include corneal edema or opacity, retinal changes (arteriolar narrowing, macular lesions, abnormal pigmentation), scotomata, optic atrophy, and visual field defects. Irreversible retinal damage (possibly due to deposition of the drug in melanin-rich retinal cells) has developed with chronic, high-dose therapy, and retinal changes and visual disturbances may progress even after cessation of therapy.

Other untoward reactions associated with 4-aminoquinolines include vertigo, tinnitus, impaired hearing, fatigue, psychic stimulation, convulsions (rare), psychotic episodes (rare), neuropathy, agranulocytosis, and other blood dyscrasias.

CONTRAINDICATIONS AND PRECAUTIONS
Use of 4-aminoquinolines is contraindicated in persons with retinal or visual field changes. A *cautious* approach to therapy is needed in patients with hepatic, neurologic or hematologic disorders, psoriasis, or porphyria, in alcoholics, in infants or small children, in pregnant women, and in nursing mothers. Knee and ankle reflexes should be tested periodically to assess any muscle weakness. These drugs can induce hemolysis in glucose-6-phosphate-dehydrogenase-deficient individuals, especially in the presence of infection or other stressful situations.

INTERACTIONS

1. Liver toxicity may be increased by combined use of other known hepatotoxic drugs.
2. Gold compounds, anti-inflammatory drugs, and other agents known to cause drug sensitization and dermatitis may increase the dermatologic side-effects of the 4-aminoquinolines.
3. Excretion of the 4-aminoquinolines may be enhanced by urinary acidifiers (*e.g.*, ammonium chloride) and reduced by urinary alkalinizers (*e.g.*, sodium bicarbonate).
4. The action of antipsoriatic drugs may be antagonized by the 4-aminoquinolines, and a severe psoriatic attack can be precipitated.
5. MAO inhibitors can increase the toxicity of 4-aminoquinolines by impairing their hepatic inactivation.
6. The GI absorption of 4-aminoquinolines may be decreased by concurrent administration of kaolin or magnesium trisilicate.

NURSING CONSIDERATIONS
A drug history is important and will alert the clinician to medical history that may warrant cautious use of chloroquine or hydroxychloroquine (see under Interactions). Any patient who takes gold compounds or anti-inflammatory medications for arthritis or anyone taking antipsoriatic drugs for psoriasis is prone to severe dermatologic side-effects from 4-aminoquinolines, and alternative therapy may be needed. The drugs should also be used with caution in any patient with a history of hepatic, renal, or hematologic dysfunction.

Table 70-1
Aminoquinolines

Drug	Preparations	Usual Dosage Range	Clinical Considerations
chloroquine (Aralen)	Tablets—phosphate—250 mg, 500 mg (equivalent to 150 mg, 300 mg of base) Injection—hydrochloride —50 mg/ml (equivalent to 40 mg/ml base)	Treatment of acute attack: Adults Oral—600 mg (base) initially followed by 300 mg (base) 6 h, 24 h, and 48 h later IM—160 mg to 200 mg (base) initially; repeat in 6 h: (maximum 800 mg base/24 h) Begin oral dosage as soon as possible and continue for 3 days. Children Oral—10 mg/kg (base) initially, followed by 5/mg/kg (base) 6 h, 24 h, and 48 h later IM—5 mg/kg (base) initially; repeat in 6 h (maximum 10 mg/kg base in a 24-h period) Suppression (oral only): Adults 300 mg (base) once weekly, beginning 2 wk before exposure, continue for 6 wk–8 wk after leaving endemic area Children 5 mg/kg (base) weekly as above Treatment of amebiasis: Oral—600 mg (base) daily for 2 days, then 300 mg (base) daily for 2 wk–3 wk IM—160 mg to 200 mg (base) injected daily for 10 days–12 days	Indicated for treatment of acute attacks and suppressive therapy of all forms of malaria; also used with an amebicide for treatment of extraintestinal amebiasis (See Chap. 72); for radical cure of vivax malaria, should be combined with primaquine; parenteral therapy should be terminated and oral therapy initiated as soon as possible; children and infants are very susceptible to adverse attacks from parenteral chloroquine; do not exceed 5 mg/kg base for any single injection in young children; may be used for treating symptoms of rheumatoid arthritis (150 mg of base in a single daily dose) but hydroxychloroquine is preferred

(continued)

Oral drugs should be taken with meals to decrease GI distress. If an individual is given suppression therapy, he will take the drug once a week for 8 weeks to 10 weeks and take it on the same day each week. He should be encouraged to use a memory jogger—such as a daily calendar page, note on the bathroom mirror, or any other device so the dose is not forgotten, an easy thing to do because the habit is not a daily one.

Ophthalmic side-effects of the drug can be devastating because the drug is cleared very slowly from the body. Drug use is contraindicated in anyone with known retinal or visual field changes. All patients should be examined thoroughly before treatment begins and periodically throughout the course of therapy. The patient should be encouraged to report immediately any blurring of vision, changes in depth perception or field of vision, or spots before the eyes, and the drug should be discontinued.

Dermatologic reactions are also quite common and may be characterized by rash, pruritis, or pigment changes. The patient should be encouraged to report symptoms, which may disappear if the drug dose is lowered. Otherwise, the drug must be discontinued.

Patients also need to know the 4-aminoquinolines may discolor urine to a yellowish brown,

Table 70-1 (continued)
Aminoquinolines

Drug	Preparations	Usual Dosage Range	Clinical Considerations
hydroxychloroquine sulfate (Plaquenil)	Tablets—200 mg (equivalent to 155 mg base)	Treatment of acute attack: Adults 620 mg (base) initially, followed by 310 mg (base) 6 h, 24 h, and 48 h later Alternately—620 mg base as a single dose Children 10 mg/kg (base) initially, followed by 5 mg/kg (base) 6 h, 24 h, and 48 h later Suppression: Adults 310 mg (base) once weekly beginning 2 wk before exposure; continue 6 wk–8 wk after leaving endemic area Children 5 mg/kg (base) weekly as above Rheumatoid arthritis: Initially 400 mg to 600 mg/day in a single dose; reduce to 200 mg to 400 mg when optimum response is observed Lupus erythematosus: Initially 400 mg once or twice a day; continue for weeks or months, but reduce to 200 mg to 400 mg/day when possible	Used for suppression and treatment of all forms of susceptible malaria and for treatment of rheumatoid arthritis and systemic lupus erythematosus; children's dose should never exceed adult dose; radical cure of vivax and malariae malaria requires concomitant therapy with primaquine; several weeks may be required to demonstrate an effect in rheumatoid arthritis; safe use in juvenile arthritis has not been established

which is harmless and will disappear when the treatment course is completed.

These drugs are especially toxic to children if an overdose is ingested. Keep out of children's reach.

Primaquine Phosphate

MECHANISM AND ACTIONS
Primaquine phosphate is a synthetic 8-aminoquinoline derivative that eliminates the tissue or exoerythrocytic forms of the malarial organism, thereby preventing relapse of vivax malaria. Primaquine is not effective alone during an acute attack, but is administered in combination with chloroquine or hydroxychloroquine, which destroys the blood or erythrocytic forms. The mechanism of

action of primaquine is not completely established. The drug appears to produce mitochondrial swelling in parasitic cells, thereby disrupting energy metabolism and impairing protein synthesis.

Some gametocytes are destroyed, while others are rendered incapable of maturation and division in the mosquito.

USES
1. Radical cure and prevention of relapse in vivax malaria or following termination of chloroquine suppressive therapy in an area where vivax malaria is endemic

ADMINISTRATION AND DOSAGE
Primaquine phosphate is used as tablets containing 26.3 mg, which is equivalent to 15 mg of base. Therapy with primaquine is begun during the last 2

weeks of, or following a course of suppression with chloroquine which quickly destroys the erythrocytic parasites. Adults are given 26.3 mg daily for 14 days or 79 mg once a week for 8 weeks. Children receive a 0.3-mg base/kg/day for 14 days or 0.9-mg base/kg/week for 8 weeks. Primaquine is also available in fixed combination with chloroquine as Aralen Phosphate with Primaquine Phosphate; the tablets contain 500 mg chloroquine phosphate and 79 mg primaquine phosphate. Adults are given 1 tablet weekly beginning at least 1 day before entering the infected area, and continuing at least 8 weeks after leaving the area.

FATE
Primaquine is well absorbed orally. Plasma levels are maximum within 2 hours to 3 hours, but fall rapidly thereafter. Relatively low levels are found in the lung, liver, heart, skeletal muscles, or brain. The drug is rapidly and completely metabolized and excreted largely in the urine.

SIDE-EFFECTS/ADVERSE REACTIONS
The most often reported side-effect with primaquine is epigastric or abdominal distress, especially at larger doses. Other adverse reactions are generally observed following high doses and may include vomiting, headache, leukopenia, hemolytic anemia (especially in glucose-6-phosphate-dehydrogenase-deficient persons) and methemoglobinemia (especially in persons deficient in NADH methemoglobin reductase activity).

CONTRAINDICATIONS AND PRECAUTIONS
Concurrent administration of quinacrine and primaquine is contraindicated (see under Interactions). Primaquine is also contraindicated in acutely ill patients with diseases that may lead to granulocytopenia (e.g., rheumatoid arthritis, lupus erythematosus) and in persons receiving other drugs that are potentially hemolytic or bone marrow depressants. Safety for use of primaquine in pregnant women has not been established. The drug should always be given in conjunction with chloroquine or hydroxychloroquine to destroy the blood (or erythrocytic) forms of the parasite.

INTERACTIONS
1. Quinacrine can potentiate the toxicity of primaquine, presumably by impairing its metabolism.

NURSING CONSIDERATIONS
Primaquine should be taken with food to minimize gastrointestinal distress. However, if symptoms persist, the physician should be notified.

The most serious side-effect is the development of hemolytic anemia which should be monitored closely, especially in dark-skinned people who are more likely to have a deficiency in erythrocytic glucose-6-phosphate-dehydrogenase. Baseline and periodic CBC with differential and urinalysis should be obtained. A drop in hemoglobin or erythrocyte count or presence of blood in urine warrants drug discontinuation. In a susceptible person, daily urine tests with Clinistix for presence of blood may be appropriate. Otherwise, the individual should be told to report immediately any chills, fever, precordial pain, fatigue, or darkening of urine, all indications that the drug should be discontinued and the patient evaluated for anemia.

Pyrimethamine
(Daraprim)

MECHANISM AND ACTION
Pyrimethamine is a folic antagonist that interferes with development of fertilized gametes in the mosquito and is used for prophylaxis of malaria due to susceptible strains. The drug selectively inhibits the enzyme dihydrofolate reductase in protozoal cells, thereby blocking conversion of dihydrofolic acid to tetrahydrofolic acid, an essential step in protozoal cell metabolism. Pyrimethamine reduces sporogony (i.e., reproduction of spores) in the mosquito, but does not destroy gametocytes. Plasmodial resistance can develop rapidly when pyrimethamine is used alone. The drug's slow onset of action reduces its usefulness in treating acute attacks. It is commonly given with a fast-acting schizonticide such as chloroquine to provide both transmission control and suppressive (not radical) cure.

USES
1. Prophylaxis of malaria due to susceptible strains of Plasmodium (usually in combination with a 4-aminoquinoline during acute attacks)
2. Treatment of toxoplasmosis, in combination with a sulfonamide

ADMINISTRATION AND DOSAGE
Pyrimethamine is used as 25-mg tablets and is also available in fixed combination with 500 mg sulfa-

doxine as Fansidar (see below). For prophylaxis of malaria, the adult dose is 25 mg once a week for at least 10 weeks after leaving the exposure area. Children may be given 6.25 mg to 12.5 mg once a week depending on age. For treating acute attacks of malaria due to susceptible plasmodia, 25 mg/day for 2 days, followed by 25 mg once weekly is given together with a rapid-acting schizonticide such as chloroquine or quinacrine.

Recommended doses for treating toxoplasmosis are as follows:

Adults: 50 mg to 75 mg/day with 1 g to 4 g/ day of a sulfapyrimidine for 1 week to 3 weeks; reduce dose by one half and continue for another 4 weeks to 5 weeks

Children: 1 mg/kg/day in two divided doses with appropriate dose of a sulfonamide for 2 days to 4 days, then reduce by one half and continue for 30 days

FATE
Pyrimethamine is well absorbed orally and has a plasma half-life of about 4 days, although suppressive levels may be maintained for up to 2 weeks. The drug appears to be excreted in the urine as several metabolites.

SIDE-EFFECTS/ADVERSE REACTIONS
At doses used for control of malaria, pyrimethamine elicits few side-effects other than occasional skin rash and GI upset. Larger doses, such as those needed for treatment of toxoplasmosis, may result in anorexia, vomiting, atrophic glossitis, megaloblastic anemia, leukopenia, thrombocytopenia, pancytopenia, and hemolytic anemia in patients with a glucose-6-phosphate-dehydrogenase deficiency. Convulsions can occur with overdosage, and treatment is usually undertaken with a parenteral barbiturate followed by leucovorin (folinic acid) in a dose of 3 mg to 9 mg IM daily for 3 days to restore depressed platelet or white blood cell counts.

CONTRAINDICATIONS AND PRECAUTIONS
Pyrimethamine should be administered with *caution* to persons with convulsive disorders or glucose-6-phosphate-dehydrogenase deficiency and to pregnant women.

INTERACTIONS
1. The action of pyrimethamine can be reduced by folic acid or para-aminobenzoic acid (PABA).

2. Pyrimethamine can increase quinine blood levels by competing for protein-binding sites.

NURSING CONSIDERATIONS
Gastrointestinal upset may be alleviated by administering the drug with food. Few other side-effects occur when the drug is used to treat malaria. However, the dosage for treatment of toxoplasmosis approaches the toxic level where adverse reactions are more likely.

In patients receiving high doses, baseline and weekly CBC with differential including platelets should be done to monitor the multiple potential blood dyscrasias which may occur. If blood levels change or the patient develops fever, sore throat, mucosal ulceration, bruising, or bleeding, the drug should be stopped immediately.

Sulfadoxine and Pyrimethamine
(Fansidar)

MECHANISM AND ACTIONS
The fixed combination of sulfadoxine and pyrimethamine blocks sequential enzymatic steps involved in the biosynthesis of folinic acid, a necessary intermediate in the parasitic cellular synthesis of purines, pyrimidines, and certain amino acids. Thus, protein and nucleic acid production is impaired in the plasmodial organisms.

USES
1. Treatment of *Plasmodium falciparum* malaria in chloroquine-resistant cases
2. Prophylaxis of malaria in travelers to areas where chloroquine-resistant *P. falciparum* is endemic

ADMINISTRATION AND DOSAGE
Sulfadoxine/pyrimethamine is available as tablets containing 500 mg/25 mg, respectively. For treating an acute malarial attack, recommended doses are:

Adults: 2 tablets to 3 tablets (500 mg/25 mg) as a single dose, either alone or in sequence with quinine

Children: ½ tablet to 2 tablets, according to age, given as outlined above

Prophylaxis against malaria can be conferred by administering the drug once a week or once every 2 weeks according to the schedule given in Table 70-2. The first dose is given 1 day to 2 days before entering the endemic area, continued during the

Table 70-2
Dosage Schedule for Sulfadoxine/Pyrimethamine

	Weekly	Every Other Week
Adults	1 tablet	2 tablets
Children (9 yr–14 yr)	¾ tablet	1½ tablets
Children (4 yr–8 yr)	½ tablet	1 tablet
Children (under 4 yr)	¼ tablet	½ tablet

stay, and then for 4 weeks to 6 weeks following return.

When travel is into endemic areas with chloroquine-resistant *Plasmodium falciparum* for extended periods of time, combined weekly prophylaxis with chloroquine and Fansidar is often beneficial. In such cases, adult doses are 300 mg of chloroquine base once weekly *plus* 1 tablet sulfadoxine/pyrimethamine once weekly during the stay and for at least 4 weeks to 6 weeks thereafter. Pediatric doses are 5 mg/kg chloroquine base once a week *plus* ⅛ tablet to 1 tablet of sulfadoxine/pyrimethamine per week depending on the child's age.

Patients receiving weekly doses of sulfadoxine/pyrimethamine must be advised to discontinue the drug if pruritus, skin rash, orogenital lesions, or pharyngitis occur, which may be early indications of more severe adverse reactions (see below).

FATE
Both drugs are well absorbed orally. Peak serum levels of sulfadoxine occur in 2 hours to 6 hours, and peak levels of pyrimethamine are observed within 2 hours to 8 hours. The elimination half-life of the drugs is quite long, averaging 150 hours for sulfadoxine and 110 hours for pyrimethamine.

SIDE-EFFECTS/ADVERSE REACTIONS
While all adverse reactions reported for the sulfonamides and pyrimethamine are theoretically possible with Fansidar, not all have been documented thus far for this combination drug. The reader should refer to the discussion of sulfonamides in Chapter 60 and to the monograph on pyrimethamine earlier in this chapter for a listing of the *potential* adverse effects with use of this drug combination.

Fatalities have occurred with use of sulfadoxine/pyrimethamine due to Stevens-Johnson syndrome and toxic epidermal necrolysis. The prophylactic dosage regimen has caused leukopenia when treatment extends 2 months or longer, but it is generally mild and reversible. Other blood dyscrasias have also been reported during therapy as well as fulminant hepatic necrosis. Prophylactic therapy should be terminated if skin rash appears, if the blood picture is altered, if an active bacterial or fungal infection occurs, or if any mucocutaneous symptoms develop, such as rash, pruritus, pharyngitis, or orogenital lesions.

The drug is teratogenic in rats at doses approximately 12 times the human weekly dose. Contraceptive measures should be undertaken to avoid pregnancy during therapy.

CONTRAINDICATIONS AND PRECAUTIONS
The drug is contraindicated in patients with megaloblastic anemia due to folate deficiency, in pregnant women or nursing mothers, and in infants under 2 months of age. Prophylactic use is contraindicated in patients with severe renal insufficiency, blood dyscrasias, or marked hepatic parenchymal damage. A *cautious* approach to use of the drug is warranted in persons with folate deficiency, severe allergies or bronchial asthma, glucose-6-phosphate-dehydrogenase deficiency, or impaired renal or hepatic function. A fluid intake of at least 2000 ml/day should be maintained during therapy to minimize the danger of crystalluria or stone formation. Contraceptive measures should be taken to avoid pregnancy during therapy.

INTERACTIONS
Drug interactions possible with use of sulfadoxine/pyrimethamine are listed under sulfonamides in Chapter 60 and under pyrimethamine earlier in this chapter.

NURSING CONSIDERATIONS
(See individual drugs.)

Quinacrine
(Atabrine)

Although quinacrine is an effective antimalarial, its use in malaria has been supplanted largely by more active and less toxic drugs. It has been used for both treatment and suppression of malaria, inasmuch as it destroys both erythrocytic forms of vivax, falciparum, and quartan malaria as well as gametocytes of vivax and quartan malaria. Quinacrine is ineffective, however, against falciparum gametocytes and all sporozoites. The drug may also be used in the treatment of tapeworm infestations and giardiasis, and this aspect is discussed more fully in Chapter 71. Quinacrine has been employed investigationally by intrapleural injection for prevention of recurrence of pneumothorax in patients at high risk, such as those with cystic fibrosis.

Quinacrine couples with DNA, rendering it unable to replicate or serve for transcription of RNA, thus impairing protein synthesis. It is readily absorbed orally, widely distributed, and highly protein-bound. Excretion is gradual by the kidney, and the drug may accumulate over time.

The drug frequently causes nausea, abdominal cramping, headache, dizziness, and a yellowing of the skin. Other adverse effects include skin eruptions, visual disturbances, nervousness, irritability, nightmares, emotional changes, hepatitis, and, rarely, blood dyscrasias, convulsions, and toxic psychosis. Quinacrine is contraindicated in the presence of psoriasis (may precipitate a severe attack), porphyria, or in conjunction with primaquine.

In treating malaria, the recommended adult dose is 200 mg (with 1 g sodium bicarbonate) every 6 hours for five doses, then 100 mg three times a day for 6 days.

Children may be given 100 mg to 200 mg three times a day for the first day, then 100 mg one or two times a day for 6 days.

Refer to Chapter 71 for additional information relative to use of quinacrine in treating cestodal infections and giardiasis.

NURSING CONSIDERATIONS

A complete history should be obtained before commencing therapy with quinacrine. It should be used with caution in patients with renal or hepatic disease, glucose-6-phosphate-dehydrogenase deficiency, during pregnancy, in small children, and in patients over 60 years old. A baseline and periodic CBC with differential should be performed throughout therapy to monitor the development of blood dyscrasias, and liver function studies should also be completed. Patients should be told to report immediately sore throat, fever, bleeding, or bruising, symptoms of hematologic changes. In addition, they should report malaise, darkening urine, or light-colored stools, which may indicate hepatitis.

Most CNS side-effects indicate the drug dose should be reduced. However, if after dosage reduc-

tion, insomnia, irritability, vertigo or emotional instability persist, the drug must be discontinued. Visual disturbances should also be immediately reported and require immediate drug discontinuation. Symptoms may be slow to abate even after drug stoppage because the drug is eliminated very slowly from the body.

Quinine Sulfate
(Legatrin, Quinamm, Quine, Quiphile, Strema)

MECHANISM AND ACTIONS

A natural alkaloid from the bark of the cinchona tree, quinine is an effective antimalarial drug that has been replaced largely by more active and less toxic drugs. However, it is used in conjunction with pyrimethamine and sulfadiazine or tetracycline for treatment of plasmodia resistant to other antimalarials, especially chloroquine-resistant falciparum strains. Due to its skeletal muscle-relaxant effects, it is also occasionally used for relief of nocturnal leg cramps. The antimalarial action of quinine appears to be due to the drug's ability to inhibit protein synthesis in malarial organisms by complexing with parasite DNA, and interfere with cellular metabolism. It also suppresses oxygen uptake and carbohydrate metabolism of plasmodia and is actively schizonticidal for all forms of malaria and gametocidal for *Plasmodium vivax* and *Plasmodium malariae* strains. Quinine also possesses an analgesic, antipyretic, skeletal muscle-relaxant, oxytocic, and hypoprothrombinemic action. Its muscle-relaxing action is due to increased refractory period of muscle cells, decreased excitability of the motor end-plate, and altered distribution of calcium within the muscle fiber.

USES
1. Adjunctive treatment of chloroquine-resistant falciparum malaria, along with pyrimethamine and sulfadiazine or tetracycline and in combination with other antimalarials for radical cure of relapsing vivax malaria
2. Relief of nocturnal leg cramps, such as those associated with arthritis, diabetes, varicose veins, thrombophlebitis, or arteriosclerosis

ADMINISTRATION AND DOSAGE
Quinine sulfate is used orally as either tablets (260 mg, 325 mg) or capsules (130 mg, 195 mg, 200 mg, 300 mg, 325 mg). For treating chloroquine-resis-

tant malaria, adult dosage is 650 mg every 8 hours for 10 days to 14 days, while children's dosage is 25 mg/kg/day in divided doses every 8 hours for 10 days to 14 days.

For relieving nocturnal leg cramps, 260 mg to 300 mg is given at bedtime.

FATE

Quinine sulfate is well absorbed from the GI tract, and peak plasma levels occur in 1 hour to 3 hours. The drug is highly (70%) protein bound and distributed throughout the body, although only small amounts enter the CNS. The drug is primarily metabolized in the liver and excreted in the urine, largely as metabolites with some unchanged drug. There is little cumulation with continued administration. The plasma half-life is 4 hours to 5 hours. Renal excretion is accelerated when the urine is acidic; increased tubular reabsorption occurs in an alkaline urine.

SIDE-EFFECTS/ADVERSE REACTIONS

Repeated use or large doses of quinine frequently result in development of cinchonism, a syndrome characterized by tinnitus, headache, nausea, disturbed vision, GI upset, and dizziness. These symptoms generally subside upon dosage reduction or discontinuation of therapy. A variety of other untoward reactions have occurred with quinine sulfate administration, particularly at high doses or with prolonged therapy, and they are listed below:

CNS—Temporary deafness, fever, apprehension, restlessness, excitement, confusion, delirium, syncope, hypothermia, convulsions

Ophthalmic—Photophobia, amblyopia, scotomata, diplopia, mydriasis, altered color perception, optic atrophy

GI—Vomiting, stomach cramps, diarrhea

Allergic—Rash, pruritus, flushing, urticaria, facial edema, asthma-like reaction

Hematologic—Hypoprothrombinemia, hemolytic anemia, thrombocytopenia, agranulocytosis

Other—(Usually observed with very large doses) hypotension, respiratory depression, muscle paralysis

Overdosage may be characterized by hypotension, depressed respiration, convulsions, paralysis, cardiovascular collapse, and coma. Fatalities have occurred. Treatment is symptomatic. Urinary acidification will hasten excretion of quinine.

CONTRAINDICATIONS AND PRECAUTIONS

Use of quinine sulfate is contraindicated in persons with optic neuritis, tinnitus, glucose-6-phosphate-dehydrogenase deficiency, and in pregnant women because fetal damage has occurred. The drug should be given with *caution* to patients with myasthenia gravis or a history of allergic reactions, and to nursing mothers.

INTERACTIONS

1. Pyrimethamine may increase quinine blood levels, possibly leading to toxic effects.
2. Quinine can enhance the effects of neuromuscular blocking agents and may increase their respiratory depressant action.
3. Quinine may potentiate the effects of oral anticoagulants by depressing the hepatic synthesis of vitamin K-dependent clotting factors.
4. The urinary excretion of quinine can be reduced by urinary alkalinizers (*e.g.*, sodium bicarbonate, acetazolamide).
5. Aluminum-containing antacids can delay or reduce the oral absorption of quinine.
6. Due to its similarity to quinidine, quinine may increase plasma levels of digoxin and digitoxin if given concurrently, as has been documented for quinidine.
7. Quinine may interfere with determination of 17-hydroxycorticosteroids and may produce elevated 17-ketogenic steroid values.

NURSING CONSIDERATIONS

A drug history should be obtained; patients taking oral anticoagulants, digitalis drugs, or neuromuscular blocking agents may need dosage adjustments in these drugs to avoid the development of toxic drug reactions.

Quinine is bitter, and the aftertaste of the drug as well as concomitant gastrointestinal distress may be relieved by taking it with food. The capsule should never be chewed or broken.

Transient dizziness or blurred vision may occur during drug therapy. Patients should be warned to use caution in driving or performing any hazardous tasks until the effect of the drug is known. If dizziness occurs, the individual should sit or lie down until the episode passes, then rise slowly. Food intake with the drug may decrease such side-effects.

All patients should be taught the symptoms of cinchonism and told to report them immediately. Headache, nausea, tinnitus, and dizziness are usually the early symptoms and may disappear if the drug dose is reduced. If not, the drug must be discontinued.

REVIEW QUESTIONS

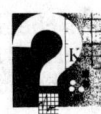

1. What species of *Plasmodium* are responsible for causing malaria?
2. Briefly describe the type of malaria caused by each of the above species.
3. How is malaria transmitted to humans?
4. Briefly describe the (a) exoerythrocytic stage and (b) erythrocytic phase of the infection.
5. What is the principal cause of relapse during a malarial infection?
6. What are the four approaches to drug therapy of malaria?
7. How do the 4-aminoquinolines act in treating malaria? What is their principal indication? In what other diseases may they be useful?
8. When is suppression therapy with 4-aminoquinolines used? How can the patient be helped to remember to take the drug?
9. List the most important adverse effects associated with the 4-aminoquinolines.
10. What is the principal indication for primaquine?
11. With what other antimalarial drug is primaquine available in fixed combination?
12. What is the most serious adverse reaction to primaquine? How should the patient be monitored to detect it early?
13. In what conditions is use of primaquine contraindicated?
14. What is the mechanism of action of pyrimethamine? What are its principal uses?
15. For treating acute malarial attacks, pyrimethamine should be given concurrently with what other type of antimalarial drug?
16. What is the rationale behind use of the fixed combination sulfadoxine and pyrimethamine? What are its principal indications?
17. List the principal adverse reactions occurring with the sulfadoxine-pyrimethamine combination.
18. For what indications is quinacrine approved?
19. What are the commonly encountered side-effects with quinacrine?
20. Briefly describe the various pharmacologic actions of quinine sulfate.
21. For what indications is quinine recommended?
22. Chronic use of quinine is frequently associated with what group of side-effects?
23. Why is a drug history essential before treatment with quinine sulfate is initiated?

BIBLIOGRAPHY

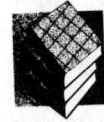

Cohen S (ed): Malaria. A Symposium. Br Med Bull 38:115, 1982
Davidson DE, Ager AL, Brown JL et al: New tissue schizonticidal antimalarial drugs. Bull WHO 59:463, 1981
Drugs for parasitic infections. Med Lett Drugs Therap 26:27, 1984
Fitch CD: Mode of action of antimalarial drugs. In Malaria and the Red Cell, p 222. Ciba Foundation Symposium 94. London, Pitman, 1983

Olansky AJ: Antimalarials and ophthalmologic safety. J Am Acad
     Dermatol 6:19, 1982
Sweeney TR: The present status of malaria chemotherapy:
     Methoquine, a novel antimalarial. Med Res Rev 1:281, 1981
Wyler DJ: Malaria: Resurgence, resistance, and research. N Engl J Med
     308:875 and 934 (2 parts), 1983
Wyler DJ: *Plasmodium* species (Malaria). In Mandell GL, Douglas
     RG, Bennett JE (eds): Principles and Practice of Infectious
     Diseases, 2nd ed, p 1514. New York, John Wiley & Sons, 1985

Anthelmintics

71

Anthelmintics are drugs used to facilitate the expulsion from the body of parasitic worms or helminths. Helminthiasis or worm infection is the most common disease in the world today, affecting over 1 billion people. Moreover, infection with *more than one type* of worm occurs frequently in tropical regions. Although endemic in many of the tropical countries, helminthiasis is by no means limited to these areas, but is found in many temperate climates as well. Poor living conditions, inadequate sanitation, contact with infected pets, lack of careful hygiene, and malnutrition are all contributory factors to the development of helminthic infections. In addition, travel has resulted in the appearance of worms in regions where they were not found previously.

Helminthic infections are caused by two principal types of worms, roundworms (nematodes), and flatworms (cestodes, trematodes). Table 71-1 lists the major species of each type of worm and the drugs that are most effective against each helminth. Most nematodal infections are confined to the intestinal tract and include parasites such as roundworms, pinworms, whipworms, hookworms, and threadworms. However, tissue-invading nematodes, such as filarial worms and pork roundworms (trichinella), can enter body organs, including the heart, liver, lungs, skeletal muscle, and CNS, in which case eradication is often quite difficult, and sequelae are usually more serious than those resulting from intestinally confined worms.

Table 71-1
Helminthiasis Classification and Treatment

Class of Helminth	Disorder	Suggested Drugs of Choice	
		Primary	Secondary
Nematodes			
Roundworm (*Ascaris lumbricoides*)	Ascariasis	mebendazole, pyrantel pamoate	piperazine, thiabendazole, diethylcarbamazine
Hookworm (*Necator americanus*) (*Ancylostoma duodenale*)	Uncinariasis	mebendazole	pyrantel pamoate, thiabendazole
Whipworm (*Trichuris trichiura*)	Trichuriasis	mebendazole	thiabendazole
Threadworm (*Strongyloides stercoralis*)	Strongyloidiasis	thiabendazole	mebendazole
Cutaneous larva migrans (*Ancylostoma braziliense*)	Creeping eruption	thiabendazole	
Capillary worm (*Capillaria philippinensis*)	Capillariasis	mebendazole	thiabendazole
Pinworm (*Enterobius vermicularis*)	Enterobiasis	mebendazole, pyrantel pamoate	thiabendazole, piperazine
Pork roundworm (*Trichinella spiralis*)	Trichiniasis, trichinosis	corticosteroids	thiabendazole, mebendazole
Filarial worms (*Wuchereria bancrofti*)	Filariasis	diethylcarbamazine	
(*Brugia malayi*)	Filariasis	diethylcarbamazine	
(*Loa loa*)	Loiasis	diethylcarbamazine	
(*Onchocerca volvulus*)	Onchocerciasis	diethylcarbamazine and suramin*	mebendazole
Guinea worm (*Dracunculus medinensis*)	Dracunculiasis	niridazole,* metronidazole	mebendazole, thiabendazole

(continued)

* Available only by request from the Parasitic Disease Drug Service, Centers for Disease Control, Atlanta, GA 30333.

Cestodal infestations can occur with several types of tapeworms, the most common being the beef tapeworm (*Taenia saginata*). These infections are usually localized in the GI tract, although larvae of the pork tapeworm (*Taenia solium*) can occasionally gain access to the systemic circulation, and eventually lodge in organs, where they can cause inflammatory and granulomatous reactions such as cysticercosis.

Trematodes which are specifically tissue invading are also known as blood flukes and are responsible for a chronic infection termed schistosomiasis, or bilharziasis, which is widespread throughout Africa and parts of South America. Complications may range from minor conditions such as rash, itching, or headache to severe damage to vital organs. Other trematodes include the lung, liver, and intestinal flukes.

Accurate diagnosis is essential for the successful treatment of the helminth infestation, because many anthelmintic drugs are highly specific for a particular infection. Diagnosis is usually accomplished by obtaining a stool specimen in which characteristic eggs or worm parts can be identified. In the case of pinworms, diagnosis may be achieved by removing eggs from the anal area in the early morning with cellophane tape. The sticky side of the tape is transferred to a slide for microscopic examination. Once the type of worm involved has been determined, selection of an appropriate anthelmintic drug can be made. Although a large number of different kinds of chemicals have been

Table 71-1 (continued)
Helminthiasis Classification and Treatment

Class of Helminth	Disorder	Suggested Drugs of Choice	
		Primary	Secondary
Nematodes (continued)			
Rat lungworm (*Angiostrongylus cantonensis*)	**Angiostrongyliasis**	thiabendazole	mebendazole
Cestodes			
Tapeworms			
Beef (*Taenia saginata*)	Taeniasis	niclosamide	praziquantel
Pork (*Taenia solium*)	**Taeniasis**	niclosamide, praziquantel	paromomycin, mebendazole
Fish (*Diphyllobothrium latum*)	Diphyllobothriasis	niclosamide	dichlorophen, praziquantel, paromomycin
Dwarf (*Hymenolepis nana*)	Hymenolepiasis	niclosamide, praziquantel	mebendazole, paromomycin
Trematodes			
Blood flukes (*Schistosoma haematobium*)	Schistosomiasis (Bilharziasis)	praziquantel, metrifonate*	niridazole*, stibocaptate*
(*Schistosoma mansoni*)	Schistosomiasis	praziquantel, oxamniquine	niridazole*, stibocaptate*
Blood flukes (*Schistosoma japonicum*)	Schistosomiasis	praziquantel, niridazole*	stibocaptate*
(*Schistosoma mekongi*)	Schistosomiasis	praziquantel	niridazole*
Lung flukes (*Paragonimus westermani*)	Paragonimiasis	praziquantel	chloroquine, bithionol*
Liver flukes (*Opisthorchis viverrini*)	Opisthorchiasis	praziquantel	mebendazole
(*Fasciola hepatica*)	Fascioliasis	praziquantel, bithionol*	metronidazole, emetine
(*Clonorchis sinensis*)	Clonorchiasis	praziquantel	mebendazole
Intestinal fluke (*Fasciolopsis buski*)	Fasciolopsiasis	niclosamide, praziquantel	tetrachloroethylene, hexylresorcinol

Table 71-2
*Anthelmintic Drugs Available by Request to Centers for Disease Control**

Drug	Principal Indications	Preparation	Usual Dosage Range	Remarks
bithionol (Bitin, Lorothidol)	Lung flukes (*Paragonimus*) and liver fluke (*Fasciola*) infections	Powder	30 mg to 50 mg/kg orally in two or three divided doses on alternate days for 10 days to 15 days	Drug of choice for treating lung fluke infections; GI side-effects are common; use with caution in children under 8 years of age
metrifonate (Bilarcil)	Schistosomiasis	Tablet—100 mg	7.5 mg to 10 mg/kg as a single dose; repeat twice at 2-wk intervals	One of the drugs of choice for *Schistosoma haematobium* infections; not effective against *S. mansoni* or *S. japonicum*; well tolerated; minimal side-effects
niridazole (Ambilhar)	Schistosomiasis, guinea worm infections	Tablets—100 mg, 500 mg	25 mg/kg/day orally in two to three divided doses for 7 days	Primary drug for *Schistosoma japonicum* and guinea worm (dracunculiasis) infections and alternate drug for other schistosomal infections; high incidence of side-effects (70%) especially GI and allergic; CNS toxicity can occur, especially at high doses; Phenobarbital (100 mg–150 mg) is given daily in divided doses to reduce the incidence of CNS side-effects; patients must be hospitalized; (continued)

* Parasitic Disease Drug Service, Bureau of Epidemiology, Centers for Disease Control, Atlanta, GA 30333.

used in the past for treating the various types of worm infestations, they have been replaced today by a few newer, more effective, and less toxic agents. Most of these newer anthelmintic drugs are not appreciably absorbed following oral administration, and thus attain high levels in the GI tract while largely avoiding systemic toxicity. Another advantage of certain of the newer drugs (mebendazole, thiabendazole, praziquantel) is that they have a broad spectrum of action and thus are effective against several types of helminths. Thus, these drugs are particularly valuable in mixed infections or when the diagnosis is uncertain.

An important aspect of successful anthelmintic therapy is proper patient education with regard to personal hygiene. Many worms are primarily transmitted by transfer of eggs (ova) by hands, food, or contaminated articles such as toilet paper, towels, clothes, or sheets, and it is imperative that patients be instructed in the necessary procedures for minimizing such spread. Important measures that should be stressed are careful washing of hands fol-

Table 71-2 (continued)
Anthelmintic Drugs Available by Request to Centers for Disease Control*

Drug	Principal Indications	Preparation	Usual Dosage Range	Remarks
niridazole (Ambilhar) (continued)				generally contraindicated in cardiac, liver, or renal disease, hypertension, epilepsy, psychiatric disorders, GI ulceration, or hemorrhage
stibocaptate (Astiban)	Schistosomiasis	Powder for injection —0.5 g/vial (5 ml saline added to prepare a 10% solution)	40 mg to 50 mg/kg total dose divided into five injections given at weekly intervals	Highly effective in treating schistosomal infections; antimony-containing compound with high incidence of side-effects, but less toxic than antimony potassium tartrate; do not use in the presence of bacterial or viral infections, hepatic, renal, or cardiac insufficiency, or anemia
suramin (Antrypol, Bayer 205, Belganyl, Germanin, Moranyl, Naganol, Naphuride)	Onchocerciasis (filarial worm infection), African trypanosomiasis (sleeping sickness)	Powder for injection —0.5 g/vial, 1 g/vial	1 g by slow IV injection weekly for 4 weeks to 7 weeks	Used to eradicate adult filariae of *Onchocerca volvulus* following treatment with diethylcarbamazine to eliminate microfilariae (see above); also viewed as drug of choice for early stages of African trypanosomiasis prior to central nervous system involvement. Proteinuria can occur; avoid extravasation, because severe pain can result

lowing each bowel movement, daily or more frequent changes of underwear, towels, and bedding especially during treatment, and avoidance of scratching of the perianal area. Nail biting should also be strongly discouraged. Diagnosis of pinworm infection, the most common helminthic infection in the United States, especially among school children, in one family member makes it imperative that all other family members be tested as well, because this infection commonly affects an entire family.

The drugs commonly used to treat the principal helminthic infections (see Table 71-1) are discussed in detail in this chapter. Other anthelminthic drugs, such as niridazole, bithionol, stibocaptate, and suramin, are used primarily for certain filarial or trematodal infections, and are currently available only upon request from the Parasitic Disease Drug Service of the Centers for Disease Control. These agents are reviewed briefly in Table 71-2. Still other drugs that are only occasionally used in certain helminthic infections (*e.g.*, emetine, chloroquine, paromomycin) have additional therapeutic actions as well; they are discussed elsewhere in this book. The term anthelmintic refers to drugs that cannot only eradicate worms from the GI tract, but also rid tissue of helminths. Although attempts have been made to categorize anthelmintic drugs into "intestinal" and "tissue" active drugs, there is considerable overlap in the actions of certain of the drugs. Therefore, the anthelmintic drugs will be considered alphabetically in this chapter.

Antimony Compounds

Antimony compounds were major antischistosomal drugs for many years, but are seldom used today because of their toxicity and the availability of other more effective drugs. Antimony potassium tartrate (tartar emetic) is an effective drug for the treatment of *Schistosoma japonicum*, *S. mansoni*, and *S. haematobium*, but because of its high toxicity (*e.g.*, dizziness, vomiting, tachycardia, arrhythmias, renal damage, blood dyscrasias), it is rarely employed today. Antimony sodium dimercaptosuccinate (stibocaptate) is an alternate drug in the treatment of schistosomal infections (see Table 71-1) and is available as Astiban from the Centers for Disease Control in Atlanta. Stibocaptate is stable in solution, can be administered IM, and is considerably less toxic than antimony potassium tartrate. The dose of stibocaptate is 40 mg/kg for *Schistosoma haematobium* and *Schistosoma mansoni* infections and 50 mg/kg for *Schistosoma japonicum* infections. The total dosage is divided into five equal parts and given once a week for 5 weeks. The course of therapy can be repeated in 2 months if necessary.

Diethylcarbamazine
(Hetrazan)

MECHANISM AND ACTIONS
Diethylcarbamazine is a piperazine derivative that is viewed as a drug of choice in treating infections caused by filarial worms (see Table 71-1). The drug causes the rapid disappearance of small worms (microfilariae) of *Wuchereria bancrofti*, *Brugia malayi*, and *Loa loa* from the blood of humans and removes microfilariae of *Onchocerca volvulus* from the skin. Diethylcarbamazine appears to immobilize the organisms as well as alter their surface membranes to render them more susceptible to destruction by host defense mechanisms.

USES
1. Treatment of Bancroft's filariasis, onchocerciasis, ascariasis, tropical eosinophilia, and loiasis

ADMINISTRATION AND DOSAGE
Diethylcarbamazine is used orally as 50-mg tablets. Recommended doses are as follows:
Filariasis, onchocerciasis, loiasis: 2 mg/kg three times a day after meals for 3 weeks to 4 weeks during the acute stage of the disease
The above dosage can be given for 3 days to 5 days to treat large numbers of patients known to harbor microfilariae, as a public health measure
Ascariasis: 13 mg/kg once daily for 7 days
    Children—6 mg to 10 mg/kg three times a day for 7 days to 10 days
Tropical eosinophilia: 13 mg/kg/day for 4 days to 7 days

SIDE-EFFECTS/ADVERSE REACTIONS
Side-effects due to diethylcarbamazine occur frequently, but are generally mild and usually disappear with continued therapy. They include headache, weakness, lassitude, malaise, nausea, and joint pain. Other adverse reactions are the result of the destruction of the parasites, and, in patients infected with *Onchocerca volvulus*, a typical reaction may include intense pruritus, skin rash, facial edema, enlargement and tenderness of the inguinal lymph nodes, tachycardia, hyperpyrexia, and headache.

Many patients undergoing therapy exhibit a leukocytosis, which peaks within the first week and gradually subsides. In addition, visual disturbances, proteinuria, abdominal pain, fever, nodular swellings, and lymphadenopathy have been reported. Corticosteroids may be utilized to minimize some of the untoward reactions occurring during therapy, and oral antihistamines may be given during therapy to reduce the severity of allergic reactions. Epinephrine should be on hand to treat severe allergic reactions.

CONTRAINDICATIONS AND PRECAUTIONS
Diethylcarbamazine should be used *cautiously* in persons having a history of allergic reactions and in persons who are malnourished or debilitated.

Mebendazole
(Vermox)

MECHANISM AND ACTIONS
Mebendazole is very effective in treating various nematodal infections. The drug blocks uptake and utilization of glucose by worms, thereby depleting endogenous glycogen and reducing the energy supply below that necessary for survival. The blood glucose levels of the host are unaffected. Clearance of the parasites from the GI tract occurs slowly, and several days may be required for complete elimination.

Mebendazole also has demonstrated effectiveness in treating some cases of trichinosis, onchocerciasis, beef and pork tapeworms, and liver flukes but should be viewed only as an alternative drug for these infections.

USES
1. Treatment of single or mixed whipworm, pinworm, roundworm, and hookworm infestations
2. Alternate therapy for trichinosis, onchocerciasis, taeniasis, and infestation with liver flukes

ADMINISTRATION AND DOSAGE
Mebendazole is used as chewable tablets containing 100 mg. Tablets may be chewed, swallowed, or crushed and mixed with food. For whipworm, hookworm, and roundworm infections, one tablet is administered morning and night for three consecutive days. If after 3 weeks a cure is not evident, a second treatment course should be given. In treating pinworm infections, 100 mg are given as a single dose. Fasting and posttreatment purging are not required.

FATE
Less than 10% of an oral dose of mebendazole is absorbed. Most of the drug is eliminated in the feces, with approximately 2% excreted in the urine within 24 hours to 48 hours.

SIDE-EFFECTS/ADVERSE REACTIONS
Side-effects are infrequent with mebendazole. In massive infections, transient abdominal pain and diarrhea have occurred, possibly due to expulsion of large numbers of worms. Fever has occurred, possibly the result of drug-induced tissue necrosis, and high doses have resulted in development of reversible neutropenia.

CONTRAINDICATIONS AND PRECAUTIONS
Mebendazole should not be given to pregnant women because it has been demonstrated to be teratogenic in laboratory animals. The drug should be used *cautiously* in nursing mothers and in children under age 2.

NURSING CONSIDERATIONS
Infected patients should be taught to avoid reinfection from possible sources. Children should be discouraged from playing in areas where soil may be contaminated with feces to avoid whipworm. In endemic areas children should play only in sandboxes which are kept covered when not in use. In areas endemic for hookworm, the population should wear shoes at all times. To avoid roundworm all cooks should be taught to wash vegetables thoroughly.

Children should be taught to avoid nail biting and putting fingers in the mouth to decrease the spread of pinworms. Nails should be cleaned daily. Hands should be washed after urinating or a bowel movement.

The patient and family should be taught to expect mild temperature elevations as a result of drug therapy and worm expulsion. Fever can be treated with acetaminophen (in children) or aspirin (in adults). Persistent fever over 101°F should be reported.

Niclosamide
(Niclocide)

MECHANISM AND ACTIONS
Niclosamide inhibits oxidative phosphorylation in the mitochondria of cestodal parasites and may also stimulate ATPase. The head (scolex) and proximal segments of the worm are killed on contact, and the parasite is released from its attachment on the intestinal wall. The partially digested worms are then expelled in the feces. The drug does not appear to produce any hematologic, renal, or hepatic abnormalities.

USES
1. Treatment of certain cestodal infections, such as beef, fish, and dwarf tapeworms, and alternative treatment of pork tapeworm

■ WARNING
In the treatment of *pork* tapeworm infections, a purgative must be given within 1 hour to 2 hours after niclosamide, because the lethal action of the drug is against the adult worm but not the ova, which can be liberated into the lumen of the gut. Subsequently, they may be absorbed and may invade other tissues, (muscles, liver, lung, brain), leading to a condition termed cysticercosis, which can produce muscle pain, weakness, nervousness, convulsions, and paralysis.

ADMINISTRATION AND DOSAGE
Niclosamide is used as chewable tablets containing 500 mg. Tablets should be thoroughly chewed and swallowed with water, and are taken after a light meal. For treating beef, pork (see Warning above), and fish tapeworm, adults receive 2 g as a single dose, whereas children are given 1 g to 1.5 g in a single dose, depending on weight. Dosage recommendations for dwarf tapeworm infections are:

Adults: 2 g as a single dose daily for 7 days
Children (over 75 lb): 1.5 g on the first day, then 1 g daily for the next 6 days
Children (25 lb–75 lb): 1 g on the first day, then 0.5 g daily for the next 6 days. For young children, tablets can be crushed and mixed with water to form a paste or mixed with food for easier administration.

Segments of worm may be present in the stool for up to 3 days after therapy. If segments or ova are present on the seventh day, a second course of therapy should be initiated. A patient is not considered cured until the stool is negative for a minimum of 3 months. Stool specimens must be examined soon after passage to determine the presence of worm segments.

FATE
Niclosamide is not appreciably absorbed from the intestines and is excreted largely in the feces.

SIDE-EFFECTS/ADVERSE REACTIONS
The most frequently occurring side-effects with niclosamide are nausea, vomiting, abdominal discomfort, anorexia, and diarrhea. Other untoward reactions resulting from use of niclosamide include oral irritation, constipation, rectal irritation or bleeding, drowsiness, dizziness, headache, weakness, skin rash, pruritus ani, alopecia, fever, sweating, backache, irritability, and palpitations. Overdosage is managed with a fast-acting laxative and enema. Vomiting should not be induced.

CONTRAINDICATIONS AND PRECAUTIONS
Niclosamide should be administered with *caution* to pregnant women or nursing mothers and to children under age 2.

NURSING CONSIDERATIONS
Anemia may occur with tapeworm infections. A CBC with differential should be drawn and iron supplements begun if hemoglobin is below normal. Anemia will slow the body's ability to fight the infection and may necessitate prolonged drug treatment, which increases the incidence of side-effects.

Oxamniquine
(Vansil)

MECHANISM AND ACTIONS
The precise mechanism of action of oxamniquine is not completely established. The drug may cause a shift in worms from the mesentery to the liver, where they ultimately will die. Oxamniquine appears to be more toxic to male schistosomes than to females, but surviving female worms no longer lay eggs.

USES
1. Treatment of all stages (acute, subacute, chronic) of *Schistosoma mansoni* infections

ADMINISTRATION AND DOSAGE
Oxamniquine is available as 250-mg capsules. Adult dosage is based on patient's weight as follows:

Weight	Dose
30 kg–40 kg	500 mg
41 kg–60 kg	750 mg
61 kg–80 kg	1000 mg
81 kg–100 kg	1250 mg

All adult doses are given as a single daily dose. Children under 30 kg should receive 20 mg/kg in two equally divided doses 2 hours to 8 hours apart.

FATE
Oral absorption is good, and peak plasma concentrations occur in 1 hour to 1.5 hours. Plasma half-life is 1 hour to 3 hours. The drug is extensively metabolized and is excreted as inactive metabolites in the urine.

SIDE-EFFECTS/ADVERSE REACTIONS
Transient drowsiness and dizziness occur in approximately one-third of patients given oxamniquine. Although the drug is otherwise well tolerated, there have been occasional reports of headache, nausea, vomiting, anorexia, abdominal pain, urticaria, EEG changes, liver enzyme elevations, and, rarely, epileptiform convulsions. The drug can be taken with food to decrease GI upset.

CONTRAINDICATIONS AND PRECAUTIONS
Oxamniquine should be given with *caution* to patients with a history of convulsive episodes or EEG abnormalities and to pregnant women or nursing mothers. The drug may color the urine a harmless orange-red.

NURSING CONSIDERATIONS
Patients should be warned that dizziness or drowsiness is likely. (Driving, climbing, or operating dangerous equipment should be avoided until the effect of the drug is known.) Taking the drug with food may reduce the severity of this side-effect.

Piperazine
(Vermizine)

MECHANISM AND ACTIONS
The major action of piperazine is on *Ascaris* worms. The drug causes a flaccid paralysis of the worms, presumably by blocking the response of the *Ascaris* muscle to acetylcholine. The paralyzed worms are then dislodged and subsequently expelled by peristalsis. The drug has little effect on larvae in the tissues.

USES
1. Treatment of pinworm and roundworm infections

ADMINISTRATION AND DOSAGE
Piperazine is available as tablets (250 mg) and syrup (500 mg/5 ml). The syrup should be well shaken before use. For roundworm infections, the adult dosage is 3.5 g in a single daily dose for 2 consecutive days. Children are given a daily dose of 75 mg/kg for 2 consecutive days; in severe infections, this dosage regimen is repeated in 1 week.

For pinworm infections, adults and children receive a single daily dose of 65 mg/kg for 7 consecutive days; this regimen may be repeated after 1 week in severe infections.

FATE
Oral absorption of piperazine is good although variable. A portion of the absorbed drug (about 25%) is metabolized and excreted in the urine. The remainder is eliminated largely in the urine as unchanged drug.

SIDE-EFFECTS/ADVERSE REACTIONS
A variety of adverse effects have been reported during piperazine therapy, especially if large doses are used. These include:
GI—Nausea, vomiting, diarrhea, abdominal cramping
CNS—Headache, vertigo, muscular weakness, hyporeflexia, blurred vision, paresthesias, tremors, choreiform movements, convulsions, impaired memory, EEG abnormalities, worsening of epileptic seizures
Allergic—Fever, urticaria, arthralgia, purpura, lacrimation, eczematous skin eruptions, rhinorrhea, bronchospasm, erythema multiforme

CONTRAINDICATIONS AND PRECAUTIONS
Piperazine is contraindicated in patients with kidney dysfunction or a history of convulsive disorders. A *cautious* approach to therapy is warranted in persons with anemia, severe malnutrition, or neurologic disorders, and in pregnant women. Prolonged or repeated use in children should be avoided because of the drug's potential neurotoxic effects.

INTERACTIONS
1. Piperazine may increase the severity of extrapyramidal reactions due to phenothiazine administration.

NURSING CONSIDERATIONS
Because children are more susceptible to the neurotoxic effects of the drug, parents should be taught to monitor closely complaints of headache, dizzi-

ness, or generalized weakness and to report such effects immediately because the drug may cause seizures. Adults taking the drug should also monitor themselves for the same symptoms.

Allergic reactions are also possible with large doses. Patients starting on the drug should be closely monitored for fever, urticaria, and arthralgia, early signs of drug hypersensitivity. Anaphylaxis or erythema multiforme may result if the allergic reaction intensifies. At the first sign of problems, the patient should be brought to an emergency room where emergency resuscitative equipment and epinephrine are available.

Gastrointestinal side-effects may be relieved by taking the drug with food, but, if not, the patient should be closely monitored. Persistent vomiting or diarrhea should be reported because dehydration and electrolyte imbalances are likely to occur, especially in children. The drug may have to be discontinued.

Praziquantel
(Biltricide)

MECHANISM AND ACTIONS
Praziquantel exhibits a rather broad spectrum of activity and a low overall incidence of serious adverse effects. It increases cell membrane permeability of susceptible worms, resulting in loss of intracellular calcium and subsequent paralysis of the worms. Praziquantel also produces vacuolization and subsequent disintegration of the surface tegumentum of the parasite, leading to phagocytosis of the parasite and death. Praziquantel is considered a first-line drug in schistosomal infections and is also active against other trematodes as well as cestodes (see Table 71-1). In addition, praziquantel also shows promise as being useful in the treatment of cysticercosis, a serious complication of *Taenia solium* infections, where the larvae of *Taenia* invade other organs of the body, leading to fatigue, muscle pain, weakness, nervousness, and possibly convulsions or general paralysis.

USES
1. Treatment of schistosomal infections (*i.e.*, *Schistosoma haematobium*, *S. mansoni*, *S. mekongi*, *S. japonicum*)—generally considered the drug of choice
2. Alternative treatment of lung, liver, and intestinal flukes and cestodal (tapeworm) infections (see Table 71-1)
3. Treatment of cysticercosis

ADMINISTRATION AND DOSAGE
Praziquantel is used as 600-mg tablets. Recommended dosage for the various indications is 20 mg/kg three times a day as a 1-day treatment. Dosing intervals should be 4 hours to 6 hours. Tablets should be swallowed whole and not chewed.

FATE
Approximately 80% of an oral dose of praziquantel is rapidly absorbed, and peak plasma levels occur in 1 hour to 3 hours. There is significant first-pass hepatic metabolism. Metabolites of the drug are excreted primarily in the urine, and have an elimination half-life of 4 hours to 5 hours.

SIDE-EFFECTS/ADVERSE REACTIONS
Side-effects with praziquantel are usually mild and transient, although they may be more serious if patients are heavily infested with worms. Reported effects include headache, malaise, abdominal discomfort, dizziness, fever, urticaria, and myalgia. Mild increases in liver enzymes have occurred in some patients. Because the tablets have a bitter taste, gagging or vomiting can occur if they are chewed or kept in the mouth too long.

CONTRAINDICATIONS AND PRECAUTIONS
Praziquantel should not be used to treat ocular cysticercosis, because destruction of parasites in the eye may lead to irreparable lesions. The drug must be given *cautiously* to pregnant or nursing women and to children under 4 years of age.

NURSING CONSIDERATIONS
Praziquantel is very bitter and can produce gagging or vomiting if chewed or kept in the mouth too long. The patient should be instructed to swallow the pill whole with liquid, preferably during a meal to decrease gastrointestinal side-effects.

Drowsiness may occur. The patient should be encouraged to limit driving or other potentially hazardous activities during the 24-hour period the drug is taken until effects are known.

Pyrantel
(Antiminth)

MECHANISM AND ACTIONS
Pyrantel exerts a depolarizing neuromuscular blocking action and inhibits cholinesterase enzymes, producing a spastic paralysis of worms. The worms are then expelled by peristalsis.

USES
1. Treatment of roundworm (ascariasis) and pinworm (enterobiasis) infections

ADMINISTRATION AND DOSAGE
Pyrantel is administered as an oral suspension containing 50 mg/ml. It is given as a single dose of 11 mg/kg (5 mg/lb) to a maximum total dose of 1 g. The drug may be taken with milk or fruit juices, and purging is not necessary.

FATE
Pyrantel is poorly absorbed orally; plasma levels are maximum in 1 hour to 3 hours, but are quite low. The drug is metabolized in the liver and greater than 50% of an oral dose is excreted unchanged in the feces, and less than 7% in the urine as both unchanged drug and metabolites.

SIDE-EFFECTS/ADVERSE REACTIONS
The most common side-effects with pyrantel are anorexia, nausea, and abdominal cramps. In addition, vomiting, diarrhea, tenesmus, gastralgia, elevated SGOT, headache, dizziness, drowsiness, insomnia, and skin rash have been reported.

CONTRAINDICATIONS AND PRECAUTIONS
Cautious use of pyrantel must be undertaken in persons with liver dysfunction, in pregnant women, and in children under 2 years of age.

INTERACTIONS
1. Pyrantel is antagonistic with piperazine in treating *Ascaris* infestation.

NURSING CONSIDERATIONS
Pinworm can be transferred from person to person so all family members should be examined once one member has been diagnosed.

Entire dose of the drug must be taken to ensure adequate dose to combat infestation. After liquid is swallowed, encourage the patient to fill the container with water, milk, or juice and drink the contents to ensure all drug has been taken.

To prevent pinworm reinfestation encourage the family to launder all undergarments, linens, and night clothes and to disinfect toilet and bathtub daily for several days after the last family member is treated. Children should be taught to avoid nail biting and putting fingers in the mouth.

To prevent roundworm reinfestation, teach all cooks to thoroughly wash vegetables.

Quinacrine
(Atabrine)

Quinacrine may occasionally be employed as an alternate drug in the management of tapeworm infections, but has largely been replaced by other, more effective, less toxic agents such as niclosamide, praziquantel, or mebendazole. It apparently acts by causing the head of the worm to detach from the intestinal wall; the worm is then expelled by use of a purgative. Because rather high doses of quinacrine are required to treat tapeworm infections, side-effects are common. Nausea and vomiting are frequently produced by the drug, as well as dizziness, headache, abdominal cramping, and signs of CNS stimulation (*e.g.*, anxiety, restlessness, confusion, aggression, and psychotic behavior). Treatment with quinacrine is best carried out in the hospital because sodium bicarbonate must be administered with the drug to decrease GI distress and alkalinize urine to reduce renal elimination of the drug. Dosage depends on the type of parasite present and is usually administered in divided amounts, followed by a saline purge to remove the worm from the intestinal tract.

For treating beef, pork, or fish tapeworm, adults are given four doses of 200 mg each, 10 minutes apart, together with 600 mg of sodium bicarbonate with each dose. Children are given a total dose of 400 mg to 600 mg in three to four divided doses at 10-minute intervals, together with 300 mg sodium bicarbonate with each dose. A saline purge is administered 1 hour to 2 hours later. The expelled worm is stained yellow.

Quinacrine is also indicated for the treatment of giardiasis, an intestinal protozoal infection caused by the flagellated protozoan *Giardia lamblia*. This disease is the most common protozoal infection in developed countries and is transmitted by cysts in contaminated food or water. Thus, travelers or campers are particularly at risk, as are persons living in crowded, unhygienic conditions. Diagnosis of giardiasis is made by identification of cysts or active trophozoites in fecal specimens. Because most infected individuals are largely asymptomatic, the disease is difficult to recognize and treat.

Adult dosage for quinacrine in giardiasis is 100 mg three times a day for 5 days to 7 days. Children are given 7 mg/kg/day in three divided doses after meals for 5 days. A repeat course may be given 2 weeks later if necessary.

Quinacrine has also been employed in the

treatment of malaria, and this application is discussed in Chapter 70.

Thiabendazole
(Mintezol)

MECHANISM AND ACTIONS

Thiabendazole is a broad-spectrum anthelmintic drug that is vermicidal against pinworm, roundworm, threadworm, hookworm, and whipworm. In addition, it suppresses egg and larvae production by *Trichinella spiralis* (pork roundworm) and reduces fever and eosinophilia, but its effect on larvae that have migrated to muscle is subject to question. The precise mechanism of action of thiabendazole is unknown, however, interference with a helminth mitochondrial enzyme system has been proposed. The drug has also been reported to have analgesic and anti-inflammatory activity. Thiabendazole is a first-line drug against threadworm and rat lungworm infections and cutaneous larva migrans (creeping eruption—see Table 71-1) but, in spite of its broad spectrum of activity, is *not* recommended as first choice in other nematodal infections.

USES

1. Treatment of threadworm (*Strongyloides*) and rat lungworm (*Angiostrongylus*) infections (drug of choice)
2. Treatment of cutaneous larva migrans (creeping eruption) (drug of choice)
3. Alternate treatment of pinworm, whipworm, hookworm, roundworm, and guinea worm infections
4. Symptomatic treatment of invasive trichinosis

ADMINISTRATION AND DOSAGE

Available preparations of thiabendazole include chewable tablets (500 mg) and an oral suspension (500 mg/5 ml). The usual adult dose is 3 g/day in two equally divided doses after meals if possible. Children and adults under 150 lb are given 10 mg/lb/dose. For pinworm infections, two doses are given for 1 day only and may be repeated in 7 days to reduce risk of reinfection. For most other infections, two doses/day are administered for two successive days (up to four successive days for trichinosis). Cleansing enemas are generally not required, nor is dietary restriction necessary.

FATE

Thiabendazole is well absorbed orally, and peak plasma levels occur in 1 hour to 2 hours. The drug is almost completely metabolized in the liver and is excreted largely (90%) within 24 hours in the urine.

SIDE-EFFECTS/ADVERSE REACTIONS

The most frequently noted side-effects during therapy are anorexia, nausea, vomiting, and dizziness. Less often, diarrhea, pruritus, lethargy, drowsiness, headache, and giddiness occur. Other infrequently reported adverse reactions with thiabendazole include:

GI—Epigastric distress, cramping, perianal rash

CNS—Tinnitus, irritability, blurred vision, numbness

Allergic—Fever, flushing, chills, angioedema, erythema multiforme, lymphadenopathy, anaphylaxis

Renal/hepatic—Enuresis, malodor of the urine, crystalluria, hematuria, cholestasis, jaundice, parenchymal liver damage, elevated SGOT

Other—Hypotension, bradycardia, hyperglycemia, leukopenia

CONTRAINDICATIONS AND PRECAUTIONS

Thiabendazole must be administered with *caution* to patients with renal or kidney dysfunction, a history of allergic disorders and to pregnant or nursing women.

NURSING CONSIDERATIONS

Taking thiabendazole with meals may decrease nausea and anorexia and may reduce dizziness. However, the patient should be cautioned to limit driving or other hazardous tasks until the effects on the body are known.

All patients should be cautioned to report immediately any early symptoms of hypersensitivity including fever, flushing, or chills. Anaphylaxis and erythema multiforme can occur with this drug and are life-threatening. The patient should be taken to an emergency room for further evaluation, and the drug will be discontinued.

REVIEW QUESTIONS

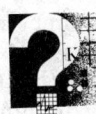

1. What are the major types of nematodes?
2. List the various types of tapeworms.
3. Give the most important types of flukes or trematodes. What is the name of the disease resulting from infection with blood flukes?
4. What adjunctive measures must be undertaken in addition to drug therapy in controlling helminthic infections?
5. What are the principal dangers associated with use of antimony compounds? For what type of infection are they occasionally used as secondary drugs?
6. Give the primary indications for diethylcarbamazine. Mention the most frequently encountered side-effects with this drug.
7. State the mechanism of action and indication for mebendazole.
8. How does niclosamide act in treating cestodal infections?
9. Why must a purgative be given within 2 hours after administering niclosamide for pork tapeworm infections?
10. What is the major indication for oxamniquine? Mention the most common side-effects with oxamniquine.
11. Describe the mechanism of action of piperazine. For what infections is it useful?
12. List the indications for praziquantel.
13. What is cysticercosis? Why is praziquantel *not* recommended for ocular cysticercosis?
14. Against what type of worm is pyrantel effective?
15. What is the mechanism of action of pyrantel?
16. For what indications is thiabendazole considered a primary drug?
17. What are the common adverse effects associated with thiabendazole?
18. What are the principal indications of the following drugs available only on request from the Centers for Disease Control? (a) bithionol, (b) niridazole, (c) stibocaptate, (d) suramin.

BIBLIOGRAPHY

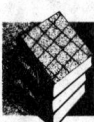

Anderson RM, May RM: Population dynamics of human helminth infections: Control by chemotherapy. Nature 297:557, 1982

Andrews P, Thomas H, Pohlke R, Seubert J: Praziquantel. Med Res Rev 3:147, 1983

Barrett-Connor E: Drugs for treatment of parasitic infection. Med Clin North Am 66:245, 1982

Cook JA: Schistosome infection in humans: Perspectives and recent findings. Ann Intern Med 97:740, 1982

Drugs for parasitic infections. Med Lett Drugs Ther 26:27, 1984

Henley M, Sears JR: Pinworms: A persistent pediatric problem. Maternal/Child Nursing 10:111, 1985

Keusch GT: Anthelmintic therapy: The worm has turned. Drug Therapy 12(8):213, 1982

Pearson RD, Guerrant RL: Praziquantel: A major advance in anthelmintic therapy. Ann Intern Med 99:195, 1983

Sinniah B, Sinniah D: The anthelmintic effect of pyrantel pamoate, oxantel-pyrantel pamoate, levamisole and mebendazole in the treatment of intestinal nematodes. Ann Trop Med Parasitol 75:315, 1981

Sotelo J et al: Therapy of parenchymal brain cysticercosis with praziquantel. N Engl J Med 310:1001, 1984

Storchler D: Chemotherapy of human intestinal helminthiasis: A review, with particular reference to community teatment. Adv Pharmacol Chemother 19:129, 1982

Van den Bossche H, Rochette F, Horig C: Mebendazole and related anthelmintics. Adv Pharmacol Chemother 19:67, 1982

Warren KS, Mahmoud AA (eds): Tropical and Geographical Medicine. New York, McGraw-Hill, 1984

World Health Organization: WHO Scientific Working Group on the Biochemistry and Chemotherapy of Schistosomiasis, p 1. Geneva, WHO, 1984

Xiao S, Catto BA, Webster LT: Effects of praziquantel on different stages of Schistosoma mansoni, in-vitro and in-vivo. J Infect Dis 151:1130, 1985

Amebicides

Carbarsone
Chloroquine
Emetine
Iodoquinol

Metronidazole
Paromomycin

Amebiasis refers to infection with the organism *Entamoeba histolytica*, a protozoan that usually invades the lower intestinal tract but may be found in the liver, lungs, brain, and other organs as well. Amebiasis affects approximately 10% of the world's population, is endemic in many tropical regions, and is present in as many as 4% of the people in the United States, especially those exposed to poor sanitary conditions.

The disease can be manifested in one of several ways:

1. *Asymptomatic intestinal amebiasis*—Presence of the organism in the intestinal tract without evidence of clinical symptoms; treatment is indicated because these patients are at risk for developing GI pathology and can serve as carriers, spreading the infection to other less resistant persons.

2. *Symptomatic intestinal amebiasis*—Presence of overt clinical symptoms ranging from mild manifestations (such as diarrhea, cramping, and flatulence) to severe dysentery with accompanying bloody diarrhea, vomiting, fever, and dehydration. Intestinal mucosal scarring and ulceration can promote systemic absorption of the protozoa, leading to the third stage of the disease, extraintestinal amebiasis.

3. *Extraintestinal (systemic) amebiasis*—Presence of organisms in other body organs, most commonly the liver and lungs; may result in liver necrosis, amebic hepatitis, lung abscesses, and empyema; organisms can also invade the heart, causing pericarditis, and the CNS, leading to brain abscesses.

The drugs used in the treatment of amebiasis can be characterized on the basis of their predominant site of action as luminal, systemic, or mixed. That is, some agents are only active against organisms present in the lumen of the intestine, others are effective against parasites found in the bowel wall and other tissues, whereas still other drugs are claimed to affect both intestinal and extraintestinal protozoa. *Luminal* amebicides include iodoquinol, carbarsone, and diloxanide, and they are used primarily to treat asymptomatic or mild intestinal forms of amebiasis. In addition, they are frequently given together with a systemic or mixed amebicide to completely eradicate an infection.

Systemic amebicides, such as dihydroemetine or chloroquine, are useful in invasive forms of amebiasis, such as amebic dysentery or hepatic abscesses. They are infrequently used today, however, because the preferred drug in most cases of symptomatic intestinal or systemic amebiasis is metronidazole, a *mixed* amebicide effective against both intestinal and systemic forms of the disease.

However, metronidazole has been demonstrated to be carcinogenic in mice and rats, and some clinicians feel that it should be reserved for use in severe acute intestinal amebiasis with hepatic abscesses. Use of metronidazole in symptomatic intestinal or systemic amebiasis is usually accompanied by the luminal drugs diloxanide or iodoquinol, because metronidazole is well absorbed and may fail to reach effective amebicidal levels in the large intestine. Emetine is also active against both intestinal and extraintestinal organisms but is a potentially dangerous drug and must be administered parenterally in a hospital setting under close supervision.

Other drugs that may be effective in intestinal forms of amebiasis are the antibiotics tetracycline, erythromycin, and paromomycin. Of these, however, only paromomycin is sometimes used as an alternative drug in chronic intestinal amebiasis, usually in conjunction with one or more other luminal amebicides.

To better understand the rationale for the use of a particular drug in the various stages of amebiasis, it is helpful to briefly review the two-stage life cycle of *Entamoeba histolytica*.

The organism is transmitted from person to person by ingestion of amebic cysts, a form in which the protozoa are extremely resistant to destruction outside the body. The cysts are likewise unaffected by gastric juice and pass intact to the small intestine where some develop into motile trophozoites that can invade the intestinal mucosa, be absorbed systemically, and find their way to other organs in the body. The remaining cysts are excreted intact, and they can thus continue the reinfective cycle in another person.

Interruption of this cycle can be accomplished in several ways. Most drugs for treating amebiasis are amebicidal, either directly killing or inhibiting the growth and maturation of the trophozoites, whereas some drugs exhibit a cystocidal action. Because most of the currently effective amebicides have the potential to elicit serious untoward reactions, their use should be undertaken only upon a definitive diagnosis of *Entamoeba histolytica* as the causative agent, and patients must be closely observed during therapy for development of adverse reactions.

The amebicides are discussed individually in this chapter. Several drugs used in amebiasis (e.g., paromomycin, chloroquine) are also effective in other disease states and have been reviewed elsewhere. Only those aspects of their pharmacology related to the treatment of amebic infections are considered here.

Carbarsone

Carbarsone is an organic arsenical compound containing approximately 30% arsenic. The drug is directly amebicidal and can eradicate cysts by destroying trophozoites. Carbarsone is rarely used today in treating intestinal amebiasis (and is *not* effective in systemic forms) because it is more toxic than the other available drugs. Adverse effects with carbarsone include nausea, diarrhea, abdominal cramping, weight loss, sore throat, skin rash, pruritus, icterus, mucosal ulceration, hepatitis, neuritis, visual disturbances, polyuria, edema, splenomegaly, liver necrosis, exfoliative dermatitis, and kidney damage.

Carbarsone is contraindicated in persons with liver or kidney diseases, amebic hepatitis, and contracted visual fields. The drug is given in a dose of 250 mg two to three times a day for 10 days; if a repeat course of therapy is needed, 10 days to 14 days rest must be allowed between treatment courses to prevent cumulation toxicity.

Chloroquine
(Aralen)

Primarily employed as an antimalarial drug, chloroquine is also effective in the treatment of amebic liver abscesses (often with emetine), because chloroquine localizes in the liver in a concentration several hundred times greater than in the plasma. The drug is largely ineffective against intestinal organisms because it is rapidly absorbed; therefore, it is always given either in combination with or following other drugs active against intestinal amebiasis. When used in hepatic amebiasis, chloroquine may also be combined with metronidazole or diloxanide or both to ensure that all protozoa are eradicated. The recommended oral dose of chloroquine phosphate for extraintestinal amebiasis is 1 g daily for 2 days, followed by 500 mg daily for 2 weeks to 3 weeks. The drug may also be given IM as the hydrochloride in a dose of 200 mg to 250 mg a day for 10 days to 12 days. Oral therapy should be substituted as soon as possible. Refer to the discussion of chloroquine in Chapter 70 for additional information pertaining to adverse effects, contraindications and interactions, and nursing considerations. At the doses utilized in treating amebiasis, the incidence of retinopathy is lower than in those instances where the drug is used for control of malaria.

Emetine
(Emetine)

MECHANISM AND ACTIONS

Emetine is a potent amebicide effective against both intestinal and extraintestinal tissue parasites. Its use is restricted to severe cases of amebic dysentery and amebic hepatitis or liver abscesses, inasmuch as the drug can cause serious untoward reactions due to cumulative toxicity as well as a wide range of milder adverse effects. The close structural analogue dehydroemetine is available as Mebadin from the Centers for Disease Control in Atlanta, and is equally effective and may be somewhat less toxic (see Table 72-1). Emetine exerts a direct lethal action on trophozoites, probably blocking protein synthesis by interfering with attachment of t-RNA to the ribosomes. The drug is more effective against motile forms than against cysts.

Emetine also possesses anticholinergic and antiadrenergic actions and may reduce serum potassium levels. Cardiac conduction and contraction may be depressed, and electrocardiographic changes have occurred.

USES
1. Symptomatic treatment of acute amebic dysentery, or acute episodes of chronic amebic dysentery, in combination with other amebicides
2. Treatment of amebic hepatitis and amebic abscesses in other tissues, in combination with an amebicide effective against intestinal parasites
3. Alternative treatment of balantidiasis, fascioliasis, and paragonimiasis

ADMINISTRATION AND DOSAGE

Emetine is available for deep SC or IM administration as an injection solution containing 65 mg/ml. The drug should *not* be given IV. Adult dosage should not exceed 65 mg/day (in a single or two divided doses) for up to 10 days. A second course of therapy should not commence in less than 6 weeks. Children over age 8 should receive a maximum of 20 mg/day while children under age 8 are given 10 mg/day. In acute fulminating amebic dysentery, the drug is usually given for 3 days to 5 days, but only long enough to control diarrhea and dysentery.

Table 72-1
*Amebicides Available by Request from the Centers for Disease Control**

Drug	Preparations	Usual Dosage Range	Remarks
dehydroemetine (Mebadin)	Injection—30 mg/ml	Adults and children—1 mg to 1.5 mg/kg/day IM or SC for up to 5 days (maximum 100 mg/day)	Clinical indications are the same as for emetine, but the incidence and severity of cardiovascular complications may be somewhat less; usually given in combination with diloxanide and a tetracycline, followed by chloroquine if hepatic amebiasis is present; daily dosage may be divided into two parts; use very cautiously in patients with cardiac disease or neuromuscular disorders
diloxanide furoate (Furamide)	Tablets—500 mg	Adults—500 mg three times a day for 10 days Children—20 mg/kg/day in three divided doses for 10 days; repeat in several weeks if necessary	A relatively nontoxic intestinal amebicide regarded by many as the drug of choice for asymptomatic and mild symptomatic intestinal amebiasis; ineffective alone against extraintestinal parasites; may be combined with metronidazole in moderate to severe intestinal disease; mild GI distress and flatulence have been reported; GI absorption is appreciable, and much of an oral dose is excreted in the urine within 48 hours, largely as metabolites

* Parasitic Disease Drug Service, Centers for Disease Control, Atlanta, GA 30333.

FATE
The drug is well absorbed from SC or IM injection sites and widely distributed in the body (e.g., kidney, spleen, lungs), with highest concentrations being found in the liver. Emetine is excreted very slowly by the kidney, and some drug is still present in the body 60 days after administration. The danger of cumulative toxicity is appreciable.

SIDE-EFFECTS/ADVERSE REACTIONS
Commonly encountered side-effects with emetine include pain, tenderness, stiffness, and local muscle weakness at injection sites, nausea, diarrhea, abdominal pain, dizziness, and fainting. Urticarial or eczematous lesions may also occur. Skeletal muscle aching and tenderness may persist during therapy. The most serious adverse effects with emetine are related to the cardiovascular system and may include hypotension, tachycardia, precordial pain, cardiac dilatation, ECG abnormalities (T-wave inversion, Q–T prolongation), dyspnea, congestive heart failure, and arrhythmias.

Overdosage is usually marked by muscle tremors, weakness and pain in the extremities, nausea, vomiting, diarrhea, and neuritis. The drug should be discontinued and symptomatic treatment initiated.

CONTRAINDICATIONS AND PRECAUTIONS
Emetine is contraindicated in patients with heart or kidney disease, in patients who have received emetine previously within the last 2 months, and in pregnant women. The drug should also not be used in children *except* those with severe dysentery not controlled by other amebicides. Emetine should be administered *cautiously* to elderly or debilitated patients, nursing mothers, persons with liver disease, and to patients with ECG abnormalities. The drug solution is very irritating and should not be allowed to contact the eye or mucous membranes.

NURSING CONSIDERATIONS
A complete history should be taken before emetine is administered because of the drug's toxic effects. Patients who are pregnant or who have preexisting

cardiovascular or kidney disease should not receive the drug, and those with liver disease should be treated with caution. All patients should have a baseline ECG, electrolytes, and renal and hepatic function studies performed before therapy is initiated. If the patient is dehydrated, which is likely with amebic dysentery, electrolyte and fluid replacements should be aggressive because emetine could cause potassium depletion.

Emetine should be given by intramuscular or deep subcutaneous injection, and sites should be rotated using a body map (see Chap. 8) to minimize the pain, tenderness, and localized weakness at the injection sites. Needle aspiration should always be performed before the injection is given regardless of route, and if blood is aspirated an alternate site should be used. Inadvertent intravenous injection can result in severe drug toxicity.

Patients will receive emetine while hospitalized to facilitate close monitoring. If dehydration and electrolyte imbalance are severe, the patient should be placed on continuous ECG monitoring. Otherwise, the patient should have an ECG performed before initiating therapy as a baseline, after the fifth dose, upon completion of treatment, and again 1 week after treatment has ended to determine the presence or extent of changes. Any arrhythmias, changes in T wave, Q–T interval, or gallop rhythms should be immediately reported. If symptoms persist or worsen the drug will be discontinued.

Renal function can also be more closely monitored while the patient is hospitalized. Intake and urinary output should be recorded and the I/O ratio measured every 24 hours. If changes occur in BUN or serum creatinine or if intake exceeds output for 24 hours, the patient develops dyspnea, rales, or peripheral edema, congestive heart failure and early renal dysfunction should be suspected. The physician should be notified and the drug discontinued.

Neuromuscular toxicity is another serious side-effect of emetine which must be evaluated. Passive range of motion of all extremities and neck rotation should be done every 4 hours while the patient is awake. The patient should be asked to report any pain, stiffness, or tenderness of muscle groups (especially of the neck and upper extremities) or feelings of fatigue or listlessness because these are all early signs of neurotoxicity based on neuromuscular effects of emetine. The physician should be notified, and further neurologic testing should be performed to determine whether the drug should be discontinued. In most cases, the drug will be stopped, because drug excretion is slow and the potential for respiratory depression exists if neuromuscular toxicity spreads to the respiratory muscles.

Emetine is very irritating to the eye and mucous membranes. Consequently, all nurses should wash their hands carefully after handling the drug during administration to avoid self-contamination.

Iodoquinol
(Moebiquin, Yodoxin)

MECHANISM AND ACTIONS
Iodoquinol (diiodohydroxyquin) is an iodinated 8-hydroxyquinoline that exerts an amebicidal action against trophozoites and cysts of *Entamoeba histolytica* in the intestine. The drug is poorly absorbed orally and is therefore *not* effective against trophozoites in the intestinal wall or extraintestinal tissues. Because iodoquinol contains approximately 60% iodine, it can interfere with certain thyroid function tests by increasing serum protein-bound iodine levels.

It is relatively nontoxic and inexpensive and has been used for mass treatment.

USES
1. Treatment of asymptomatic or mild to moderate acute or chronic intestinal amebiasis
2. Treatment of giardiasis (investigational use)

ADMINISTRATION AND DOSAGE
Iodoquinol is used orally as tablets containing either 210 mg or 650 mg. The usual adult dosage is 650 mg two to three times a day for 20 days. Children may receive 40 mg/kg/day in three divided doses for 20 days. The drug should be taken after meals to decrease gastrointestinal discomfort.

FATE
The drug is poorly absorbed from the GI tract (approximately 5%–10%) and is eliminated largely in the feces.

SIDE-EFFECTS/ADVERSE REACTIONS
Gastric distress is the most often reported side-effect with iodoquinol, and is usually manifested as nausea, diarrhea, and abdominal discomfort. In addition vomiting, pruritus ani, fever, chills, headache, vertigo, thyroid enlargement, skin eruptions, urticaria, and itching have occurred during therapy. Long-term therapy with iodoquinol has re-

sulted in neurotoxicity, such as peripheral neuropathy, optic neuritis, and optic atrophy, but these effects are rare when the drug is used at recommended doses for 20 days.

CONTRAINDICATIONS AND PRECAUTIONS

Iodoquinol should not be given to persons with iodine hypersensitivity, and safety for use in pregnant women and nursing mothers has not been established. The drug must be given *cautiously* to persons with thyroid disorders. Iodoquinol can interfere with certain thyroid function tests by increasing protein-bound serum iodine levels.

NURSING CONSIDERATIONS

Patients should be asked about allergy to iodine or previous reaction to diagnostic dyes (which contain iodine) before the drug is given. Hypersensitivity is not uncommon. Patients should be told to report pruritis, urticaria, chills, or fever immediately to avoid serious hypersensitivity. The drug will be discontinued, and appropriate treatment, usually with antihistamines, will be used to alleviate symptoms.

Although rare, optic neuritis and atrophy can occur with this drug, especially in young children. Baseline and periodic ophthalmologic examinations should be performed throughout drug treatment. Patients should be told to report immediately any eye pain, blurring of vision, or black spots in the field of vision, and the drug should be discontinued.

Metronidazole

(Femazole, Flagyl, Metizole, Metro I.V., Metryl, Protostat, Satric)

Metronidazole exerts a direct amebicidal and trichomonacidal action against *Entamoeba histolytica* and *Trichomonas vaginalis*, respectively. It is considered the drug of choice for oral treatment of trichomoniasis in both women and men. In addition, it is employed in treating acute intestinal amebiasis, both symptomatic and asymptomatic as well as amebic liver abscess. The drug has been reported to be carcinogenic in mice and rats, and *unnecessary* use should be avoided. However, metronidazole remains a valuable drug for the therapy of both amebiasis and trichomoniasis.

In addition to its use as both an amebicide and trichomonacide, metronidazole is also available both orally and IV for the treatment of serious infections caused by susceptible anaerobic bacteria.

Parenteral metronidazole has demonstrated clinical activity against the following organisms: anaerobic gram-negative bacilli, including *Bacteroides* and *Fusobacterium* species, anaerobic gram-positive bacilli, including *Clostridium* species; anaerobic gram-positive cocci, including *Peptococcus* and *Peptostreptococus* species. Necessary surgical procedures should always be performed in conjunction with drug treatment, and in mixed aerobic–anaerobic infections, appropriate antibiotics should be included in the drug regimen. The principal hazard connected with parenteral metronidazole therapy is the possibility of convulsive seizures and development of peripheral neuropathy. The benefit-to-risk ratio must be critically evaluated in patients who show evidence of abnormal neurologic signs.

MECHANISM AND ACTIONS

The mechanism of action of metronidazole is not entirely established. It appears to enter the cells of the organism, where it is converted to unstable intermediate compounds which disrupt the structure of DNA in susceptible organisms, causing strand breakage and loss of helical structure. Metronidazole destroys most organisms within 24 hours to 48 hours.

USES

1. Treatment of acute intestinal amebiasis (amebic dysentery) and amebic liver abscess
2. Treatment of symptomatic and asymptomatic trichomoniasis in both sexes (oral only)
3. Treatment of serious infections caused by susceptible anaerobic bacteria, especially *Bacteroides*, *Clostridium*, *Eubacterium*, *Peptococcus*, and *Peptostreptococcus* species (IV)
4. Preoperative, intraoperative, or postoperative prophylaxis of infection in patients undergoing surgery classified as potentially contaminated, such as colorectal, abdominal, or gynecologic surgery.
5. Investigational uses include (a) hepatic encephalopathy, (b) treatment of giardiasis or *Gardnerella vaginalis* infections, (c) Crohn's disease, (d) antibiotic-induced pseudomembranous colitis, and (e) as a radiosensitizer to render tumors more susceptible to radiation.

ADMINISTRATION AND DOSAGE

Metronidazole is available as 250-mg and 500-mg tablets, powder for injection (500 mg/vial), and an injection solution containing 500 mg/100 ml. Recommended doses for the various indications are as follows:

Amebiasis:
Acute intestinal
  Adults: 750 mg three times/day for 5 days
    to 10 days (combined with
    iodoquinol—650 mg three times/day for
    20 days)
  Children: 35 mg to 50 mg/kg/day in three
    divided doses for 10 days.
Amebic liver abscess
  Adults: 500 mg to 750 mg three times/day
    for 5 days to 10 days
Trichomoniasis
  250 mg three times a day orally for 7 days
    for males and females; alternately 2 g in a
    single dose or two divided doses. Allow 4
    weeks to 6 weeks between courses of
    therapy when repeat therapy is required.
    Both partners must be treated to avoid
    reinfection.
Anaerobic infections
  Initially 15 mg/kg infused over 1 hour;
    followed by maintenance doses of 7.5
    mg/kg infused over 1 hour every 6 hours
    for 7 days to 10 days. Maximum dose is 4
    g/24-hour period. A change to oral
    therapy (7.5 mg/kg every 6 hours) should
    be made as condition warrants.
Prophylaxis of postoperative infection
  15 mg/kg infused over 30 minutes to 60
    minutes and completed at least 1 hour
    before surgery, followed by 7.5 mg/kg
    infused over 30 minutes to 60 minutes at
    6 hours and 12 hours after the initial dose.

FATE

Metronidazole is well absorbed from the GI tract; peak serum levels occur in 1 hour to 2 hours. The drug is widely distributed in the body and diffuses well into all tissues and is only slightly (20%) bound to plasma proteins. The plasma half-life is approximately 6 hours to 10 hours. Metronidazole is excreted largely in the urine, both as unchanged drug (20%) and metabolites. Both the parent compound and a 2-hydroxymethyl metabolite have antibacterial activity.

SIDE-EFFECTS/ADVERSE REACTIONS

The most common side-effects encountered during oral metronidazole therapy are nausea, anorexia, diarrhea, epigastric distress, and abdominal cramping. In addition, metallic taste, constipation, proctitis, glossitis, and stomatitis have occurred, frequently accompanied by a local monilial infection. A variety of neurologic effects have been reported with metronidazole and range from mild reactions such as dizziness, vertigo, incoordination, ataxia, irritability, confusion, weakness, insomnia, headache, and paresthesias to more serious effects like peripheral numbness or neuropathy and seizures. These neurologic effects are seen primarily with extended therapy and occur rarely with short courses of low dose therapy.

A mild leukopenia has been noted in some patients but is reversible upon discontinuation of therapy, and no persistent hematologic abnormalities have occurred. Other adverse effects attributable to metronidazole include:

  Allergic—Pruritus, flushing, urticaria, fever
  Urinary—Dysuria, cystitis, polyuria,
    incontinence, darkened urine
  Other—Nasal congestion, xerostomia,
    dyspareunia, decreased libido, pyuria,
    flattened T wave, joint pain, pancreatitis

Thrombophlebitis has developed after IV infusion and may be minimized by avoiding prolonged use of indwelling catheters. Metronidazole has been implicated in paradoxically *causing* pseudomembranous colitis as well as being effective in treating this condition.

Chronic oral administration of metronidazole in rodents has resulted in an increased incidence of neoplastic tumors, especially hepatic and mammary. Unnecessary use of the drug should therefore be avoided.

Overdosage may be characterized by nausea, vomiting, and ataxia. Treatment is generally of a supportive nature.

CONTRAINDICATIONS AND PRECAUTIONS

Use of metronidazole is contraindicated in patients with organic CNS disease and during the first trimester of pregnancy unless *absolutely* necessary. Metronidazole should be used *cautiously* in patients with hepatic dysfunction, persistent fungal infections, kidney disease, in pregnant women or nursing mothers, alcoholics (see under Interactions), and in young children. In addition, some infusion solutions contain substantial amounts of sodium and should be given with care to persons requiring sodium restriction.

INTERACTIONS

1. Alcohol ingestion during metronidazole therapy may elicit a disulfiram-like reaction (abdominal cramps, vomiting, severe headache, hypotension; see Chap. 26).
2. Metronidazole may potentiate the effects of

oral anticoagulants, prolonging prothrombin time.

3. The effectiveness of metronidazole may be reduced if given concurrently with phenobarbital or phenytoin, drugs that may increase its rate of metabolism.
4. Cimetidine may inhibit the metabolism of metronidazole.

NURSING CONSIDERATIONS

See also Nursing Process for patients on anti-infective therapy, Chapter 59.

A drug history should be obtained. If the patient is taking oral anticoagulants, doses may need reduction because metronidazole will potentiate effects and may result in bleeding episodes. Use of phenobarbital or phenytoin should also be noted because these drugs interfere with metronidazole effectiveness; cimetidine may enhance the drug by inhibiting its metabolism. The patient needs to be questioned about alcohol use, because any alcohol ingestion may result in a disulfiram reaction (see Chap. 26). The patient should be cautioned to read all labels and to avoid using cough preparations, mouthwashes, or other substances which might result in inadvertent alcohol ingestion and subsequent reaction. If vomiting, diarrhea, flushing, dizziness (from hypotension), or abdominal pain occur, the patient should seek immediate medical attention. The patient who is a known alcoholic may not be an appropriate candidate for this drug.

Careful history taking should also attempt to rule out pregnancy, renal, hepatic or central nervous system disease, or persistent fungal infections, all of which warrant cautious use. If pregnancy is confirmed by laboratory evaluation, the risks of treatment (possible fetal damage) must be carefully weighed against benefits to the mother and discussed with her before treatment begins.

Laboratory data may include a CBC, total and differential leukocyte counts in all patients, and renal or hepatic function studies and electrolytes in patients who have a history of renal or hepatic problems or diseases necessitating sodium restriction, such as hypertension or congestive heart failure.

Oral drug forms are usually given without complication if the drug is taken with food to decrease the chance of gastrointestinal distress. Intramuscular doses are irritating to the tissue and must be administered in a large muscle mass to decrease pain. Sites should be rotated using a body map (see Chap. 8) and assessed before each injection for pain, swelling, hardness, or induration, all evidence of tissue damage. If symptoms develop, alternate sites or an alternate route should be used. Intravenous administration is associated with thrombophlebitis because the drug is very irritating. IV sites should be changed at least every 48 hours or whenever pain, swelling, or redness of a site develops. Appropriate mixing to neutralize the drug will decrease irritation. The drug will usually be mixed in the pharmacy or be purchased in a premixed form. However, if the nurse must mix the drug on the nursing unit, the sequence of steps given in the manufacturer's instructions must be followed exactly to decrease the chance of precipitate formation. During administration, the IV line should be checked for precipitate, and the infusion rate should be closely monitored. Slow infusion, over 60 minutes, also decreases the risk of thrombophlebitis, but if the drug is not infused in the set time frame, precipitation may have occurred. The solution should be examined and removed if particulate matter is found in the lines.

Mild leukopenia may develop as a side-effect of the drug, necessitating periodic evaluation of total and differential leukocyte counts but is usually asymptomatic. However, if fever, lymph node swelling, or superinfection develop, or if the patient's leukocyte count drops drastically, the patient may need to be placed on protective (reverse) isolation and the drug discontinued until immune resistance is restored.

Superinfection from a secondary fungal overgrowth may occur during metronidazole therapy and will not respond to treatment by that drug. Glossitis, stomatitis, vaginitis, proctitis, or "furry" tongue must be treated with other antifungal medication.

Neurologic side-effects are more common with intravenous therapy and long-term administration. Mild symptoms such as dizziness and vertigo may disappear as the patient adjusts to the drug. Until effects are known, the patient should be cautioned against driving or engaging in any potentially hazardous tasks which may cause injury. More serious effects such as confusion, headache, incoordination, or pain, tingling or numbness of fingers, hands, feet or toes should be immediately reported because they signal CNS toxicity and peripheral neuropathy and warrant drug discontinuation.

Patients should be informed that metronidazole releases an azo metabolite which turns urine a dark reddish-brown but that it is harmless and does not indicate bleeding.

Paromomycin
(Humatin)

MECHANISM AND ACTIONS
Paromomycin is an aminoglycoside that exhibits an antibacterial action resembling that of neomycin. In addition, it exerts an amebicidal action in the intestinal tract, but is not appreciably absorbed orally; therefore it is ineffective in extraintestinal amebiasis. Paromomycin has a direct amebicidal action *in vivo* and *in vitro* and may also reduce the population of intestinal microbes essential for proliferation of protozoa. It is also effective against *Salmonella* and *Shigella*.

USES
1. Treatment of acute and chronic intestinal amebiasis, usually as an alternative drug to other more potent and specific amebicides
2. Adjunctive therapy in management of hepatic coma

ADMINISTRATION AND DOSAGE
Paromomycin is used as 250-mg capsules. In intestinal amebiasis, 25 mg to 35 mg/kg are given daily in three divided doses with meals for 5 days to 10 days. For management of hepatic coma, 4 g/day are administered in divided doses at regular intervals for 5 days to 6 days.

FATE
Paromomycin is not significantly absorbed orally and is excreted almost completely in the stool.

SIDE-EFFECTS/ADVERSE REACTIONS
Untoward reactions are generally limited to the GI tract, and doses above 3 g/day have resulted in nausea, diarrhea, abdominal cramps, vomiting, heartburn, and increased motility. Rarely, vertigo, headache, and skin rash have occurred. Overgrowth of nonsusceptible organisms has resulted from prolonged or repeated therapy. Systemic absorption of the drug, for example through ulcerated areas of the bowel, can lead to tinnitus, hearing impairment, and renal damage.

CONTRAINDICATIONS AND PRECAUTIONS
Paromomycin should not be used in the presence of ulcerative bowel lesions or intestinal obstruction. A *cautious* approach to therapy must be undertaken in patients with preexisting hearing loss, vestibular damage, or renal dysfunction.

NURSING CONSIDERATIONS
See Nursing Process for aminoglycosides in Chapter 65.

REVIEW QUESTIONS

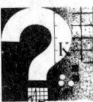

1. Briefly distinguish between intestinal and extraintestinal amebiasis.
2. How may drugs used to treat amebiasis be classified?
3. Describe the two-stage life cycle of *Entamoeba histolytica*.
4. What are the principal disadvantages of carbarsone?
5. What are the indications for chloroquine as an amebicide? Why is the drug largely ineffective against intestinal organisms?
6. Give the mechanism of action of emetine. What other pharmacologic actions does the drug possess?
7. Why must emetine be given IM or SC? Why must needle aspiration be performed with every injection?
8. List the major adverse effects of emetine. How will the patient be monitored for them while receiving the drug?
9. What are the indications for iodoquinol? The drug contains approximately 60% of what element?
10. List the common side-effects of iodoquinol.
11. Why is a drug history essential before metronidazole administration? What information must be obtained in a medical history?
12. Briefly give the major uses for metronidazole.

13. Outline the steps a nurse should follow to ensure careful IV administration of metronidazole.
14. What are the principal dangers associated with metronidazole? What are its most common side-effects?
15. Why must alcohol be avoided during metronidazole therapy?
16. In what forms of amebiasis is paromomycin used?
17. For what condition is diloxanide frequently viewed as the drug of choice?

BIBLIOGRAPHY

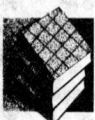

Finegold SM: Metronidazole. Ann Intern Med 93:585, 1980

Goldman P: Metronidazole. N Engl J Med 303:1212, 1980

Gupte S: Phenobarbital and metabolism of metronidazole. N Engl J Med 308:529, 1983

Harries J: Amebiasis: A review. J R Soc Med 75:190, 1982

Knight R: The chemotherapy of amebiasis. J Antimicrobial Chemotherap 6:577, 1980

Molavi A, Le Frock JL, Prince RA: Metronidazole. Med Clin North Am 66:121, 1982

Neal RA: Experimental amebiasis and the development of antiamebic compounds. Parasitology 86:175, 1983

Oldenburg B, Speck WT: Metronidazole. Pediatr Clin North Am 30:71, 1983

Ralph ED: Clinical pharmacokinetics of metronidazole. Clin Pharmacokinet 8:43, 1983

Salvio K, Apuzzio JJ: New antibiotics in the treatment of pelvic infections. JOGN Nursing 13:308, 1984

Warren KS, Mahmoud AAF (eds): Tropical and Geographic Medicine. New York, McGraw-Hill, 1984

Antifungal Drugs

73

Fungal, or mycotic, infections are responsible for a number of pathologic conditions in humans that, with few exceptions, remain a difficult-to-treat group of diseases. Fungal diseases are conventionally categorized as either topical (cutaneous, superficial) or deep (systemic) infections.

Topical infections commonly involve the skin, hair, nails, or vaginal tract and are usually readily treatable with a variety of topical antifungal drugs. Systemic fungal infections are of a more serious nature and may rapidly progress to an acute emergency state. Systemic infections often develop in persons with weakened or compromised host defense mechanisms, such as those situations resulting from disease (*e.g.*, AIDS), trauma, or use of immunocompromising drugs like the cancer chemotherapeutic agents. In addition, organisms responsible for *local* infections of the skin, nails, vagina, or GI tract (such as *Candida*) can also invade deeper body organs, resulting in systemic involvement and serious complications. Because there are only a few effective systemic antifungal drugs, most of which are relatively toxic in the doses needed to eliminate deep mycotic infections, successful treatment of systemic fungal diseases is one of the most difficult tasks in chemotherapy. The need for specific, safe, and effective systemic antifungal agents is acute; until such drugs become available, it is imperative that the currently available drugs be prescribed properly and monitored closely.

Reflecting the classification of fungal diseases into topical or deep infections, antifungal drugs can be categorized in much the same way, although it should be noted that some drugs are utilized in treating both superficial and systemic infections. A useful classification of antifungal agents is given in the box entitled Antifungal Drugs.

The various organisms responsible for the common fungal infections, together with the preferred drugs for treating each disease, are listed in Table 59-1. Most systemic fungal infections respond best to amphotericin B, but it is a highly toxic drug. Flucytosine is indicated for serious candidal or cryptococcal infections and is synergistic with amphotericin B against these organisms. Miconazole and ketoconazole are viewed as rather broad-spectrum antifungal agents, but some questions exist as to their clinical efficacy in many fungal diseases. In addition, relapses have frequently occurred with use of these agents. Oral nystatin is indicated solely for intestinal candidiasis. Topical or vaginal monilial infections due to *Candida* species can be effectively controlled by several antifungal drugs, such as butoconazole, clotrimazole,

---

Antifungal Drugs

A. Drugs for treating systemic infections only
   · flucytosine
B. Drugs for treating both systemic and topical infections
   · amphotericin B
   · ketoconazole
   · miconazole
   · nystatin
C. Drugs for treating topical infections only
   1. Oral administration only
      · griseofulvin
   2. Cutaneous administration only
      · ciclopirox
      · econazole
      · haloprogin
      · iodochlorhydroxyquin
      · tolnaftate
      · triacetin
      · undecylenic acid
   3. Vaginal administration only
      · butoconazole
   4. Cutaneous and vaginal administration
      · clotrimazole
D. Drugs for treating ophthalmic infections only
   · natamycin

---

miconazole, and nystatin. Cutaneous dermatophytal infections (*e.g.*, tinea) of the skin, hair, or nails (such as ringworm, athlete's foot, or jock itch) can be controlled either by oral griseofulvin (severe ringworm) or one of the topically effective antifungal drugs such as ciclopirox, econazole, haloprogin, tolnaftate, triacetin, or undecylenic acid. Natamycin is an antifungal agent used locally in the eye for treatment of fungal conjunctivitis, blepharitis, and keratitis.

The systemic antifungal agents are reviewed individually in detail in this chapter. The topically effective drugs are then listed in Table 73-1, along with their indications, dosage ranges, and specific information relating to each drug.

Systemic Antifungal Agents

Amphotericin B
(Fungizone)

MECHANISM AND ACTIONS
Amphotericin B is an antibiotic produced by a strain of *Streptomyces nodosus* that is active against many species of fungi producing systemic mycotic disease. It has no effect on bacteria, vi-

ruses, or rickettsiae. The drug may be fungistatic or fungicidal depending on the organism and concentration of drug. It binds to sterols (e.g., ergosterol) in the fungal cell membrane, thus increasing cell permeability and allowing leakage of cellular constituents which irreversibly damages the fungal cell. Amphotericin potentiates the effects of flucytosine and other antibiotics by allowing penetration of these drugs into the fungal cell. Because mammalian cell membranes also contain sterols, the drug can damage human cells as well.

Amphotericin is a first-line drug for many severe progressive and potentially fatal systemic fungal infections, but because of its serious toxicity, it should never be used to treat trivial or clinically insignificant fungal diseases. It is also used topically to treat cutaneous or mucosal candidal (i.e., monilial) infections.

USES
1. Treatment of serious and potentially fatal systemic fungal infections, such as aspergillosis, blastomycosis, coccidioidomycosis, cryptococcosis, disseminated candidiasis (moniliasis), histoplasmosis, mucormycosis, and sporotrichosis (see Table 59-1)
2. Alternative treatment of American mucocutaneous leishmaniasis (IV only)—not drug of choice.
3. Treatment of cutaneous and mucocutaneous candidal (monilial) infections (topically only)

ADMINISTRATION AND DOSAGE
Amphotericin is used by slow IV infusion as a solution prepared from lyophilized powder (50 mg/vial) mixed with sterile water for injection only. The infusion solution is then obtained by further dilution (1:50) with 5% dextrose injection of pH above 4.2. The drug is also available as a 3% cream ointment or lotion for topical use. A test dose of 1 mg may be infused slowly to determine patient tolerance. Dosage is individualized and given as follows:

IV infusion: initially 0.25 mg/kg/day infused over 6 hours; increase gradually to 1 mg/kg/day or 1.5 mg/kg every other day as tolerance permits; total treatment time is usually several months, although some serious infections (e.g., sporotrichosis, aspergillosis) can require 9 months to 12 months of therapy

The maximum daily dose is 1.5 mg/kg; total dosage can range from 1.5 g for blastomycosis up to 4 g for life-threatening infections such as rhinocerebral

phycomycosis, although the risk of toxicity is extremely high at these levels

Intrathecal/intraventricular: 0.1 mg initially, increased gradually up to 0.5 mg every 48 hours to 72 hours (investigational use only—drug does not penetrate CNS when given IV)

Topical: apply liberally to lesions two to four times a day for 1 week to 4 weeks depending on response

FATE
Amphotericin is poorly absorbed from the GI tract and is not given orally. Following IV infusion, the drug is highly (90%–95%) bound to plasma proteins and has a plasma half-life of 24 hours. Amphotericin diffuses well into inflamed pleural and peritoneal cavities and joints, but poorly into most other body tissues. It is slowly excreted by the kidneys (elimination half-life is 15 days), a small fraction in a biologically active form. Drug can be detected in the urine for at least 7 weeks after termination of therapy.

SIDE-EFFECTS/ADVERSE REACTIONS

■ WARNING
Because amphotericin B is frequently the only drug effective in potentially fatal fungal diseases, the high likelihood of adverse effects must be viewed in the context that this is a potentially life-saving drug.

IV administration of amphotericin B is associated with the frequent occurrence of a variety of untoward reactions, such as fever, chills, nausea, vomiting, diarrhea, headache, dyspepsia, impaired renal function (hypokalemia, azotemia, renal tubular acidosis, nephrocalcinosis), anorexia, weight loss, malaise, muscle and joint pain, abdominal cramping, pain at injection site, phlebitis, and normochromic-normocytic anemia.

Less commonly noted reactions include maculopapular rash, pruritus, tinnitus, hearing loss, blurred vision, vertigo, flushing, peripheral neuropathy, blood pressure alterations, arrhythmias, cardiac arrest, blood dyscrasias, coagulation defects, anuria, oliguria, hemorrhagic gastroenteritis, convulsions, anaphylactic reaction, and acute liver failure.

Permanent renal damage has occurred in patients receiving large doses (e.g., greater than 5 g).

Decreased renal blood flow and glomerular filtration rate and increased serum creatinine are noted in many patients, and electrolyte disturbances (*e.g.,* hypokalemia, hypomagnesemia) can develop.

Many of the adverse reactions can be minimized by giving aspirin, antihistamines, antiemetics, corticosteroids, and sodium supplementation. Alternate day therapy may decrease the incidence of anorexia and phlebitis. Meperidine may be useful in reducing fever and shaking chills, while heparin has been used to minimize the incidence of thrombophlebitis.

Topical application of amphotericin B has resulted in drying of the skin, irritation, pruritus, erythema, burning, contact dermatitis, and skin discoloration.

CONTRAINDICATIONS AND PRECAUTIONS

There are no absolute contraindications to amphotericin B if the situation being treated is potentially life-threatening. A *cautious* approach to use of amphotericin B is necessary in patients with renal impairment, blood dyscrasias, neurologic disorders, peptic ulcer, and in pregnant women.

INTERACTIONS

1. Hypokalemia produced by amphotericin B may be increased by diuretics or corticosteroids, and poses a danger in patients receiving digitalis drugs.
2. Amphotericin B can enhance the effect of peripherally acting muscle relaxants, for example, curare, gallamine, or succinylcholine.
3. Concomitant use of corticosteroids, antibiotics, or antineoplastics with amphotericin B can increase the incidence of superinfections and blood dyscrasias.
4. Aminoglycosides and other nephrotoxic or ototoxic drugs can have additive toxic effects with amphotericin B.
5. Flucytosine, minocycline, and rifampin can potentiate the antifungal activity of amphotericin B.

■ Nursing Process

□ ASSESSMENT

□ Subjective Data

Although the benefits of therapy will always be weighed against the risks, amphotericin B is used to treat fungal infections for which there are few or no alternatives. However, data collection can help

identify the patients at greatest risk for problems. A drug history should be obtained (see under Interactions). Patients on digitalis drugs are at greater risk for digitalis toxicity while taking amphotericin B because of the chance of drug-induced hypokalemia. Therefore, the patient on digitalis may need a potassium supplement throughout treatment. Likewise, patients receiving thiazide diuretics or corticosteroids which deplete body potassium may also need supplements for the same reason. All patients should be asked about use of nephrotoxic or ototoxic drugs such as furosemide or aminoglycosides and, if possible, these should be discontinued because the risk of toxicity increases with such combinations.

Medical history usually does not rule out any patient who needs the drug, but amphotericin B should be used cautiously in patients who are pregnant or who have known renal, blood, or neurologic disorders or peptic ulcer disease. Close laboratory monitoring and dosage adjustments are essential in such patients.

□ Objective Data

Physical assessment includes examination of the site of infection as well as baseline measurements of temperature, pulse, respiration, blood pressure, weight, and urinary output, all of which can change as a result of drug side-effects.

Diagnostic work-up should include a baseline ECG because cardiac arrhythmias may occur during drug therapy. Laboratory data should include CBC with differential, serum and urine electrolytes, especially sodium, potassium, and chloride, hepatic function studies (amphotericin can alter SGOT and SGPT), serum creatinine, BUN, and urinalysis.

□ NURSING DIAGNOSIS

Actual nursing diagnoses for the patient receiving amphotericin B include:

Knowledge deficit related to the drug's action and side-effects (and application if the topical formulation is used)

Potential nursing diagnoses for common drug side-effects may include:

Alteration in body temperature: a drug side-effect

Alteration in bowel elimination: diarrhea

Alteration in comfort: nausea, vomiting, headache

Alteration in tissue perfusion related to thrombophlebitis at IV site or renal dysfunction

Alteration in skin integrity related to effects of topical applications to skin

□ *PLAN*

Nursing care goals focus on

1. Safe, correct administration of the drug
2. Close monitoring of major side-effects, including electrolyte imbalance, renal toxicity, gastrointestinal and thermoregulation dysfunction, and hypersensitivity as well as the less frequent problems of cardiac arrhythmias, ototoxicity, blood dyscrasias, liver failure, and peripheral neuropathy
3. Teaching the patient correct topical administration and most frequent side-effects to monitor

□ *INTERVENTION*

Topical amphotericin B should be applied liberally to the infected site and rubbed well into the lesions. These preparations can stain all fabrics, but the stain is easily removed by washing with soap and water or using a commercial stain remover. The cream formulation may stain skin and is more likely to cause skin drying; the lotion can stain nail lesions. Topical amphotericin B may cause local hypersensitivity reactions but is not likely to cause significant systemic side-effects unless the therapy is prolonged or systemic absorption through an open lesion is significant. In such cases the patient should be closely monitored as described below.

Intravenous amphotericin B must be administered slowly (usually over 6 hours) by intermittent infusion and monitored by an infusion pump or other rate control device. The drug solution will aggregate in a 0.22-micron final filter; therefore, if filtering is desired, the mean pore diameter must be at least 1.0 micron to ensure drug passage. Amphotericin B is physically incompatible with normal saline and potassium chloride; it must be mixed with 5% dextrose and water as the infusion fluid. In general, amphotericin B is incompatible with most drugs and should be infused separate from other intravenous medications. However, certain drugs are frequently prescribed with the antifungal agent to decrease the incidence of side-effects and may be administered intravenously with amphotericin B. These include chlorpheniramine maleate, diphenhydramine hydrochloride, hydrocortisone sodium succinate, methylprednisolone sodium succinate, and heparin. The manufacturer recommends covering the bag or bottle containing amphotericin B, but institutional policy may vary because recent studies indicate little change in drug stability in hospital light. The infusion container should be agitated every hour to ensure the drug remains dispersed in solution.

Initial IV therapy usually begins with a test dose of 1 mg administered over 2 hours to 6 hours. Vital signs should be monitored every 30 minutes to 60 minutes during this infusion to catch early the development of high fever or pulse changes. Vital signs should then be taken at least every 4 hours throughout the course of drug therapy because adverse reactions can happen at any time.

Thrombophlebitis occurs frequently during intravenous administration. Sites must be rotated at least every 48 hours or more frequently if redness, pain, or swelling occur. The danger of thrombophlebitis can be decreased by using small bore needles such as a 22-gauge scalp vein type, but if persistent problems occur the physician may order low dose heparin, usually 500 U to 1500 U to each 500-ml bottle of 5% dextrose and water.

To decrease the frequent side-effects of headache, fever, and chills associated with amphotericin B as a result of hypersensitivity to the drug, the physician may order premedication with acetaminophen or aspirin; antiemetics may be ordered to counteract nausea and vomiting; antidiarrheals may be used to treat diarrhea. If these measures do not work, antihistamines and corticosteroids may be added. However, the nurse must be aware that addition of significant doses of corticosteroids increases the risk of superinfection by other organisms not susceptible to amphotericin B.

Nephrotoxicity, a danger of amphotericin B with the majority of patients, must be monitored closely to avert irreversible damage. Laboratory evaluations of BUN, serum creatinine, and urinalysis must be done weekly throughout therapy and more often when dosage is being increased. If BUN exceeds 40 mg/dl or if serum creatinine is greater than 3.0 mg/dl, the drug dose should be lowered or the drug should be discontinued. Other signs of renal dysfunction include oliguria (monitor intake and urinary output closely), hematuria, cloudy urine, or azotemia (identifiable on urinalysis) and should be immediately reported. Most renal problems are reversible unless the daily dose exceeds 4 g, which may permanently damage the renal tubules.

Renal changes during drug therapy lead to tubule acidosis, which may cause potassium depletion. Signs of hypokalemia include muscle weakness, cramping, drowsiness, and paresthesias and should be reported. Supplemental potassium may be needed. Sodium and chloride deficiencies can also occur as a result of renal changes. To identify problems early, the patient should have weekly serum and urine electrolyte levels drawn.

Other side-effects are less common, but most are potentially dangerous. High-pitch hearing should be tested weekly with a tuning fork, and the patient should be told to report immediately any dizziness, tinnitus, or changes in hearing because amphotericin B is potentially ototoxic especially as renal function becomes impaired. Cardiovascular changes should be closely monitored by frequent pulse and blood pressure checks every 4 hours during therapy and by a weekly ECG. Patients should be told to report any dizziness or palpitations. Blood dyscrasias can be monitored by a weekly CBC with differential, and the patient needs to report any sore throat, bleeding, bruising, or petechiae. Peripheral neuropathies can develop. Pain, pressure, temperature, and strength testing of fingers, hands, toes, and feet should be completed weekly, and the patient should report numbness, tingling, or weakness of any extremities. Acute liver failure can also occur. Weekly liver enzymes and bilirubin should be monitored, and the patient should be checked for signs of weakness, malaise, fever, darkening of urine, and light-colored stools.

□ *EVALUATION*

Outcome criteria which may be used to judge the effectiveness of drug therapy include resolution of infection; correct administration in the prescribed time frame; no evidence of thrombophlebitis; adequate control of headache, fever, chills, and diarrhea with adjunctive drug therapy; BUN below 40 mg/dl and serum creatinine below 3.0 mg/dl for duration of therapy with no other evidence of renal toxicity; timely monitoring of electrolytes with replacement before depletion occurs; no evidence of significant side-effects such as ototoxicity, cardiovascular abnormalities, blood dyscrasias, peripheral neuropathies, or acute liver failure. For the patient using topical amphotericin B, the outcomes sought include evidence that the patient knows how to apply the drug correctly, and that the patient verbalizes an understanding of possible hypersensitivity reaction to the drug and reports any problems promptly.

Flucytosine

(Ancobon)

MECHANISM AND ACTIONS

Flucytosine is a synthetic pyrimidine that is structurally related to the antineoplastic drug fluorouracil. Flucytosine is an orally effective systemic antifungal drug that is considered a secondary agent in treating deep-seated mycotic infections due to *Candida* and *Cryptococcus* species. It is less toxic than amphotericin B, but is less effective as well, and resistance frequently develops rapidly. Thus, it is used mainly in combination with amphotericin B for treating cryptococcal infections such as meningitis and pulmonary infections.

Flucytosine is probably converted to 5-fluorouracil in fungal cells (but not normal mammalian cells) and acts as a competitive inhibitor of nucleic acid synthesis. Host cells apparently lack the enzyme that converts drug to the active metabolite and are thus unaffected.

USES

1. Treatment of serious systemic candidal infections (endocarditis, septicemia, urinary) or cryptococcal infections (meningitis, septicemia, pulmonary, urinary). Flucytosine appears to have a synergistic effect with amphotericin B against *Candida* and *Cryptococcus*.

ADMINISTRATION AND DOSAGE

Available preparations of flucytosine include 250-mg and 500-mg capsules. The usual dosage is 50 mg to 150 mg/kg/day in divided doses at 6-hour intervals. If large doses are required, capsules may be taken a few at a time over 15 minutes to minimize nausea and vomiting. The dosage must be lowered if BUN or serum creatinine is elevated.

FATE

Flucytosine is well absorbed orally, and peak plasma concentrations occur within 1 hour to 2 hours. The drug is minimally bound to plasma proteins. Flucytosine is widely distributed in the body, and drug levels in cerebrospinal fluid reach 50% to 100% of those in the serum. It is not significantly metabolized, but excreted largely unchanged (90%) in the urine; the serum half-life is 3 hours to 6 hours.

SIDE-EFFECTS/ADVERSE REACTIONS

Flucytosine is reasonably well tolerated, and untoward reactions appear to be the result of conversion of the drug to 5-fluorouracil (see under Mechanism and Actions). The most often encountered side-effects are nausea, diarrhea, vomiting, and skin rash. Among the other reported adverse reactions are anemia, leukopenia, thrombocytopenia, pancytopenia, hepatomegaly, enterocolitis, elevation of SGOT, SGPT, BUN, and serum creatinine. Headache, vertigo, drowsiness, confusion, and hallucinations have occurred rarely.

CONTRAINDICATIONS AND PRECAUTIONS

There are no absolute contraindications to flucytosine. The drug should be used *cautiously* in patients with renal impairment, bone marrow depression, hematologic disorders, hepatic dysfunction, in pregnant women or nursing mothers, and in persons receiving radiation or cancer chemotherapy.

INTERACTIONS

1. Flucytosine can potentiate the antifungal effects and the toxicity of amphotericin B.
2. Concurrent use with other bone marrow-depressing drugs (*e.g.,* antineoplastics, phenylbutazone) may increase the toxic effects of both drugs.

NURSING CONSIDERATIONS

Baseline and periodic evaluations of BUN, creatinine, liver enzymes, and CBC with differential should be performed to identify early any renal, hepatic, or hematologic dysfunction. A periodic culture and drug sensitivity of the infected site must be done to determine if drug resistance has developed, which may occur with prolonged therapy.

Nausea and vomiting may be minimized by having the patient take the capsules a few at a time over a 15-minute period for each dose. Small frequent meals and limiting fluids with drug dose may also help. Antidiarrheal agents may be taken if diarrhea develops. However, if symptoms persist, the physician should be notified.

Urinary output and the ratio of intake to output should be closely monitored in addition to BUN and serum creatinine throughout therapy as an indicator of renal function. Serum drug level of flucytosine should also be drawn at intervals to determine whether the drug is being excreted normally. A decrease in urinary output or a significant change in serum drug level may be the first signs of renal failure and must be reported immediately.

Griseofulvin

Microsize (Fulvicin-U/F, Grifulvin V, Grisactin)
Ultramicrosize (Fulvicin P/G, Grisactin Ultra, Gris-PEG)

MECHANISM AND ACTIONS

Griseofulvin is an orally administered fungistatic antibiotic derived from a species of *Penicillium*. It is *only* effective against dermatophyte infections of the skin, hair, and nails. Griseofulvin is available as either a microsize or ultramicrosize particle formulation. Ultramicrosize griseofulvin exhibits approximately 1.5 times the biologic activity of microsize griseofulvin, largely because of improved GI absorption; thus a 330-mg dose of ultramicrosize yields antifungal activity comparable to a 500-mg dose of the microsize formulation. However, there is no evidence that the ultramicrosize formulation is clinically superior with regard to efficacy or safety. The drug localizes in keratin precursor cells in skin, nails, and hair and disrupts the mitotic spindle, thus arresting cell division. New keratin that is subsequently formed strongly binds griseofulvin and becomes resistant to fungal invasion. Griseofulvin has no effect on bacteria, yeasts, or fungi other than dermatophytal organisms.

USES

1. Treatment of fungal infections of the skin, hair, or nails caused by the following dermatophytes: *Epidermophyton, Microsporum,* or *Trichophyton* (Griseofulvin is *not* effective in systemic mycotic infections, candidiasis, tinea versicolor, or bacterial infections—it should not be used in trivial infections which respond to topical agents alone.)

ADMINISTRATION AND DOSAGE

The microsize formulations of griseofulvin include capsules (125 mg, 250 mg), tablets (250 mg, 500 mg), and an oral suspension (125 mg/5 ml). The ultramicrosize preparations are tablets containing either 125 mg, 165 mg, 250 mg, or 330 mg of griseofulvin. Adult dosage is 500 mg to 1 g microsize or 330 mg to 750 mg ultramicrosize daily in a single dose or divided doses. Treatment is continued until the organism is completely eradicated, as determined by clinical and laboratory evaluation and may range from 2 weeks to 4 weeks for infections of the scalp to at least 6 months for infections of the toenails.

Children over 2 years may be given 11 mg/kg/day of the microsize or 7.3 mg/kg/day of the ultramicrosize in divided doses. Dosage has not been established for children under 2 years of age.

FATE

Oral absorption is somewhat variable, the ultramicrosize preparation being absorbed more efficiently than the microsize formulation. Peak plasma levels occur in about 4 hours, and drug is detectable in the skin within 4 hours to 8 hours. Griseofulvin exhibits a greater affinity for diseased skin than normal skin. Its plasma half-life is approximately 24 hours, and it is metabolized in the liver and slowly excreted in the urine, mainly as metabolites.

SIDE-EFFECTS/ADVERSE REACTIONS

Skin rash and urticaria are the most commonly encountered side-effects with griseofulvin. Less frequently, nausea, vomiting, diarrhea, epigastric distress, headache, fatigue, dizziness, insomnia, confusion, psychomotor impairment, oral thrush, paresthesias, photosensitivity, proteinuria, leukopenia, and acute intermittent porphyria have been reported. A systemic lupus-like syndrome has occurred during griseofulvin therapy.

CONTRAINDICATIONS AND PRECAUTIONS

Griseofulvin should not be used in patients with porphyria, severe liver disease, and systemic lupus erythematosus. The drug is teratogenic in rats and should not be given to pregnant women unless absolutely necessary. Griseofulvin should be administered *cautiously* to patients with a history of penicillin allergy, to alcoholics (see under Interactions), and to patients with renal dysfunction.

INTERACTIONS

1. Griseofulvin can reduce the activity of oral anticoagulants.
2. The activity of griseofulvin may be diminished through enzyme induction by barbiturates, glutethimide, diphenhydramine, orphenadrine, and phenylbutazone.
3. The effects of alcohol may be potentiated by griseofulvin, producing tachycardia and flushing.

NURSING CONSIDERATIONS

A drug history should be obtained (see under Interactions). The patient should be asked about allergy to penicillin as cross-hypersensitivity to griseofulvin may occur. However, patients allergic to penicillin have been successfully treated with griseofulvin without allergic reactions.

Griseofulvin should be taken with meals to decrease the chance of gastrointestinal distress. Diet during therapy should contain moderate amounts of fat which increase absorption of the drug. Alcohol should be avoided completely during treatment.

Drug therapy must be taken for a complete course to be effective and will be prolonged until the infecting organism is completely eradicated as indicated by clinical and laboratory examinations.

The process is slow because hair and nails generally grow slowly and, consequently, the infected cells are removed slowly.

A weekly CBC with differential should be performed during extended therapy to monitor possible blood dyscrasias. In addition, the patient should be told to report immediately fever, sore throat, mucosal ulceration, or extreme malaise.

Local hypersensitivity reactions are common but should be reported immediately. The physician may opt to treat urticaria with antihistamines and continue the drug treatment. If symptoms persist or worsen, the drug must be discontinued.

Photosensitivity may occur in some patients. Patients should be told of the potential for severe sunburn and be advised to avoid midday sun and to wear protective clothing and sunscreens as much as possible.

Superinfection with nonsusceptible fungi may develop when a patient is taking griseofulvin. Diarrhea, perianal itching, stomatitis, or black "furry" tongue should be immediately reported. Treatment with appropriate antifungals will usually alleviate the problem.

Ketoconazole

(Nizoral)

MECHANISM AND ACTIONS

Ketaconazole is an orally effective antifungal agent used for treating a variety of oral and systemic fungal infections. It is less toxic than amphotericin B, but somewhat less effective as well. Gastrointestinal complaints are common, and serious hepatotoxicity has been reported. The mechanism of action is not completely established; however, the drug impairs the synthesis of ergosterol, which is a vital component of fungal cell membranes, resulting in increased permeability and subsequent leakage of cellular components. The clinical response to ketoconazole is slow, and the drug is usually more suited to chronic suppressive therapy than treatment of acute, severe fungal infections. Penetration of the drug into the CNS is negligible, and it is of limited usefulness in fungal meningitis (except in very high doses) and in urinary tract infections, because it is extensively metabolized before excretion.

USES

1. Treatment of the following systemic fungal infections: candidiasis, oral thrush, chronic mucocutaneous candidiasis, candiduria, histo-

plasmosis, blastomycosis, coccidioidomycosis, paracoccidioidomycosis, and chromomycosis
2. Treatment of severe, resistant, cutaneous dermatophytal infections not responding to topical therapy or oral griseofulvin
3. Investigational uses include treatment of onychomycosis (due to *Trichophyton* or *Candida* species), pityriasis versicolor (tinea versicolor), recurrent vaginal candidiasis, and advanced prostatic carcinoma

ADMINISTRATION AND DOSAGE

Ketoconazole is available as oral tablets containing 200 mg, an oral suspension containing 100 mg/5 ml, and as a 2% topical cream (see Table 73-1). The recommended adult dosage is 200 mg once daily; this may be increased to 400 mg once daily if the response is insufficient. Children over 2 years of age may be given 3.3 mg to 6.6 mg/kg/day as a single daily dose. Minimum treatment is 1 week to 2 weeks for candidiasis, 4 weeks for recalcitrant dermatophyte infections, and 6 months for other systemic mycotic infections.

FATE

Ketoconazole is usually well absorbed orally, and peak serum levels occur in 1 hour to 2 hours. Tablet dissolution and absorption of drug require an acidic environment, and absorption can be impaired by alkalinizing agents (see under Interactions). This drug is highly (95%–99%) protein-bound. Cerebrospinal fluid penetration is negligible. Ketoconazole undergoes extensive hepatic metabolism and is excreted largely (80%–90%) in the bile and feces (by enterohepatic circulation) with about 10% to 15% of drug excreted in the urine. The *rate* of elimination is dose dependent.

SIDE-EFFECTS/ADVERSE REACTIONS

Nausea, GI upset, and vomiting are the most common side-effects with ketoconazole, but their incidence can be reduced by administering the drug with food. Other reported untoward reactions include diarrhea, headache, dizziness, photophobia, somnolence, pruritus, fever, chills, impotence, gynecomastia, urticaria, rash, paresthesias, thrombocytopenia, oligospermia (with doses above 400 mg), and hepatic dysfunction. Elevated transaminase occurs in 5% to 10% of patients, however it is usually mild and asymptomatic. *Serious* hepatic toxicity with ketoconazole is relatively rare, and hepatic injury is reversible upon discontinuation of the drug. The drug should be stopped if signs of liver dysfunction occur, such as fatigue, anorexia, nausea, vomiting, darkened urine, pale stools, and jaundice.

CONTRAINDICATIONS AND PRECAUTIONS

Ketoconazole is not appropriate for treating fungal meningitis because it penetrates poorly into the CNS. The drug must be administered *cautiously* to persons with hepatic dysfunction, and to pregnant women or nursing mothers and children under 2 years of age.

INTERACTIONS

1. GI absorption of ketoconazole may be impaired by antacids, cimetidine, ranitidine, famotidine, anticholinergics, and other drugs that reduce stomach acidity.
2. Ketoconazole can enhance the anticoagulant effect of coumarins and may elevate the plasma level of cyclosporine.
3. Rifampin can reduce blood levels of ketaconazole if given concurrently.
4. Use of ketoconazole and phenytoin may alter the metabolism of one or both drugs.

NURSING CONSIDERATIONS

A drug history should be obtained, and the patient should be asked specifically about the use of antacids, cimetidine, or anticholinergics, which will decrease stomach acidity and interfere with drug absorption.

Gastrointestinal side-effects can be reduced or eliminated by taking the drug with a small amount of food, but if possible the drug should be taken before meals. Persistent vomiting or diarrhea should be reported to the physician. Ketoconazole may cause dizziness; therefore, the patient should be warned to limit driving or other potentially hazardous activities until the effects on his body are known. Hypersensitivity reactions are also common, so the patient should be told to report pruritus, urticaria, fever, or chills.

Blood dyscrasias and hepatic dysfunction are uncommon (see under Side-Effects/Adverse Reactions), but patients on extended therapy should have a periodic CBC with differential and hepatic enzymes drawn. They should be told to report bleeding, sore throat, fever, or bruising (signs of blood dyscrasias), as well as fatigue, nausea, darkened urine, or light-colored stools (liver dysfunction).

Miconazole

(Monistat IV)

MECHANISM AND ACTIONS

Miconazole is a broad-spectrum antifungal agent that can be used intravenously for treatment of severe systemic fungal infections as well as topically and vaginally for control of cutaneous and mucocutaneous candidal and dermatophytal infections. The discussion that follows focuses on the systemic use of miconazole; its topical application is considered in Table 73-1. Miconazole alters the permeability of the fungal cell membrane, resulting in loss of cell constituents and ultimately cellular death. The drug is less effective than amphotericin B in severe systemic fungal infections and is not a drug of choice for any systemic infection but represents an alternative to amphotericin B.

USES

1. Alternative treatment of coccidioidomycosis, paracoccidioidomycosis, cryptococcosis, petriellidiosis, and chronic mucocutaneous candidiasis (not effective alone in fungal meningitis or urinary bladder infections)
2. Topical treatment of cutaneous and mucocutaneous candidal and dermatophytal infections (see Table 73-1)

ADMINISTRATION AND DOSAGE

Miconazole is available as an injectable solution containing 10 mg/ml as well as several topical dosage forms listed in Table 73-1. The drug solution is diluted in at least 200 ml of fluid (0.9% sodium chloride or 5% dextrose) and infused over 30 minutes to 60 minutes. The total daily dosage listed below may be divided over three infusions; the average duration of therapy is indicated below for the various infections.

   Coccidioidomycosis—1800 mg to 3600 mg/
      day for 3 weeks to 20 weeks
   Cryptococcosis—1200 mg to 2400 mg/day for
      3 weeks to 12 weeks
   Petriellidiosis—600 mg to 3000 mg/day for 5
      weeks to 20 weeks
   Candidiasis—600 mg to 1800 mg/day for 1
      week to 20 weeks
   Paracoccidioidomycosis—200 mg to 1200
      mg/day for 2 weeks to 15 weeks

   Longer treatment may be necessary in severe or resistant infections, and the drug should be continued until clinical and laboratory tests indicate that the organism has been eradicated.

   Children may be given a dose of 20 mg to 40 mg/kg/day in divided infusions, not to exceed a dose of 15 mg/kg per infusion.

   Miconazole may also be administered intrathecally as an undiluted solution in a dosage of 20 mg (2 ml) every 3 days to 7 days as an adjunct to IV treatment in fungal meningitis. Injections should be rotated between the lumbar, cervical, and cis-

teral sites with each dose. Urinary bladder mycoses may be treated with instillation of 200 mg of diluted solution into the bladder.

FATE

Miconazole is highly bound to plasma protein, and penetration into cerebrospinal fluid is poor. The drug does attain significant levels in the peritoneal cavity, eye, and inflamed joints. It is rapidly metabolized in the liver and excreted both in the urine and feces, mainly as inactive metabolites. The elimination half-life is 20 hours to 25 hours.

SIDE-EFFECTS/ADVERSE REACTIONS

Following IV administration, there is a frequent occurrence of nausea, vomiting, phlebitis, pruritus, rash, and fever. Other untoward reactions are diarrhea, anorexia, thrombocytopenia, drowsiness, flushing, hyponatremia, and anaphylactic reactions. Reversible hyperlipemia has occurred and is probably due to the vehicle (Cremophor EL, which is PEG 40 and castor oil). Too rapid injection of undiluted miconazole may produce transient tachycardia or arrhythmias.

CONTRAINDICATIONS AND PRECAUTIONS

Miconazole must be administered with *caution* to pregnant women or nursing mothers, young children, and to persons with hyperlipemia or anemia (drug can decrease hematocrit).

INTERACTIONS

1. The effects of oral anticoagulants may be enhanced by IV miconazole.
2. Miconazole and amphotericin B are mutually antagonistic and the antifungal activity of the combination is less than that of either drug used alone.
3. Miconazole may potentiate the hypoglycemic action of the oral antidiabetic drugs.
4. The metabolism of phenytoin may be reduced by concurrent use of miconazole.

NURSING CONSIDERATIONS

Miconazole should be infused slowly to minimize side-effects and decrease the risk of phlebitis. Cardiac arrest has occurred with too rapid administration. The IV site should be rotated every 48 hours or more frequently if redness, pain, or swelling occur. The infusion should be monitored with an infusion pump to prevent rapid administration. The patient should be placed on a cardiac monitor for the first dose especially if there is a history of cardiac problems.

Nausea and vomiting may be severe unless pretreatment antiemetics are administered. Slowing the infusion rate, decreasing the dose, and avoiding mealtime drug administration may also help minimize gastrointestinal upset.

Baseline and periodic hemoglobin, hematocrit, and serum electrolytes should be performed to detect the development of hyponatremia which may occur rapidly if vomiting has been persistent. Early symptoms such as headache, malaise, and lethargy will proceed to seizures and coma if sodium is not replaced. If serum sodium drops below 135 mEq/L or hematocrit drops or hemoglobin increases (reflecting hemoconcentration from inadequate plasma volume), the patient should be given some hypertonic fluids, and oral fluid intake should be limited to the amount of the output for the previous 24 hours until serum sodium increases. Water intake should be limited; other fluids rich in electrolytes, such as fruit juices and bouillion, should be substituted.

Serum lipids should be drawn periodically; hyperlipemia may occur in some patients and warrants a reduction in dose or discontinuation of therapy. Likewise, hepatic enzymes and renal function studies should be performed at regular intervals on all patients receiving therapy beyond 4 weeks or in any patient suspected of liver or kidney dysfunction to ensure toxicity is not developing.

Nystatin, Oral
(Mycostatin, Nilstat)

MECHANISM AND ACTIONS
Nystatin is a fungicidal antibiotic obtained from a species of *Streptomyces* and is used primarily in the treatment of candidal infections of the skin, mucous membranes, and intestinal tract. The drug binds to sterols in the membrane of fungal cells, altering cellular permeability; the resultant leakage of intracellular components leads to cellular death. Following oral administration, nystatin is poorly absorbed and thus is only effective against candidal infections of the oral cavity and intestinal tract. The drug is available as an oral tablet (which is swallowed whole) for the treatment of intestinal candidiasis and also as an oral suspension (which is retained in the mouth as long as possible before swallowing) for the treatment of candidiasis of the oral cavity. Those indications are discussed here, while the topical use of nystatin is considered in Table 73-2.

USES
1. Treatment of intestinal candidiasis (oral tablet)
2. Treatment of candidiasis of the oral cavity (oral suspension)
3. Treatment of cutaneous and mucocutaneous candidal infections (for topical and vaginal application, see Table 73-1)

ADMINISTRATION AND DOSAGE
Nystatin is available as oral tablets (500,000 units), an oral suspension containing 100,000 units/ml, and several topical dosage forms as listed in Table 73-1.

In treating intestinal candidiasis, a dose of 500,000 U to 1,000,000 U (1 tablet to 2 tablets) is given three times a day and continued for at least 48 hours after a clinical cure has been obtained.

For oral candidiasis, adults and children are given 400,000 U to 600,000 U (4 ml–6 ml oral suspension) four times a day (one half dose in each side of mouth which should be retained for as long as possible before swallowing). Continue for at least 48 hours after symptoms have disappeared. The oral retention of the drug may be improved by the use of nystatin "popsicles," which are formulated to contain 250,000 U. Alternately, nystatin vaginal tablets may be given orally and dissolved in the mouth.

Infants should receive 200,000 U four times a day, with one-half of each dose inserted into each side of the mouth. Cotton swabs can be used to paint the lesions in the infant's mouth to ensure drug contact.

FATE
Nystatin given orally is not appreciably absorbed and is eliminated largely unchanged in the stool.

SIDE-EFFECTS/ADVERSE REACTIONS
Oral nystatin is usually well tolerated, and untoward reactions are infrequent. Occasionally, large doses can produce nausea, vomiting, GI distress, and diarrhea.

NURSING CONSIDERATIONS
The patient should be asked about allergy to streptomcyin because cross-hypersensitivity can occur but is usually minimal because mycostatin is not systemically absorbed to any extent.

Nystatin administration for oral candidiasis can be difficult because the drug must make contact with all affected lesions. Patients should be told to plan to take the drug during times when they can sit quietly, without talking, to allow maximum contact on dissolving. They can also paint the lesions with cotton swabs to ensure contact. This may be especially important with children. Mycostatin contains 50% dextrose which can damage teeth if left on; therefore, teeth should be cleaned after each dose by careful brushing with water or wiping with swabs or a cloth.

Topical/Vaginal Antifungal Agents

Amphotericin B, Butoconazole, Ciclopirox, Clotrimazole, Econazole, Haloprogin, Iodochlorhydroxyquin, Ketoconazole, Miconazole, Nystatin, Tolnaftate, Triacetin, Undecylenic acid

A number of drugs possessing antifungal activity are employed topically or intravaginally for the treatment of cutaneous infections, such as ringworm, athlete's foot, or jock itch, or for mucocutaneous infections, such as vulvovaginal moniliasis. They are listed alphabetically in Table 73-1 along with dosage and other relevant information. Griseofulvin, an orally administered drug discussed earlier in the chapter, is also employed for treating ringworm (tinea) infections of the skin, hair, or nails. Ketoconazole, a systemic antifungal agent, is also used in recurrent, resistant vaginal candidal infections.

Nurses may encounter many women with vaginal monilia and may see these drugs used frequently. Susceptibility seems to increase during the first few months after initial sexual encounters, during treatment with antibiotic medications for systemic infections, and in menopausal women. Drug therapy should not be delayed, and symptoms usually respond well to antifungal agents. Encourage all women to report any unusual vaginal discharge immediately.

Ophthalmic Antifungal Agent

Natamycin
(Natacyn)

MECHANISM AND ACTIONS
Natamycin is an antibiotic obtained for *Streptomyces natalensis* that possesses fungicidal activity against a variety of fungi and yeasts, including *Candida, Aspergillus, Cephalosporium, Fusarium,* and *Penicillium.* Natamycin appears to bind to sterols in fungal cell membranes, altering the cell permeability and allowing escape of essential cell constituents. It is not effective against bacteria. Natamycin is not absorbed orally and is only used in the eye for treatment of localized fungal infections.

USES
1. Treatment of fungal blepharitis, conjunctivitis, and keratitis due to susceptible organisms. It is the initial drug of choice for *Fusarium solani* keratitis.

ADMINISTRATION AND DOSAGE
Natamycin is used as a 5% ophthalmic suspension. For fungal keratitis, 1 drop is instilled into the eye every 1 hour to 2 hours for 2 days to 4 days, then six to eight times a day thereafter for 14 days to 21 days, or until there is complete resolution of the infection. Dosage frequency may be reduced gradually at 4-day to 7-day intervals.

In fungal blepharitis or conjunctivitis, 1 drop four to six times a day is usually adequate.

FATE
There is little systemic absorption following ophthalmic instillation. Effective concentrations are attained in the corneal stroma but generally not in the intraocular fluid.

SIDE-EFFECTS/ADVERSE REACTIONS
Ophthalmic administration of natamycin is well tolerated, and adverse effects are minimal. There have been occasional reports of blurred vision, increased sensitivity to light, hyperemia, and conjunctival chemosis (*i.e.,* corneal swelling).

CONTRAINDICATIONS AND PRECAUTIONS
If clinical improvement is not observed within 7 days to 10 days, the patient's status should be reevaluated and additional laboratory tests performed to determine if other organisms are present.

NURSING CONSIDERATIONS
Hypersensitivity reactions are rare, but the patient should report immediately any sudden eye itching, swelling, or redness. An eye wash may be done, and the drug must be discontinued.

Table 73-1
Topical/Vaginal Antifungal Agents

Drug	Preparations	Usual Dosage Range	Clinical Considerations
amphotericin B, topical (Fungizone)	Cream—3% Ointment—3% Lotion—3%	Apply liberally two to four times a day; duration of therapy ranges from 1 wk–2 wk for simple infections (e.g., candidiasis) up to several months for onychomycoses	Used for treating cutaneous and mucocutaneous candidal infections; similar to nystatin in activity; cream may have a drying effect and may discolor the skin; lotion and ointment may stain nail lesions; redness, itching, and burning have occurred with all preparations; discoloration of clothing or fabrics is removable by washing in soap and water or cleaning fluid; also used parenterally (see separate discussion).
butoconazole (Femstat)	Vaginal cream—2%	1 applicatorful into vagina at bedtime for 3 days; may administer for 6 days if necessary	Used for vulvovaginal candidiasis. A 3-day course of therapy is usually sufficient except in pregnant women, who should receive the drug for 6 days. Avoid during the first trimester of pregnancy. Vulvar and vaginal itching and burning can occur.
ciclopirox (Loprox)	Cream—1%	Apply twice a day	Broad-spectrum antifungal used for tinea pedis, tinea cruris, tinea corporis, candidiasis, and tinea versicolor due to *Malassezia furfur*; disrupts integrity of fungal cell membrane, allowing leakage and cell death; penetrates hair, hair follicles, sebaceous glands, and dermis; do not use occlusive dressings; if no clinical improvement occurs within 4 wk, reevaluate therapy; very low incidence of irritation, sensitization, or phototoxicity; safety and efficacy in children less than 10 yr of age have not been established.
clotrimazole (Gyne-Lotrimin, Lotrimin, Mycelex)	Cream—1% Solution—1% Lotion—1% Troches—10 mg Vaginal tablets—100 mg, 500 mg Vaginal cream—1%	Topical—massage into infected area twice a day Vaginal—one 100 mg tablet inserted at bedtime for 7 days or 1 applicatorful of vaginal cream inserted at bedtime for 7 days to 14 days. Alternately: two 100-mg tablets intravaginally for 3	Broad-spectrum antifungal used topically for dermatophytal infections, candidiasis, and tinea versicolor, vaginally for vulvovaginal candidiasis and orally for oropharyngeal candidiasis; topical application may cause burning, stinging, peeling, *(continued)*

Table 73-1 (continued)
Topical/Vaginal Antifungal Agents

Drug	Preparations	Usual Dosage Range	Clinical Considerations
clotrimazole (Gyne-Lotrimin, Lotrimin, Mycelex) (*continued*)		nights *or* one 500-mg tablet used *once only* Oral—one troche dissolved slowly in the mouth five times a day for 14 days.	itching, urticaria, and edema; clinical improvement usually occurs within 7 days; discontinue if severe irritation or hypersensitivity reactions occur; vaginal application has resulted in mild burning, rash, urinary frequency, bloating, and lower abdominal cramping; use of sanitary pad will prevent staining of clothing; in case of treatment failure, presence of other pathogens (*e.g.*, Trichomonas, Hemophilus vaginalis) should be suspected; stress importance of taking full course of therapy; oral use results in prolonged salivary levels of drug; 3-h dosing maintains effective salivary drug concentration; nausea, vomiting, and abnormal liver function tests (*e.g.*, elevated SGOT) occur in approximately 15% of patients using troches.
econazole (Spectazole)	Cream—1%	Apply once or twice a day	Broad-spectrum antifungal with good activity against dermatophytes, yeasts, and some gram (+) bacteria; following application, inhibitory concentrations of drug were found as deep as the middle region of the dermis; low incidence of burning, itching, and erythema; apply after cleansing affected area; treat candidal infections, tinea cruris, and tinea corporis for 2 wk, and tinea pedis for 4 wk.
haloprogin (Halotex)	Cream—1% Solution—1%	Apply liberally two times a day for 2 wk–4 wk	Indicated for superficial fungal infections of the skin and for tinea versicolor; side-effects include irritation, burning, vesicle formation, and pruritus, may worsen preexisting lesions; avoid contact with eyes; if no improvement is noted *(continued)*

Table 73-1 (continued)
Topical/Vaginal Antifungal Agents

Drug	Preparations	Usual Dosage Range	Clinical Considerations
haloprogin (Halotex) (*continued*)			within 4 wk, patient's condition should be re-evaluated.
iodochlorhydroxyquin–clioquinol (Torofor, Vioform)	Cream—3% Ointment—3%	Apply two to three times a day for a maximum of 1 wk	Antibacterial and antifungal agent used in treatment of cutaneous fungal infections and inflammatory skin conditions (*e.g.,* eczema); do not use in the presence of superficial viral conditions, tuberculosis, vaccinia, or varicella; infrequently elicits skin irritation, but can stain skin, hair, or fabrics; may be absorbed systemically if used on widespread areas, and can interfere with thyroid function tests, because drug contains iodine; available in combination with hydrocortisone (Vioform-HC) as prescription only, but can be sold over the counter when used alone.
miconazole (Micatin, Monistat-Derm, Monistat-3, Monistat 7)	Cream—2% Lotion—2% Powder—2% Spray—2% Vaginal cream—2% Vaginal suppositories—100 mg, 200 mg	Topical—apply twice a day for 2 wk–4 wk Vaginal—1 applicatorful or 1 suppository (100 mg) vaginally at bedtime for 7 days *or* 1 suppository (200 mg) once daily for 3 days	Indicated for cutaneous dermatophytal and candidal infections, tinea versicolor, and vulvovaginal candidiasis; rarely causes burning or irritation topically; avoid contact with eyes; use lotion rather than cream between the toes or fingers to avoid maceration effects; clinical improvement should occur in 1 wk–2 wk; diagnosis should be re-evaluated after 4 wk if good response is not evident; pathogens other than *Candida* should be ruled out before using drug for vaginitis, because it is only effective against candidal vulvo-vaginitis; 100 mg suppository (Monistat 7) is given for 7 days while 200 mg suppository (Monistat-3) is only used for 3 days; advise patient to insert suppository high into vagina, to use sanitary napkin to prevent

(continued)

Table 73-1 (continued)
Topical/Vaginal Antifungal Agents

Drug	Preparations	Usual Dosage Range	Clinical Considerations
miconazole (Micatin, Monistat-Derm, Monistat-3, Monistat 7) (continued)			staining, to complete full course of therapy, and to avoid sexual intercourse during treatment to prevent reinfection; if burning, itching, or irritation occur, advise physician; use cautiously during pregnancy, especially the first trimester; perform urine and blood glucose studies in patients who do not respond to treatment, because persistent candidal vulvovaginitis may result from unrecognized diabetes mellitus; also used IV for severe systemic fungal infections; see separate discussion.
nystatin (Mycostatin, Mykinac, Nilstat, Nystex, O-V Statin)	Cream—100,000 U/g Ointment—100,000 U/g Powder—100,000 U/g Vaginal tablets—100,000 U Troches—200,000 U	Topical—apply two to three times a day until healing is complete Vaginal—1 tablet inserted vaginally daily for 14 days Oral—1 or 2 troches dissolved in the mouth 4 to 5 times a day for up to 14 days	Used in treating cutaneous and vaginal infections due to *Candida* species; troches and oral suspension (see Nystatin, Oral) are used to treat oral candidiasis; no detectable blood levels are noted following topical application; irritation is rare, and drug does not stain skin or mucous membranes; avoid contact with eyes; powder may be dusted into shoes and socks as well as onto feet; symptomatic relief of cutaneous infections usually occurs within 72 h; vaginal application should be continued for entire 14 days, even though clinical symptoms disappear within a few days; lack of response suggests presence of other pathogens besides *Candida*; no adverse effects or complications have been reported when drug is used during pregnancy; also available in oral tablets for treatment of intestinal candidiasis; see separate discussion.
tolnaftate (Aftate, Footwork, Fungatin, Genaspor, NP-27, Tinactin, Zeasorb-AF)	Cream—1% Gel—1% Solution—1%	Apply small amount two to three times a day for 2 wk–6 wk as necessary	Effective in treating cutaneous dermatophytal infections (*e.g.*, athlete's foot,

(continued)

Table 73-1 (continued)
Topical/Vaginal Antifungal Agents

Drug	Preparations	Usual Dosage Range	Clinical Considerations
tolnaftate (Aftate, Footwork, Fungatin, Genaspor, NP-27, Tinactin, Zeasorb-AF) (continued)	Liquid aerosol—1% Powder—1% Powder aerosol—1%		jock itch, or ringworm); inactive systemically, virtually nontoxic, nonirritating, and nonsensitizing; serious or chronic fungal infections may require concomitant use of griseofulvin; powder is only used as adjunctive therapy; whereas liquids or solutions are preferred for primary therapy or in hairy areas; not effective against Candida, therefore if patient does not improve within several weeks, additional antifungal therapy is indicated; discontinue treatment if irritation occurs or condition worsens; available over the counter
triacetin (Enzactin, Fungacetin, Fungoid)	Cream—25% Ointment—25% Liquid (Fungoid)—with cetylpyridinium and chloroxylenol	Apply twice a day for at least 1 wk after symptoms have subsided	Indicated for milder superficial fungal infections (e.g., athlete's foot); cleanse affected area with alcohol or soap and water before application; cover treated areas; avoid contact with eyes; use cautiously in patients with impaired circulation; may stain certain fabrics; available over the counter, except Fungoid, which contains additional antiseptics
undecylenic acid and salts (Caldesene, Cruex, Desenex, Quinsana, Ting, and various other manufacturers)	Ointment—5% undecylenic acid and 20% zinc undecylenate Cream—20% Solution—10% undecylenic acid and 47% isopropyl alcohol Powder and aerosol powder—10% calcium undecylenate or 20% zinc undecylenate plus 2% undecylenic acid Soap—2% undecylenic acid Foam—10% undecylenic acid and 35% isopropyl alcohol	Apply as needed several times a day	Fungistatic and weak antibacterial activity; mainly used for athlete's foot, jock itch, or ringworm, exclusive of nails and hairy areas; also employed for relief or prevention of diaper rash, prickly heat, groin irritation, and other minor skin irritations; do not use if skin is broken or severely abraded; area should be cleansed well before application; use with caution in patients with impaired circulation; powder is recommended only as adjunctive therapy; ointments, creams, and liquids are used as primary therapy in most areas.

REVIEW QUESTIONS

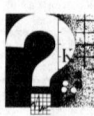

1. What are the *major* categories of antifungal drugs?
2. Briefly describe the mechanism of action of amphotericin B. What are its principal indications?
3. List the principal adverse effects associated with use of amphotericin B.
4. Are there any absolute contraindications to use of amphotericin B? Why or why not?
5. Why must a drug history be obtained before amphotericin B is given?
6. Why is baseline and periodic laboratory evaluation essential with amphotericin B?
7. List some administration rules for intravenous amphotericin B?
8. Discuss the mechanism of action of flucytosine. How is the drug primarily used?
9. What are the two product formulations of griseofulvin? How do they differ?
10. For what indications is griseofulvin used?
11. What dietary information should the patient taking griseofulvin be given?
12. List the uses for ketoconazole.
13. What is the major danger with ketoconazole? Give the most frequently encountered side-effects.
14. In what dosage forms is miconazole available?
15. What are the most common side-effects with miconazole? How should they be monitored? Why may hyperlipemia occur with IV use of the drug?
16. For what uses is nystatin employed (a) topically and (b) orally? How should oral nystatin be administered?
17. What antifungal drug is used as an ophthalmic suspension? For what conditions is it used?
18. What vaginal antifungals may be administered effectively for only 3 days?
19. Which antifungals may be administered topically, intravaginally, and orally?
20. What dosage forms of topically applied antifungals are preferred on hairy areas of the body?

BIBLIOGRAPHY

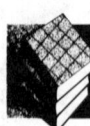

Bennett JE: Antifungal Agents. In Mandell GL, Douglas RG, Bennett JE (eds): Principles and Practice of Infectious Diseases, 2nd ed, p 263. New York, John Wiley & Sons, 1985

Borelli D: Treatment of pityriasis versicolor with ketoconazole. Rev Infect Dis 2:592, 1980

Cantanzaro A et al: Ketoconazole for treatment of disseminated coccidioidomycosis. Ann Intern Med 96:436, 1982

Craven PC, Graybill JR: Combination of oral flucytosine and ketoconazole as therapy for experimental cryptococcal meningitis. J Infect Dis 149:584, 1984

Drouhet E, DuPont B: Laboratory and clinical assessment of ketoconazole in deep-seated mycoses. Am J Med 74:30, 1983

Drugs for the treatment of systemic fungal infections. Med Lett Drugs Ther 26:36, 1984

Drutz DJ: Amphotericin B in the treatment of coccidioidomycosis. Drugs 26:337, 1983

Drutz DJ: Newer antifungal agents and their use, including an update on amphotericin B and flucytosine. In Remington JS, Swartz MN (eds): Current Clinical Topics in Infectious Diseases, vol 3, p 97. New York, McGraw-Hill, 1982

Gever LN: Giving amphotericin B for systemic fungal infections. Nursing 84 14(7):8, July 1984

Hume AL, Kerkering TM: Ketoconazole. Drug Intell Clin Pharm 17:169, 1983

Janssen PA, Symoens JE: Hepatic reactions during ketoconazole treatment. Am J Med 74:80, 1983

Koldin MH, Medoff G: Antifungal chemotherapy. Pediatr Clin North Am 30:49, 1983

Medoff G, Brajtburg J, Kobayashi GS, Bolard J: Antifungal agents useful in the therapy of systemic fungal infection. Annu Rev Pharmacol Toxicol 23:303, 1983

Meunier-Carpentier F: Treatment of mycoses in cancer patients. Am J Med 74:74, 1983

New topical antifungal drugs. Med Lett Drugs Ther 25:98, 1983

Norris SM: Amphotericin B—how safe and effective? Infec Control 6:243, 1985

Odds FC: Interactions among amphotericin B, 5-fluorocytosine, ketoconazole and miconazole against pathogenic fungi *in vitro*. Antimicrob Agents Chemother 22:763, 1982

Owens NJ et al: Prophylaxis of oral candidiasis with clotrimazole troches. Arch Intern Med 144:290, 1984

Shechtman LB et al: Clotrimazole treatment of oral candidiasis in patients with neoplastic disease. Am J Med 76:1, 1984

Soh CA: Evaluation of ketoconazole. Clin Pharm 1:217, 1982

Stevens DA: Miconazole in the treatment of coccidioidomycosis. Drugs 26:347, 1983

Sud IJ, Feingold DS: Effect of ketoconazole on the fungicidal action of amphotericin B in *Candida albicans*. Antimicrob Agents Chemotherap 23:185, 1983

Van Cutsem J: The antifungal activity of ketoconazole. Am J Med 74:9, 1983

Waldorf AR, Polak A: Mechanisms of action of 5-fluorocytosine. Antimicrob Agents Chemotherap 23:79, 1983

Ward MD: Amphotericin B. Crit Care Nurs 4(6):7, Nov/Dec 1984

Antiviral Agents

Acyclovir   Zidovudine
Amantadine
Idoxuridine
Ribavirin
Trifluridine
Vidarabine

74

Although viruses are responsible for a large number of diseases, only a few clinically effective antiviral drugs are currently available, and these have a rather limited therapeutic application. The principal obstacle to effective antiviral treatment is the fact that virus particles are intracellular parasites and replicate within host (*i.e.*, human) cells by utilizing the enzyme systems of the invaded cell. Thus, drugs interfering with intracellular viral replication are likely to damage the host cell as well, and are therefore usually quite toxic if given systemically. In addition, in many viral infections, the replication of viral particles is already proceeding at a maximal rate by the time clinical symptoms first appear. Thus, viral diseases are often asymptomatic until the infectious process within the host cells is well advanced, by which time the body's own defense mechanisms have already come into play. Thus, in order to be maximally effective, drugs that block viral replication should be administered before the onset of the disease. Such is the case with use of amantadine as a prophylactic agent against influenza A virus. On the other hand, some viral infections, such as herpes virus, continue to manifest viral replication even after symptoms have appeared. In these diseases, inhibition of further viral replication may speed healing and thus serves as the basis for use of drugs such as acyclovir, idoxuridine, and vidarabine in herpetic infections.

Most therapeutically effective antiviral drugs act either to interfere with penetration of the host cells by the viral particles or to inhibit the synthesis of viral-directed proteins and nucleic acid following the entrance of the virus into the cell.

Viral diseases are best managed prophylactically, either by active (attenuated or killed virus vaccines) or in some cases passive (viral antibodies) immunization (see Chap. 81). Once the disease has appeared, however, immunization is of no value, and most common viral infections (such as colds or "flu") are usually best treated symptomatically. Specific antiviral drugs have a limited therapeutic application, largely for the reasons outlined above. Only a handful of viral infections have been shown to be responsive to the few available antiviral agents which are discussed in this chapter.

The recent surge in cases of acquired immune deficiency syndrome (AIDS) has spawned great interest in the development of antiviral drugs that may be useful in either slowing the progression of this deadly disease or perhaps even providing a cure. The first such useful antiviral agent, which became available in early 1987, is zidovudine (formerly known as azidothymidine or AZT) and while far from the ideal drug in terms of its potentially serious side-effects, it has afforded a ray of hope that eventual control and perhaps even eradication of this dread disease are attainable. A review of zidovudine is given at the end of this chapter.

Acyclovir
(Zovirax)

MECHANISM AND ACTIONS

Acyclovir is a nucleoside of guanine with *in vitro* antiviral activity against herpes simplex types 1 and 2 (HSV-1; HSV-2), varicella-zoster, Epstein-Barr, and cytomegalovirus.

Acyclovir is converted by herpes simplex virus-coded thymidine kinase into acyclovir monophosphate, which is further transformed into the diphosphate and triphosphate, the latter representing the active form of the drug. Acyclovir triphosphate interferes with herpes simplex virus DNA polymerase, thus blocking viral replication, and can also be incorporated into growing chains of DNA by viral DNA polymerase, thereby terminating further growth of the DNA chain.

Normal cellular thymidine kinase enzyme does not utilize acyclovir; hence, the drug selectively inhibits viral cell replication with minimal toxicity for normal uninfected cells. Thus, the drug is well tolerated by most patients. In herpes genitalis, acyclovir can reduce healing time and may decrease the duration of pain and viral shedding. In patients with *frequent* recurrences, oral acyclovir can reduce the frequency and severity of recurrences in up to 95% of patients. Topical application of the drug can also shorten healing time and reduce pain when applied to primary lesions, but generally has no significant beneficial effect on *recurrent* genital lesions.

USES

Ointment
1. Management of initial episodes of herpes genitalis and limited, non-life-threatening mucocutaneous herpes simplex infections in immunocompromised patients

Intravenous infusion
1. Treatment of initial and recurrent mucosal and cutaneous herpes simplex (HSV-1 and HSV-2) infections in immunocompromised patients
2. Treatment of severe initial episodes of herpes genitalis in patients who are not immunocompromised

Oral

1. Treatment of initial episodes of genital herpes (HSV-2)
2. Management of recurrent episodes of genital herpes

ADMINISTRATION AND DOSAGE

Acyclovir may be administered topically as a 5% ointment, orally as 200-mg capsules, and by IV infusion as a diluted solution prepared from powder for injection containing 500 mg/vial. Recommended doses for the different preparations are:

Topical:

Apply sufficient ointment using a finger cot or rubber glove to cover all lesions every 3 hours six times a day for 7 days

Oral:

Initial infections: 200 mg every 4 hours while awake for a total of five capsules a day for 10 days

Recurrent infections: 200 mg three to five times a day for up to 6 months

Oral dosage must be reduced to 200 mg twice a day in patients with renal impairment if creatinine clearance is less than 10 ml/min/1.73 m².

Parenteral:

The drug is given by *IV infusion only.* Avoid SC, IM, or bolus IV injections. Adult dosage is 5 mg/kg infused over 1 hour every 8 hours for 7 days. Children under age 12 are given 250 mg/m² infused over 1 hour every 8 hours for 7 days. The IV dosage and dosing interval must also be reduced if the creatinine clearance is less than 50 ml/min/1.73 m² according to the values given in the package literature. Recommended diluents are sterile water for injection or bacteriostatic water for injection containing benzyl alcohol. Solutions containing parabens as preservatives should *not* be used because precipitation can occur.

FATE

Oral acyclovir is slowly and incompletely absorbed, and absorption is unaffected by food. Peak plasma levels occur in 1.5 hours to 2 hours. Protein binding is low (10%–30%). With both oral and IV administration, the drug is widely distributed into most body tissues. Concentrations in cerebrospinal fluid are approximately one half those in the plasma. The plasma half-life is 2 hours to 3 hours in patients with normal kidney function, but this increases if renal function is impaired. Up to 90% of an IV dose is eliminated unchanged by the kidney. Renal excretion of unchanged drug following oral administration is less than 20%.

Following topical application, systemic absorption is minimal.

SIDE-EFFECTS/ADVERSE REACTIONS

Commonly encountered side-effects following oral administration include headache, nausea, vomiting, and diarrhea. With IV infusion, there is frequently inflammation and phlebitis at the site of infiltration, elevated serum creatinine, rash, and urticaria. Topical application often results in mild pain and transient stinging or burning at the site of administration.

Other untoward reactions with acyclovir include:

Oral: dizziness, vertigo, fatigue, insomnia, irritability, depression, skin rash, acne, accelerated hair loss, anorexia, arthralgia, fever, sore throat, palpitations, muscle cramping, lymphadenopathy, edema, menstrual abnormalities, and superficial thrombophlebitis

IV: nervousness, sweating, hypotension, headache, nausea, hematuria, thrombocytosis, and rarely, tremor, clonic contractions, seizures, hallucinations, cerebral edema, and coma

Topical: Pruritus, rash, and vulvitis

Overdosage can result in precipitation of acyclovir in the renal tubules, especially if the solubility in intratubular fluid is exceeded. Elevations in BUN and serum creatinine and subsequent renal failure have occurred. Treatment is by hemodialysis; a 6-hour dialysis can reduce plasma acyclovir levels by 60%.

CONTRAINDICATIONS AND PRECAUTIONS

Although there are no absolute contraindications to acyclovir, the safety and efficacy of the oral form have not been established in children. A *cautious* approach to therapy is indicated in persons with underlying neurologic abnormalities, hypoxia, renal or hepatic dysfunction, electrolyte abnormalities, dehydration, and in pregnant or nursing women. Bolus IV injection must be avoided, because precipitation of acyclovir crystals in the renal tubules can occur if the maximum solubility of free acyclovir is exceeded. Patients should be made aware that acyclovir does *not* eliminate latent

HSV-2 virus and cannot be considered a cure. The recommended dosage and duration of therapy should not be exceeded, and dosage adjustment must be made in patients with renal dysfunction (see under Administration and Dosage).

INTERACTIONS

1. Probenecid increases the half-life of acyclovir and reduces the rate of urinary elimination by retarding tubular secretion.

NURSING CONSIDERATIONS

For all types of administration, acyclovir should be initiated as early in the disease process as possible. The drug is not considered a cure; it does not eliminate the latent HSV-2 virus from the body. In addition, patients should also be aware that they may still be contagious even during remission when no lesions are evident. This information is very disheartening to the patient with herpes. Time for verbalization about fears, anger, and guilt over the disease process is needed. The goal with acyclovir therapy is to reduce pain, facilitate healing of lesions, and stop an outbreak once it begins.

The topical formula is used only for initial lesions. It is usually not effective against recurrent outbreaks, and it will not prevent transmission to others during an outbreak. The nurse needs to emphasize the importance of wearing a finger cot or glove when applying the ointment to prevent transmittal of the virus to the fingers and subsequently to other body sites. Local hypersensitivity reactions are not uncommon, but most patients will attempt to tolerate mild irritation in order to derive the drug benefit. The patient should be told to report any localized swelling, diffuse rash, or severe pruritis.

Intravenous acyclovir should be administered using an infusion pump to ensure that the dose is given slowly. The patient must be well hydrated before the dose is given, and fluids must be encouraged in the patient able to swallow. Otherwise intravenous fluid hydration must be undertaken. Urine output must be sufficient to prevent precipitation of acyclovir crystals in the urine. If urinary output drops, if BUN or serum creatinine increase, or if hematuria develops, the physician should be notified because the drug may have to be discontinued due to renal toxicity.

IV sites should be rotated every 48 hours or more frequently if pain, redness, or swelling develops. Phlebitis is a common side-effect of the drug, which is strongly alkaline. Ample dilution and slow rate of infusion will decrease the risk of phlebitis. The IV site must be monitored every hour for signs of extravasation because tissue irritation and inflammation can occur.

The oral dosage form should be started in the prodromal phase of the herpes infection, if possible, to increase the chance the infectious process will be halted early. Patients usually describe tingling, itching, and pain at the site at the beginning of an episode. Patients should be reminded that even the oral drug form does not make them less contagious, although some patients believe that the oral form is able to do so. Transient dizziness may occur; therefore, patients should be cautioned against driving or engaging in any hazardous activities until the effects of the drug are known. A baseline and midtreatment CBC with differential should be performed each time the drug is used to monitor the patient for the development of blood dyscrasias. The patient should also be told to report any fever, sore throat, bleeding, or fatigue.

Amantadine
(Symmetrel)

MECHANISM AND ACTIONS

Amantadine is a tricyclic amine that is effective in *preventing* infection with strains of type A influenza virus, but is *not* effective against type B influenza. Although the mechanism of action is not completely understood, the drug appears to inhibit viral replication at an early stage, probably by preventing the uncoating of viral nucleic acid and blocking the release of nucleic acids into host cells. It may also interfere with penetration of the virus itself into cells. Amantadine is up to 90% effective in preventing illnesses caused by type A influenza virus. In addition, when given within 24 hours to 48 hours *after* onset of influenza viral illness, the drug can reduce the duration of symptoms (e.g., fever) and result in a more rapid recovery.

The antiviral activity of amantadine appears to be specific for A virus strains, and there is no evidence that the drug is effective for either prophylaxis or treatment of other viral diseases.

In addition to its antiviral activity, the drug can facilitate the release of dopamine from nerve endings in the CNS and is also used as adjunctive therapy for Parkinson's disease and drug-induced extrapyramidal reactions.

The antiparkinsonian actions of the drug are discussed in detail in Chapter 31, and only its antiviral activity is considered here.

USES

1. Prevention and symptomatic management of Asian (A) influenza infections, especially in high-risk patients (*e.g.*, those with cardiovascular, pulmonary, neuromuscular, or immunodeficiency diseases) or in cases in which contact with the virus is likely, for example, in hospital wards or infected households. Although early immunization is the preferred method for preventing influenza viral disease, amantadine may be used for chemoprophylaxis when immunization is contraindicated or not available.
2. Adjunctive treatment of Parkinson's disease or drug-induced extrapyramidal reactions (see Chap. 31)

ADMINISTRATION AND DOSAGE

Amantadine is used as capsules (100 mg) or syrup (50 mg/5 ml). For prophylaxis or symptomatic management of influenza A viral illness, the following doses are recommended.

Adults: 200 mg/day, in a single dose or two divided doses

Children (1 year–9 years): 4.4 mg to 8.8 mg/kg/day (maximum 150 mg/day) in a single or two equally divided doses

Children (9 years–12 years): 100 mg twice a day

Prophylactic therapy should begin prior to anticipated contact or as soon as possible after exposure and continued for at least 10 days following a known exposure. When vaccine is not available, amantadine may be given for up to 50 days if exposure to virus is likely. When influenza viral vaccine is used, amantadine should be given for 2 weeks to 3 weeks after administration of the vaccine until a sufficient antibody level develops.

In treating a viral illness once infection has occurred, amantadine should be started as soon as possible after onset of symptoms and continued for at least 24 hours after symptoms disappear.

Dosage and dosing frequency should be reduced in persons with renal disease according to instructions supplied with the product.

FATE

Amantadine is readily absorbed orally, and peak serum levels occur in 2 hours to 4 hours, but 48 hours are required for drug to reach maximal tissue concentrations. The drug is excreted largely unchanged in the urine, primarily by tubular secretion. Elimination half-life in persons with normal renal function is 16 hours to 20 hours. The excretion rate is increased if the urinary *p*H is acidic.

SIDE-EFFECTS/ADVERSE REACTIONS

The most common side-effects observed with amantadine are dizziness, lightheadedness, anxiety, irritability, confusion, anorexia, mild depression, orthostatic hypotension, urinary hesitancy, nausea, constipation, peripheral edema, difficulty in concentration, and livedo reticularis (skin mottling). In addition, hallucinations and psychotic behavior have been reported, especially in older patients or patients with renal impairment. Other untoward reactions occurring less frequently with amantadine are:

Cardiovascular—Congestive heart failure

Neurologic—Fatigue, weakness, headache, nervousness, insomnia, tremors, convulsions, slurred speech, blurred vision, oculogyric crisis, seizures

GI—Vomiting, dry mouth

Other—Leukopenia, neutropenia, skin rash, eczematoid dermatitis, dyspnea

Overdosage may be characterized by vomiting, anorexia, excitability, tremors, blurred vision, slurred speech, lethargy, depression, and convulsions, probably the result of increased dopamine activity in the CNS. Treatment is supportive, along with gastric lavage or induction of emesis. Urinary acidification can increase the rate of elimination. Anticonvulsants, vasopressors, or antiarrhythmics may be employed as necessary.

CONTRAINDICATIONS AND PRECAUTIONS

Amantadine should not be used in pregnant women unless absolutely necessary because fetal abnormalities have occurred in a few instances. The drug must be given with *caution* to persons with epilepsy or a history of convulsive disorders, psychoses, or psychoneuroses; congestive heart failure, peripheral edema, renal impairment, orthostatic hypotension, liver disease, history of skin rash, or other allergic dermatoses, and to elderly or debilitated patients.

Persons with active seizure disorders should be given reduced doses (*i.e.*, 100 mg/day) as higher doses increase the risk of seizures. Abrupt discontinuation of amantadine has resulted in a sudden worsening of symptoms in patients with Parkinson's disease.

INTERACTIONS

1. Amantadine may exhibit additive atropine-like effects with anticholinergic drugs, tricyclic antidepressants, or antihistamines.

2. Excessive CNS stimulation may occur with combined use of amantadine and other CNS stimulants (e.g., amphetamines, methylphenidate).
3. Decreased urinary excretion of amantadine has occurred when hydrochlorothiazide plus triamterene was administered concurrently

NURSING CONSIDERATIONS

Patients should be cautioned against driving or engaging in any hazardous activity until the effect of the drug is known because dizziness, confusion, and blurred vision may occur. This is particularly important in industrial settings where the drug may be given prophylactically. Orthostatic hypotension may persist for several days; therefore, the patient needs to rise from sitting or lying positions slowly.

Other side-effects of the drug may be bothersome but are not serious.

Amantadine may cause constipation. The patient should be encouraged to increase fluid intake and roughage foods; a mild laxative may be used if necessary. The drug should not be taken close to bedtime because insomnia can result. Livedo recticularis, skin mottling which usually occurs in the lower extremities, is usually self limiting and will subside when the dose is decreased or the drug is discontinued. However, the patient should report immediately changes in temperature or sensation to the extremities as well as tingling, pain, or numbness because these may signal more serious consequences.

Idoxuridine

(Herplex, Stoxil)

MECHANISM AND ACTIONS

Idoxuridine (IDU) is a structural analogue of thymidine, an essential intermediate in DNA synthesis. Because it is rapidly inactivated by enzymes, IDU is used only locally in the eye for the treatment of herpes simplex keratitis, a viral disease that affects the cornea. The drug is incorporated into viral DNA, producing a faulty molecule incapable of reproduction, thus blocking herpes viral cell replication in the cornea. Herpes virus can proliferate in the avascular cornea and idoxuridine remains localized in the structure due to its avascular nature.

USES

1. Treatment of herpes simplex keratitis (epithelial infections respond better than stromal infections)

Idoxuridine will control the infection but has no effect on accumulated scarring or progressive loss of vision.

ADMINISTRATION AND DOSAGE

Idoxuridine may be used as either a 0.5% ophthalmic ointment or a 0.1% ophthalmic solution.

One drop of the solution is placed into the infected eye every hour during the day and every 2 hours at night until definite improvement is noted, as evidenced by loss of staining with fluorescein. Dosage frequency is then reduced to every 2 hours during the day and every 4 hours at night and continued for at least 3 days to 5 days after healing is complete.

The ophthalmic ointment is instilled into the infected conjunctival sac every 4 hours five times a day and continued for at least 5 days to 7 days after healing is complete to prevent recurrent infection. Light pressure should be applied to the lacrimal sac for 1 minute after drug instillation to decrease systemic absorption. All forms, except Herplex Liquifilm should be refrigerated.

In epithelial infections, improvement is usually noted within 7 days to 8 days. Therapy should be continued no longer than 21 days. Antibiotics or corticosteroids may be used concurrently with idoxuridine as the condition warrants.

SIDE-EFFECTS/ADVERSE REACTIONS

Localized irritation, burning, or lacrimation have occurred upon instillation of idoxuridine into the eye. Other adverse effects include pain, inflammation, pruritus, and edema of eyes and eyelids, photophobia, local allergic reactions and corneal clouding, vascularization or stippling. Prolonged use can result in follicular conjunctivitis, blepharitis, conjunctival hyperemia, and corneal epithelial staining. Squamous cell carcinoma has been noted at the site of topical treatment. Idoxuridine is potentially carcinogenic and mutagenic and is not employed systemically.

CONTRAINDICATIONS AND PRECAUTIONS

Idoxuridine should be used with caution in pregnant women, because systemic absorption can occur. Some strains of herpes simplex are resistant, and if no response is noted after 14 days of treatment, alternate therapy should be considered. Corticosteriods can extend the spread of a viral infection and should never be used without concomitant idoxuridine therapy.

INTERACTIONS
1. Boric acid-containing solutions may cause increased irritation in the presence of idoxuridine.

Ribavirin
(Virazole)

MECHANISM AND ACTIONS
Ribavirin has demonstrated antiviral activity against respiratory syncytial virus (RSV), influenza A and B viruses, and herpes simplex virus. The drug appears to interfere with guanidine monophosphate formation and subsequent nucleic acid synthesis. When administered as an aerosol, ribavirin retards replication of RSV in infants and reduces the severity and duration of the illness. Aerosol ribavirin has also been shown to be effective against influenza A and B, and oral ribavirin (an investigational dosage form) has been reported to be active in other viral diseases such as acute and chronic hepatitis, herpes genitalis, measles, and Lassa fever.

USES
1. Treatment of selected hospitalized infants and young children with *severe* lower respiratory tract infections due to respiratory syncytial virus
2. Investigational uses include aerosol treatment of influenza A and B virus infection and oral therapy of hepatitis virus, herpes genitalis virus, measles, and Lassa fever.

ADMINISTRATION AND DOSAGE
Ribavirin is available as powder for reconstitution for aerosol use containing 20 mg/ml in 100-ml vials. Treatment should be initiated within 3 days of onset of RSV lower respiratory tract infection. The drug is solubilized with sterile water for injection and diluted to a final volume of 300 ml. The aerosol is delivered to an infant oxygen hood using the Viratek Small Particle Aerosol Generator (SPAG). Treatment is carried out for 12 hours to 18 hours per day for 3 days to 7 days. Use of a face mask or oxygen tent may be necessary if a hood cannot be used.

FATE
Administration by aerosol results in significant systemic absorption. The plasma half-life is 8 hours to 10 hours. Ribavirin and its metabolites accumulate in red blood cells.

SIDE-EFFECTS/ADVERSE REACTIONS
A number of adverse effects have occurred during ribavirin therapy, especially in severely ill infants and in adults with chronic obstructive pulmonary disease. Deterioration of respiratory status marked by dyspnea, chest soreness, bacterial pneumonia, pneumothorax, and apnea has occurred, and the drug should be stopped if there is a sudden worsening of respiratory function. In patients requiring assisted ventilation, precipitation of drug within the ventilatory apparatus and accumulation of fluid in tubing have resulted in increased inspiratory and expiratory pressure which can markedly interfere with safe and efficient operation.

Other adverse reactions associated with use of ribavirin include rash, conjunctivitis, hypotension, reticulocytosis, and, rarely, cardiac arrest.

Aerosol administration of ribavirin has resulted in cardiac lesions in mice and rats, and oral dosing of ribavirin in rats has led to development of mammary, pancreatic, adrenal, and pituitary tumors, as well as testicular lesions. The human significance of these findings remains to be established. Ribavirin may cause fetal damage, and the drug should not be given to pregnant women (see below).

CONTRAINDICATIONS AND PRECAUTIONS
Use of ribavirin is contraindicated in pregnant women or in women who may become pregnant during use of the drug and in nursing mothers. The drug must be used *cautiously* in persons with chronic obstructive lung disease and in persons taking digitalis drugs because ribavirin can increase the likelihood of digitalis toxicity.

NURSING CONSIDERATIONS
The nurse should be familiar with the functioning of a Viratek Small Particle Aerosol Generator (SPAG) before administration of the drug begins. A complete respiratory assessment of all lung fields should be done at therapy onset and periodically during treatment to determine changes. The patient should be observed for increasing dyspnea, labored breathing, apnea, or evidence of pneumothorax (uneven chest movement on inspiration), all of which indicate the need for respiratory assis-

tance resulting from a drug side-effect or worsening of the patient's condition. If respiratory problems result in the patient being placed on a mechanical ventilator the ribavirin must be immediately discontinued.

A CBC with differential should be performed frequently during therapy, especially if treatment is prolonged. Ribavirin may precipitate a drop in hemoglobin, hematocrit, and red blood cells. Changes in laboratory values should be reported immediately.

Cardiac rhythm should be monitored continuously and frequent vital signs taken to catch early any cardiac arrhythmias or hypotension which could lead to cardiac arrest.

Trifluridine
(Viroptic)

MECHANISM AND ACTIONS
Trifluridine is a fluorinated pyrimidine that has *in vivo* antiviral activity against herpes simplex virus, types 1 and 2 and vaccinia virus, as well as *in vitro* activity against adenovirus. The drug appears to interfere with DNA synthesis. Its clinical application is presently restricted to ophthalmic infections due to sensitive organisms, and the drug is often effective in patients unresponsive to idoxuridine and vidarabine.

USES
1. Treatment of primary keratoconjunctivitis and recurrent epithelial keratitis due to herpes simplex viruses 1 and 2
2. Treatment of epithelial keratitis in patients intolerant of or unresponsive to idoxuridine or vidarabine
3. Treatment of ophthalmic infections due to vaccinia virus or adenovirus (clinical efficacy not definitely established)
4. Prophylaxis of herpes simplex virus keratoconjunctivitis and epithelial keratitis (efficacy not definitely established)

ADMINISTRATION AND DOSAGE
Trifluridine is used as a 1% ophthalmic solution. One drop is placed onto the cornea every 2 hours while awake (maximum nine drops a day) until corneal ulcer has completely re-epithelialized, then one drop is instilled every 4 hours (maximum five drops a day) for an additional 7 days.

If improvement is not noted within 7 days or *complete* re-epithelialization has not occurred

after 14 days of therapy, other forms of therapy should be considered.

FATE
Intraocular penetration following topical application is good, and systemic absorption is negligible. Increased penetration of drug into the aqueous humor can occur if corneal integrity is reduced.

SIDE-EFFECTS/ADVERSE REACTIONS
Transient burning or stinging in the eye often accompanies use of trifluridine. Palpebral edema is also a common occurrence. Other adverse reactions may include superficial punctate keratopathy, epithelial keratopathy, stromal edema, irritation, hypersensitivity reactions, hyperemia, and increased intraocular pressure.

CONTRAINDICATIONS AND PRECAUTIONS
Trifluridine must be given with *caution* in the presence of glaucoma and to pregnant or nursing women. The drug should not be used unless a clinical diagnosis of herpetic keratitis has been established because the drug is not effective against bacterial, fungal, or chlamydial infections. The recommended dosage and frequency of administration should not be exceeded, and the drug should not be used for longer than 21 days except in very severe cases.

NURSING CONSIDERATIONS
A complete ophthalmic examination should be done including test for ocular pressure as a baseline and periodically throughout therapy to measure treatment effectiveness and onset of edema or intraocular pressure.

The patient must be taught to direct the drop of medication directly onto the cornea. He must hold the upper and lower lid firmly to prevent blinking on instillation, a natural reflex. The lacrimal sac should be compressed for 1 minute to ensure even distribution of the drug and minimize systemic absorption.

Trifluridine should be refrigerated to decrease the rate of drug degradation.

Vidarabine
(Vira-A)

MECHANISM AND ACTIONS
Vidarabine or adenine arabinoside is a pyrimidine derivative that possesses *in vivo* antiviral activity

against herpes simplex virus types 1 and 2. Vidarabine is phosphorylated to a triphosphate derivative in the cell, which inhibits viral DNA polymerase to a much greater extent than mammalian DNA polymerase. It may be used systemically in the treatment of herpes simplex virus encephalitis, or ophthalmically for keratoconjunctivitis and epithelial keratitis. Prompt diagnosis of herpes encephalitis, a frequent complication of cancer immunosuppressive therapy, and treatment by vidarabine can reduce mortality from 70% to approximately 25%. However, many survivors exhibit a severe neurologic deficit. Patients already in a comatose state at the time therapy is initiated do not appear to benefit significantly from the drug. When applied locally in the eye, vidarabine is often effective in patients resistant to or intolerant of idoxuridine.

USES

1. Treatment of herpes simplex virus encephalitis (IV only)
2. Treatment of superficial and recurrent epithelial keratitis and acute keratoconjunctivitis due to herpes simplex virus types 1 and 2 (ophthalmic only)
3. Reduce complications of herpes zoster in immunocompromised patients and inhibit viremia in chronic active hepatitis (investigational uses for IV dosage form)

ADMINISTRATION AND DOSAGE

Vidarabine is available as a 3% ophthalmic ointment and as a suspension for injection containing 200 mg/ml, which is diluted for administration by IV infusion. For IV use, the drug is given by slow infusion *only*; bolus IV injection is to be avoided as is IM or SC injection, because of the low solubility of the drug and poor absorption. The recommended IV dose is 15 mg/kg/day, given over a 12-hour to 24-hour period for 10 days.

For ophthalmic application, one-half inch of ophthalmic ointment is placed into the lower conjunctival sac five times a day at 3-hour intervals until reepithelialization has occurred, then treatment is continued twice a day for an additional 7 days.

The solubility of vidarabine in IV fluids is minimal. Each liter of infusion solution can solubilize 450 mg of the drug. Most IV solutions are suitable except biologic or colloidal fluids such as protein solutions and blood products. The infusion solution should be prewarmed to facilitate solution of the drug, and final filtration with an in-line membrane filter of 0.45 micron or smaller is required.

FATE

Following IV infusion, vidarabine is rapidly deaminated to hypoxanthine arabinoside, its principal metabolite, which is quickly distributed in the body but possesses only one-tenth the *in vitro* antiviral activity of vidarabine. The half-life of vidarabine is 1 hour; that of hypoxanthine arabinoside is 3.5 hours. The drug is excreted primarily by the kidneys. Following ophthalmic application, only trace amounts of the drug or metabolite are detectable in the aqueous humor. Systemic absorption following ocular administration is negligible.

SIDE-EFFECTS/ADVERSE REACTIONS

Following IV infusion, reported adverse effects include anorexia, nausea, vomiting, diarrhea, hematemesis, tremor, dizziness, ataxia, confusion, hallucinations, psychosis, decreased hemoglobin and hematocrit values, reduced white blood cell count and platelet count, weight loss, malaise, rash, pruritus, pain at injection site, and elevated total bilirubin and SGOT. Because the drug is relatively insoluble, its administration is usually associated with a large fluid load, which may be harmful to patients with cardiac disease, renal impairment, or cerebral edema. IV doses greater than 20 mg/kg/day have resulted in bone marrow depression, thrombocytopenia, and leukopenia.

When used locally in the eye, the following adverse effects have occurred: temporary visual haze, irritation, ocular pain, photophobia, lacrimation, burning, superficial punctate keratitis, punctal occlusion, foreign body sensation, and hypersensitivity reactions.

CONTRAINDICATIONS AND PRECAUTIONS

Vidarabine should not be used to treat trivial infections, and the recommended dose and duration of therapy should not be exceeded because vidarabine has exhibited a mutagenic and carcinogenic potential in laboratory animals. The significance of these findings in humans remains to be assessed.

IV infusion should be used very cautiously during pregnancy and lactation, in patients with impaired renal or liver function, or in CNS infections other than herpes encephalitis because vidarabine has not demonstrated effectiveness against pathogens other than herpes simplex.

INTERACTIONS

1. Concurrent use of allopurinol may interfere with vidarabine metabolism.

NURSING CONSIDERATIONS

Ophthalmic application of vidarabine must be used exactly as directed in order to achieve therapeutic levels capable of eradicating the virus. However, frequent administration means the patient may suffer photophobia and blurred vision during much of the therapy. The patient must avoid driving or engaging in any hazardous activity while blurring occurs. Sunglasses may be worn, even in the house, to decrease the pain and glare from light sensitivity.

Intravenous infusions of vidarabine must be closely monitored to ensure the drug remains in solution. IV bags should be agitated periodically, and the final filter should be checked for clogging. If particulate matter is noted in the IV line, the infusion should be discontinued and a new bag started. The IV site should be examined hourly for signs of pain, redness, and swelling, and the site should be rotated every 48 hours or more frequently if phlebitis or extravasation occur.

Baseline and periodic laboratory values should be measured to detect any adverse reactions. A CBC with differential should be taken weekly, and hemoglobin, hematocrit, white blood cells, and platelet count should be noted. Any changes should be reported immediately. Liver enzymes and bilirubin levels should also be measured because these may be the first indication of hepatic dysfunction.

Neurologic status should be evaluated frequently. Dizziness, confusion, and changes in motor function should be reported immediately as indicators of neurologic toxicity. Hallucinations and psychosis have been reported with this drug.

Nausea, vomiting, and anorexia are not uncommon. The patient may benefit from pretreatment and routine administration of antiemetic medications. Meals should be small and frequent; fluids should be offered in small amounts, between meals. If vomiting is persistent, electrolyte levels and hydration status must be closely monitored.

Anti-AIDS Drug

Zidovudine
(Retrovir)

Zidovudine, previously known as azidothymidine (AZT), is the first in what is expected to be a long list of antiviral drugs employed in an attempt to stem the alarming increase of acquired immune deficiency syndrome (AIDS) and the AIDS-related complex (ARC). Although there is no conclusive evidence that zidovudine destroys the AIDS virus, the drug does appear to inhibit its reproduction and bring about some immunologic reconstruction. Unfortunately, the effects of the drug are entirely palliative, and, to date, no cures have been reported.

Before discussing the current status of zidovudine in more detail, it must be noted that the chemotherapy of AIDS is undergoing constant change at a rapid pace. Today's therapy may be totally outmoded in a matter of months. Thus, the information presented below, while topical at the time of writing, must be viewed in the context that it may be largely dated by the time it is read. Hopefully, better and safer drugs for treating this dread disease will be available by the time this monograph appears in print.

MECHANISM AND ACTIONS

Zidovudine is a thymidine analog that is converted by thymidine kinase into the monophosphate and ultimately into the triphosphate derivative, which is the active form. Zidovudine triphosphate inhibits replication of the human immunodeficiency virus (HIV) by blocking viral RNA-dependent DNA polymerase (reverse transcriptase). The drug is incorporated into growing chains of DNA by viral reverse transcriptase, and thus terminates the incorporation of the DNA chain. Treatment with zidovudine does *not* reduce the risk of transmission of the virus through sexual contact or blood contamination.

USES

1. Management of patients with symptomatic HIV infection (*i.e.*, AIDS or advanced AIDS-related complex [ARC]) who have a history of cytologically confirmed *Pneumocystis carinii* pneumonia *or* an absolute CD4 (T$_4$ helper/induced) lymphocyte count of less than 200/mm^2.

■ NOTE

The above conditions for usage were those in effect at the time of writing; as supplies of the drug become more readily available and as the epidemiology of the disease changes, the parameters for use of zidovudine may be dramatically altered.

ADMINISTRATION AND DOSAGE

Zidovudine is used as capsules containing 100 mg. The initial dose is 200 mg every 4 hours around the clock. If anemia or granulocytopenia (see Side-Effects/Adverse Reactions) occur, dose reduction or temporary interruption in dosing may be necessary. Upon recovery of marrow function, the drug may be reinitiated cautiously and dosage increased gradually.

FATE
Oral absorption is rapid and peak plasma levels occur within 1 hour. Plasma protein binding is 35% to 40%. The drug is quickly metabolized in the liver; plasma half-life is approximately 1 hour. The metabolites and some unchanged drug are eliminated in the urine.

SIDE-EFFECTS/ADVERSE REACTIONS

■ WARNING
The most frequent adverse effects occurring with zidovudine are anemia and granulocytopenia. The frequency of occurrence is directly related to dose and duration of therapy, and inversely related to T_4 lymphocyte number, hemoglobin, and granulocyte count at the outset of therapy. Anemia usually occurs within 4 to 6 weeks of therapy and frequently requires blood transfusion. Myelosuppression is generally reversible, but often recurs even with dosage reduction, which may necessitate repeated transfusions.

Other adverse effects seen frequently during zidovudine therapy are headache, nausea, GI pain, skin rash, fever, asthenia, insomnia, and myalgia. Many other untoward reactions have been reported in patients taking zidovudine, but cannot always be directly related to the drug; they are listed below by organ system.

GI: anorexia, diarrhea, vomiting, dysphagia, flatulence, mouth ulcers, bleeding gums, edema of the tongue, rectal bleeding
CNS: dizziness, paresthesia, somnolence, anxiety, confusion, nervousness, syncope, depression
Respiratory: dyspnea, cough, nosebleed, sinusitis, pharyngitis, hoarseness, rhinitis
Urinary: dysuria, polyuria, urinary frequency
Dermatologic: pruritus, urticaria, acne
Other: vasodilation, arthralgia, muscle spasm, tremor, photophobia, hearing loss, amblyopia, chills, body odor, hyperalgesia, lymphadenopathy, altered taste

CONTRAINDICATIONS AND PRECAUTIONS
There are no absolute contraindications to use of zidovudine. The drug should be administered with *caution* to patients with liver or kidney dysfunction, compromised bone marrow function (*e.g.*, granulocyte count less than 1000/mm^3 or hemoglobin less than 9.5 g/dl), and to pregnant women or nursing mothers.

INTERACTIONS
1. Use of drugs that are nephrotoxic or cytotoxic (*e.g.*, amphotericin B, flucytosine, dapsone, pentamidine, vincristine, vinblastine) may increase the risk of toxicity during zidovudine administration.
2. Drugs that are likely to produce hematologic toxicity (chloramphenicol, carbamazepine, adriamycin, interferon) will increase the likelihood of such effects with zidovudine.
3. Drugs that can inhibit the metabolism (glucuronidation) of zidovudine (such as probenecid, indomethacin, aspirin, acetaminophen) by competitive antagonism may potentiate the toxic effects of the drug.

A major point of controversy concerning use of zidovudine is the suitability for administration of the drug to the large numbers of patients who have not developed AIDS disease, but who suffer from AIDS-related complex (ARC) with T_4 cell counts *greater* than 200; these patients are at increased risk for developing AIDS. The high cost of the drug, and the risk of hematologic toxicity and subsequent need for and cost of blood transfusions in these ARC patients must be carefully balanced with the potential benefit that the majority of ARC patients might ultimately derive from zidovudine therapy.

In summary, zidovudine is the forerunner for what is hoped to be a spate of new drugs that will provide improved quality and length of life to AIDS victims and perhaps ultimately a cure for this dread disease. As many as 50 antiviral and immunomodulating drugs are currently undergoing clinical trials for the treatment of AIDS, ARC, and AIDS-associated diseases, such as pneumocystis pneumonia and Kaposi's sarcoma. Among these investigational drugs are ampligen, eflornithine, alpha- and beta-interferons, interleukin-2, ribavirin (see earlier discussion), thymopentin, and thymostimuline.

REVIEW QUESTIONS

1. Why are viral diseases often asymptomatic until the course of the infection is well advanced?
2. In what two ways do most antiviral drugs work?
3. Against which viruses is acyclovir effective?
4. For what indications is (a) oral and (b) IV acyclovir used?
5. What are the most frequently encountered side-effects following (a) topical and (b) oral administration of acyclovir?
6. Outline guidelines for intravenous administration of acyclovir.
7. How can the risk of renal toxicity from acyclovir be minimized?
8. What are the major pharmacologic actions of amantadine?
9. Give the principal indications for amantadine.
10. List the most common side-effects encountered during amantadine therapy.
11. What are the indications for use of idoxuridine?
12. Briefly describe the mechanism of action of ribavirin. Against which viruses does the drug demonstrate effectiveness?
13. How is ribavirin administered in treating RSV?
14. What are the major dangers associated with use of ribavirin aerosol?
15. For what indications is trifluridine approved?
16. What are the uses for (a) IV and (b) ophthalmic vidarabine?
17. Why are large IV doses of vidarabine hazardous?
18. What are the major side-effects of vidarabine? How should they be monitored and managed?
19. In what patients is use of zidovudine approved?
20. Briefly describe the major toxicity of zidovudine.

BIBLIOGRAPHY

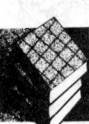

Bennett JA: What we know about AIDS. Am J Nurs 86:1016, 1986

Corey L, Holmes KK: Genital herpes simplex virus infections: Current concepts in diagnosis, therapy and prevention. Ann Intern Med 98:973, 1983

deMiranda P, Blum MR: Pharmacokinetics of acyclovir after intravenous and oral administration. J Antimicrob Chemother 12(suppl. B):29, 1983

Douglas RG: Antiviral drugs. Med Clin North Am 67:1163, 1983

Elion CB: Mechanism of action and selectivity of acyclovir. Am J Med 73:7, 1982

Halpern JS: Acyclovir: A respite, not a cure for primary genital herpes. J Emer Nursing 10:268, 1984

Hayden FG, Douglas RG: Antiviral agents. In Mandell GL, Douglas RG, Bennett JE (eds): Principles and Practice of Infectious Diseases, 2nd ed, p 270. New York, John Wiley & Sons, 1985

Hirsch MS, Schooley RT: Treatment of herpes virus infections. N Engl J Med 309:963, 1983

Hirsch MS, Swartz MN: Antiviral agents. N Engl J Med 302:903, 1980

Keeney RE, Kirk LE, Bridgen D: Acyclovir tolerance in humans. Am J Med 75(suppl):176, 1983

Laskin OL: Acyclovir. Ration Drug Ther 18(5):1, 1984

Oral acyclovir for genital herpes simplex infections. Med Lett Drugs Ther 27:41, 1985

Sasso CS: Acyclovir for herpes infections. MCN 8:433, 1983

Schinazi RF, Prusoff WH: Antiviral agents. Pediatr Clin North Am 30:77, 1983

Scott TM, Parish LC, Witkowski JA: Herpes simplex virus infections. II, Diagnosis and treatment. Drug Ther 15:135, 1985

Stuart-Harris CH, Oxford JS (eds): Problems of Antiviral Therapy: The Fifth Beecham Colloquium. p 71. London, Academic Press, 1983

Wade JC, Newton B, Flournoy N, Meyers JD: Oral acyclovir for prevention of herpes simplex virus reactivation after marrow transplantation. Ann Intern Med 100:823, 1984

Antineoplastic Drugs

Alkylating Agents
Busulfan, Carmustine,
Chlorambucil,
Cisplatin,
Dacarbazine,
Lomustine,
Mechlorethamine,
Melphalan,
Pipobroman,
Streptozocin,
Triethylenethio-
phosphoramide,
Uracil mustard

Antimetabolites
Cytarabine, Floxuridine,
Fluorouracil,
Mercaptopurine,
Methotrexate,
Thioguanine

Natural Products
Asparaginase, Bleomycin,
Dactinomycin,
Daunorubicin,
Doxorubicin,
Etoposide,
Mitomycin,
Mitoxantrone,
Plicamycin,
Vinblastine,
Vincristine

**Hormonal, Antihormonal, and
Gonadotropin-Releasing
Hormone Analogue Agents**

Miscellaneous Agents
Hydroxyurea, Interferon,
Procarbazine

Combination Chemotherapy

75

Cancer ranks second in mortality to heart disease in the United States, claiming more than 440,000 lives in 1986. The exact etiology of most cancers is still unknown; but infections as well as environmental (chemicals, fiber particles, radiation) and genetic factors are all capable of inducing a normal cell to become neoplastic.

There are more than 250 different types of malignant diseases which may be classified into four major groups based on tissue origin:
1. Carcinomas—Epithelial tissue
2. Sarcomas—Connective tissue
3. Leukemias—Hematopoietic tissue
4. Lymphomas—Lymphoreticular system

All of the different types of cancer may be characterized by the following:
1. Excessive cell growth due to permanent impairment of normal growth-controlling mechanisms
2. Cells and tissues are undifferentiated.
3. Cells exhibit invasiveness and have the ability to metastasize (i.e., establish themselves at sites distant from their original location).
4. Cells have acquired heredity (i.e., properties of the original cancerous cells).
5. Cells demonstrate increased synthesis of macromolecules from nucleosides and amino acids.

The treatment options for cancer include surgery, radiation, immunotherapy, and chemotherapy. Until recently, chemotherapy with antineoplastic drugs was used primarily as an adjunct to surgery or radiation therapy, primarily to eradicate any remaining metastatic tumor cell foci. Today, however, there are more than 40 commercially available antineoplastic agents, and some neoplastic diseases are treated primarily with chemotherapy, with many patients achieving a significantly prolonged survival time and, in some cases, complete remission (see Table 75-1).

To understand how chemotherapy works at the cellular level, it is important to review the phases of cell division:

G_1 (Gap one)—Postmitotic phase; various enzymes necessary for DNA synthesis are manufactured (several hours to several days)

S—Period of DNA synthesis for chromosomes; content of DNA doubles (10 hours–20 hours)

G_2 (Gap two)—Premitotic phase; specialized protein and RNA synthesis and formation of mitotic spindle (2 hours–10 hours)

M—Mitosis (½ hour–1 hour)

G_0 (Gap zero)—Temporarily nondividing

cells, cell differentiation, or cell death (variable duration)

Some antineoplastic agents inhibit cells during a specific phase of the above cycle and are referred to as cell-cycle specific (CCS). The therapeutic response to cell-cycle specific agents is usually schedule dependent (i.e., therapeutic blood levels must be maintained for a sufficient period of time to allow large numbers of cells to enter the S phase, thus producing a larger cell kill). Other antineoplastic agents are cytotoxic during any phase of the cell cycle and are referred to as cell-cycle nonspecific (CCNS). Cell-cycle nonspecific agents are dose dependent and are usually more effective if given in large intermittent doses. The various cell-cycle specific and cell-cycle nonspecific agents are listed in Table 75-2.

Before addressing the complex pharmacology of the antineoplastic agents, it is necessary to review the general principles of cancer chemotherapy.
1. The goal of cancer therapy is to destroy or remove all neoplastic cells with minimal effect on normal host cells.
2. The maximum chance for cure exists when the tumor cell burden is at a minimum and tumors have a high growth fraction (i.e., a high proportion of tumor cells are actively dividing). Debulking procedures (surgery, radiation) should be performed prior to the start of chemotherapy whenever possible.
3. A given dose of antineoplastic agent kills a constant percentage of cells, not a constant number.
4. Cell-cycle specific agents are more effective than cell-cycle nonspecific agents in tumors with a large bulky mass.
5. Before a change to another agent, treatment with an antineoplastic agent should continue until either the desired response is obtained or toxicity occurs. Cell-cycle specific agents are more effective when given in a prolonged and continuous schedule. Cell-cycle nonspecific agents are schedule independent and appear to be most effective when given in large intermittent doses.
6. Toxicity is often the limiting factor in the usefulness of an antineoplastic agent, and the risk of toxicity is increased if the patient has received prior chemotherapy or radiation treatment. However, the highly fatal nature of the disease makes the risk of serious toxicity relatively acceptable in most instances.

Table 75-1
Neoplastic Diseases Showing a Good Response to Chemotherapy

Disease	Antineoplastic Agents*
Acute lymphocytic leukemia (pediatric)	Induction—vincristine + prednisone ± asparaginase or doxorubicin Maintenance—methotrexate + 6-mercaptopurine
Acute myelogenous leukemia (adult)	doxorubicin or daunorubicin + cytarabine or cytarabine + thioguanine or cytarabine + vincristine + prednisone
Breast cancer	Estrogens, progestins, and tamoxifen cyclophosphamide + methotrexate + fluorouracil ± prednisone or cyclophosphamide + doxorubicin ± fluorouracil
Burkitt's lymphoma	cyclophosphamide or cyclophosphamide + methotrexate + vincristine
Choriocarcinoma	methotrexate ± dactinomycin
Diffuse histiocytic lymphoma	CHOP (cyclophosphamide, doxorubicin, vincristine, prednisone) or BACOP (bleomycin, doxorubicin, cyclophosphamide, vincristine, prednisone) or COMA (cyclophosphamide, vincristine, methotrexate, cytarabine) or MACOP-B (methotrexate, bleomycin, doxorubicin, cyclophosphamide, vincristine, prednisone) or Pro MACE-MOPP (prednisone, methotrexate, doxorubicin, cyclophosphamide, etoposide-mechlorethamine, vincristine, procarbazine, prednisone) or COP-BLAM (cyclophosphamide, vincristine, prednisone, bleomycin, doxorubicin, procarbazine)
Ewing's sarcoma	Cyclophosphamide + doxorubicin + vincristine
Hairy cell leukemia	Interferon
Hodgkin's disease	MOPP (mechlorethamine, vincristine, procarbazine, prednisone) or ABVD (doxorubicin, bleomycin, vinblastine, dacarbazine)
Lung cancer (small cell)	CAV (cyclophosphamide, doxorubicin, vincristine) or etoposide + cisplatin
Retinoblastoma	cyclophosphamide
Rhabdomyosarcoma	VAC (vincristine, dactinomycin, cyclophosphamide) ± doxorubicin
Testicular cancer	vinblastine + bleomycin + cisplatin or BEP (bleomycin, etoposide, cisplatin)
Wilm's tumor	dactinomycin + vincristine ± doxorubicin

* (±) indicates a possibly beneficial addition.

Table 75-2
Cell-Cycle Specific and Cell-Cycle Nonspecific Agents

Cell-Cycle Specific	Cell-Cycle Nonspecific
Antimetabolites	Alkylating agents
cytarabine	busulfan
floxuridine	carmustine
fluorouracil	chlorambucil
mercaptopurine	cisplatin
methotrexate	cyclophosphamide
thioguanine	dacarbazine
Natural products	lomustine
asparaginase	mechlorethamine
bleomycin	melphalan
etoposide	pipobroman
vinblastine	streptozocin
vincristine	triethylenethiophosphoramide
Miscellaneous	Natural products
hydroxyurea	dactinomycin
	daunorubicin
	doxorubicin
	mitomycin
	mitoxantrone
	Antimetabolites
	floxuridine
	fluorouracil
	Miscellaneous
	procarbazine

7. Malignant cells may exhibit resistance to some antineoplastic agents, thus limiting their usefulness. Resistance may be natural or acquired, that is, either the tumor is resistant from the start of therapy (natural), or resistance occurs after therapy has begun and results from drug-induced adaptation or mutation of malignant cells (acquired).

8. Drug scheduling is very important. High-dose intermittent therapy is usually more effective, less toxic, and less immunosuppressive than low-dose, continuous therapy. Toxicity may be reduced and cell resistance may be delayed by administering combinations of drugs in cycles or sequence (see discussion of combination chemotherapy at the end of this chapter).

9. Patient factors such as age, sex, physical condition, prior treatment, and altered renal or hepatic function can influence the outcome of chemotherapy.

10. When dosage of antineoplastic agents is based on weight, children tolerate relatively larger doses of drugs than do older patients. Dosage may be more accurately calculated in adults and children using body surface area; mg/kg

doses may be conveniently converted to mg/m² doses by multiplying by 40.

■ Nursing Process for Antineoplastic Drugs

The nursing care of patients undergoing chemotherapy is a complex and challenging task. It requires a thorough understanding of drugs, expected side-effects, appropriate symptom management, and patient responses to illness and treatment. Prior to the initiation of chemotherapy, a thorough assessment is essential. This section will detail information necessary for general assessment and care of the patient receiving chemotherapy.

□ *ASSESSMENT*

□ *Subjective Data*

1. Assess risk factors for developing cancer: drug, environmental and occupational exposure to toxins, diet, smoking, alcohol history.

2. Explore personal and social history: family members, social support systems, economic status, educational level, social and leisure activities, patterns of daily living, sleeping patterns. Identify the impact of cancer diagnosis and treatment on daily living.

3. Assess understanding of disease and expectations for treatment.

4. Examine medication history prior to starting chemotherapy.

□ *Objective Data*

1. Physical Assessment—A comprehensive and systematic physical assessment is essential prior to the initiation of chemotherapy as well as prior to each treatment. The major goal is to identify and minimize adverse side-effects of treatment. Therefore, knowledge of the potential problems, specific data which must be collected, and the drug and dose limiting factors must be available to the nurse. A tool, developed by Engelking and Steele to assist the nurse in pretreatment assessment of patients receiving chemotherapy, serves as an excellent framework for the systematic assessment of patients (see Table 75-3).

In addition to those parameters mentioned in Table 75-3, examination should also include the following:

Oral cavity: Note hygiene characteristics; condition of the mouth, gums, teeth, buccal

(Text continues on p. 1391.)

Table 75-3
*Prechemotherapy Nursing Assessment Model: Guidelines for Nursing Assessment
of the Patient Receiving Cancer Chemotherapy**

Part I: Physical Status

Potential Problems	Assessment Parameters/Signs and Symptoms	Drug and Dose-Limiting Factors
Hematopoietic System		
1. Impaired tissue perfusion related to chemotherapy-induced anemia	· Hgb g/dl (norms 12–14, 14–16) · Hct % (norms 32–36, 36–40) · Vital signs (↓BP ↑pulse ↑respiration) · Pale skin color (face, palms, conjunctiva) · Fatigue or weakness · Vertigo	Hgb < 8 g Hct < 20% and blood transfusions not initiated
2. Potential for infection related to chemotherapy-induced leukopenia	· WBC (norm 4500–9000/mm³) · Pyrexia/rigor, erythema, swelling, pain any site · Abnormal discharges, draining wounds, skin/mucous membrane lesions · Productive cough, shortness of breath, rectal pain, urinary frequency	WBC < 3000/mm³ Fever 101°F · Hold all myelosuppressive agents (Exceptions may include leukemia and lymphoma)
3. Potential for bleeding related to chemotherapy-induced thrombocytopenia	· Platelet count (150,000–400,000/mm³) · Spontaneous gingival bleeding or epistaxis · Presence of petechiae or easy bruisability · Hematuria, melena, hematemesis, hemoptysis · Hypermenorrhea · Signs and symptoms of intracranial bleed (irritability, sensory loss, unequal pupils, headache, ataxia)	Platelet count ≤ 100,000/mm³ · Hold all myelosuppressive agents (Exceptions may include leukemia and lymphoma)
Integumentary System		
Impairment of skin integrity related to chemotherapy-induced mucositis of mouth, nasopharynx, esophagus, rectum, anus, or ostomy stoma	Mucositis Scale 0 = pink, moist, intact mucosa; absence of pain or burning +1 = generalized erythema with or without pain or burning +2 = isolated small ulcerations and/or white patches +3 = confluent ulcerations with white patches on 25% mucosa +4 = hemorrhagic ulcerations	+ 2 mucositis · Hold antimetabolites (especially methotrexate, 5-fluorouracil) · Hold antitumor antibiotics (especially adriamycin, dactinomycin)
Gastrointestinal System		
Discomfort, nutritional deficiency or fluid and electrolyte disturbances related to chemotherapy-induced: A. Anorexia	· Lab values: albumin and total protein · Normal weight/present weight (% of body weight loss) · Normal diet pattern/changes in diet pattern · Presence of alterations in taste sensation · Presence of early satiety	

B. Nausea and vomiting	· Lab values: Electrolytes
	· Pattern of nausea and vomiting (incidence, duration, severity)
	· Antiemetic plan
	  Drug(s), dosage(s), schedule, efficacy
	  Other (dietary adjustments, relaxation techniques, environmental manipulation)
		Intractable nausea and vomiting for 24 h if IV hydration not initiated

(continued)

Table 75-3 (continued)
Prechemotherapy Nursing Assessment Model: Guidelines for Nursing Assessment
*of the Patient Receiving Cancer Chemotherapy**

Part I: Physical Status

Potential Problems	Assessment Parameters/Signs and Symptoms	Drug and Dose-Limiting Factors
Gastrointestinal System (continued)		
C. Bowel disturbances 1. Diarrhea	· Normal pattern of bowel elimination · Consistency (loose, watery/bloody stools) · Frequency and duration (no./day and no. of days) · Antidiarrheal drug(s), dosage(s), efficacy	Diarrheal stools for 3h to 24 h · Hold antimetabolites (especially methotrexate, 5 fluorouracil)
2. Constipation	· Normal pattern of bowel elimination · Consistency (hard, dry, small stools) · Frequency (hours or days beyond normal pattern) · Stool softener(s)/laxative(s), efficacy	No BM for 48 h past normal bowel patterns · Hold vinca alkaloids

D. Hepatotoxicity	· Lab values: LDH, SGOT, SGPT, Alk Phos, Bilirubin
	· Pain/tenderness over liver, feeling of fullness
	· Increase in nausea/vomiting or anorexia
	· Changes in mental status
	· Presence of jaundice
	· Presence of high-risk factors:
	   Hepatic metastasis
	   Viral hepatitis
	   Abdominal radiation therapy
	   Concurrent hepatotoxic drugs
	   Graft vs host disease
	   Blood transfusions
		Evidence of chemical hepatitis
		· Hold hepatotoxic agents (especially methotrexate, 6-mercaptopurine) until differential diagnosis is established

Respiratory System		

Respiratory dysfunction related to chemotherapy-induced pulmonary fibrosis	· Lab values: pulmonary function tests; chest x-ray
	· Respiration (rate, rhythm, depth)
	· Chest pain
	· Nonproductive cough
	· Progressive dyspnea
	· Wheezing/stridor
	· Presence of high-risk factors:
	   Total cumulative dose of bleomycin
	   Age 60 yr
	   Concomitant use of other pulmonary toxic drugs
	   Pre-existing lung disease
	   Prior/concomitant radiation therapy
	   Smoking history
		Acute unexplained onset respiratory symptoms
		· Hold all antineoplastic agents until differential diagnosis established

Cardiovascular System		
Decreased cardiac output related to chemotherapy-induced: A. Cardiac arrhythmias B. Congestive heart failure (CHF)	· Lab values: cardiac enzymes, electrolytes, ECG, echocardiography, MUGA scan · Vital signs · Presence of arrhythmia (irregular radial/apical) · Signs and symptoms of CHF (dyspnea, ankle edema, nonproductive cough, rales, cyanosis)	Acute symptoms of CHF or cardiac arrhythmia · Hold all antineoplastic agents until differential diagnosis is established Total dose adriamycin or daunomycin 550 mg/m² · Hold anthracyclines

(continued)

Table 75-3 (continued)
Prechemotherapy Nursing Assessment Model: Guidelines for Nursing Assessment of the Patient Receiving Cancer Chemotherapy*

Part I: Physical Status

Potential Problems	Assessment Parameters/Signs and Symptoms	Drug and Dose-Limiting Factors

Cardiovascular System (continued)

| | · Presence of high-risk factors: Total cumulative doses anthracyclines Pre-existing cardiac disease Prior/concurrent mediastinal XRT Bolus administration higher drug doses | |

Genitourinary System

| Impaired renal function related to chemotherapy-induced: A. Hemorrhage B. Glomerular or renal tubule damage C. Hyperuricemic nephropathy | · Lab values: BUN, creatinine clearance, serum creatinine, uric acid, electrolytes, urinalysis · Color, odor, clarity of urine · 24-h fluid intake and output (estimate/actual) · Presence of hematuria; proteinuria · Development of oliguria or anuria · Presence of high-risk factors: Pre-existing renal disease Concurrent treatment with nephrotoxic drugs (especially aminoglycoside antibiotics) | Hematuria · Hold cytoxan Serum creatinine 2.0 or creatinine clear 70 ml/min · Hold cisplatin, streptozocin Anuria for 24 h · Hold all antineoplastic agents |

Nervous System

| 1. Impaired sensory/motor function related to chemotherapy-induced A. Peripheral neuropathy B. Cranial nerve neuropathy | Presence of: · Paresthesias (numbness, tingling in feet, fingertips) · Trigeminal nerve toxicity (severe jaw pain) · Diminished or absent deep tendon reflexes (ankle and knee jerks) · Motor weakness/slapping gait/ataxia · Visual and auditory disturbances | Presence of any neurologic signs and symptoms · Hold vinca alkaloids, cisplatin, hexamethylamine, procarbazine until differential diagnosis is established |
| 2. Impaired bowel and bladder elimination related to chemotherapy-induced autonomic nerve dysfunction | Presence of: · Urinary retention · Constipation/abdominal cramping and distention · Presence of high-risk factors: Changes in diet or mobility Frequent use narcotic analgesics Obstructive disease process | Presence of any neurologic signs and symptoms · Hold vinca alkaloids until differential diagnosis is established |

Part II: Performance Status: Modified Zubrod Scale

Patient Classification	Defining Characteristics
0	Normal activity; no evidence of disease
1	Disease symptoms present, but able to carry out activities of daily living
2	out of bed 50% of time; requires occasional assistance
3	out of bed 50% of time; requires specialized care
4	Bedridden, requires complete care or assistance with all aspects of care

(continued)

Table 75-3 (continued)
Prechemotherapy Nursing Assessment Model: Guidelines for Nursing Assessment
of the Patient Receiving Cancer Chemotherapy*

Part III: Psychosocial/Cognitive Functioning

Potential Problem	*Assessment Parameters*

Anxiety related to disease and treatment	· *Potential etiology*
	Fear of treatment procedure (*e.g.,* pain of injection)
	Fear of potentially life-threatening complications; poor treatment response
	Concern about potential/actual changes in body image (*e.g.,* alopecia)
	Concern about potential/actual changes in life-style or role
	Communication difficulty with health-care provider(s)
	Financial/occupational concerns
	· *Subjective data*
	Verbalization of fears, concerns, feeling nervous
	· *Objective data*
	Physiologic manifestations:
	  Voice tremors/pitch changes
	  Increased vital signs
	  Increased muscle tension
	  Diaphoresis
	  Tremors/headaches
	  Anticipatory nausea/vomiting
	Behavioral manifestations:
	  Fixed perceptual focus (excessive attention to treatment detail)
	  Pacing, crying, handwringing
	  Scattered perceptual focus (inability to concentrate)
	  Increased verbalization

Ineffective individual coping secondary to the need for cancer chemotherapy	· *Potential etiology* See under Potential etiology for "Anxiety . . ." and "Knowledge deficit . . ." History of ineffective problem-solving abilities or coping behaviors Lack of kinship and social support network(s) · *Subjective data* Verbalization of inability to cope with chemotherapy-related fears or side-effects · *Objective data* Inability to request or accept information or assistance in coping with chemotherapy-related fears or side-effects Inappropriate or exaggerated behaviors (*e.g.,* anger, hostility, agitation, apathy, dependency) Deterioration of established pattern of communication with health-care providers/significant others Demonstrated withdrawal from social relationships or activities, occupational/role responsibilities
Ineffective family coping secondary to their family member's need for cancer chemotherapy	· *Potential etiology* See under Potential etiology for "Ineffective individual coping . . ." Preestablished pattern of family conflict Impaired family communication pattern · *Subjective data* Patient expresses or confirms concern or complaint about significant other's response to patient's illness or treatment Significant person describes or confirms inadequate understanding or knowledge base regarding chemotherapy which interferes with effective supportive behaviors · *Objective data* See under Objective data for "Ineffective individual coping . . ." Exacerbation, family conflicts or tension Display of disproportionate protective behavior to patient's abilities or need for autonomy

(continued)

Table 75-3 (continued)
Prechemotherapy Nursing Assessment Model: Guidelines for Nursing Assessment
*of the Patient Receiving Cancer Chemotherapy**

Part III: Psychosocial/Cognitive Functioning

Potential Problem	Assessment Parameters
Knowledge deficit related to chemo-therapy	· *Potential etiology* Lack of exposure Lack of recall Cognitive/perceptual limitation Difficulty communicating with health-care provider(s) Information misinterpretation Conflicting information given Impaired readiness for learning related to fear, anxiety, denial, disinterest · *Subjective data* Verbalization of lack of knowledge/understanding of chemotherapy regimen or required self-management activities · *Objective data* Inadequate performance of self-management activities: Inaccurate follow-through on instruction for management of drug-induced side-effects Failure to obtain prescribed tests/keep appointments

* *Note:* Because this is a general guide, not all assessment parameters will apply to every patient. Some may weigh more heavily than others depending upon the disease itself, the particular drugs and dosages, as well as individual factors. Therefore, the nurse using these guidelines to assess a patient prior to chemotherapy administration must modify her assessment to address each individual situation. (Adapted from Engelking, C, Steele, N: A model for pretreatment nursing assessment of patients receiving cancer chemotherapy. Cancer Nursing 7(3):203, 1984; The Oncology Nursing Society Clinical Practice Committee: Guidelines for nursing care of patients with altered protective mechanisms; and Kin MJ, Moritz DA (eds): Classification of Nursing Diagnoses: Proceedings of Third and Fourth National Conferences. New York, McGraw-Hill, 1982)

mucosa, and tongue; taste changes; evidence of infection or stomatitis.
Genitourinary: Note frequency, urgency, dysuria, hesitancy, narrowing of stream, hematuria, nocturia, or polyuria.
Musculoskeletal: Note pain, fractures, swelling, range of motion
Other:
   Male: Note evidence of testicular pain, change in size of scrotum
   Female: Note breast lumps, discharge, asymmetry of breasts, skin changes, menstrual history, vaginal bleeding; also date of last pap smear
2. Laboratory data and diagnostic tests
   · CBC, platelets, and differential prior to each treatment
   · BUN, creatinine
   · Liver function tests: SGOT, SGPT, alkaline phosphatase, bilirubin
   · Electrolytes

□ *NURSING DIAGNOSIS*
Actual nursing diagnoses for the patient receiving antineoplastic agents include:

Knowledge deficit related to administration and side effects of the antineoplastic agents.
Potential nursing diagnoses include:
   Potential for infection: neutropenia
   Potential for injury: thrombocytopenia and anemia
   Fluid volume deficit related to nausea and vomiting
   Alteration in nutrition; less than body requirement
   Disturbance in body image/self-concept related to alopecia
   Sexual dysfunction
   Alterations in oral mucous membranes; stomatitis

□ *PLAN*
The nursing care of the patient receiving any antineoplastic agent is directed toward (1) minimizing any side-effects experienced, (2) fostering self-care behaviors, (3) ensuring identification of early signs and symptoms of toxicities by the patient, and (4) implementing appropriate interventions.

□ INTERVENTION

Nursing care for the patient undergoing chemotherapy will frequently be directed toward the management of drug-induced side-effects which may be unavoidable. The education provided the patient to prepare him for dealing with these side-effects will greatly influence the response to treatment. The following section will deal with strategies for patient education and for management of side-effects such as neutropenia, thrombocytopenia, anemia, nausea and vomiting, stomatitis, alopecia, nutritional deficits, and infertility.

□ Patient Education

Education for both the patient undergoing chemotherapy and the family is a critical role for nurses. It not only involves the exchange of information but it influences the knowledge, attitudes, and behavior of the patient and persons associated with him. Therefore, the major goals in an effective education program are to facilitate adaptation and adjustment to the cancer process, to minimize complications, and to identify toxicities of therapy.

A thorough cognitive assessment will help the nurse develop a realistic teaching plan. Assessment parameters should include: patient's past experience with cancer, current physical and emotional response to cancer, developmental stage preference for information (i.e., written material, discussion, audiovisual aids), and phase of illness. Identification of myths and misconceptions regarding treatment is an important part of the nurse's role. In addition, the nurse must recognize that the phase of illness and overall goals of treatment will affect the learning needs of the patient and family members. Information and teaching goals will vary depending on whether the patient is in the initial diagnosis and treatment phase, the adjuvant therapy and remission phase, or the supportive treatment phase.

The nurse and patient will formulate learning needs together in a successful teaching plan. Lauer has identified the five most important learning needs of patients during chemotherapy: purpose of treatment, schedule for treatment, length of time for therapy, expected side-effects, and self-care behaviors to minimize the side-effects of therapy.

Implementation of the educational program should include both written and verbal information. The use of multiple media sources is recommended whenever possible, such as materials available from the American Cancer Society, National Cancer Institute, drug companies, and private vendors.

Evaluation of the teaching plan involves eliciting feedback from the patient that the information is helpful and meets his learning needs. The process of patient education for the patient receiving cancer chemotherapy is a challenging opportunity for nurses. The quality of life experienced by patients undergoing chemotherapy may be greatly influenced by the information and guidance they receive.

□ Neutropenia

Neutropenia is defined as a white blood cell count containing less than $1000/m^3$ granulocytes and substantially less than the normal granulocyte count. The nadir or low point of the white blood cell count occurs approximately 7 days to 10 days after administration of chemotherapy. Recovery of the white blood cell count can be anticipated 14 days to 21 days after chemotherapy.

The patient experiencing neutropenia is at great risk for infection. The risk is increased by the degree of neutropenia and the length of time to recovery. During this time even seemingly mild infections and low-grade temperatures may develop into life-threatening conditions. During the period of neutropenia the patient needs to be instructed to maintain mucous membrane and skin integrity. Any trauma, however mild, may be an entry point for bacteria into the bloodstream which, when coupled with a lack of white blood cells to limit the infection, may result in sepsis.

The patient should be taught to report any of the following temperature alterations: any temperature greater than 101°F, temperature greater than 100°F for more than 4 hours, or any temperature less than 96°F. Patients should also be instructed to report immediately any shaking chills and areas of pain or discomfort, particularly if there is redness, or warmth. Because of the lack of granulocytes, there will be little if any pus formation. Cutaneous infections may manifest themselves as areas of redness or warmth. Pain inconsistent with area involved should be of particular concern, particularly in the rectal area. Any new cough or shortness of breath should also be reported immediately.

To minimize potential for infection, patients should avoid all potential trauma. This includes use of indwelling catheters (i.e., urinary, intravenous), rectal thermometers, enemas, suppositories, and tampons. Patients should report any discomfort urinating or with bowel movements. Patients should be instructed to avoid large crowds particularly during the cold or flu season. Patients should also avoid constipation or diarrhea and should pay careful attention to cleansing the rectal area after a bowel movement. Patients should pay particular attention to development of mouth sores.

□ Thrombocytopenia

The degree of thrombocytopenia experienced by the patient relates to the types and doses of the drugs used in his therapy. The patient should be instructed to recognize and report signs and symptoms of a low platelet count including easy bruising, petechiae, bleeding from body orifices, blood in urine and stool, and hypermenorrhea.

Close monitoring of the platelet count prior to administering chemotherapy is essential. There is an increased risk for bleeding when the platelet count falls below 50,000/mm^3. Therefore, patients should be instructed to avoid trauma that may precipitate bleeding (e.g., by using an electric razor and soft toothbrush, and wearing shoes at all times), to eliminate aspirin-containing medications, and to prevent constipation.

Excessive venipunctures should be discouraged because easy bleeding and bruising may result. Applying pressure to venipuncture sites for 3 minutes to 5 minutes should be instituted. Avoid IM injections or taking of rectal temperatures if possible.

Platelet transfusions may be required if thrombocytopenia is severe.

□ Anemia

Anemia refers to the depression of hemoglobin and the red cell portion of the blood. Signs of this occurrence include easy fatigability, headache, lightheadedness, fainting, pallor, palpitations, tachycardia, and shortness of breath.

Hemoglobin and hematocrit results must be examined closely because the state of dehydration may cause the hematocrit to rise and hide an underlying anemia.

Causes of anemia vary, and the exact cause for this syndrome should be determined. Common etiologies for anemia, besides bone marrow depression secondary to chemotherapeutic agents, include iron deficiency, hemorrhage, or tumor invasion of the bone marrow.

Blood transfusions of packed red blood cells together with oxygen therapy may be required if the RBC count falls to an abnormally low level.

Interventions are directed at symptom control as well as blood transfusions. Patients should be aware of signs and symptoms of anemia and instructed to adjust level of activity to conserve energy by allowing for frequent rest periods. If short-

ness of breath or palpitations are experienced, the physician should be notified immediately.

□ Nausea and Vomiting

Nausea and vomiting are common side-effects of many antineoplastic agents. Noncompliance with therapy or refusal of additional therapies is often related to the inability to control this phenomenon. In fact, uncontrolled nausea and vomiting may lead to a syndrome known as anticipatory nausea and vomiting in which nausea and vomiting occur before the chemotherapy administration. Patients find this to be extremely distressing.

The severity of the nausea and vomiting is correlated with the antineoplastic agents used and with previous responses to other chemotherapy. (See box entitled Antineoplastic Drugs Associated with Nausea and Vomiting.) The nurse needs to inform the patient of the possibility of this side-effect, as well as the availability of premedication with an antiemetic to prevent or reduce its severity. However, antiemetic therapy is often adjusted or changed in response to the patient's tolerance.

Antineoplastic Drugs Associated With Nausea and Vomiting

L-asparaginase	5-fluorouracil
5-azacytidine	hydroxyurea
bleomycin	methotrexate
cisplatin	mithramycin (plicamycin)
cyclophosphamide	mitomycin
dacarbazine	mitoxantrone
dactinomycin	nitrogen mustard
daunorubicin	procarbazine
doxorubicin	streptozocin

The inability to control chemotherapy-induced nausea and vomiting can produce an impaired nutritional intake, leading to weight loss, fluid and electrolyte imbalances, and weakness. Therefore, control of symptoms is an important nursing function.

Nursing actions to combat nausea and vomiting must be individualized to each patient. Interventions can be both pharmacologic and behavioral and may include the following:

· Treating the patient in a well-ventilated, calm environment, free of foul smells
· Having an emesis basin at close range, but out of patient's sight
· Obtaining a complete history of previous nausea and vomiting experiences as well as helpful measures used to alleviate these symptoms in the past

- Administering antiemetics as ordered and giving proper instructions for home use, including possible side-effects (suppository forms of various antiemetics are very useful when nausea and vomiting are especially severe)
- Providing thorough dietary instruction, encouraging small frequent meals and the avoidance of fried or greasy foods
- Encouraging adequate nutritional intake (including supplements)
- Using distraction techniques to attempt to minimize the degree of nausea and vomiting experienced (e.g., radio, headphones, relaxation techniques, self-hypnosis)

☐ *Stomatitis*

Stomatitis, the inflammation of the mucous membranes of the oral cavity, occurs with various antineoplastic agents, but the severity of the symptom depends greatly on the dose and schedule of the drugs being used.

Early detection and management of this side-effect may prevent worsening of the symptoms and possible infection of the oral cavity.

Comfort measures should be instituted immediately to ensure adequate nutrition is maintained.

Nursing interventions include:

- Ongoing assessment of the oral cavity
- Ensuring a dental evaluation is performed prior to the initiation of therapy
- Instructing the patient in proper oral hygiene
- Instituting saline rinses on a p.r.n. basis
- Instructing the patient to report promptly any symptoms of oral discomfort or ulceration
- Stressing the importance of informing the oncologist of any dental work planned while on therapy
- Advising the patient to ingest cold liquids and soft foods which may be more easily tolerated than spicy foods or alcohol

☐ *Alopecia*

The alopecia which results from chemotherapy is one of the most distressing side-effects experienced by patients and may affect body image, relationships, and social interactions. Nurses need to be sensitive to this issue and provide patients with information and suggestions to anticipate this side-effect of chemotherapy.

Hair loss may be complete or partial. The degree of hair loss is related to the type of drugs administered, the dosage, and duration of therapy. The two drugs most often associated with hair loss are doxorubicin and cyclophosphamide. Other agents that commonly cause hair loss include actinomycin D, bleomycin, daunorubicin, 5-fluorouracil, cytarabine, etoposide, busulphan, vincristine, dacarbazine, streptozocin, nitrogen mustard, mitomycin, and methotrexate. Several methods have been used to minimize loss of scalp hair during treatment, including use of a scalp tourniquet, scalp hypothermia, or a combination of both; these have had varying success in minimizing hair loss. These measures should not be used, however, in leukemia, lymphoma, or the presence of scalp metastasis from solid tumors.

Although loss of scalp hair is most common, patients may also experience hair loss from the face, eyebrows, eyelashes, axillary, pubic, and body areas. It is important to reassure patients that hair will grow back, although it may be a different color or texture. New hair growth usually begins within 1 month to 2 months after the last treatment.

☐ *Nutritional Concerns*

Adequate nutrition is essential in patients undergoing any chemotherapy. Patients who are well nourished seem to tolerate chemotherapy and its side-effects better and seem to recover quicker from side-effects. Conversely, patients who are poorly nourished tend to respond more slowly to supportive measures.

Patients who have lost more than 10% of their body weight should be evaluated for nutritional supplementation and must be monitored closely. Supplemental measures may include oral nutrients, tube feedings, or parenteral hyperalimentation.

Patients should discuss strategies to maintain adequate nutrition with their health-care provider. Many patients prefer cold, soft foods such as milkshakes, soft fruit, and yogurt, and they should be encouraged to eat any and all foods that are appealing. The nurse needs to remind the patient that appetite may vary so eating should take place whenever appetite is present. A pleasant social atmosphere, particularly eating with others, is also helpful. Foods, such as frozen dinners or made-at-home frozen meals, are helpful because they require little time or energy to prepare.

Some patients may feel there is no desire or reason to eat. Frequent encouragement, not nagging, is needed to help these patients eat, and should focus on maximizing their sense of well-being rather than on the volume of food they consume. Instructions should focus on the need for high-calorie, high-protein foods. Food choices should reflect this need, such as flat soda or juice rather than water. Many suggestions are available in a booklet entitled *Eating Hints* available from the U.S. Department of Health and Human Services.

Small frequent meals should be encouraged to maximize food intake and limit a bloated feeling. Patients should be urged to taste different foods—food taste and preference change over time and with chemotherapy.

□ *Infertility*

Chemotherapy affects the reproductive organs as well as other body systems. This is a critical issue for many patients and should be addressed prior to the initiation of chemotherapy. In particular, women of childbearing age must be assessed for the possibility of pregnancy because chemotherapy affects the fetus as well as the women's reproductive function. In the presence of pregnancy, therapy may be delayed until after delivery. If delay is not possible, a therapeutic abortion may be necessary. Men should be given the option to bank their sperm prior to the initiation of chemotherapy so future homologous insemination may be possible.

A variety of chemotherapeutic agents affect reproduction potential in both men and women. The alkylating agents have a profound effect on both ovarian and testicular function. Other agents likely to cause dysfunction include vinblastine, bleomycin, actinomycin D, daunorubicin, doxorubicin, mitomycin, and procarbazine. These agents often cause temporary or permanent sterility. The loss of reproductive capacity tends to be progressive, occurring over time, rather than abruptly. The reversibility of damage is related to age, drug dosage, and length of treatment. Permanent damage is more likely in women over age 30 and with treatment courses longer than 6 months in duration.

It is imperative that nurses become aware of the effect of disease and treatment on the reproductive function of patients. Contraceptive information should be provided during the initial phases of treatment. Ongoing assessment and information may be necessary to ensure compliance. It is recommended that contraceptives be used during treatment and for 2 years following the discontinuation of treatment to allow adequate time for repair of spermatogenesis. Family planning is another important part of follow-up treatment.

Patients should be advised that normal children have been born to patients who have undergone treatment with chemotherapy. Close follow-up of children with an oncologist is recommended however. There is little information presently available on the long-term effects of chemotherapy on offspring. Alternative parenting options may also be explored.

□ *EVALUATION*

The evaluation of these interventions will be measured by

1. The patient's ability to report adverse effects, as they first appear, to health-care providers
2. The patient's ability to perform intervention necessary to minimize side-effects
3. The patient's ability to function as independently as possible without endangering himself relative to actual side-effects

The nursing process for the patient receiving antineoplastic chemotherapy is summarized in Nursing Care Plan 75-1.

□ *PREVENTION AND EARLY MANAGEMENT OF EXTRAVASATION*

Proper and safe administration of antineoplastic agents is a challenging and important role of the oncology nurse. Several agents used to treat cancer patients are potentially irritating or sclerosing to veins. For this reason, special care must be used when administering these drugs. Before administering the agent, the nurse must verify that informed consent has been obtained and that the patient is aware of the possible risks involved in receiving these agents. The nurse and physician should discuss the entire procedure with the patient.

Depending on the specific drug, it may act as an irritant or as a sclerosing agent. An irritant produces pain at the IV site or along the vein, with or without an inflammatory reaction. A sclerosing agent is capable of causing blistering and tissue destruction of skin, nerves, tendons, and muscles in the affected area. (See box entitled Agents That Can Cause Sclerosing or Vein Irritation.) The best way

(*Text continues on p. 1399.*)

Agents That Can Cause Sclerosing or Vein Irritation

Sclerosing Agents

dactinomycin
dacarbazine
daunorubicin
doxorubicin
mithramycin
mitomycin C
mechlorethamine
vinblastine
vincristine

Irritant Agents

carmustine
etoposide
streptozocin

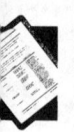

Assessment

Subjective Data

1. Medication history: Refer to Interactions section in each class to formulate pertinent questions.
   a. Identify use of aspirin or any nonsteroidal anti-inflammatory agents which may precipitate bleeding in a compromised patient.
   b. Identify use of alcohol.
   c. Drug allergies/hypersensitivity or reactions to any drugs in the class
2. Medical history
   a. Present site of malignancy and its manifestations as a rationale for proposed drug therapy.
   b. Dietary history: nutritional status, appetite, ingestion of foods which may adversely react to certain drugs
   c. Pre-existing medical problems that may complicate therapy and require cautious administration. See under Contraindications and Precautions and Nursing Process for each drug class.
   d. Patient's description of symptoms and effect on activities of daily living (*e.g.*, pain, appetite, activity, bowel habits)
3. Personal history/compliance issues
   a. Perception of problem, attitude toward cancer, and attitude about chemotherapy as a treatment
   b. Past compliance with complex regimens
   c. Financial resources, ability to work, insurance coverage
   d. Personal support systems

Objective Data

1. Physical assessment: A complete physical examination should be performed on every patient prior to receiving antineoplastic therapy. For examples of systems most affected by certain drugs see the *Nursing Process* section for each drug class.
2. Laboratory Data: See *Nursing Process*, Objective Data, for each drug class. However, all patients should have the following:
   · CBC, with differential and platelet count
   · Complete liver function tests
   · BUN, serum creatinine
   · PT, PTT, fibrinogen

Nursing Diagnoses	Client Goal/Expected Outcome	Intervention
Knowledge deficit related to administration and side-effects of chemotherapy	Will demonstrate appropriate drug administration	Assess patient understanding of current drug regimen including drugs, dose, schedule, time of administration, route, and length of treatment.
	Will verbalize early signs and symptoms of discomfort during administration of irritants or vesicants	Instruct patient to report any signs and symptoms of discomfort during administration especially with vesicants or irritants.
	Will comply with the current drug regimen as instructed	Discuss drug, dietary, alcohol concerns related to specific drug regimens.
		Provide written information regarding specific drug regimen.
	Will verbalize an understanding of the side-effects of therapy, methods to prevent or control symptoms, and when to contact the health-care team	Discuss anticipated side-effects of drug therapy.
		Provide written information about specific side-effects.
		Discuss appropriate interventions to prevent or minimize potential side-effects.

(continued)

Nursing Diagnoses	Client Goal/Expected Outcome	Intervention
		Instruct patient to report adverse signs and symptoms of drugs to health-care providers immediately.
Potential for infection related to neutropenia	Will state signs and symptoms of infection which should be reported	Instruct patient about potential risk for infection.
		Assess areas of body for signs/symptoms of infection *Mouth*—Lesions, soreness, swelling *Rectum*—tenderness, redness, induration, hemorrhoids *GI*—Constipation/diarrhea, pain *Skin*—Redness, swelling, induration, lesions, pain *GU*—Pain, burning, odor *Respiratory*—Pain, cough
	Will identify measures to prevent or minimize infection	Avoid performing invasive procedures—rectal temps, IM injections, enemas, suppositories, tampons, urinary catheters
		Instruct patient to avoid trauma—use electric razor, wear shoes, avoid straining
		Instruct patient to report signs/symptoms of infection including T 101°F at any time T 100°F on two occasions T 96 °F and chills or other symptoms noted above
Potential for injury: thrombocytopenia	Will recognize factors that increase risk of bleeding and will report early signs of bleeding	Avoid invasive procedures, IM injections, rectal temps, enemas, tampons, prolong BP cuff pressure, suppositories.
		Apply pressure to puncture sites for at least 5 min.
		Restrict activity if platelet count < 10,000 or active bleeding.
		Do not administer any aspirin compounds.
		Instruct patient to use soft toothbrush; use electric razor, no straight edges; report any bruising or bleeding; wear shoes out of bed; apply pressure to sites of any bleeding.
Potential for injury: anemia	Will verbalize an understanding of the symptoms of anemia, methods to prevent or control symptoms, and when to contact the health-care team	Instruct patient regarding risk for anemia.
		Discuss signs and symptoms of anemia.
		Suggest frequent rest periods during the day.
		Pace patient's activities.
		Discuss potential need for transfusions and if needed, nurse will administer according to established guidelines.

(continued)

Nursing Diagnoses	Client Goal/Expected Outcome	Intervention
		Teach the patient to report syncope, palpitations, chest pain, and dizziness to health-care providers.
Potential alteration in oral membranes	Will learn to recognize the signs and symptoms of stomatitis which should be reported	Assess oral cavity twice a day. Teach patient signs and symptoms of stomatitis, erythema, burning, pain, ulcerations.

	Will implement measures to minimize the risk of developing stomatitis	Begin normal saline solution rinses.
		Discuss importance of daily oral hygiene
		  Brush after each meal and before bed
		  Use of soft toothbrush
		  Avoid commercial mouthwash containing alcohol
		Teach patient to avoid hot spicy foods; to use bland, moderate-temperature soft foods; to maintain adequate hydration and nutrition.
		If mouth sores develop notify health-care providers
		  Increase frequency of mouth care
		  May use local anesthetics and pain medications
		  May use nystatin (antifungal) and/or oral antibiotic for infection

Potential fluid volume deficit related to nausea and vomiting	Will state the degree of risk for the development of nausea and vomiting with chemotherapy	Discuss the anticipated degree of nausea and vomiting re: therapy. Assess previous experience with chemotherapy
	Will obtain relief from prescribed antiemetic therapy	Administer antiemetics prior to therapy and appropriate to anticipated degree of nausea and vomiting post-treatment.
	Will verbalize an understanding of the undesirable effects of nausea and vomiting, how to prevent them, and when to notify the health-care team	Teach patient to monitor actual episodes of nausea, to report inability to maintain adequate hydration, to report bleeding in vomitus. Discuss signs and symptoms of dehydration. Instruct patient to drink 2 L–3 L noncarbonated beverages/day.
	Will state recommended strategies to avoid or minimize nausea and vomiting	Avoid fried and greasy food. Encourage bland high-carbohydrate foods. Encourage small frequent meals.
Potential disturbance in body image/self-concept	Will verbalize an understanding of the risk for hair loss and perception of changes in self-image resulting from such loss	Discuss degree of risk for hair loss. Discuss potential use of wigs/scarves/caps. Reassure patient that hair will grow back. It may come back different color or different texture.
	Will identify measures to minimize hair loss during therapy	Implement measures to minimize hair loss Mild shampoo.

(continued)

Nursing Diagnoses	Client Goal/Expected Outcome	Intervention
		Avoid use of dyes and perms on hair.
		Avoid vigorous brushing.
		Explore use of hypothermia cap, scalp tourniquet.
		Identify written and audiovisual materials available.
Potential alterations in sexual patterns	Will state the risks to reproductive potential as a result of chemotherapy and will discuss alternatives available	Obtain a pregnancy test on all women of child-bearing age prior to initiation of chemotherapy.
		Explore issues related to sperm banking in men before the initiation of chemotherapy.
		Discuss potential for temporary or permanent sterility.
		Explore alternatives for parenthood.
	Will implement use of effective contraception during treatment	Discuss need for contraceptive measures during and for 2 years after chemotherapy for both men and women.
		Normal children have been born to parents who have undergone chemotherapy but no data exist on long-term effects. These children should be followed by an oncologist.
Potential alteration in nutrition: Less than body requirements	Will state strategies to minimize the risk of weight loss during therapy	Discuss potential changes in taste perceptions, appetite, and GI function.
		Discuss factors that may affect ability to eat: stomatitis, nausea/vomiting, fatigue, depression.
		Encourage small, frequent meals with increased calorie and protein content.
		Implement use of nutritional supplements if unable to meet calorie requirements.
		Monitor weight.
		Obtain a dietary consult if weight loss is more than 2 lb/week.

to avoid irritation or sclerosing is to prevent extravasation. Extravasation is leakage of the drug from the vein into the subcutaneous tissue.

Prior to administration of the antineoplastic agent, the nurse must critically examine each patient's access sites and choose an acceptable vein. The vein should have the following properties: (1) it should travel a straight course long enough to accept the needle; (2) it should not be sclerosed or inflamed.

The superficial or cutaneous veins of the dorsum of the hand and forearm are those most commonly used (Fig. 75-1). These consist of the metacarpals, cephalic, basilic, and median cubital veins. The use of the antecubital fossa should be avoided, because these veins tend to be fibrosed and not easily visible and therefore early signs of extravasation may be difficult to detect.

Due to the possibility of impaired circulation and drainage, the nurse should also avoid using an

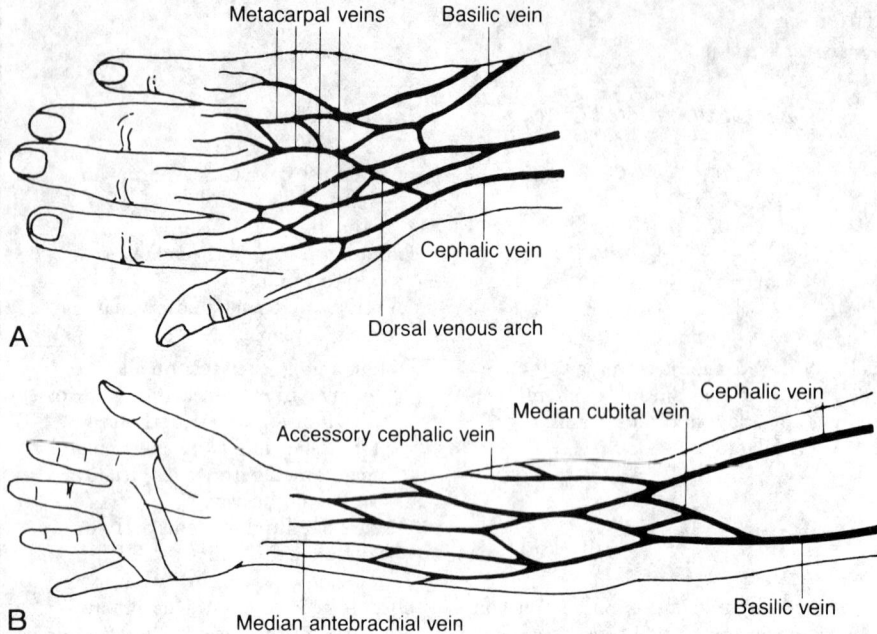

Figure 75-1. Veins of (A) the hand and (B) the forearm that may be used for intravenous administration of chemotherapeutic drugs.

arm where axillary node dissection or mastectomy have been performed. When a sclerosing drug is being administered, there should be no previous venipuncture above the potential injection site within the past 6 hours to 12 hours.

After choosing the proper vein, the skin should be prepared with alcohol or povidone-iodine solution. According to the size of the vein, a 21-, 23-, or 25-gauge butterfly needle is inserted into the vein and secured, allowing maximal visibility of the area. To ensure proper placement of the needle, normal saline solution should be infused and its flow rate closely observed. The presence of a blood return should be verified. When all the above criteria are met, the agent may then be administered. The patient should be instructed to inform the nurse of any burning, tingling, numbness, or unusual sensations at the injection site at any time during the infusion. If there is any question of IV patency, the injection infusion should be stopped and the drug administered at another site.

Despite the utmost care exercised by the nurse, extravasation of a sclerosing or irritant agent can occur and accounts for approximately 2% to 5% of all adverse side-effects from antineoplastic drugs.

Recognizing an extravasation is sometimes difficult. Careful monitoring of the patient during the entire administration is essential. The most common signs of extravascular infiltration include increased edema at the injection site; redness, burning, stinging, or pain; loss of or change in the blood return; or a slowing or change in the drip rate of the main line of normal saline.

Immediate action by trained personnel must be instituted for any suspicious or actual infiltration. Therefore, the nurse should possess a clear understanding of the institutional emergency procedures in this situation.

Whenever an extravasation is suspected, the antineoplastic agent should be discontinued immediately. The nurse or physician should attempt to draw back any residual drug present in the tubing or blood from the injection site. Based on the drug that was used, a specific antidote should be administered (see Table 75-4).

After the antidote is given, ice or warm compresses should be applied to the affected area for 24 hours to 48 hours. Close observation of the area is needed during the treatment. The nurse should monitor the area for any signs of increased redness, swelling, tenderness, dryness, or skin ulceration. A photograph and thorough descriptive documentation of the area, at the time of the extravasation and at subsequent intervals, will provide a helpful form of follow-up. If pain, erythema, enduration, or necrosis occurs, surgery may be needed to prevent muscle, tendon, or nerve damage in the area.

□ PROPER HANDLING OF ANTINEOPLASTIC AGENTS

Proper handling and disposal of antineoplastic agents should be practiced by all health-care pro-

Table 75-4
Known Antidotes for Sclerosing Agents

Sclerosing Agent	Antidote	Dose	Method of Administration	Additional Action
doxorubicin	hydrocortisone (100 mg/ml)	100 mg (not to exceed 100 mg)	Inject thru IV, if able and SC around site with multiple injections	Apply ice or cold compresses for 24h–48 h
daunorubicin	dexamethasone	2 mg–4 mg (not to exceed 4 mg)		May apply topical hydrocortisone 1% sparingly to affected area
	sodium bicarbonate 1 mEq/ml	1.0 mEq–3.0 mEq		
vinblastine vincristine etoposide	Hyaluronidase	150 U–900 U	Multiple SC injections around affected area	Apply *warm* compresses *Note:* Cooling or corticosteroids may worsen the toxicity.
nitrogen mustard	Thiosulfate	0.2 g–0.24 g	Inject thru IV and also SC around affected area with multiple injections	Apply ice or cold compresses to area for 24 h–48 h

(Adapted from Wolfe CA, Linkewich JA: Preparation of guidelines for the avoidance and treatment of extravasation due to antineoplastic agents. Hospital Pharm 22: 125, Feb 1987)

viders to decrease any environmental or personal hazards associated with these potentially toxic agents.

The nurse should become familiar with the institutional policies for handling the drugs. Currently, general recommendations include the following:

· Preparation of antineoplastic agents should be performed by trained personnel in a vertical flow hood. The preparer should wear protective clothing consisting of vinyl gloves, long-sleeved gown, and goggles unless a plastic shield is on the hood cabinet.

· Prior to the administration of any agent, correct drug, dose route, and expiration date should be verified.
· Vinyl gloves should always be worn while administering and discontinuing any antineoplastic agent. Because most of the agents discussed in this chapter are excreted in the urine, gloves should also be worn by the nurse when disposing any urine up to 48 hours after the completion of the therapy.
· Any unused drug or equipment used to prepare or administer the drug should be disposed in easily identified "hazardous waste" receptacles.

Antineoplastic Drugs

Antineoplastic agents may be classified in a variety of ways. The broadest classification and the one used for this discussion is based on mechanism of action and source of the drug. Thus, the antineoplastic drugs include the following:
    Alkylating agents
    Antimetabolites
    Natural products
    Hormones
    Miscellaneous agents

Alkylating Agents

Busulfan, Carmustine, Chlorambucil, Cisplatin, Cyclophosphamide, Dacarbazine, Lomustine, Mechlorethamine, Melphalan, Pipobroman, Streptozocin, Triethylenethiophosphoramide (Thiotepa), Uracil mustard

The alkylating agents used in chemotherapy may be divided into six different chemical groups as follows:
 1. Nitrogen mustards—chlorambucil, cyclophosphamide, mechlorethamine, melphalan, uracil mustard
 2. Ethylenimines—thiotepa
 3. Alkyl sulfonates—busulfan
 4. Triazenes—dacarbazine
 5. Nitrosoureas—carmustine, lomustine, streptozocin
 6. Miscellaneous alkylator-like agents—cisplatin, pipobroman

Although the alkylating agents represent a diverse group of chemical structures, each agent has the capacity to contribute alkyl groups to molecules such as DNA, which produces breaks and instability in the DNA molecule; they may also cross-link the twin strands of DNA thereby causing abnormal DNA replication and RNA transcription. A more detailed explanation follows.

MECHANISM AND ACTIONS

Alkylating agents are polyfunctional compounds that produce highly reactive carbonium ions that form covalent linkages with nucleophilic centers such as amino, carboxyl, hydroxyl, imidazole, phosphate, and sulfhydryl groups. The most important site of alkylation is the number 7 nitrogen in the purine base guanine. This may cause cross-linking of DNA strands and miscoding of the genetic message, resulting in abnormal base pairing. Destruction of the imidazole ring of guanine and actual breaking of DNA strands caused by depurination leads to inhibition of DNA replication, transcription of RNA and normal nucleic acid function. Cross-linking of DNA strands thus appears to be the major cytotoxic effect of the alkylating agents.

Nitrogen Mustards

Chlorambucil, mechlorethamine, melphalan, uracil mustard—Activity due to formation of unstable ethylenimmonium ion which alkylates with nucleic acids, causing cross-linking of DNA and RNA strands and inhibition of protein synthesis.

Cyclophosphamide—A metabolite, phosphoramide mustard, alkylates with nucleic acids with action similar to chlorambucil

Ethylenimines

Thiotepa—Same as chlorambucil above

Alkylsulfonates

Busulfan—Exact mechanism unknown; causes little cross-linking and main action is due to myelosuppression

Triazenes

Dacarbazine—Exact mechanism unknown; major activity is probably due to alkylation by an activated carbonium ion. Additional activity is due to antimetabolite activity as a purine precursor and interaction with sulfhydryl groups in proteins.

Nitrosoureas

Carmustine, lomustine—Exact mechanism of action is not known, but carmustine, lomustine, and their metabolites act by alkylating DNA and RNA and also by carbamylation of amino acids to inhibit some enzymes.

Streptozocin—Exact mechanism of action is unknown, but streptozocin undergoes spontaneous decomposition to produce reactive methylcarbonium ions which alkylate DNA causing cross-linking. Streptozocin has little effect on RNA and has weak activity compared to carmustine and lomustine.

Miscellaneous Alkylator-like Agents
Cisplatin—A heavy metal inorganic complex whose exact mechanism of action is unknown. Because of its neutral charge and *cis* configuration, cisplatin is able to enter cells by diffusion. Within the cell, the two chloride molecules of the platinum complex are displaced by water, resulting in a positively charged active complex which produces intrastrand and interstrand cross-links in DNA which inhibits DNA synthesis. An alternative mechanism of action may be the ability of cisplatin to alter neoplastic cells to enhance immunogenicity, making the neoplastic cells more susceptible to destruction by the body's normal immune mechanisms.

Pipobroman—Exact mechanism of action is unknown.

USES
See Table 75-5.

ADMINISTRATION AND DOSAGE
See Table 75-5.

FATE
See Table 75-6.

SIDE-EFFECTS/ADVERSE REACTIONS
The side-effects and adverse reactions of chemotherapeutic agents are for the most part unavoidable and are due to the pharmacologic action of the agents; the potential benefits should always outweigh the risks before such agents are used. The adverse reactions and side-effects most frequently seen are the result of damage to the most rapidly and actively dividing normal cells such as the hematopoietic system, cells of hair follicles, and cells lining the gastrointestinal tract and oral cavity. Some toxicities (leukopenia and thrombocytopenia) are actually used to measure a particular agent's effectiveness and also as a basis to calculate subsequent doses of the agent.

Because not all side-effects and adverse reactions are observed with all drugs, Table 75-7 indicates the common toxicities for the alkylating agents. For a complete list of side-effects and adverse reactions of each agent, refer to the manufacturer's product information.

CONTRAINDICATIONS AND PRECAUTIONS
All alkylating agents have been shown to be teratogenic, carcinogenic (due to a direct cellular action or immunosuppression), and to cause testicular and ovarian suppression. The exact effect of dose and duration of therapy is unknown, but the risk is increased by long-term therapy.

All alkylating agents are to be used with caution in patients with leukopenia, thrombocytopenia or anemia caused by previous chemotherapy or radiation therapy, hepatotoxicity, renal toxicity, and known hypersensitivity.
1. Busulfan is contraindicated in the "blastic" phase of chronic myelogenous leukemia.
2. There may be cross-hypersensitivity between chlorambucil and melphalan.
3. Cyclophosphamide tablets and uracil mustard capsules contain tartrazine which may cause allergic asthma-like reactions in some patients.
4. Pipobroman is not recommended for use in children under 15 years of age due to a lack of proof of clinical efficacy.

INTERACTIONS
1. The toxicity of chlorambucil and cyclophosphamide may be increased when used concurrently with barbiturates, chloral hydrate, or phenytoin due to induction of liver microsomal enzymes.
2. Cisplatin used concurrently with aminoglycosides may increase nephrotoxicity and ototoxicity.
3. Allopurinol and chloramphenicol may increase the toxicity of cyclophosphamide.
4. Corticosteroids may decrease the activity of cyclophosphamide due to inhibition of microsomal enzymes.
5. Cyclophosphamide and thiotepa may decrease serum pseudocholinesterase and therefore enhance the effect of succinylcholine.
6. Cyclophosphamide used concurrently with daunorubicin or doxorubicin may increase cardiotoxicity.
7. Dacarbazine may potentiate the activity of allopurinol by inhibiting xanthine oxidase.

(*Text continues on p. 1416.*)

Table 75-5
Alkylating Agents

Drug	Preparations	Usual Dosage Range
bulsulfan (Myleran)	Tablets—2 mg	Initially—4 mg–12 mg/day Maintenance—2 mg once or twice a week to 1 mg–4 mg/day Children—Induction: 0.06 mg–0.12 mg/kg/day or 1.8 mg–4.6 mg/m²/day
carmustine (BiCNU, BCNU)	Injection—100 mg/vial	75 mg–100 mg/m² by IV infusion over 1 h–2 h for 2 consecutive days or 200 mg/m² in a single dose no more frequently than every 6 weeks–8 weeks A suggested guide for subsequent dosage adjustment is the following:
chlorambucil (Leukeran)	Tablets—2 mg	Initially—0.1 mg–0.2 mg/kg/day for 3 weeks–6 weeks (4 mg–12 mg/day for the average patient) Maintenance—2 mg–6 mg/day, not to exceed 0.1 mg/kg/day; may be as low as 0.03 mg/kg/day Children—0.1 mg–0.2 mg/kg/day or 4.5 mg/m² day Nephrotic syndrome—0.1 mg–0.2 mg/kg/day for 8 weeks–12 weeks Macroglobulinemia—2 mg–10 mg/day or 8 mg/m²/day for 10 days repeated every 6 weeks–8 weeks
cisplatin (Platinol)	Injection—10 mg/vial, 50 mg/vial	As a single agent—100 mg/m² IV once every 4 weeks Testicular tumors—20 mg/m² IV for 5 days every 3 weeks for three courses in combination with · bleomycin—30 U IV on day 2 of each week for 12 doses + · vinblastine—0.15 mg–0.2 mg/kg IV on days 1 and 2 of each week every 3 weeks for four courses · Maintenance for patients who respond—vinblastine 0.2 mg/kg IV every 4 weeks for 2 years Ovarian tumors—50 mg/m² IV once very 3 weeks on day 1 in combination with · doxorubicin—50 mg/m² IV once every 3 weeks on day 1 A repeat dose should not be given until serum creatinine is below

Within the carmustine row:

Nadir After Prior Dose		% of Prior Dose to Be Given
Leukocytes	Platelets	
Above 4,000	Above 100,000	100
3,000–3,999	75,000–99,999	100
2,000–2,999	25,000–74,999	70
Below 2,000	Below 25,000	50

Uses	Clinical Considerations

Chronic myelogenous leukemia (DOC*)
Polycythemia vera

May increase uric acid levels in blood and urine; pulmonary fibrosis usually occurs with long-term therapy; onset after 8 months to 10 years (average 4 yr); treatment is usually unsatisfactory and death usually occurs within 6 months of diagnosis

Brain tumors (DOC)
Multiple myeloma (in combination with prednisone) (DOC)
Hodgkin's disease (in combination with other approved drugs in patients who relapse while on primary therapy or fail to respond to the primary therapy)
Non-Hodgkin's lymphomas (in combination with other drugs; see above)
Hepatic tumors by intra-arterial injection
May also be useful in Burkitt's tumor, Ewing's sarcoma, malignant melanoma, mycosis fungoides

Unopened vials of dry powder must be stored under refrigeration; oily film on bottom of the vial is sign of decomposition, and vial should be discarded. *Preparation of solutions:* Dissolve contents of vial with 3 ml absolute alcohol diluent and then add 27 ml of sterile water for injection. The resulting solution contains 3.3 mg/ml. Further dilution in 500 ml of dextrose 5% or sodium chloride 0.9% results in a solution stable for 48 h when refrigerated and protected from light. Contact with skin may cause transient hyperpigmentation; may increase bilirubin, alkaline phosphatase, SGOT, and BUN levels; a 0.1%–0.4% solution in 95% alcohol applied topically one to two times/day for 6 weeks–8 weeks has been used to treat mycosis fungoides. Pulmonary fibrosis and pneumonitis occur primarily with high cumulative dose (1200 mg–1400 mg/m^2) or long-term therapy (5 months) but may also occur with short-term, low-dose therapy.

Chronic lymphocytic leukemia (DOC)
Malignant lymphomas
Hodgkin's disease
Choriocarcinoma
Ovarian carcinoma
Breast carcinoma
Macroglobulinemia
Nephrotic syndrome

Give dose 1 h before breakfast or 2 h after evening meal; may increase serum and urine uric acid levels

Metastatic testicular tumors (DOC)
Metastatic ovarian tumors (DOC)
Lymphoma
Squamous cell carcinoma of head and neck
Advanced bladder carcinoma (DOC)
Cervical cancer (DOC)
Prostate carcinoma (DOC)
Non-small cell lung carcinoma

Unopened vials of dry powder must be stored under refrigeration. *Preparation of solution:* Dissolve contents of vial in 10 ml sterile water for injection. Solution is stable for 20 h at room temperature. Do *not* refrigerate. Hydrate patient with 1 L–2 L fluid infused over 8 h–12 h before treatment. Dilute drug in 1 L–2 L 5% dextrose in 0.3% or 0.45% saline containing 37.5 g mannitol, and infuse over 6 h–8 h. Maintain urinary output of 100 ml/h for 24 h after therapy to reduce danger of nephrotoxicity. Do not use needles, IV sets, or equipment containing aluminum to administer cisplatin; a black precipitate of platinum will form. May increase BUN, serum creatinine, SGOT, and serum uric acid levels
May decrease creatinine clearance and serum calcium, magnesium, and potassium levels. High frequency hearing loss may occur in one or both ears; more common in children

(continued)

Table 75-5 (continued)
Alkylating Agents

Drug	Preparations	Usual Dosage Range
cisplatin (Platinol) (continued)		1.5 mg/100 ml or BUN is below 25 mg/100 ml, platelets are over 100,000/mm^3, and WBCs are over 4000/mm^3
		Advanced bladder carcinoma—50 mg–70 mg/m^2 IV once every 3 weeks–4 weeks; patients receiving prior radiation or chemotherapy should start at 50 mg/m^2 IV once every 4 weeks
		Non-small cell lung carcinoma—75 mg–120 mg/m^2 IV once every 3 weeks–6 weeks
		Renal impairment—
		Creatinine clearance 10 ml–50 ml/min · 75% of usual dose
		Creatinine clearance < 10 ml/min · 50% of usual dose
cyclophosphamide (Cytoxan, Neosar)	Tablets—25 mg, 50 mg Powder for injection—100 mg/vial, 200 mg/vial, 500 mg/vial, 1 g/vial, 2 g/vial Lyophilized injection—500 mg/vial, 1 g/vial 2 g/vial	*Oral:* Adult—1 mg–5 mg/kg/day Children—induction: 2 mg–8 mg/kg or 60 mg–250 mg/m^2 for 6 or more days Maintenance—2 mg–5 mg/kg or 50 mg–150 mg/m^2 twice a week Immunosuppressant, nephrotic syndrome—2 mg–2.5 mg/kg/day Rheumatoid arthritis—1.5 mg–3 mg/kg/day *IV:* Adult—induction: 40 mg–50 mg/kg in divided doses over 2 days–5 days Maintenance—10 mg–15 mg/kg every 7 days–10 days or 3 mg–5 mg/kg twice a week or 1.5 mg–3 mg/kg daily Children—induction: 2 mg–8 mg/kg or 60 mg–250 mg/m^2 in divided doses for 6 or more days Maintenance—10 mg–15 mg/kg every 7 days–10 days or 30 mg/kg every 3 weeks–4 weeks Reduce induction dose by ⅓ to ½ in patients with bone marrow depression Hepatic impairment—bilirubin 3.1 mg%–5.0 mg% or SGOT > 180, reduce dose by 25%, bilirubin > 5.0 mg%, omit dose Renal impairment—glomerular filtration rate < 10 ml/min, decrease dose by 50%
dacarbazine (DTIC-Dome)	Injection—100 mg/vial, 200 mg/vial	IV—2 mg–4.5 mg/kg/day for 10 days, repeated every 28 days or 250 mg/m^2/day for 5 days, repeated every 21 days

Uses	Clinical Considerations

Hodgkin's disease
Non-Hodgkin's lymphomas (DOC)
Follicular lymphomas
Lymphocytic lymphosarcoma
Reticulum cell sarcoma
Lymphoblastic lymphosarcoma
Burkitt's lymphoma (DOC)
Multiple myeloma (DOC)
Leukemias:
   Chronic lymphocytic leukemia
   Chronic granulocytic leukemia
   Acute myelogenous and monocytic leukemia
   Acute lymphoblastic leukemia
Mycosis fungoides
Neuroblastoma (DOC)
Adenocarcinoma of ovary (DOC)
Retinoblastoma (DOC)
Carcinoma of breast or lung (DOC)
Ewing's sarcoma (DOC)
Other uses: Immunosuppressant to prevent transplant rejection, rheumatoid arthritis, nephrotic syndrome, systemic lupus erythematosus

Preparation of solution: Reconstitute powder with sterile water for injection or bacteriostatic water for injection (paraben preserved only). Use 5 ml for the 100-mg vial, 10 ml for the 200-mg vial, 25 ml for the 500-mg vial, 50 ml for 1-g vial, and 100 ml for 2-g vial. Reconstitute the lyophilized injection with the same diluents as above as follows: use 20 ml–25 ml for the 500-mg vial, 40 ml–50 ml for the 1-g vial, 80 ml–100 ml for the 2-g vial. Solution is stable for 24 h at room temperature or 6 days refrigerated. Solution may be given IM, IV push, intraperitoneally, intrapleurally, or by IV infusion in 5% dextrose in 0.9% saline, or 0.9% saline. May suppress positive reactions to skin tests. May increase uric acid levels of urine and serum. May produce false-positive PAP test. Secondary malignancies have been observed, most frequently of the urinary bladder. May cause syndrome of inappropriate antidiuretic hormone secretion (SIADH) manifested as tiredness, weakness, confusion, agitation. An oral solution may be prepared by dissolving the powder for injection in aromatic elixir to a concentration of 1 mg–5 mg/ml; refrigerate and use within 14 days; tablets contain tartrazine

Metastatic malignant melanoma (DOC)
Hodgkin's disease
Investigational uses:
   Soft-tissue sarcomas
   Neuroblastoma

Preparation of solution: add 9.9 ml sterile water for injection to 100-mg vial or 19.7 ml sterile water for injection to 200-mg vial giving a concentration of 10 mg/ml; solution colorless or clear yellow, is stable 8 h at room temperature or 72 h refrigerated, protected from light; a change in color to pink indicates decomposition; may be given by IV push

(continued)

Table 75-5 (continued)
Alkylating Agents

Drug	Preparations	Usual Dosage Range
lomustine (CCNU, CeeNU)	Capsules—10 mg, 40 mg, 100 mg	*Oral:* Adults and children—100 mg–130 mg/m² as a single dose, repeated every 6 weeks A suggested guide for subsequent dosage adjustment is the following:

Nadir After Prior Dose		% of Prior Dose to Be Given
Leukocytes	*Platelets*	
Above 4,000	Above 100,000	100
3,000– 3,999	75,000– 99,999	75–100
2,000– 2,999	25,000– 74,999	50–75
Below 2,000	Below 25,000	0–50

Drug	Preparations	Usual Dosage Range
mechlorethamine (Mustargen, nitrogen mustard)	Injection—10 mg/vial	IV—0.4 mg/kg as a single dose or in divided doses of 0.1 mg–0.2 mg/kg/day; repeat every 3 weeks–6 weeks Intracavitary—0.4 mg/kg diluted in 50 ml–100 ml 0.9% saline; 0.2 mg/kg may be used intrapericardially Ointment and solution—Apply once a day (four times/day in severe cases) to entire skin surface for 6 months–12 months until response occurs, then every 2 days–7 days for 3 years
melphalan (Alkeran, PAM, L-PAM, phenylalanine mustard, L-Sarcolysin)	Tablets—2 mg	0.15 mg/kg/day for 7 days followed by a rest period of 2 weeks–6 weeks then 0.05 mg/kg/day maintenance or 0.1 mg–0.15 mg/kg/day for 2 weeks–3 weeks or 0.25 mg/kg/day for 4 days followed by a rest period of 2 weeks–4 weeks, then 2 mg–4 mg a day maintenance or 0.2 mg/kg/day for 5 days followed by a rest period of 4 weeks–5 weeks (for ovarian carcinoma) or

Uses	Clinical Considerations
Polycythemia vera Chronic myelocytic leukemia	May increase uric acid levels in blood and urine; may increase serum potassium Not recommended for children under 15 years of age

Metastatic islet cell carcinoma of the pancreas (DOC)
Investigational uses:
   Malignant carcinoid tumors
   Advanced Hodgkin's disease
   Colorectal cancer
	Dry powder must be refrigerated and protected from light. *Preparation of solution:* reconstitute with 9.5 ml or 5% dextrose in water or 0.9% sodium chloride; solution is stable for 12 h at room temperature, according to manufacturer, however, studies show solution is stable 48 h at room temperature and 96 h refrigerated; solution is preservative-free and should not be used for more than one dose; a change in color from pale gold to brown indicates decomposition; adequate patient hydration may reduce renal toxicity; hypophosphatemia may be first sign of renal toxicity

Superficial papillary carcinoma of the urinary bladder (DOC) Adenocarcinoma of the breast and ovary Intracavitary injection to control malignant effusions Lymphomas Bronchogenic carcinoma Investigational use: To prevent pterygium recurrence, malignant meningeal neoplasms	Dry powder must be refrigerated. *Preparation of solution:* reconstitute with 1.5 ml sterile water for injection; solution should be clear to slightly opaque; if grossly opaque, discard; solution is stable 5 days under refrigeration; compatible with procaine 2% and epinephrine HCl 1:1000 for local injection; dehydrate patients 8 h–12 h before bladder instillation; may increase uric acid levels in blood and urine; has been used IM, although not approved by the FDA
Chronic lymphocytic leukemia Non-Hodgkin's lymphomas Chronic myelocytic leukemia Polycythemia vera (early stage) Mycosis fungoides	May increase uric acid levels in blood and urine Total dosage of 1 mg/kg greatly increases the risk of irreversible bone marrow depression. Capsules contain tartrazine.

Table 75-6
Fate of Alkylating Agents

Drug	Absorption/Distribution/ Half-Life	Metabolism	Excretion
busulfan	Well absorbed from GI tract Half-life—2 h–3 h	Hepatic and plasma to at least 12 metabolites including methanesulfonic acid	Renal, slow, as metabolites
carmustine	Well distributed; crosses blood–brain barrier with good concentration in cerebrospinal fluid Half-life of intact drug—5 min; biologic effect, 15 min–30 min; metabolites remain in plasma 3 days–4 days due to enterohepatic circulation	Hepatic to active metabolites	Renal—30% in 24 h, 60%–70% in 96 h Feces—≤1% Respiratory—6%
chlorambucil	Rapidly and completely absorbed from GI tract Highly protein bound; not known if it crosses blood-brain barrier; does cross placental barrier Half-life—1.5 h active drug; 2.5 h for amino-phenylacetic acid metabolite	Hepatic to active metabolite amino-phenylacetic acid	Renal—primarily as metabolites; probably not dialyzable
cisplatin	Highly protein bound with wide distribution; does not readily cross blood–brain barrier Half-life—biphasic Initial—25 min–50 min Terminal—58 h–96 h	Intracellular to inactive metabolites	Renal—27%–45% over 3 days–5 days; may be dialyzed only within 3 h after administration
cyclophosphamide	Well absorbed from GI tract Active drug has low protein-binding; active metabolites exhibit 50% protein binding Well distributed throughout body and crosses blood–brain barrier in low concentrations Half-life Adults—1.8 h–12.4 h (average 6.5 h) Children—2.4 h–6.5 h (average 4.1 h)	Hepatic by microsomal enzymes to active and inactive metabolites	Renal—≤25% as unchanged drug, balance as metabolites; may be dialyzed.
dacarbazine	Crosses blood–brain barrier to a limited extent Protein binding very low (≤5%)	Hepatic by microsomal enzymes to active and inactive metabolites	Renal by tubular secretion —40% of a dose excreted in 6 h, 50% unchanged

(continued)

Table 75-6 (continued)
Fate of Alkylating Agents

Drug	Absorption/Distribution/Half-Life	Metabolism	Excretion
	Half-life—biphasic Initial—19 min Terminal—5 h		
lomustine	Rapidly and completely absorbed from GI tract Well distributed; crosses blood–brain barrier with good concentrations in cerebrospinal fluid Half-life— Intact drug = 15 min Biologic effect = 94 min Metabolites have biphasic half-life Initial—4 h–5 h Terminal—30 h–50 h	Hepatic to active cyclohexyl, carbenyl, and chloroethyl metabolites	Renal—60% as metabolites after 48 h Feces—≤5% Respiratory—10%
mechlorethamine	Distributes to water and body fluids Half-life—15 min	Plasma—rapidly hydrolyzed to active ions	Renal—50% as inactive metabolites in 24 h
melphalan	Absorption from GI tract is erratic and incomplete Rapidly distributed throughout body water Protein binding initially 50%–60% increasing to 80%–90% in 4 h–12 h Half-life—90 min	Hydrolyzed in plasma and body fluids to monohydroxy and dihydroxy metabolites	Renal—20%–35% as unchanged drug and metabolites in 24 h Feces—20%–50%
pipobroman	Well absorbed from the GI tract	Unknown	Unknown
streptozocin	Rapidly cleared from plasma and concentrated in liver, kidney, intestine, and pancreas Metabolites readily cross blood–brain barrier within 2 h Half-life: Initial—6 min Intermediate—3.5 h (as metabolite) Terminal—40 h (as metabolite)	Hepatic and renal to active metabolites whose structures have not been determined	Renal—10% unchanged drug, 60%–70% metabolites in 24 h Respiratory—5% Feces—≤1%
triethylenethiophosphoramide	Variable absorption following local administration to bladder, or pleura, and after IM injection Rapidly cleared from plasma Half-life—7 days	Hepatic	Renal—60%–85% in 24 h–72 h as metabolites
uracil mustard	No data available on absorption in humans	Probably hepatic	Renal

Table 75-7
Side-Effects/Adverse Reactions of Alkylating Agents

Drug	Alopecia/Dermatologic	Gastrointestinal	Hepatic
busulfan	Hyperpigmentation of intertriginous areas	Some nausea and vomiting Diarrhea	
carmustine	Vesicant, some alopecia	Severe nausea and vomiting occur within minutes and may last 6 h	Mild and reversible
chlorambucil	Rash, alopecia rare		Rare
cisplatin		Severe nausea and vomiting within 1 h–4 h and may last 24 h	
cyclophosphamide	alopecia—frequently	Severe nausea and vomiting with high IV dose therapy	Rare
dacarbazine	Extravasation will cause tissue necrosis Alopecia—rare	Severe nausea and vomiting lasting 1 h–12 h Stomatitis—rare	Hepatic vein thrombosis and hepatocellular necrosis are rare
lomustine	Alopecia—rare Hyperpigmentation	Stomatitis Severe nausea and vomiting within 3 h–6 h and may last 24 h	Rare
mechlorethamine	Vesicant, alopecia	Severe nausea and vomiting within 1 h–3 h; vomiting lasts up to 8 h and nausea up to 24 h	Rare

Myelosuppression	Neurologic	Renal	Other
Leukopenia, thrombocytopenia Nadir 10 days–30 days Recovery 1 month to 2 years			Pulmonary interstitial fibrosis
Leukopenia Nadir 35 days–40 days Thrombocytopenia Nadir 28 days–35 days Recovery 6 weeks–12 weeks		Decreased kidney size, progressive azotemia, renal failure	Pulmonary fibrosis
Leukopenia, thrombocytopenia Nadir 7 days–28 days Recovery 14 days–28 days	Seizures in children being treated for nephrotic syndrome		Rare pulmonary fibrosis
Leukopenia, thrombocytopenia Nadir 18 days–23 days Recovery 21 days–39 days	Peripheral neuropathy may occur after a single dose or prolonged therapy	Tubular necrosis	Ototoxicity in high frequency range (more severe in children) Hypomagnesemia and hypocalcemia may develop during or following therapy Anaphylactoid reactions usually following four to five previous doses of drug
Leukopenia Nadir 7 days–12 days Recovery 17 days–21 days		Hemorrhagic cystitis	Pulmonary fibrosis following high dose prolonged therapy. Cardiac toxicity (high dose therapy has caused hemorrhagic myocardial necrosis and acute myopericarditis)
Leukopenia Nadir 21 days–25 days Recovery 24 days–29 days Thrombocytopenia Nadir 16 days Recovery 19 days–24 days			Influenza-like syndrome begins 7 days after therapy and lasts 1 week–3 weeks and may occur with each course of therapy. Anaphylactoid reaction
Leukopenia Nadir 28 days–42 days Recovery 42 days–49 days Thrombocytopenia Nadir 28 days Recovery 35 days–42 days		Decreased kidney size, progressive azotemia, renal failure	Pulmonary fibrosis or pneumonitis rare after long-term and high cumulative dose
Leukopenia Nadir 6 days–8 days Recovery 20–22 days Thrombocytopenia Nadir 10 days–16 days Recovery 24 days–30 days	Neurotoxicity has occurred with high dose intra-arterial or regional perfusion therapy		Allergic reaction rare

(continued)

Table 75-7 (continued)
Side-Effects/Adverse Reactions of Alkylating Agents

Drug	Alopecia/Dermatologic	Gastrointestinal	Hepatic
melphalan		Mild nausea and vomiting after high doses	
pipobroman	Rash—transient	Mild nausea and vomiting	
streptozocin	Tissue necrosis may occur following extravasation	Severe nausea and vomiting within 1 h–4 h and lasting 24 h; antiemetics have little effect; diarrhea	Rare
triethylenethio-phosphoramide		Mild to moderate nausea and vomiting are infrequent; stomatitis	
uracil mustard	Some alopecia	Nausea, vomiting, and diarrhea; severity dose related	Rare

8. The metabolism of dacarbazine may be enhanced by phenobarbital and phenytoin due to induction of liver microsomal enzymes.
9. Most alkylating agents may antagonize the effects of antigout medications (probenecid, sulfinpyrazone) by increasing serum uric acid levels; dosage adjustment of the antigout medications may be necessary.
10. Alkylating agents cause immunosuppression, which may result in a patient developing a viral disease following immunization with a live virus vaccine.
11. Corticosteroids used concurrently with streptozocin may increase the hyperglycemic effect of streptozocin.
12. Streptozocin should not be used concurrently with nephrotoxic medications such as aminoglycoside antibiotics, cephalothin, cisplatin, or polymyxins.
13. Phenytoin may protect pancreatic beta cells from the cytotoxic effects of streptozocin, thus reducing its therapeutic effect in patients with islet cell tumors.
14. Carmustine used concurrently with cimetidine may cause increased myelosuppression.
15. Chlorambucil used concurrently with immunosuppressants such as corticosteroids, azathioprine, cyclophosphamide, cyclosporine, or mercaptopurine may increase the risk of infection and development of secondary neoplasms.

■ Nursing Process for Alkylating Agents

□ **ASSESSMENT**

□ *Subjective Data*
Eliciting a thorough medication history is essential during the assessment process. Particular attention should be focused on the following drugs:

Myelosuppression	Neurologic	Renal	Other
Leukopenia, thrombocytopenia Nadir 10 days–21 days Recovery 35 days–42 days or longer			Pulmonary fibrosis rare; anaphylactic reaction
Leukopenia, thrombocytopenia Nadir 28 days Recovery rapid after discontinuation of drug			
Mild leukopenia and thrombocytopenia Nadir 7 days–14 days Recovery 21 days		Tubular necrosis	
Leukopenia, thrombocytopenia Nadir 10 days–14 days and up to 30 days Recovery 28 days			
Leukopenia, thrombocytopenia Maximum depression may not occur until 2 weeks–4 weeks after cessation of therapy. As dose (cumulative) approaches 1 mg/kg, irreversible bone marrow suppression may occur.			

1. Aminoglycosides and cephalosporins—Concurrent use of these agents with cisplatin and streptozocin increase the risk of drug-induced nephrotoxicity.
2. Vitamin A, barbiturates, steroids, and allopurinol—Concurrent use of these agents with cyclophosphamide increases the incidence of adverse side-effects.
3. Daunorubicin and doxorubicin—Concurrent use with cyclophosphamide increases the cardiotoxicity of these agents.
4. Busulfan and carmustine—The pulmonary toxicity associated with these drugs increases significantly with increased doses or following prolonged therapy.

The identification of risk factors assists the nurse in identifying individuals who may experience an increased incidence of the following adverse side-effects:

Carmustine, lomustine, busulfan—Pulmonary toxicity

· Previous thoracic radiation treatments
· Pre-existing lung disease
· Tobacco use
· Industrial exposure

Cisplatin, streptozocin—Nephrotoxicity
· Pre-existing renal disease
· Age ≥ 70 years and unable to maintain adequate hydration

During each contact with the patient, the nurse should assess the patient's level of understanding regarding the treatment schedule and provide written instructions if necessary.

The nausea and vomiting associated with cisplatin, dacarbazine, streptozocin, and nitrogen mustard are severe and may affect patient compliance. Therefore, it is essential to institute aggressive antiemetic therapy and to continually evaluate patient response to this therapy. The degree of nausea and vomiting experienced and the length of time these symptoms persist should be noted throughout the course of treatment.

□ **Objective Data**
1. Physical Assessment—A *complete* physical assessment is necessary prior to initiation of chemotherapy. This section, however, will highlight the essential systems to be reviewed and the associated toxicities of drug therapy.

   Pulmonary—carmustine, lomustine, busulfan, cyclophosphamide

   Hepatic—carmustine, dacarbazine, lomustine, streptozocin

   Renal—carmustine, cisplatin, streptozocin

   Genitourinary—cyclophosphamide

   Neurologic—cisplatin

   Hematopoietic—All drugs

2. Laboratory Data and Diagnostic Tests
   · Pulmonary function tests (PFTs)—busulfan
   · 24-hour creatinine clearance—cisplatin, streptozocin
   · Audiogram—cisplatin, nitrogen mustard
   · Calcium levels—cisplatin, streptozocin

□ **NURSING DIAGNOSIS**

Actual nursing diagnoses for the patient receiving alkylating agents include:

   Knowledge deficit with regard to chemotherapy side-effects

Potential nursing diagnoses include:

   Anxiety

   Fluid volume deficit related to nausea and vomiting

   Impaired gas exchange

   Sensory-perceptual alterations

   Alteration in nutrition: less than body requirement

   Altered sexuality patterns

   Disturbance in body image/self-control

   Potential for infection

□ **PLAN**

The nursing care plan is directed toward minimizing the side-effects of chemotherapy and promoting self-care behavior so the patient can identify early signs and symptoms of toxicities and can implement appropriate interventions.

□ **INTERVENTION**

The appropriate route of administration and drug dosages have been discussed in the previous pharmacology section. Therefore, this section will discuss nursing considerations during administration of specific agents

1. Carmustine is administered by the intravenous route. The dose should be diluted in 100 ml to 250 ml of D5/W or normal saline solution and infused over a period of ½ hour to 2 hours. Infusion must be completed within 2 hours because the drug tends to decompose after 2 hours. Rapid administration of the drug may cause pain at the IV site and intense flushing of the skin and conjunctiva. This side-effect may occur up to 2 hours after administration of the drug and last for 4 hours. If this occurs during the infusion, the rate of infusion should be slowed and the patient should be reassured that this is an expected side-effect of the drug.

2. Although cisplatin is administered as an intravenous infusion, the rate of infusion varies according to the proposed protocol. The most common protocol infusion times include 15-minute to 30-minute infusion, 6-hour to 8-hour infusion or 24-hour infusion.

   During the administration of cisplatin, an aluminum needle should not be used because this could induce precipitation and thus inactivation of the drug.

   A major consideration in preparing the patient for administration of cisplatin is adequate hydration. The amount and duration of pretreatment hydration will be determined by the dose of cisplatin to be administered. In addition, aggressive diuresis may be indicated with furosemide or mannitol to maintain an adequate urine output during the cisplatin treatment.

3. Cyclophosphamide may be administered by either the oral or IV route. Cyclophosphamide should be administered in the morning to prevent the development of hemorrhagic cystitis. Oral hydration (2 L–3 L per day) is important during treatment with cyclophosphamide especially if the patient receives a dose greater than 500 mg. If the patient is unable to take fluids by mouth, IV hydration is indicated with doses above 500 mg.

4. Dacarbazine and streptozocin are administered as IV infusions over 15 minutes to 1 hour. Burning may occur at the site during infusion. To reduce the intensity of burning, the rate of infusion should be decreased or ice packs should be used above the infusion site. Caution must be exercised during administration of dacarbazine because it is classified as a vesicant. Extravasation of this drug could result in tissue damage. If infiltration is suspected, the infusion should be stopped immediately and agency guidelines for extravasation instituted. See under Extravasation.

5. Lomustine is administered as an oral agent. It

should be given on an empty stomach, preferably prior to bedtime. Premedication with antiemetics is essential.

6. Mechlorethamine is administered as an IV bolus over 2 minutes to 3 minutes. Care should be exercised during administration because it is a vesicant drug and extravasation results in severe tissue necrosis. Thrombophlebitis may occur with the infusion.

7. Thiotepa may be administered IV, IM, or as an intracavitary instillation. It is usually given rapidly by the IV route, either as an IV bolus or infusion. It may be instilled in the bladder. The patient is given nothing by mouth for 8 hours to 12 hours prior to instillation. The drug is diluted in 30 ml to 60 ml of sterile water and instilled by means of a catheter. The patient should be instructed not to void for at least 2 hours after instillation and to change position every 15 minutes for 1 hour to distribute the drug throughout the bladder.

The administration of alkylating agents results in three major types of side-effects: nausea and vomiting, bone marrow depression, and impaired fertility. The nursing management of these side-effects is discussed under Nursing Process for Antineoplastic Drugs. Alkylating agents can also cause multiple other side-effects (see Table 75-7). The following section will highlight the side-effects of these drugs and the necessary patient education.

1. *Pulmonary fibrosis* is associated with busulfan, carmustine, lomustine, and cyclophosphamide. The nurse should be alert for the development of dyspnea, rales, and nonproductive cough. The onset of these symptoms is often insidious, developing over several weeks to months. This side-effect may be reversible if detected at an early stage and with the prompt initiation of steroid treatment. Therefore, ongoing pulmonary assessment is a critical nursing intervention; educating patients to report pulmonary symptoms promptly is vital.

2. *Nephrotoxicity* is associated with cisplatin, streptozocin, and carmustine. The nephrotoxicity resulting from cisplatin can be a dose-limiting side-effect. However, the advent of aggressive hydration and diuresis during treatment has significantly decreased this side-effect. The nurse must carefully assess the patient's renal status prior to administering the drug. Attention to fluid balance and urine output is critical. Intake and output should be checked every hour, and urine output must be between 100 ml and 150 ml/h prior to administering the drug. Urine output must be assessed every hour and maintained at 100 ml/h after cisplatin administration for 4 hours to 12 hours depending on the dosage. The intake and output should be monitored continually for 24 hours after the administration, and the intake must remain greater than the output. The physician should be notified immediately if the urine output becomes less than 100 ml/h or if the patient exhibits negative fluid balance. With streptozocin, the patient's intake and output should be monitored during the treatment period. Oral hydration should be encouraged during and for at least 24 hours after treatment. In addition, the urine should be monitored daily for protein and glucose.

3. *Hemorrhagic cystitis* may result from cyclophosphamide metabolites in the urine. It is usually a cumulative, dose-related phenomenon and may be severe. It may develop during any time of cyclophosphamide use as well as after it is discontinued. It is essential to provide patient education regarding prevention of this complication. Adequate fluid intake is critical. Patients should drink 2 L to 3 L of fluid the day of treatment and the day after treatment. If unable to tolerate fluids by mouth especially with high IV doses ($\geq 1.5 \ g/m^2$), they should receive 2 L to 3 L of IV hydration. If patients are hospitalized and receive high IV doses, they should be on intake and output for 48 hours after cyclophosphamide. Attention to urine output should be noted because the development of *inappropriate ADH secretion* may occur, which is manifested by the retention of water and decreased serum sodium. The use of IV diuretics may be indicated. In addition, the urine should be checked for occult blood. It is strongly suggested to administer cyclophosphamide early in the day rather than in the evening because frequent emptying of the bladder is important. Patients should be encouraged to void every 2 hours during the day and empty the bladder before retiring for bed. Instruction in the signs and symptoms of hemorrhagic cystitis, which include painful urination and bloody urine, will allow patients to report these symptoms promptly to healthcare providers. If cystitis occurs, therapy should be discontinued immediately.

4. *Nasal stuffiness, congestion,* and *sneezing* may occur with the rapid IV infusion of cyclophosphamide. Decreasing the rate of infusion will help reduce these side-effects. The patient

should be reassured that these are expected side-effects.

5. *Flu-like syndrome* may occur with dacarbazine. It usually occurs 7 days to 10 days after treatment and may persist for several weeks. Patients should be informed of this side-effect, and appropriate symptom management should be implemented after evaluation.

6. *Metabolic disturbances* have been noted with streptozocin and cisplatin.
   · Streptozocin—Hypoglycemia may result during the first 24 hours of treatment with higher doses. However, with longer therapy, glucose intolerance has been noted together with increased serum glucose levels. Patients should be instructed about the signs and symptoms of hypoglycemia/hyperglycemia. They should wear a Medic-Alert bracelet describing their condition.
   · Cisplatin—Electrolyte imbalances tend to occur with cisplatin. Hypomagnesemia is the most common and can lead to tetany. In addition, decreases in calcium, potassium, and phosphorus may also occur. Replacement of these electrolytes is often necessary.

7. *Neurotoxicity* appears to be a dose-limiting side-effect of cisplatin because the nephrotoxicity usually can be controlled with adequate hydration and diuresis. Neurotoxicity tends to occur with cumulative doses of 775 mg/m^2. The concurrent use of neurotoxic drugs such as vincristine may increase the incidence of neurotoxicity. Common manifestations are peripheral neuropathies in the upper and lower extremities, lower extremity weakness, and loss of taste. Seizures may also be seen. This is usually a transient situation and does not require antiepileptic medication. Patients should be instructed to report immediately numbness and tingling in fingers and toes.

8. *Ototoxicity* occurs frequently in patients receiving cisplatin and also appears to be a cumulative effect. Tinnitus, loss of high-frequency hearing, and vestibular toxicity have been reported. Auditory changes may be transient; however, in some cases they may be permanent. Patients should be instructed to report auditory changes such as ringing in the ears or decreased hearing acuity. Hearing loss has also been noted with high doses of mechlorethamine.

9. *Anaphylaxis* has occurred during administration of cisplatin. The physician should be notified immediately. Prompt discontinuation of the infusion and the administration of epinephrine, hydrocortisone, and diphenhydramine are necessary.

□ *EVALUATION*

Outcome criteria to measure treatment effectiveness include:

1. Patient will report adverse side-effects promptly to health-care providers.
2. Patient will maintain adequate hydration during treatment and for 24 hours after treatment.
3. Patient will report adequate control of nausea and vomiting through the use of appropriate antiemetic treatment.
4. Patient will identify appropriate/effective methods for contraception during and for 2 years after chemotherapy.

Antimetabolites

Cytarabine, Floxuridine, Fluorouracil, Mercaptopurine, Methotrexate, Thioguanine

The antimetabolites are structural analogues of normally occurring metabolites which interfere with the synthesis of nucleic acids by competing with purines and pyrimidines in metabolic pathways. The antimetabolites themselves may also be incorporated into nucleic acids, resulting in a cell product that fails to function. Antimetabolites act during the S phase of the cell cycle. They can be divided into three groups: folic acid antagonists (methotrexate); purine antagonists (mercaptopurine, thioguanine); and pyrimidine antagonists (floxuridine, fluorouracil, cytarabine).

MECHANISM AND ACTIONS

1. Folic acid antagonists—Methotrexate binds to the enzyme dihydrofolate reductase, the enzyme necessary to reduce folic acid to tetrahydrofolic acid, thus limiting the availability of one-carbon fragments necessary for purine and thymidine synthesis. This relatively irreversible binding thus inhibits DNA, RNA and protein synthesis, and subsequent cell replication.
2. Purine antagonists—Mercaptopurine and thioguanine compete with hypoxanthine and guanine, due to their similarity of structure, for the enzyme hypoxanthine-guanine phosphoribosyl transferase, and are converted to

the active nucleotide forms thioinosinic acid and 6-thioguanylic acid, respectively. These nucleotides then act by a variety of mechanisms to inhibit purine biosynthesis, DNA and RNA synthesis, chromosomal replication, and protein synthesis thereby causing their cytotoxic effect.

3. Pyrimidine antagonists—Floxuridine and fluorouracil inhibit the enzyme thymidylate synthetase which is necessary for the formation of thymidine, a substrate necessary for the synthesis of DNA. Floxuridine, after conversion to fluorouracil, and fluorouracil may also act by two additional mechanisms; fluorouracil may be incorporated, in small amounts, into RNA, thereby producing fraudulent RNA; and fluorouracil inhibits the utilization of uracil in RNA synthesis by blocking uracil phosphorylase.

Cytarabine is metabolized by deoxycytidine kinase to the nucleotide cytarabine triphosphate (ara-CTP), an inhibitor of DNA polymerase, an enzyme necessary for the synthesis of DNA.

USES
See Table 75-8.

ADMINISTRATION AND DOSAGE
See Table 75-8.

FATE
See Table 75-9.

SIDE-EFFECTS/ADVERSE REACTIONS
(See under Side-Effects/Adverse Reactions for alkylating agents.)

Table 75-10 indicates the common toxicities of the antimetabolites. For a complete list of all side-effects and adverse reactions on each agent, see the manufacturer's product information.

CONTRAINDICATIONS AND PRECAUTIONS
All antineoplastic agents have the potential to be carcinogenic (due to a direct cellular action or immunosuppression) and to cause testicular and ovarian suppression. The exact effect of dose and duration of therapy is unknown; however, the risk is increased by long-term therapy.

All antimetabolites are to be used with caution in patients with leukopenia, thrombocytopenia or anemia caused by previous chemotherapy or radiation therapy, hepatotoxicity, renal toxicity, and known hypersensitivity.

1. Cytarabine and mercaptopurine may cause chromosome abnormalities in humans.
2. Floxuridine is mutagenic in animals.
3. There is usually complete cross-resistance between mecaptopurine and thioguanine.
4. Methotrexate is excreted in breast milk.

INTERACTIONS
1. Cytarabine and methotrexate used concurrently can have either a synergistic or antagonistic effect.
2. Fluorouracil is incompatible with cytarabine, diazepam, doxorubicin, and methotrexate. Complete flushing of IV line between injections is recommended.
3. The absorption of fluorouracil when given orally is decreased by the presence of food.
4. Concomitant administration of mercaptopurine and allopurinol increases both the antineoplastic and toxic effects of mercaptopurine. The dosage of mercaptopurine should be reduced to one third to one fourth the usual dosage.
5. Alcohol may enhance the possibility of methotrexate-induced hepatotoxicity.
6. Chloramphenicol, phenylbutazone, phenytoin, para-aminobenzoic acid, salicylates, sulfonamides, and tetracyclines can displace methotrexate from binding sites and cause increased toxicity.
7. Probenecid and salicylates can block the tubular secretion of methotrexate and thus increase its toxicity.
8. Pyrimethamine used concurrently with methotrexate can cause increased toxicity because of similar folic acid antagonist actions.
9. Methotrexate may enhance the hypoprothrombinemic effect of oral anticoagulants such as warfarin.
10. Concurrent use of methotrexate and asparaginase may block the antineoplastic action of methotrexate by inhibiting cell synthesis. Asparaginase should be administered 9 days to 10 days before or within 24 hours after administering methotrexate; the toxic effect of methotrexate may also be reduced.
11. Vitamin preparations containing folic acid may decrease the effect of methotrexate.
12. Most antimetabolite agents may antagonize the effects of antigout medications (probenecid, sulfinpyrazone) by increasing serum uric acid levels; dosage adjustments of the antigout medications may be necessary.
13. Antimetabolite agents cause immunosuppres-

(Text continues on p. 1428.)

Table 75-8
Antimetabolites

Drug	Preparations	Usual Dosage Range
cytarabine (cytosine arabinoside, ARA-C, Cytosar-U)	Injection—100-mg vial, 500-mg vial	Induction—*IV infusion:* 100 mg–200 mg/m²/day or 3 mg/kg/day as a continuous IV infusion over 24 hours (or in divided doses by rapid IV injection) for 5 days–10 days and repeated approximately every 2 weeks Maintenance—*IM, SC:* 1 mg–1.5 mg/kg once or twice a week at 1-week to 4-week intervals or 70 mg–100 mg/m²/day by rapid IV injection in divided doses or continuous IV infusion for 2 days–5 days repeated every 30 days Investigational use for refractory acute myelogenous leukemia—3 g/m² IV infusion over 1 h–2 h every 12 h for four to twelve doses Combination therapy 1. cytarabine and doxorubicin: cytarabine, 100 mg/m²/day continuous IV infusion on days 1 and 10 doxorubicin, 30 mg/m²/day IV infusion over 30 min on days 1 and 3 2. cytarabine, daunorubicin, and thioguanine: cytarabine, 100 mg/m²/day IV infusion over 30 min every 12 h days 1–7 daunorubicin, 60 mg/m²/day IV infusion days 5–7 thioguanine, 100 mg/m² every 12 h days 1–7 3. cytarabine, doxorubicin, prednisolone, and vincristine cytarabine 100 mg/m²/day IV infusion days 1–7 doxorubicin 30 mg/m²/day IV infusion days 1–3 prednisolone 40 mg/m²/day IV infusion every 12 h days 1–5 vincristine 1.5 mg/m²/day IV infusion days 1 and 5 4. cytarabine and daunorubicin cytarabine 100 mg/m²/day IV infusion days 1–7 daunorubicin 45 mg/m²/day IV push days 1–3 5. cytarabine, daunorubicin, prednisone, thioguanine, and vincristine cytarabine 100 mg/m²/day IV every 12 h days 1–7 daunorubicin 70 mg/m²/day IV infusion days 1–3 prednisone 40 mg/m²/day days 1–7 thioguanine 100 mg/m²/day every 12 h days 1–7 vincristine 1 mg/m²/day IV infusion days 1 and 7 6. cytarabine and thioguanine cytarabine 3 mg/kg every 12 h by in-

Uses	*Clinical Considerations*

Acute myelogenous leukemia (DOC)*
Also useful for:
  Acute lymphocytic leukemia
  Chronic myelogenous leukemia
	Store freeze-dried powder under refrigeration; reconstitute vials with bacteriostatic water for injection (0.9% benzyl alcohol) 5 ml/100-mg vial; 10 ml/500-mg vial. Use 5 ml–10 ml Elliott's B solution, lactated Ringer's solution or patient's own cerebrospinal fluid to reconstitute for intrathecal injection; solution may be stored at room temperature for 48 h; discard any hazy or cloudy solution; infusion solutions may be prepared in 0.9% sodium chloride or dextrose 5%; solutions are stable at room temperature for 7 days; reconstitute with smaller volumes (1 ml–2 ml) for SC injection; may increase SGOT levels and uric acid levels in blood and urine; usual pediatric dose is equivalent to the adult dose; less nausea, vomiting, diarrhea if given IV infusion rather than IV injection, but danger of hematologic toxicity is increased

(continued)

Table 75-8 (continued)
Antimetabolites

Drug	Preparations	Usual Dosage Range
cytarabine (cytosine arabinoside, ARA-C, Cytosar-U) (continued)		jection + thioguanine 2.5 mg/kg every 12 h; give both drugs until bone marrow depression occurs; repeat cycle after 10 days–20 days rest Stop therapy if leukocyte count falls below 1000 or platelet count below 50,000; resume usually after 5–7 drug-free days, when above levels are reached *Intrathecal injection* 5 mg–75 mg/m² or 30 mg–100 mg every 2 days–7 days or once a day for 4 days until CSF findings are normal, plus one additional dose
floxuridine (FUDR)	Injection—500 mg/vial	*Intra-arterial infusion only:* 0.1 mg–0.6 mg/kg/day by continuous infusion; 0.4 mg–0.6 mg/kg/day for hepatic artery infusion; continue therapy until toxicity occurs, usually 14 days–21 days, with 2 weeks rest between each course *IV* (investigational only)—0.5 mg–1 mg/kg/day IV infusion for 6 days–15 days or until toxicity occurs By single IV injection—30 mg/kg/day for 5 days then 15 mg/kg/day every other day for up to 11 days or until toxicity occurs
fluorouracil (5-fluorouracil, 5-FU, Adrucil)	Injection—500 mg/10 ml, 5000 mg/100 ml	Initially, 12 mg/kg IV injection over 1 min–2 min once daily for 4 days; maximum daily dose 800 mg; if no toxicity, give 6 mg/kg on days 6, 8, 10, and 12 or 7 mg–12 mg/kg/day IV for 4 days and if no toxicity 7 mg–10 mg/kg/day every 3 days–4 days for 2 weeks (For poor-risk patients, reduce dose 50%) Maintenance—Repeat above schedule every 30 days after last day of previous treatment or 10 mg–15 mg/kg IV once a week, not to exceed 1 g/week; or 300 mg–500 mg/m²/day for 4 days–5 days repeated every 30 days; dosage based on actual body weight unless patient is obese or has fluid retention Oral—15 mg–20 mg/kg/day for 5 days–8 days; dilute in water or bicarbonate buffer solution rather than juice
mercaptopurine (6-mercaptopurine, 6-MP, Purinethol)	Tablets—50 mg	Adult—Initially 2.5 mg/kg or 80 mg–100 mg/m² daily in single or divided doses; if no response and no toxicity after 4 weeks increase to 5 mg/kg/day Maintenance—1.5 mg–2.5 mg/kg or 50 mg–100 mg/m² daily Children—2.5 mg/kg or 75 mg/m² daily

Uses	Clinical Considerations
Palliative management of GI adenocarcinoma metastatic to liver, pancreas, or biliary tract Head and neck tumors	Reconstitute with 5 ml sterile water for injection; solution stable for 14 days under refrigeration; further dilution in 0.9% sodium chloride or dextrose 5% is necessary for infusion; dilution is stable for 24 h; may increase serum alkaline phosphatase, LDH, SGOT, SGPT, and bilirubin levels
Palliative management of carcinoma of colon, rectum, stomach, and pancreas (DOC) Treatment of breast, ovarian, cervical, and liver carcinomas	Solution may discolor slightly during storage, but may still be used safely; crystal precipitate may be redissolved by heating to 60°C; allow to cool to body temperature before using; infusions may be prepared using 0.9% sodium chloride or dextrose 5%; solutions are stable for 24 h; incompatible with cytarabine, doxorubicin, and methotrexate; may increase 5-hydroxyindole acetic acid (5-HIAA) in urine; may decrease plasma albumin. FDA has not approved the drug for oral use. Oral dose should be given 2 h before or after food.
Acute lymphocytic (DOC) and myelogenous leukemia Chronic myelogenous leukemia Has been used investigationally in the treatment of many autoimmune diseases (ulcerative colitis, Crohn's disease)	Decrease dose of mercaptopurine to ½ to ¼ usual dose if given concurrently with allopurinol; may increase uric acid levels in blood and urine; rarely used as a single agent for maintenance of remissions in acute leukemia; may falsely increase serum glucose and uric acid levels when the SMA (sequential multiple analyzer) is used

(continued)

Table 75-8 (continued)
Antimetabolites

Drug	Preparations	Usual Dosage Range
		Inflammatory bowel disease—1.5 mg/kg/ day; if no improvement in 2 months–3 months, gradually increase to 2.5 mg/kg/day
		(Calculate all doses to nearest 25 mg)
methotrexate (Abitrexate, Amethopterin, Folex, MTX, Mexate, Mexate-AQ, Methotrexate LPF)	Tablets—2.5 mg Injection—2.5 mg/ml, 25 mg/ml Powder for injection—20 mg/vial, 50 mg/vial, 100 mg/vial, 250 mg/vial Liquid (preservative free)—25 mg/ml	Choriocarcinoma—15 mg–30 mg/day orally or IM for 5 days; repeat for three to five courses with 1 week–2 weeks rest between each course
		Leukemia—induction: 3.3 mg/m^2 IM, IV, or orally daily for 4 weeks–6 weeks combined with prednisone 60 mg/m^2 daily
		Maintenance—30 mg/m^2 orally or IM twice a week or 2.5 mg/kg IV every 14 days
		Children—20 mg–30 mg/m^2 orally or IM once a week
		Meningeal leukemia—10 mg–15 mg/m^2 intrathecally every 2 days–5 days; maximum 15 mg; maximum pediatric dose 12 mg
		Burkitt's lymphoma—Stage I–II: 10 mg–25 mg orally daily for 4 days–8 days then rest 1 week
		Stage III: Up to 1 g/m^2/day combined with cyclophosphamide and vincristine
		Mycosis fungoides:
		Oral—2.5 mg–5 mg/day for weeks or months as needed
		IM—50 mg once a week or 25 mg twice a week
		Psoriasis:
		Oral—Three schedules may be used: 1. 10 mg–25 mg once a week to a maximum of 50 mg/week 2. 2.5 mg every 12 h for three doses or every 8 h for four doses once a week, to a maximum of 30 mg/week 3. 2.5 mg/day for 5 days, skip 2 days, and repeat; maximum 6.25 mg/day (this schedule may cause increased liver toxicity)
		IM, IV—10 mg–25 mg once a week to a maximum of 50 mg/week
		Rheumatoid arthritis—2.5 mg–25 mg/ week orally or 7.5 mg–15 mg IM once a week
		High dose methotrexate:
		IV infusion—100 mg/m^2 to 10 g/m^2 over 6 h–24 h every 1 week–3 weeks; follow with calcium leucovorin rescue
		Calcium leucovorin dose: *Oral, IV, IM*—10 mg–15 mg/m^2 every 6 h starting 1 h–24 h after methotrexate and continue for 24 h–72 h (dosage and schedule vary according to protocol and methotrexate dose)

Uses	Clinical Considerations
Trophoblastic tumors such as gestational choriocarcinoma, chorioadenoma destruens, or hydatidiform mole (DOC) Acute lymphocytic leukemia (DOC); prophylaxis of meningeal leukemia (DOC); breast, lung, and epidermoid cancers of head and neck; Burkitt's lymphoma (DOC); lymphosarcoma; mycosis fungoides; severe psoriasis; rheumatoid arthritis (investigational use)	Monitor urinary chorionic gonadotropin to determine effectiveness of therapy in choriocarcinoma; level should return to less than 50 IU/24 h after three to four courses of therapy; use preservative-free solution in treating meningeal leukemia; reconstitute with Elliott's B solution, 0.9% sodium chloride, lactated Ringer's solution, or patient's own cerebrospinal fluid; powders may be reconstituted with sterile water for injection, 0.9% sodium chloride injection, or dextrose 5% in water; solution is stable for 7 days at room temperature but should be used within 24 h because it is not preserved; for high-dose methotrexate therapy, use preservative-free solution and dilute in 0.9% sodium chloride or dextrose 5% in water; patient should be well hydrated and urine alkalinized with sodium bicarbonate (3 g every 3 h for 12 h before therapy) to prevent renal toxicity; may increase uric acid levels in blood and urine. Calcium leucovorin is used as "rescue" because it is metabolized to tetrahydrofolic acid, which blocks the effect of methotrexate; CNS toxicity is commonly associated with intrathecal injection; methotrexate is excreted in breast milk.

(continued)

Table 75-8 (continued)
Antimetabolites

Drug	Preparations	Usual Dosage Range
thioguanine (TG, 6-thioguanine)	Tablets—40 mg	Induction: Adults and children—2 mg/kg/day or 75 mg–100 mg/m²/day as single dose; if no response in 3 weeks–4 weeks and no toxicity, increase dose to 3 mg/kg/day (calculate dose to nearest 20 mg) Maintenance Adults and children—2 mg–3 mg/kg/day or 75 mg–400 mg/m²/day

*DOC, Drug of choice (alone or in combination with other drugs).

sion, which may result in a patient developing a viral disease following immunization with a live virus vaccine.

14. Concurrent use of fluorouracil and allopurinol may reduce the hematologic toxicity of fluorouracil.
15. Mercaptopurine may increase or decrease the anticoagulant effect of warfarin.
16. Mercaptopurine used concurrently with immunosuppressants such as corticosteroids, azathioprine, chlorambucil, cyclophosphamide, and cyclosporine may increase the risk of infection and development of secondary neoplasms.
17. Mercaptopurine and methotrexate cause hepatotoxicity, and concurrent use of other hepatotoxic agents should be avoided.
18. Concurrent use of intrathecal methotrexate and parenteral acyclovir may result in CNS toxicity.

■ Nursing Process for Antimetabolites

□ ASSESSMENT

□ Subjective Data

Obtaining a thorough medication history prior to administering methotrexate or 6-mercaptopurine is essential. The following drugs are likely to increase the toxicity associated with methotrexate: sulfonamides; antibacterial, hypoglycemic and diuretic agents; tetracycline; chloramphenicol; chloral hydrate; phenytoin; para-aminobenzoic acid; and salicylates. In addition to these agents,

vitamin preparations containing folic acid should be avoided because they may interfere with the effectiveness of methotrexate.

The concomitant use of allopurinol with 6-mercaptopurine may increase the toxicities. Therefore, if these drugs are used together, the patient should receive a 75% reduction in the allopurinol dose.

The identification of risk factors assists the nurse in identifying individuals who may experience increased incidence of adverse side-effects.

High dosages of cytarabine may cause neurologic toxicity. Dosages greater than 24 g/m² are implicated in increased development of neurologic toxicity. There also seems to be an increased incidence of neurologic symptoms in patients over 50 years of age. Symptoms of neurologic toxicity include lethargy, expressive aphasia, unsteady tandem gait, and nystagmus followed by ataxia.

High dose methotrexate may cause severe systemic side-effects if it is not administered with leucovorin rescue. Patients with altered renal function or presence of extra third space fluid are at increased risk. Particular attention to serum methotrexate levels is important in these individuals.

Patient compliance with leucovorin rescue is a critical issue. The nurse should reinforce the importance of proper and prompt administration of this drug. Written instructions providing the correct dosage and time for administration should be given to the patient. The patient may need to set an alarm clock to get up for a morning dose. Exploration of sleeping patterns is necessary. If the patient has difficulty waking up, an alternate plan such as setting two alarm clocks or asking a relative or a friend to assist with administration of the medication may be necessary.

Uses	Clinical Considerations
Acute lymphocytic and myelogenous leukemia (DOC) Chronic myelogenous leukemia	May increase uric acid levels of blood and urine

During each contact with the patient, the nurse should assess the patient's level of understanding regarding the treatment schedule and provide written instructions if necessary.

□ **Objective Data**
1. Physical Assessment

    A *complete* physical assessment is necessary prior to initiation of chemotherapy. This section, however, will highlight the essential systems to be reviewed and the associated toxicities of drug therapy.

    Pulmonary—methotrexate

    Hepatic—methotrexate, cytarabine, thioguanine, 6-mercaptopurine

    Renal—methotrexate, cytarabine

    Neurologic—cytarabine (high dose), methotrexate (intrathecal), fluorouracil

    Integumentary—methotrexate, cytarabine, fluorouracil

    Gastrointestinal—methotrexate, cytarabine, fluorouracil

    Hematopoietic—All drugs
2. Laboratory Data and Diagnostic Tests
    · Intravenous pyelogram—methotrexate
    · 24-hour urine for creatinine clearance—methotrexate

□ **NURSING DIAGNOSIS**
Actual nursing diagnoses for the patient receiving antimetabolites include:

    Knowledge deficit with regard to chemotherapy side-effects
Potential nursing diagnoses include:
    Anxiety
    Fluid volume deficit related to nausea and vomiting

Alteration in bowel elimination: diarrhea
Alteration in comfort: pain
Impaired verbal communication
Potential for infection
Alteration in nutrition: less than body requirements
Alterations in oral mucous membrane
Self-care deficit
Disturbance in body image/self-concept
Altered sexuality patterns
Impairment of skin integrity

□ **PLAN**
The nursing care plan is directed toward minimizing the side-effects of chemotherapy and promoting self-care behaviors so the patient can identify early signs and symptoms of toxicities and implement appropriate interventions.

□ **INTERVENTION**
The appropriate route of administration and drug doses have been discussed in the previous pharmacology section. Therefore, this section will discuss nursing considerations during administration of specific agents.
1. Cytarabine can be administered by the intravenous, intrathecal or subcutaneous route.

    Low and medium dosages of cytarabine are usually administered by IV infusion. The patient may receive an IV bolus injection of cytarabine followed by a 5-day or greater continuous infusion depending on the protocol.

    High dosages of cytarabine are given as a 1-hour to 2-hour infusion twice a day for 6 days. It appears that the rate of infusion of high dosage cytarabine is important in helping to minimize the neurologic toxicity of this drug.

Table 75-9
Fate of Antimetabolites

Drug	Absorption/Distribution/Half-Life	Metabolism	Excretion
cytarabine	20% absorption after an oral dose (ineffective and not used by oral administration) Widely distributed—crosses blood-brain barrier and reaches levels 40%–50% of plasma concentration Low protein binding Half-life—biphasic Initial—10 min–15 min Terminal—1 h–3 h	Rapid hepatic, also metabolized in blood, kidneys, and other tissues	Renal—10% unchanged, 90% as inactive metabolite ARA-U
floxuridine	Fair distribution, some penetration of blood–brain barrier	Hepatic—Slow infusion causes conversion to active monophosphate metabolite FUDR-MP Rapid infusion causes conversion to fluorouracil	Respiratory—60% Renal—10%–13% unchanged and as metabolites
fluorouracil	Wide distribution—crosses blood-brain barrier Protein binding is low Erratic oral absorption 50%–80% Half-life—biphasic Initial—10 min–20 min Terminal—20 h (due to storage in tissue)	In tissues to active metabolite FUDR-MP Catabolized in liver to inactive metabolites	Respiratory—60%–80% as CO_2 Renal—15%
mercaptopurine	Oral absorption is variable and incomplete only up to 50% Crosses blood–brain barrier only in low concentrations Protein binding—low Half-life—biphasic or triphasic Initial—30 min–90 min Secondary—2 h–3 h Terminal—10 h	Hepatic—Either by oxidation by enzyme xanthine oxidase or by methylation of sulfhydryl group	Renal—May be dialyzed
methotrexate	Oral absorption at doses < 30 mg/m² is good; doses > 30 mg/m² may be poorly absorbed Widely distributed—crosses blood-brain barrier in low concentrations Protein binding—moderate (60%) Half-life—biphasic or triphasic Initial—30 min–60 min Secondary—2 h–3 h Terminal—8 h–10 h (up to 27 h)	Hepatic	Renal—Primarily unchanged
thioguanine	Oral absorption is slow and variable only 30% Wide distribution—crosses blood-brain barrier in low concentrations Protein binding—30%	Hepatic	Renal—Primarily as metabolites

Therefore, careful attention to the dosage and rate of infusion is important. In the event of adverse side-effects, the drug should be discontinued and the physician should be notified immediately.

The administration of intrathecal agents should be diluted with a preservative free solution.

When cytarabine is administered subcutaneously the white blood count should be checked prior to administration. If the patient is neutropenic, proper preparation of the site with betadine will minimize infection.

2. Methotrexate can be administered by mouth or by intravenous, intramuscular, subcutaneous, or intrathecal routes.

The intravenous method of administration may vary depending on the protocol. However, the most common methods are 5 mg to 149 mg administered by slow intravenous push; 150 mg to 499 mg are administered by IV infusion over 20 minutes; 500 mg to 1500 mg are administered according to protocol.

It is especially important to know the dose of methotrexate being used. High doses of methotrexate (≥ 100 mg/m^2) must be administered with caution, because the resulting systemic toxic effects can be lethal and must be counteracted by the administration of calcium leucovorin rescue. Leucovorin rescue spares normal cells from the toxic side-effects of methotrexate (see Chap. 38). The physician will prescribe the dosage and specific times the patient must take this drug, either during or following treatment with high-dose methotrexate. The patient *must* take this medication. If the patient is unable to tolerate it by mouth, it must be administered IM or IV. The nurse must ascertain the patient's level of understanding and provide written instructions describing the correct time for administration of leucovorin. The patient must contact healthcare providers immediately if unable to tolerate oral doses.

Adequate hydration and alkalization of urine are important treatment considerations in high-dose methotrexate. Renal toxicity may occur during the first 30 hours of treatment. Therefore, oral or intravenous administration of sodium bicarbonate may be ordered to maintain urine pH at or higher than 6.5 throughout therapy. Hydration should be maintained at 2 L to 3 L/day.

Serum levels of methotrexate should be monitored to minimize toxicity. High-risk individuals include those with an elevated BUN or creatinine or patients who have extra third space fluids, such as ascites or effusions.

Intrathecal drugs must be diluted with a preservative-free solution.

3. Fluorouracil is administered intravenously or as an arterial infusion. It can also be applied as a topical agent.

Intravenous doses may be given once a week or by continuous infusion for 5 days.

Hepatic artery infusion is performed according to protocol.

The nurse must wear gloves when applying fluorouracil as a topical agent. The use of occlusive dressings should be avoided because this may increase the inflammatory response of adjacent normal tissue.

☐ *Side-Effects and Patient Education*
The administration of antimetabolites results in three principal types of side-effects in the majority of patients: nausea and vomiting, stomatitis, and bone marrow depression. The nursing management of these side-effects is discussed under Nursing Process for Antineoplastic Drugs.

Antimetabolites also cause multiple other side-effects (see Table 75-10). The following section will highlight the side-effects of these drugs and the necessary patient education.

1. *Neurologic toxicity* may occur with cytarabine (high dose), intrathecal methotrexate, and fluorouracil. The neurologic side-effects of cytarabine are more common in doses greater than 24 g/m^2 and in patients over 50 years of age. Nursing interventions include identification of high risk patients, and procedures to assess and document the baseline neurologic exam prior to administration of the drug. The drug should be withheld if signs of toxicity are noted. Patients usually receive vitamin B$_6$ to minimize toxicity during treatment. In addition, the rate of IV infusion should be monitored closely and should occur over 1 hour to 2 hours.

Central nervous system symptoms, such as increased temperature, nausea, vomiting, headache, drowsiness, or blurred vision, may occur 2 hours to 4 hours after intrathecal administration of methotrexate and may last for 72 hours. The patient should report these symptoms to health-care providers immediately.

Table 75-10
Side-Effects/Adverse Reactions of Antimetabolites

Drug	Alopecia/Dermatologic	Gastrointestinal	Hepatic
cytarabine	Alopecia Skin ulceration Rash (6 h–10 h after dose) Freckling	Moderated nausea and vomiting Stomatitis	Rare
floxuridine	Alopecia Rash Localized erythema	Mild nausea and vomiting Diarrhea Stomatitis Enteritis	Rare
fluorouracil	Alopecia Rash Hyperpigmentation and photo- sensitivity	Mild nausea and vomiting Diarrhea Stomatitis Enteritis	Rare
mercapto- purine	Hyperpigmentation, rash, and itching are rare.	Occasional nausea and vomiting	Hepatic necrosis and fibrosis Jaundice in 10%–40% patients High dose >2.5 mg/kg/day asso- ciated with hepatic toxicity
methotrexate	Alopecia—less common Acne Depigmentation Photosensitivity Rash Reddening of skin with high dose therapy	Occasional nausea and vomiting Stomatitis GI ulceration Diarrhea	Atrophy, cirrhosis, necrosis, fi- brosis more common with daily prolonged therapy
thioguanine	Dermatitis Rash	Occasional nausea and vomiting Stomatitis	Jaundice

Myelosuppression	Neurologic	Renal	Other

Leukopenia
  Nadir 7 days–9 days and 15 days–24 days
  Recovery—24 days–35 days
Thrombocytopenia
  Nadir 12 days–15 days
  Recovery 22 days–25 days
	Cerebral and cerebellar dysfunction with high dose therapy (dysarthria, ataxia)		Acute pancreatitis has occurred in patients previously treated with asparaginase.
			Cytarabine syndrome—Fever, myalgia, bone pain, rash, conjunctivitis, malaise, chest pain, 6 h–12 h after dose—treat with corticosteroids

Leukopenia
  Nadir 9 days–14 days
  Recovery 30 days
Thrombocytopenia
  Nadir 7 days–17 days
  Recovery 30 days
  (Myelosuppression less frequent than fluorouracil)
	Lethargy, malaise		Local reactions due to intra-arterial administration include: arterial ischemia, thrombosis, embolism, bleeding at catheter site, infection, abscess, thrombophlebitis

Leukopenia
  Nadir 9 days–14 days (as long as 25 days)
  Recovery 30 days
Thrombocytopenia
  Nadir 7 days–17 days
  Recovery 30 days
	Ataxia—Rare		Myocardia ischemia—usually after repeated doses

Leukopenia and thrombocytopenia (usually mild)
  Nadir 7 days–14 days
  Recovery 21 days
		Uric acid nephropathy	Interstitial pneumonitis (rare)

Leukopenia
  Nadir 4 days–7 days and 12 days–21 days
  Recovery 7 days–13 days and 15 days–29 days
Thrombocytopenia
  Nadir 5 days–12 days
  Recovery 15 days–27 days
	More frequent with intrathecal administration and classified as: Chemical arachnoiditis—Headaches, back pain, nuchal rigidity, fever
	Transient paresis—One or more spinal nerve roots
	Leukoencephalopathy—Confusion, ataxia, irritability, somnolence, dementia, occasional seizures
		Tubular obstruction due to drug precipitation
		Uric acid nephropathy
			Alveolitis (rare)—More frequent with prolonged daily therapy

Leukopenia and thrombocytopenia
  Nadir 14 days
  Recovery 21 days
	Unsteady gait (rare)		Hyporuricemia

Reversible cerebellar ataxia may occur with the administration of fluorouracil. This complication may persist for several weeks after discontinuation of therapy. Common symptoms include dizziness, nystagmus, and lack of coordination. The patient should be instructed to report these symptoms immediately.

2. *Hepatic toxicity* may occur with cytarabine, thioguanine, and 6-mercaptopurine. The patient should report yellowing of skin, dark urine, clay-colored stools, and pruritis to health-care providers.

3. *Skin changes* may occur with cytarabine, methotrexate, and fluorouracil.

Cytarabine may induce several skin changes. A rash may occur on the palms and feet; this is more common in children. In addition, a "cytarabine syndrome" may occur 6 hours to 12 hours after administration with high dosages of cytarabine and is manifested by fever, malaise, myalgia, bone pain, rash, conjunctivitis, and chest pain. The patient should be informed this may occur, and the nurse should intervene with appropriate symptom management.

A skin rash and hyperpigmentation of the veins treated with fluorouracil may occur. The patient should be reassured that these side-effects are expected, and the nurse should institute appropriate symptom management.

Increased sensitivity to sunlight can occur as a result of treatment with methotrexate and fluorouracil. The patient should be cautioned to avoid excessive and extreme exposure to the sun. Sunscreen with #15 or higher skin protection factor (SPF) should be suggested, as well as use of protective clothing and sunglasses.

4. *Gastrointestinal* side-effects are associated with cytarabine, methotrexate, and fluorouracil.

Diarrhea may occur with cytarabine, methotrexate, and fluorouracil. Daily monitoring of bowel function, consistency, and frequency should be assessed by the nurse. Appropriate symptom management for diarrhea should be implemented, such as local or systemic antidiarrheals (see Chap. 45). Local care, such as sitz baths or application of protective ointments, may also be necessary.

Stomatitis is common with cytarabine, methotrexate, and fluorouracil. Daily oral assessment is suggested. The patient should be started on a preventive oral care regimen, such

as normal saline solution rinses. Attention to meticulous oral hygiene is also important. The patient should report the development of mouth sores to health-care providers, so that appropriate symptom management can be implemented (see Nursing Care Plan 75-1). Because stomatitis is an *early* sign of methotrexate toxicity, patients should inform the health-care team *immediately* if it occurs.

5. *Nephrotoxicity* may occur with methotrexate and cytarabine.

Renal toxicity seen with methotrexate may be enhanced by many other drugs. Therefore, it is essential to be aware of any other drugs the patient is receiving. High doses of methotrexate may precipitate in the renal tubules at acidic pH. Alkalization of the urine is necessary with doses greater than 1 g/m^2; oral or intravenous sodium bicarbonate may be administered. Urinary pH should be checked at least four times a day and maintained above 6.5. Hydration will minimize nephrotoxicity. Fluids should be encouraged to at least 2 L to 3 L per day. The patient's intake and output should be monitored. The physician should be notified if urine output decreases below the level of intake for 1 hour to 4 hours.

Uric acid nephrotoxicity may occur with cytarabine. Uric acid should be monitored closely during the first several days of treatment. Allopurinol may be ordered to minimize this toxicity. Hydration therapy of 2 L to 3 L of fluid per day should be encouraged prior to starting treatment and throughout the course of treatment. Intake and output should be monitored during treatment and for 24 hours after treatment is discontinued.

6. *Ocular toxicity* may occur with high dose cytarabine, and excessive lacrimation may occur with fluorouracil.

Conjunctivitis, ocular pain, photophobia, burning, lacrimation, and decreased visual acuity may occur with high dose cytarabine. Patients should be informed of these potential side-effects. Steroid-containing eye drops may be administered to minimize these side-effects. Patients should be instructed to wear sunglasses if photophobia occurs. The patient's room should be darkened to minimize discomfort if ocular toxicity occurs. Patients should be reassured that this is a transient side-effect which will improve with time.

Excessive lacrimation may occur with fluorouracil but usually will completely resolve 1 week to 2 weeks after treatment is discontinued.

□ EVALUATION
Outcome criteria to measure treatment effectiveness include:
1. The patient will report adverse side-effects promptly to health-care providers.
2. The patient will implement appropriate preventive oral hygiene measures prior to and during administration of chemotherapy.

Natural Products

Asparaginase, Bleomycin, Dactinomycin, Daunorubicin, Doxorubicin, Etoposide, Mitomycin, Mitoxantrone, Plicamycin, Vinblastine, Vincristine

The natural products commercially available are used to treat a wide range of malignant diseases and include an enzyme, six antibiotics, and three plant derivatives with several more products under investigation. Asparaginase, an enzyme isolated from *Escherichia coli*, is used to treat acute lymphocytic leukemia. Most antibiotics are isolated from different strains of the *Streptomyces* fungus, and include bleomycin, dactinomycin, daunorubicin, doxorubicin, mitomycin, and plicamycin. Mitoxantrone is a synthetic anthracenedione. The plant derivatives include vinblastine and vincristine, which are plant alkaloids isolated from periwinkle (*Vinca rosea*), and etoposide, a semisynthetic podophyllotoxin derived from the root of the May apple or mandrake plant (*Podophyllum*). For the indications and uses of the natural products see Table 75-11.

MECHANISM AND ACTIONS
1. *Asparaginase*—Asparaginase breaks down the essential amino acid asparagine, which is necessary for the synthesis of DNA and essential proteins, to aspartic acid and ammonia. Normal cells are able to synthesize their own asparagine; some malignant cells are unable to produce their own asparagine and thus are not able to survive. Asparaginase is cell-cycle specific for the G_1 phase of cell division.
2. *Bleomycin*—The exact mechanism of action of bleomycin is unknown. Bleomycin causes scission of both single- and double-stranded DNA, and also appears to inhibit the incorporation of thymidine into DNA, thus inhibiting DNA synthesis. Bleomycin is cell-cycle specific for the G_2 and M phases of cell division.
3. *Dactinomycin*—The exact mechanism is unknown, however, dactinomycin appears to inhibit DNA-dependent RNA synthesis by intercalating with guanine cytosine base pairs of DNA to form a complex which impairs the template activity of DNA. Dactinomycin is cell-cycle nonspecific.
4. *Daunorubicin and doxorubicin*—The exact mechanism of action of these two anthracycline antibiotics is still unknown. Both agents inhibit DNA synthesis and DNA-dependent RNA synthesis by intercalating with base pairs of DNA to form a complex which inhibits the template activity of DNA and slightly uncoils the DNA helix. Doxorubicin also inhibits protein synthesis. Both agents are primarily cell-cycle nonspecific.
5. *Etoposide*—The exact mechanism of action is unknown; etoposide is cell-cycle specific at the S and G_2 phases of cell division. Etoposide inhibits mitosis at high concentrations (>10 mcg/ml) by causing lysis of cells entering mitosis, and at low concentrations (0.3 mcg–10 mcg/ml) by inhibiting cells from entering prophase; the net effect is inhibition of DNA synthesis.
6. *Mitomycin*—After intracellular enzymatic reduction, mitomycin functions as an alkylating agent, causing DNA cross-linking and inhibiting DNA synthesis. At high concentrations mitomycin also inhibits RNA and protein synthesis.
7. *Mitoxantrone*—Although not completely established, the mechanism of action of mitoxantrone appears to be related to its effects on DNA. It possesses a cytocidal action on both proliferating and nonproliferating human culture cells.
8. *Plicamycin*—The antineoplastic mechanism of action is the same as dactinomycin. The exact mechanism by which plicamycin lowers serum calcium is unknown, however, plicamycin blocks the hypercalcemic action of vitamin

(*Text continues on p. 1444.*)

Table 75-11
Natural Products

Drug	Preparations	Usual Dosage Range

asparaginase (Elspar, L-asparaginase)	Injection—10,000 IU/vial	Children—
		 · Regimen I
		   asparaginase—1000 IU/kg/day IV for 10 days starting day 22
		   vincristine—2 mg/m² IV once a week on days 1, 8, 15; maximum single dose is 2 mg
		   Prednisone—40 mg/m²/day in three divided doses for 15 days, then 20 mg/m² for 2 days, 10 mg/m² for 2 days, 5 mg/m² for 2 days, and 2.5 mg/m² for 2 days
		 · Regimen II
		   asparaginase—6000 IU/m² IM every 3 days for nine doses starting day 4
		   vincristine—1.5 mg/m² IV for four doses on days 1, 8, 15, 22
		   Prednisone—40 mg/m²/day in three divided doses for 28 days, then taper over 14 days
		 Sole induction agent—200 IU/kg IV daily for 28 days
		 Adult induction—10,000 IU/m² every 1 week–2 weeks
		 Intra-arterial—20,000 IU/day for 7 days–10 days

bleomycin (Blenoxane)	15 U/ampule	Squamous cell carcinoma, lymphosarcoma, reticulum cell sarcoma, testicular carcinoma—0.25 U–0.5 U/kg (10 U–20 U/m²) IV, IM, or SC, weekly or twice a week to a total of 300 U–400 U IV infusion—0.25 U/kg/day or 15 U/m²/day over 24 h for 4 days–5 days Hodgkin's disease—As above until 50% response occurs, then 1 U daily or 5 U weekly IV or IM Intra-arterial infusion for squamous cell carcinoma of head, neck, and cervix—30 U–60 U/day over 1 h–24 h Malignant effusions— *Intrapleural*—15 U–120 U/100 ml 0.9% sodium chloride allowed to dwell for 24 h; up to 240 U have been used *Intraperitoneal*—60 U–120 U/100 ml 0.9% sodium chloride allowed to dwell for 24 h Warts—0.2 U–0.8 U intralesionally of a solution of 15 U/15 ml 0.9% sodium chloride injection every 2 weeks–4 weeks to a maximum of 2 U Reduce dose in patients with impaired renal function

Uses	Clinical Considerations

Acute lymphocytic leukemia (DOC)*
Investigational uses—Lymphosarcoma, chronic lymphocytic leukemia, hypoglycemia due to pancreatic islet cell tumors

Adult usage is primarily investigational; may be administered by way of the hepatic artery for insulin-secreting pancreatic islet cell tumors; store intact vial under refrigeration; for IV use, reconstitute with 5 ml 0.9% sodium chloride and inject over at least 30 min into running IV of 0.9% sodium chloride or dextrose 5%; for IM use reconstitute with 2 ml 0.9% sodium chloride; do not inject more than 2 ml into one site; avoid vigorous shaking during reconstitution; solution is stable for 8 h at room temperature; discard solution if cloudy; not recommended as the sole induction agent unless combined chemotherapy is inappropriate due to toxicity or other factors; intradermal skin test is recommended prior to initiation of therapy and when more than 7 days have elapsed between doses (up to 35% of patients exhibit hypersensitivity reactions); give 0.1 ml (2 IU) of test solution and observe for at least 1 h for erythema or wheal; to prepare skin test solution, reconstitute vial with 5 ml 0.9% sodium chloride; withdraw 0.1 ml (200 IU) and inject into 9.9 ml 0.9% sodium chloride injection giving test solution of 20 IU/ml; desensitization should be used on any positive reactors; inject 1 IU IV and double the dose every 10 min, provided there is no reaction, until total accumulated dose is equal to the dose for that day; may increase blood ammonia, glucose, and uric acid levels; may increase urine uric acid levels and decrease serum albumin and calcium; gelatinous fiber-like particles may develop in IV infusion on standing; solution may be administered through a 5-μ filter to remove particles without loss of potency; do not administer thru a 0.2-μ filter because loss of potency may result. Asparaginase derived from *Erwinia carotovora* (investigational) may be used in patients allergic to commercial preparation

Squamous cell carcinoma of head and neck (DOC), mouth, tongue, nasopharynx, oropharynx, sinus, palate, lip, buccal mucosa, gingiva, epiglottis, skin, larynx, penis, cervix (DOC), vulva
Lymphomas—
  Hodgkin's disease
  Reticulum cell sarcoma
  Lymphosarcoma
  Testicular carcinomas (DOC)
  Embryonal cell carcinoma
  Choriocarcinoma
  Teratocarcinoma (DOC)
  Malignant effusions
  Warts (verucca vulgaris)

For IM or SC use, reconstitute with 1 ml–5 ml of sterile water for injection, 0.9% sodium chloride, 5% dextrose or bacteriostatic water for injection; for IV use, reconstitute with 5 ml 0.9% sodium chloride or 5% dextrose and administer slowly over 10 min; solution is stable 14 days at room temperature and 28 days refrigerated; give test dose of 2 U for first two doses in lymphoma patients because of possibility of anaphylactoid reaction; pneumonitis occurs in 10%–40% of patients at total doses of 200 U–400 U; if bleomycin has been used to treat malignant effusions, half of the administered dose should be counted toward this total; be alert for symptoms such as dry cough, dyspnea, and fine rales; fatal in 10% of patients; cutaneous allergic reactions are also common; hypothermia occurs in 25% of patients 3 h–6 h after administration and lasts 4 h–12 h; becomes less frequent with continued use

(continued)

Table 75-11 (continued)
Natural Products

Drug	Preparations	Usual Dosage Range
bleomycin (Blenoxane) *(continued)*		Serum Creatinine / Dosage 1.5–2.5 — ½ normal dosage 2.5–4.0 — ¼ normal dosage 4.0–6.0 — ⅛ normal dosage 6.0–10.0 — ¹⁄₁₀ to ¹⁄₂₀ normal dosage
dactinomycin (actinomycin D, Cosmegen)	Injection—0.5 mg/vial	Adults—0.01 mg–0.015 mg/kg/day IV for 5 days every 4 weeks–6 weeks, or 0.5 mg/m² (maximum 2 mg) IV once a week for 3 weeks Children—0.01 mg–0.015 mg/kg/day IV for 5 days or a total dose of 2.5 mg/m² IV in divided doses over 7 days; may repeat every 4 weeks–6 weeks Isolation perfusion: Upper extremity—0.035 mg/kg Lower extremity or pelvis area—0.05 mg/kg Dosage should be based on body surface area in obese or edematous patients
daunorubicin (Cerubidine)	Injection—20 mg/vial	Single agent: 30 mg–60 mg/m²/day IV on days 1, 2, and 3 every 3 weeks–4 weeks or 0.8 mg–1 mg/kg/day IV for 3 days–6 days repeated every 3 weeks–4 weeks Combination: daunorubicin—45 mg/m²/day IV on days 1, 2, 3 of first course and days 1 and 2 of subsequent courses cytarabine—100 mg/m²/day IV infusion daily for 7 days for the first course and daily for 5 days for subsequent courses Children— Combination: daunorubicin—25 mg–45 mg/m² IV once a week for 4 weeks–6 weeks Vincristine—1.5 mg/m² IV once a week for 4 weeks–6 weeks Prednisone—40 mg/m² daily po Children under 2 years of age or <0.5 m² body surface area—dosage based on body weight Total cumulative dose of daunorubicin should not exceed 550 mg/m² or 450 mg/m² in patients who received previous chest radiation therapy Reduce dose in patients with impaired hepatic or renal function. Serum Bilirubin / Serum Creatinine / Dosage 1.2 mg–3 mg/dl — — ¾ normal dosage above 3 mg/dl — above 3 mg/dl — ½ normal dosage
doxorubicin (Adriamycin-RDF, Adriamycin PFS)	Injection—10 mg/vial, 20 mg/vial, 50 mg/vial, 150 mg/vial	Adults—60 mg–75 mg/m²/day IV repeated every 21 days or 25 mg–30 mg/m²/day IV for 3 days repeated every 4 weeks

Uses	Clinical Considerations

Wilms' tumor (DOC)
Rhabdomyosarcoma (DOC)
Carcinoma of testis and uterus
Ewing's sarcoma
Investigational uses—Kaposi's sarcoma, malignant melanoma, Paget's disease, to manage acute organ rejection in kidney and heart transplants

Reconstitute with 1.1 ml sterile water for injection (preservative-free); administer directly into tubing of running IV of 0.9% sodium chloride or 5% dextrose; may dilute and infuse over 10 min–15 min; an in-line cellulose ester membrane filter should *not* be used, because it may remove some of the drug; **avoid extravasation; never administer IM or SC**; solution is theoretically stable at room temperature for long periods but should be discarded within 24 h to prevent bacterial contamination; may increase uric acid levels of blood and urine; hyperpigmentation occurs if skin has been previously irradiated; nausea and vomiting are common during first few hours and may persist for up to 24 h, hyperbilirubinemia may require dosage reduction by $^1/_3$ to $^1/_2$

Acute myelogenous leukemia (DOC)
Acute lymphocytic leukemia
Investigational uses—Non-Hodgkin's lymphomas

Reconstitute with 4 ml sterile water for injection; solution is stable for 24 h at room temperature and 48 h under refrigeration; protect from exposure to sunlight; administer into the tubing of a rapidly flowing IV of 0.9% sodium chloride or 5% dextrose; **avoid extravasation; never administer IM or SC**; may increase uric acid levels of blood and urine

Acute lymphocytic and myelogenous leukemia
Wilms' tumor
Neuroblastoma (DOC)

Reconstitute with 0.9% sodium chloride injection (5 ml/10-mg vial, 10 ml/20-mg vial and 25 ml/50-mg vial); solution is stable for 24 h at room temperature and 48 h under re-
(continued)

Table 75-11 (continued)
Natural Products

Drug	Preparations	Usual Dosage Range
		IV—20 mg/m² once a week may cause lower cardiotoxicity
		Bladder instillation—30 mg/30 ml of a 0.9% sodium chloride instilled and retained for 30 min; repeat monthly
		Children—30 mg/m²/day IV for 3 days repeated every 4 weeks
		Total cumulative dose should not exceed 550 mg/m²
		Reduce dosage in patients with impaired hepatic function.

Serum Bilirubin	*Dosage*
1.2 mg–3 mg/dl	½ normal dosage
above 3 mg/dl	¼ normal dosage

Drug	Preparations	Usual Dosage Range
etoposide (VePesid, VP-16-213)	Injection—100 mg/5 ml Capsules—50 mg	IV—50 mg–100 mg/m²/day for 5 days repeated every 3 weeks–4 weeks In combination with other agents: 100 mg/m²/day on days 1, 3, and 5 repeated every 3 weeks–4 weeks Kaposi's sarcoma in patients with AIDS—150 mg/m²/day IV for 3 days repeated every 4 weeks Oral (for small cell lung cancer)—Two times the IV dose, rounded to the nearest 50 mg.
mitomycin (Mutamycin)	Injection—5 mg/vial, 20 mg/vial	IV—10 mg–20 mg/m² as a single dose repeated every 6 weeks–8 weeks or 2 mg/m²/day IV for 5 days, skip 2 days, and repeat 2 mg/m²/day for 5 days; cycle may be repeated every 6 weeks–8 weeks Bladder instillation—20 mg–40 mg of a solution of 1 mg/ml in water retained for 2 h–3 h, repeated weekly for 8 weeks A suggested guide for subsequent dosage adjustment is the following:

Nadir After Prior Dose		*% of Prior Dose to Be Given*
Leukocytes	*Platelets*	
Above 4,000	Above 100,000	100
3,000–3,999	75,000–99,999	100
2,000–2,999	25,000–74,999	70
Below 2,000	Below 25,000	50

Drug	Preparations	Usual Dosage Range
		Doses greater than 20 mg/m² are no more effective than lower doses, but increase toxicity
Mitoxantrone (Novantrone)	Injection—2 mg/ml	Acute nonlymphocytic leukemia—Initially, 12 mg/m²/day on days 1 to 3, as an IV infusion with 100 mg/m² of cytosine arabinoside for 7 days as a continuous 24-h infusion on days 1 to 7. A second course may be given if response is incomplete, consisting of mitoxantrone, 12 mg/m² on days 1 and 2, and 100 mg/m² cytosine arabinoside on days 1 to 5.

Uses	Clinical Considerations

Soft-tissue and bone sarcomas (DOC)
Thyroid carcinoma
Hodgkin's disease
Non-Hodgkin's lymphomas (DOC)
Breast and ovarian carcinoma (DOC)
Bronchogenic carcinoma (DOC)
Bladder carcinoma (DOC)
Endometrial carcinoma
Gastric carcinoma
Retinoblastoma (DOC)

frigeration; protect from exposure to sunlight; administer into the tubing of a rapidly flowing IV of 0.9% sodium chloride or 5% dextrose; local erythematous streaking along the vein or facial flushing may indicate too rapid administration; **avoid extravasation; never administer IM or SC**; may increase uric acid levels of blood and urine; cardiotoxic effects can occur at cumulative doses above 550 mg/m^2 in most patients, but may be seen at lower doses in patients who have received previous mediastinal irradiation or cyclophosphamide, dactinomycin, or mitomycin therapy; dose should not exceed 400 mg/m^2

Refractory testicular tumors
Small cell lung carcinoma (DOC)
Investigational uses—Acute myelogenous leukemia
Hodgkin's disease
Non-Hodgkin's lymphomas
Kaposi's sarcoma

Do not give by rapid IV push; severe hypotension may result; IV infusion prepared in 5% dextrose or 0.9% sodium chloride injection may be given over 30 min–60 min; infusion concentrations of 0.2 mg/ml are stable for 96 h at room temperature, and concentrations of 0.4 mg/ml are stable for 48 h in both glass and plastic containers; oral form is *not* indicated for testicular tumors due to insufficient data.

Adenocarcinoma of stomach, pancreas, colon, rectum, and breast
Squamous cell carcinoma of head, neck, lungs, and cervix (DOC)
Malignant melanoma
Chronic myelogenous leukemia
Bladder carcinoma

Reconstitute with sterile water for injection: 10 ml/5-mg vial, 40 ml/20-mg vial; solution is stable 7 days at room temperature and 14 days if refrigerated; protect from light; may be diluted for IV infusion (5% dextrose, stable for 3 h at room temperature; 0.9% sodium chloride, stable 12 h; sodium lactate, stable 24 h). **Avoid extravasation; never administer IM or SC**; may increase BUN and serum creatinine levels; vomiting is usually transient (3 h–4 h), but nausea may persist up to 72 h; if disease shows no response after two courses of therapy, discontinue because likelihood of response is minimal

Acute nonlymphocytic leukemia

Solution is diluted with sodium chloride injection or 5% dextrose injection. Extravasation reactions are rare. Avoid contact with skin (rinse immediately if contact occurs); do not mix in same syringe with heparin, as precipitate may form.

(continued)

Table 75-11 (continued)
Natural Products

Drug	Preparations	Usual Dosage Range
plicamycin (Mithracin; former generic name—Mithramycin)	Injection—2.5 mg/vial	Testicular carcinoma—0.025 mg–0.03 mg/kg/day IV infusion for 8 days–10 days or 0.025 mg–0.05 mg/kg/day IV on alternate days for three to eight doses; repeat every 4 weeks Hypercalcemia and hypercalciuria—0.025 mg/kg/day for 3 days–4 days; may repeat at 1-week intervals or 0.015 mg–0.025 mg/kg IV over 4 h–6 h as a single dose; if no response in 24 h–48 h then 0.015 mg–0.025 mg/kg/day for 2 days–4 days (see Chap. 53); reduce dose (by 25%–50%) in patients with impaired hepatic and renal function Paget's disease—0.015 mg/kg/day IV for 10 days
vinblastine (Alkaban-AQ, Velban, Velsar)	Injection—1 mg/ml, 10 mg/vial	Adults—initially, 0.1 mg/kg or 3.7 mg/m^2 once every 7 days; increase in increments of 0.05 mg/kg or 1.8 mg–1.9 mg/m^2 until tumor size decreases, leukocyte count falls to 3,000, or a maximum dose of 0.5 mg/kg or 18.5 mg/m^2 is reached (usual range is 0.15 mg–0.2 mg/kg or 5.5 mg–7.4 mg/m^2); maintenance dose is one increment smaller than final initial dose repeated every 7 days–14 days or 10 mg once or twice a month Children—Initially, 2.5 mg/m^2 once every 7 days; increase in increments of 1.25 mg/m^2 until leukocyte count falls to 3,000, tumor size decreases, or maximum dose of 7.5 mg/m^2 is reached; maintenance dose is one increment smaller than final initial dose repeated every 7 days–14 days; subsequent maintenance doses should not be given to adults or children until leukocyte count exceeds 4,000.
vincristine (Oncovin, Vincasar PFS)	Injection—1 mg/ml, 2 mg/2 ml, 5 mg/5 ml	Adults—0.01 mg–0.03 mg/kg or 0.4 mg–1.4 mg/m^2 IV every 7 days as a single dose Children—1.5 mg–2 mg/m^2 IV every 7 days as a single dose Small daily doses are not recommended because severe toxicity occurs with no increased benefits.

* DOC, Drug of choice (alone or in combination with other drugs).

Uses	Clinical Considerations
Testicular carcinoma Hypercalcemia and hypercalciuria (not responsive to conventional treatment) associated with advanced neoplasms (see Chap. 53) Investigational uses—Paget's disease, glioblastomas	Store intact vial under refrigeration; alternate-day dosing may reduce toxicity; delayed toxicity may occur up to 72 h after medication has been discontinued following daily administration but not alternate-day therapy; reconstitute with 4.9 ml sterile water for injection; stable 24 h at room temperature and 48 h refrigerated; dilute in 5% dextrose or 0.9% sodium chloride, and infuse over 4 h–6 h; **Avoid extravasation**; may increase SGOT, SGPT, LDH, BUN, serum creatinine levels; may decrease serum calcium, phosphorus, and potassium levels; be alert for epistaxis or hematemesis, early signs of possible hemorrhagic diathesis; advise physician immediately

Frequently responsive—
  Hodgkin's disease (DOC)
  Lymphosarcoma
  Reticulum cell sarcoma
  Neuroblastoma
  Advanced mycosis fungoides
  Histiocytosis X (Letterer-Siwe disease)
  Kaposi's sarcoma
  Testicular carcinoma (DOC)
Less responsive—
  Choriocarcinoma
  Breast carcinoma
  Chronic myelogenous leukemia
Investigational uses—Idiopathic thrombocytopenic purpura, auto-immune hemolytic anemia
	Store unopened vial under refrigeration; reconstitute with 10 ml 0.9% sodium chloride; solution is stable 30 days under refrigeration; administer by IV push or through tubing of a running IV (0.9% sodium chloride or 5% dextrose) over 1 min; **avoid extravasation**; rinse syringe and needle with venous blood before withdrawing. If extravasation occurs, damage may be minimized by local injection of hyaluronidase and by following guidelines for treatment of extravasation outlined at the beginning of this chapter; may increase uric acid levels of blood and urine; Raynaud's phenomenon is seen with combined use of vinblastine and bleomycin for testicular carcinoma; response may not be seen in some patients until 4 weeks–12 weeks of therapy have been completed

Acute lymphocytic leukemia (DOC) Burkitt's lymphoma (DOC) Hodgkin's disease (DOC) Lymphosarcoma Rhabdomyosarcoma (DOC) Neuroblastoma (DOC) Wilms' tumor (DOC) Carcinoma of lung and breast Cervical carcinoma Investigational uses—Ewing's sarcoma, multiple myeloma idiopathic thrombocytopenic purpura, auto-immune hemolytic anemia	Store unopened vial under refrigeration; protect from light, administer by IV push or through tubing of running IV (0.9% sodium chloride or 5% dextrose) over 1 min; for IV use only; intrathecal administration will cause death; **avoid extravasation** (see Vinblastine); neurotoxicity (numbness, weakness, myalgia, jaw pain, loss of deep tendon reflexes, motor difficulties, visual disturbances) can occur as soon as 2 months after start of therapy and is usually progressive as long as treatment is continued; paralytic ileus can occur, more commonly in young children; syndrome of inappropriate antidiuretic hormone secretion has been noted, resulting in hyponatremia

D_1 and may also act directly on osteoclasts to inhibit full response to parathyroid hormone.

9. *Vinblastine and vincristine*—Vinblastine and vincristine block mitosis during the metaphase (cell-cycle specific M phase) by binding to or crystallizing microtubular proteins of the mitotic spindle, thus preventing proper polymerization. At high concentrations both drugs may inhibit nucleic acid and protein synthesis; both agents may also interfere with amino acid metabolism.

USES
See Table 75-11.

ADMINISTRATION AND DOSAGE
See Table 75-11.

FATE
See Table 75-12.

SIDE-EFFECTS/ADVERSE REACTIONS
(See under Side-Effects/Adverse Reactions for alkylating agents.) Table 75-13 indicates the common toxicities of the natural products. For a complete list of all side-effects and adverse reactions on each agent, see the manufacturer's product information.

CONTRAINDICATIONS AND PRECAUTIONS
All antineoplastic agents have the potential to be carcinogenic (due to a direct cellular action or immunosuppression) and to cause testicular and ovarian suppression. The exact effect of dose and duration of therapy is unknown, however, the risk is increased by long-term therapy.

All natural products are to be used with caution or are contraindicated in patients with leukopenia, thrombocytopenia, or anemia caused by previous chemotherapy or radiation therapy, hepatotoxicity, renal toxicity, and known hypersensitivity.

1. *Asparaginase* can cause serious allergic reactions, and cross-sensitivity has been reported between the commercial product and the investigational product derived from *Erwinia carotovora*. A negative skin test *does not* preclude the possibility of an allergic reaction. Asparaginase is contraindicated in patients with pancreatitis or a history of pancreatitis.
2. *Bleomycin* has caused idiosyncratic reactions, similar to anaphylaxis, in lymphoma patients. The reaction consists of hypotension, confusion, fever, chills, sweating, and wheezing and may be immediate or delayed but usually occurs after the first or second dose.
3. *Bleomycin* sensitizes lung tissue to oxygen; caution should be observed in patients receiving general anesthesia who were previously treated with bleomycin, because pulmonary fibrosis may occur postoperatively even at safe oxygen concentrations.
4. *Dactinomycin* should be used only in infants older than 6 months due to an increased incidence of adverse effects in infants.
5. Dosage of *daunorubicin* should be reduced in patients with impaired hepatic and renal function (see Table 75-11). The cardiotoxicity of daunorubicin increases with high cumulative doses (see Table 75-13).
6. *Doxorubicin* produces greater and more frequent cardiotoxicity in children under 2 years of age and adults over 70 years of age (see Table 75-13).
7. The dosage of *doxorubicin* should be reduced in patients with impaired hepatic function (see Table 75-11).
8. *Etoposide* is excreted in breast milk, and breast-feeding is not recommended.
9. *Plicamycin* is contraindicated in patients with thrombocytopenia, thrombocytopathy, coagulation disorders, and any conditions that increase hemorrhagic tendencies.
10. *Mitoxantrone* can cause cardiac toxicity (congestive heart failure, decreased left ventricular ejection fraction) and must be given with caution to patients with pre-existing cardiac disease.

INTERACTIONS
1. Most natural products may antagonize the effects of antigout medications (probenecid, sulfinpyrazone) by increasing serum uric acid levels; dosage adjustment of the antigout medications may be necessary.
2. Concurrent use of asparaginase and methotrexate may block the antineoplastic action of methotrexate by inhibiting cell synthesis. Administer asparaginase 9 days to 10 days before or within 24 hours after administering methotrexate; the toxic effect of methotrexate may also be reduced.
3. The concurrent administration of asparaginase, vincristine, and prednisone may enhance the hyperglycemic effect, neurotoxicity, and myelosuppression of asparaginase. Toxicity

does not appear to be enhanced when asparaginase is administered after vincristine and prednisone.

4. Because asparaginase causes hyperglycemia, dosage adjustment of hypoglycemic medications may be necessary during asparaginase therapy.

5. Raynaud's phenomenon has occurred in patients with testicular carcinoma being treated with a combination of bleomycin and vinblastine. It is unknown whether the cause is the disease, the chemotherapeutic agents, or a combination of these factors.

6. Dactinomycin may decrease the effect of vitamin K, requiring an increase in the dose of vitamin K and close observation of the patient.

7. Daunorubicin is incompatible with heparin sodium and dexamethasone phosphate when mixed together.

8. Concurrent use of cyclophosphamide, dactinomycin, or mitomycin with doxorubicin may result in increased cardiotoxicity. The total dose of doxorubicin should not exceed 400 mg/m^2.

9. Doxorubicin is incompatible in solution with aminophylline, cephalothin, dexamethasone, fluorouracil, hydrocortisone, and sodium heparin.

10. Concurrent use of cyclophosphamide or radiation therapy to the mediastinal area with daunorubicin or doxorubicin may increase cardiac toxicity. The total dose of daunorubicin should not exceed 400 mg to 450 mg/m^2, and the total dose of doxorubicin should not exceed 400 mg/m^2.

11. Administration of doxorubicin to a patient who has received daunorubicin, or vice versa, increases the risk of cardiotoxicity. Neither agent should be used in a patient who has previously received complete cumulative doses of the other agent.

12. Concurrent use of vincristine with doxorubicin and prednisone can increase myelosuppression; this combination must be avoided.

13. Patients receiving natural product antineoplastic agents may develop a viral disease following immunization with a live virus vaccine for that disease.

14. Asparaginase may interfere with the interpretation of thyroid function tests by causing a rapid decrease of serum thyroxine-binding globulin within 2 days of administration of the drug; concentrations return to pretreatment

levels within 4 weeks following the last dose of asparaginase.

15. Concurrent use of dactinomycin and radiation therapy may potentiate the effects of both and increase the toxicities of both; lower doses of both are suggested.

16. Concurrent use of doxorubicin with streptozocin may prolong the half-life of doxorubicin, therefore a reduction in dosage of doxorubicin is recommended.

17. The elimination of etoposide may be impaired in patients who have been previously treated with cisplatin.

18. Plicamycin can cause hypoprothrombinemia and inhibit platelet aggregation and therefore increase the risk of hemorrhage in patients receiving warfarin, heparin, thrombolytic agents, aspirin, dextran, dipyridamole, or valproic acid.

19. Concurrent use of vincristine with other neurotoxic drugs and spinal cord radiation therapy may produce increased neurotoxicity.

■ Nursing Process for Natural Products

□ ASSESSMENT

□ Subjective Data

1. Prior to administration of any antineoplastic a complete medication history should be taken. Natural products may alter the effectiveness of antigout medication even if patient has previously been stabilized.

2. Patients receiving asparaginase should be alerted to possible changes in response to hypoglycemic agents. This includes patients who may have a history of hyperglycemia controlled by diet.

3. Several drugs in this classification, including asparaginase, dactinomycin, and plicamycin, may directly affect clotting abilities. These may interfere with factors necessary for effective clotting, and an alteration in anticoagulant dosage may be necessary. Most drugs in this class also cause thrombocytopenia. Other drugs affecting platelet count and function, such as aspirin, should be carefully evaluated for potential harm to the patient due to hemorrhage. Concurrent narcotic use may potentiate the development of constipation due to vin-

(Text continues on p. 1454.)

Table 75-12
Fate of Natural Products

Drug	Absorption/Distribution/Half-Life	Metabolism	Excretion

asparaginase	Distributed primarily in plasma; only 1% crosses blood–brain barrier
	Low protein binding
	Half-life
	   Intramuscular—39 h–49 h
	   Intravenous—8 h–30 h
		Hepatic sequestration by the reticuloendothelial system	Uncertain—Only trace amount in urine

bleomycin	Distributed primarily to skin, lungs, kidneys, peritoneum, and lymphatics following IV injection
	Very low protein binding
	45%–50% of intrapleural or intraperitoneal dose is systemically absorbed
	Half-life
	   Initial—10 min–20 min
	   Terminal—2 h–4 h
	Continuous IV infusion increases half-life
		Inactivated in liver and kidney tissue by the enzyme bleomycin-hydrolase (skin and lung tissue do not contain this enzyme)	Renal—50%–80% in 24 h primarily unchanged

dactinomycin	Widely distributed into tissues; does not cross blood–brain barrier Highly bound in tissue Half-life—36 h	Minimal	Renal—10%–30% Biliary—50%

daunorubicin	Widely and rapidly distributed to spleen kidney, liver, lungs, and heart; does not cross blood–brain barrier
	Half-life
	   Initial—45 min
	   Terminal—18 h
	   Daunorubicinol (active metabolite) has terminal half-life of 26 h
		Rapidly metabolized in liver to active metabolite daunorubicinol	Renal—14%–23% over 72 h
			Biliary—40%

doxorubicin	Widely distributed to liver, lungs, heart, kidneys, and other tissues but does not cross blood–brain barrier
	Half-life
	doxorubicin
	   Initial—30 min
	   Terminal—17 h
	adriamycinol (active metabolite)
	   Initial—3 h
	   Terminal—32 h
		Rapidly metabolized in liver and other tissues to adriamycinol, an active metabolite	Bile and feces—40%–50% in 7 days
			Renal—5% in 5 days unchanged

(continued)

Table 75-12 (continued)
Fate of Natural Products

Drug	Absorption/Distribution/Half-Life	Metabolism	Excretion

etoposide	Distributed into intestine, lung, liver, kidney, thyroid, skin, bone marrow, and low and variable concentrations in CSF
	Highly protein bound
	Half-life
	  Initial—½ h–3 h
	  Terminal—3 h–19 h
		Probably hepatic	Renal—40%–60% primarily unchanged
			Fecal—2%–16%

mitomycin	Distributed into kidneys, muscles, eyes, lungs, intestines, and stomach; does not cross blood–brain barrier
	Half-life
	  Initial—5 min–15 min
	  Terminal—50 min
		Rapidly inactivated in liver and somewhat in kidney	Renal—Primarily as metabolites
			Biliary—Small amount

mitoxantrone	Tissue distribution is extensive, but does not cross blood-brain barrier Half-life—5–6 days Protein binding—75%–80%	Hepatic—converted to two inactive metabolites	Biliary—at least 25% Renal—5%–10%
plicamycin	Distributed to Kupffer's cells of the liver, renal tubular cells, along formed bone surfaces and may localize in areas of active bone resorption. Crosses the blood–brain barrier Half-life unknown Duration of action—3 days–3 weeks or longer	Unknown	Renal

vinblastine	Rapidly distributed to body tissues and concentrated in platelets and leukocytes
	Does not cross blood–brain barrier
	Highly protein bound
	Half-life
	  Initial—1 h
	  Terminal—20 h
		Metabolized in liver to active metabolite desacetylvinblastine	Biliary primary
			Renal secondary

vincristine	Rapidly and widely distributed; crosses blood–brain barrier in very low concentrations
	Highly protein bound
	Half-life—triphasic
	  alpha—4 min–5 min
	  beta—1 h–3 h
	  gamma—23 h–85 h
		Hepatic	Biliary—60%–70%
			Renal—10% excreted as active drug and metabolites

Table 75-13
Side-Effects/Adverse Reactions of Natural Products

Drug	Alopecia/Dermatologic	Gastrointestinal	Hepatic
asparaginase	Rash Rarely alopecia	Mild nausea and vomiting Stomatitis	Occurs in up to 80% of patients within 2 weeks Liver function tests may be increased and liver shows fatty changes
bleomycin	Diffuse alopecia usually several weeks after therapy Mucocutaneous toxicity characterized by hyperpigmentation, thickening of skin, pruritis, rash, urticaria on fingertips, elbows, palms, skin tenderness, erythematous swelling of fingers—occurs in 25%–50% of patients 2 weeks–4 weeks after first dose and usually after cumulative dose of 150 U–200 U	Stomatitis Mild nausea and vomiting	Rare
dactinomycin	Alopecia usually 7 days–10 days after dose Skin necrosis if extravasation occurs Rash Erythema from previous radiation therapy may be reactivated	Severe nausea and vomiting usually within 1 h–3 h lasting 4 h–20 h Stomatitis Diarrhea	Rare
daunorubicin	Alopecia (complete) Extravasation causes skin necrosis	Moderate to severe nausea and vomiting starting soon after dose and lasting 24 h–48 h Stomatitis Diarrhea	Rare
doxorubicin	Alopecia Extravasation causes skin necrosis Hyperpigmentation of nailbeds, soles and, palms Erythema from previous radiation therapy may be reactivated	Moderate to severe nausea and vomiting Stomatitis Esophagitis Occasional diarrhea Ulceration and necrosis of colon have occurred in patients receiving doxorubicin and cytarabine for acute myelogenous leukemia	Rare

Myelosuppression	Neurologic	Renal	Other
Rare	CNS—confusion, drowsiness, hallucinations, depression, nervousness, tiredness Usually in adults (30%–60%) occurs with first day of treatment and subsides 1 day–3 days after treatment ends	Azotemia—Rare	Anaphylaxis; pancreatitis; hypofibrinogenemia due to decrease in Factors V and VIII and some decrease in Factors VII and IX Low fibrinogen levels cause prolonged thrombin, prothrombin, and partial prothrombin times; however, bleeding is only rarely a problem
Mild leukopenia and thrombocytopenia Nadir—10 days Recovery—18 days			Pneumonitis progressing to pulmonary fibrosis—occurs in 10%–40% of patients usually after 4 weeks–10 weeks of therapy. More frequent in patients over age 70 or who received >400 U; has been reported in patients who received as low as 30 U–60 U Fever and chills—frequent; usually 3 h–6 h after dose and lasts 4 h–12 h; less frequent after repeated doses
Leukopenia, thrombocytopenia Nadir—14 days–21 days Recovery—21 days–25 days		Uric acid nephropathy	Anaphylactoid reactions have occurred
Leukopenia and thrombocytopenia Nadir—10 days–14 days Recovery—21 days		Uric acid nephropathy	Cardiotoxicity—usually CHF; more frequent if adult dose > 550 mg/m^2 or children >2 yrs dose >300 mg/m^2 or children <2 yrs dose >10 mg/kg or patient has a history of cardiac disease or mediastinal radiation Usually occurs 1 month–6 months after initiation of therapy and onset may be sudden
Leukopenia and thrombocytopenia Nadir—10 days–14 days Recovery—21 days		Uric acid nephropathy	Cardiotoxicity—Acute, transient with abnormal ECG findings and arrhythmias or chronic, cumulative progressing to CHF as doses approach 550 mg/m^2. Usually occurs 1 month–6 months after initiation of therapy and onset may be sudden; may *(continued)*

Table 75-13 (continued)
Side-Effects/Adverse Reactions of Natural Products

Drug	Alopecia/Dermatologic	Gastrointestinal	Hepatic
doxorubicin *(continued)*			
etoposide	Alopecia Rash (rare)	Moderate nausea and vomiting Diarrhea Stomatitis—More likely to occur with high dose or previous radiation therapy to head and neck	Rare
mitomycin	Alopecia Extravasation causes skin necrosis Rash Purple-colored bands on nails with repeated doses	Mild to moderate nausea and vomiting Stomatitis	Rare
mitoxantrone	Alopecia Rash/urticaria (rare)	Nausea, vomiting, diarrhea Stomatitis, mucositis Abdominal pain (rare)	Rare
plicamycin	Extravasation causes skin necrosis Rash Hyperpigmentation	Severe nausea and vomiting occurs within 1 h–2 h and lasts 12 h–24 h (severity is increased by rapid administration) Stomatitis Diarrhea	Daily dosing commonly hepatic toxicity Discontinue therapy if AST (SGOT) concentration >600 units/ml or LDH >2000 units/ml
vinblastine	Alopecia (partial) Extravasation causes skin necrosis Phototoxicity	Moderate nausea and vomiting Diarrhea, constipation, abdominal pain, adynamic ileus, stomatitis, rectal bleeding, bleeding from old peptic ulcer	

Myelosuppression	Neurologic	Renal	Other
			be irreversible and fatal, responds to treatment if detected early Anaphylaxis (rare)

Leukopenia
  Nadir—7 days–14 days
  Recovery—21 days
Thrombocytopenia
  Nadir—9 days–16 days
  Recovery—20 days
	CNS—Weakness, somnolence, peripheral neuropathy in <1% of patients		Hypotension following rapid IV administration (infuse slowly over 30 min–60 min)
			Anaphylaxis in up to 2% of patients (fever, chills, bronchospasm, dyspnea, tachycardia, hypo- or hypertension)

Appears to be cumulative; more profound and prolonged after repeated doses
Leukopenia
  Nadir—42 days
  Recovery—70 days–84 days
Thrombocytopenia
  Nadir—28 days–42 days
  Recovery—70 days–84 days
About 25% of patients do not recover to pretreatment levels
		Occurs in 2% of patients with rise in BUN or serum creatinine	Pulmonary toxicity (hypertrophy of alveolar cells)
			Syndrome of microangiopathic hemolytic anemia with thrombocytopenia; renal failure and pulmonary hypertension has occurred with long-term (6 months–12 months) therapy.

Has been reported	Seizures (rare) Headache		Cough/dyspnea in up to 15% of patients Cardiotoxicity—congestive heart failure (5%), arrhythmias (3%–4%) Conjunctivitis Fever is very common (75%) Sepsis and other infections can occur

Mild leukopenia and thrombocytopenia
  Nadir—14 days
  Recovery—21 days–28 days
	CNS toxicity (infrequent) headache, irritability, akathesia, lethargy	Tubular necrosis (more frequent with daily therapy) may occur in 20% of patients	Hemorrhagic diathesis—Facial flushing, epistaxis, thrombocytopenia, prolonged prothrombin time, hematemesis, and generalized GI hemorrhage—much more frequent in patients receiving doses >0.03 mg/kg/day or more than 10 doses

Leukopenia
  Nadir—5 days–10 days
  Recovery—7 days–14 days
Thrombocytopenia—Mild and rapid recovery
	High-dose, long-term therapy can cause toxicity of autonomic, central, and peripheral nervous systems in 10% of patients (numbness, paresthesia, depression, loss of deep tendon reflexes, headache, malaise, weakness, dizzi-		Bronchospasm may occur a few minutes to several hours after administration to patients previously treated with mitomycin.

(continued)

Table 75-13 (continued)
Side-Effects/Adverse Reactions of Natural Products

Drug	Alopecia/Dermatologic	Gastrointestinal	Hepatic
vinblastine (continued)			
vincristine	Alopecia (20%–70% of patients) Rash Extravasation causes skin necrosis	Mild nausea and vomiting Stomatitis (infrequent) Constipation—May be upper colon impaction Paralytic ileus—More common in children	

Myelosuppression	Neurologic	Renal	Other
	ness, double vision, seizures, face and jaw pain, urinary retention, orthostatic hypotension, pain in fingers, toes, or testicles		
Leukopenia and thrombocytopenia rarely occur at usual doses and are mild with rapid recovery if they do occur	Peripheral nervous system toxicity may occur in 90%–100% of patients—earliest sign is loss of the Achilles reflex, followed by loss of other deep tendon reflexes; numbness, pain, tingling. Long-term, high-dose therapy may cause wrist drop, foot drop, atrophy, cramps, ataxia, a slapping gait, difficulty walking, cranial nerve palsies (facial and jaw pain, hoarseness or vocal cord paresis, ptosis, double vision, optic atrophy, blindness, transient cortical blindness) Autonomic nervous system toxicity may occur in 50% of patients—Constipation, adynamic ileus, cramps, incontinence, urinary retention, nocturia, oliguria, dysuria, polyuria, orthostatic hypotension, abnormal Valsalva response, defective sweating. Central nervous system toxicity may occur in 50% of patients—Altered consciousness, depression, agitation, insomnia, hallucinations, seizures (frequently with hypertension), progressive encephalopathy, respiratory problems, coma Recovery from neurotoxicity occurs with discontinuance of drug—paresthesias are reversible, deep tendon reflexes may not recover and other neurologic problems may persist for months	Uric acid nephropathy	Syndrome of inappropriate antidiuretic hormone (SIADH) secretion may occur rarely. Bronchospasm may occur a few minutes to several hours after administration to patients previously treated with mitomycin.

cristine. Several factors have been associated with increased risk of toxicity from this classification of drug. Patients known to have such risk factors should be closely monitored.

4. Cumulative drug administration may result in more frequent occurrence of side-effects. With vincristine, neuropathies become more frequent at higher doses. Cardiac complications are seen more frequently with total doses over 550 mg/m^2 with daunorubicin and 450 mg/m^2 with doxorubicin. Pre-existing cardiac disease may result in more frequent congestive heart failure with these drugs. Pulmonary fibrosis increases with dose escalations more than 300 mg/m^2 of bleomycin. Interstitial pneumonitis is seen more frequently in patients receiving bleomycin who are older than age 70 and those who have pre-existing pulmonary disease.

5. A family or personal history of hyperglycemia may increase the likelihood of hyperglycemia related to asparaginase.

□ *Objective Data*

1. Physical Assessment—As always, a thorough physical assessment must precede administration of any antineoplastic agent. The following systems are potentially affected by this class of drug:

    Neurologic—vincristine, vinblastine
    CNS—vincristine, vinblastine
    Pulmonary—bleomycin, mitomycin
    Hematopoietic—All drugs (rare with asparaginase)
    GI—All drugs
    Mouth—bleomycin, dactinomycin, plicamycin, vincristine, vinblastine
    Cardiac—doxorubicin, daunorubicin, daunomycin
    Dermatologic—bleomycin, dactinomycin, doxorubicin, mitomycin
    Renal—plicamycin, mitomycin
    Hepatic—Metabolized doxorubicin, mitomycin, plicamycin, asparaginase

2. Laboratory Data and Diagnostic Tests
    Baseline studies
    · CBC, differential, platelet count
    · BUN, creatinine
    · Liver function tests, especially with doxorubicin and daunorubicin
    · EKG
    · Prior to treatment with daunorubicin or doxorubicin if question of cardiac function—cardiac ejection fraction
    · Pulmonary function tests—bleomycin

□ *NURSING DIAGNOSIS*

Actual nursing diagnoses for the patient receiving natural products include:
    Knowledge deficit related to chemotherapy regimen
Potential nursing diagnoses include:
    Potential for infection
    Potential for injury related to thrombocytopenia or extravasation
    Potential for physical injury related to neurologic deficits
    Alteration in nutrition: less than body requirements
    Alteration in oral mucous membranes
    Potential fluid volume deficit
    Potential impairment of skin integrity
    Alteration in bowel elimination: constipation
    Impaired gas exchange
    Alteration in cardiac output: decreased
    Alteration in comfort: pain

□ *PLAN*

The main goals of nursing care focus on the following:

1. To teach the patient to follow necessary treatment

2. To provide the patient with information about the early symptoms of side-effects which require notification of the health team.

3. To develop and use strategies to minimize side-effects of drug therapy

□ *INTERVENTIONS*

It is very important that natural products are administered appropriately.

The most serious concern is proper administration of sclerosing agents (vesicants), including dactinomycin, daunorubicin, doxorubicin, mitomycin, plicamycin, vinblastine, and vincristine. Improper technique, resulting in tissue infiltration of drug, can cause severe tissue destruction, including the nerves and tendons. These drugs can permanently impair function and potentially result in loss of a limb. For proper administration, care of extravasation and antidotes, see section on extravasation earlier in this chapter.

Anaphylaxis during administration is also a concern with several drugs in this classification. Asparaginase can cause anaphylactic shock. This is more common with IV than IM administration, on repeated doses, and when administered over a prolonged period of time. Some sources recommend intradermal skin testing prior to initiation of therapy or when more than 7 days have elapsed, but a negative skin test does not preclude the development of an anaphylactic response.

Prior to administration of intravenous antihistamines (e.g., diphenhydramine), steroids, epinephrine, and oxygen should be on hand. Drug administration should be discontinued if urticaria, pruritus, or respiratory difficulty develops, and the physician should be notified immediately. For IM administration, use of an upper extremity may decrease the severity of reaction and enable better control. The patient should be observed closely for at least 1 hour after administration by any route.

Some patients may receive asparaginase derived from *Erwinia* after development of hypersensitivity reactions. These patients should be watched closely, but cross-sensitivity is not expected.

Anaphylactic reaction is also reported in 1% of lymphoma patients receiving bleomycin for the first time. This reaction may occur immediately or several hours later. This should *not* be confused with the frequently occurring fever and chills. The anaphylactic reaction includes fever, urticaria, wheezing, and shock. Some sources recommend that the patient receive a test dose before the first dose. Prior to the first administration intravenous diphenhydramine, epinephrine, steroids, and oxygen should be readily available. The physician should evaluate the patient because life hemodynamic support may be necessary.

Anaphylaxis has also been rarely noted with etoposide and dactinomycin.

Hypotension with too-rapid infusion has occurred with etoposide. Infusions must be monitored closely. Vital signs, particularly pulse and blood pressure, should be observed closely for change indicating hypotension. The rate of infusion should be decreased if signs of hypotension develop. The patient should be encouraged to change position slowly, immediately after infusion.

□ *Side-Effects and Patient Education*

Many of the natural products cause similar side-effects. These drugs can cause varying degrees of nausea, vomiting, alopecia, and myelosuppression. The nursing management of these side-effects is discussed under Nursing Process for Antineoplastic drugs.

The following are side-effects that commonly occur with a few of these drugs.

Pulmonary pneumonitis leading to pulmonary fibrosis can occur with bleomycin, particularly when the dose is greater than 300 U/m^2. The patient should be instructed to report any increase in shortness of breath, change in exercise tolerance, or dry unproductive cough. Careful respiratory assessment and attention to any change in symptomatology are essential.

Cardiac toxicity can occur with doxorubicin or daunorubicin. This toxicity is demonstrated by acute congestive heart failure (CHF) and EKG abnormalities. The patient should be taught to report immediately any new signs of CHF (leg or ankle swelling, cough, shortness of breath, or sudden weight gain) or rhythm disorders (palpitations, new dizziness). Patients at high risk for developing cardiac toxicity should be taught to take their pulse and report abnormalities. Family members of those at high risk should be taught how to perform cardiopulmonary resuscitation and how to obtain emergency care if necessary. Patients who develop early signs of CHF should be instructed to keep legs raised and not obstructed by crossing when sitting, to avoid tight socks, and to limit sodium intake.

Hyperpigmentation is medically harmless but alarming to the patient and his self-image. Similar to loss of hair, hyperpigmentation may have different degrees of meaning to various patients. Daunorubicin can cause hyperpigmentation limited to the soles of the feet, hands, and nailbeds. Plicamycin can cause a generalized pigmentation as can bleomycin, which may also cause darkening along vein of administration and possibly rash characterized by pruritus and urticaria. Mitomycin can cause purple-colored bands on the nails. The patient should be reassured that with the exception of generalized rash due to bleomycin, these discolorations are not permanent and will fade over time.

If the patient develops generalized pruritus and rash, the physician should be notified. Patients should be taught to report any rash, redness or tightness of skin, particularly on hands. Supportive measures to relieve pruritus and swelling should be implemented until rash subsides. The patient should be taught to report immediately any ulcerations or inability to move joints, particularly in the fingers.

Hypofibrinogenemia is a serious side-effect which can occur with asparaginase and plicamycin. This side-effect is marked by inability or marked slowness in appropriate clotting due to lack of clotting factors. The patient should be taught to report immediately any bleeding, such as bruising of the skin, epistaxis, or bleeding from old injury sites. The patient should be taught to test the stool for blood and to be alert for prolonged menstrual bleeding. Family members should be advised to be alert for any change in consciousness or function which may indicate central nervous system bleeding. Patients should be made aware of potential need for transfusion of supplemental clotting factors.

Patients who receive daunorubicin or doxorubicin during or after radiation therapy may experience erythema of the radiated site. The patient should be instructed that this reaction will subside. Cooling, nonirritating solutions may provide symptomatic relief. The patient should be instructed to avoid prolonged direct sun exposure to these areas.

Patients receiving bleomycin may experience fever and shaking chills 3 hours to 6 hours after administration. Patients should be instructed to take diphenhydramine and acetaminophen every 4 hours for approximately 12 hours and advised to report high temperature or chills that persist more than 24 hours after administration.

Severe neurotoxicity can occur with vincristine or vinblastine. Patients should be instructed to report any numbness or tingling, however slight. Patients should also be taught proper bowel regimens to ensure daily stools. This may require stool softeners, bulk laxatives, and instruction on dietary fiber. Failure to maintain adequate bowel management may result in development of constipation and paralytic ileus. Family members should be taught to watch for signs of changes in dexterity while dressing or changes in gait while walking. The patient should be taught that neurotoxicity may be progressive until the drug is stopped. The effect on peripheral nerves may limit ability to perform routine tasks, such as buttoning buttons or using eating utensils. Gait may also be affected. If the neurotoxicity is debilitating, physical therapy may be necessary. The patient should be reassured that recovery will occur but paresthesias will disappear slowly over several months.

In more severe neurotoxicity, central nervous system dysfunction may occur, resulting in altered consciousness, seizures, agitation, and loss of deep tendon reflexes. Patient and family should be instructed to report any changes in consciousness, mood, and personality immediately. These effects may take months to disappear after cessation of drug.

Hyperglycemia may occur with asparaginase. The patient should be taught signs and symptoms of hyperglycemia, how to test urine, and how to eat a no concentrated sweets diet.

□ *EVALUATION*

The outcome criteria to measure the effectiveness of treatment may include:

1. The patient will report adverse side-effects promptly to health-care providers.
2. Patient will perform interventions necessary to minimize side-effects.

Hormonal, Antihormonal, and Gonadotropin-Releasing Hormone Analogue Agents

Hormonal agents are of value in the treatment of a number of neoplastic diseases, primarily prostatic and breast carcinomas. Carcinomas arising from the prostate or mammary glands often retain some of the hormonal requirements of the normal glands for a period of time; altering the hormonal environment of such carcinomas by the administration of natural or synthetic hormonal agents makes it possible to alter the neoplastic process and delay tumor growth. Hormonal agents are not curative, however, because most lack cytotoxic action. Still, they may provide the patient with prolonged palliation without major toxicities.

The principal hormones used as antineoplastic agents are the sex hormones (androgens, estrogens, progestins) and the corticosteroids. Androgens, derivatives of testosterone, are used for the palliative treatment of advanced or disseminated breast cancer in postmenopausal women when hormonal therapy is indicated. The androgens discussed in this section include the oral preparations (fluoxymesterone, methyltestosterone, testolactone) and long-acting injectables (dromostanolone propionate, testosterone cypionate, testosterone enanthate, testosterone propionate).

Estrogens are used for the palliative treatment of postmenopausal breast cancer, advanced prostatic cancer, and male breast cancer in selected patients. The estrogens reviewed in this section include the estradiol compounds whose steroidal structures closely resemble the natural hormone, estramustine, a phosphorylated combination of estradiol and mechlorethamine, and several nonsteroidal agents possessing estrogenic activity, such as chlorotrianisene and diethylstilbestrol (DES).

Progestins are steroidal compounds related to the natural hormone progesterone. Progestins have been used in the palliative treatment of carcinoma of the breast, endometrium, and renal cells. The progestational agents discussed in this section include hydroxyprogesterone caproate, medroxyprogesterone acetate, and megestrol acetate.

Corticosteroids are synthetic steroidal agents derived from the natural adrenal hormone cortisol (hydrocortisone). Corticosteroids, primarily prednisone, are used frequently in combination chemotherapy regimens for the treatment of acute and chronic lymphocytic leukemia, Hodgkin's and non-Hodgkin's lymphomas, multiple myeloma, and some breast cancers.

In addition to the hormonal agents, four other agents are considered in this section as well. Aminoglutethimide is an antiadrenal agent used in the palliative treatment of postmenopausal breast carcinoma and prostatic carcinoma. Mitotane, a derivative of the insecticide DDT, is an antineoplastic agent with antiadrenal action used in the palliative treatment of inoperable adrenocortical carcinoma. Tamoxifen, a nonsteroidal antiestrogen, is used for the palliative treatment of advanced breast cancer in postmenopausal women with estrogen receptor (ER) positive tumors. Leuprolide is a gonadotropin-releasing hormone analogue used in the palliative treatment of advanced prostatic cancer when orchiectomy or estrogen therapy is either not indicated or is unacceptable to the patient.

MECHANISM AND ACTIONS

Hormones

Androgens—The exact mechanism of the antitumor effect of androgens is unknown. It is thought that exogenous administration of androgens inhibits the release of endogenous testosterone by feedback inhibition of pituitary luteinizing hormone (LH). The lack of endogenous testosterone, an immediate precursor of estrogens in the biosynthetic pathway, results in an androgen-induced estrogen depletion, the most highly favored mechanism of action.

In most cases, hormone receptors must be present in the tumor cell cytosol for androgens to be effective. A second mechanism of action suggests that androgens may bind to the hormonal receptor site, competitively inhibiting the binding of estrogen. The androgen complex is transported into the cell nucleus and blocks normal cell growth by inhibiting the transport of estrogen into the cell.

Estrogens—The exact mechanism of the antitumor effect of estrogens is unknown. It is known that estrogen-responsive tissues contain intracellular cytosol-binding proteins which bind estrogen;

these estrogen-binding protein complexes translocate into the cell nucleus and block normal growth of the cell. Estrogens can also cause regression of some tumors by suppressing normal pituitary function. In males with prostatic cancer, estrogens decrease the amount of LH secreted by the pituitary, which in turn decreases the amount of androgen secreted by the testes. The antitumor effects of estramustine may be due to (1) estradiol, (2) the alkylating activity of mechlorethamine, (3) a direct effect of estramustine, or (4) a combination of these effects.

Progestins—The exact mechanism of progestin antitumor activity is unknown. Progestins may have a direct local effect on hormonally sensitive endometrial cells and may also decrease the amount of LH secreted by the pituitary gland. The antineoplastic effect of progestins on carcinoma of the breast is unknown.

Corticosteroids—Corticosteroids produce their antitumor effects by binding to corticosteroid receptors present in high numbers on lymphoid tumors. This binding appears to inhibit both cellular glucose transport and phosphorylation, which decreases the amount of energy available for mitosis and protein synthesis, ultimately resulting in cell lysis.

Antihormonal Agents

Aminoglutethimide blocks the conversion of cholesterol to pregnenolone by inhibiting the desmolase complex enzyme system in adrenal mitochondria, thus blocking the biosynthesis of all steroid hormones. Additionally, aminoglutethimide blocks the conversion of androgens to estrogens in peripheral tissues by blocking the aromatase enzyme. The net result is a medical adrenalectomy due to the complete suppression of the adrenal cortex by aminoglutethimide.

Mitotane—The exact mechanisms of action of mitotane are not known. A direct cytotoxic effect may be due to the covalent bonding of mitotane metabolites to mitochondrial proteins causing focal lesions in the fascicular and reticular zones of the adrenal cortex with resultant atrophy. Mitotane may also cause adrenal inhibition without cellular destruction; levels of adrenocorticoids and their metabolites are decreased, and the extra-adrenal metabolism of endogenous and exogenous steroids is altered.

Tamoxifen is a nonsteroidal estrogen antagonist with weak estrogenic effects. Tamoxifen competitively inhibits estradiol uptake by binding to estrogen receptor sites in the cytosol of the cell. This complex is translocated to the nucleus of the cell where it acts as a false messenger and ultimately inhibits DNA synthesis. Tamoxifen is unlikely to cause a response in patients who have had a negative estrogen receptor (ER) assay.

Gonadotropin-Releasing Hormone Analogue
Leuprolide is a gonadotropin-releasing hormone (GnRH) analogue that has the same action as the naturally occurring hormone. Long-term administration of leuprolide causes inhibition of gonadotropin secretion and suppression of ovarian and testicular steroidogenesis. Leuprolide produces a decrease in the number of pituitary GnRH or testicular luteinizing hormone (LH) receptors, which causes pituitary or testicular desensitization, respectively. Leuprolide may also inhibit the enzymes necessary for steroidogenesis.

In males, leuprolide decreases serum LH, follicle-stimulating hormone (FSH), testosterone, and dihydrotestosterone levels, with serum testosterone levels reaching castration levels after 2 weeks to 4 weeks of continuous therapy. In females, leuprolide decreases serum LH, FSH, progesterone, and estrogen levels by suppressing ovarian estrogen and androgen production by inhibiting pituitary gonadotropin release; serum estrogen levels in premenopausal women may be reduced to postmenopausal levels after 2 weeks to 4 weeks of therapy.

USES
See Table 75-14.

ADMINISTRATION AND DOSAGE
See Table 75-16.

FATE
The fate of the androgen, estrogen, progestin, and corticosteroid agents are reviewed in Chapters 58, 56, and 55, respectively. Only those androgen, estrogen, and progestin agents used primarily as antineoplastic agents will be reviewed in Table 75-15 along with the antihormonal and gonadotropin-releasing hormone analogue agents.

SIDE-EFFECTS/ADVERSE REACTIONS
The common side-effects and significant adverse reactions of the androgen, estrogen, progestin, and corticosteroid agents are reviewed in Chapters 58, 56, and 55, respectively. Only those side-effects of androgen, estrogen, and progestin agents used *primarily* as antineoplastic agents will be reviewed in

Table 75-16 along with the antihormonal and gonadotropin-releasing hormone analogue agents. For a complete list of all side-effects and adverse reactions of each agent, see the manufacturer's product information.

CONTRAINDICATIONS AND PRECAUTIONS
All antineoplastic agents have the potential to be carcinogenic (due to direct cellular action or immunosuppression) and to cause testicular and ovarian suppression. The exact effect of dose and duration of therapy is unknown, however, the risk is increased by long-term therapy. The contraindications and precautions listed apply to the use of these agents as antineoplastic drugs.

1. Androgens are contraindicated in carcinoma of the male breast, known or suspected prostatic cancer, and premenopausal women.
2. Estrogens are contraindicated in men or women with known or suspected cancer of the breast, except in appropriately selected patients being treated for metastatic disease.
3. Estrogen usage is contraindicated in known or suspected estrogen-dependent neoplasia.
4. Estrogen and progestin usage is contraindicated in active thrombophlebitis or thromboembolic disorders and in markedly impaired liver function.
5. The progestins hydroxyprogesterone and medroxyprogesterone are contraindicated in known or suspected breast carcinoma, known or suspected genital malignancy, and undiagnosed vaginal bleeding.

(See Chaps. 55, 56, and 58 for additional information on contraindications of hormonal agents.)

6. Dromostanolone should be used with caution in patients with liver disease, cardiac decompensation, nephritis, and nephrosis.
7. The use of progestins during the first 4 months of pregnancy is contraindicated because they may cause fetal harm.
8. Aminoglutethimide has been designated FDA pregnancy category D, indicating there is positive evidence of increased fetal deaths and teratogenic effects.
9. Aminoglutethimide is contraindicated in patients with a hypersensitivity to glutethimide (Doriden).
10. Aminoglutethimide should be used with caution in children because it may induce precocious sexual development in males and masculinization and hirsutism in females.

11. Mitotane should be administered with caution to patients with liver disease other than metastasis of adrenal carcinoma; the metabolism of mitotane may be reduced resulting in accumulation of the drug.

12. It may be advisable to stop mitotane therapy following shock, severe trauma, or infection and to administer steroids due to the adrenocortical insufficiency caused by mitotane.

13. Leuprolide should be used with extreme caution in patients with life-threatening disease, because exacerbation of signs and symptoms may have resulted in rapid death of two patients receiving *another* GnRH analogue for prostatic carcinoma.

14. Patients receiving leuprolide who have vertebral metastasis or urinary obstruction should be observed closely during the first few weeks of therapy for weakness and paresthesias of the legs or worsening of hematuria and urinary obstruction.

15. Erythema and induration may occur at the injection site of leuprolide in patients with known hypersensitivity to benzyl alcohol used as a preservative in the vehicle.

INTERACTIONS

1. The androgens, particularly fluoxymesterone and methyltestosterone, may increase sensitivity to anticoagulants. The dosage of the anticoagulant may have to be decreased.

2. Androgens may enhance the hypoglycemic effect of antidiabetic agents.

3. Estrogens may reduce the effect of oral anticoagulants by increasing certain clotting factors in the blood.

4. The anticonvulsants carbamazepine, phenobarbital, phenytoin, and primidone may reduce the effect of estrogens due to increased estrogen metabolism caused by the induction of liver enzymes.

5. Concurrent use of rifampin and estrogens may result in decreased estrogenic activity due to enzyme induction.

6. Large doses of estrogens may enhance the side-effects of tricyclic antidepressants and decrease their antidepressant effect.

7. Corticosteroids, when used concurrently with amphotericin B, may cause increased potassium depletion leading to hypokalemia.

8. Corticosteroids may increase or decrease the response to oral anticoagulants.

9. Corticosteroids cause hyperglycemia and thus may increase requirements for insulin or oral hypoglycemic agents.

10. Ephedrine, phenobarbital, phenytoin, and rifampin enhance the metabolism of corticosteroids through enzyme induction, thus decreasing corticosteroid activity.

11. Patients taking potassium-depleting diuretics and corticosteroids concomitantly may develop hypokalemia.

12. Corticosteroids may decrease blood salicylate levels by increasing glomerular filtration rate and by decreasing tubular reabsorption of water.

13. Mitotane alters corticosteroid metabolism, and higher doses of corticosteroids may be needed to treat adrenal insufficiency.

14. Mitotane and CNS depressants used concurrently may cause additive CNS depression.

15. Aminoglutethimide may decrease the effects of medroxyprogesterone, digitoxin, and theophylline, due to hepatic enzyme induction.

16. Concurrent use of rifampin and progestins may result in decreased progestin activity due to enzyme induction. This interaction may even occur for several days after the discontinuation of rifampin.

17. Aminoglutethimide may decrease the effects of warfarin due to hepatic enzyme induction.

18. Aminoglutethimide accelerates the metabolism of dexamethasone, thereby decreasing the pharmacologic effects of dexamethasone.

19. Mitotane may decrease the effects of phenobarbital, warfarin, and phenytoin due to hepatic microsomal enzyme induction.

20. Concurrent administration of spironolactone with mitotane may block the action of mitotane.

■ *Nursing Process for Hormones, Antihormonals, and Gonadotropin-Releasing Hormone Analogue Agents*

□ *ASSESSMENT*

□ *Subjective Data*

1. Prior to administration of any hormones, antihormones, or gonadotropin-releasing hormones, a thorough medication history should be taken. Many of these drugs may change the effectiveness of anticoagulant therapies. Read-

(Text continues on p. 1464.)

Table 75-14
Hormonal, Antihormonal, and Gonadotropin-Releasing-Hormone Analogue Agents

Drug	Preparations	Usual Dosage Range
Androgens		
dromostanolone proprionate (Drolban)	Injection—50 mg/ml	IM—100 mg three times a week
fluoxymesterone (Android-F, Halotestin, Ora-Testryl)	Tablets—2 mg, 5 mg, 10 mg	10 mg–40 mg/day in divided doses (0.05 mg–1 mg/kg/day)
testolactone (Teslac)	Tablets—50 mg	Oral—250 mg four times a day up to a maximum of 2 g/day
methyltestosterone (Android, Oreton Methyl, Metandren, Testred, Virilon)	Tablets—10 mg, 25 mg Buccal tablets—5 mg, 10 mg	Oral—50 mg–200 mg/day Buccal—25 mg–100 mg/day
testosterone cypionate (Andro-Cyp, Andronate, Depo-Testosterone, Depotest, Duratest, Testoject, and others)	Injection—50 mg/ml, 100 mg/ml, 200 mg/ml	IM—200 mg–400 mg every 2 weeks–4 weeks
testosterone enanthate (Andro-LA, Andryl 200, Delatestryl, Everone, Testrin PA, and others)	Injection—100 mg/ml, 200 mg/ml	IM—200 mg–400 mg every 2 weeks–4 weeks
testosterone propionate (Testex)	Injection—25 mg/ml, 50 mg/ml, 100 mg/ml	IM—50 mg–100 mg three times a week
Estrogens		
chlorotrianisene (Tace)	Capsules—12 mg, 25 mg, 72 mg	Oral—12 mg–25 mg/day
diethylstilbestrol (DES)	Tablets—0.1 mg, 0.25 mg, 0.5 mg, 1 mg, 5 mg (plain and enteric-coated tablets)	Breast cancer: Oral—1 mg–5 mg three times a day Prostatic cancer: Oral—1 mg–3 mg/day initially, then decrease to 1 mg/day
diethylstilbestrol diphosphate (Stilphostrol)	Tablets—50 mg Injection—250 mg/5 ml	Oral—50 mg–200 mg three times a day IV—500 mg on day 1, 1000 mg on days 2 to 5, then 250 mg–500 mg one to two times a week Maintenance—250 mg–500 mg IV once or twice a week
estradiol (Estrace)	Tablets—1 mg, 2 mg	Breast cancer: 10 mg three times a day Prostatic cancer: 1 mg–2 mg three times a day
estradiol cypionate (Depo-Estradiol, Depestro, DepGynogen, Depogen, Dura-Estrin, Estra-D, Estro-Cyp, Estrofem, Estroject-LA, Estronol-LA, Hormogen-Depot)	Injection—1 mg/ml, 5 mg/ml	IM—initially, 1 mg–5 mg/wk Maintenance—2 mg–5 mg every 3 weeks–4 weeks
estradiol valerate (Delestrogen, Dioval, Duragen, Estradiol-LA, Estraval, Gynogen LA, Valergen)	Injection—10 mg/ml, 20 mg/ml, 40 mg/ml	IM—30 mg or more every 1 week–2 weeks

Uses	Clinical Considerations
Advanced breast carcinoma	Indicated for women with inoperable cancer who are 1-year to 5-year postmenopausal; continue treatment 8 weeks–12 weeks to determine efficacy; if disease progresses during first 6 weeks–8 weeks of therapy, consider alternate therapy; fewer androgenic side-effects than testosterone; do not refrigerate; precipitation may occur
Advanced breast carcinoma	See under dromostanolone; higher incidence of biliary stasis and jaundice than other androgens; Halotestin tablets contain tartrazine.
Advanced breast carcinoma in women only	See under dromostanolone; may be used in premenopausal women whose ovarian function has been terminated; devoid of androgenic activity in normal doses
Advanced breast carcinoma	See under dromostanolone; androgenic side-effects are more common; painful, erythematous local reactions can occur at injection site; hypercalcemia may result if patient is immobilized or if bony metastases are present; crystals may develop at low temperatures but warming and shaking will redissolve them; moisture from wet needle or syringe may cloud the solution but potency is not affected
Advanced prostatic carcinoma (DOC)*	Also used for symptomatic treatment of menopausal symptoms and relief of postpartum breast engorgement (72-mg capsules); (see Chap. 56)
Advanced breast and prostatic carcinoma (DOC)	Dosage may be increased in advanced prostatic carcinoma, but incidence of thromboembolic complications increases with doses above 1 mg
Advanced prostatic carcinoma (DOC)	Mix drug in 300 ml 5% dextrose or normal saline solution; administer slowly for 10 min–15 min at 20 drops–30 drops/min; then increase rate to run entire infusion in over 1 h
Advanced breast and prostatic carcinoma	Continue breast cancer treatment for a minimum of 3 months to determine efficacy
Advanced prostatic carcinoma (DOC)	
Advanced prostatic carcinoma (DOC)	

(continued)

Table 75-14 (continued)
Hormonal, Antihormonal, and Gonadotropin-Releasing-Hormone Analogue Agents

Drug	Preparations	Usual Dosage Range
estramustine phosphate sodium (Emcyt)	Capsules—140 mg	14 mg/kg/day in three or four divided doses; maintenance therapy 10 mg–16 mg/kg/day in divided doses

estrogens, conjugated (Estrecon, Premarin, Progens) and estrogens, esterified (Estratab, Menest)	Tablets—0.3 mg, 0.625 mg, 1.25 mg, 2.5 mg	Breast cancer:
		  10 mg three times a day
		Prostatic cancer:
		  1.25 mg–2.5 mg three times a day

estrone (Bestrone, Estrone-A, Estronol, Femogen, Gynogen, Theelin Aqueous)	Injection—2 mg/ml, 5 mg/ml	IM—2 mg–4 mg two to three times a week

ethinyl estradiol (Estinyl, Feminone)	Tablets—0.02 mg, 0.05 mg, 0.5 mg	Breast cancer:
		  1 mg three times a day
		Prostatic cancer:
		  0.15 mg–2 mg/day

polyestradiol phosphate (Estradurin)	Injection—40 mg	IM—40 mg every 2 weeks–4 weeks, may increase to 80 mg

Progestins

hydroxprogesterone caproate (Delalutin, Duralutin, Gesterol LA, Hylutin, Hyprogest, Hyproval P.A., Hyroxon, Pro-Depo)	Injection—125 mg/ml, 250 mg/ml	IM—1 g–7 g/week
medroxyprogesterone acetate (Amen, Curretab, Cycrin, Provera, Depo-Provera)	Tablets—2.5 mg, 5 mg, 10 mg Injection—100 mg/ml, 400 mg/ml	Oral, IM—400 mg–1000 mg/week Maintenance—400 mg/month or adjusted to patient's needs

megestrol acetate (Megace)	Tablets—20 mg, 40 mg	Breast cancer:
		  40 mg four times a day
		Endometrial cancer:
		  40 mg–320 mg/day in four divided doses

Corticosteroids

prednisone (Deltasone, Orasone Liquid Pred, Pediapred, Prednisone Intensol)	Tablets—1 mg, 2.5 mg, 5 mg, 10 mg, 20 mg, 50 mg
	Syrup—5 mg/5 ml
	Solution—5 mg/5 ml
	Solution concentrate—5 mg/ml
		Acute and chronic lymphocytic leukemia:
		  40 mg–60 mg/m^2/day
		Hodgkin's disease and non-Hodgkin's lymphomas:
		  40 mg–100 mg/m^2/day
		Multiple myeloma:
		  75 mg/m^2/day
		Breast cancer:
		  40 mg/m^2/day

Antihormonal Agents

aminoglutethimide (Cytadren)	Tablets—250 mg	Antiadrenal—250 mg two or three times a day for 2 weeks
		  Maintenance—250 mg four times a day every 6 h to a maximum of 2 g/day
		Breast and prostatic cancer—250 mg two or three times a day for 2 weeks
		  Maintenance—250 mg four times a day every 6 h in combination with hydrocortisone 40 mg/day (10 mg in AM, 10 mg at 5 PM, 20 mg at bedtime)

Uses	Clinical Considerations
Advanced prostatic carcinoma	Store in refrigerator and protect from light; continue treatment 1 month–3 months to determine efficacy; may increase serum bilirubin, LDH, and SGOT concentrations
Advanced breast and prostatic carcinoma (DOC)	Continue breast cancer treatment 8 weeks–12 weeks to determine efficacy; determine effectiveness in prostatic cancer by monitoring serum phosphate levels, which should decrease
Advanced prostatic carcinoma (DOC)	Continue treatment for 3 months to determine efficacy
Advanced breast and prostatic carcinoma (DOC)	
Advanced prostatic carcinoma (DOC)	Continue treatment for 3 months to determine efficacy, reconstitute with sterile diluent provided; do not agitate violently; store at room temperature away from light for 10 days and discard at first sign of cloudiness or precipitate
Advanced endometrial carcinoma (stage III or IV)—DOC	Stop therapy when relapse occurs or after 12 weeks with no objective response
Endometrial and renal carcinoma (DOC)	Recommended only as adjunctive and palliative therapy in advanced inoperable cases; usually well tolerated even in large doses; gluteal abscesses have occurred
Breast and endometrial carcinoma (DOC)	Continue treatment at least 2 months to determine efficacy; relatively nontoxic in doses up to 800 mg/day
Acute and chronic lymphocytic leukemia (DOC) Hodgkin's disease (DOC) Non-Hodgkin's lymphomas (DOC) Multiple myeloma (DOC) Some breast cancers	Never used alone but always as a part of combination chemotherapy regimens; side-effects are minimized by alternate-day or intermittent therapy; concentrate solution is 30% alcohol
Cushing's syndrome associated with adrenal carcinoma Investigational uses—Postmenopausal metastatic breast cancer and prostatic carcinoma	Serum acid phosphatase levels should decrease in patients with prostatic cancer if aminoglutethimide is producing a positive clinical response; replacement glucocorticoid therapy is usually required in patients with breast and prostatic cancer; replacement mineralocorticoid (fludrocortisone) may be necessary in 20%–50% patients with Cushing's syndrome to prevent reduction of aldosterone which could lead to hyponatremia and orthostatic hypotension; monitor thyroid function tests in patients on prolonged therapy

(continued)

Table 75-14 (continued)
Hormonal, Antihormonal, and Gonadotropin-Releasing-Hormone Analogue Agents

Drug	Preparations	Usual Dosage Range
mitotane (Lysodren)	Tablets—500 mg	Adult—Initially, 8 g–10 g/day in three to four divided doses; adjust dosage to maximum tolerated dose (usually 2 g–16 g/day); maximum dose 18 g–19 g/day Children—1 g–2 g/day in divided doses; may be gradually increased to 5 g–7 g/day Cushing's syndrome—Initially, 3 g–6 g/day in three to four divided doses; Maintenance—500 mg twice a week to 2 g/day
tamoxifen (Nolvadex)	Tablets—10 mg	10 mg–20 mg twice a day

Gonadotropin-Releasing Hormone Analogue Agents

leuprolide (Lupron)	Injection—5 mg/ml, 2.8-ml and 5.6-ml kits (14-day and 28-day)	SC—1 mg/day

* DOC, Drug of choice (alone or in combination with other drugs).

justment of anticoagulant therapy may be necessary. Androgens may increase the hypoglycemic effects of antihyperglycemic agents. Careful monitoring of blood sugars and adjustment of medications may be necessary.

2. History of any previous antineoplastic therapies may indicate previous malignancies. Great care is necessary to evaluate the existence of hormone-dependent tumors other than the tumor under current treatment (see specific contraindications and precautions).

3. Risk factors—Several conditions increase the risk of adverse reactions to this class of drugs.

   The risk of pregnancy should be stressed prior to initiation of therapy, due to possible harm to the fetus from these drugs.

   The risk of development of additional malignancy should be considered, because several drugs may put patient at risk.

   Hepatic abnormalities may result in further liver damage and possible failure to metabolize drug appropriately.

4. There is the possibility of worsening of symptoms for up to 4 weeks to 6 weeks after beginning the therapy. This is of particular concern where disease progression places patient in a life-threatening position.

5. The nurse should evaluate patient's degree of understanding of drug regimen. Absolute compliance in taking the drug as ordered is necessary.

□ *Objective Data*

1. Physical Assessment—A thorough physical assessment should precede administration of any antineoplastic agent. However, specific drugs in this class affect specific systems and warrant careful review. The following are systems potentially affected by drugs in this class:

   Dermatologic—Most drugs
   GI—Most drugs
   Neurologic—tamoxifen
   Sexual characteristics—Most drugs
   Cardiovascular—estrogens, steroids, tamoxifen, leuprolide
   Urologic—mitotane

Uses	Clinical Considerations
Functional and nonfunctional adrenal cortical carcinoma (DOC) Investigational uses—Cushing's syndrome	Continue therapy 3 months to determine efficacy; may decrease protein-bound iodine and urinary 17-hydroxycorticosteroid levels; adrenocortical insufficiency can occur; replacement therapy may be necessary; periodic neurologic assessments are recommended for patients on therapy longer than 2 years
Advanced breast carcinoma (DOC)	May increase serum calcium levels; transient "flaring" of disease may occur during initial therapy, usually subsides rapidly; ocular toxicity is associated with long-term, high-dose therapy; induces ovulation which puts patient at risk of becoming pregnant
Advanced prostatic carcinoma (DOC) Investigational uses—Premenopausal breast cancer	Patients may experience an increase in testosterone levels and worsening of signs and symptoms early in treatment; refrigerated prior to dispensing but may be stored at room temperature while in use. Serum testosterone and prostatic acid phosphatase (PAP) should be done periodically to monitor therapeutic response

2. Laboratory Data and Diagnostic Tests
Diagnostic tests which should be performed before any of the hormonal agents are given include:
 · Pregnancy tests
 · Liver function studies
 · BUN and creatinine levels
 · Electrolytes—serum calcium and serum potassium levels, serum cholesterol
 · Coagulation studies and blood sugar level

□ NURSING DIAGNOSIS
Actual nursing diagnoses for the patient receiving hormones, antihormonals, and gonadotropin-releasing hormone analogue agents include:
 Lack of knowledge related to chemotherapy
Potential nursing diagnoses include:
 Alteration in comfort: pain
 Potential fluid volume deficit
 Alteration in fluid volume: excess
 Alteration in cardiac output: decreased
 Alteration in tissue perfusion
 Noncompliance related to drug administration
 Sensory-perceptual alterations—input deficit
 Self-esteem disturbance—sexual dysfunction

□ PLAN
Nursing care focuses on the following goals:
 1. To teach patient to follow necessary treatment
 2. To provide patient with information to notify health-care providers of early development of side-effects
 3. To develop and utilize strategies to minimize side-effects of drug therapy

□ INTERVENTIONS
The single most important concern when administering most of the drugs of this classification is compliance. Because many of these drugs are administered orally on a daily basis, the patient must be an active participant in the therapy. Unpleasant side-effects, appearance of secondary sexual characteristics of the opposite sex, or worsening of symptoms may result in the patient being unwilling to take a medication as prescribed. Careful teaching of all anticipated side-effects will result in

Table 75-15
Fate of Hormonal, Antihormonal, and Gonadotropin-Releasing Hormone Analogue Agents

Drug	Absorption/Distribution/ Half-Life	Metabolism	Excretion
Androgens			
dromostanolone	Highly bound to testosterone—estradiol-binding globulin	Hepatic	Urine—90% Feces—6%
testolactone	Well absorbed from GI tract, widely distributed	Hepatic	Renal
Estrogens			
diethylstilbestrol diphosphate	Moderate protein binding, widely distributed	Hepatic	Renal
estramustine phosphate sodium	Well absorbed from GI tract, widely distributed Half-life—multiphasic Terminal—20 h	Hepatic	Feces (primarily) Urine (minor)
polyestradiol phosphate	Widely distributed 50% protein bound Duration of action—14 days–28 days	Hepatic	Renal
Progestins			
megestrol acetate	Well absorbed from GI tract Widely distributed	Hepatic	Renal (57%–78%)
Antihormonal Agents			
aminoglutethimide	Well absorbed from GI tract Low protein binding Half-life—13 h reduced to 7 h after prolonged therapy due to enzyme induction	Hepatic to N-acetyl-aminoglutethimide	Renal (50%)
mitotane	35%–40% absorbed from GI tract Widely distributed; stored in fat; very small amounts of metabolite have been found in CSF Half-life—18 days–159 days	Hepatic and renal	Renal—10%–25% as metabolites Biliary—15%
tamoxifen	Well absorbed from GI tract Distribution unknown Half-life Initial—7 h–14 h Terminal—7 days	Hepatic to desmethyl tamoxifen, an active metabolite	Feces—Primarily as metabolites Renal—Very small amounts
Gonadotropin-Releasing Hormone Analogue Agents			
leuprolide	Readily absorbed following SC administration Distribution has not been determined Half-life—3 h	Unknown	Unknown

the patient being less apprehensive. It must be impressed on the patient to call a health-care professional prior to discontinuing the drug. Also the possibility of worsening of symptoms, including pain, must be discussed with the patient. Increased pain, inability to void, and onset of numbness and tingling are reasons for the patient to contact the physician.

The patient also needs to know the importance of continuing medication when symptoms begin to decrease. The need to continue the medication daily as long as ordered should be emphasized.

Pain and burning may appear at injection sites, particularly with leuprolide and testolactone. The patient should be reassured that this will disappear and taught to report prolonged redness, drainage, or fever.

□ *Side-Effects and Patient Education*

The nursing management of nausea, vomiting, and alopecia is discussed under Nursing Process for Antineoplastic Drugs earlier in the chapter. There is much information the patient must possess to knowledgeably take this class of drug and work with the health-care provider.

Development of secondary sexual characteristics of the opposite sex is very disconcerting to many patients. See Table 75-16 for specific reactions with each drug. The patient should be taught to maximize unaffected attributes (with make-up, clothes). The patient should be reassured that these effects will decrease when the drug is discontinued. The patient should eat a limited calorie and low sodium diet to limit potential weight gain.

Menstrual irregularity or suppression and impotence may be caused by alteration in hormone levels. Teaching should include a review of anticipated side-effects with the patient as well as family members. Patients experiencing suppression of ovarian function should actively practice effective birth control.

Patients receiving leuprolide may experience CNS symptoms including anxiety, headache, and paresthesias. Patients should be taught to report immediately any new onset of symptoms or change in existing symptoms, such as headaches. The family should be taught to report any unusual behavior.

The cardiovascular system can be affected with different manifestations by several drugs. Most drugs of this class cause fluid retention, characterized by swollen ankles or rapid weight gain. The patient should report these signs or any other swelling or bloatedness. Estrogens may increase the possibility of myocardial infarction. The patient should be told to report any chest tightness, pain, or pressure immediately. Estrogens and leuprolide have been implicated in development of thrombophlebitis and pulmonary emboli. The patient must avoid tight, constrictive clothing or crossing legs when sitting. The patient should report immediately any extremity pain, swelling, or warmth, or any acute shortness of breath or chest pain.

Changes in hormonal balance may result in behavioral changes which may vary among patients. Unusual bizarre behavior or signs of depression should be reported to the physician. The patient must be periodically reassured if the health-care team or family begin to feel he is a danger to himself or others. Patients should be informed that their mood will return to baseline as medication is discontinued. In severe cases, anti-anxiety drugs or antidepressants may be ordered.

Androgens and tamoxifen have been known to cause hot flashes. The patient should be instructed to dress normally and avoid chills. Patients should take their temperature if chills are present before "hot flashes." The patient should be reassured that "hot flashes" are related to specific medications.

Hypercalcemia has been known to occur during treatment with hormones, especially during initial period of disease exacerbations. Patients should drink plenty of fluids at all times (at least eight glasses of water per day).

□ *EVALUATION*

The outcome criteria to measure treatment effectiveness include:

1. The patient will report adverse effects as they first appear
2. The patient will implement appropriate measures to prevent or minimize side-effects.

Miscellaneous Agents

Hydroxyurea, Interferon, Procarbazine

The agents discussed in this section, hydroxyurea; interferon alfa-2a, recombinant; interferon alfa-2b, recombinant; and procarbazine, are classified as miscellaneous agents because their mechanism(s) of action or source does not correspond with the other classes of antineoplastic drugs.

The interferons, the newest antineoplastic

Table 75-16
Side-Effects/Adverse Reactions of Androgen, Estrogen, Progestin, Antihormonal
and Gonadotropin-Releasing Hormone Analogue Agents

Drug	Alopecia/Dermatologic	Gastrointestinal	Hepatic
Androgens			
dromostanolone	In females acne, facial hair growth (unusual hair loss; virilism)	Anorexia, nausea and vomiting Glossitis	
testolactone	Alopecia and nail growth disturbance with prolonged high dose therapy	Nausea, vomiting, diarrhea Glossitis	
Estrogens			
diethylstilbestrol diphosphate		Nausea, vomiting Anorexia	
estramustine phosphate sodium	Rash, pruritis, dry skin, thinning hair	Moderate nausea, vomiting, diarrhea, anorexia, flatulence	Rare
polyestradiol phosphate (see diethylstilbestrol diphosphate)			
Progestins			
megestrol acetate	Alopecia	Nausea and vomiting	
Antihormonal Agents			
aminoglutethimide	Measles-like rash or itching usually appears 10 days–15 days after therapy started and persists for 5 days–7 days. Stop medication if rash is severe or persists for more than 5 days–8 days. Darkening of skin.	Anorexia, nausea, vomiting	
mitotane	Maculopapular rash (15%) transient and may disappear without stopping or adjusting dose of drug Hyperpigmentation	Nausea, vomiting, diarrhea, anorexia in 80% of patients	

Myelosuppression	Neurologic	Renal	Other
	Paresthesia Rare CNS adverse effects		Edema Deepening voice Clitoral enlargement Hypercalcemia Aches of extremities
	Peripheral neuropathies		Aches Edema of extremities Hot flashes
	Dizziness, headaches		Increased risk of myocardial infarction, pulmonary embolism, thrombophlebitis, congestive heart failure Gynecomastia Hot flashes Impotence
Rare	Insomnia Anxiety		Breast tenderness or enlargement, edema of extremities. Increased risk of myocardial infarction, pulmonary embolism, thrombophlebitis, or congestive heart failure Thrombophlebitis, carpal tunnel syndrome, breast tenderness
Rare	CNS—Clumsiness, dizziness, drowsiness, lethargy, uncontrolled eye movements occur in 30% of patients; usually reduced in 2 weeks–6 weeks even with continued therapy. Depression Headache		Hypotension due to reduced aldosterone production Hypothyroidism and goiter are rare (due to blockage of iodination of tyrosine). Myalgia Rare hypersensitivity reaction of cholestatic jaundice, fever, skin eruptions, increased AST(SGOT).
	CNS—40% of patients; primarily lethargy and somnolence, also dizziness or vertigo, depression, headache, tremors, confusion, lethargy may		Hemorrhagic cystitis Blurred or double vision due to lens opacity or toxic retinopathy

(continued)

Table 75-16 (continued)
Side-Effects/Adverse Reactions of Androgen, Estrogen, Progestin, Antihormonal and Gonadotropin-Releasing Hormone Analogue Agents

Drug	Alopecia/Dermatologic	Gastrointestinal	Hepatic
	Alopecia, perinasal scaling, facial swelling are rare.		
tamoxifen	Rash (rare)	Nausea and vomiting Anorexia	

Gonadotropin-Releasing Hormone Analogue Agent

Drug	Alopecia/Dermatologic	Gastrointestinal	Hepatic
leuprolide	Rash, itching (rare), hair loss (rare) Erythema and ecchymosis at injection site (rare)	Nausea, vomiting, anorexia, constipation, GI bleeding, diarrhea, sour taste in mouth are infrequent.	

agents approved by the FDA, are synthetic protein chains consisting of 165 amino acids produced by recombinant DNA technology using genetically engineered *Escherichia coli*. Interferon alfa-2a, recombinant, has lysine group at position 23, and interferon alfa-2b, recombinant, has an arginine group at position 23.

MECHANISM AND ACTIONS
Hydroxyurea—The exact mechanism of action of hydroxyurea is unknown, but the drug may function as an antimetabolite by interfering with the enzyme ribonucleoside diphosphate reductase which is necessary for the conversion of ribonucleotides to deoxyribonucleotides. Hydroxyurea may also inhibit the incorporation of thymidine into DNA and may directly damage DNA. The net result is that hydroxyurea interferes with the synthesis of DNA without interfering with the synthesis of RNA or protein and is cell-cycle specific for the S phase of cell division.

Interferon—The exact mechanism of action of the interferons is unknown; however, it is known that interferons have antiviral, antiproliferative,

1471

Myelosuppression	Neurologic	Renal	Other
	occur; ataxia, speech difficulty, neuropathy, hallucinations, and psychosis are rare.		
Transient thrombocytopenia	Mental depression Confusion Lethargy		Increased bone and tumor pain at initiation of therapy may be associated with a good response. Vaginal bleeding or discharge and menstrual irregularities are infrequent. Peripheral edema Hot flashes are frequent Retinopathy, corneal opacities, and decreased visual acuity have occurred in patients on high-dose (240 mg–320 mg/day), long-term therapy Hypercalcemia may occur in patients with bone metastasis. Pulmonary embolism and thrombophlebitis are rare.
	CNS—Anxiety, dizziness, pain, headache, paresthesia, blurred vision, lethargy, insomnia, irritability, memory disorder, numbness are infrequent.		Congestive heart failure, thrombophlebitis, myocardial infarction, and pulmonary embolism are rare. Hot flashes (50%) Gynecomastia and breast tenderness (3%) Peripheral edema Myalgia (less than 3%) Increased bone or tumor pain at start of therapy usually subsides in 2 weeks–4 weeks Impotence (less than 3%)

and immunomodulatory activities, and any or all of these activities play important roles in the antitumor action of the interferons.

The interferons bind to specific membrane receptors on the surface of the cell and initiate a complex sequence of intracellular events that includes the induction of several enzymes (synthetases, protein kinases, and endonucleases). This process, in part, is responsible for the cellular responses to interferon: inhibition of virus replication in virus-infected cells, suppression of cell proliferation, and enhancement of the phagocytic activity of macrophages and augmentation of the specific cytotoxicity of lymphocytes for target cells.

Procarbazine—The exact mechanism of antineoplastic action of procarbazine is unknown. The action of procarbazine may resemble that of the alkylating agents after metabolism in the liver by the cytochrome P-450 system to cytoxic alkylating and methylating metabolites. Procarbazine also inhibits mitosis by prolonging the interphase of cell division and has also been reported to cause chromosomal breakage. All of these actions ultimately result in the inhibition of DNA, RNA, and protein synthesis. No cross-resistance with other alkylating agents has been demonstrated, and procarbazine is cell-cycle specific for the S phase of cell division. Procarbazine also has weak monoamine oxidase (MAO) inhibiting properties which are not related to its antineoplastic action.

USES
See Table 75-17.

ADMINISTRATION AND DOSAGE
See Table 75-17.

FATE
See Table 75-18.

SIDE-EFFECTS/ADVERSE REACTIONS
The side-effects and adverse reactions of chemotherapeutic agents are for the most part unavoidable and are due to the pharmacologic action of the agents; the potential benefits should outweigh the risks before such agents are used. The adverse reactions and side-effects most frequently seen are the result of damage to the most rapidly and actively dividing normal cells such as the hematopoietic system, cells of hair follicles, and cells leaving the gastrointestinal tract and oral cavity. Some toxicities (leukopenia and thrombocytopenia) are actually used to measure a particular agent's effectiveness and also as a basis to calculate subsequent doses of the agent.

Not all side-effects and adverse reactions are observed with all drugs. Table 75-19 lists the common side-effects of the miscellaneous agents. For a complete list of all side-effects and adverse reactions of each agent see the manufacturer's product information.

CONTRAINDICATIONS AND PRECAUTIONS
All antineoplastic agents have the potential to be carcinogenic (due to a direct cellular action or immunosuppression) and to cause testicular and ovarian suppression. The exact effect of dose and duration of therapy is unknown, but the risk is increased by long-term therapy.

The miscellaneous agents are to be used with caution or are contraindicated in patients with leukopenia, thrombocytopenia, or anemia caused by previous chemotherapy or radiation therapy, hepatotoxicity, renal toxicity, and known hypersensitivity.

1. *Hydroxyurea* is teratogenic in animals, and although information is limited, the risks and benefits must be considered prior to use during pregnancy.
2. Patients hypersensitive to any alfa interferon may also be intolerant of *recombinant interferon alfa-2a, or alfa-2b.* Also patients hypersensitive to mouse immunoglobulin may also be hypersensitive to *interferon alfa-2a, recombinant.*
3. *Procarbazine* is teratogenic in animals, and minor malformations and premature births have been reported when it is given later in pregnancy in humans.

INTERACTIONS
1. Hydroxyurea may antagonize the effects of antigout medications (probenecid, sulfinpyrazone) by increasing serum uric acid; dosage adjustment of the antigout medications may be necessary.
2. Procarbazine and ethanol ingestion may cause a disulfiram-like reaction and have an additive CNS depressant effect.
3. Concurrent use of procarbazine with tricyclic antidepressants, carbamazepine, cyclobenzaprine, maprotiline, or other MAO inhibitors could cause hyperpyretic crises or severe seizures and is not recommended on an outpatient basis.
4. Thiazide diuretics, antihypertensives, and other hypotension-producing medications such as general anesthetics, spinal anesthetics, nitrates, or trazodone, administered concurrently with procarbazine may cause enhanced hypotension.
5. CNS depressants, such as narcotic analgesics and barbiturates, used concurrently with procarbazine may cause enhanced CNS depression and hypotension in some patients but may cause excitation, rigidity, sweating, hyperpyrexia, and hypertension in others; the use of meperidine should be avoided within 2 weeks to 3 weeks of procarbazine therapy; caution should also be used when using alfentanil, fentanyl, or sufentanil in patients who have received procarbazine in prior 2 weeks.
6. Procarbazine may enhance the effects of insulin and oral hypoglycemic medications; dosage adjustment of hypoglycemic agent may be necessary.
7. Guanethidine, guanadrel, levodopa, methyldopa, or reserpine used concurrently with pro-

carbazine may result in hypertension and excitation.

8. Sympathomimetics such as amphetamines, epinephrine, ephedrine, pseudoephedrine, isoproterenol, methylphenidate, and phenylpropanolamine used concurrently with procarbazine may cause hyperpyrexia and a severe hypertensive crisis.

9. Ingestion of foods with a high tyramine content (see Chap. 29) may cause a severe hypertensive crisis in a patient on procarbazine therapy.

10. Concurrent use of the miscellaneous agents with live virus vaccines may potentiate the replication of the vaccine virus, increase the side-effects and adverse reactions of the vaccine virus, or decrease the patient's antibody response to the vaccine because the patient's normal defense mechanisms are suppressed.

11. Concurrent use of procarbazine with dextromethorphan (a cough suppressant found in many nonprescription cough preparations) may cause excitation and hyperpyrexia.

12. The gastrointestinal absorption of digoxin may be decreased by bleomycin, carmustine, cyclophosphamide, cytarabine, doxorubicin, methotrexate, procarbazine, and vincristine. Serum digoxin levels should be monitored and the patient should be checked for worsening congestive heart failure and the dose should be adjusted accordingly.

■ Nursing Process for Miscellaneous Antineoplastic Agents

□ ASSESSMENT

□ Subjective Data

1. Besides performing the preassessment previously addressed under Nursing Process for Antineoplastic Drugs, there are some specific nursing assessments related to the drugs included in this category.

2. When assessing a patient who will be receiving procarbazine, it is extremely important to obtain a complete medication history. Because procarbazine can cause symptoms associated with CNS depression, all CNS depressants, barbiturates, narcotics, and phenothiazines should be used cautiously, if at all.

3. Procarbazine also posesses weak MAO inhibi-

tor activity; therefore, any foods containing high amounts of tyramine should be avoided (see Chap. 29). These foods include many beers and wines, aged cheese, yogurt, pickled herring, chicken liver, canned figs, yeast extract, broad beans, and soy sauce. In addition, chocolate, meat tenderizers, and excessive amounts of caffeine should be avoided. Use of any of these can precipitate a hypertensive crisis, intracranial bleeding, or headache.

4. Thorough assessment of the patient's performance status is essential when initiating interferon (see Table 75-3) due to the various side-effects this drug may produce. With a good baseline of the patient's level of activity, any abnormal fatigue or depression can be noted easily and corrected with a readjustment of the dose of interferon by the physician.

□ Objective Data

A complete physical assessment is recommended before drug therapy is initiated. In addition, frequent monitoring of vital signs is recommended when interferon is initiated and throughout therapy because of the high probability of fevers and fluctuations in vital signs. These symptoms tend to lessen as treatment continues.

Close monitoring of blood work including CBC and hepatic and renal functions is essential before treatment and throughout therapy. All three of the miscellaneous drugs can cause some degree of bone marrow depression which may be dose limiting.

□ NURSING DIAGNOSIS

Actual nursing diagnoses for the patient receiving hydroxyurea, interferon, or procarbazine include:
 Knowledge deficit related to administration of chemotherapy
 Knowledge deficit related to side-effects of the antineoplastic agents

Potential nursing diagnoses include:
 Anxiety
 Fluid volume deficit related to nausea and vomiting
 Alteration in nutrition, less than body requirements
 Potential for infection: neutropenia
 Potential for injury: thrombocytopenia
 Alteration in bowel elimination: diarrhea
 Disturbance in body image/self-concept related to alopecia
 Alteration in comfort (secondary to flu-like symptoms associated with interferon therapy)

Table 75-17
Miscellaneous Antineoplastic Agents

Drug	Preparations	Usual Dosage Range
hydroxyurea (Hydrea)	Capsules—500 mg	Solid tumors: Intermittent therapy—80 mg/kg as a single dose every third day Continuous therapy—20 mg–30 mg/kg daily as a single dose Carcinoma of head and neck—80 mg/kg as a single dose every third day; used concomitantly with radiation Myelocytic leukemia—20 mg–30 mg/kg daily as a single dose
interferon alfa-2a, recombinant (Roferon-A)	Injection— Solution— 3 million IU/ml (SDV) 18 million IU/3 ml (MDV) Lyophilized powder— 3 million IU/vial (MDV) 18 million IU/vial (MDV)	Hairy cell leukemia: IM, SC— Induction—3 million IU per day for 16 weeks–24 weeks Maintenance—3 million IU three times/week Reduce dose by 50% if severe adverse effects occur. *Some dosage regimens for investigational uses:* Chronic myelogenous leukemia— IM—5 million U/m^2/day Kaposi's sarcoma— IM—36–50 million U/day for 4 weeks–8 weeks, then three times/week Non-Hodgkin's lymphomas— IM—50 million U/m^2 three times/week; reduce a dose as needed due to side-effects Renal cell carcinoma— IM—20 million U/m^2/day, or five times a week, or three times a week Malignant melanoma— IM—12 million U–50 million U/m^2 three times/week Mycosis fungoides— IM—50 million U/m^2 three times/week Multiple myeloma— IM—2 million U–100 million U/m^2/day
interferon alfa-2b, recombinant (Intron A)	Injection— lyophilized powder: 3 million IU/vial 5 million IU/vial 10 million IU/vial 25 million IU/vial	IM, SC—2 million IU/m^2 three times/week Reduce dose by 50% if severe adverse effects occur.
procarbazine (Matulane)	Capsules—50 mg	Adults—initially 2 mg–4 mg/kg/day (to the nearest 50 mg) in single or divided doses the first week; then 4 mg–6 mg/kg/day until leukocytes fall below 4,000, platelets below 100,000, or a maximum clinical response is obtained

Uses	Clinical Considerations

Chronic myelocytic leukemia
Malignant melanoma
Ovarian carcinoma
Squamous cell carcinoma of head and neck (excluding the lip)
Investigational uses—
    Advanced prostatic carcinoma
    Lung carcinoma
    Psoriasis
    Hypereosinophilic syndrome

Discontinue therapy if leukocytes are less than 2,500 and platelets are less than 100,000; drowsiness occurs with large doses; hydroxyurea should be started at least 7 days before radiation therapy; contents of capsules may be emptied into a glass of water and taken immediately if patient is unable to swallow capsules (some inert material may not dissolve and may float on the surface); may increase serum uric acid, BUN, and creatinine levels; dysuria may occur, but is usually temporary; intermittent therapy causes less toxicity; continue therapy 6 weeks to determine efficacy

Hairy cell leukemia in patients 18 years of age or older
Investigational uses—
    Renal carcinoma
    Bladder carcinoma (instillation)
    Non-Hodgkin's lymphomas
    Malignant melanoma
    Mycosis fungoides
    AIDS–Kaposi's sarcoma
    Condylomata accuminata (genital warts)—by intralesional injection
Chronic myelogenous leukemia
Multiple myeloma

Interferon alfa-2a and 2b are *not* interchangeable.
Store solution in refrigerator; do *not* shake or freeze
Patients should be well hydrated during initiation of therapy to prevent hypotension due to fluid depletion.
Patients should be treated for 6 months to determine efficacy of therapy; maintenance therapy may be continued for up to 20 months.
Neutralizing antibodies to alfa-2a have been detected in 27% of patients but *no* clinical significance has been determined.
Patients with platelet counts less than 50,000/mm^3 should receive SC injection *not* IM injection.
Premedicate patient with acetaminophen to minimize flu-like syndrome and administer at night to minimize persistent fatigue.

Hairy cell leukemia in patients 18 years and older
Investigational uses—
    Laryngeal papillomas
    Renal cacinoma
    Bladder carcinoma (instillation)
    Non-Hodgkin's lymphomas
    Malignant melanoma
    Mycosis fungoides
    Kaposi's sarcoma
    Chronic hepatitis

See interferon alfa-2a recombinant. In addition, store injection both before and after reconstitution in refrigerator
Preparation of solution—

Vial Strength	Amount of Diluent	Final Concentration
3 million IU	1 ml	3 million IU/ml
5 million IU	1 ml	5 million IU/ml
10 million IU	2 ml	5 million IU/ml
25 million IU	5 ml	5 million IU/ml

After reconstitution with bacteriostatic water for injection the clear, colorless to light yellow solution is stable for 30 days when refrigerated. Prothrombin time (PT) and partial thromboplastin time (PTT) may be increased.

Hodgkin's disease (DOC)*
Non-Hodgkin's lymphomas (DOC)
Investigational uses—
    Lung carcinoma
    Malignant melanoma
    Brain tumors

Tolerance to GI side-effects usually develops within several days; fever, chills, and sweating are most common during early stages of therapy; use in children is limited; undue toxicity such as tremors, coma, and convulsions have occurred; dosage must be individualized.

(continued)

Table 75-17 (continued)
Miscellaneous Antineoplastic Agents

Drug	Preparations	Usual Dosage Range
procarbazine (Matulane) (continued)		Following recovery from hematologic toxicity, 1 mg–2 mg/kg/day; maintenance —1 mg–2 mg/kg/day
		Children—initially, 50 mg/day for 1 week; then 100 mg/m^2 daily (to the nearest 50 mg) until hematologic toxicity occurs or maximum response occurs, then 50 mg/day after recovery; maintenance—50 mg/day

* DOC, Drug of choice (alone or in combination with other drugs).

Potential activity intolerance
Potential for noncompliance with regimens as
  prescribed, due to drug side-effects
Self-care deficit related to all activities of
  daily living
Sexual dysfunction
Sleep pattern disturbances

☐ **PLAN**
Nursing care focuses on the following goals:
1. To minimize side-effects of these chemotherapeutic agents
2. To promote self-care behaviors so that the patient will promptly identify any unusual signs

and symptoms and report them to appropriate
health-care workers

☐ **INTERVENTION**
Nursing intervention strategies will vary in response to the patient's drug regimen and the side-effects experienced.

Refer to Nursing Process for Antineoplastic Drugs for nursing actions related to side-effects common to all chemotherapy.

Procarbazine and hydroxyurea are taken orally, and the patient should be instructed to never open capsules before ingesting.

Dividing doses of procarbazine throughout the

Table 75-18
Fate of Miscellaneous Antineoplastic Agents

Drug	Absorption/Distribution/Half-Life	Metabolism	Excretion
hydroxyurea	Very well absorbed from GI tract Crosses blood–brain barrier with peak concentration in 2 h–3 h Also distributed to gut, kidneys, and lungs	Hepatic	Respiratory as carbon dioxide Renal—50% unchanged
interferon	Greater than 80% absorption from IM or SC injection sites Distributed primarily to blood and kidneys Half-life— Interferon alfa-2a, recombinant 3.7 h–8.5 h Interferon alfa-2b, recombinant 6 h–7 h	Renal	Negligible— Products of renal catabolism are almost completely reabsorbed.
procarbazine	Very well absorbed from GI tract Rapidly crosses blood–brain barrier Distributed also to liver, kidney, intestine, and skin Half-life—7 min–10 min	Hepatic to active metabolites	Renal—70% (primarily as metabolites) Respiratory as carbon dioxide and methane

Uses	Clinical Considerations

Investigational uses (continued)
Multiple myeloma
Polycythemia vera
Mycosis fungoides

day may help reduce the nausea and vomiting commonly associated with this drug. The nurse should be alert for flu-like symptoms which may occur during the initiation of procarbazine therapy. These symptoms may abate after 7 days to 10 days.

Particular attention must be shown in teaching and assisting the patient receiving procarbazine in instituting proper dietary changes while on therapy (see under Assessment).

The nurse should discuss the interaction of CNS depressants and alcohol with procarbazine and stress the importance of notifying the physician immediately if any signs or symptoms of CNS depression, hypertensive crisis, or "disulfiram-like" reaction occur.

The patient receiving procarbazine and hydroxyurea may be drowsy or dizzy, or may have blurred vision and must exercise caution while driving or performing other tasks requiring mental alertness.

The diabetic patient on procarbazine must be closely monitored for signs of hypoglycemia.

Exacerbation of postirradiation erythema may occur while on hydroxyurea therapy, if previous radiation therapy was performed.

The route of administration for interferon varies greatly; the nurse must become familiar with the various methods used. Subcutaneous self-administration is a common form of home therapy. Thorough instruction of proper subcutaneous injection techniques and body sites, as well as storage requirements for interferon must be done with patients and family members involved in their care.

Maintaining adequate fluid and electrolyte balance is essential for the patient receiving interferon. Severe flu-like symptoms can occur 2 hours after treatment, lasting for most of the day. These symptoms include fevers, chills, malaise, headache, loss of appetite, nausea and vomiting, fatigue, and diarrhea. Patients should be instructed to push oral fluids and monitor temperature closely. Avoidance of aspirin and nonsteroidal anti-inflammatory agents should be stressed. Acetaminophen is suggested to control fever.

Encouragement may be needed through this very difficult and uncomfortable time. Noncompliance with the therapy may occur; therefore, the nurse should monitor closely and inform the patient that many side-effects tend to dissipate or improve as the treatment continues.

Any signs of diminished mental alertness, depression, visual disturbances, or sleep disturbances while on interferon therapy should be reported quickly.

□ EVALUATION
Outcome criteria to judge the effectiveness of therapy include:
1. Side-effects of drugs were minimal, with early detection of any adverse reactions.
2. Dietary modifications were followed.
3. Accurate doses of drugs were taken using proper administration techniques specific to the agent being used.

Combination Chemotherapy

Combination chemotherapy is used widely today in many neoplastic diseases to produce higher response rates and longer remission periods than obtained with single-agent therapy. Combinations of
(Text continues on p. 1494.)

Table 75-19
Side-Effects/Adverse Reactions of Miscellaneous Antineoplastic Agents

Drug	Alopecia/Dermatologic	Gastrointestinal	Hepatic
hydroxyurea	Alopecia—rare Mild rash, facial erythema, pruritis in some patients	Mild nausea and vomiting Stomatitis Anorexia Constipation or diarrhea	Elevation of hepatic enzymes
interferon*	Partial alopecia usually after prolonged therapy (>4 months) Skin rash (15%)—Maculopapular eruptions on trunk and extremities; usually transient Reactivation of herpes labialis (8%) Mild pruritis	Anorexia (40%) Nausea (32%) Vomiting (10%) Diarrhea (29%) Change in taste (13%) Nausea and vomiting due to interferon alfa-2a usually resolves within 4 weeks after therapy is stopped. Nausea and vomiting due to interferon alfa-2b usually resolves within 3 days–5 days after therapy is stopped. Dryness of mouth and throat (16%)	Elevated serum alkaline phosphatase (48%), serum alanine aminotransferase (ALT[SGPT]), serum aspartate aminotransferase (AST[SGOT]) (78%), serum lactic dehydrogenase (LDH) (47%), and bilirubin (31%) Hepatitis—rare
procarbazine	Alopecia, dermatitis, pruritis, herpes, hyperpigmentation, flushing, and photosensitivity are infrequent.	Diarrhea, constipation, stomatitis, and anorexia are infrequent. Nausea and vomiting may be moderate but toleration may develop to continued therapy.	

* Interferon is being evaluated for the treatment of many other types of cancers (see Table 75-17). The doses generally used (12–50 million IU/m²) are much higher than those indicated for the treatment of hairy cell leukemia. The *incidence* of adverse reactions with high-dose therapy was the same as those described above for hairy cell leukemia but *more severe* with high-dose therapy.

Myelosuppression	Neurologic	Renal	Other

Leukopenia
  Nadir—10 days
  Recovery—rapid after cessation of therapy
Thrombocytopenia—less common; usually follows leukopenia with rapid recovery after cessation of therapy
	Headaches, drowsiness, dizziness, disorientation, hallucinations, and convulsions are rare.
	Large doses may cause drowsiness.
		Renal tubular function may be suppressed with elevated serum uric acid, BUN, and creatinine levels.	Fever, chills, malaise, increased inflammation of mucous membranes may occur in patients receiving concurrent radiation therapy.
			Self-limiting megaloblastic erythropoiesis may occur at start of therapy but becomes less pronounced as therapy continues.

Leukopenia and thrombocytopenia occur frequently but are mild.
Interferon alfa-2a—
  Leukopenia—
  Nadir—22 days–38 days
  Recovery—2 weeks–4 weeks after withdrawal
  Thrombocytopenia—
  Nadir—17 days–19 days
  Recovery—2 weeks–4 weeks after withdrawal
Interferon alfa-2b
  Leukopenia and thrombocytopenia
  Nadir—3 days–5 days
  Recovery—3 days–5 days after withdrawal
	Dizziness (21%)
	Paresthesias (6%)
	Numbness (6%)
	Decreased mental status, depression, visual disturbances, sleep disturbances, and nervousness have occurred rarely.
	Seizures, obtundation, coma, hallucinations have occurred with high-dose therapy (12 to 50 million IU/m²).
		Proteinuria (25%)
		Elevated uric acid (15%)
		Elevated serum creatinine and BUN (10%)
			Flu-like syndrome of fatigue (89%), fever (98%), chills (64%), myalgias (73%), and headache (71%) occurs in majority of patients but diminishes with continued therapy.
			Decreased libido
			Transient impotence
			Cardiovascular adverse reactions—Hypotension edema, angina, arrhythmia, tachycardia, CHF and myocardial infarction are associated primarily with high-dose therapy.
			Interferon alfa-2b increases prothrombin time (PT) and partial thromboplastin time (PTT).

Leukopenia and thrombocytopenia are moderate. Nadir—21 days–28 days Recovery—35 days–42 days	CNS reactions may occur in up to 30% of the patients and include: paresthesias, neuropathies, depression, acute exogenous psychosis, manic reactions, hallucinations, dizziness, headache, apprehension, nervousness, nightmares, insomnia, falling, unsteadiness, ataxia, disorientation, foot drop, decreased reflexes, tremor, coma, confusion, delirium, and seizures.		Pulmonary toxicity (alveolitis) rare with delayed onset Flu-like syndrome of fever, chills, sweating, lethargy, myalgia, and arthralgia usually limited to initial therapy Cough and shortness of breath due to allergic pneumonitis Infrequent to rare adverse effects include hoarseness, tachycardia, nystagmus, hypotension, photophobia, diplopia, inability to focus, papilledema, and altered hearing.

Table 75-20
Combination Chemotherapeutic Regimens

Acronym	Drug	Dosage	Indications
ABVD	A—doxorubicin B—bleomycin V—vinblastine D—dacarbazine	25 mg/m² IV days 1 and 14 10 U/m² IV days 1 and 14 6 mg/m² IV days 1 and 14 375 mg/m² IV days 1 and 14 Repeat every 28 days for six to eight cycles.	Hodgkin's disease
AC-BCG	A—doxorubicin C—cyclophosphamide BCG—bacille Calmette Guérin	40 mg/m² IV days 1 and 14 200 mg/m² IV days 3–6 1 vial by scarification on days 8 and 15 Repeat every 3–4 weeks.	Ovarian carcinoma
A Ce (AC)	A—doxorubicin Ce—cyclophosphamide	40 mg/m² IV day 1 200 mg/m² PO days 3–6 Repeat every 21 days–28 days.	Breast carcinoma
ACMF	A—doxorubicin C—cyclophosphamide M—methotrexate F—fluorouracil	40 mg/m² IV day 1 1 g/m² IV day 1 30 mg to 40 mg/m² IV days 21, 28, and 35 400 mg to 600 mg/m² IV days 21, 28, and 35 Repeat every 42 days.	Breast carcinoma
A-COPP	A—doxorubicin C—cyclophosphamide O—vincristine P—procarbazine P—prednisone	60 mg/m² IV day 1 300 mg/m² IV days 14 and 20 1.5 mg/m² IV days 14 and 20 (maximum 2 mg) 100 mg/m² PO days 14–28 40 mg/m² PO days 1–27 (first and fourth cycles) days 14–27 (second, third, fifth, and sixth cycles) Repeat every 42 days for six cycles.	Hodgkin's disease
ACV	A—doxorubicin C—cyclophosphamide V—vincristine	75 mg/m² IV days 1 and 43 40 mg/kg IV day 21 0.04 mg/kg IV day 22	Ewing's sarcoma
AD	A—doxorubicin D—dacarbazine	60 mg/m² IV day 1 (adequate marrow) 45 mg/m² IV day 1 (inadequate marrow) 250 mg/m² IV days 1–5 (adequate marrow) 200 mg/m² IV days 1–5 (inadequate marrow)	Soft tissue and bony sarcomas
Ad-OAP (AOAP)	Ad—doxorubicin O—vincristine A—cytarabine P—prednisone	40 mg/m² IV day 1 2 mg IV day 1 70 mg/m² continuous infusion days 1–7 or 100 mg/m² continuous infusion days 5–9 100 mg/day on days 1–5 Repeat after 2 weeks.	Acute myelocytic leukemia
Adria + BCNU	Adria—doxorubicin BCNU—carmustine	30 mg/m² IV day 1 30 mg/m² IV day 1 Repeat every 21 days –28 days.	Multiple myeloma
AMV	A—doxorubicin M—mitomycin V—vinblastine	30 mg/m² IV every 4 weeks 10 mg/m² IV every 8 weeks 6 mg/m² IV every 4 weeks	Breast carcinoma
AP	A—doxorubicin P—cisplatin	50 mg/m² IV every 21 days 50 mg/m² IV every 21 days	Ovarian carcinoma

(continued)

Table 75-20 (continued)
Combination Chemotherapeutic Regimens

Acronym	Drug	Dosage	Indications
Ara-C + ADR	Ara-C—cytarabine	100 mg/m² continuous IV infusion for 7 days–10 days	Acute myelocytic leukemia
	ADR—doxorubicin	30 mg/m² IV days 1–3	
Ara-C + DNR + PRED + MP	Ara-C—cytarabine	80 mg/m² IV days 1–3	Acute myelocytic leukemia (in children)
	DNR—daunorubicin	25 mg/m² IV day 1	
	PRED—prednisolone	40 mg/m² PO daily	
	MP—mercaptopurine	100 mg/m² PO daily	
		Repeat weekly until remission, then monthly for maintenance.	
Ara-C + 6-TG	Ara-C—cytarabine	100 mg/m² IV every 12 h for 10 days	Acute myelocytic leukemia
	6-TG—thioguanine	100 mg/m² PO every 12 h for 10 days	
		Repeat every 30 days until remission, then repeat monthly for 5 days for maintenance.	
AV	A—doxorubicin	60 mg–75 mg/m² day 1	Breast carcinoma
	V—vincristine	1.4 mg/m² days 1 and 8	
		Repeat every 3 weeks.	
BACON	B—bleomycin	30 U IV (6 h after vincristine)	Squamous cell carcinoma of lung
	A—doxorubicin	40 mg/m² IV day 1; repeat every 4 weeks	
	C—lomustine	65 mg/m² PO day 1; repeat every 4 weeks–8 weeks	
	O—vincristine	0.75 mg–1 mg IV day 2; repeat every week for 6 weeks	
	N—mechlorethamine	8 mg/m² IV day 1 (30 min after lomustine); repeat every 4 weeks	
BACOP	B—bleomycin	5 U/m² IV days 15 and 22	Non-Hodgkin's lymphomas
	A—doxorubicin	25 mg/m² IV days 1 and 8	
	C—cyclophosphamide	650 mg/m² IV days 1 and 8	
	O—vincristine	1.4 mg/m² IV days 1 and 8	
	P—prednisone	60 mg/m² PO days 15–28	
		Repeat every 28 days for six cycles.	
BCAP	B—carmustine	50 mg/m² IV day 1	Multiple myeloma
	C—cyclophosphamide	200 mg/m² IV day 1	
	A—doxorubicin	20 mg/m² IV day 2	
	P—prednisone	60 mg/m² PO days 1–5	
		Repeat every weeks.	
B-CAVe	B—bleomycin	5 U/m² IV days 1, 28, 35	Hodgkin's disease
	C—lomustine	100 mg/m² PO day 1	
	A—doxorubicin	60 mg/m² IV day 1	
	Ve—vinblastine	5 mg/m² IV day 1	
		Repeat every 6 weeks for nine cycles.	
BCMF	B—bleomycin	7.5 U/m² continuous infusion days 1–3	Squamous cell carcinoma of head and neck
	C—cyclophosphamide	300 mg/m² IV day 5	
	M—methotrexate	30 mg/m² IV day 5	
	F—fluorouracil	300 mg/m² IV day 5	
		Repeat every 3 weeks.	
BCNU + 5-FU	BCNU—carmustine	40 mg/m² IV days 1–5	Gastric carcinoma
	5-FU—fluorouracil	10 mg/kg IV days 1–5	
		Repeat every 6 weeks.	
BCOP	B—carmustine	100 mg/m² IV day 1	Non-Hodgkin's lymphomas
	C—cyclophosphamide	600 mg/m² IV day 1	

(continued)

Table 75-20 (continued)
Combination Chemotherapeutic Regimens

Acronym	Drug	Dosage	Indications
BCOP (continued)	O—vincristine P—prednisone	1 mg/m² IV days 1 and 14 40 mg/m² PO days 1–7 Repeat every 28 days.	
BCVPP	B—carmustine C—cyclophosphamide V—vinblastine P—procarbazine P—prednisone	100 mg/m² IV day 1 600 mg/m² IV day 1 5 mg/m² IV day 1 100 mg/m² PO days 1–10 60 mg/m² PO days 1–10 Repeat every 28 days for six cycles.	Hodgkin's disease
B-DOPA	B—bleomycin D—dacarbazine O—vincristine P—prednisone A—doxorubicin	4 U mg/m² IV days 2 and 5 150 mg/m² IV days 1–5 1.5 mg/m² PO days 1 and 5 40 mg/m² PO days 1–6 60 mg/m² IV day 1 Repeat every 21 days.	Hodgkin's disease

BEP	B—bleomycin
	E—etoposide
	P—cisplatin
		30 U IV weekly
		100 mg/m²/day IV days 1–5
		20 mg/m²/day IV days 1–5
		Repeat every 3 weeks for 4 cycles
		Reduce dose of etoposide by 20%
		   if patient received prior radio-
		   therapy
			Testicular carcinoma

BHD	B—carmustine
	
	H—hydroxyurea
	
	D—dacarbazine
		100 mg or 150 mg/m²/day IV day
		   1; repeat every 6 weeks
		1480 mg/m²/day PO days 1–5; re-
		   peat every 3 weeks
		100 mg or 150 mg/m²/day IV
		   days 1–5; repeat every 3 weeks
			Malignant melanoma

BLEO-MTX	BLEO—bleomycin MTX—methotrexate	15 U IV every 4 days–14 days 15 mg/m² IV every 4 days–14 days	Head and neck carci- noma
B-MOPP	B—bleomycin M—mechlorethamine O—vincristine P—procarbazine P—prednisone	2 U/m² IV days 1 and 8 6 mg/m² IV days 1 and 8 1.4 mg/m² IV days 1 and 8 100 mg/m² PO days 1–4 50 mg/m² PO days 1–14 cycles 1 and 4 only Repeat every 28 days	Hodgkin's disease
BM	B—bleomycin M—mitomycin	5 U/day IV days 1–7 10 mg IV day 8 Repeat every 2 weeks.	Carcinoma of cervix
BOPP	B—carmustine O—vincristine P—procarbazine P—prednisone	80 mg/m² IV day 1 1.4 mg/m² IV days 1 and 8 50 mg PO day 1; 100 mg PO day 2; 100 mg/m²/day PO days 3–14 40 mg/m²/day PO days 1–14 Repeat every 28 days for six cycles.	Hodgkin's disease
BVD	B—carmustine V—vincristine D—dacarbazine	65 mg/m² IV days 1, 2, 3 1 mg–1.5 mg IV weekly 250 mg/m² IV days 1, 2, 3 Repeat every 6 weeks	Malignant melanoma

CAF	C—cyclophosphamide
	A—doxorubicin
	F—fluorouracil
		100 mg/m² PO days 1–14
		30 mg/m² IV days 1 and 8
		500 mg/m² IV days 1 and 8
		Repeat every 4 weeks until total
		   dose of 450 mg/m² doxorubicin
		   is administered; then discon-
			Breast carcinoma

(continued)

Table 75-20 (continued)
Combination Chemotherapeutic Regimens

Acronym	Drug	Dosage	Indications
CAF *(continued)*		tinue doxorubicin and replace with methotrexate 40 mg/m² IV and increase fluorouracil to 600 mg/m² IV.	
CAM	C—cyclophosphamide A—doxorubicin M—methotrexate	600 mg/m² IV day 1 40 mg/m² IV day 1 15 mg/m² PO days 9, 13, 16, 20 Repeat every 21 days.	Prostatic carcinoma (advanced)
CAMP	C—cyclophosphamide A—doxorubicin M—methotrexate P—procarbazine	300 mg/m² IV days 1 and 8 20 mg/m² IV days 1 and 8 15 mg/m² IV days 1 and 8 100 mg/m² PO days 1–10 Repeat every 28 days.	Lung carcinoma (non-oat cell)
CAP	C—cyclophosphamide A—doxorubicin P—cisplatin	400 mg/m² IV day 1 40 mg/m² IV day 1 60 mg/m² IV day 1 Repeat every 4 weeks for 10 cycles	Adenocarcinoma of lung
CAV	C—cyclophosphamide A—doxorubicin V—vincristine	500 mg/m² IV day 1 50 mg/m² IV day 1 1.4 mg/m² IV day 1 (not to exceed 2 mg) Repeat every 28 days.	Non-small cell lung carcinoma
	OR C—cyclophosphamide A—doxorubicin V—vincristine	750 mg/m² IV day1 50 mg/m² IV day1 2 mg IV day 1 Repeat every 21 days.	Small cell lung carcinoma
CAVe	C—lomustine A—doxorubicin Ve—vinblastine	100 mg/m² PO day 1 60 mg/m² IV day1 5 mg/m² IV day 1 Repeat every 6 weeks for nine cycles.	Hodgkin's disease
CCV	C—cyclophosphamide C—lomustine V—vincristine	700 mg/m² IV days 1 and 22 70 mg/m² PO day 1 2 mg IV days 1 and 22 Repeat every 6 weeks.	Oat-cell carcinoma of lung
CCV-AV	C—lomustine C—cyclophosphamide V—vincristine AV—doxorubicin	100 mg/m² PO day 1 1 g/m² IV days 1 and 22 2 mg IV days 1, 22, 42, 63 75 mg/m² IV days 42 and 63 Repeat every 12 weeks.	Oat-cell carcinoma of lung
CD	C—cisplatin D—doxorubicin	50 mg–60 mg/m² IV day 1 50 mg–60 mg/m² IV day 1 Repeat every 21 days–28 days.	Prostatic carcinoma (advanced)
	OR C—cytarabine D—daunorubicin	100 mg/m² IV infusion over 24 h daily for 7 days 45 mg/m² IV days 1, 2, and 3	Acute myelocytic leukemia
CDV	C—cyclophosphamide D—dacarbazine V—vincristine	750 mg/m² IV day 1 250 mg/m² IV days 1–5 1–5 mg/m² IV day 1 Repeat every 22 days	Neuroblastoma
CFD	C—cyclophosphamide F—fluorouracil D—doxorubicin	500 mg/m² IV day 1 500 mg/m² IV day 1 50 mg/m² IV day 1 Repeat every 21 days.	Prostatic carcinoma (advanced)

(continued)

Table 75-20 (continued)
Combination Chemotherapeutic Regimens

Acronym	Drug	Dosage	Indications
CHL + PRED	CHL—chlorambucil	0.4 mg/kg PO 1 day every other week, increase by 0.1 mg/kg every 2 weeks until toxicity or control	Chronic lymphocytic leukemia
	PRED—prednisone	100 mg/PO days 1 and 2 every other week	
CHOP	C—cyclophosphamide	750 mg/m^2 IV day 1	Non-Hodgkin's lymphoma
	H—doxorubicin	50 mg/m^2 IV day 1	
	O—vincristine	1.4 mg/m^2 IV day 1 (maximum 2 mg)	
	P—prednisone	60 mg/day PO days 1–5 Repeat every 21 days–28 days for six cycles.	
CHOP-BCG	CHOP—(as above) plus BCG—bacille Calmette Guérin	1 vial by scarification days 7 and 14	Non-Hodgkin's lymphoma
CHOP-Bleo	C—cyclophosphamide	750 mg/m^2 IV day 1	Non-Hodgkin's lymphoma
	H—doxorubicin	50 mg/m^2 IV day 1	
	O—vincristine	1.4 mg/m^2 IV day 1 (maximum 2 mg)	
	P—prednisone	100 mg/m^2/day days 1–5	
	Bleo—bleomycin	4 U IV days 1 and 8 or 15 U IV days 1 and 5 Repeat every 21 days–28 days.	
CHOR	C—cyclophosphamide	750 mg/m^2 IV days 1 and 22	Lung carcinoma
	H—doxorubicin	50 mg/m^2 IV days 1 and 22	
	O—vincristine	1 mg IV days 1, 8, 15, 22	
	R—radiation	3000 rad total dose in daily fractions over 2 weeks starting day 36	
CISCA	CIS—cisplatin	100 mg/m^2 IV infusion over 2 h day 2	Urinary carcinoma
	C—cyclophosphamide	650 mg/m^2 IV day 1 Increase to 1000 mg/m^2 when doxorubicin is discontinued.	
	A—doxorubicin	50 mg/m^2 IV day 1; discontinue at 450 mg/m^2 total dose; repeat every 21 days	
CMC-High dose	C—cyclophosphamide	1000 mg/m^2 IV days 1 and 29	Lung carcinoma
	M—methotrexate	15 mg/m^2 IV twice a week for 6 weeks	
	C—lomustine	100 mg/m^2 PO day 1	
CMC-V	C—cyclophosphamide	700 mg/m^2 IV day 1	Small-cell carcinoma of the lung
	M—methotrexate	20 mg/m^2 PO days 18 and 21	
	C—lomustine	70 mg/m^2 PO day 1; repeat every 28 days	
	V—vincristine	2 mg IV days 1, 8, 15, 22; then 1.3 mg/m^2 IV every 4 weeks	
CMF	C—cyclphosphamide	100 mg/m^2 PO days 1–14	Breast carcinoma
	M—methotrexate	40 mg–60 mg/m^2 IV days 1 and 8	
	F—fluorouracil	600 mg/m^2 IV days 1 and 8 Repeat every 28 days; above age 60, reduce methotrexate dose to 30 mg/m^2 and fluorouracil dose to 400 mg/m^2.	

(continued)

Table 75-20 (continued)
Combination Chemotherapeutic Regimens

Acronym	Drug	Dosage	Indications
CMFP	C—cyclophosphamide M—methotrexate F—fluorouracil P—prednisone	100 mg/m² PO days 1–14 60 mg/m² IV days 1 and 8 700 mg/m² IV days 1 and 8 40 mg/m² PO days 1–14 Repeat every 28 days.	Breast carcinoma
CMFVP (Cooper's regimen)	C—cyclophosphamide M—methotrexate F—fluorouracil V—vincristine P—prednisone	2 mg/kg PO daily 0.75 mg/kg IV weekly for 8 weeks, then every other week 12 mg/kg IV weekly for 8 weeks, then every other week 0.035 mg/kg IV weekly (maximum 2 mg) 0.75 mg/kg PO days 1–10 then taper	Breast carcinoma
COMA or COMLA	C—cyclophosphamide O—vincristine M—methotrexate A—cytarabine	1.5 g/m² IV 1.4 mg/m² IV days 1, 8, 15 120 mg/m² PO Give leucovorin 25 mg PO every 6 h for four doses starting 6 h after methotrexate. 300 mg/m² IV bolus 16 h after methotrexate Repeat every 7 days–14 days for eight cycles through days 22–71.	Non-Hodgkin's lymphoma
COAP	C—cyclophosphamide O—vincristine A—cytarabine P—prednisone	100 mg/m² IV days 1–5 1 mg IV days 1, 8, 15, 22 200 mg/m² IV days 1–5 or 100 mg/m² IV days 1–10 100 mg/day PO days 1–5 Repeat after 2-week interval.	Acute myelocytic leukemia
COP	C—cyclophosphamide O—vincristine P—prednisone	1,000 mg/m² IV day 1 1.4 mg/m² IV day 1 (maximum 2 mg) 60 mg/m² PO days 1–5 Repeat every 21 days for six cycles.	Non-Hodgkin's lymphoma
COP-BLAM	C—cyclophosphamide O—vincristine P—prednisone BL—bleomycin A—doxorubicin M—procarbazine	400 mg/m² day 1 1 mg/m² IV day 1 40 mg/m² PO days 1–10 15 U IV day 14 40 mg/m² IV day 1 100 mg/m² PO days 1–10 Repeat every 21 days.	Histiocytic lymphoma
COPP or C-MOPP	C—cyclophosphamide O—vincristine P—procarbazine P—prednisone	650 mg/m² IV days 1 and 8 1.4 mg/m² IV days 1 and 8 (maximum 2 mg) 100 mg/m² PO days 1–14 40 mg/m² PO days 1–14 Repeat every 28 days for six cycles.	Non-Hodgkin's lymphoma
CP	C—carmustine P—prednisone	150 mg/m² IV day 4 60 mg/m² PO days 1–4 Repeat every 42 days.	Multiple myeloma
Hi-CP	C—cyclophosphamide P—prednisone	1000 mg/m² IV day 1 60 mg/m² days 1–4 Repeat every 42 days.	Multiple myeloma
CT	C—cytarabine	1 mg–3 mg/kg IV daily for 8 days–32 days	Acute myelocytic leukemia

(continued)

Table 75-20 (continued)
Combination Chemotherapeutic Regimens

Acronym	Drug	Dosage	Indications
CT *(continued)*	T—thioguanine	2 mg–2.5 mg/kg PO daily for 8 days–32 days Thioguanine usually given in morning and cytarabine 8 h–10 h later	
CV	C—cyclophosphamide V—vincristine	10 mg/kg IV every other week 0.05 mg/kg IV on the alternate weeks Continue treatment 12 weeks or longer	Neuroblastoma
CVB	C—cisplatin V—vinblastine B—bleomycin	20 mg/m² IV days 1–5; repeat every 3 weeks for three cycles 0.2 mg/kg IV days 1 and 2; repeat every 3 weeks for 12 weeks; then 0.3 mg/kg IV every 4 weeks for 2 years 30 U IV weekly for 12 weeks	Testicular carcinoma
CVB	C—lomustine V—vinblastine B—bleomycin	100 mg/m² PO day 1 6 mg/m² IV days 1 and 8 15 U/m² IV days 1 and 8 Repeat every 28 days.	Hodgkin's disease
CVP	C—cyclophosphamide V—vincristine P—prednisone	400 mg/m² PO days 2–6 1.4 mg/m² IV day 1 (maximum 2 mg) 40 mg/m² PO days 1–14 Repeat every 28 days for 6 cycles.	Non-Hodgkin's lymphoma
CVPP	C—cyclophosphamide V—vinblastine P—procarbazine P—prednisone	300 mg/m² IV days 1 and 8 10 mg/m² IV days 1, 8, 15 100 mg/m² PO days 1–15 40 mg/m² PO days 1–15 (cycles 1 and 4 only) Repeat every 28 days.	Hodgkin's disease
CVPP/CCNU	C—cyclophosphamide V—vinblastine P—procarbazine P—prednisone CCNU—lomustine	600 mg/m² IV day 1 6 mg/m² IV day 1 100 mg/m² PO days 1–14 40 mg/m² days 1–14 75 mg/m² day 1 (alternate cycles) Repeat every 28 days.	Hodgkin's disease
CY-VA-DIC	CY—cyclophosphamide V—vincristine A—doxorubicin DIC—dacarbazine	500 mg/m² IV day 1 1.4 mg/m² IV days 1 and 5 (maximum 2 mg) 50 mg/m² IV day 1 250 mg/m² IV days 1–5 Repeat every 21 days.	Soft-tissue sarcomas
DA	D—daunorubicin A—cytarabine	45 mg/m² IV days 1–3 100 mg/m² IV days 1–10 Repeat as needed.	Acute myelocytic leukemia
DAT	D—daunorubicin A—cytarabine (Ara-C) T—thioguanine	60 mg/m² IV days 5, 6, 7 100 mg/m² IV over 30 min twice a day for 7 days 100 mg/m² PO every 12 h for 7 days Repeat every 30 days with 5 days therapy of cytarabine and thioguanine alternating with a single dose of daunorubicin.	Acute myelocytic leukemia

(continued)

Table 75-20 (continued)
Combination Chemotherapeutic Regimens

Acronym	Drug	Dosage	Indications
DMC	D—doxorubicin	2.5 mg/kg/day IV days 1–3	Osteogenic sarcoma
	M—methotrexate	200 mg–750 mg/kg/24 h IV infusion day 14	
	C—citrovorum factor (calcium leucovorin)	9 mg PO every 6 h for 12 doses starting 12 h after methotrexate infusion	
		Repeat every 28 days	
DOAP	D—daunorubicin	60 mg/m² IV day 1	Acute myelocytic leukemia
	O—vincristine	1 mg IV days 1, 8, 15, 22	
	A—cytarabine	200 mg/m² IV days 1–5 or 100 mg/m² IV days 1–10	
	P—prednisone	100 mg/day PO days 1–5	
		Repeat after 2-week interval.	
FAC	F—fluorouracil	500 mg/m² IV days 1 and 8	Breast carcinoma
	A—doxorubicin	50 mg/m² IV day 1	
	C—cyclophosphamide	500 mg/m² IV day 1	
		Repeat every 3 weeks.	
FAM	F—fluorouracil	600 mg/m² IV days 1, 2, 28, 36	Lung or gastric carcinoma
	A—doxorubicin	30 mg/m² IV days 1 and 28	
	M—mitomycin	10 mg/m² IV day 1	
		Repeat every 8 weeks	
	OR		
	F—fluorouracil	600 mg/m² IV week 1, 2, 5, 6, 9	Pancreatic carcinoma
	A—doxorubicin	30 mg/m² IV week 1, 5, 9	
	M—mitomycin	10 mg/m² IV week 1 and 9	
FAP	F—fluorouracil	500 mg/m² IV day 1	Bladder carcinoma
	A—doxorubicin	50 mg/m² IV day 1	
	P—cisplatin	100 mg/m² IV day 1; reduce to 50 mg–75 mg/m² after three doses	
		Repeat every 4 weeks.	
FCP	F—fluorouracil	8 mg/kg/day IV for 5 days	Breast carcinoma
	C—cyclophosphamide	4 mg/kg/day IV for 5 days	
	P—prednisone	30 mg/day PO tapered to 10 mg/day	
	(±)vincristine	1.4 mg/m² IV days 1 and 5	
FIVB (FDVB)	F—fluorouracil	10 mg/kg IV days 1–5	Colorectal carcinoma
	I—dacarbazine	3 mg/kg IV days 1 and 2	
	V—vincristine	0.025 mg/kg IV day 1	
	B—carmustine	1.5 mg/kg IV day 1	
		Repeat every 4 weeks–6 weeks.	
FOMi	F—fluorouracil	300 mg/m² IV days 1–4	Lung carcinoma (non-small cell)
	O—vincristine	2 mg IV day 1	
	Mi—mitomycin	10 mg/m² IV day 1	
		Repeat every 3 weeks for three cycles then every 6 weeks.	
HOP	H—doxorubicin	80 mg/m² IV day 1	Non-Hodgkin's lymphoma
	O—vincristine	1.4 mg/m² IV day 1 (maximum 2 mg)	
	P—prednisone	100 mg/m² PO days 1–5	
		Repeat every 3 weeks.	
M-2 Protocol	vincristine	0.03 mg/kg IV day 1 (maximum 2 mg)	Multiple myeloma
	carmustine	0.5 mg/kg IV day 1	
	cyclophosphamide	10 mg/kg IV day 1	
	melphalan	0.25 mg/kg PO days 1–14	

(continued)

Table 75-20 (continued)
Combination Chemotherapeutic Regimens

Acronym	Drug	Dosage	Indications
M-2 Protocol (continued)	prednisone	1 mg/kg PO days 1–7, then taper to day 21 Repeat every 35 days.	
MA	M—mitomycin A—doxorubicin	10 mg/m^2 IV day 1 50 mg/m^2 IV days 1 and 22 Repeat every 6 weeks.	Breast carcinoma Adenocarcinoma of lung
MAC	M—methotrexate A—dactinomycin C—chlorambucil	15 mg IM days 1–5 8 mcg–10 mcg/kg IV days 1–5 8 mg–10 mg PO days 1–5 Repeat every 10 days–14 days.	Choriocarcinoma
MACC	M—methotrexate A—doxorubicin C—cyclophosphamide C—lomustine	40 mg/m^2 IV day 1 40 mg/m^2 IV day 1 400 mg/m^2 IV day 1 30 mg/m^2 PO day 1 Repeat every 21 days.	Lung carcinoma (non-oat cell)
MACM	M—mitomycin A—doxorubicin C—lomustine M—methotrexate	8 mg/m^2 IV day 1 60 mg/m^2 IV day 1 60 mg/m^2 PO day 1 40 mg/m^2 IV day 1 Repeat every 4 weeks.	Squamous cell carcinoma of lung
MACOP-B	M—methotrexate A—doxorubicin C—cyclophosphamide O—vincristine P—prednisone B—bleomycin Co-trimoxazole	400 mg/m^2 IV weeks 2, 6, 10 given as 100 mg/m^2 IV bolus and 300 mg/m^2 IV infusion over 4 h followed in 24 h by leucovorin calcium 15 mg PO every 6 h for 6 doses 50 mg/m^2 IV weeks 1, 3, 5, 7, 9, 11 350 mg/m^2 IV weeks 1, 3, 5, 7, 9, 11 1.4 mg/m^2 IV weeks 2, 4, 6, 8, 10, 12 75 mg/day PO daily; dose tapered over the last 15 days 10 U/m^2 IV weeks 4, 8, 12 Two tablets twice a day throughout 12-week course of therapy	Non-Hodgkin's lymphoma
MAP	M—melphalan A—doxorubicin P—prednisone	6 mg/m^2 PO days 1–4 25 mg/m^2 IV day 1 60 mg/m^2 PO days 1–4 Repeat every 4 weeks.	Multiple myeloma
M-BACOD	M—methotrexate B—bleomycin A—doxorubicin C—cyclophosphamide O—vincristine D—dexamethasone	3 g/m^2 IV day 14 followed by leucovorin calcium 10 mg/m^2 IV in 24 h and 10 mg/m^2 PO every 6 h for 72 h 4 U/m^2 IV day 1 45 mg/m^2 IV day 1 600 mg/m^2 IV day 1 1 mg/m^2 IV day 1 6 mg/m^2 PO days 1–5 Repeat every 21 days	Non-Hodgkin's lymphoma
MBD	M—methotrexate B—bleomycin D—cisplatin (cis-diamminedichloroplatinum)	40 mg/m^2 IM days 1 and 15 10 U IM weekly 50 mg/m^2 IV day 4 Repeat every 21 days.	Head and neck carcinoma
MCBP	M—melphalan C—cyclophosphamide	4 mg/m^2 PO days 1–4 300 mg/m^2 IV day 1	Multiple myeloma

(continued)

Table 75-20 (continued)
Combination Chemotherapeutic Regimens

Acronym	Drug	Dosage	Indications
MCBP (continued)	B—carmustine	30 mg/m² IV day 1	
	P—prednisone	60 mg/m² PO days 1–4	
		Repeat every 4 weeks.	
MCC	M—methotrexate	10 mg/m² PO two times a week	Non-small cell lung carcinoma
	C—cyclophosphamide	500 mg/m² IV every 21 days	
	C—lomustine (CCNU)	50 mg/m² PO every 42 days	
MCP	M—melphalan	6 mg/m² PO days 1–4	Multiple myeloma
	C—cyclophosphamide	500 mg/m² PO day 1	
	P—prednisone	60 mg/m² PO days 1–4	
		Repeat every 4 weeks.	
MF	M—mitomycin	15 mg–20 mg/m² IV day 1; repeat every 8 weeks; reduce dose 50% after second dose	Colorectal carcinoma
	F—fluorouracil	1 g/m² continuous IV infusion over 24 h days 1–4	
		Repeat every 4 weeks.	
M-F	M—methotrexate	125 mg–250 mg/m² IV	Head and neck carcinoma
	F—fluorouracil	600 mg/m² IV 1 h later	
	Leucovorin rescue	10 mg/m² IV or PO at 24 h then 10 mg/m² PO every 6 h for five doses	
		Repeat every 7 days.	
MOB	M—mitomycin	20 mg/m² IV day 1	Squamous cell carcinoma of cervix
	O—vincristine	0.5 mg/m² IV twice a week for 12 weeks	
	B—bleomycin	6 U/m² IM or IV 6 h after vincristine twice a week for 12 weeks	
		Repeat every 6 weeks.	
MOPP	M—mechlorethamine	6 mg/m² IV days 1 and 8	Hodgkin's disease
	O—vincristine	1.4 mg/m² IV days 1 and 8 (maximum 2 mg)	
	P—procarbazine	100 mg/m² PO days 1–14	
	P—prednisone	40 mg/m² PO days 1–14	
		Repeat every 28 days for six to eight cycles	
MOPP-LO BLEO	M—mechlorethamine	6 mg/m² IV days 1 and 8	Hodgkin's disease
	O—vincristine	1.5 mg/m² IV days 1 and 8 (maximum 2 mg)	
	P—procarbazine	100 mg/m² PO days 2–7, 9–12	
	P—prednisone	40 mg/m² PO days 2–7, 9–12	
	BLEO—bleomycin	2 U/m² IV days 1 and 8	
		Repeat every 28 days for 6 cycles.	
MP	M—melphalan	0.25 mg/kg PO days 1–4	Multiple myeloma
	P—prednisone	2 mg/kg PO days 1–4	
		Repeat every 6 weeks.	
MPL + PRED (MP)	MPL—melphalan	8 mg/m² PO days 1–14	Multiple myeloma
	PRED—prednisone	75 mg/m² PO days 1–7	
MTX + MP	MTX—methotrexate	20 mg/m² IV weekly	Acute lymphocytic leukemia
	MP—mercaptopurine	50 mg/m²/day PO	
		Continue until relapse or remission for 3 years.	
MTX + MP + CTX	MTX—methotrexate	20 mg/m² IV weekly	Acute lymphocytic leukemia
	MP—mercaptopurine	50 mg/m²/day PO	
	CTX—cyclophosphamide	200 mg/m² IV weekly	
		Continue until relapse or remission for 3 years.	

(continued)

Table 75-20 (continued)
Combination Chemotherapeutic Regimens

Acronym	Drug	Dosage	Indications
MV	M—mitomycin V—vinblastine	20 mg/m² IV day 1 0.15 mg/kg IV days 1 and 22 Repeat every 6 weeks–8 weeks	Breast carcinoma
MVPP	M—mechlorethamine V—vinblastine P—procarbazine P—prednisone	6 mg/m² IV days 1–8 6 mg/m² IV days 1 and 8 100 mg/m² PO days 1–14 40 mg/day PO days 1–14 Rest 28 days and repeat for six or more cycles.	Hodgkin's disease
MVVPP	M—mechlorethamine V—vincristine V—vinblastine P—procarbazine P—prednisone	0.4 mg/kg IV day 1 1.4 mg/m² IV days 1, 8, 15 6 mg/m² IV days 22, 29, 36 100 mg/m² PO days 22–43 40 mg/m² PO days 1–22 (taper over 14 days) Repeat every 57 days.	Hodgkin's disease
OAP	O—vincristine A—cytarabine P—prednisone	1 mg IV days 1, 8, 15, 22 200 mg/m² IV days 1–5 or 100 mg/m² IV days 1–10 100 mg PO days 1–5 Repeat after 2-week interval.	Acute myelocytic leukemia
PA	P—cisplatin A—doxorubicin	50 mg–60 mg/m² IV 50 mg–60 mg/m² IV Repeat every 3 weeks–4 weeks.	Adenocarcinoma of prostate

PAC-5	P—cisplatin
	
	A—doxorubicin
	
	C—cyclophosphamide
		20 mg/m² IV days 1–5 (total dose
		  300 mg/m²)
		50 mg/m² IV day 1 (total dose
		  450 mg/m²)
		750 mg/m² IV day 1 (increase
		  dose 20% after stopping cispla-
		  tin and doxorubicin)
		Repeat every 3 weeks.
			Ovarian carcinoma

PCV	P—procarbazine C—lomustine V—vincristine	60 mg/m² PO days 8–21 110 mg/m² PO day 1 1.4 mg/m² IV days 8 and 29 Repeat every 6 weeks–8 weeks.	Primary malignant brain tumors
POCC	P—procarbazine O—vincristine C—cyclophosphamide C—lomustine	100 mg/m² PO days 1–14 2 mg IV days 1 and 8 600 mg/m² IV days 1 and 8 60 mg/m² PO day 1 Repeat every 28 days.	Lung carcinoma
POMP (low dose)	P—prednisone O—vincristine M—methotrexate P—mercaptopurine	150 mg/day PO days 1–5 2 mg/day IV day 1 5 mg/m²/day IV days 1–5 500 mg/m²/day IV days 1–5 Repeat every 2 weeks–3 weeks as tolerated.	Acute myelocytic leukemia

Pro-MACE-MOPP	Pro—prednisone
	M—methotrexate
	
	A—doxorubicin
	C—cyclophosphamide
	E—etoposide
		60 mg/m² PO days 1–14
		1500 mg/m² IV day 14 followed
		  in 24 h by leucovorin calcium
		  50 mg/m² PO every 6 h for 5
		  doses
		25 mg/m² IV days 1 and 8
		650 mg/m² IV days 1 and 8
		120 mg/m² IV days 1 and 8
		Repeat every 28 days.
			Non-Hodgkin's lym-
			phomas

(continued)

Table 75-20 (continued)
Combination Chemotherapeutic Regimens

Acronym	Drug	Dosage	Indications
Pro-MACE-MOPP (continued)	MOPP	Standard MOPP therapy after remission and repeated every 28 days	
SCAB	S—streptozocin C—lomustine A—doxorubicin B—bleomycin	500 mg/m^2 IV days 1 and 15 100 mg/m^2 PO day 1 45 mg/m^2 IV day 1 15 U/m^2 IV days 1 and 8 Repeat every 28 days.	Hodgkin's disease
SMF	S—streptozocin M—mitomycin F—fluorouracil	1000 mg/m^2 IV days 1, 8, 29, 35 10 mg/m^2 IV day 1 600 mg/m^2 IV days 1, 8, 29, 35 Repeat every 8 weeks.	Pancreatic carcinoma

T-2 protocol	*Cycle No. 1*
	Month 1
	  dactinomycin
	  doxorubicin
	  radiation
	Month 2
	  doxorubicin
	  vincristine
	
	  cyclophosphamide
	  radiation
	Month 3
	  vincristine
	
	  cyclophosphamide
	Cycle No. 2
	  Repeat Cycle No. 1 without radiation.
	Cycle No. 3
	Month 1
	  dactinomycin
	  doxorubicin
	Month 2
	  vincristine
	
	  cyclophosphamide
	Month 3
	  No drugs given for 28 days
	Cycle No. 4
	  Repeat Cycle No. 3.
		
		0.45 mg/m^2 IV days 1–5
		20 mg/m^2 IV days 20–22
		Days 1–21, then rest 2 weeks
		
		20 mg/m^2 IV days 8–10
		1.5 mg–2 mg/m^2 IV day 24 (maximum 2 mg)
		1200 mg/m^2 IV day 24
		Days 8–28
		
		1.5 mg–2 mg/m^2 IV days 3, 9, 15 (maximum 2 mg)
		1200 mg/m^2 IV day 1
		
		0.45 mg/m^2 IV days 1–5
		20 mg/m^2 IV days 20–22
		
		1.5 mg–2 mg/m^2 IV days 8, 15, 22, 28 (maximum 2 mg)
		1200 mg/m^2 IV days 8 and 22
			Ewing's sarcoma

TODD	T—thioguanine O—vincristine D—pyrimethamine D—dexamethasone	2 mg/kg PO days 1–5 2 mg/m^2 IV day 1 1.5 mg/kg PO days 1–5 2 mg/m^2 PO three times a day on days 1–5 Repeat every 11 days with 6 days' rest period.	Acute lymphocytic leukemia
TRAMPCO(L)	T—thioguanine R—daunorubicin A—cytarabine M—methotrexate	100 mg/m^2 PO days 1–3 Increase to 4 days–5 days after first course. 40 mg/m^2 IV day 1 100 mg/m^2 IV days 1–3 Increase to 4 days–5 days after first course. 7.5 mg/m^2 IV or IM days 1–3	Acute leukemias

(continued)

Table 75-20 (continued)
Combination Chemotherapeutic Regimens

Acronym	Drug	Dosage	Indications
TRAMPCO (L) (*continued*)		Increase to 4 days–5 days after first course.	
	P—prednisolone	200 mg PO days 1–3 Increase to 4 days–5 days after first course.	
	C—cyclophosphamide	100 mg/m² IV days 1–3 Increase 4 days–5 days after first course.	
	O—vincristine	2 mg IV day 1	
	L—L-asparaginase	8,000 U/m² IV days 1–28 in first two courses Repeat every 2 weeks, 3 weeks, or 4 weeks with wider spacing in patients with good response.	
TRAP	T—thioguanine	100 mg/m²/day PO days 1–5	Acute myelocytic leukemia
	R—daunorubicin (rubidomycin)	40 mg/m²/day IV day 1	
	A—cytarabine	100 mg/m²/day IV or IM days 1–5	
	P—prednisone	30 mg/m²/day PO days 1–5	
VAC	V—vincristine	1.5 mg/m² IV every week for 10 weeks–12 weeks	Ovarian carcinoma
	A—dactinomycin	0.5 mg/day IV days 1–5; repeat every 4 weeks	
	C—cyclophosphamide	5 mg–7 mg/kg/day IV days 1–5; repeat every 4 weeks	
VAC Pulse	V—vincristine	2 mg/m² IV weekly for weeks 1–12 (maximum 2 mg)	Sarcoma
	A—dactinomycin	0.015 mg/kg IV days 1–5 of weeks 1 and 13, then every 3 months for five to six courses (maximum 0.5 mg a day)	
	C—cyclophosphamide	10 mg/kg IV or PO for 7 days Repeat every 6 weeks for 2 years.	
VAC Standard	V—vincristine	2 mg/m² IV weekly for weeks 1–12 (maximum 2 mg)	Sarcoma
	A—dactinomycin	0.015 mg/kg IV days 1–5; repeat every 3 months for five to six courses (maximum 0.5 mg a day)	
	C—cyclophosphamide	2.5 mg/kg PO daily for 2 years	
VBAP	V—vincristine	1 mg IV day 1	Multiple myeloma
	B—carmustine	30 mg/m² IV day 2	
	A—doxorubicin	30 mg/m² IV day 2	
	P—prednisone	60 mg/m² PO days 2–5 Repeat every 3 weeks.	
VBD	V—vinblastine	6 mg/m² IV days 1 and 2	Melanoma
	B—bleomycin	15 U/m² IV days 1–5 by 24-h infusion	
	D—cisplatin	50 mg/m² IV day 5 Repeat every 28 days.	

(continued)

Table 75-20 (continued)
Combination Chemotherapeutic Regimens

Acronym	Drug	Dosage	Indications
VBP	V—vinblastine	0.2 mg/kg IV days 1 and 2; repeat every 3 weeks for five courses	Testicular carcinoma
	B—bleomycin	30 U/week IV 6 h after vinblastine on the second day of each week for 12 weeks until total dose of 360 U	
	P—cisplatin	20 mg/m² IV days 1–5, 6 h after vinblastine	
		Repeat every 3 weeks for three courses	
VCAP	V—vincristine	1 mg VI day 1	Multiple myeloma
	C—cyclophosphamide	100 mg/m² PO days 1–4	
	A—doxorubicin	25 mg/m² IV day 2	
	P—prednisone	60 mg/m² PO days 1–4	
		Repeat every 4 weeks.	
VCR-MTX-CF or VMC	VCR—vincristine	2 mg/m² IV for one dose (maximum 2 mg)	Osteogenic sarcoma
	MTX—methotrexate	3000 mg–7500 mg/m² IV 6-h infusion starting 30 min after vincristine	
	CF—citrovorum factor (calcium leucovorin)	15 mg IV every 3 h for eight doses, then 15 mg PO every 3 h for eight doses	
VM	V—vinblastine	5 mg/m² IV	Adenocarcinoma of lung
	M—mitomycin	6 mg/m² IV	
		Repeat every 2 weeks.	
VMCP	V—vincristine	1 mg IV day 1	Multiple myeloma
	M—melphalan	5 mg/m² PO days 1–4	
	C—cyclophosphamide	100 mg/m² PO days 1–4	
	P—prednisone	60 mg/m² PO days 1–4	
		Repeat every 3 weeks.	
VP	V—vincristine	2 mg/m² IV every week for 4 weeks–6 weeks (maximum 2 mg)	Acute lymphocytic leukemia
	P—prednisone	60 mg/m² PO daily for 4 weeks, then taper weeks 5–7	
VP-L-Asparaginase	V—vincristine	2 mg/m² IV every week for 4 weeks–6 weeks (maximum 2 mg)	Acute lymphocytic leukemia
	P—prednisone	60 mg/m² PO daily for 4 weeks–6 weeks, then taper	
	L-asparaginase	10,000 U/m² IV days 1–14	
VP plus Daunorubicin	V—vincristine	1.5 mg/m² IV weekly for 4 weeks–6 weeks	Acute lymphocytic leukemia
	P—prednisone	40 mg/m² PO daily for 4 weeks–6 weeks	
	daunorubicin	25 mg/m² IV weekly for 4 weeks–6 weeks	

agents are also used to delay or prevent the emergence of resistance in the tumor cells and to obtain a synergistic therapeutic effect with minimal toxicity.

The general principles used for the selection of agents to be used for a combination chemotherapeutic regimen are as follows:
1. Each agent used in the regimen must be clinically active in the specific disease.
2. To obtain synergism, each agent must have a different mechanism of action. Agents are used to block different sites in biochemical pathways or to inhibit critical cell functions. Three different types of blockade have been described:
   a. Sequential blockade—Inhibition of two different steps of the same biochemical pathway
   b. Concurrent blockade—Blockade of parallel metabolic pathways leading to a common end product
   c. Complementary inhibition—Inhibition at different sites by agents with entirely different modes of inhibitory action, in the synthesis of large polymeric molecules (most common basis for design of combination chemotherapeutic regimens)

3. Agents with different toxicities or different timing of a similar toxicity are used to reduce cumulative toxicity to a single organ system and allow individual agents to be used in full clinical doses.
4. Agents are scheduled with respect to tumor cell kinetics to potentiate the effect of each agent in the regimen. Both cell-cycle specific and cell-cycle nonspecific agents are used in regimens to simultaneously kill both dividing and nondividing cell fractions in the tumor. Careful intermittent scheduling has also proved to be less immunosuppressive and less toxic than continuous daily therapy.
5. Each agent should be administered at the maximum dose tolerated by the patient and such dose should be close to, or beyond, the minimum effective *dosage* of each agent as a single agent.

Table 75-20 lists a number of currently used combination chemotherapeutic regimens. Individual drug components of each combination are given along with the recommended dosage and indications. Continuing research constantly reveals new dosages, regimens, and combinations of antineoplastic agents (for specific and current indications consult the literature).

CASE STUDY

Jim, an 18-year-old college freshman, presented 2 months ago to his college infirmary with complaints of fever, night sweats, weight loss, and an enlarging right neck mass. The nurse sent him to the local hospital, where a chest x-ray revealed a mediastinal mass. A biopsy of his neck mass showed lymphoblastic lymphoma.

Since his diagnosis, he has been treated with the CHOP regimen (cyclophosphamide, doxorubicin, vincristine, and prednisone) (see Table 75-20) given every 3 weeks, with weekly vincristine, and six doses of asparaginase.

Jim presents today, 7 days after his fifth course of chemotherapy, with complaints of chills and moderate amounts of "tingling" in his fingers and toes. Oral temperature is 101°F. CBC was drawn and revealed a WBC of 800 and platelets of 295,000.

Discussion Questions

1. Which drugs that Jim is receiving are causing myelosuppression?
2. What nursing actions would be instituted in the care of this patient with neutropenia?
3. Which drug included in Jim's therapy would be most likely to cause neuropathies?

4. Would the nurse expect to see Jim experience constipation? What are some nursing measures to prevent constipation?

REVIEW QUESTIONS

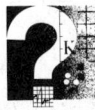

1. Describe the characteristics common to all types of cancer.
2. Briefly discuss the phases of cell division.
3. What do the terms CCS and CCNS mean in regard to cancer chemotherapeutic agents?
4. Indicate the differences between CCS and CCNS antineoplastic drugs. List three examples of each.
5. What is the primary goal of cancer therapy?
6. Briefly describe the general principles of cancer chemotherapy.
7. What type of patient education is appropriate with regard to the development of the following untoward reactions: (1) thrombocytopenia, (2) anemia, (3) alopecia, and (4) nausea and vomiting?
8. How may extravasation of drug solutions be prevented? How may the local tissue reactions that occur upon extravasation be managed?
9. What is the mechanism of action of the alkylating agents? List five examples of drugs classified as alkylating agents.
10. Indicate the principal contraindications and precautions associated with the use of alkylating agents.
11. What is the basic mechanism of action of the antimetabolites used in cancer chemotherapy?
12. List the three groups of antimetabolites. Give an example of each.
13. Briefly discuss the major adverse reactions associated with use of antimetabolites, and what types of teaching the nurse must provide to patients receiving these drugs.
14. List the types of natural products used as antineoplastic agents. Give an example of each.
15. What is the mechanism of action of (1) vinblastine and vincristine, (2) asparaginase, and (3) etoposide?
16. Describe the toxicity associated with doxorubicin that may occur several months after initiating therapy. What nursing interventions are necessary in this situation?
17. What toxicity may occur in 90% to 100% of patients receiving vinblastine or vincristine? What are some signs of this toxicity?
18. What are the indications for the use of androgens and estrogens in the therapy of breast carcinoma? List two different agents in each category.
19. What is the mechanism of action of tamoxifen? In what type of patient is this agent *unlikely* to be effective?
20. What is the mechanism of action of leuprolide? For what types of carcinomas is it used?
21. What are interferons? How are they being used in cancer treatment? What actions contribute to the antitumor activity of this agent?
22. What action of procarbazine causes this agent to have

many potential drug interactions? List three different drug interactions observed with procarbazine.
23. Discuss the rationale and general principles of combination cancer chemotherapy.

BIBLIOGRAPHY

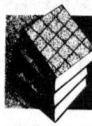

Akahoski M: High dose methotrexate with leucovorin in rescue. Cancer Nursing 1(4):319, 1978

Aronin PA, Mahaley MS, Rudnick S et al: Prediction of BCNU pulmonary toxicity in patients with malignant gliomas: An assessment of risk factors. N Engl J Med 303(4):183, 1980

Barnett M, Waxman J, Richards M et al: Central nervous system toxicity of high dose cytosine arabinoside. Semin Oncol 12(2):133, 1985

Baxley K, Erdman L, Henry E, Roof B: Alopecia: Effect on cancer patient's body image. Cancer Nursing 7:499, 1984

Becker T: Cancer Chemotherapy: A Manual for Nurses. Boston, Little Brown, 1981

Benner P: From Novice to Expert: Excellence and Power in Clinical Nursing Practice. Menlo Park CA, Addison-Wesley, 1984

Brager B, Yasko J: Care of the Client Receiving Chemotherapy. Reston, Reston Publishing, 1984

Brandt B: A nursing protocol for the client with neutropenia. Oncol Nurs Forum 11(2):24, 1984

Burkhalter D, Donley D: Dynamics of Oncology Nursing. New York, McGraw-Hill, 1978

Calabresi P, Schein PS, Rosenberg SA (eds): Medical Oncology. New York, MacMillan, 1985

Cancer chemotherapy. Med Lett Drug Ther 29:29, 1987

Cline B: Prevention of chemotherapy-induced alopecia: A review of the literature. Cancer Nursing 7(3):221, 1984

Conrad K: Cerebellar toxicities associated with cytosine arabinoside: A nursing perspective. Oncol Nurs Forum 13(5):57, 1986

Cooley M, Cobb S: Sexual and reproductive issues for women with Hodgkins disease: I. Overview of issues. Cancer Nursing 9(4):188, 1986

Dellefield ME: Caring for the elderly patient with cancer. Oncol Nurs Forum 13(3):19, 1986

DeVita VT, Hellman S, Rosenberg SA (eds): Cancer: Principles and Practice of Oncology, 2nd ed. Philadelphia, JB Lippincott, 1985

Dorr RT, Fritz WL: Cancer Chemotherapy Handbook. New York, Elsevier, 1980

Engelking C, Steele N: A model for pretreatment nursing assessment of patients receiving cancer chemotherapy. Cancer Nursing 7(3):203, 1984

Fasley K, Ignoffo RJ: Manual of Oncology Therapeutics. St. Louis, CV Mosby, 1981

Furr BJ, Jordan VC: Pharmacology and clinical uses of tamoxifen. Pharmacol Ther 25:127, 1984

Glazer RI (ed): Developments in Cancer Chemotherapy. Boca Raton, CRC Press, 1984

Goodman M: Cisplatin: Outpatient and office hydration regimens. Semin Oncol Nurs 3(1, Suppl 1):36, 1987

Goodman M: Management of nausea and vomiting induced by outpatient cisplatin therapy. Semin Oncol Nurs 3(1, Suppl 1):23, 1987

Griffiths MJ, Murray KH, Russo DC: Oncology Nursing: Pathophysiology Assessment and Intervention. New York, MacMillan, 1985

Hacker MP, Douple EB, Krakoff IH (eds): Platinum co-ordination complexes in cancer chemotherapy. Boston, Martinus Nijhoff, 1984

Holden S, Felde G: Nursing care of patients experiencing cisplatin-related peripheral neuropathy. Oncol Nurs Forum 14(1):13, 1987

Hughes CB: Giving cancer drugs IV: Some guidelines. Am J Nurs 86(1):34, Jan 1986

Hunter R: Hodgkin's disease: A critical review. Cancer Chemotherapy Update 1(2): Sept/Oct 1983

Ignoffo RJ: Oncology. In Kotcher BS, Young LY, Koda-Kimble MA (eds): Applied Therapeutics—The Clinical Use of Drugs, p 899. Spokane, Applied Therapeutics, Inc, 1983

Ignoffo RJ, Friedman MA: Therapy of local toxicities caused by extravasation of cancer chemotherapeutic drugs. Cancer Treat Rev 7:17, 1980

Kaempfer S: The effects of cancer chemotherapy on reproduction: A review of the literature. Oncol Nurs Forum 8(1):11, 1981

Kaempfer S, Wiley F, Hoffman D, Rhodes E: Fertility considerations and procreative alternatives in cancer care. Semin Oncol Nurs 1(1):25, 1985

Knoben JE, Anderson PO: Handbook of Clinical Drug Data, 5th ed. Hamilton, IL, Drug Intelligence Publications, 1983

Knobf MK, Fischer DS, Welch-McCaffrey D: Cancer Chemotherapy: Treatment and Care. Boston, GK Hall Medical Publishers, 1984

Knobf MK, Lewis KP, Fischer DS et al: Cancer Chemotherapy: Treatment and Care. Boston, GK Hall Medical Publishers, 1981

Lauer P: Learning needs of cancer patients: A comparison of nurse and patient's perceptions. Nursing Research 31(1):11, 1982

Lydon J: Nephrotoxicity of cancer treatment. Oncol Nurs Forum 13(2):68, 1986

Marsh JC, Fischer DS: Combination chemotherapy. In Marsh JC, Fischer DS (eds): Cancer Therapy. Boston, GK Hall Medical Publishers, 1982

Miller S, Dodd M, Goodman M, et al: Cancer Chemotherapy: Guidelines and Recommendations for Nursing Education and Practice. Oncology Nursing Society, 1984

Miller S: Considerations in the outpatient and office administration of cisplatin. Semin Oncol Nurs 3(1, Suppl 1):3, 1987

Muggia EM, Nishoff M (eds): Cancer Chemotherapy, Vol II. Boston, Martinus Nijhoff, 1985

O'Dwyer PJ, Leyland-Jones B, Alonso MT et al: Etoposide (VP-16-213): Current status of an active anticancer drug. N Engl J Med 312:692, 1985

Riggs CE: Combination Chemotherapy. In Moossa AR, Robsen MC, Schimpf SC (eds): Comprehensive Testbook of Oncology. Baltimore, Williams & Wilkins, 1986

Rubin P: Clinical Oncology, 6th ed. New York, American Cancer Society, 1983

Solimando DA: Myelosuppressive effects of antineoplastic agents. Highlights on Antineoplastic Drugs 4(2):1, May/June 1986

Watson P: Patient education: The adult with cancer. Nurs Clin North Am 17(4):735, 1982

Welch-McCaffrey D: Evolving patient education needs in cancer. Oncol Nurs Forum 12(5):62, 1985

Welch-McCaffrey D (ed): Nursing Considerations in Geriatric
    Oncology. Columbus, OH Adria Laboratories, 1986
Wickham P: Pulmonary toxicity secondary to cancer treatment. Oncol
    Nurs Forum 13(5):69, 1986
Wojciechowski NJ, Carter CA, Skoutakis VA et al: Leuprolide: A
    gonadotropin-releasing hormone analog for the palliative
    treatment of prostatic cancer. Drug Intell Clin Pharm 20:746, 1986
Wolfe CA, Linkewich JA: Preparation of guidelines for the avoidance
    and treatment of extravasation due to antineoplastic drugs.
    Hospital Pharm 22:125, 1987
Yarbo C, Perry M: The effect of cancer therapy on gonadal function.
    Semin Oncol Nurs 1(1):3, 1985

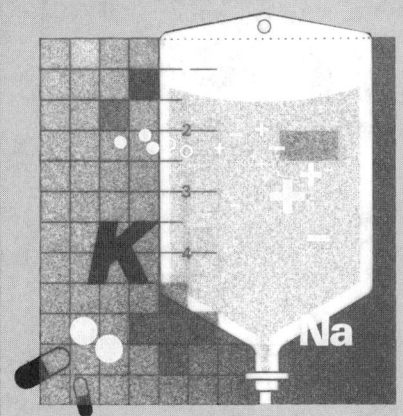

Nutrients, Fluids, and Electrolytes

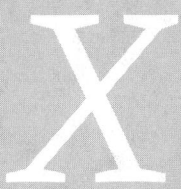

X

Water-Soluble Vitamins: Vitamins B and C

76

Vitamins are commonly classified as either water soluble (B complex, C) or fat soluble (A, D, E, K). The water-soluble vitamins are reviewed in this chapter and the fat-soluble vitamins are discussed in Chapter 76.

Vitamins: General Considerations

Vitamins are organic substances required by the body for synthesis of essential cofactors that catalyze metabolic reactions. The body does not have the capacity to provide enough of all the essential vitamins, and hence dietary sources are necessary. Since the average diet is usually more than adequate in supplying most required vitamins, the majority of people rarely have a need for additional vitamins and indiscriminate use of single- or multiple-vitamin preparations should be discouraged.

There are, however, certain situations in which vitamin supplementation can be justified. Vitamin-deficiency states can result from inadequate nutritional intake; impaired absorption; increased requirements; malnutrition (*e.g.*, from starvation, anorexia, extreme diets, food faddism); pathologic conditions (gastrointestinal disorders, hyperthyroidism, intestinal surgery, carcinomas); alcoholism; prolonged stress; dialysis; and a variety of other conditions. Provided that a definite vitamin deficiency can be demonstrated based on clinical symptoms, selective replacement of those vitamins that are lacking is indicated. Use of multivitamin formulations for replacement therapy, however, is usually unnecessary and can become a significant expense as well. A much more reasonable approach is to supply the deficient vitamins in the amounts required to eliminate the symptoms of the vitamin-deficiency state. For example, thiamine is indicated for beriberi, niacin for pellagra, ascorbic acid for scurvy, and cyanocobalamin for pernicious anemia. It is important, however, to regard vitamins as drugs, and as such they should only be used where there is valid indication. Injudicious or excessive intake of vitamins is at best wasteful and can lead to untoward reactions, especially in the case of the fat-soluble vitamins (A, D, E, K). Moreover, continued self-medication with vitamin preparations may delay recognition or mask the symptoms of a more serious underlying disease. Vitamin supplementation should only be undertaken following consultation with a health-care professional, and the type and amount of individual vitamins prescribed should be based on a thorough clinical assessment of the patient's diet, health status, and presenting symptoms.

The Food and Nutrition Board of the National Academy of Sciences periodically provides guidelines for recommended intake of individual nutrients, including vitamins. The recommended dietary allowances (RDAs) are *not* requirements but are suggested daily intakes of vitamins and other nutrients that, based on current scientific data, are believed to be adequate for the nutritional needs of most healthy persons under normal environmental conditions. RDAs will vary with sex and age, and additional allowances are made for special circumstances, such as during pregnancy and lactation. As noted, RDA values apply to *healthy* persons and are not intended to cover nutritional requirements in disease or other abnormal situations. RDAs are subject to periodic revision (the latest values were released in 1980) and values do change as population subgroups with unique nutritional requirements emerge.

The U.S. Food and Drug Administration regulates the labeling of vitamin and mineral products sold as foods or drugs and has designated an "official" U.S. RDA for each substance, which serves as the legal standard for nutritional labeling of those products controlled by the U.S. Food and Drug Administration. In general, U.S. RDAs represent the highest male or female RDA for each nutrient. Previously, these U.S. RDAs were labeled *minimum daily requirements* (MDRs), but this term has become obsolete.

The current RDAs for the B complex and C vitamins are listed in Table 76-1 and those for the fat-soluble vitamins (A, D, E, K) are listed in Table 77-1 in Chapter 77.

Although millions of people regularly ingest quantities of vitamins greatly in excess of the RDA, there is no convincing evidence that use of excessive amounts (*i.e.*, megadoses) of vitamins can cure or prevent non-nutritional diseases. Despite the many, usually anecdotal, claims made by proponents of megadose vitamin therapy for beneficial effects in diseases ranging from alopecia to warts, use of quantities of vitamins beyond those needed for normal body functioning is at the very least wasteful and can be potentially quite hazardous.

General Nursing Considerations

Despite the lack of evidence that megadoses of vitamins are beneficial, many people routinely take

Table 76-1
Water-Soluble Vitamins

| Vitamin | Major Dietary Sources | Recommended Dietary Allowances | | | | Principal Symptoms of Deficiency States |
| | | Infants | Children | Adults | | |
				Males	Females	
B-Complex						
Thiamine (B₁)	Liver, whole grain, enriched bread and cereals, pork	0.3 mg– 0.5 mg	0.7 mg– 1.2 mg	1.2 mg– 1.4 mg	1.0 mg– 1.1 mg	Anorexia, constipation, beriberi (cardiac complications, peripheral neuritis)
Riboflavin (B₂)	Organ meats, milk, eggs, green vegetables, enriched bread and flour	0.4 mg– 0.6 mg	0.8 mg– 1.4 mg	1.4 mg– 1.7 mg	1.2 mg– 1.3 mg	Stomatitis, glossitis, ocular itching or burning, photophobia, facial dermatitis, cheilosis, corneal vascularization
Nicotinic acid (niacin, B₃)	Liver, fish, poultry, red meat, enriched bread and cereals	6 mg– 8 mg	9 mg– 16 mg	16 mg– 19 mg	13 mg– 15 mg	Pellagra (nervousness, insomnia, dermatitis, diarrhea, confusion, delusions)
Pantothenic acid (B₅)	Organ meats, egg yolks, peanuts, whole grains, cauliflower	*	*	*	*	Weakness, fatigue, mood changes, dizziness, "burning-foot" syndrome
Pyridoxine (B₆)	Red meat, liver, yeast, whole grains, soy beans, green vegetables	0.3 mg– 0.6 mg	0.9 mg– 1.6 mg	1.8 mg– 2.2 mg	1.8 mg– 2.0 mg	Anemia, CNS lesions, epileptic convulsions in children
Cyanocobalamin (B₁₂)	Red meat, milk, liver, egg yolk, oysters, clams	0.5 mcg– 1.5 mcg	2 mcg– 3 mcg	3 mcg	3 mcg	Pernicious anemia, glossitis, paresthesias, muscle incoordination, confusion
Vitamin C						
Ascorbic acid	Citrus fruits, tomatoes, green vegetables, potatoes, strawberries, green peppers	35 mg	45 mg	50 mg– 60 mg	50 mg– 60 mg	Scurvy (petechiae, bleeding gums, bruising, impaired wound healing, loosened teeth)

* RDA is not established.

them daily for a variety of reasons. Consequently, the nurse must include questions about vitamin use in any drug history and must assume a nonjudgmental attitude to determine the patient's rationale for use, dose taken, and the length of therapy. If the patient has strong beliefs about the effectiveness of the vitamin, has been taking the dose for an extended period of time with no side-effects, and the vitamin is unlikely to interfere with the proposed therapy, the nurse may be more successful in gaining the patient's trust by not making an issue of vitamin use. However, sometimes vitamin intake does interfere with drug therapy; for example, vitamin C and oral anticoagulants in combination may seriously reduce prothrombin time and increase the risk of bleeding.

In such cases the patient's cooperation must be enlisted to prevent such adverse effects. In general, the doses of most vitamins patients take, although above the recommended daily allowances, are well below the levels that produce toxicity. However, patients should be warned to be moderate in intake of fat-soluble vitamins because these can be stored in the body and are therefore potentially dangerous. Patients with liver or kidney problems should take vitamins only on the advice of a physician since changes in metabolism and excretion may increase the risk of toxicity.

Pregnant patients should receive careful instruction about vitamin intake because although needs increase during pregnancy they can be met by proper food intake as well as by supplement.

Megadoses of vitamins, especially of fat-soluble ones, can cause fetal problems.

A complete nutrition history is essential for anyone about to receive vitamins therapeutically or who takes megadose vitamin therapy. Gaps in nutrition intake should be identified to determine potential deficiencies or toxicities. Patients who follow strict vegetarian diets or weight-reduction diets below 1000 calories/day or who are starving because of poverty, famine, bulimia, or anorexia are likely to have multiple vitamin deficiencies, as are chronic alcoholics. Children between 6 months to 4 years of age or who are in a growth spurt are at risk of vitamin deficiencies if their diets are not consistently balanced. Women who take oral contraceptives, people who smoke, and anyone who uses laxatives to excess, especially mineral oil, are at risk for vitamin deficiencies. These patients should be identified early and appropriate measures taken to reduce the risk of permanent damage from vitamin deficiencies.

Water-Soluble Vitamins

Certain vitamins are readily soluble in water and are found together in many of the same foods. They are therefore usually grouped together as the water-soluble vitamins. They include the B-complex group and ascorbic acid (vitamin C). These substances are readily excreted in the urine and thus are potentially much less toxic following large doses than are the fat-soluble vitamins, which are metabolized slowly and can be stored in significant amounts in the body. Table 76-1 lists the water-soluble vitamins together with their RDAs, dietary sources, and other pertinent information.

B-Complex Vitamins

The vitamin B-complex group is composed of a number of compounds that differ in structure and biological activity, but that are obtained from many of the same sources, most notably liver and yeast. Of the 11 members of the B-complex family, the need for four—biotin, choline, inositol, and p-aminobenzoic acid (PABA)—in human nutrition has not been established. These substances are not considered here; they are discussed briefly in Chapter 78. Two others, cyanocobalamin (vitamin B_{12}) and folic acid (vitamin B_9) have been reviewed in Chapter 38, because they are primarily indicated in the treatment of pernicious anemia; cyanocobalamin is discussed here only as a nutritional supplement. The remaining five B-complex vitamins are examined individually in this chapter.

Patients may report the use of B-complex vitamins to reduce stress and decrease premenstrual symptoms. Other uses advocated for B-complex vitamins by lay health groups are to decrease the symptoms of acne, cancer, atherosclerosis, hypertension, diabetes, and arthritis. Conclusive evidence for the effectiveness of the B vitamins in these conditions is lacking, however.

Vitamin B_1 (Thiamine)
(Betalin S, Biamine)

MECHANISM AND ACTIONS
Thiamine, or vitamin B_1, is an organic molecule that is essential for carbohydrate metabolism. It combines with ATP to form thiamine pyrophosphate, a coenzyme that functions in the decarboxylation of alpha keto acids, such as pyruvate, and in the utilization of pentose in the hexose monophosphate shunt. Thiamine may also serve as a modulator of neuromuscular transmission, since transmission is impaired by pyrithiamine, a thiamine antagonist.

Thiamine requirements are closely linked to caloric intake, and clinical manifestations of thiamine deficiency can range from mild (anorexia, weakness, paresthesias, hypothermia, hypotension) to moderate (polyneuritis, sensory and motor defects, cardiovascular disease) to severe (Wernicke's encephalopathy, Korsakoff's psychosis) (see Disease Briefs in Chap. 26). Beriberi is a thiamine deficiency with several manifestations (see Disease Brief) and is frequently observed in Far Eastern countries where the diet consists largely of polished rice, which is very low in thiamine. Alcoholism, on the other hand, is the most common cause of thiamine deficiency in the United States.

DISEASE BRIEF

■ Beriberi

Beriberi is a thiamine-deficiency disease characterized by neurologic and musculoskeletal symptoms such as paresthesias, muscle weakness ("wrist-drop" and "foot-drop" syndromes) and cramping, fatigue, memory loss, personality changes, and depression. This type, termed *dry beriberi*, is generally present in older adults. A second form, known as *wet beriberi*, is associated with cardiovascular complications such as tachycardia, palpitations, dyspnea on exertion, electrocardiographic abnormalities (T wave inversion, prolonged Q-T interval), and high-output cardiac failure. Edema may be extensive, largely the result of hypoproteinemia (from inadequate protein intake) and failing ventricular function.

Treatment consists of thiamine administration plus maintenance of a balanced diet. In milder cases, the biochemical abnormalities are usually rapidly reversible and signs of heart failure disappear within several days, with the heart returning to normal size within several weeks. If the disease is advanced, restoration of cardiovascular and neurologic function to normal may be impossible although improvement is often significant.

USES
1. Prevention and treatment of thiamine-deficiency states (*e.g.*, beriberi).
2. Oral thiamine has been investigated as a mosquito repellant.

ADMINISTRATION AND DOSAGE
Thiamine is used orally as tablets (5 mg, 10 mg, 25 mg, 50 mg, 100 mg, 250 mg, 500 mg) or by injection (100 mg/ml, 200 mg/ml). The dietary supplement dose is 5 mg to 30 mg/day. For symptoms of beriberi, 10 mg to 20 mg is given IM three times/day for 2 weeks, supplemented with a daily oral multivitamin containing 5 mg to 10 mg thiamine for one month to achieve body tissue saturation.

Wet beriberi with myocardial failure is treated as an emergency condition and up to 30 mg thiamine is given IV 3 times/day. Thiamine is also added to total parenteral nutrition solutions. (See Chap. 79.)

FATE
Oral absorption is limited to 8 mg to 15 mg/day. As intake exceeds the minimal requirement (1 mg–2 mg), tissue stores become saturated, and the excess appears in the urine, either as unchanged thiamine or as a pyrimidine metabolite. With normal renal function, up to 95% of an IV dose is also excreted in the urine.

SIDE-EFFECTS/ADVERSE REACTIONS
Adverse reactions with thiamine are infrequent and generally result from high doses. They can include a feeling of warmth, pruritus, urticaria, sweating, nausea, restlessness, weakness, cyanosis, dyspnea, tightness of the throat, angioedema, pulmonary edema, and gastrointestinal (GI) hemorrhage.

Sensitivity reactions can occur and deaths have resulted from IV use. An intradermal sensitivity test should be performed prior to IV injection in patients with suspected thiamine sensitivity.

INTERACTIONS
1. Thiamine can enhance the response to peripherally acting muscle relaxants.
2. Thiamine is unstable in alkaline solutions, for example, with carbonates, citrates, or barbiturates.
3. Thiamine-deficient patients may experience a sudden worsening of the symptoms of Wernicke's encephalopathy (*e.g.*, ataxia, diplopia, tremor, agitation) following IV glucose administration. Administer thiamine before a glucose load.

NURSING CONSIDERATIONS
Thiamine deficiency is common among chronic alcoholics in the United Staes and is usually part of a multiple-deficiency state requiring supplements of multiple vitamins, minerals, and nutrients. Symptoms of thiamine deficiency can occur within 3 weeks of total absence of dietary thiamine and must therefore be considered in any patient on a very low-calorie diet or who has been on an extended drinking binge. Therapy should include a diet rich in foods containing thiamine (see Table 76-1).

If thiamine is given IV an intradermal sensitivity test will be performed prior to injection to determine presence of hypersensitivity. However, emergency resuscitative equipment to support respiration and drugs such as epinephrine, antihistamines, and corticosteroids should be immediately available to deal with anaphylaxis should it occur.

If thiamine is given IM it should be injected deep into a large muscle mass such as the gluteus. The injection is usually very painful and ice may be applied if swelling and pain are severe. Sites should be rotated using a body map (see Chap. 8) if multiple injections are required.

Patients being treated for this or other self-inflicted dietary insufficiencies should receive counseling and follow-up care to prevent repeated episodes.

Vitamin B₂ (Riboflavin)

MECHANISM AND ACTIONS
Riboflavin, or vitamin B₂, is converted to one of two riboflavin-containing biologically active coenzymes, flavin mononucleotide (FMN) and flavin adenine dinucleotide (FAD), which play a vital metabolic role in the action of tissue respiratory flavoproteins. The compound derives its name from the presence of the sugar ribose as a component of the molecule and from the fact that the remainder of the structure is a yellow-pigmented compound termed a *flavin*.

USES
1. Prevention and treatment of riboflavin deficiency (*i.e.*, ariboflavinosis)

ADMINISTRATION AND DOSAGE
Riboflavin is available as tablets containing 5 mg, 10 mg, 25 mg, 50 mg, 100 mg, and 250 mg. The recommended dosage in deficiency states is 5 mg to 10 mg/day.

FATE
Riboflavin is well absorbed orally and widely distributed in the body; however, very little is stored. In small amounts, approximately 10% is excreted in the urine; larger doses are eliminated in increasing proportion in the urine. The drug is present in the feces, but probably represents vitamin synthesized by intestinal microorganisms.

SIDE-EFFECTS/ADVERSE REACTIONS
Riboflavin is virtually free of side-effects. The drug imparts a harmless yellowish color to the urine.

INTERACTIONS
1. Riboflavin may inhibit the activity of tetracyclines when mixed together in solution.
2. Riboflavin can reduce chloramphenicol-induced bone marrow depression and optic neuritis.

NURSING CONSIDERATIONS
Riboflavin deficiency rarely occurs as a single entity but usually is a part of a multiple-deficiency state, frequently occurring in chronic alcoholics in the United States. Symptoms of deficiency include sore throat, stomatitis, glossitis, photophobia, and seborrheic dermatitis. Corneal vascularization, cheilosis, and blepharospasm may also occur. All symptoms will usually disappear with prompt replacement therapy. Patients should be informed that the vitamin causes urine to turn a dark yellowish color, which is harmless.

Vitamin B₃ (Nicotinic Acid)
(*Niac, Niacels, Nico-400, Nicobid, Nicolar, Nicotinex, Span-Niacin*)

Nicotinic acid, or niacin (vitamin B₃), is a B-complex vitamin that serves as a constituent of two important coenzymes, nicotinamide-adenine dinucleotide (NAD; coenzyme I) and nicotinamide-adenine dinucleotide phosphate (NADP; coenzyme II). These coenzymes function in various oxidation–reduction reactions required for cellular and tissue respiration. In addition to its function in the above reactions, niacin possesses several other pharmacologic actions that can vary according to dose. For example, large doses exert a hypolipemic effect, presumably by reducing triglyceride synthesis and blocking the release of very-low-density lipoproteins (VLDL) from the liver. The drug may also increase cholesterol oxidation and inhibit mobilization of fatty acids, and may exert a direct, although relatively weak, relaxing effect on peripheral vascular smooth muscle.

Niacin is an essential dietary constituent, the lack of which results in pellagra, a condition that primarily affects the skin, GI tract, and central nervous system (CNS) (see Disease Brief). In addition to its value in treating pellagra and other nicotinic acid–deficiency states, niacin is also employed in large doses as adjunctive therapy in various forms of hyperlipidemia and hypercholesterolemia. These latter indications are reviewed in detail in Chapter 37. Finally, its vasodilatory action has led to its use as a circulatory aid in peripheral vascular diseases, but there is no conclusive evidence that the drug has a clinically beneficial effect in patients with circulatory impairment.

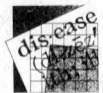

DISEASE BRIEF

■ Pellagra

Pellagra is a nicotinic acid–deficiency disease characterized by symptoms involving the skin, GI tract, and CNS, a triad that is referred to as the *three Ds*, that is, dermatitis, diarrhea, and dementia. The early signs of pellagra are nonspecific, and include anorexia, weakness, GI disturbances, anxiety, irritability, and depression. As the disease progresses, there is the appearance of glossitis, stomatitis, nausea, diarrhea, and excessive salivary secretion. The tongue may become so swollen and painful that swallowing becomes difficult. Chronic dermatitis frequently resembles the reaction from extensive exposure to sunlight. Symptoms of CNS involvement include delusions, disorientation, hallucinations, and dementia. Motor and sensory disturbances of peripheral nerves can also occur. Megaloblastic anemia from associated folic acid deficiency is common.

Treatment consists of administration of niacin, together with a diet adequate in niacin as well as tryptophan, the precursor of niacin. Acute symptoms generally improve within a few days, but complete recovery from the deficiency state may require several weeks. Anemia, if present, requires either folic acid or iron therapy, or both.

Finally, large doses of nicotinic acid have been employed in treating schizophrenia, as part of what has been termed *orthomolecular psychiatry*. There is no convincing evidence that such treatment is effective, and use of high doses of nicotinic acid may be associated with significant toxicity, including liver damage, arrhythmias, peptic ulceration, sensory neuropathy, hyperglycemia, dermatoses, and GI distress.

USES

1. Prevention and treatment of pellagra and other niacin-deficiency states
2. Adjunctive therapy of hypercholesterolemia and hyperbetalipoproteinemia (types IIb, III, IV, and V); see Chapter 37.
3. Symptomatic treatment of peripheral vascular disorders; see Chapter 36.

ADMINISTRATION AND DOSAGE

Niacin is available in several dosage forms, including tablets (25 mg, 50 mg, 100 mg, 250 mg, 500 mg), timed-release tablets (150 mg), timed-release capsules (125 mg, 250 mg, 300 mg, 400 mg, 500 mg), elixir (50 mg/5 ml), and injection (100 mg/ml). Recommended initial doses for the various indications are as follows:

Niacin deficiency—10 mg to 20 mg daily
Pellagra—Up to 500 mg daily depending on symptoms
Hyperlipidemia—1 g to 2 g three times/day to a maximum of 6 g/day

Niacin may be given IV for vitamin deficiencies where oral therapy is impractical. A slow IV injection is recommended, although the drug can be given intramuscularly or subcutaneously if necessary.

FATE

Niacin is readily absorbed orally and widely distributed. Peak serum concentrations occur in 45 minutes. The elimination half-life is approximately 45 minutes to 60 minutes. Nearly one third of a normal oral dose is excreted unchanged in the urine; with very large doses, the principal urinary excretory product is the unchanged drug.

SIDE-EFFECTS/ADVERSE REACTIONS

The most common side-effects with niacin are cutaneous flushing (especially in the areas of the face, neck, and ears), pruritus, and GI distress. Other untoward reactions that can occur, especially at high doses, include severe and generalized flushing, headache, tingling, skin rash, dryness of the skin, keratosis nigricans, jaundice, activation of peptic ulcer, abdominal pain, vomiting, diarrhea, hypotension (orthostatic), dizziness, hyperuricemia, toxic amblyopia, and decreased glucose tolerance.

CONTRAINDICATIONS AND PRECAUTIONS

Niacin use is contraindicated in patients with active peptic ulcer, severe hypotension, hepatic dysfunction, and hemorrhaging. The drug must be given *cautiously* to persons with a history of jaundice, liver disease, or peptic ulcer; to persons with gallbladder disease, diabetes, gout, or angina; to children; and to pregnant or lactating women.

INTERACTIONS

1. Niacin may have additive blood-pressure-lowering effects with antihypertensive drugs.
2. Niacin can reduce the effectiveness of oral antidiabetic agents by elevating blood glucose levels.
3. Niacin may reduce the uricosuric action of sulfinpyrazone or probenecid.

NURSING CONSIDERATIONS

In addition to treatment of schizophrenia, lay health publications have advocated the use of niacin to treat acne, cancer, diabetes, and hypertension. All claimed benefits are currently unsubstantiated by research; however, the nurse must be aware of such claims when obtaining a history of niacin ingestion. Since most side-effects are dose related, especially when doses are high, it is important to determine the amount a patient takes daily.

The patient should be encouraged to take niacin with meals and cold water to reduce gastrointestinal upset and vasodilation. Symptoms of vasodilation such as tingling, headache, or flushing may occur shortly after ingestion but usually subside almost immediately and may disappear with prolonged therapy. If symptoms persist niacinamide may be used instead.

Nicotinamide (Niacinamide)

An amide of nicotinic acid, nicotinamide provides a source of niacin that can be utilized by the body, but that is devoid of hypolipidemic and vasodilatory effects. Thus, it is only indicated for treatment of niacin-deficiency states, where it is preferred by many patients who find the flushing and paresthesias resulting from niacin itself unpleasant. Nicotinamide is available for oral or parenteral administration, and the dose is highly individualized based on symptoms and response. The usual oral dosage range is 50 mg three to ten times a day. Parenteral dosage is 100 mg to 200 mg one to five times/day. Other than a reduced incidence of circulatory side-effects, the pharmacology of nicotinamide is essentially similar to that of nicotinic acid.

Vitamin B₅ (Calcium Pantothenate)

MECHANISM AND ACTIONS

Pantothenic acid, occasionally referred to as vitamin B_5, is a precursor of coenzyme A, which catalyzes a variety of metabolic reactions such as oxidative metabolism of carbohydrates, gluconeogenesis, synthesis and degradation of fatty acids, and synthesis of sterols and steroid hormones. Because pantothenic acid is found abundantly in the normal diet, deficiency states are quite rare. Although it is a necessary nutrient, the daily requirement is not precisely known and no RDAs are available. Pantothenic acid in the form of its calcium salt is commonly found in multivitamin preparations, but its presence is probably unnecessary.

USES

1. Treatment of pantothenic acid deficiency, although this condition has not been recognized in humans with an ordinary diet

ADMINISTRATION AND DOSAGE

Pantothenic acid is available as calcium pantothenate as tablets containing 25 mg, 30 mg, 100 mg, 200 mg, 218 mg, 250 mg, 500 mg, and 545 mg. The usual dosage range is 25 mg/day to 100 mg/day, although up to 10 g/day has been given without apparent adverse effects.

FATE

Pantothenic acid is readily absorbed orally and widely distributed in the body. The drug is not metabolized to any extent, and is excreted largely unchanged in the urine.

Use of pantothenic acid is virtually devoid of side-effects. There are no known contraindications to its use.

Vitamin B₆ (Pyridoxine)

(Beesix, Hexa-Betalin, Nestrex, Pyroxine)

MECHANISM AND ACTIONS

Pyridoxine (vitamin B_6) is a naturally occurring substance that can be converted to pyridoxal and pyridoxamine.

All three forms of vitamin B_6 are converted *in vivo* to pyridoxal phosphate or pyridoxamine phosphate, the physiologically active forms that serve as coenzymes for a number of essential metabolic reactions, including decarboxylation, transamination, and transsulfuration of amino acids, conversion of tryptophan to serotonin or niacin, and glycogenolysis. The need for pyridoxine increases with the amount of protein in the diet. Its RDAs are listed in Table 76-1.

USES

1. Treatment of pyridoxine deficiency, as seen, for example, with inadequate dietary intake, inborn errors of metabolism (*e.g.,* pyridoxine-dependent convulsions, pyridoxine-responsive anemia), or drug-induced depletion (*e.g.,* from isoniazid, alcohol, oral contraceptives)
2. Control of nausea and vomiting in pregnancy or resulting from radiation (effectiveness not conclusively demonstrated)
3. Investigational uses include reversal of the neurologic symptoms of hydrazine poisoning, symptomatic treatment of the premenstrual syndrome, and treatment of oxalate kidney stones.

ADMINISTRATION AND DOSAGE

Pyridoxine may be used as tablets (10 mg, 25 mg, 50 mg, 100 mg, 200 mg, 250 mg, and 500 mg) and injection (100 mg/ml). Recommended doses are as follows:

Dietary deficiency—10 mg to 20 mg/day orally for 3 weeks, followed by an oral multivitamin containing 2 mg to 5 mg pyridoxine daily

Pyridoxine dependency syndrome—up to 600 mg/day initially, reduced to 25 mg to 50 mg/day for life

Isoniazid overdosage (10 g or more)—Give an equal amount of pyridoxine (4 g IV by direct injection or infusion at a rate of 50 mg/minute, followed by 1 g IM every 30 minutes)

FATE

Pyridoxine is well absorbed orally and converted to pyridoxal phosphate and pyridoxamine phosphate. The half-life is 15 days to 20 days. The drug is metabolized in the liver to 4-pyridoxic acid, which is excreted in the urine.

SIDE-EFFECTS/ADVERSE REACTIONS

Side-effects that may occasionally be encountered, especially at high doses, include paresthesias, somnolence, flushing, and reduced serum folic acid levels. Pain may occur at the injection site when the drug is given parenterally.

CONTRAINDICATIONS AND PRECAUTIONS

Pyridoxine should be used cautiously in nursing mothers, because it may inhibit lactation by suppressing prolactin release. Persons taking very large daily doses (500 mg–6 g) have developed ataxia and sensory neuropathy.

INTERACTIONS

1. Pyridoxine can reduce the effectiveness of levodopa by accelerating its peripheral metabolism.
2. Pyridoxine requirement may be increased in patients taking isoniazid, cycloserine, oral contraceptives, hydralazine, or penicillamine, and in alcoholics.
3. Chloramphenicol-induced optic neuritis can be prevented by pyridoxine.
4. Concomitant administration of pyridoxine may decrease serum levels of phenobarbital and phenytoin.

NURSING CONSIDERATIONS

In addition to the accepted uses of pyridoxine, lay health literature has advocated its use in alleviating the symptoms of atherosclerosis, painful finger joints, and Parkinson's disease, most of which is unsubstantiated by clinical research. However, excessive intake of pyridoxine by the patient taking levodopa may actually increase symptoms since vitamin B_6 accelerates levodopa metabolism. Careful history taking is essential to uncover a patient's reasons for vitamin use and a drug history that may be adversely affected by pyridoxine intake.

Pyridoxine deficiency is usually part of a multiple-deficiency state and is common in chronic alcoholics. Replacement therapy is usually successful in removing symptoms of deficiency and follow-up should include diet instruction to increase intake of foods rich in vitamin B_6 (see Table 76-1) and a multiple vitamin preparation.

Vitamin B_{12} (Cyanocobalamin)

Cyanocobalamin, or vitamin B_{12}, is essential for normal growth and development, cell reproduction, hematopoiesis, and nucleoprotein and myelin synthesis. Insufficient GI absorption of cyanocobalamin, due primarily to decreased availability of the intrinsic factor, leads to pernicious anemia and is treated with large oral or parenteral doses (see Chap. 38). Oral preparations containing less than 500 mcg cyanocobalamin are not indicated for pernicious anemia, but are employed solely as a nutritional supplement, especially in persons on strict vegetarian diets. The recommended dosage range is 25 mcg to 250 mcg/day, although it should be remembered that the RDA for cyanocobalamin is only 3 mcg in adults.

Vitamin C (Ascorbic Acid)

Vitamin C, or ascorbic acid, is an essential dietary substance that plays a major role in many metabolic reactions as well as in the formation and maintenance of collagen and intracellular ground substance. The name *ascorbic acid* is a condensation of the term *antiscorbutic vitamin*, and is derived from the compound's ability to prevent scurvy, the principal ascorbic acid–deficiency state. In normal therapeutic doses, ascorbic acid elicits few demonstrable pharmacologic effects except in the scorbutic person (*i.e.*, the patient with symptoms of scurvy). This disease is occasionally observed in elderly or debilitated persons, drug addicts, alcoholics, and others with poor diets. It is characterized by degenerative changes in connective tissue, bones, and capillaries. The symptoms of ascorbic acid deficiency (swollen and bleeding gums, petechiae, easy bruising, delayed wound healing, loosened teeth, joint pain, and bloody stools) are usually readily relieved by 200 mg to 400 mg ascorbic acid daily for several days; they can be prevented from recurring by small (50 mg–100 mg) daily supplemental doses of the vitamin. Although very large amounts (megadoses) of ascorbic acid have been advocated for a wide variety of disease states, ranging from prophylaxis of the common cold to treatment of carcinomas, conclusive evidence for the vitamin's effectiveness in megadose quantities for any of the proposed indications is lacking.

MECHANISM AND ACTIONS
Vitamin C participates in a number of essential biological functions, for example, formation of collagen and intracellular ground substance, cellular respiration, microsomal drug metabolism, steroid synthesis, tyrosine metabolism, and conversion of folic acid to folinic acid. It is also important for the maintenance of tooth and bone matrix and capillary integrity, and may aid wound healing. Vitamin C reduces the pH of the urine, especially at high doses, and is occasionally used as a urinary acidifier.

USES
1. Prevention and treatment of scurvy and other ascorbic acid–deficiency states
2. Adjunctive therapy in extensive or deep burns, delayed wound healing, chronic or severe illnesses, and a variety of other disease states and stressful situations (effectiveness has not been conclusively demonstrated)
3. Acidification of the urine, usually in conjunction with a urinary anti-infective such as methenamine

ADMINISTRATION AND DOSAGE
Ascorbic acid is available in a variety of dosage forms, including oral tablets (25 mg–1500 mg), chewable tablets (100 mg–500 mg), timed-release tablets (500 mg–1500 mg), effervescent tablets (1000 mg), timed-release capsules (500 mg), syrup (100 mg/5 ml–500 mg/5 ml), solution (100 mg/ml), liquid (35 mg/0.6 ml), powder and injection (100 mg/ml–500 mg/ml). The sodium and calcium salts of ascorbic acid are also available, but are infrequently employed.

The usual oral dosage ranges for the various indications are as follows:
Deficiency states—300 mg to 1 g/day (maintenance dose is 75 mg–150 mg/day)
Children—100 mg to 300 mg/day (maintenance dose is 30 mg/day)
Wound healing—300 mg to 500 mg/day for 7 to 10 days, although much larger amounts have been used
Burns—1 g to 2 g/day
IM, SC, IV—Up to 2 g/day may be given as needed for severe deficiency states; maintenance dose is 100 mg to 250 mg once or twice a day.

FATE
Vitamin C is readily absorbed orally or parenterally and widely distributed. The drug is partly metabolized and excreted in the urine both as metabolites and unchanged drug. The amount excreted markedly increases with large doses.

SIDE-EFFECTS/ADVERSE REACTIONS
Side-effects are rare with use of vitamin C preparations in recommended doses. Large doses may cause diarrhea and may result in precipitation of oxalate or urate renal stones if the urine is acidic. IM or SC injection can be followed by transient soreness at the injection site. Too-rapid IV admin-

istration may cause temporary faintness or dizziness.

CONTRAINDICATIONS AND PRECAUTIONS
Large doses of vitamin C must be used with *caution* in pregnant or nursing mothers, and in diabetics, patients prone to recurrent kidney stones, persons taking anticoagulants (see Interactions), and persons undergoing occult blood tests for the stool.

INTERACTIONS
1. Large doses of ascorbic acid lower urinary pH and thus may reduce excretion of acidic drugs (*e.g.*, salicylates, barbiturates) and increase excretion of basic drugs (*e.g.*, quinidine, atropine, amphetamines, tricyclic antidepressants, and phenothiazines).
2. Ascorbic acid increases the possibility of crystalluria with the sulfonamides.
3. Large doses of ascorbic acid may shorten the prothrombin time in patients receiving oral anticoagulants.
4. Ascorbic acid can interfere with the effectiveness of disulfiram when it is used in the alcoholic patient (see Chap. 26).
5. Ascorbic acid in large doses may enhance the absorption of oral iron.
6. Mineral oil can retard absorption of ascorbic acid.
7. Ascorbic acid is chemically incompatible with

penicillin G potassium and should not be mixed in the same syringe.
8. Large doses of ascorbic acid may result in false readings of urine glucose, serum uric acid, and urinary steroids.
9. Intermittent administration of ascorbic acid may increase the risk of oral contraceptive failure.
10. Smoking may slightly reduce ascorbic acid serum levels; conversely, ascorbic acid can enhance excretion of nicotine, perhaps resulting in an increased desire to smoke.

NURSING CONSIDERATIONS
In addition to the accepted uses of vitamin C patients may report use to treat or prevent the common cold, cancer, heat rash, thrombophlebitis, heart disease, stress, arthritis, and stroke; to increase athletic performance; and as an added replacement if the patient smokes. Patients who take high doses of vitamin C usually believe strongly in its benefit and are unlikely to discontinue use unless it interferes with another prescribed regimen. Even then they may manipulate the drug therapy and include vitamin intake. In most cases such use will be harmless. However, the nurse should take a thorough drug history to determine any potentially adverse interactions and determine if a history of diabetes or kidney stones exists, which may contraindicate use.

Oral forms should be used as much as possible since IV injection may cause dizziness and fainting and IM injection may result in tissue necrosis.

REVIEW QUESTIONS

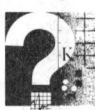

1. What are vitamins?
2. List several possible causes of vitamin-deficiency states.
3. Distinguish between the water-soluble and the fat-soluble vitamins.
4. What is meant by recommended dietary allowances (RDAs) of vitamins?
5. How do RDAs differ from U.S. RDAs?
6. Which patients are at greatest risk of vitamin deficiencies?
7. What are the potential problems for the patient who takes megadoses of vitamins? What approach should the nurse use when dealing with this individual?
8. Which other uses may patients claim for vitamins other than those substantiated by clinical research?
9. What are the major dietary sources of (1) thiamine, (2) nicotinic acid, and (3) pyridoxine?
10. What are the symptoms of thiamine deficiency?
11. Distinguish between "dry" beriberi and "wet" beriberi.

12. What is the major cause of thiamine deficiency in the United States?
13. What is the principal physiologic role of riboflavin (vitamin B_2)?
14. List the major pharmacologic actions of nicotinic acid (vitamin B_3).
15. What is pellagra? Describe the major symptoms of this condition.
16. Give the common side-effects noted with nicotinic acid.
17. For what indications may pyridoxine (vitamin B_6) be used?
18. What are the symptoms of ascorbic acid (vitamin C) deficiency?
19. In what essential biologic functions is ascorbic acid believed to participate?
20. What are the approved indications for ascorbic acid? For what conditions have very large doses (*i.e.*, megadoses) been used?

BIBLIOGRAPHY

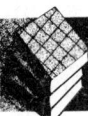

Cerrato PL: When to worry about vitamin overdose. RN 48(10):69, Oct, 1985

Food and Nutrition Board, National Research Council: Recommended Dietary Allowances, 9th ed. Washington, DC. National Academy of Sciences, 1980

Goodhart RS, Shils ME (eds): Modern Nutrition in Health and Disease, 6th ed. Philadelphia, Lea & Febiger, 1980

Halpern JS: Megavitamins: Therapeutic or a threat to health. J Educ Nurs 9:346, 1983

Luke B: Megavitamins and pregnancy: A dangerous combination. Maternal Child Nursing 10:18, 1985

Miller DR, Hayes KC: Vitamin excess and toxicity. In Nutritional Toxicology, vol 1, p 18. New York, Academic Press, 1982

Rivlin RS (ed): Riboflavin. New York, Plenum Press, 1975

Toxic Effects of Vitamin Overdosage. Med Lett Drugs Ther 26:73, 1984

Fat-Soluble Vitamins: Vitamins A, D, E, and K

77

Unlike the B-complex and C vitamins discussed in Chapter 76, vitamins A, D, E, and K are poorly soluble in water but dissolve readily in fats. This property is responsible for certain characteristics that distinguish the fat-soluble vitamins from their water-soluble counterparts. While the B and C vitamins are readily absorbed orally, the fat-soluble vitamins require the presence of sufficient amounts of bile salts in the gastrointestinal (GI) tract for adequate absorption. However, their absorption may be impaired by the presence of mineral oil or other fatty vehicles that can sequester the vitamins in the lumen of the intestine. Compared to the water-soluble vitamins, vitamins A, D, E, and K are stored in much larger amounts in various body tissues, such as adipose tissue, liver, and muscles. From these storage depots, small amounts are released over extended periods of time to meet nutritional needs; hence symptoms of a fat-soluble vitamin deficiency usually develop only after long periods of inadequate intake; that is, until body stores are depleted. Loss of fat-soluble vitamins in the urine is minimal and excretion proceeds at a very slow rate. The inefficient excretion of most fat-soluble vitamins can result in accumulation to toxic levels if excessive quantities of the vitamins are ingested to supplement the diet, and such a practice should be discouraged.

Characteristics of the fat-soluble vitamins are listed in Table 77-1, along with their recommended dietary allowances where available. The four vitamins making up the fat-soluble group are reviewed individually below.

In addition, two vitamin D metabolites, calcifediol and calcitriol, as well as a synthetic sterol, dihydrotachysterol, which is structurally and func-

Table 77-1
Fat-Soluble Vitamins

Vitamin	Major Dietary Sources	Recommended Dietary Allowances				Principal Symptoms of Deficiency States
		Infants	Children	Adults		
				Males	Females	
vitamin A	Fish liver oils, eggs, milk, butter, green and yellow vegetables, tomatoes, squash	2000 IU–2100 IU	2000 IU–3500 IU	5000 IU	4000 IU	Night blindness, xerophthalmia, keratinization of epithelial tissues, increased susceptibility to infection, retarded growth and development
vitamin D (ergocalciferol, cholecalciferol)	Fish liver oils, egg yolk, milk, butter, margarine, salmon, sardines	400 IU	400 IU	200 IU–400 IU	200 IU–400 IU	Rickets, osteomalacia
vitamin E	Wheat germ, vegetable oils, green leafy vegetables, nuts, cereals, eggs, dairy products	4 IU–6 IU	7 IU–10 IU	12 IU–15 IU	12 IU	Not established in humans; possibly hemolytic anemia, muscular lesion and necrosis, creatinuria
vitamin K	Green leafy vegetables, liver, cheese, egg yolks, tomatoes, meats, cereals	*	*	*	*	Hypoprothrombinemia, hemorrhage

* RDAs are not established.

tionally related to ergocalciferol, are also considered in this chapter.

Several compounds related to vitamin A (etretinate, isotretinoin, tretinoin) may be used in treating various skin disorders, such as acne vulgaris, excessive keratinization, and recalcitrant psoriasis. These drugs, especially those administered systemically, are quite toxic and must be used with extreme caution. They are considered in detail in Chapter 83.

Vitamin A
(Aquasol A)

The term vitamin A is commonly used to refer to a group of several biologically active compounds. Vitamin A_1 (retinol) is the principal naturally occurring substance and is formed from precursors termed *carotenes*, the most important of which is beta-carotene (provitamin A). The average adult receives about one half of his daily dietary intake of vitamin A as preformed retinol and the remainder as carotene precursors (*i.e.*, carotenoids). Vitamin A_2 (3-dehydroretinol) occurs mixed with retinol in many dietary sources. Most currently used preparations are synthetic retinol esters, which have largely replaced the natural vitamin A products previously extracted from fish liver oils, inasmuch as they are generally better absorbed and provide more consistent blood levels of the vitamin.

The potency of vitamin A preparations is expressed as international units (IU), 1 IU being equal to 0.3 mcg retinol or 0.6 mcg beta-carotene. Vitamin A is required for growth of bones and teeth, integrity of epithelial tissue, normal functioning of the retina (especially visual adaptation to darkness), reproduction, and embryonic development. Deficiencies are rarely observed when reasonable dietary practices are followed, and liver stores of vitamin A are usually sufficient to satisfy up to a 2-year requirement of the vitamin.

MECHANISM AND ACTIONS
The mechanism of action of vitamin A is complex and incompletely understood. Among the actions ascribed to vitamin A are increased synthesis of ribonucleic acid (RNA), proteins, steroids, mucopolysaccharides, and cholesterol. The vitamin prevents growth retardation and preserves the integrity of epithelial cells. Retinol combines with opsin, the rod pigment in the retina, to form rhodopsin, a photosensitive pigment necessary for visual adaptation to darkness. Vitamin A may play a role in wound healing. Deficiency of the vitamin can result in night blindness (nyctalopia), keratomalacia (corneal necrosis), drying of the skin, lowered resistance to infection, growth retardation, thickening of bone, decreased adrenal cortical production, and fetal malformations.

USES
1. Treatment of vitamin A–deficiency states (*e.g.*, biliary or pancreatic disease, colitis, hepatic cirrhosis, celiac disease, regional enteritis)
2. Prophylaxis of vitamin A deficiency during periods of increased requirements, for example, infancy, pregnancy, lactation, or severe illness

ADMINISTRATION AND DOSAGE
Available preparations of vitamin A include capsules (10,000 IU, 25,000 IU, 50,000 IU), drops (5,000 IU/0.1 ml), and an injection containing 50,000 IU/ml. Recommended dosage schedules are as follows.

Adults
　Oral—100,000 IU to 500,000 IU/day for 3 days, then 50,000 IU/day for 2 weeks, then 10,000 IU to 20,000 IU/day for 2 months
　IM—100,000 IU/day for 3 days, then 50,000 IU/day for 2 weeks

Children
　Oral—10,000 IU to 15,000 IU/day as a dietary supplement
　IM (1 year–8 years)—17,500 IU to 35,000 IU/day for 10 days

Infants
　IM—7500 IU to 15,000 IU/day for 10 days

FATE
GI absorption of vitamin A preparations is good in the presence of bile acids, pancreatic lipase, and dietary fat. Peak plasma concentrations occur in about 3 hours to 4 hours. Most of a dose is stored in the liver, with smaller amounts stored in many other body tissues. Vitamin E increases tissue storage of vitamin A. Plasma levels increase substantially when hepatic storage sites are saturated. It is slowly released from the liver, and serum concentrations of vitamin A can be maintained for months by hepatic stores. Vitamin A is transported in the plasma as retinol bound to retinol-binding protein. The excretion of vitamin A probably occurs primarily in the bile as a glucuronide, with small amounts appearing in the urine.

SIDE-EFFECTS/ADVERSE REACTIONS

Side-effects are rare with normal doses of vitamin A. Chronic overuse of the vitamin, however, can result in a hypervitaminosis A syndrome that may be characterized by the following symptoms:

Central nervous system—Fatigue, irritability, malaise, lethargy, night sweats, vertigo, headache, increased intracranial pressure (may manifest as papilledema)

Dermatologic—Drying and fissuring of skin and lips, alopecia, gingivitis, pruritus, desquamation, increased pigmentation, tender swellings on the extremities

Musculoskeletal—Retarded growth, arthralgia, premature closure of the epiphyses, bone pain

GI—Abdominal pain, vomiting, anorexia

Other—Liver and spleen enlargement, jaundice, leukopenia, hypomenorrhea, polydipsia, polyuria, hypercalcemia

CONTRAINDICATIONS AND PRECAUTIONS

Use of oral vitamin A supplements is contraindicated in patients with malabsorption syndrome and hypervitaminosis A. Vitamin A should not be administered by the IV route. The drug must be given *cautiously* to pregnant women and to patients with impaired renal or hepatic function.

INTERACTIONS

1. Mineral oil, cholestyramine resin, and colestipol may impair absorption of vitamin A.
2. Increased plasma vitamin A levels have occurred in women taking oral contraceptives.

NURSING CONSIDERATIONS

Vitamin A administration during pregnancy should not exceed the recommended daily allowance (RDA) of 5000 IU per day. Fetal abnormalities such as cleft palate, kidney abnormalities, and eye and ear malformations have been reported, as well as subtle changes to the nervous system, which may result in behavioral and learning disabilities. All women who are pregnant should be warned of the danger involved in taking vitamin A. Women taking large doses of any form of vitamin A for acne or other skin disorders should be told to discontinue treatment *before* conception.

In addition to the accepted clinical uses of vitamin A, patients may report use for asthma, tumors, to increase sexual potency, and to control premenstrual symptoms, although such uses have no clinical research base. Patients who insist on supplementation should be warned to watch for hypervitaminosis (see Side-Effects/Adverse Reactions), which may take 6 months to 15 months to become apparent with daily doses of 4000 IU/kg. Since vitamin A can be sold over the counter in capsules containing 25,000 IU each, it is possible for an individual to take toxic doses. Since the drug is stored in fat and the liver, excretion is slow even when the drug is discontinued. Therefore, symptomatic treatment may be necessary until the vitamin levels drop and may include analgesics for headache, antiemetics for nausea and vomiting, rest, and bland diet with increased fluids. The gravest danger with hypervitaminosis A is increased intracranial pressure, which may be treated with osmotic diuretics if severe.

Patients taking vitamin A should be told to avoid use of mineral oil as a laxative, since absorption is impaired. In addition, women using oral contraceptives should be warned to avoid vitamin A supplementation if dietary intake is adequate, since increased plasma levels of the vitamin may occur, increasing the risk of hypervitaminosis.

Vitamin D Preparations

Calcifediol, Calcitriol, Cholecalciferol, Dihydrotachysterol, Ergocalciferol

Vitamin D is a term commonly applied to two related fat-soluble substances, ergocalciferol (D_2) and cholecalciferol (D_3), which are formed from the provitamins ergosterol and 7-dehydrocholesterol, respectively, by ultraviolet irradiation. The principal source of endogenous vitamin D in humans is the synthesis of vitamin D_3 from 7-dehydrocholesterol on exposure to the ultraviolet rays of the sun. Vitamin D_3 is then converted by hepatic microsomal enzymes to calcifediol (25-hydroxycholecalciferol), the principal transport form of vitamin D_3. Calcifediol possesses minor intrinsic vitamin D activity, and is further metabolized in the kidney to calcitriol (1,25-dihydroxycholecalciferol), the most active form of vitamin D_3. Both calcifediol and calcitriol are now available for clinical use, and are reviewed separately in this chapter. Vitamin D_2 is the form usually found in commercial vitamin preparations and in fortified milk, bread, and cereals. Because in humans there is no difference in activity between vitamin D_2 and vitamin D_3, vitamin D will be used as the collective term for all substances, natural and synthetic, having similar activity. The following is a general discussion of vitamin D; the individual vitamin D products are listed in Table 77-2. A further discussion of the interrelationships among vitamin D, parathyroid hormone, and calcitonin is found in Chapter 53.

MECHANISM AND ACTIONS
Vitamin D substances enhance the active absorption of calcium and phosphorus from the small intestine, facilitating their resorption from bone, and promote the reabsorption of phosphate by the renal tubules. Plasma levels of calcium and phosphorus are therefore maintained at levels adequate for neuromuscular activity, mineralization of bone, and other calcium-dependent functions.

USES
1. Prevention or treatment of vitamin D deficiency (cholecalciferol)
2. Treatment of refractory (vitamin D–resistant) rickets (ergocalciferol)
3. Treatment of familial hypophosphatemia and hypoparathyroidism (ergocalciferol, dihydrotachysterol)
4. Treatment of metabolic bone disease or hypocalcemia in patients on chronic renal dialysis (calcifediol, calcitriol)
5. Treatment of acute, chronic, or latent forms of postoperative tetany or idiopathic tetany (dihydrotachysterol)

ADMINISTRATION AND DOSAGE
See Table 77-2.

FATE
Vitamin D is well absorbed from the small intestine; the D_3 form appears to be more rapidly and more completely absorbed than the D_2 form. Bile is essential for vitamin D absorption. The vitamin is stored chiefly in the liver, and is also found in many other body tissues, including fat, skin, muscle, brain, and bones. Vitamin D is bound to plasma proteins. The plasma half-life of the various derivatives varies from 24 hours for ergocalciferol up to 20 days for calcifediol. The primary route of excretion of vitamin D is the bile; very small amounts are found in the urine.

SIDE-EFFECTS/ADVERSE REACTIONS
Side-effects encountered early in a course of therapy with vitamin D can include headache, drowsiness, weakness, nausea, vomiting, dry mouth, constipation, muscle or bone pain, and a metallic taste. Other adverse reactions associated with administration of vitamin D, especially in large doses or over prolonged periods of time, are polyuria, nocturia, elevated blood urea nitrogen, hypercalciuria, hypercalcemia, azotemia, nephrocalcinosis, proteinuria, urinary casts, renal insufficiency, anorexia, acidosis, anemia, irritability, photophobia, conjunctivitis, pancreatitis, hypertension, arrhythmias, vascular and soft tissue calcification, bone demineralization, mental retardation in children, dwarfism, hyperthermia, and elevated serum glutamic-oxaloacetic transaminase (SGOT) and serum glutamic-pyruvic transaminase (SGPT).

CONTRAINDICATIONS AND PRECAUTIONS
Vitamin D preparations are contraindicated in patients with hypercalcemia, hypervitaminosis D syndrome, or evidence of vitamin D toxicity. Vitamin D must be given with *caution* to patients with a history of renal stones, to pregnant or nursing mothers, and to children.

INTERACTIONS
1. Mineral oil and cholestyramine resin can impair vitamin D absorption.
2. Phenytoin, primidone, and barbiturates may reduce the effectiveness of vitamin D by increasing its metabolic inactivation.
3. Thiazide diuretics may potentiate vitamin D-induced hypercalcemia in hypoparathyroid patients.
4. Vitamin D may increase the likelihood of cardiac arrhythmias with digitalis drugs.
5. The effects of verapamil and possibly other calcium channel blockers may be reduced by vitamin D-induced hypercalcemia.
6. Magnesium-containing antacids used together with vitamin D may result in development of hypermagnesemia.

NURSING CONSIDERATIONS
Vitamin D administration during pregnancy should not exceed the RDA of 400 IU to 600 IU per day. Fetal abnormalities such as aortic stenosis and conditions such as elevated blood cholesterol and infantile hypercalcemia syndrome characterized by damage to brain, heart, and kidneys have been reported. Women who drink vitamin D-fortified milk during pregnancy in quantities of 3 to 4 cups per day need little or no vitamin D supplementation.

Table 77-2
Vitamin D Preparations

Drug	Preparations	Usual Dosage Range	Clinical Considerations
calcifediol (Calderol)	Capsules—20 mcg, 50 mcg	Initially, 300 mcg–350 mcg/week, on a daily or alternate-day schedule; may increase at 4-week intervals as needed Usual maintenance range, 50 mcg–100 mcg/day	Hydroxylated metabolite of cholecalciferol; principal serum transport form of vitamin D_3; converted in the kidney to calcitriol; increases serum calcium and decreases alkaline phosphatase and parathyroid hormone levels.
calcitriol (Calcijex, Rocaltrol)	Capsules—0.25 mcg, 0.5 mcg Injection—1 mcg/ml, 2 mcg/ml	Initially, 0.25 mcg/day; increase by 0.25 mcg/day increments at 4-week–8-week intervals. Hemodialysis patients generally require doses of 0.5 mcg–1 mcg/day *Hypoparathyroidism:* 0.5 mcg–2.0 mcg daily	Most active metabolite of vitamin D; potent hypercalcemic agent primarily used for treating hypocalcemia in patients undergoing renal dialysis. Avoid magnesium-containing antacids, because hypermagnesemia may occur, and do not give other vitamin D supplements during therapy. Advise patients to note occurrence of weakness, vomiting, or muscle or bone pain, as these may indicate hypercalcemia.
cholecalciferol (Delta-D)	Tablets—400 IU, 1000 IU	400 IU–1000 IU daily	Used as a dietary supplement in vitamin D–deficiency states. It is a precursor of calcifediol and calcitriol.
dihydrotachysterol (DHT, Hytakerol)	Tablets—0.125 mg, 0.2 mg, 0.4 mg Capsules—0.125 mg Oral solution—0.25 mg/ml, 0.2 mg/5 ml	Initially, 0.8 mg–2.4 mg daily for several days Maintenance doses are 0.2 mg–1 mg daily as needed to maintain normal serum calcium levels.	Potent vitamin D preparation that is more effective than ergocalciferol in mobilizing calcium from bone but shorter acting; primarily used in treating tetany and symptoms of hypoparathyroidism; maximal hypercalcemic effects require 1 week–2 weeks to develop. Safety margin with drug is rather small. Be alert for symptoms of hypercalcemia.
ergocalciferol (Calciferol, Drisdol)	Capsules—50,000 IU Tablets—50,000 IU Liquid—8,000 IU/ml Injection—500,000 IU/ml	*Vitamin D-resistant rickets* 50,000 IU–500,000 IU daily depending on severity of disease *Hypoparathyroidism* 50,000 IU–200,000 IU daily *plus* 4 g calcium lactate 6 times/day	IM administration is necessary in patients with GI, liver, or biliary disease associated with malabsorption of vitamin D. The range between therapeutic and toxic doses is small. Serum calcium concentration is maintained between 9 mg and 10 mg/dl. Use with caution in patients with impaired kidney function or kidney stones.

In addition to the accepted clinical uses of vitamin D, patients may report using it to prevent or treat aging, cancer, gallstones, cirrhosis, emphysema, and arthritis. There is little or no clinical research to support such use. However, patients who insist on supplementation should be warned that doses 10 to 20 times the normal RDA of 200 IU daily may result in symptoms of overdosage (see Side-Effects/Adverse Reactions). Vitamin D has a very narrow margin of safety.

The most serious adverse effects of vitamin D are changes in urine and serum calcium, phosphate, potassium, and urea. If overdosage occurs with hypercalcemia, the patient may exhibit weakness, vomiting, constipation, and calciuria, and may progress to sensory loss and coma. The vitamin should be discontinued immediately and the patient placed on a low-calcium diet.

Supportive measures such as increased fluid intake, acidification of the urine, and administration of IV saline, sodium citrate, or diuretics may facilitate calcium excretion. Safety measures should be taken to protect the patient if changes in consciousness occur.

Vitamin E

(Aquasol E and various other manufacturers)

Vitamin E is commonly used as a generic term to describe eight naturally occurring tocopherols possessing vitamin E activity. Alpha-tocopherol comprises about 90% of the tocopherols found in animal tissues, is the most biologically active of the eight, and is available both naturally in vegetable oils and other foods as well as synthetically. Because the potencies of the various forms of vitamin E vary somewhat, dosage is standardized in international units (IUs) based on activity. The following list indicates relative potencies of 1 mg of the various clinically available tocopherols:

d-alpha tocopherol = 1.49 IU
dl-alpha tocopherol = 1.1 IU
d-alpha tocopheryl acetate = 1.36 IU
dl-alpha tocopheryl acetate = 1.0 IU
d-alpha tocopheryl acid succinate = 1.21 IU
dl-alpha tocopheryl acid succinate = 0.89 IU

Although RDAs have been published for vitamin E, there is little conclusive evidence that it is of significant nutritional or therapeutic value. Deficiencies of vitamin E in humans are rare, inasmuch as adequate amounts are supplied in the ordinary diet (see Table 77-1). Low levels have occasionally been noted in severely malnourished infants and in

patients with prolonged fat malabsorption or acanthocytosis. Based on occasional relief of experimentally produced deficiency symptoms in laboratory animals, vitamin E has been advocated by some for treatment of an imposing array of human ills, including sterility, habitual abortion, muscular dystrophy, cardiovascular and peripheral vascular disorders, fever blisters, psoriasis, menopausal hot flashes, menstrual pain, and schizophrenia, as well as for the improvement of athletic performance. These claims have *not* been substantiated and use of vitamin E supplementation, other than in clearly established deficiency states, cannot be justified. Topical forms of vitamin E (creams, ointments, lotions, and so on) are also available for temporary relief of minor skin disorders.

MECHANISM AND ACTIONS

The precise biochemical mechanisms of action of vitamin E are unclear, although its effects appear to be due to its antioxidant properties. The vitamin may stabilize cell membranes by protecting them against peroxidation, preserve the cell wall integrity of red blood cells (thus preventing hemolysis), and act as a cofactor in many enzyme systems. Other actions attributed to vitamin E include interference with platelet aggregation, enhanced utilization of vitamin A, and increased hematopoiesis.

USES

1. Prevention or treatment of vitamin E deficiency states
2. Control of dry or chapped skin and temporary relief of minor skin disorders, for example, itching, sunburn, diaper rash, and abrasions (topical use only)
3. Investigational uses include reduction of the toxic effects of oxygen therapy on lung parenchyma (bronchopulmonary dysplasia) and the retina (retrolental fibroplasia) in premature infants, adjunctive treatment of hemolytic anemia in infants, and prevention of periventricular hemorrhage in premature infants.

ADMINISTRATION AND DOSAGE

Vitamin E for systemic use is available as capsules or tablets whose potency may either be expressed in units (100, 200, 400, 500, 600, 1000) when the form of vitamin E present is not known or in milligrams (74, 165, 294, 331) when the particular form of vitamin E is stated. Drops containing 50 mg/ml are also used. Vitamin E is available for topical application as a cream, ointment, liquid, or oil containing varying amounts of vitamin E preparations.

In treating vitamin E–deficiency states, a wide range of dosages has been employed, although the adult RDA for vitamin E is only 12 IU to 15 IU. Vitamin E should never be administered IV; a number of deaths have occurred in infants given vitamin E IV. For topical application, a thin layer of ointment, cream, or liquid is applied to the affected area.

FATE

Vitamin E is readily absorbed from the GI tract if fat absorption is adequate. It is widely distributed in the body and stored in tissues for extended periods of time, providing a continual source of the vitamin. Placental transfer is poor. Vitamin E is largely excreted in the feces by way of the bile, with smaller amounts appearing as metabolites in the urine.

SIDE-EFFECTS/ADVERSE REACTIONS

Untoward reactions are rare with vitamin E; occasional GI distress and muscle weakness are noted. A hypervitaminosis E syndrome has been noted, and is characterized by fatigue, headache, nausea, weakness, diarrhea, flatulence, blurred vision, and dermatitis.

INTERACTIONS

1. Vitamin E may enhance the action of oral anticoagulants by reducing levels of vitamin K-dependent clotting factors.
2. Vitamin E can reduce the efficacy of oral iron preparations.
3. Vitamin E requirements may be *increased* in patients taking large doses of oral iron and *decreased* in persons receiving selenium, antioxidants, or sulfur-amino acids.

NURSING CONSIDERATIONS

Vitamin E requirement during pregnancy is approximately the same as the adult RDA of 12 IU to 15 IU and is easily obtained in foods. Although no birth defects have been reported with high doses of the vitamin, megadoses of vitamin E have been linked to thrombophlebitis, elevated blood pressure, and skin changes. Therefore, cautious use is warranted.

Women who require extra iron during pregnancy should be told to limit vitamin E supplementation since the vitamin decreases iron absorption. Likewise, patients taking oral anticoagulants should also limit vitamin E supplementation since the vitamin may enhance drug action, thus increasing the risk of bleeding.

Vitamin K

Menadiol Sodium Diphosphate (K_4), Phytonadione (K_1)

Vitamin K refers to several structurally similar compounds that all possess the ability to promote hepatic synthesis of certain blood clotting factors. The primary source of vitamin K in humans is through absorption of phytonadione (vitamin K_1) synthesized in the gut by intestinal bacteria. In addition, vitamin K is found in many foods (see Table 77-1), although in most cases these represent a minor source of utilizable vitamin. Vitamin K_1 (phytonadione) is the only naturally occurring vitamin K used clinically; however, this lipid-soluble derivative is also prepared synthetically. The other synthetic vitamin K compound employed therapeutically is menadiol sodium diphosphate (vitamin K_4), a water-soluble analogue that is approximately one-half as potent as vitamin K_3 (menadione), to which it is converted *in vivo*. Phytonadione is the preferred drug for treating hypoprothrombinemia, because it is the most potent of the derivatives and exhibits the fastest onset and longest duration of action. However, adequate absorption of phytonadione occurs only in the presence of bile salts, whereas K_4 can be adequately absorbed without bile salts.

The available vitamin K derivatives are discussed below as a group and listed individually in Table 77-3. Phytonadione has been reviewed previously in Chapter 39 as an antidote to overdosage with oral anticoagulants and is considered only briefly here.

MECHANISM AND ACTIONS

Vitamin K promotes hepatic synthesis of blood clotting factors II, VII, IX, and X, probably by functioning as an essential cofactor for microsomal enzyme systems that activate the precursors of these clotting factors.

USES

1. Treatment of vitamin K deficiency due to antibacterial therapy
2. Treatment of hypoprothrombinemia secondary to impaired absorption or synthesis of vitamin K, for example, due to obstructive jaundice, biliary fistulas, ulcerative colitis, sprue,

Table 77-3
Vitamin K Preparations

Drug	Preparations	Usual Dosage Range	Clinical Considerations
K$_1$ phytonadione (Aquamephyton, Konakion, Mephyton)	Tablets—5 mg Injection—2 mg/ml, 10 mg/ml	*Hypoprothrombinemia and anticoagulant-induced prothrombin deficiency* 2.5 mg–25 mg initially; repeat in 6 h–8 h after parenteral injection or 12 h–48 h after oral administration until prothrombin time is in desired range *Hemorrhagic disease of newborn* Prophylaxis—0.5 mg–2 mg IM or (less desirable) 1 mg–5 mg to the mother 12 h–24 h before delivery Treatment—1 mg–2 mg SC or IM daily	Fat-soluble derivative that is the preferred antidote to oral anticoagulant overdose; only vitamin K preparation indicated for hemorrhagic disease of the newborn; requires bile salts for oral absorption; injection is available as an aqueous colloidal solution (Aquamephyton) for IV, SC, or IM use and as an aqueous dispersion (Konakion) for IM use only; do not exceed 1 mg/minute when injecting IV; preferred route is intermittent IV infusion diluted in normal saline, 50% normal saline, or 50% water and infused slowly. Use smaller doses for antidoting short-acting anticoagulants and larger doses for longer-acting anticoagulants; protect solutions from light.
K$_4$ menadiol sodium diphosphate (Synkayvite)	Tablets—5 mg Injections— 5 mg/ml, 10 mg/ml, 37.5 mg/ml	Oral—5 mg–10 mg/day Parenteral (SC, IM, IV) Adults—5 mg–15 mg 1 to 2 times a day Children—5 mg–10 mg 1 to 2 times/day	Water-soluble derivative of vitamin K, well absorbed orally, and does not require presence of bile salts; primarily used for hypoprothrombinemia due to obstructive jaundice, biliary fistulas, or administration of salicylates or antibiotics; single dose usually restores prothrombin time within 8 hours to 24 hours; may induce hemolysis of erythrocytes in glucose 6-phosphate dehydrogenase–deficient patients; incompatible with other drugs, so infuse separately; may be given with any IV fluid.

celiac disease, regional enteritis, intestinal resection, cystic fibrosis, or salicylate therapy

3. Treatment of oral anticoagulant-induced prothrombin deficiency (phytonadione only)
4. Prophylaxis and treatment of hemorrhagic disease of the newborn (phytonadione only)

ADMINISTRATION AND DOSAGE
See Table 77-3.

FATE
Phytonadione is absorbed from the GI tract by way of the lymph and only in the presence of bile salts. Menadione and menadiol are absorbed directly into the bloodstream even in the absence of bile. Bleeding is controlled within 6 hours to 12 hours following oral administration and within 3 hours to 6 hours following parenteral injection. The drug is initially concentrated in the liver but levels decline very rapidly. There is little accumulation in other tissues and the drug is rapidly metabolized and excreted both in the bile and urine.

SIDE-EFFECTS/ADVERSE REACTIONS
Gastric upset, nausea, vomiting, and headache have occurred after oral doses of vitamin K. Occasional allergic reactions such as rash, urticaria, or pruritus have been noted as well. Anaphylactic reactions can also occur, especially following IV injection, and shock and cardiac arrest have resulted from IV use of phytonadione. Parenteral administration (IM, SC, IV) can also lead to dizziness, tachycardia, weak pulse, chills, fever, sweating, hypotension, dyspnea, cyanosis, pain and swelling

at the injection site, and erythematous skin reactions.

Hyperbilirubinemia has been reported in newborns following injection, especially with menadione or menadiol, and may result in kernicterus, which can lead to brain damage and death; larger infants appear to exhibit greater tolerance to vitamin K than premature or very small infants.

CONTRAINDICATIONS AND PRECAUTIONS

Menadiol is contraindicated in infants and in women during the last few weeks of pregnancy and during labor, as a prophylactic measure against hypoprothrombinemia or hemorrhagic disease in the newborn. Vitamin K must be given *cautiously* to persons with liver disease, as hypoprothrombinemia due to hepatocellular damage is *not* corrected by vitamin K and repeated large doses can further impair hepatic function. The smallest dose that is effective in restoring normal prothrombin time (*i.e.*, 12 seconds–14 seconds), should be used, because large doses can provide the same conditions that previously increased the risk of clotting. Prothrombin time should be monitored frequently. IV injection should be undertaken only when other routes of administration are not appropriate, because severe hypersensitivity reactions, some fatal, have occurred following IV injection of phytonadione. Only normal saline or 5% dextrose solutions should be used as diluent and the injection performed very slowly.

INTERACTIONS

1. Vitamin K antagonizes the anticoagulant action of coumarins and indandiones, but not the anticoagulant action of heparin.
2. Mineral oil or cholestyramine may impair GI absorption of K_1 but not GI absorption of K_4.
3. Antibiotics may reduce endogenous vitamin K activity by decreasing its synthesis by intestinal flora. Increased bleeding can result.

NURSING CONSIDERATIONS

Vitamin K is usually administered parenterally when a patient is bleeding in an attempt to slow or stop the process. The drug takes 1 hour to 2 hours to change the prothrombin time even when administered intravenously. Therefore, if bleeding is profuse, fresh whole blood must also be administered until the drug takes effect.

Parenteral administration should be reserved for serious bleeding episodes and administered with caution since allergic reactions may occur. The drug should be infused slowly and blood pressure monitored every 2 minutes to 5 minutes during infusion since severe hypotension can occur. Allergic reactions can be mild, characterized by rash, urticaria, and pruritus, or severe, leading to anaphylactic shock and cardiac arrest. Emergency resuscitative equipment to manage respiration and emergency drugs such as epinephrine, corticosteroids, and antihistamines, as well as defibrillation and various cardiac drugs, should be immediately available. At the first sign of drug sensitivity, the infusion should be stopped and the physician notified. The patient's vital signs should be carefully monitored since fever, tachycardia, weak pulse, and dyspnea are possible in addition to hypotension.

Prothrombin time (PT) and partial thromboplastin time (PTT) should be obtained as a baseline and monitored throughout therapy. When these values return to normal limits, the drug therapy is considered effective. However, one of the adverse effects of large doses of vitamin K, especially menadiol, is prolongation of PT, the opposite of the effect desired. Therefore, if symptoms of hypoprothrombinemia persist, characterized by bleeding of gums or from nose or vagina, blood in stool or urine, or petechiae or ecchymosis, the physician should be notified and laboratory values checked. Vitamin K may need to be discontinued or an alternate form utilized.

Patients who are stabilized on vitamin K should limit intake of vitamin K-rich foods (see Table 77-1), since increasing such food intake may increase the risk of side-effects or adverse reactions from the drug. Patients who require further anticoagulation while taking vitamin K must be treated with heparin because they will be unresponsive to oral anticoagulants.

REVIEW QUESTIONS

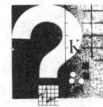

1. Why do symptoms of vitamin A deficiency only develop after an extended period of inadequate intake?
2. What are the principal dietary sources of (1) vitamin A, (2) vitamin D, and (3) vitamin E?
3. How is vitamin A synthesized?
4. Give the principal symptoms of vitamin A deficiency.

5. Chronic overconsumption of vitamin A can result in what major symptoms? What measures are taken to treat overconsumption?
6. What reasons may a patient give for taking large doses of vitamin A?
7. What fetal abnormalities are possible with overconsumption of vitamin A or D during pregnancy?
8. List the five substances possessing vitamin D activity.
9. What is the principal transport form of vitamin D? What is the most active form of the vitamin?
10. Briefly describe the mechanisms of action of vitamin D.
11. Give the major uses for vitamin D.
12. In what conditions are vitamin D preparations contraindicated?
13. What are the symptoms of vitamin D overconsumption? How is overdosage treated?
14. What reasons may a patient give for taking large doses of vitamin D?
15. What is the principal form of vitamin E found in animal tissues?
16. Describe the possible mechanisms of action of vitamin E.
17. In what different dosage forms is vitamin E available?
18. List the clinically available vitamin K preparations.
19. What are the major indications for vitamin K?
20. What is the danger in giving vitamin K to premature and newborn infants?
21. Describe the possible hazards associated with IV administration of vitamin K.
22. What precautions should be taken when administering parenteral vitamin K? What laboratory values should be monitored?

BIBLIOGRAPHY

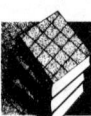

Bieri JG, Corash L, Hubbard VS: Medical uses of vitamin E. N Engl J Med 308:1063, 1983

Bieri JG, McKenna MC: Expressing dietary values for fat-soluble vitamins: Changes in concepts and terminology. Am J Clin Nutr 34:289, 1981

Cerrato PL: When to worry about vitamin overdose. RN 48(10):69, Oct, 1985

Deluca HF, Schnoes HK: Vitamin D: Recent advances. Annu Rev Biochem 52:411, 1983

Herbert V: Toxicity of 25,000 IU vitamin A supplements in "health" food users. Am J Clin Nutr 36:185, 1982

Kodicek E: The story of vitamin D. From vitamin to hormone. Lancet 1:325, 1974

Leo MA, Lieber CS: Hepatic vitamin A depletion in alcoholic liver injury. N Engl J Med 307:597, 1982

Luke B: Megavitamins and pregnancy: A dangerous combination. MCN 10:18, 1985

Machlin LJ (ed): Vitamin E: A comprehensive treatise. New York, Marcel Dekker, 1980

O'Connor ME, Livingstone DS, Hannah J, Wilkins D: Vitamin K deficiency and breast feeding. Am J Dis Child 137:601, 1983

Spron MB, Roberts AB, Goodman DS (eds): The Retinoids, Vols I and II. New York, Academic Press, 1984

Oral Nutrients, Fluids, and Electrolytes

Oral Nutritional Supplements

Systemic Alkalizers

78

The fluid composition of the body is normally maintained reasonably constant despite the many stresses placed on it. Significant alterations in the volume and composition of the internal fluid environment can, however, result from disease, trauma, or drug therapy, as well as from a number of other external factors. Disturbances in fluid and electrolyte balance may involve changes in *p*H, volume, osmolarity, or concentrations of individual ions, and can seriously impair the normal metabolic activity of body organs. Although abnormalities of a *single* parameter occasionally occur, multiple disturbances in several of the above properties are more often encountered. Thus, the various chemical constituents of the body (*i.e.*, electrolytes, minerals, amino acids, fluids, proteins, lipids) are often administered concurrently to correct acute or chronic deficiency states, and such a procedure is termed *nutritional replacement therapy.*

This chapter considers those nutrients, fluids, and electrolytes that are commonly used orally to supply the nutritional needs of patients suffering from a deficiency state of one or more of these substances. Not all of the substances used as nutritional supplements are considered here, inasmuch as several have a specific relationship with the functioning of a particular organ or body system. These substances are therefore considered in other chapters dealing with drugs affecting specific organs with which a particular mineral or electrolyte is intimately associated. Thus, calcium is discussed with parathyroid hormone and calcitonin in Chapter 53; iron is reviewed along with other drugs used to treat anemia in Chapter 38; and iodine and iodide salts are considered in Chapter 52 with the thyroid hormones. The vitamins are discussed individually in Chapters 76 and 77.

Oral Nutritional Supplements

The substances used orally for correcting nutritional deficiency states include minerals, electrolytes, amino acids, proteins, and lipids, as well as a few other miscellaneous drugs. Perhaps the most widely used oral electrolytes are potassium and fluoride, and these preparations are considered individually in detail below. The remaining oral nutritional supplements are listed in Table 78-1.

Potassium
(Various Manufacturers)

MECHANISM AND ACTIONS
Potassium is the principal intracellular cation and is essential for many vital physiologic processes, including cellular metabolism; acid–base balance; enzymatic reactions; nerve impulse transmission; skeletal, cardiac, and smooth muscle contraction; maintenance of intracellular tonicity; and proper renal function. Normal serum potassium levels range from 3.8 mEq/liter to 5 mEq/liter.

The usual adult dietary intake of potassium is 40 mEq to 150 mEq per day. Despite this variability in intake, plasma potassium levels are normally maintained within the narrow range noted above by renal regulatory mechanisms.

Potassium depletion occurs most frequently as a result of diuretic therapy, but may also be due to hyperaldosteronism, severe diarrhea, or diabetic ketoacidosis. It is usually accompanied by chloride loss as well, and is therefore frequently associated with metabolic alkalosis. Symptoms of potassium depletion (hypokalemia) include muscle weakness, cramping, fatigue, disturbances in cardiac rhythm, and inability to concentrate urine.

USES
1. Prevention and treatment of hypokalemia, for example, resulting from diuretic therapy, prolonged vomiting or diarrhea, diabetes, hepatic cirrhosis, inadequate dietary intake, malabsorption, hyperaldosteronism, or nephropathy

ADMINISTRATION AND DOSAGE
The dosage of potassium is given in milliequivalents (mEq) of the ion. Clinically available salts of potassium (with the potassium content) are as follows:

potassium acetate 10.2 mEq K^+/g
potassium bicarbonate 10 mEq K^+/g
potassium chloride 13.4 mEq K^+/g
potassium citrate 9.25 mEq K^+/g
potassium gluconate 4.3 mEq K^+/g

Potassium is available in a variety of different dosage forms as listed below (with potassium content given in milliequivalents):

Liquid—10 mEq/15 ml, 15 mEq/15 ml, 20 mEq/15 ml, 30 mEq/15 ml, 40 mEq/15 ml, 45 mEq/15 ml
Tablets—1.33 mEq, 2 mEq, 2.5 mEq, 5 mEq, 8 mEq, 10 mEq, 20 mEq, 25 mEq

Chew tablets—1 mEq, 2.5 mEq
Enteric-coated tablets—4 mEq
Controlled-release tablets—6.7 mEq, 8 mEq,
    10 mEq, 20 mEq
Controlled-release capsules—8 mEq, 10 mEq
Effervescent tablets—20 mEq, 25 mEq, 50 mEq
Powder packets—15 mEq, 20 mEq, 25 mEq

The usual dosage range for preventing hypokalemia (as may occur with diuretic therapy) is 16 mEq/day to 24 mEq/day, in divided doses. For treatment of potassium depletion, dosages of 40 mEq/day to 100 mEq/day have been used.

When hypokalemia is associated with alkalosis, the chloride salt should be used. When acidosis is present, one of the other salts is indicated. When oral replacement therapy is not feasible (as with severe vomiting, prolonged diuresis, marked diabetic acidosis), parenteral (IV infusion) therapy is indicated (see Chap. 79).

FATE
Oral potassium is well absorbed. Renal excretion of potassium occurs primarily by secretion in the distal portion of the nephron. Most of the filtered load of potassium is reabsorbed in the proximal tubule. Fecal excretion is minimal and does not play a significant role in potassium hemostasis.

SIDE-EFFECTS/ADVERSE REACTIONS
The most commonly encountered side-effects with oral potassium are nausea, diarrhea, abdominal discomfort, and vomiting. These effects may be minimized by taking the drug with meals or diluting the liquid preparations with juice or other beverage. Other adverse effects attributable to oral potassium include gastrointestinal (GI) bleeding, ulceration, or perforation; skin rash; and hyperkalemia (characterized by paresthesias, flaccid paralysis, confusion, weakness, hypotension, respiratory distress, arrhythmias, cardiac depression, and heart block). With normal kidney function, it is difficult to elicit potassium intoxication with oral dosage, since renal excretion increases with increasing serum levels. However, use in patients with renal impairment should be undertaken cautiously and at reduced dosage, and intake-to-output ratio should be monitored.

Potassium chloride tablets have produced ulcerative lesions of the small bowel, resulting in obstruction, hemorrhage, and perforation. The incidence of small bowel lesions is least with controlled-release wax-matrix tablets, and lower with enteric-coated tablets than with uncoated

tablets. Patients at greatest risk for developing potassium-induced gastrointestinal (GI) lesions include those with diabetes mellitus, cardiomegaly, esophageal stricture, or scleroderma, and elderly patients.

CONTRAINDICATIONS AND PRECAUTIONS
Potassium replacement products are contraindicated in patients with severe renal impairment (with oliguria, anuria, or azotemia), Addison's disease, acute dehydration, heat cramps, or hyperkalemia from any cause, including patients receiving potassium-sparing diuretics. In addition, solid dosage forms of potassium are contraindicated in patients in whom there is delayed passage of contents through the GI tract.

Potassium supplementation must be undertaken with caution in patients with systemic acidosis, acute dehydration, chronic renal dysfunction, cardiac disease, adrenal insufficiency, or peptic ulcer. Safety for use during pregnancy and lactation and in children has not been established. Acid–base balance, serum electrolytes, and the electrocardiogram should be closely monitored during treatment of hypokalemia with potassium salts to avoid potassium intoxication, which can result in arrhythmias and cardiac depression.

INTERACTIONS
1. Combinations of potassium salts with potassium-sparing diuretics can result in severe hyperkalemia.
2. Increased serum potassium decreases both toxicity and effectiveness of digitalis drugs.
3. Concurrent use of salt substitutes with potassium supplements can lead to hyperkalemia.
4. Concomitant administration of anticholinergics and oral potassium products may increase the likelihood of GI erosion due to slowed GI motility and delayed gastric emptying.
5. Captopril can cause potassium retention leading to hyperkalemia.

NURSING CONSIDERATIONS
Oral potassium comes in many forms; therefore, administration is dependent on the form ordered. The advantage of multiple forms is that if one is not palatable, another can be tried. The disadvantages are that preparation and administration can vary widely among forms, may be confusing to the patient, and can lead to incorrect dosage and subsequent hyperkalemia, a serious side-effect. Con-

(Text continues on p. 1532.)

Table 78-1
Oral Nutritional Supplements

Drug	Preparations	Usual Dosage Range	Clinical Considerations
Minerals and Electrolytes			
magnesium (Almora, Magonate, Magnate, Nephro-Mag)	Tablets—27 mg (as magnesium gluconate), 100 mg (as magnesium–amino acids chelate), 250 mg magnesium carbonate	27 mg–100 mg 2 to 4 times/day depending on requirement	RDAs are 200 mg (children 4 years–6 years), 300 mg–400 mg (adults), and 450 mg (pregnant or lactating women); excessive amounts may produce diarrhea; necessary for a number of enzyme systems and for nerve conduction and muscle contraction; deficiency is rare in well-nourished persons.
manganese	Tablets—20 mg, 50 mg (chelated manganese)	20 mg/day–50 mg/day	Need in human nutrition is not established; functions as a cofactor in many enzyme systems; stimulates cholesterol and fatty acid synthesis in the liver; localized primarily in mitochondria.
oral electrolyte mixture (Gastrolyte Oral, Infalyte, Lytren, Pedialyte, Resol, Rehydralyte)	Solution or powder (containing various electrolytes and dextrose or glucose)—Use solution as is, or dissolve 1 packet of powder in water	*Estimated daily requirements* Infants and young children —1500 ml–2500 ml/m² Children (5 years–10 years) —1000 ml to 2000 ml/ day Children (over 10 years) and adults—2000 ml–3000 ml/day	Used to replace water and electolytes when food and fluid intake is sharply reduced (*e.g.*, postoperatively, starvation) or when fluid loss is excessive (*e.g.*, diarrhea, severe vomiting); severe continual diarrhea requires additional parenteral replacement therapy; use only in recommended volumes to prevent electrolyte overload; reduce intake when other electrolytes are reinstituted; do not use in the presence of intestinal obstruction, intractable vomiting, adynamic ileus, perforated bowel, or impaired renal function; avoid mixing with other electrolyte-containing liquids (milk, fruit juice).
phosphorus (K-Phos Neutral, Neutra-Phos, Neutro-Phos-K, Uro-KP-Neutral)	Tablets—250 mg (with sodium and potassium) Capsules—250 mg (with sodium and potassium) Powder for solution—250 mg/75 ml (reconstituted solution with sodium and potassium)	1 to 2 tablets 4 times/day *or* Contents of 1 capsule mixed with 75 ml water 4 times/day *or* 75 ml reconstituted solution 4 times/day	Used as dietary supplement where diet is deficient, needs are increased, or GI absorption is impaired; RDAs are 800 mg (adults and children 4 years–6 years) and 1200 mg (children 11 years–18 years *(continued)*

Table 78-1 (continued)
Oral Nutritional Supplements

Drug	Preparations	Usual Dosage Range	Clinical Considerations
Minerals and Electrolytes (*continued*)			
phosphorus (K-Phos Neutral, Neutra-Phos, Neutro-Phos-K, Uro-KP-Neutral) (*continued*)			and pregnant or lactating women); phosphate can lower urinary calcium levels; a laxative effect is common early in therapy; it is contraindicated in hyperkalemia and Addison's disease.
sodium chloride (Slo-Salt)	Tablets—650 mg, 1 g, 2.25 g Tablets (slow release)—600 mg Enteric-coated tablets—1 g	0.5 g–1 g 3 to 6 times/day for prevention of dehydration and heat cramps (maximum is 4.8 g/day)	Used to replace excessive loss of sodium and chloride (*e.g.*, resulting from perspiration or extreme diuresis) and to counteract excessive salt restriction; use cautiously in patients with congestive heart failure, renal disease, circulatory insufficiency, or electrolyte disturbances; it is also available with dextrose and vitamin B_1 (sodium chloride with dextrose) and in fixed combination with potassium chloride, calcium phosphate, and magnesium carbonate (Heatrol).
zinc sulfate (Orazinc, Scrip-Zinc, Verazinc, Zinc-220, Zincate, Zinkaps)	Tablets—66 mg, 200 mg, (equivalent to 15 mg, and 47 mg elemental zinc, respectively) Capsules—110 mg, 220 mg (equivalent to 25 mg and 50 mg elemental zinc, respectively)	25 mg–50 mg elemental zinc a day	Important mineral for normal growth and repair of body tissues; symptoms of zinc deficiency include anorexia, loss of taste and olfactory sensation, mood changes, and growth retardation; used investigationally to treat delayed wound healing, acne, and rheumatoid arthritis; to improve the immune response in the elderly; and to delay onset of dementia in patients genetically at risk; RDAs are 10 mg for children 1 year–10 years, 15 mg for adults, 20 mg–25 mg for pregnant or lactating women; excessive doses may produce severe vomiting, dehydration, and restlessness; GI upset can occur and can be minimized by taking drug with food or milk; zinc can impair absorption of tetracyclines.
zinc gluconate	Tablets—10 mg, 15 mg, 35 mg, 50 mg, 105 mg (equivalent to 1.4 mg, 2 mg, 5 mg, 7 mg, and 15 mg elemental zinc, respectively)		

(continued)

Table 78-1 (continued)
Oral Nutritional Supplements

Drug	Preparations	Usual Dosage Range	Clinical Considerations
Miscellaneous Nutritional Factors			
bioflavonoids (Ascorbin II, C Speridin, Citro-Flav 200, C.V.P., duo-C.V.P., Flavons 500, Pan C-500, Peridin-C, Span-C, Super-C)	Tablets—100 mg, 150 mg, 300 mg, 500 mg Capsules—100 mg, 200 mg	100 mg–500 mg/day	Derived from green citrus fruits; many products also contain vitamin C; previously used to reduce capillary fragility and referred to as vitamin P ("permeability"); there is no evidence that they are effective and no need in human nutrition has been established.
calcium caseinate (Casec)	Powder—Containing 88% protein, 2% fat, and 4.5% minerals	Variable according to patient's requirments	Used as an infant formula modifier or as a diet supplement
l-carnitine (Carnitor, Vitacan)	Tablets—330 mg Capsules—250 mg Liquid—100 mg/ml	Adults—1 g to 3 g a day Children—50 to 100 mg/kg/day	Naturally occurring amino acid derivative synthesized from methionine and lysine; acts to facilitate fatty acid metabolism and subsequent energy production; used in patients with primary carnitine deficiency, which can result in elevated triglycerides and free fatty acids, impaired ketogenesis, and in children, reduced growth and development; GI distress is common; drug may also produce an unpleasant body odor; has been used experimentally to improve athletic performance.
choline	Tablets—250 mg, 500 mg, 520 mg, 650 mg Powder	250 mg–1 g/day	A component of lecithin that has a lipotropic action, and is essential for the formation of acetylcholine; average diet provides sufficient choline for body needs; has been used to treat fatty liver and cirrhosis and to relieve symptoms of CNS disorders such as Huntington's disease, Gilles de la Tourette's syndrome, Friedreich's ataxia, and tardive dyskinesias; can cause GI disturbances and imparts an odor of decaying fish to the feces and occasionally the breath due to its metabo- *(continued)*

Table 78-1 (continued)
Oral Nutritional Supplements

Drug	Preparations	Usual Dosage Range	Clinical Considerations
Miscellaneous Nutritional Factors (continued)			
choline *(continued)*			lism to trimethylamine; it is used as free choline as well as bitartrate, chloride, and dihydrogen citrate salts.
corn oil (Lipomul Oral)	Liquid—10 g/15 ml	Adults—45 ml 2 to 4 times/day Children—30 ml 1 to 4 times/day	Used to increase caloric intake in malnourished or debilitated patients; use cautiously in persons with diabetes and gallbladder dysfunction; each dose contains 270 cal and 30 g fat.
glucose polymers (Moducal, Polycose, Pro-Mix Carbohydrate Liquid, Sumacal)	Liquid or powder—Containing various amounts of carbohydrates, sodium, chloride, potassium, calcium, and phosphorus	Add to foods or beverages and give in small, frequent feedings	Derived from cornstarch; supplies calories in patients unable to meet caloric needs with usual food intake, or in patients on protein-, electrolyte-, and fat-restricted diets; not intended as the sole nutritional source; it may be used for extended periods of time with diets containing all other essential nutrients or as an oral adjunct to IV nutrients.
inositol	Tablets—250 mg, 500 mg, 650 mg Powder	1 g–3 g/day in divided doses	An isomer of glucose possessing lipotropic activity in animals; physiologic role in humans is obscure and there is no evidence that it is clinically effective, although it has been used to treat liver disorders and disordered fat metabolism; dietary sources include mainly vegetables.
lactase (Lact-Aid, Lactrase)	Liquid—1000 neutral lactase units per 5-drop dose Capsules—125 mg of standardized lactase enzyme Tablets—3300 lactase units	5–10 drops per quart of milk or 1–2 capsules or tablets either added to a quart of milk or taken along with milk or dairy products	Powdered enzyme preparation used to facilitate digestion of milk lactose in patients with lactose intolerance.
lecithin	Capsules—520 mg, 1.2 g Granules	1–2 capsules/day	A source of choline, inositol, phosphorus, and linoleic and linolenic acids employed as a dietary supplement (see choline, above).
l-lysine (Enisyl)	Tablets—312 mg, 325 mg, 334 mg, 500 mg	312 mg–1500 mg/day	An essential amino acid, used as a dietary supple-

(continued)

Table 78-1 (continued)
Oral Nutritional Supplements

Drug	Preparations	Usual Dosage Range	Clinical Considerations
Miscellaneous Nutritional Factors (continued)			
l-lysine (Enisyl) (continued)			ment to increase utilization of vegetable proteins; used investigationally for prophylaxis and treatment of herpes simplex infections, although efficacy is questionable; it is available in combination with other amino acids, vitamins, and minerals in a variety of combination products.
medium-chain triglycerides (MCT Oil)	Oil—consisting primarily of the triglycerides of C_8 and C_{10} saturated fatty acids	15 ml 3 to 4 times/day	A dietary supplement for persons who cannot efficiently digest and absorb conventional long-chain fatty acids; medium-chain triglycerides are more rapidly hydrolyzed than conventional food fat, and are not dependent on bile salts for emulsification; may be mixed with juices, poured on salads or other foods, incorporated into sauces, or used in cooking and baking; use with caution in persons with hepatic cirrhosis; one dose (15 ml) contains 115 cal.
para-aminobenzoic acid (PABA, Potaba)	Tablets—30 mg, 100 mg, 500 mg Capsules—500 mg Powder	Adults—12 g/day in 4 to 6 divided doses Children—1 g/10 lb daily in divided doses	A substance found naturally associated with the B-complex vitamins and essential for the functioning of a number of important biologic processes; considered "possibly effective" for scleroderma, dermatomyositis, morphea, pemphigus, and Peyronie's disease; dissolve tablets in liquid to minimize GI

(continued)

Table 78-1 (continued)
Oral Nutritional Supplements

Drug	Preparations	Usual Dosage Range	Clinical Considerations
Miscellaneous Nutritional Factors (continued)			
para-aminobenzoic acid (PABA, Potaba) (*continued*)			upset; drug should be taken with food; adverse reactions include anorexia, nausea, fever, and rash; use cautiously in patients with kidney impairment; do not give concurrently with sulfonamides, because PABA interferes with the antibacterial action; has no known human nutritional value; it acts as a sunscreen when applied topically.
protein hydrolysates (A/G-Pro, PDP Liquid Protein)	Tablets—542 mg (45% amino acids with minerals) Capsules—292 mg protein (with vitamins and minerals) Liquid—15 g protein/30 ml Powder—Containing carbohydrates, fats, and electrolytes	2 tablets 3 times/day *or* 1 capsule 3 times/day *or* 30 ml liquid/day *or* 1 tbsp–5 tbsp powder in liquid/day	Preparations of amino acids and peptides obtained by hydrolysis of larger proteins; used as dietary supplement to correct or prevent protein deficiency; optimum daily intake of dietary protein is 1 g/kg.
safflower oil (Microlipid)	Emulsion—50% fat	1 tbsp—2 tbsp several times a day as necessary or may be added to formula for tube feeding	A caloric and fatty-acid supplement used in malnourished patients and other persons with fatty-acid deficiencies; it contains 4500 cal and 500 g fat per liter.
l-tryptophan (Trofan, Typtacin)	Tablets—300 mg, 500 mg, 667 mg, 1 g	500 mg–2 g/day in divided doses	An essential amino acid that serves as a precursor for serotonin; has been used experimentally as an antidepressant and hypnotic, although its clinical efficacy in this regard remains to be established; doses of 4 g–5 g reduce sleep latency and increase sleep time.

sequently, if a patient has difficulty managing preparation and administration of potassium or has an impaired memory, a family member should be taught the procedure to ensure safe drug taking.

Liquids, powders, and effervescent tablets should be completely dissolved in 4 oz to 8 oz of a cold beverage such as fruit juice or water. Effervescent tablets should be allowed to stop fizzing before they are ingested. Liquids should be measured by drops exactly as ordered to avoid overdosage. These forms are frequently prescribed because they are relatively inexpensive and easily swallowed, and come in a wide variety of dosage forms, which makes management of the potassium level easy. These forms can also be administered by way of a nasogastric tube. However, some patients find the salty taste unappealing and are unable to tolerate them. Others develop gastrointestinal symptoms, which may be minimized by taking the drug with meals. However, if problems persist other dosage forms are available.

All tablets, except for chewable tablets, must *not* be chewed or broken but must be swallowed whole. The tablet should not be allowed to dissolve in the mouth where it can cause mucosal ulceration. If the patient has difficulty swallowing, another form may be used. The advantage of some of the controlled-release and enteric-coated tablets is reduced GI irritability.

The patient receiving potassium supplementation should have frequent electrolyte levels drawn. If the potassium level is higher than normal, dosage should be reduced immediately. While hyperkalemia is unlikely from potassium supplements taken at prescribed dosage, the side-effect may occur if renal function is diminished or if the patient is unreliable in remembering to take the drug. Patients and family should be told to report immediately any muscle weakness, numbness or tingling of extremities, shortness of breath, or changes in pulse rate, which are symptoms of drug overdosage. Hyperkalemia can be life threatening and must be treated immediately with hydrating fluids. It may be treated with intravenous dextrose and insulin solution, sodium bicarbonate, calcium gluceptate, calcium chloride, or calcium gluconate, or with Kayexalate retention enemas. If necessary, peritoneal or hemodialysis may be performed to remove potassium.

Patients should also be taught to monitor for GI side-effects since GI bleeding and perforation can occur. The patient should report immediately any vomiting, blackened stools, bloody stools,

weakness, or abdominal pain or distention. If any of these occur, the drug must be discontinued.

Fluoride
(Luride, Pediaflor, Phos-Flur, and various other manufacturers)

MECHANISM AND ACTIONS
The fluoride ion is used orally as sodium fluoride and topically (in the form of a mouth rinse or gel) as either sodium fluoride, stannous fluoride, or acidulated phosphate fluoride.

Fluoride is incorporated into the external layer of dental enamel, where it appears to increase tooth resistance to acid dissolution, promote remineralization through increased osteoblastic activity, and inhibit the development of caries. Acidification promotes greater topical fluoride uptake by dental enamel than neutral solutions.

USES
1. Prevention of dental caries where community water supplies are low in fluoride (*i.e.*, less than 0.7 parts per million) or following radioactive therapy of head or neck tumors, which can result in extreme dryness of the mouth and increased tooth decay
2. Topical desensitization of exposed tooth root surfaces
3. Investigational use is in preventing or treating osteoporosis in menopausal women, in conjunction with calcium, vitamin D, or estrogen supplementation.

ADMINISTRATION AND DOSAGE
Oral fluoride preparations include regular or chewable tablets (0.25 mg, 0.5 mg, 1 mg) or drops (0.125 mg/drop, 0.25 mg/drop, 0.5 mg/ml). Topical preparations include solutions (0.01%, 0.02%, 0.09%) and gels (0.1%, 0.5%, 1.23%) for rinsing of the oral cavity.

Oral dosage ranges from 0.25 mg/day to 1.0 mg/day depending on the patient's age and the fluoride content of drinking water. Tablets or drops should be taken with meals. Dairy products can slow the absorption of fluoride tablets. The tablets may be dissolved in the mouth, chewed, swallowed whole, or added to water or other beverage.

Mouth rinses are used in volumes of 5 ml to 10 ml once a day, after brushing or flossing. The rinse should be retained in the mouth for one minute and then expectorated (and not swallowed). Gels are squeezed into the mouth, swirled for one minute, then expectorated. Eating or drinking should be discouraged for at least 30 minutes after use of either the rinse or gel.

FATE

Fluoride is rapidly absorbed orally and widely distributed in the body. Calcium, iron, or magnesium ions can delay fluoride absorption. The ion is quickly deposited in teeth and bone. Excretion is primarily by way of the kidney.

SIDE-EFFECTS/ADVERSE REACTIONS

Side-effects are infrequent with oral fluoride preparations. Occasional nausea, gastric distress, headache, weakness, and allergic rash have been reported. Mouth rinses or gels containing stannous fluoride may produce surface staining of teeth. Chonic overdosage may lead to mottling or brown discoloration of tooth enamel and softening of tooth enamel. Acute ingestion of large doses of fluoride may cause excessive salivation, GI disturbances, irritability, tetany, hyperreflexia, seizures, and cardiac failure.

CONTRAINDICATIONS AND PRECAUTIONS

Supplemental fluoride should not be given when fluoride content of drinking water exceeds 0.7 parts per million or to patients on low-sodium or sodium-free diets. Tablets or rinses containing 1 mg are not recommended in children under 3 years of age or when the drinking water contains more than 0.3 parts per million of fluoride.

INTERACTIONS

1. Absorption of fluorides may be impaired by concurrent ingestion of dairy products containing calcium, or by the presence of iron or magnesium in the stomach.

NURSING CONSIDERATIONS

Fluoride is frequently an ingredient in liquid vitamins and minerals given to young children, especially those who are breast-feeding and may be receiving insufficient fluoridated water on a daily basis. It is important to ask the mother what sources of fluids a baby receives to determine the need for fluoride supplementation. Once the child receives juices mixed with fluoridated water or drinks water on a daily basis, the need for fluoride supplementation is reduced. If the family drinks only bottled water or lives in an area where the fluoride content is less than 0.7 parts per million,

fluoride supplementation may be necessary for several years. The nurse can help a family make decisions on fluoride supplementation by being aware of which communities add fluoride to the water. Such information should be available from the county health department and the water companies in the area.

As with other medications, fluoride supplements should be kept out of the reach of children. Acute fluoride overdosage will usually result in excessive salivation, GI upset, and vomiting, which serves as a protective mechanism to the body. However, emergency treatment should be sought.

Systemic Alkalizers

Oral products containing sodium bicarbonate, potassium citrate, sodium citrate, or citric acid may be used as gastric, systemic, or urinary alkalizers. Potassium citrate and sodium citrate are metabolized to potassium bicarbonate and sodium bicarbonate, respectively. Citric acid is metabolized to CO_2 and water and merely functions as a temporary buffer.

The agents can be used to correct the metabolic acidosis resulting from renal tubular disorders or other causes and for maintenance of an alkaline urine, for example, to prevent uric acid crystallization.

Preparations containing potassium citrate (*e.g.,* Polycitra-K) are preferred in patients requiring sodium restriction, whereas solutions containing sodium citrate (*e.g.,* Bicitra, Oracit) are useful where hyperkalemia is present. Other products containing both potassium citrate *and* sodium citrate (*e.g.,* Polycitra) may be employed where electrolyte restriction is not necessary. The usual adult dosage of these citrate products is 15 ml to 30 ml diluted with water after meals and before bedtime. Children may be given 5 ml to 15 ml in water.

Diarrhea, nausea, abdominal pain, and vomiting can occur with potassium citrate; GI distress can be minimized by dilution in water and following a dose with additional water if necessary.

Sodium bicarbonate is available as tablets (325 mg, 650 mg) and as powder. The recommended dose is 325 mg to 2 g four times a day to a maximum of 16 g a day in patients under 60 years of age and 8 g a day in older patients. Sodium bicarbonate preparations must be given with caution to patients requiring sodium restriction, such as those with congestive heart failure, hypertension, or renal impairment.

REVIEW QUESTIONS

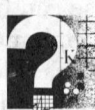

1. In what physiologic processes does potassium play a vital role?
2. What conditions may lead to potassium depletion? Describe the principal symptoms of potassium loss.
3. In what different dosage forms is potassium available? What instructions should be given with each of them?
4. What are the common side-effects associated with potassium administration?
5. Potassium replacement products should not be used in the presence of what conditions?
6. Briefly describe the function of fluoride in the body.
7. List the major uses for oral fluoride preparations.
8. What is the danger of chronic excessive use of fluoride?
9. Give the principal indications for use of oral electrolyte mixtures, such as Lytren and Pedialyte.
10. List several potential uses for oral zinc.
11. What are the possible indications for choline?
12. How is lactose used?
13. For what applications may para-aminobenzoic acid (PABA) be useful?
14. How has l-tryptophan been used experimentally?
15. What products are utilized as systemic alkalizers? What are their principal indications?

BIBLIOGRAPHY

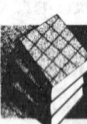

Agranoff BW (ed): Inositol triphosphate (symposium). Fed Proc 45(11):2627, 1986

Bia MJ, DeFronzo RA: Extrarenal potassium homeostasis. Am J Physiol 240:F257, 1981

Levander OA, Cheng L (eds): Micronutrient interactions: Vitamins, minerals and hazardous elements. Ann NY Acad Sci 355:1, 1980

Massry SG: Pharmacology of magnesium. Annu Rev Pharmacol Toxicol 17:67, 1977

Munro HN (ed): Placental transport of nutrients (symposium). Fed Proc 45(10):2500, 1986

Pardridge WM (ed): Blood-brain transport of nutrients (symposium). Fed Proc 45(7):2047, 1986

Rude RK, Singer FR: Magnesium deficiency and excess. Annu Rev Med 32:245, 1981

Young DB: Relationship between plasma potassium concentration and renal potassium excretion. Am J Physiol 242:F599, 1982

Parenteral Fluids and Electrolytes: Total Parenteral Nutrition

79

Parenteral nutritional supplementation is provided for a number of reasons, ranging from correction of simple acute dehydration to chronic treatment of serious nutritional deficiencies resulting from such conditions as severe gastrointestinal (GI) disorders, prolonged kidney failure, and extensive burns.

Substances provided in parenteral nutritional supplements include electrolytes, carbohydrates, fats, proteins, and vitamins. Administration of solutions by way of peripheral veins (*i.e.*, peripheral parenteral nutrition) is generally adequate if caloric requirements are minimal and can be partially satisfied with oral supplements and if nutritional therapy will only be required for 1 week to 2 weeks. Conversely, in severely depleted patients or in patients who will require prolonged supplemental nutrition, total parenteral nutrition (TPN) using a central venous catheter is usually indicated. TPN, sometimes referred to as hyperalimentation, is used to maintain an anabolic state when conventional oral or tube feeding is inappropriate and when peripheral IV therapy cannot meet the nutritional demands of the patient.

This chapter will consider the various types of substances used for parenteral nutrition. Individual carbohydrate, protein, lipid, and electrolyte solutions will be reviewed first, followed by an in-depth discussion of TPN.

Protein (Amino Acid) Products

The protein products employed as parenteral nutrients include protein hydrolysates and mixtures of crystalline amino acids, with or without added electrolytes. Most products are used for TPN (see following discussion of TPN), but some amino acid preparations can be employed as dilute solutions for peripheral parenteral feeding. These products provide a concentrated form of utilizable amino acids for protein synthesis as well as varying amounts of electrolytes, but they require addition of sufficient dextrose to provide for full caloric energy requirements when used for chronic hyperalimentation.

Crystalline Amino Acid Infusions

(Aminosyn, Branch Amin, FreAmine III, Neopham, Novamine, ProcalAmine, Travasol, TrophAmine)

Crystalline amino acids are hypertonic solutions of essential and nonessential l-amino acids or low-molecular-weight peptides with varying proportions of electrolytes that provide a substrate for protein synthesis and exert a protein-sparing effect. Preparations differ in degree of osmolarity, amino acid ratios, and content of nitrogen. In addition to the general amino acid formulations listed in the above heading, specialized formulations are available for use in patients with renal failure, hepatic failure/encephalopathy, or acute metabolic stress. These latter products are considered after the review of the general formulations.

MECHANISM AND ACTIONS
Amino acid infusions provide replacement of deficient amino acids and electrolytes and possess a nitrogen-sparing effect when used with a nonprotein caloric source. They can promote a positive nitrogen balance and increase protein synthesis.

USES
1. Prevention of nitrogen loss or treatment of negative nitrogen balance
2. Adjuncts in providing adequate total parenteral nutrition, as a component product of total parenteral nutrition in full strength or peripheral parenteral nutrition in diluted form

ADMINISTRATION AND DOSAGE
Crystalline amino acid infusions contain between 3% and 11.4% of both essential and nonessential amino acids in varying proportions, together with various electrolytes. The solutions are supplied in volumes ranging from 250 ml to 1000 ml. Generally, solutions containing 3.5% of amino acids or less are *not* used for central TPN. Solutions used for peripheral parenteral nutrition are usually diluted prior to infusion.

Dosage is flexible and depends on daily protein requirements, patient's clinical response, and metabolic activity. Refer to the individual package instructions.

SIDE-EFFECTS/ADVERSE REACTIONS
Side-effects with infusion of crystalline amino acid solutions include nausea, flushing, and a sensation of warmth, especially on too-rapid infusion.

Other adverse reactions associated with these preparations are vomiting, chills, headache, abdominal pain, dizziness, allergic reactions, phlebitis, venous thrombosis, skin rash, and papular eruptions; metabolic disturbances include acidosis, alkalosis, hypocalcemia, hypophosphatemia, hyperglycemia, glycosuria, hypovitaminosis, and other electrolyte imbalances.

CONTRAINDICATIONS AND PRECAUTIONS

Amino acid infusions should not be administered in the presence of anuria, oliguria, severe liver or kidney impairment, metabolic disorders involving impaired nitrogen utilization, decreased circulating blood volume, inborn errors of amino acid metabolism, hepatic coma or encephalopathy, and hyperammonemia.

INTERACTIONS

1. Antianabolic drugs and tetracyclines may reduce the protein-sparing effects of amino acids.
2. Addition of calcium to the infusion may precipitate the phosphate ion.

Amino Acid Formulation for Renal Failure

(Aminosyn R.F., NephrAmine, RenAmin)

Amino acid formulation for renal failure is indicated to provide nutritional support for uremic patients where oral nutrition is impractical and dialysis is not feasible. The products are used in conjunction with dextrose, electrolytes, and vitamins, and are administered by central venous injection. Amino acid formulation for renal failure supplies only essential amino acids, thus allowing urea nitrogen to be recycled to glutamate, which serves as a precursor for synthesis of nonessential amino acids. Therefore, use of these products in uremic patients results in utilization of retained urea and amelioration of azotemic symptoms. To promote urea reutilization, however, it is essential to provide adequate calories and to restrict intake of nonessential nitrogen.

Amino Acid Formulation for High Metabolic Stress

(FreAmine HBC)

Amino acid formulation for high metabolic stress is a mixture of essential and nonessential amino acids with high concentrations of the branched-chain amino acids isoleucine, leucine, and valine. Metabolic stress is often characterized by increased urinary excretion of nitrogen and by hyperglycemia, with decreased plasma levels of branched-chain amino acids. As a result, glucose utilization and fat mobilization are impaired. By supplying branched-chain amino acids, this formulation provides the substrates needed to meet the energy requirements of muscle and brain tissue.

Amino Acid Formulation for Hepatic Failure or Hepatic Encephalopathy

(HepatAmine)

Amino acid formulation for hepatic failure is very similar to the formulation for high metabolic stress, above, being a mixture of essential and nonessential amino acids with high concentrations of branched-chain amino acids. It is used for treating hepatic encephalopathy in patients intolerant of general-purpose amino acid injections. Replenishment of stores of branched-chain amino acids can reverse the abnormal plasma amino acid pattern seen in hepatic encephalopathy, with resultant improvement in mental status and electroencephalogram (EEG) pattern. Nitrogen balance is also significantly improved.

NURSING CONSIDERATIONS

Most amino acid infusions are indicated for TPN and should be administered by way of a central vein if possible. However, Aminosyn 3.5%, FreAmine III 3% with electrolytes, ProcalAmine, and Travasol 3.5% with electrolyte 45 can be used for peripheral vein infusion. Large veins should be used as much as possible for infusions, and peripheral sites must be rotated every 48 hours or more frequently if pain, redness, or swelling occur at the IV site. All amino acid solutions are hypertonic and may produce phlebitis. Peripheral solutions should be administered using an infusion pump.

Amino acid infusions are physically incompatible with blood, blood products, many antibiotics, and electrolytes. Therefore, no drugs should be piggybacked into a TPN or peripheral amino acid infusion without checking with a pharmacist knowledgeable about IV compatibilities. If the amino acid solutions cannot be premixed with fat emulsions, they can be infused simultaneously by means of a Y connector located near the infusion site (but below any inline filter). Check with the pharmacist before doing this. The infusions should be observed for clumping or particulate matter, and if any are seen the infusion should be discontinued immediately and the physician notified.

Amino acid solutions should be used cautiously in patients with impaired liver function, and liver enzymes and ammonia level should be closely monitored. If ammonia level rises or if the patient exhibits reduced body temperature, weak pulse, or GI distress, the infusion must be discontinued and the physician notified. Special amino acid formulations such as HepatAmine may be required for patients with hepatic problems.

Likewise, if symptoms of renal failure, such as elevated blood urea nitrogen or serum creatinine, or azotemia or uremia develop, the amino acid solution must be discontinued. If appropriate, a special formulation for patients in renal failure will be used.

The amino acids in these solutions are converted to glucose by way of gluconeogenesis in the liver and add substantially to the glucose available to the body. Consequently, urine and blood glucose levels must be monitored throughout therapy and the patient should be observed for signs of hypoglycemia or hyperglycemia.

As with other solutions containing nutrients, careful asepsis must be maintained to prevent bacterial or fungal growth in the solution container or tubing. Opening of the infusion system must be kept to a minimum. Portal connectors should be used whenever possible to add drugs or solutions and tubing should be changed at least every 24 hours according to institution policy.

Carbohydrate Products

Parenteral carbohydrate solutions are indicated primarily as a source of calories and fluid in patients with nutritional deficiencies who are unable to obtain the necessary nutrients orally. The available preparations include dextrose in water, alcohol in dextrose infusion, fructose in water, and invert sugar (dextrose and fructose) in water.

Dextrose in Water Injection

($D_{2.5}W$, D_5W, $D_{10}W$, $D_{20}W$, $D_{25}W$, $D_{30}W$, $D_{38.5}W$, $D_{50}W$, $D_{60}W$, $D_{70}W$)

Dextrose in water injection is available as solutions of varying concentrations of dextrose (D-glucose) in water for injection. Caloric content ranges from 85 cal/liter (2.5%) to 2380 cal/liter (70%). The 5% solution is isotonic and along with the 2.5% and 10% solutions may be given by IV infusions into peripheral veins to provide calories where nonelectrolytic fluid is required. The 20% solution provides adequate calories in a minimal volume of water. The more concentrated solutions provide even greater caloric content with less fluid volume and may be

irritating if given by peripheral infusion; they are usually administered by central venous catheters as a component of TPN. Dextrose is also available in several electrolyte solutions in various concentrations for IV infusion in patients having both a carbohydrate and an electrolyte deficit. Principal electrolytes used in fixed combination with dextrose are sodium, chloride, potassium, calcium, magnesium, phosphate, lactate, and acetate.

MECHANISM AND ACTIONS
Dextrose in water injection provides a source of calories and fluid volume where nutritional or fluid deficiencies (or both) exist. Parenterally administered dextrose is oxidized to CO_2 and water and provides 3.4 cal per gram of D-glucose. Dextrose injections may induce diuresis. Dextrose promotes glycogen deposition, decreases protein and nitrogen loss, and therefore in sufficient amounts can prevent ketosis.

USES
1. Provides nonelectrolytic fluid and caloric replacement (usually 5% or 10% solution)
2. Component of total parenteral nutrition, in conjunction with other solutions of proteins, electrolytes, fats, and vitamins (usually 40%, 50%, 60%, or 70% solution)
3. Treatment of insulin hypoglycemia to restore blood glucose levels (50% solution)
4. Treatment of acute symptomatic hypoglycemia in the neonate or older infant to restore depressed blood glucose levels (25% solution)

ADMINISTRATION AND DOSAGE
Dextrose in water injection is available in solutions containing 2.5%, 5%, 10%, 20%, 25%, 30%, 38.5%, 40%, 50%, 60%, and 70% dextrose. Dosage is dependent on the patient's age, weight, and clinical condition. The maximum rate at which dextrose can be infused without producing glycosuria is 0.5 g/kg/hour. In treating insulin-induced hypoglycemia, adults may be given 10 g to 25 g. Children may receive 250 mg/kg/dose, up to 600 mg/kg/dose.

FATE
Approximately 95% is retained if infusion rate is 800 mg/kg/hour. Essentially 100% retention occurs at 400 mg to 500 mg/kg/hour.

SIDE-EFFECTS/ADVERSE REACTIONS
Adverse effects resulting from use of dextrose in water infusions include thrombophlebitis (with prolonged infusion), irritation, tissue necrosis, in-

fection at injection site, hypervolemia, mental confusion, hyperglycemia, glycosuria (especially with concentrated solutions or too-rapid administration), overhydration, congestion, and pulmonary edema.

CONTRAINDICATIONS AND PRECAUTIONS

Dextrose in water injection is contraindicated in diabetic coma. In addition, *concentrated* solutions should not be used in patients with intracranial or intraspinal hemorrhage, delirium tremens, or glucose–galactose malabsorption syndrome.

These solutions should be used *cautiously* in patients with renal insufficiency, cardiac decompensation, hypervolemia, diabetes mellitus, carbohydrate intolerance, or urinary tract obstruction.

INTERACTIONS

1. Dextrose infusions may alter insulin or oral anti-diabetic drug requirements, and cause vitamin B-complex deficiency.
2. Hyperglycemia and glycosuria may be intensified by diuretics that decrease glucose tolerance.

Alcohol in Dextrose Infusion

Alcohol in dextrose infusions are solutions of 5% dextrose in water containing 5% or 10% ethyl alcohol that provide a source of carbohydrate calories. They are not as commonly used as plain dextrose in water infusions due to the adverse effects of alcohol in many patients. These solutions supply a source of carbohydrate calories and may result in liver glycogen depletion. They can also exert a protein-sparing action. Alcohol can prevent premature labor, presumably by inhibiting release of oxytocin from the posterior pituitary.

Alcohol in dextrose infusion may be used as an aid in increasing caloric intake in nutritional deficiencies and to prevent premature labor, which is an investigational use of the 10% solution.

The usual adult dosage is 1 liter to 2 liters of a 5% solution in a 24-hour period, given by slow infusion. Children may be given 40 ml/kg/24 hours.

Too-rapid infusion can be associated with vertigo, flushing, sedation, disorientation, and an alcoholic odor on the breath. Other adverse reactions include fever, local pain at infusion site, and venous phlebitis or thrombosis. Alcohol in dextrose infusions should be avoided in patients with epilepsy, alcohol addiction, diabetic coma, urinary tract infections, severe kidney or liver impairment, shock, and following cranial surgery.

The following interactions may occur:

1. Alcohol may shorten the effects of phenytoin, warfarin, and tolbutamide.
2. Alcohol can potentiate the postural hypotensive effects of antihypertensive drugs, vasodilators, and diuretics.
3. Additive central nervous system (CNS)-depressive effects can occur between alcohol and other CNS depressants, such as barbiturates, benzodiazepines, meprobamate, glutethimide, narcotics, phenothiazines, and so forth.
4. An acute alcohol intolerance syndrome (*e.g.*, flushing, sweating, tachycardia, nausea) has occurred with concurrent administration of disulfiram, metronidazole, moxalactam, cefamandole, cefoperazone, and sulfonylurea antidiabetic drugs.
5. Increased GI bleeding can occur with combined use of salicylates or other anti-inflammatory drugs.

Fructose in Water

A 10% solution of fructose (levulose) in water provides approximately 375 cal/liter. Unlike dextrose, it does not require insulin for ultimate conversion to utilizable glucose, and produces lower serum and urinary glucose levels. In addition, it is more readily converted to glycogen than is dextrose. Thus, it may be preferred to dextrose in diabetic patients. However, it is of no value for treating hypoglycemia. It is principally an alternative source of calories and fluid, and the dosage must be adjusted to the caloric needs of the patient. Electrolyte and vitamin supplementation should be provided as needed.

Infusion rates should not exceed 1 g/kg/hour to minimize the danger of metabolic acidosis, especially in infants and small children. Fructose should not be given to patients with gout, because it may increase the serum uric acid level. Use with caution in patients with renal insufficiency, frank cardiac decompensation, hypervolemia, or urinary tract obstruction. The suitability of long-term fructose infusions is questionable, because significant depletion of liver adenosine triphosphate (ATP) can occur.

Invert Sugar in Water

A solution containing equal parts of dextrose and fructose, invert sugar in water is available as a 10%

concentration. The fructose reportedly enhances the utilization of dextrose and the combination represents an alternative to use of either agent alone. Refer to the respective discussions of each sugar for additional information.

NURSING CONSIDERATIONS
Dextrose solutions up to 10% to 15% in concentration are relatively isotonic and cause little venous irritation if infused at the prescribed rate. They are among the most common of the IV solutions used in all forms of intravenous therapy and are frequently used for administration of drugs by intermittent infusion. Higher concentrations of dextrose are irritating to the vein and must be given through a central line. However, the patient should be closely observed for signs of phlebitis, such as pain, redness, and swelling of adjacent tissues, especially when the solutions are part of TPN therapy.

All dextrose solutions provide the body with an instantly usable source of glucose. At low concentrations, in most patients, the body will produce sufficient insulin to accommodate this increase. However, if the patient is diabetic, or if concentrated solutions are used, urine and blood glucose levels should be monitored closely and additional insulin provided as needed. Clinical signs of hyperglycemia such as confusion, thirst, and tachycardia should also be monitored. When a highly concentrated glucose infusion has been administered for over 1 week it should be gradually discontinued over a 24-hour period to reduce the risk of marked hypoglycemia resulting from sudden cessation of therapy.

Overinfusion of dextrose solutions can cause fluid overload, which will lead to dilution of electrolytes, cardiac decompensation, and possible pulmonary edema. Prolonged IV infusions of dextrose solutions should be avoided whenever possible. Serum electrolytes should be monitored and intake and output should be carefully recorded.

Lipid Products

Intravenous Fat Emulsion
(Intralipid 10%, 20%; Liposyn 10%, 20%; Liposyn II 10%, 20%; Soyacal 10%, 20%; Travamulsion 10%, 20%)

MECHANISM AND ACTIONS
Intravenous fat emulsions are prepared from either soybean or safflower oil and contain a mixture of neutral triglycerides, which are largely polyunsaturated fatty acids. In addition, these products also contain 1.2% egg yolk phospholipids as an emulsifier and glycerin to adjust tonicity. Caloric content of the 10% IV fat emulsion is 1.1 cal/ml and that of the 20% emulsion is 2.0 cal/ml. These IV emulsions are isotonic and may be given by either peripheral or central venous routes. They are used to provide a source of calories and essential fatty acids in parenteral nutrition regimens.

USES
1. Supplemental source of calories and fatty acids for patients requiring total parenteral nutrition for extended periods of time, whose caloric requirements cannot be met by glucose
2. Prevention and treatment of fatty-acid deficiency states

ADMINISTRATION AND DOSAGE
Intravenous fat emulsions contain either 10% or 20% safflower or soybean oil together with varying proportions of unsaturated fatty acids (linoleic, oleic, palmitic, linolenic, stearic), egg yolk phospolipids, and glycerin. Fat emulsion should comprise no more than 60% of the total caloric intake of the patient, with amino acids and carbohydrates comprising the rest.

To correct fatty-acid deficiency states, 8% to 10% of the caloric intake should be supplied by IV fat emulsion.

For total parenteral nutrition (see following discussion), recommended doses are

Adults
  10%—Initially 1 ml/minute for 15 minutes to 30 minutes; gradually increase rate to 83 ml/hour to 125 ml/hour; infuse only 500 ml first day, then gradually increase dose.
  20%—Initially 0.5 ml/minute for 15 minutes to 30 minutes; gradually increase rate to 62 ml/hour; infuse only 250 ml first day.
  Do not exceed 3 g/kg/day.
Children (see Side-Effects/Adverse Reactions)
  10%—Initially 0.1 ml/minute for 10 minutes to 15 minutes
  20%—Initially 0.05 ml/minute for 10 minutes to 15 minutes; gradually increase rate of each to 1 g/kg/4 hours.
  Do not exceed 4 g/kg/day.

SIDE-EFFECTS/ADVERSE REACTIONS

■ WARNING

Infusion of IV fat emulsion in premature infants has resulted in fatalities, presumably due to fat accumulation in the lungs. Follow dosage guidelines strictly; infusion rate should be as slow as possible, not to exceed 1 g/kg/4 hours. Carefully monitor the infant's ability to clear the fat from the circulation between infusions, for example, by measurement of triglyceride or free fatty-acid levels. Lipemia must clear between daily infusions.

The most frequently encountered side-effects with IV fat emulsion are thrombophlebitis due to vein irritation and sepsis due to contamination of the emulsion.

Other adverse reactions noted with IV fat emulsion are dyspnea, cyanosis, allergic reactions, nausea, vomiting, flushing, headache, fever, sweating, insomnia, dizziness, chest or back pain, hyperlipemia, hypercoagulability, irritation at injection site, transient increase in liver enzymes; with *prolonged* administration, adverse reactions are hepatomegaly, jaundice, leukopenia, thrombocytopenia, splenomegaly, seizures, and shock.

CONTRAINDICATIONS AND PRECAUTIONS

IV fat emulsion should not be used in patients with disturbed fat metabolism such as acute pancreatitis, lipoid nephrosis, or pathologic hyperlipidemia. The use of the emulsion is also contraindicated in patients with severe egg allergies, since egg yolk phospholipids are present. The product must be given with *caution* to patients with liver damage, pulmonary disease, anemia, or coagulation disorders, or where there is danger of fat embolism. Safety for use in pregnancy has not been established. Because free fatty acids can displace bilirubin bound to albumin, cautious use is necessary in jaundiced or premature infants.

NURSING CONSIDERATIONS

Prior to administration of lipids, the patient should be asked about egg allergies because lipids contain a 1.2% egg yolk phospholipid base. The emulsion should also be infused cautiously in any patient with a history of liver dysfunction, pulmonary disease, anemia, or coagulation disorders.

Lipids should be used cautiously in any patient who is at high risk for the development of fat embolism, such as the immobilized patient, the debilitated patient, or the patient recovering from a broken bone.

Baseline and periodic complete blood counts with differential and coagulation, platelet, and hepatic function studies should be completed, since lipid administration can alter these blood values. Neonates are especially prone to a decrease in platelets during lipid infusions, which can induce a coagulation disorder. Preinfusion serum triglycerides should be obtained and drawn again 8 hours after the infusion is completed to determine the effectiveness of infusion and to ensure levels do not remain abnormally elevated. If the patient cannot clear fat from the circulation after infusion, future administration is contraindicated.

Some patients may complain of a metallic or fishy taste in the mouth, and this will usually disappear when the infusion is slowed. If the patient exhibits itching, rash, nausea, vomiting, or diarrhea, an intolerance to the infusion is developing; the lipids should be discontinued and the physician notified.

Lipids are not usually mixed with TPN solutions but are administered concurrently by means of a Y connector located near the infusion site. The lipid infusion container and line must be kept higher than the TPN infusion line to prevent backflow and the lipids should be infused below the final inline filter because the molecules will clog the filter. Some institutions prohibit concurrent lipid administration with TPN solutions for infection-control reasons. In such cases the lipids are infused separately in a peripheral vein as needed.

Electrolytes

Ammonium, Bicarbonate, Calcium, Chloride, Magnesium, Phosphate, Potassium, Sodium, Tromethamine

An electrolyte is an element or compound that, when dissolved in water or other solvent, dissociates into ions and is able to conduct an electric current. Electrolytes are present in blood plasma, interstitial fluid, and cell fluid and affect the movement of substances between those compartments.

Parenteral electrolytes are sometimes supplied individually to correct a specific known deficiency (*e.g.*, hyponatremia, hypokalemia), but more commonly they are used as combination electrolyte solutions for adjunctive treatment of nutritional disorders, dehydration, severe burns, trauma, and other emergency situations. Combined electrolyte solutions are also employed as part of the TPN regimen. Serum electrolyte levels must be monitored closely during treatment, and the composition of the infusion solution as well as the rate of administration should be adjusted to provide as nearly optimal blood levels of each electrolyte as possible.

The various parenteral electrolytes as listed in Table 79-1 with available preparations, dosage, and clinical considerations. Although the discussion afforded these preparations here is rather brief, anyone using these products routinely should become thoroughly familiar with their pharmacology and toxicology, because serious untoward reactions have occurred with improper selection or administration of parenteral electrolytes. In addition, a number of *trace metals* are used as a supplement to IV solutions in total parenteral nutrition, and these are listed in Table 79-4.

Total Parenteral Nutrition

Total parenteral nutrition (TPN) is a balanced diet of liquid nutrients in a highly concentrated, hypercaloric solution administered by parenteral (intravenous) infusion through a central line, usually entering one of the vena cavae or the right atrium of the heart. TPN can be utilized as a nutritional supplement to an oral diet or it can replace oral intake for an indefinite period.

The idea of supplying nutrients parenterally is not a new concept. In Toronto, in 1873, milk was administered intravenously to combat cholera. During the First World War, intravenous infusions of 5% dextrose solutions were administered. But the first significant step toward successful use of intravenous nutrients occurred in 1967, when Drs. Dudrick, Rhoads, and Wilmore infused dogs with solutions containing glucose, amino acids, vitamins, and minerals, which maintained nutritional balance and normal growth and development. Subsequently, improvements in solution preparation and techniques for administration allowed the safe use of TPN in humans. Patients who previously were unable to eat and who might have died of starvation while recovering from illness now had a safe and complete method of achieving the parameters of normal nutrition. Initially, TPN was referred to as administration of "Dudrick's

solution." In the early 1970s the name *hyperalimentation* was used to describe the procedure; currently, the preferred term is *total parenteral nutrition.*

In order to understand how TPN can provide the body with sufficient nutrition, it is important to understand the body's energy sources and the mechanism by which energy depletion leads to starvation.

The human body has three primary energy sources: carbohydrates, fats, and protein. Each gram of carbohydrate provides 4 calories; each gram of fat provides 9 calories; and each gram of protein provides 4 calories. Calories, which are the body's energy source, are essential for all of its metabolic functions. The body maintains a carbohydrate reserve, in the form of glycogen, of approximately 1200 calories. This reserve is expended within 12 hours of fasting or stress. After the body has depleted its carbohydrate reserve, fat will begin to be utilized. However, the central nervous system as well as granulation tissue and leukocytes are glucose dependent and breakdown of fat reserves will not satisfy their energy requirements. Therefore, another source of glucose will be sought.

While the body has minimal reserves of carbohydrates and fats, it has no reserves of protein and every molecule of protein is essential. Body proteins can be divided into two compartments; the somatic compartment, which consists of actin and myosin in the muscles, and the visceral compartment, which is composed of antibodies, albumin, white cells, and transferrin. When glucose is no longer available, the body will convert protein (amino acids) into glucose through a process called *gluconeogenesis* in the liver. However, protein utilization will result in immediate functional deficits such as a decrease in plasma proteins, muscle wasting, and other symptoms of malnutrition, as well as alterations in serum electrolytes and acid–base balance. These deficits help the clinician identify the malnourished or starving patient who may be a candidate for TPN.

Malnutrition is classified into three categories: marasmus, kwashiorkor, and marasmus/kwashiorkor mixed (Table 79-2, p. 1549).

Marasmus is defined as protein–calorie malnutrition and is characterized by the patient who is thin, emaciated, and severely cachectic. This condition is caused by inadequate protein and nonprotein calorie intake. Deficiencies will exist in the fat stores as well as somatic (muscle) protein compartments. The patient exhibits a true picture of a malnourished patient, with no fat stores and severe muscle wasting.

Kwashiorkor is defined as protein malnutrition whereby a person's caloric supply is inadequate or devoid of protein. The individual appears well nourished and may even be overweight. Careful scrutiny of visceral, nonmuscle proteins will show evidence of major deficits. These patients will utilize visceral proteins and preserve fat stores and somatic or muscle proteins. Kwashiorkor is most often an iatrogenic disease resulting from prolonged intravenous infusions of dextrose solutions as the main caloric source, since 1 liter of 5% dextrose solution provides an insufficient 200 calories.

Kwashiorkor/marasmus mix consists of deficits in both somatic and viseral protein compartments.

Uses of TPN

Assessment of nutritional deficits is usually coupled with a medical history to determine the appropriateness of TPN therapy. If a patient requires hydration therapy but needs less than 750 calories in 24 hours, peripheral parenteral nutrition (PPN) should be considered. A standard peripheral formula contains a 10% dextrose solution and a 3.5% amino acid solution, plus appropriate additives, and may be given in 1 liter to 2 liters per day.

Patients who require 1000 calories or more to maintain or improve nutritional status are candidates for TPN. Included in this group are patients who cannot receive adequate nutrition by mouth or peripheral vein because of surgical complications, underlying disease, or increased metabolic needs. Some specific indications for TPN include the following:

1. Crohn's disease, ulcerative colitis, or intractable diarrhea, where bowel rest is often essential to heal irritated areas in the bowel
2. Preoperative nutritional build-up for patients who will be NPO postoperatively for longer than 7 days; since peripheral solutions cannot provide adequate calories or nutrition, TPN should be employed to prevent malnutrition.
3. Enterocutaneous fistulas, pancreatitis, short bowel syndrome, and any malabsorption syndrome—TPN provides adequate nutrition during the healing process
4. Large and small bowel obstructions and paralytic ileus—where TPN provides adequate nutrition postoperatively during the healing phase
5. Adjunct therapy for patients receiving chemotherapy and radiation therapy—TPN helps build strength and improve the function of the immune system prior to and during therapy.
6. Severe burns and sepsis—TPN assists in adequate wound healing and improves the status of the immune system in order to fight infection.
7. Anorexia nervosa—TPN provides supportive therapy during the acute phase, in conjunction with psychiatric care.
8. Hyperemesis gravidarum—TPN provides adequate nutrition and hydration during acute hyperemesis; it is supportive therapy for both fetus and mother.
9. Acquired immunodeficiency syndrome (AIDS) with intractable diarrhea due to *Cryptosporidium*, a protozoal bacterium—TPN will supply adequate nutrition and may improve the patient's compromised immune system.

Components of TPN Solutions

Based on the patient's nutritional needs and the desired outcome of TPN therapy, which may range from maintenance of body stores to increased weight gain, the physician will vary the order for TPN solution and additives. A typical liter of TPN solution will contain 500 ml of amino acid solution and 500 ml of a dextrose solution. The strength of the dextrose, 15% to 70%, depends on the patient's requirement for carbohydrates. An additional 75 ml to 100 ml will be added to the solution in the form of vitamins, electrolytes, and trace elements depending on the patient's needs. Table 79-3 shows several typical TPN solutions. Lipids are not administered in the TPN solutions but are given separately based on the patient's needs. Lipid therapy is discussed earlier in this chapter.

Dextrose, one of the major components of the TPN solution, yields large quantities of nonprotein calories (carbohydrates). This provides the body with an essential energy source, prevents protein catabolism, and permits the body to utilize amino acids (protein) properly. A discussion of various dextrose solutions is found earlier in this chapter.

Protein, which is provided in the form of amino acids, yields protein calories. Amino acids assist the body in wound healing, enable the body to produce indispensable enzymes and antibodies, and

(Text continues on p. 1548.)

Table 79-1
Parenteral Electrolytes

Drug	Preparations	Usual Dosage Range	Clinical Considerations
calcium chloride	Injection—10% (1 g = 13.6 mEq)	Slow IV injection only Hypocalcemia—500 mg–1 g at 1-day to 3-day intervals Magnesium intoxication—500 mg at once; repeat as necessary Cardiac resuscitation—200 mg–800 mg into the ventricular cavity or 500 mg–1 g IV	Indicated for treatment of hypocalcemia requiring a prompt elevation in serum calcium levels (*e.g.*, neonatal tetany, parathyroid deficiency, alkalosis); also used to prevent hypocalcemia during exchange transfusions, as adjunctive therapy in treating serious insect bites, for managing lead colic and magnesium intoxication, and for cardiac resuscitation (calcium chloride only) when epinephrine therapy is ineffective; calcium chloride is highly irritating and severe necrosis and sloughing can occur; other calcium salts are preferred where possible; IM administration of calcium salts (except chloride—IV only) should be done only where IV administration is impractical or technically too difficult; do not mix calcium salts with sulfates, phosphates, carbonates, or tartrates in solution, because precipitation can occur; IV solutions should be warmed to body temperature and given slowly (0.5 ml–2 ml/minute). Side-effects are infrequent at recommended doses; use with caution in digitalized patients and in patients with arrhythmias; calcium may antagonize the effects of calcium-channel blockers.
calcium gluceptate	Injection—1.1 g/5 ml (1.1 g = 4.5 mEq)	*Hypocalcemia* IM—2 ml–5 ml IV—5 ml–20 ml *Exchange transfusions in newborn* 0.5 ml after each 100 ml of blood is exchanged	
calcium gluconate (Kalcinate)	Injection—10% (1 g = 4.5 mEq)	*Hypocalcemia* Adults—5 ml–20 ml as needed by infusion Children—500 mg/kg/day in divided doses	
magnesium sulfate	Injection—10% (0.8 mEq/ml), 12.5% (1 mEq/ml), 25% (2 mEq/ml), 50% (4 mEq/ml)	*Mild magnesium deficiency* 1 g (2 ml 50% solution) IM every 6 h for 4 doses *Severe magnesium deficiency* IM—2 mEq/kg within 4 h IV—5 g (40 mEq)/1000 ml infused over 3 h *Total parenteral nutrition* Adults—8 mEq–24 mEq/day	Indicated for replacement therapy in magnesium-deficiency states, especially when accompanied by signs of tetany, and for treating hypomagnesemia resulting from hyperalimentation; may also be employed in certain acute convulsive states, for example, tox-

(continued)

Table 79-1 (continued)
Parenteral Electrolytes

Drug	Preparations	Usual Dosage Range	Clinical Considerations
magnesium sulfate (*continued*)		Infants—2 mEq–10 mEq/day	emia, eclampsia, pre-eclampsia, epilepsy (1 g–4 g 10%–20% solution IV) although other more effective and less toxic drugs are available (see Chap. 30); use with extreme caution in patients with renal impairment and observe closely for signs of overdosage (hypotension, respiratory depression, absence of patellar reflex); have respiratory assistance available; urine output should be maintained at a minimum of 100 ml/4 hours; do not exceed 1.5 ml/minute when infusing the 10% concentration (or equivalent volume of higher concentrations); dilute 50% solution to a concentration of 20% or less before infusing; however, the full-strength solution may be injected IM in adults; effects of CNS depressants can be potentiated by magnesium.
phosphate (potassium phosphate, sodium phosphate)	Injection—3 mM phosphate/ml and either 4 mEq sodium/ml or 4.4 mEq potassium/ml	*Total parenteral nutrition* Adults—10 mM–15 mM phosphorus (310 mg–465 mg elemental phosphorus) per liter of TPN solution Infants—1.5 mM–2 mM/kg/day	Primarily used to prevent or correct hypophosphatemia in patients undergoing hyperalimentation; contraindicated in diseases with high phosphate or low calcium levels; used IV only, diluted in a larger volume of fluid and slowly infused; monitor serum phosphorus, calcium, and sodium or potassium levels depending on which phosphate salt is used; be alert for symptoms of hypocalcemic tetany; use cautiously in patients with renal impairment, cardiac disease, arrhythmias, or adrenal insufficiency; symptoms of overdosage include weakness, confusion, paresthesias, hypotension, arrhythmias, flaccid paralysis, and ECG abnormalities.

(continued)

Table 79-1 (continued)
Parenteral Electrolytes

Drug	Preparations	Usual Dosage Range	Clinical Considerations
potassium chloride potassium acetate	Injection—10 mEq, 20 mEq, 30 mEq, 40 mEq, 60 mEq, 90 mEq, in various volumes; 1,000 mEq/500 ml Injection—40 mEq/20 ml, 120 mEq/30 ml	Dependent on patient's status and governed by serum potassium level and ECG pattern; if serum potassium is less than 2 mEq/liter, maximum infusion rate is 40 mEq/h to a total of 400 mEq/day; if serum potassium is greater than 2.5 mEq/liter, maximum infusion rate is 10 mEq/h to a maximum of 200 mEq/day.	Indicated for the prevention or treatment of moderate to severe potassium deficiency states and as adjunctive therapy in the management of cardiac arrhythmias, especially those due to digitalis overdosage; contraindicated in patients with anuria, oliguria, azotemia, adrenocortical insufficiency, acute dehydration, hyperkalemia, and severe hemolytic reactions; dilute injections with large volumes of parenteral solutions and administer slowly IV; direct injection of undiluted solution may be fatal; use cautiously in patients with cardiac disease, especially those taking digitalis drugs; monitor serum potassium levels, ECG, and urine flow frequently during therapy; be aware that toxic effects of potassium on the heart may be increased if serum sodium or calcium levels decrease or serum pH is reduced; most frequent adverse reactions are nausea, vomiting, diarrhea, and abdominal pain; avoid extravasation because irritation is often severe and tissue necrosis can occur.
sodium acetate sodium bicarbonate sodium lactate	Injection—2 mEq sodium and 2 mEq acetate/ml Injection—4% (0.48 mEq/ml), 4.2% (0.5 mEq/ml), 5% (0.595 mEq/ml), 7.5% (0.892 mEq/ml), 8.4% (1.0 mEq/ml) Injection—0.167 mEq/ml, 5 mEq/ml	*Metabolic acidosis* Initially 2 mEq–5 mEq/kg by IV infusion over 4 h–8 h; adjust dose as necessary depending on clinical response. *Cardiac arrest* Adults—Initially 1 mEq/kg, followed by 0.5 mEq/kg every 10 minutes of arrest; use 7.5% or 8.4% solution Children (under 2 years)—Initially 1 mEq–2 mEq/kg over 1 minute to 2 minutes, followed by 1	Indicated for acute treatment of metabolic acidosis, such as resulting from cardiac arrest, shock, or other circulatory insufficiency states, severe dehydration, or diabetic or lactic acidosis; also used to alkalinize the urine for treating certain drug intoxications and adjunctively in severe diarrhea to replace loss of bicarbonate; sodium lactate and sodium acetate are metabolized to bicar- *(continued)*

Table 79-1 (continued)
Parenteral Electrolytes

Drug	Preparations	Usual Dosage Range	Clinical Considerations
sodium lactate (*continued*)		mEq/kg every 10 minutes of arrest; use 4.2% solution.	bonate, although conversion of lactate to bicarbonate is impaired in patients with hepatic disease; contraindicated in hypochloremia, metabolic or respiratory alkalosis, and hypocalcemia; use cautiously in patients with congestive heart failure, kidney impairment, edema, hypertension, or arrhythmias; do not exceed 8 mg/kg/day in small children, and infuse slowly because rapid injection or use of hypertonic solutions has resulted in decreased CSF pressure and intracranial hemorrhage; closely monitor serum *p*H and blood gases and electrolytes; avoid over-dosage and subsequent production of alkalosis by giving repeated small doses; observe for signs of developing alkalosis (hyperirritability, restlessness, tetany) and discontinue drug; sodium bicarbonate is incompatible in solution with a wide variety of other drugs; administer *alone* to avoid undesirable interaction.
sodium chloride intravenous infusion	Infusion solution—0.45% (77 mEq/liter), 0.9% (154 mEq/liter), 3% (513 mEq/liter), 5% (855 mEq/liter)	(Dependent on patient's status and preparation being used) 0.9% solution—1.5 liters to 3 liters/24 h	Used IV in various concentrations as a source of fluid and electrolytes; the 0.45% solution (hypotonic) is used when fluid loss exceeds electrolyte depletion; the 0.9% solution (isotonic) is most commonly used as replacement for fluid and sodium loss and as a diluent for many other drugs and nutrients; the 3% and 5% solutions (hypertonic) are indicated for hyponatremia and hypochloremia, extreme dilution of body fluids due to excessive water intake, and treatment of severe salt depletion; use with cau-
sodium chloride injection for admixtures	Injection—50 mEq/vial, 100 mEq/vial, 625 mEq/vial	0.45% solution—2 liters to 4 liters/24 h	
sodium chloride diluents	Injection—0.9% in various volumes	3% or 5% solution—Maximum of 100 ml over 1 h	

(continued)

Table 79-1 (continued)
Parenteral Electrolytes

Drug	Preparations	Usual Dosage Range	Clinical Considerations
sodium chloride diluents (continued)			tion in patients with congestive heart failure, severe renal impairment, and edema with sodium retention; the 3% and 5% solutions should not be used when plasma sodium and chloride are elevated, normal, or even slightly decreased; monitor intake–output ratio and serum electrolytes; also use cautiously in patients with decompensated cardiovascular or nephrotic diseases and in patients receiving corticosteroids; infuse higher-strength solutions very slowly to avoid pulmonary edema.
tromethamine (Tham, Tham-E)	Infusion solution—18 g (150 mEq/500 ml) Powder for injection—36 g (300 mEq/150 ml) with sodium, potassium, and chloride (Tham-E)	*Acidosis associated with cardiac arrest* 2 g–6 g (62 ml–185 ml) injected into ventricular cavity *or* 3.6 g–10.8 g (111 ml–333 ml) injected into a large peripheral vein; additional amounts as needed *Acidosis during cardiac bypass surgery* 9.0 ml/kg (2.7 mEq/kg) to a maximum of 500 ml (up to 1000 ml in severe cases)	A highly alkaline, sodium-free organic amine that acts as a proton acceptor, combining with hydrogen ions to prevent or correct systemic acidosis associated with, for example, cardiac arrest or cardiac bypass surgery; also added to ACD priming blood to elevate pH; may function as an osmotic diuretic and increase urine flow and excretion of fixed acids, carbon dioxide, and electrolytes; *(continued)*

also afford the body an additional energy source. Amino acid solutions are also discussed earlier in this chapter.

Vitamins assist the body in effective utilization of intravenously administered nutrients, and are essential for normal cell growth, function, and maintenance. Fat-soluble and water-soluble vitamins may be added to the TPN solution on a daily or semi-daily basis depending on the patient's need. See Chapters 76 and 77 for a discussion of these vitamin supplements.

Electrolytes may be added to the solution based on the patient's serum levels. Electrolytes typically added to a TPN solution include sodium, chloride, potassium, phosphate, calcium, and magnesium. A discussion of parenteral electrolyte additives is also found earlier in this chapter.

Trace minerals are a necessary component of the TPN solution, especially if the patient is on prolonged therapy. They are normally found in the whole blood, plasma, and plasma fraction, and assist in several body functions. Trace minerals and symptoms of deficiency appear in Table 79-4. Laboratory assays of trace minerals will help determine specific patient requirements.

Several other drugs may also be added to TPN

Table 79-1 (continued)
Parenteral Electrolytes

Drug	Preparations	Usual Dosage Range	Clinical Considerations
tromethamine (Tham, Tham-E) (continued)		*Correct acidity of ACD priming blood* 0.5 g–2.5 g (15 ml–77 ml) added to each 500 ml of ACD blood (usually 2 g is adequate)	contraindicated in anuria or uremia; should be administered slowly IV to avoid overdosage and alkalosis; may also be given by injection into ventricular cavity during cardiac arrest and by addition to pump oxygenator, ACD blood or other priming fluid; treatment should not continue longer than a 24-hour period; determine blood values (pH, P_{CO_2}, P_{O_2}, glucose), electrolytes, and urinary output before treatment and frequently during drug administration to assess progress of treatment; adjust dose so that blood pH does not increase above normal (7.35–7.45); drug may depress respiration; have respiratory assistance available; avoid extravasation, because severe inflammation, vascular spasm, and tissue necrosis can result; transient hypoglycemia may occur, especially in infants; use cautiously in children, in patients with impaired renal function, and in pregnant women.

Table 79-2
Types of Malnutrition

Type	Symptoms	Deficits
Marasmus	Emaciated Thin extremities No fat stores	Protein, calories, somatic protein compartment
Kwashiorkor	Well-nourished Overweight	Protein, visceral protein compartment
Kwashiorkor/ marasmus mix	Appears nutritionally sound	Visceral and somatic protein compartments

Table 79-3
Typical TPN Formulations

Type A

Amino acid solution 8-1/2%	1000 ml
Dextrose 50%	1000 ml
Sodium chloride	40 mEq
Sodium acetate	40 mEq
Potassium chloride	20 mEq
Phosphate (as potassium)	30 mM
Magnesium sulfate	16 mEq
Calcium gluconate	9.6 mEq
M.V.I.-12	10 ml
Multiple trace elements	1 ml
Heparin sodium	2000 U

Type B

Dextrose 50%	1000 ml
Amino acid solution 8-1/2%	1000 ml
Potassium chloride	16 mEq
Phosphate (as potassium)	30 mM
Sodium acetate	16 mEq
Sodium chloride	50 mEq
Magnesium sulfate	10 mEq
Calcium gluconate	8 mEq
M.V.I.-12	10 ml
$CuSO_4$	2 mg
$MnSO_4$	0.5 mg
$ZnSO_4$	5 mg

Type C

Amino acid solution 8-1/2%	1000 ml
Dextrose 30%	1000 ml
Sodium chloride	54 mEq
Sodium acetate	16 mEq
Potassium chloride	16 mEq
Phosphate (as potassium)	30 mM
Magnesium sulfate	10 mEq
M.V.I.-12	10 ml
Multiple trace elements	1 ml
Regular insulin	20 U

solutions. *Heparin*, an anticoagulant, is often employed to prevent the formation of fibrin sheaths or blood clots in the catheter. It has also been shown to enhance the body's utilization of fat particles by releasing lipoprotein lipase. The normal dose is 2000 U/liter. *Insulin* can be added directly to the solution to control glucose intolerance as needed. Careful monitoring of both serum and urine glucose is essential for all patients throughout therapy because the patient's insulin needs may vary.

Cimetidine, a histamine-2 antagonist, is often added to TPN to prevent stress ulcers in the patient who is NPO. The drug reduces hydrochloric acid formation in the stomach, thereby decreasing the chance of ulcer formation. The normal dose is 300 mg/liter (see Chap. 18).

Many other medications can be safely added to TPN solutions. However, physical compatibility, drug interactions, and patient comfort should be considered prior to any drug addition.

The TPN solution is aseptically prepared by a pharmacist, under a horizontal laminar flow hood. The hood blows sterilized air around the additives to prevent contaminated air from reaching the bottle opening. Dextrose and amino acid solutions are combined in one bag, and all electrolyte additions are filtered into the main solution.

Methods of TPN Administration

The high osmolarity of TPN solutions would cause phlebitis if administered in a peripheral vein. Consequently, the solution must be administered through a large vein such as the superior vena cava where the dilution will be 1 part TPN to 1000 parts blood. A catheter is inserted into the subclavian vein and threaded into the superior vena cava by one of three methods: a subclavian (central) line; a Hickman, Broviac, or Groshong catheter; or an implantable port. The advantages and disadvantages of these three methods are outlined in Table 79-5.

A Hickman catheter is a Silastic catheter that is tunneled along the chest wall and feeds into the subclavian vein. The catheter has a 1-mm Dacron cuff that surrounds it. Scar tissue adheres to the Dacron cuff, which produces a barrier to bacteria within 5 days. Alternately, a central (subclavian) line may be established by insertion of a Teflon catheter, 6 to 8 inches long, directly into the subclavian vein. Both catheters are used for long-term TPN maintenance. However, infection in a subclavian line usually develops within 30 days, and the line must be removed. A Hickman catheter can remain in place safely for years and the incidence of infection with strict aseptic technique is usually very low.

Another, less than optimal, route of venous access for TPN is the totally implantable port (Porta-Cath). A port is composed of two parts; a subcutaneous injection portal, which is a cone-shaped stainless-steel chamber with a self-sealing silicone septum, and a Silastic catheter. It is usually inserted in the operating room. Insertion requires that a subcutaneous pocket be prepared in the midclavicular area. A cutdown is made into the subcla-

Table 79-4
Trace Minerals Used in TPN

Trace Minerals	Function	Symptoms of Deficiency
Iron	Assists in iron transport by way of hemoglobin in red blood cells Essential in the immune system	Low blood hemoglobin level Pale, weak, tired
Zinc	Essential for wound healing, the immune system, and cell growth	Skin rash, alopecia Intestinal disorders Night blindness Impaired taste perception
Copper	Essential for lymphocyte function and skeletal mineralization Promotes cardiac function and glucose metabolism Essential for transferrin production	Microcytic anemia Pale skin Neutropenia
Manganese	Essential for energy production	No deficiency reported in literature
Selenium	Helps improve absorption of vitamin E	Cardiomyopathy Muscle tenderness (myositis) Muscle weakness
Chromium	Potentiates insulin Regulates lipoprotein metabolism Essential for peripheral nerve functioning	Impairment of glucose tolerance
Molybdenum	Important factor in metabolism	Intermittent headache Nausea and vomiting Disorientation

vian vein into which the catheter is inserted, and the steel chamber is seated into the pocket and sutured into place. A port must be accessed with noncoring Huber needles. The device is excellent for intermittent infusion therapy, when the needles can be removed and no daily maintenance is required. However, Huber needle changes can be traumatic to the patient and can cause tissue tenderness over the access chamber. Therefore, for continuous long-term TPN, a Hickman catheter is the venous access device of choice.

Once a central venous catheter is inserted, a sterile saline solution is infused at a rate of approximately 40 ml/hour until a chest x-ray study can be performed. If a saline solution is infused for a *short* period of time, the body readily reabsorbs it. The x-ray film verifies catheter tip placement in the subclavian vein or vena cava. Pneumothorax can occur during insertion and must be identified before TPN is initiated. If TPN solutions were infused into lung tissue, the results could be devastating. Consequently, an x-ray study must be performed immediately after catheter insertion and *before* any TPN solution is infused.

Once catheter placement is established, gradual infusion of TPN begins. In the first 24 hours of therapy, the patient usually receives about 1000 ml of solution to determine tolerance to the hyperosmolar, concentrated glucose source. If blood glucose remains normal, up to 2000 ml is given in the next 24 hours, again testing blood glucose every 4 to 6 hours. Insulin can be added to the solution or given by subcutaneous injection if needed. If 3000 ml are required, and the patient can tolerate the solution, a third liter is added 24 hours later. TPN solution quantity must be increased gradually to

Table 79-5
Advantages and Disadvantages of Central Lines
Used for TPN Administration

Device	Advantages	Disadvantages
Subclavian (central line)	Inexpensive Quicker insertion Less traumatic insertion	Insertion site is under clavicle; poor location for patients with tracheostomies Higher infection rate Potential for insertion complications such as pneumothorax, venous or arterial lacerations. Requires daily care and is difficult to dress and maintain
Hickman, Broviac, Groshong	Infection rate considerably less, due to Dacron cuff acting as a bacterial barrier Exit site is mid-chest; easier to dress and maintain Silicone tends to cause less foreign body reaction. Insertion complications are reduced.	Some care and maintenance is required External catheter may break. Visible catheter may alter patient's self-image.
Implanted ports	No daily care and maintenance Good patient self-image; no visible catheter Excellent for monthly bolus injection	Infection can occur. Access can be painful. Limited port access—long-term accessing may cause skin necrosis. Must use special Huber needles to access ports

allow the body time to adjust to the changed insulin requirements resulting from the increased glucose load.

Complications of TPN Therapy

The most serious complication of TPN therapy is hyperosmolar, hyperglycemic, nonketotic dehydration (HHND), which occurs when serum, and thus urinary, glucose remains elevated for 48 hours or longer. The glucose in the urine acts as a diuretic that draws sodium and water out of the renal tubules, resulting in severe dehydration. The patient's serum glucose is usually over 1000 and serum acetone and urine ketones are negative. The patient will usually appear weak and disoriented and will rapidly develop seizures that may progress to coma. Treatment includes stopping the TPN so-

lution, rapid infusion of a hypotonic solution such as 5% dextrose and half normal saline to rehydrate the patient, and administration of insulin once rehydration begins. Emergency equipment and drugs such as diazepam (for seizures) and vasopressors (for hypotension) should be on hand, since respiratory or cardiac arrest is possible. This complication can be prevented with careful monitoring of serum and urinary glucose with appropriate adjustment of infusion rate and glucose content.

Other metabolic complications of TPN therapy include essential fatty-acid deficiency, hypoglycemia, zinc deficiency, dehydration, and overhydration. Nonmetabolic complications include air embolism, sepsis (secondary to infected insertion site or bottle contamination), and thrombophlebitis. Table 79-6 outlines the symptoms of these complications and appropriate treatment and prevention strategies.

Table 79-6
Complications of TPN and Methods for Prevention and Treatment

Complication	Clinical Signs	Treatment	Prevention
Metabolic			
Essential fatty-acid deficiency (EFAD)	Dry, flaky skin on extremities and torso	Administer lipids twice/week.	Monitor serum lipids weekly.
Hyperosmolar hyperglycemic, nonketotic dehydration (HHND)	Two-plus urinary glucose level for over 48 h Acetone negative Serum glucose over 1000 Neurologic symptoms, coma	Stop TPN. Infuse hyperosmolar solution of D_5/NSS Replace lost body water and sodium.	Monitor blood glucose and urine glucose every 6 hours.
Hypoglycemia due to excess insulin administration	Lightheadedness, dizziness, apprehension, chills, hunger	Increase oral sugar. Increase TPN glucose. *or* Decrease amount of insulin in the TPN solution.	Monitor blood glucose and urine glucose every 6 hours.
Zinc deficiency	Skin blisters, open oozing	Add zinc to solution.	Monitor serum zinc levels weekly.
Dehydration	Urine output of less than 900 ml/24 h Dry mouth	Increase fluid therapy. Monitor kidney for possible failure.	Maintain accurate intake–output record and ratio.
Low albumin Overhydration	Edema of extremities Sacral edema	Monitor central venous pressure. Reduce fluid intake.	Maintain accurate intake–output record. Monitor serum albumin weekly.
Nonmetabolic			
Endophlebitis: infection of vein lining *or* Thrombophlebitis: clot formation in the vein	Pain at catheter exit side (endophlebitis) *or* Pain radiating up neck or arm on side of catheter, swollen (thrombophlebitis)	Documented on venogram Pull the line.	Monitor patient's temperature and check insertion site daily for redness, swelling, drainage.
Air embolus: usually 30 ml–40 ml; may occur at tubing change, during catheter insertion or catheter removal	Disorientation, cyanosis, chest pain, dyspnea, hypoxia; may progress to seizures, hypotension, and coma	Trendelenburg position Turn on left side. Call physician.	Have patient perform Valsalva maneuver during catheter insertion, catheter removal, or tubing change. Keep hub of catheter capped at all times except when necessary for tubing change.
Infection of central line; *Candida albicans* or *Staphylococcus epidermidis*	Drainage of serosanguinous fluid from around the exit site of catheter	Rule out other infection sources. Culture central line. Pull the line. Administer amphotericin B.	Maintain sterile technique when changing dressing. Maintain dressing change schedule every 48 hours in acute-care setting or 3 times/week at home. Use sterile technique when mixing fluid preparations.

■ *Nursing Process*

□ *ASSESSMENT*

□ *Subjective Data*

The decision to start TPN may be based on medical history, medical diagnosis, or clinical condition (see Uses of TPN, above), as well as the patient's nutritional status. For example, a burn patient might be able to eat but be unable to consume sufficient calories to maintain his metabolic needs during recovery. Although he may be treated initially with oral supplements and a regular diet, if weight loss occurs, TPN may be added to facilitate adequate caloric intake. Therefore, data collected by the nurse, dietitian, and physician may be used to determine a patient's need for TPN. Patients with known diabetes or renal or hepatic disease should be identified because adjustments in solutions or insulin administration may be needed.

If the patient will receive TPN at home, the patient's perception of the effects of home therapy must be explored. Home TPN requires the patient's active participation and agreement about the appropriateness of treatment. Without patient agreement, the treatment is likely to fail. Family support, the physical home environment, and financial resources must also be explored. A family member or other resource should learn all the procedures for home therapy as a backup to the patient or as the primary care giver if the patient is too ill to operate the equipment independently. Physical environment must include refrigeration and some storage as well as adequate electrical wiring to accommodate the machinery. Financial resources play a part in therapy but much of the cost is covered under major medical insurance plans, special program grants by the companies providing TPN, and Medicare and Medicaid. However, resource availability differs across the country so a plan for financial management of the program must be initiated early, since this therapy is very expensive.

If the patient is to have a central catheter, such as a Hickman, inserted in the operating room, perceptions about the procedure must be explored. Allergy to any of the local anesthetic drugs should also be identified, since insertion will probably be done under local anesthesia.

□ *Objective Data*

A complete physical examination should be completed. Baseline temperature, pulse, respiration, blood pressure, height, and weight should be recorded. A complete nutritional assessment will be done, including current caloric intake, assessment of protein compartments and fat distribution, hydration, ability to masticate and swallow, and ability to tolerate fluids and solid food. Renal function will be assessed by measuring urinary output and comparing it to total intake.

Laboratory data should include a baseline complete blood count with differential, serum electrolytes, serum glucose, renal function studies (blood-urea nitrogen and serum creatinine), and hepatic function studies (liver enzymes, bilirubin). If cardiac status is questionable (*e.g.*, presence of congestive heart failure) an electrocardiogram may be performed.

□ *NURSING DIAGNOSES*

Actual nursing diagnoses for the patient receiving TPN may include

    Knowledge deficit related to TPN, administration, monitoring techniques, side-effects, and therapeutic effects

    Anxiety related to the effectiveness of the treatment, insertion of the catheter, consequences of long-term therapy, or learning home management

Potential nursing diagnoses may include

    Alteration in respiratory function related to air embolism (a serious complication of TPN therapy)

    Alteration in family process related to long-term TPN therapy at home

    Alteration in fluid volume: Excess, related to overhydration

    Fluid volume deficit related to inadequate or incorrect fluid infusion

    Potential for infection at the catheter insertion site related to poor aseptic technique

    Alteration in nutrition: Either less than or greater than body requirements (must be reassessed periodically to prevent either problem)

    Disturbance in body image and self-esteem related to an inability to eat normally, isolation from family patterns, presence of catheter, prolonged infusion times

    Impaired skin integrity related to fatty acid deficiency or micro-mineral deficiencies

    Sexual dysfunction related to altered body image and presence of mechanical devices

□ *PLAN*

Nursing care focuses on three areas: preparation for insertion, acute care, and home management.

The major nursing goals for catheter insertion are
1. To prepare the patient for the sequence of events to occur
2. To support the patient whether the procedure is done at the bedside or in the operating room

The major nursing goals for the patient receiving TPN in the acute-care setting are
1. To administer TPN correctly to facilitate nutritional goals (usually weight gain)
2. To monitor accurately laboratory values indicating changes in need, nutritional changes, and side-effects of therapy
3. To use sterile technique to change dressings and tubing according to institution policy
4. To provide emotional support for the patient who cannot eat

The major nursing goals for the patient and family learning to manage home TPN are
1. To teach the patient/family about nutritional requirements and how TPN provides them
2. To help the patient/family learn to
   a. Follow correct techniques for administering TPN at home
   b. Complete home TPN monitoring sheet accurately on a daily basis, including intake and output, weight, temperature, urinary sugar, and acetone
   c. Recognize early signs of trouble, including indications of hyper- and hypoglycemia, infection, fluid overload, and electrolyte deficiencies
   d. Understand the importance of the TPN infusion schedule
3. To provide opportunities for the patient/family to discuss concerns and fears about home management, changes in body image, family functioning, sexuality, and so forth, as appropriate
4. To set up a support network between the patient, home care providers, and equipment suppliers
5. To assist the patient/family to incorporate the TPN regimen into their daily lives with the least amount of interruption

□ INTERVENTION

□ Catheter Insertion

If a subclavian line is inserted at the bedside, the procedure will be performed using a local anesthetic, but it may be uncomfortable for a debilitated patient who must lay flat in bed, with head tilted to the left and hyperextended for a considerable period of time. If a venous port or Hickman (or Broviac or Groshong) catheter is inserted, preoperative preparation must be completed so the patient understands what will happen in the operating room. Regardless of the type of catheter used, initial fluid infusion after insertion should be sterile saline solution and a chest x-ray film must document catheter tip placement before TPN solution is infused. The major complications of insertion are arterial puncture resulting in hemorrhage, pneumothorax, and air embolus. Refer to Chapter 8 for further discussion of these complications and appropriate nursing strategies to handle them. Once a central line has been designated for infusion of TPN, it may not be used to measure central venous pressure (CVP), draw blood, or administer intermittent intravenous drug therapy or blood, all of which can increase the risk of infection and phlebitis.

□ Acute Care

TPN is infused at a prescribed rate, usually at a maximum of 125 ml/hour when 3000 ml are ordered every 24 hours, but, as described earlier, the infusion rate is gradually increased over a 3-day period according to patient tolerance and blood glucose levels. The infusion is usually administered through a 0.22-micron, final inline filter designed to remove particulate matter, bacteria, and fungi and to reduce the possibility of infusing air, thus decreasing the risk of air emboli. Controversy exists over the use of such filters; some physicians believe the filters will trap bacteria but release harmful endotoxins into the venous system. The nurse should follow institutional guidelines usually outlined by infection-control personnel or an intravenous therapy committee.

TPN bags will usually be mixed in the pharmacy under a laminar flow hood, but the nurse should compare the infusion label to the physician's order to ensure all additives requested have been included. Most institutions have specific protocols for TPN orders and additives; the nurse using TPN should become familiar with these protocols. The bag is hung for no longer than 24 hours and is infused through a volumetric infusion pump. TPN solution infusion should never be speeded up once the rate is set, since doing so increases the glucose supply but may overtax the body's ability to produce enough insulin to meet the supply.

The TPN tubing and filter are usually changed every 24 hours, but institution policy may vary. Each time the tubing is changed the patient should be asked to perform a Valsalva maneuver to decrease the chance of air entering the line and forming an air embolus. To perform a Valsalva maneuver, the patient takes a deep breath and bears down as if having a bowel movement. The maneuver increases venous pressure in the intrathoracic veins and will prevent air from entering the system while the tubing is being changed.

A sterile dressing must be maintained over the catheter insertion site and is changed every 48 hours to 72 hours, depending on institutional guidelines. Most dressing protocols include the use of Betadine as an antifungal agent and many use occlusive dressings. Aseptic technique must be strictly followed during the dressing change to reduce the chance of infection at the catheter insertion site and possible sepsis.

The patient receiving TPN must be carefully monitored throughout therapy but especially during the early stages when individual response to the formula is unknown. A flow sheet may facilitate close monitoring and should include spaces for multiple entries. Table 79-7 identifies appropriate parameters and the rationale for monitoring them.

In addition, documentation of dressing changes, catheter site condition, and the patient's tolerance to TPN should be recorded. All monitoring is designed to detect any untoward reactions to TPN at an early stage. (See Table 79-6 for the major complications, symptoms, treatment, and prevention.)

The patient who cannot eat at all while on TPN therapy may have a difficult time adjusting to the therapy, especially once he discovers how much activity and conversation are directed toward food and eating. The nurse may begin to facilitate the process of management by providing frequent oral care, by encouraging ambulation if possible, and by encouraging verbalization about not being able to eat. If other patients on TPN are strong enough and available a small support group can be started in the hospital. For the patient on long-term therapy, a support group with other patients facing the same problems may be valuable in helping the patient to develop coping strategies.

□ *Home TPN Management*
Once the health team determines a patient must remain on TPN for an extended period of time and physical condition otherwise warrants discharge, plans are made for the patient and family to learn

Table 79-7
Parameters for Monitoring TPN

Monitoring Parameter	Frequency	Rationale
Temperature	Every 4 h	Elevation may indicate line infection, sepsis
Pulse, blood pressure	Every 4 h	Hydration, fluid volume status
Weight	Daily	Indication of effective nutrition
Height (in children)	Monthly	Indication of growth (TPN effectiveness)
Intake (fluid and oral)	Continuous	Measure of nutritional status
Output	Continuous	Measure of renal function (minimum 900 ml/24 h—adults)
Urine sugar and acetone	Every 6 h	Measure of insulin use; first sign of hypo- or hyperglycemia
Blood glucose (finger stick)	Every 6 h	Measure of insulin use; first sign of hypo- or hyperglycemia
Electrolytes	Daily	Determine electrolyte needs
Serum albumin	Twice/ week	Visceral protein status
Blood urea nitrogen, serum creatinine	Weekly	Renal function
Serum lipids	Weekly	Determine need for lipid administration to provide essential fatty acids

the necessary procedures. Patients on home TPN usually receive the same solution given in the acute-care setting. The oral diet is advanced as patient and diagnosis warrant; laboratory values, weight, and caloric counts are closely evaluated. However, TPN is most commonly infused by way of a Hickman catheter, not a subclavian line, since it is easier to maintain, and the incidence of infection is greatly reduced due to the Dacron cuff. Home TPN is infused cyclically instead of continuously. A typical home TPN solution usually infuses over 12 hours to 16 hours, at a rate of about 160 ml to 180 ml/hour, anywhere from 5 days to 7 days per week. Patients are usually connected to the TPN while they sleep, so that they may maintain a normal life in the daytime. Many people take care of families and hold down full-time jobs.

The one significant difference between hospital TPN and home TPN is that the patient or a designated care giver is the "primary nurse." This person is taught to perform the procedures that are normally relegated to nurses in hospitals. Nurses will do home visits on a weekly or monthly basis to collect nutritional assessment data and reestablish

---

Guidelines for Teaching Home Management of TPN

Day 1

1. Brief overview of the TPN therapy and what will be required of the primary care giver
2. Teaching of one basic skill such as cap change procedure with return demonstration by the care giver. Hickman, Broviac, Groshong, and central line caps should be changed at least once a week when an "indirect connect" is utilized, meaning the needle on the end of the pump tubing is inserted *through* the cap. When "direct connect" is employed, that is, the tubing is directly connected to the catheter (no needle is used), a new cap is needed daily. Mastery of one skill will help the care giver feel an immediate sense of accomplishment and satisfaction.
3. If the patient can absorb more information, teaching should also begin on changing the catheter site dressing with a return demonstration. Hickman, Broviac, and Groshong catheter dressings can be changed once or twice per week. After the catheter has been in place for 5 days, and the Dacron cuff is securely in place, clean technique is all that is required.

Day 2

1. Return demonstration of procedures from day 1.
2. Teaching the catheter flush procedure. Hickman, Broviac, and central lines should be flushed at the completion of the infusion with a heparin flush solution of 2.5 ml to 3.0 ml with a concentration of 10 U/ml to prevent the catheter from clotting.
3. Teaching the care giver how to draw up and add vitamins to a TPN bag. Vitamins are unstable in solution for longer than 24 hours and must be added on a daily basis.
4. Overview of the infusion pump, what it does, and how it works

Day 3

1. Return demonstration of procedures from days 1 and 2
2. Teaching how to set up and disconnect the infusion pump and how to troubleshoot the alarm system. A new TPN bag, line, and filter should be used daily.
3. Return demonstration of priming the infusion pump

Day 4

1. Return demonstration of procedures from days 1, 2, and 3, especially the pump
2. Teaching how to test urine sugar and acetone and finger stick blood glucose if appropriate
3. Discussion of importance of completing the TPN flow sheet, including weight, intake and output, temperature, and sugar and acetone
4. Instruction on how to recognize complications, that is, hyper- or hypoglycemia, electrolyte disturbances, fluid overload, infection, dehydration

Day 5

1. Procedure instruction is complete. Review and return demonstrations should be performed in correct sequence so that the care giver demonstrates correct set-up, administration, and disconnection from the TPN infusion.
2. Support network for home care should be firmly established with telephone numbers and contacts for the care giver available 24 hours a day, 7 days a week in case of emergency.
3. Family needs to discuss concerns about the effects of home management on family life, work, and play. Patient needs an opportunity to explore body image and self-esteem. These can be done initially and as the therapy is progressing at home.

goals for the patient. The support nurse is present to fit the TPN into the patient's life-style. The main long-term goal for home TPN patients is self-sufficiency. The patient should be in control of TPN, not the TPN in control of the patient.

Patients who require long-term TPN at home will need to learn procedures usually in a very short period of time. The patient and care giver should be given a written manual complete with all the procedures they will need to know and methods for dealing with emergencies. Sometimes the procedures are put on an audio tape recording so the patient can listen and perform tasks in sequence. The tape must be timed to the patient's speed of performance. TPN regimens can be initiated at home, but are usually started in the acute-care setting where early reaction to the solution can be closely monitored. The patient is discharged when he can return-demonstrate procedures needed to administer the TPN and when the TPN formula is stabilized.

Guidelines for Teaching Home Management of TPN are given here for teaching a patient or care giver home TPN management. Institutions may vary in the methods used. However, as with all teaching plans, in order to achieve success the patient or care giver must be a willing participant; must be made to feel he can achieve success; must be able to remember the sequence of steps in a procedure; and must know how to read directions in a manual or be able to follow taped instructions to perform the sequence of steps. He must also have the manual dexterity to perform the procedures required. The patient should anticipate frequent changes in his solution "recipe," which alters his mixing procedure slightly each time.

The home TPN infusion nurse serves multiple functions when visiting the patient and usually sees the patient on a weekly basis. Home visits may include taking blood for complete blood count with differential, electrolytes, and renal function studies, which are evaluated weekly; performing a pulmonary assessment and checking catheter tip placement to ensure infusion is not going into the lung; providing exercises ranging from passive to active to ensure proper utilization of amino acids; and evaluating weights and caloric counts to ensure proper weight gain and correct TPN formula for the patient's needs. The nurse also provides counseling and may help the family work out household problems surrounding management of the TPN infusion.

☐ EVALUATION

Outcome criteria that can be used to evaluate TPN success in the acute-care setting include steady weight gain of 1 lb to 2 lb per week, normal vital signs, laboratory parameters within normal limits, no signs of infection or phlebitis at catheter site, no signs of hypoglycemia or hyperglycemia, and no evidence of fluid overload or dehydration.

Outcome criteria that can be used to determine successful home management of TPN include successful return demonstrations of procedures for administering TPN and caring for the catheter line and catheter insertion site, maintenance of weight or increase in weight as desired, normal laboratory values including glucose, lack of side-effects, return for appointments as scheduled, early reporting of problems, accurate recording of required home monitoring, and family interactions that demonstrate incorporation of the regimen into daily life. Nursing Care Plan 79-1 provides guidelines for developing a nursing care plan for the patient receiving TPN.

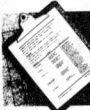

Nursing Care Plan 79-1
The Patient Receiving TPN

Assessment

Subjective Data	1. Medication history
	  a. Refer to the Interactions sections for amino acid infusions and carbohydrate solutions to formulate a list of drugs and solutions that may adversely interact with TPN.
	  b. Use pharmacist or incompatibility chart to determine physical incompatibilities.
	  c. Assess all drugs patient currently takes that may influence TPN.
	  d. General rule is that nothing is injected into line once TPN is infusing.
	  e. Drug/food allergies: especially to egg yolks, proteins, or any carbohydrate intolerance.
	2. Medical history
	  a. Present problem and its relationship to dietary needs; will provide rationale for TPN.
	  b. Dietary history: dietary intake, ability to ingest sufficient calories
	  c. Pre-existing medical problems that may complicate therapy and require cautious administration, such as diabetes mellitus, hepatic or renal dysfunction, cardiac decompensation, metabolic imbalances involving nitrogen utilization, ammonia excretion, or carbohydrate intolerance.
	3. Personal history/compliance issues
	  a. Perception of problem, attitude toward eating, ability to self-manage a complex regimen
	  b. Financial resources
	  c. Personal support system
	  d. Home environment if home TPN is anticipated: refrigeration, storage, electrical wiring, water

Objective Data	1. Physical assessment
	  a. Cardiovascular: heart rate, rhythm, peripheral edema, presence of a patent central catheter line
	  b. Renal: urinary output; I/O ratio
	  c. Head and neck, and GI system: ability to swallow, ability to masticate, presence of functioning GI system
	  d. Musculoskeletal: height, weight, muscle mass, strength, presence of fat pads (part of protein assessment)
	2. Laboratory/diagnostic data
	  a. CBC with differential
	  b. Serum electrolytes
	  c. Serum protein
	  d. Renal and hepatic function studies
	  e. Blood glucose level
	  f. ECG if cardiac status is questionable

Nursing Diagnosis	*Expected Client Outcome*	*Intervention*
Alteration in nutrition: less than body requirements related to increased metabolic needs	Weight will return to (or remain within) normal limits with minimal adverse effects	Administer TPN as prescribed. Check the additives label against the physician's order before hanging a new bag to ensure accuracy. Infusion at pre-set rate on an infusion pump. Rate should not be increased unless physician orders changes. Monitor patient closely to ensure metabolic needs are met but adverse side-effects do not occur. Develop a flow sheet using criteria from Table 79-7 to collect data systematically. *(continued)*

Nursing Diagnosis	Expected Client Outcome	Intervention
Alteration in nutrition: less than body requirements related to increased metabolic needs (*continued*)		Monitor for side-effects as outlined in Table 79-6. Follow preventive/treatment strategies as described, according to physician's orders. Hyperglycemia and hypoglycemia are the most critical metabolic side-effects and must be monitored at least every 6 hours.
Knowledge deficit related to the action and rationale for TPN, duration of therapy, and potential side-effects	Will verbalize an understanding of the rationale for TPN therapy and frequent monitoring to prevent side-effects	Explain how TPN actually improves nutrition and can do so for an indefinite period of time. Explain why frequent monitoring is important to ensure patient gets appropriate nutrients and to catch early any adverse reactions to the infusion. Be realistic about the expected length of therapy. If home TPN is anticipated, develop a day-by-day teaching plan using the Guidelines for Teaching Home Management of TPN.
Potential for infection related to poor aseptic technique	Will remain free of infection in acute care and in home management	Take patient's temperature every 4 hours during acute care. Teach patient to take temperature daily at home. Change IV lines and filters at least every 24 hours according to institution policy. Teach patient to do the same. If temperature is high, notify physician immediately. Use strict sterile technique when changing dressing over catheter site. If patient has a long-term central catheter (i.e., Hickman) he can use aseptic technique at home. Monitor insertion site for redness, swelling, and discharge. Notify physician of any changes.
Potential disturbance in body image related to inability to eat and presence of equipment	Will be allowed food as soon as possible	Encourage discussion, fantasy about food and its importance in life. Encourage increased ambulation as tolerated and diversional activity to reduce focus of attention on food. Provide "sham" feedings as prescribed to provide sucking for a child or mastication for an adult. (Feedings are not swallowed, or if swallowed are diverted to outside by tubing.)
Potential alteration in family process related to long-term TPN therapy at home	Will verbalize concerns and develop plans to manage problems	Include family from outset; identify primary supports and allow time throughout to discuss anger, guilt, fears, financial concerns, and changed roles. Set up a support network for family through visiting nurse, specialty support groups, equipment provider resources.

REVIEW QUESTIONS

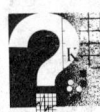

1. What strength amino acid infusions are available clinically? Which strengths are not suitable for total parenteral nutrition?
2. In what conditions are amino acid infusions contraindicated?
3. List the various uses for dextrose in water injections. In what concentrations are the solutions used?
4. For what indications is intravenous fat emulsion employed?
5. What side-effects are most often encountered with intravenous fat emulsion?
6. Give the principal indications for the parenteral use of (1) ammonium chloride, (2) magnesium sulfate, (3) sodium bicarbonate, and (4) tromethamine.
7. Briefly outline the body's three main energy sources and the order in which they are utilized.
8. Define the two body protein compartments. How are these compartments used in identifying a malnourished person?
9. Under what circumstances can a patient receive peripheral parenteral nutrition? What are the components of such a solution? At what point would a patient be classified as needing total parenteral nutrition (TPN) instead?
10. What are the components of a typical TPN solution?
11. What is the rationale for adding (1) heparin, (2) insulin, or (3) cimetidine to a TPN solution?
12. What precautions must be taken immediately after a central line is inserted and before a TPN solution is infused?
13. What are the major metabolic and nonmetabolic complications of TPN? How can they be prevented?
14. What data must the nurse collect before initiating administration of TPN?
15. Nursing intervention focuses on three main areas for the patient about to receive TPN. What are they?
16. What IV equipment is essential when administering TPN?
17. What parameters must be closely monitored during TPN therapy to avert the development of side-effects and ensure optimal treatment? How can the nurse remember to check these parameters?
18. What memory joggers can be used to help the patient going home on TPN remember the sequence of steps to mix and infuse the solution?
19. What learning abilities must the nurse assess before beginning teaching for home TPN?
20. What is the role of the home care nurse when visiting the patient on TPN?
21. What outcomes can be used to measure therapy success?

BIBLIOGRAPHY

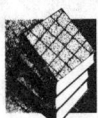

Atkins J, Oakley C: A nurse's guide to TPN. RN, June, 1986
Baker DJ: Ten years of TPN at home. Am J Nurs 84:1248, 1984
Brill E, Kitts D: Foundation for Nursing. New York, 1980
Exton JH: Gluconeogenesis. Metabolism 21:945, 1975
Fischer JE (ed): Total Parenteral Nutrition. Boston, Little, Brown & Co, 1976

Foltz A: Evaluation of implanted infusion devices. Journal of the National Intravenous Therapy Association, January–February, 1987

Gardner C: Home I.V. therapy: Part II. Journal of the National Intravenous Therapy Association, May–June, 1986

Grant JP: Handbook of Total Parenteral Nutrition. Philadelphia, WB Saunders, 1980

Hutchinson MM: Administration of fat emulsions. Am J Nurs 82:275, 1982

Johnson I: Advances in Parenteral Nutrition. Lancaster, England, MTP Press, 1977

Maki DG, McCormick KN: Acetone defatting in cutaneous antisepsis. Crit Care Med 9:200, 1981

Managing I.V. Therapy. Nursing Photobook. Horsham, PA, Intermed Communications, 1980

Marein C et al: Home parenteral nutrition. Nutrition in Clinical Practice, August, 1986

Masoorli S: Tips for trouble-free subclavian lines. RN 38, February, 1984

Masoorli S, Giordano C, Conly D: Taking the worry out of hyperal, Part I. RN 42, June, 1981

Masoorli S, Giordano C, Conly D: Taking the worry out of hyperal, Part II. RN 50, July, 1981

Mullen JL: Consequences of malnutrition in the surgical patient. Surg Clin North Am 61:465, 1981

Plumer ADA: Principal and Practices of I.V. Therapy. Boston, Little, Brown & Co, 1987

Rombeau J, Caldwell M: Enteral Nutrition: Clinical Nutrition, Vol I. Philadelphia, WB Saunders, 1986

Rombeau J, Caldwell M: Parenteral Nutrition: Clinical Nutrition, Vol II. Philadelphia, WB Saunders, 1986

Schmidt A, Williams D: The amazing Hickman and its easy home care. RN 56, February, 1982

Vandersalm TJ: New techniques for placement of long-term venous catheters. JPEN 5:326, 1981

Wilkes G, Vannicola P, Starck P: Long-term venous access. Am J Nurs 85:793, 1985

Winters V: Implantable vascular access devices. Oncology Nursing Forum 11:25, 1984

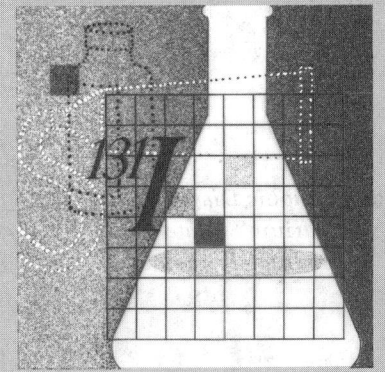

Miscellaneous Drug Products

XI

Diagnostic Agents

80

Effective treatment of many disease states depends on a critical assessment of the underlying pathology. To accomplish this, a number of diagnostic agents are available that assist the clinician in evaluating the clinical status of the patient as well as the functional capacity of many body organs. In most instances, proper use of diagnostic agents requires specially trained personnel and a thorough knowledge of the agent being employed. The extensive array of available diagnostic drugs precludes an in-depth discussion of each agent. Thus, this chapter presents a brief review of the principles of diagnostic drug use and tabular listings of the various categories of diagnostic agents. It is imperative, however, that health-care personnel using these drugs familiarize themselves thoroughly with the pharmacology and toxicology of the particular diagnostic agent being employed.

For purposes of discussion, the various diagnostic agents can be grouped into one of the four following categories:

1. *In vitro* diagnostic aids—Agents usually employed at home or in the physician's office to monitor blood or urine levels of various substances such as glucose, proteins, or ketones, as well as *p*H; also included in this category are the pregnancy-screening tests, as well as tests for the presence of occult blood in the urine or feces.
2. Intradermal diagnostic biologicals—Agents used to skin test for sensitivity to certain diseases, notably tuberculosis, coccidioidomycosis, histoplasmosis, and mumps
3. *In vivo* diagnostic aids—Agents usually employed to evaluate the functional status of various body organs, such as the liver, kidney, heart, pancreas, stomach, adrenal cortex, or pituitary; used in a hospital setting and require skilled personnel for administration and interpretation
4. Radiographic diagnostic agents—Opaque contrast substances, usually barium or iodinated compounds, that are impenetrable by x-rays; used to visualize internal structures such as the GI tract, kidneys, gallbladder, and bronchial tree; used in a hospital setting and require skilled personnel for administration and interpretation

In Vitro *Diagnostic Aids*

A large number of preparations are used to screen the urine, feces, or blood rapidly for the presence of certain substances. These *in vitro* diagnostic aids commonly employ either (1) a reagent or tablet that is mixed in a test tube or on a slide with the sample to be analyzed or (2) a reagent-impregnated strip or tape that is dipped into the sample. Most are available over the counter and complete instructions for performing the test and analyzing the results are provided with the package. A few of these aids, however, such as tests for diagnosing mononucleosis, sickle cell anemia, and the presence of beta-hemolytic streptococci, are prescription-only items and require someone familiar with use of the product for proper interpretation. Pregnancy tests may be employed either in the home or in the physician's office and generally employ a reagent to be added to a urine sample. Although home test kits are certainly valuable as a preliminary screening method, confirmation of pregnancy should always be obtained professionally by use of one of the more established pregnancy-screening procedures performed in the physician's office, which measure the presence of chorionic gonadotropin in the urine.

The various *in vitro* diagnostic aids are listed alphabetically by trade name in Table 80-1 with information regarding the types of preparation and their diagnostic uses.

Intradermal Diagnostic Biologicals

The ability of selected biological products to elicit a local allergic reaction following intradermal injection is used to assess sensitivity to, but not necessarily the active presence of, certain diseases. The most commonly employed skin test is the tuberculin test, although sensitivity to mumps, histoplasmosis, and coccidioidomycosis can also be determined by intradermal testing. Interpretation of the tests is based on the appearance of local hypersensitivity reaction at the site of intradermal injection, usually consisting of induration (tissue hardening) and, in some cases, erythema in those patients previously exposed to the infecting organism.

Since *systemic* allergic reactions can occur with the use of many of the intradermal diagnostic solutions, in certain patients appropriate antidotal measures should be immediately available. These may include cold packs, topical steroids, and epinephrine.

Information relating to the available intradermal diagnostic drugs is presented in Table 80-2.

(Text continues on p. 1570.)

Table 80-1
In Vitro *Diagnostic Aids*

Trade Name	Preparation	Diagnostic Uses
Abbott HTLV III EIA	Kit	Antibody to human T-lymphotropic virus, Type III
Accusens T	Liquid	Taste dysfunction
Acetest	Tablets	Serum/urinary ketones
Advance-Test	Reagent	Pregnancy
Albustix	Strips	Urinary proteins
Answer	Reagent	Pregnancy
Azostix	Strips	Blood urea nitrogen
Bili-Labstix	Strips	Urinary glucose, proteins, pH, blood, ketones, bilirubin
Biocult-GC	Swab	Gonorrhea (cervical, pharyngeal, rectal, urethral)
Chemstrip bG	Strips	Blood glucose
Chemstrip GP	Strips	Urinary glucose, protein
Chemstrip K	Strips	Urinary ketones
Chemstrip LN	Strips	Urinary leukocytes, nitrite
Chemstrip uG	Strips	Urinary glucose
Chemstrip uGK	Strips	Urinary glucose, ketones
Chemstrip 5L	Strips	Urinary glucose, protein, pH, blood, ketones, leukocytes
Chemstrip 6L	Strips	Urinary glucose, protein, pH, blood, ketones, bilirubin, leukocytes
Chemstrip 7L	Strips	Urinary glucose, protein, pH, blood, ketones, bilirubin, urobilinogen, leukocytes
Clearblue Pregnancy	Kit	Pregnancy
Clearplan	Kit	Predict time of ovulation
Clinistix	Strips	Urinary glucose
Clinitest	Tablets	Urinary glucose
Clinitest 2-Drop	Tablets	Urinary glucose
Coloscreen	Kit	Fecal blood
Combistix	Strips	Urinary glucose, protein, pH
CS-T ColoScreen	Pad	Fecal blood
Culturette 10 min. Group A Strep ID	Slide	Group A streptococcal antigen
Daisy 2	Reagent	Pregnancy
Dextrostix	Strips	Blood glucose
Diastix	Strips	Urinary glucose
Early Detector	Kit	Fecal blood
Entero-Test	Capsule	Upper intestinal bleeding, duodenal parasites
Entero-Test Pediatric	Capsule	Screening of gastroesophageal reflux
e.p.t.	Reagent	Pregnancy
EZ-Detect	Pad	Fecal blood
Fact	Reagent	Pregnancy
First Response	Reagent	Pregnancy
First Response Ovulation Predictor	Kit	Monoclonal immunoassay for hLH in urine
Fleet Detecatest	Slide	Fecal blood
Fortel Ovulation	Kit	Pregnancy
Gastroccult	Reagent	Blood in gastric contents
Gastro-Test	Kit	Stomach pH
Glucostix	Strips	Blood glucose
Gonodecten	Kit	Gonorrhea
Hema-Chek	Slide	Fecal blood
Hema-Combistix	Strips	Urinary glucose, protein, pH, blood
Hemastix	Strips	Urinary blood
Hematest	Tablets	Fecal blood
Hemoccult	Slide	Fecal blood
Ictotest	Reagent	Urinary bilirubin
Insta-Kit	Slide	Group A Streptococci
Keto-Diastix	Strips	Urinary glucose, ketones
Ketostix	Strips	Urinary/blood ketones
Kyodex	Strips	Blood glucose
Kyotest GPB	Strips	Urinary glucose, protein, blood
Kyotest UG	Strips	Urinary glucose

(continued)

Table 80-1 (continued)
In Vitro *Diagnostic Aids*

Trade Name	Preparation	Diagnostic Uses
Kyotest UK	Strips	Urinary ketones
Kyotest UGK	Strips	Urinary glucose ketones
Kyotest 2V	Strips	Urinary glucose, protein
Kyotest 3V	Strips	Urinary glucose, protein, *p*H
Kyotest 4V	Strips	Urinary glucose, protein, *p*H, blood
Kyotest 5V	Strips	Urinary glucose, protein, *p*H, blood, ketones
Kyotest 6V	Strips	Urinary glucose, protein, *p*H, blood, ketones, bilirubin
Kyotest 7V	Strips	Urinary glucose, protein, *p*H, blood, ketones, bilirubin, urobilinogen
Kyotest 8V	Strips	Urinary glucose, protein, *p*H, blood, ketones, bilirubin, urobilinogen, nitrite
Labstix	Strips	Urinary glucose, protein, *p*H, blood, ketones
LA-test-ASO	Kit	Antistreptolysin O antibodies
LA-test-CRP	Kit	C-reactive protein in serum (acute inflammation)
LA-test-RF	Kit	Rheumatoid factor in blood
Microstix-3	Strips	Urinary nitrite, total bacteria, gram-negative bacteria
Microstix-Nitrite	Strips	Urinary nitrite
MicroTrak Chlamydia	Slide	*Chlamydia trachomatis* in tissue culture
MicroTrak HSV 1/HSV 2 culture confirmation	Kit	Typing of herpes simplex in tissue culture
Mono-Chek	Reagent	Mononucleosis
Mono-Diff Test	Reagent	Mononucleosis
Monospot	Reagent	Mononucleosis
Monosticon Dri-Dot	Reagent	Mononucleosis
Mono-Sure	Reagent	Mononucleosis
Mono-Test	Reagent	Mononucleosis
MPS Papers	Strips	Urinary acid mucopolysaccharides
Multistik	Strips	Urinary glucose, protein, *p*H, blood, ketones, bilirubin, urobilinogen
Multistix SG	Strips	Urinary glucose, protein, *p*H, blood, ketones, bilirubin, urobilinogen, specific gravity
Nimbus	Liquid	Monoclonal antibody immunoassay
Nitrazine Paper	Strips	Urinary *p*H
N-Multistix	Strips	Urinary glucose, protein, *p*H, blood, ketones, bilirubin, urobilinogen, nitrite
N-Multistix-C	Strips	As above, plus ascorbic acid
N-Multistix SG	Strips	As above, plus specific gravity
Ovu Stick	Strips	Urinary test to predict ovulation
Phenistix	Strips	Phenylketonuria
Pregnolisa	Reagent	Pregnancy
Pregnosis	Slide	Pregnancy
Pregnospia	Reagent	Pregnancy
Pregnosticon Dri-Dot	Slide	Pregnancy
Rapid Test Strep	Slide	Group A Streptococci
Respiracult	Swab	Group A beta-hemolytic streptococci
Respiralex	Slide	Group A beta-hemolytic streptococci
Respirastick	Strip	Group A Streptococci
Rheumanosticon Dri-Dot	Slide	Rheumatoid factor in blood
Rotalex	Slide	Rotavirus in feces
Rubacell II	Reagent	Rubella virus in serum or plasma
Sickledex Test	Strips	Hemoglobin S (sickle cells)
Stix	Strips	Urinary ascorbic acid
Streptonase-B	Reagent	Serum-B antibodies (streptococcal infection)
Strepto-Sec	Slide	Beta-hemolytic streptococci, groups A, B, C, and G
Tes-Tape	Strips	Urinary glucose
UCG-Slide Test	Slide	Pregnancy
Uricult	Strips	Urinary bacteriuria/uropathogens
Uristix	Strips	Urinary glucose, protein
Urobilistix	Strips	Urinary urobilinogen
Visidex II	Strips	Blood glucose

Table 80-2
Intradermal Diagnostic Biologicals

Diagnostic Agent	Preparations	Uses	Clinical Considerations
coccidioidin (Spherulin)	Injection—1:10, 1:100	Diagnosis of coccidioido-mycosis Differentiation of cocci-dioidomycosis from other diseases with similar clinical findings (*e.g.*, histo-plasmosis, sarcoidosis)	Diluted with sodium chloride injection; 0.1 ml of 1:10,000 is injected intradermally; if negative, repeat with 1:1000 and finally 1:100; positive reaction is appearance of area of induration measuring 5 mm or greater; erythema without induration is considered negative; reaction is readable at 24 hours and maximal at 36 hours, and indicative that contact with the fungus has occurred in the past but patient does not necessarily have an active infection; false-positive skin reactions do not occur; sensitive individuals may exhibit an intense local response.
diphtheria (diphtheria toxin for Schick test)	Injection—1 vial of toxin and 1 vial of control	Diagnosis of serologic immunity to diphtheria	Injected intradermally on flexor surface of forearm, control solution on one arm and toxin on other arm; results are read on day 4 or 5; positive reaction is appearance of circumscribed area of redness and slight infiltration measuring 1 cm or more in diameter, and indicates person has little or no antitoxin to diphtheria and is susceptible to infection; aspirate prior to injection to ensure needle is not in blood vessel.
histoplasmin (histoplasmin diluted; Histolyn-CYL)	Injection—1.0 ml/vial in 10 0.1-ml doses, 1.3-ml multidose vial	Diagnosis of histoplasmosis Differentiation of histo-plasmosis from other mycotic or bacterial infections (*e.g.*, coccidioido-mycosis, sarcoidosis)	A sterile filtrate from cultures of *Histoplasma capsulatum*; 0.1 ml is injected intradermally into flexor surface of the forearm and reaction is read in 48 hours to 72 hours; induration of 5 mm or greater is considered positive and may indicate a previous mild, subacute, or chronic infection with *Histoplasma capsulatum* or immunologically related organisms; little value in diagnosing acute, fulminating infections *(continued)*

Table 80-2 (continued)
Intradermal Diagnostic Biologicals

Diagnostic Agent	Preparations	Uses	Clinical Considerations
histoplasmin (histoplasmin diluted; Histolyn-CYL) (continued)			because a negative reaction usually occurs; large doses can produce severe erythema and induration with ulceration and necrosis; systemic allergic reactions can occur; it is an infrequently used test.
mumps skin test antigen	Injection—1 ml (10 tests)	Determination of sensitivity to mumps virus	Suspension of killed mumps virus used to determine skin sensitivity to mumps; effectiveness has not been conclusively established; may be useful in adolescence for identifying those who should be protected against the disease; however, most of the population have had contact with mumps virus and will demonstrate a delayed cutaneous hypersensitivity to the antigen; following injection of 0.1 ml intradermally on inner surface of forearm, reaction is read in 24 hours to 36 hours; erythema of 1.5 cm or more indicates sensitivity to virus and probable immunity; negative reaction suggests probable susceptibility; do not use in persons sensitive to chicken, eggs, or feathers because preparation is cultivated in chicken embryo.
skin test antigens, multiple (Multitest CMI)	Eight single-dose applications preloaded with seven delayed hypersensitivity skin test antigens and glycerin control	Detection of nonresponsiveness to antigens by means of delayed hypersensitivity skin testing	Applicator has 8 test heads preloaded with delayed hypersensitivity skin test antigens to tetanus toxoid, diphtheria toxoid, *Streptococcus*, old tuberculin, *Candida*, *Trichophyton*, and *Proteus*; reactivity may be reduced in patients receiving drugs that suppress immunity or in patients with acute viral infections. Test results are read at 24 hours and 48 hours; positive reaction is induration of 2 mm or greater at antigen site provided there is *no* in-

(continued)

Table 80-2 (continued)
Intradermal Diagnostic Biologicals

Diagnostic Agent	Preparations	Uses	Clinical Considerations
skin test antigens, multiple (Multitest CMI) (continued)			duration at control site. Do not apply on infected or inflamed skin. If periodic testing is done, rotate sites of application.
tuberculin purified protein derivative—tuberculin PPD (Aplisol, Tubersol)	Injection—1 U/0.1 ml, 5 U/0.1 ml, 250 U/0.1 ml	Aid in diagnosis of tuberculosis	Aqueous solution of a purified protein fraction from filtrates of cultured human strains of *Mycobacterium tuberculosis*; use only fresh tuberculin preparations for testing; injected intradermally (5 U) on the flexor or dorsal surface of the forearm; reaction is read in 48 hours to 72 hours; induration of 10 mm or more is a positive reaction, whereas induration of 5 mm or less is negative; erythema is not of diagnostic significance, but may indicate incorrect administration; retesting is indicated if induration measures 5 mm–9 mm; positive reaction does not indicate an active infection, but suggests further evaluation is necessary; positive reaction may also indicate previous BCG vaccination; preferred over old tuberculin (OT) test due to greater-(continued)

Further information describing proper methods of administration and interpretation is provided with the individual drugs and should be consulted before performing the test.

In Vivo *Diagnostic Aids*

The diagnostic agents used to assess the functional capacity of internal body organs are termed *in vivo* diagnostic aids and are administered either orally or parenterally. Frequently, these compounds are designed to be concentrated in or excreted by the organ to be evaluated. Since they are administered systemically, a potential for untoward reactions does exist, and although these are generally mild and transient, patients should be observed carefully during, and for some time following, the testing procedure for development of more serious adverse reactions.

Several compounds that may be used for diagnostic purposes have been discussed in other chapters (*e.g.*, edrophonium for myasthenia gravis in Chap. 13; phentolamine for pheochromocytoma in Chap. 16; radioiodide 131 for thyroid function in Chap. 52) and are not considered here. Table 80-3 lists the important *in vivo* diagnostic drugs, together with their preparations, uses, and pertinent remarks. It should be recognized that the consideration given to the agents in this chapter is

Table 80-2 (continued)
Intradermal Diagnostic Biologicals

Diagnostic Agent	Preparations	Uses	Clinical Considerations
tuberculin purified protein derivative—tuberculin PPD (Aplisol, Tubersol) (*continued*)			purity; highly sensitive-persons may experience vesiculation, ulceration, and necrosis, and persons suspected of being highly sensitive should receive an initial dose of only 1 U; the 250-U injection is only used for persons who do not react to 5 U, although individuals not reacting to 5 U may be considered tuberculin negative.
tuberculin PPD, multiple puncture device (Apli-test, Sclavo Test-PPD, Tine Test PPD)	Cylindrical plastic units	See tuberculin purified protein derivative	A single-use device consisting of 4 stainless-steel tines coated with tuberculin PPD, standardized to give reactions equivalent to 5 U of intradermal tuberculin PPD.
old tuberculin, multiple puncture devices (Tuberculin, Mono-Vacc Test, Tuberculin, Old, Tine Test)	Individual units	See tuberculin purified protein derivative	Single-use, multiple puncture device standardized to give reactions equivalent to 5 U of standard solution of old tuberculin administered intradermally; test is read 48 hours to 96 hours after administration; positive reaction is vesiculation or induration of 1 mm or greater but further diagnostic tests are necessary to establish presence of infection; it is an infrequently used preparation.

brief and is not intended to provide comprehensive information regarding their safe and effective use. Experienced personnel and proper facilities are necessary to derive maximum benefit from use of these diagnostic agents and to deal with any untoward reaction that may occur.

Radiographic Diagnostic Agents

With the exception of barium sulfate, substances used for radiographic diagnostic procedures are primarily iodine-containing compounds. These agents are opaque chemicals that are employed as contrast media to enhance visualization of internal structures by x-ray examination. Localization of a substance to a particular area to be visualized is accomplished either through direct instillation into an organ (*e.g.*, uterus, colon, bronchioles, spinal column) or by incorporation of the radiopaque drug into an organic compound whose properties determine its distribution in the body (*e.g.*, excretion by way of the bile or urine or plasma protein binding).

In addition to barium sulfate and iodine-containing radiopharmaceuticals, a few other radioactively labeled drugs may be employed in various diagnostic tests (Table 80-4, p. 1580).

(*Text continues on p. 1580.*)

Table 80-3
In Vivo Diagnostic Aids

Diagnostic Agent	Preparations	Uses	Clinical Considerations
aminohippurate sodium (PAH)	Aqueous solution—20%	Assessment of renal blood flow and tubular secretory mechanisms	Occasionally used to study certain aspects of kidney function; used by IV injection; not metabolized, and excreted solely by the kidney; low plasma concentrations (1 mg–2 mg/dl) are used to measure renal blood flow; higher concentrations (40 mg–60 mg/dl) are employed to determine maximal tubular secretory capacity; may elicit nausea, feelings of warmth, and urge to defecate.
L-arginine (R-Gene 10)	Solution—10% in sterile water for injection for IV infusion	Determination of pituitary human growth hormone reserve; diagnosis of panhypopituitarism, pituitary dwarfism, pituitary trauma, and other hypopituitary conditions	Stimulates pituitary to release growth hormone; dosage is 300 ml in adults and 5 ml/kg in children; rate of false-positive reactions is 32% and false-negative is 27%; do not use in patients with strong allergic tendencies; excessive infusion rates can result in irritation, nausea, vomiting, and flushing; have antihistamine available in case of allergic reactions; do not use if solution is not clean or if bottle lacks a vacuum; refer to package literature for interpretation of results.
bentiromide (Chymex)	Solution—500 mg/7.5 ml	Screening test for pancreatic exocrine insuffiency	A peptide containing 170 mg para-aminobenzoic acid (PABA) per 500-mg dose; following oral administration, bentiromide is hydrolyzed by pancreatic chymotrypsin, liberating PABA, which is excreted in the urine; if exocrine pancreatic function is normal, over 50% of the PABA contained in bentiromide appears in the urine within 6 hours and can be detected using the Smith modification of the Bratton-Marshall test for arylamines; patients should fast at least 8 hours before receiving a test dose; diarrhea, headache, nausea, flatulence,

(continued)

Table 80-3 (continued)
In Vivo *Diagnostic Aids*

Diagnostic Agent	Preparations	Uses	Clinical Considerations
bentiromide (Chymex) (continued)			and weakness can occur; instruct patient to urinate immediately before receiving bentiromide; falsely elevated readings can occur if the patient is taking other drugs metabolized to arylamines, such as acetaminophen, chloramphenicol, lidocaine, procaine, procainamide, sulfonamides, or thiazide diuretics.
benzylpenicilloylpolylysine (Pre-Pen)	Ampules	Skin test for penicillin hypersensitivity in patients who have previously received penicillin and demonstrated a clinical hypersensitivity reaction	May be applied either by scratching forearm (preferred method) or by intradermal injection on upper outer arm surface; positive reaction consists of whealing, erythema, and itching; occurs usually within 10 minutes, and is associated with an incidence of allergic reactions to systemic benzylpenicillin or penicillin G of greater than 20%; a negative skin test response predicts a less than 5% incidence of allergic complications; of doubtful value in assessing sensitivity to semisynthetic penicillins or cephalosporins; it may produce an intense local inflammatory response and occasionally systemic allergic reactions.
cosyntropin (Cortrosyn)	Vials with diluent—0.25 mg with 10 mg mannitol	Diagnosis of adrenal cortical insufficiency	Synthetic subunit of human ACTH used IM or by IV infusion to differentiate primary (adrenal) from secondary (pituitary) adrenocortical insufficiency; in primary Addison's disease, 24-hour urinary 17-hydroxycorticosteroid levels fail to rise following IV infusion and plasma cortisol levels do not increase significantly within 30 minutes following IM injection; secondary pituitary failure is characterized by a slow increase in urinary steroids following IV in-

(continued)

Table 80-3 (continued)
In Vivo Diagnostic Aids

Diagnostic Agent	Preparations	Uses	Clinical Considerations
cosyntropin (Cortrosyn) (continued)			fusion; it produces fewer allergic reactions than ACTH injection.
gonadorelin (Factrel)	Powder for injection—100 mcg/vial, 500 mcg/vial	Evaluation of hypothalamic–pituitary–gonadotropic function Evaluation of residual gonadotropic function following hypophysectomy Investigational uses include induction of ovulation and treatment of precocious puberty	A synthetic luteinizing-hormone-releasing hormone (LHRH) structurally identical to natural LHRH possessing a gondotropin-releasing effect on the anterior pituitary; used SC or IV; in females, test should be performed in early follicular phase of the menstrual cycle; do not give concurrently with gonadal hormones, glucocorticoids, or spironolactone, because pituitary secretion of gonadotropins can be affected; SC injection can result in localized pain, swelling, and itching; use during pregnancy only where clearly needed; refer to package prescribing information for testing methodology.
histamine phosphate	*Injection* Gastric test—0.55 mg (0.2 mg base/ml); 2.75 mg (1 mg base/ml)	Assessment of gastric acid secretory capacity	Basal acid secretion is measured, then 0.01 mg–0.04 mg histamine base/kg is injected SC and gastric contents are collected in 4 15-minute specimens and analyzed for volume, *p*H, and acidity; an antihistamine should be administered IM before histamine; many side-effects noted and severe allergic reactions (*e.g.*, asthma) can occur; it has largely been replaced by other, safer diagnostic measures (*e.g.*, pentagastrin).
	Pheochromocytoma—0.275 mg (0.1 mg/base)/ml	Presumptive diagnosis of pheochromocytoma	Once used for diagnosis of pheochromocytoma (positive response was at least a 60 mm/40 mm rise in blood pressure above the baseline or an increase of at least 20 mm/10 mm above that obtained in the cold pressor test); very hazardous procedure; phentolamine must be readily available to (*continued*)

Table 80-3 (continued)
In Vivo *Diagnostic Aids*

Diagnostic Agent	Preparations	Uses	Clinical Considerations
histamine phosphate (*continued*)			control excessive increases in blood pressure; it is rarely employed today with the availability of more accurate and less dangerous procedures.
hysteroscopy fluid (Hyskon)	Solution—32% w/v dextran 70 in 10% w/v dextrose	Aid in distending the uterine cavity and visualizing its surfaces	Introduced into the uterine cavity by means of a cannula under low pressure until uterus is sufficiently distended to permit adequate visualization; volume usually required is 50 ml–100 ml; allergic reactions, including anaphylaxis, can result if drug is absorbed systemically; do not exceed 150 mm Hg infusion pressure.
indocyanine green (Cardio-Green)	Vials—25 mg, 50 mg Disposable units—10 mg, 40 mg	Determination of cardiac output, hepatic function, and liver blood flow Aid in ophthalmic angiography	A water-soluble dye that is injected IV, is quickly bound to plasma proteins, and is taken up almost exclusively by hepatic parenchymal cells; dilution of dye in blood samples obtained from different sites at various times following administration is an indication of blood flow in a particular area; adverse effects are minimal; drug contains a small amount of sodium iodide and may interfere with radio-active iodine-uptake studies.
inulin	Injection—100 mg/ml	Measurement of glomerular filtration rate	Polymer of fructose given by IV infusion; drug is rapidly filtered by the kidney, and neither secreted nor reabsorbed; following a loading dose, samples of urine are collected at regular intervals and concentration of inulin in each sample is determined colorimetrically; normal adult inulin clearance is 100 ml–160 ml/minute.
mannitol	Solution—5%, 10%, 15%, 20%, 25%	Measurement of glomerular filtration rate	An osmotic diuretic (see Chap. 41) that is also used to measure glomerular filtration rate (GFR); *(continued)*

Table 80-3 (continued)
In Vivo *Diagnostic Aids*

Diagnostic Agent	Preparations	Uses	Clinical Considerations
mannitol (continued)			100 ml of a 20% solution is diluted with 180 ml normal saline and infused at a rate of 20 ml/minute; urine is collected by a catheter for a specific time period and a blood sample is drawn at the beginning and end of the collection period; mannitol concentrations (mg/ml) are determined for each sample and the GFR is calculated as milliliters of plasma that must be filtered to yield the amount of mannitol excreted per minute in the urine.
methacholine (Provocholine)	Powder for dilution—100 mg/5-ml vial	Assessment of bronchial airway hyperactivity	Cholinergic agent that is administered by inhalation in solutions of increasing concentration; pulmonary function (forced expiratory volume —FEV) is measured after each dose; requires trained personnel and emergency equipment, and medications must be readily available; may cause headache, throat irritation, lightheadedness, and itching; do not inhale powder; response in patients receiving beta blockers may be exaggerated.
metyrapone (Metopirone)	Tablets—250 mg	Diagnosis of hypothalamic–pituitary function	Used to test whether pituitary secretion of ACTH is adequate; ability of adrenals to respond to ACTH should be demonstrated by ACTH or cosyntropin test before giving metyrapone; following a 2-day rest period, 15 mg/kg is administered orally every 4 hours for 6 doses, then urinary 17-hydroxycorticosteroids (17-OHCS) are collected for 24 hours; normal pituitary function is indicated by a 2- to 4-fold increase in 17-OHCS over control levels obtained before drug ad-*(continued)*

Table 80-3 *(continued)*
In Vivo *Diagnostic Aids*

Diagnostic Agent	Preparations	Uses	Clinical Considerations
metyrapone (Metopirone) (continued)			ministration; excessive excretion of 17-OHCS suggests Cushing's syndrome (adrenal hyperplasia), while subnormal excretion indicates hypopituitarism.
pentagastrin (Peptavlon)	Injection—0.25 mg/ml	Evaluation of gastric acid secretory capacity	Action resembles that of natural gastrin; following SC injection of 6 mcg/kg, acid secretion begins within 10 minutes, peaks in 20 minutes to 30 minutes, and lasts 60 minutes to 90 minutes; elicits fewer and less intense side-effects than either histamine or betazole, and is the preferred drug for measuring gastric acid secretion; children's doses have not been established; use with caution in patients with hepatic, biliary, or pancreatic disease.
protirelin (Relefact TRH, Thypinone)	Injection—0.5 mg/ml	Adjunct in the evaluation of thyroid function Adjunct for adjustment of thyroid hormone dosage in hypothyroid patients	Synthetic peptide similar in action to thyrotropin-releasing hormone (TRH); following IV injection (adults—500 mcg; children—7 mcg/kg), protirelin causes release of thyroid-stimulating hormone (TSH) from anterior pituitary; TSH blood levels are determined before injection and again 30 minutes after injection; thyroid function is characterized by comparing baseline TSH serum levels to those obtained following drug injection; if test is repeated, allow an interval of 7 days; discontinue thyroid drugs at least 7 days before performing test; most common side-effects are nausea, urinary urgency, flushing, lightheadedness, headache, dry mouth, and abnormal discomfort; patient should be supine during testing to minimize changes in blood pressure.

(continued)

Table 80-3 (continued)
In Vivo Diagnostic Aids

Diagnostic Agent	Preparations	Uses	Clinical Considerations
secretin (Secretin-Kabi)	Injection—10 U/ml when reconstituted according to package instructions	Diagnosis of pancreatic exocrine disease or gastrinoma (Zollinger-Ellison syndrome) Adjunct in obtaining pancreatic cells for pathologic study	Hormone obtained from porcine duodenal mucosa that increases volume and bicarbonate content of pancreatic secretions; powder is dissolved in 10 ml sodium chloride injection and administered by slow IV injection (5 min) at a dose of 1 U–2 U/kg; samples are collected with a gastric tube and analyzed for volume, enzyme and bicarbonate content, occult blood, and biliary pigment; cautious use in acute pancreatitis; it is frequently given with sincalide (see below).
sincalide (Kinevac)	Injection—5 mcg/vial for reconstitution to 1 mcg/ml	Stimulate pancreatic or gallbladder secretions	Synthetic subunit of cholecystokinin that produces gallbladder contraction following IV injection; also enhances pancreatic secretions when given in combination with secretin; to contract gallbladder, 0.02 mcg/kg is given by rapid (30 sec–60 sec) IV injection, which may be repeated in 15 minutes at 0.04 mcg/kg; for secretin–sincalide test of pancreatic function, 0.02 mcg/kg is infused over a 30-minute period beginning 30 minutes after the secretin infusion; safety not established in children or pregnant women; abdominal discomfort and urge to defecate frequently occur.
teriparatide (Parathar)	Powder for injection— 200 U hPTH activity	Differentiation of hypoparathyroidism from pseudohypoparathyroidism	Synthetic polypeptide hormone consisting of the 1-34 fragment of human parathyroid hormone; hypercalcemia may develop; systemic allergic reactions have occurred; does *not* discriminate between hypoparathyroidism and normal.

(continued)

Table 80-3 (continued)
In Vivo *Diagnostic Aids*

Diagnostic Agent	Preparations	Uses	Clinical Considerations
thyrotropin (Thytropar)	Powder for injection—10 IU thyrotropic activity/ vial	Diffential diagnosis of thyroid failure and decreased thyroid reserve	Purified, lyophilized thyroid-stimulating hormone obtained from bovine anterior pituitary; increases iodine uptake by gland and formation and release of thyroid hormones; thyroid hyperplasia can occur; administered IM or SC (10 IU for 1–3 days), followed by radioiodine study 24 hours after last dose; no response is indicative of thyroid failure; nausea, vomiting, headache, urticaria, tachycardia, and hypotension can occur, anaphylactic reactions have been reported; use cautiously in presence of coronary artery disease or heart disease.
tolbutamide sodium (Orinase Diagnostic)	Injection—1 g/vial with 20 ml diluent	Aid in the diagnosis of pancreatic islet cell adenoma or diabetes	Patients with pancreatic cell insulinomas show a sharp, intense drop in blood glucose following IV injection of 1 g tolbutamide sodium; hypoglycemia may persist for several hours, and may require treatment if symptoms are too intense; diabetic patients show a gradual decrease in blood glucose, whereas normal persons evidence a prompt reduction (15 min–20 min) associated with an elevation in serum insulin.
D-xylose (Xylo-Pfan)	Powder	Test for intestinal malabsorption states	Nonmetabolizable sugar given orally (25 g) to assess absorptive capacity of GI tract; normal values are 5 g–8 g in urine within 5 hours and 40 mg/100 ml blood within 2 hours.

Table 80-4
Radiolabeled Agents Used
for Diagnostic Purposes

Agent	Diagnostic Use
^{14}C-labeled triglycerides	Triglyceride absorption
^{51}Cr (sodium chromate)	Red cell volume and survival time
	GI blood loss
^{57}Co (cyanocobalamin)	Vitamin B_{12} absorption
^{197}Hg (chlormerodin)	Kidney function
^{99m}Tc (sodium pertechnetate)	Localization of brain tumors
^{32}P (sodium phosphate)	Localization of brain tumors

Barium Sulfate

Barium sulfate is the most commonly used substance for visualization of the gastrointestinal (GI) tract. It is a highly insoluble compound; thus, only minimal amounts are absorbed systemically and toxicity is quite low. Barium sulfate can be administered orally as a thick paste for examination of the esophagus or as a more dilute suspension for visualization of the stomach and upper intestinal tract. X-ray studies of the lower GI tract and colon may be performed following a cleansing enema and rectal instillation of barium sulfate suspension. Barium sulfate may be constipating, and complete expulsion of the suspension from the GI tract following the examination usually requires the use of a laxative or enema. The various barium-containing diagnostic agents are listed in Table 80-5.

Iodinated Radiopaque Agents

A variety of iodine-containing organic compounds can be used either orally or parenterally to visualize a number of different body organs. The opacity of these agents depends on the percentage of iodine in the molecule and the amount of drug concentrated at a particular site. Patients should be questioned concerning iodine hypersensitivity before administration of one of these compounds. Severe, sometimes fatal, allergic reactions have occurred with use of these agents, and patients with a history of bronchial asthma or other allergies must be closely monitored during and at least 1 hour following administration. Appropriate antidotal measures, including respiratory aids, epinephrine, and corticosteroids, should be available.

Adverse reactions are uncommon, but the possibility of their occurrence must not be overlooked. Among the untoward reactions reported with use of the radiographic contrast media are urticaria,

(Text continues on p. 1585.)

Table 80-5
Barium-Containing Diagnostic Agents

Trade Name	Preparations	Uses	Dosage
Baricon	Powder for suspension—95% barium sulfate	Upper and lower GI studies	Prepare 60% suspension
Baro-Cat	Suspension—1.5% barium sulfate	Upper and lower GI studies	300 ml at 2 hr and again at 15 min before exam
Baroflave	Powder—100% barium sulfate	Upper and lower GI studies	50 g–500 g suspended in water
Barosperse	Powder for suspension—95% barium sulfate in single-dose cups, disposable enemas, and air-contrast units	Esophageal, upper and lower GI, and colon studies Air-contrast studies	Esophageal—45 g in 15 ml water to yield 75% suspension Upper/lower GI, air contrast—225 g in 150 ml water to yield a 60% suspension Colon—dilute 500 ml 60% suspension with 1,500 ml water to make 20% suspension; use by enema
Barosperse 110	Powder for suspension—95% barium sulfate	Upper and lower GI and colon studies	Upper GI/colon—add 600 ml water to make a 60% suspension Low-density upper GI—add 875 ml water to make a 50% suspension

Table 80-6
Iodinated Radiographic Diagnostic Agents

Trade Name	Dosage Form	Iodine Content	Composition	Diagnostic Uses
Amipaque	Injection	48.25%	13.5%, 18.75% metrizamide	Myelography Computed tomography of intracranial subarachnoid spaces Peripheral arteriography Pediatric angiocardiography
Angio-Conray	Injection	48%	80% iothalamate	Angiocardiography Aortography
Angiovist 282	Injection	28%	60% diatrizoate meglumine	Angiography Arthrography Cholangiography Diskography Excretory urography Peripheral arteriography Pyelography Splenoportography Venography
Angiovist 292	Injection	29.2%	52% diatrizoate meglumine and 8% diatrizoate sodium	See Angiovist 282, above
Angiovist 370	Injection	37%	66% diatrizoate meglumine and 10% diatrizoate sodium	See Angiovist 282, above
Bilivist	Capsules	61.4%	500 mg ipodate sodium	Cholangiography Cholecystography
Bilopaque	Capsules	57.4%	750 mg tyropanoate sodium	Cholecystography
Cholebrine	Tablets	62%	750 mg iocetamic acid	Cholecystography
Cholografin	Injection	5.1%	10.3% iodipamide meglumine	Cholecystography Cholangiography
Cholografin	Injection	26%	52% iodipamide meglumine	Cholecystography Cholangiography
Conray	Injection	28.2%	60% iothalamate meglumine	Cerebral angiography Drip-infusion pyelography Peripheral arteriography Urography Venography
Conray-30	Injection	14.1%	30% iothalamate meglumine	Infusion urography
Conray-43	Injection	20.2%	43% iothalamate meglumine	Lower extremity venography
Conray-325	Injection	32.5%	54.3% iothalamate sodium	Excretory urography
Conray-400	Injection	40%	66.8% iothalamate sodium	Angiocardiography Aortography Excretory urography IV pyelography Renal arteriography
Cysto-Conray	Instillation solution	20.2%	43% iothalamate meglumine	Cystography Cystourethrography Retrograde pyelography
Cysto-Conray II	Instillation solution	8.1%	17.2% iothalamate meglumine	Cystography Cystourethrography Retrograde pyelography
Cystografin	Instillation solution	14.1%	30% diatrizoate meglumine	Cystourethrography Retrograde pyelography
Cystografin-Dilute	Instillation solution	8.5%	18% diatrizoate meglumine	Retrograde cystourethrography

(continued)

Table 80-6 (continued)
Iodinated Radiographic Diagnostic Agents

Trade Name	Dosage Form	Iodine Content	Composition	Diagnostic Uses
Diatrizoate-60	Injection	29.2%	52% diatrizoate meglumine and 8% diatrizoate sodium	See Angiovist 282, above Computed tomography
Diatrizoate meglumine 76%	Injection	35.8%	76% diatrizoate meglumine	Aortography Excretory urography Pediatric angiocardiography Peripheral arteriography
Ethiodol	Injection	37%	Ethiodized oil	Hysterosalpingography Lymphography
Gastrografin	Oral/rectal solution	37%	66% diatrizoate meglumine and 10% diatrizoate sodium	GI radiography
Gastrovist	Oral/rectal solution	37%	66% diatrizoate meglumine and 10% diatrizoate sodium	GI radiography
Hexabrix	Injection	32%	39.3% ioxaglate meglumine and 19.6% ioxaglate sodium	Cerebral angiography Coronary arteriography Peripheral arteriography Visceral arteriography Digital angiography Peripheral venography Excretory urography Computed tomography
Hypaque 20%	Instillation solution	12%	20% diatrizoate sodium	Retrograde pyelography
Hypaque 25%	Injection	15%	25% diatrizoate sodium	Drip-infusion pyelography (excretory urography)
Hypaque 50%	Injection	30%	50% diatrizoate sodium	Angiography (cerebral and peripheral) Aortography Cholangiography Hysterosalpingography Intraosseous venography Splenoportography
Hypaque-M 75%	Injection	38.5%	50% diatrizoate meglumine and 25% diatrizoate sodium	Abdominal aortography Angiocardiography Arteriography (coronary, peripheral, and renal) Urography
Hypaque-M 90%	Injection	46.2%	60% diatrizoate meglumine and 30% diatrizoate sodium	Abdominal aortography Angiocardiography Arteriography (coronary and peripheral) Hysterosalpingography Urography
Hypaque-Cysto	Instillation solution	14.1%	30% diatrizoate meglumine	Retrograde cystourethrography
Hypaque Meglumine 30%	Injection	14.1%	30% diatrizoate meglumine	Infusion urography Computed tomography
Hypaque Meglumine 60%	Injection	28.2%	60% diatrizoate meglumine	Arthrography Cerebral angiography Cholangiography Diskography

(continued)

Table 80-6 (continued)
Iodinated Radiographic Diagnostic Agents

Trade Name	Dosage Form	Iodine Content	Composition	Diagnostic Uses
Hypaque Meglumine 60% (continued)				Excretory urography Peripheral arteriography and venography Splenoportography
Hypaque Sodium	Liquid	24.9%	2.4 g diatrizoate sodium/ml	GI radiography
Hypaque Sodium	Powder for oral solution	59.8%		GI radiography
Hypaque-76	Injection	37%	66% diatrizoate meglumine and 10% diatrizoate sodium	See Angiovist 282, above
Isovue 300	Injection	30%	61% iopamidol	Angiography Arteriography IV contrast enhancement
Isovue 370	Injection	37%	75.5% iopamidol	See Isovue 300, above
Isovue-M 200	Injection	20%	40.8% iopamidol	Contrast enhancement Intrathecal neuroradiology Ventriculography
Isovue-M 300	Injection	30%	61.2% iopamidol	See Isovue-M 200, above
MD-50	Injection	30%	50% diatrizoate sodium	See Hypaque 50%, above
MD-60	Injection	29.2%	52% diatrizoate meglumine and 8% diatrizoate meglumine	See Angiovist 282, above
MD-76	Injection	37%	66% diatrizoate meglumine and 10% diatrizoate sodium	See Angiovist 282, above
MD-Gastroview	Injection	37%	66% diatrizoate meglumine and 10% diatrizoate sodium	See Angiovist 282, above
Omnipaque	Injection	——	Iohexol equivalent to 18%, 24%, 30%, or 35% iodine	Intrathecal or intravascular radiography
Oragrafin Calcium	Granules for oral suspension	61.7%	3 g ipodate calcium/8-g packet	Cholangiography Cholecystography
Oragrafin Sodium	Capsules	61.4%	500 mg ipodate sodium	Cholecystography
Renografin-60	Injection	29%	52% diatrizoate meglumine and 8% diatrizoate sodium	Arthrography Cerebral angiography Cholangiography Computed tomography Diskography Excretory urography Peripheral arteriography

(continued)

Table 80-6 (continued)
Iodinated Radiographic Diagnostic Agents

Trade Name	Dosage Form	Iodine Content	Composition	Diagnostic Uses
Renografin-60 (continued)				Pyelography Splenoportography Venography
Renografin-76	Injection	37%	66% diatrizoate meglumine and 10% diatrizoate sodium	See Renografin-60, above
Reno-M-30	Instillation solution	14%	30% diatrizoate meglumine	Retrograde or ascending pyelography
Reno-M-60	Injection	28%	60% diatrizoate meglumine	Arthrography Cerebral angiography Cholangiography Diskography Excretory urography Peripheral arteriography Pyelography Splenoportography Venography
Reno-M-Dip	Injection	14%	30% diatrizoate meglumine	Computed tomography Drip-infusion pyelography
Renovist	Injection	37%	34.3% diatrizoate meglumine and 35% diatrizoate sodium	Angiocardiography Aortography Excretory urography Peripheral arteriography and venography Venocavography
Renovist II	Injection	31%	28.5% diatrizoate meglumine and 29.1% diatrizoate sodium	See Renovist, above
Renovue-65	Injection	30%	65% iodamide meglumine	Excretory urography
Renovue-Dip	Injection	11.1%	24% iodamide meglumine	Excretory urography
Sinografin	Injection	38%	52.7% diatrizoate meglumine and 26.8% iodipamide meglumine	Hysterosalpingography
Telepaque	Tablets	66.7%	500 mg iopanoic acid	Cholecystography
Urovist Cysto	Instillation solution	14.1%	30% diatrizoate meglumine	Cystourethrography Retrograde pyelography
Urovist Meglumine DIU/CT	Injection	14.1%	30% diatrizoate meglumine	Drip-infusion pyelography Computed tomography Venography
Urovist Sodium 300	Injection	30%	50% diatrizoate sodium	See Hypaque 50%, above
Vascoray	Injection	40%	52% iothalamate meglumine and 26% iothalamate sodium	Angiocardiography Aortography Arteriography (coronary and renal) Excretory urography

wheezing, dyspnea, angioneurotic edema, laryngeal spasm, anaphylaxis, hyperthermia, headache, chest tightness, and tremor. Reactions that are probably attributable to volume, speed, and site of injection are flushing, dizziness, nausea, generalized vasodilation, and hypotension. Pain and irritation at the injection site have been noted, as well as paresthesias, numbness, hematomas, ecchymoses, and thrombophlebitis.

The various iodinated radiographic contrast agents are listed in Table 80-6, along with their dosage forms, iodine content, composition, and diagnostic use. Because their dose and route of administration depend on their diagnostic intent, the information included with each drug must be consulted before administration.

An adjunctive drug that is sometimes used in lymphography to facilitate visualization of the lymphatic system is isosulfan blue (Lymphazurin 1%). Following subcutaneous injection of 0.5 ml into three interdigital spaces of each extremity per study, isosulfan is selectively concentrated in the lymphatic vessels, which are colored a bright blue. Adverse reactions are relatively infrequent (1%–2%) and are largely of an allergic nature, ranging from itching and swelling of the hands to generalized edema and respiratory distress in rare instances.

Another adjunctive agent that is used in certain radiographic studies is potassium perchlorate (Perchloracap). This agent provides perchlorate ion (ClO_4), which suppresses accumulation of pertechnetate ion (TcO_4) in the choroid plexus and salivary and thyroid glands of patients receiving radioactive sodium pertechnetate (^{99m}Tc) for brain imaging and placenta localization. Perchlorate competes for plasma protein-binding sites with TcO_4, with a resultant shift of a portion of TcO_4 from the plasma to the red blood cell. The drug is given orally as capsules in a dose of 200 mg to 400 mg 30 minutes to 60 minutes before a dose of sodium pertechnetate.

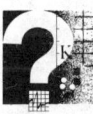

REVIEW QUESTIONS

1. What are the major categories of diagnostic agents?
2. In what dosage forms are *in vitro* diagnostic aids employed?
3. What are the principal diagnostic uses for *in vitro* diagnostic aids?
4. For what diseases are *intradermal* diagnostic aids employed as a screening method?
5. Against which antibodies are the multiple skin test antigens (Multitest CMI) useful?
6. List the various preparations useful in skin testing for tuberculosis.
7. What are the principal uses for the following *in vivo* diagnostic aids?
   (1) bentiromide
   (2) betazole
   (3) cosyntropin
   (4) gonadorelin
   (5) inulin
   (6) methacholine
   (7) pentagastrin
   (8) protirelin
   (9) sincalide
8. What two substances are most commonly used as radioactive diagnostic agents?
9. For what diagnostic purposes are barium-containing agents used?
10. What are the major hazards associated with administration of iodinated radiopaque agents?
11. Briefly describe the adjunctive use of (1) isosulfan blue and (2) potassium perchlorate in radiologic studies.

12. List several of the major diagnostic uses of iodinated radiographic agents.

BIBLIOGRAPHY

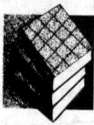

Bentiromide—A test for pancreatic insufficiency. Med Lett Drugs Ther 26:50, 1984

Berger ME, Hubner KF: Hospital hazards: Diagnostic radiation. Am J Nurs 83(8):1155, 1983

Early PJ, Sodee DB: Principles and Practice of Nuclear Medicine. St Louis, CV Mosby, 1985

Hermann CS: Performing intradermal skin tests the right way. Nursing '83 13(10):50, 1983

Rayudu CVS: Radiotracers for Medical Applications. Boca Raton, FL, CRC Press, 1983

Sincalide for cholecystography. Med Lett Drugs Ther 19:36, 1977

Synthetic LH-RH. Med Lett Drugs Ther 25:106, 1983

Serums and Vaccines

81

The ability of circulating antibodies to render a person resistant to a particular disease is known as *immunity*. Immunity may be of two types, natural or acquired. Persons born with resistance to a certain disease state are said to have natural immunity; however, this is a relatively rare occurrence. Most types of immunity are acquired, that is, attained during the person's lifetime, either by production of antibodies in response to an invasion by foreign microorganisms (active acquired immunity) or by utilization of antibodies obtained from an animal or another human immunized against a particular disease (passive acquired immunity). Active immunity, therefore, is acquired through contact with the antigen itself, which stimulates the body to produce its own specific antibodies to combat it. If the antibodies develop in response to exposure to an actual disease state, whether clinical symptoms are present or not, the active immunity is said to be *naturally acquired*. Conversely, if the antibodies form in response to inoculation into the body of killed or attenuated microorganisms or their toxic by-products, the active immunity is referred to as *artificially acquired*.

The various biological preparations used to confer immunity may be categorized in the following manner:

I. Agents for active immunity
   A. Toxoids (*e.g.*, diphtheria, tetanus)
   B. Vaccines
      1. Bacterial (*e.g.*, BCG, cholera, hemophilus, typhoid)
      2. Viral (*e.g.*, influenza, measles, hepatitis B, poliovirus)
II. Agents for passive immunity
   A. Antitoxins/antivenins (*e.g.*, diphtheria, tetanus, black widow spider)
   B. Human immune serums (*e.g.*, immune globulins)
III. Rabies prophylaxis products (*e.g.*, antirabies serum, rabies immune globulin, rabies vaccine)

Agents for Active Immunity

Agents used for active immunization contain specific antigens that induce the formation of antibodies when injected into the body. These antigenic substances are of two types, toxoids and vaccines. Toxoids are toxins derived from microorganisms that have been modified (*i.e.*, detoxified), usually with formaldehyde, so they are no longer toxic but are still antigenic, and thus are capable of stimulating antibody production. Vaccines are suspensions of whole microorganisms, either killed or chemically attenuated to reduce their virulence, which are capable of inducing the formation of antibodies without causing an outbreak of the disease. Active immunity with toxoids or vaccines requires several days or even weeks to develop, because sufficient antibody levels need to be attained. In some cases, more than one dose may be required. Thus, toxoids and vaccines are of limited value in treating active infections. Once acquired, however, active immunity can usually be made to last a lifetime, especially if reinforced by periodic "booster" doses at appropriate intervals.

Toxoids

Diphtheria, Diphtheria and Tetanus, Diphtheria and Tetanus Toxoids and Pertussis Vaccine, Tetanus

Toxoids are generally prepared by treating exotoxins with formaldehyde, which renders them nontoxic but still antigenic. Stimulation of antibody production by toxoids can be increased by precipitating the toxoid with alum or adsorbing it onto colloids such as aluminum hydroxide. The precipitated or adsorbed products are absorbed and excreted more slowly, and persist in tissues a longer period of time than do plain toxoids, resulting in higher antibody production. The principal disadvantage of these precipitated or adsorbed toxoids is that their use is frequently associated with pain, swelling, and tenderness at the injection site, especially in older children and adults. These reactions are sometimes quite severe. The most commonly employed toxoids are diphtheria and tetanus, which are frequently given in combination with pertussis vaccine as DTP for routine immunization in preschool children. Table 81-1 lists the various toxoids.

Vaccines

BCG; Cholera; Hemophilus b; Hepatitis B; Influenza Virus; Measles; Measles and Rubella; Measles, Rubella, and Mumps;

Table 81-1
Toxoids

Preparations	Administration	Clinical Considerations
diphtheria toxoid, adsorbed, pediatric	2 injections (0.5 ml) IM 6 weeks–8 weeks apart, then a third dose 1 year later Booster: 5-year–10-year intervals	Used in infants and children under 6 years; do not administer subcutaneously; avoid giving during active infections or in patients receiving corticosteroids or other immunosuppressive agents because antibody response is diminished; cautious use in children with neurologic or convulsive disorders; begin with very low doses in these patients.
diphtheria and tetanus toxoids, combined, pediatric	Infants (6 wk–1 yr)—3 injections (0.5 ml) IM at least 4 wk apart. A fourth injection is given after 6 mo–12 mo. Children (1 yr–6 yr) 2 injections (0.5 ml) at least 4 wk apart. A third dose is given after 6 mo–12 mo. Booster: 0.5 ml at 4 yr to 6 yr	Used only in children 6 years or under; indicated only where the triple antigen (DTP) is contraindicated; do not administer during acute infection or in patients receiving immunosuppressant drugs; note that pediatric preparation is 3–8 times as potent as adult preparation with respect to diphtheria toxoid. Side-effects include localized pain, swelling, and tenderness; drowsiness, fretfulness, and anorexia.
diphtheria and tetanus toxoids, combined, adult	2 injections (0.5 ml) IM 4 weeks–6 weeks apart, then a third dose 6 months–12 months later Booster: 10-year intervals	Reduced amount of diphtheria toxoid 2 U/0.5 ml provides adequate immunization in adults with minimal risk of hypersensitivity reactions; tetanus toxoid content is identical in pediatric and adult preparations; cautious use during pregnancy and in debilitated individuals
diphtheria and tetanus toxoids and pertussis vaccine, adsorbed-DTP (Tri-Immunol)	3 injections (0.5 ml) IM at 4-week–8-week intervals, beginning at 2 months then a fourth dose 1 year thereafter Booster: At 4 years–6 years of age	Most commonly used preparation for routine immunization of young children; not recommended in adults or children over 7 years; use with extreme caution in children with history of CNS disease or convulsions because pertussis has caused neurologic side-effects in a small percent of children; defer administration during an acute febrile illness, shock, alterations in consciousness, extremely agitated behavior, or if patient is receiving immunosuppressive therapy; slight fever, malaise, and injection site pain frequently occur following injection.
tetanus toxoid, fluid or adsorbed	Fluid—0.5 ml at 4-week–8-week intervals for 3 doses, then a fourth dose 6 months–12 months later Adsorbed—0.5 ml at 4-week–8-week intervals for 2 doses, then a third dose 6–12 months later Booster: Every 10 years for each	Adsorbed toxoid gives higher antibody levels and longer protection than fluid toxoid and is the preferred agent; adsorbed preparation is given IM only, but fluid preparation can be administered IM or SC; do not use in patients with acute respiratory infection, convulsive disorders, or in persons receiving immunosuppressive therapy; local soreness, erythema, and swelling are common, especially in adults; lumps may develop at injection site and will gradually disappear over a period of weeks.

Meningitis; Mixed Respiratory; Mumps; Plague; Pneumococcal; Poliovirus; Rubella; Rubella and Mumps; Staphage Lysate; Typhoid; Yellow Fever

Vaccines are suspensions of killed or attenuated microorganisms of bacteria or viruses that are capable of stimulating antibody production but that are in themselves nonpathogenic. The live, attenuated vaccines are claimed to provide longer-lasting immunity in most cases than the killed or inactivated vaccines, although both types are quite effective in increasing antibody levels. Caution must be observed, however, in using a vaccine grown and cultivated in living tissues, for example, chick embryo, because allergic reactions can occur in patients hypersensitive to the specific animal proteins. However, influenza virus vaccine, although grown in embryonated eggs, is highly purified, and is much less likely to elicit hypersensitivity reactions than other vaccines. Conversely, live viral vaccines prepared by growing viruses in human cell culture (*e.g.*, rubella) are much less antigenic than animal-derived products.

Viral replication following administration of live attenuated virus vaccines can be enhanced in persons with immunodeficiency diseases or suppressed immune response, for example, persons with leukemia or malignancies or persons receiving corticosteroids or cancer chemotherapeutic agents. Such patients should not be given live, attenuated virus vaccines.

In the case of certain viral vaccines, a subclinical disease state may be induced by the vaccine itself, accompanied by fever, myalgia, and other manifestations of the particular viral disease (*e.g.*, rash, urticaria, parotitis). These symptoms are generally mild and transient and usually require nothing more than symptomatic management with medications such as antipyretics or analgesics. Vaccines do not afford immediate protection, because several days or occasionally weeks are required to produce sufficient serum antibody levels. A second and occasionally a third injection at 4-week to 8-week intervals are frequently given with certain vaccines to ensure adequate antibody levels. Active or imminent infections, therefore, require administration of one of the immune serums or antitoxins.

The various bacterial and viral vaccines are listed in Table 81-2, along with dosage guidelines and pertinent remarks.

In addition to the commercially available vaccines listed in Table 81-2, several other vaccines are available from the Centers for Disease Control in Atlanta for nonemergency use in persons at high risk for exposure in the laboratory. These vaccines include botulinum toxoid (pentavalent), eastern equine encephalitis (EEE) vaccine (live, attenuated), Japanese encephalitis vaccine, smallpox vaccine, tularemia vaccine (live, attenuated), and Venezuelan equine encephalitis (VEE) vaccine.

Agents for Passive Immunity

Substances used to confer passive immunity are termed *immune serums* and consist of preformed antibodies derived from either human or animal sources. Human immune serums contain globulins possessing antibodies against a number of bacterial and viral diseases and are derived from human serum or plasma. Conversely, immune serums obtained by actively immunizing an animal against a specific disease, then removing and purifying the serum, which contains antibodies against that disease, are generally termed *antitoxins* or *antivenins*. Although both types of immune serums are effective in protecting against certain diseases, the human immune serums are much less likely to elicit hypersensitivity reactions, inasmuch as they do not contain foreign (*i.e.*, animal-derived) proteins.

Antitoxins/Antivenins

Black Widow Spider Antivenin, Crotalidae Antivenin, Diphtheria Antitoxin, North American Coral Snake Antivenin, Tetanus Antitoxin

Antitoxins and antivenins are prepared by repeatedly inoculating an animal, usually a horse, with a toxoid (*e.g.*, diphtheria, tetanus) or a venom (*e.g.*, from a snake or black widow spider), then bleeding the animal and concentrating the antibody-containing fraction of the plasma. The partially purified antibodies or antitoxins can then be administered to humans to neutralize toxins produced by invading microorganisms or introduced by a bite.

It is imperative that a skin or conjunctival hypersensitivity test be performed before adminis-

(*Text continues on p. 1600.*)

Table 81-2
Vaccines

Vaccine	Preparations	Administration	Clinical Considerations
Bacterial			
BCG vaccine (BCG)	Injection (intradermal)—8 million U–26 million U/ml of standardized BCG bacillus prepared from culture Injection (percutaneous)—50 mg/vial of Tice-Chicago strain	0.1 ml intradermal: (0.05 ml in infants) Percutaneous: 0.2 ml–0.3 ml dropped onto skin, followed by application of a multiple puncture disc	Live, attenuated vaccine used in tuberculin-negative patients exposed to persons with active tuberculosis; contraindicated in tuberculin-positive patients, burn patients, and persons receiving chronic corticosteroid therapy; low incidence of untoward reactions, but can produce skin ulceration and abscesses; do not expose vaccine to light; sterilize unused portion before disposal.
cholera vaccine	Injection—Suspension of killed *Vibrio cholerae* organisms	Adults—0.5 ml SC or IM followed in 1 week–4 weeks by a second 0.5-ml dose Children—0.2 ml–0.3 ml SC or IM (or 0.2 ml intradermally); repeat in 1 week–4 weeks Booster—0.2 ml–0.5 ml (depending on age) given every 6 months as long as protection is desired	Used to protect travelers to or residents of countries where cholera is endemic or epidemic or for mass immunization *prior* to a cholera outbreak; *not* indicated for treatment of acute cholera infection; vaccine does not prevent development of a carrier state; immunity is short-lived (3 months–6 months); therefore, repeated doses are necessary to confer long-lasting protection; protection is not absolute, and disease can still be contracted if exposure occurs; injections often cause local pain, erythema, swelling, and a febrile reaction; intradermal route may be used in children over 5; for mass immunization during epidemics, a single dose of 1.0 ml can be used.
hemophilus b polysaccharide vaccine (b-Capsa I, Hib-Imune)	Powder for injection—25 mcg Hib polysaccharide/0.5 ml when reconstituted	0.5 ml (25 mcg) SC. Do *not* give IV or intradermally.	Used for immunization of children 18 months–6 years against disease caused by *H. influenzae* b; children under 18 mon. may not be adequately protected; acute febrile reaction, erythema, and induration of injection site can occur; do not give during acute febrile illness or active infection.
hemophilus b conjugate vaccine (ProHIBiT)	Powder for injection—25 mcg (with 18 mcg conjugated diphtheria toxoid protein) per 0.5 ml when reconstituted	0.5 ml (25 mcg) IM	

(continued)

Table 81-2 (continued)
Vaccines

Vaccine	Preparations	Administration	Clinical Considerations
meningitis vaccine (Meno-mune-A/C/Y/W-135)	Powder for injection—Suspensions of polysaccharides from meningococcus, groups A, C, Y, and W-135	0.5 ml (50 mcg meningococcal isolated product) SC as a single injection; do not give intradermally or IV	Stimulates antibody production against *Neisseria meningitidis* groups A, C, Y, and W-135; used in persons 2 years of age and older at risk in epidemic or endemic areas (*e.g.*, travelers, medical and laboratory personnel, household or institutional contacts); adverse reactions include chills, fever, malaise, local soreness; it is contraindicated in presence of active infections, in persons taking corticosteroids, and in pregnant women.
mixed respiratory vaccine (MRV)	Injection—Suspensions of several strains of bacterial organisms present in common respiratory infections (*e.g.*, *Staphylococcus aureus*, *Streptococcus pneumoniae*, *Klebsiella pneumoniae*, *Hemophilus influenzae*, and so forth)	Initially, 0.05 ml SC; increase by 0.05 ml–0.1 ml at 4-day–7-day intervals until a maximum of 1 ml is given; maintenance dose 0.5 ml every 1 week–2 weeks	Used to prevent bacterial hypersensitization in respiratory infections that can lead to asthma, urticaria, rhinitis, and so forth; effectiveness has *not* been conclusively demonstrated; repeat doses should not be given until all local reactions from previous dose have disappeared; frequency of administration is highly individualized; children's dose is the same as that for adults; observe for symptoms of allergic reaction and, if severe, administer epinephrine, corticosteroids, or antihistamines; local hypersensitivity reactions are common and are not a cause for alarm.
plague vaccine	Injection—2 billion killed plague bacilli/ml	Adults—1.0 ml IM, followed in 1 month–3 months by 0.2 ml IM; third injection of 0.2 ml IM after 3 months to 6 months is recommended. Booster: 0.1 ml–0.2 ml at 6-month intervals during active exposure Children (Under 1 year) $^1/_5$ adult dose (1 year–4 years) $^2/_5$ adult dose (5 years–10 years) $^3/_5$ adult dose	Suspension of inactivated *Yersinia pestis* organisms grown in artificial media; repeated injections increase the likelihood of adverse reactions, especially local allergic effects; common initial side-effects are malaise, headache, fever, local erythema, and mild lymphadenopathy; vaccine is recommended for those persons who must be in known plague areas (*e.g.*, Asia, South America, (*continued*)

Table 81-2 (continued)
Vaccines

Vaccine	Preparations	Administration	Clinical Considerations
Viral (continued)			
hepatitis B vaccine, recombinant (Recombivax HB) (continued)			transfusions; hepatitis B infections have also been linked to hepatocellular carcinoma; effectiveness of vaccine in preventing hepatitis B when given *after* exposure to virus is not conclusively established, but vaccine has been given with hepatitis B immune globulin with no deleterious effects. Infants born to mothers who are Hepatitis B Surface Antigen (HBsAg) positive are at high risk of becoming carriers of hepatitis B virus and of developing chronic infection sequelae; they should be treated beginning at birth according to the schedule given under Administration.
influenza virus vaccine (Fluogen, Fluzone)	Injection—Suspension of inactivated influenza virus particles of the currently prevailing type	Over 13 years—0.5 ml IM in a single dose 3 years–12 years—2 doses of 0.5 ml IM at least 4 weeks apart Under 3 years—2 doses of 0.25 ml IM at least 4 weeks apart	Composition of vaccine changes yearly depending on prevalent virus strains; recommended in persons at high risk for adverse reactions from lower respiratory infections, such as those with heart disease, chronic pulmonary disease, renal dysfunction, diabetes, or debilitation; also recommended in all persons over 65 yr; contraindicated during first trimester of pregnancy, in persons with severe neurologic disorders, and in patients with a history of Guillain-Barre syndrome; use with caution in hypersensitive persons, because vaccine is egg-grown; defer immunization in patients with acute respiratory disease or other active infection; not effective against all influenza viruses; available as "whole-virus" or "split-virus" preparations; split virus associated with fewer adverse *(continued)*

Table 81-2 (continued)
Vaccines

Vaccine	Preparations	Administration	Clinical Considerations
Viral (continued)			
influenza virus vaccine (Fluogen, Fluzone) (continued)			effects in children and is preferred in patients under 12 years; a single dose is sufficient for persons inoculated within the previous 2 years; vaccine may reduce elimination of drugs metabolized by cytochrome P-450 system in the liver (_e.g._, theophylline, warfarin).
measles vaccine—rubeola (Attenuvax)	Injection—Suspension of Enders' attenuated Edmonston strain of measles virus in single-dose vials with diluent	Administer total volume of reconstituted vaccine SC Booster: not necessary	Live, attenuated strain of measles virus grown in chick embryo tissue culture; most often given together with mumps and rubella vaccines as a single preparation (see below); produces a mild measles infection (_e.g._, fever, rash 7 days–10 days after immunization and lasts 1 day–2 days), which induces immunity in 97% of susceptible individuals; recommended in children 15 months or older; revaccination is not required if child was over 12 months when initially vaccinated; contraindicated in pregnancy and in immunocompromised patients; use cautiously in children with a history of febrile convulsions or cerebral injury; discard if not used within 8 hours; store reconstituted vaccine in a dark place.
measles and rubella vaccine (M-R Vax II)	Injection—Single-dose vials with diluent containing a combination of live, attentuated strains of measles and rubella viruses	Administer total volume of reconstituted vaccine SC Booster: Not necessary	Indicated for simultaneous immunization against measles and rubella (German measles) in children over 15 months; see measles vaccine and rubella vaccine for additional information; it is most frequently given together with mumps vaccine as a single preparation (see below).

(continued)

Table 81-2 *(continued)*
Vaccines

Vaccine	Preparations	Administration	Clinical Considerations
measles, mumps, and rubella vaccine (M-M-R II)	Injection—Single-dose vials, with diluent containing live, attenuated strains of measles, mumps, and rubella viruses	Administer total volume of reconstituted vaccine SC Booster: Not necessary	Indicated in children over 15 months for simultaneous immunization against measles, mumps, and rubella; highly effective (95%–98% of children develop effective antibody levels to all three viruses) and generally well tolerated; hypersensitivity reactions can occur; widely used preparation; immunity persists for at least 8 years–10 years; thus, revaccination is not required; see measles, mumps, and rubella vaccines, individually, for other considerations.
mumps vaccine (Mumpsvax)	Injection—Single-dose vials with diluent containing live, attenuated mumps virus	Administer total volume of reconstituted vaccine SC Booster: Not necessary	Used for immunization of children over 15 months and adults; immunity is produced in 97% of children and 93% of adults with a single dose, and persists for at least 10 years; do not use in pregnant women; allergic reactions can occur (vaccine is derived from chick embryo); be prepared with epinephrine and antihistamines; fever and parotitis have occurred but are generally mild.
poliovirus vaccine, inactivated—IPV (Poliomyelitis Vaccine—Purified)	Injection—Suspension of 3 types of polio-virus (types 1, 2, 3) grown in monkey kidney cell cultures	3 doses (1.0 ml each) given SC at 4-week–6-week intervals, followed by a fourth dose (1.0 ml) 6 months–12 months after the third dose Booster: Every 5 years	Indicated for polio immunization in persons with compromised immune system either due to disease (*e.g.*, malignancy) or to drugs (*e.g.*, steroids, antimetabolites); oral polio vaccine (Sabin) is vaccine of choice in other persons; dosage schedule is often integrated with that of DTP immunization and begun at 6 weeks–12 weeks of age; vaccine should be clear red; do not use if cloudy, discolored, or precipitated; defer injections during periods of other active infections; hyper- *(continued)*

Table 81-2 (continued)
Vaccines

Vaccine	Preparations	Administration	Clinical Considerations
***Viral** (continued)*			
poliovirus vaccine, inactivated—IPV (Poliomyelitis Vaccine—Purified) *(continued)*			sensitivity reactions can occur; have epinephrine injection available.
poliovirus vaccine, live oral trivalent—TOPV, Sabin (Orimune)	Dispettes—Single-dose (0.5 ml) containing types 1, 2, and 3 poliovirus grown in monkey kidney cell cultures	3 doses (0.5 ml each) given orally at 6 weeks–12 weeks of age, 8 weeks later, and 8 months after the second dose Booster: 5 years of age	Vaccine of choice for primary immunization against poliovirus; advantages over Salk vaccine are ease of administration, longer-lasting immunity, protection against infection by wild polioviruses, and lack of need for periodic booster doses; do not administer if persistent vomiting or diarrhea is present; store in a freezer, thaw before use; when live virus is used for polio immunization, a nonimmunized parent of the child has a *very small risk* of developing polio by handling the feces of a newly immunized infant. The parent may wish to receive the IPV vaccine concurrently as a precautionary measure.
rubella vaccine (Meruvax II)	Injection—Single-dose vials with diluent, containing Wistar RA 27/3 strain of rubella virus propagated in human diploid cell culture	Administer total volume of reconstituted vaccine SC	Live, attenuated rubella virus strains used to immunize against rubella in children from 15 months to puberty; antibody levels persist for at least 6 years; useful in adolescents and adults to prevent outbreaks in high-risk situations; do not administer to pregnant women and use cautiously in women of childbearing age, because congenital abnormalities *(continued)*

Table 81-2 (continued)
Vaccines

Vaccine	Preparations	Administration	Clinical Considerations
Viral (continued)			
rubella vaccine (Meruvax II) (*continued*)			can occur; usually given combined with measles and mumps vaccines (see MMR); side-effects are uncommon, but can include symptoms of the disease (rash, urticaria, sore throat, malaise, fever, headache, lymphadenopathy); arthralgia is fairly common in women (12%–20%). Side-effects are more common in older children and adults.
rubella and mumps vaccine (Biavax-II)	Injection—Single-dose vials with diluents, containing a mixture of mumps and rubella virus strains	Administer total volume of reconstituted vaccine SC	Combination vaccine yielding effective antibody levels in 97%–100% of susceptible children; may be given as early as 1 year of age; not as frequently used as measles, mumps, and rubella vaccine (MMR); see Clinical Considerations for rubella and mumps vaccines, above.
yellow fever vaccine (YF-Vax)	Injection—Vials with diluent, for needle injection, containing a live, attenuated 17D strain virus cultured in chick embryo	0.5 ml SC for adults and children	Indicated for immunization of persons traveling to countries requiring vaccination against yellow fever; immunity develops within 7 days and can last for up to 10 years; administer at least 1 month apart from other live viruses; fever and malaise occur in about 10% of patients; keep frozen until reconstituted and then use within 1 hour; do not use if vaccine has been exposed to temperatures above 5°C.

tering any of the horse serum antitoxins to determine if the patient might exhibit an allergic reaction to the foreign serum. Package literature describing the appropriate hypersensitivity testing procedure should always be consulted before utilizing one of these products. Even a negative sensitivity test result, however, does not completely rule out the possibility of an allergic reaction and epinephrine injection should always be available when an antitoxin is administered. Adverse reactions to antitoxins range from local pain and erythema at the injection site, to serum sickness and anaphylaxis; the incidence of the more serious allergic reactions is approximately 5% to 10%.

Information pertaining to the commercially available antitoxins and antivenins is presented in Table 81-3. In addition, botulism equine antitoxin is available by request from the Centers for Disease Control in Atlanta.

Human Immune Serums

Hepatitis B Immune Globulin; Immune Globulin, Human; Lymphocyte Immune Globulin; Pertussis Immune Globulin; $Rh_o(D)$ Immune Globulin; Tetanus Immune Globulin; Varicella Zoster Immune Globulin

Immune globulins containing antibodies against certain diseases can be obtained from human serum, and these products are generally preferred over animal-derived globulins because of the lower incidence of hypersensitivity reactions. Human immune globulins may be obtained from pooled plasma of human donors, in which case the preparation contains antibodies against a number of diseases (e.g., hepatitis, rubella, varicella) or from the blood of persons recently recovered from or hyperimmunized against a particular disease, in which case the globulins contain high antibody titers against that particular disease. These human immune serums should be used cautiously in individuals with immunoglobulin A deficiency, thrombocytopenia, or coagulation disorders, and in pregnant women. Skin testing for hypersensitivity is meaningless with human immune serums, be-

cause intradermal injections frequently give rise to a local inflammatory response that can be misinterpreted as an allergic reaction. True hypersensitivity reactions to human immune globulins are extremely rare.

The human immune serums are listed in Table 81-4 along with dosages and other pertinent information. In addition, western equine encephalitis (WEE) immune globulin is available by request from the Centers for Disease Control in Atlanta.

Rabies Prophylaxis Products

Antirabies Serum, Equine; Rabies Immune Globulin; Rabies Vaccine, Human Diploid Cell Culture

Rabies is an acute viral disease of animals that can be transmitted to other animals and humans by the bite of an infected animal. Although many animals are susceptible to rabies, it occurs most commonly in dogs, cats, raccoons, skunks, coyotes, and wolves. The virus has a high affinity for the nervous system, and is inevitably fatal unless appropriate immunologic therapy is instituted quickly.

Products used for rabies prophylaxis include the following:

1. Human diploid cell vaccine (HDCV)—Suspension of Wistar rabies virus strain grown in human diploid cell cultures
2. Rabies immune globulin (RIG)—Human immune globulin obtained from plasma of hyperimmunized donors
3. Antirabies serum, equine origin (ARS)—Concentrated serum obtained from hyperimmunized horses

Postexposure treatment is best accomplished by a combination of active and passive immunization, that is, vaccine and immune globulin. For passive immunization, rabies immune globulin is the drug of choice. The equine antirabies serum should only be used when the immune globulin is unavailable. For active immunization, HDCV is used.

The various rabies prophylaxis products are briefly reviewed in Table 81-5. It is important, however, that anyone using any of the products become thoroughly familiar with the indications, precautions, and general handling procedures of each particular preparation by consulting the product literature.

Nursing Process for Patients Receiving Toxoids and Vaccines

□ ASSESSMENT

□ *Subjective Data*
A complete history is the health team's most effective tool in identifying patients at risk for adverse reactions to these vaccines. Information about allergies and previous experience with immunizations can identify the patient likely to have an allergic reaction. Check the manufacturer's insert to determine components used in making the drug. Examples of components include egg protein, horse serum, duck embryo, and neomycin, among others. Patients allergic to these products or animals or who list multiple food and drug allergies should be brought to the attention of the physician before the drug is given.

History taking should also focus on evidence of immunosuppression, presence of gastrointestinal or neurologic disease, or current pregnancy. Immunosuppression can result if the patient has a malignant disease such as leukemia or lymphoma, has advanced acquired immunodeficiency syndrome (AIDS), a prolonged illness such as mononucleosis or hepatitis, is receiving radiation treatments, or is taking immunosuppressive drugs such as corticosteroids or antineoplastic agents. The immunosuppressed individual has an inadequate immune defense system to react to the injected virus and consequently is likely to have a severe reaction to the drug. Patients who are immunosuppressed should not receive any live virus vaccine that includes BCG, measles, mumps, rubella, yellow fever, or polio. Likewise, pregnant women should not receive these vaccines, which may harm the fetus, nor should they receive influenza vaccines during the first trimester of pregnancy. Poliovirus vaccine may be given. Any woman of childbearing age not using contraception should have a pregnancy test before the immunization is given. The woman should refrain from conceiving for 2 months after receiving the vaccination.

The patient with gastroenteritis should not receive oral polio vaccine (OPV). This infection will interfere with the viral colonization in the intestines that is needed to develop an immune response. This intestinal colonization can lead to an acute case of polio if an unimmunized person has contact with the vaccine recipient's feces, such as in the case of a child and his unimmunized parent. Parents and caretakers must be warned of this prior to the child's vaccination. The parent should be immunized first.

The patient with a neurologic disorder should have a complete check-up before the decision is made to give pertussis vaccine or influenza vaccine, and benefits of immunization should be carefully weighed against the risks. Loss of consciousness and seizures are potential problems for the neurologically impaired patient who receives these vaccines.

Any patient with an acute febrile infection such as flu or upper respiratory infection should have immunization postponed until the infection is resolved. Administration during such an episode may decrease the body's defenses, making the reaction to the infection more pronounced or prolonging the infection. In addition, the presence of a fever masks any febrile reaction from the immunization, making correct diagnosis difficult if a severe reaction occurs.

Patients at high risk for developing severe respiratory infections from influenza viruses should be identified and administered the vaccine in the early fall before the "flu season" begins. These include patients with heart disease, chronic pulmonary disease, renal disorders, endocrine diseases such as diabetes, and any patient suffering a debilitating illness.

□ *Objective Data*
Each patient should have a current temperature recorded to rule out a febrile infection. Patients with a history of immunosuppression should have a complete blood count with differential drawn to determine white blood cell levels. The patient scheduled to receive BCG vaccine should have a PPD test performed prior to vaccine administration.

□ NURSING DIAGNOSES
Actual nursing diagnoses may include
  Knowledge deficit related to the drug, its effect, and side-effects
  Anxiety related to injection
Potential nursing diagnoses may include
  Alteration in respiratory function related to a severe hypersensitivity reaction

(Text continues on p. 1606.)

Table 81-3
Antitoxins/Antivenins*

Antitoxin/Antivenin	Preparations	Administration	Clinical Considerations
Antivenins			
Crotalidae antivenin, polyvalent	Injection—Vial of lyophilized serum with diluent plus vial of normal horse serum for sensitivity testing	*Dosage depends on severity of bite.* Mild—2–4 vials IV Moderate—5–9 vials IV Severe—10–20 vials IV (Children and small adults may require larger doses; children's dosage is *not* based on weight.)	Preparation of serum globulins containing protective antibodies against a number of crotalids, including pit vipers, rattlesnakes, cottonmouths, copperheads, bushmasters (see package instructions); administer as soon as possible after bite and immobilize patient to minimize spread of venom; do not administer at or around the site of the bite; children have less resistance and require proportionately larger doses than adults; subsequent injections depend on clinical response; use barbiturates, narcotics with caution, because increased respiratory depression can result; test for sensitivity to horse serum prior to injecting.
North American coral snake antivenin (Antivenin *Micrurus fulvius*)	Injection—Vial with diluent	3–5 vials (30–50 ml) slowly injected directly into IV infusion tubing or added to reservoir bottle of IV drip	Concentrated solution of serum globulins obtained from horses immunized against eastern coral snake venom; bitten area should be completely immobilized; first several milliliters of antivenin should be administered over a 5-minute period and patient carefully observed for evidence of allergic reaction; up to 10 vials have been required in some persons with severe or multiple bites; drugs that depress respiration should be used cautiously because snake venom itself produces respiratory depression and paralysis; test for sensitivity to horse serum prior to injecting.

(continued)

* See also Table 81-8.

Table 81-3 (continued)
Antitoxins/Antivenins

Antitoxin/Antivenin	Preparations	Administration	Clinical Considerations
black widow spider species antivenin (Antivenin *Latrodectus mactans*)	Injection—6000 U/vial with diluent plus vial of normal horse serum for sensitivity testing	Adults and children—2.5 ml reconstituted antivenin IM or 2.5 ml in 10 ml–50 ml saline by IV infusion	Used to treat persons bitten by black widow spider; prompt administration yields most effective results; use of muscle relaxants appears to be most important during early reaction phase; test for sensitivity to horse serum prior to injecting.

Antitoxins

diphtheria antitoxin	Injection—10,000 or 20,000 U/vial	Adults and children— 20,000 U–120,000 U IM or slow IV infusion depending on severity and duration of infection; repeat in 24 hours if clinical improvement is not apparent. Prophylaxis—10,000 U IM if sensitivity test is negative	Concentrated solution of purified globulins obtained from the serum of horses immunized against diphtheria toxin; delay in beginning therapy increases dosage requirements and reduces beneficial effects; continue treatment until all symptoms are controlled; appropriate antimicrobial agents should be used concurrently; nonimmunized patients exposed to diphtheria should receive a low dose (see Administration) to produce a temporary passive immunity; sensitivity testing is necessary before administration.
tetanus antitoxin	Injection—1500 U or 20,000 U/vial	Treatment—50,000 U–100,000 U IV or partly IV and the remainder IM Prophylaxis—1500 U–5000 U IM or SC depending on body weight	Concentrated solution of serum globulins from horses immunized against tetanus toxin; indicated *only* when tetanus immune globulin is not available; protection lasts about 2 weeks with a single prophylactic dose; tetanus toxoid, adsorbed, is usually given with the antitoxin to initiate active immunization; most children are routinely immunized against tetanus and the need for the antitoxin seldom occurs.

Table 81-4
Human Immune Serums

Immune Serum	Preparations	Administration	Clinical Considerations
hepatitis B immune globulin (H-BIG, Hep-B-Gammagee, HyperHep)	Injection—1-ml, 4-ml, 5-ml vials	0.06 ml/kg IM as soon after exposure as possible; repeat in 1 month *Prevention of carrier state*—0.5 ml IM no later than 24 hours after birth; repeat in 3 months *Prophylaxis of infants born to HB$_s$Ag-positive mothers*—0.5 ml IM at birth, and again at 3 months and 6 months	Solution of immunoglobulins containing a high titer of antibodies to hepatitis B surface antigen (HB$_s$Ag); indicated for prophylaxis following accidental oral, parenteral, or direct mucous membrane exposure to antigen-containing materials such as blood or serum; also for prophylaxis of infants born to HB$_s$Ag-positive mothers who are at risk of being infected or becoming chronic carriers; may be given at the same time or up to 1 month preceding hepatitis B vaccine without altering the resultant immune response; solution should be stored at 2°C–8°C but not frozen.
immune globulin—intramuscular (ISG) (gamma globulin, Gamastan, Gammar, Immuglobin)	Injection—2-ml, 10-ml vials	*IM injection only* Hepatitis A—0.02 ml/kg Immunoglobulin deficiency—1.3 ml/kg initially, then 0.66 ml/kg every 3 weeks–4 weeks Measles—0.2 ml/kg (do *not* give with measles *vaccine*) Rubella—0.55 ml/kg (pregnant women only) Varicella—0.6 ml–1.2 ml/kg (only if zoster immune globulin is unavailable)	Solution of globulins obtained from pooled human serum, containing antibodies to a number of organisms; used to decrease the severity of certain diseases (hepatitis, measles, varicella) in persons exposed to an active infection; also indicated as replacement therapy for immunoglobulin deficiency states; may be of benefit in pregnant women exposed to rubella virus to lessen possibility of fetal damage, but routine use in early pregnancy cannot be justified; injections can be very painful.
immune globulin, intravenous (Gamimune N, Gammagard, Sandoglobulin)	Injection—5% (in 10% maltose) Powder for injection—1-g, 2.5-g, 3-g, 5-g, and 6-g vials with diluent	*IV infusion only:* 100 mg/kg–300 mg/kg once a month by IV infusion (0.01 ml/kg–0.04 ml/kg/min for 30 minutes) *Idiopathic thrombocytopenic purpura*—400 mg/kg for 5 consecutive days	Provides immediate antibody levels; half-life is approximately 3 weeks; preferred to immune globulin, IM, in patients requiring rapid increase in IgG antibodies, in patients with a small muscle mass, and in patients with bleeding tendencies; maltose or sucrose is added to stabilize the *(continued)*

Table 81-4 (continued)
Human Immune Serums

Immune Serum	Preparations	Administration	Clinical Considerations
immune globulin, intravenous (Gamimune N, Gammagard, Sandoglobulin) (continued)			protein, reducing the incidence of adverse effects; may cause a precipitous drop in blood pressure, especially at rapid infusion rates; monitor vital signs carefully during infusion; have epinephrine available for allergic reactions.
lymphocyte immune globulin—antithymocyte globulin (Atgam)	Injection—50 mg/ml	IV infusion only (over 4 hours–8 hours) Adults—10 mg/kg–30 mg/kg/day Children—5 mg/kg–25 mg/kg/day Drug is usually given daily for 14 days, then every other day for a total of 21 doses	A lymphocyte-selective immunosuppressant that reduces the number of circulating, thymus-dependent lymphocytes; used by experienced personnel only for management of allograft rejection in renal transplant patients and as an adjunct to other immunosuppressive therapy to delay onset of first rejection; discontinue if anaphylaxis or severe thrombocytopenia or leukopenia occurs; frequently encountered adverse reactions are fever, chills, rash, pruritus, urticaria, leukopenia, and mild thrombocytopenia; drug must be diluted in saline before infusion; do not dilute with dextrose solutions or highly acidic solutions, because precipitation can occur; a dose should not be infused in less than 4 hours; have resuscitative materials available (e.g., epinephrine, antihistamines, steroids, and so forth); injection solution should be kept refrigerated but not frozen; following dilution, use within 12 hours.
tetanus immune globulin (Homo-Tet, Hu-Tet, Hyper-Tet)	Injection—250 U/vial or disposable syringe	Treatment—500 U–6000 U IM Prophylaxis—250 U–500 U IM	Usually indicated for passive tetanus prophylaxis in persons not actively immunized or whose immunization status is uncertain; not generally necessary if person has had at least two doses of tetanus toxoid; produces effective levels of circulat- (continued)

Table 81-4 (continued)
Human Immune Serums

Immune Serum	Preparations	Administration	Clinical Considerations
tetanus immune globulin (Homo-Tet, Hu-Tet, Hyper-Tet) (continued)			ing antibodies for much longer periods of time than tetanus antitoxin; does *not* interfere with immune response to tetanus toxoid given at the same time; thorough cleansing of wounds and removal of all foreign particles are important to prevent infection; do *not* inject IV; store injection solution between 2°C and 8°C.
Rh₀ (D) immune (Gamulin Rh, HypRho-D, Rho-GAM)	Injection—vial with diluent	Inject contents of 1 vial IM for every 15 ml fetal packed red cell volume within 72 hours following delivery, miscarriage, abortion, or transfusion (See package instructions for mixing and injecting directions)	Used to prevent sensitization in a subsequent pregnancy to the Rh₀(D) factor in an Rh-negative mother who gave birth to an Rh-positive infant by an Rh-positive father; also may be employed to prevent Rh₀(D) sensitization in Rh-negative patients accidentally transfused with Rh-positive blood; consult product information for blood typing and drug administration procedures; do not give IV; also available *(continued)*

Alteration in tissue perfusion related to a severe hypersensitivity reaction
Alteration in comfort: Pain at injection site
Hyperthermia related to febrile reaction to the vaccine or serum

□ *PLAN*

Nursing care goals focus on
1. Safe, correct drug administration
2. Teaching the patient and family the side-effects to monitor during the first 24 hours to 48 hours

□ *INTERVENTION*

Once the immunization is judged appropriate by the health team, the patient's or parent's informed consent must be obtained. The potential side-effects of the immunization must be explained in light of the benefits of the drug. Literature may be made available in advance but the physician or nurse should explain how immunizations protect the child and the community from communicable diseases. Parents with small children may express some concern about the value of the DTP series of shots since recent media attention has focused on the adverse neurologic reactions of several toddlers to the pertussis component. The risk of a small child dying of pertussis is ten times greater than the risk of developing encephalitis or brain damage (secondary to the vaccine). However, the parent will make a judgment on accepting immunization for the child. The health-care team can only provide information.

Societal pressure to conform to a standardized immunization schedule exists in the form of school admission standards. Most nursery schools, day-

Table 81-4 (continued)
Human Immune Serums

Immune Serum	Preparations	Administration	Clinical Considerations
Rh_o (D) immune (Gamulin Rh, HypRho-D, RhoGAM) (continued)			in microdose form (MICRhoGAM, Mini-Gamulin Rh) to prevent maternal Rh-immunization following miscarriage or abortion up to 12-weeks' gestation unless father is Rh-negative; beyond 13 weeks' gestation, Rh_o (D) immune globulin is used.
varicella-zoster immune globulin (human)—VZIG	Injection—10%–18% solution of the globulin fraction of human plasma containing 125 U of antibody to varicella-zoster virus in a single-dose vial	IM injection only: 125 U/10 kg body weight, to a maximum of 625 U; do not give fractional units	Globulin fraction of adult human plasma (primarily immunoglobulin G) with high titer of varicella-zoster antibodies; used for passive immunization of immunodeficient children following exposure to varicella; most effective if given within 96 hours after exposure; not indicated prophylactically; do not administer IV; no more than 2.5 ml should be injected at a single IM site (1.25 ml maximum if patient weighs less than 10 kg); VZIG must be requested from regional distribution centers of American Red Cross Blood Services.

care centers, and kindergartens require children to have completed certain immunizations before they are admitted. The recommended schedule of immunizations is listed in Table 81-6. Table 81-7 shows an immunization schedule for children not inoculated at recommended intervals during infancy.

Administration of vaccines and toxoids is by intramuscular or subcutaneous injection (see individual drugs). The site chosen for injection should have sufficient muscle mass to reduce pain and swelling. When injections known to be painful are given the site used should be one least likely to affect the patient's mobility. For example, a tetanus toxoid injection should be given in a deltoid site in the nondominant arm in older children and adults. DTP vaccine is usually given in the vastus lateralis of the thigh in small children but may reduce mo-

bility of the leg if the reaction is severe. See Chapter 8 for a complete discussion on administering injections.

Patients may call health-care providers when planning travel to foreign countries to determine the necessity of receiving certain vaccines. Information about vaccine requirements may be obtained from the local health department or from a pamphlet prepared by the Centers for Disease Control entitled *Health Information for International Travel*, distributed by the Superintendent of Documents, U.S. Government Printing Office, Washington, D.C. 20402.

The most serious side-effect from most vaccines and toxoids is a hypersensitivity reaction. Local reactions may include pain, swelling, urticaria, and rash around the site and are usually self-limiting. They may be treated with antihistamines

Table 81-5
Rabies Prophylaxis Products

Drug	Preparations	Administration	Clinical Considerations
antirabies serum, equine (ARS)	Injection—125 units/ml	40 U/kg (1000 U/55 lb) IM in a single dose. Usually given together with HDVC, although not at the same site nor in the same syringe	Used in conjunction with HDVC (see below) to promote passive immunity to rabies when rabies immune globulin is unavailable; delays propagation of virus, thus allowing time for rabies vaccine to induce sufficient antibodies; give as soon as possible after exposure; sensitivity testing (intradermal or conjunctival) should be done before administration; up to 50% of the dose should be infiltrated into the tissue around the wound; adverse reactions include local pain, erythema, and urticaria and occasionally serum sickness.
rabies immune globulin, human—RIG (Hyperab, Imogam)	Injection—150 U/ml	20 U/kg (9.1 U/lb) at the time of the initial HDVC dose; give ½ the dose IM and ½ the dose to infiltrate the wound	Used to provide rabies antibodies immediately; given in conjunction with rabies vaccine; should be given as soon as possible following exposure, but regardless of interval, immune globulin is still recommended; do not give repeated doses once vaccine has been administered; side-effects include local tenderness or soreness and low-grade fever.
rabies vaccine, human diploid cell cultures— HDVC (Imovax)	Injection—single dose lyophilized preparation with diluent; contains 2.5 units rabies antigen/ml	Preexposure—3 injections, IM, of 1.0 ml each on days 0, 7, and 21 or 28. Boosters—every 2 years in high-risk individuals. Postexposure—5 injections, IM, of 1.0 ml each on days 0, 3, 7, 14, and 28 with a dose of rabies immune globulin on day 0	Preferred rabies vaccine due to greater efficacy and safety compared to duck embryo vaccine; antibody response is virtually 100% with recommended 5 doses; preexposure vaccination is indicated for persons in contact with rabid animals or patients or those handling rabies virus or contaminated articles; post-exposure treatment should also include rabies immune globulin; adverse reactions to vaccine are infrequent; local swelling and erythema have occurred; corticosteroids and other immunosuppressive agents can interfere with development of active immunity to vaccine; do not administer together.

Table 81-6
Recommended Schedule for Active Immunization
of Normal Infants and Children

Recommended Age	Immunization(s)	Comments
2 months	DTP*, OPV†	Can be initiated as early as 2 weeks of age in areas of high endemicity or during epidemics
4 months	DTP, OPV	2-month interval desired for OPV to avoid interference from previous dose
6 months	DTP (OPV)	OPV is optional (may be given in areas with increased risk of poliovirus exposure)
15 months	Measles, mumps, rubella (MMR)‡	MMR preferred to individual vaccines; tuberculin testing may be done
18 months	DTP§,‖ OPV‖	
24 months	HBPV#	
4 years–6 years**	DTP, OPV	At or before school entry
14 years–16 years	Td††	Repeat every 10 years throughout life

* DTP—Diphtheria and tetanus toxoids with pertussis vaccine
† OPV—Oral, poliovirus vaccine contains attenuated poliovirus types 1, 2, and 3
‡ MMR—Live measles, mumps, and rubella viruses in a combined vaccine
§ Should be given 6 to 12 months after the third dose
‖ May be given simultaneously with MMR at 15 months of age
Hemophilus b polysaccharide vaccine
** Up to the seventh birthday
†† Td—Adult tetanus toxoid (full dose) and diphtheria toxoid (reduced dose) in combination
For all products used, consult manufacturer's package insert for instructions for storage, handling, and administration. Biologics prepared by different manufacturers may vary, and those of the same manufacturer may change from time to time. Therefore, the physician should be aware of the contents of the package insert.
(Report of the Committee on Infectious Diseases, American Academy of Pediatrics, 20th ed, p 9. Copyright American Academy of Pediatrics, 1986)

and acetaminophen or aspirin. Systemic reactions are extremely rare but may occur in patients allergic to the components used in making the drug. Sensitivity tests may be done on such patients to determine the potential for reaction, and desensitizing doses or divided doses may be given to attempt to avert anaphylaxis if the immunization is considered essential. However, such a patient should be inoculated only under direct supervision and should be closely monitored for increased blood pressure, respiratory distress, flushing, and angioedema. Emergency resuscitative equipment including oxygen, intubation, and tracheostomy equipment and mechanical ventilation, as well as emergency drugs such as epinephrine, corticosteroids, and vasopressors, should be on hand.

The most common reactions to immunizations are low-grade fever (101°F or less) and injection site pain. Acetaminophen (for children) and aspirin (for adults only) may be used every 4 hours to re-

Table 81-7
Recommended Immunization Schedules for Children
Not Immunized in First Year of Life

Recommended Time	Immunization(s)	Comments
Less Than 7 Years Old		
First visit	DTP, OPV, MMR	MMR if child ≥ 15 months old; tuberculin testing may be done
Interval after first visit		
1 month	HBPV*	For children 24 months–60 months
2 months	DTP, OPV	
4 months	DTP (OPV)	OPV is optional (may be given in areas with increased risk of poliovirus exposure)
10–16 months	DTP, OPV	OPV is not given if third dose was given earlier
Age 4 years–6 years (at or before school entry)	DTP, OPV	DTP is not necessary if the fourth dose was given after the fourth birthday; OPV is not necessary if recommended OPV dose at 10 months–16 months following first visit was given after the fourth birthday
Age 14 years–16 years	Td	Repeat every 10 years throughout life
7 Years Old and Older		
First visit	Td, OPV, MMR	
Interval after first visit		
2 months	Td, OPV	
8–14 months	Td, OPV	
Age 14 years–16 years	Td	Repeat every 10 years throughout life

* *Hemophilus* b polysaccharide vaccine can be given, if necessary, simultaneously with DTP (at separate sites). The initial three doses of DTP can be given at 1- to 2-month intervals; so, for the child in whom immunization is initiated at 24 months old or older, one visit could be eliminated by giving DTP, OPV, MMR at the first visit; DTP and HBPV at the second visit (1 month later); and DTP and OPV at the third visit (2 months after the first visit). Subsequent DTP and OPV 10 to 16 months after the first visit are still indicated.
(Report of the Committee on Infectious Diseases, American Academy of Pediatrics, 20th ed, p 11. Copyright American Academy of Pediatrics, 1986)

lieve both. Pediatricians frequently advise parents to begin giving a child acetaminophen within 2 hours of an immunization such as DTP to decrease the risk of fever and minimize pain. When the child or adult receives MMR vaccine he or she should be told to watch for fever and possible mild rash 7 days to 10 days after the vaccine. Although most symptoms are mild and self-limiting, the parent or patient should be told to call immediately if a temperature elevation above 101°F occurs, if pain at the site is severe, or if respiratory flu-like or other symptoms occur. Any persistent symptoms beyond 48 hours should be reported.

Parents of children receiving DTP shots may want to know what neurologic problems can occur as a result of the injection. The incidence of such side-effects is rare but may include fever greater than 102°F, persistent crying or high or unusual pitch, irritability, and periods of limpness. Seizures may occur, usually as a result of high fever. Encephalopathy and permanent brain damage have occurred but are extremely rare.

☐ *EVALUATION*

Outcome criteria that may judge success include verbalization by the parent (or adult) of the need for immunizations and return to clinic for immunizations as scheduled; minimal side-effects or adequate management of side-effects by family; absence of hypersensitivity reactions; and effective immunity against diseases for which inoculation was administered. The nursing process for the child receiving a vaccine is summarized in Nursing Care Plan 81-1.

PATIENTS RECEIVING ANTITOXINS/ ANTIVENINS

All antivenins and antitoxins are developed from horse serum. Therefore, any patient allergic to horses or who lists multiple allergies should have a sensitivity test performed before these drugs are given. Sensitivity testing may be intradermal injection, skin scratch, or conjunctival scratch of small amounts of normal horse serum. Reactions may range from local redness and swelling to generalized urticaria, angioedema, and anaphylaxis to the sensitivity test.

The decision to treat the patient in spite of sensitivity may be made in light of the risks of severe reaction or death from the bite or from the disease.

Desensitizing doses of the drugs may gradually be given if necessary. However, in all cases, antitoxins and antivenins work best when given as soon as possible after the event is diagnosed to minimize escalation of symptoms and lingering side-effects. The amount of drug given depends on the severity of symptoms, number of bites, and size of the person, or in the case of snakebite, the size of the snake known. The child or small-statured adult may actually require higher doses of antivenins than a larger adult because the amount of venom is distributed over a smaller body weight. Allergic reactions and serum sickness may occur several hours or days to weeks after therapy and is frequently related to the amount of drug administered. Epinephrine and emergency respiratory equipment must be available while the drugs are infusing to respond to the respiratory depression that may occur as a result of allergic reaction. The patient should be told to report any swelling lymph glands, skin rash, fever, or joint or muscle pain after treatment is completed, which are symptoms of serum sickness.

Identifying the symptoms of an allergic reaction to the drugs may be difficult since many of the symptoms of venom poisoning or toxin reaction are similar to those of anaphylaxis. The health-care team needs to identify the patient's symptoms clearly before drug therapy is initiated and to compare those to symptoms exhibited once drug therapy is started. Symptoms of anaphylaxis are usually sudden in onset and revolve around the respiratory, cardiovascular, and integumentary systems, whereas symptoms of snake or spider bites, tetanus, and diphtheria have a much wider range. Table 81-8 lists the symptoms of the various snake and spider bites, tetanus, and diphtheria, and outlines some specific supportive therapies that may be used.

All patients must be closely monitored. The frequency and amount of drug given will depend on response of symptoms to the drug. Improvement is the best method by which to judge if the drug is working. However, supportive care, especially for respiratory and general muscle weakness, may be prolonged even after other symptoms have subsided.

PATIENTS RECEIVING RABIES PROPHYLAXIS PRODUCTS

See Table 81-5. The patient who appears for emergency treatment after being bitten by an animal is usually frightened by the experience, and if he knows anything about the treatment he is frightened by the prospect of multiple painful injections. Therefore, it is essential that the health team determine the risk of rabies infection before the decision is made to treat the patient with a prophylaxis regimen.

Factors used to determine the risk of infection include prevalence of the infection in the geographic area, type of animal bite, nature of the attack, and type of wound. The danger of rabies infection is most prevalent in bites from dogs, cats, skunks, raccoons, bats, coyotes, and bobcats. Although people are usually equally afraid of bites by rats, mice, squirrels, hamsters, gerbils, chipmunks, and rabbits there has been no known transmission of rabies by these animals in the United States in recent years. However, the best way to determine the risk is to catch the animal and test it for rabies. If this cannot be accomplished the next factor to consider is the nature of the attack. An unprovoked attack is more likely to be rabid. However, attempted feeding or interruption of feeding is considered provocation. The last element to consider is

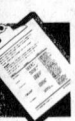

Subjective Data	1. Medication history
	  a. History of allergies to substances used in vaccine preparation (see package inserts for additives in specific products)
	  b. Reactions to previous immunization, particularly pertinent with pertussis vaccine
	  c. Use of immunosuppressive drugs, antimicrobials, anticonvulsants, and blood or blood products give clues to diseases that may be contraindications for concurrent immunization
	2. Medical history
	  a. Preexisting conditions that may contraindicate immunization, such as neurological disease, immune system disease such as AIDS, leukemia, or lymphoma, malignancy, and pregnancy
	  b. Presence of acute febrile illness, such as respiratory infection or gastroenteritis
	  c. Chronic disease for which some immunizations are recommended, such as heart and pulmonary disease, renal disorder, diabetes, debilitating illness
	3. Personal history/compliance: Child's schedule of immunizations, parent's concern about immunization, family finances, and access to health facilities. These factors may influence compliance with future recommended immunizations.

Objective Data	1. Physical assessment highlighting
	  a. Temperature
	  b. Acute febrile illness
	  c. Neurologic behavioral data
	2. Laboratory data
	  a. CBC with differential for child with potential for immunosuppression
	  b. PPD prior to BCG administration

Nursing Diagnosis	Expected Client Outcome	Intervention
Knowledge deficit related to drug effect and side-effects	Will verbalize knowledge of purpose and schedule of immunization.	Teach purpose of each immunization. Obtain written and verbal informed consent. Teach data of recommended return to health facility for future immunization. Instruct parents to maintain clear records of child's immunization for future reference and school records.
	Will verbalize knowledge of common side-effects and their treatment.	Teach common side-effects for each immunization. Teach treatment for side-effects such as use of cold on injection site, use of analgesics, comfort measures.
	Will differentiate common side-effects from rare, serious side-effects.	State manifestation, occurrence, and incidence of rare, serious side-effects. Teach family to contact a health facility immediately for serious side-effects. Answer questions and concerns related to potential serious effects of immunization. Contrast risks of immunization with risks of the diseases they prevent. *(continued)*

Nursing Diagnosis	Expected Client Outcome	Intervention
Anxiety related to injection	Child will verbalize anxiety related to injection.	State purpose of immunization. Allow verbalization of fears. Allow child to make some choices if old enough (*i.e.*, which arm to use, reward to receive after injection). Allow crying.
	Injection will be received with minimal psychological and physical trauma.	Restrain child securely. Explain procedure concisely and clearly. Allow comfort following procedure (*i.e.*, parent holding, bandage, reward such as sticker or balloon). Praise child for bravery and behavior.
Potential alteration in respiratory function and tissue perfusion related to a severe hypersensitivity reaction	Child will be free of hypersensitivity reaction.	Examine allergy history. Have epinephrine 1:1000 and other emergency drugs and equipment immediately available. Have written protocols for dosages of emergency drugs if administering immunizations in a clinic without a physician present. Observe child for several minutes following immunization administration.
Potential alteration in comfort: pain at injection site	Child will experience minimal pain and discomfort.	Instruct parents in administration and dosage of analgesic (usually acetaminophen). Encourage other comfort measures such as holding child, avoiding constricting clothing on injection site, and applying a cool cloth to a reddened injection site.
Potential hyperthermia related to febrile reaction to the vaccine	Child will have temperature within the normal range.	Instruct parents in administration and dosage of antipyretic (usually acetaminophen). Instruct parents in other temperature-reducing measures such as limiting clothing, lowering room temperature, and giving baths in tepid water.

the degree of penetration into the skin by the animal's teeth and saliva. An open wound, one with deep penetration, or one where animal saliva is present is more likely to be contaminated.

The wound should be vigorously scrubbed with soapy water and an antiseptic solution such as benzalkonium chloride (Zephiran), and a deep wound may be flushed with a syringe containing antiseptic. A decision to treat should be made as soon as possible since the incubation period for rabies is 20 days to 60 days although symptoms may start sooner. Once the decision is made to treat the patient for rabies, a dose of RIG will be given. One half the dose will be used to infiltrate the wound and the other half will be given IM. HDVC, 1.0 ml, will also be given IM at the same time in a different syringe. HDVC will be given again on days 3, 7, 14, and 28 after exposure. Sites should be rotated with each injection using any site with adequate muscle mass including the deltoid, vastus lateralis, and ventral gluteal area. Warm or cool compresses can be used to reduce injection site pain.

Table 81-8
Symptoms of Various Toxins and Venoms and Supportive Care

Venom/Toxin	Onset of Symptoms	Symptoms	Specific Supportive Care*
black widow spider venom	15 minutes–several hours	Paralysis and destruction of the peripheral nerves leading to pain, weakness and spasm of thigh, shoulder, and back muscles initially but progressing to abdomen and thorax, leading to respiratory distress, nausea, vomiting, restlessness, hypotension, tachycardia, and pallor, which can lead to shock or coma	Warm baths to alleviate spasms Calcium gluconate 10% IV for spasms Analgesia and sedation for pain and anxiety but must monitor for signs of respiratory distress and hypotension
Crotalidae (pit viper) venom	Within 5 minutes	Local edema around bite, which spreads along the affected extremity, gradually producing ecchymosis, vesicles, hemorrhagic blebs, and petechiae Systemic symptoms include numbness and tingling in face, scalp, toes, fingers, and bite site; muscle spasms; alterations in clotting time resulting in multiple bleeding sites such as hematuria, hematemesis, epistaxis, melena, and pulmonary edema from capillary destruction leading to respiratory arrest; hypotension, which may lead to shock	Tetanus prophylaxis Monitor urine for cells, blood for clotting time, and monitor progression of edema since changes in these parameters indicate the need for more drug. Analgesia and sedation for pain but must monitor for signs of respiratory distress; frequent vital signs
North American coral snake toxin	1 hour–7 hours	Local mild to moderate edema, pain, redness, and paresthesia at bite site	Tetanus prophylaxis; frequent vital signs; monitor closely for respiratory *(continued)*

Table 81-8 (continued)
Symptoms of Various Toxins and Venoms and Supportive Care

Venom/Toxin	Onset of Symptoms	Symptoms	Specific Supportive Care*
North American coral snake toxin (*continued*)		Systemic responses include nausea, vomiting, salivation, cranial nerve dysfunction, abnormal reflexes, and generalized motor weakness, which may progress to respiratory paralysis.	distress and keep analgesia at a minimum.
diphtheria toxin	2 days–4 days after exposure	Sore throat, fever, extreme weakness, cough, difficulty swallowing Inflammation of the oropharynx with thin, patchy red exudate (early), which changes to a thick gray membrane within hours Oropharyngeal and laryngeal swelling can lead to respiratory distress. Myocarditis characterized by hypotension and arrhythmias may occur.	Monitor respiration, speech, and swallowing as indicators of increasing oropharyngeal edema. Have emergency equipment available. Antibiotic therapy with penicillin or erythromycin in addition to antitoxin therapy
tetanus toxin	3 days–21 days but can occur within 24 hours	Jaw stiffness (trismus) and stiffness of the muscles of the throat and tongue causing difficulty in speech and swallowing; painful tonic contractions of voluntary muscles, which can cause anoxia and death if prolonged since respiratory muscle action will be limited	Try to give antitoxin before symptoms begin for best results; penicillin will be given; diazepam for muscle spasm. Pancuronium may be given to induce respiratory paralysis; then artificial respiration is provided until acute tetanus toxicity passes.

* See also text.

CASE STUDY

Steven Michaels, aged 18 months, is brought to the pediatrician's office by his mother to receive a well-baby check-up, OPV vaccine, and his fourth DTP shot. Steven is getting over an upper respiratory infection that started 7 days ago. Mrs. Michaels says he still has a runny nose but no other symptoms.

Discussion Questions

1. What data should be collected before Steven receives these vaccines?
2. What information should Mrs. Michaels receive about monitoring Steven after he receives the two vaccines?
3. Steven wakes up from his afternoon nap crying and refuses to stand on his left leg, the one where the shot was given. Mrs. Michaels calls the physician for advice. What information should she be given?

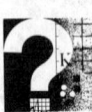

REVIEW QUESTIONS

1. Distinguish between natural and acquired immunity.
2. What types of products may be used to confer (1) *active* immunity and (2) *passive* immunity?
3. What are toxoids? How do they differ from vaccines?
4. How may the available vaccines be categorized?
5. What are the most frequently encountered side-effects with viral vaccines?
6. Why should immunosuppressed patients not receive live virus vaccines?
7. What information should be provided to a parent before asking for consent to administer a vaccine to a child?
8. What should a parent be taught to monitor when a child receives a vaccine? What actions should the parent take if symptoms develop?
9. What are immune serums? How do they differ from antitoxins?
10. What procedure should be performed before administering an antitoxin?
11. What are the various types of rabies prophylaxis products? Which are used for (1) passive immunization and (2) active immunization?
12. What factors are reviewed when determining whether to initiate rabies prophylaxis?
13. How should a wound from a potentially rabid animal be treated?
14. List the various toxoids available for clinical use.
15. What cautions must be observed with use of diphtheria and tetanus toxoids and pertussis vaccine (DTP)?
16. What data should be collected from any patient about to receive a DTP shot?
17. For what age group is hemophilus B vaccine recommended?
18. What are the indications for pneumococcal vaccine?
19. Describe the two types of hepatitis B vaccine.
20. Distinguish between the composition of monovalent versus trivalent influenza virus vaccine.

21. What are the various types of "high-risk" patients to whom the influenza virus vaccine should be given?
22. In which children is the injectable polio virus vaccine recommended over the oral form?
23. What are the indications for hepatitis B immune globulin?
24. Give the principal use for lymphocyte immune globulin.
25. How is $Rh_o(D)$ immune globulin utilized?
26. What is the preferred rabies vaccine?

BIBLIOGRAPHY

Austrian R: A reassessment of pneumococcal vaccine. N Engl J Med 310:651, 1984
Bernard KW et al: Human diploid cell rabies vaccine. JAMA 247:1138, 1982
Fulginite VA: Immunization. In Kempe CH, Silver HK, O'Brien D (eds): Current Pediatric Diagnosis and Treatment, 8th ed. Los Altos, Lange Medical Publications, 1984
Gurevich J: Viral hepatitis. Am J Nurs 83(4):571, 1983
Halpern JS: Rabies vaccine: Reduced risks and fears. Journal of Emergency Nursing 10(2):101, 1984
Immunization Practices Advisory Committee: Monovalent influenza A (H1N1) vaccine, 1986–1987. MMWR 35:517, 1986
Immunization Practices Advisory Committee: Prevention and control of influenza. MMWR 35:317, 1986
Kirkman-Liff B, Dandoy S: Hepatitis B: What price exposure? Am J Nurs 84:988, 1984
Nichols AO: Taking the fear out of rabies treatment. Nursing 83 13(6):42, June, 1983
Robbins JB, Hill JC, Sadoff JC: Bacterial Vaccines. New York, Thieme-Stratton, 1987
Williams A: Hepatitis B virus vaccine. Nurse Pract 8:30, 1983

Prostaglandins and Other Eicosanoids

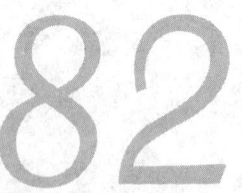

Prostaglandins are a family of 20-carbon essential fatty acids found in every major organ and body fluid and capable of eliciting a wide range of physiologic effects. They are produced in response to an extremely wide diversity of stimuli and in very minute amounts can markedly alter the functioning of most bodily organs. In addition to the prostaglandins, other structurally related biologically active lipids may be derived from the same precursors as the prostaglandins. These other lipids include the thromboxanes, leukotrienes, hydroperoxyeicosatetraenoic acids (HPETEs) and hydroxyeicosatetraenoic acids (HETEs). Collectively, these lipid families, including the prostaglandins, have been termed "eicosanoids," because they all derive from the same eicosaenoic acid precursors.

In the 1930s, several laboratories described the uterine smooth muscle-contracting action of human semen, and somewhat later, the active material was identified as a lipid-soluble acid and named *prostaglandin* because it was assumed that it was derived from prostate gland secretions. Many years later, *prostaglandin* was in fact shown to be a family of substances of similar structures and the first two crystalline compounds to be isolated were termed prostaglandin E (PGE) and prostaglandin F (PGF). In time, other prostaglandins were characterized so that today, there are at least nine groups recognized and they are designated by the letters of the alphabet A through I.

In the mid 1970s, a substance released by aggregating platelets was shown to be derived from the same precursors as the prostaglandins. This substance contained a different ring structure (*i.e.*, oxane), however, and was given the name *thromboxane*. Other substances structurally related to prostaglandins, but formed by way of an alternate enzymatic pathway (see Fig. 82-1), are the leukotrienes, HPETEs, and HETEs mentioned above.

Synthesis of the Eicosanoids

Eicosanoids are synthesized at a cellular membrane level in response to a variety of stimuli. Arachidonic acid is the principal precursor for the eicosanoids and is derived from the diet. Arachidonate is esterified and forms a component of the phospholipids in cell membranes. In response to various hormonal, chemical, or mechanical stimuli, enzymes such as phospholipase are activated and result in cleavage of arachidonic acid from the glycerophospholipids that comprise part of the lipid bilayer of cellular membranes. Upon its release, arachidonic acid is acted upon by various enzyme systems, depending on the particular type of cell involved, and is converted ultimately to one of the eicosanoids.

The overall scheme of eicosanoid synthesis is presented in Figure 82-1. Upon cleavage from membrane phospholipids, arachidonic acid may be acted upon by two primary groups of enzymes, *cyclooxygenases* and *lipooxygenases*. Cyclooxygenase converts arachidonic acid into the highly unstable intermediates PGG_2 and PGH_2, which display half-lives under 5 minutes. These substances are termed "cyclic endoperoxides" and are rapidly changed to one of several groups of prostaglandins (PGD_2, PGE_2, PGF_2, PGI_2) by the action of various enzymes as indicated in Figure 82-1. In addition, thromboxane A_2 (TXA_2) is also synthesized from the cyclic endoperoxides. The prostaglandins E can be converted further into prostaglandins A, B, and C during chemical extraction procedures, but formation of PGA, PGB, or PGC is probably of minimal importance biologically.

The formation of PGI_2, also known as prostacyclin, occurs as a result of the action of the enzyme prostacyclin synthetase on PGH_2 and occurs primarily in vascular endothelium. PGI_2 is also a very unstable compound, with a half-life of 3 minutes to 4 minutes. PGH_2 is also converted to thromboxane A_2 (TXA_2) by the action of the enzyme thromboxane synthetase, and this reaction is largely limited to the platelet cell. TXA_2 is an extremely short-lived substance (half-life of 30 seconds) and is quickly converted to the stable but inactive thromboxane B_2 (TXB_2).

Another group of enzymes known as lipooxygenases interact with free arachidonic acid in cells to form hydroperoxyeicosatetraenoic acids (HPETEs) which are then further converted to hydroxyeicosatetraenoic acids (HETEs) or leukotrienes. The most important of these lipooxygenases is 5-lipooxygenase, which converts arachidonic acid into 5-HPETE, which in turn is acted upon by a dehydrase enzyme to form leukotriene A_4 (LTA_4). LTA_4 is then transformed by different enzymes into either leukotriene B_4 (LTB_4) or leukotriene C_4 (LTC_4). LTC_4 may then be converted sequentially into leukotrienes D_4, E_4, and F_4. It is now known that a mixture of LTC_4 and LTD_4 is the substance that was previously known as the "slow-reacting substance of anaphylaxis" (SRS-A), an endogenous allergen contained within bronchiolar mast cells (see Pharmacologic Effects of Eicosanoids, below).

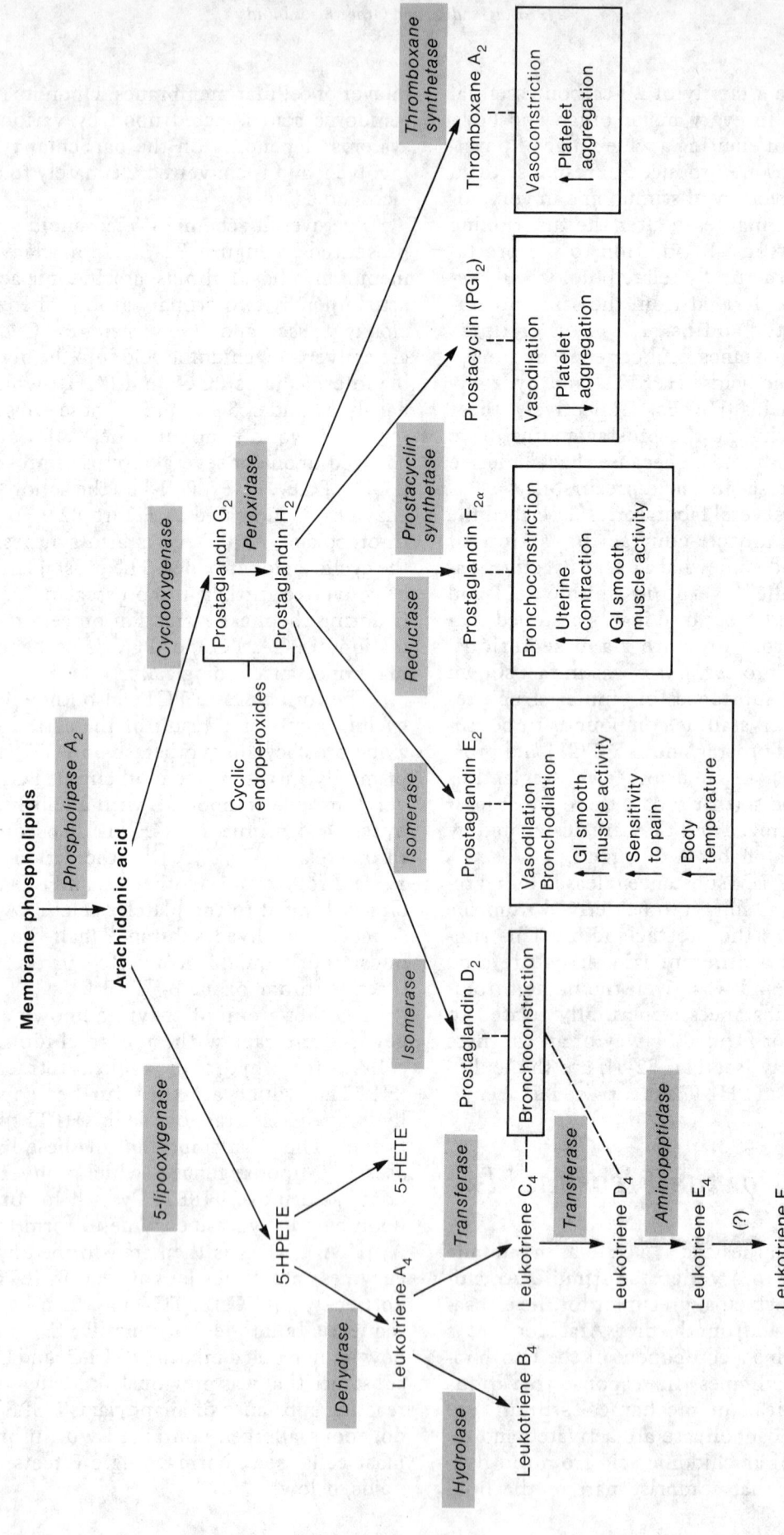

Figure 82-1. *Synthesis of eicosanoids and their principal pharmacologic actions. See text for a more detailed discussion.*

Synthesis of the various eicosanoids varies among different tissues in the body. While most tissues appear capable of forming PGG_2 and PGH_2, the cyclic endoperoxides, from arachidonic acid, subsequent metabolism to the different prostaglandins or thromboxanes is dependent on the presence of enzymes in specific tissues. For example, lung and spleen appear to be able to synthesize the whole range of products, whereas blood vessel walls synthesize primarily PGI_2 and platelets form mainly TXA_2.

Inhibition of Eicosanoid Formation

Several different drug groups have been shown to interfere at various stages with the synthesis of different eicosanoids. Corticosteroids enhance formation of a protein that can inhibit the activity of phospholipases, thereby preventing the initial cleavage and release of arachidonic acid from the membrane phospholipids. These drugs can therefore reduce formation of *all* eicosanoids.

Aspirin and the nonsteroidal anti-inflammatory drugs (*e.g.*, ibuprofen, indomethacin, naproxen, piroxicam) inhibit cyclooxygenase activity and thus block synthesis of prostaglandins and thromboxane. However, these drugs do *not* block the lipooxygenase pathway. In fact, inhibition of cyclooxygenase can lead to *increased* formation of leukotrienes presumably by making more arachidonic acid available for lipooxygenases.

As indicated in Figure 82-1, different eicosanoids produce different, and in some instances, opposing pharmacologic effects. For example, PGE_2 is a bronchodilator, while PGD_2 and PGF_2 are bronchoconstrictors. PGI_2 (prostacyclin) is a vasodilator and inhibits platelet aggregation, whereas TXA_2 is a vasoconstrictor and facilitates platelet aggregation. Therefore, development of *selective inhibitors*, which would interfere with the formation of individual prostaglandins, would be a significant contribution toward eliminating undesirable effects (*e.g.* platelet aggregation, bronchoconstriction) and maximizing desirable ones, such as bronchodilation or reduced platelet aggregation. In this regard, imidazole derivatives, such as dazoxiben, have shown promise as selective inhibitors of TXA_2 synthesis. Other substances may interfere with the interaction of individual prostaglandins or thromboxanes at the tissue receptor sites.

Pharmacokinetics of Eicosanoids

The naturally occurring eicosanoids are relatively short-acting substances which are rapidly inactivated by enzymes present on many body tissues, including the spleen, kidney, plasma, liver, intestines, and adipose tissue. The half-life of most prostaglandins in the plasma is less than 1 minute. Eicosanoid metabolites are excreted largely in the urine.

Pharmacologic Effects of Eicosanoids

Prostaglandins and related eicosanoids exhibit a wide spectrum of effects on the body. Moreover, different compounds may display different activities, both qualitatively and quantitatively, depending on their tissue site of action. The following discussion will focus on the more important actions of the various eicosanoids on different body organs.

Mechanisms of Action

Prostaglandins appear to regulate the formation of cyclic AMP and cyclic GMP by activating or inhibiting enzymes necessary for their synthesis. This action is believed to result from an interaction of the prostaglandins (or related eicosanoids) on specific membrane-bound receptors on various body tissues. Further, these receptors are *not* blocked by conventional autonomic blocking agents. For example, PGE_2 stimulates formation of steroid hormones in the adrenal cortex by activating the enzyme adenylate cyclase, thereby increasing cyclic AMP formation. Similarly, PGE_2 produces vasodilation, presumably by elevating cyclic AMP levels. On the other hand, vasoconstriction produced by PGF_2 appears to be due to increased levels of cyclic GMP.

Another mechanism of action that has been demonstrated for certain eicosanoids is facilitation of intracellular movement of calcium. For example, the uterine spasmogenic action of PGE_2 is the result of increased calcium influx into myometrial cells. Increased platelet clumping in response to TXA_2 has also been associated with increased release of intracellular calcium. Conversely, platelet aggregation is inhibited by PGI_2 (prostacyclin) due to increased levels of cyclic AMP, which appears to promote calcium sequestration.

Although much interest is centered on development of selective receptor antagonists of the various eicosanoids, there are presently no clinically useful, potent eicosanoid receptor antagonists. Several types of chemical substances have been shown to interfere presumably with eicosanoid receptor activity in selected *in vitro* tests; however, their *in vivo* action remains to be determined. For example, certain prostanoic acid derivatives can selectively antagonize the response of platelets and smooth muscle cells to TXA_2; still other substances have demonstrated an antagonistic action against both PGF_2- and PGD_2-induced bronchoconstriction. Finally, a carboxylic acid derivative is a potent and specific leukotriene antagonist but is of little clinical use because its half-life is only about 30 seconds.

Effects of Eicosanoids on Smooth Muscle

Eicosanoids exhibit diverse effects on smooth muscle, the responses being dependent on factors such as species, location, and type of eicosanoid.

Vascular Smooth Muscle

In most vascular beds, PGE_2, PGI_2, and PGA_2 are vasodilators, especially of the resistance vessels, whereas PGF_2 and TXA_2 generally elicit vasoconstriction. The leukotrienes have little effect on major blood vessels but may exert a constrictive effect on the microvasculature.

Respiratory Smooth Muscle

In general, PGFs contract and PGEs relax tracheal and bronchial smooth muscle. PGI_2 is a bronchodilator, although to a lesser degree than PGE_2. PGD_2 may exert a bronchoconstrictive effect when produced by human lung tissue. TXA_2 is a potent bronchial spasmogen, but its role in physiologically induced bronchospasm is uncertain. Finally, the leukotrienes can result in marked bronchoconstriction, especially in the peripheral airways, and these substances appear to be far more potent than histamine in causing bronchospasm.

Uterine Smooth Muscle

Uterine smooth muscle is uniformly contracted by $PGF_{2\alpha}$, and increased levels of $PGF_{2\alpha}$ in myometrial smooth muscle at the time of menses is responsible for development of uterine cramping or dysmenorrhea. The effects of PGE_2 on the uterus appear to be concentration-dependent, with contraction noted at low levels but relaxation occurring at higher levels. PGI_2 can also relax uterine smooth muscle. Infusion of either PGE_2 or $PGF_{2\alpha}$ to pregnant women elicits a dose-dependent increase in the frequency and intensity of myometrial contraction, and this action has led to their use clinically as abortifacients (see below). The effects of other eicosanoids on uterine contractility are not well established.

Gastrointestinal Smooth Muscle

The responses of GI smooth muscle to eicosanoids vary widely with species, type of muscle, segment of the GI tract, and particular eicosanoid. In general, longitudinal muscle is contracted by PGE_2 and $PGF_{2\alpha}$, whereas circular muscle is contracted by $PGF_{2\alpha}$ but relaxed by PGE_2. PGAs, PGDs, PGI_2, and TXA_2 exhibit little activity on intestinal smooth muscle. Leukotrienes appear to exert a contractile effect on gastrointestinal smooth muscle *in vitro*, although the effect of these agents on human function is less well established.

PGA, PGE_2, and PGI_2 inhibit gastric acid secretion, reducing the volume, acidity, and pepsin content. In addition, they may increase mucus secretion in the stomach and small intestine.

Effects of Eicosanoids on Blood

The two eicosanoids that play principal roles in platelet function are PGI_2 and TXA_2. PGI_2 is synthesized in vascular endothelium and is a powerful inhibitor of platelet aggregation. Conversely, TXA_2 is formed within the platelets and is a potent inducer of platelet aggregation and the platelet-release reaction. Generation of PGI_2 by vascular endothelium plays a principal role in maintaining continuous blood flow through the vasculature. Interruption in this flow, for example due to a wound or partial obstruction of the vessel, results in adherence of platelets and increased synthesis of

TXA$_2$, which promotes additional platelet aggregation. Thus, PGI$_2$ and TXA$_2$ appear to represent a biologically important control mechanism for regulating blood flow and platelet–vessel wall interactions. Interference with platelet synthesis of TXA$_2$, as seen with aspirin and some other agents, may play a beneficial role in preventing circulatory disturbances and protecting against stroke and other ischemic vascular phenomena. More specific inhibition of the TXA$_2$ synthetase enzyme in platelets has been reported with the investigational compounds dazoxiben and 9,11-azoprosta-5,13-dienoic acid, but their role in clinical therapy remains to be established.

Effects of Eicosanoids on the Nervous System

PGE$_2$ and possibly PGI$_2$ can sensitize afferent nerve endings to the noxious effects of chemical or mechanical stimuli. This action can intensify the reaction to painful stimuli, and inhibition of the synthesis of PGE$_2$ underlies the pain-relieving effects of aspirin and other related analgesics. In addition, release of PGE$_2$ during the inflammatory process is related to the increased vascular permeability and capillary leakage, as well as the pain and erythema accompanying an inflammatory reaction. In addition, LTB$_4$ is a very potent chemotactic substance and promotes attraction of polymorphonuclear leukocytes to the inflamed area.

The central nervous system effects of eicosanoids remain to be definitively established. Attention has been focused on the role of PGE$_2$ in the generation of elevated body temperatures, although its precise role is uncertain.

Effects of Eicosanoids on the Kidney

PGE$_2$ and PGI$_2$ can improve renal blood flow and elicit diuresis accompanied by sodium and potassium loss. They also can cause release of renin from the renal cortex. TXA$_2$, on the other hand, reduces renal blood flow and glomerular filtration rate. Synthesis of PGE$_2$ and PGI$_2$ may be increased in response to reduced renal blood flow. The action of antidiuretic hormone (ADH) can be antagonized by PGE$_2$.

Effects of Eicosanoids on the Endocrine System

A variety of endocrine effects have been associated with the prostaglandins, for example, PGE$_2$ can elevate circulating levels of ACTH, growth hormone, prolactin, and the gonadotropins. In addition, adrenal steroid production can be increased, insulin secretion may be enhanced, and progesterone release from the corpus luteum can be impaired, leading to luteal regression (especially with PGE$_{2\alpha}$).

Clinical Uses of Prostaglandins

To date, prostaglandins have a limited clinical application, although the potential for their beneficial use in a variety of pathologic states is enormous. The principal limiting factors to their widespread clinical applicability are their short duration of action, their susceptibility to rapid metabolism, and their substantial range of side-effects. The approved therapeutic applications for the prostaglandins are for the production of therapeutic abortion based on their uterine spasmogenic properties, and for therapy of neonates with congenital heart defects. In addition, synthetic analogues of prostaglandin E are being investigated for their antiulcer action (by virtue of inhibition of gastric acid secretion), for their bronchodilator action in the management of chronic obstructive pulmonary disease, and for their vasodilating action in the treatment of severe peripheral vascular disease. Prostaglandin I$_2$ derivatives have been shown also to reduce gastric acid secretion, to prevent platelet aggregation on extracorporeal circulatory systems, and to increase pulmonary blood flow and oxygenation of blood in infants with reduced pulmonary or systemic blood flow. PGE$_2$ and PGF$_{2\alpha}$ may be useful in inducing labor at term, while PGI$_2$ has been reported to limit the ischemic damage to the myocardium following coronary artery ligation on experimental animals.

Prostaglandin Abortifacients

Carboprost Tromethamine
(Prostin/15 M)

Dinoprost Tromethamine
(Prostin F₂ Alpha)

Dinoprostone
(Prostin E₂)

Termination of pregnancy can be accomplished by both mechanical and pharmacologic methods. During the early weeks of pregnancy, there is no safe and reliable method for pharmacologically inducing fetal expulsion, and suction curettage is the commonly performed procedure. Beginning at about the start of the second trimester, however, pharmacologic methods are usually employed; these usually consist of injections of either hypertonic saline solution or prostaglandins (F_2 alpha) into the amniotic sac, IM administration of a prostaglandin salt, or use of a prostaglandin (E_2) vaginal suppository. Certain prostaglandins (PGE_2, $PGF_{2\alpha}$) have been detected in amniotic fluid during labor or spontaneous abortion and appear to play a role in fetal expulsion by facilitating myometrial contractions. These observations have led to the development of several prostaglandin preparations indicated for the induction of second trimester elective abortion. Currently available drugs can be used by intra-amniotic or IM injections or insertion of a vaginal suppository. These agents are preferable to intra-amniotic injection of hypertonic sodium chloride (see Chap. 57) because they have a more rapid onset of action and a lower incidence of side-effects. The prostaglandins used as abortifacients are reviewed as a group, followed by a listing of individual drugs and dosages in Table 82-1.

MECHANISM AND ACTIONS
Prostaglandins E_2 (dinoprostone) and $F_{2\alpha}$ (carboprost, dinoprost tromethamine) elicit contractions of the gravid uterus, probably by a direct stimulation of the myometrium. They may also produce a regression of corpus luteum function. These agents increase contractile activity of the GI tract and other smooth muscle, an action probably responsible for the vomiting and diarrhea common with use of the prostaglandins. *Large doses* of $PGF_{2\alpha}$ can elevate the blood pressure, presumably by contracting vascular smooth muscle, but a clinically significant hypertensive effect is rare at recommended doses. Conversely, PGE may lower blood pressure. Elevation of body temperature has also occurred during treatment with the prostaglandin abortifacients.

The abortifacient action of the prostaglandins in the *early weeks* of pregnancy is inconsistent and often incomplete and may be accompanied by a high incidence of disturbing side-effects.

USES
1. Termination of pregnancy from the 12th through the 20th gestational week
2. Production of abortion during second trimester in the event of premature rupture of the membranes in the presence of a previable fetus (carboprost *only*)
3. Production of uterine evacuation in cases of missed abortion or fetal death up to 28 weeks (dinoprostone *only*)
4. Management of nonmetastatic gestational trophoblastic disease (benign hydatidiform mole)—dinoprostone only
5. Induction of labor and initiation of cervical ripening prior to induction of labor (dinoprostone vaginal suppositories—investigational use only)

ADMINISTRATION AND DOSAGE
See Table 82-1.

FATE
The drugs are widely distributed in both the fetal and maternal circulation. Their half-life in amniotic fluid is several hours, but is much shorter in plasma. The prostaglandins are metabolized by the maternal liver and excreted largely in the urine.

SIDE-EFFECTS/ADVERSE REACTIONS
The most frequently encountered side-effects with prostaglandin abortifacients are nausea, diarrhea, and vomiting (25%–75% incidence), headache, chills, shivering, hyperthermia (up to 50% of patients receiving *dinoprostone*), flushing, and abdominal cramping. Systemic effects occur more frequently with IM injection of *carboprost* than with intra-amniotic injection of *dinoprost* or intravaginal use of *dinoprostone*.

Other adverse effects observed during use of the prostaglandin abortifacients are listed below:

GI—Hiccups, dry throat, choking sensation, pharyngitis, laryngitis, taste alterations

CNS—Paresthesia, weakness, drowsiness, tremor, dizziness, lethargy, anxiety, blurred vision, tinnitus, vertigo, sleep disorders

CV—Hypertension, hypotension with *dinoprostone*, chest pain, arrhythmias, bradycardia, palpitations, congestive heart failure, cardiac arrest

Respiratory—Coughing, wheezing, dyspnea, hyperventilation, asthmatic-like reactions, pulmonary embolism

Genitourinary—Endometritis, urinary tract infection, perforated cervix or uterus,

Table 82-1
Prostaglandin Abortifacients

Drug	Preparations	Usual Dosage Range	Clinical Considerations
carboprost tromethamine (Prostin/15 M)	Injection—250 mcg/ml	*Abortion* Initially 250 mcg IM; repeat at 1½-h–3½-h intervals; may increase to 500 mcg per dose if necessary; maximum dose, 12 mg. *Refractory postpartum bleeding* Initially, 250 mcg IM; if necessary, additional doses may be given at 15 min–90 min intervals to a maximum of 2 mg	Administer deeply IM; abortion is incomplete in about 20% of cases; may produce transient elevation in body temperature (1°–3°F), which persists only as long as drug is being given; forced fluids are recommended during hyperpyrexia; an optional test dose of 100 mcg (0.4 ml) may be given initially to ascertain hypersensitivity to drug.
dinoprost tromethamine (Prostin F2 Alpha)	Injection—5 mg/ml	Inject 40 mg slowly into the amniotic sac; may repeat in 24 h with 10 mg to 40 mg if abortion is not established or complete	A transabdominal tap of the amniotic sac should be performed before drug injection and at least 1 ml of fluid should be withdrawn; do not inject drug if tap is bloody; if abortion is incomplete, other measures should be taken to ensure complete fetal expulsion (*e.g.*, hypertonic sodium chloride)
dinoprostone (Prostin E2)	Vaginal suppository— 20 mg	Insert 1 suppository high into vagina; repeat at 3-h–5-h intervals until abortion occurs	Keep patient supine for at least 10 min following insertion; vomiting occurs in about two thirds of all patients, and diarrhea in approximately half; provide assistance as needed; nausea, headache, chills, and hypotension (20 mm Hg–30 mm Hg) have also been noted frequently

uterine or vaginal pain, urinary incontinence, hematuria

Other—Sweating, hot flashes, muscle pain, leg cramps, joint pain, stiff neck, diplopia, polydipsia, rash, aggravation of diabetes, uterine infections (1%–5% with dinoprost)

CONTRAINDICATIONS AND PRECAUTIONS

Prostaglandin abortifacients are contraindicated in patients with acute pelvic inflammatory disease and active cardiac, pulmonary, hepatic, or renal disease. They should *not* be employed if the fetus has reached a stage of viability. Dinoprost should *not* be administered if the amniocentesis is bloody.

A *cautious* approach to therapy must be under-taken in patients with asthma, hypertension, cardiovascular disease, renal or hepatic impairment, anemia, jaundice, diabetes, epilepsy, adrenal disorders, scarred uterus, cervicitis or vaginitis (especially dinoprostone suppositories), and glaucoma.

Prostaglandins have the capacity to damage the fetus; therefore, when abortion is incomplete (up to 20% incidence with carboprost), other measures should be taken to ensure complete abortion. Hypertonic saline solution (see Chap. 57) should not be given, however, until the uterus is no longer contracting.

INTERACTIONS

1. The activity of oxytocin may be enhanced by prostaglandin abortifacients.

NURSING CONSIDERATIONS

Prior to administration of a prostaglandin abortifacient, the patient will have a CBC with differential to assess any bleeding, as indicated by a decrease in hemoglobin or hematocrit, or infectious process, as indicated by a increase in white blood cell count, and renal and hepatic function studies to evaluate the function of those organ systems. An ultrasound of the uterus will also be completed, especially in a late second-trimester abortion, to determine the viability of the fetus. If the fetus is viable, prostaglandin should not be administered. The physician will also perform a transabdominal tap to withdraw approximately 1 ml of amniotic fluid, which is examined for blood. If blood is present, prostaglandin should not be given and the source of the bleeding should be determined.

Time should be taken to determine the woman's and partner's feelings about the abortion and whether the pregnancy was desired or not. This information can be used to determine the type and amount of supportive information and care that will be needed during drug administration.

The prostaglandin abortifacients are most frequently given by intra-amniotic injection through a catheter inserted into the amniotic sac through the vagina. The first milliliter is injected slowly over 5 minutes, and the patient is observed for vasomotor response such as bradycardia and severe hypotension. If no adverse effects occur, the remainder of the dose is injected slowly over 5 minutes to 10 minutes. Labor pains usually begin within one-half hour of injection, and delivery of the fetus is usually complete within 24 hours.

Intramuscular injections are occasionally used, especially if vaginal bleeding prevents administration of suppositories, but are extremely painful. If multiple injections are necessary, sites should be rotated using a body map (see Chap. 8) to minimize discomfort and trauma. Intra-amniotic injection and vaginal suppositories are the preferred technique.

The side-effects produced by these drugs are numerous and unpleasant. The most common side-effects from these drugs are nausea, vomiting, and diarrhea, which occur in almost two-thirds of all patients receiving them. Pretreatment with antiemetics and antidiarrheal agents may reduce the smooth muscle stimulation which causes these problems and reduce the intensity of symptoms. Patients should be warned about the potential for their development, and bathroom facilities should be close at hand. If the patient is bedridden or in a weakened condition, close monitoring is essential to prevent aspiration of vomitus.

Hyperthermia and chills may occur, although temperature rarely exceeds 101°F and will usually return to normal once the drug is discontinued. However, temperature should be monitored every 1 hour to 2 hours during drug administration.

Headache is a very common side-effect, especially with dinoprostone. Mild analgesics, usually acetaminophen, may be helpful in relieving pain. Headache will usually disappear once the drug is discontinued.

Blood pressure changes, arrhythmias, wheezing, and dyspnea are more likely to occur early in the drug administration period, but may occur at any time. Dizziness may result; therefore, the patient should be encouraged to ambulate only with assistance if such symptoms occur. Vital signs, including respiratory rate, should be monitored every hour during treatment, and emergency equipment and drugs to deal with respiratory or cardiac arrest should be immediately available. Diabetic patients will require additional monitoring of urine and blood glucose.

When labor pains intensify, contractions should be monitored and the woman must be coached in breathing and relaxation techniques to facilitate delivery of the fetus. Analgesia may be required in some patients.

Throughout the procedure and especially after delivery of the fetus, the woman and her partner will need emotional support whether the pregnancy was desired or not. Prostaglandin abortifacients force the woman to go through an entire delivery process without the usual expected outcome of a viable child. The procedure is emotionally traumatic and physically draining. The patient may want to know the sex of the baby, to view the fetus, or to have some time alone with it. The nurse who can provide positive support during this period can ease the patient's emotional burden and facilitate some closure on the event.

Once delivery by means of prostaglandin is complete, the patient may face a dilation and curettage (D and C) to ensure complete evacuation of placenta.

Alprostadil

(Prostin VR Pediatric)

MECHANISM AND ACTIONS

Alprostadil (prostaglandin E_1) is a solution for IV infusion that is used in neonates with congenital heart defects to temporarily maintain the patency of the ductus arteriosus until corrective surgery can be performed. The drug relaxes smooth muscle of the ductus arteriosus, thereby providing for adequate blood oxygenation. Other actions of PGE_1 include vasodilation, increased tone of intestinal and uterine smooth muscle, and inhibition of platelet aggregation.

USES
1. Palliative therapy of neonates with congenital heart defects (e.g., pulmonary stenosis, tricuspid atresia, tetralogy of Fallot, aortic coarctation) to maintain patency of the ductus arteriosus until corrective surgery can be performed

ADMINISTRATION AND DOSAGE
Alprostadil (PGE_1) is used as an injection solution containing 500 mcg/ml, which is diluted with sodium chloride injection or dextrose injection to provide solutions ranging from 2 mcg/ml to 20 mcg/ml. The drug is then infused continuously into a large vein. The initial dosage is 0.1 mcg/kg/min. Once a desired therapeutic response is obtained (i.e., increased pO_2 in infants with restricted pulmonary blood flow or increased systemic blood pressure and blood pH in infants with restricted systemic blood flow), the infusion rate is reduced to the lowest rate that maintains the response (usually 0.01 mcg–0.05 mcg/kg/min). The maximum recommended dose is 0.4 mcg/kg/min.

FATE
Alprostadil is rapidly metabolized, and over 75% may be metabolized in one pass through the lungs. The metabolites are excreted in the urine, and excretion is virtually complete within 24 hours.

SIDE-EFFECTS/ADVERSE REACTIONS
Side-effects occurring most frequently with alprostadil infusion include fever (12%–15%), apnea (10%–12%), flushing (10%), and bradycardia (7%–8%). Apnea is especially prominent in neonates weighing less than 2 kg and usually appears within the first hour of infusion.

Other untoward reactions associated with use of alprostadil include:

Cardiovascular—Tachycardia, hypotension, peripheral edema, second-degree heart block, hyperemia, shock, congestive heart failure, ventricular fibrillation, cardiac arrest

CNS—Seizures, hyperirritability, lethargy, hypothermia, cerebral bleeding, hyperextension of the neck

Hematologic—Disseminated intravascular coagulation, anemia, thrombocytopenia, bleeding

GI—Diarrhea, regurgitation, hyperbilirubinemia

Respiratory—Wheezing, hypercapnia, respiratory depression

Other—Anuria, hematuria, sepsis, peritonitis, hypokalemia, hypoglycemia, cortical proliferation of long bones

Overdosage may be characterized by marked fever, hypotension, flushing, bradycardia, and apnea. If significant bradycardia or apnea occurs, the nurse should discontinue infusion and provide supportive therapy. If fever or hypotension is noted, the nurse should reduce infusion rate and monitor the patient carefully.

CONTRAINDICATIONS AND PRECAUTIONS
Alprostadil should not be used in patients with respiratory distress syndrome (hyaline membrane disease). The drug should be given cautiously to neonates with bleeding tendencies. Alprostadil must be administered only by personnel trained in settings providing intensive pediatric care.

NURSING CONSIDERATIONS
The neonate receiving this drug should be in a neonatal intensive care nursery. Cardiac and apnea monitors should be in place and, if possible, an umbilical artery catheter should be inserted to monitor blood pressure. The infant needs constant attention while the drug is infusing to ensure prompt response to fever, hypothermia, bradycardia, seizures, or other dysrhythmias, apnea, and hypotension. If any of these symptoms develops, the drug will be discontinued or slowed down until the symptoms are successfully treated. Therapy is maintained at the lowest effective dose only until surgery can be performed to correct the defect. These patients should be carefully monitored for signs of congestive heart failure (e.g., rales, dyspnea, tachypnea).

To measure treatment effectiveness in improving pulmonary circulation, frequent monitoring of pulmonary artery wedge pressure and of arterial blood gas values for pO_2 are reviewed. To measure improvement in system blood flow, blood pH and systemic blood pressure are reviewed.

REVIEW QUESTIONS

1. What is meant by the term "eicosanoid"?
2. How were prostaglandins first isolated?
3. How are the various groups of prostaglandins named?
4. From what cellular constituents are eicosanoids formed?
5. What are leukotrienes?
6. Briefly describe the steps in the synthesis of (a) leukotrienes, (b) thromboxanes, and (c) prostaglandins.
7. What drugs can interfere with the synthesis of eicosanoids?
8. Describe the opposing effects of (a) PGE_2 and $PGF_{2\alpha}$ on the bronchioles and (b) PGI_2 and TXA_2 on platelets.
9. Discuss briefly the mechanisms of action proposed for the prostaglandins.
10. Outline the major actions of prostaglandins on (a) vascular smooth muscle, (b) respiratory smooth muscle, (c) uterine smooth muscle, and (d) gastrointestinal smooth muscle.
11. What is the proposed role of PGE_2 in pain and inflammation?
12. Describe the principal actions of eicosanoids on the kidney.
13. What are the approved clinical indications for prostaglandins?
14. List the important adverse effects of prostaglandin abortifacients.
15. What are the contraindications to the use of prostaglandin abortifacients?
16. For what indications is alprostadil (Prostin VR Pediatric) approved?

BIBLIOGRAPHY

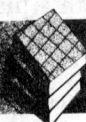

Belch JJ et al: Epoprostenol (prostacyclin) and severe arterial disease. A double-blind trial. Lancet 1:315, 1983

Berkowitz BA, Zabko-Potapovich B, Valocik R et al: Effects of the leukotrienes on the vasculature and blood pressure of different species. J Pharmacol Exp Ther 229:105, 1984

Busse R, Trogisch G, Bassenge E: The role of the endothelium in the control of vascular tone. Basic Res Cardiol 80:475, 1985

Chan WY: Prostaglandins and nonsteroidal antiinflammatory drugs in dysmenorrhea. Annu Rev Pharmacol Toxicol 23:131, 1983

Feuerstein G: Leukotrienes and the cardiovascular system. Prostaglandins 27:781, 1984

Feuerstein G, Hallenbeck JM: Prostaglandins, leukotrienes and platelet-activating factor in shock. Ann Rev Pharmacol Toxicol 27:301, 1987

Furchgott RF: The role of the endothelium in the responses of vascular smooth muscle to drugs. Annu Rev Pharmacol Toxicol 24:175, 1984

Kaley G, Hintze TH, Panzenbeck M et al: Role of prostaglandins in microcirculatory function. Adv Prostaglandin Thromboxane Res 13:27, 1985

Kennedy I et al: Studies on the characterization of prostanoid receptors: A proposed classification. Prostaglandins 24:667, 1982

Larsen GL, Henson PM: Mediators of inflammation. Annu Rev Immunol 1:335, 1983

Lefer A, Darius H: A pharmacological approach in thromboxane receptor antagonism. Fed Proc 46:144, 1987

Lefer A, Gee M (eds): Leukotrienes in Cardiovascular and Pulmonary Function. New York, Liss Co, 1985

McGiff JC: Prostaglandins, prostacyclin, and thromboxanes. Annu Rev Pharmacol Toxicol 21:479, 1981

Ogletree ML: Overview of physiological and pathophysiological effects of thromboxane A_2. Fed Proc 46:133, 1987

Owen PR: Prostaglandin synthetase inhibitors in the treatment of primary dysmenorrhea. Am J Obstet Gynecol 148:96, 1984

Peters SP et al: Effect of prostaglandin D_2 in modulating histamine release from human basophils. J Pharmacol Exp Ther 228:400, 1984

Piper PJ: Pharmacology of leukotrienes. Br Med Bull 39:255, 1983

Samuelsson B: Leukotrienes: Mediators of immediate hypersensitivity reactions and inflammation. Science 220:568, 1983

Smith JB: Pharmacology of thromboxane synthetase inhibitors. Fed Proc 46:139, 1987

Smith WL: Prostaglandin biosynthesis and its compartmentation in vascular smooth muscle and endothelial cells. Annu Rev Physiol 48:251, 1986

Vane JR: Prostacyclin: A hormone with a therapeutic potential. J Endocrinology. 95:3P, 1982

Wolfe LS: Eicosanoids: Prostaglandins, thromboxanes, leukotrienes and other derivatives of carbon-20 unsaturated fatty acids. J Neurochem 38:1, 1982

Dermatologic Drugs

83

Drugs are applied to the skin and mucous membranes for a variety of reasons and in a number of different dosage forms. This chapter will consider those drugs that have *not* been reviewed previously and that are used topically for their local effects.

Although topical therapy is quite effective in treating many dermatologic disorders, systemic administration of drugs is occasionally necessary to treat severe or constant conditions. A few systemically administered drugs will also be considered in this chapter.

Anatomy and Physiology of the Skin

Structurally, the skin has two principal components: an outer epithelial layer or *epidermis*, and a deeper connective tissue layer termed the *dermis* or *corium*.

The epidermis and dermis are firmly joined together, forming a cohesive membrane that varies in thickness in different parts of the body. Collagenous fibers extending downward from the dermis anchor the skin to an underlying subcutaneous tissue layer, alternatively called the superficial fascia or hypodermis. The loose organization of the subcutaneous tissue provides a certain latitude of movement to the skin, and it also permits the introduction of a considerable volume of fluid, as in the case of subcutaneous injection of drugs.

Skin is often classified into two types: *thick* and *thin*, these terms generally referring to the thickness of the epidermal layer, rather than that of the whole skin. The cells in the deepest layer of the avascular epidermis are living cells which proliferate through mitosis. As the epithelial cells are displaced toward the surface by the formation of new cells, they are pushed away from the dermis and their source of nutrients. Consequently, the cells die and become transformed into keratin-rich scales which desquamate from the surface.

The constantly changing appearance of the cells in the epidermis allows this layer, histologically classified as *keratinizing stratified squamous epithelium*, to be subdivided into five layers:

1. *Stratum germinativum epidermidis*
   This deepest layer of the epidermis, also known as the *stratum basale*, consists of essentially columnar cells which proliferate through continued cell division.
2. *Stratum spinosum epidermidis*
   This layer contains eight to ten rows of poly-

hedral cells which fit closely together by means of desmosomes.

3. *Stratum granulosum epidermidis*
   This third layer of the epidermis consists of two to four rows of roughly diamond-shaped cells which contain deeply staining *keratohyalin* granules.
4. *Stratum lucidum epidermidis*
   This epidermal layer, notably absent in thin skin, consists of several rows of clear, flat cells containing droplets of *eleidin*, which presumably is a transformation product of the keratohyalin found in cells of the stratum granulosum epidermidis.
5. *Stratum corneum epidermidis*
   This outermost layer of the epidermis consists of many rows of flat, dead scale-like cells characterized by the presence of *keratin*. Keratin is a tough fibrous protein which serves as a barrier against water loss and limits entry of microorganisms.

The principal pigment of the skin is *melanin*. The relative amount of melanin in the epidermis accounts for the varying skin color in different races. Melanin is produced in cells called melanocytes, which are found just beneath or between the cells of the stratum germinativum. Melanocytes synthesize the enzyme tyrosinase which converts amino acid substrates into melanin. Exposure to ultraviolet radiation stimulates melanin production and dispersion, thereby protecting the deep layers of the epidermis and the underlying dermis from its harmful effects. (In some individuals, epidermal melanin occurs in small patches—freckles). An inherent inability of an individual to produce melanin results in albinism. In such cases, the melanin pigment is absent from the hair and eyes, as well as from the skin.

The *dermis* is composed of two merging layers of connective tissue. The outer, thinner portion, known as the *papillary* layer, consists of loose connective tissue containing fine elastic fibers. Finger-like projections called dermal papillae extend into the epidermis. These dermal papillae are richly supplied with blood capillaries which provide nourishment for the avascular epidermis, and which also participate in heat regulation.

The deeper, thicker reticular layer of the dermis consists of dense, irregularly arranged connective tissue containing interlacing bundles of collagenous and coarse elastic fibers. Functionally important structures located in the dermis include sebaceous glands, sweat (sudoriferous) glands, hair follicles, and nerves. The skin is a dynamic organ which responds to a variety of environmental stimuli and which performs several other important functions.

The skin protects underlying tissues from various chemical and mechanical assaults, from invasion by microorganisms, and from potentially harmful ultraviolet light. The waterproofing action of keratin minimizes dehydration and water loss. The regulation of body temperature is greatly facilitated by adaptations in cutaneous blood flow and sweat gland activity. Through the sweat glands, the skin plays a minor excretory role, eliminating water, salts, and certain waste products. The skin also serves as a source of vitamin D upon exposure to ultraviolet light.

Dermatologic Vehicles

Topically applied drugs are usually incorporated into a vehicle for the purposes of ease of application and to facilitate the percutaneous absorption of the drug. Vehicles that are used include creams, ointments, gels, pastes, aerosols, lotions, wet dressings, and tinctures.

The selection of an appropriate vehicle for a particular drug depends on several factors such as (1) the solubility and stability of the drug in the vehicle, (2) the efficiency with which the drug is released from the vehicle, (3) the ability of the vehicle to enhance percutaneous absorption of the drug, and (4) the action of the vehicle itself on the skin. Vehicles are frequently chemically and pharmacologically inert; however, some vehicles can exhibit either beneficial or deleterious effects depending on the condition being treated.

In general, drug penetration through the skin is increased when the stratum corneum is well hydrated. Vehicles providing the best hydration are occlusive preparations, such as ointments or creams, whereas tinctures and wet dressings provide little hydration. Therefore, dermatologic conditions associated with oozing or vesiculation are best managed with drying preparations such as tinctures, wet dressings, and some lotions. Conversely, when scaling or extreme dryness is present, ointments or creams are generally preferred. For application of drugs to hairy areas, aerosols, tinctures, or lotions provide for good skin contact. Skin hydration can also be enhanced by wrapping the treated area with an occlusive dressing, such as plastic wrap. Of course, abraded or denuded skin provides an area for rapid absorption of topically applied drugs, and drugs must be applied with care if the skin is broken.

Types of Dermatologic Drugs

A variety of different drugs are used topically for treating dermatologic disorders, and a general classification of these drugs is presented in Table 83-1. The dermatologic drugs are discussed below by groups, except where they have been considered in a previous chapter, in which case an appropriate reference is made.

Acne Aids

Topical preparations used in treating acne vulgaris include tretinoin (an acid form of vitamin A), benzoyl peroxide, sulfur, the anti-infectives erythromycin, clindamycin and tetracycline, and various keratolytics and astringents. In addition, isotretinoin, a synthetic retinoid, is used orally for severe resistant forms of acne and is discussed below. Systemic administration of tetracycline or erythromycin has also been employed in treating more severe forms of acne.

Tretinoin
(Retin-A)

MECHANISM AND ACTIONS
Tretinoin (retinoic acid) promotes epidermal cell turnover, facilitates desquamation, suppresses keratin synthesis, and prevents formation of comedones. Its effectiveness approaches that of steroid–antibiotic combinations and generally surpasses that of most other currently available topical acne preparations. Its use is frequently associated with erythema and desquamation, however, and some patients do not tolerate the drug.

Table 83-1
Drugs Used For Dermatologic Disorders

Drug Type	Examples
Acne aids	benzoyl peroxide, tretinoin
Antibacterials	bacitracin, neomycin, tetracycline
Antifungals	clotrimazole, econazole, nystatin
Antihistamines	diphenhydramine, pyrilamine
Antipsoriatics	anthralin, coal tar
Antiseptics	chlorhexidine, hexachlorophene
Antivirals	acyclovir, idoxuridine
Corticosteroids	betamethasone, fluocinolone
Enzymes	collagenase, sutilains
Keratolytics	cantharidin, podophyllum resin
Local anesthetics	benzocaine, lidocaine
Pigmenting/depigmenting agents	methoxsalen, hydroquinone
Scabicides/pediculicides	lindane, permethrin
Sunscreens	PABA, padimate, oxybenzone

USES
1. Treatment of acne vulgaris, especially grades I, II, and III; not effective against acne conglobata (*i.e.*, deep cystic nodules and extensive pustules)
2. Treatment of several forms of skin cancer (investigational use)
3. Retard premature skin aging and wrinkling (investigational use)

ADMINISTRATION AND DOSAGE
Tretinoin is available as a cream (0.05%), gel (0.025%), and liquid (0.05%). The drug is applied once a day at bedtime for 4 weeks to 6 weeks; the entire area should be covered lightly. Once the lesions have responded, therapy should be maintained with less frequent applications.

SIDE-EFFECTS/ADVERSE REACTIONS
Common side-effects with tretinoin include stinging, feeling of warmth, dryness, peeling, and erythema. In addition, the drug may elicit edema, blistering, pigmentary changes, photosensitivity, and contact dermatitis (rare).

CONTRAINDICATIONS AND PRECAUTIONS
Tretinoin should be used with caution in patients with eczema, because severe irritation can occur. The drug should be kept away from the eyes, mouth, and other mucous membranes. Use during pregnancy or nursing is not recommended.

INTERACTIONS
1. Increased skin peeling can occur if tretinoin is used with sulfur, resorcinol, benzoyl peroxide, or salicylic acid.
2. Excessive skin drying can result from concomitant use of tretinoin and products containing high concentrations of alcohol, astringents, or lime.

NURSING CONSIDERATIONS
The individual with acne has probably tried a variety of over-the-counter remedies before seeking medical advice. Therefore it is essential to determine what the patient is currently using and to encourage him to eliminate the use of any skin care products containing alcohol, astringents, or lime or any other products that dry the skin and will result in increased skin effects from tretinoin (see under Interactions). The clinician should help the patient establish a skin care regimen which includes washing the affected area two to three times a day with mild soap, using nondrying creams or cosmetics sparingly, and applying a light film of tretinoin once a day at bedtime. The patient should be discouraged from attempting to apply the drug more frequently because such use will increase side-effects.

The patient should be informed what to expect as a typical drying action. Tretinoin generally produces a mild erythema early in therapy along with a stinging sensation and feeling of warmth. Dryness and peeling of treated skin are expected. Initially, a temporary worsening of acne lesions may occur as the drug acts on deeper lesions which were previously invisible. However, within 3 weeks, some improvement should be evident, and erythema, stinging, and skin dryness, while still present, will stabilize. If symptoms worsen at any time during the treatment the drug should be withheld and the physician notified. The treatment may be reduced in frequency or temporarily discontinued depending on severity of symptoms.

Tretinoin imparts photosensitivity, which can cause a severe sunburn and rash especially if the patient lays in the sun. Frequently, patients with acne use sunlamps, tanning lamps, or sunshine in an attempt to clear lesions. The patient must be instructed to avoid such activity during the entire course of treatment and, if the patient must be outdoors for an extended period, to wear a hat or other protective clothing over the skin to minimize exposure.

Tretinoin should be used with caution in women of childbearing age. A sexual history can be taken to determine if the woman is or intends to be sexually active during treatment. If the history is positive the woman should be encouraged to use contraception during treatment and told that the drug is potentially dangerous to a fetus. Any woman who suspects she is pregnant should stop taking the drug immediately and contact the physician.

Isotretinoin

(Accutane)

MECHANISM AND ACTIONS

Isotretinoin is an isomer of retinoic acid, a metabolite of retinol (Vitamin A). The mechanism of action of isotretinoin is not completely established; the drug may reduce sebum secretion and inhibit sebaceous gland differentiation. Keratinization is also inhibited, and plasma triglycerides and cholesterol may be elevated. Due to its potential for eliciting serious untoward reactions, isotretinoin should be used with utmost caution and only under close supervision. Women who are pregnant or who intend to become pregnant must *not* use isotretinoin (see below).

USES

1. Treatment of severe, recalcitrant cystic acne in patients unresponsive to conventional therapy, including antibiotics (*e.g.*, tetracyclines)
2. Treatment of disorders of excessive keratinization (*e.g.*, ichthyosis, pityriasis, rubra pilaris, hyperkeratosis palmaris et plantaris)
3. Treatment of cutaneous T-cell lymphoma (mycosis fungoides)

ADMINISTRATION AND DOSAGE

Isotretinoin is used as capsules containing 10 mg, 20 mg, or 40 mg. The initial dose is 0.5 mg to 1 mg/kg/day, which may be increased up to 2 mg/kg/day in two divided doses for 15 weeks to 20 weeks. A second course of therapy may be initiated after a 2-month drug holiday. Doses as small as 0.05 mg/kg/day have been effective in some patients, but relapses are more common.

FATE

Oral bioavailability of the capsule dosage form is approximately 25%. Peak plasma levels occur in about 3 hours. The drug is almost completely protein-bound, and the elimination half-life averages 10 hours (range 7 hours–35 hours). Isotretinoin is excreted in the urine and feces in approximately equal amounts.

SIDE-EFFECTS/ADVERSE REACTIONS

■ *WARNING*
Isotretinoin should not be used in women who are pregnant or who intend to become pregnant, because numerous fetal abnormalities and spontaneous abortions have occurred. An effective means of contraception must be employed during therapy and for at least 1 month before *and* after therapy.

Most adverse effects with isotretinoin are dose-related. The most frequently reported side-effects are cheilitis, eye irritation, conjunctivitis, dry skin, skin fragility, pruritus, nosebleed, dryness of the nose and mouth, nausea, vomiting, abdominal pain, lethargy, white cells in urine and elevated sedimentation rate. Increased triglyceride and cholesterol and decreased high-density lipoprotein levels occur in up to 25% of patients but are reversible upon cessation of therapy. Many other untoward reactions have occurred in persons taking isotretinoin and these are listed below:

Dermatologic—Facial skin desquamation, nail brittleness, rash, alopecia, photosensitivity, skin infections, erythema nodosum, pigmentary changes, urticaria
GI—Anorexia, regional ileitis, mild GI bleeding, inflammatory bowel disease, weight loss
CNS—Insomnia, fatigue, paresthesias, headache, dizziness, visual disturbances, papilledema, corneal opacities
Musculoskeletal—Arthralgia, joint and muscle pain and stiffness
Urinary—Proteinuria, hematuria
Other—Bruising, edema, respiratory infections, abnormal menses, herpes simplex infections, increased SGOT, SGPT, alkaline phosphatase and fasting serum glucose, elevated platelet counts, hyperuricemia, elevated cholesterol, decreased high-density lipoproteins

CONTRAINDICATIONS AND PRECAUTIONS

Isotretinoin is contraindicated during pregnancy. *Cautious use* is recommended in obese, alcoholic, or diabetic patients, because elevated serum triglycerides occur more frequently and levels are generally higher. A transient worsening of acne may occur during the initial stages of therapy.

INTERACTIONS

1. Vitamin A supplements together with isotretinoin may result in increased toxicity.
2. Tetracyclines and isotretinoin can lead to pseudotumor cerebri or papilledema.
3. Concomitant ingestion of alcohol may further increase serum triglyceride levels.

■ Nursing Process

□ ASSESSMENT

□ Subjective Data

The patient who is about to start treatment with isotretinoin has usually tried, unsuccessfully, a wide range of products to control acne. The therapy and skin care regimen the individual currently uses must be determined because antibiotic therapy with tetracyclines must be discontinued. In addition, the use of skin-drying agents frequently found in many over-the-counter (OTC) acne remedies and skin care products must be discontinued because their use in combination with isotretinoin may cause excessive dryness and skin breakdown. Patients with acne frequently take OTC vitamin A supplements in the belief that this will also help their skin. Ingestion of supplements must also be discontinued before treatment with isotretinoin because the danger of hypervitaminosis A exists when such a combination is taken. By obtaining a thorough history the nurse can avert potentially serious problems from drug or product combinations.

A woman of childbearing age should be asked about sexual activity before treatment begins. Any woman who is sexually active should be encouraged to begin using contraception one menstrual cycle before beginning treatment until at least one cycle after treatment is discontinued. If a woman suspects she might be pregnant a pregnancy test should be performed before isotretinoin is prescribed. The drug is highly teratogenic and is linked to such congenital abnormalities as hydrocephalus, microcephalus, cardiac abnormalities, and abnormalities of the external ear, in addition to an increased incidence of spontaneous abortions. Any woman who suspects she has become pregnant while taking isotretinoin should stop the drug immediately and contact the physician.

□ Objective Data

A skin assessment should be performed and the extent and number of acne lesions, especially cystic sites, should be recorded. This information will be used to determine drug effectiveness during the treatment course. Liver and spleen should be palpated because enlargements may occur as drug side-effects. The patient should be weighed to determine an accurate dosage range.

Laboratory data should include serum lipids (triglyceride and high-density lipoprotein levels), CBC with differential, and liver enzymes (SGOT, SGPT, LDH, and alkaline phosphatase). A fasting blood sugar may be drawn if the patient is diabetic because the drug may cause an increase, which could be dangerous.

□ NURSING DIAGNOSES

Actual nursing diagnoses may include:

Knowledge deficit related to the drug action, administration, side-effects and potential for adverse interactions from other drugs and skin products

Disturbance in self concept: body image related to the extent of acne lesions

Potential nursing diagnoses may include:

Alteration in comfort: musculoskeletal pain from drug therapy

Impaired skin integrity related to the excess drying effect of the drug or photosensitivity

Sensory-perceptual alteration in vision related to eye irritation or conjunctivitis, a drug side-effect

□ PLAN

Nursing care goals focus on:

1. Teaching the patient appropriate drug-taking techniques, a safe skin care regimen, and side-effects to monitor and report
2. Providing the patient with an opportunity to express concerns about body image, hopes for the success of drug treatment, and ways to improve self-concept

□ INTERVENTIONS

The patient should be aware of what to expect from the drug's action. The dose will be gradually increased to the maximum tolerable dose for the patient's weight or until a response to the drug is noted or side-effects begin to appear. During the initial stages of therapy, the patient may notice a transient worsening of acne lesions as the drug begins to act on deep lesions which were previously invisible. Gradually, lesions will begin to respond, and the patient will begin to see improvements.

The patient will usually be required to return for follow-up on a biweekly basis. During each visit the lesions will be assessed for improvement. If no change is noted, the drug will be increased. An ophthalmologic exam should be performed on each visit to determine the extent of eye irritation or development of conjunctivitis, common side-effects of the drug which the patient should be told to report immediately. Laboratory data should also be collected at each visit, including a CBC with differential, serum lipids, and liver enzymes. Treatment with isotretinoin can cause elevated sedimentation rate, elevated platelet counts, increased triglycerides and cholesterol, and decreased high-density lipoprotein levels. Liver enzymes may be increased. Changes in any of these levels should be immediately reported.

The patient should also have an opportunity to discuss self-concept and reaction of peers to acne problems. Many people, especially teenagers, are very self-conscious about acne and may decrease social interaction, leading to isolation and depression. Others become defensive and irritable. The patient needs time to explore his concerns, how drug therapy is changing his image of himself, and how to build confidence.

The patient should be told to monitor the drying effects of the drug. The most common one, cheilitis, is dry, cracking, inflammation of the lips which may be severe enough to warrant discontinuation. Frequent use of lubricating creams on all dry skin sites may slow or decrease dryness, but any persistent or cracking site must be reported because the risk of subsequent inflammation and infection is high. Dryness of the mucous membranes can also occur, which may range from simple dry mouth to nasal mucosa cracking resulting in epistaxis. Dry mouth may be relieved by sucking hard candies and increasing water intake. Epistaxis should be reported to the physician.

Serum lipid levels may increase dramatically, especially in patients who are overweight, who drink alcohol, who have a family history of elevated lipids, or who are diabetic. Diet should be modified to reduce fat intake and eliminate alcohol in all patients on the drug; if the patient is overweight, calorie intake should be reduced as well.

The patient who is diabetic should be monitored closely. Usually, lipid values will return to pretreatment levels once the drug is discontinued.

Side-effects are generally related to dose, and increasing doses make the patient more susceptible to drug adverse reactions. In addition to the drug effects already noted, the patient should be told to report any of the untoward reactions listed under Side-Effects/Adverse Reactions, especially muscle or joint pain, fatigue, insomnia, headache, nausea, or any excessive drying or fissuring of skin which indicates hypervitaminosis A. Fever, jaundice, malaise, or bruising should also be reported because it indicates potential hepatotoxicity.

□ **EVALUATION**

The outcome usually used to measure drug effectiveness is a reduction in the extent of acne lesions, especially of cystic formations. Drug therapy will usually be discontinued once the lesions have been reduced approximately 70% or when the maximum time frame for therapy (usually 20 weeks) has been reached. Other measures of treatment success include return of the patient for clinical follow-up as advised, laboratory values within normal limits, and absence of significant or adverse side-effects.

Benzoyl Peroxide

(Benzac, Desquam-X, Fostex, Persa-Gel, and various other manufacturers)

Benzoyl peroxide is used as a liquid, soap, lotion, cream, or gel for treating mild to moderate acne. Its effectiveness appears to be due to its antibacterial activity against *Propionibacterium acnes*, the major organism found in sebaceous follicles and comedones. It may be applied once or twice a day after cleansing the skin. Drying, scaling, or erythema usually occurs with benzoyl peroxide, but if it becomes excessive, the dose should be reduced. The various preparations are available in strengths ranging from 5% to 10%.

Sulfur Preparations

(Acne-Aid, Liquimat, Xerac, and various other manufacturers)

Sulfur is used as a lotion, gel, or cream in strengths of 2% to 5% as an aid in treating mild acne and oily skin. A thin film is applied one to three times a day following a thorough cleansing of the skin. Reddening and scaling of the skin occur frequently, and, if severe, the drug should be discontinued.

Antibiotics

Various antibiotics (tetracycline, erythromycin, clindamycin) are useful for the control of acne and may be applied topically as alcoholic solutions or as a cream. These uses are reviewed in Chapters 63, 64, and 68, respectively.

Antibacterials

Topical antibacterials are generally used to prevent infection in minor skin wounds or abrasions and to treat superficial infections of the skin due to susceptible organisms. The selection of an appropriate antibacterial agent should be based, wherever possible, on *in vitro* culture and sensitivity testing, although in most instances, empirical prescribing is employed for minor wounds. Antibacterial drugs most commonly used topically are bacitracin, neomycin, polymyxin B, and gentamicin. These agents may be given alone, together in combination, or in conjunction with corticosteroids. Antibiotic–corticosteroid combinations are frequently employed in treating diaper rash and eczema.

As indicated above, tetracycline, clindamycin, and erythromycin are active against *Propionibacterium acnes* and are useful in the management of acne vulgaris.

The various antibacterial agents that are employed topically are discussed in the Anti-infective section earlier in the text.

Antifungals

Superficial fungal infections generally respond quite well to topical antifungal agents. Many different antifungal drugs are available for topical application in treating dermatophyte and yeast infections of the skin and mucous membranes, and the various preparations are listed in Table 73-1. In addition, oral administration of griseofulvin or ketoconazole may be useful in the treatment of cutaneous fungal infections not responsive to the topically applied drugs. These latter two agents are also discussed in Chapter 73.

Antihistamines

Topical antihistamines, in the form of creams or lotions, are sometimes employed to relieve itching due to minor skin disorders. These drugs possess some local anesthetic activity but may cause localized irritation and sensitization, especially with prolonged use. Most preparations for topical application contain either diphenhydramine or pyrilamine, frequently combined with a local anesthetic or an astringent. These products should not be applied to raw, blistered, or oozing areas. A complete discussion of antihistamines is presented in Chapter 18.

Antipsoriatics

A variety of drugs have been employed in the treatment of psoriasis, including topical use of corticosteroids, salicylic acid, coal tar, and anthralin, as well as systemic administration of corticosteroids, methotrexate, or etretinate (the latter agents being primarily used for severe, recalcitrant forms of the disease). Topical and systemic corticosteroids are considered in Chapter 55, salicylic acid is discussed in Chapter 23, and methotrexate is reviewed in detail in Chapter 75. The remaining antipsoriatic drugs are considered below.

Anthralin

(Anthra-Derm, DrithoCreme, Lasan)

Anthralin is a mild irritant that reduces the proliferation of epidermal cells in psoriatic lesions by inhibiting synthesis of nucleic protein. The drug is used as an ointment or cream (0.1% to 1%) and applied as a thin layer once or twice a day, which is then covered by a protective film of petrolatum. Treatment is continued until scales are removed or lesions are flattened. The patient should avoid applying drug to the face and should discontinue use if an allergic reaction or inflammation develops.

Anthralin will cause erythema and irritation of unaffected skin. Therefore, gloves should be worn when applying the drug to protect skin on hands, and care must be taken to avoid applying the drug to unaffected skin.

The drug will stain fabric; therefore, the patient should be told to keep the affected site exposed if possible, or to wear old clothing which can be later discarded. The patient with white or gray hair should be told the drug may cause temporary discoloration and that hair rinses should be avoided during treatment.

Coal Tar Preparations

Shampoo—Denorex, Polytar, Tegrin

Bath oils—Balnetar, Cutar, Polytar Bath, Zetar Emulsion

Gel—Aquatar, Estar, P and S Plus, Psori Gel

Ointment—Pragmatar

Lotion/Cream—Alphosyl, Fototar, Mazon, Tegrin Medicated

Soap—Packer's Pine Tar, Polytar

Coal tar-containing products possess antipruritic, antieczematous, and keratoplastic activity and are used adjunctively for a variety of dermatologic disorders, including psoriasis, seborrheic dermatitis, atopic dermatitis, and other chronic skin disorders. Available preparations include shampoos, bath emulsion, gels, creams, ointments, lotions, and soaps. These coal-tar preparations should not be used when acute inflammation is present and should not be applied near the eyes nor to the genital or rectal areas. Shampoos should be applied liberally, then rinsed after 5 minutes. Frequency of use depends on condition and can range from once daily to once weekly.

Etretinate

(Tegison)

MECHANISM AND ACTIONS

Etretinate is related to retinoic acid (vitamin A) and is effective in certain forms of severe, recalcitrant psoriasis. The drug decreases erythema and thickness of lesions and promotes normalization of epidermal differentiation. There is also decreased inflammation of the epidermis and dermis. Etretinate can produce a wide range of adverse effects, and its use is restricted to patients unresponsive to or intolerant of conventional modes of antipsoriatic therapy.

USES

1. Treatment of severe, recalcitrant psoriasis in patients unresponsive to systemic corticosteroids, methotrexate, psoralens plus UV light, or topical tar plus UV light.

ADMINISTRATION AND DOSAGE

Etretinate is available as capsules (10 mg, 25 mg). Dosage is usually initiated at 0.75 mg to 1.0 mg/kg/day in divided doses, although erythrodermic psoriasis may respond to lower initial doses (0.25 mg/kg/day).

Maintenance doses of 0.5 mg to 0.75 mg/kg/day may be used generally after 8 weeks to 16

weeks of therapy. Therapy may eventually be terminated in patients whose lesions have sufficiently resolved.

FATE

Oral absorption is good and may be increased by a high-lipid diet. The drug undergoes significant first-pass hepatic metabolism. Etretinate is more than 99% protein bound. The drug has an extremely long half-life, and elimination is very slow. Chronic dosing has resulted in the maintenance of detectable serum levels up to 3 years after therapy was discontinued. Excretion is by way of both the urine and bile.

SIDE-EFFECTS/ADVERSE REACTIONS

■ *WARNING*
Etretinate must not be used by women who are pregnant during therapy or for some time following discontinuation of therapy (perhaps up to 2 years due to the drug's extremely slow elimination). Fetal abnormalities have been reported (see also under Isotretinoin).

The most frequently reported side-effects during therapy with etretinate are dry nose, chapped lips, sore mouth, thirst, nosebleed, cheilitis, hair loss, peeling of palms, soles or fingertips, itching, rash, dry skin, bruising, sunburn, bone or joint pain, muscle cramping, fatigue, headache, fever, eye irritation, visual disturbances, altered appetite, and nausea. Increased triglycerides, SGOT, SGPT, alkaline phosphatase, and cholesterol also occur frequently, as do changes in serum potassium, calcium, phosphorus, and WBC in the urine. Use of etretinate can result in an extensive array of other untoward reactions, the most important of which are listed below:

CNS—Dizziness, lethargy, pain, anxiety, depression, emotional lability, flu-like symptoms, abnormal thinking, pseudotumor cerebri (benign intracranial hypertension)

Sensory—Earache, otitis externa, lacrimation, hearing changes, photophobia, decreased night vision, scotoma

GI—Constipation, diarrhea, weight loss, oral ulcers, altered taste, tooth cavities

CV—Chest pain, postural hypotension, phlebitis, syncope, arrhythmias

Dermatologic—Bullous eruption, urticaria,

pyogenic granuloma, onycholysis, hirsutism, impaired wound healing, herpes simplex infections, skin odor, fissures, skin atrophy, gingival bleeding, decreased mucus secretion, rhinorrhea

Musculoskeletal—Myalgia, gout, hyperostosis (see under Contraindications and Precautions), hyperkinesia

Other—Coughing, dysphonia, pharyngitis, proteinuria, glycosuria, urinary casts, hemoglobinuria, kidney stones, abnormal menses, atrophic vaginitis, dysuria, polyuria or urinary retention, hepatotoxicity (see under Contraindications and Precautions).

CONTRAINDICATIONS AND PRECAUTIONS

Etretinate is contraindicated in women who are pregnant, who intend to become pregnant, or who do not use contraceptive measures during treatment. Serious fetal abnormalities can occur. Etretinate use is frequently associated with development of extraspinal tendon and ligament calcification (hyperostosis), commonly involving the ankles, pelvis, and knees; however, there were no bone or joint symptoms in approximately one-half of affected patients.

Hepatotoxicity can occur with etretinate and is usually indicated by elevated levels of SGOT, SGPT, or LDH. Hepatitis has developed during and following discontinuation of therapy. If hepatotoxicity is suspected during treatment, the drug should be discontinued and the patient should be observed closely.

Etretinate must be given cautiously to patients with hypertension, visual disturbances, or elevated serum lipids. Because most untoward reactions resemble those of a hypervitaminosis A syndrome, patients should refrain from taking vitamin A supplements during therapy.

INTERACTIONS
1. The oral absorption of etretinate may be increased by the presence of milk.

NURSING CONSIDERATIONS
See Nursing Process for Isotretinoin because most measures are similar. Although oral absorption of the drug may be enhanced by a high-lipid diet, dietary fat intake should be limited during treatment to decrease the risk of elevated serum lipids and potential development of cardiovascular problems. The patient may be advised to take the drug with regular milk, which contains 4% milk fat and may facilitate drug absorption.

A sexual history is very important because the patient taking etretinate may maintain detectable serum levels of the drug for several years after it is discontinued. The patient must understand the need for contraception during and after treatment to avoid conceiving a child with congenital abnormalities. The woman facing this decision may need time and a forum to discuss how treatment will affect the other parts of her life before therapy begins.

The list of side-effects and adverse reactions for this drug is even more extensive than for isotretinoin. Therefore, the patient must be monitored closely and be told to report early any flu-like symptoms, earache or changes in hearing, or changes in vision. The patient should have frequent dental check-ups to monitor the development of caries.

Periodic radiologic evaluation of the ankles, pelvis, and knees should be performed during treatment to detect early hyperostoses. Evidence of emerging calcification of tendons or ligaments warrants immediate drug discontinuation.

Antiseptics

Several different types of compounds are useful as topical antiseptics or germicides for cleansing the skin preoperatively or for treatment of minor skin wounds or abrasions.

Benzalkonium Chloride
(Benza, Germicin, Zephiran)

Benzalkonium chloride is a cationic, surface-active agent that is either bactericidal or bacteriostatic (depending on concentration) toward a variety of bacteria as well as some viruses, fungi, and protozoa. The drug is available as a solution (1:750), concentrate (17%), and a tincture spray (1:750). The aqueous solutions are used in an appropriate dilution for antisepsis of skin, mucous membranes, and wounds; for preoperative preparation of the skin; for preservation of ophthalmic solutions; for irrigation of the eye, body cavities, bladder, and urethra; and for vaginal douching. The tincture spray is useful for preoperative skin preparation and for treatment of abrasions and minor superficial wounds.

The drug is rapid acting and has a relatively long duration of action. The drug may be inactivated by soaps or anionic detergents, and the area should be rinsed thoroughly prior to application of benzalkonium if these substances have been used previously. Solutions can be irritating, and the drug should not be used in occlusive dressings, casts, and anal or vaginal packs. Avoid use of concentrations stronger than 1:5000 on mucous membranes.

Chlorhexidine

(Hibiclens, Hibistat)

Chlorhexidine is an effective antimicrobial agent against a wide range of gram-positive and gram-negative microorganisms, including *Pseudomonas aeruginosa*. It may be used as a sudsing cleanser (4%), a drug-impregnated sponge (4%), a topical rinse (0.5%), or an oral rinse (0.12%). The cleanser is primarily used as a surgical scrub or skin wound cleanser; the hand rinse may be used as a germicidal rinse. The drug should be kept out of the eyes and ears; deafness can occur if the drug reaches the middle ear through a perforated eardrum. Irritation and dermatitis are infrequent with topical use.

Hexachlorophene

(pHisoHex, Septi-Soft, Septisol)

Hexachlorophene is bacteriostatic against many gram-positive microorganisms. It may be used as a liquid (0.25%, 3%), sponge (3%), or foam (0.23%), as a surgical scrub, or bacteriostatic skin cleanser. Hexachlorophene is not intended for use on open cuts, burns, wounds, or mucous membranes, or as an occlusive dressing, wet pack, or lotion. Rapid absorption can occur if hexachlorophene is applied to areas of lesioned skin, and toxic blood levels can ensue. Infants are particularly likely to absorb hexachlorophene, and systemic toxicity is often manifested as CNS stimulation (*e.g.*, irritability, seizures). The drug must not be used for routinely bathing infants. Occasional adverse reactions include dermatitis, photosensitivity, mild peeling, and dryness of the skin.

Povidone-Iodine

(Betadine, Pharmadine, and various other manufacturers)

Povidone-iodine is a water-soluble complex of iodine with povidone, which liberates approximately 10% free iodine. The complex provides the germicidal action of iodine without irritation to the skin and mucous membranes. Povidone-iodine is available in a multitude of dosage forms, which may be used as a surgical scrub, skin cleanser, perineal disinfectant, mouthwash/gargle, or whirlpool concentrate.

Thimerosal

(Mersol, Merthiolate)

Thimerosal is an organomercurial containing approximately 50% mercury. It possesses prolonged bacteriostatic and fungistatic activity against many common pathogens. Available preparations include a tincture, solution, and aerosol containing a concentration of 1:1000. Thimerosal may be used for treating contaminated wounds after cleansing, for antisepsis of intact skin, for pre- and postoperative use, and for local application to the eye, nose, throat, vagina, or genitourinary tract. Thimerosal should not be used with or immediately following strong acids, salts of heavy metals, potassium permanganate, or iodine, because it is incompatible with these substances. Side-effects are infrequent with topical application of thimerosal.

Antivirals

Antiviral drugs used topically include idoxuridine, trifluridine, and vidarabine, which may be instilled in the eye for local viral infections, and acyclovir, which is used as an ointment for the management of initial episodes of herpes genitalis or other mucocutaneous herpes simplex viral infections. These agents are reviewed in detail in Chapter 74.

Corticosteroids

A number of different corticosteroids are available for topical application for the treatment of inflammatory dermatoses. The relative potency of the various agents is dependent on several factors including the concentration of drug applied, the type of vehicle employed, and whether or not an occlusive dressing was applied. The topical corticosteroids are considered in Chapter 55. A relative potency ranking of the available topical corticosteroids is found in Table 55-2. Dermatologic disorders that generally respond well to topical corticosteroids include atopic, contact, eczematous, irritant, and seborrheic dermatitis, as well as pruritus ani, lichen simplex, and mild psoriasis of the face and genitalia. Dermatologic conditions that respond less well include discoid lupus erythematosus, sarcoidosis, pemphigus, vitiligo, acne cysts, keloids, hypertrophic lichen planus, and alopecia areata. Local side-effects of topical corticosteroid application include persistent erythema, telangiectatic vessels, "wrinkled" skin, steroid acne, pustules and papules on the central facial area, and hypertrichosis.

Enzymes

Several different enzymes are used topically for debriding surface ulcers, surgical or other types of wounds, and second- or third-degree burns. Their effectiveness varies with the condition of the wound or ulcer. To enhance their effectiveness, the lesion should be cleansed of debris, and any dry, dense eschar should be removed if possible prior to application of the enzyme. Generally, once daily application is sufficient, but the drug may be applied more frequently if the dressing becomes too soiled. The different topical enzyme preparations are listed in Table 83-2.

Keratolytics

Keratolytics are desquamating agents that cause degeneration and sloughing of epidermal cells. They are used for various indications, such as removal of epithelial growths (*e.g.*, warts), excessive keratin in hyperkeratotic skin disorders, and psoriatic lesions.

Salicylic acid, used as a gel, cream, liquid, ointment, transdermal patch, or plaster, has long been employed as a keratolytic in concentrations of between 3% and 6%, and in concentrations up to 40% for removal of warts and corns. The various salicylic acid preparations used in this manner may be found in Table 23-1.

Cantharidin

(Cantharone, Verr-Canth)

Cantharidin is an irritant substance isolated from *Cantharis vesicatoria*, also known as *Spanish fly* or dried blister beetles. Its acantholytic action results from changes in epidermal cell membranes leading to blister formation. This effect is confined to epi-

dermal cells, and there is no scarring from topical application. The major clinical uses are for removal of benign epithelial growths, such as ordinary, periungual, subungual, or plantar warts, and molluscum contagiosum. The drug is not recommended for use in anogenital areas because it is a strong irritant. Application of the drug to the skin may result in tingling, itching, or burning within several hours. Cantharidin may produce blisters on normal skin or mucous membranes and should be wiped or rinsed off at once if the drug is spilled on the skin. Use of a mild antibacterial is recommended with cantharidin until tissue re-epithelialization occurs. Patients must be warned to keep the drug away from the eyes; if the drug is spilled in the eyes, they must be flushed with water immediately.

Podophyllum Resin

(Podoben, Pod-Ben-25, Podofin)

Podophyllum resin is a mixture of several substances that are cytotoxic to embryonic and tumor cells. Following application there is degeneration of epithelial cells and mitotic arrest with distortion of the nuclear pattern. The principal clinical applications of podophyllum resin are for the treatment of condylomata acuminata, verrucae, and multiple superficial epitheliomatoses and keratoses. Neuropathy has resulted from podophyllum application, usually when large amounts are applied to multiple or widespread lesions. Other untoward effects associated with the drug are nausea, vomiting, lethargy, tachycardia, stupor, flaccid paralysis, paresthesias, pyrexia, leukopenia, thrombocytopenia, and coma. Podophyllum resin should not be used by diabetics or others with compromised circulation, or by pregnant women. The drug should not be applied to moles, birthmarks, inflamed or irritated warts, or to the area around the eyes because severe corneal damage can result.

Urea

(Aquacare, Carmol, and various other manufacturers)

Urea (or carbamide) possesses a softening or moisturizing effect on the stratum corneum and can increase the solubilization of keratin, possibly by disrupting its hydrogen bond structure. Urea promotes removal of excess keratin in dry skin or hyperkeratotic conditions. It is available as a cream (2%–40%) or lotion (2%–25%). The 40% cream

(Text continues on p. 1644.)

Table 83-2
Topical Enzyme Preparations

Drug	Preparations	Indications	Administration and Dosage	Clinical Considerations
collagenase (Biozyme-C, Santyl)	Ointment—250 U/g	Debridement of dermal ulcers and severe burns	Apply once daily or once every other day	Digests collagen and promotes formation of granulation tissue and epithelialization of ulcers and burns; optimal pH range for enzymatic activity is 6 to 8; cleanse lesion before application and cover wound with sterile gauze after using ointment each time a dressing is changed; a suitable antibacterial ointment is used when infection is present; avoid soaks or washing with solutions containing metal ions or acidic substances, because they reduce enzymatic activity.
fibrinolysin and desoxyribonuclease (Elase)	Ointment—30 U fibrinolysin and 20,000 U DNAase per 30 g Powder—25 U fibrinolysin and 15,000 U DNAase per 30-ml container with thimerosal	Topical—debridement of inflamed, ulcerative, or infected lesions, general surgical wounds, or burns Intravaginal—adjunctive treatment of vaginitis and cervicitis	Topical—apply as ointment or solution prepared from powder in the form of a spray or wet dressing Change dressing two to three times a day, removing debris and exudates each time Vaginal—instill 5 g of ointment or 10 ml of solution (1 vial/10 ml) deep into vagina at bedtime for 5 days	Combination of two enzymes that attack both DNA and fibrin, thus breaking down necrotic tissue and fibrinous exudates; do not use parenterally because bovine fibrinolysin may be antigenic; solutions from dry powder must be used within 24 h; following instillation of solution into vagina, wait 1 min–2 min, then insert a tampon for 12 h–24 h; affected area must be cleaned, and dense, dry, escharotic tissue removed before application of drug, because enzymes must be in contact with the tissue to

(continued)

Table 83-2 (continued)
Topical Enzyme Preparations

Drug	Preparations	Indications	Administration and Dosage	Clinical Considerations
fibrinolysin and des-oxyribonuclease (Elase) *(continued)*				be removed to be effective; also available as ointment with 10 mg/g chloramphenicol as Elase-Chloromycetin, which is indicated in infected lesions where a topical antibiotic is required
papain (Panafil)	Ointment—10% with 10% urea	Debridement of surface lesions	Apply directly to lesion one to two times a day	Enzyme derived from *Carica papaya*; cover with gauze and remove accumulated necrotic tissue at each redressing; hydrogen peroxide may inactivate papain; itching or stinging can occur with topical application.
sutilains (Travase)	Ointment—82,000 casein U/g	Debridement of burned areas, decubitus ulcers, incisional or traumatic wounds and surface ulcers resulting from peripheral vascular diseases	Apply in a thin layer to moistened wound area three to four times a day	Proteolytic enzyme that digests necrotic tissue thus facilitating formation of granulation tissue; avoid contact of ointment with eyes; a moist environment is essential for optimal enzymatic activity; action of enzyme is reduced by iodine, thimerosal, hexachlorophene, benzalkonium chloride, and nitrofurazone; side-effects include mild pain, paresthesias, dermatitis, and possibly bleeding
trypsin (Granulex)	Aerosol—0.1 mg trypsin/0.82 ml with balsam of Peru and castor oil	Treatment of decubitus and varicose ulcers, wounds, and severe sunburn	Spray twice daily	Used as a spray for debriding necrotic areas; do not use on fresh arterial clots; avoid contact with eyes; balsam of Peru may improve circulation to the wound site

may be employed to remove dystrophic nails without local anesthesia or surgery. Concentrations of the drug in excess of 10% may be associated with a stinging sensation upon application.

Local Anesthetics

Topically applied local anesthetics are used for a variety of skin disorders, as well as for preparation for minor surgical procedures. The drugs are applied to both the skin and mucous membranes in a variety of dosage forms, including creams, ointments, solutions, and jellies. The various local anesthetics available for topical use are discussed in Chapter 20.

Pigmenting/Depigmenting Agents

Normal skin pigmentation is due to the presence of melanocytes in the basal layer of the epidermis. These cells have the ability to form the pigment melanin by oxidation of tyrosine. Subsequent activation of melanin occurs by exposure to radiant energy in the form of UV light.

Pigmenting Agents

Psoralens
(Oxsoralen, Trisoralen)

Two psoralen compounds, methoxsalen and trioxsalen, have the ability to increase the deposition of the pigment melanin in the skin in response to ultraviolet (UV) radiation. They may be employed either orally or topically to facilitate repigmentation in patients with vitiligo, a disorder characterized by patchy areas of nonpigmented skin. The oral dosage form of these two drugs can also be used to increase tolerance to sunlight in persons with fair complexions who suffer severe reactions upon exposure. Finally, much interest is centered around the possible beneficial effects of these drugs in treating severe psoriasis, when followed by controlled exposure to long-wavelength UV light (320 nm–400 nm). Such treatment, known as PUVA therapy, shows promise of being a very effective, albeit potentially toxic, form of therapy.

In vitiligo, repigmentation varies in time of onset, degree of completeness, and duration. Although some effect may be evident within several weeks after beginning therapy, significant repigmentation may take 6 months to 12 months. The psoralens are only effective in enhancing pigmentation when followed by exposure of affected skin areas to UV light, either artificial or natural (sunlight). The two drugs are reviewed together and listed individually in Table 83-3.

MECHANISM AND ACTIONS
The precise mechanism of action is not established. The drugs may increase the number of functional melanocytes and activate resting or dormant cells. They can also initiate a local inflammatory response and increase the synthesis of melanosome and activity of tyrosinase, an enzyme involved in conversion of tyrosine to dihydroxyphenylalanine, a precursor of melanin. Activity is dependent on the presence of functional melanocytes *and* activation of the melanin by UV radiation, either artificial or natural.

USES
1. Repigmentation of idiopathic vitiligo
2. Aid to increasing tolerance to sunlight (trioxsalen only)
3. Treatment of severe recalcitrant, disabling psoriasis not responsive to other forms of therapy —given only in conjunction with controlled doses of long-wavelength UV radiation (see Nursing Alert below)

ADMINISTRATION AND DOSAGE
See Table 83-3.

FATE
Oral absorption is 95% complete. Food appears to increase serum concentrations. Following oral ingestion, skin sensitivity to UV radiation is maximal in 2 hours and disappears within 8 hours. Psoralens are metabolized in the liver and excreted primarily (90%) in the urine. Topical application produces a rapid sensitivity.

SIDE-EFFECTS/ADVERSE REACTIONS
Nausea is common with oral administration of the psoralens. Pruritus and erythema can also occur with topical application.

Other adverse reactions include skin irritation and blistering following topical use, and GI upset, nervousness, insomnia, depression, edema, dizziness, headache, hypopigmentation, vesiculation, nonspecific rash, urticaria, folliculitis, leg cramps, and hypotension with oral use.

Table 83-3
Psoralens

Drug	Preparations	Usual Dosage Range	Clinical Considerations
methoxsalen (Oxsoralen)	Lotion—1% Capsules—10 mg	Topical—apply once weekly to small, well-defined lesions, then expose area to UV light for 1 min; subsequent exposure times should be increased with caution. Oral—2 capsules/day in a single dose, followed in 2 h–4 h by a 5-min exposure to UV light; gradually increase exposure time to 30 min–35 min; therapy should only be given on alternate days	Pigmentation may begin within several weeks, but significant repigmentation may require treatment for 6 months to 9 months; do not increase dosage of oral preparation; perform liver function tests periodically during therapy, and stop drug if liver impairment occurs; topical preparation is only used on small, well-defined vitiliginous lesions that can be protected from excessive exposure; use of bandages or sunscreens or both may be necessary
trioxsalen (Trisoralen)	Tablets—5 mg	Vitiligo—10 mg/day followed in 2 h–4 h by UV exposure ranging from 15 min–30 min. Sunlight tolerance—10 mg/day, 2 h before exposure to sun, for a maximum of 14 days	More active than methoxsalen, yet its median lethal dose is six times higher; do not increase dosage and only lengthen exposure time in gradual increments; discontinue drug if repigmentation is not evident within 3 months to 4 months.

■ WARNING
Use of psoralens together with UV radiation must be undertaken only by healthcare personnel experienced in photochemical treatment of psoriasis and vitiligo. Severe adverse reactions can occur (burns, ocular damage, skin aging, skin cancer), and patients must be informed of the risks inherent in such treatment. There exists an approximate tenfold increase in the risk of squamous cell carcinoma among PUVA-treated patients and approximately a twofold increase in basal cell carcinoma.

CONTRAINDICATIONS AND PRECAUTIONS
Psoralens are contraindicated in patients with melanoma, invasive squamous cell carcinoma, aphakia, albinism, porphyria, acute lupus erythematosus, leukoderma of infectious origin, in children under 12 years of age, and with concurrent use of a photosensitizing drug.

Patients must be instructed to shield the lens of the eye from sunlight for at least 24 hours following ingestion of methoxsalen, because cataracts have developed due to irreversible binding of methoxsalen to proteins and the DNA components of the lens in the presence of UV light.

INTERACTIONS
1. An increased danger of severe burns exists if psoralens are used together with known photosensitizing agents, such as anthralin, coal tar derivatives, griseofulvin, nalidixic acid, phenothiazines, sulfonamides, tetracyclines, and thiazide diuretics.

NURSING CONSIDERATIONS
A thorough drug history must be obtained to determine if the patient takes any photosensitizing drugs (see under Interactions). These must be discontinued before PUVA therapy is initiated. In addition, the patient should be asked to describe the current treatment being used for psoriasis. Patients using anthralen or coal tar derivatives must discontinue use during PUVA therapy to decrease the

danger of burns. A history of renal or hepatic problems should be noted. Patients with impaired function may not be appropriate candidates for treatment because psoralens are metabolized in the liver and excreted in the urine. Diagnostic studies before treatment should include a CBC, renal and liver function studies, and a complete ophthalmologic examination. These should be repeated periodically throughout therapy to detect early any changes. Liver dysfunction may occur and may be first detected by elevations in liver enzymes. The patient should be told to report any jaundice, fever, malaise, darkened urine, or light-colored stools—later signs of hepatic problems. Renal dysfunction is rare but may be characterized by a decrease in urine output, peripheral edema, and a feeling of fullness which should be reported immediately.

Oral psoralens commonly cause gastrointestinal distress, which can be minimized by taking the drug with food or milk. However, food enhances absorption and, in some patients, may not relieve GI distress. In such cases, the patient can divide the oral dose into two portions taken one-half hour apart.

Immediately after topical application and 2 hours after oral administration, the patient receives phototherapy with UV radiation. The patient should always be supervised in the treatment and timer-controlled lights (if done under lights), or a digital timer (if sunlight is used) should be used so the patient gets only the amount of light prescribed. Light exposure time is gradually increased during the course of therapy but only as the patient shows ability to tolerate such increases. PUVA therapy can cause severe burns and rash. Lips should be protected with sunblock, and eyes should be covered with opaque lid covers during therapy. The patient should be reminded to keep the treated lesions out of sunlight, except during therapy times, to avoid overexposure and the possibility of severe burns and blistering. This is especially important during the first few days of therapy when sensitivity to light is greatest.

Oral psoralens can cause cataract formation. The patient should minimize time out in bright sunlight during therapy and always wear dark sunglasses with side blinders if possible whenever outdoors. Any blurring of vision or appearance of spots before the eyes should be immediately reported.

Depigmenting Agents

Two agents are available for reducing hyperpigmentation of skin, but they differ in that one of the drugs, hydroquinone, generally produces a temporary lightening of skin areas whereas the other drug, monobenzone, produces irreversible depigmentation.

Hydroquinone
(Eldopaque, Esoterica Regular, Porcelana, and various other manufacturers)

Hydroquinone is capable of interfering with the formation of melanin by inhibiting the enzymatic oxidation of tyrosine. Skin color begins to lighten usually after 3 weeks to 4 weeks, but a good response may require up to 6 months. The drug may be applied twice a day as a cream (2%, 4%), lotion (2%), solution (3%), or gel (4%), often in combination with a sunscreening agent to minimize repigmentation upon exposure to sunlight. Hydroquinone should only be applied to limited areas of the face, neck, hands, or arms; the drug is not to be used on irritated, denuded, or damaged skin. Because the effect of the drug is temporary, treated skin areas will return to their original color when the drug is discontinued. Principal uses for hydroquinone are for reversible bleaching of hyperpigmented skin areas, such as freckles, chloasma, melasma, or senile lentigines.

Monobenzone
(Benoquin)

Monobenzone is employed as a 20% cream for permanent depigmentation in patients with extensive vitiligo. It is not to be used on freckles, melasma, pigmented nevi, or hyperpigmentation resulting from photosensitization, inflammation, or other causes. It is a *potent* depigmenting agent. Depigmentation occurs within 1 month to 4 months after initiation of therapy. Safety for use in pregnant women, nursing mothers, and children under age 12 has not been established. The cream is applied two to three times a day. If irritation, burning, or dermatitis occurs upon application, the drug should be discontinued.

Scabicides/Pediculicides

Crotamiton
(Eurax)

Crotamiton is a scabicide with antipruritic properties. It is effective in the eradication of scabies

(*Sarcoptes scabiei*) and for treatment of pruritic skin. Crotamiton may be used as a 10% cream or lotion. In treating scabies, two applications are made 24 hours apart, and a cleansing bath is taken 48 hours following the second application. The drug should not be applied to the area of the eyes or mouth, nor to inflamed or weeping skin areas. Crotamiton is viewed as an alternative to lindane (see below).

Lindane
(G-Well, Kwell, Kwildane, Scabene)

Lindane is an effective pediculicide and scabicide that is useful in the treatment of *Pediculus humanus capitis* (head lice) and *Phthirus pubis* (crab lice) as well as scabies (*Sarcoptes scabiei*). It may be applied as a 1% cream, lotion, or shampoo. The cream or lotion is applied in a sufficient quantity to cover the affected area, rubbed in, left in place for 8 hours to 12 hours, and then thoroughly washed off. Reapplication is only necessary if living lice are detected 7 days later. The shampoo is applied to dry hair, thoroughly worked through the hair, and allowed to remain for 5 minutes. Small quantities of water are then added to form a good lather, and the hair is then rinsed and dried. A fine-tooth comb may then be run through the hair to remove any remaining nit shells.

Concern about possible neurotoxicity or hepatomas, if significant percutaneous absorption occurs, have led to warnings that the drug should *not* be used in premature neonates and used *with caution* in infants, pregnant women, and patients with known seizure disorders. The drug should not be applied to the face, nor to open wounds or abrasions, and unnecessary skin contact should be avoided. When used properly, the risk of adverse reactions is quite small. Oils may enhance the percutaneous absorption of lindane; use of oil-based hair dressings or lotions should be avoided during application of lindane.

Permethrin
(Nix)

Permethrin is active against lice, mites, ticks, and fleas, because it acts on the nerve cell membranes of the parasites to cause paralysis. The drug is available as a 1% liquid for treatment of head lice and its nits (*i.e.*, eggs). Application is made to the hair and scalp, and the drug is allowed to remain in contact with the area for 10 minutes before it is rinsed off.

A single treatment is up to 99% effective in eliminating head lice infestation. Pruritus may be temporarily exacerbated by application of permethrin, and burning, stinging, and numbness of the scalp can occur. Systemic absorption is minimal. Safety and efficacy for use in children under age 2 have not been established.

Pyrethrins

Pyrethrins are available in combination with piperonyl butoxide and petroleum distillate in a number of over-the-counter pediculocides, such as A-200 Pyrinate, RID, or R & C shampoo. The combination exerts a synergistic action against head lice, body lice, and pubic lice and is applied either as a gel, liquid, or shampoo. The product is allowed to remain in contact with the area no longer than 10 minutes, then the area is washed thoroughly with warm water. Two applications may be required 24 hours apart.

NURSING CONSIDERATIONS FOR SCABICIDES/PEDICULICIDES

The topical agents discussed above are extremely effective in ridding the victim of the parasites. However, the patient should be examined 7 days to 10 days after initial treatment because any untreated eggs (nits) will hatch at that time, necessitating retreatment. If parents are to do the re-examination, they must be taught to differentiate nits and parasites from hair debris and dandruff. The side-effects from these agents occur most frequently when the patient has been *overtreated* for an infestation.

To systematically remove the threat of infestation from the whole family whose member has been identified as having lice or scabies, all members should be thoroughly examined and all infected persons should be treated at the same time. In addition, all bedding and clothing should be washed in hot (150°F) water or run through the hottest cycle in the clothes dryer for at least 20 minutes. Any item of clothing or bedding that cannot be washed by this method should be dry cleaned or placed in a sealed plastic bag for 10 days. All combs and brushes should be soaked in hot (150°F) water or in a solution containing a pediculicide shampoo. Rugs and upholstered furniture should be thoroughly vacuumed, and the dust bag should be discarded or cleaned.

To prevent infestation, children attending any school should have an assigned coat hook with a place for a hat; clothing should never be piled together. Children should be discouraged from sharing combs, hats, towels, or other clothing.

Sunscreens

Preparations useful as sunscreens provide either a chemical or physical barrier to sunlight. *Chemical* sunscreens absorb UV radiation in the medium wavelength range of 290 nm to 320 nm which is the spectrum of UV light most responsible for sunburning. *Physical* sunscreens reflect or scatter light in the spectrum of 290 nm to 700 nm and prevent its skin penetration.

Available sunscreens in each category are:

Chemical

1. Benzophenones (oxybenzone, dioxybenzone)
2. PABA and esters (PABA, octyldimethyl PABA [Padimate-O], glyceryl PABA)
3. Cinnamates (cinoxate, ethylhexyl-p-methoxycinnamate)
4. Salicylates (octylsalicylate, homosalate)
5. Methyl anthranilate
6. Digalloyl trioleate

Physical

1. Titanium dioxide
2. Red petrolatum
3. Zinc oxide

PABA (para-aminobenzoic acid) and its ester are among the most effective absorbers of UV light in the dangerous range of 270 nm to 320 nm and are found in many of the commercially available sunscreens. The benzophenones provide a somewhat broader range of protection (250 nm to 360 nm) but are somewhat less effective than PABA.

Effectiveness of a sunscreen preparation is given by its sun protection factor (SPF) which indicates the relative resistance to sunburning afforded by the product. For example, an SPF of 6 means that use of the product will permit six times as much sun exposure as use of no sunscreen. Fair-skinned individuals should use products with SPF of at least 10; persons with darker skins may safely use a sunscreen with a lower SPF rating.

Sunscreens should be applied to all exposed areas and reapplied periodically to maintain an even film, especially after swimming or excessive sweating.

Contact dermatitis may develop with PABA or its esters, benzophenones, and cinnamates. PABA may impart a permanent yellow stain on clothing. Contact with the eyes should be avoided, and use of the product should be discontinued if rash or other signs of irritation appear.

REVIEW QUESTIONS

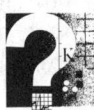

1. What are the two principal components of the skin?
2. Briefly describe the five layers of the skin.
3. Where is melanin produced, and what are its functions?
4. What are the components of the dermis?
5. List the various types of vehicles in which dermatologic drugs may be incorporated?
6. Which types of vehicles provide the best skin hydration?
7. Which types of vehicles are best for application to hairy areas?
8. How does tretinoin act in treating acne?
9. What baseline information is needed before a patient is treated with tretinoin?
10. What are the indications for isotretinoin?
11. Why is a drug/treatment history important for a patient about to receive isotretinoin?
12. What monitoring is essential in the patient receiving isotretinoin to detect early any adverse effects?
13. What is the most common side-effect of isotretinoin? How can it be managed?
14. In what conditions is use of isotretinoin contraindicated?
15. What kinds of topical drugs may be useful in treating acne?
16. What antibacterial drugs are effective for chronic treatment of acne?

17. List the different (a) topical and (b) systemic drugs useful for the symptomatic management of psoriasis.
18. What is the mechanism of action of etretinate? How is it used?
19. What monitoring is essential for the patient receiving etretinate to detect early any adverse effects?
20. Describe the major adverse reactions associated with etretinate.
21. Briefly discuss the actions of (a) benzalkonium chloride, (b) chlorhexidine, and (c) hexachlorophene.
22. Which types of dermatologic disorders generally respond best to topical corticosteroids?
23. For what indication are topical enzymes used?
24. Describe the action of keratolytics. List several drugs useful as keratolytics.
25. What is the principal action of psoralens?
26. Briefly discuss PUVA therapy. What protective measures should be used to prevent adverse effects of therapy?
27. What are the major side-effects of PUVA therapy?
28. Distinguish between the actions of hydroquinone and monobenzone as depigmenting agents.
29. What are the principal indications for (a) crotamiton and (b) permethrin?
30. In what forms is lindane used as a pediculicide?
31. What are the potential systemic effects of lindane following percutaneous absorption?
32. How can families prevent reinfestation with lice once a member has been successfully treated?
33. Briefly describe the various mechanisms of action of the different sunscreen agents.
34. What is the "SPF" in relation to sunscreens?

BIBLIOGRAPHY

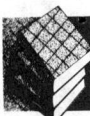

Berry ARC, Walt B, Goldacre MJ et al: A comparison of the use of povidone-iodine and chlorhexidine in the prophylaxis of postoperative wound infection. J Hosp Infect 3:55, 1982

Block SS (ed): Disinfection, Sterilization and Preservation, 3rd ed. Philadelphia, Lea & Febiger, 1983

Bronaugh R, Maibach HI: Percutaneous Penetration: Principles and Practices. New York, Marcel Dekker, 1985

Ehmann CW, Voorhees JJ: International studies of the efficacy of etretinate in the treatment of psoriasis. J Am Acad Dermatol 6:692, 1982

Isotretinoin. Med Lett Drugs Ther 24:79, 1982

Kaidbey KH, Kligman AM: An appraisal of the efficacy and substantivity of the new high-potency sunscreens. J Am Acad Dermatol 4:566, 1981

Leigh DA, Strange JL, Marriner J et al: Total body bathing with Hibiscrub (chlorhexidine) in surgical patients: A controlled trial. J Hosp Infect 4:229, 1983

McLaury P: Head lice: Pediatric social disease. Am J Nurs 83:1300, 1983

Neuberger GB, Reckling JB: A new look at wound care. Nursing 15:34, 1981

Orkin M et al (eds): Scabies and Pediculosis. New York, Marcel Dekker, 1985

Pathak MA: Topical and systemic approaches to protection of human skin against harmful effects of solar radiation. J Am Acad Dermatol 7:285, 1982

Peck GL et al: Isotretinoin versus placebo in the treatment of cystic acne. J Amer Acad Dermatol 6:735, 1982

Pegg SP: The role of drugs in management of burns. Drugs 24:256, 1982

Robertson DB, Maibach HI: Topical corticosteroids: A Review. Int J Dermatol 21:59, 1982

Rogers DM, Blouin GS, O'Leary JP: Povidone-iodine wound irrigation and wound sepsis. Surg Gynecol Obstet 57:426, 1983

Schachner L: The treatment of acne: A contemporary review. Ped Clin North Am 30:501, 1983

Schacter B: Treatment of scabies and pediculosis with lindane preparation: An evaluation. J Am Acad Dermatol 5:517, 1981

Sunscreens. Med Lett Drug Ther 26:56, 1984

Susong CR, Nordlung JJ: Vitiligo: Guidelines for successful therapy. Drug Ther 15:133, 1985

Miscellaneous Drugs

84

Several pharmacologic agents cannot be conveniently classified into any of the drug categories previously discussed. These agents will be considered in this chapter.

Antidotes

Most drugs employed as specific antidotes (i.e., narcotic antagonists, acetylcysteine, protamine sulfate, digoxin immune FAB, vitamin K, physostigmine, leucovorin) have been considered previously in the individual chapters dealing with the pharmacologic agents that they specifically antagonize. Certain other drugs are also useful as antidotes for certain types of poisonings.

Activated Charcoal

(Acta-Char, CharcoalantiDote, Liquid-Antidose, SuperChar)

Activated charcoal is a carbon residue with a very large surface area due to a fine network-like structure. This results in a great adsorptive capacity per unit of weight. The amount of drug or other substance which can be adsorbed by activated charcoal is approximately 100 mg to 1000 mg per gram of charcoal. The drug is used as a powder or liquid for the emergency treatment of poisoning by most drugs and chemicals, *except* cyanide, alkalis, and mineral acids. It is also largely ineffective against poisoning with ethanol, methanol, and iron salts.

The initial dosage would be 1 g/kg or approximately five to ten times the amount of poison ingested. The charcoal powder is given as a suspension in 6 oz to 8 oz of water, as soon as possible (ie, within 30 min) after the poisoning. Although the black solution does not appear palatable, it is odorless and tasteless. It may be mixed with sweet syrup to enhance palatability. Emesis should be induced if possible prior to administration of charcoal except in cases of poisoning with strong acids or alkalis, petroleum distillates, or other caustic substances. Concurrent use of syrup of ipecac or laxatives with charcoal should be avoided because charcoal can adsorb and inactivate these agents as well.

Either constipation or diarrhea may occur, and the stools will be blackened.

Heavy Metal Antagonists

Deferoxamine Mesylate
Dimercaprol
Edetate Calcium Disodium

Several agents have the ability to complex with various heavy metals (such as iron, lead, gold, mercury) and are employed to treat poisoning with these substances. Such poisoning can occur either from drug overdosage, for example, with use of gold salts for rheumatoid arthritis or iron for severe anemias, or accidental ingestion, such as lead-containing paints, insecticides, or pesticides. Heavy metal intoxication often results in impaired enzymatic functions, which, if severe, can lead to cellular anoxia, shock, coma, and possibly death.

Table 84-1 lists the various heavy metal antidotes, together with their indications, dosage, and clinical considerations.

■ Nursing Process for Patients Being Treated for Poisoning

See also Poisons and Antidotes in Appendix.

□ ASSESSMENT

□ Subjective Data
Antidotes and heavy metal antagonists are most frequently used in the treatment of poisoning. To determine appropriate treatment with the correct substance certain initial data must be collected. The first encounter with the patient may be a frantic telephone call from a concerned parent or significant other or the patient may be brought to the emergency room. If a telephone contact is made, it is useful to obtain the following information:

1. Name, address, and telephone number of the caller so that contact can be reestablished if the situation becomes more serious during the conversation and the caller leaves the phone or hangs up
2. The substance ingested, quantity ingested, time ingested, age and weight of the victim
3. Condition of the victim; level of consciousness and presence of gastrointestinal symptoms
4. If victim is alert: availability of home remedies

(*i.e.*, syrup of ipecac, milk, eggs, antacids, charcoal) that may be used before transporting the patient to a health-care facility (see Appendix for direction on first aid for specific poisons)

5. The availability of the bottle in which substance was contained. This should be brought to the health-care facility with the patient for identification.

6. The availability of safe transportation to an emergency facility, if necessary. Arrangements should be made if the caller is unable to do so.

Once the patient is brought in for emergency treatment other useful information includes a brief medical history, especially of problems in cardiovascular, neurologic, or renal function and any medications the patient is taking currently.

□ *Objective Data*

Physical assessment will focus on cardiovascular status and respiratory function. Vital signs should be taken and weight obtained to facilitate calculation of dosages. Renal output should be measured, and a brief neurologic examination should be performed. A flow sheet for vital signs, intake, output, and level of consciousness should be established.

Laboratory and diagnostic evaluation will include renal function studies, serum electrolytes, acid–base levels, arterial blood gases, and may include analysis of gastric contents if gastric lavage is performed.

□ *NURSING DIAGNOSIS*

Actual nursing diagnosis will usually include:

Anxiety related to potential complications of poisoning and guilt on the part of parents or significant others who find the victim
Knowledge deficit related to the effects of the poison and the proposed treatment and potential outcomes of treatment

The nurse will collaborate with other health professionals in managing the complications of poisoning and subsequent treatment.

□ *PLAN*

Nursing goals focus on
1. Assisting in correct identification of the poison and correct initial treatment
2. Providing supportive care to minimize damage from the poison

□ *INTERVENTION*

Once the poison substance is identified, appropriate management can begin and substances such as specific antidotes, charcoal, or syrup of ipecac can be initiated. Administration of antidotes or heavy metal antagonists does not preclude the advance of symptoms, which will depend on the quantity of substance already absorbed by the time treatment begins. Consequently, nursing care will be directed at observing for and managing symptoms as they occur.

A clear airway must be maintained. Ingestion of narcotics, barbiturates, salicylates, iron, caustics and corrosives, and large amounts of lead among others may lead to apnea or increased secretions. Emergency equipment, such as airways, oxygen, intubation equipment, Ambu bag, and mechanical ventilators, should be on hand until the patient's condition is stabilized. The patient should be suctioned as needed and turned frequently to prevent respiratory infection. Respiration and character of breath sounds should be assessed frequently, and changes should be reported immediately.

Cardiovascular status must also be monitored. Hypotension may occur as an effect of the poison or during administration of deferoxamine. Hypertension can occur with dimercaprol (BAL). In addition, myocardial depression or irritation can occur as a result of the poison or the antidote causing a variety of arrhythmias and cardiac arrest. Cardiac monitoring is essential, and, if possible, an arterial line for continuous arterial blood pressure monitoring is useful in the acute phase of treatment. Vasopressors and antiarrhythmics should be on hand.

Metabolic (acid–base) balance and serum electrolyte levels may be adversely affected by the presence of poisonous compounds or by the substances produced when heavy metal antagonists are given. Such changes may be produced by acute renal dysfunction resulting from the poisoning. Therefore, frequent monitoring of the serum levels of the poison, serum electrolytes, acid–base levels, and arterial blood gases is essential to detect early any problems. Intravenous fluids will be ordered, and electrolytes are administered based on these levels. Fluid intake and urinary output should be monitored on an hourly basis during the acute phase because renal failure is a potential problem with many poisonings and particularly with dimercaprol (BAL) and EDTA administration.

(*Text continues on p. 1656.*)

Table 84-1
Heavy Metal Antidotes

Drug	Preparations	Indications	Usual Dosage Range	Clinical Considerations
deferoxamine mesylate (Desferal)	Powder for injection—500 mg/vial	Acute iron intoxication Chronic iron overload (e.g., multiple transfusions) Management of aluminum accumulation in bone in renal failure and in aluminum-induced dialysis encephalopathy (investigational uses)	Acute intoxication: 1 g IM, followed by 0.5 g every 4 h for two doses, then every 4 h–12 h as needed IV infusion—same as IM dose at rate of 15 mg/kg/h Chronic overload: IM—0.5 g to 1 g/day IV—2 g at a rate of 15 mg/kg/h SC—1 g to 2 g/day over 8 h–24 h with a mini-infusion pump Children—50 mg/kg IM or IV every 6 h or up to 15 mg/kg/h by IV infusion	Chelates iron in the ferric state, forming a stable, water-soluble, readily excretable complex; no effect on electrolyte or trace metal excretion; contraindicated in severe renal disease; should be used in conjunction with other appropriate antidotal measures (emesis, lavage, correction of acidosis, control of shock, respiratory assistance); pain on injection, allergic reactions, blurred vision, diarrhea, abdominal pain, tachycardias, and fever have been reported; Urine may be colored red. Use an infusion pump to conrol drip rate, and monitor BP every 5 min until stable. Too rapid infusion can cause hypotension, urticaria, erythema and shock.
dimercaprol (BAL in Oil)	Injection—100 mg/ml	Arsenic, gold, and mercury poisoning Acute lead poisoning (in combination with calcium EDTA)	IM only: Arsenic/gold poisoning—2.5 mg to 3 mg/kg four to six times a day for 2 days, then two to four times a day on the third day, then one to two times a day for 10 days Mercury poisoning—5 mg/kg initially, then 2.5 mg/kg one to two times a day for 10 days Lead poisoning—4 mg/kg at 4-h intervals in combination with calcium sodium EDTA at a different site	Complexes with various heavy metals forming stable, water-soluble chelates that are readily excreted by the kidney; sulfhydryl enzymes are thus protected from the toxic action of the metals; do not use in iron, cadmium, or selenium poisoning, because resultant complexes are more toxic than the metals; most effective when given as soon as possible after metal ingestion; urine should be kept alkaline to minimize kidney

(continued)

Table 84-1 (continued)
Heavy Metal Antidotes

Drug	Preparations	Indications	Usual Dosage Range	Clinical Considerations
dimercaprol (BAL in Oil) *(continued)*				damage as chelate is being excreted; local pain is frequent at site of injection; contraindicated in hepatic insufficiency; large doses may increase blood pressure and heart rate; other adverse effects include fever in children (30% frequency), nausea, vomiting, headache, burning in the mouth and throat, chest constriction, lacrimation, salivation, and paresthesias; other supportive measures are necessary (fluids, electrolytes, respiratory assistance)
edetate calcium disodium (Calcium Disodium Versenate, Calcium EDTA)	Injection—200 mg/ml	Acute and chronic lead poisoning and lead encephalopathy	IV—1 g diluted to 250 ml to 500 ml and infused over 1 h; administer twice a day for up to 5 days, stop 2 days to allow adequate renal excretion of drug, then resume for another 5 days if necessary IM (preferred in children)—50 mg to 75 mg/kg/day in two equally divided doses for 3 days to 5 days	Calcium in the compound is displaced by a heavy metal (*e.g.*, lead), resulting in formation of a stable metal–drug complex that is removed by the kidneys; potentially a very toxic compound; recommended dosage levels should not be exceeded; do not infuse rapidly in patients with lead encephalopathy; increased intracranial pressure can be fatal; IM is the preferred route of administration but procaine hydrochloride should be added to the solution to reduce pain; closely monitor renal function; do not give to patients with impaired kidney function; refer to package instructions for mixing and administering directions

Neurologic function also must be closely monitored. A standard flow sheet such as the Glasgow Coma Scale or other systematic assessment of neurologic function is essential because coma, convulsions, or cerebral edema is a potential outcome of poison ingestion. Parenteral diuretics and corticosteroids and solutions such as mannitol or urea should be on hand to treat cerebral edema. Diazepam or other anticonvulsants may be used to treat convulsions.

If the patient has been poisoned by skin contact with organophosphate (insecticide) or other hazardous chemical, the nurse must wear a gown and gloves when removing clothing or cleansing the skin in order to avoid self-contamination. The patient's contaminated clothing should be removed and placed in a *labeled* plastic bag. All personnel dealing with the patient should exercise caution.

Parents or significant others need an opportunity to discuss events that led to the poisoning. They may feel anger, guilt, or overwhelming fear that the patient will die as a result of ingesting the poison. Many patients are left with residual side-effects, especially if a large amount of poison was ingested or a prolonged time period elapsed before treatment was initiated. Therefore, family members may need help in sorting out their feelings about the event and in learning to cope with the demands of the care that their loved one may require during recovery.

□ EVALUATION

The outcome sought is reversal of the symptoms and effects of the ingested poison. In addition, treatment effectiveness is also measured by early management or prevention of side-effects of the poison and the drugs used as antidotes.

Binding/Chelating Agents

Drugs capable of binding or chelating others substances, such as metals, are useful in treating certain diseases characterized by excessive body levels of these various substances. One such drug, penicillamine, is an effective copper chelating agent useful in treating Wilson's disease (see Disease Brief in Chap. 23) and also in the symptomatic management of rheumatoid arthritis. It is reviewed in detail with other anti-inflammatory drugs in Chap. 23. A second chelating drug also useful in treating Wilson's disease is trientine.

Trientine
(Cuprid)

MECHANISM AND ACTIONS
Trientine is a copper chelating agent that is able to remove excess copper from the body by chemically complexing with the metal.

USES
1. Treatment of patients with Wilson's disease who are intolerant of penicillamine, which is normally the drug of choice

Note: Unlike penicillamine, trientine is not recommended for use in cystinuria, rheumatoid arthritis, or biliary cirrhosis.

ADMINISTRATION AND DOSAGE
Trientine is available as 250-mg capsules. The initial adult dose is 750 mg to 1250 mg daily in two to four divided doses. The maximum dose in adults is 2 g/day.

Children should receive an initial dose of 500 mg to 750 mg daily in two to four divided doses; the maximum dose in children is 1500 mg/day. Trientine should be given on an empty stomach, at least 1 hour before or 2 hours after meals.

The average duration of therapy is approximately 4 years, with a range of 2 months to 160 months. Long-term dosage should be reevaluated every 6 months by measurement of urinary and serum copper levels.

SIDE-EFFECTS/ADVERSE REACTIONS
Adverse effects reported during trientine therapy are iron defiency, dermatitis, heartburn, epigastric distress, malaise, anorexia, cramps, muscle pain or weakness, and systemic lupus-like symptoms.

CONTRAINDICATIONS AND PRECAUTIONS
There are no absolute contraindications to use of trientine. *Cautious use* must be undertaken in patients with iron deficiencies and in pregnant women, nursing mothers, and children under age 6.

NURSING CONSIDERATIONS
A baseline urinalysis, serum copper level, and CBC with differential should be obtained at the beginning of therapy. These parameters will be measured throughout treatment. Changes in copper level will indicate the drug is working. A decrease in hemoglobin or hematocrit may indicate iron deficiency anemia, and iron supplements may be nec-

essary. The patient should be encouraged to eat foods rich in iron including red meats, dark green vegetables, eggs (especially egg yolk), whole grains, legumes, raisins, prunes, brewer's yeast, and nuts. Appearance of protein or casts in urine may indicate early renal changes from the drug.

An administration schedule should be established whereby the patient takes the drug on an empty stomach, at least 1 hour apart from any food, other drug, milk, or antacid. Unfortunately, trientine may cause heartburn and epigastric distress, which will usually be relieved by food. Persistent problems or inability to take the drug should be immediately reported to the physician.

Systemic lupus-like symptoms which may develop with trientine administration include malaise, anorexia, arthralgia, and fever and may include a decrease in urine output. All symptoms should be reported immediately because the drug may need to be discontinued.

Cellulose Sodium Phosphate
(Calcibind)

MECHANISM AND ACTION
Cellulose sodium phosphate (CSP) is a phosphorylated cellulose that is capable of exchanging sodium for calcium. It is capable of binding calcium by the ion-exchange mechanism, and the complex of calcium and cellulose phosphate is then excreted in the feces. The complex also binds dietary magnesium and may increase urinary phosphorus and oxalate. There is no apparent alteration in serum levels of copper, zinc, or iron. The drug is used for the treatment of absorptive hypercalciuria (type I), with recurrent calcium oxalate or calcium phosphate nephrolithiasis. New stone formation is substantially reduced.

ADMINISTRATION AND DOSAGE
The drug is used as powder packets containing approximately 34% inorganic phosphate and 11% sodium. The initial dosage is 5 g with each meal; dosage may be reduced to 10 g/day (5 g with supper and 2.5 g with the other two meals) when urinary calcium falls below 150 mg/day.

Each dose is suspended in a glass of water, juice, or soft drink to mask the unpleasant taste. Magnesium supplementation should be provided because CSP binds to dietary magnesium. The recommended supplement is 1 g to 1.5 g of magne-

sium gluconate twice a day taken at least 1 hour before or after CSP to prevent binding.

SIDE-EFFECTS/ADVERSE REACTIONS
Diarrhea and dyspepsia are the most frequently encountered side-effects. The sodium content of the preparation may be dangerous in patients with congestive heart failure or ascites. Dietary sodium restriction is usually encouraged. Contraindications to use of cellulose sodium phosphate are primary or secondary hyperparathyroidism, hypomagnesemia, osteoporosis, osteomalacia, hypocalcemia, and hyperoxaluria.

Intake of calcium, sodium, oxalate (*i.e.*, dark green vegetables), and vitamin C should be moderated during therapy.

Chymopapain
(Chymodiactin, Discase)

MECHANISM AND ACTIONS
Chymopapain is a proteolytic enzyme derived from *Carica papaya*. It is injected into the nucleus pulposus of lumbar intervertebral discs, where it hydrolyzes the polypeptides and proteins that serve to maintain the structural integrity of chondromucoprotein. As a result, the osmotic pressure within the disc is lowered, fluid absorption is decreased, and the intradiscal pressure is relieved.

USES
1. Treatment of herniated lumbar intervertebral discs that have not responded to other conventional means of therapy (approximately 75% of patients respond successfully)

ADMINISTRATION AND DOSAGE
Chymopapain is used as powder for injection (2 units/ml, 2.5 units/ml) which is reconstituted with 5 ml sterile water for injection. Dosage is 2 units to 5 units injected into each herniated disc in a volume of 1 ml to 2 ml. The maximum dose in a patient with multiple herniated discs is 10 units. Each disc should receive only a single injection.

Subarachnoid injection must be avoided (see Warning below).

FATE
Chymopapain or its reactive fragments are detectable in the plasma at 30 minutes and decline over 24 hours. Small amounts of fragments are also found in the urine. The liquefied nucleus diffuses

into the circulation, where the enzyme is inactivated.

SIDE-EFFECTS/ADVERSE REACTIONS

■ *WARNING*
Serious and sometimes fatal anaphylaxis has occurred following chymopapain injection. In addition, paraplegia, cerebral hemorrhage, and other serious neurologic changes have also been reported after chymopapain injection. The drug is toxic when injected into the subarachnoid space. Great care must be taken to inject the drug only within the nucleus of the disc. The drug is only to be used in a hospital setting by physicians trained in its proper use.

The most frequently reported side-effects with chymopapain are back spasm, pain, stiffness, and soreness. Less commonly occurring untoward reactions are headache, dizziness, leg pain, hyperalgesia, paresthesias, nausea, rash, itching, urticaria, urinary retention, and paralytic ileus.

Anaphylaxis may occur in as many as 1% of treated patients. Females, especially those with elevated erythrocyte sedimentation rate, are especially prone to develop such a reaction. Because chymopapain is a foreign protein, it can cause an immunologic response. Patients who have received chymopapain once should *not* be reinjected a second time.

CONTRAINDICATIONS AND PRECAUTIONS
Chymopapain is contraindicated in patients with progressing paralysis, spinal cord tumors, or cauda equina lesions. The drug should not be injected into any spinal region other than the lumbar area. Safety for use in pregnant women and children has not been established. *Cautious use* must be observed in persons with a history of allergies. Prompt management of any allergic reaction is essential. Symptoms may be of immediate onset or delayed as long as 2 weeks following injection.

NURSING CONSIDERATIONS
In addition to standard OR preparation of the patient, the OR nurse should make sure epinephrine and other emergency drugs, as well as equipment to manage respiratory or cardiac arrest, are immediately on hand should the patient develop anaphylaxis. The danger of allergic reaction is greatest 1

minute to 1 hour after injection, but allergic reaction may occur as long as 2 weeks later. Patients at discharge should be told to report immediately any swelling, pain, or redness at the injection site or any pruritis, dyspnea, or urticaria.

Postoperative assessment of neurologic function, motor strength, and circulatory status of the lower extremities is essential to determine any problems. Status checks should be made every 15 minutes for 1 hour, every ½ hour for 2 hours, every hour for 8 hours, then every 4 hours.

Dexpanthenol
(Ilopan, Panol, Panthoderm)

MECHANISM AND ACTIONS
Dexpanthenol is a derivative of pantothenic acid, a precursor of coenzyme A, which serves as a cofactor in the synthesis of acetylcholine (ACh). ACh exerts a range of functions in the body, including maintenance of intestinal tone and peristalsis. The drug acts as a GI stimulant for treating adynamia and also functions topically as an emollient to relieve skin itching and aid in the healing of minor skin lesioning.

USES
1. Prevention of paralytic ileus and intestinal atony following abdominal surgery (IM)
2. Treatment of adynamic ileus (IM)
3. Relief of itching and to assist healing of skin lesions in minor skin conditions (topical)

ADMINISTRATION AND DOSAGE
Dexpanthenol is available for injection in a solution containing 250 mg/ml and as a 2% topical cream. Dosage is as follows:

Prevention of paralytic ileus: 250 mg to 500 mg IM; repeat in 2 hours, then every 6 hours until danger of adynamic ileus has passed

Treatment of adynamic ileus: 500 mg IM; repeat in 2 hours and again every 6 hours as needed

Skin lesions: apply topically one to four times a day

SIDE-EFFECTS/ADVERSE REACTIONS
Systemic administration of dexpanthenol has resulted in itching, erythema, dermatitis, urticaria, dyspnea, intestinal colic, hypotension, vomiting, and diarrhea.

CONTRAINDICATIONS AND PRECAUTIONS

Dexpanthenol is contraindicated in persons with hemophilia or ileus due to a mechanical obstruction. The drug should be given with *caution* to pregnant women or nursing mothers.

INTERACTIONS

1. Concomitant use of antibiotics, barbiturates, or narcotics may increase the likelihood of allergic reactions to dexpanthenol.
2. Respiratory difficulty has occurred when dexpanthenol has been administered following succinylcholine. It should not be given within 1 hour of succinylcholine.

NURSING CONSIDERATIONS

A complete abdominal assessment should be performed before the drug is given. Baseline information to be recorded includes abdominal girth; auscultation of bowel sounds noting location, frequency, and pitch; palpation of the abdomen noting rigidity, softness, and location of pain or tenderness. A record of the frequency of stools should also be kept. These parameters must be reassessed periodically during the course of therapy. The physician should be notified of any changes.

Hypersensitivity reactions to parenteral dexpanthenol may occur. The patient should be told to report immediately any itching, redness, or urticaria.

Dimethyl Sulfoxide

(Cryoserv, Rimso-50)

MECHANISM AND ACTIONS

Dimethyl sulfoxide (DMSO) is a clear, colorless solvent possessing a wide range of pharmacologic actions, but only a very limited clinical applicability, because the compound has not been adequately tested and its potential toxicity is rather high. It is approved for use as a bladder irrigant for the treatment of interstitial cystitis; it appears to exert an anti-inflammatory and local anesthetic action. In addition, it has been used experimentally by topical application for treatment of various musculoskeletal disorders and collagen diseases. Dimethylsulfoxide can also serve as a vehicle to enhance percutaneous absorption of other drugs and has been reported to possess diuretic, local anesthetic, vasodilatory, muscle relaxant, and bacteriostatic activity, although data to support these claims are insufficient. Principal adverse effects are a garlic-like odor on the breath and skin, topical irritation, and allergic reactions due to histamine release. Ocular disturbances have been noted in experimental animals. The following discussion is limited to the use of dimethyl sulfoxide as a bladder irrigant. Its topical application should be discouraged until the efficacy and safety of the drug have been conclusively established.

USES

1. Symptomatic treatment of interstitial cystitis (no evidence of effectiveness in bacterial urinary infections)
2. Investigational uses include topical treatment of a variety of musculoskeletal disorders and to enhance the percutaneous absorption of other drugs.

ADMINISTRATION AND DOSAGE

DMSO is available as 50% and 99% solutions. The solution is instilled into the bladder in a volume of 50 ml by a catheter or syringe and allowed to remain 15 minutes. Elimination occurs with voiding. Treatment is repeated every 2 weeks until maximum relief is obtained.

SIDE-EFFECTS/ADVERSE REACTIONS

Side-effects following bladder instillation of DMSO are a garlic-like taste and discomfort in the bladder. Topical application can result in local dermatitis, nausea, vomiting, sedation, headache, and burning eyes. Hypersensitivity reactions can occur, presumably due to release of histamine.

CONTRAINDICATIONS AND PRECAUTIONS

DMSO must be used with *caution* in pregnant or nursing women and in patients with liver or kidney disease. Patients should seek approval from the physician for use of any other drug during treatment with DMSO because bladder irritability may occur.

Immunosuppressants

Drugs that suppress the immune response are extremely valuable agents in preventing rejection of transplanted tissues and in treating diseases believed to result from overactivity of the body's immune system. The various clinically available immune suppressant drugs are reviewed below.

Azathioprine

(Imuran)

MECHANISM AND ACTIONS

Azathioprine is an immunosuppressive agent used to prevent rejection in renal transplantations. It is a potent bone marrow depressant, and frequent blood counts are necessary during therapy. Although its mechanism of action is not completely established, the drug is converted to 6-mercaptopurine, which appears to interfere with nucleic acid and protein synthesis and coenzyme function (see under Mercaptopurine, Chap. 75). Azathioprine may also alter cellular metabolism.

Azathioprine has been used experimentally in treating other disorders believed to be the result of altered immunologic function, such as severe rheumatoid arthritis, systemic lupus erythematosus, and idiopathic thrombocytopenic purpura.

USES

1. Adjunct for prevention of rejection in renal homotransplantation
2. Treatment of severe, active rheumatoid arthritis in patients not responsive to conventional therapy (i.e., aspirin, nonsteroidal anti-inflammatory drugs, corticosteroids, gold)
3. Treatment of chronic ulcerative colitis (investigational use only)

ADMINISTRATION AND DOSAGE

Azathioprine is available as tablets (50 mg) and a powder for injection containing 100 mg/vial. Recommended doses are as follows:

Prevention of rejection: Initially 3 mg to 5 mg/kg/day IV beginning at the time of transplant; switch to oral therapy as soon as feasible; usual maintenance range is 1 mg to 3 mg/kg/day.

Rheumatoid arthritis: Initially 1 mg/kg as a single dose or two divided doses; increase stepwise in 0.5-mg/kg/day increments at 4-week to 6-week intervals if response is not satisfactory and no serious toxicity is noted; maximum dose is 2.5 mg/kg/day.

For IV administration, 10 ml sterile water for injection is added to the vial, and the solution is used within 24 hours. Further dilution into sterile saline or dextrose may be made for IV infusion, which is administered over 1 hour to 2 hours. Dosage should be reduced one-third to one-fourth if given concurrently with allopurinol (see under Interactions).

FATE

Azathioprine is largely converted to 6-mercaptopurine (6-MP) following administration. Both compounds are metabolized in the liver and erythrocytes. No azathioprine or 6-MP is detectable in the urine after 8 hours. Renal clearance is not critical in determining the drug's effectiveness or toxicity although dosage reduction is probably warranted in patients with poor renal function.

SIDE-EFFECTS/ADVERSE REACTIONS

The most commonly encountered side-effects with azathioprine are leukopenia, infections (fever, chills, sore throat, cold sores), nausea, and vomiting. Other adverse effects encountered during therapy are anemia, thrombocytopenia, bleeding, jaundice, diarrhea, alopecia, oral mucosal lesions, pancreatitis, arthralgia, steatorrhea, severe secondary infections, toxic hepatitis, and biliary stasis.

CONTRAINDICATIONS AND PRECAUTIONS

Use of azathioprine is contraindicated for treatment of rheumatoid arthritis in pregnant women or in patients previously treated with alkylating agents. The drug should be used with caution in patients with liver or kidney disease, during an active infection, and in pregnant women or nursing mothers and women of childbearing age.

INTERACTIONS

1. Allopurinol inhibits azathioprine and mercaptopurine metabolism and can increase the toxic effects of these drugs.
2. Azathioprine may reverse the neuromuscular blocking activity of nondepolarizing muscle relaxants (e.g., pancuronium).

NURSING CONSIDERATIONS

Baseline and periodic laboratory data will provide clues to the development of many of the drug's side-effects. The patient who accepts long-term therapy with this drug must recognize the need to maintain consistent clinical follow-up for early detection of problems. Laboratory tests should be done at least every 2 weeks to 3 weeks throughout the course of treatment.

A CBC with differential is essential to detect any leukopenia, thrombocytopenia, anemia, or other blood dyscrasias. Rapid fall or persistent decrease in leukocyte count warrants a dosage reduction or drug withdrawal. The patient should be told to monitor and report any fever, sore throat, malaise, abnormal bleeding, petechiae, or mucosal ulceration as these are indicative of changes in blood count. Patients on long-term therapy with azathioprine have developed leukemia and lymphoma. Therefore, early reporting of symptoms is essential.

Liver enzymes and bilirubin levels should also be monitored regularly because the drug can be hepatotoxic. The patient should report immediately any pruritus, darkened urine, light-colored stools, or yellowing of skin or sclera which may indicate the development of hepatitis.

Renal function studies and serum electrolytes should also be performed regularly because renal excretion of the drug may become compromised during long-term therapy.

As with other immunosuppressant drugs the patient taking azathioprine is very susceptible to infection. The patient should be encouraged to maintain good nutrition, get adequate sleep, avoid getting run down, use good oral and perianal hygiene techniques, and avoid contact with anyone in the acute stage of infection. If the patient does become ill, even with flu symptoms or a cold, he should contact the physician immediately. Likewise, any cut or abrasion should be treated immediately using sterile technique to avoid infection. Venipuncture, catheterization, nasotracheal suctioning, or any other invasive procedures should be kept to a minimum to decrease the risk of infection. Oral assessments should be performed periodically, and the patient should be told to report immediately any lesions which may indicate viral or fungal infections.

Azathioprine may cause nausea and vomiting. If this is a persistent problem, the patient may be given an antiemetic prior to meals and be encouraged to have small frequent meals evenly spaced throughout the day.

Cyclosporine
(Sandimmune)

MECHANISM AND ACTIONS
Cyclosporine (cyclosporin A) is an immunosuppressant which may be employed to prolong and assist survival of allogeneic transplants involving the heart, kidney, liver, and possibly also the bone marrow, pancreas, and lung. The drug can inhibit immunocompetent lymphocytes in the G_0 or G_1 phase of the cell cycle. It appears to specifically and reversibly inhibit T-lymphocytes, including the T-helper cell and T-suppressor cell. Lymphokine pro-

duction is also impaired, and release of interleukin-2 or T-cell growth factor may be reduced.

USES
1. Prevention of organ rejection in kidney, liver, or heart transplants, in conjunction with adrenal corticosteroids
2. Treatment of chronic rejection in patients previously treated with other immunosuppressive drugs

ADMINISTRATION AND DOSAGE
Cyclosporine is used as an oral solution (100 mg/ml) or as an IV solution (50 mg/ml). Recommended doses are as follows:

Oral: initially 15 mg/kg/day, 4 hours to 12 hours prior to transplantation; continue for 1 week to 2 weeks postoperatively, then taper by 5% each week to a maintenance level of 5 mg to 10 mg/kg/day.

The oral solution may be mixed with milk or orange juice in a glass container (not styrofoam) preferably at room temperature. This will mask the unpleasant taste. The mixture is stirred well and drunk *immediately* (solution should not be allowed to stand before drinking). The mixing container should be rinsed with milk or juice, and the patient should drink the second glass to ensure all of the drug has been taken.

IV: initially 5 mg to 6 mg/kg/day 4 hours to 12 hours prior to transplantation, as a slow (2 hour–6 hour) infusion of dilute solution (50 mg per 20 ml to 100 ml of sodium chloride injection or 5% dextrose injection). Continue the single daily dosing until the patient can tolerate the oral solution.

FATE
Oral absorption is erratic and incomplete; cyclosporine blood levels must be closely monitored to ensure adequate levels. Peak serum levels are attained in 3 hours to 4 hours. The drug distributes to erythrocytes, granulocytes, leukocytes, and plasma, where it is approximately 90% protein bound. It is extensively metabolized and excreted primarily by the bile, with only about 60% of the dose eliminated in the urine.

SIDE-EFFECTS/ADVERSE REACTIONS
The most often encountered side-effect during cyclosporine therapy is nephrotoxicity. Elevated serum creatinine and BUN levels are common and

generally respond to dosage reduction. Renal function must be closely monitored. If BUN and serum creatinine remain persistently high and are unresponsive to dosage adjustments another immunosuppressive should be considered.

Other commonly occurring side-effects with cyclosporine are hypertension, hirsutism, and tremor. Many other adverse reactions have been reported on occasion and are listed below.

CNS—Headache, confusion, convulsions, flushing, paresthesias

GI—Diarrhea, vomiting, abdominal pain, gastritis, peptic ulcer, anorexia, hepatotoxicity

Dermatologic—Acne, brittle nails

Other—Anxiety, depression, muscle weakness, joint pain, chest pain, visual disturbances, gynecomastia, difficulty in swallowing, upper GI bleeding, pancreatitis, mouth sores, constipation, night sweats, leukopenia, lymphoma, anemia, thrombocytopenia

Infections develop in approximately 75% of patients on cyclosporine. Care must be taken to treat infections promptly.

CONTRAINDICATIONS AND PRECAUTIONS

Cyclosporine should not be used with any other immunosuppressive drugs (except adrenal steroids), because serious toxicity and infection can result (see under Interactions). The drug must be given with *caution* to patients with hypertension, renal or liver dysfunction, seizure disorders, and to pregnant women or nursing mothers.

INTERACTIONS

1. Cyclosporine can enhance the nephrotoxicity of aminoglycosides, loop diuretics, and other drugs that can damage the kidney.
2. Ketoconazole and amphotericin B can elevate the plasma levels of cyclosporine.
3. Concurrent use of phenytoin, phenobarbital, rifampin, or sulfamethoxazole-trimethoprim may reduce plasma levels of cyclosporine.
4. Concomitant use of cyclosporine with other immunosuppressive drugs can result in increased susceptibility to infection and possible development of lymphoma.

NURSING CONSIDERATIONS

The patient on cyclosporine must be prepared for regular clinical follow-up, close monitoring of laboratory values, and must learn a series of symptoms to monitor and report. In addition, the therapy is expensive and may cost up to $6,000 the first year and approximately $3,000 in following years. This cost may not be reimbursed under normal health-care insurance coverage. Financial resources must be evaluated, and special programs may be needed to underwrite the cost of therapy.

Drug dosage must be carefully calculated to ensure the patient gets the full benefit of the drug. The patient on home therapy must learn accurate dosing. Cyclosporine radioimmunoassay levels are drawn frequently to ensure adequate blood drug levels are maintained. Even small variations in the drug can result in transplant rejection. Early symptoms of rejection include elevated temperature, malaise, and a decrease in organ function (e.g., a decrease in urine output, decrease in respiratory volume, or change in pulse rate), all of which should be reported immediately. Transplant rejection is treated with corticosteroids because cyclosporine is ineffective once the process begins.

Hospital personnel and the patient and family should follow good infection control at all times. Thorough handwashing, use of sterile technique when handling dressings, and good skin care are essential to reduce the risk of contamination. The patient should avoid contact with anyone in the acute stage of infection and should maintain good nutrition, sleep, and hygiene.

Blood pressure should be monitored every 1 hour to 4 hours during acute treatment because hypertension can occur. Allergic reactions are also possible especially in early stages, and anaphylaxis can develop rapidly. Emergency equipment and drugs such as epinephrine should be immediately available if needed.

Nephrotoxicity is the most serious side-effect of cyclosporine and can usually be managed by decreasing the drug dose if detected early. Monitoring should include daily serum BUN, electrolyte, and creatinine levels, urinalysis, and urine creatinine clearance tests while the patient is hospitalized. Hourly urine output measurements should be taken in the hospital. Renal function studies may be reduced to weekly tests once the patient is discharged. The patient must be taught to keep a record of fluid intake and to measure urine output with each voiding. Any changes in laboratory values or decrease in urine output in an 8-hour period or change in I/O ratio must be reported immediately. In addition, the patient should learn to weigh himself daily and report weight gain of 3 lb to 5 lb overnight, edema, or puffiness.

Liver function studies should also be performed daily during the acute phase of treatment and periodically after discharge. Changes in liver enzymes or bilirubin should be reported immediately. The patient should report any fever, malaise, darkened urine, light-colored stool, or yellowing of skin or sclera; these are indications of hepatotoxicity.

The woman of childbearing age who takes cyclosporine should be encouraged to use an effective form of contraception because the drug is teratogenic.

Muromonab-CD3
(Orthoclone OKT3)

MECHANISM AND ACTIONS
Muromonab-CD3 is a monoclonal antibody to the T_3 (CD3) antigen of human T-cells. The drug blocks T-cell function (which plays a major role in acute renal rejection) by reacting with and blocking the action of a molecule (CD3) in the membrane of human T-cells that is essential for signal transduction. A rapid decrease in circulating T-cell number is observed within minutes after administration. Muromonab-CD3 reacts with most peripheral T-cells in blood and body tissues.

USES
1. Treatment of acute allograft rejection in renal transplant patients

ADMINISTRATION AND DOSAGE
Muromonab-CD3 is used by IV injection as a 1-mg/ml solution. The recommended dosage is 5 mg/day for 10 days to 14 days, begun once the acute renal rejection has been diagnosed. Methylprednisolone (1 mg/kg, IV) is given prior to the first dose of muromonab-CD3, and hydrocortisone (100 mg, IV) is administered 30 minutes after muromonab-CD3 to minimize the incidence of reactions to the first dose. Acetaminophen and antihistamines are also useful in reducing early reactions.

The drug is given as an IV bolus in less than 1 minute. It should *not* be administered by IV infusion nor in combination with other drug solutions.

FATE
Mean serum levels of drug will rise over the first 3 days and then level off during the remaining 7 days to 10 days. Antibodies to muromonab-CD3 have occurred and generally appear after approximately 21 days.

SIDE-EFFECTS/ADVERSE REACTIONS
The majority of patients receiving muromonab-CD3 experience a slight rise in body temperature during the first 2 days of therapy. Other commonly noted side-effects in the early stages of therapy include chills, wheezing, dyspnea, chest pain, vomiting, nausea, diarrhea, and tremor. Severe pulmonary edema has been reported following the first dose of muromonab-CD3, primarily in patients with pre-existing fluid overload.

These "first-dose" side-effects can be minimized by concurrent use of steroids (see under Administration and Dosage) and acetaminophen and weight restriction to less than 3% weight gain over the 7 days prior to injection. A chest x-ray taken 24 hours prior to administration must be clear of fluid. The first-dose effects are markedly reduced on successive days of therapy.

Infections may develop during muromonab-CD3 treatment, the most common being cytomegalovirus and herpes simplex. A few patients have developed serum sickness, anaphylactic reactions, or lymphoma during therapy, although the causal relationship is unclear.

CONTRAINDICATIONS AND PRECAUTIONS
Muromonab-CD3 is contraindicated in patients with fluid overload. The drug should be used *cautiously* if the patient's temperature is elevated. Cautious use is also warranted in pregnant women. A second course of therapy should be undertaken with care, because the drug induces antibody formation in the majority of patients which may limit its effectiveness on repeat administration. Antibodies normally develop within several weeks of the start of therapy.

NURSING CONSIDERATIONS
To monitor the "first-dose" side-effects of muromonab-CD3, the patient's vital signs should be assessed every 15 minutes for the first hour, every half hour for the next hour, then every 2 hours progressing to every 4 hours for the duration of therapy. As mentioned under Administration and Dosage, methylprednisolone, acetaminophen, and antihistamines may be ordered. Breath sounds should be auscultated frequently to monitor the development of fluid. Any changes in breathing or character of breath sounds should be reported immediately to the physician.

Because muromonab-CD3 acts on all T-cells, the patient has an increased susceptibility to infection. The patient should be encouraged to maintain good oral hygiene and report immediately any mouth sores because herpes simplex infection is common. Patients should also be advised to avoid contact with anyone in an acute stage of infection, regardless of cause. If the patient develops a cold or flu symptoms, he should contact the physician immediately. Likewise, any cut or abrasion should be treated immediately using sterile technique to avoid infection. Venipuncture, catheterization, nasotracheal suctioning, or other invasive procedures should be kept to a minimum to decrease the risk of infection during hospitalization.

Mesalamine

(Rowasa)

MECHANISM AND ACTIONS
Mesalamine is 5-aminosalicylic acid, one of the hydrolytic products of sulfasalazine (see Chap. 60). Mesalamine exerts an antiinflammatory action in the colon, presumably by inhibiting production of prostaglandins and possibly leukotrienes. Following rectal instillation, it provides a topical action to reduce pain and discomfort associated with chronic bowel inflammatory conditions.

USES
1. Treatment of distal ulcerative colitis, proctitis, or other inflammatory bowel syndromes

ADMINISTRATION AND DOSAGE
Mesalamine is available as a rectal suspension enema containing 4 g per 60 ml. The usual dosage is 4 g once daily, preferably at bedtime, which should be retained for 8 hours. Therapy is usually continued over 3 to 6 weeks.

FATE
Mesalamine is poorly absorbed rectally, with approximately 15% to 25% of the dose recovered in the urine in 24 hours. Excretion is primarily by way of the feces.

SIDE-EFFECTS/ADVERSE REACTIONS
The most frequently encountered side-effects with mesalamine are abdominal pain or cramping, flatulence, nausea, and headache. Other adverse reactions encountered during therapy include weakness, malaise, fever, diarrhea, dizziness, skin rash, rectal pain, hemorrhoids, bloating, leg pain, peripheral edema, and urinary infections.

CONTRAINDICATIONS AND PRECAUTIONS
Mesalamine should be given with caution to patients with renal dysfunction, sulfa allergies, and to pregnant or nursing mothers. Safety for use in children has not been established.

Plasma Expanders

Dextran 40, Dextran 70, Dextran 75, Hetastarch

Dextran, a synthetic polysaccharide of varying molecular weights, and hetastarch, a chemically modified corn starch, are employed to expand reduced plasma volume, which can occur in hypovolemic shock resulting from hemorrhage, extensive burns, surgery, sepsis, or other forms of trauma. Their principal advantages over whole blood or plasma for volume replacement are their relatively low cost, wide availability, and lack of incompatibility problems, as well as the fact that they are not associated with the danger of transmitting diseases such as viral hepatitis or AIDS. However, these synthetic polysaccharides can produce allergic reactions, occasionally severe, and may also interfere with platelet function, resulting in increased bleeding tendencies. Prior IV injection of dextran-1 (Promit), a monovalent hapten, may prevent severe anaphylactic reactions to dextran infusion.

The agents used as plasma expanders are considered as a group, and then are listed individually in Table 84-2.

MECHANISM AND ACTIONS
Plasma expanders elevate the osmotic pressure of the blood, thus drawing water from extravascular spaces into the bloodstream. Plasma volume expands slightly in excess of the volume of drug solution infused. The drugs also decrease blood viscosity and reduce erythrocyte aggregation and rouleau formation, thus improving microcirculation. They reduce platelet adhesiveness and can alter the structure of fibrin clots, thus reducing the likelihood of thrombus formation. Secondary cardiovascular effects include increased blood pressure, venous return, cardiac output, and urine flow, and decreased heart rate and peripheral resistance.

Table 84-2
Plasma Expanders

Drug	Preparations	Usual Dosage Range	Clinical Considerations
dextran 40—low molecular weight (Gentran 40, 10% LMD, Rheomacrodex)	Injection—10% in either sodium chloride or 5% dextrose	Shock—20 ml/kg/24 h by IV infusion the first day; thereafter, 10 ml/kg/day for a maximum of 5 days Extracorporeal circulation—10 ml to 20 ml/kg added to perfusion circuit Prophylaxis of venous thromboses—10 ml/kg on day of surgery, then 500 ml/day for 2 days to 3 days, then 500 ml every 2 days to 3 days for 2 weeks	Low-molecular-weight dextran is effective in reducing erythrocyte clumping and sludging and is reported to be able to disrupt thrombi; bleeding time can be prolonged and platelet function may be depressed by large doses; monitor coagulation time closely during therapy and observe for early signs of bleeding (epistaxis, petechiae)
dextran 70, 75—high molecular weight (Gentran 75, Macrodex)	Injection—6% in either sodium chloride or 5% dextrose	Shock: Adults—10 ml to 20 ml/kg/24 h by IV infusion; usually, 500 ml is given at a rate of 20 ml to 40 ml/min for emergency treatment Children—Maximum dose 20 ml/kg	High-molecular-weight dextran is slower in onset, but more prolonged acting than low-molecular-weight dextran; be alert for allergic reactions, which most often develop in first few minutes of infusion; may adversely affect capillary flow by increasing blood viscosity; can interfere with platelet aggregation, and can transiently prolong bleeding time
hetastarch (Hespan)	Injection—6% in sodium chloride	Volume expansion—500 ml to 1000 ml/day (maximum 1500 ml/day); in acute situations, infusion rate is 20 ml/kg/h Leukapheresis—250 ml to 700 ml infused at a fixed ratio (e.g., 1:8) to venous whole blood	Synthetic polymer prepared from amylopectin; similar to dextran in action and can also increase erythrocyte sedimentation rate; thus is used to improve efficiency of granulocyte collection by centrifugation; may elevate bilirubin levels; use with caution in patients with liver disease; during leukapheresis, hemoglobin and platelet counts may be temporarily reduced due to volume expanding effects of hetastarch; blood counts, hemoglobin determinations, and prothrombin times should be performed during therapy

USES

1. Adjunctive treatment of shock due to hemorrhage, burns, surgery, sepsis, or other trauma (*not* to be viewed as a substitute for blood or plasma)
2. Priming fluid in pump oxygenators during extracorporeal circulation (dextran 40 only)
3. Prophylaxis against venous thrombosis and pulmonary embolism in patients undergoing high-risk procedures, for example, hip surgery (dextran 40 only)
4. Adjunctive use in leukapheresis to increase granulocyte yield (hetastarch only)

ADMINISTRATION AND DOSAGE
See Table 84-2.

FATE
Onset of volume-expanding action varies from several minutes (dextran 40) to about 1 hour (dextran 75); hemodynamic status is improved for at least 12 hours (dextran 40) to over 24 hours (dextran 75, hetastarch) with a single infusion. Molecules less than 50,000 molecular weight are eliminated by the kidneys, 40% to 75% within 24 hours; larger molecular weight molecules are slowly metabolized to smaller sugars and either excreted in the urine or eliminated as breakdown products (*e.g.*, carbon dioxide and water). Small amounts of drugs are excreted in the feces.

SIDE-EFFECTS/ADVERSE REACTIONS
Untoward reactions associated with use of plasma expanders include allergic reactions (nasal congestion, urticaria, wheezing, dyspnea, hypotension), anaphylactic reactions (rare), nausea, vomiting, headache, fever, joint pain, infection at injection site, phlebitis, hypervolemia, pulmonary edema, osmotic nephrosis, renal failure (rare), and prolongation of bleeding time; hetastarch can also cause submaxillary and parotid gland enlargement, flu-like symptoms, and edema of the lower extremities. (See also Table 84-2.)

CONTRAINDICATIONS AND PRECAUTIONS
Contraindications to use of the plasma expanders include severe cardiac decompensation, renal failure, and marked hemostatic defects (hyperfibrinogenemia, thrombocytopenia).

Plasma expanders should be used *cautiously* in patients with liver or kidney disease, severe dehydration, active bleeding or bleeding tendencies, or a history of allergic reactions, and in pregnant women. Solutions containing sodium chloride should not be given to patients with congestive heart failure or renal insufficiency or to persons receiving corticosteroids. Excessive doses can precipitate renal failure; the patient should adhere to recommended dosage guidelines.

INTERACTIONS

1. Dextran may cause false elevations in blood glucose, urinary proteins, bilirubin, and total protein assays, and can give unreliable readings in blood-typing and cross-matching procedures.
2. Abnormally prolonged bleeding times can occur if plasma expanders are used together with anticoagulants or antiplatelet drugs.

NURSING CONSIDERATIONS
The patient receiving plasma expanders usually needs extra volume in the cardiovascular system to compensate for a large loss. Therefore, the nurse's first responsibility is to monitor the patient's response to the infusion to determine treatment effectiveness. Parameters which indicate the plasma expander is working include an elevation in blood pressure with a concurrent drop in pulse rate and respiratory rate and effort, a decrease in pulmonary wedge pressure (PWP) or central venous pressure (CVP) if PWP is not available, an increase in urine output to at least 30 ml/h and a decrease in urine specific gravity as urinary output increases. All of these factors indicate a re-equilibration of the plasma volume.

However, plasma expanders do not replace the proteins, cells, and plasma products, and consequently can change the laboratory values of a number of tests (see under Interactions), giving false values. Consequently, the patient should be typed and cross-matched prior to receiving these fluids if blood product administration is anticipated. In addition, the danger of too much hemodilution exists, which may occur if hematocrit falls below 30 mg/dl. If this occurs, the infusion should be slowed or stopped, the physician should be notified immediately, and the patient should be closely observed for signs of cardiac failure from fluid overload. Symptoms include a drop in blood pressure, an increase in pulse rate and respiratory rate and effort, coughing, presence of rales, an increase in PWP or CVP, and a decrease in PO_2. All of these are the opposite of signs of drug effectiveness and require immediate intervention by the physician. Emergency equipment and drugs should be on hand to deal with cardiac or respiratory arrest if it should occur.

The most serious side-effect of these fluids is the potential for anaphylaxis. Although allergic reactions are generally mild and are characterized by nasal congestion, urticaria, wheezing, dyspnea, and hypotension, they must be recognized as such and vigorously treated to avoid anaphylaxis. Epinephrine, antihistamines, corticosteroids, and emergency resuscitative equipment should be on hand at all times during infusion. The patient should be most closely observed during the first hour of *each* infusion which is when an allergic response is most likely to occur. Tolerance to one infusion does not preclude allergic reaction to later infusions.

Because plasma expanders affect platelet aggregation, erythrocyte formation and various aspects of the coagulation process, the potential for bleeding episodes exists during the course of therapy. A CBC with differential and coagulation studies should be obtained for baseline information and periodically throughout the infusion. Changes in platelet count, prothrombin time, or bleeding time should be immediately reported to the physician. Incisions, venipunctures, and invasive procedures should be kept to a minimum to reduce the potential sites of bleeding. All orifices, incisions, catheters, and venipuncture sites should be monitored closely, and any oozing or frank bleeding should be reported. Bleeding is characterized by a decrease in blood pressure, increase in pulse rate, and diaphoresis, and may be the first signs of internal bleeding.

Changes in hemodynamics from shock or from volume overload with plasma expanders can lead to renal failure. Serum BUN and creatinine levels should be drawn daily, but the early signs of failure may be a drop in the hourly urine output to less than 30 ml/h and an increase in urine specific gravity to greater than 1.030. Such changes seen together warrant discontinuation of the infusion and contacting the physician immediately. Hydrating solutions such as 5D/W, Ringer's, lactate, or normal saline are continued.

Partially used containers of plasma expanders should be discarded because they contain no bacteriostatic agent. Fluids should be stored at room temperature to prevent crystallization. Solution and container should be examined prior to use and discarded if the solution is not clear or the container seal is broken.

Plasma Protein Fractions

Albumin (Human) Plasma Protein Fraction

The plasma protein fractions are obtained by fractionating human plasma, and include normal serum albumin and plasma protein fraction. These products are primarily employed to expand plasma volume, as they raise the osmotic pressure of the blood. Because both preparations are heat treated to destroy hepatitis B virus, they are considered somewhat safer than whole blood or plasma as volume expanders.

These albumin preparations do not appear to interfere with normal coagulation mechanisms and do not require cross-matching. The absence of cellular elements, moreover, greatly reduces the risk of sensitization with repeated administration.

The plasma protein fractions will be discussed together, then listed individually in Table 84-3.

MECHANISM AND ACTIONS
Plasma protein fractions increase intravascular osmotic pressure, thereby drawing extracellular fluid into the bloodstream and expanding plasma volume. They also bind bilirubin in the plasma.

USES
1. Adjunctive emergency treatment of hypovolemic shock
2. Temporary replacement of blood loss to prevent hemoconcentration following severe burns
3. Treatment of hypoproteinemia due to nephrotic syndrome, hepatic cirrhosis, toxemia of pregnancy, and tuberculosis, and in postoperative patients and premature infants
4. Adjunctive therapy during exchange transfusions in hyperbilirubinemia and erythroblastosis fetalis
5. Adjunctive treatment of acute liver failure, adult respiratory distress syndrome, acute peritonitis, pancreatitis, or mediastinitis and during cardiopulmonary bypass or renal dialysis

ADMINISTRATION AND DOSAGE
Normal serum albumin is available in two concentrations, a 5% solution, which is approximately osmotically and isotonically equivalent to human plasma, and a 25% solution, osmotically equivalent

Table 84-3
Plasma Protein Fractions

Drug	Preparations	Usual Dosage Range	Clinical Considerations
albumin, human (Albuminar, Albutein, Buminate, Plasbumin)	Injection—5%, 25%	Variable, depending upon diagnosis, severity of condition, patient's age, and concentration of solution; usually, the equivalent of 25 g to 100 g albumin per day is given by slow IV infusion (1 ml–4 ml/min depending on concentration); maximum recommended dose is 250 g/48 h	Available in two strengths, 5% and 25%, both containing 130 mEq to 160 mEq/L; the 25% solution allows administration of large amounts of albumin quickly, and 100 ml provides as much plasma protein as 500 ml plasma or 2 pints whole blood; concentrated solution usually requires supplemental fluids in dehydrated patients; thus 5% solution may be preferred for routine use, because maximum osmotic effect is attained without additional fluids; preparations may cause an elevation of alkaline phosphatase levels; the 25% solution is preferred in most patients requiring sodium restriction
plasma protein fraction (Plasmanate, Plasma-Plex, Plasmatein, Protenate)	Injection—5%	Hypovolemic shock: Adults—250 ml to 500 ml by IV infusion Children—20 ml to 30 ml/kg Hypoproteinemia—1000 ml to 1500 ml/day	Rate of infusion is determined by condition and patient's age and body weight; maximum infusion rate is 10 ml/min in shock and 5 ml to 8 ml/min in hypoproteinemia; do not give more than 250 g in 48 h; monitor patients carefully for signs of volume overload; slow infusion if blood pressure declines; use cautiously in sodium-restricted patients; solution contains 130 mEq to 160 mEq/L; if edema is present, or if large amounts of protein are lost, use 25% albumin solution

to five times the volume of plasma. Plasma protein fraction is a 5% solution of human plasma proteins (83%–90% albumin with small amounts of alpha and beta globulins) that is osmotically equivalent to human plasma.

The usual dosage range and other clinical considerations are presented in Table 84-3.

SIDE-EFFECTS/ADVERSE REACTIONS
Adverse reactions associated with administration of plasma protein fractions are hypotension, allergic reactions (fever, chills, flushing, urticaria, rash), headache, nausea, vomiting, tachycardia, salivation, back pain, and respiratory irregularities. In addition, vascular overload and pulmonary edema can occur with too rapid infusion.

CONTRAINDICATIONS AND PRECAUTIONS
Plasma protein fractions are contraindicated in patients with cardiac failure, severe anemia, and normal or increased intravascular volume. In addition, plasma protein fraction is contraindicated in patients on cardiopulmonary bypass.

These agents must be given with *caution* to patients with mild anemia, low cardiac reserve, hepatic or renal failure, or congestive heart failure. Albumin preparations are not a substitute for whole blood, and large volume requirements should be satisfied with supplemental whole blood or plasma. Additional fluids should be given to patients with marked dehydration to minimize excessive depletion of tissue fluid.

NURSING CONSIDERATIONS
Plasma protein fractions (PPF) must be infused slowly (see Table 84-3) to reduce the risk of fluid overload. Infusion should be controlled by an infusion pump and checked at regular intervals. PPFs are usually piggybacked into an IV infusion solution but should not be given with any solutions containing alcohol or protein hydrosylates because precipitation may occur, nor should any drugs be infused in the same line at the same time. PPF must be infused within 4 hours once the container is opened because the products do not contain any preservative or bacteriostatic agents. Any solution which appears cloudy or contains sediment should be discarded. New IV tubing should be used with each container.

Successful therapy with PPFs depends on adequate hydration and cardiac functioning. Fluid therapy must be started in the patient who is dehydrated and a measure of circulatory volume should be established by insertion of a central venous pressure (CVP) catheter or pulmonary artery catheter (Swan-Ganz) to measure pulmonary wedge pressure (PWP). As circulatory volume improves, PWP or CVP will increase, however, the physician should set a numeric goal for these pressures after which the PPFs should be titrated downward. The potential for cardiac failure from fluid overload exists during this therapy and can be prevented through close adherence to circulatory volume goals. Symptoms of cardiac failure include increased pulse, increased blood pressure, increased respiratory rate and effort, onset of a third or fourth heart sound, and distended neck veins, which should be reported to the physician immediately. Emergency resuscitative equipment and drugs should be on hand at all times should cardiac arrest occur.

Allergic reactions to PPF are not uncommon, and patients should be closely monitored during infusion. Temperature, pulse, respiration, and blood pressure should be taken every ½ hour to 1 hour according to institution policy. If symptoms such as fever, chills, flushing, urticaria, or rash develop, the infusion should be stopped and the physician should be notified immediately.

PPFs do not provide clotting factors and are not a substitute for blood products. Therefore, as blood pressure increases from volume expansion, hemorrhage may occur at incision sites or sites of catheter or venipuncture insertion. If bleeding is noted from any site, the physician should be notified immediately.

Sclerosing Agents

Morrhuate Sodium
Sodium Tetradecyl Sulfate

MECHANISM AND ACTIONS
Sclerosing agents are primarily used to treat varicose veins. They produce their effects by irritating the vessel lining, producing a thrombus that occludes the damaged vessel. As a result, fibrous tissue develops, resulting in obliteration of the vein.

USES
1. Treatment of small, uncomplicated varicose veins of the lower extremities

2. Supplement to venous ligation to obliterate residual varicosed veins or reduce risk of surgery
3. Treatment of internal hemorrhoids (effectiveness is not conclusively established)
4. Treatment of esophageal varices (investigational use)

ADMINISTRATION AND DOSAGE
See Table 84-4.

SIDE-EFFECTS/ADVERSE REACTIONS
Local burning at the injection site is common with use of sclerosing agents. Other adverse reactions that have been reported with use of these agents are cramping sensations, urticaria, and tissue sloughing and necrosis. Rarely, drowsiness, headache, hypersensitivity reactions, dizziness, weakness, respiratory difficulty, GI upset, vascular collapse, pulmonary embolism, and anaphylaxis have occurred.

CONTRAINDICATIONS AND PRECAUTIONS
Among the contraindications to use of the sclerosing agents are acute thrombophlebitis, uncontrolled diabetes, sepsis, blood dyscrasia, thyrotoxicosis, tuberculosis, neoplasms, asthma, acute respiratory or skin disease, varicosities due to abdominal or pelvic tumors, bedridden patients, and persistent occlusion of deep veins.

Safety for use of these drugs in pregnancy has not been established. Inadvertent intra-arterial injection may result in severe ischemic damage.

NURSING CONSIDERATIONS
Patient sensitivity to the drug must be determined by administering a test dose as outlined in Table 84-4. While this procedure will be performed by the physician, the nurse must have emergency drugs such as antihistamines, epinephrine, and corticosteroids as well as resuscitative equipment should a hypersensitivity reaction or anaphylaxis occur. Patients should be advised that following injection the vein will become hard and swollen, and will be tender to touch. Aching and a feeling of stiffness will occur and may persist for up to 48 hours. Persistent burning, cramping, or change in tissue color should be reported to the physician immediately.

Table 84-4
Sclerosing Agents

Drug	Preparations	Usual Dosage Range	Clinical Considerations
morrhuate sodium (CMC)	Injection—50 mg/ml	50 mg to 250 mg IV (1 ml–5 ml) depending on size of vein, given as multiple injections at the same time, or a single dose; repeat at 5-day to 7-day intervals as needed	To determine patient sensitivity, 0.25 ml to 1 ml is given into a varicosity 24 h before administration of a large dose; vial should be warmed before injecting; use a large-bore needle to fill syringe, because solution froths easily; however, a small-bore needle is used for injection; pulmonary embolism has occurred
sodium tetradecyl sulfate (Sotradecol)	Injection—10 mg/ml, 30 mg/ml	0.5 ml to 2 ml of either strength solution depending on size of varicosity	Initially 0.5 ml of 1% solution should be given to determine patient sensitivity; observe for several hours before giving a larger amount; may *permanently* discolor vein at injection site; do *not* use for injecting veins for cosmetic purposes; caution in patients taking oral anticoagulants

Yohimbine

(Yocon, Yohimex)

Yohimbine is an alkaloid that chemically resembles reserpine. The drug is primarily an alpha$_2$-adrenergic blocker and can enhance the release of presynaptic stores of norepinephrine. Yohimbine can also block peripheral serotonin receptors. In addition, it readily enters the CNS, where it elicits a complex pattern of events, including central excitation, increased blood pressure and heart rate, release of antidiuretic hormone, irritability, and tremor.

Yohimbine has no FDA-sanctioned indications, but has been used with some success in overcoming male erectile impotence, as it can improve vasodilation of penile vessels, resulting in engorgement of blood in erectile tissue. The drug is used as 5.4-mg tablets in a dosage of 1 tablet three times a day if tolerated. Lower doses may be necessary. The occurrence of orthostatic hypotension has been reduced by yohimbine, and it may also act as an aphrodisiac.

The adverse effects associated with yohimbine are largely due to the CNS actions of the drug. They include elevated blood pressure and heart rate, irritability, increased motor activity, dizziness, headache, skin flushing, sweating, nausea, and vomiting. It should not be used in persons with renal disease, in pregnant women, or in children.

REVIEW QUESTIONS

1. How is activated charcoal utilized as an antidote?
2. What drugs may be used as heavy metal antidotes? Why is heavy metal intoxication hazardous?
3. What initial data should be collected from a caller who identifies a poison victim? What arrangements should be made?
4. What monitoring is essential for any poison victim who becomes acutely ill?
5. What are some of the side-effects of treatment of poisons with heavy metal antagonists?
6. What is the mechanism of action of trientine? For what indications is it used.
7. What baseline and periodic laboratory data should be collected to monitor the effects of trientine?
8. With which substances is cellulose sodium phosphate capable of binding?
9. Briefly describe the actions and uses of chymopapain. What are the major dangers associated with its use?
10. List the principal indications for dexpanthenol.
11. What are the (a) approved and (b) investigational uses for dimethyl sulfoxide (DMSO)?
12. Give the major uses for azathioprine.
13. What laboratory data must be closely monitored during long-term therapy with azathioprine? What side-effects must the patient be taught to monitor and report immediately?
14. What infection precautions should be taken with any patient on immunosuppressant therapy?
15. Describe the mechanism of action and indications for cyclosporine.
16. What are the principal adverse effects of cyclosporine?
17. What administration techniques must be used to ensure a patient receives the total amount of an oral dose of cyclosporine?
18. How does muromonab-CD3 function as an immunosuppressant? What are its common side-effects?
19. What are the indications for mesalamine? How is the drug administered?

20. What are the advantages of dextran and hetastarch over whole blood or plasma for volume replacement?
21. What physiologic parameters indicate therapy effectiveness with plasma expanders? What changes in these indicate cardiac failure from fluid overload?
22. What anaphylaxis precautions must be taken when a patient receives plasma expanders or plasma protein fractions?
23. For what indications are the plasma protein fractions used?
24. What is the mechanism of action of the sclerosing agents? For what conditions are they useful?
25. Briefly describe the uses and adverse effects of yohimbine.

BIBLIOGRAPHY

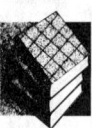

Beveridge T: Cyclosporin A: An evaluation of clinical results. Transplant Proc 15:433, 1983

Canafax DM, Ascher NC: Cyclosporine immunosuppression. Clin Pharm 2:515, 1983

Cantilena LR, Klaassen CD: The effect of chelating agents on the excretion of endogenous metals. Toxicol Appl Pharmacol 63:344, 1982

Clinical news: Enthusiastic cyclosporine consensus. Am J Nurs 85:861, 1985

Diehl JT, Lester JL, Cosgrove DM: Clinical comparison of hetastarch and albumin in postoperative cardiac patients. Ann Thorac Surg 34:674, 1982

Golden D et al: Understanding the magic of cyclosporine. RN 48(6):53, June 1985

Greenhouse AH: Heavy metals and the nervous system. Clin Neuropharmacol 5:45, 1982

Gunby P: Chymopapain: Tropical tree to surgical suite. JAMA 249:1115, 1983

Haddad LM, Winchester JF (eds): Clinical Management of Poisoning and Drug Overdose. Philadelphia, WB Saunders, 1983

Kahan BD (ed): First International Congress on Cyclosporine. Transplant Proc 15(suppl 1 and 2):2207, 1983

Lafferty KJ, Borel JF, Hodgkin P: Cyclosporine-A (CsA): Models for the mechanism of action. Transplant Proc 15(suppl 1):2230, 1983

Levine WG (ed): The Chelation of Heavy Metals. New York, Pergamon Press, 1979

Levy RS, Fisher M, Alter JN: Penicillamine: Review of cutaneous manifestations. J Am Acad Dermatol 8:548, 1983

Montefusco C et al: Cyclosporine immunosuppression in organ graft recipients: Nursing implications. Crit Care Nurse 4:117, 1984

Scherer P: New drugs: Hands-on experience, Part 1. Am J Nurs 87:448, 1987

Sodium cellulose phosphate (Calcibind). Med Lett Drugs Ther 25:67, 1983

Thomson AW: Immunobiology of cyclosporin—A review. Aust J Exp Biol Med Sci 61:147, 1983

Wagner H: Cyclosporin A: Mechanism of action. Transplant Proc 15:523, 1983

Weil C: Cyclosporin A: Review of results in organ and bone-marrow transplantation in man. In deStevens G (ed): Medicinal Research Reviews, vol 4, p 221. New York, John Wiley & Sons, 1984

Wenger R: Synthesis of cyclosporine and analogues: Structure activity relationships of new cyclosporine derivatives. Transplant Proc 15(suppl 1):2230, 1983

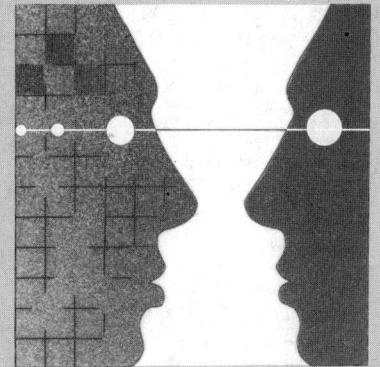

Drug Dependence
and Addiction

XII

Drug Abuse: Recognition and Treatment

85

The abuse of drugs, a part of cultures from the beginnings of recorded medical history, has in recent years reached near-epidemic proportions in certain segments of the population and shows no signs of abating. Rather, improper use of mind-altering substances, whether legally prescribed or illegally obtained, has risen significantly in the last decade, and it is likely that the incidence of drug abuse will continue to increase in the foreseeable future in spite of the many legal and educational efforts being made to reverse the trend.

Drug abuse is a nebulous term, broadly applied to the use of any drug in a manner that deviates from the generally accepted medicosociologic norm. The precise interpretation of this definition, however, is dependent on the variability from culture to culture regarding acceptable behavioral patterns in drug-taking individuals. For example, chronic cigarette smokers are not usually viewed in the same light as chronic narcotic users in terms of drug abuse, yet both forms of behavior may be considered a misuse of a drug substance. Thus, the term *drug abuse* does not necessarily connote legally or socially unacceptable behavior, and therein frequently lies a significant deterrent to its eradication.

Drug abuse has many origins and an equal number of perpetuating factors. Precipitating circumstances include indiscriminate prescribing and inadequate monitoring of psychoactive drugs, emotional instability, peer pressure, and an environment that permits or encourages drug usage. However, a most important indicator of future substance abuse is a person's self-image. It is generally agreed by many drug counselors that those teenagers with a negative self-concept are more likely to demonstrate antisocial behavior than children who think about themselves in a positive manner. The role of the family is crucial regarding development of a positive self-image; love, respect, and discipline must be provided. The compulsion to continue one's drug-taking habit may be reinforced by a number of factors, including availability, parental behavior patterns, stressful demands of everyday life, and desire for social acceptance. Drug abuse, therefore, is an extremely complex phenomenon involving environmental, sociologic, and psychologic aspects.

Drug testing is another complex issue. Detection of a psychoactive substance or its metabolites in urine means *only* that use has occurred at some point in the immediate past. There are, however, several problems with even this interpretation.

First, a nonuser may passively inhale enough marijuana smoke of others to give a positive urine test (this is *not* likely but it can happen). Second, because some drugs and their respective metabolites have extremely long half-lives (*e.g.*, delta-9-THC [major psychoactive component of marijuana] has a half-life ranging from approximately 25 hours to 60 hours), they will appear in the urine from 1 day to 6 days *after* use! Third, depending upon both the lab and the test kit used, there can be a 4% to 10% error rate (*i.e.*, 4% to 10% of all persons tested may show up as *false* positive). Fourth, substances other than those being looked for can give a false reading of an abused substance (*e.g.*, decongestants in over-the-counter cold medications can show up as amphetamine in some tests). Fifth, and most important, is the simple fact that the degree of impairment can be accurately correlated only to *blood* levels (or, in the case of alcohol, also to breath levels); it is scientifically invalid to measure the amount of drug in the urine and then attempt to determine the extent to which the person is impaired!

The discussion that follows focuses primarily on the pharmacology of the various drugs of abuse and reviews methods for proper recognition and treatment of the drug-intoxicated state. An extensive listing of "street" names of abused drugs is provided at the end of this chapter to acquaint the reader with some of the terminology used by many drug abusers.

A useful, but by no means complete, classification of drugs subject to abuse is as follows:

    I. CNS depressants
      A. Alcohol
      B. Barbiturates
      C. Nonbarbiturate sedatives and antianxiety agents
    II. CNS stimulants
      A. Amphetamines
      B. Anorectics
      C. Cocaine
   III. Narcotics
   IV. Psychotomimetics (*e.g.*, LSD, DOM, STP, psilocybin, DMT, mescaline)
    V. Phencyclidine (PCP)
   VI. Volatile inhalants (*e.g.*, acetone, benzene, trichloroethylene, toluene)
  VII. Marijuana
 VIII. Nicotine

In discussing the drugs of abuse, frequent reference is made to the various schedules in which controlled drugs are categorized. These schedules reflect the different regulations governing the prescribing and dispensing of each agent and the penalties for illegal possession. Descriptions of the various schedules for controlled substances and a listing of drugs in each schedule are found in Table 7-1, Chapter 7.

Before reviewing the pharmacology of abused drugs, it is necessary to describe briefly a few terms that appear throughout the discussion, recognizing, of course, that the following descriptions are by no means complete or universally accepted:

Habituation—A pattern of repeated drug usage, although the actual physical need for the drug is minimal. There is no desire to increase the amount taken, and removal of the drug is usually not accompanied by withdrawal symptoms or by a compulsive need to obtain the drug at any cost.

Tolerance—A reduced effect of a drug resulting from repeated exposure to that particular drug or to a similar drug. The latter condition is also known as cross-tolerance.

Drug dependence—A state of reliance on a drug's effects to such an extent that absence of the drug impairs the ability to function continually in a socially acceptable manner; often interchanged with habituation; two distinct types are recognized.

1. Psychologic dependence—A compulsive need to experience a pleasurable drug reaction, ranging from a mild desire for the drug on a routine basis to an overwhelming need to have the drug at any cost; very similar to habituation and often used interchangeably; with many drugs, can lead to a more severe type of dependence, namely:

2. Physical dependence—An altered physiologic state resulting from prolonged use of a drug; regular drug usage is necessary to avoid precipitation of withdrawal reactions that are often severe depending on the drug and duration of use

Addiction—A vague term that can refer to compulsive drug usage, the necessity of obtaining the drug at any cost, and the appearance of withdrawal symptoms if the drug is unavailable; a quantitative term that is usually applied to severe habituation or physical dependence

CNS Depressants

Alcohol

Alcohol abuse is the major drug problem in the United States in terms of damaged health, accidents, family strife, business interruptions, and socially unacceptable behavior. The characteristics of acute alcohol intoxication depend largely on the blood level, and range from euphoria and altered judgment (50 mg/dl) to impaired motor coordination, concentration, and memory (100 mg–150 mg/dl) to profound respiratory and cardiovascular depression and coma (300 mg–400 mg/dl). More insidious and dangerous, however, are the consequences of prolonged alcohol consumption. Chronic alcohol abuse is associated with GI disturbances, liver damage, pancreatitis, neuronal damage, cardiac impairment, malnutrition, and psychotic disturbances (e.g., Wernicke's encephalopathy and Korsakoff's psychosis). In addition, alcohol in combination with other CNS depressants creates the most frequently observed drug-related hospital emergency and is responsible for more fatalities than any other drug or combination of drugs.

Chronic alcohol ingestion results in development of tolerance and ultimately physical dependence similar to that seen with barbiturates. Cessation of alcohol after several weeks of steady consumption may result in tremors, GI disturbances, anxiety, confusion, weakness, insomnia, and possibly delusions. Longer periods of alcohol abuse can, upon abrupt termination, lead to delirium tremens (fever, tachycardia, tremors, profuse sweating), agitation, disorientation, intense hallucinations, and convulsions.

Treatment of acute alcohol withdrawal is largely symptomatic and usually involves use of sedatives or anticonvulsants (e.g., diazepam, barbiturates) or both, along with necessary supportive therapy. Effective management of chronic alcoholism, on the other hand, often requires a combination of supportive social interaction (e.g., Alcoholics Anonymous), psychiatric counseling, and appropriate pharmacotherapy, such as antianxiety agents or disulfiram (see Chap. 26).

Barbiturates

The barbiturates, although declining in therapeutic use, remain valuable agents for induction of general anesthesia and in epilepsy. Members of the drug subculture, however, frequently employ these agents for their anxiety-reducing effects, often to quell the central excitatory action resulting from excessive stimulant abuse. The various barbiturates are classified into either Schedule II, III, or IV, depending on their potency, duration of action, and tendency to produce dependence. The shorter acting drugs (amobarbital, pentobarbital, secobarbital, and combinations thereof) are sought most by abusers because they produce a degree of euphoria following ingestion. These agents are all Schedule II drugs.

Symptoms of barbiturate intoxication closely resemble those of alcohol intoxication and depend primarily on the blood level of the drug. Slurred speech, disorientation, impaired motor coordination, poor judgment, confusion, and emotional instability are frequent occurrences with excessive barbiturate usage. Serious overdosage may be associated with decreased respiration, rapid and weak pulse, cyanosis, mydriasis, and ultimately coma and respiratory paralysis. The CNS effects of barbiturates are additive to those of other CNS depressants, and combinations with alcohol or narcotics often prove fatal. Regular barbiturate use reduces the amount of time spent in rapid eye movement (REM) sleep and can lead to irritability and possibly to personality and behavioral changes.

Withdrawal reactions occur upon abrupt termination of excessive barbiturate use, and range from anxiety, weakness, confusion, anorexia, insomnia (due to rebound REM sleep), and mild tremors, to delirium, disorientation, hallucinations, and convulsions. Symptoms are generally more severe with the shorter acting derivatives. Management of the withdrawal state is symptomatic. Treatment of chronic barbiturate dependence may be accomplished by substituting phenobarbital for the barbiturate being abused at a dose that initially provides a similar effect, then gradually reducing the phenobarbital dose over a period of weeks. (See also Chap. 24.)

Nonbarbiturate Sedatives and Antianxiety Agents

Chronic use of a number of other hypnotic, sedative, and antianxiety drugs can result in dependence and an abstinence syndrome resembling that of the barbiturates. Glutethimide, methyprylon, and ethchlorvynol are among the hypnotic drugs employed as barbiturate alternatives, but they offer no significant advantages. Habituation commonly results from their prolonged use. Glutethimide, in particular, is an undesirable agent, inasmuch as convulsions and toxic psychoses have occurred during its continued administration; and its long duration of action makes reversal of acute overdosage extremely difficult. (See also Chap. 25.)

Methaqualone has been withdrawn from the market but nevertheless remains one of the "street drugs of choice" and is widely abused by a large number of persons. The number of medical emergencies resulting from methaqualone has risen dramatically. Methaqualone is used orally and produces effects resembling those of the barbiturates; in addition, paresthesias are experienced by many persons before the onset of the hypnotic effect. Although acute toxicity is usually not accompanied by severe respiratory and cardiovascular depression, other effects such as convulsions, rigidity, and coma can occur. Prolonged use invariably leads to dependence. A combination of methaqualone and the antihistamine diphenhydramine is marketed in Great Britain as Mandrax and is a more dangerous preparation than methaqualone alone, because the antihistamine can produce excitation, ataxia, and psychotic behavior in large doses. Withdrawal symptoms noted following cessation of methaqualone use include nausea, headache, cramping, insomnia, and occasionally toxic psychoses and severe convulsions.

Meprobamate is viewed as a minor tranquilizer and is used mainly for relief of anxiety, tension, and accompanying muscle spasms. It is somewhat less potent than the barbiturates and correspondingly less toxic, although tolerance occurs rather easily and physical dependence has been reported with as little as 3 g/day for several weeks. Meprobamate withdrawal is usually characterized by insomnia, anxiety, and tremors, but can include hallucinations, convulsions, and coma. Fatalities have occurred with meprobamate overdosage.

The benzodiazepines are the most widely used antianxiety drugs, primarily because their margin of safety is greater than with other sedatives or hypnotics. Diazepam is the most frequently prescribed benzodiazepine and is involved in more reported emergency room cases than any other drug, with the exception of alcohol. Although not preferred as "street" drugs, benzodiazepines are frequently misused by patients being treated for anxiety neuroses or other psychosomatic disorders. A principal hazard with these drugs is the possibility of serious intoxication when they are combined with other depressants, most notably alcohol; deaths have resulted from this combination. Prolonged use of the benzodiazepines has resulted in both psychologic and physical dependence; abrupt discontinuation of treatment (60 mg–120 mg/day) after 2 months has resulted in the appearance of cramping, sweating, agitation, disorientation, confusion, tremors, depression, auditory and visual hallucinations, and paranoia. Some patients exhibit these effects after withdrawing from even lower doses. (See Chap. 28 for further discussion.)

Flurazepam, temazepam, and triazolam are benzodiazepine analogues used for short-term treatment of insomnia and are claimed to have several advantages over the barbiturates (no hangover, no depression of REM sleep, greater safety margin). They are habituating drugs, nevertheless, and therefore should be accorded the same respect as any other hypnotic agent.

CNS Stimulants

Amphetamines

The three amphetamines (DL-amphetamine, dextroamphetamine, methamphetamine), as well as the structural analogues phenmetrazine and methylphenidate, are classed as Schedule II drugs. Their approved clinical indications are limited and currently include only treatment of the attention deficit disorder syndrome in children, short-term treatment of obesity, and symptomatic control of narcolepsy. They are, however, a widely abused group of drugs, and together with the anorectics (see next discussion) are misused for their CNS-stimulating effects. Students, truck drivers, housewives, executives, athletes, and health professionals (e.g., doctors, nurses, pharmacists) have all employed amphetamines in therapeutic doses to suppress fatigue, increase alertness, enhance psychomotor performance, and generally induce a temporary state of well-being. While potentially hazardous, and in some instances illegal, this type of amphetamine use is usually not labeled abuse. Amphetamine abuse refers to the parenteral or oral administration of large doses of the drugs to attain the intense "rush" or rapid "high" characteristic of these agents. Methamphetamine or "speed" is a favorite among drug abusers, because an IV injection elicits an almost instantaneous euphoria or orgasmic-like reaction. However, tolerance to this effect develops rapidly, so that increasingly larger doses must be administered to experience the same sensation. Whereas normal therapeutic doses are in the 5-mg to 15-mg/day range, "speed freaks" have been known to use as much as 5000 mg/day. Obviously this behavior cannot continue for long, and after a period of several days to, occasionally, weeks, the person becomes exhausted to the point of lapsing into long periods of sleep and depression—the so-called crash.

Symptoms of mild amphetamine intoxication include insomnia, increased blood pressure and pulse rate, excitation, hyperactive reflexes, mydriasis, anorexia, and palpitations. More severe overdosage is reflected by extreme agitation, hostility, impulsiveness, hallucinations, confusion, bizarre behavior, aggressiveness, paranoid ideation, convulsions, and possibly death. The social implications of amphetamine abuse are obvious. Methamphetamine abuse, moreover, can result in cerebral vascular spasm, systemic necrotizing angiitis, cerebral hemorrhaging (cerebrovascular accident; CVA), arrhythmias, and severe abdominal pain. Effects of acute amphetamine intoxication have been treated with haloperidol, a dopamine antagonist with minimal anticholinergic effects.

Amphetamines are now believed to induce physical dependence; abrupt withdrawal results in the appearance of fatigue, muscle pain, lethargy, and depression. Withdrawal should be accomplished by allowing the patient to remain in a quiet environment and providing support of vital functions where necessary. Diazepam may be employed if sedation is needed; however, caution must be exercised to avoid adding to the subsequent depression. Acidification of the urine (e.g., with ammonium chloride) markedly increases the excretion of amphetamines and is frequently used to facilitate their removal. Conversely, the amphetamine "high" can be prolonged by concurrent use of urinary alkalinizers that slow renal excretion of the drug.

Although the legal production of amphetamines has been sharply curtailed, clandestine laboratories are currently providing vast amounts of these drugs, especially methamphetamine, for the street market. Amphetamine abuse remains a serious sociologic and medical problem.

Phenmetrazine, an anorectic, and methylphenidate, a drug principally used in attention deficit disorder, are two structurally related compounds classified as Schedule II drugs that possess pharmacologic and toxicologic actions similar to the amphetamines. Although administered orally for their clinical indications, the tablets are frequently dissolved in water by abusers and injected IV. A major danger associated with parenteral use of these drugs is the presence of insoluble talc particles in the injection solution, which can result in circulatory impairment and talc deposits in the lungs and eye. (See also Chap. 32.)

Anorectics

A number of other amphetamine-related drugs termed anorectics are employed as adjuncts in the treatment of obesity and are discussed in Chapter 32. Their pharmacology in most cases is similar to that of the amphetamines, but they are less potent CNS stimulants and generally not as desirable as street drugs. They are, however, frequently misused as appetite suppressants, and chronic ingestion of these agents produces many of the symptoms of prolonged amphetamine use, namely insomnia, elevated blood pressure, tachycardia, and anxiety. Severe overdosage can result in a syndrome resembling amphetamine intoxication; these drugs should never be used continuously for longer than several weeks at a time. Most of these drugs are found in Schedule III, while phentermine and fenfluramine are listed in Schedule IV.

Cocaine

Cocaine is a natural product extracted from the leaves of the coca plant and has been employed clinically as a local anesthetic, especially for the nose and oral cavity. It is currently a very popular drug of abuse; its systemic effects resemble those of amphetamine, but are of much shorter duration. The powdered drug is most commonly administered by inhalation or "snorting" through the nasal passages, although it has been injected IV as well. Crack, a new, hardened form of cocaine, is heated in a glass pipe and smoked; it produces an intense euphoria within minutes. Irrespective of its mode of administration, cocaine quickly elicits a pleasurable high that may be accompanied by tachycardia, elevated blood pressure, restlessness, and mydriasis. Repeated use can lead to an overwhelming psychologic dependence, characterized by an extreme involvement in procuring and using the drug on a daily basis. Cocaine powder is commonly adulterated with various sugars as well as with local anesthetics at every level of distribution; clinical studies have shown that cocaine users are unable to distinguish between lidocaine and cocaine.

Chronic use of cocaine is now associated with the following effects:

Cardiovascular
  Arrhythmias
  Acute myocardial infarction
  Rupture of the ascending aorta
  Cerebrovascular accident (CVA)
Respiratory
  Pulmonary edema
  Pneumomediastinum
  Rhinorrhea
  Rhinitis
  Ulceration and perforation of the nasal
    septum
Gastrointestinal
  Intestinal ischemia (may cause gangrene,
    requiring resection)
  Weight loss
  Nausea
Central Nervous System
  Anxiety
  Irritability
  Tactile hallucinations (imaginary skin
    insects or "cocaine bugs")
  Visual disturbances (flashing lights, "snow
    effect")
  Paranoia
  Insomnia
  Assertive behavior
Genitourinary
  Difficulty in maintaining erection
  Delay in orgasm for both men and women

Overdosage with cocaine can lead to arrhythmias, tremors, convulsions, respiratory failure, and death. Treatment of acute intoxication requires use of sedatives along with appropriate supportive therapy, and must include careful monitoring of cardiovascular and respiratory function.

Narcotics

The narcotic drugs, including the natural alkaloids of the opium plant (morphine and codeine) and the many semisynthetic and synthetic derivatives (see Chap. 22), are widely used for their potent analgesic, antitussive, and antidiarrheal actions. The alleviation of pain induced by these drugs frequently results in a temporary state of euphoria and relief from the accompanying anxiety and is a very pleasurable sensation. However, despite the fact that healthy, well-adjusted persons do not always experience the euphoric effects of opiates, it is precisely the desire to repeat this effect when it occurs that leads to opiate abuse.

Heroin, a Schedule I narcotic, is a widely abused street opiate. Pure heroin is rarely obtainable, and most illicit heroin usually contains only 1% to 10% active drug, the remainder consisting of fillers such as sugars, starches, or quinine. This variable composition is a major cause of overdosage (i.e., when the percentage of opiate is significantly larger than expected). Most other narcotics are qualitatively if not quantitatively similar in their effects, and are variously classified as Schedule II, III, IV, or V. Other favorite narcotics of abuse are hydromorphone (Dilaudid), a potent, short-acting opiate used either orally or parenterally, and oxycodone, available for oral administration alone or in combination with either aspirin as Percodan or acetaminophen as Percocet or Tylox.

IV injection of heroin and other potent narcotics results in a sensation of exquisite pleasure (orgasmic effect, "rush") and a feeling of extreme contentment. Oral use of narcotics does not produce the rush, but usually leads to relaxation, euphoria, and a feeling of detachment or indifference to anxiety or pain. Other effects of narcotic drugs unrelated to their abuse potential are miosis, drowsiness, constipation, nausea, vomiting, and depression of vital functions.

Repeated use of narcotics invariably results in tolerance to the pleasurable effects of the drugs, resulting in the compulsion to continually increase the dosage. Eventually, a state of physical dependence ensues, and the abuser soon requires the drug, not to provide the euphoric effect, but to prevent development of withdrawal symptoms. Overdosage leading to respiratory paralysis is a common cause of opiate fatalities, because the dosage is pushed to extreme limits in the desire to continue to experience the rush. Other related hazards of narcotic addictions are malnutrition, infections due to unsterile injection equipment and poor hygiene, toxic reactions to contaminants injected along with the narcotic, hepatitis, vasculitis, thromboembolic complications, and AIDS (acquired immune deficiency syndrome).

Acute opiate overdosage is marked by stupor, slow and shallow respiration, pinpoint pupils (patients may present with dilated pupils due to activation of the sympathoadrenal system in cases of extreme overdosage), cold and clammy skin, hypotension, bradycardia, and possibly coma. Treatment involves a narcotic antagonist (naloxone) along with necessary supportive treatment (respira-tory assistance, vasopressors). Dosage of the narcotic antagonist must be carefully controlled to avoid precipitation of acute withdrawal symptoms.

When narcotics are unavailable to a physically dependent individual, withdrawal symptoms usually begin within 8 hours to 12 hours, reach a maximum intensity in 36 hours to 72 hours, and can persist for up to 7 days to 10 days. The severity of these symptoms depends on the degree of dependence, a function of the length of time the drugs have been used, and the average amount administered. Initial signs of withdrawal include yawning, perspiration, lacrimation, sneezing, and restlessness. Progressively severe symptoms encompass anorexia, irritability, insomnia, anxiety, vomiting, generalized body aches, stomach cramping, diarrhea, fever, chills, tremors, jerking movements, muscle spasms, tachycardia, and elevated blood pressure. Although frightening to the patient, symptoms experienced during narcotic withdrawal are not usually life-threatening, in contrast to those associated with barbiturate withdrawal, which have resulted in fatalities.

Withdrawal symptoms can be suppressed by administration of another narcotic, frequently oral methadone, in an initial stabilizing amount, 20 mg once or twice a day, then a gradual reduction of the dose. Methadone's long duration of action (up to 24 hours) also permits single daily dosing. However, it should be recognized that methadone is also a potent narcotic, and methadone abuse has now become a significant problem as well. Withdrawal from methadone is more prolonged than from opiates, but symptoms are often less severe. Methadone and a newer chemically related compound, levo-alpha-acetylmethadol (LAAM), an even longer acting drug (48 hours–72 hours), are being used for management of narcotic addiction. This procedure involves stabilizing a patient on a regular oral dose of one of the compounds, resulting in development of cross-tolerance to the abused opiate, for example, heroin. Thus, the addict no longer experiences the rush or euphoria characteristic of heroin, and theoretically at least, can now slowly be withdrawn from methadone or LAAM.

Naltrexone (Trexan) is a long-acting antagonist which is now available for treatment of narcotic addiction; effects of heroin can be blocked for up to 3 days (depends on naltrexone dose). The patient must be narcotic-free for at least 7 days and have normal liver function prior to receiving naltrexone.

Detoxification programs work best in conjunction with psychiatric and social counseling. Because the addict's daily behavior is usually structured completely around obtaining and using narcotic drugs, withdrawal alone is rarely entirely successful in overcoming narcotic dependence.

Psychotomimetics

Psychotomimetic drugs, often termed hallucinogens, are a group of both naturally occurring compounds (such as psilocybin, mescaline) and synthetic compounds (e.g., LSD, DOM) capable of producing profound distortion of reality. Psychotomimetics are Schedule I drugs that can cause serious psychologic harm to the occasional, as well as the habitual, user. They have the capacity to distort mental function, often resulting in confusion, delirium, amnesia, and a distorted sense of direction, time, and distance. In large doses, delusions and hallucinations are common, and seriously impaired judgment and severe depression have frequently resulted from ingestion of these drugs. While the drugs are usually employed in a desire to experience the "pleasant" psychic alterations such as euphoria, elation, vivid color imagery, and synesthesias ("hearing" colors, "seeing" sounds), the psychologic state induced by these agents depends on many variables, most importantly the personality and expectations of the user and the environmental situation. Some persons experience the opposite type of effects, such as anxiety, dysphoria, panic, severe depression, despair, and suicidal tendencies, the so-called bad trip. These latter effects tend to occur following ingestion of large doses by inexperienced, nontolerant persons, especially those persons with pre-existing psychologic disturbances. Unpleasant reactions are also observed more commonly in threatening, hostile, or disturbing surroundings. Treatment of such bad trips may be accomplished by placing the patient in a nonthreatening, supportive environment, and maintaining reassuring verbal contact ("talking down"). Mild sedatives (such as benzodiazepines) are recommended, but use of phenothiazines should be avoided.

Recurrences of the various perceptual distortions are experienced in a large number of psychotomimetic drug users, especially with LSD, and can occur up to 5 years after initial usage. These "flashbacks" vary in duration from seconds to minutes, and although occasionally spontaneous, are most frequently triggered by periods of stress or anxiety or by use of other psychotropic drugs, such as marijuana. These flashback episodes may be po-

tentially harmful to the person depending on their severity and place of occurrence.

While a degree of tolerance to the behavioral and psychologic effects of LSD develops within a short period of time, marked psychologic dependence is rare, and physical dependence does not occur. There are no characteristic symptoms following abrupt discontinuation of drug usage.

Chronic episodes of psychotic behavior are not uncommon following use of psychotomimetic drugs. Most occur in persons who exhibit underlying emotional instability. The extent to which use of hallucinogens contributes to the protracted disturbed behavior of these people is difficult to assess accurately. Unfortunately, it is just such unstable persons who frequently become involved with use of psychotomimetic agents.

The most commonly used hallucinogens are the following:

LSD—The most potent hallucinogen currently available; effects usually last 8 hours to 12 hours; tolerance develops quickly and effects usually cannot be duplicated for several days; sold as tablets, thin squares of gelatin ("window panes"), or impregnated paper ("blotter acid"); average effective oral dose is 25 mcg to 50 mcg.

Mescaline—Active ingredient of the flowering heads of the peyote cactus; oral doses of 250 mg to 500 mg produce hallucinations lasting 6 hours to 12 hours.

DOM—Structural analogue of mescaline, also known as STP, an acronym for "serenity, tranquility, and peace"; a potent, synthetic psychotomimetic producing intense, prolonged psychic alterations at a dose of 5 mg, occasionally lasting for several days following a single oral dose; frequently sold on the illicit market as mescaline.

DMT—A naturally occurring hallucinogen, N,N-dimethyltryptamine is not effective orally, and must be inhaled or smoked; produces a rapid, brief alteration in perception and mood.

Psilocybin and psilocin—Active ingredients of Psilocybe mushrooms, chemically related to LSD, although much less potent and shorter acting; usually administered orally.

There are many other substances used for their hallucinogenic effects, many being amphetamine derivatives or centrally acting anticholinergics. One compound in particular, phencyclidine, is chemically related to the dissociative anesthetic ketamine and has become a very dangerous, widely misused drug in the United States. It is discussed separately below.

Phencyclidine (PCP)

Phencylidine (PCP, "angel dust"), a potent psychotomimetic that is the most dangerous of all drugs of abuse, is no longer legally manufactured in the United States. Related to ketamine, PCP had been used as a veterinary anesthetic, but the PCP available on the street is a product of clandestine laboratories, often highly contaminated, and frequently misrepresented as LSD, THC, cocaine, or mescaline. Although occasionally administered orally or IV, it is most often used by smoking or nasal inhalation (snorting).

Effects of PCP are dependent on the dose and route of administration. Small amounts elicit euphoria, numbness of the extremities, and a sense of detachment. Larger amounts can result in analgesia, impaired speech, loss of coordination, agitation, muscle rigidity, tachycardia, elevated blood pressure, exaggerated gait, auditory hallucinations, acute anxiety, self-destructive behavior, and severe mood disorders, including paranoia, violent hostility, and feelings of depersonalization or doom. A psychotic state indistinguishable from paranoid schizophrenia is often a result of prolonged use of the drug, but has occurred after only one dose. Delayed psychologic reactions have been observed for up to several weeks following administration.

Undesirable reactions ("bad trips") have become a significant problem with PCP, and the drug is capable of producing severe behavioral disturbances, frequently prolonged. Treatment of overdosage is best carried out by use of sedatives to control agitation and urinary acidifiers to facilitate excretion, and by isolation of the patient. Verbal contact should be avoided during the acute recovery stage, which is frequently accompanied by involuntary movements, facial grimacing, torticollis, and catatonic-like posturing. Although usually rapid, recovery can take several days or even weeks, and patients should be kept under close observation during this time.

Volatile Inhalants

Volatile hydrocarbons such as acetone, benzene, carbon tetrachloride, trichloroethane, trichloroethylene, and toluene are present in many household products, including glue, paint, lighter fluid, nail polish remover, and varnish thinner, and are frequently abused by young persons. These volatile liquids are commonly placed on a rag or handkerchief or in a bag, and inhaled. The initial effects are CNS excitation, characterized by a sense of exhilaration, dizziness, and occasionally auditory or visual hallucinations, accompanied by tinnitus, blurred vision, slurred speech, and a staggering gait. These effects generally last 30 minutes to 60 minutes. Larger amounts of inhaled vapors can lead to drowsiness, hypotension, delirium, stupor, unconsciousness, and possibly coma. Amnesia frequently follows recovery. Fatalities have resulted, either from drug-induced respiratory failure or due to suffocation from the plastic bags placed over the face. Cardiac arrest has also been reported.

Recent reports indicate that several deaths among teenagers resulted from inhalation of correction fluid (e.g., Liquid Paper, White-Out); the halogenated hydrocarbons in these products appear to induce ventricular fibrillation.

Psychologic dependence can develop, but physical dependence is rare, primarily due to the rather brief duration of action. Chronic misuse of volatile hydrocarbons can result in significant organ damage, especially to the liver, kidneys, heart, and CNS, and it is this dangerous aspect of volatile inhalant abuse that is frequently overlooked by youthful users.

Treatment of acute intoxication resembles that of barbiturate overdosage and employs oxygen and respiratory assistance along with other supportive care as needed. Injections of vasopressors (such as epinephrine) should be avoided, however, due to the danger of myocardial sensitization by the volatile hydrocarbon, resulting in precipitation of arrhythmias in the presence of adrenergic amines.

Marijuana

Marijuana is obtained from the hemp plant, Cannabis sativa, and constitutes a mixture of dried leaves, flowering tops, and other parts of the plant. The biologically active constituents of marijuana are termed cannabinoids and among the more than 60 known compounds, delta-9-tetrahydrocannabinol (THC) appears to be the major psychoactive derivative. Marijuana may be administered orally, but it is several times more potent when the powder is rolled loosely into cigarettes ("joints") and smoked. Depending on the potency, peak psychopharmacologic effects occur within 10 minutes to 20 minutes of inhalation and persist for 1 hour to 4 hours. The average "joint" contains between 2% and 4% THC (approximately 10 mg–20 mg), of which approximately one-half is usually absorbed.

The resinous secretions from the flowering tops of the cannabis plant are also available as hashish. These secretions are usually dried and then either smoked or compressed into a variety of other dosage forms, such as cookies, cakes, or candies. While hashish ranges in potency depending upon the source, it is generally between five and ten times more potent than marijuana itself. Hashish oil, a concentrated liquid extract of cannabis plant materials, contains a high percentage of THC (10%–50%), and several drops are equivalent to a single "joint" of marijuana. Hashish oil has also been administered IV, but this procedure is associated with a significant mortality rate.

The psychic and perceptual effects of marijuana vary widely among individuals and depend on the mental status, mood, previous experience, and expectations of the users, as well as the environment and circumstances surrounding its use. Typical psychic reactions include a sense of relaxation and well-being, perhaps even euphoria, impaired time and space orientation, altered sensory perception (especially sound and color), and spontaneous, often uncontrolled laughter. Short-term memory may be affected, psychomotor performance may be somewhat impaired, and attention span can be reduced, driving ability compromised, and perceptual difficulties can prove hazardous to a person behind the wheel. Large doses may result in image distortion, depersonalization, disorganized thought and speech, fantasies, and, rarely, hallucinations.

Physiologic changes accompanying marijuana usage can include elevated pulse rate and conjunctival congestion, which occur routinely, and erythema, enhanced appetite, disturbed equilibrium, xerostomia, oropharyngeal irritation, tinnitus, paresthesias, and vomiting, all of which may or may not be present.

Adverse reactions may appear to be minimal with occasional use in emotionally stable persons. Reported untoward reactions to marijuana comprise mild depression, anxiety, agitation, and a "panic" state, most frequently observed in first-time users. Acute intoxication from high doses (toxic psychosis) is manifested by hallucinations, severe agitation, and paranoia. Acute intoxication can occur even in patients currently being treated with antipsychotic medication, and usually resolves within 24 hours. It is seen most frequently in patients prone to schizophrenia. THC can disrupt pituitary production of gonadotropic hormones and is excreted in breast milk. Further, new evidence suggests that marijuana-induced teratogenicity may occur; these data need confirmation, however. Therefore, pregnant and lactating women should refrain from marijuana use.

Prolonged usage of marijuana has been implicated in pulmonary toxicity (precancerous cellular changes), suppression of cellular-mediated immune responsiveness, and personality and behavioral changes. Severe psychic disturbances, however, occur primarily in persons with pre-existing emotional disorders.

Chronic use of marijuana may result in psychologic dependence, but physical dependence is rare. A phenomenon of "reverse" tolerance has been reported in some marijuana users, whereby smaller amounts of the drug are able to elicit the desired psychic effects with repeated administration. This may be due in part to cumulation effects of the drug with frequent use.

Although acute overdosage with marijuana is rare, episodes can be managed by appropriate support of respiration, blood pressure, and other vital functions as required. A quiet environment and reassuring attitude are quite helpful during the acute psychotic phase, and extreme agitation is best treated with benzodiazepines such as diazepam.

Potential clinical applications are receiving much attention. Two areas of potential therapeutic benefit for the cannabinoids, especially THC, are the control of nausea and vomiting produced by chemotherapeutic agents and reduction of elevated intraocular pressure in glaucoma. A THC product (Marinol) is now available in the United States for the former purpose (see Chap. 46). Other properties of THC currently being investigated for possible clinical use are its analgesic, anti-inflammatory, tranquilizing, bronchodilatory, and anticonvulsant actions.

Nicotine

Nicotine is an alkaloid found in tobacco in a concentration usually between 1% and 2%. It is rapidly absorbed by the lungs and has a mild central stimulatory effect. At the same time, there is decreased skeletal muscle tone, reduced appetite, and, in naive users, occasionally nausea, vomiting, dizziness, and irritability. Tolerance usually develops to these latter effects but is of a very variable nature and duration. Withdrawal from nicotine can result in nausea, diarrhea, increased appetite, headache, drowsiness, insomnia, irritability, and poor concentration. Following extended abstinence, blood pressure and heart rate decrease, peripheral blood flow increases, and respiratory difficulties are reduced, but weight gain is common, because food is often used as a substitute form of oral gratification. Gradual reduction in nicotine consumption is usually less effective over the long term than abrupt cessation.

The other major risk factors associated with cigarette smoking (e.g., lung and bladder cancer, coronary artery disease, emphysema, and other chronic pulmonary disorders) cannot be exclusively linked to the nicotine content of the tobacco, but probably result from constant exposure to the many carcinogenic products found in cigarette smoke. (See also Chap. 17.)

■ Nursing Process for Patients Who Abuse Drugs

Refer to Chapter 26 regarding nursing education for the patient who ingests alcohol and helping impaired professional colleagues.

The nurse needs to focus on multiple levels for drug abuse as well as alcohol abuse: prevention of abuse by educating target populations, identification of the patient in an acute care setting who may go through withdrawal while receiving treatment for other problems, treatment of withdrawal and rehabilitation. In addition, nurses need to be aware that colleagues may be abusing drugs; statistics indicate that 10% to 20% of all health-care workers may be involved in drug or alcohol abuse. Consequently, nurses need some guidelines to help identify individuals with potential problems and strategies to cope with such individuals.

□ ASSESSMENT

□ Subjective Data
Identifying a patient who abuses drugs may be difficult because the patient is unlikely to share the information readily or, as a defense mechanism, denies that drug use is a problem. When taking a medication history, the nurse should ask about street drugs and alcohol use which may provide an opening for obtaining some information. The attitude conveyed to the patient must be nonjudgmental, and the nurse must assure confidentiality. The nurse should never promise not to share information about street drug or alcohol use with the patient's physician because drug use may alter therapy plans.

If the patient admits to using street drugs or alcohol, the nurse needs to identify the type, quantity, and frequency of use. This may be stated in street terms by the patient. The Glossary at the end of this chapter lists some of the terms used. The nurse may need to clarify others with the patient or pharmacist. The social or family network involved in drug taking should also be identified, if possible. The patient whose entire circle of significant others is associated with drug taking will have difficulty breaking drug habits unless a change in environment can be established. The extent of use and its effect on the patient's treatment may determine what the nurse does with the information. For example, the patient who reports occasional marijuana use in social situations is engaging in illegal drug taking, but such information may not be relevant to treatment and the health-care team may elect to do nothing. On the other hand, the patient who reports daily heroin use for the last 7 months and who is scheduled for surgery with general anesthesia requires further evaluation, and plans must be made to reduce the risks of anesthesia and manage the addiction with drugs to prevent withdrawal in the postoperative period.

Many times patients who abuse drugs or alcohol deny the problem on interview. In such cases, the nurse may have to rely on interactions and physical symptoms to identify the problem. The nurse may note a patient to be distrustful of staff or the proposed regimen and to be secretive about visits from friends or family. The patient may appear tense, anxious, or become angry with little provocation. The nurse may find the patient is frequently manipulative about requests, especially for pain medication. Narcotic addicts are very fearful of pain and are usually very sensitive to it. Unrecognized drug abusers may initially be labeled as simply "problem patients."

□ Objective Data
Some physical signs of abuse are easy to identify. The patient who is hallucinating clearly reveals the problem although the source of the drug may be difficult to identify. The patient who is actively engaged in drug taking when first seen will have characteristic symptoms identified under each drug heading in this chapter.

Other general characteristics may be apparent in a chronic drug abuser. The individual may appear cachectic, malnourished, and pale, which usually reflects poor eating habits during drug taking. Poor teeth, dental care, or swollen gums also indicate poor nutrition. Frequently these individuals complain of a lingering upper respiratory infection that won't go away or a sore that won't heal.

If the patient injects drugs, needle marks may be apparent. If dirty needles have been used the patient may be first seen because of abscess formation, cellulitis, hepatitis, or bacterial endocarditis and may be very ill.

Blood and urine samples may be obtained. Urine samples are frequently inaccurate as discussed earlier in this chapter. Blood levels will accurately reflect most of the drugs discussed above but only during times of ingestion. Diagnosis of a drug abuse problem is best made by thorough history taking.

☐ **NURSING DIAGNOSIS**[1]

Actual nursing diagnoses for the patient who abuses drugs may include:

Knowledge deficit related to effect of drug use on life and family and treatment available

Ineffective individual coping: Anger, dependence, or denial related to inability to constructively manage stressors without drugs/alcohol

Disturbance in self-concept, related to guilt, mistrust, or ambivalence

Anxiety related to loss of control

Potential nursing diagnoses may include:

Alteration in nutrition: less than body requirements related to anorexia (narcotics, CNS stimulants, hallucinogens)

Potential fluid volume deficit related to fluid loss secondary to vomiting and diarrhea (CNS depressants, CNS stimulants)

Potential for infection related to use of nonsterile needles and syringes (all IV drug abuse)

Potential for injury related to disorientation, tremors, or impaired judgment

Potential for violence related to impulsive behavior, disorientation, tremors, or impaired judgment

Sleep pattern disturbance related to irritability, tremors, nightmares

Sensory perceptual alterations related to confusion, memory loss, impaired judgment, overdose/withdrawal

[1] Adapted from Carpenito L: Handbook of Nursing Diagnoses, pp. 201–202. Philadelphia, JB Lippincott, 1985.

Impaired social interactions, related to emotional immaturity, irritability, anxiety, impulsive behavior, aggressive responses

Sexual dysfunction related to impotence or loss of libido

Alteration in family processes related to disruption in marital dyad and inconsistent limit setting

☐ **PLAN**

Nursing care goals vary depending on whether the nurse is providing educational information, managing an addicted patient suffering from an acute illness, caring for a patient going through withdrawal, or helping a patient through a rehabilitation process. However, in general the nurse:

1. Provides relevant, clear information about drug and alcohol abuse
2. Sets limits for acceptable behavior while the patient is engaged in a therapeutic interaction either as an inpatient or an outpatient
3. Identifies local resources and methods of utilizing them to assist patients who want help
4. Administers prescribed drugs correctly and safely to the patient who requires drug intervention during acute illness or the withdrawal stage of addiction
5. Monitors the addicted patients for the side-effects of the abused drug, the side-effects of withdrawal, and the adverse effects that may result from street or prescribed drug combinations
6. Provides support, counseling, and referral according to ability and patient need

☐ **INTERVENTION**

The first step in establishing effective intervention strategies is for the nurse to become aware of the perceptions he or she has about alcohol and drug abusers. Perceptions may range from open disgust and condemnation to the idea that if the patient just wanted to quit he could. Such attitudes will be obvious to the patient and will be counterproductive in establishing any therapeutic relationship. Information should also be conveyed as nonjudgmentally as possible. Addictive patients are frequently hostile and paranoid and become more so when faced with judgmental staff.

The nurse needs to establish what is acceptable behavior in any therapeutic interaction and that, as well as the rules of the institution, should be clearly explained to the patient. For example, it is not acceptable for the patient to take any illegal drugs while in the hospital. The nurse needs to establish an honest relationship with this patient, to complete tasks he or she agrees to do, and to refuse to do that which compromises patient care. A nurse who promises to contact a physician about the patient's pain medication needs to make sure the promise is kept. On the other hand, if the patient asks the nurse to keep a discovered indiscretion while hospitalized a secret (*i.e.*, smoking marijuana), the nurse must refuse. In addition, the nurse needs to recognize that drug abuse is the patient's problem, a complex problem that is not easily solved and one which the nurse may not be able to help with during a specific period of time. Nurses who accept this can reduce the guilt they frequently feel for not getting the patient to accept treatment for an addiction.

Documentation is essential when dealing with a patient suspected of abusing drugs. Suspicions about drug taking should be charted and shared with other nursing staff, supervisors, and the patient's physicians. Referrals should be made to appropriate resources and documented. However, the nurse is not a police officer in the process of investigating abuse and should refuse requests to illegally search the patient's room or possessions. In an acute care facility, such action is the responsibility of the security department or outside law enforcement agencies.

Nurses are responsible for monitoring the patient's behavior and watching for changes. The patient who abuses IV drugs and who has an IV may be a particular problem because many street drugs can easily be injected through an IV line. The nurse should suspect problems if the patient is euphoric soon after visiting hours are over, if the IV line becomes clogged or infiltrated frequently, or the patient resists having an IV discontinued. Such drug use can be lethal.

Once a patient who abuses drugs is identified, nursing care is somewhat easier. Decisions must be made about withdrawal from the drug, and delay or change in the course of treatment may occur while the patient is detoxified. For example, the patient who uses amphetamines or barbiturates should be withdrawn slowly and under supervision before anesthesia is used for surgery. On the other hand, the heroin addict may be placed on a methadone regimen approximately equivalent to the street dose until surgery and immediate recovery are passed.

During withdrawal from drugs or alcohol, the patient should be placed in a room where environmental stimuli are minimal. Psychologic support will vary, but the patient must be continually reoriented to reality. Nursing staff should anticipate hostility, verbal abuse, and occasionally violence. Cardiac, respiratory, and neurologic function should be monitored at regular intervals because arrhythmias, respiratory changes, and seizures or coma are frequently possible. Attempts should be made to improve the patient's nutritional status. A flow sheet should be used to facilitate accurate, consistent monitoring. See specific chapters and drug headings in this chapter for clinical considerations for patients withdrawing from alcohol, narcotics, and barbiturates.

Once acute withdrawal has passed, nursing staff expect the patient will accept rehabilitation because the pain and symptoms of withdrawal are usually horrible. However, most patients remember very little of the physical withdrawal episode but may already know what the long-term psychologic withdrawal will be like. Therefore, frequently the patient will refuse rehabilitation. However, if the patient shows interest, referrals should be made immediately. Nurses must know the variety of community resources available, how to tap them, what funding is available, and the waiting period for admission. All facilities should have this information readily available. Lists can be obtained from the state department of health but specific facilities should be contacted to determine admission requirements. Giving the patient the name of a facility and telephone number is insufficient. A contact must be made before discharge.

□ **EVALUATION**

The long-term outcome sought is that the patient refrains from drug use. This may be unrealistic. Suitable short-term outcomes may include admission of a problem by the patient, absence of or adequate control of major physiologic side-effects during withdrawal, establishment of an agreement about interactions between the patient and staff, lack of illegal drug use while in the hospital, and agreement by the patient to enter a rehabilitation program. Many others are possible depending on the patient and the abused drug.

Glossary of "Street Names" for Drugs of Abuse

Acapulco gold	Marijuana
Acid	LSD
Angel dust	Phencyclidine
Beans	Amphetamines

Bennies	Amphetamines	Hazel	Heroin
Big H	Heroin	Hearts	Dextroamphetamine
Black beauties	Amphetamines	Heaven dust	Cocaine
Black mollies	Amphetamines	Hemp	Marijuana
Blockbusters	Barbiturates	Herb	Marijuana
Blotter acid	LSD	Hero	Heroin
Blow	Cocaine	Hog	Phencyclidine, chloral hydrate
Bluebirds	Barbiturates		
Blue devils	Barbiturates	Hombre	Heroin
Blues	Barbiturates	J	Marijuana
Boy	Heroin	Jay	Marijuana
Brown	Heroin	Joint	Marijuana
Brownies	Amphetamines	Junk	Heroin
Brown sugar	Heroin	Lady	Cocaine
Buttons	Peyote	Log	Marijuana
C	Cocaine	Ludes	Methaqualone
Caballo	Heroin	Mary Jane	Marijuana
Cactus	Peyote	Mesc	Peyote, mescaline
California sunshine	LSD	Mescal	Peyote
Cannabis	Marijuana	Meth	Methamphetamine
Charley	Cocaine	Mexican mud	Heroin
Christmas tree	Barbiturates	Mexican reds	Barbiturates, secobarbital
Chiva	Heroin		
Coca	Cocaine	Microdots	LSD
Coke	Cocaine	Minibennies	Amphetamines
Colombian	Marijuana	Morf	Morphine
Copilots	Amphetamines	Morpho	Morphine
Crack	Cocaine	Morphy	Morphine
Crank	Methamphetamines	Mota	Marijuana
Crap	Heroin	Mud	Morphine
Crossroads	Amphetamines	Mujer	Cocaine
Crystal	Methamphetamine, phencyclidine	Mutah	Marijuana
		Nebbies	Barbiturates, pentobarbital
Cube	Morphine, LSD		
Cubes	LSD	Nimbies	Barbiturates, pentobarbital
Cyclone	Phencyclidine		
Dexies	Dextroamphetamine	Nose candy	Cocaine
Dillies	Dilaudid	Oranges	Amphetamines
Dollies	Methadone	Panama red	Marijuana
Double cross	Amphetamines	Paper acid	LSD
Downers	Barbiturates	Paradise	Cocaine
Estuffa	Heroin	PCP	Phencyclidine
First line	Morphine	Peace pill	Phencyclidine
Flake	Cocaine	Pep pills	Amphetamines
Footballs	Amphetamines	Perico	Cocaine
Ganga	Marijuana	Pink ladies	Barbiturates
Giri	Cocaine	Pinks	Barbiturates, secobarbital
Goma	Morphine		
Grass	Marijuana	Polvo	Heroin
Green dragons	Barbiturates	Polvo blanco	Cocaine
Griffa	Marijuana	Pot	Marijuana
H	Heroin	Purple haze	LSD
Hash	Hashish	Quacks	Methaqualone
Haze	LSD	Quads	Methaqualone

Rainbows	Barbiturates, Tuinal	Stumblers	Barbiturates
Reds and blues	Barbiturates, Tuinal	Stuff	Heroin
Redbirds	Barbiturates, secobarbital	Sunshine	LSD
		Supergrass	Phencyclidine
Red devils	Barbiturates, secobarbital	T's and blues	Pentazocine and tripelennamine
Reefer	Marijuana	Tea	Marijuana
Roach	Marijuana	THC	Tetrahydrocannabinol
Rock	Cocaine	Thing	Heroin
Rocket fuel	Phencyclidine	Thrusters	Amphetamines
Roses	Amphetamines	Tic tac	Phencyclidine
Sativa	Marijuana	Truck drivers	Amphetamines
Scag	Heroin	Uppers	Amphetamines
Sleeping pills	Barbiturates	Wake-ups	Amphetamines
Smack	Heroin	Wedges	LSD
Smoke	Marijuana	Weed	Marijuana
Snow	Cocaine	Whites	Amphetamines
Soapers	Methaqualone	Window panes	LSD
Soles	Hashish	Yellow jackets	Barbiturates, pentobarbital
Sparklers	Amphetamines		
Speed	Methamphetamine	Yellows	Barbiturates, pentobarbital
Stick	Marijuana		

REVIEW QUESTIONS

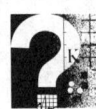

1. List several possible precipitating circumstances that can lead to drug abuse.
2. Briefly discuss the limitations of urine testing for drug use.
3. Distinguish between the terms habituation and physical dependence.
4. What are the principal consequences of chronic alcohol abuse?
5. Describe the symptoms of barbiturate intoxication. How may chronic barbiturate dependence be treated?
6. What symptoms can occur following abrupt discontinuation of benzodiazepine drugs following prolonged use?
7. Describe the symptoms of amphetamine intoxication. Abrupt withdrawal from amphetamines can lead to what reactions?
8. List the major effects of chronic cocaine use.
9. What is "crack"? What symptoms may be associated with overdosage?
10. Describe the effects of an IV injection of potent narcotic drugs.
11. Give the principal symptoms of acute opiate overdosage.
12. What are the various symptoms that may occur during opiate withdrawal in a dependent person?
13. What means are available to manage the opiate withdrawal syndrome?
14. How is naltrexone used in managing the narcotic addict?
15. What are the major effects of psychotomimetic drugs?
16. List the most commonly used hallucinogens.

17. What is considered the *most dangerous* of all drugs of abuse? Why?
18. How is phencyclidine overdosage managed?
19. What are some volatile inhalants that have been abused by inhalation of their vapors?
20. Give the dangers associated with inhalation of volatile hydrocarbons.
21. Describe the typical acute effects of smoking marijuana.
22. What reactions can occur with chronic use of marijuana?
23. Briefly discuss the potential *clinical uses* for the active constituents of marijuana.
24. What are the immediate *and* long-term effects of nicotine inhaled in cigarette smoke?
25. What information can the nurse use to help detect a patient who abuses drugs or alcohol?
26. What are realistic goals for a nurse working with a drug abuse patient in an acute care setting during a five-day hospital admission?
27. What are some perceptions health care staff have about patients who abuse drugs? How might these perceptions influence delivery of care?
28. What guidelines can the nurse use to establish a therapeutic relationship with a manipulative patient as part of a drug-taking personality?
29. What additional documentation is necessary when caring for a drug-abusing patient?
30. What are the goals for safe withdrawal from most street drugs?

BIBLIOGRAPHY

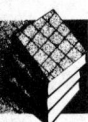

Benowitz NL, Jacob P: Daily intake of nicotine during cigarette smoking. Clin Pharmacol Ther 35:499, 1984

Chasnoff IJ, Burns WJ, Schnoll SH et al: Cocaine use in pregnancy. N Engl J Med 313:666, 1986

Cregler LL, Mark H: Medical complications of cocaine abuse. N Engl J Med 315:1495, 1986

Edwards G, Littleton J (eds): Pharmacological Treatments for Alcoholism. London, Croom Helm, 1984

Fultz JM, Senay EC, Pray BJ et al: When a narcotic addict is hospitalized. Am J Nurs 80:478, 1980

Gavin FH, Kleber HD: Cocaine abuse treatment. Open pilot trial with desipramine and lithium carbonate. Arch Gen Psychiatry 41:903, 1984

Gay GR: Clinical management of acute and chronic cocaine poisoning. Ann Emerg Med 11:562, 1982

Goldstein FJ: Cocaine: Clinical pharmacology and toxicology. Med Times 116(3):123, 1988

Goldstein FJ: Substance abuse in the health professions. Compend Contin Educat in Dentistry 8(6):438, 1987

Grabowski J (ed): Cocaine: Pharmacology, Effects, and Treatment of Abuse. National Institute of Drug Abuse Research Monograph Series, Publication 84-1326, Washington, D.C., U.S. Government Printing Office, 1984

Green PL: The impaired nurse: Chemical dependency. Focus on Critical Care 11(2):42, 1984

Hollister LE: Health aspects of cannabis. Pharmacol Rev 38:1, 1986

Jacobs BL (ed): Hallucinogens: Neurochemical, Behavioral and Clinical Perspectives. New York, Raven Press, 1984

Jones RT: Cannabis and health. Annu Rev Med 34:247, 1983

Kandel DB: Marijuana users in young adulthood. Arch Gen Psychiatry 41:200, 1984

Leporati NC, Chychula LH: How can you *really* help the drug abusing patient? Nursing 82 12(6):46, 1982

Maykut MO: Health consequences of acute and chronic marihuana use. Prog Neuropsychopharmacol Biol Psychiatry 9:209, 1985

Mendelson JH, Mello NK (eds): The Diagnosis and Treatment of Alcoholism. New York, McGraw-Hill, 1984

Mittleman HS, Mittleman RE, Elser B: Cocaine. Am J Nurs 84:1092, 1984

Redmond DF, Krystal JH: Multiple mechanisms of withdrawal from opioid drugs. Annu Rev Neurosci 7:443, 1984

Smart RC et al (eds): Research Advances in Alcohol and Drug Problems, vol 8. New York, Plenum Press, 1984

Zamora LC: The client who generates anger. In Haber J, Lead A, Schudy S et al (eds): Comprehensive Psychiatric Nursing. New York, McGraw-Hill, 1978

Appendix

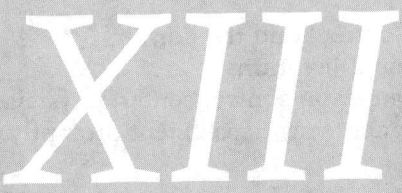

Poisons and Antidotes

Common Non-pharmaceutical and Pharmaceutical Agents Resulting in Human Poison Exposures

The lists below are compiled from data collected by the American Association of Poison Control Centers. The agents listed are those in which at least 5000 exposures were reported or in which poison exposure resulted in at least 10 reported deaths for the time frame of data collection.

Poison exposures may be accidental, intentional, or the result of an adverse drug reaction. Many exposures occur in children under 6 years old and in the elderly. These lists may provide useful checklists for adults to remind them to place such items out of reach of anyone who may use them inappropriately.

Nonpharmaceutical Agents

Adhesives (*i.e.*, glues, cements, pastes)
*Alcohol, ethanol (*not* rubbing alcohol)
Art, craft, and office supplies
Bee, wasp, or hornet bites
*Carbon monoxide
*Chemicals, total
  Acid chemicals
  Glycol products (excluding automotive products)
Cleaning substances
  Ammonia cleaners
  Bleaches containing hypochlorite
  Hand dishwashing detergents
Miscellaneous cleaners
  Alkali
  Anionic/nonionic
Cosmetics
  Hair care products
  Perfume, cologne, aftershave
Fertilizers
Food products/food poisoning
Hydrocarbons
  Gasoline

Insecticides/pesticides
  Organophosphate type
Mushrooms
Paints and stripping agents
Plants
  Gastrointestinal irritants
  Nontoxic varieties
  Oxalate
Rodenticides
  Anticoagulant type

Pharmaceutical Agents

Acetaminophen, adult and pediatric formulations
*Aspirin, adult formulation and combination products
*Amitriptyline
Antihistamines
Antibiotics
*Benzodiazepines
Calcium salts
*Cardiovascular drugs (all types but especially beta-blockers)
Cold and cough preparations
Diaper care products
Eye/ear/nose/throat preparations
Ibuprofen
*Imipramine
Laxatives
Oral contraceptives
*Phenothiazines
*Street drugs (especially amphetamines, cocaine, and heroin)
Vitamins, adult and pediatric formulations

* Indicates poison exposures in which at least 10 reported incidences resulted in death.(1985 Annual Report of the American Association of Poison Control Centers National Data Collection System)

Poisoning First Aid

1. Separate the patient and the poison.
2. Keep the patient breathing.
3. Always call a poison control center, physician, or hospital emergency department promptly.

The following are safe first aid measures for various types of poisoning.

Swallowed Poisons

This is an emergency—any nonfood substance is a potential poison.

Call physician, poison control center, or hospital emergency department promptly for advice.

Do *not* make the patient vomit if:
- Patient is unconscious or drowsy.
- Patient is convulsing or having tremors (or "twitching" of the arms or legs or having uncontrolled body movements).
- Patient swallowed a strong corrosive (such as drain cleaner, oven cleaner, toilet bowl cleaner, strong acids).
- Patient swallowed furniture polish, kerosene, gasoline, or other petroleum products (except after specific medical advice).

Directions for making a patient vomit:
- Use syrup of Ipecac. (Do not give salt water.)
- For children under 12 months of age, obtain medical advice.
- For children 1 year to 10 years of age, give 3 teaspoons (1 tablespoon or ½ oz) syrup of Ipecac followed by 4 oz to 8 oz of water. If no vomiting occurs in 20 minutes, may repeat dose once only.
- For children over 10 years of age, give 2 tablespoons (1 oz) Ipecac syrup followed by 4 oz to 8 oz of water.

If instructed, drive carefully to medical facility. Take pan to collect vomitus. Bring package or container with intact label of material ingested or whatever leftover material there is.

Fumes or Gases

FUEL GASES, AUTO EXHAUST, DENSE SMOKE FROM FIRES, OR FUMES FROM POISONOUS CHEMICALS
- Get victim into fresh air.
- Loosen clothing.
- If victim is not breathing, start artificial respiration promptly. Do not stop until patient is breathing well, or help arrives.
- Have *someone else* call a physician, poison control center, hospital, or rescue unit.
- Transport victim to a medical facility promptly.

Eye

- Holding lids open, flush out eye immediately with water.
- Remove contact lenses if worn.
- Irrigate eye for 15 minutes with a gentle continuous stream of water from a pitcher.
- Never permit eye to be rubbed or use eye drops.
- Call physician, poison control center, or emergency department for further advice.

Skin

ACIDS, LYE, OTHER CAUSTICS, AND PESTICIDES
- Brush off dry material gently. Then immediately wash off skin with a large amount of water; use soap if available.
- Remove any contaminated clothing.
- Call physician, poison control center, or emergency department for further advice.

Bites and Stings

SNAKE

Nonpoisonous
- Treat as a puncture wound. Consult physician.

Poisonous
- Put patient and injured part at rest. Keep quiet.
- Do not apply ice. May use cool compress for pain.
- Immediate suction without incision may be beneficial.
- Apply loose (allow two fingers under) constricting band above the bite (not around fingers or toes) if cannot get to medical help in one hour.
- Transport victim promptly to a medical facility.

INSECTS

Spiders, Scorpions, or Unusual Reaction to Other Stinging Insects Such as Bees, Wasps, Hornets
- Remove stinger if present with a scraping motion of a plastic card or fingernail to reduce injection of more toxin. Do not pull out.
- Use cold compresses on bite area to relieve pain.

- If victim stops breathing, use artificial respiration and have someone call rescue unit and physician for further instructions.
- If any reactions such as hives, generalized rash, pallor, weakness, nausea, vomiting, "tightness" in chest, nose, or throat, or collapse occurs, get patient to physician or emergency department immediately.
- For scorpion sting, get immediate medical advice.
- For spider bites, obtain medical advice. (Save live specimen if safe and possible.)

Ticks

- Always thoroughly inspect child after time in woods or brush. Ticks carry many serious diseases and must be completely removed.
- Use tweezers placed close to the head or protected fingers to pull tick away from point of attachment.
- If head breaks off, victim should be taken without delay for medical removal.

ANIMAL

- Bat, raccoon, skunk, and fox bites as well as unprovoked bites from cats and dogs may be from a rabid animal.
- Call physician or medical facility.
- Wash wound gently but thoroughly with soap and water for 15 minutes.

POISONOUS MARINE ANIMALS

Stingray, Lionfish, Catfish, and Stonefish Stings
- Put victim at rest and submerge sting area in hot water.

Other Marine Stings
- Flush with water, remove any clinging material.
- Apply cold compress to relieve pain.
- Call physician or medical facility.

(Used with permission from the American Academy of Pediatrics, Elk Grove Village, Illinois, 1987)

Normal Laboratory Values and Pulmonary Function Tests

Representative Laboratory Values

The following table lists laboratory values according to traditional units and, whenever possible, according to the International System of Units. Readers are advised to determine the system used in their institution's laboratory before comparing values to those given in this chart. The values are often dependent on the method used and "normal values" may differ between laboratories.

Laboratory Test	Traditional Units	International (SI*) Units
ACTH, 8 AM, plasma	<80 pg/ml	<3.8 pmol per liter
Albumin, serum	3.5 g–5.5 g/100 ml	35 g–55 g per liter
Aldosterone, 8 AM (patient supine, 100 mEq Na and 60 mEq–100 mEq K intake)	1 ng–5 ng/dl	0.03 nmol–0.15 nmol per liter
Ammonia, urine	30 mEq–50 mEq in 24 h	30 mmol–50 mmol per day
Ammonia, whole blood venous	80 μg–110 μg/dl	47 μmol–65 μmol per liter
Amylase, serum	60–180 Somogyi units/dl 0.8 U–3.2 U/Liter	13 nmol–53 nmol per second per liter
Amylase, urine	35–260 Somogyi units per hour	
Arterial blood gases (sea level)		
Bicarbonate (HCO_3^-)	21 mEq–28 mEq per liter	21 mmol–28 mmol per liter
Carbon Dioxide (pCO_2)	35–45 mmHg	4.7 kPa–6.0 kPa

(continued)

Laboratory Test	Traditional Units	International (SI*) Units
pH (arterial blood)	7.38–7.44	
Oxygen (pO₂)	80–100 mmHg	11 kPa–13 kPa
Oxygen saturation (SₐO₂)	95% to 99%	
Base excess (BE)	0 ± 2 mEq/L	
Ascorbic acid, serum	0.4 mg–1.0 mg/dl	23 μmol–57 μmol per liter
Ascorbic acid, leukocytes	25 mg–40 mg/dl	1420 μmol–2270 μmol per liter
Base, total, serum	145 mEq–155 mEq/L	145 mmol–155 mmol per liter
B (beta)- Hydroxybutyrate, plasma	<0.5 mmol/L	
Bilirubin, total, serum	0.3 mg–1.0 mg/dl	5.1 μmol–17 μmol per liter
Direct serum	0.1 mg–0.3 mg/dl	1.7 μmol–5.1 μmol per liter
Indirect serum	0.2 mg–0.7 mg/dl	3.4 μmol–12 μmol per liter
Bleeding time, (Ivy) 5-mm wound	1 min–9 min	
Bromides, serum toxic levels	>17 mEq/L	17 mmol per liter
Calcitonin, plasma	0–28 pg/ml	0–8.2 pmol/L
Calcium, ionized	2.3 mEq–2.8 mEq/L	
	8.5 mg–10.5 mg/dl	2.2 mmol–2.7 mmol per liter
Calcium, urine	<7.5 mEq/24 h or <150 mg/24 h	<3.8 mmol per day
Carbon dioxide content, plasma (at sea level)	21 mEq–30 mEq/L or 50–70 volume %	21 mmol–30 mmol per liter
Carcinoembryonic antigen (CEA)	0 ng–2.5 ng/ml (healthy nonsmokers)	0 μg–2.5 μg per liter
Carotenoids, serum	50 μg–300 μg/dl	0.9 μmol–5.6 μmol per liter
Catecholamines, urinary excretion		
Free catecholamines	<100 μg per day	<590 nmol per day
Epinephrine	<50 μg per day	<295 nmol per day
Metanephrines	<1.3 mg per day	<6.2 μmol per day
Vanillylmandelic acid (VMA)	<8 mg per day	<40 μmol per day
Chlorides, serum (Cl⁻)	98 mEq–106 mEq/L	98 mmol–106 mmol per liter
Copper, serum	80 μg–140 μg/dl	12 μmol–24 μmol per liter
Cortisol		
8 AM	5 μg–24 μg/dl	140 nmol–662 nmol per liter
4 PM	3 μg–12 μg/dl	82 nmol–331 nmol per liter
Creatine phosphokinase, serum (CPK)	10 U–70 U/ml (females)	0.17 mmol–1.18 mmol per second per liter
	25 U–90 U/ml (males)	0.42 mmol–1.51 mmol per second per liter
Isoenzymes serum	Fraction 2 (MB) <5% total	
Creatinine, serum	0.6 mg–1.5 mg/dl	53 μmol–133 μmol/L
Creatinine clearance, urine	91 ml–130 ml/min	1.5 ml–2.2 ml/s
Digoxin, serum		
Therapeutic level	1.2 ± 0.4 ng/ml	1.54 ± 0.5 nmol per liter
Toxic level	>2.4 ng/ml	>3.2 nmol per liter
Dilantin, plasma		
Therapeutic level	10 μg–20 μg/ml	40 μmol–79 μmol per liter
Toxic level	>30 μg/ml	>119 μmol per liter
Estradiol, plasma		
Women (higher at ovulation)	20 pg–60 pg/ml	0.07 nmol–0.22 nmol per liter
Men	<50 pg/ml	<0.18 nmol per liter
Ethanol, blood		
Mild to moderate intoxication	80 mg–200 mg/dl	17 mmol–43 mmol per liter
Marked intoxication	250 mg–400 mg/dl	54 mmol–87 mmol per liter
Severe intoxication	>400 mg/dl	>87 mmol per liter
Fatty acids, free (nonesterified), plasma	<0.7 mmol/L	
Ferritin, serum	15 ng–200 ng/ml	15 μg–200 μg per liter
Fibrinogen, plasma	160 mg–415 mg/dl	0.5 μmol–1.4 μmol per liter
Fibrinogen split products	titer 1:4 or less	
Folic acid, serum	6 ng–15 ng/ml	14 nmol–34 nmol per liter
Folic acid, red blood cell	150 ng–450 ng/ml of cells	340 nmol–1020 nmol per liter cells
Gastrin, serum	40 pg–200 pg/ml	40 ng–150 ng per liter
Globulins, serum	2.0 g–3.0 g/dl	20 g–30 g per liter
Glucagon, plasma	50 pg–200 pg/ml	14 pmol–56 pmol per liter

(continued)

Laboratory Test	Traditional Units	International (SI*) Units
Glucose (fasting) plasma		
Normal	75 mg–105 mg/dl	4.2 mmol–5.8 mmol per liter
Diabetes mellitus	>140 mg/dl (on more than one occasion)	>7.8 mmol per liter
Glucose, 2-h postprandial, plasma		
Normal	<140 mg/dl	<7.8 mmol per liter
Impaired glucose tolerance	140 mg–200 mg/dl	7.8 mmol–11.1 mmol per liter
Diabetes mellitus	>200 mg/dl on more than one occasion	>11.1 mmol per liter
Glucose, true, urine	50 mg–300 mg/24 h	0.3 mmol–1.7 mmol per day
Gonadotropins, plasma		
Women, mature, premenopausal (except during ovulation)		
FSH	5 mU–30 mU/ml	5 units–30 units per liter
LH	5 mU–25 mU/ml	5 units–25 units per liter
Women, ovulatory surge		
FSH	5 mU–20 mU/ml	5 units–20 units per liter
LH	15 mU–40 mU/ml	15 units–40 units per liter
Women, postmenopausal		
FSH	>40 mU/ml	>40 units per liter
LH	>40 mU/ml	>40 units per liter
Men, mature		
FSH	5 mU–20 mU/ml	5 units–20 units per liter
LH	5 mU–20 mU/ml	5 units–20 units per liter
Children, both sexes, prepubertal		
FSH	<5 mU/ml	<5 units per liter
LH	<5 mU/ml	<5 units per liter
Growth hormone (after 100 g glucose by mouth)	<5 ng/dl	<230 pmol per liter
Haptoglobin, serum	103 mg–153 mg/dl	1.3 ± 0.2 g per liter
Hemoglobin, blood		
Adult males	14 g–18 g/dl	8.7 mmol–11.2 mmol per liter
Adult females	12 g–16 g/dl	7.4 mmol–9.9 mmol per liter
Infant: Days 1–13	14.5 g–24.5 g/dl	
Days 14–60	11.3 g–17.3 g/dl	
Child: 3 months–10 years	9.9 g–14.5 g/dl	
11 years–15 years	13.4 g/dl	
Hemoglobin A	up to 6% of total hemoglobin	
Immunoglobulins, serum		
IgA	90 mg–325 mg/dl	0.9 g–3.2 g per liter
IgE	<0.025 mg/dl	<0.00025 g per liter
IgG	800 mg–1500 mg/dl	8.0 g–15 g per liter
IgM	45 mg–150 mg/dl	0.45 g–1.5 g per liter
Insulin, serum or plasma, fasting	6 μU–26 μU/ml	43 pmol–186 pmol per liter
Iron, serum (mean ± 1 SD)	105 ± 35 mcg/dl	19 ± 6 μmol per liter
Iron binding capacity, serum (mean ± 1 SD)	305 ± 32 mcg/dl	55 ± 6 μmol per liter
saturation	20%–45%	
Ketones, total, plasma	0.5 mg–1.5 mg/dl	5.0 mg–15.0 mg per liter
Ketones, total, urine	19.8 mg–81.2 mg/24 h	
Lactate dehydrogenase, serum	200 units–450 units/ml (Wrobleski)	
	60 units–100 units/ml (Wacker)	
	25 units–100 units/L	0.4 μmol–1.7 μmol per second per liter
Lactic acid, blood	<1.2 mmol/L	
Lead, serum	<20 μg/dl	<1.0 μmol per liter
Leukocytes, total	4,300 to 10,000 per mm^3 (avg. 7,000)	
Neutrophils, juvenile and band	100 to 2,100 per mm^3 (avg. 520)	
Neutrophils, segmented	1,100 to 6,050 per mm^3 (avg. 3,000)	
Eosinophils	0 to 700 per mm^3 (avg. 150)	
Basophils	0 to 150 per mm^3 (avg. 30)	
Lymphocytes	1,500 to 4,000 per mm^3 (avg. 2,500)	
Monocytes	200 to 950 per mm^3 (avg. 430)	

(continued)

Laboratory Test	Traditional Units	International (SI*) Units
Lipase, serum	1.5 units (Cherry Crandall)	
Lipids, total	400 mg–1000 mg/dl	
Total plasma cholesterol	150 mg–250 mg/dl	
Triglycerides	40 mg–150 mg/dl	
Phospholipids	150 mg–250 mg/dl	48 mmol–81 mmol per liter
Lithium, serum		
Therapeutic level	0.6 mEq–1.5 mEq/L	0.5 mmol–1.5 mmol/L
Toxic level	>2.0 mEq/L	>2 mmol per liter
Magnesium, serum	1.5 mEq–2.5 mEq per liter	
	2 mg–3 mg/dl	0.8 mmol–1.3 mmol per liter
Nitrogen, nonprotein, serum	15 mg–35 mg/dl	0.15 g–0.35 g per liter
Oxygen content: (see also arterial blood gases)		
Arterial blood (sea level)	17 to 21 volume percent	
Venous blood, arm (sea level)	10 to 16 volume percent	
Oxytocin, plasma		
Men, preovulatory women	0.5 μU–2 μU/ml	0.5 mU–2 mU per liter
Ovulating women	2 μU–4 μU/ml	2 mU–4 mU per liter
Lactating women	5 μU–10 μU/ml	5 mU–10 mU per liter
Partial thromboplastin time (PTT)	(Standard) 68 to 82 seconds	
	(Activated) 32 to 46 seconds	
Phosphatase, alkaline, serum	21 to 91 IU per liter at 37°C	0.4 μmol–1.5 μmol per second per liter
Phosphorus, inorganic, serum	3 mg–4.5 mg/dl	1.0 mmol–1.4 mmol per liter
Platelets (Brecher-Cronkite method)	150,000 to 440,000 per cubic ml	2.9×10^{11} per liter
Potassium, serum	3.5 mEq–5.0 mEq/L	3.5 mmol–5.0 mmol per liter
Potassium, urine	25 mEq–100 mEq/24 h	25 mmol–100 mmol per day
Progesterone		
Men, prepubertal girls, postmenopausal women	<2 ng/ml	6 nmol per liter
Women, luteal, peak	>5 ng/ml	>16 nmol per liter
Prolactin, serum	2 ng–15 ng/ml	0.08 nmol–6.0 nmol/L
Protein, total, serum	5.5 g–8.0 g/dl	55 g–80 g per liter
Protein, urine	<150 mg/24 hr	<0.05 g per day
Protein fractions, serum (see albumin, globulin)		
Prothrombin time	11 seconds–15 seconds	
Quinidine, serum		
Therapeutic level	1.5 μg–3 μg/ml	4.6 μmol–9.2 μmol per liter
Toxic level	5 μg–6 μg/ml	15.4 μmol–18.5 μmol per liter
Reticulocytes	0.5%–2.0% of red blood cells	
Salicylate, plasma		
Therapeutic level	20 mg–25 mg/dl	1.4 mmol–1.8 mmol per liter
Toxic level	>30 mg/dl	>2.2 mmol per liter
Sedimentation rate (Westergren)		
Men	≤15 mm/h	
Women	≤20 mm/h	
Children	≤10 mm/h	
Sodium, serum	136 mEq–145 mEq/L	136 mmol–145 mmol per liter
Sodium, urine	100 mEq–260 mEq/24 h	100 mmol–260 mmol per day
Specific gravity, urine		
After 12-h fluid restriction	1.025 or more	
After 12-h deliberate water intake	1.003 or less	
Testosterone		
Women	<100 ng/dl	<3.5 nmol per liter
Men	300 ng–1000 ng/dl	105 nmol–350 nmol per liter
Prepubertal boys and girls	5 ng–20 ng/dl	0.175 nmol–0.702 nmol per liter
Thyroid function tests		
Radioactive iodine uptake 24 hr.	5%–30% (range varies in different areas of the thyroid due to variable uptake)	
Reverse triiodothyronine (rT$_3$), serum	10 ng–40 ng/dl	0.128 nmol–0.512 nmol per liter
Thyroxine (T$_4$), serum radioimmunoassay	4 μg–12 μg/dl	50 nmol–154 nmol per liter

(continued)

Triiodothyronine (T$_3$), serum radio-immunoassay	80 ng–100 ng/dl	1.2 nmol–1.5 nmol per liter
Thyroid-stimulating hormone (TSH)	<5 μU/ml	<5 mU per liter
Transaminase, serum glutamic oxalo-acetic (SGOT)	10 to 40 Karmen units/ml 6 units–18 units/L	0.10 μmol–0.30 μmol per second per liter
Transaminase, serum glutamic pyru-vic (SGPT)	10 to 40 Karmen units/ml 3 units–26 units/L	0.05 μmol–0.43 μmol per second per liter
Urea nitrogen, whole blood (BUN)	10 mg–20 mg/dl	3.6 mmol–7.1 mmol per liter
Uric acid, serum		
Males	2.5 mg–8.0 mg/dl	0.15 mmol–0.48 mmol per liter
Females	1.5 mg–6.0 mg/dl	0.09 mmol–0.36 mmol per liter
Vitamin A, serum	20 μg to 100 μg/dl	0.7 μmol–3.5 μmol per liter
Vitamin B$_{12}$, serum	200 pg–600 pg/ml	148 pmol–443 pmol per liter
White blood cells (see leukocytes)		
Zinc, serum	100 μg–140 μg/dl	15 μmol–21 μmol per liter

* From the French name, Système International d'Unités.

Pulmonary Function Tests

The following table lists values for pulmonary function tests. Normal values are listed for men and women.

	Normal Values	
Test Name (symbol)	Men	Women
Spirometry		
Forced vital capacity (FVC)	≥4.0 L	≥3.0 L
Forced expiratory volume in 1 second (FEV)	>3.0 L	>2.0 L
FEV/FVC (FEV, %)	>60%	>70%
Lung volumes		
Total lung capacity (TLC)	6 L–7 L	5 L–6 L
Functional residual capacity (FRC)	2 L–3 L	2 L–3 L
Residual volume (RV)	1 L–2 L	1 L–2 L
Inspiratory capacity (IC)	2 L–4 L	2 L–4 L
Expiratory reserve volume (ERV)	1 L–2 L	1 L–2 L
Vital capacity (VC)	4 L–5 L	3 L–4 L

Common Abbreviations

a̅a̅	of each (equal parts)	dr.	dram
abd.	abdomen	dsg./dssg.	dressing
a.c.	before meals	d.t.d.	dispense such doses
A.D.	right ear	DTR	deep tendon reflexes
ad	up to	Dx.	diagnosis
ad lib	as much as needed		
Adm.	admission, admitted	ECG (EKG)	electrocardiogram
alb.	albumin	ECR	Emergency Chemical Restraint
alk.	alkaline	EEG	electroencephalogram
AM	morning	*e.g.*	for example
amp.	ampule	elix.	elixir
amt.	amount	EMG	electromyogram
appt.	appointment	ENT	ear, nose, throat
aq. (dest.)	water (distilled)	EOM	extraocular movements
A.S.	left ear	ER	Emergency Room
A.U.	both (each) ear(s)	etc.	et cetera
aur.	ear	eval.	evaluation
		ex.	example
bid	twice daily	extrem.	extremity
bm	bowel movement		
BP	blood pressure	FBS	fasting blood sugar
BR	bathroom	Fe	iron
B.S.A.	body surface area	fl.	fluid
		ft	foot; feet
c̄	with	FUO	fever of unknown origin
Ca	calcium		
Cal.	calories	gal	gallon
caps	capsule	GC	gonorrhea, gonococcus
CBC	complete blood count	GI	gastrointestinal
cc	cubic centimeter	gm (g)	gram
Cl	chloride	gr	grain
CNS	central nervous system	gtt.	drop
c/o	complained of	GU	genitourinary
col. ct.	colony count	gyn	gynecology
comp.	compound		
conc.	concentrated	H_2O	water
CP	cerebral palsy	H_2O_2	hydrogen peroxide
CPR	cardiopulmonary resuscitation	hct	hematocrit
		hgb	hemoglobin
diarr.	diarrhea	HEENT	head, eyes, ears, nose, and throat
dil.	dilute	Hosp.	hospital
disch.	discharge	hr (h)	hour
disp.	dispense	H-S	hepato-spleno
dist.	distilled	h.s.	hour of sleep, bedtime
DOA	date of admission	hx.	history
DOB	date of birth		
DPT/DTP	diphtheria, pertussis, tetanus immunization	IA	intra-arterial
		IM	intramuscular

I&O (I/O)	intake and output	PMH	past medical history
IPV	inactivated polio vaccine	p.o.	by mouth
IV	intravenous	PPD	Purified Protein Derivative
		ppm	parts per million
K	potassium	prn	when necessary
		PT	physical therapy
L	liter (quart)	pulv.	a powder
Ⓛ	left		
Lab.	laboratory	q	every
Lat.	lateral	q2h	every 2 hours
lb	pound(s)	q4h	every 4 hours
LDH	lactic dehydrogenase	qd	every day
LE	lower extremities	qh	every hour
liq.	liquid; a solution	qid	four times a day
LLQ	left, lower quadrant	qod	every other day
LMP	last menstrual period	qs.	quantity sufficient
ltd.	limited		
LUQ	left, upper quadrant	r	rectal
		Ⓡ	right
mcg	microgram	RBC	red blood cell
Med.	medical	RDA	recommended dietary allowance
mg	milligram	re	that is; regarding; in reference to
min	minute	rep.	repeat; may refill
mixt.	mixture	RLQ	right, lower quadrant
ml	milliliter	R/O	rule out
mo	month	ROM	range of motion
mx.	minim	RUQ	right, upper quadrant
		Rx	prescription
n/c/o	no complaint of		
neg.	negative	s̄	without
Neuro.	neurology	sens.	sensitive
noct.	night	S.G.	specific gravity
non rep. (NR)	do not repeat	SGOT	serum glutamic oxaloacetic transaminase
NPO	nothing by mouth		
Nsg.	nursing	SGPT	serum glutamic pyruvic transaminase
NSR	normal sinus rhythm		
N&V (N/V)	nausea and vomiting	sig.	give directions; label
		sl (SL)	under tongue; sublingual
OCP	oral contraceptive pills	sol.	solution
OD	right eye	span.	spansule
oint.	ointment	s̄s̄	half
OPV	oral polio vaccine immunization	STAT	immediate
OS	left eye	STS	serologic test for syphilis
OT	occupational therapy	sub.q. (SC)	subcutaneous
OU	each eye	suppos.	suppository
oz	ounce	sx.	symptoms
		syr.	syrup
p.c.	after meals		
per (os)	through *or* by (mouth)	t, tsp	teaspoon
PERLA	Pupils equal and reactive to light and accommodation	T, tbsp	tablespoon
		tab.	tablet
PERRLA	Pupils equal, round and reactive to light and accommodation	TB	tuberculosis
		tet-tox.	tetanus toxoid
plt.	platelet	tid	three times daily
PM	afternoon; evening	TM	tympanic membrane

TNTC	too numerous to count	vag.	vaginal
TPR	temperature, pulse, respirations	VD	venereal disease
tinc.	tincture	VDRL	venereal disease test
tr.	trace or tincture	V/S	vital signs
Tx.	treatment		
		WBC	white blood count
UA	urinalysis	wk	week
UE	upper extremities	WNL	within normal limits
ung.	ointment	w/o	without
ut dict (UD)	as directed	wt	weight

Drug Compatibility Guide

The following table presents a compilation of drug compatibility information obtained from several sources. It is intended to be used as a *general guide* to drug compatibilities rather than as a definitive information source, inasmuch as the compatibility of two or more drugs in solution is dependent on a number of variables, such as the solution itself, the concentration of drugs present, and the method of mixing (bottle, syringe, or Y-site).

Drugs reported to be compatible in solution are indicated by Y in the table, while drugs documented to be incompatible as reflected by the development of cloudiness, turbidity, or precipitation within the solution, are indicated by an N. Where no information was found on the compatibility of two drugs, the corresponding space was left blank.

With some drug combinations, conflicting information was obtained about their compatibility, especially where different parameters were used in obtaining the data. In such cases, a conservative approach was followed, and the combination was indicated as *not compatible* in the table, although compatibility may be dependent on solution strength, vehicle, time after mixing before used, or any number of other factors.

Before mixing any two drugs, it is imperative that health-care personnel ascertain with certainty if a potential incompatibility problem exists by referring to an appropriate information source or by contacting the pharmacist. The accompanying table is solely intended to provide a handy guide from which one can quickly obtain a general idea of drug solution compatibility.

BIBLIOGRAPHY

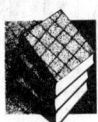

Allen LV, Levinson RS, Phisutsinthop D: Compatibility of various admixtures with secondary additives at Y-injection sites of intravenous administration sets. Am J Hosp Pharm 34: 939, 1977

Allen LV, Stiles ML: Compatibility of various admixtures with secondary additives at Y-injection sites of intravenous administration sets (Part 2). Am J Hosp Pharm 38:380, 1981

Misgen R: Compatibilities and incompatibilities of some intravenous solution admixtures. Am J Hosp Pharm 22: 92, 1965

Ng P: Compatibility guide for combining IV medications. Am J Nurs 79: 1292, 1979

Trissel CA: Handbook of Injectable Drugs, 4th ed. Washington, DC, Amer. Soc. Hosp. Pharmacists 1986

	aminophylline	amphotericin B	ampicillin	atropine	calcium gluconate	carbenicillin	cefazolin	cimetidine	clindamycin	diazepam	dopamine	epinephrine	erythromycin	fentanyl	furosemide	gentamicin	glycopyrrolate	heparin sodium	hydrocortisone	hydroxyzine	levarterenol	lidocaine	meperidine	morphine	nitroglycerin	pentobarbital	potassium chloride	sodium bicarbonate	tetracycline	vancomycin	verapamil	vitamin B & C complex
aminophylline	*		Y		Y	N	N		N	Y	Y	Y	N	N				Y	Y	N	N	Y	N	N	Y	Y	Y	Y	Y	N	Y	N
amphotericin B		*	N		N	N		N			N					N		Y	Y			N					N	Y	N		N	
ampicillin	Y	N	*	N	N	Y	Y		N		N		N			N		Y	N		Y					Y		N	Y		Y	Y
atropine			N	*			Y		N		N		Y				Y	N		Y	N		Y	Y		N	Y	N			Y	Y
calcium gluconate	Y	N	N		*		N		N		Y	N	Y					Y	Y		Y	Y					Y	N	N	Y	Y	Y
carbenicillin	N	N	Y			*		Y	Y		Y	N	N		N			N	Y			Y				Y		Y			Y	N
cefazolin	N		Y	N	N		*	N			Y					Y			N		Y					N	Y				Y	
cimetidine		N		Y		Y	N	*	Y			Y	Y		Y	Y		Y			Y	Y				N			Y	Y	Y	Y
clindamycin	N		N		N	Y		Y	*							Y		Y	Y				N	N		Y					Y	Y
diazepam	Y		N				Y			*		N				N		N	N		N	N	N	N		N	N	N			Y	N
dopamine	Y	N	N		Y	Y					*					N		Y	Y		Y				Y		Y		Y		Y	Y
epinephrine	N		N	N	N	N		Y		N		*	N		N			Y			N	N	Y				N	N			Y	Y
erythromycin	N		N	Y	Y	N	N	Y				N	*					N	Y			Y					N	Y	N	Y	Y	N
fentanyl				Y										*						Y			Y	Y		N						
furosemide								Y	N		N				*	N		Y			N				Y		Y		N		Y	Y
gentamicin		N	N			N	N	Y			Y				N	*		N													Y	Y
glycopyrrolate				Y							N						*		Y		Y	Y	Y		N	N						
heparin sodium	Y	Y	Y	N	Y			Y	Y	N	Y	Y	N		Y	N		*	N	N	Y	N	N	N			Y	Y	N	N	N	Y
hydrocortisone	Y	Y	N		Y	Y	Y		Y		Y		Y					N	*		Y	Y				N	Y	Y	Y	N	Y	Y
hydroxyzine	N		Y								N		Y				Y	N		*	Y	Y	Y		N							N
levarterenol	N		N		Y	N	N	Y			N	N						Y	Y		*					N	Y				Y	Y
lidocaine	Y	N	Y		Y	Y	N	Y		N	Y	N	Y				Y	Y	Y	Y		*		Y	Y	Y	Y	Y	Y		Y	Y
meperidine	N		Y	Y						N		Y		Y			Y	Y	N				*	N		N					N	
morphine	N		Y	Y						N		Y		Y				Y	N				N	*		N					Y	Y
nitroglycerin	Y							Y			Y								Y			Y			*						Y	
pentobarbital	Y		N			N	N	N	N			N	N				N		N	N		N	N	N	Y	*	N	N	N		N	Y
potassium chloride	Y	N	Y	Y	Y	Y	Y	Y	Y	Y	N	Y	N	Y	Y			Y	Y		Y	Y				Y	*	Y	Y	Y	Y	
sodium bicarbonate	Y	Y	N	N			Y	N			N	Y	Y					N	Y	Y		Y	N	N		N	Y	*	N	Y	N	N
tetracycline	N	N	N		N	N	N	Y			Y		N					N	Y	Y						N	Y	N	*			Y
vancomycin	N				Y		Y	Y					Y					N	Y							N	Y	N		*	Y	Y
verapamil	Y	N	Y	Y	Y	Y	Y	Y	Y	Y	Y	Y	Y		Y	Y		Y	Y		Y	Y	Y	Y	Y	Y	Y	N		Y	*	Y
vitamin B & C complex	N		Y	Y	Y	N	Y	Y	Y	N	Y	Y	N		Y	Y		Y	Y	N	Y	Y			Y			N	Y	Y	Y	*

Answers to Practice Problems in Chapter 11

NOTE: Some answers given may vary slightly depending on the conversion values used.

Page 158

a. 500,000 mg
b. 0.1 L
c. 3000 mcg
d. 2500 ml
e. 500 ml
f. 3000 mg
g. 100 cc
h. 0.004 g
i. 50 mcg
j. 0.5 kl

Page 159

1. a. 12 dr
   b. 32 minims
   c. 6 fl oz
   d. 30 gr
   e. $2\frac{1}{2}$ fl dr
   f. 4 pt

2. a. 240 gr
   b. 4 fluid dr
   c. 7680 minims
   d. 2 dr
   e. 0.25 gallon
   f. 240 gr
   g. 8 fluid dr
   h. 0.5 qt
   i. 192 dr
   j. 12 scruples

Page 159

a. 4 tsp
b. 120 gtt
c. 2 fluid oz
d. 4 tsp
e. 2 fluid dr

Page 160

NOTE: Some answers are approximations.

1. a. 0.5 gr
   b. $1\frac{1}{2}$ fluid dr
   c. $\frac{1}{12}$ gr
   d. 16 fluid oz
   e. 120 minims
   f. 1.5 gr
   g. 1/100 gr
   h. 32 fluid dr
   i. 10 minims
   j. 0.75 dr
   k. 0.67 fluid oz
   l. 1/60 gr

2. a. 8 ml
   b. 120 ml
   c. 30 g or 32 g
   d. 0.12 mg
   e. 0.33 g
   f. 2 L
   g. 15 ml
   h. 5000 mg
   i. 450 mcg
   j. 0.2 g
   k. 60 mg
   l. 120 ml

3. a. 1 tsp
   b. 8 fluid dr
   c. 30 gtt
   d. 8 tsp
   e. 0.5 L
   f. 1 tsp

4. a. 30 ml; 0.03 qt
   b. 120 minims; 8 ml
   c. 30,000 mcg; 30 mg
   d. 4 dr; 0.5 oz
   e. 4 fluid dr; 16 ml
   f. 4 dr; 32 dr
   g. $\frac{1}{15}$ gr; 0.004 g
   h. 800 fluid dr; 6 pt
   i. 10 gtt; 10 minims

1704 XIII: Appendix

Page 162

a. 1:50
b. 0.5%
c. 0.25 mg/ml
d. 0.67 gr/ml
e. 1:10,000

Page 163

1. a. 0.25%
b. 0.01%
c. 33%
d. 4%
e. 4%
f. 60%
g. 0.8%
h. 0.4%

2. a. 1:5
b. 1:250
c. 1:1.25
d. 1:2000
e. 1:100
f. 1:500
g. 1:250
h. 1:500

3. 0.42%

4. 6.4%

5. a. 0.125%; 1:800
b. 0.1%; 1:1000
c. 3%; 1:33
d. 10%; 1:10
e. 0.04%; 1:2500

Page 164

1. a. 8 g
b. 15 g
c. 0.1 g
d. 0.06 g
e. 100 g
f. 2 g

2. $1\frac{1}{2}$ gr

3. 9 ml

Page 164–165

1. 30 ml

2. 180 ml

3. 2 fl oz

4. 900 ml

Page 165

1. 600 ml

2. 1170 ml

3. 0.24 ml

4. $2\frac{1}{2}$ fl oz

5. 5 minims

Page 167

1. 14 tablets

2. 6 tablets

3. 4 tablets

4. 28 capsules

5. 10 g

6. $\frac{1}{8}$ gr

7. 75 ml

8. 1200 mg

9. 300 mg

10. 21.6 gr

Page 168–169

1. 1.2 ml

2. 1.6 ml

3. 1 ml

4. 2.5 ml

Page 169

1. 3.33 ml

2. 62.5 mg

3. 3,000,000 units

Page 170

1. 8.3 drops/min

2. 31 drops/min

3. 25 drops/min

Page 172

1. 126 mg
2. 1500 mg
3. $\frac{1}{2}$ gr
4. 30 mg/kg/day
5. 16 mg (Young's rule)
6. 3 mg (Fried's rule)
7. 0.8 g to 1.6 g (Clark's rule)
8. 100 mg/day (Fried's rule)
9. 1 gr (Young's rule)
10. 40 mg (Young's rule)
   56 mg (Clark's rule)
   89 mg (Body Surface Area)

General Bibliography

Pharmacology and Nursing

Abrams AC: Clinical Drug Therapy—Rationales for Nursing Practice, 2nd ed. Philadelphia, JB Lippincott, 1987

Albanese JA: Nurses' Drug Reference, 2nd ed. New York, McGraw-Hill, 1982

Albanese JA, Bond T: Drug Interactions: Basic Principles and Clinical Problems. New York, McGraw-Hill, 1978

Alfaro R: Application of the Nursing Process. Philadelphia, JB Lippincott, 1986

American Drug Index (yearly): Philadelphia, JB Lippincott, 1988

Annual Review of Pharmacology and Toxicology (yearly). Palo Alto, CA, Annual Reviews, Inc.

Asperheim MK, Eisenhauer LA: The Pharmacologic Basis of Patient Care, 4th ed. Philadelphia, WB Saunders, 1981

Avery GS: Drug Treatment, 3rd ed. Baltimore, Williams & Wilkins, 1985

Beeson PB, McDermott W, Wyngaarden J (eds): Cecil-Loeb Textbook of Medicine, 15th ed. Philadelphia, WB Saunders, 1979

Bevan JA, Thompson JH (eds): Essentials of Pharmacology, 3rd ed. Philadelphia, Harper & Row, 1983

Bowman WC, Rand MJ: Textbook of Pharmacology, 2nd ed. Oxford, England, Blackwell Scientific Publications, 1980

Brunner LS, Suddarth DS: Textbook of Medical-Surgical Nursing, 5th ed. Philadelphia, JB Lippincott, 1984

Carpenito LJ: Handbook of Nursing Diagnosis, 2nd ed. Philadelphia, JB Lippincott, 1987

Clark JB, Queener SF, Karb VB: Pharmacological Basis of Nursing Practice, 2nd ed. St. Louis, CV Mosby, 1986

Cooper JR, Bloom FE: The Biochemical Basis of Neuropharmacology, 5th ed. New York, Oxford University Press, 1986

Craig CR, Stitzel RE (eds): Modern Pharmacology, 2nd ed. Boston, Little Brown & Co. 1986

Csaky TZ, Barnes BA: Cutting's Handbook of Pharmacology, 7th ed. Appleton-Century-Crofts, 1984

Eisenhauer LA, Gerald MC: The Nurse's Guide to Drug Therapy. Englewood Cliffs, NJ, Prentice-Hall, 1984

Facts and Comparisons. Philadelphia, JB Lippincott (updated monthly)

Feldman RS, Quenzer LF: Fundamentals of Neuropsychopharmacology. Sunderland, MA, Sinauer Associates, 1984

Gahart BL: Intravenous Medications, 4th ed. St. Louis, CV Mosby, 1984

Gilman AG, Goodman LS, Rall TW, Murad F (eds): The Pharmacological Basis of Therapeutics, 7th ed. New York, Macmillan, 1985

Goth A: Medical Pharmacology, 11th ed. St. Louis, CV Mosby, 1984

Govoni LE, Hayes JE: Drugs and Nursing Implications, 5th ed. New York, Appleton and Lange, 1985

Haber J, Leach A, Schudy S, et al: Comprehensive Psychiatric Nursing, 3rd ed. New York, McGraw-Hill, 1987

Hahn AB, Barkin RL, Oestreich SJ: Pharmacology in Nursing, 16th ed. St. Louis, CV Mosby, 1986

Hamilton HK (ed): Procedures. Springhouse, PA, Intermed Communications, Inc., 1983

Handbook of Nonprescription Drugs, 8th ed. Washington, DC, American Pharmaceutical Association, 1986

Hansten PD: Drug Interactions, 5th ed. Philadelphia, Lea & Febiger, 1985

Howry LB, Bindler RM, Tso Y: Pediatric Medications. Philadelphia, JB Lippincott, 1981

Irons PD: Psychotropic Drugs and Nursing Intervention. New York, McGraw-Hill, 1978

Iversen SD, Iversen LL: Behavioral Pharmacology, 2nd ed. New York, Oxford University Press, 1981

Jensen MD, Benson RC, Bobak IM: Maternity Care: The Nurse and the Family, 3rd ed. St. Louis, CV Mosby, 1985

Katzung BC (ed): Basic and Clinical Pharmacology, 3rd ed. Los Altos, CA, Appleton and Lange, 1987

Long JW: The Essential Guide to Prescription Drugs, 4th ed. New York, Harper & Row, 1985

Malseed RT: Pharmacology: Drug Therapy and Nursing Considerations, 2nd ed. Philadelphia, JB Lippincott, 1985

Martin EW: Hazards of Medication, 2nd ed. Philadelphia, JB Lippincott, 1978

Mathewson MK (ed): Pharmacotherapeutics. Philadelphia, FA Davis, 1986

The Medical Letter on Drugs and Therapeutics. New Rochelle, NY, Medical Letter, Inc. (biweekly)

Melmon KL, Morrelli HF (eds): Clinical Pharmacology, 2nd ed. New York, Macmillan, 1978

Pagana KD, Pagana TJ: Diagnostic Testing and Nursing Implications: A Case Study Approach, 2nd ed. St. Louis, CV Mosby, 1985

Pagliaro AM, Pagliaro LA: Pharmacologic Aspects of Nursing. St. Louis, CV Mosby, 1986

Physicians' Desk Reference, 42nd ed. Oradell, NJ, Medical Economics, 1988

Poe WD, Holloway DA: Drugs and the Aged. New York, McGraw-Hill, 1980

Rodman MJ, Karch AM, Boyd EH, Smith DW: Pharmacology and Drug Therapy in Nursing, 3rd ed. Philadelphia, JB Lippincott, 1985

Russell H: Pediatric Drugs and Nursing Intervention. New York, McGraw-Hill, 1980

Sager DP, Bomar SK: Intravenous Medications. Philadelphia, JB Lippincott, 1980

Scherer JC (ed): Lippincott's Nurses' Drug Manual. Philadelphia, JB Lippincott, 1985

Schmidt RM, Margolin S: Harper's Handbook of Therapeutic Pharmacology. Philadelphia, Harper & Row, 1981

Spencer RT, Nichols LW, Waterhouse HP et al: Clinical Pharmacology and Nursing Management. Philadelphia, JB Lippincott, 1983

United States Pharmacopeia Dispensing Information. St. Louis, CV Mosby, 1988

Waechter EH, Phillips J, Holaday B: Nursing Care of Children, Philadelphia, JB Lippincott, 1985

Wardell SC, Bousard LB: Nursing Pharmacology: A Comprehensive Approach to Drug Therapy. Monterey, CA, Wadsworth, Inc., 1985

Wiener MB, Pepper GA: Clinical Pharmacology and Therapeutics in Nursing, 2nd ed. New York, McGraw-Hill, 1985

Physiology

Annual Review of Physiology (yearly). Palo Alto, CA, Annual Reviews, Inc.

Ganong WF: Review of Medical Physiology, 10th ed. Los Altos, CA, Lange Medical Publications, 1981

Guyton AC: Human Physiology and Mechanisms of Disease, 4th ed. Philadelphia, WB Saunders, 1987

Hole JW: Human Anatomy and Physiology, 4th ed. Dubuque, IA, WC Brown, 1987

Tortora GJ: Principles of Human Anatomy, 4th ed. New York, Harper & Row, 1986

Tortora GJ, Anagnostakos NP: Principles of Anatomy and Physiology, 5th ed. New York, Harper & Row, 1987

Vander AJ, Sherman JH, Luciano DS: Human Physiology: The Mechanisms of Body Function, 4th ed. New York, McGraw-Hill, 1985

Generic Drug Index

Most drugs are listed by their generic names; brand names are listed in parentheses following the generic name. Over-the-counter products are listed by their brand names. Additional material about specific drugs may be found under the drug type. Trade names are listed in the *Trade Name Index* on page 1739.

Page numbers in italics indicate figures; page numbers followed by *t* indicate tabular material.

direct-acting, *188,* 188–196, 189t
effect on cholinergic function, 188, *188*
indirect-acting, 196–208
  antidote to, 206–208
  antimyasthenic, 198t, 199, 200–201t, 202–204
  contraindications and precautions with, 202
  fate of, 202
  interactions of, 202–203
  mechanism of action of, 199
  nursing process and, 203
  side-effects/adverse reactions with, 202
  uses of, 199, 202
  cholinesterase inhibitor antidote and, 206–208
  effect on cholinergic function, 188, *188*
  irreversible, 196, 204–206
  reversible, 196–204
Cholinergic system, 177
Choline salicylate (Arthropan), 409t
Cholinesterase inhibitors. *See* Cholinergic drugs, indirect-acting
Cholinomimetic agents. *See* Cholinergic drugs
Cholografin, 1581t
Choriocarcinoma, response to chemotherapy, 1385t
Christmas disease, 794
Chromaffin cells, 1050
Chromium, in total parenteral nutrition formulations, 1551t
Chromophobes, 963
Chronic disease, in elderly, 150
Chylomicrons, 739
Chymopapain (Chymodiactin; Discase), 1657–1658
  administration and dosage of, 1657
  contraindications and precautions with, 1658
  fate of, 1657–1658
  mechanism of action of, 1657
  nursing considerations and, 1658
  side-effects/adverse reactions with, 1658
  uses of, 1657
Chymotrypsin, 858t
Ciclopirox olamine (Loprox), 1353t
Cilastatin. *See* Imipenem-cilastatin
Cimetidine (Tagamet), 304–306, 1550
Cinoxacin (Cinobac), 1262
Ciprofloxacin (Cipro), 1280–1281
  common infections and, 1141–1145t
Cisplatin (*cis*-diamminedichloroplatinum), 1386t, 1393, 1480t, 1482t, 1483t, 1486–1488t, 1490t, 1492t, 1493t
  fate of, 1412t
  mechanism of action of, 1403
Citrocarbonate, 846–847t
Citrovorum factor (calcium leucovorin), 1487t, 1493t
Clark's rule, 172
Clavulanic acid, common infections and, 1140t, 1144t
Cleaning substances, 1692

Clearblue Pregnancy, 1566t
Clearplan, 1566t
Clemastine (Tavist), 296t
Clidinium bromide (Quarzan), 222t
Clindamycin (Cleocin), 1281–1285
  common infections and, 1140t, 1141t, 1143–1145t
Clinical use, classification of drugs by, 6–7
Clinistix, 1566t
Clinitest, 1566t
Clinitest 2-Drop, 1566t
Clioquinol [iodochlorohydroxyquin] (Torofor; Vioform), 1355t
Clobetasol propionate (Temovate), 1056t, 1060t
Clocortolone pivalate (Cloderm), 1057t, 1060t
Clofazimine (Lamprene), 1285–1286
Clofibrate (Atromid-S), 742–743
Clomiphene (Clomid; Serophene), 1108–1109
Clonazepam (Klonopin), 575–577
Clonidine (Catapres), 687–689, *688*
Clonidine transdermal therapeutic system (Catapres-TTS), 689–690
  nursing considerations and, 689–690
Clorazepate (Tranxene), 519–520t, 577
Clostridium, antimicrobial drugs of choice for, 1141t
Clotrimazole (Gyne-Lotrimin; Lotrimin; Mycelex), 1353–1354t
  common infections and, 1141t
Cloxacillin (Cloxapen; Tegopen), 1170t, 1175t
Coagulation factors, 765, 766t
Coal tar preparations (Alphosyl; Aquatar; Balnetar; Cutar; Denorex; Estar; Fototar; Mazon; Packer's Pine Tar; P and S Plus; Polytar; Polytar Bath; Psori Gel; Pragmatar; Tegrin; Tegrin Medicated Lotion; Zetar Emulsion), 1638
Cocaine, 349t
  abuse of, 1679
  street names for, 1687t, 1698t
Coccidioides immitis, antimicrobial drugs of choice for, 1141t
Coccidioidin (Spherulin), 1568t
Coccidioidomycosis, miconazole in, 1365
Codeine (codeine phosphate; codeine sulfate), 385–386t, 913, 915t
  kaodene with, 886t
  nursing considerations and, 915–916
Code name, 3
Colchicine, 436–438
Cold and cough preparations, 1692. *See also* Antitussives
Colestipol (Colestid), 741–742
Colistimethate (Coly-Mycin M), 1254–1256
  common infections and, 1140t
Colistin sulfate (Coly-Mycin S), 1256–1257
  common infections and, 1140t
Collaborative problems, 65
Collagenase (Biozyme-C; Santyl), 1642t
Collegial relationships, 73, 75
Coloscreen, 1566t

Combistix reagent strips, 1566t
Community education, about alcohol, 478–479
Competence, in elderly, 152
Competitive antagonist, 23
Comprehensive Drug Abuse Prevention and Control Act of 1970 (Controlled Substances Act), 81, 96
Concentration, in solution, oral absorption and, 14
Conduction velocity, digitalis glycosides and, 627
Conformational distortion theory, of general anesthesia, 358
Congestive heart failure (CHF), 623–625, *624,* 624t, 625t
  captopril in, 694
Conjugated estrogens (Estrocon; Premarin; Progens), 1084t
Conjugation, 18
Conn's syndrome, 1053
Conray, 1581t
Conray–30, 1581t
Conray–43, 1581t
Conray–325, 1581t
Conray–400, 1581t
Constipation, 866, 868
Content labeling, 79
Contraceptives, steroid, 1099–1105, 1100t, 1692t
Controlled substances. *See* Narcotics
Controlled Substances Act (Comprehensive Drug Abuse Prevention and Control Act of 1970), 81, 96
Controller, intravenous infusion and, 119
Convulsions. *See* Seizures; Anticonvulsants
Coombs' test, methyldopa and, 691
Copper
  serum, test for, 1695t
  in total parenteral nutrition formulations, 1551t
Corium, 1631
Corneal deposits, 45
Corn oil (Lipomul Oral), 1529t
Coronary circulation, angina and, 714
Corpora quadrigemina, 184
Corpus callosum, 184
Corpus striatum, 184
  in parkinsonism, 582
Corrective Mixture with Paregoric, 886t
Corticoids, 1053–1070
Corticosteroids, 928, 1462–1463t
  adverse effects on fetus and neonate, 128t
  antineoplastic, mechanism of action of, 1457
  dermatologic, 1640–1641
  inhaled, 944–945
  nursing considerations and, 945
  topically applied, relative potencies of, 1056t
Corticotropin (adrenocorticotropic hormone; ACTH), 966–967, 977–979
  plasma, test for, 1694t

Trade Name Index

Page numbers in italics indicate figures; page numbers followed by *t* indicate tabular material. The generic and chemical names for these drugs are found in the generic drug index on page 1707.

Abbokinase, 785–787
Abitrexate, 128t, 1386t, 1393, 1426–1427t, 1430t, 1432–1433t, 1480–1485t, 1487–1493t
Accutane, 1634–1636
Achromycin, 128t, 1140–1145t, 1215t, 1215–1217, 1218–1221t, 1222–1224
Acidulin, 859
Aclovate, 1057t, 1059t
Acne-Aid, 1636
ACSH, 966, 1116
ACTH, 966–967, 977–979, 1694t
Acthar, 977–979
ACTH Gel, 977–979
Actidil, 299t
Actinomycin D, 1386t, 1393, 1395, 1438–1439t, 1488t, 1448–1449t, 1491t, 1492t
Activase, 787–790
Acutrim, 250t, 611t
Adalat, 730t
Adapin, 538
Adriamycin-RDF, 1386t, 1393, 1395, 1401t, 1435, 1438–1441t, 1444, 1446t, 1449–1451t, 1480–1488t, 1490–1493t
Adrin, 260, 734
Adrucil, 1386t, 1393, 1424–1425t, 1430t, 1432–1433t, 1480t, 1481t, 1483–1485t, 1487t, 1489t, 1491t
Adsorbocarpine, 193–194
Advil, 428t, 1692
AeroBid, 945t, 1061–1062t
Aerolate, 931t, 934–935t
Aerolone, 240–244
Aerosporin, 1140t, 1257–1258
Afrin, 250t
Afrinol, 250–251t
Aftate, 1141t, 1356–1357t
Agoral Plain, 871–872t
A/G-Pro, 1531t
AHA, 1261, 1272–1273
Akarpine, 193–194
AK-Chlor, 1140–1145t, 1277–1280
AK-Con, 253t, 250t
AK-Dilate, 248–249, 250t, 253t
AK-Homatropine, 223t
Akineton, 221t, 592t
Akmycin, 1228t
AK-Nefrin, 248–249, 250t, 253t
Akne-mycin, 1228t
AK-Pentolate, 220t
AK-Ramycin, 1140t, 1218–1219t
Akshun, 875t
Ak-Sulf, 1154t
Ak-taine, 351t
AK-Tracin, 1253–1254
Ak Zol, 577–578, 814t
Alatone, 826–827
Alazine, 640t, 699–700

Albalon, 253t, 250t
Albamycin, 1290–1291
Albuminar, 1668t, 1669
Albutein, 1668t, 1669
Alcaine, 351t
Aldactone, 826–827
Aldomet, 682–684, 690–692
Alfenta, 391t
Alkaban-AQ, 1386t, 1395, 1401, 1442–1443t, 1444, 1447t, 1450–1453t, 1480–1483t, 1486t, 1490–1493t
Alka-Mints, 842–843t, 1013t
Alkeran, 1402, 1408–1411t, 1413t
Allerest, 250t, 253t
Almocarpine, 193–194
Almora, 1526t
Alophen, 875–876t
Alphaderm, 1055t, 1063t, 1401t
Alphamul, 875t
AlphaRedisol, 760
Alphatrex, 1056t, 1060t
Alphosyl, 1638
ALterna GEL, 842t
Alu-Cap, 842t
Alupent, 256–257
Alurate, 451t
Alu-Tab, 842t
Ambilhar, 1330–1331t
Amcill, 1140–1145t, 1170t, 1178–1179t
Amen, 1092t, 1462–1463t
Amethopterin, 128t, 1386t, 1393, 1426–1427t, 1430t, 1432–1433t, 1480–1485t, 1487–1493t
Amicar, 790–792
Amidate, 371–372
Amikin, 1140t–1144t, 1237t, 1238t, 1240t
Aminosyn, 1536–1537
Aminosyn R.F., 1537
Amitone, 842–843t, 1013t
Amitril, 537t, 1692
Amoline, 933t
Amoxil, 1142–1145t, 1170t, 1177–1178t
Amphojel, 842t
Amytal, 451t
Anabolin, 1121t
Anabolin LA, 1120–1121t
Anadrol-50, 1121t
Anaprox, 430t
Anaspaz, 217t
Anavar, 1121t
Ancef, 1197–1199t
Ancobon, 1140t, 1141t, 1361–1362
Andro-Cyp, 1120t, 1460–1461t
Andro L.A., 1120t, 1460–1461t
Andro 100, 1119t
Android, 1119t, 1460–1461t
Android-F, 1119t, 1460–1461t
Androlone, 1121t
Androlone-D, 1120–1121t

1739